QM Medical Libraries

KU-627-396

ORGANIC PSYCHIATRY

...MEW'S AND THE ROYAL LONDON
MEDICINE AND DENTISTRY
...STREET, LONDON E1 2AD

24 1006945 9

WITHDRAWN
FROM STOCK
QMUL LIBRARY

ORGANIC PSYCHIATRY

The Psychological Consequences of Cerebral Disorder

William Alwyn Lishman

MD, DSc, FRCP, FRCPsych, DPM

Emeritus Professor of Neuropsychiatry,
Institute of Psychiatry, London;
Emeritus Consultant Psychiatrist,
The Bethlem Royal and Maudsley Hospitals, London;
Honorary Senior Research Fellow,
Institute of Neurology, London;
Honorary Life President,
British Neuropsychiatry Association

THIRD EDITION

Blackwell
Science

© 1987, 1988 by William Alwyn Lishman
© 1978 by Blackwell Science Ltd

Editorial Offices:
Osney Mead, Oxford OX2 0EL
25 John Street, London WC1N 2BL
23 Ainslie Place, Edinburgh EH3 6AJ
350 Main Street, Malden
  MA 02148 5018, USA
54 University Street, Carlton
  Victoria 3053, Australia
10, rue Casimir Delavigne
  75006 Paris, France

Other Editorial Offices:
Blackwell Wissenschafts-Verlag GmbH
Kurfürstendamm 57
10707 Berlin, Germany

Blackwell Science KK
MG Kodenmacho Building
7–10 Kodenmacho Nihombashi
Chuo-ku, Tokyo 104, Japan

Iowa State University Press
A Blackwell Science Company
2121 S. State Avenue
Ames, Iowa 50014-8300, USA

The right of the Author to be
identified as the Author of this Work
has been asserted in accordance
with the Copyright, Designs and
Patents Act 1988.

All rights reserved. No part of
this publication may be reproduced,
stored in a retrieval system, or
transmitted, in any form or by any
means, electronic, mechanical,
photocopying, recording or otherwise,
except as permitted by the UK
Copyright, Designs and Patents Act
1988, without the prior permission
of the copyright owner.

First published in 1978
Reprinted 1980
Second edition 1987
Reprinted 1998, 1999, 2001, 2002, 2003

Set by Excel Typesetters Co., Hong Kong
Printed and bound in Great Britain
at the Alden Press Limited,
Oxford and Northampton

The Blackwell Science logo is a
trade mark of Blackwell Science Ltd,
registered at the United Kingdom
Trade Marks Registry

For further information on
Blackwell Science, visit our website:
www.blackwell-science.com

DISTRIBUTORS

Marston Book Services Ltd
PO Box 269
Abingdon, Oxon OX14 4YN
(*Orders*: Tel: 01235 465500
     Fax: 01235 465555)

USA
Blackwell Science, Inc.
Commerce Place
350 Main Street
Malden, MA 02148 5018
(*Orders*: Tel: 800 759 6102
     781 388 8250
 Fax: 781 388 8255)

Canada
Login Brothers Book Company
324 Saulteaux Crescent
Winnipeg, Manitoba R3J 3T2
(*Orders*: Tel: 204 224-4068)

Australia
Blackwell Science Pty Ltd
54 University Street
Carlton, Victoria 3053
(*Orders*: Tel: 3 9347 0300
     Fax: 3 9347 5001)

A catalogue record for this title
is available from the British Library

ISBN 0-86542-842-5 (hardback)
    0-86542-820-4 (paperback)

Library of Congress
Cataloging-in-publication Data

Lishman, William Alwyn.
    Organic psychiatry: the psychological consequences of cerebral
disorder / William Alwyn Lishman.—3rd ed.
        p.   cm.
    Includes bibliographical references and index.
    ISBN 0-86542-842-5 (hardback). ISBN 0-86542-820-4 (limp)
    1. Neuropsychiatry. 2. Neurobehavioral disorders—
Etiology. 3. Brain—Diseases—Complications. I. Title.
    [DNLM: 1. Organic Mental Disorders, Psychotic—etiology.
2. Brain Diseases—complications.   WM 220 L769o 1997]
RC386.L57   1997
616.89′071—DC21
DNLM/DLC   97-7107
for Library of Congress   CIP

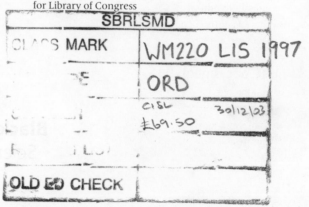
SBRLSMD

CLASS MARK   WM220 LIS 1997

            ORD

            CISL   30/12/03
            £69.50

OLD ED CHECK

Contents

Foreword to the First Edition

Since medicine began there has been the belief that there are two main categories of mental disorder, those due to natural or medical causes and those due to supernatural or 'moral' causes. Throughout history either the one or the other gained the greater recognition and attention. Medicine had little responsibility for the mentally ill throughout many centuries, and apart from the belief among medieval physicians in the Greek notions of the humoral pathology of mental disorder, the prepotence of moral or supernatural causes was accepted by most educated persons. The great advances in physical and biological science during the last century led to the recognition of man's place in nature as a biological entity. The development of medicine and particularly pathology led, in Europe, to the intensive study of the mentally ill from the point of view of the natural sciences. This phase in the development of organic psychiatry was limited by the concept of different forms of degeneration in the brain which was associated with the emergence of neuropathology, and by the absence of any knowledge or techniques for other types of enquiry. By the turn of the century it was overtaken by the immense influence of psychoanalysis which directed attention once again, particularly in Europe and in USA, to the 'moral' and psychological causes of mental disorder. Mental disorder was seen not so much as a disturbance of man's place in nature, but as a disorder of man as an individual. Psychopathology became for many a disorder of intrapsychic or interpersonal relationships.

It is only in the present century that psychiatry has begun to break free from the constraints of philosophy. The essential nature of the relationships between mental events and physical events in the nervous system remains as much as ever an unresolved mystery, but the amount of knowledge relevant to our understanding has increased vastly in the last few decades. This applies not only to the cerebral mechanisms upon which such fundamental functions as consciousness, memory, emotion, attention and learning are dependent but also to the ways in which pathological processes can alter them. The application of techniques of investigation based upon discoveries in the neurosciences and psychology has made this possible. This too has been paralleled by greater precision in the recognition and description of the clinical phenomena of organic cerebral disease. The tools of clinical diagnosis and investigation have been refined and extended.

Many emphasise that the approach to every patient should remain a holistic one. Above all his essential individuality as a person in all respects is our concern. It is necessary to investigate the patient's psychic reality and experience and the bearing this has on his disorder. It is also necessary to investigate the psychosocial environment and culture within which the patient lives and works. But it is equally necessary to examine the patient as a biological organism and in this the psychiatrist needs the knowledge and skills of modern medicine. If this is not understood and accepted there is no reason why psychiatrists should be medically trained. It is very difficult, and indeed impossible, to think about all three avenues to understanding and explanation at the same time, but they are not mutually exclusive, and they are equally important. The psychiatrist's capacity to know, after the initial interview, to which area he should in the main direct his attention is dependent upon his clinical experience and training, his skill in examination, but above all upon his detailed knowledge of the clinical phenomena which mental disorder presents, and their significance.

The author of this book sets out to examine and to describe in detail the psychological phenomena associated with the various organic disorders of the nervous system, and the psychological consequences of those numerous extracerebral diseases, toxic, metabolic and endocrine, which affect the brain indirectly. He describes how the clinician can go about identifying them; his extended treatment of this neglected field of clinical enquiry is more complete than any hitherto available. He has provided a textbook in which the clinical manifestations of various pathological processes affecting the brain are examined in the light of knowledge derived from the applications of the neurosciences and psychology, and has critically evaluated the evidence. The task has been a major one, for knowledge in the various fields has greatly increased in the last few decades, as the selected references, more than 2000 in number, show. The book is therefore a comprehensive text from the point of view of the clinician of the state of knowledge of organic psychiatry at the present time.

In the first part of the book, four chapters are concerned with the principles underlying our understanding of the relation between specific psychological deficits and brain function, methods of clinical assessment and differential diagnosis. In the second part of the book a series of chapters describe the clinical, psychiatric and psychological consequences of the different pathological processes. A final chapter summarises what is known from the point of view of numerous neurological disorders of diverse pathogenesis.

The appearance of this work at the present time comes to fill a much required need. There is no comparable book in the English-speaking world. The importance of organic psychiatry, if it was ever in doubt, has been emphasised by the movement of psychiatry into the general medical scene, and by the large numbers of physically ill patients presenting with disorder of behaviour for whom the psychiatrist's help is now sought. The work will no doubt become standard reading not only for postgraduate students of psychiatry and neurology, but also for neuropsychologists and for specialists engaged in continuing education and across a wide spectrum of medical specialties. Above all it provides a reference source book which will prove invaluable for clinicians and medical scientists alike whose enquiries direct them to some aspect of this large clinical field.

Institute of Psychiatry   DENIS HILL
University of London

Preface to the First Edition

The impetus for writing a book on organic psychiatry has come largely from clinical practice and teaching. Both reveal the lack of focused knowledge concerning the overlapping territories between psychiatry and neurology —a gap manifested in the paucity of textbook literature on the subject. Clearly, as with any borderland zone, there has been a risk of relative neglect as each separate discipline has proceeded on its specialised way, leaving, perhaps inevitably, an uneasy interface between.

Neurology deals directly with the apparatus of mind by investigating malfunction of the brain. Yet paradoxically it has often paid scant attention to mental disorder itself. Psychiatry on its part deals essentially with mental disorder, yet has had little in relative terms to do with the hardware upon which mind depends. The rich complexity of human behaviour, and the multitude of factors which can shape and distort it, have clearly demanded a multifaceted growth of clinical psychiatry; the subject had profited from psychodynamic, psychosocial and pharmacological approaches to mental disorder, but with the expert neurologist waiting in the wings the factor of brain malfunction has sometimes tended to be eclipsed. Sir Denis Hill, in his Foreword to the book, has touched on the dilemma and set it in much wider historical perspective.

It has therefore seemed worthwhile to attempt a comprehensive review of the cognitive, behavioural and emotional consequences of cerebral disorder, and the problems in this area which are encountered in clinical practice. The task proved greater than at first envisaged. In the first place neurology and psychiatry with their attendant disciplines have both proceeded apace, sometimes drawing closer together and sometimes further apart in their different approaches to disease. The literature on their common ground has correspondingly flourished, but in a scattered manner. Secondly it soon became obvious that a text devoted to psychiatric disorders associated with structural brain disease would be unduly restrictive, and that certain metabolic, toxic and other systemic disorders must also be considered if brain malfunction was to be the central theme.

Others could have argued for the inclusion of a good deal more than is here presented. Very little will be found on mental subnormality or child psychiatry since such fields are beyond the author's competence. And the temptation to speculate in detail on possible 'cerebral' contributions to the major functional psychoses has been resisted. Boundaries have in general been drawn short of hypothetical situations, and the work is mainly confined to disorders of cerebral function which are indubitable and well established.

Within the selected field coverage of different topics will no doubt be found inequitable. An avowed preoccupation with focal cerebral disorder, and the light which disease has thrown on regional brain function, will be apparent to the reader. But other considerations have also been at work. Some very rare disease processes are given considerable attention when their psychiatric components can on occasion be important or when important lessons have been learned from them. Similarly the selection of case reports will sometimes illustrate rare conditions or phenomena, if case presentation seems much better than lengthy description for communicating the essence of the matter. In the sections on treatment, physical approaches will often be described in more detail than psychotherapeutic or social interventions, without any necessary assumption that these have less important parts to play in overall management of the patient. Thus in many respects the emphases in the book must be construed, not as reflecting the absolute importance of a topic, but rather the particular slant indicated in a work devoted to organic aspects of psychiatry. Finally if scant attention seems to have been paid to purely psychological reactions to physical disorder this in no sense implies that such aspects are less intriguing or practically important. Matters of space and time, and the patience of the reader, have dictated that lines must be drawn, however arbitrarily and painfully.

Acknowledgements for the help of others are traditionally given, but the list would be long indeed if I were to pay tribute to all the teachers, colleagues and students

who have fostered my interest and guided my thinking on
the subjects dealt with herein. I will list instead those who
have been directly concerned with the book and have
often spent generous hours in detailed discussion and the
reading of drafts. The late Sir Aubrey Lewis took a keen
and encouraging interest in the earlier stages of the work.
Sir Denis Hill has given both detailed criticism and constant helpful support. I am greatly indebted to him for
generously providing a Foreword to the book. Special
thanks must go to Dr Richard Pratt for reading large parts
of the manuscript and allowing me to draw on his exceptional knowledge of the literature. Those who have criticised individual sections and chapters include Professor
Frank Benson, Professor Robert Cawley, Dr Elaine Drewe,
Dr Griffith Edwards, Professor George Fenton, Dr John
Gunn, Dr Derek Hockaday, Dr Raymond Levy, Professor
David Marsden, Dr David Parkes, Dr Felix Post and Dr
Sabina Strich. Others who have helped in innumerable
ways include Dr Christopher Colbourn, Mrs Isobel Colbourn, Dr John Cutting, Dr May Monro, Dr Maria Ron

and Dr Brian Toone. Miss Helen Marshall put at my disposal her unrivalled expertise in guiding me to the rich
store of information in the Institute of Psychiatry library.
To all of these kind friends and colleagues I am very
deeply grateful.

Finally I must record my gratitude to the two people
who have been most intimately concerned of all. Mrs
Dorothy Wiltshire has not only collaborated on an
arduous task, but has positively welcomed the burden
and done much to sustain my enthusiasm. Her expert secretarial skills and untiring patience have, in effect, made
the venture possible. My wife, Marjorie, deserves the
warmest thanks of all—meticulous help with the manu-
scripts and with problems of the English language have
been but a tiny part; over several years she has paved the
way, deflected obstacles and taken over numerous
burdens in an ever-helpful manner which is most affec-
tionately acknowledged.

June 1977   ALWYN LISHMAN

Preface to the Second Edition

This new edition has entailed a considerable amount of rewriting, particularly in the clinical sections, and the addition of material which had been overlooked before. Meanwhile, pruning has been attempted to ensure that the book remains reasonable in size.

The preparation for the updating has been a rewarding exercise, involving new reading in the psychiatric, neurological, neuropsychological and medical literature. The necessary library research was facilitated by the award of a 6-month Visiting Fellowship at Green College, Oxford, and I am much indebted to Sir Richard Doll and the Fellows of the College for their generous hospitality. It was a special delight to work once more in the Radcliffe Science Library division of the Bodleian Library, where my first clinical papers were written some 25 years ago.

The most remarkable advances since the first edition have come from developments in brain imaging. Such is the present pace of progress in the imaging field that no doubt the information contained herein will soon appear as rudimentary as that of the previous edition. Progress with dementia, particularly in the neurochemical aspects, is also a welcome sign, betokening a new courage to tackle the fundamentals of a long-neglected problem. New information concerning the brain damage associated with alcoholism has been a personal interest in recent years, accounting for the emphasis placed on the topic in several places. The movement disorders, with their special fascination and lessons for both psychiatrists and neurologists have now earned a chapter of their own. Altogether, to my surprise, almost as many new references were consulted for this new edition as appeared in the first, and over a thousand of them have been incorporated.

I have sometimes been questioned about the title 'Organic Psychiatry' and this perhaps deserves a word of explanation. Some might have preferred 'Biological Psychiatry' or 'Neuropsychiatry' to define the area of specialised interest. Biological psychiatry would, I think, be inappropriate. It represents, not a circumscribed clinical field, but rather a particular approach to the understanding of mental illness generally; it is concerned with mechanisms and pathophysiologies of a biological nature which can be sought out and studied in relation to virtually all forms of psychiatric disorder—organic conditions certainly, but also the major psychoses, the personality disorders and the neuroses. Biological psychiatry has many achievements but this book does not seek to encompass them.

The appeal of 'Neuropsychiatry' as a title is more difficult to dispel. Neuropsychiatry defines a territory within the corpus of mental disorder, *viz.* that which can be demonstrated to owe its origins to brain malfunction of clearly identifiable nature. (Research in biological psychiatry seems, incidentally, to be bent on extending this territory.) The term might therefore have seemed admirable for delineating the areas surveyed in this book. The decision not to use it came from two main considerations. First, neuropsychiatry is often regarded as the interface between neurology and psychiatry, which indeed it is, clinical neurology constituting by far the most relevant discipline additional to psychiatry itself. But my aim was to broaden the scope somewhat further by considering endocrine, toxic and metabolic disorders as well. These may also operate to disturb brain function, but they are the concern of general medicine rather than of neurology *per se*.

The second consideration has historical and conceptual roots though it emerges as immensely important in clinical practice. The term neuropsychiatry has sometimes earned for itself pejorative connotations. It has been regarded as narrow in approach and eschewing the rich diversity of psychiatric progress. At the worst it has been seen as the provenance of amateurs in both neurology and psychiatry, an imperfect chimera poorly endowed with the fruits of either discipline. This could scarcely be further from my conception of what neuropsychiatry entails. The study and treatment of those psychiatric disorders deriving from brain malfunction must capitalise on all that psychiatry has to offer. There are psychodynamic, social and cultural aspects of neuropsychiatry to be considered; exploration of conflict must take its place alongside the physical examination in differential diagnosis, psychotherapy alongside pharmacotherapy in treatment. To circumscribe a particularly complex and multidimensional segment of mental disorder, then to discard much that we have learned from psychiatry generally would be absurd. Neuropsychiatric practice requires a widening, not a narrowing, of psychiatric skills and interests.

Altogether it seemed a neat side-stepping of several pitfalls to choose a title not widely employed before — 'Organic Psychiatry' — though no doubt this still raises problems of its own.

Among those friends and colleagues thanked in the previous preface I have lost the two who perhaps did most to sustain early efforts with the book—Sir Denis Hill and Dr Richard Pratt. Their passing has been an immense blow to psychiatry and to medicine generally. For help with this second edition I must especially thank Dr Maria Ron, also Dr Peter Fenwick, Dr Simon Fleminger, Dr Robin Jacobson, Dr Eileen Joyce, Dr Michael Kopelman and Dr Brian Toone. Dr Maria Wyke has kept me in touch with the fascination of neuropsychology. It must also be appropriate to thank those patients from whom I have learned continually. The appearance, regularly over the horizon, of students with new talents and ideas has perhaps done most of all to help keep me abreast of progress.

Mrs Patsy Mott deserves my warmest gratitude for her untiring and expert secretarial skills. By ensuring the smooth running of day-to-day affairs she has made time available for the work to go ahead. The typing of drafts and extensive work with the bibliography and proofreading have proceeded steadily despite the demands of other activities. As with the first edition I have been singularly fortunate to have had such enthusiastic and meticulous secretarial help. In this connection I must record my gratitude to Mrs Dorothy Wiltshire once again, who gave further invaluable help in her retirement.

Finally my wife Marjorie, and children Victoria and William, have played an enthusiastic part in the preparation of this book—checking of the manuscript and cross-referencing in particular. Victoria gave willing and extensive help in the library. More than this they have provided the domestic background against which to mix long hours of work with diversion, sustenance and affection. I thank them for their forbearance. The generosity of a lively family has made the appearance of this new edition possible.

June 1985   ALWYN LISHMAN

Preface to the Third Edition

This third edition represents a more substantial revision than before, largely due to the availability of the entire manuscript for modification on disc. Though retaining the format of previous editions much of the text has been redrafted in accordance with newer conceptions and advances. Sizeable new sections have been added, particularly in the chapters dealing with the dementias and toxic disorders and with respect to the expanding range of rarer neurodegenerative disorders. The problems of HIV infection now receive extensive coverage as befits their clinical importance, likewise the accumulating evidence pointing towards a neuropsychiatric basis for schizophrenia. In the process almost as many new references have been added as remain from the previous edition. Radical pruning has meanwhile been carried out to maintain a book of manageable size while attempting to retain earlier material of lasting value or historical importance.

A main reward from the rewriting has been the realisation of the enormous amount achieved during the past decade, both in the clarification of disease mechanisms and also in the purely clinical field. Fundamental discoveries in, for example, cellular biology and molecular genetics, have developed alongside astonishing advances in aspects of brain imaging. The sophistication of neuropsychology has increasingly been harnessed to the latter, especially in the realm of functional neuroimaging. But equally striking has been progress in the clinical arena. Research into the psychiatric concomitants of cerebral disorder now proceeds with a degree of scientific rigour and exactitude which rivals the finesse of neurology. Disease entities within the domain of organic psychiatry have been more closely defined, with careful explorations of their nosology and epidemiology. New disorders, for example Lewy body dementia and frontal lobe dementia, have been brought into prominence and the range of prion-related disorders extended. Indeed the author has been led at times to look back with some dismay at his clinical practice and wonder how often his diagnoses may have been seriously adrift.

Psychiatrists and neurologists have drawn closer in recent years in efforts to clarify the pathophysiology and the phenomenology of the consequences of brain affections. Perhaps it is not too optimistic to see in this an increasing respect by each discipline for the endeavours of the other. The movement disorders in particular seem to emerge as a focal point in this interaction. For example, the recasting of a wide range of dystonic manifestations as markedly psychosensitive but basically organic in origin may be more than a swing of the pendulum. If so these fascinating disorders will demand even closer collaborative efforts for their further elucidation and management. Advances also clarify those psychiatric manifestations which are *not* the result of brain disease — leading to appropriate attempts at treatment and understanding.

A word may be needed to defend the territory encompassed by the book from its beginning. It has become somewhat unfashionable to seek to distinguish between organic and non-organic influences in the pathogenesis of mental disorder. The human being, his brain, his relationships and his social context add up to a formidable array of interacting systems with fragilities at many points in the totality of functioning. Meanwhile the biological basis of much of psychiatric disorder is becoming increasingly apparent, so that the dividing line between what may ultimately reflect disturbed cerebral functioning and what may not is often hard to discern. This suggests to some that the distinction between organic and non-organic in psychiatry is destined to become blurred if not entirely obsolete.

This could perhaps be argued on theoretical grounds and it doubtless presents a problem for neat classificatory systems. ICD-10 and DSM-IV have wrestled with the issue and come up with rather different solutions. But *practical* issues remain as ever to confront the clinician — how far in the individual patient should an organic component be suspected as the primary event in the development of a psychiatric disturbance, and even more importantly how urgently must this possibility be explored if optimal care is to be given? Organic psychiatric disorders may be defined as *those in which there is a high probability that appropriate examination and investigation will uncover some cerebral or systemic pathology responsible for, or contributing significantly to, the mental condition.* Thus it is the exigencies of the clinical situation which commend the perpetuation of the term 'organic psychiatry', and since the present book is firmly clinical in orientation the justification for its existence still appears to hold essential force.

I sincerely thank many of the colleagues listed in previous editions for giving their help once more, in valuable discussion, criticism and pointers towards the literature. On this occasion I am additionally indebted to Professor Tony David, Dr Ian Everall, Dr Laura Goldstein, Professor Peter Lantos, Professor Charles Polkey and Dr Mary Robertson. As with the last edition I must record the sad loss of a close friend who gave much assistance with the book at its inception — Professor Frank Benson from UCLA, whose contributions to knowledge in the field can scarcely be rivalled.

The librarians of the Institute of Psychiatry have been unfailingly helpful and I thank them for their hospitality

in setting space aside for me after my retirement. The resources of the splendid library at the Royal Society of Medicine have also been invaluable.

Peter Saugman at Blackwell Science skilfully manoeuvred me into willingness to attempt a third edition. Stuart Taylor and Edward Wates from Blackwells have given steadfast, friendly support throughout its preparation, not least by persuading me to embrace the rewards of modern word processing technology. Jane Andrew's expertise as production editor is very much appreciated.

Most sincere thanks must again go to Mrs Patsy Mott for unwavering secretarial support, and even more importantly for a calm enthusiasm for the project which did more than she will know to sustain my efforts. My wife, Marjorie, who has been a principal impetus for the book from the time of its conception, has once again supported and facilitated the preparation of this new edition and guided me on innumerable points. It is impossible to overstate the debt that I, and the book, owe to her.

November, 1996   ALWYN LISHMAN

While every effort has been made to ensure the accuracy of drug dosages and side effects described in this book, the author and publishers make no representation, express or implied, that they are correct. The reader is therefore urged to consult the drug company's printed instructions before implementing treatments recommended herein.

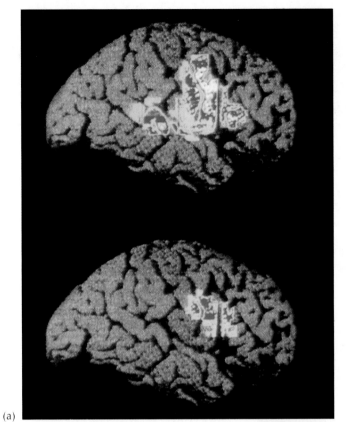

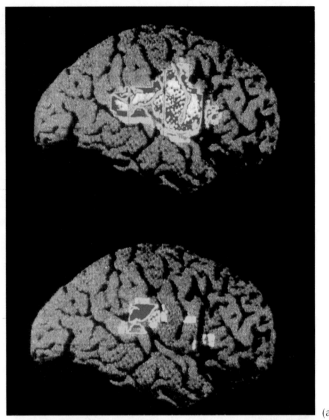

(a)

Developmental dyslexics   Normal controls

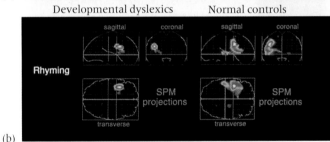

(b)

Plate 1

(a)

Developmental dyslexics   Normal controls

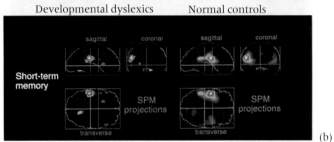

(b)

Plate 2

Plates 1 & 2. ^{15}O-PET scans showing the site of increases in regional cerebral blood flow during the performance of phonological tasks, areas of significant activation being transcribed onto lateral views of the brain (Plate 1a, rhyming task; Plate 2a, phonological short-term memory task). See text, pp. 48–9. Comparisons between normal controls (upper images) and subjects with developmental dyslexia (lower images) show the more restricted brain areas activated in the latter. Plates 1b and 2b represent integrated projections through sagittal, coronal and transverse views of the brain, in order to demonstrate the areas involved more precisely. (Apapted from *Brain* (1996), **119**, 143–157, courtesy of Oxford University Press. Images kindly made available by Professors Uta and Chris Frith.)

Plate 3. Regional cerebral blood flow measured by ^{133}Xe inhalation in normal controls and schizophrenic patients. The latter fail to activate the prefrontal cortex while performing an analogue of the Wisconsin Card Sorting Test (right images), in comparison to flows while performing a number-matching task (left images). See text, p. 87. (Reproduced from *Archives of General Psychiatry* (1986), **43**, 126–135, courtesy of Dr Daniel Weinberger.)

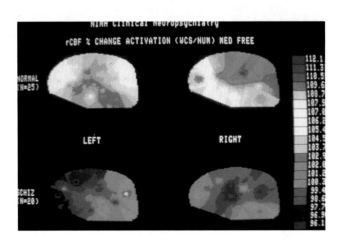

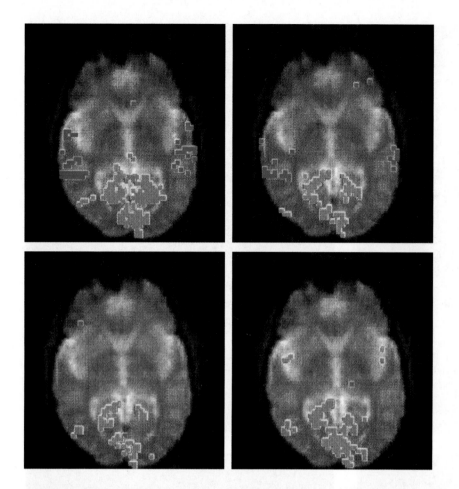

Plate 4. Functional MRI scans obtained from a schizophrenic patient while auditory verbal hallucinations were absent (upper images) or in progress (lower images). Pixels activated by visual stimulation (shown in red) are little affected during the occurrence of the auditory hallucinations, whereas those activated by auditory stimulation (shown in blue) are markedly suppressed. Left images, patient on medication; right images, patient off medication. See text, p. 88. (Reproduced from *NeuroReport* (1996), **7**, 932–936, courtesy of Dr Anthony David and Rapid Science Publishers Ltd.)

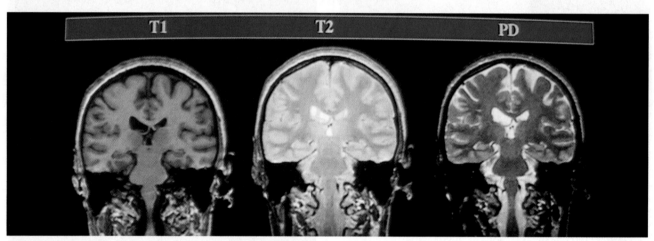

Plate 5. Coronal magnetic resonance brain images illustrating different scanning sequences. T_1, inversion recovery; T_2, spin-echo; PD, proton density. See text, p. 141. (Image kindly supplied by Dr Nancy Andreasen.)

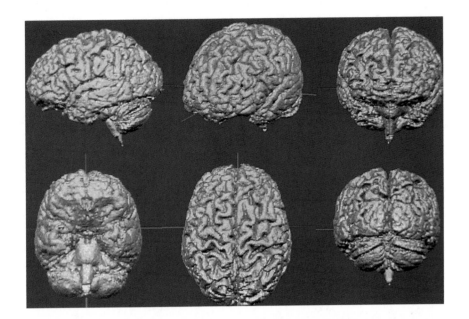

Plate 6. Three-dimensional surface-rendered images of the brain derived by computer reconstruction from MRI scans. See text, p. 142. The images can be enlarged and rotated to permit viewing of the sulci and gyral patterns from any angle. See *Journal of Neuropsychiatry and Clinical Neurosciences* (1993), **5**, 121–130. (Courtesy of Dr Nancy Andreasen.)

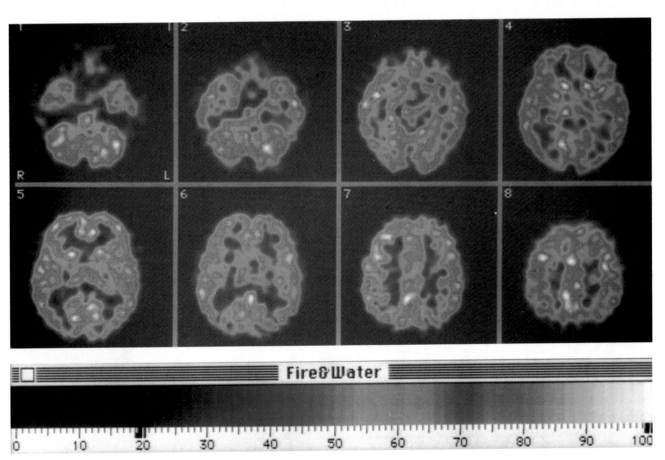

Plate 7. An HMPAO-SPECT scan from a normal subject, using a Strichman Medical Equipment multislice, head-dedicated scanner. See text, p. 148. The slices are orientated parallel to the orbitomeatal plane. (Courtesy of the Department of Nuclear Medicine, King's College Hospital, London.)

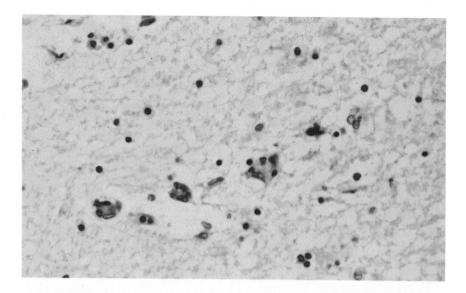

Plate 8. Large multinucleated giant cells in cerebral white matter of a patient with HIV encephalitis and dementia (haematoxylin and eosin). See text, p. 322. Magnification ×250. (Courtesy of Dr Ian Everall.)

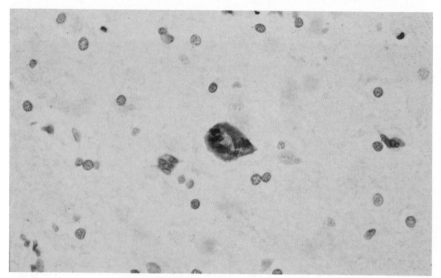

Plate 9. A multinucleated giant cell from a patient with HIV encephalitis immunostained for the glycoprotein gp 41, revealing viral particles. See text, p. 322. Magnification ×400. (Courtesy of Dr Ian Everall.)

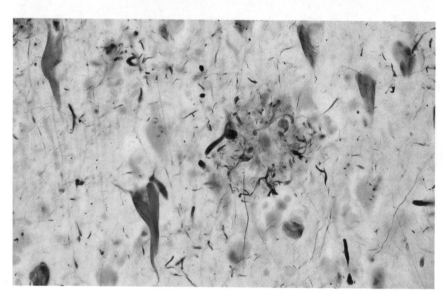

Plate 10. A senile (neuritic) plaque with dystrophic neuronal processes at the margin, and numerous neurofibrillary tangles within or replacing neuronal cell bodies. See text, pp. 440 and 441. From the CA1 area of the hippocampus in a patient with Alzheimer's disease (Glees and Marsland silver impregnation). Magnification ×400. (Courtesy of Dr Nigel Cairns.)

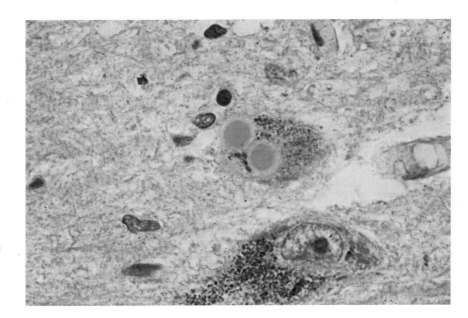

Plate 11. Lewy bodies in the substantia nigra (haematoxylin and eosin). See text, pp. 452 and 647. Magnification ×600. (Courtesy of Professor Peter Lantos.)

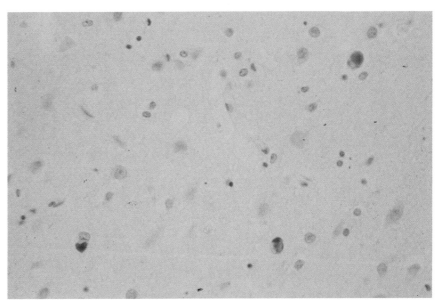

Plate 12. Lewy bodies in the cerebral cortex, immunostained for ubiquitin (ABC method). See text, p. 452. Magnification ×250. (Courtesy of Professor Peter Lantos.)

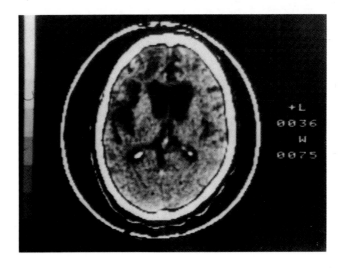

Plate 13. CT scan of patient with advanced Pick's disease, confirmed at autopsy. See text, p. 461.

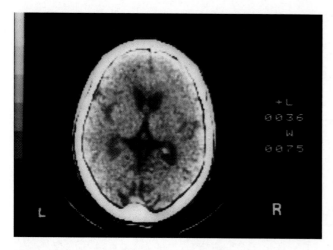

Plate 14. CT scan of a patient with Huntington's disease, confirmed at autopsy (see p. 470). The patient is described on p. 471.

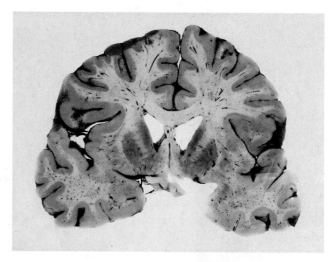

Plate 15. Autopsy appearances of the patient shown in Plate 14, confirming shrinkage of the heads of the caudate nuclei. (Plates 14 and 15 are reproduced from Brooks, D.S., Murphy, D., Janota, I. & Lishman, W.A., *British Journal of Psychiatry* (1987), **151**, 850–852.)

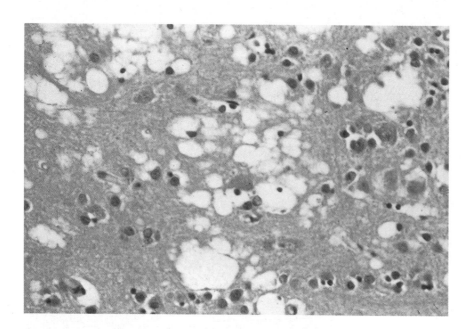

Plate 16. Severe spongiform degeneration in a patient with Creutzfeldt–Jakob disease, as described on p. 478 (haematoxylin and eosin). Magnification ×325. (Courtesy of Professor Peter Lantos.)

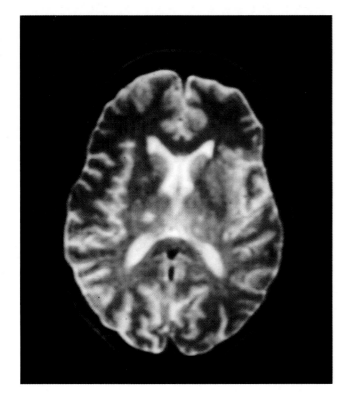

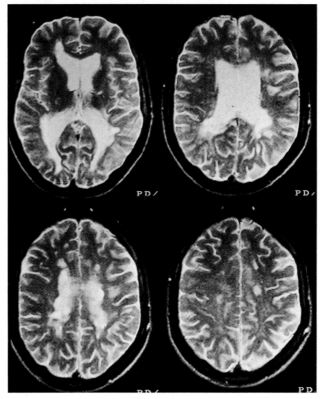

Plate 17. MRI scan of a patient with acute Wernicke's encephalopathy, showing discrete lesions in both thalamic regions. See text, p. 579. (Courtesy of Dr Eileen Joyce.)

Plate 18. MRI scans showing plaques in the periventricular white matter in a patient with multiple sclerosis (see p. 690). The patient is described on p. 694. (Reproduced from Hotopf, M.H., Pollock, S. & Lishman, W.A., *Psychological Medicine* (1994), **24**, 525–528, courtesy of Cambridge University Press.)

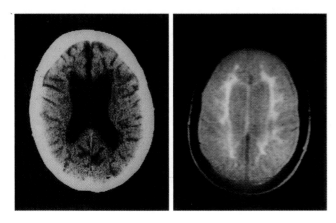

Plate 19. CT and MRI scans from a patient with metachromatic leucodystrophy. The patient is described on pp. 758–9. (Reproduced from Fisher, N.R., Cope, S.J. & Lishman, W.A., *Journal of Neurology, Neurosurgery and Psychiatry* (1987), **50**, 488–489, courtesy of BMJ Publishing Group.)

PART 1
PRINCIPLES

Chapter 1: Cardinal Psychological Features of Cerebral Disorder

In most psychiatric illnesses the clinical picture is profoundly coloured and sometimes decisively shaped by factors specific to the individual and his environment. Hence the notorious difficulty in identifying separate disease processes in psychiatry. This is compounded still further by the lack of collateral evidence by way of tissue pathology where most mental disorders are concerned. Organic psychiatric illnesses escape in some degree from both of these constraints. The psychological disturbances which result from brain pathology often share common ground which cuts across differences in background, personality and social situation. They are related to pathological processes within the brain, or acting on the brain, which can often be identified by the techniques of medical investigation. In these respects organic psychiatry draws closer to the rest of medicine, and should at least in theory be amenable to a similar approach in leading towards useful clinicopathological correlations.

In large measure this is so. However, psychological symptoms are hard to identify objectively and can rarely be measured accurately. Difficulties of assessment increase abruptly as we ascend from basic motor and sensory processes to mental phenomena, and especially when we move from simple cognitive impairments to changes in emotion, personality and other complex aspects of behaviour. Moreover when symptoms characteristic of the neuroses or major psychoses emerge in the brain-damaged person it is necessary to consider the possibility that he may have been specially predisposed to their development. Ultimately, indeed, we are often forced back again to the problems of the main body of psychiatry, since the more complex effects of cerebral disorder can be properly assessed only when the whole individual is viewed in the context of his personal history and environment. The situation is therefore a good deal more complex than in most other branches of medicine, and the opportunities for relating abnormalities of behaviour to precise aspects of cerebral pathology are limited in several important respects.

Fortunately for the diagnostic process, organic psychiatric disorders tend to have certain features in common which usually allow them to be distinguished from non-organic mental illnesses. Different varieties of pathological change are often associated with similar forms of impairment. Bonhoeffer (1909, 1910) deserves the credit for recognising this and discarding the Kraepelinian view that each noxious agent affecting the brain evokes a specific psychiatric picture. Impairment of consciousness, for example, may result from a number of toxic processes acting on the brain or from raised intracranial pressure; dementia may result from anoxia, from trauma or from primary degenerative disease. It is therefore possible to extract important symptoms and syndromes which indicate the possibility of cerebral disorder whatever the basic pathology and despite the colouring lent by pathoplastic features. Such symptoms form the cornerstone of diagnosis in organic psychiatry and it is essential to recognise their earliest and most minor manifestations. Many disease processes affecting the brain will come to attention with psychological symptoms alone and well before the appearance of definite neurological signs, and it is often by the correct appreciation of these common forms of reaction that a mistaken diagnosis of non-organic (or so-called 'functional') psychiatric disorder will be avoided.

Other forms of presentation may indeed occur with change of personality, affective disturbance, neurotic symptoms or even pictures indicative of schizophrenia. The clinician must remain aware that occasionally a mental illness presenting in this way may be related to the early stages of cerebral disease. Such cases are not infrequent; however, as the condition progresses organic mental symptoms will usually appear.

Nosology and the use of terms

The present chapter will describe the cardinal psychological symptoms and signs of cerebral disorder.* The principal accent will be on the shared forms of reaction common to most individuals and to different pathological processes, though features particular to individuals will also be briefly described where appropriate.

The recognition of common forms of reaction has led to the widespread use of all-embracing terms. A main division into acute and chronic forms of reaction is customary. In addition a number of syndromes have been delineated, such as clouding of consciousness, delirium and dementia. These terms are clinically useful for purposes of broad classification, and for shorthand description of groups of clinical phenomena. They are not, however, diagnoses in themselves, and must be appreciated as interim judgements which await clarification by further observation and investigation of the patient.

Unfortunate tendencies have developed in the use of some of these terms. Some are used to refer interchangeably to symptoms, syndromes or to disease entities; others have had restrictions placed upon them by virtue of aetiological or prognostic considerations. 'Dementia', for example, may refer to a syndrome in which failing intellect is prominent, or to a number of specific disease entities. In addition it has acquired implications for irreversibility of the process. 'Confusion' may refer to a lack of clarity in thinking, or be used as in 'acute confusional state' to indicate a broad nosological category of disorders. The term 'toxic confusional state' is similarly widely used but can properly be applied only when toxic influences on the brain have been established.

'*Acute organic reaction*' and '*chronic organic reaction*' are the terms best used for the first major division of organic psychiatric illnesses, each functioning as no more than a pointer to a class of problems, and serving only as starting points for further enquiries into aetiology. These terms carry implications for abruptness and onset and to some extent for the constellation of symptoms which are most in evidence. Each may show features not seen in the other, and requiring specific approaches for their identification. The terms also carry implications for likely duration, but not directly for ultimate prognosis. It is more usual for acute than for chronic organic reactions to recover, but the prognosis in each case will depend upon the precise aetiology at work. A separate category of 'subacute organic reactions' is sometimes demarcated, and

---

* The distinction between symptoms and signs which is customary in general medicine is often difficult to make where psychological phenomena are concerned. To avoid repetition, 'symptoms' will often be used alone when both the patient's complaints and the psychological abnormalities detected by the examiner are being considered together. For similar reasons 'he' or 'his' will often be used when 'he/she' or 'his/her' would be more appropriate and correct.

merely implies less sudden onset than the acute disorders, somewhat longer continuation, and an admixture of clinical symptoms characteristic of acute and chronic reactions. It must be accepted, however, that both acute and chronic reactions will vary in the degree of their acuteness or chronicity, and that in some cases the former will, with time, prove to merge into the latter.

'*Confusion*' refers to symptoms and signs which indicate that the patient is unable to think with his customary clarity and coherence. It is seen in both organic and nonorganic mental disturbances, and the term is useful merely as a shorthand clinical description of an important aspect of such mental states. In acute organic reactions confusion is due largely to impairment of consciousness. In chronic organic reactions it betrays the disruption of thought processes due to structural brain damage. In a whole range of psychiatric disorders confusion of thinking may be much in evidence without any identifiable brain pathology whatever, similarly when powerful emotions from any cause interfere with the efficient ordering of cognitive processes.

It is unfortunate therefore that 'confusion' has sometimes been made the hallmark of organic mental states and incorporated into terms denoting categories of organic mental disorder. Victor and Adams (1962), for example, recognised three syndromes within the class of 'confusional state', depending on the associated increase or decrease of psychomotor activity or the presence of associated degenerative brain disease ('delirium', 'primary mental confusion' and 'beclouded dementia'). Such classifications are cumbersome and of uncertain clinical usefulness. It would seem preferable to restrict the use of the term confusion to denote phenomena as defined above, and to avoid its use in nosological classifications.

'*Clouding of consciousness*' denotes the mildest stage of impairment of consciousness, which is detectable clinically, on the continuum from full alertness and awareness to coma. As such it is manifest as slight impairment of thinking, attending, perceiving and remembering, in other words as mild global impairment of cognitive processes in association with reduced awareness of the environment. The patient will frequently, though not always, appear to be drowsy. As Lipowski (1967) points out, clouding of consciousness is not exactly synonymous with reduced wakefulness. The one is a stage on the way to coma, the other on the way to sleep which is very different (p. 6). In clouding of consciousness the patient's awareness of himself and his surroundings is impaired, but his activity may vary from drowsiness and lethargy on the one hand to increased excitability on the other.

Unfortunately the term has sometimes been endowed with broader meaning. Jaspers (1963) distinguished between torpor and clouding, only the former representing a stage on the continuum from full alertness to unconsciousness. Clouding in this view has additionally the hallmarks of fragmentation of psychic experience and florid subjective events in the form of fantasies, vivid affects and hallucinations. In such a conception 'clouding of consciousness' embraces additional phenomena and describes a complete mental state rather than one definable component. It would seem preferable to restrict its use in the manner described above.

'Delirium'. There are many meanings and definitions of this term, sometimes embracing all varieties of acute organic reaction, sometimes referring to the degree of overt disturbance, and sometimes confining its use to clinical pictures with certain specific features. Special characteristics have included wakefulness with ability to respond verbally, increased psychomotor activity, pronounced disturbance of affect, defective reality testing, or the appearance of productive symptoms in the form of illusions and hallucinations. Delirium tremens is often taken as a prototype for delirium, and contrasted with the 'simple confusion' of subdued cognitive impairment in other illnesses.

In the DSM-III classification 'delirium' was effectively synonymous with 'acute organic reaction', and included all varieties of the latter (Diagnostic & Statistical Manual of Mental Disorders 1980; Lipowski 1980a). The DSM-IV revision retains this broad definition, dividing the syndrome into delirium due to a general medical condition, substance-induced delirium, and delirium due to multiple aetiologies (Diagnostic & Statistical Manual of Mental Disorders 1994). Fundamental to all is a *disturbance of consciousness* (i.e. reduced clarity of awareness of the environment) coupled with a *reduced ability to focus, sustain or shift attention*. Additional requirements are a change in cognition (such as memory deficit, disorientation or language disturbance) or the development of a perceptual disturbance (misinterpretations, illusions or hallucinations, mainly visual), with the proviso that these are not better accounted for by a pre-existing or evolving dementia. The disturbance develops over a short period of time (usually hours to days) and tends to fluctuate during the course of the day.

The ICD-10 classification (World Health Organization 1992) similarly stresses concurrent disturbances of consciousness and attention, along with changes in cognition, perception, psychomotor behaviour, sleep–wake cycle and emotion. The disorder is usually rapid in onset, with diurnal fluctuations, most cases recovering within 4 weeks or less but sometimes continuing for up to 6 months.

For a definite diagnosis of delirium ICD-10 requires symptoms in each one of the following areas:

(a) Impairment of consciousness and attention, with reduced ability to direct, focus, sustain, and shift attention.
(b) Global disturbance of cognition—perceptual distortions, illusions and hallucinations, mostly in the visual modality; impairment of abstract thinking and comprehension; impairment of immediate recall and recent memory; disorientation for time and sometimes place and person as well.
(c) Psychomotor disturbance which may consist of hypo- or hyperactivity or unpredictable shifts between the two.
(d) Disturbance of the sleep–wake cycle—insomnia, daytime drowsiness, sleep reversal; nocturnal worsening of symptoms; or disturbing dreams and nightmares which may continue as hallucinations on awakening.
(e) Emotional disturbances—depression, anxiety, fear, irritability, euphoria, apathy or perplexity.

In the UK it was formerly traditional to reserve the term for patients whose acute cerebral disorder resulted in some degree of disturbed or disruptive behaviour, i.e. to emphasise the restless hyperactivity and emotional disturbance which is so commonly part of the picture. It is clear, however, that not all patients who meet current criteria for delirium present like this, some showing predominant listlessness, inertia and dulling of the senses. In a daily evaluation of 125 patients who met DSM-III criteria for delirium in a general hospital, Liptzin and Levkoff (1992) classified 15% as hyperactive, 19% as hypoactive, 52% as mixed and 14% as neither.

It is important to appreciate that consciousness is not merely quantitatively reduced in delirium, but also qualitatively changed. Typically the patient becomes preoccupied with his own inner world which is distorted by illusions, hallucinations and delusions, and sometimes by powerful affective changes derived therefrom or more directly from dysfunction of specific brain systems. Even though awareness of external events is impaired, arousal may be high enabling these productive symptoms to occur. The fluctuations in severity are commonly accompanied by fluctuations in content, manifesting as a continuously changing clinical picture. Many different disturbances of cerebral function can lead to delirium, with little that can be regarded as specific in the clinical pictures that result. Toxic and metabolic disturbances are perhaps prone to be associated with listlessness and apathy, and infective processes and alcohol withdrawal syndromes with hyperactivity, fearfulness and prominent hallucinations.

'Twilight states'. Among Bonhoeffer's 'forms of exogenous reaction' due to pathogenic factors acting on the brain, twilight states and delirium were separately demarcated along with hallucinosis, epileptiform excitement and amentia. The last three terms have mostly been discarded in this context, but 'twilight state' continues to be used. The essential features appear to include abrupt onset and ending, variable duration from hours to weeks, and the interruption of quiet periods of behaviour by unexpected and sometimes violent acts or outbursts of rage or fear. Thereafter clinical descriptions are often divergent. Consciousness is sometimes said to be severely impaired, with profound slowness of reaction and monotonous stereotyped movements, while others stress relatively normal outward behaviour between episodes of disturbance. Other descriptions include dream-like 'oneiroid' states, vivid hallucinations and delusional ideas which dictate powerful affective disturbance. Clearly, therefore, the term is used to cover a variety of syndromes and can now have little useful meaning. It is, moreover, widely employed to describe hysterical manifestations in addition to acute organic reactions. In the organic field current practice appears increasingly to be to restrict its use to a type of complex partial seizure as considered on p. 255.

'*Coma*' represents the extreme of a graded continuum of impairment of consciousness, at the opposite pole of the spectrum from full alertness and awareness of the environment. The patient is incapable of sensing or responding adequately to external stimuli or inner needs, shows little or no spontaneous movement apart from respiration, and no evidence whatever of mental activity.

Coma is itself a graded phenomenon. At its deepest there is no reaction to stimuli of any intensity, and corneal, pupillary, pharyngeal, tendon and plantar reflexes are absent. Respiration is slow and sometimes periodic (Cheyne–Stokes respiration) and cardiovascular regulating processes may show signs of failure. Lighter degrees of coma ('semicoma') allow partial response to stimulation, though this is incomplete, mostly non-purposive and usually consists of ineffectual movements or rubbing and scratching of the stimulated area. Bladder distension may call forth groaning or ill-coordinated motor stirring but the patient is still incontinent. Tendon reflexes may or may not be obtainable, and the plantars may be either flexor or extensor. The Glasgow Coma Scale which has proved its usefulness for the grading of depth of coma is described on p. 167.

Coma needs to be distinguished from deep sleep and from stupor. In deep sleep and in coma the pictures may be closely similar on superficial observation. But the sleeper can be roused again to normal consciousness by the efforts of the examiner. He may wake spontaneously to unaccustomed stimuli, or in response to inner sensations such as hunger or bladder distension. In sleep there is sporadic continuing mental activity in the form of dreams which leave traces in memory. Coma is more difficult to demarcate from stupor which is described below. The distinguishing features usually accepted are that in coma the eyes remain shut even in response to strong arousal stimuli, do not resist passive opening, and do not appear to be watchful or follow moving objects; movements in response to stimulation are never purposeful, and there is no subsequent recall of events or inner fantasies from the time in question.

'*Stupor*' is an exceedingly difficult term to define, principally because it has been used widely in neurological and psychiatric practice to refer to conditions with markedly different causation. Sometimes it is used loosely and wrongly to refer to an intermediate stage on the continuum of impairment of consciousness which leads ultimately to coma; sometimes to refer to a syndrome characteristic of lesions in the neighbourhood of the diencephalon and upper brain stem ('akinetic mutism'); and sometimes to clinical states superficially similar to this but due to hysterical, depressive or schizophrenic illness.

Stupor is thus a term without definite nosological status, but valuable when properly used in referring, in essence, to a clinical syndrome of akinesis and mutism but with evidence of relative preservation of conscious awareness. It would appear that with the exception of 'akinetic mutism' due to brain damage, stupor may be a non-specific general reaction of the central nervous system, with some individuals presumably predisposed towards its development. In some cases at least stupor appears to be experienced as a quasi-volitional act, sometimes delusionally motivated.

There is a profound lack of responsiveness, and evidence of impairment, or at least putative or apparent impairment, of consciousness. Speech and spontaneous movement are absent or reduced to a minimum, and the patient is inaccessible to the great majority of external stimuli. Unlike coma and semicoma, however, the patient may at first sight appear to be conscious, since the eyes may be open and seem to be watchful. The patient may direct his gaze towards the examiner and the eyes may follow moving visual stimuli in a manner which appears to be purposeful rather than random. When the eyes are shut they may resist passive opening. Relative preservation of consciousness is also betrayed by the response to stimulation—strong painful stimuli may induce blinking or purposeful coordinated efforts to dislodge the noxious agent. Moreover in some cases there is subsequent recall of events or delusional fantasies occurring in the stuporose state.

Typically, spontaneous movements are absent but there may be tremors, coarse twitching or, in light stupor, restless stereotyped motor activity. The latter may seem to occur in response to hallucinatory experiences, or to display special meaning in stupors due to psychotic illness. Here also the resting posture may be awkward or bizarre, or it may be meaningful in the context of the patient's delusions. Reflexes are usually entirely normal.

Complete mutism is the rule, but again there may sometimes be partially coherent muttering, or arousal may be possible to the extent of brief stereotyped exclamations. In light stupor there may be no sphincter disturbance, and even feeding may be possible with coaxing. Simple responses to commands may then be obtained, though these are slow, inaccurate and often ill-coordinated. The least severe examples may merge indefinably with severe psychomotor retardation in psychotic depression, or with severe blocking of thought and volition in catatonic schizophrenia. The causes of stupor and their differential diagnoses are considered on p. 155.

'Dementia' is used in two contexts which must be clearly distinguished; first to label a group of specific disease entities, namely the 'presenile and senile dementias', and secondly to refer to a clinical syndrome which can have many other causes.

The specific diseases for which the term is used are considered in Chapter 10. They are characterised by progressive and widespread brain degeneration with, at the moment, a hopeless prognosis. When denoting a syndrome, however, the term may validly be used more widely, and can be defined very simply as *an acquired global impairment of intellect, memory and personality, but without impairment of consciousness*. As such it is almost always of long duration, usually progressive and often irreversible, but these features are not included as part of the definition.

For an ICD-10 research diagnosis of dementia (World Health Organization 1993) there must be evidence of:
1 A decline in memory affecting both verbal and non-verbal material, sufficient at least to interfere with everyday activities.
2 A decline in other cognitive abilities, characterised by deterioration in judgement and thinking and in the general processing of information. Deterioration from a previously higher level of performance should be established.
     For a confident diagnosis both 1 and 2 must have been present for at least 6 months.
3 Preserved awareness of the environment during a period sufficiently long to allow the unequivocal demonstration of the symptoms in 1 and 2; when there are superimposed episodes of delirium the diagnosis of dementia should be deferred.
4 Decline in emotional control or motivation, or a change in social behaviour manifest as at least one of emotional lability, irritability, apathy or coarsening of social behaviour.

DSM-IV specifies individual criteria for dementia of the Alzheimer-type, vascular dementia, etc., the common elements being as follows:
a The development of multiple cognitive deficits manifested by both:
    1 memory impairment;
    2 one or more of aphasia, apraxia, agnosia or disturbance of executive function (planning, organising, sequencing, abstracting).
b Such cognitive deficits cause significant impairment in social or occupational functioning, and represent a significant decline from a previous level of functioning.
c The deficits do not occur exclusively during the course of a delirium.
Further inclusion and exclusion criteria then apply to the several varieties of dementia specified in DSM-IV.

The syndrome therefore consists of a constellation of symptoms which suggest chronic and widespread brain dysfunction. Global impairment of intellect is the central and essential feature, manifest as difficulty with memory, attention, thinking and comprehension. Other mental functions are usually affected concurrently, and changes of mood, personality and social behaviour may sometimes be the outstanding or even presenting features. Nevertheless 'dementia' should not be used to describe such changes unless intellectual deterioration can be identified.

Historically the term has acquired implications for inevitable decline and irreversibility. This remains true for the disease entities of dementia, but not for all the settings in which the syndrome may appear. The dementia accompanying general paresis can be arrested, and that due to head injury or normal-pressure hydrocephalus may improve with time or treatment. Thus when matters of prognosis are kept out of the definition the term can be used whatever the cause of the syndrome and whatever future therapeutic discoveries may bring.

It is also important that the syndrome be defined in terms of global impairment of *functions*, and not in terms of diffuse cerebral damage. Focal brain damage can sometimes lead to global impairment of intellect, memory and personality in addition to regional deficits. Frontal lobe tumours are notorious in this regard, and can produce a picture of dementia indistinguishable at first sight from other causes. In such cases it remains logical to use the term to describe the clinical picture which presents for attention, even though diffuse affection of brain tissue is not the immediate cause. Indeed some forms of dementia are best regarded as the end result of multiple focal pathologies which coalesce and combine to impair functions globally, as in the vascular dementias. It is essential, therefore, to avoid defining the syndrome in terms of a pathology which has yet to be displayed.

The term is thus reserved for the description of a group of clinical symptoms, while all considerations of prognosis and aetiology are excluded from the definition. This has a certain practical importance, in that once the syndrome has been identified it must always dictate a search for ultimate causes. These may be focal or diffuse, within or without the brain, and may have possibilities for treatment.

'Organic personality change'. Brain damage often results in changes of temperament, or changed patterns of reac-

tion to events and to other people. As a result behavioural tendencies which have previously been enduring characteristics of the individual are found to be altered. Areas typically affected include the control of emotions and impulses and aspects of motivation and social judgement (Lipowski 1980a). Such 'change of personality' is usually prominent in dementia, as already described, and is then seen along with cognitive defects. But sometimes brain damage may operate more directly by disruption of regional cerebral systems upon which the synthesis of the personality depends. This situation is compatible with excellent preservation of intellect to formal testing, yet the personality change is nonetheless organic in origin. Thus when disturbance of cognitive processes cannot be identified, the term 'organic personality change' is preferable to 'dementia'. Most examples occur with strictly focal brain damage, the best known being with lesions of the frontal lobes of the brain.

'Chronic amnesic syndrome'. Disorder of memory, especially for recent events, is an integral part of dementia, but can also exist without global impairment of intellect. Such memory disturbance may emerge as the sole defect, as after bilateral hippocampal lesions, or more commonly may stand out as the obtrusive defect while other cognitive processes are but little affected. Such a syndrome may ensue on an acute organic reaction which clears to reveal a relatively isolated defect of memory, as when Wernicke's encephalopathy leads on to Korsakoff's syndrome.

The term 'chronic amnesic syndrome' usefully describes the essential features of disorder in all such cases, and emphasises the distinction from dementia. It may be defined as an organic impairment of memory out of all proportion to other cognitive changes. A focal rather than a diffuse brain pathology can be confidently predicted as described on pp. 25–8.

Unfortunately the terms 'chronic amnesic syndrome' and 'Korsakoff's amnesic syndrome' are sometimes used interchangeably, the territory of the latter being allowed to expand considerably. Strictly speaking the term Korsakoff's syndrome should be restricted to those patients whose amnesia depends on lesions in the hypothalamus and diencephalon and is consequent upon thiamine deficiency. A broader conception allows inclusion of all amnesic syndromes deriving from brain damage in this location, as described on p. 25. Chronic amnesic syndromes due to damage elsewhere, for example in the medial temporal lobe structures, should not be labelled as korsakovian.

'Organic hallucinosis' refers to a syndrome of recurrent or persistent hallucinations, occurring in a setting of full preservation of consciousness and awareness of the envi-

ronment yet attributable to organic factors. The patient is not disorientated and proves capable of thinking with normal clarity throughout. The hallucinations occur mostly in the auditory or visual modalities but any sensory modality can be affected. Insight into the unreal nature of the phenomena may vary markedly in degree, but any delusions that occur are secondary to the hallucinatory experiences. Such a syndrome may be occasioned by circumscribed brain lesions, strategically placed to irritate cortical or subcortical areas, but is more commonly seen as a result of toxic processes. The hallucinations occurring during the early phase of alcohol withdrawal (pp. 598–9) or after lysergic acid diethylamide (LSD) (p. 621) are typical examples.

In the DSM-III classification of mental disorders it was proposed that further organic syndromes should be recognised, to take account of those patients who show predominantly non-cognitive psychopathological features in the presence of brain malfunction (Diagnostic & Statistical Manual of Mental Disorders 1980; Lipowski 1980b). Thus an 'organic affective syndrome', an 'organic anxiety syndrome' and an 'organic delusional syndrome' were recognised when such disturbances were judged to be the direct consequence of a cerebral disorder rather than a reflection of the subjective meaning of an event or situation for the person. Before applying such labels it was necessary to establish the provoking organic condition, usually with a definable temporal relationship to the development of the mental disturbance. Examples of organic affective disorder included the depression seen with Cushing's disease or induced by rauwolfia alkaloids; and organic delusional disorders included certain psychoses seen with epilepsy and the acute paranoid psychoses following amphetamine intoxication. In DSM-IV there is no longer a need for such categories, since mood disorders and psychoses arising in such contexts are listed under their respective general headings and specified as being due to a general medical condition or arising from substance abuse.

Contemporaneously, however, ICD-10 has introduced equivalent terms—'organic catatonic disorder', 'organic delusional (schizophrenia-like) disorder', 'organic mood disorder', 'organic anxiety disorder', 'organic dissociative disorder' and 'organic emotionally labile (asthenic) disorder' (World Health Organization 1992). Such diagnoses are made when there is evidence of cerebral disease, damage or dysfunction, or of systemic physical disease, known to be associated with one of the listed syndromes; when there is a temporal relationship between the development of such disease and the onset of the mental syndrome; and absence of delirium or dementia. The justification for applying the label is increased when recovery from the mental disorder follows improvement of the underlying presumed cause, and in the absence of evidence of a strong family history or of precipitating stress.

Generalised versus focal cerebral disorder

A great number of organic psychiatric disorders are due to widespread disturbance of brain function. This may be the result of diffuse disease processes within the brain, as in certain degenerative diseases, or of systemic disturbances, for example those leading to anoxia which impair brain function indirectly. Moreover, well localised brain lesions may declare themselves only when secondary diffuse effects supervene, as with raised intracranial pressure in association with cerebral tumour. The majority of acute and chronic organic reactions therefore reflect widespread disorder of cerebral activity and contain symptoms of defective function in many spheres.

It has become customary to talk of 'generalised cerebral disorder' and to distinguish this from the effects of strictly focal pathology. It must, however, be appreciated that both generalised and focal disturbances of brain function represent theoretical extremes which are rarely if ever encountered in practice. It is most unlikely that intrinsic brain disease is ever uniformly distributed throughout the brain, and some degree of focal emphasis can usually be discerned with careful observation. Extrinsic factors which impair brain function are likewise selective in their effects, sparing some neural or neurochemical systems while disrupting others. Impairment of consciousness, for example, represents interference with brain stem alerting functions while cardiovascular and respiratory functions are little affected. Similarly disruption of cortical and subcortical functions very rarely occurs to an equivalent extent.

Strictly focal disorder, on the other hand, is also very rare except when purposely produced by surgical procedures. In naturally occurring disease we merely see a focal emphasis of pathology, which in greater or lesser degree is complicated by the additional effects of damage elsewhere.

Nevertheless it is of great importance in practical clinical terms to preserve the distinction between clinical pictures which result from widely disseminated or from relatively circumscribed brain dysfunction. The distinction is essential in the formulation of likely causes and thence in deciding on the lines which investigation must follow. Each, in practice, contains different symptoms of fundamental importance.

The plan in the present chapter will be first to describe in broad terms the characteristic clinical pictures seen in 'generalised' acute and chronic reactions, and then to summarise the salient features seen with focal damage or focal emphasis of pathology in specific brain regions. The focal significance of certain symptoms and symptom complexes will be dealt with in more detail in Chapter 2.

Clinical picture in acute organic reactions
(acute brain syndrome, acute confusional state, acute organic psychosis, acute psycho-organic syndrome, 'delirium')

The acute organic reactions are called forth by a great number of different pathological processes affecting the brain, including trauma, cerebral anoxia, epilepsy, metabolic derangements such as uraemia, or the toxic effects of drugs or alcohol. A list of causes is presented in Table 3 on p. 153. The onset is always fairly abrupt, though when slight in degree the disorder may not declare itself in an obvious fashion from the outset. The majority of acute organic reactions are reversible when the underlying pathology can be remedied, but some may progress directly to a chronic organic syndrome, as when an acute post-traumatic psychosis clears to reveal dementia or when Wernicke's encephalopathy results in an enduring amnesic syndrome.

The clinical pictures which result are essentially due to disruption of normal brain function by virtue of biochemical, electrical or mechanical disturbances. The symptomatology follows a surprisingly constant pattern despite these various causes. To some extent there are specific features depending on rate of development, the intensity and perhaps the nature of the noxious agent, but this variability is small in relative terms. The personality and background of the patient will also colour the picture, especially in minor affections and particularly where matters such as intensity of emotional disturbance or content of delusional thinking are concerned. The main emphasis in what follows, however, will be on shared and common forms of reaction.

Impairment of consciousness

Impairment of consciousness is the primary change in acute organic reactions, and in some degree is universal. It therefore holds a fundamentally important place in the detection of acute disturbances of brain function and in the assessment of their severity. Other features, such as disordered psychomotor activity, perception and emotion, may be more striking but are less constantly found and are also more variable in their manifestations.

Impairment of consciousness ranges on a single continuum from barely perceptible dulling of awareness to profound coma. Characteristically the impairment fluctuates when mild in degree, often worsening at night with fatigue and with decreased environmental stimulation. The fluctuations and the appearance of lucid intervals are observations of great clinical importance in the differential diagnosis of organic from non-organic psychiatric disorders, also in distinguishing acute from chronic organic reactions. Daytime visits may find the patient at his best, and it is thus essential to pay attention to reports of changed behaviour as nightfall approaches.

Considerable difficulties can surround the conception of levels of consciousness in patients with acute organic reactions, partly because of problems inherent in the use of certain terms and partly because of the expectation that impaired consciousness must necessarily be accompanied by decreased responsiveness to stimuli. In fact surprising instances may be seen. In most conditions impairment of consciousness is accompanied by diminished arousal and alertness which become clinically apparent at some stage of the disorder. But in others, as in delirium tremens, the patient may be hyperaroused and hyperalert. Arousal and alertness, in this context, refer to the readiness with which the patient responds to environmental stimuli, 'arousal' being best used to describe the physiological state of the organism and 'alertness' to describe the observational data from which this state is inferred.

Preserved alertness is not, however, the sole yardstick by which preservation of normal consciousness is assessed. To be useful alertness must be coupled with an ability to select discriminatingly between those stimuli which are important and meaningful and those which are not. Moreover, the relevant stimuli must gain access to conscious awareness where they can be related to past experience and present needs. For these purposes alertness must be accompanied by a capacity to attend. When consciousness is impaired certain qualities of attention will invariably be found to be defective—qualities referred to as *phasic, modulated, selective* or *directed* attention.

They involve the capacity not merely to allow a stimulus to elicit a response, but to mobilise, focus, sustain and shift attention in a fluid and changing manner according to the needs of the moment. Whether the patient is hypo- or hyperalert it will often soon become apparent that such mechanisms are at fault. Failure to be selective can result in indiscriminate, often excessive, responses to stimuli with the result that the patient is *distractible*; failure to mobilise and sustain attention is seen in *impaired concentration*; inability to shift attention can lead to *perseveration*. The examiner's difficulty in engaging with the patient may owe much to all of these factors. A more pervasive change may also occur, whereby internal percepts, thoughts and images come to hold attention more readily than percepts from the environment, allowing them to become elaborated in an unrestrained manner. This would appear to be important in the genesis of the vivid affects, fantasies and hallucinations of 'delirium', as described on pp. 600–1.

A true appreciation of the patient's level of consciousness must therefore include assessment, not only of alertness and responsivity, but also of capacity to attend in a discriminating manner to what is going on around.

A minor degree of impairment of consciousness may present merely with complaints of vague malaise and feelings of uncertainty. It may escape detection at the time, and be revealed only in retrospect by the amnesic gap left for the period in question. Other sensitive indicators are minor difficulties in judging the passage of time, in focusing attention as described just above, or in thinking coherently. The latter again may initially be more apparent subjectively than to external observation. Sometimes there may be neglect of appearance and of needs, or an episode of incontinence may be an early sign. The sleep–wakefulness cycle is almost universally disturbed in some degree, with various combinations of insomnia, vivid dreams and dream-like mentation (Lipowski 1980a, 1990). The diurnal rhythm of activity is sometimes clearly disordered, with a tendency to somnolence by day and excitability at night.

With more severe degrees of impairment, the patient is observed to be slow in responding, loses the thread in conversation, and attention to outside events is hard to arouse and sustain. Responses to requests may betray inadequate understanding or lack of volition to carry them out. Later still the patient is clearly drowsy, sleeps excessively and, if rousable shows only a torpid and muddled awareness.

Psychomotor behaviour

Motor behaviour usually diminishes progressively as impairment of consciousness increases. When left alone the patient shows little spontaneous activity and habitual acts such as eating are carried out in an automatic manner. The capacity for purposive action is diminished. When pressed to engage in activities the patient is slow, hesitant and often perseverative. He responds to external stimuli apathetically if at all, though highly charged subjective events such as hallucinatory experiences may still call forth abrupt and even excessive reactions. Speech is slow and sparse, answers stereotyped or incoherent, and difficult questions are usually ignored. There is often slurring, perseveration, or dysphasic difficulties. In severe cases there may be no more than incoherent muttering.

While the above is the rule with most acute affections of the brain, some show the reverse with restless hyperactivity and noisy disturbing behaviour. Delirium tremens and the deliria which accompany certain systemic infections are the well-known examples. Not surprisingly these florid cases figure disproportionately highly in most published accounts of acute organic reactions. Psychomotor activity is greatly increased with an excessive tendency to startle reactions. Typically the overactivity consists of repetitive, purposeless behaviour, such as ceaseless groping or picking movements. Behaviour may be dictated by hallucinations and delusions, the patient turning for example to engage in imaginary conversation, or ransacking the bedclothes for objects thought to be hidden there. More rarely he may perform complex stereotyped movements, re-enacting the driving of a car or miming his usual work ('occupational delirium'). Sometimes there is dangerously belligerent behaviour. When purposive, the activities are usually misdirected, inappropriate or bizarre, and voluntary movements are often jerky and uneven. The overactivity is often accompanied by excitement with noisy shouting, laughing or crying. There may be pressure of speech with incoherent flight of ideas. Most of the behaviour is obviously dictated by the patient's own internal world, and alertness to external stimuli is seen to be impaired. Not uncommonly the clinical picture shows rapid changes from phases of overactivity to periods of apathy and aspontaneity.

Thinking

Thought processes show characteristic changes when consciousness is impaired. In the early stages there is subjective slowing, with difficulty in focusing thoughts or formulating complex ideas. Mental fatigue may be obvious in the course of examination. Later, reasoning becomes less clear and coherent, logic is impaired and thinking is more concrete and literal. Even when speeded by high arousal the thought content is seen to be banal and impoverished. Trains of thought become chaotic, showing in speech as fragmentation and incoherence.

An important change is in the relative importance of the internal and external worlds, and in the decreasing ability to preserve the distinction between the two. Thus perceptions and thoughts become inextricably interwoven (defective 'reality testing'). Comprehension of events is impaired, with inability to embrace the elements of experience and relate them meaningfully to one another (impaired 'grasp'). The patient may be unaware of the most obvious features of his situation, whether he is standing or lying, whether indoors or in the street. At the same time increased significance is attached to subjective experiences, ideas or false perceptions, which come to dominate the content of consciousness. Bizarre thoughts and fantasies intrude into awareness, and false significance is attached to external cues. Illusions and hallucinations readily arise, and vivid dream material may be carried over into waking life.

Ideas of reference and delusion formation may become prominent, depending to some extent on qualities in the premorbid personality. Delusions of persecution are especially common, and may well up suddenly with conviction. They usually betray their organic origin in being poorly elaborated, vague, transient and inconsistent. When consciousness is relatively clear, however, the delusions may be more coherently organised, with a picture more closely resembling schizophrenia. In rare cases delusions may persist when the patient has recovered from the acute illness, with an obstinate belief in the reality of the hallucinatory experiences that occurred.

Insight is typically lost early, but may vary with fluctuations in the level of consciousness. Sometimes even in moderately severe affections the patient may be briefly roused to self awareness and to a better appreciation of reality.

Memory

With impairment of consciousness there is disturbance of registration, retention and recall. Registration of current experience is hampered by defects in attention, perception and comprehension. Accordingly the immediate memory span for digits or similar material is found to be reduced. Defective retention leads to difficulty with new learning which is a sensitive clinical indicator in mild stages of disorder. Recent memories prove to be faulty while long-term memories are reasonably intact, though with moderate impairment of consciousness both are found to suffer.

An early change is defective appreciation of the flow of time, and the jumbling of time sequences for recent events. This quickly leads to disorientation in time, which is sometimes regarded as the hallmark of acute organic reactions. Disorientation may, however, be transient in the early stages, and a normally orientated patient may prove later to be amnesic for all that passed during the interview in which he was examined.

Disorientation for place, and later still for person, follow with worsening of perceptual and cognitive disorganisation. Patterson and Zangwill (1944) have drawn attention to the way in which patients may maintain two incompatible attitudes towards their orientation without seeming aware of the inconsistency. This can emerge strikingly where orientation for place is concerned, the patient saying quite correctly, for example, that he is in hospital in one town, yet interpreting his surroundings and behaving in every other way as though he were at home in another part of the country ('reduplicative paramnesia'). Such correct and incorrect orientations may exist side by side in a vacillating and unrelated manner, or be reconciled by shallow rationalisations. The patient may insist that the two places are the same, or contiguous with each other, or confabulate a recent journey between the two.

Reduplicative paramnesias may take a number of forms and are sometimes associated with misrecognition or reduplication of persons. They can be seen with chronic organic reactions as well, perhaps particularly in association with right hemisphere pathology.

In the above example the reduplicative paramnesia consists of a false and internally inconsistent orientation between two places. In others the faulty orientation is internally consistent, as when the patient claims that the house he is in is not the real one but a duplicate with every feature correctly reproduced. In this it resembles the Capgras syndrome (p. 15). Kapur *et al.* (1988) describe such an example, suggesting that the substrate for its development is a particular combination of memory impairment, attentional/spatial deficit and impaired reasoning capacity. In Fleminger's (1992a) example it seemed likely that preconscious processing of percepts played a part, in that manipulation of the patient's expectations could cause the paramnesia to disappear. His conviction that the house he was in was not his real home could be broken by walking him to a nearby bus stop and getting a bus back to the house which was his habitual method of coming home: the sense of familiarity aroused on alighting from the bus restored the normal affective colouring of the perception of his house.

A third variety consists of false memories rather than faulty orientation, the patient believing for example that he was admitted from a house identical to his own but in another place, or believing that he has been in numerous different hospitals, perhaps all with identical layout but in different parts of the country. Patterson and Mack (1985) describe an interesting example of the latter following a right hemisphere infarct, the reduplicative memories persisting for several months. A combination of perceptual and memory deficits appeared to be responsible along with impaired ability to integrate information.

False memories and confabulation may occasionally be in evidence, and misidentifications, including pseudo-recognition, are facilitated by the perceptual abnormalities described below.

On recovery there is typically a dense amnesic gap for the period of the acute illness, though where fluctuation has been marked islands of memory may remain. Sometimes sensory impressions, and especially vivid hallucinations, stand out clearly and are remembered in great detail when all else is forgotten, attesting again to the importance of subjective experience over external reality in severe stages of the disorder.

Perception

Quite commonly it is the more florid perceptual abnormalities which draw attention to the presence of an acute organic reaction in a patient suffering from some physical disease. However, these are not essential features in every case, and the diagnosis should be made by seeking out the subtle deficits in thinking, memory and attention which betray impairment of consciousness.

Early on the patient may be aware that perception requires unusual effort, particularly where vision is concerned. Sometimes, by contrast, perceptions appear subjectively to be hyperacute. Disturbances of vision include micropsia, macropsia or distortions of shape and position. Disordered auditory perception may hinder clear communication. There may be distortions of weight and size, or bizarre disorders of the body image in which body parts feel shrunken, enlarged, misplaced or even disconnected. The whole body may feel as though it is tilted or floating. Disordered perception of internal bodily sensations lead sometimes to bizarre complaints. Genuine physical symptoms such as vertigo, headache and paraesthesiae are likewise often reported in distorted fashion.

Depersonalisation and derealisation are common, though usually incompletely expressed. Dissolution of the perceptual boundaries between the self and the environment may give rise to terrifying feelings of imminent dissolution or loss of bodily and personal integrity.

Perceptual abnormalities readily lead to misinterpretations and illusions which are typically fleeting and changeable. The visual modality is affected most often. Difficulty with visual recognition combines with faulty thinking and memory to produce false recognitions and faulty orientation in place. The unfamiliar tends to be mistaken for the familiar, or may be interpreted as hostile or persecutory. Thus the patient may misidentify a nurse as a relative, or the doctor as an old friend or enemy. The hospital ward may be mistaken for home or prison. Chance noises may similarly be misinterpreted, contributing to delusion formation. The whole is often reinforced by disordered affects of fear and suspicion.

Hallucinations are also commonest in the visual modality, though tactile and auditory hallucinations occur as well. They probably derive partly from failure to distinguish inner images from outer percepts, and partly from vivid dreams carried over into the waking state as consciousness waxes and wanes. Simple visual hallucinations consist of flashes of light, geometrical patterns or colours. More complex phenomena, sometimes kaleidoscopic in nature may occur, with fully-formed hallucinations of scenes, people and animals. A bizarre fantastic quality is not uncommon. The hallucinated material may be grossly distorted, as with Lilliputian hallucinations where objects and people appear to be minute in size. The reality of the phenomena is fully accepted by the patient, who may react with fear and alarm but sometimes with interest or even amusement.

Hallucinations appear to be particularly characteristic of the acute organic reactions occasioned by certain pathological processes. Delirium tremens remains the classic example with extremely florid hallucinations as described on pp. 600–1. Toxic agents such as LSD are also notorious for the wealth of formed and unformed hallucinations that occur. Animals are said to feature particularly frequently in the hallucinations of delirium tremens, and visual hallucinations of 'nets' were said to characterise the organic reactions seen in bromide intoxication when this was common.

Emotion

In early stages mild depression, anxiety and irritability may be expected, though typically the affect is shallow. With deeper impairment, and further impoverishment of mental processes, apathy usually becomes the striking feature, and the whole course of the illness may pass with indifference and emotional withdrawal. More lively affects are seen in conjunction with increased psychomotor activity when affective disturbance may become intense. Anxiety and fear are especially common, increasing sometimes to terror and panic. A state of wondering perplexity forms a common background to other affective states. Depression is frequent, elation or anger less so. Paranoid attitudes may show in marked hostility and suspicion. The affective reactions are often fleeting and changeable with changing delusional ideas. Sudden displays of primitive and highly charged emotion are often called forth by hallucinatory experiences.

In part the emotional state is likely to be determined by the stress of the physical illness, and in part by a vague awareness of cognitive impairments. The individual's personality structure may contribute in considerable measure, some patients being predisposed to react by apathetic withdrawal and others by projection of fantasised dangers onto the environment. The extent of such influences has not been determined, nor the degree to which the picture is shaped by different pathogenic agents. There are strong clinical impressions that delirium tremens tends to be accompanied by intense fear, hepatic encephalopathy by euphoria or depression, and uraemia by apathy, but reliable and systematic comparisons have not been made. It is clear, moreover, that several factors are often operative together in leading to delirium in the individual patient, particularly in the elderly (Francis *et al.* 1990).

Other features

In the milder stages in particular, the definitive organic features may be less in evidence than those which depend on individual traits and characteristics. Psychological reactions to early cognitive impairment, or to the stress of the underlying physical disease, may dominate the picture and emerge in the form of neurotic symptoms. Similarly, vulnerable aspects of personality may be exaggerated, with the appearance of depressive, hypochondriacal or phobic features. Histrionic and importunate behaviour may sometimes be much in evidence. Hysterical conversion symptoms, usually transient but sometimes persistent, may lead to mistakes in diagnosis. Paranoid developments occur frequently, and can become the overriding feature at an early stage in susceptible individuals. A distinct schizophrenic colouring to the total clinical picture is likewise not uncommon. With progression of cognitive disorganisation the true situation usually becomes apparent, but mild self-limiting acute organic reactions can be misdiagnosed for some time as non-organic psychiatric illness.

Clinical picture in chronic organic reactions (chronic brain syndrome, chronic confusional state, chronic organic psychosis, chronic psycho-organic syndrome, 'dementia')

Chronic like acute organic reactions, result from many different pathological processes, yet the clinical picture shows a large measure of similarity from one condition to another. A focal emphasis of pathology may produce special patterns of impairment, but the purpose in what follows is to describe the general clinical picture and to emphasise the shared and common forms of reaction that occur.

While the majority of chronic organic reactions are due to diffuse and widespread affections of the brain, some owe their origins to focal pathology, so careful examination for signs of localising value must always be undertaken. The principal causes are listed in Table 4 on p. 153. Most of the illnesses concerned are slowly progressive with increasing disablement, but static pictures may be seen as with arrested general paresis, or gradual improvement may occur as after head injury. In a small but extremely important group therapeutic intervention can decisively reverse the process, for example with myxoedema or normal-pressure hydrocephalus, or when a frontal meningioma is discovered to be the cause.

Mode of presentation

Some chronic organic reactions follow upon acute episodes such as trauma or anoxia, and are then revealed in full when the patient recovers consciousness, or else emerge by a process of transition from an acute organic reaction. The great majority, however, develop insidiously from the start.

The commonest mode of onset is with evidence of impairment of memory or more general disorganisation of intellect. Failures of memory are usually noted earlier by relatives and workmates than by the patient himself. They show in missed appointments, apparent unawareness of recent happenings, a tendency to mix up times or to lose things. More general cognitive failure emerges in slipshod work and loss of overall efficiency. The patient may be noticed to think and speak less coherently than usual, to muddle money or to fail to grasp essentials.

Change in personality as the first manifestation is much less common, but when it occurs the patient is especially likely to come before the psychiatrist. Here intellectual deficits are mild or absent in the early stages, or pass unnoticed because of curtailment of activities and the use of props and evasions. Deterioration of manners may be the earliest sign, or diminished awareness of the needs and feelings of others. Some social blunder may disclose the problem, such as stealing or disinhibited behaviour out of character for the individual. Sometimes the earliest change is merely the exaggeration of long-standing personality traits such as suspiciousness or egocentricity. Neurotic traits may be elaborated with the production of depressive, obsessional, hysterical or hypochondriacal symptoms. More rarely the illness presents with the picture of a psychotic illness of depressive, paranoid or schizophrenic type in especially predisposed individuals. It is then only by careful examination that the intellectual deterioration is revealed.

Whatever the form of presentation, the illness may declare itself abruptly even though its evolution has been insidious. Some episode of acute mental disturbance may bring the disease to attention. Or relatives may have adjusted to the slow decline until some dramatic instance forces their attention to the true situation. Not infrequently a tenuous adjustment is concealed until new demands must be met, for example on the death of a partner or a move to a new environment. Admission to hospital may be the step which reveals the disorder, and only careful retrospective enquiry then establishes that the onset has been gradual. Intercurrent illness may bring the situation to light by pushing the patient below the threshold at which the brain was previously coping, especially infection, anoxia or postoperative metabolic derangements.

General behaviour

Although impairment of intellectual ability is the hallmark of chronic organic reactions this may be manifest only indirectly by way of behavioural change. Typical early signs are loss of interest and initiative, inability to perform up to the usual standard, or minor episodes of muddle and confusion. Episodes of bizarrely inappropriate behaviour may occur, as when the housewife unloads her shopping in the oven or prepares a meal at an inappropriate time. As described just above, some cases present with changes in the field of social behaviour well before impairment of cognitive processes is overt.

As the disorder progresses the same division is seen, some aspects of behaviour reflecting the intellectual disorganisation, and some the change in emotional control and social awareness. Intellectual impairment shows as incapacity for decisive action, loss of application and inability to persist in a consistent course of conduct. Despite full alertness and the preservation of normal levels of consciousness the patient fatigues readily on mental effort. He responds appropriately to stimuli within his limited range of comprehension and is capable of directed attention as the need arises, but powers of concentration are impaired. Goldstein (1939, 1942) has stressed the various behavioural changes which reflect the attempts of the personality to cope with such defects. There is often restlessness, with purposeless overactivity. Typically this occurs within a diminishing sphere of interests and activities ('shrinkage of the milieu'), with rigid adherence to routines and stereotyped organisation of behaviour ('organic over-orderliness'). In this manner the patient may be enabled to cope for a while. When taxed beyond his ability, however, he may become evasive and sullen, or react abruptly with an explosion of primitive affect such as anger, anxiety or tears ('catastrophic reaction'). Social interaction is often marked by lack of concern towards others, stubborn egocentricity or withdrawal from social contact ('self exclusion').

In the later stages hygiene and personal appearance are neglected and ritualistic hoarding may develop. Food is eaten sloppily, habits deteriorate and there is indifference to urinary or faecal incontinence. In contrast, however, some patients preserve superficial social competence until surprisingly late in the course of the disease.

Eventually, behaviour becomes futile and aimless, often with stereotypies and mannerisms. Impoverishment of thought is reflected in lack of purposive activity, and physical deterioration follows with increasing weakness and emaciation.

Thinking

Thinking is impaired both qualitatively and quantitatively. It becomes slowed with reduced powers of concentration and ready mental fatigue. The content of thought is impoverished with fewer associations, inability to produce new ideas, and a tendency to dwell on set topics and memories from the past. Themes are banal and perseveration usually marked. The ability to reason logically and to manipulate concepts is impaired, likewise the ability to keep in mind various aspects of a situation simultaneously. Specific skills such as calculation are usually impaired from an early stage.

Intellectual flexibility is lost, leading to difficulty in shifting from one frame of reference to another. The lack of effective counter-ideas leads the patient to become tied to the immediate situations that arise, so that he is distracted by accidental impressions and events and becomes 'stimulus bound' to them. Such difficulties are compounded by inability to extract the essentials of a situation or experience ('disturbance of figure–ground relationships'). Abstract ideas present especial difficulty and concepts tend to be given their most literal interpretation ('concretisation').

Judgement is impaired early. The patient's insight is poor and there may be little awareness of illness at all. False ideas readily gain ground and paranoid ideation is particularly common. Ideas of reference may reflect an exaggeration of premorbid tendencies. Delusions are typically persecutory in nature and may owe much to limbic dysfunction (Cummings 1992a). The complexity of their content tends to be inversely proportional to the severity of cognitive impairment, patients with severe dementia usually harbouring only simple and loosely structured false beliefs. Occasionally, however, they become entrenched and unshakeable. As Roth and Myers (1969) point out they may be delusions in the technical sense, in that the beliefs are held in the face of evidence of their falsehood, but this is largely because the evidence fails to be understood, not because it is rejected. Delusional themes are often crude and bizarre, typically of being robbed, poisoned, threatened or deprived.

Major theme-specific delusions may sometimes stand out in relative isolation, as with the reduplicative paramnesias described on p. 12. Delusions involving the reduplication of persons, as opposed to places, can also emerge with brain disease. The *Capgras syndrome* ('illusion de sosies'), in which the patient believes that a relative or friend has been replaced by an impostor who resembles the original exactly, was associated with evidence of brain damage in almost two-thirds of the cases reviewed by Malloy *et al.* (1992). Right frontotemporal dysfunction appeared often to be involved. Related disorders include the *Fregoli syndrome*, in which a persecutor is believed to have adopted multiple disguises; thus while a number of people around the patient are recognised as having different appearances they are all thought to represent a single familiar person who is bent on harming the patient. With *intermetamorphosis* individuals are believed to have changed appearance to look like

others, particularly enemies, and in the *doppelgänger delusion* the patient believes that he himself has a double or impersonator. All are rare.

In the later stages thinking appears to be restricted to circumscribed reiterative themes, and becomes grossly fragmented, incoherent and disorganised.

Speech

The disturbances in thinking are mirrored in speech. The most characteristic disturbance is poverty of speech with excessive employment of clichés and set phrases. The pool of vocabulary is greatly reduced, and speech initiative is poor. Sentences are often simple, incomplete and poorly constructed, with perseveration, stereotyped utterances and echolalia.

Paraphasic errors, and nominal dysphasia, are not uncommon. Barker and Lawson (1968) suggest that difficulty in word finding is a general feature in dementia if care is taken to test with words of low frequency of usage. Stengel (1964) has described special characteristics of nominal dysphasia in patients with diffuse brain lesions. There may be little evidence of disability until the patient is pressed to name an object, whereupon he may show little awareness of his errors. This is in contrast to the situation in nominal dysphasia due to focal brain lesions. Sometimes he may improvise to produce new words, showing perseveration and 'clang' associations. Stengel also describes 'lowering of the speech conscience', in which words are used as fancy dictates, all being part of the disregard of language as a code of communication. Concretisation shows in the excessive use of words which refer to the self and the tendency for external stimuli to influence the words that are chosen — 'the situation and the self tend to intrude excessively into the process of naming'.

Ultimately, speech becomes grossly disorganised and fragmented, and used exclusively in the service of bodily needs. The patient may become mute or capable only of a restricted range of semicoherent ejaculations.

Memory

Memory disturbance is frequently the earliest sign of a developing chronic organic reaction, and at first may be intermittent. Allison (1962) makes the important point that with diffuse as opposed to focal cerebral lesions the onset of memory disturbance can rarely be dated accurately because it has been of such gradual evolution. The onset may be marked by minor forgetfulness and 'absent mindedness', or by more definite episodes in which new impressions fail to register and striking lapses of memory occur. Loss of topographical memory is often seen, with the patient losing his way when away from home. Disorientation in time is a frequent early sign; disorientation for place and person are found much later in development.

The memory defect is typically global, affecting all categories of material and remote as well as recent events, as described on pp. 32–3. Failure at new learning is usually the most conspicuous sign, but there is rarely the sharp demarcation between remote and recent memory which characterises the purer amnesic syndromes. Recall is affected as well as registration and retention, as shown by increased success with prompting and better performance at recognition than at free recall. Memory for names is sometimes particularly affected. Temporal sequences are disorganised early, with faulty appreciation of the flow of time and mislocation of past events. Berlyne (1972) found that over a third of an unselected group of demented patients showed unequivocal confabulation, sometimes representing a true memory displaced in time, but sometimes consisting of more sustained and elaborate productions.

Characteristically the patient's awareness of his memory difficulties is impaired, or there may even be an apparently motivated desire to hide the deficits with facile excuses and shallow confabulations. In the early stages the patient may show surprising ingenuity in covering up his failures, and may compensate by means of a rigid daily routine and the use of a notebook. Ultimately, however, memory for current events may fail completely and the patient may be able produce only a few jumbled recollections from the past.

Emotion

Emotional changes form an integral part of the clinical picture in chronic organic reactions and deterioration of emotion and intellect frequently pursue a parallel course.

Early emotional changes probably reflect the struggle to cope with incipient intellectual deficits, and are coloured by premorbid personality characteristics. Anxiety is common, likewise depression with agitation and hypochondriacal features. Serious suicidal attempts may occur at this stage. Irritability leads to querulous morose behaviour, and sometimes to outbursts of anger and hostility. Perplexity and suspicion are other common early developments, leading on to paranoid beliefs and attitudes.

Further deterioration produces emotional changes of a distinctive organic type. Affective blunting and shallowness may progress to states of apathy or empty euphoria.

Emotions may take on a child-like aspect, with petulant importunate behaviour and short-lived excessive responses to trivial annoyances. Thus the death of a spouse may leave the patient unmoved, yet interference with some simple routine may provoke outbursts of anger.

Emotional control may show a characteristic threshold effect in which there is little response to mild stimulation but thereafter an excessive and prolonged disturbance. Emotional lability may be extreme, with episodes of pathological laughing and crying for little or no cause. The 'catastrophic reaction' may be observed when the patient is taxed beyond his ability to cope, as described on p. 97.

The ultimate picture in progressive disease represents a combination of these various emotional changes, but characterised above all by increasing emptiness of affect, shallowness, dullness and lack of emotional response.

Other features

The impact of chronic diffuse brain disease is not entirely unaffected by features specific to the individual. As already mentioned, neurotic manifestations may be conspicuous in mild stages of disorder. Hysterical conversion symptoms and obsessional disorders may figure prominently, the former perhaps by virtue of increased suggestibility and the latter as a mode of coping with reduced resources. A predisposition towards affective or schizophrenic psychosis may lend a distinctive colouring to the clinical picture and lead to mistaken diagnosis in the early stages. Hallucinations can occur in visual, auditory and tactile modalities, and are typically paranoid in content. With progressive disease all such manifestations are usually ultimately engulfed in the general pattern of intellectual and social decline.

Clinical picture in focal cerebral disorder

Strictly focal brain damage can be responsible for both acute and chronic organic reactions. Symptoms and signs of localizing significance may then be much in evidence, and must be kept in mind in the clinical assessment of all patients who show organic psychiatric illnesses.

Epileptic phenomena, and especially those of temporal lobe epilepsy, are clear examples of acute psychological disturbances due to focal brain dysfunction, also some of the disturbances seen after small acute cerebrovascular accidents. Wernicke's encephalopathy is another classic example, with its own distinctive chronic end-state in the chronic amnesic syndrome. For obvious reasons, however, focal brain disorder has been most comprehensively studied in slowly progressive or static lesions of long duration, which allow the focal components to be disentangled from any generalised deficits that coexist.

In Chapter 2 the complex problems of the focal significance of psychological symptoms will be dealt with in detail. Here, those which emerge with fair consistency after lesions of different parts of the brain will be described in summary form. Neurological defects are in general more reliable than psychological symptoms in pointing to the site of focal pathology, and these too will be included. The content of focal epileptic seizures, as discussed on pp. 249–57, provides additional clinical information which must also be taken into account.

In general focal signs and symptoms serve only to indicate the site of likely pathology, and are of relatively little value in themselves in suggesting the nature of the lesion.

Frontal lobes

Frontal lesions may confer distinctive changes of disposition and temperament subsumed under the term 'change of personality'. Most characteristic is disinhibition, with expansive over-familiarity, tactlessness, over-talkativeness, childish excitement ('moria') or prankish joking and punning ('Witzelsucht'). Social and ethical control may be diminished, with lack of concern for the future and for the consequence of actions. Sexual indiscretions and petty misdemeanours may occur, or gross errors of judgement with regard to financial and interpersonal matters. Sometimes there is marked indifference, even callous unconcern, for the feelings of others. Lack of insight on the part of the patient is characteristic. Elevation of mood is often seen, mainly as an empty and fatuous euphoria rather than as a true elation which communicates itself to the observer. In other cases the principal changes are lack of initiative, aspontaneity and profound slowing of psychomotor activity, particularly with frontal lobe tumours. This may progress to a state of extreme aspontaneity amounting virtually to stupor.

Concentration, attention and ability to carry out planned activity are impaired by these changes, but performance on tests of formal intelligence is often surprisingly well preserved once the patient's cooperation has been secured. Even with sharply circumscribed frontal lesions, however, the overall picture may at first sight strongly resemble a generalised dementing process. The hazards of misdiagnosis are increased by the 'silent' nature of frontal lobe lesions, which can allow them to grow large before declaring themselves with neurological signs.

When frontal lesions encroach upon the motor cortex or motor projections there will be contralateral spastic paresis, usually seen earliest in the face and more obvious on voluntary movement than emotional expression. Paresis may be extremely slight, and show only as slowness of repeated movements or falling away of the outstretched arm. A grasp reflex may be the only definite sign. Firmer evidence may be found in hyperactive tendon reflexes and a positive Babinski response. Characteristic decomposition of gait may be seen, with trunk ataxia or awkward postures.

Lesions affecting the orbital part of the frontal lobes may be associated with the 'forced utilisation' of objects presented to the patient, as described on p. 106. This appears to be an extension of the more commonly observed forced grasping. Posterior lesions of the dominant lobe may produce a primary motor dysphasia, a motor agraphia or an apraxia of the face and tongue. Ipsilateral optic atrophy or anosmia may result from orbital lesions of the lobe, the latter being commonly overlooked in clinical examination. Sphincteric incontinence may occur surprisingly early in view of the reasonable preservation of intellect, and is a valuable added indication.

Parietal lobes

Parietal lobe lesions are associated with a rather bewildering variety of complex cognitive disturbances, including defects of language and number sense, defective appreciation of external space, and disorders of the body image. Where some are concerned it is uncertain how far the lesions of the parietal lobe are alone responsible, or how far adjacent lesions in the temporal and occipital lobes contribute to the total picture. These matters are dealt with in Chapter 2, but the following is presented as a brief clinical guide.

Lesions of either parietal lobe may result in visuospatial difficulties and topographical disorientation. Visuospatial difficulties are most readily revealed by asking the patient to copy simple drawings or construct patterns from coloured blocks or matchsticks ('visuospatial agnosia', 'constructional dyspraxia'). Defective performance is seen more commonly with lesions of the non-dominant than dominant lobe but may occur with either. Difficulty in locating objects in space, or in describing the relationships between different objects by vision alone, may also be observed. Topographical disorientation is revealed by difficulty in learning or remembering the way about, with the result that the patient mislocates his bed in the ward, fails to find the bathroom or loses himself even in familiar surroundings.

Dominant parietal lobe lesions are associated with various forms of dysphasia, primary motor dysphasia being most in evidence with anterior lesions and primary sensory dysphasia with posterior lesions. The latter may include alexia in association with agraphia. Motor apraxia similarly accompanies dominant parietal lobe lesions, and usually affects the limbs of both sides of the body. Various components of Gerstmann's syndrome may be seen, namely finger agnosia, dyscalculia, right–left disorientation and agraphia. The syndrome is rarely seen in its entirety and individual components often occur along with other parietal lobe symptoms. Bilateral tactile agnosia is occasionally seen, as are various forms of visual agnosia when the lesion lies posteriorly in the parieto-occipital region.

Non-dominant parietal lobe lesions may produce disturbed appreciation of the body image and of external space, particularly involving the contralateral side. The left limbs may fail to be recognised or may be disowned by the patient. If paralysed or hemianaesthetic the disability may be ignored or refuted ('anosognosia'), a part of the body may be felt to be absent ('hemisomatognosia'), or in rare cases there may be phantom reduplication of body parts. Neglect of the left half of external space may show in the omission of left-sided details when drawings are copied, or in the crowding of writing into the right-hand part of the paper. Left-hand turnings may be overlooked when finding the way about. 'Dressing dyspraxia' consists of muddle when inserting limbs into garments or putting garments over the head. In addition to visuospatial agnosia there may be a marked defect of the recognition of faces ('prosopagnosia') when the lesion is posterior and involves the occipital lobe.

Neurological signs indicative of a parietal lobe lesion include cortical sensory loss and the phenomena of extinction and inattention. Cortical sensory loss consists not of analgesia but of a more complex impairment of sensation and difficulty with discrimination; objects cannot be identified by palpation ('astereognosis'), figures written on the hand cannot be named ('agraphaesthesia'), two point discrimination is impaired, and the localisation of sensory stimuli is inaccurate. Sensory extinction (sensory inattention) is shown when two parts of the body are lightly touched simultaneously and that on the side contralateral to the lesion is not perceived. Visual inattention may be demonstrated by asking the patient to point to moving objects in both half-fields of vision; when two objects move simultaneously that in the contralateral half-field is ignored.

Sensory deficits are often accompanied by evidence of mild hemiparesis in the limbs contralateral to the lesion. Deep lesions affecting the optic radiation produce a contralateral homonymous hemianopia, usually more fully developed in the lower than the upper quadrants.

Temporal lobes

Lesions restricted to the poles of the temporal lobes can be entirely asymptomatic. More commonly, however, temporal lobe lesions are associated with disturbance of intellectual functioning—lesions of the dominant lobe more so than those of the non-dominant lobe.

Dominant temporal lesions may produce language difficulties alone. This is typically a sensory dysphasia, resulting in severe cases in jargon productions. More posterior lesions on the dominant side may also impair visual aspects of language in the form of alexia and agraphia. Parietal lobe symptomatology may then also appear by way of motor apraxia, constructional apraxia and aspects of the Gerstmann syndrome.

Non-dominant temporal lobe lesions often show a paucity of symptoms and signs. Sometimes, however, visuospatial difficulties are in evidence, also prosopagnosia and hemisomatognosia.

Bilateral lesions of the medial temporal lobe structures can produce amnesic syndromes of great severity and virtually uncontaminated by other intellectual disturbances (p. 31). Unilateral temporal lobe lesions lead to a more restricted disturbance of memory for certain classes of material along with related perceptual deficits, but this is rarely a spontaneous complaint and is usually revealed only by special testing. Lesions on the dominant side impair the learning and retention of verbal material even in the absence of overt dysphasia. Non-dominant lesions impair the learning and retention of non-verbal patterned stimuli, such as music, or faces and drawings to which a name cannot be attached.

Personality disturbances identical with those accompanying frontal lesions may occur, but will more commonly be associated with intellectual and neurological deficits. Chronic temporal lobe lesions are notorious for their association with disturbance of personality, and particularly with emotional instability and aggression. Similarly lesions of the temporal lobe appear to carry an increased risk of psychotic disturbances akin to schizophrenia (p. 84). Depersonalisation may be prominent, also disturbance of sexual function. Epileptic phenomena are common with temporal lobe lesions and give important evidence of localisation (pp. 250–2).

The most reliable neurological sign of deep temporal lobe lesions is a contralateral homonymous upper quadrantic visual field defect, caused by interruption of the visual radiation in the central white matter. This sign alone may occasionally betray the presence of a temporal lobe lesion in a dementing process which has been attributed to diffuse brain damage. Deep lesions may also result in a mild contralateral hemiparesis or sensory loss due to encroachment upon fibres in the corona radiata. Equilibrium and hearing are not impaired, even by extensive unilateral lesions of the temporal neocortex.

Occipital lobes

Occipital lobe lesions lack well-established focal symptomatology except where vision is concerned. Complex disturbances of visual recognition characterise lesions of the parastriate areas. Agnosia for written or printed material ('alexia without agraphia'), colour agnosia and 'simultanagnosia' are characteristic of dominant occipital or occipitotemporal lesions, whereas bilateral pathology is usually present with visual object agnosia or prosopagnosia. Visuospatial agnosia occurs more commonly from non-dominant than from dominant occipitoparietal lesions, likewise metamorphopsia in which the appearance of objects is distorted. Complex visual hallucinations are said to occur more commonly from non-dominant than dominant occipital lesions.

Lesions of the striate cortex produce homonymous defects in the opposite half-field of vision. Extensive bilateral lesions may produce cortical blindness, distinguished from peripheral blindness by the normal appearance of the optic fundi and the preservation of pupillary light reflexes.

Corpus callosum

Expanding corpus callosum lesions typically extend laterally into adjacent parts of the hemispheres, producing a picture of severe and rapid intellectual deterioration along with changes specific to the lobes involved. Anterior tumours produce marked frontal lobe disturbance, often with extreme psychomotor retardation and aspontaneity. Dysphasia, apraxia and asymmetrical pyramidal signs are common when the parietal lobes are affected. Involvement of diencephalic structures leads to somnolence, stupor and akinesis. Bizarre postural motor abnormalities may strongly resemble the pictures seen in catatonia. Disruption of communication between the two hemispheres may result in lack of access of the non-dominant hemisphere to the speech mechanisms in the dominant hemisphere; there will then be left-sided apraxia to verbal commands, with agraphia and astereognosis in the left hand (Geschwind & Kaplan 1962). Lesions restricted to the posterior part, in association with lesions of the left occipital lobe, may result in dyslexia (without agraphia) for similar reasons (Geschwind 1962).

Diencephalon and brain stem

The most characteristic symptoms of lesions in the deep midline structures of the brain are amnesia of the Korsakoff type and hypersomnia. These may stand out against a background of progressive intellectual deterioration or present initially as the sole disturbance. Amnesia which is strikingly more marked for recent than remote events, and is sometimes accompanied by confabulation, is characteristic of lesions in the neighbourhood of the third ventricle, aqueduct and posterior hypothalamus. Somnolence and hypersomnia suggest a lesion of the posterior diencephalon and upper midbrain. It may fluctuate in intensity, or occur in brief attacks suggestive of narcolepsy. Sometimes it may progress to states of profound stupor or coma. 'Akinetic mutism' ('coma vigil') is a characteristic syndrome in which the patient lies immobile and mute, though the eyes may be open and follow moving objects (p. 229).

Intellectual deterioration may occur by virtue of raised intracranial pressure consequent upon obstruction of the cerebrospinal fluid circulation. Some focal lesions, however, produce rapidly progressive dementia without such generalised disturbance, particularly those originating within the thalamus (p. 755). Features closely akin to the 'frontal lobe syndrome' may occur with diencephalic and brain stem lesions—disinhibition, indifference, carelessness and euphoria. Insight into the changes is said to be better preserved than with the equivalent pictures produced by frontal lobe lesions. Swings of mood and sudden outbursts of violent emotion are also held to be characteristic. Bilateral lesions within the upper brain stem and diencephalon, seen for example with pseudobulbar palsy, are associated with extreme emotional lability and 'emotional incontinence'. The patient laughs or cries excessively in response to trivial stimuli, yet if questioned he denies experiencing the degree of emotion he displays, and may well be distressed at his inability to control the response.

Focal neurological signs may be surprisingly absent in the early stages of progressive diencephalic lesions. Raised intracranial pressure with headache and papilloedema are found with the majority of obstructive lesions, though even here mental symptoms may be severe before this develops. Visual field defects will betray lesions such as craniopharyngiomas which grow upwards from the sella turcica and compress the optic chiasma. However, the patient who has considerable intellectual loss may make no complaint of the visual field disturbance, and testing can sometimes be impossible.

Disturbance of hypothalamic function can result in

polydypsia, polyuria, obesity or elevation of temperature. Amenorrhoea or impotence may occur in the adult, delayed or precocious sexual development in the child. Involvement of the pituitary gland will result in a wide variety of endocrine changes, which may, however, be overlooked for a time when psychiatric disturbance is prominent.

Thalamic lesions cause the sensory disturbances characteristic of parietal lobe lesions with, in addition, hypalgesia or analgesia to painful stimuli. Brain stem lesions cause characteristic cranial nerve palsies, along with evidence of dense long-tract motor and sensory disturbances.

Chapter 2: Symptoms and Syndromes with Regional Affiliations

Certain psychological manifestations deserve particular attention because they are sometimes found in association with relatively circumscribed brain lesions. In every case they can also be seen with pathology which involves the brain diffusely or disturbs its functions widely, so their presence is not by any means a certain indication of a single localised lesion. Nevertheless when they emerge as isolated defects, or stand out prominently against a background of mild impairment of other cerebral functions, they command especial care in the search for focal pathology.

What we ask of psychological symptoms as guides to focal pathology must be considerably less than we expect of neurological signs. The latter will often point with fair precision to the site of the lesion, but psychological symptoms can often tell us little more than that the pathology is unlikely to be diffuse. The careful analysis of dysphasia or of visual perceptual deficits may take us some way towards assessing the site of the lesion, but even here we must usually be content with rather broad indications of the areas of brain that fail to function. Thus with rare exceptions there remains uncertainty about the 'regional' as opposed to the 'focal' implications of most of the syndromes considered in this chapter. Some of them will be found to owe their origin, in different patients, to focal lesions in a variety of sites.

The majority of focal psychological symptoms represent defects of cognitive functioning. Less can be said with certainty about the focal significance of emotional, motivational or 'personality' abnormalities. 'Psychotic' symptoms in particular elude clear ties to focal brain pathology, and here other determinants are known to be more important. Nevertheless, certain non-cognitive disorders and even some psychotic manifestations do show interesting regional affiliations, and these will also be briefly reviewed.

Strictly focal brain damage or dysfunction is rare, except when produced by operations on the brain. In naturally occurring disease we see merely a focal emphasis in pathology, with effects which are then compounded by the effects of damage elsewhere. Focal head injury, for example, is usually accompanied by brain damage remote from the site of principal destruction; epileptic disturbances which originate focally disrupt other cerebral systems more or less widely; and circumscribed tumours produce distant effects by distortion of brain tissue, vascular complications or raised intracranial pressure. It is not surprising, therefore, that knowledge of regional cerebral disorder has been slow to accumulate and raises many areas of controversy. Brain imaging by computerised tomography (CT) or magnetic resonance imaging (MRI), and the more recent development of sophisticated functional imaging techniques, now hold promise of clarifying some of the problems in this area. Evidence from work with animals has given important leads, but even so has obvious limitations. It has also sometimes produced results which have appeared to undermine the supposition that discrete lesions can produce discrete defects of function. Thus both laboratory work and clinical observation have taken part in determining the swings of the pendulum between holistic and atomistic theories of brain function which have characterised progress during the past 100 years.

Historical development

Holistic views of brain function fitted well with early humoral theories of the mind and appeared to be upheld by the early experiments of Flourens (1824) in the first part of the 19th century. It was shown that piecemeal removal of the pigeon's cerebral hemispheres produced a decline in many abilities, so that by the time they were blind the birds were also unable to learn. In the 20th century the influential work of Lashley (1929) again led to an holistic orientation, this time specifically in relation to the acquisition of new knowledge. In tests of maze learning in rats it was shown that the size but not the location of the lesion was related to impairment of learning. Lashley's law of mass action expressed the view that learning ability is determined by the total mass of normally functioning cortex, and his law of equipotentiality that no part could be considered prepotent in this regard. In the clinical field, Goldstein (1939) was the most determined antagonist of mosaic theories of brain function, claiming that clinical reporting often highlighted the rare and exceptional in pointing to focal functions, and that the techniques of clinical examination had led to spurious findings where many clinicopathological correlations are concerned.

Radically opposite views have meanwhile flourished alongside these opinions. Strict localisationist views gained impetus in the early 19th century from the widespread credibility accorded to Franz Joseph Gall and his followers. Though a leading neuroanatomist, Gall propounded the doctrines of phrenology, which ultimately reached the fantastic lengths of claiming cerebral centres for such functions as 'hope', 'patriotism' and 'attraction to wine'. The reaction and counter-reaction to such excesses has perhaps continued to influence the building of theories where definitive information is lacking. As recently as 1937, Kleist was still attempting elaborate diagrams which partitioned functions such as 'skills', 'efficiency of thought' and 'personal and social ego' to discrete parts of the cerebral cortex.

Focal representation of function has, of course, been firmly established for basic sensory and motor functions. Early notable observations were those of Hughlings Jackson (1869) who saw that motor seizures developed on the side opposite the cerebral lesion, and Fritsch and Hitzig (1870) who showed that discrete motor movements followed discrete stimulation of the cortex. Knowledge of the cerebral representation of such 'lower level' functions is now extensive, though even here it is important to recognise the immense complexities and intricacies which have proved to be involved.

The symbolic functions of language were also recognised at an early stage to depend on circumscribed regions of the brain. Dax (1836) and Broca (1861) noted that articulated speech was disturbed by left posterior frontal pathology, and shortly thereafter Wernicke (1874) found disturbance of comprehension of speech with a left superior temporal lesion. Since this time there has been a steady though far from smooth accumulation of evidence concerning the cerebral representation of language and of other symbolic 'gnostic' functions. Unfortunately much of this initially depended upon uncritical compilations of case material, and at the turn of the century the 'diagram makers' were frequently in confusion. Hughlings Jackson's theory of *levels* of functional organisation within the nervous system, and the emergence of symptoms by a process of dissolution of such levels, received little attention at the time. Progress even now remains bedevilled by

the complexities of the issues involved in analysing impairment of higher cognitive functions, quite apart from the difficulty of finding suitable case material on which detailed pathological observations can be made.

Luria (1964) set forth some of the problems in the way of clearer understanding, and the fallacies which led to error both in the hands of over-localisers and the hands of those who held an over-holistic view. His arguments have such general significance that they will be dealt with in some detail:

Luria pointed out that even so elementary a process as the knee jerk has in fact a complex structure which can be affected by lesions at many points in a chain. Even simple visual recognition requires eye movements to investigate the object, the registration of its most informative signs, and the participation of language to relate it to a certain class. More complex mental functions will have a correspondingly more complex structure, involving many functional systems and many hierarchically arranged localisations within the nervous system. Destruction of any one of many links may impair performance, and it is therefore not surprising that the symptoms of deficit may follow from lesions at very different points in the brain. Observations which remain restricted to the level of gross functional deficits will therefore tend towards holistic views of brain function. But careful qualitative analysis of the nature of the deficits may still allow localisation, because the particular way in which the function is disturbed will depend upon which particular link is broken. The accomplishment of writing, for example, may be disturbed in a number of ways and by several factors, with a net result superficially the same but in fact with a variety of underlying disturbances of function. Agraphia may prove to be due to defective acoustic analysis of speech, in which case consonants close to each other in sound will be especially confused and copying of a clear visual image of well-known words will be relatively preserved (left temporal lesion); or the patient may handle separate sounds well but easily lose the correct ordering of sequences (premotor lesion); or the essential difficulties may lie in the visuospatial analysis of letters and the motor act of writing (parieto-occipital lesion). Here then the detailed analysis of the symptom may still allow disturbance of a complex mental function to be used in regional diagnosis.

A related task is to search for common factors in a series of seemingly disparate symptoms, since a single functional defect may have issue in many forms. A left parietal lesion may disturb orientation in space and numerical schemes together, which at first sight appear to be very different functions. But Luria suggests that detailed analysis shows a common factor in that both represent disturbance of the organisation of elements into simultaneous spatially orientated schemes.

All such analyses are of course harder because strictly focal damage is rarely seen, and usually the lesion touches on several zones and damages several overlapping systems together. Moreover, the plasticity of organisation is such that the structure of a psychological function may vary with the particular mental task involved; for example the recall of one series may utilise a mnemonic logical path, and the recall of another series, a path based on visual images.

Finally Luria underlined Hughlings Jackson's important warning that a clear distinction must always be maintained between the localisation of the pathology accounting for symptoms, and the localisation of the functions whose disturbance the symptoms represent. The undisturbed function may emanate from the central nervous system in a much more complex manner and may have a completely different organisation.

In the field of new learning, Lashley's views of mass action and equipotentiality in rats have had to be decisively modified for man. Whilst the cortex as a whole is undoubtedly involved in learning and in the storage of information, lesions in different parts do not have equivalent effects. Left temporal lesions impair verbal learning, and right temporal lesions non-verbal learning to a special extent. Highly discrete lesions in the hypothalamic–diencephalic region, or damage restricted to the hippocampal areas, may virtually abolish new learning in any modality. Thus we now have clear evidence that the proper organisation of memory functions involves to some considerable degree discrete systems within the brain.

The search for focal deficits has also been extended into matters other than cognitive function. In animals focal brain lesions can lead to dramatic changes of temperament—rage reactions or placidity—depending on the site of the lesion. In the split-brain monkey, Downer (1962) showed that the emotional disposition could vary according to the hemisphere which processed information; visual information fed to an amygdalectomised hemisphere elicited a mild response, whereas in the same animal information fed to the intact hemisphere met with the animal's usual ferocity. Papez (1937) proposed that the limbic system constituted an essential mechanism for the elaboration of emotional experience and emotional expression, and MacLean (1955) has reviewed the evidence suggesting that this applies to man as well as to lower animals.

With special parts of the brain involved in cognitive functions and emotional regulation, what of higher functions still such as 'personality' and social behaviour? Certainly in monkeys interesting results can follow focal extirpations of brain tissue. Removal of the temporal lobes leads not only to placidity, but also to strong oral tendencies in examining available objects, tendencies to attend and react to every visual stimulus, and an increase in sexual behaviour (Klüver & Bucy 1939). The human counterpart of such a syndrome has been reported in certain patients (Pilleri 1966; Marlowe et al. 1975; Lilly et al. 1983). Cingulectomy in monkeys leads to inquisitiveness, loss of shyness for man and loss of 'social conscience' in interaction with other monkeys (Ward 1948; Glees et al. 1950). In man the hope for further discoveries has

been spurred on by the observation of frontal lobe deficits which can clearly involve profound disturbance of aspects of personality and social behaviour. The temporal lobe has also frequently come under suspicion, especially in view of the personality disturbances which may accompany epilepsy arising within the temporal lobes (pp. 266–8).

However, systematic attempts to investigate the relationship between location of brain damage and such matters as personality or social behaviour have often given disappointing results. In view of the foregoing discussion this should perhaps not be surprising, since the complexity of structure of such higher order functions must be immense. Chapman and Wolff (1959), for example, carried out a thorough survey of the life patterns and behaviour of patients in whom circumscribed cortical excisions had been performed:

Four categories of 'highest integrative function' were measured by detailed interview and rating procedures. They comprised: the capacity to express needs, appetites and drives, such as ability to express affect, to interact with the environment and to engage in purposive activity; the mechanisms for goal achievement, including learning, memory and the categorisation of information; the capacity to initiate, organise and maintain appropriate adaptive reactions, as evidenced by the deployment of psychological defence mechanisms such as projection and denial; and the capacity to maintain organisation during stress and to recover promptly from its effects. For a given amount of tissue loss, impairment was less in those who premorbidly had shown a high order of adaptive versatility, but as the amount of tissue loss increased this individual variation was seen to a diminishing extent. Overall, the degree of impairment in such functions was directly related to the mass of cerebral cortex which had been lost, but was entirely without regard to side or site.

Chapman and Wolff concluded that where highest level integrative functions were concerned, impairment due to brain damage is likely to be related to the total number of neurones lost but not to the area from which the loss occurs. Other evidence indicated that it was immaterial whether the loss was aggregated in one place or distributed diffusely throughout the hemispheres.

The verdict concerning focal brain dysfunction in relation to personality and social behaviour therefore remains 'unproven'. It remains possible that with less ambitious design, and a closer focusing on predetermined areas of 'higher function', some focal effects may yet emerge to supplement what we already know about the frontal lobes.

Finally, the most ambitious development is to carry the debate into the field of mental pathologies, such as affective disorders and schizophrenia. Focal biochemical pathology has been suspected in some depressive illnesses, with indications of disturbed monoamine levels in certain hindbrain structures in patients who have committed suicide (Bourne *et al.* 1968; Pare *et al.* 1969). The consensus, however, is that depression is biochemically heterogeneous in terms of the anatomical sites and precise neurochemistry involved (Delgado *et al.* 1992). Schizophrenia has proved more interesting with respect to regional brain disorder, appearing to show a special relationship with temporal lobe disturbance and with patterns of hemispheric lateralisation. These latter developments are discussed at the end of the present chapter.

Disorder of memory

Memory disorder is a symptom of the utmost importance in psychiatric practice, in that it is often the decisive clinical feature which indicates the presence of underlying cerebral disease. It is, in fact, one of the most sensitive indicators of brain damage or dysfunction, regardless of the ultimate pathology.

Organic amnesias can be divided into two broad categories which are not mutually exclusive—those due to focal and those due to diffuse cerebral disorder. In the former, amnesic defects can result from lesions in highly discrete parts of the brain and stand out against the relative preservation of other cognitive functions. In the latter, amnesic defects form an integral part of acute or chronic generalised organic reactions but may nonetheless be for some time the most intrusive psychological symptom. It is possible that memory disorder in these two categories depends on different fundamental disturbances of the memory mechanisms of the brain, and this may to some extent be reflected in the detailed nature of the amnesic deficits that are produced. In both, moreover, the form of memory loss is different from that seen in amnesias of psychogenic origin where brain damage does not exist. Two aspects of memory disorder will therefore be considered below—first the cerebral systems which appear to be mainly involved, and then the psychological structure of common amnesic states.

Cerebral systems involved in memory

The relationship between disorder of memory and cerebral pathology has repaid detailed study, and clinico-pathological correlations have here reached firmer ground than where most other psychological symptoms are concerned. This is largely because many aspects of memory are amenable to objective measurement by simple testing procedures, and can often be studied in lower animals as well as in man himself. These are both features that are rarely encountered in symptoms and syndromes of key importance in psychiatry.

What we have learned in the clinical field, however,

still leaves unanswered the more fundamental question of the mechanisms of memory storage itself. The various possibilities that have been considered all remain highly speculative and unsatisfactory. Physiological theories which postulate changes in electrical activity of neurones and their interconnections serve to explain very short-term storage, but for the establishment of durable memories there must be the ability to withstand profound derangement of electrical activity as in anaesthesia, hypothermia or convulsions. Connectionist theories, which propose anatomical changes in synaptic relationships between cells, fail to explain why focal extirpation of brain tissue does not lead to loss of detailed memories for particular past events (while paradoxically punctate stimulation of the brain may sometimes evoke specific recall of past experiences (Penfield 1968)).

The development of biochemical theories, which suggest changes in the synthesis of neurotransmitters and intracellular proteins, or changes in gene expression within the neurone, may perhaps offer more hope for explanation when taken in conjunction with earlier ideas.

Squire (1987), Kandel and Hawkins (1992) and Tranel and Damasio (1995) discuss some of the more recent and exciting findings in this area. Studies of the mollusc, *Aplysia*, for example, have shown unequivocal evidence both of changes in transmitter release and morphological alterations in synapses during learning.

The discovery that brief high frequency stimulation can alter the excitability of postsynaptic cells in the hippocampus for several hours or even weeks ('long-term potentiation', LTP) has also been shown to have relevance to learning. The initiation of LTP is subserved by the binding of glutamate to receptors on target cells; whereas its maintenance appears to depend on some factor, possibly nitric oxide, which acts in a retrograde manner on presynaptic terminals to enhance transmitter release. And both electrical and biochemical theories are brought together by the discovery that the *N*-methyl-D-aspartate (NMDA) glutamate receptor has a channel that opens to extracellular ions only when the cell is depolarized. This dual requirement for both receptor binding and electrical depolarization suggests that NMDA receptors may act as conjunction detectors in the hippocampus with a role in associative learning.

Perhaps of equal significance, it has been shown in *Aplysia* that the adenylate cyclase of the cell can be activated by dual chemical mechanisms (serotonin and calcium), such that exposure to the one predisposes to greater production of cyclic adenosine monophosphate (AMP) in response to the other; this provides a close biochemical model for the principle of contiguity in classic conditioning.

The problems of coding for storage are, however, only less baffling than the possible mechanisms of recall, which can allow near-instantaneous retrieval of the required information from the past.

The two main regions of the brain that have emerged as specially significant in relation to amnesia are the hypothalamic–diencephalic region and the hippocampal apparatus. Damage to either of these relatively circumscribed areas can selectively impair the capacity to form durable records of experience. It is associated also with a variable retrograde gap for memories laid down before the damage occurred, whilst beyond this the majority of remote memories remain substantially intact. Thus although these are the sites where the smallest lesions can have the most devastating effect they do not represent the 'repositories' or storehouses of memories. They appear rather to be concerned with adding to the store and perhaps with retrieval from the store, as will be considered further below. The whereabouts as well as the mechanism of memory storage remains unknown. Phylogenetic considerations point to the participation of the cerebral cortex in the storage of past experience, but no one part of it can be singled out as pre-eminent in this function.

Besides these parts of the brain, other neural systems must be implicated in the processes of remembering. We preserve in memory mainly those things towards which attention is directed, and the alerting mechanisms of the brain must therefore be involved. The emotional connotations of material can also influence its recall (Lishman 1972, 1974; Master et al. 1983, 1986; Dunbar & Lishman 1984), and here the emotional apparatus of the brain must play a part. Other complex variables normally affect the detailed content of what is available for future recall, such as interest in the material perceived, its relevance, importance, and consistency with existing frames of reference for the subject (Bartlett 1932; Edwards 1942). These complexities can be carried even further by consideration of the highly individual determinants of specific amnesias as revealed by psychoanalytic study. Clearly therefore the clinicopathological correlations outlined below reveal but a small part of the total mechanisms involved in remembering. They perhaps reveal something of the mechanisms which determine the distinction between memory for remote and recent events, but very little indeed about the neural basis which underlies other more complex features. Fortunately our appraisal of amnesia as a symptom in cerebral disease depends principally on the temporal sequence by which memories are impaired, and very little on higher order distinctions.

Hypothalamic–diencephalic system

Lesions in the posterior hypothalamus and nearby midline structures were the first to be firmly linked with amnesia. They constitute the principal pathological basis of Korsakoff's syndrome, and involve areas around the third ventricle, the periaqueductal grey matter, the upper brain stem, certain thalamic nuclei, and the posterior hypothalamus. The mamillary bodies along with the terminal portions of the fornices are nearly always affected, and certain publications reviewed by Brierley (1966) have suggested that damage confined almost exclusively to the mamillary bodies can account for the Korsakoff memory defect. Victor (1964), however, in a particularly careful study suggested that lesions in the medial dorsal nuclei of the thalamus were of more critical importance and may in fact be crucial for the development of amnesic symptoms in Korsakoff's syndrome. The importance of the thalamus has been reinforced by the remarkable example of patient 'N.A.', who became severely amnesic after a stab wound from a miniature fencing foil; CT scans showed damage apparently restricted to the left dorsal thalamus, in a region corresponding to the dorsomedial nucleus (Squire & Moore 1979).

Debate continues, nonetheless, over the relative importance of the mamillary bodies and the thalamic nuclei in Korsakoff patients, or indeed whether both must be involved together (Mair et al. 1979). Lesion studies in animals, as reviewed by Squire (1987), may ultimately help to resolve the problem. Kopelman (1995) reviews recent evidence suggesting that a circuit involving the mamillary bodies, the mamillothalamic tracts and the *anterior* (rather than the medial dorsal) nuclei of the thalamus may be particularly critical for memory function.

The common cause for lesions in this situation is thiamine deficiency, the amnesic difficulties developing as a sequel to Wernicke's encephalopathy (p. 575). Chronic alcoholism is the usual prelude to the vitamin deficiency, but other established causes include carcinoma of the stomach, pregnancy, severe malnutrition, or persistent vomiting from any cause.

Some authorities reserve the term 'Korsakoff's syndrome' for cases with such an aetiology, while others employ it more widely to include the similar amnesic states which may follow other forms of damage to the same brain regions. Tumours in the neighbourhood of the hypothalamus and third ventricle may produce a closely similar picture (p. 227). Subarachnoid haemorrhage may occasionally be followed by a pronounced amnesic syndrome, due to local haemorrhage or organisation of the clot in the basal regions of the brain (p. 394). In the severe stages of tuberculous meningitis a picture closely similar to Korsakoff's syndrome may be witnessed over many weeks (p. 367). With recovery normal memory function gradually returns, leaving only an amnesic gap for the acute phase of the illness and a retrograde amnesia for a variable period before it (Williams & Smith 1954). The characteristic pathology of tuberculous meningitis in the amnesic phase is an inflammatory process with organisation of exudate, largely limited to the anterior basal cisterns of the brain and involving the mamillary region and the floor of the third ventricle. There is evidence to suggest that these regions have escaped the main impact of the infective process in those few cases where memory difficulties do not appear.

While the importance of diencephalic and hypothalamic lesions in relation to amnesia cannot be doubted, it is important to remember that the pathology of Korsakoff's syndrome involves additional brain regions, including those which contain important neurochemical nuclei. Thus the locus caeruleus may be implicated, leading to monoaminergic depletion in the cortex, likewise the basal forebrain including the nucleus basalis of Meynert. Arendt *et al.* (1983) were able to demonstrate severe loss of neurones in the Meynert nucleus in a small group of alcoholic Korsakoff patients. This has led to the suggestion that loss of cholinergic inputs to cortical and limbic structures may play an important part in adding to the memory difficulties of Korsakoff patients (Butters 1985). Animal models, created by prolonged alcohol consumption in rodents, have confirmed cholinergic depletion in the cortex and hippocampus accompanied by memory deficits, both being reversible by cholinergic-rich foetal brain transplants (Arendt *et al.* 1988; Hodges *et al.* 1991). Unfortunately, however, such biochemical hypotheses have not led to clearcut therapeutic strategies in man, as outlined on pp. 484–5.

Hippocampal system

Long after the description of Korsakoff's syndrome, the opportunity arose to study an amnesic syndrome closely similar in phenomenology to that of the korsakovian defect, but which surprisingly stems from lesions in quite different parts of the brain. This results from bilateral lesions of the hippocampus and hippocampal gyrus, which lie on the inferomedial margins of the temporal lobes. That such regions should be closely implicated in amnesia is all the more remarkable in that the hippocampal areas are usually free from damage in the typical case of Korsakoff's syndrome. The responsible lesions can be demarcated with some precision because the condition was first fully recognised after surgical extirpation of brain tissue for the relief of psychotic illness and epilepsy (Scoville 1954; Scoville & Milner 1957).

Lesions of the temporal neocortex have no effect on memory, similarly damage restricted to the uncus and amygdaloid region of the archipallium. It is essential that the lesions should extend far enough posteriorly to damage portions of the hippocampus and hippocampal gyrus, and the extent of their removal then appears to be roughly proportional to the severity of the memory disorder (Milner 1966). It is also fairly certain that bilateral lesions are required before global amnesia will appear and persist. When amnesic symptoms have followed unilateral temporal lobe resection there has usually been evidence that the remaining hippocampal zone was already defective. Thus, in occasional patients global amnesia has followed unilateral temporal lobectomy, but only when bilateral temporal lobe damage has been suspected. Serafetinides and Falconer (1962a) found that mild subjective forgetfulness sometimes followed unilateral right lobectomy, but in all such cases there was evidence of a postoperative spike discharging focus at the opposite temporal lobe, indicating dysfunction if not a lesion there.

These clear examples produced by circumscribed surgical lesions almost certainly reveal the mechanism responsible for other naturally occurring amnesic states. Cerebrovascular accidents may sometimes be followed by the acute onset of similar amnesic difficulties, as in the patient described by Victor *et al.* (1961) who suffered occlusion of each posterior cerebral artery in turn, and at autopsy was found to have lesions in the inferomedial portions of each temporal lobe. Two years intervened between the two strokes and it was only after the second episode that the amnesic syndrome appeared. Glees and Griffith (1952) reported a patient with sudden onset of dementia in whom amnesic symptoms figured very prominently, and who at autopsy showed cystic degeneration, consistent with old infarction, in the medial temporal lobe structures. The enduring memory difficulties which follow some cases of encephalitis (Rose & Symonds 1960) may also depend upon pathology in this distribution, since encephalitis due to the herpes simplex virus is known to have a predilection for the 'limbic lobe' which includes the hippocampus and the hippocampal gyrus (Fields & Blattner 1958; Brierley *et al.* 1960). Evidence from epilepsy similarly points to the importance of the hippocampal areas for memory, since these are the regions implicated in complex partial seizures where amnesia constitutes an essential feature of the attacks.

Some debate has centred on whether damage to the hippocampus alone is sufficient to produce amnesia, or whether there must be conjoint damage to the hippocampus and amygdala. In the lesions described above both structures are almost invariably involved together, and animal experimental work has shown that damage to both leads to a more severe deficit than hippocampal lesions alone (Mishkin 1978). However, the issue appears to have been resolved by the patient reported by Zola-Morgan *et al.* (1986), who developed a marked and persistent anterograde amnesia after ischaemic damage restricted to the CA1 fields of the hippocampus bilaterally.

High resolution MRI has proved capable of visualising hippocampal damage during life in amnesic patients. Press *et al.* (1989) reported three patients with circumscribed amnesic states, one due to respiratory arrest and the others of unknown aetiology, all of whom showed bilateral hippocampal abnormalities on coronal T_1-weighted images taken perpendicularly to the long axis of the hippocampus. The area of the hippocampal formation (including the fimbria, dentate gyrus, hippocampus proper and subiculum) was approximately half that seen in control subjects, whereas the total temporal lobe area was virtually identical. It was possible on occasion to see that components such as the pyramidal cell layers of the subiculum or hippocampus were less distinct, and to detect marked reduction in size of the dentate gyrus. Squire *et al.* (1990) have further used MRI to detect the size of the mamillary bodies in patients with alcoholic Korsakoff's syndrome, thus aiding distinctions during life between amnesias of hippocampal or diencephalic origin.

Other clinicopathological correlations

It is tempting to see a unitary mechanism for memory functions in the two brain regions described above. However, early reports suggested that the fornix bundles, which provide the main connection between the hippocampi and the hypothalamic structures, could be cut bilaterally without disturbing memory (Dott 1938; Cairns & Mosberg 1951). Such patients, however, were not subjected to formal neuropsychological evaluation. More recently memory deficits have been documented after lesions of the fornix, even in the absence of CT or MRI evidence of damage to other key memory structures (Grafman *et al.* 1985; Hodges & Carpenter 1991). The patient reported by Tucker *et al.* (1988) was particularly interesting in that a small focal astrocytoma of the left fornix led to a memory deficit confined to verbal material, much as would be expected from a left hippocampal lesion.

Damage to the fornix may also be chiefly responsible for the examples of 'retrosplenial amnesia' reported after vascular accidents or with tumours of the splenium of the corpus callosum (Valenstein *et al.* 1987; Rudge & Warrington 1991). The fornix is closely applied to the splenium during this part of its course. However, the retrosplenial cortex, situated in the cingulate gyrus just above and posterior to the splenium, also contains relays between the anterior nucleus of the thalamus and the medial temporal lobe and may be directly involved itself.

With regard to the neocortex, difficulty with memory appears to be related to size rather than locus of cortical lesions (McFie & Piercy 1952; Chapman & Wolff 1959), but it is difficult to obtain firm evidence because damage must be widespread before generalised memory impairment results. The accompanying intellectual disturbance then hampers careful analysis of the memory disorder.

The frontal lobes have been increasingly highlighted where memory functions are concerned. Operations on the frontal lobes rarely produce enduring memory disorders, though in the early postoperative period there may be a striking deficit of retention of current experience together with patchy retrograde amnesia (Klein 1952; Kral & Durost 1953). Whitty and Lewin (1960) described a transient memory disorder involving especially the temporal sequence of events following limited ablations of the anterior cingulate cortex. The early amnesic patient recorded by Mabille and Pitres (1913) was found to have symmetrical areas of infarction in the frontal white matter, strategically placed to interrupt long association fibres from the frontal lobes to other parts of the brain. However, this isolated though fascinating case has remained something of a medical curiosity.

It remains a matter of controversy whether the frontal lobes play a primary role in memory *per se*, or merely influence it by virtue of their involvement in such functions as attention, problem solving and the general organisation of behaviour. There are numerous pathways between the prefrontal cortex and the medial temporal lobe structures through which such influences could be exerted, without needing to postulate neural mechanisms for memory in the frontal lobes themselves (Goldman-Rakic 1987). Evidence accumulates, nonetheless, for frontal involvement in relation to special aspects of the memory process, for example in the suppression of irrelevant associations, in memory for temporal order and spatiotemporal context ('source memory'), and in the efficient retrieval of memories from the past (Mayes *et al.* 1985; Schacter 1987; Mayes 1988; Kopelman 1991). The role of superadded frontal lobe damage in Korsakoff's syndrome has been especially closely studied (pp. 582–3).

Special parts of the brain appear to be related to memory for special types of experience as displayed in verbal, visuospatial or motor learning, though it remains uncertain how far deficits in such individual functions should be regarded as failures of memory rather than defects in perception or in the categorisation of ideas. A temporal lobe (hippocampal) lesion in the hemisphere dominant for speech impairs the learning and retention of verbal material, resulting for example in forgetfulness for names, for material read in newspapers or material heard in lectures. Conversely, patients with non-dominant temporal lobe lesions are impaired in the memorising of matters which cannot be categorised in words, such as tunes, faces and meaningless drawings. There is now a considerable body of experimental data available on such distinctions between left and right hemisphere lesions. These specific disorders are, however, relatively trivial, often requiring special testing for their detection, and seem not to affect the recall of events. They are considered further on p. 312.

Some forms of dysphasia, apraxia or agnosia can be regarded as 'limited amnesias' consequent upon focal cortical damage, but as their manifestations are so specific they are best considered quite separately from amnesia.

Functional brain imaging techniques have recently been applied to examine anatomical aspects of memory processing in normal subjects. A particularly fascinating result has been the differential implication of the left and right prefrontal cortex during encoding and retrieval of memories, respectively. Such laterality effects had scarcely been expected from the extensive experience gained from examining patients with brain lesions.

Fletcher *et al.* (1995), for example, have used positron emission tomography (PET) scans to follow changes in regional cerebral blood flow during performance on a paired-associate learning task. Subtraction techniques were employed to pinpoint the brain areas involved in memory processing as distinct from those concurrently activated by other cognitive processes involved in the task. During the phase of encoding the regions activated were the left prefrontal cortex and the retrosplenial area of the posterior cingulate cortex; during retrieval, by contrast, there was activation of the right prefrontal cortex and the precuneus. These, then, appear to be the regions critically involved in auditory–verbal episodic memory. Tulving *et al.* (1994) review other PET scan studies utilizing rather different memory tasks which support prefrontal asymmetry in encoding and retrieval.

In parallel experiments, Fletcher *et al.* (1995) tested retrieval from semantic memory (p. 29). This was found to engage a different though overlapping neural system compared to that involved in retrieval from episodic memory, lending anatomical support to the distinction between the two.

The absence of demonstrable activation of medial temporal lobe structures in these studies is surprising. It could be that the hippocampus was continually active during both the memory and the control tasks, and therefore failed to be highlighted with the subtraction technique employed. Or the PET scan may be insufficiently sensitive to reveal activation in circumscribed groups of hippocampal neurones. Squire *et al.* (1992) were nevertheless able to demonstrate activation of the right hippocampus and parahippocampal gyrus during PET scan studies of word recall.

Clinical picture in amnesia

The detailed structure of amnesic states has been most comprehensively studied in patients who are relatively free from other intellectual impairments, namely in patients with focal lesions in the hypothalamic–diencephalic or hippocampal systems. This has provided important clinical guides which help in distinguishing them from amnesia due to diffuse brain damage and from psychogenic amnesia. In clinical practice a complex admixture of causes will sometimes be seen, but first the classic pictures may be outlined.

For purposes of clinical description a somewhat arbitrary division is made into 'immediate', 'recent' and 'remote' memory. The *immediate memory span* (or 'ultra short-term memory') is reflected in the reproduction of material such as brief digit sequences which fall within the span of attention. It appears to represent the functioning of short-term storage mechanisms, which need not, even in normal circumstances, lead on to an enduring record. Clinically it provides evidence that registration is intact. *Recent memory* is reflected in ability to acquire and retain new knowledge ('current memorising', 'new learning') and requires a process of consolidation in addition to registration. Clinically it is assessed by noting ability to learn or retain material over short spans of time, usually by testing ability to repeat simple information after several minutes have elapsed. *Remote memory* is reflected in the ability to recall information acquired at a considerable distance in time, and certainly before the onset of the memory difficulties. It therefore represents a process of retrieval of material which has been held in long-term storage.

In everyday clinical practice it is convenient to employ the terms 'immediate', 'recent' and 'remote' as outlined just above. Unfortunately, however, considerable confusion can arise over some of the terms used in referring to memory mechanisms, and particularly when attempting to translate the experimental literature to clinical practice. 'Short-term memory', for example, is often used by psychologists as synonymous with immediate memory, and often in medical practice as broadly congruent with recent memory.

An important division is recognised between short- and long-term memory mechanisms (STM and LTM, respectively) both in animal and human experimental work. STM is also referred to as *'primary memory'* and LTM as *'secondary memory'*. Each has certain characteristics not shared by the other. Primary memory (STM) has a strictly limited capacity, being able to hold only a small number of unrelated items of information at a time. Decay from it is rapid when rehearsal is prevented. This is the aspect of memory tested by the digit span. The material held in primary memory is retained in a form closely tied to the qualities of the initial percepts (timbre, visual detail, precise verbal content, etc.); it is non-selective, and material can be reproduced from it without comprehension of the meaning. Subsequent entries to the system displace what is already there. Primary memory thus acts as a short-term back-up to perceptual experience, giving time for selective attention to focus on what is meaningful and valuable for transfer into secondary memory.

Secondary memory (LTM) has very different properties. Material held in secondary memory is encoded mainly in semantic terms, i.e. in the form of meaningful concepts, and the primary qualities of the percepts involved become obscured. The result is a far more durable record. There is no known limit to the amount that can be stored. Secondary memory thus encompasses all material retained beyond a period of several seconds, and includes both the recent and the remote memory of the usual clinical terminology.

Studies carried out both in normal subjects and in patients with amnesia have in general upheld these broad divisions, though complex interrelationships clearly exist between the two memory storage systems. Valuable reviews of more recent experimental work in the area are to be found in Cermak (1982), Squire (1987) and Parkin (1987).

A number of further terms are in vogue for defining different aspects of memory. *'Working memory'* (Baddeley 1976; Hitch 1984) is an elaboration of the concept of primary memory described above. It emphasises those components which can hold information in short-term storage and manipulate it while performing on-going cognitive tasks, and recognises the existence of different subsystems dealing with specialised forms of material. The 'articulatory loop', for example, deals with phonological information, and the 'visuospatial scratch pad' with visual images. Suitable experimental paradigms, and studies in patients with brain lesions, can show the relative independence of the one from the other (Vallar & Papagno 1995).

The *'episodic–semantic' distinction* was introduced by Tulving (1972) and can be useful in describing the detailed content of losses from the long-term memory store. Episodic memory refers to memory for specific, personally experienced events or episodes from the individual's past; thus its content accumulates along with the individual's day-to-day experiences, and it is usually recalled in the form of temporally dated episodes. Semantic memory or 'knowledge memory' is less personally orientated and deals essentially with organised knowledge about the world—knowledge of objects, labels, vocabulary, principles and concepts. As such it is shared with others, not held in temporally specific order, and is largely acquired early in life. Both episodic and semantic aspects of memory can be affected (or spared) in amnesic states. Thus episodic memory for long-distant events may remain unaffected, whereas the disruption of new learning may prevent the addition of new facts to the semantic store. Nevertheless episodic memory appears to be the more vulnerable of the two in most amnesic syndromes.

A further distinction is made between *'declarative'* and *'procedural'* memory, and has particular relevance to the classic amnesic syndrome. Declarative ('explicit') memory refers to knowledge of facts and data acquired by processing information, and is directly accessible to conscious awareness by a process of recall (Squire 1987). It thus embraces both episodic and semantic memory as defined above. Procedural ('implicit') memory, by contrast, is shown by the capacity to perform a particular task, without necessarily knowing when or where one learned to do it. This 'knowing how' is expressed only in performance, not in the form of detailed conscious recollection. The various forms of procedural memory include skill memory (e.g. how to ride a bicycle or tie shoe laces), and the capacity for certain cognitive operations (e.g. how to solve certain types of puzzle). The phenomenon of 'priming' probably also falls within the domain of procedural memory, i.e. the capacity to profit from prior exposure to cues, such as previously perceived or partially completed words, in the execution of a task. Again this represents 'unconscious memory', manifest only in behaviour. Procedural memory is typically preserved when declarative memory is severely disrupted by hippocampal or diencephalic lesions.

Thus there appear to be several independent memory systems, possibly tied to different neural networks within the brain. Declarative memory is clearly closely associated with hippocampal and diencephalic structures; and there is some evidence that skill learning may be related to the striatum, and priming effects to the neocortex (Squire 1986).

Amnesia due to diencephalic and hippocampal lesions

There are many important respects in which the memory deficits are closely similar, whether produced by lesions in the hypothalamic–diencephalic system or in the hippocampal regions. Thus perception is unimpaired, the immediate memory span is well preserved, and beyond a variable retrograde gap remote memories are substantially intact. The principal defect with both types of cerebral lesion emerges in the field of recent memory (current memorising) so that current events become less available for future recall. More recent detailed studies have served to qualify the view that all amnesic syndromes are identical, as described on pp. 37–8, but in broad outline they can be described together as follows.

The preservation of the immediate memory span is a point of great importance clinically. Performance on a test of digit span is usually normal, and therefore will fail to reveal the existence even of a severe amnesic syndrome. The cases with bilateral temporal lobe resection, in whom good ability to cooperate is well preserved, have shown that in the absence of distraction such brief information can be retained for several minutes by dint of constant verbal rehearsal. Forgetting occurs, however, as soon as new activity demands a shift away from the task in hand. Moreover, the learning of a list which slightly exceeds the normal digit span is markedly impaired, revealing the essential difficulty in getting new material into longer term store (Drachman & Arbit 1966).

Recent memory is thus defective, and disorientation at least in time is almost universal. New learning is impaired, and in the most extreme cases may be reduced to nil, so that as time goes by there is a continuing and extending anterograde amnesia. If recovery subsequently occurs, a dense and permanent gap will be left for the period of the illness. In less severe examples the problem shows as uncertainty about events which occurred minutes, days or weeks before, some being vaguely recalled and others having made no lasting impression at all. The retelling of simple stories is marked by gross omissions, incorrect juxtapositions and condensations of material. More careful testing shows that the problem affects all types of material, both verbal and non-verbal, such as word associations, drawings and numbers.

It seems clear also that these defects of memory are to a large extent independent of the significance of the material involved. In mild cases it is sometimes found that memory for personal matters is better preserved than for impersonal, and for concrete matters better than for abstract. Events of high emotional significance may sometimes appear to be remembered especially well. But within this framework there will usually be exceptions and surprising instances. Victor (1964), in a group of alcoholic Korsakoff patients, was unable to discern any factors that governed what was remembered and what was forgotten. A patient might fail to retain news of a bereavement which shocked him profoundly at the time, yet retain other matters of no significance whatever. The most severe case following bilateral hippocampal resection described by Milner (1966), 'H.M.', showed a failure of retention which cut across all factors of vividness or emotional significance: '. . . His initial emotional reaction may be intense, but it will be short-lived, since the incident provoking it will soon be forgotten. Thus, when informed of the death of his uncle, of whom he was very fond, he became extremely upset, but then appeared to forget the whole matter and from time to time thereafter would ask when his uncle was coming to visit them; each time, on hearing anew of his uncle's death, he would show the same intense dismay, with no sign of habituation.'

Despite such pervasive deficits *procedural memory* (p. 29) *is well preserved*, even in the most severely affected patients. Milner's (1966) patient, for example, showed a normal learning curve for a task of mirror drawing, even though on each test occasion he was completely unaware that he had tried the task before. Other tests of motor and perceptual skills, such as pursuit-rotor tasks or the reading of mirror-reversed words, have also revealed

learning and retention over considerable periods of time (Corkin 1968; Starr & Phillips 1970; Cohen & Squire 1980). 'Priming effects' are largely preserved, as when prior presentation of a word increases the tendency to produce that word when its initial letters are shown some minutes later (Squire *et al.* 1987). Thus the forms of memory which are accessible only in performance, and not as acts of conscious recollection or recognition, appear to be spared in the classic amnesic syndrome.

The *retrograde amnesia* often covers a period of months or years before the onset of the illness. This is usually dense for events just prior to the onset, but may be incomplete and patchy where the parts most distant in time are concerned. Time sense is characteristically disordered within the retrograde gap, with jumbling of the sequential ordering of those events which are recalled. In patients with Korsakoff's syndrome of alcoholic origin the retrograde amnesia is often of particularly long duration, extending even over several decades but showing a clearcut temporal gradient. In discrete amnesic syndromes of other aetiologies the difficulties with recall seem rarely to exceed 2–4 years. The careful experimental studies which have addressed such issues are described on pp. 36–7. Over the course of time many retrograde amnesias may shrink considerably, especially those seen after temporal lobe resection or when the pathology resolves as in tuberculous meningitis.

Disturbance of time sense and of the ordering of events is an outstanding characteristic, particularly in Korsakoff's syndrome. The patient may allocate some recent remembered event to the distant past, or bring up a past event as a recent happening. He may condense long periods of time or telescope repeated happenings into one. This affects recent memory and the period of the retrograde gap particularly, but may be observed for more remote happenings as well. Talland (1965) suggested that the problem is due not to loss of appreciation of the flow of time, but rather to 'contextual isolation'; that is to say, events within the memory store appear to lose relationship with the totality of experience which surrounds them and in which they would normally be framed sequentially.

Remote memory, for matters beyond the retrograde gap, is much better preserved. In severe amnesias after temporal lobe resection, remote events are often reported to be perfectly preserved, though in Korsakoff's syndrome the distinction is less clear-cut and remote memories are often found to be somewhat impaired when opportunities arise to check them in detail. It is, of course, difficult to assess the competence of remote memory in any comprehensive way, as discussed on p. 99.

Confabulation can be a striking feature in amnesias due

to lesions of the hypothalamic–diencephalic structures, but seems to be rare in those which follow bilateral hippocampal destruction. Traditionally it seems to have been greatly overstressed. When present, it is commoner in the early stages than in the chronic phases of Korsakoff's syndrome, but it is certainly not universal (Victor *et al.* 1971). It may appear as an evanescent phenomenon, or in rare cases may last for many years.

Typically, the patient gives a reasonably coherent but false account of some recent event or experience, usually in relation to his own activities and often in response to suggestion by the examiner. Berlyne (1972), who provided a useful review of the subject, defined confabulation as 'a falsification of memory occurring in clear consciousness in association with an organically derived amnesia'. He upheld Bonhoeffer's early distinction between two varieties. The common 'momentary type' is brief in content, has reference to the recent past and has to be provoked. The content can sometimes be traced to a true memory which has become displaced in time or context. Much rarer is the 'fantastic type' in which a sustained and grandiose theme is elaborated, usually describing far-fetched adventures and experiences which clearly could not have taken place at any time. This form tends to occur spontaneously even without a provoking stimulus, and the content is often related to wish fulfilment and the seeking of prestige. Kopelman (1987a) prefers a classification simply into 'provoked' and 'spontaneous' confabulation, and has shown that the former appears in the context of efforts at recall by both Korsakoff and Alzheimer patients.

There is probably not a unitary mechanism underlying the appearance of confabulation. It occurs in a setting of amnesic difficulties, but the memory disorder itself is unlikely to be the complete explanation otherwise it would be seen a great deal more commonly. Often, as already stated, it appears to represent fragments of genuine past experience which are dislocated in time. As Barbizet (1963) pointed out, the patient who is unable to retain new material will tend to live on his stock of old memories, and will react to a new situation with what he has available.

Sometimes confabulation may represent the residue of abnormal and confused experiences, including misidentifications and misinterpretations which occurred in the delirium of the initial Wernicke's encephalopathy. Thus it commonly sets in as clouding of consciousness is receding and persists thereafter while insight into the unreal nature of the delirious experiences is lacking. Others have sought to explain it in terms of unawareness or even motivated denial of the memory disorder, though this is likely to have only limited application.

Kopelman (1987a) was able to demonstrate examples of 'provoked' confabulation in healthy subjects when asked to recall prose passages after a considerable interval of time; these were similar in nature to those sometimes observed in Korsakoff and Alzheimer patients when tested shortly after exposure, consisting mainly of additions of inaccurate or irrelevant material or changes in the sense of the passage. This type can thus be regarded as a 'normal' response to a faulty memory.

In many well-established and persistent cases a strong iatrogenic component can often be discerned, and the symptoms may then reflect in considerable measure the patient's suggestibility and desire to please. Interesting evidence has also come forward to link confabulation to the presence of frontal lobe dysfunction in certain instances, particularly confabulation of the expansive or 'fantastic' type. Stuss *et al.* (1978) reported five patients in whom frontal deficits, superadded to their memory problems, appeared to account for their persistent and extraordinary confabulation. Kapur and Coughlan (1980) were able to chart the change from fantastic to momentary confabulations in a patient with left frontal damage following subarachnoid haemorrhage, and to show that this change was paralleled by improvement in performance on frontal lobe tests. It seems possible, therefore, that a special combination of deficits may be the essential prerequisite for the more elaborate and striking instances of confabulation in association with memory disorder.

Other cognitive functions are relatively well preserved, and the above amnesic deficits are out of all proportion to other disturbances of intellect or behaviour. In particular the patients are alert, responsive to their environments and without any evidence of clouding of consciousness. The amnesic states following temporal lobe resection are in all respects astonishingly pure, with no evidence of other cognitive deficits and with good preservation of insight into the memory difficulties. Where premorbid personality has been sound there is no disturbance of social behaviour, of motivation or of emotional control.

In Korsakoff's syndrome, however, the situation is less straightforward. Other cognitive functions are usually found to be disordered when carefully examined (Talland 1965; Zangwill 1966; Victor *et al.* 1971). There is often difficulty in sustaining mental activity, coupled with inflexibility of set and reduced capacity to shift attention from one task or train of thought to another. Thinking is usually stereotyped, perseverative and facile, with inadequate concept formation and defective ability to categorise. Butters and Cermak (1980) review the visuoperceptual impairments which are almost universally revealed when sought out by special tests, for example the digit–symbol substitution test, hidden figures test, or tests requiring the sorting and discrimination of complex visual stimuli. All of these deficiencies are nonetheless overshadowed by the prominence of the memory disorder. It is this disproportion between memory deficits and other cognitive deficits which is the hallmark of the condition. The likelihood that there may be transitional forms between the classic picture and patients with more global cognitive impairment is discussed on p. 584.

Even superficial acquaintance with Korsakoff patients also reveals certain marked disturbances of personality.

There is often a pronounced degree of apathy and loss of initiative, a bland or even fatuous disposition, and a tendency towards self neglect. Left to himself the patient occupies himself poorly, makes few demands or enquiries from those around, and obeys instructions in a passive and indifferent manner. A virtual disinterest in alcohol may represent a particularly striking change. Lack of insight is also almost universal; few Korsakoff patients appreciate that they are ill, and in those who do the gravity of their defects is minimised or explained away by facile rationalisations.

Thus while surgical resection of the medial temporal lobe structures produces clear evidence of circumscribed memory disorder, the neuropathological picture seen in Korsakoff's syndrome must account for a good deal more than the memory deficits alone. In the latter, the admixture of motivational and attitudinal deficits probably accounts for the somewhat capricious nature of the memory disorder and leads to difficulties in attempts to analyse it with the same degree of precision.

Amnesia in diffuse cerebral disorder

When associated with diffuse cerebral disorder, amnesia lacks the definitive structure described above. In addition it is often submerged among more widespread impairments of intellectual function, which make precise analysis of the memory deficits extremely difficult if not impossible. In acute organic reactions some of the memory difficulties can be traced directly to impairment of consciousness and to the problems with attention and perception that result. In chronic organic reactions amnesia often represents no more than the earliest manifestation to come to light of general cognitive failure, in the sense that memory difficulties tend to be more readily spotted than other aspects of intellectual loss.

The general picture of the memory difficulties in acute organic reactions has been discussed on pp. 11–12 and in chronic organic reactions on pp. 15–16. Certain distinctive features may, however, be summarised here for comparison with the picture in focal amnesic states.

The amnesic defects of diffuse brain disease are commonly global, affecting both recent and remote events to an obvious degree. Only rarely is there a clear-cut disturbance of recent memory along with a retrograde gap beyond which remote events are found to be well preserved.

Recent events may be the most obviously affected, but in part at least this may be due to lack of interest and involvement in current experiences. Remote memories may appear to be relatively intact, but often prove in fact to be banal, stereotyped and lacking in detail. Using structured tests, Wilson *et al.* (1981) were unable to demonstrate relative preservation of very remote memories in a group of patients with dementia. To a marked extent performance may be variable from one occasion to another, and capricious in that some events are easily recalled while others, apparently equally trivial or unimportant, are not. Indeed much of the difficulty can often be seen to lie in failure to sustain attention and concentration on the general task of directed recall.

It is on evidence such as this that the memory disorder in dementia is thought to reflect the diffuse pathology which exists throughout the cortex and elsewhere. Thus deficits are attributed to losses within the memory store, and to disruption of the mechanisms of association and of access to the store which must follow upon reduction of interconnections between one cortical region and another. It is also clear that primary as well as secondary memory functions (p. 28) are implicated in dementia. The immediate memory span is impaired (Miller 1973; Kaszniak *et al.* 1979), unlike the situation in patients with circumscribed amnesic syndromes, and losses occur more rapidly from the primary memory store (Corkin 1982; Kopelman 1985a). It is interesting, however, that once material is acquired into secondary memory, forgetting rates have emerged as essentially normal, as is also the case with Korsakoff's syndrome (Corkin *et al.* 1984; Kopelman 1985a). Kopelman (1985b, 1986) and Kopelman and Corn (1988) review the evidence that depletion within the cholinergic system in dementia (pp. 444 and 504) can account only partially for the memory disorder encountered in such patients.

The evidence with regard to implicit (procedural) memory in dementia has been conflicting, and proves to be closely tied to the specific test paradigms employed. The general picture that emerges in Alzheimer's disease is of preserved motor skill learning, as on pursuit-rotor tasks (Eslinger & Damasio 1986), and relatively normal curves of improvement on perceptual tasks such as mirror reading (Deweer *et al.* 1993); by contrast a variety of priming tasks can be shown to be impaired, as revealed by word-stem completion or semantic association tests (Shimamura *et al.* 1987; Brandt *et al.* 1988).

It would, however, be premature to conclude that diffuse brain damage is always the complete explanation for the amnesic symptoms in dementing illnesses. In Alzheimer's disease there may be a relative intensity of pathological change in the hippocampal regions and mamillary bodies, and perhaps particularly when memory deficits have been severe (Brierley 1961; Corsellis 1970). Conversely in Pick's disease the pathological process may spare in large degree the hippocampal regions, and here striking memory problems are rarely an early manifestation. It is therefore probable that when amnesia is pronounced in relation to other disabilities, the pathological changes may have progressed especially far in the cerebral systems which are particularly concerned with memory functions.

The common memory deficits of old age may likewise depend in part on generalised and in part on focal degenerative changes. Huppert (1994) reviews the attempts made to specify those aspects of memory most vulnerable to the ageing process, and the difficulty in generalising about the pathological substrates which may be responsible. One of the firmer strands of evidence centres on the presence of retention deficits in healthy elderly subjects; in comparison with younger controls they show slightly but significantly faster forgetting of material even after careful matching for initial level of performance (Huppert & Kopelman 1989). This contrasts with the normal forgetting rates observed in Alzheimer's dementia and Korsakoff's syndrome when compared with age-matched controls (*vide supra*), and implies a distinct pathological basis.

There is also evidence that substantial deficits occur with 'working memory' with age, i.e. the ability not merely to hold information in short-term storage, but concurrently to manipulate and combine it with further incoming information. Other problems highlighted in the elderly concern 'prospective memory' (i.e. remembering to carry out a task some time later while engaged in other activities) and deficits in memory for context (Huppert 1994). Grady *et al.* (1995) have shown certain differences on PET scans during the performance of memory tasks in young and old people, indicative of impaired cortical and hippocampal activation during the encoding of material in the elderly.

Beyond this it is hard to draw firm conclusions. The pathological changes characteristic of ageing occur so frequently and so diffusely that clinicopathological correlations are again hard to obtain. The hippocampal regions have sometimes been found to be particularly affected (Gellerstedt 1933), and Busse (1962) reported a relatively high incidence of electroencephalographic abnormalities in the temporal lobes of elderly people, more markedly so when learning ability was deficient.

Similar uncertainty surrounds the pathogenesis of the amnesic phenomena which accompany closed head injury, as discussed on p. 162.

Psychogenic amnesia

Psychogenic amnesia is commonly either dense and global, or alternatively restricted to circumscribed themes or events. When global it may involve the blotting out of long periods of past life, or even loss of personal identity, in a manner which is inconsistent with the general preservation of intellect. Amnesias of this severity do not occur in organic states unless at the same time there is abundant evidence of disturbance of consciousness or of severe disruption of cognitive functions generally. Interestingly, even with dense psychogenic amnesias there may sometimes be 'islands' of preserved memories which can be uncovered by careful questioning (Schacter *et al.* 1982).

Inconsistencies in the account may also be noted. The subject with hysterical amnesia, for example, may insist that certain events could not have occurred during the period covered by the amnesic gap, while at the same time he is in no position to refute the proposition. More restricted psychogenic amnesias will usually be found to centre on a related constellation of events or circumscribed areas such as the patient's work or marriage. Repeated episodes of psychogenic amnesia will frequently betray stereotyped themes or settings, as with the patient described on p. 416.

Psychogenic amnesia is suspected when from the outset profound difficulty with recall of past events is coupled with normal ability to retain new information, or alternatively when there is total inability to retain information even for the few seconds required for the immediate memory span. A delayed curve of forgetting, which during the course of some days or weeks leads to complete extinction of important and significant material, is likewise sometimes seen in psychogenic but not in organic amnesias.

Kopelman (1987b) discusses factors which appear to predispose to psychogenic amnesia, notably precipitating stress, depressed mood or the experience of an earlier organic amnesia due to head injury, epilepsy or alcoholism. In the medicolegal field amnesia for offending is commonest with homicide, occurring in 30–40% of cases, but may also be seen in connection with other violent and non-violent offences. The amnesic episodes are typically fairly brief and knowledge of personal identity usually remains intact.

Special difficulties, of course, arise when psychogenic and organic aspects of memory loss occur together. Psychogenic factors may sometimes be obtrusive in amnesias which are clearly due primarily to brain damage, or an organic memory defect may come to be selectively reinforced or perpetuated on a psychogenic basis. Such difficulties are well illustrated by the celebrated dispute, reviewed by Zangwill (1967), which surrounded the Grünthal–Störring case for more than 30 years. A more recent example, illustrating the need to search carefully for organic factors in patients who appear to manifest purely psychogenic amnesia, is described by Kopelman *et al.* (1994b). Difficult problems may equally surround attempts at distinguishing between psychogenic amnesia and simulated amnesia, as in the patient reported by Kopelman *et al.* (1994a).

Memory disorder in the 'functional' psychoses

While it is traditionally held that memory disorder is the hallmark of organic brain damage, there are indications that memory may sometimes be defective in the so-called 'functional' psychoses. At an anecdotal level it is not infrequently noted that patients lack detailed knowledge of key features of their abnormal beliefs and experiences on recovery from schizophrenia or severe affective disorder. Depression, moreover, has been shown to have a marked effect upon the selective processes normally operative in memory, leading to readier recall and more accurate recognition of unpleasant compared to pleasant material (Lloyd & Lishman 1975; Dunbar & Lishman 1984). Among normal subjects such selectivity operates in the reverse direction.

However, until recently little attention had been given to overall memory efficiency in patients with depression or schizophrenia. Cutting's (1979) survey was therefore of considerable interest. Groups of patients with acute schizophrenia, chronic schizophrenia and depressive illness were compared with normal subjects and patients with organic psychosyndromes. Verbal learning and pattern recognition memory were separately assessed. The most prominent finding was that patients with chronic schizophrenia were impaired on both types of task, being sometimes comparable in performance to patients with confusional states, dementia or Korsakoff's syndrome. The depressives were also impaired on both tasks but to a less marked degree. Acute schizophrenic patients performed poorly on verbal memory alone. It seemed unlikely that coincidental brain damage could be the explanation, but the possible effects of medication were harder to discount.

McKenna *et al.* (1990) evaluated a large group of acute and chronic schizophrenic patients on the Rivermead Behavioural Memory Test battery (p. 117), and found that poor performance was common and sometimes substantial. The level of memory impairment appeared occasionally to approach that of patients with overt brain damage. Tamlyn *et al.* (1992) confirmed such deficits in a more detailed neuropsychological study of the same sample, finding that the pattern of impairment was similar to that of the classic amnesic syndrome. However, virtually all of the patients were receiving neuroleptic medication and many were also taking anticholinergic drugs, which may have contributed substantially to their poor performance. Saykin *et al.* (1991) nevertheless demonstrated a disproportionate and apparently selective deficit on memory and learning tasks in 36 non-medicated acute schizophrenic patients.

Duffy and O'Carroll (1994) have recently reported a detailed study of 40 schizophrenic patients, using the Rivermead Behavioural Memory Test battery, paired associate learning and other memory tests. This was a heterogeneous sample of acute and chronic patients, all screened to exclude those with a history of alcohol or drug abuse, head injury or other brain disease. Poor performance was demonstrated on several tests; and on the Rivermead battery the group was as likely to show significant memory impairment as the brain-damaged sample upon which the battery was originally validated. The severity of impairment was related to age and chronicity of illness, but not to measures of motivation, severity of psychotic symptoms or amount of neuroleptic medication. Of particular interest were comparisons with a group of chronic Korsakoff patients. On the tests of episodic memory the schizophrenics were less impaired than the Korsakoff patients, but on a test of semantic memory (i.e. judgements of whether a series of factual sentences were true or false) they were significantly worse. Further work will be required to substantiate this possible double dissociation. McKenna *et al.* (1995) provide a comprehensive review of research into this and other aspects of memory in the disorder, including the apparent sparing of procedural memory. Rizzo *et al.* (1996) produce evidence that memory for temporal context may be especially disrupted.

Such findings dictate a measure of caution in placing too great a reliance on tests of memory alone in deciding whether a patient with schizophrenia may harbour a brain lesion. It is important to recognise, nonetheless, that Duffy and O'Carroll's schizophrenic patients were less impaired to a very considerable degree than their Korsakoff sample on standard tests of memory, only 5% scoring within the severely impaired range.

Unresolved problems in amnesic states

Consolidation defect, encoding deficit or failure of inhibition?

The amnesic syndrome was for many years regarded as reflecting a failure of consolidation of new experience. Thus while the immediate memory span is normal, and old memories may remain substantially intact, current experience cannot gain proper access to the long-term store.

Evidence has, however, come forward to challenge this straightforward view, despite the appeal that it holds on first acquaintance. A simple consolidation hypothesis is hard pressed to explain why some forms of cueing can improve performance, or why patients can achieve better results on recognition tests than when tested by free recall. More strikingly, it has been possible, using the Huppert–Piercy technique outlined on p. 38, to show that rates of forgetting from the memory store are not accelerated in Korsakoff's syndrome or Alzheimer's disease once material has been learned to a constant criterion (Huppert & Piercy 1978, 1979; Kopelman 1985a). Normal forgetting rates of this nature were observed for intervals as long as 7 days.

Butters and co-workers have stressed the role of *deficient encoding of information* in leading to the poor performance of amnesic subjects (Cermak & Butters 1972; Butters & Cermak 1980). This, it seems, may account in considerable degree for their failure to store material adequately. Thus Korsakoff patients were found to rely unduly on simple acoustic encoding of the information they receive, rather than analysing it more deeply in terms of semantic meaning. Experiments have shown in addition that they use inappropriate strategies for the rehearsal and 'chunking' of information, all rendering it more susceptible to interference and rapid decay. When specifically instructed to attend to semantic features of the words presented, for example when forced to analyse them in terms of categories, attributes or meaning, the Korsakoff patient is found to achieve a somewhat improved performance on memory tasks.

Other approaches have emphasised difficulties at the level of retrieval, occasioned perhaps by failure to inhibit the intrusion of irrelevant material. This *'retrieval–interference' theory* holds that amnesics encode and store with reasonable efficiency, though the items in memory are poorly insulated from one another; in consequence they are in constant competition when retrieval is attempted. Support for such a mechanism came from experiments using the 'technique of partial information' (Warrington & Weiskrantz 1968, 1970; Warrington 1971):

A technique was elaborated for testing learning and retention by the presentation of graded clues. A word or picture may, for example, be prepared in several forms, ranging from a very indistinct image through progressively clearer forms until the word or picture emerges with full clarity. When such a graded series is presented to the subject, the point at which recognition occurs can be established; on subsequent presentations of the same material recognition occurs earlier in the course of the series if learning has occurred. With this technique it was shown that severely amnesic subjects, both with hippocampal damage and with Korsakoff deficits, displayed learning and retention over considerable periods of time, when such was not the case with conventional test material. Moreover there was evidence that it was in the processes of retrieval that the technique of partial information allowed the amnesic subject to demonstrate that learning had occurred. Thus conventional tasks of rote learning could also emerge as unimpaired when recall was tested by this special means.

This evidence suggests that the amnesic patient is continuing to store information, but in such a manner that the usual processes of retrieval cannot demonstrate that this is so. Stored material is perhaps not inhibited or dissipated in the normal manner, and as a result intrudes disruptively into the processes of recall. Such a view would be consistent with other anomalous findings in amnesic patients, such as the tendency in verbal learning experiments for items learned in one list to re-occur as intrusion errors in subsequent lists ('proactive interference'). Retrieval by the technique of partial information could thus produce superior results because it restricts the choice of possible responses available to the subject, and helps him to eliminate incorrect false–positive responses. In essence, far from storing too little, the amnesic patient may store or retrieve too much.

This fascinating suggestion has come under criticism, as reviewed by Piercy (1977) and Butters and Cermak (1980). Warrington and Weiskrantz (1978) have themselves reported experiments which necessitate a recasting of the theory in considerable degree. In particular it now seems difficult to uphold response competition as accounting directly for the amnesic patients' retrieval difficulties. And it can be shown that partial information techniques enhance recall in normal as well as in amnesic subjects, so the demonstration may be of a general effect, not of a special problem arising with amnesia (Woods & Piercy 1974). Furthermore, it is difficult to account for the temporal gradient seen in retrograde amnesias on such a basis. The observations of Warrington and Weizkrantz have, nonetheless, emphasised yet another aspect of the memory apparatus which must be taken into account. The naïve view of a consolidation defect alone obviously requires extensive qualification.

It has emerged, indeed, that any theory concerning the underlying deficits in amnesia can only provide a partial explanation of the phenomena encountered. Some observations emphasise the encoding aspect, some the storage difficulties, and others the problems with retrieval processes. All of these stages, however, are highly interactive and interdependent, one upon the other. It is clear that they are not neatly separable in normal memory, so it would be unreasonable to expect to pinpoint the source of the difficulties in amnesic patients with great precision.

The long retrograde amnesia

The short retrograde amnesia (RA) of several minutes' duration, such as commonly occurs after head injury, can be plausibly explained on the view that new learning requires a period of consolidation for stable long-term memory to be established. It is difficult, in contrast, to provide an explanation for the very long RAs which may extend for months or years prior to the onset of an amnesic syndrome.

If regarded as a failure of the mechanisms of retrieval, this cannot be a general defect of the recall apparatus. RAs are often patchy, and in any case the patient continues to retrieve well for events prior to the retrograde gap. Furthermore, recovered cases after head injury or tuberculous meningitis may be left with long RAs when current memorising ability has returned virtually to normal, so that here retrieval can be observed to operate well on both sides of the retrograde gap.

An explanation in terms of loss of retention for events within the retrograde gap is equally unsatisfactory. To explain very long RAs on this basis it would be necessary to suppose that full consolidation takes months or even years before the memory trace becomes resistant to extinction. Moreover, RAs may sometimes shrink with the passage of time, showing that the memory trace must have been intact all along.

It is probably a fault in principle to try to partition the blame too rigidly between primary faults in recall or in consolidation. Symonds (1966) put forward a hypothesis which may help towards resolving the dilemma of the long RA. He suggested that certain amnesic syndromes should be viewed in terms of excess, or acceleration, of the natural process of forgetting. This might normally be opposed by an activating system situated mainly in the hippocampal system. When the operation of the activating system ceases from any cause decay will prevail, affecting most severely the memory units most recently established, and progressively less those which have existed, perhaps with structural modification within the central nervous system, over a period of time. Decay, or forgetting, is thus seen as a graded process: some of the more recent memories will decay to zero potential and will then be included in the dense RA that persists, even in those cases where current memorising ability is again restored; beyond this will be a zone in which memory units have decayed to a non-functional level but can gradually recover their function if activation is restored. On such a basis the long RA which ultimately shrinks becomes more readily explainable.

An alternative escape from the dilemma is to discount the long RA as an artefact of clinical examination. It is hard to assess the preservation, or loss, of memories for personal events far back in time, and most impressions of long, temporally graded RAs are based on anecdotal or unsystematic observations. Sanders and Warrington (1971), in a pioneering experiment, appeared to obtain

support for the view that retrograde memory difficulties extended over virtually the whole of past experience, and affected all time periods equivalently. Using a standardised questionnaire concerning distant public events, and a recognition test of well-known public figures, they found that recall ability was steadily lowered in amnesic subjects for periods of up to 40 years. No clear onset to the retrograde gap could be discerned. More recent studies, however, have reinstated the temporal gradient and shown that the RA in circumscribed amnesic syndromes is truly a time-linked phenomenon:

Albert *et al.* (1979) developed tests concerning previous public events and recognition tests of famous faces. Patients with Korsakoff's syndrome showed retrograde memory deficits extending over several decades, but with clear-cut temporal gradients and relative preservation for the remote past. More events and pictures, for example, were recognised from the 1930s and 1940s than from the 1960s. An especially interesting feature was the inclusion in the tests of pictures of well-known individuals both early and late in their careers, for example of Marlon Brando from the 1950s and the 1970s; whereas normal subjects were more accurate at identifying the later pictures, Korsakoff patients showed precisely the reverse.

Squire and Slater (1975) produced a test based on titles of television programmes which had been broadcast for one season or less and were equivalently matched for public exposure. These showed that the transient RA following electroconvulsive therapy (ECT) was limited to several years, with normal performance beyond such a gap. Other tests derived from the procedures of Albert *et al.* have also confirmed temporal gradients in Korsakoff patients (Cohen & Squire 1981; Squire & Cohen 1982).

Meudell *et al.* (1980) used voices of famous people recorded over the past 50 years. Again this demonstrated poor recognition extending over several decades in Korsakoff subjects, but with relative preservation of memories for the more remote past. Other tests suited to British subjects include the News Events Test covering the period from 1935 to 1984 (Kopelman 1989), the Famous Personality Test (Stevens 1979), and the Personal Semantic Memory Schedule and Autobiographical Incidents Schedule which cover past aspects of the individual's life (Kopelman *et al.* 1989).

Carefully conducted and controlled studies have shown therefore that RAs, however long, tend to spare memories dating from childhood and early adulthood. Moreover they have emphasised that the RA in patients with alcoholic Korsakoff's syndrome is remarkably severe and extensive, in contrast to that seen with other amnesic syndromes. In Squire's studies, for example, Korsakoff patients showed deficits extending over several decades, whereas patients tested very shortly after ECT showed gaps limited to 4 years or less (Cohen & Squire 1981; Squire & Cohen 1982) Milner's patient 'H.M.' who had suffered hippocampal resection, and Squire's patient

'N.A.' who had sustained a focal lesion in the thalamus, also showed retrograde gaps covering no more than a few years or months.

Butters and Albert (1982) discuss the possibility that the very extensive RAs in alcoholic Korsakoff patients may derive, in part at least, from their poor acquisition of material into long-term memory throughout their alcoholic careers. The anterograde memory difficulties of the typical alcoholic will have led to tenuous storage of material even before the Korsakoff syndrome supervenes; and the progressive increase in severity of such difficulties over the years might account for the temporally graded nature of the RA once the Korsakoff syndrome is established. Alternatively, it may be that earlier memories are relatively well preserved simply because these are particularly salient and well rehearsed (Kopelman 1989).

Meudell (1992) discusses the further possibility that much may depend on 'contextual isolation'. Both the anterograde and retrograde memory deficits may stem from a failure to employ contextual features in a normal manner during the process of remembering. And it is likely that as memories age they become less dependent on context for their recall, thus contributing to the tendency for distant memories to be spared.

In a series of exceptionally careful studies, Kopelman (1989, 1991) has shown that in both Korsakoff and Alzheimer patients the retrograde memory loss improves significantly when cues are provided, for example in comparisons between free recall and recognition in the News Events Test. This was observed across all time intervals sampled, confirming that a retrieval deficit contributes to the difficulties encountered. Moreover the severity of the RA in both patient groups was related to defective performance on tests of frontal lobe function. It is therefore possible that frontal dysfunction, when added to hippocampal or other pathology, may produce the disorganisation of retrieval processes which has issue in the temporally extensive RA.

Finally, it is noteworthy that the temporal gradient characteristic of the RA in patients with amnesic syndromes is not so evident in patients with dementia. When the remote memory tests of Albert *et al.* were applied to patients with presumed Alzheimer's disease, uniformly poor performance was observed for items throughout the whole 40-year span of the tests (Wilson *et al.* 1981). There was no discernible trend towards relative preservation of memories from the earliest decades. A similarly 'flat' curve has been observed in patients with Huntington's chorea (Albert *et al.* 1981). Kopelman (1989), however, found evidence of a temporal gradient in both Alzheimer and Korsakoff patients, though the slope was significantly more gentle in the dements. Thus it would seem that

with diffuse cerebral pathology retrieval is more evenly impaired for all parts of past experience, albeit with some indications of a gradient with particularly careful testing. Other ways in which the memory disorder seen with diffuse brain dysfunction differs from that of the classic amnesic syndrome have already been discussed (p. 32).

Certain rare patients have been described in whom there is an extensive RA coupled with only minimal impairment on tests of anterograde memory ('isolated retrograde amnesia'). Such a dissociation is commonplace in the context of psychogenic amnesia, but a number of reasonably convincing cases have now been reported in whom the pattern appears to have an organic basis. Kapur *et al.*'s (1986, 1989) patient experienced numerous episodes of transient global amnesia, during the course of which he developed an extensive retrograde loss covering significant material extending over the past two or three decades. He performed very badly on tests of retrograde memory, but by contrast performed well on the Wechsler Memory Scale with only mild impairment on certain subtests.

A second patient (Kapur *et al.* 1992) was injured during a riding accident, suffering contusions in both frontal lobes and the anterior portions of the temporal lobes. Eighteen months later she showed only mild and patchy anterograde impairment; but tests of retrograde memory for both public and autobiographical events showed extremely poor performance extending back to childhood. Hodges (1995) describes further examples, concluding that there is evidence to implicate damage to the anterior temporal structures (the pole, entorhinal and parahippocampal cortices) in most cases. Such patients suggest that one must be cautious in attributing extensive RAs to psychogenic mechanisms solely because new learning is relatively intact, and underline the importance of full investigation including neuroimaging when the situation is unclear.

Interesting dissociations have also been described between RA for personal and impersonal information. De Renzi *et al.* (1987), for example, reported a patient who was severely impaired after herpes encephalitis on a wide range of general information — knowledge about World War II, Hitler or Mussolini and other historical and geographical facts. She also performed poorly on formal tests of semantic memory such as classifying animal names or detecting incorrect sentences. Yet she remembered personal events well from both before and after her illness, was correctly informed about current family matters, and performed adequately on a questionnaire concerning autobiographical events from her schooldays onwards. Conversely, Dalla Barba *et al.* (1990) have described a patient with Korsakoff's syndrome whose RA was severe and selective for autobiographical matters, while knowledge about famous people and events appeared to be reasonably intact. These examples serve as a reminder of the complexity underlying the organisation of memory, and the anomalies likely to be encountered when it is dissected in an ever more detailed manner.

Amnesic syndrome or syndromes?

It is commonly assumed that amnesic syndromes of varying aetiology are fundamentally similar. The alcoholic Korsakoff syndrome may have superadded deficits, in subtle aspects of cognitive function and personality, as mentioned on pp. 31–2, and the RA in such cases tends to be exceptionally long as described above. Nevertheless the 'core' structure of the amnesic deficits themselves has been viewed as identical whatever the causative process.

This assumption has now been challenged in certain respects. There is evidence, for example, that the amnesias seen with hippocampal and diencephalic pathology may not be entirely congruous.

A first pointer in this direction was provided by Lhermitte and Signoret (1972), who compared three postencephalitic patients (with presumed hippocampal damage) with a group of Korsakoff patients. The former performed at a lower level on a test of memory for spatial position, whereas the latter were worse on tests of temporal sequence. This was interpreted as indicating that the postencephalitic patients had a more profound failure of retention, whereas the Korsakoff patients were more impaired with regard to the organisation of material and with recall.

Firmer evidence has come from studies of speed of forgetting. Huppert and Piercy (1978, 1979) designed an ingenious method for examining forgetting rates over long time spans after ensuring that material had been learned to a constant criterion. A large number of pictures were exposed to the subjects, then recognition rates were tested at 10 minutes, 1 day and 7 days. By 'titrating' the time of initial exposure, recognition performance at the 10-minute interval was brought to a constant level in different groups. Using this technique it was possible to show that forgetting over the subsequent week was indistinguishable between Korsakoff patients and normal controls; in other words, provided the Korsakoff patients had been given enough time to analyse the stimuli thoroughly they were able to display normal recognition memory over an extended period of time. Milner's patient 'H.M.', by contrast, showed abnormally rapid forgetting when tested similarly. His amnesic syndrome had resulted from bilateral hippocampal resection.

Squire (1981) reinforced this distinction by applying the technique to Korsakoff patients, to patient 'N.A.' who had sustained focal damage to the thalamus, and to patients tested shortly after electroconvulsive therapy (ECT). The diencephalic amnesics (Korsakoff patients and 'N.A.') showed normal rates of forgetting, whereas the ECT patients forgot at an accelerated rate. The amnesia following ECT is presumed to derive from dysfunction in the medial temporal regions.

Taken together these studies provide support for the view that the underlying amnesic difficulties may be qualitatively different, depending on the brain regions affected. The normal rate of forgetting in patients with diencephalic lesions suggests that their deficit must lie at the stage of registration or encoding, or in acquiring information into the long-term store. Rapid forgetting in patients with hippocampal damage implies a deficit in the consolidation occurring after initial learning has been achieved.

Other distinctions have also been claimed on tests of proactive interference and in terms of rates of forgetting from the primary memory store. These are reviewed by Butters and Cermak (1980), Squire (1982) and Parkin (1987). When taken in conjunction with differences between groups in the duration of RA (see above), the unitary character of the amnesic syndrome can be seen to be under question. There is not, however, a firm consensus on the issue, and further detailed studies will be necessary to clarify the situation.

Possible mechanisms in psychogenic amnesia

Traditionally a rather rigid distinction is maintained between psychogenic and organic disturbances of memory, with indeed quite separate systems of explanation for the one and the other. This may be convenient in the present state of knowledge, but is perhaps a somewhat artificial dichotomy. It may fairly be presumed that a pathophysiology of some kind accompanies psychogenic amnesia, just as there must be a physiological basis for the influence of emotional and motivational factors on the normal processes of remembering and forgetting.

The mechanisms may vary somewhat from case to case. Faulty encoding of information may explain some examples as discussed below, while others may represent 'motivated forgetting' or 'repression'. A third possibility, discussed by Kopelman (1987b), is of a primary retrieval deficit reflecting mood-dependent phenomena. Sometimes there may indeed be a substrate in transient organic memory dysfunction which dictates the form the psychogenic reaction takes, as in the alcoholic patient reported by Gudjonsson and Taylor (1985).

It may be asked whether the study of organic amnesic states and their neuropathology leads us any nearer to understanding the physiological basis of these psychologically induced phenomena. Certainly the neurological structures important in committing new experience to memory turn out to be strategically situated for allowing an integration between affective and cognitive aspects of experience. The hippocampal system forms part of the neural substrate proposed by Papez (1937) for the experiencing and expression of emotion; and the mamillary bodies, as Kral (1959) pointed out, lie at the intersection of Papez's emotional circuit and the reticular formation upon which arousal depends. Such observations suggest possible mechanisms which may account for the emotional determinants of what is committed to memory and what is not. In states of profound emotional disturbance, perhaps also in dissociative states, it is possible that the total apparatus fails to function harmoniously, so that a durable memory trace cannot be established in the usual way. A simple explanation will not, however, suffice, and very often it appears that in psychogenic amnesias the principal fault lies with mechanisms for subsequent voluntary recall. Thus, behaviour during dissociative states often indicates that memorising, at least in the short term, must still be taking place, and much may later be accessible to recall under hypnosis or drug abreaction.

It is possible, furthermore, that certain cases of psychogenic amnesia may depend, at least in part, on failure in the initial processing of experience, rather than on a process of forgetting or repression (Kopelman 1985b, 1987b). Thus Taylor and Kopelman (1984) found that inability to recall a criminal offence was frequent when this had been committed in a state of very high emotional arousal, in the context of florid psychotic delusions, or under heavy alcoholic intoxication. All such factors would be liable to impair normal registration of what was happening at the time.

The mechanisms which may underlie psychogenic disturbances of *recall* receive little clarification from the study of organic memory syndromes. Organically determined RAs are to a large extent time related and tend to cover all experiences, whether significant emotionally or not. Psychogenic amnesia, on the other hand, may cover a circumscribed period in the distant past, and classically affects a system of related ideas or experiences. However, certain observations by Zangwill (1961) on the shrinkage of RAs after head injury are very interesting. Careful anamnesis in such cases sometimes shows that vulnerability during the retrograde gap is not wholly a function of recency, but that what is disturbed above all is the temporal coherence of the memory train. Shrinkage later occurs by the emergence in sporadic fashion of islands of memory, at first without firm context, which are later amplified and linked by rearousal of associative links. Zangwill suggested that this is not so very dissimilar from what is seen in psychogenic amnesia. Here again there is functional isolation of memory systems, with failures of associative linkage.

Lucchelli *et al.* (1995) further illustrate the blurring of the distinction between organic and psychogenic RAs, describing two patients who experienced a sudden resolution of their extensive RAs. Both had sustained brain insults at onset, and one had an accompanying anterograde memory impairment which persisted after the RA

had recovered. In both patients there was an abrupt flooding back of the lost memories while they were engaged in a situation closely similar to one experienced before. Once a single autobiographical past experience had emerged the whole framework of past memories resurfaced into consciousness, in a manner suggesting the 'unblocking' of a retrieval deficit. Lucchelli *et al.* favour an interaction of organic and psychogenic factors in their patients, with recovery dependent on the resetting of distorted 'patterned matrices' subserving memory.

Our understanding of the mechanisms which underlie retrieval is, however, too fragmentary to allow more detailed speculation regarding possible distinctions, or analogies, between psychogenic and organic disturbances of recall in examples such as these.

Disorder of language functions

Disturbance of language is an important source of evidence of focal brain disorder and, indeed, historically provided the chief impetus for attempts at correlating focal psychological deficits with regional brain pathology. Dysphasic symptoms probably remain more useful clinically than any other cognitive defect in indicating the approximate site of brain pathology. Yet despite 100 years of careful enquiry and observation the analysis of dysphasia remains a controversial area, and beyond certain broad limits its relationship to regional cerebral disorder remains in many respects uncertain. This should not be surprising in view of the complex interrelationships that exist between different aspects of language processes, and the intimate way in which language must enter into many other cognitive functions. The parts of the brain concerned with language are extensive, and necessarily diffused over a considerable territory so that auditory, visual and motor mechanisms can be subserved. Consequently cerebral lesions which produce dysphasia can lead to many forms of deficit, and at the same time to other defects which render the appraisal of clinicopathological correlations difficult. It is moreover likely that individual variation is considerable where the anatomical substrate for language is concerned.

Cerebral dominance for language

The earliest observation of a relationship between anatomy and psychology to gain universal acceptance was that dysphasia was overwhelmingly more common after lesions of the left hemisphere than the right. Later right hemisphere lesions were reported to produce dysphasia in left-handed subjects, and the general rule was proposed that the hemisphere contralateral to handedness governed speech. This has been upheld in large measure where right-handed subjects are concerned; Piercy (1964) reviews the evidence that the incidence of dysphasia in right-handed subjects is 67% when the lesion is in the left hemisphere and only 1% when the lesion is right sided. But it is now known from large unselected series of patients with brain lesions that left-handers also suffer dysphasia more often from left than from right hemisphere lesions, in fact in a ratio of approximately 2:1. Bilateral speech representation appears to be more common in left-handers than right-handers, though remaining rare in both.

The most direct confirmation of these relationships has come from observing the transient effect on speech of injecting sodium amytal into the carotid arteries of the left and right sides separately by the Wada technique (Wada & Rasmussen 1960; Rasmussen & Milner 1977). Sodium amytal, 175 mg as a 10% solution, is injected over 2–3 seconds into the internal carotid artery. This results in a contralateral flaccid paralysis lasting for several minutes during which the preservation or disruption of language can be briefly assessed. Rasmussen and Milner (1977) have reported 396 epileptic patients examined under such conditions. Among the right-handers 92% were found to have left hemisphere speech, 6% to have right hemisphere speech and in 2% there was bilateral representation. Among left-handers and ambidextrous patients (without early brain damage) 70% had left hemisphere speech, 15% right hemisphere speech and 15% had bilateral speech representation. In subjects with evidence of bilateral speech representation the speech defects were mild, from both the right- and left-sided injections.

An alternative method for assessing language laterality involves the use of dichotic listening. Verbal information in the form of groups of spoken digits or monosyllabic words is fed through earphones to the two ears, but in such a way that different information arrives at each ear simultaneously. The subject must report whatever he hears, and is found to report more accurately and comprehensively from the ear contralateral to the hemisphere subserving language. The results are less clear-cut than with the Wada technique, but dichotic listening has the advantage that it can readily be applied to a non-selected sample of subjects, including those in whom there is no reason to suspect the presence of brain damage. Satz *et al.* (1967) used this method to explore the relationship between handedness and language laterality in 123 healthy volunteers.

First it was shown that the situation in left-handed subjects becomes more complicated the more carefully left-handedness is evaluated. Handedness in fact proves to be a relative term, many 'left-handed' subjects showing a division of hand preferences and skills for different operations between the right and left hands. Thus a significant proportion of subjects who are left-handed in the ordinary sense of the term prove to prefer the right hand for certain tasks, and sometimes even for a greater number of activities than the left. With objective tests of manual dexterity, Satz *et al.* found that almost half showed better performance with the right hand than the left. On a composite score derived from all such evidence 17% of left-handed subjects emerged with strong right hand superiority, 22% as ambidextrous, and only 61%, could be judged as strongly left-handed in practice. All of this was in contrast to right-handed subjects who showed more consistency across preferences and tasks, 97% being confirmed in right hand superiority.

Interesting findings emerged when a dichotic listening technique was used to assess the hemisphere subserving language in these subjects. The self-reported right-handers showed strong evidence of left hemisphere dominance for language; so also did the 17% of left-handers who had proved to have right-handed superiority and the 22% who were ambidextrous. The 61% who were truly strongly left-handed were divided approximately equally, half showing left hemisphere dominance and half right hemisphere dominance.

In a similar though smaller study, Lishman and McMeekan (1977) found evidence of a progressively decreasing incidence of left hemisphere dominance for language in right-handed, mixed-handed and left-handed individuals (100, 67 and 60%, respectively). Moreover, among strong left-handers a family history of sinistrality appeared to be another significant variable; the ear difference scores on dichotic testing were then smaller, indicating reduced lateralization or bilateral representation of language in such individuals.

Electroconvulsive therapy has also been used as a means of determining language laterality, again in subjects who are free from any evidence of cerebral disease (Pratt & Warrington 1972; Warrington & Pratt 1973, 1981). By testing for dysphasia shortly after unilateral ECT to each side of the head, in patients undergoing treatment for depressive illness, it was shown that right hemisphere speech existed in only one of 55 right-handed subjects and in about 25% of 24 left-handed subjects.

Some two-thirds of normal adults are strongly right-handed and approximately 90% use the right hand for writing (Subirana 1969; Annett 1970). For this there appear to be strong genetic determinants. Even so, environmental pressures seem to be capable of altering the genetically determined preference, likewise damage to the upper limb or to the brain in childhood. The age of 10–12 years is generally accepted as the upper limit beyond which brain damage will not alter handedness and beyond which the second hemisphere will not develop fully adequate language skills by way of compensation. But that shifts in cerebral dominance do occur in relation to early left hemisphere damage is strongly upheld by Rasmussen and Milner's (1977) results of intracarotid amytal injection already mentioned above. Where left-handedness or ambidexterity was accompanied by a history of early left hemisphere damage there was, in contrast to all other groups, a large percentage of cases with language representation in the right hemisphere (28% left hemisphere speech, 53% right hemisphere speech, 19% bilateral speech representation).

Anatomical evidence has now come forward to complement the frequency with which language is represented in the left hemisphere. Yakovlev and Rakic (1966) reported that in foetal and newborn brains the corticospinal tract from the left hemisphere usually begins to decussate higher in the medulla than that coming from the right, and the corticospinal tract is usually larger on the right side of the cord than the left. Right hand preference, therefore, probably develops on the basis of the increased motor innervation available to the right side of the body. More directly Geschwind and Levitsky (1968), examining 100 adult human brains at postmortem, reported marked differences between the two hemispheres in the size of the planum temporale which lies on the superior surface of the temporal lobe immediately behind Heschl's gyrus. This is the region which contains the auditory association cortex, and represents the classic Wernicke's area known to be important for language. This area was found to be larger on the left in 65 brains, larger on the right in 11, and equal on the left and right in 24. These findings have been confirmed by others, as reviewed by Le May and Geschwind (1978).

Further interesting evidence has come from neuroradiological studies which have displayed a number of differences between right- and left-handers. Le May, for example, showed that in right-handers the occipital lobe was usually wider on the left than the right, whereas the frontal lobe was wider on the right than the left; these asymmetries were less striking in left-handers who, moreover, quite commonly show a reversal of the normal situation (Le May 1976, 1977; Galaburda *et al.* 1978). Such differences were readily detectable on the CT scan, also differences in the degree of forward or backward extension of the left and right hemispheres of the brain. The configuration of the lateral ventricles is likewise revealing, with a tendency for the occipital horns to be longer on the left in right-handers but less regularly so in left-handers (McRae *et al.* 1968). Arteriography has given indications of further differences, for example in the relative levels of the posterior ends of the Sylvian fissures and of the disposition of the transverse sinuses (Le May & Geschwind 1978). Witelson and Kigar (1988) review numerous other anatomical studies of this nature and discuss their possible relevance to hemispheric asymmetries of function. Kertesz and Naeser (1994) describe

further indices of asymmetry which can be derived from MRI images, including assessment of asymmetries in the region of the planum temporale.

Certain differences in brain configuration, with possible relevance to language, are also evident in postmortem comparisons between male and female brains (Witelson 1991). Thus the posterior part of the Sylvian fissure turns upwards more posteriorly on the left than the right side of the brain, and this asymmetry is more marked in men than women. Greater asymmetry in this regard is found in right-handed than non-right-handed men. Secondly, the isthmus of the corpus callosum, representing the part that contains fibres connecting the posterior parietal and superior temporal regions of the left and right hemispheres, is significantly smaller by some 20% in right-handed men than in women, and smaller in right-handed than non-right-handed men.

Such anatomical differences are consistent with evidence from numerous sources that language is more strongly lateralised to the left hemisphere in males than females, and more so in right-handed than non-right-handed subjects. Greater bilaterality of language representation may require less marked anatomical asymmetry but a greater degree of cross hemispheric communication between language-related brain areas. It remains puzzling, however, that the anatomical differences discerned between right- and non-right-handers have so far been observed in males alone.

Evidence with regard to cerebral dominance for language has also come from observations after section of the corpus callosum for the relief of intractable epilepsy (Sperry 1966; Sperry & Gazzaniga 1967; Gazzaniga & Sperry 1967). As a result of the operation the two hemispheres are virtually isolated from each other and information can be fed tachistoscopically to either hemisphere alone by brief exposures in the opposite half-field of vision. When a picture of an object is exposed to the dominant hemisphere it can be named promptly or recorded in writing; but similar exposures to the non-dominant hemisphere meet with no such response. If pressed to answer after information has been fed to the non-dominant hemisphere, the patient may deny seeing anything, or alternatively the speaking hemisphere may resort to pure guesswork and produce a random response. Nonetheless the patient can select the appropriate matching object, by means of palpation with the left hand, from among a group of objects concealed behind a screen, indicating that the non-dominant hemisphere has correctly perceived the picture despite the patient's inability to name it. In a similar way an object concealed from view can be named when palpated by the right hand but not when palpated by the left hand. The non-dominant hemisphere is therefore mute as would have been expected.

In some of these patients, however, it seems certain that limited comprehension of language can take place in the non-dominant hemisphere. The left hand can correctly select or point to an object which corresponds to a name exposed briefly to the non-dominant hemisphere alone. That the dominant hemisphere can have played no part is shown by the failure of the right hand to perform accurately in this situation; moreover the subject cannot name the matching object if this has been selected by the left hand but remains concealed from view. Auditory comprehension can be demonstrated by flashing a picture to the non-dominant hemisphere then asking the patient to signal when the matching word is read aloud to him; this he can do by signalling with the left hand but not with the right. Alternatively a word can be spoken out loud, and the patient asked to signal when the corresponding printed word is exposed visually to the non-dominant hemisphere. In such experiments it appears that even short phrases can be comprehended, the word 'clock' being selected in response to the spoken phrase 'used to tell time'.

Ingenious research techniques have allowed further exploration of the language capacities of the non-dominant hemisphere as described by Zaidel (1977, 1978) and Gazzaniga (1983). It has become apparent that such capacities are present in only a small proportion of patients, and that these usually have a history of early left hemisphere brain damage. The degree of sophistication varies widely from primitive levels of comprehension to the ability to detect semantic incongruities in sentences and to understand syntactic rules. In exceptional instances, patients have developed a limited degree of *expressive* speech controlled by the right hemisphere some months or years after callosal section, for example being capable of producing verbal descriptions of stimuli presented to the left visual field. Nevertheless even in such patients it seems clear that the right hemisphere remains severely limited in general cognitive skills, and does not compare with the left in its capacity for inferential reasoning or simple mathematical computations (Gazzaniga & Smylie 1984; Gazzaniga 1985).

It is not known how far these fascinating results have general application. It is possible that the patients reported to date have been unusual in the extent to which language was already represented bilaterally within the brain, and definite conclusions on the issue still cannot be drawn.

Some exceedingly rare observations have been made on patients after total surgical removal of the dominant hemisphere. One such patient was investigated by Smith (1966a) after left hemispherectomy for recurrence of a glioblastoma. The patient had previously been strongly right-handed. In the immediate postoperative period there was, as expected, a severe sensory and motor dysphasia along with right hemiplegia and hemianopia. Even then, however, he could follow some simple commands, indicating some preservation of comprehension of

speech. He could also utter emotional expletives such as 'Goddamit' with good articulation, at a time when single words could not be repeated and when there was no ability at all to communicate in propositional speech. Suddenly in the 10th postoperative week he asked his nurse 'What does "B.M." mean?' in response to her enquiry about his bowel movements. Thereafter the occasional use of fragments of propositional speech increased, along with ability to repeat progressively longer sentences on command, though most of the time the patient remained incapable of speaking voluntarily. Comprehension of speech, by contrast, appeared to reach approximately normal levels at 1 year postoperatively before the tumour recurred (Smith 1972). Of particular interest in view of the evidence linking musical functions with the minor hemisphere (p. 64), was the patient's eventual ability to sing familiar songs and hymns with little hesitation and few errors of articulation, even though speaking remained very severely impaired. A remarkably similar postoperative course has been documented in a second patient (Burklund & Smith 1977). Other scattered examples in the literature are reviewed by Searleman (1977).

The rarity of such cases again makes it difficult to estimate how far the results may have been due to an unusual degree of bilaterality of language already present before operation, or how far new capacities to organise language were developed in the non-dominant hemisphere. The complex effects of hemispherectomy on language development following brain damage in childhood are described by Vargha-Khadem *et al.* (1991).

Finally, there is now considerable evidence that the affective components of language, including prosody and emotional gesturing, are the special prerogative of the right hemisphere (Ross & Mesulam 1979; Ross 1981). Thus patients with right hemisphere strokes may lose the ability to express emotion by voice or gesture, or to perceive the affective colouring in the speech or gestures of others, while formal propositional aspects of language remain intact. Ross (1981) suggests, indeed, that the functional organisation of the affective components of language in the right hemisphere may closely mirror that of propositional language in the left, and has produced evidence of a similar range of 'aprosodic' subsyndromes to that encountered among the dysphasias ('motor aprosodia', 'sensory aprosodia', etc.).

The concept of 'auditory affective agnosia' in relation to language is considered on p. 65.

Language functions within the dominant hemisphere

We have little direct knowledge about the physiological

mechanisms which underlie language functions in the healthy intact brain. Since language is unique to man there is no paradigm which can be studied in animals, and evidence has had to accumulate slowly from the study of the damaged human brain. Inferences about normal from abnormal function are notoriously dangerous, and not surprisingly numerous theories abound on psychological, physiological and anatomical levels. Many of the most eminent neurologists have struggled to provide a functional conception of language organisation, against which to arrive at a rational classification of the dysphasias. But even recent authorities can offer little more than speculations which serve to guide future enquiry. It is, however, useful to have a framework against which to view the phenomena of dysphasia, and the theoretical background will therefore be briefly reviewed before the clinical data are considered.

The detailed history of past endeavours was outlined by Brain (1965). Early and primitive localisationist views postulated 'speech centres' for speaking, reading and writing, which contained the repositories for word images and could be disturbed either directly by lesions or by damage to various connecting pathways. Such views became discredited by more careful neuropathology and by more detailed clinical appraisal of the range of deficits shown by dysphasic patients. The need was seen for a more dynamic explanation in terms of impairment of symbolic functions as a whole. Freud was one of the first to attack the 'diagram makers' and propose a more holistic view of the functions of the speech territory in the dominant hemisphere. Head further developed the dynamic concepts of Hughlings Jackson and proposed a classification of dysphasia which depended primarily on symptoms of deficit rather than locus of lesion.

In recent years linguists and psychologists have joined increasingly in the debate and have produced objective evidence to countermand or support the impressions of clinicians. Linguistic aspects of dysphasia are discussed by Lesser and Reich (1982) and summarised concisely by Benson and Ardila (1996). The psycholinguistic classification of the dyslexias is discussed by Newcombe and Marshall (1981) and Shallice and Warrington (1987). Intriguing forms of dyslexic error have been highlighted, for example in 'deep dyslexia' in which words are misread yet in a manner that betrays understanding at some level of their meaning (Marshall & Newcombe 1973). For example, *dinner* may be read as 'food', *close* as 'shut', or *dog* as 'animal'. Observations such as these have led to speculation and experimentation in attempts to clarify the various 'routes' whereby the written word image is translated into meaning (Coltheart *et al.* 1987).

Psychologists have used batteries of tests and factor analysis of the results to refine major categories of language disorder. From this and other evidence, Piercy (1964) was led to conclude: 'The language areas of the brain are not mutually undifferentiated, nor can they be envisaged as a collection of discrete centres. Rather one discerns gradients of specialisation in the neural substrata of language; gradients which are steeper in some areas and for some functions than others, and perhaps steepest for verbal articulation and for reading.'

Two major contributions attempt to reach beyond the objective evidence and present a partial theory of language function from which the phenomena of dysphasia can be derived. The first, by Brain, is largely psychological and physiological in emphasis, the second, by Geschwind, is slanted towards an anatomical explanation. Both start with 'naming' as the essential function upon which language comes to be built.

Brain (1965) suggested that the physiological basis for the recognition of words must rest with the acquisition of 'schemas', which operate as enduring physiological standards of comparison but do not enter consciousness. The development of naming during childhood implies increasing accuracy in the recognition and abstraction of the precise elements of the concept for which the name stands; furthermore the elements which constitute 'the name' must come to be recognised without conscious effort despite variations in the pitch, speed and intonation with which the name is pronounced. Simple 'phoneme schemas' must be built into 'word schemas' at a higher level of organisation, since the second phoneme of a word may influence the recognition accorded to the first. Word schemas are linked to the physiological bases of perception and thought connected with that which the word symbolises, and so enable the word to be endowed with meaning. At the same time 'word-meaning schemas' must be capable of modification when the grammar or syntax of the sentence containing the word is altered. At a higher level of organisation still there must therefore be 'sentence schemas'. Similarly on the efferent side there must be schemas for the motor production of speech. And to serve the purposes of reading and writing there must be visual and graphic schemas superimposed upon the fundamental schemas of speech. This complex physiological organisation may be damaged in whole or in part; to the extent that each type of schema is organised anatomically in relative isolation from others, it may be possible to move towards an explanation of some of the varieties of dysphasia.

Thus word schemas are regarded in Brain's formulation as the basic element both in the comprehension and expression of words, and their disorganisation will result in defective understanding and expression in both spoken and written modalities. Word-meaning schemas, when disorganised, may leave words freely available but their power to evoke or express meaning will be impaired. Disorganisation of sentence schemas will impair meaning derived from syntactical relationships while leaving the meaning of individual words relatively intact.

Pure word-deafness may be regarded as a disorder restricted to auditory phoneme schemas, pure word-dumbness as a disorder of motor phoneme schemas. Disturbances of higher order schemas are more difficult to illustrate from clinical material, since all appear to depend on a comparatively limited area of the temporal and parietal lobes in the dominant hemisphere. However, word schemas appear to be principally disturbed in 'central' dysphasias, in which both comprehension and expression are impaired, and word-meaning schemas in nominal dysphasia. The predominantly motor dysphasias may represent a breakdown in the relationship between the word schemas and the motor schemas for the production of articulated speech. In pure alexia the perception of words fails to arouse the visual word schemas which serve to evoke their meaning, whereas in agraphia the graphic schemas fail to arouse the motor schemas organised in relation to the parts of the motor cortex which control the hand in writing.

This suggested organisation, while necessarily at a theoretical level, serves to emphasise the complexities inherent in conceptualising the anatomical–physiological basis for language functions. It has the virtue of attempting to bring together a psychological and a physiological interpretation of the processes which underlie speech, and of insisting on a dynamic approach towards the understanding of dysphasic disturbances. In clinical practice, however, it clearly suffers from attempting to impose a philosophical theory upon the facts, instead of allowing observed phenomena to generate the explanatory theory.

Geschwind (1967) provided a model based upon the learning and arousal of associative links. He pointed out that the distinctive element in human language, which is not present in animal communication, derives from man's ability to form higher-order associations between one sensory stimulus and another. In subhuman primates the principal outflow from sensory association areas is to the limbic system, enabling the animal to learn which stimuli have importance with regard to drives for food, sex or aggression; interconnections between the sensory association regions for different sensory modalities are meagre by comparison. The impressive advance in the human brain lies in the expansion of the zone in the region of the angular gyrus at the junction of the temporal, parietal and occipital lobes, which is an area strategically situated with respect to the association cortices for hearing, touch and vision. This may constitute the neural substrate which allows the human being readily to form linkages between two or more 'non-limbic' stimuli, and achieve the higher-order associations which underlie the acquisition of language skills. It is noteworthy that inputs to this part of the brain are almost exclusively from other cortical regions, and furthermore that it is one of the last brain regions to myelinate during development.

In Geschwind's model for naming, an object which is seen stimulates the visual association cortex, and thereafter connections via the angular gyrus arouse associations with regard to the 'heard name' in the auditory association cortex of the first temporal convolution (Wernicke's area). This in turn is transmitted via the arcuate fasciculus to the motor association cortex in the posterior part of the frontal lobe (Broca's area), where the 'rules' are contained for turning the output from Wernicke's area into the motor acts of speech. At each way-station there is not only transmission of the 'message', but certain operations are carried out on it so that coding is reorganised in distinctive ways. The two crucial processes therefore consist first of comprehension, then of repetition by which we learn to reproduce the auditory stimulus. Each has a different anatomical location. Thus the type of disturbance of speech produced by circumscribed lesions will change as we move from one region to another.

A lesion in Wernicke's area will impair verbal comprehension. Comprehension is developmentally a process by which we learn to associate the auditory stimulus of a word with a visual or other sensory stimulus. A lesion here will prevent the incoming auditory signals from being classified into patterns as a prelude to recognition, and from being conveyed elsewhere in the brain to arouse meaningful associations. Reading will likewise be impaired since this is learned by the child in association with the spoken language, the essence of which has already been mastered; when visual language can no longer excite auditory associations it will fail to be comprehended. Writing will also be impaired because the first step in writing consists of the reverse act of arousing visual associations from the auditory forms of the word. Speaking is impaired because this depends first upon the arousal of auditory associations which are then transmuted into motor speech by Broca's area. Since Broca's area remains intact, however, it may 'run on' to some extent autonomously and produce a fluent flow of faulty speech; overlearning has occurred there for many of the sequences of language, and when deprived of the control of higher functional levels the output of speech may even be excessive while faulty.

Lesions of the arcuate fasciculus also allow a fluent dysphasia, since Broca's area remains intact, and comprehension is relatively preserved because Wernicke's area is intact. But the speech is abnormal and repetition markedly defective because Broca's area normally 'repeats' the messages which arrive from the temporal lobe.

Lesions in Broca's area itself leave comprehension relatively well preserved because Wernicke's area remains intact. The output of speech is sparse, laboured and with poor articulation, because the rules for translating the message into motor speech are damaged.

Geschwind's scheme does not attempt to explain how meaning can be derived from the relationships between words in their syntactical context. It adheres remarkably closely, though with more persuasive evidence, to the essence of the theory put forward by Wernicke in 1874.

Neuroimaging and language

The various syndromes of language impairment have been derived from the noting of clusters of clinical symptoms and relating these where possible to neuroanatomical information. In general, structural neuroimaging has tended to support the traditional syndrome localisations for the main subvarieties—Broca's, Wernicke's and conduction dysphasia—likewise for the principal subdivisions of alexia and agraphia (Benson & Ardila 1996). However, functional imaging techniques have shown additional complexities, revealing areas of hypometabolism extending beyond or even distant from the areas of known structural damage. Sometimes they have seemed to argue for a return towards holistic views of language representation in the brain.

Metter and Hanson (1994), for example, report PET scan studies which show that hypometabolism in the left temporoparietal cortex appears to be critical for the development of dysphasia, being present in all the dysphasics they studied irrespective of the location of structural damage. The severity, and many of the characteristics of the dysphasia, appeared to depend on the combined effects of the focal lesion and its functional consequences in the temporoparietal region. Rather more than half of the subjects examined also showed hypometabolism in the left prefrontal regions, anterior and superior to the classic Broca's area, often with damage extending subcortically. In this there was some correlation with the type of dysphasia displayed—the frontal regions were more markedly hypometabolic in Broca's than in Wernicke's dysphasia or conduction dysphasia, and Wernicke patients showed the most severe temporoparietal hypometabolism.

Activation studies, coupled with neuroimaging, have so far contributed little to the understanding of dysphasia, but by contrast are illuminating the brain regions involved in language processing in the intact brain:

Petersen et al. (1988) used PET scanning to explore linguistic functions in an interesting experimental paradigm. Seventeen right-handed normal volunteers were given repeated brief PET scans, using ^{15}O-labelled water, under a succession of experimental conditions arranged hierarchically. By subtraction, the effects of each extra task demand on regional cerebral blood flow could be discerned. In the first comparison nouns were presented (visually or auditorily) without task demands, and compared with a control state of simple visual fixation. Involuntary word-form processing was targeted by this subtraction. Next the subject was required to speak each word, revealing areas involved in output coding and motor control. Finally the subject was asked to give a use for each presented word, revealing the cerebral substrate for noun–verb associations (semantic processing).

The passive processing of words activated regions bilaterally in the sensory association regions appropriate to the modality in which the words were presented—striate and peristriate cortex with visual presentations and superior temporal cortex, more extensively on the left, for auditory presentations. Speaking the words activated similar regions whether the presentations had been visual or auditory—the mouth region of the Rolandic cortex on the left, Rolandic cortex superior to this bilaterally, Sylvian regions close to Broca's area (but also bilaterally), and supplementary motor cortex. The semantic word generation task activated inferior frontal cortex, only on the left, and anterior cingulate cortex known to be implicated in 'attention for action' (p. 146). It is noteworthy that Wernicke's area and the region of the left angular gyrus were unaffected during the process of reading words, implying that written stimuli do not require phonological recoding prior to semantic access. The results thus supported multiple route models for language processing, in which visual and auditory inputs pursue separate pathways of access to articulatory and semantic centres.

The complexities inherent in attempting to dissect language mechanisms in this fashion are, however, shown by an analogous PET scan study by Wise et al. (1991). They imaged brain activity by the inhalation of ^{15}O-labelled carbon dioxide during a series of language tasks, comparing each with images obtained during a rest condition. Listening to non-words activated precisely the same brain areas as comparisons between words, namely neural networks along both superior temporal gyri in primary and association auditory cortex, suggesting that the loci for acoustic processing and semantic processing of heard material are congruous with one another. It is hard to be certain, however, that an element of semantic processing is not involved when listening to non-words.

When the subjects were asked to think, without vocalisation, of as many verbs as possible in relation to a given noun, activation was confined to the left hemisphere and involved frontal as well as temporal brain regions. These included the superior temporal gyrus (Wernicke's area), posterior parts of the middle and inferior frontal gyri (including Broca's area), and the supplementary motor cortex. The implication of Wernicke's area during word generation differed from Petersen et al.'s (1988) finding, which the authors attempt to explain in terms of the differing experimental paradigms employed. The involvement of the supplementary motor cortex during word generation without vocalisation suggests that the act of retrieving words from memory results automatically in 'inner speech', and that the supplementary motor area contains neural pathways concerned in this process.

A surprising result of PET activation studies has been the demonstration that the cerebellum is activated not only during word repetition and spontaneous speech, but also during the generation of word associations and the making of semantic decisions (Chertkow & Bub 1994). The posterior lobule of the cerebellum appears to be especially involved in such cognitive activities as verbal encoding and decision making.

Finally Binder and Rao (1994) discuss the possible value of functional MRI in studies of language processing. The technique has already demonstrated that the perception of speech activates larger areas of the superior temporal gyrus bilaterally than the perception of white noise; and that the performance of a semantic task (detecting particular classes of animals in a list) then activates additional areas in the left hemisphere alone — in lateral frontal, parieto-occipital and temporo-occipital regions.

Dysphasia and other aspects of intelligence

Opinion has differed about the extent to which dysphasia can be regarded merely as 'loss of a linguistic tool' while other aspects of intellect remain intact. Language is, of course, an integral part of conceptual thinking and of problem solving in many areas; but it may be that some dysphasic patients retain in large degree the automatic and subconscious use of words in thinking processes. The question of the preservation or loss of internal speech is very hard to assess.

Quite apart from this it is likely that the cerebral structures subserving language also subserve other functions, so that lesions will almost always impair more than language alone. Some aspects of dysphasia can be seen as reflecting the general difficulties of brain-injured patients as stressed by Goldstein (1936): a difficulty in differentiating 'figure from background' may contribute to inability to pronounce a word in isolation while it can still be produced as part of a series, or general difficulties in categorisation may contribute to problems in naming objects. Impairment of the ordered perception of space or time may worsen dysphasic difficulties, since a proper conception of such matters is essential for symbolic thought.

Psychological testing has helped to some extent to clarify the subject, and is discussed by Piercy (1964), Newcombe (1969) and Zangwill (1969). Dysphasic patients are certainly impaired on language-based intelligence tests to a greater degree than brain-injured patients without dysphasia. Performance is also inferior on certain non-verbal tests when compared to normals, and some-

times even when compared to non-dysphasic brain-injured subjects. In particular Weinstein et al. (1955) reported difficulty with a test of conditional reactions to combinations of visual shapes and backgrounds, and Teuber and Weinstein (1956) with a test of perceiving hidden figures. In both of these it is hard to blame any hypothetical difficulty with internal speech or impaired comprehension of instructions. The often difficult question of assessing legal competency in dysphasic patients is discussed by Benson and Ardila (1996).

Subcortical dysphasia

The possibility that subcortical pathology might contribute to, or even be responsible for, certain dysphasic syndromes has a considerable history. Renewed attention has been directed to the issue now that neuroimaging is capable of revealing discrete subcortical infarcts, and certain syndromes such as 'thalamic' and 'striatal' dysphasia have been proposed. Benson and Ardila (1996) review the still uncertain status of such syndromes, and the difficulty in deciding whether the language disturbance reflects the direct effects of the subcortical lesion or derives from distant effects induced elsewhere in the brain. Functional imaging techniques have shown that secondary involvement of cortical language areas is common, presumably in consequence of 'diaschisis' subsequent upon disruption of subcortical–cortical mechanisms (Perani et al. 1987). Instances of 'subcortical neglect' may similarly owe much to secondary effects on right hemisphere cortical activity.

The picture usually described is of mutism following an acute intracerebral haemorrhage, followed by hypophonia and slow, amelodic output. This may evolve to a combination of severely paraphasic speech with relatively well-preserved capacity for repetition, which appears to be the characteristic pattern. The subcortical structures involved are virtually always situated in the hemisphere dominant for language.

Thalamic dysphasia begins with mutism but generally changes to a fluent, paraphasic, jargon output. Difficulty with naming is often dramatically severe, but comprehension and repetition are comparatively well preserved. In most cases the language disorder is transient, showing improvement over the course of weeks or months. The puzzling feature is the rarity of such a development among the considerable number of persons who develop thalamic lesions.

Striatal (striatocapsular) dysphasia appears to derive chiefly from lesions of the putamen and internal capsule. The patients reported by Damasio et al. (1982a) had prominent involvement of the anterior limb of the capsule and also the head of the caudate nucleus. Speech remains sparse, fluent but hesitant, dysarthric and paraphasic, though again comprehension and repetition are usually good. The ability to name is better preserved than with thalamic dysphasia. Naeser *et al.* (1982) have pointed to subdivisions within the syndrome according to the precise site of the lesion and its extension into neighbouring territories.

Developmental dyslexia (specific reading retardation)

Some children experience unusual difficulty in learning to read and to spell, despite normal or even superior intelligence and equivalent educational opportunities to their peers. The proportion so affected has varied in different surveys and according to the criteria employed, but has been judged to involve just under 4% of 10-year-olds on the Isle of Wight compared with almost 10% in inner London boroughs (Rutter *et al.* 1970; Berger *et al.* 1975; Rutter & Yule 1975). Such disorder has been labelled as 'developmental dyslexia', or alternatively as 'specific reading retardation' to distinguish it from the reading difficulties associated with generally poor intellectual endowment.

Important distinctions from the latter have emerged in group comparisons, including a 3–4-fold preponderance in boys, an association with speech and language impairment as opposed to a wider range of developmental delays, and less frequent evidence of brain damage as judged from birth history, neurological examination or electroencephalography (Rutter 1978; Maugham & Yule 1994). Rather strikingly, the Isle of Wight study showed that children with specific reading retardation made significantly *less* progress with reading or spelling than children with 'general reading backwardness', between the ages of 10 and 14, despite their superior intelligence, whereas their progress with mathematics was superior as expected (Yule 1973; Rutter *et al.* 1976). Distinctions between the two groups have traditionally relied on identifying the size of the discrepancy between reading attainment as predicted on the basis of age and IQ scores and the actual level of attainment observed. Though criticised because of the doubtful predictive value of IQ for literacy attainment, such a formula permits the identification of children with disproportionate reading difficulty across a wide range of levels of intelligence, including those whose intelligence is below the average.

The disorder is now increasingly recognised among those engaged in education, and specialist courses designed to upgrade the knowledge and expertise of teachers are slowly being established. However, the problems not uncommonly persist into adult life as a continuing source of handicap and social embarrassment. With effort and specialist teaching some affected individuals appear to overcome their reading problems, proceeding successfully to higher education, though poor spelling usually persists as an aftermath.

Different theories abound as to the basis of the condition. Genetic influences are quite strongly apparent from twin studies, and in the frequent occurrence of reading difficulties in family members from one generation to another, as reviewed by Maugham and Yule (1994). Environmental influences such as poor family circumstances or inadequate schooling clearly also make a contribution, at least to the extent of rendering difficulties of this nature more readily overt. But increasing attention has focused on the possible pathophysiological mechanisms that may underlie the special difficulties in learning to decode the written word or sentence into articulated speech and meaning. It has been noted, *inter alia*, that such children often show sequencing difficulties, right–left confusions, and in some cases varying degrees of motor clumsiness and incoordination. In a small proportion there seem to be problems with aspects of visual perception, but more commonly the difficulties are essentially linguistic and appear to lie with problems in phonological decoding and syntactical processes. It remains uncertain whether the condition can be regarded as a homogeneous syndrome or whether different subvarieties exist.

Traditionally the disorder has been viewed by neurologists as 'maturational' in nature, perhaps resulting from delayed myelination or other problems in crucial neural systems. Recent studies have, however, given support to the proposition that definable abnormalities of cerebral structure or function may sometimes persist even in adults who have largely compensated for their early deficits. Three such areas of investigation will be briefly outlined.

Galaburda and colleagues have reported certain unusual features in the brains of dyslexic subjects examined at autopsy (Galaburda & Kemper 1979; Galaburda *et al.* 1985; Humphreys *et al.* 1990; Galaburda 1992). In the four male and three female brains examined there was a consistent and notable lack of asymmetry in the size of the planum temporale of the two hemispheres. Moreover, all showed areas of architectonic dysplasia by way of disruption of the normal laminar organisation of the cortex, along with neuronal 'ectopias' consisting of abnormal nests of cells in the cortex and subjacent white matter. These were often closely associated with the dysplasic areas, resulting in the appearance of small nodules ('brain warts'). It is perhaps noteworthy, however, that at least some of these subjects had suffered from epilepsy (see p. 244).

Such changes were most common in the inferior frontal and superior temporal cortex, clustering particularly in the peri-Sylvian region and affecting the left hemisphere predominantly. These probably derived from the mid gestational period, at the time of peak migration of neurones from the germinal matrix to the cortical plate. Polymicrogyria was observed in two of the male cases, in the left planum temporale and the left temporal lobe. Additionally two of the females and one of the males showed multiple foci of cortical glial scarring; and since most such scars were myelinated they had probably arisen later during gestation or in the early postnatal period.

The tentative view was proposed that a familial predisposition to dyslexia could be manifest as the lack of asymmetry with respect to the planum temporale, with the ectopias, dysplasias and glial scars then leading to further disruption of cerebral organisation. Both sets of factors could thus be necessary before the dyslexia became overt.

MRI studies have confirmed that an unusual degree of symmetry of the planum is significantly more common in dyslexic subjects than controls (Hynd *et al.* 1990; Larsen *et al.* 1990). Moreover in Larsen *et al.*'s study of 19 adolescent dyslexics, there was a close relationship between abnormal symmetry of the planum and measures of phonological dysfunction. Hynd and Hiemenz (1997) summarise more recent interesting findings concerning posterior peri-Sylvian morphology in dyslexia. Duara *et al.* (1991) have further demonstrated with MRI that the splenium of the corpus callosum, which connects the regions of the angular gyri of the two hemispheres, is larger in dyslexic subjects than in normal controls, this being particularly marked in female dyslexics.

Along different lines, Livingstone *et al.* (1991) have pursued the hypothesis that there are problems with the perception of visual material in developmental dyslexia, perhaps attributable to deficits in the 'magnocellular' component of the visual pathways. This subdivision of the perceptual system is concerned with the detection of fast, low-contrast visual information, and also carries information about motion, stereopsis and perhaps figure–ground separation. The magnocellular and parvocellular subdivisions of the visual pathways are largely segregated from the retinal level onwards, the distinction being most apparent in the lateral geniculate bodies. Several studies have shown that subjects with developmental dyslexia do poorly on tasks requiring rapid visual processing, for example on flicker-fusion tests.

In five dyslexic subjects Livingstone *et al.* demonstrated impairment of visual evoked potentials to rapid low-contrast stimuli, but normal responses to slow or high-contrast stimuli, in a manner consistent with defects in the magnocellular pathway. Furthermore, in a study of the structure of the lateral geniculate bodies in dyslexic subjects they found abnormalities in the magnocellular but not the parvocellular layers. Livingstone *et al.* hypothesise that other cortical systems may similarly be divided into fast and slow subdivisions, including the auditory system; if so, this could be relevant to the linguistic problems of dyslexia, since phonemic discriminations involve the processing of rapid auditory transitions.

Finally, Uta Frith and her colleagues have devised elegant strategies for exploring the role of defective phonological decoding in dyslexia, using PET scanning to detect the brain regions involved (Paulesu *et al.* 1996). Problems in the domain of phonology are currently strongly favoured as a core problem in developmental dyslexia (Stanovich 1991; Snowling *et al.* 1994; Snowling 1996), and phonological strategies appear to be especially effective with many dyslexics in attempts at remediation. Moreover among those dyslexics who attain academic success, this is often largely achieved through acquiring a large 'sight vocabulary', and underlying deficits in phonology may persist throughout adulthood.

Paulesu *et al.* used a rhyming task for examining phonological similarity judgements, also a phonological short-term memory task, both presented visually. PET scans using ^{15}O-labelled water were carried out during performance on the tasks to detect the brain regions activated. These paradigms had previously been used to explore the cerebral correlates of subvocal rehearsal and short-term storage of verbal material in normal volunteers (Paulesu *et al.* 1993). The subjects were five adults with a clear past history of developmental dyslexia but who had ultimately succeeded academically, and in this sense were 'compensated' dyslexics. On a variety of demanding tasks involving phonological processing they were nonetheless still considerably impaired. Control subjects without a history of reading difficulties were matched in terms of educational level.

In the rhyming task the subject had to judge whether pairs of letters presented on a screen rhymed with each other or not (e.g. BG vs. BL). This requires segmentation of each letter name into its consonant and vowel (viz. 'buh-ee' vs. 'buh-el') by a process of subvocal rehearsal ('segmented phonology'). A control task of shape similarity judgements (with letters from the Korean alphabet) was used, subtraction of PET images between the two allowing the regions activated by rhyme judgements to be discerned.

The phonological short-term memory task involved testing for the recall of consonants presented visually ('whole word phonology'), the control task then being short-term memory for visual shapes. The simplicity of the tasks was such that the dyslexics could perform them virtually as well as the control subjects.

During the phonological similarity judgement (rhyming) task the controls activated the peri-Sylvian structures of the left hemisphere widely, including Broca's and Wernicke's areas and much of the insula, also the left caudate nucleus and other left hemisphere structures. By contrast the dyslexics activated a much more restricted domain, involving Broca's area and the left caudate alone (Plate 1). During the phonological short-term memory task the controls showed a similar pattern of activation to that of the rhyming task, with additional activations in the left supramarginal gyrus and certain regions of the right hemisphere. Again the dyslexics showed more restricted activation, including Wernicke's area and the left supramarginal gyrus, but Broca's area only weakly. Right hemisphere activations were scarcely seen (Plate 2). Thus the dyslexics could activate Broca's area (segmented phonology), Wernicke's area (whole word phonology) and the supramarginal gyrus, but unlike the controls did not activate these regions in concert. Moreover, in noteworthy fashion activations of the insula region were not apparent.

Paulesu et al. (1996) interpret their findings as revealing something of the difficulties dyslexics experience in associating between the different 'codings' involved in acquiring reading skills. Thus the sound of the heard word, the sight of the written word and the articulatory sequences of the spoken word must be mapped one upon another, including the mapping of both segmented phonological codes and whole word codes. The insula appears to constitute a bridge between posterior and anterior language areas, and Paulesu et al. speculate that it may perform the function of converting between such dissimilar codes. In effect there appeared to be a 'disconnection' in their dyslexic subjects, with problems in translating directly from the written word to its associated phonology in segmented form. This would result in a lack of support for recoding, and difficulty in holding both segmented and unsegmented codes simultaneously in working memory.

Clinical syndromes of language impairment

For purposes of clinical evaluation it is useful to consider a broad division into defective understanding of speech or written material, and defective production of speech or writing. However, the great majority of patients with language disturbance show a complicated mixture of deficits. This was well illustrated by Brown and Simonson's (1957) review of 100 dysphasic patients who were examined without reference to conventional categories and simply scored in terms of disorder of speaking, listening, reading and writing. Only nine had a deficit limited to one function and this was always slight in degree. Sixteen had deficits in two components, 14 in three, and the remaining 61 had deficits in all components of language. Many of the patients with disordered appreciation of spoken speech had severe impairment of all four components and

appeared most commonly to represent the cases of 'global dysphasia'.

The syndromes considered below represent no more than approximations which may be regarded as clinically useful. The first four syndromes, pure word-deafness, word-blindness, word-dumbness and pure agraphia, though all rare, are outlined first because they represent the purest forms of defect. All are produced by lesions near the areas of association cortex for vision, hearing or motor function. Lesions in such locations will more commonly be sufficiently extensive to produce widespread dysphasic difficulties, resulting for example in combinations of primary motor dysphasia with pure word-dumbness. The next three syndromes, 'primary sensory dysphasia', 'primary motor dysphasia' and 'nominal dysphasia', represent the more commonly occurring clinical pictures and show deficits in more than one component of language. The terms 'sensory' and 'motor' are used as a guide to the source of primary breakdown of language function, since this has implications for site of pathology. The terms must not be taken to indicate the nature of functional impairment, for of course primary sensory dysphasia has itself a marked defect in motor expression. Finally, certain other clinical syndromes are briefly outlined.

Table 1 on p. 103 summarises the rather bewildering array of disturbances of function found in these different syndromes. For an extended presentation and discussion of the various disorders Benson and Ardila (1996) should be consulted. At least partial support for the principal subvarieties and their anatomical localisation has come from neuroimaging studies as described on p. 45, though many authorities argue against the neatness with which language disturbance can be subdivided (Smith 1978). Critchley (1987) in reviewing the subject presents a balanced position between over-holistic and over-localisationist points of view. The syndromes outlined below are clearly to a considerable extent abstractions from a very complex whole.

Pure word-deafness (subcortical auditory dysphasia, verbal auditory agnosia)

The patient can speak fluently and virtually without error, and similarly can write normally. He can also read and comprehend what he reads. The defect is restricted to the understanding of spoken speech, even though other aspects of hearing are intact. In fact the patient hears words as sounds but fails to recognise these sounds as words. Hemphill and Stengel's (1940) patient said: 'Voice comes but no words. I can hear, sounds come, but words don't separate. There is no trouble at all with the sound.

Sounds come. I can hear, but I cannot understand it.' As a result the patient cannot repeat words spoken to him and cannot write to dictation.

Such a defect can equally be regarded as an agnosia for spoken words. It is extremely rare, but there is general agreement that the lesion is in the dominant temporal lobe, closely adjacent to the primary receptive area for hearing—Heschl's gyrus of the first temporal convolution. Geschwind suggests that it is caused by interruption of the auditory pathway to the dominant temporal lobe together with a lesion of the corpus callosum. The patient can still hear because the auditory pathway to the non-dominant cortex is intact, but incoming auditory information cannot gain access to the speech-receiving mechanisms of the dominant lobe. The disorder is rare because a lesion in this situation will usually extend far enough to the surface to damage the speech-receiving mechanisms themselves, resulting in the more widespread disabilities of a primary sensory dysphasia.

Pure word-blindness (alexia without agraphia, agnosic alexia, subcortical visual aphasia, occipital alexia)

The patient can speak normally and has no difficulty with comprehension of the spoken word. His difficulties with language are entirely restricted to his understanding of what he reads. In the most severe examples even letters cannot be comprehended, while in less severe cases occasional words are understood. The patient can still describe or copy letters even though he cannot recognise them, showing that the defect is not due to loss of the visual images of the letters. Some patients manage better with written script than printed material, presumably because they can more readily reproduce the letters in imagination with the right hand and thereby obtain kinaesthetic cues. Occasionally, numbers continue to be recognised when letters are not, perhaps again via kinaesthetic cues derived from early associations between counting and manual activities.

The patient can write spontaneously and to dictation, though subsequently he cannot read what he has written. The writing is usually entirely normal, though it may contain minor errors of reduplication or misalignment of letters. He may be able to copy written material slowly and laboriously.

An almost invariable accompaniment is a right homonymous hemianopia. Colours cannot be named, even though colour perception can be shown to be intact by sorting tests. Here it is probably significant that colour naming represents a purely visual–verbal association process and cannot derive support from other cues.

Essentially, word-blindness is a failure to recognise the language values of the visual patterns which make up letters and words, although there is no disturbance of the symbolic function of the words themselves. This is confirmed when the patient can spell out loud and recognise words that are spelled out loud. The lesion is of the left visual cortex together with the splenium of the corpus callosum; thus visual input is possible only to the right hemisphere, and cannot gain access to the language systems of the left. The situation is therefore analogous to that of the lesion causing pure word-deafness. Pure word-blindness is commoner, however, because the lesion does not so readily impinge on the language areas themselves. The usual cause is occlusion of the left posterior cerebral artery.

Pure word-dumbness (apraxic anarthria, subcortical motor dysphasia, aphemia)

The patient can comprehend both spoken speech and written material without difficulty, and shows this by his ability to respond to complex commands. He can express himself normally in writing, which also serves to demonstrate that inner speech is perfectly preserved. The defect is restricted to the production of spoken speech, which is marked by slurring and dysarthria. The patient cannot speak normally at will, cannot repeat words heard and cannot read aloud. In severe cases he may be totally unable to articulate. Yet for other purposes the muscles of the tongue and lips function without impairment.

The condition may thus be regarded as an apraxia restricted to the movements required for speech. The exact site of pathology is uncertain, but the lesion is probably beneath the region of the insula, interrupting the pathway from the cortical centres responsible for motor schemas for words to the motor systems used in articulated speech. It is extremely rare because the lesion usually also involves the former at the same time, resulting in a primary motor dysphasia.

Pure agraphia (agraphia without alexia)

Agraphia may accompany almost any form of generalised dysphasia, or be a component of generalised apraxia. As an isolated defect, however, it may be seen as the graphic equivalent of pure word-dumbness. Comprehension of written and spoken material is normal, and the patient's own speech is unimpaired. However, he is unable to write either spontaneously or to dictation, though he may fare rather better at the copying of written material.

Brain (1965) pointed out that writing is a considerably more complex process than articulated speech, since after the processes leading up to speech there must then be evocation of visual graphic schemas in the posterior parts of the brain, and of motor schemas in close relation to the motor cortex. The lesion in pure motor agraphia is thought to interrupt the pathway from the left angular gyrus to the hand area of the left motor cortex, and to lie usually in the second frontal gyrus anterior to the hand area, or sometimes in the parietal lobe.

Primary sensory dysphasia (receptive dysphasia, Wernicke's dysphasia)

The primary deficit is in the comprehension of spoken speech. There is defective appreciation of the meaning of words, and in particular of meaning conveyed by grammatical relations. The patient has corresponding difficulty in repeating what is said to him and in responding to commands. In less severe examples the difficulty in responding to commands can be observed to increase with the complexity of instructions, though interestingly quite complex 'whole-body' commands can prove to be surprisingly well performed (Benson & Geschwind 1971). Other aspects of hearing are intact, as with pure word-deafness, but unlike the latter there are also impairments of spontaneous speech, writing and reading. These added difficulties are attributable to the fact that the cortical mechanisms for analysing incoming speech are directly implicated by the lesion, not merely cut off from input as in pure word-deafness.

Thus ability to speak is also impaired, presumably because auditory associations or schemas must first be aroused before the efferent speech mechanisms can produce speech in a normal manner. Words are used wrongly, paraphasic errors and neologisms are frequent, and sentences tend to be poorly constructed with errors of grammar and syntax. However, the faulty speech is produced fluently and without effort. Normal rhythm and inflexion are preserved and there are no articulatory defects. The speech may even be excessive in flow or under pressure, perhaps because the effector mechanisms 'run on' to a large degree autonomously when freed from the control of higher functional levels.

A patient reported by Brain (1965) responded as follows: When asked 'Do you have headaches?' he replied 'No. I've been fort in that way. I haven't been headache troubled not for a long time'. When shown a picture of an elephant he was unable to name it, but pointed to the mouth and said 'That's his sound, he is making his sound—seems to have got his voice opened there'. When shown a picture of a penguin he said 'A kind of little ver (bird)—machinery—a kind of animal do for making a sound'. When shown a tape measure he called it 'A kind of machinery', and when immediately afterwards shown a bunch of keys and asked to name it he said 'Indication of measurement of piece of apparatus or intimating the cost of apparatus in various forms'.

Reiterative errors are obvious in the above example, in that the speech is contaminated by words which the patient has once used but then cannot easily discard. The patient is usually unaware of his mistakes and makes no attempt to correct them. Unlike the patient with nominal dysphasia (see below) he is often unable to recognise the correct name for an object when this is told to him.

Reading and writing are also impaired since these are presumably also dependent on the cortical areas involved in comprehending spoken speech (and developmentally they are learned in association with spoken language). Single words may be read aloud correctly, but reading out of sentences becomes jumbled and contaminated by paraphasic errors. Written instructions, even if correctly read, may not be carried out, indicating that the patient has failed to understand what he has read. Generally the degrees of disability in understanding spoken and written language parallel each other closely. The disturbances of writing also closely mirror those of spoken speech, except that a copious fluent flow is much less common in writing than in speaking.

The lesion is in the auditory association cortex of the superior and middle temporal gyri of the dominant hemisphere (Wernicke's area), presumably preventing the recoding of auditory messages for recognition, and debarring the arousal of auditory associations as a necessary step for reading, writing and the production of spoken speech. According to Brain's conception outlined above, the complex deficit is due to impaired utilisation of word schemas, which constitute the physiological link between the various neural processes connecting the sensory stimuli of words to their meaning.

Primary motor dysphasia (cortical motor dysphasia, expressive dysphasia, Broca's dysphasia)

The primary defect is on the effector side of speech, thus involving the mechanisms by which words are chosen and articulated and sentences constructed. Unlike pure word-dumbness, however, writing is affected in parallel with speaking, and while comprehension is relatively intact there may be difficulty in carrying out complex instructions. This may be on account of apraxia or because the instructions require complex internal verbalisation for their efficient execution.

Speech is characteristically sparse, slow and hesitant, with marked disturbances of rhythm, inflexion and articulation, unlike the fluent expressive speech of primary sensory dysphasia. Moreover the patient is clearly under stress while trying to speak. Word finding provides obvious difficulty, wrong words are often chosen and the words that are chosen are often mispronounced. Marked reiteration and perseveration are common. However, the patient usually recognises his mistakes, attempts to correct them and becomes impatient about them. Moreover, he can select the correct word when this is offered to him. There is a marked impairment of syntax ('agrammatism'), with a relative decrease in syntactical structural words and grammatical word endings. This further impairs the patient's ability to transmit meaning. He often tries to compensate for his speech defects by means of pantomime and gesture, all again in contrast to the patient with primary sensory dysphasia.

The phrase length is short, and the style may be abbreviated and 'telegraphic' with omissions of words, but the speech that does emerge is meaningful. Ability to repeat what the examiner says to him may be an improvement on what the patient can produce spontaneously, but nevertheless is always profoundly impaired. In the most severe examples the patient may have only one or two words at his command, or there may be stereotyped repetition of some word or phrase ('reiteration', 'recurring utterance'). Total loss of ability to speak is not seen, however, and an occasional speech sound can usually be discerned.

Among these marked expressive difficulties it may be noted that the automatic repetition of serials, such as numbers or days of the week, is relatively well preserved even though they are not well articulated. Also, in severe cases, emotional ejaculations may be surprisingly intact when voluntary utterance is reduced to the minimum. Sometimes an object exposed to view can be named when the same name cannot be found in spontaneous speech. Similarly an habitual situation may call forth a word such as 'goodbye' when the patient is quite unable to produce it on request.

Comprehension of written and spoken instructions may be relatively intact but is rarely normal. Particular difficulty is encountered over the comprehension of grammatically significant structures. Quite often the patient may be well aware of the meaning of a word which he reads even though he cannot pronounce it aloud. Reading out loud will show a halting, jerky flow, with slurring and occasional mispronunciations. In a high proportion of cases the features of 'anterior alexia' will also be present (p. 54), often in severe degree. Disturbances of writing may be closely similar to those of speaking.

The lesion is in the posterior two-thirds of the third frontal convolution, i.e. the pars triangularis and opercu-lum of the premotor cortex, the classic Broca's area. Sometimes this extends also onto the lower part of the precentral convolution.

Nominal dysphasia (amnesic aphasia, anomic aphasia)

Though this is one of the commonest forms of aphasia it is the least understood in terms of pathophysiology. The principal difficulty lies in evoking names at will. This may vary from total inability to name any object on confrontation to a mild disorder demonstrable only where uncommon words are concerned. Rochford and Williams (1962, 1965) showed that there was a close parallel between the difficulty presented by a name and the frequency with which the word appears in language. The patient can describe the object and give its use, even when the name eludes him, and like the patient with primary motor dysphasia can usually recognise the correct name when this is offered to him. He can often use the same word without difficulty a moment later in spontaneous connected speech.

Conversational speech is fluent, with no difficulty in articulation and little or no paraphasic interference, but circumlocutions are used and word-finding pauses may be evident. 'Empty words' such as *thing* or *these* may be frequently employed, and there is a notable lack of substantive words. Otherwise, the grammatical structure of sentences is usually well preserved. The patient can repeat fluently what is said to him, and he usually performs relatively well on well-learned serials such as numbers or days of the week.

Comprehension is relatively preserved in most instances, but internal speech is often affected so there may be difficulty in understanding or executing some oral or written commands.

It is not generally agreed whether nominal dysphasia represents a distinct form of defect. Some view it merely as a mild form of primary sensory dysphasia, since with expanding lesions one may merge progressively into the other. Brain considers the essential fault to lie in the use of words in their capacity as symbols, resulting from a break in the link between word schemas and meaning schemas. Geschwind views it as the consequence of difficulty in evoking intermodal associations, which normally allow the auditory associations of a word to be found from some of its other attributes. This explains the good preservation of grammatical structure, since grammar develops entirely within the linguistic system and does not, like naming, depend on intermodal associations.

This is the type of dysphasia which in mild degree has most often been attributed to diffuse rather than focal brain damage. Certainly it may occur with diffuse brain dysfunction due to toxic or degenerative conditions. However, it may also be found with focal brain lesions, perhaps particularly (though not exclusively) with dominant temporoparietal lesions in the neighbourhood of the angular gyrus. Acalculia and other components of Gerstmann's syndrome often occur as associated deficits.

Conduction dysphasia (central dysphasia, syntactical dysphasia)

Under the above headings many authorities separate a further category of dysphasia, while others regard it merely as a further variant of primary sensory dysphasia. Essentially, conduction dysphasia consists of a grave disturbance of language function in which speech and writing are impaired in the manner described above for primary sensory dysphasia, but in which comprehension of spoken and written material is nonetheless relatively well preserved, as shown for example by simple yes/no responses. Repetition of speech is very severely impaired. Errors of grammar and syntax are a marked feature in cases designated 'syntactical dysphasia'.

According to Geschwind it results from a lesion which spares both Wernicke's and Broca's areas but disrupts the major connections between them. Thus Wernicke's area can function relatively well in analysing incoming information, though it can no longer act to guide the patient's own productions. There are contending views about the site of the responsible lesion (see Benson & Ardila 1996). One view, which accounts for the essential features of the disorder, blames a lesion of the arcuate fasciculus as it passes from the temporal to the frontal lobe by way of the parietal lobe. The more the lesion comes to implicate Wernicke's area itself the more will comprehension be impaired, and the closer will the picture approximate to that of primary sensory dysphasia.

The repetition defect in conduction dysphasia has come under closer scrutiny as a result of the work by Warrington and Shallice (1969) and Warrington et al. (1971), who consider that in a subgroup of these patients there is a highly specific impairment of immediate verbal memory. Three patients were reported who showed a marked repetition defect for verbal material presented in the auditory modality. This appeared on analysis to be a selective impairment of the immediate memory span for auditory verbal material which was directly related to the 'memory' load of the task. There was much less difficulty when comparable material was presented visually. Moreover, auditory verbal learning and verbal long-term memory were relatively intact, indicating that material could nonetheless gain access to the long-term memory store.

Syndromes of the isolated speech area

Under this title Goldstein (1948) and Geschwind et al. (1968) describe further variants of dysphasia, which though rare demand an alternative explanation in terms of mechanism. Comprehension is profoundly disturbed, but in contrast to primary sensory dysphasia the patient can easily repeat what is said to him, and the ability to learn new verbal material is retained. Moreover, spontaneous speech is slow and laboured and lacks the fluency of primary sensory dysphasia. It is postulated that both Wernicke's and Broca's areas, and the connections between them, remain intact but the whole system is cut off from other parts of the cortex. It is the lack of these widespread connections which leads to impaired comprehension and defects of propositional speech.

Though in pure form the syndrome is extremely rare, two variants are well recognised. 'Transcortical (or extrasylvian) motor dysphasia' differs in that the patient can comprehend spoken speech, and is ascribed to a lesion anterior and/or superior to Broca's area, or in some cases in the supplementary area of the medial frontal cortex. 'Transcortical (or extrasylvian) sensory dysphasia' differs in that the fluency of output is preserved. Echolalia is often prominent. The facility with which the patient repeats the examiner's statements, and the fluent jumbled output of speech, stand in contrast to the patient's lack of comprehension. This may lead to misinterpretation of the syndrome as an acute psychotic disturbance, especially since obvious neurological deficits can be lacking (Benson & Ardila 1996). The lesion usually involves either the parieto-occipital or temporo-occipital border zone areas.

Alexia with agraphia (visual asymbolia, parietotemporal alexia)

The patient is unable to read as with pure word-blindness, but in addition he is unable to write. However, the execution and comprehension of spoken speech are substantially unimpaired.

The difficulty in reading is similar to that described for pure word-blindness. The difficulty in writing varies from complete inability to form letters to preservation of partial attempts at writing words. Copying is better than spontaneous writing, which is the converse of the situation in pure word-blindness. Moreover the patient cannot understand words that are spelled out loud, revealing that he is truly illiterate, unlike the patient with pure word-blindness.

The condition may be the predominant symptom from the outset but this is rare. Usually it is found as the residual disturbance when a more global dysphasia clears up. It is usually accompanied by some degree of nominal dysphasia, dyscalculia, spatial disorganisation or visual object agnosia.

The defect results from disturbance of those parts of the brain which deal with the visual symbolic components of language, in Brain's terminology with 'visual word schemas'. The lesion is usually extensive within the parietal or parietotemporal region of the dominant hemisphere, but the angular and supramarginal gyri are always involved.

Anterior alexia

Benson (1977) and Benson and Ardila (1996) draw attention to a third form of alexia, differing from those seen with occipital or parietotemporal lesions. This occurs in association with Broca's dysphasia and presumably depends on analogous frontal pathology. Hitherto such a combination had sometimes been used to argue in favour of holistic views of language organisation within the brain, but Benson was able to highlight features that distinguished this form of alexia from the others. It therefore seems probable that the anterior lesion producing Broca's dysphasia also interferes with certain aspects of reading ability.

Distinctive features include the ability to read occasional words, characteristically nouns or action verbs, but not to grasp the meaning of whole sentences. If a word can be read aloud it is understood, but the ability to interpret grammatical structures is severely undermined. Moreover the patient cannot name the individual letters that make up a word even though he may manage to read the word by 'gestalt' ('literal alexia'), and he usually fails to recognise words that are spelled out to him. Severe agraphia is usually present, including impairment in copying written material.

Such alexia occurred in severe degree in more than half of the Broca aphasics reported by Benson, and appeared to be the rule rather than the exception in some degree. It is usually associated with right hemiparesis and sometimes with disordered control of ocular movements, but visual field defects are comparatively rare. The reading difficulties tend to remain severe, often persisting as the most disabling symptom following good recovery from the dysphasia itself.

Jargon aphasia

Jargon aphasia is the term used when speech is produced freely, volubly and clearly, but with such semantic jumble and misuse of words that meaning cannot be discerned. Typically there are phonetic distortions, neologisms, words put together in meaningless sequence, and sequences which are entirely irrelevant. The intonation and rhythm of formal speech are nevertheless preserved. Jargon aphasia is conventionally regarded as representing a severe example of primary sensory dysphasia, perhaps with superadded difficulties due to pure word-deafness, or perhaps with a marked degree of generalised intellectual impairment. Kertesz and Benson (1970) have reported typical severe neologistic jargon in patients both with Wernicke's dysphasia and conduction dysphasia.

Weinstein et al. (1966) were led to conclude quite differently that jargon aphasia represents dysphasia in conjunction with anosognosia, rather than a distinctive pattern of breakdown in the intrinsic speech structure. In their patients receptive difficulties were rarely severe, and the distinctive accompanying feature was disturbance of consciousness sufficient to produce confabulation, disorientation and reduplicative delusions. In conformity with their observations on anosognosia generally (p. 70), the jargon often appeared selectively when the patient was questioned about his disabilities, and more coherent speech was produced in relation to neutral topics. The pathological basis was a lesion of the dominant hemisphere along with additional brain damage elsewhere, and all patients had bilateral cerebral involvement. However, in favour of the conventional view that jargon represents a primary receptive defect, with failure to monitor speech productions, is the finding that patients who display it are not disturbed in the normal fashion when made to listen to delayed auditory feedback of their own speech productions.

Psychiatric disturbance and dysphasia

Benson and Geschwind (1971) and Benson (1973) summarise the common forms of reaction which may be seen in dysphasic patients. These differ considerably in the different forms of language defect.

In primary motor dysphasia (Broca's dysphasia), frustration and depression are frequently seen, or more rarely the 'catastrophic reaction' in which tension and embarrassment culminate in a sudden outburst of weeping or anger with the patient's realisation of his failings. Indeed the absence of distress among such patients is usually indicative of widespread cerebral damage and consequent impairment of general intellectual ability. Both frustration and depression are considered to indicate a more favourable prognosis for recovery with therapy, representing as they do an awareness of the speech difficulties. On the other hand, angry negativism with hostile responses and refusal to participate in treatment can sometimes emerge and seriously complicate rehabilitation.

By contrast, the patient with primary sensory dysphasia (Wernicke's dysphasia) typically shows a lack of interest in, or even unawareness of, his language problems. Such patients often act as though they believe their own speech to be normal and as though they feel that people around them fail to speak normally. Agitation and sometimes severe paranoid reactions may ensue, with suspicions that others are talking about them, plotting against them or deliberately using unintelligible jargon to prevent them from understanding. Outbursts of impulsive, aggressive behaviour may be seen. In Benson's experience almost every patient who had needed custodial care during recovery from dysphasia had suffered a paranoid reaction secondary to severe comprehension disability.

Over and above specific problems of this nature, Benson and Ardila (1996) stress the psychosocial difficulties encountered by dysphasic patients generally. Dysphasia is frequently followed by calamitous alterations in life-style and economic status, along with disruption of simple pleasures such as conversation, reading or watching television. Social and family status are often undermined, irrespective of the presence of other handicaps such as hemiparesis, likewise confidence in sexual functioning.

From the diagnostic point of view the disordered language productions of certain schizophrenic patients, and the phenomena of dysphasia due to brain damage, need to be very carefully distinguished from one another. This can only be done by careful attention to the *form* of language output and by comprehensive tests of language function. The 'word salad' of the chronically deteriorated schizophrenic may sometimes closely resemble dysphasic speech; conversely some patients with dysphasia are mistakenly diagnosed as psychotic for long periods of time, especially those with primary sensory dysphasia or transcortical sensory dysphasia who produce a wealth of paraphasic neologisms. The neurological examination is often negative in such patients, their output is vague and apparently 'confused', and they may react negatively to the examiner's speech in a manner suggestive of psychosis. Any *sudden* onset of speech disorder must therefore always dictate caution, even in the established chronic schizophrenic patient.

Gerson et al. (1977) have analysed tape-recorded interviews with groups of posterior aphasic and schizophrenic patients in order to determine the features most useful in making the clinical distinction. Paraphasic substitutions of incorrect words and perseverative responses at some point in the interview were common among the dysphasics but absent among the schizophrenics. The length of verbal responses to open-ended questions was consider-

ably shorter among the dysphasics, and these did not show the bizarre reiterative themes frequently encountered among the schizophrenics. The dysphasic patients showed at least some awareness of their language difficulties, and used gestures or pauses to enlist the examiner's aid, whereas the schizophrenic patients were impervious to the adequacy or otherwise of their communication. Vagueness of response arose from word-finding difficulties in the dysphasic patients but was apparently attributable to shifts of attention in the schizophrenics. The 'circumlocution' of dysphasia could thus often be contrasted with the 'circumstantiality' of schizophrenic speech.

It is only on rare occasions that difficulty arises in distinguishing between psychogenic and organic disturbances of language function. The most common hysterical speech disorder consists of complete aphonia or mutism; or if sounds are produced there are usually no recognisable words at all. A very rare example of dyslexia and dysgraphia of psychogenic origin has been described by Master and Lishman (1984).

Apraxia (dyspraxia) and related executive disorders

Apraxia is notoriously difficult to define. In essence it refers to an inability to carry out learned voluntary movements, or movement complexes, when this cannot be accounted for in terms of paresis, incoordination, sensory loss or involuntary movements. The patient cannot at will set the movement in train or guide a series of consecutive movements in their correct spatial and temporal sequence, even though the same muscles can be used and analogous movements performed in other contexts.

Geschwind and Damasio (1985) point out that apraxia is often overlooked on clinical examination since it is unlikely to be complained of by the patient or his family. The patient who is apraxic on testing will usually perform learned movements normally in a natural setting, and especially when he can see and manipulate objects in their proper environment. In consequence the disorder is probably a good deal commoner than is usually appreciated.

The essential nature of apraxic disturbances is incompletely understood. Dysphasia is an accompanying defect in the great majority of cases and deficient comprehension of commands may sometimes play a part. Agnosia for an object may hinder the patient from carrying out purposive movements appropriate to its use, while agnosia for spatial relationships will similarly interfere with the copying of a movement by imitation. Over and above such complications, however, one must in many cases postulate some higher-order difficulty with aspects of cerebral organisation which have a specific bearing on motor functions.

The difficulties for any explanatory system include the observation that movements which cannot be performed to command can sometimes be performed in imitation of the examiner, or a movement which cannot be initiated is performed a moment later when the patient's attention is not directed towards it. Sometimes simple discrete movements are affected, and sometimes complex coordinated sequences as in the lighting of a candle or the use of a tool. Frequently, performance is much better in the actual presence of the tool than when the patient is asked to demonstrate its use in imagination. Finally, and to a surprising extent, whole body movements to command are often found to be perfectly preserved, while limb and facial movements are defective. Simple hierarchies of difficulty do not provide an explanation for these anomalies, and systems which attempt to classify the pictures meet with many exceptions. The precise details of the test situation can obviously have a considerable influence on the assumptions that are drawn.

Brain (1965) suggested that purposive movements are organised by 'schemas' which may or may not enter consciousness depending on the context of the movement. The more practised the act, and the more automatic it has become, the more it will be carried out without conscious awareness and conscious volition. Apraxia may be regarded as the result of disorganisation of such schemas and as taking place at various levels of complexity. At the highest level will be found disturbance where the schemas are involved in the formulation of the idea of a movement, and at the lowest where the schema consists of a motor pattern which regulates the selection of the appropriate muscles.

Geschwind (1965) put forward a simpler model which viewed the apraxias as failures of connection between certain cortical regions. Lesions which disrupt connections between the auditory association cortex and motor association cortex of the dominant hemisphere will result in inability to carry out motor commands with the limbs of either side of the body, since this depends on impulses carried forward to the left motor cortex and thence across the corpus callosum to equivalent regions on the right. A lesion of the left motor cortex itself may produce a right hemiplegia together with apraxia limited to the left arm, when the origin of the transcallosal pathway has been destroyed. The dysphasia accompanying both of these lesions is of a type which leaves comprehension perfectly adequate for the understanding of the commands. Lesions of the corpus callosum itself result in apraxia to command without dysphasia, and limited to the left limbs, since the motor cortex of the right hemisphere is now isolated from the speech mechanisms of the left. When imitation of movements is also disrupted this is presumed to depend on loss of essential connections between the visual and the motor association cortices. Geschwind made the further interesting point that the patient's own explanations for his defects are often quite inadequate, because he cannot introspect in the usual way and produce verbal reports about the failures of right hemisphere function.

Ajuriaguerra and Tissot (1969) reviewed these and other theories of apraxia and found them to be inadequate. They presented instead a view of apraxia derived from the developmental psychology of Piaget, with apraxia closely linked to the processes involved in the mastery of space. The child begins with understanding the space involved in the manipulation of objects, then proceeds to master space centred on his body, and finally external and 'objective' space. This process is intimately bound with extensions outwards of the developing body schema. Experience in manipulating objects leads to progressive dissociation of the concept of time from that of space, and finally the spatial schema of 'action' becomes conceivable independently of time. Disintegration of this process may result variably in different classic syndromes, namely disordered appreciation of spatial relationships (constructional apraxia), disturbance of body gestures, disturbance of spatial and temporal relationships in movement, or inability to utilise tools and objects. The forms of apraxia may thus depend upon the type of space in which the movements are realised, whether external space, space centred on the body, or the 'concrete space of manipulation'.

The relationship of apraxia to intellectual impairment must also be considered. Apraxia is perhaps more often seen with diffuse than with strictly focal brain lesions, so that other intellectual processes are frequently also impaired. With focal lesions, however, other cognitive processes may prove to be largely intact, even though at first sight the severely apraxic patient is sometimes misdiagnosed as demented. Nonetheless such patients are severely handicapped in many tasks requiring the demonstration of intelligence, and it is likely that schemas for purposive movement are so interwoven in cognitive processes that their disruption is bound to have an adverse effect.

The chief varieties of apraxia that are recognised in clinical practice are outlined below.

Limb kinetic apraxia

In this type of apraxia the skill and delicacy of movements is disturbed, both for complex and simple actions. Thus the patient may have difficulty in doing up buttons or opening a safety pin. The difficulty that the patient experiences is a function of the muscular complexity rather than the psychomotor complexity involved. It may be confined to particular muscle groups, and even to certain fingers of a hand. This form has characteristics intermediate between paresis and apraxia and is therefore often excluded from the apraxias proper. It results from a relatively small lesion of the contralateral premotor cortex.

Also of frontal origin is the 'magnetic syndrome', in which a grasp reflex is coupled with an irrepressible tendency to follow objects with the hands when they are touched or when they enter the field of vision. This fixation interferes with the execution of other movements, since the hand adheres to the paper when the patient wishes to write, or the foot to the ground when he wishes to walk. Once the foot is lifted a complete step follows immediately. The 'utilisation behaviour' which may also accompany a frontal lesion is described on p. 106.

Ideomotor apraxia

In essence ideomotor (or 'ideokinetic') apraxia refers to the inability to carry out a requested movement properly (Geschwind & Damasio 1985). It may be regarded as a disturbance of voluntary movement at a fairly low level of motor organisation, or alternatively as a disturbance in the use of space centred on the body. The patient can often formulate to himself the idea of the movement that he wishes to perform, but finds that he cannot execute it. Thus the voluntary impulse does not evoke the appropriate organisation of the movement in space and time. For example, the patient cannot raise his hand or wave it to command, even though the instructions are understood. In some cases he can copy equivalent movements, but this too may fail. Yet essentially the same movements can be performed automatically, as in signalling goodbye, or in the course of other activities to which his attention is not directed. In general the greater the volitional nature of the act, and the less it has become automatic, the more it is disrupted.

The disorder is usually bilateral and most commonly involves the upper limbs. Unilateral apraxia almost always involves the left upper limb, and is then typically seen with right hemiplegia and aphasia. In facial apraxia the patient cannot smile or produce tongue movements to order, and this too may be bilateral or unilateral. In truncal apraxia the patient cannot organise at will the movements required for sitting or lying. This, however, is relatively rare and whole body movements are usually well preserved in the other forms.

There is general agreement that lesions of the dominant left hemisphere are much commoner than non-dominant lesions in apraxia. The parietal lobe has been chiefly incriminated, especially lesions involving the angular and supramarginal gyri (Geschwind & Damasio 1985). With apraxia of the face and tongue the lesion is usually situated at the base of the precentral motor cortex. In cases of left unilateral apraxia, a lesion of the corpus callosum or of its lateral extension into the left motor association cortex is likely to be responsible.

Ideational apraxia

The patient is unable to carry out coordinated sequences of actions, such as taking a match from a box and striking it, or to perform the complex movements involved in using such tools as a comb or a pair of scissors. Ideomotor apraxia may coexist, or by contrast the patient may be capable of straightforward imitation of simple movements. Sometimes performance is clearly better when the tool is held by the patient than when he attempts to demonstrate the action in the abstract. Variability may be seen from one task to another and on different occasions.

In ideational apraxia the concepts of the required movements appear to be disturbed, together with the planning of the act to be accomplished. This may represent a disturbance of the 'schemas' at a high level of their organisation, while lower levels remain comparatively intact. The conception of the movements as a whole can be seen to be faulty, with disruption of the relationships between their spatial and temporal components. It may be regarded as a 'programming' apraxia, whereas ideomotor apraxia is a more basic executory defect.

Others, however, discount such a distinction based on functional levels, and base it rather on the nature of the task. In ideomotor apraxia the essential disorder lies in the formation of gestures in space, while tools are used normally. In ideational apraxia the problem lies not with the complexity of the task but in the requirement that tools should be used to a purpose; it is thus an 'agnosia of utilisation'. Still others doubt the validity of any distinction between the two forms when patients are investigated with due attention to detail, and view ideational apraxia merely as a more severe form of ideomotor apraxia.

Ideational apraxia is always bilateral. If based on circumscribed pathology the lesion usually involves the dominant hemisphere, and again usually the parietal or temporal lobes. It is in fact mostly seen with bilateral or diffuse brain lesions, and is usually accompanied by severe dysphasia or a considerable degree of generalised intellectual impairment.

Apraxia for dressing

The patient has obvious difficulty in putting on clothes. He cannot relate the spatial form of garments to that of his body, puts the jacket on back to front or the arm into the wrong sleeve. Buttons and laces present particular difficulty and are often left undone.

Clinically, the concept of dressing apraxia is useful in drawing attention to a dramatic symptom when more refined tests of apraxia and agnosia have yet to be performed. It is improbable, however, that it represents a distinct form of apraxia, and the symptoms probably depend on a variety of deficits which differ from case to case. There is often a mixture of apraxia and agnosia, the latter with visuospatial components. In many cases, right–left disorientation, unilateral inattention, neglect of the left limbs and other disturbances of the body image are likely to contribute to the picture. Generalised cognitive impairment can also often be detected.

The disorder is seen more commonly with right-sided or bilateral lesions than with left-sided lesions. The parieto-occipital regions are usually involved.

Constructional apraxia

Constructional apraxia is identified when the spatial disposition of actions is altered without any apraxia for individual movements. It thus becomes apparent in tasks which involve the use, and more particularly the representation, of space, for example in the construction or copying of patterns under visual control. It is obvious that such disorders will have a profound effect on many conventional tests of non-verbal intelligence, and this is how they sometimes come to light. Raven's matrices and Kohs' block test will be particularly affected along with the assembly items of the Wechsler performance scale.

The defect is clearly not purely motor in nature, but involves perceptual functions as well. This may be immediately apparent in the patient's satisfaction with a grossly imperfect copy of presented test material. For many authorities constructional apraxia is broadly synonymous with visuospatial agnosia, and this form of defect is therefore further considered on pp. 61–2.

Other forms of executive defect

Executive deficits of a more minor degree, and not amounting to formal apraxias, were investigated by Wyke (1968). Detailed measurements were made of motor skills which required timing and precision of movement in patients with a variety of focal brain lesions. Patients with right hemisphere lesions showed unilateral deficits with the opposite hand only, whereas patients with left hemisphere lesions showed bilateral deficits, albeit more severe in the contralateral limb. These interesting findings support the view that left hemisphere lesions result in some higher order executive defect which cannot be explained in terms of paresis or incoordination alone.

Agnosia and related defects of perception

The term 'agnosia' was introduced by Freud (1891), although the condition had been described much earlier than this. It may be defined as 'an impaired recognition of an object which is sensorially presented while at the same time the impairment cannot be reduced to sensory defects, mental deterioration, disorders of consciousness and attention, or to a non-familiarity with the object' (Frederiks 1969). Agnosia thus implies a disorder of perceptual recognition which takes place at a higher level than the processing of primary sensory information. Even though elementary sensory processes are themselves unimpaired there is an inability to interpret sensory information, to recognise its significance and endow it with meaning on the basis of past experience. Lissauer (1890), on the basis of his early case, divided the process of recognition into two stages—first a stage of processing whereby elementary physical stimuli are integrated to form a conscious percept ('apperception'), then the stage of associating the percept with other notions such as memory traces which endow it with meaning ('association'). Thus distinct forms of apperceptive and associative agnosia have come to be recognised.

Clinically, the situation is identified when there is a failure of recognition which cannot be attributed to a primary sensory defect or to generalised intellectual impairment. A patient may, for example, fail to recognise an object by sight and be unable to name it, demonstrate its use or relate it to a matching picture, even though vision is intact for other purposes. Nevertheless the same object is readily recognised by means of touch, showing that the patient is suffering from a modality-specific defect of higher cerebral function, and not from aphasia or apraxia. The several types of agnosia related to vision have received most attention, but agnosias are also described in relation to hearing and to touch.

Brain (1965) pointed out that the underlying disorder of function must have something in common with both aphasia and apraxia, since a patient can only demonstrate that he recognises an object by using speech or action; in effect agnosia represents an isolated aphasia and apraxia related to a particular object when it is perceived through a particular sensory channel. During development an object is presented to more than one sense and thereby comes to be perceived as an entity. Thereafter, perception via one channel alone is able to evoke a large number of sensorimotor experiences in relation to the object, and, moreover, to allow its identification whether seen from one aspect or another or even when represented in two-dimensional form. Brain therefore postulated physiological sensory 'schemas' which represent the bases of patterns common to manifold presentations, and which allow recognition. Separate schemas for vision, touch and hearing must be to some extent anatomically distinct, since we do not lose recognition through all sensory channels by any focal brain lesion but only in dementia due to diffuse brain disease. Equally this means that the actual process of recognition to which the schema gives access is a function of the brain as a whole.

The whole concept of agnosia has, however, come under increasingly critical discussion. Lesions producing so restricted a form of defect are rare (with the exception of visuospatial agnosia), and the examples reported in the literature have often been open to argument. A formidable amount of controversy has surrounded such questions as the independence of agnosic defects from subtle aspects of primary sensory defects, and the rarity of cases without some degree of dementia has made such questions hard to resolve. Geschwind (1965) suggested that most agnosias are, in fact, no more than modality-specific defects resulting from the isolation of the primary sensory cortex from the areas subserving language. Benson and Greenberg (1969) pointed out, in the case of the visual agnosias, that the number of suggested mechanisms very nearly equals the number of recorded cases. This confusion is often paralleled by conflicting claims about the site of the responsible pathology. For detailed discussion of these points Fredericks' (1969) comprehensive review should be consulted.

Neuropsychology has therefore come to concern itself less with the search for examples of pure agnosic defects and arguments over their significance, but to concentrate instead on an operational analysis, in large numbers of subjects, of the correlations between site of lesion and the form of the deficits that follow. Such deficits may be absolute or relative in degree, sometimes involving simple perceptual processes and sometimes implicating other higher mental mechanisms. Their precise nature is thus amenable to dissection by means of standardised examination techniques.

In the sections which follow the classic agnosic syndromes will be described, and also the more common forms of related perceptual defect.

Visual agnosias and visual perceptual defects

Visual object agnosia

In visual object agnosia an object cannot be named by sight but is readily identified by other means such as touch or hearing. There is equally failure to select a matching picture from a group, or to indicate the appropriate use of the object, showing that this is not a naming defect alone. Sometimes the patient may describe a use appropriate to an incorrect recognition. The difficulty may vary from day to day, and sometimes an object may be recognised from other cues in its familiar surroundings but not elsewhere. Usually the problem is restricted to small objects, but in severe examples it may extend to larger objects, with consequent difficulty in finding the way about.

In general, the more complex the visual information the more difficulty the patient experiences. Greater problems may be encountered with two-dimensional representations, such as line drawings or photographs, than with the actual objects themselves. Commonly, though not invariably, faces continue to be recognised. In many reported examples there has been difficulty in describing objects from memory and in drawing them (i.e. loss of visual images of objects), also difficulty with colour recognition, dyslexia and dysgraphia.

In keeping with the distinction between apperceptive and associative forms of agnosia described on p. 58, subdivisions have been attempted in the field of visual object agnosia (Warrington 1985; Warrington & James 1988). Patients with visual apperceptive agnosia are particularly sensitive to difficulties surrounding perceptual aspects of identification and fail when these are increased—for example when the perceptual characteristics of an object are partially obscured, or distorted by photographing it from unusual angles. By contrast, visual associative agnosics fail on tests where objects must be matched according to common functions as opposed to physical identity (e.g. a watch and a clock), or when asked to pick out clear pictures of objects which belong to a particular class (e.g. objects found in a kitchen). In this they betray a lack of recognition of the essential meaning of the objects. Interestingly, associative agnosia can sometimes appear to be category specific, with particular difficulty centring on animate or inanimate objects, pictorial representations of concrete or abstract items, or even categories as specific as animals or foods.

Apperceptive agnosics cannot copy objects or drawings, whereas associative agnosics can perhaps make reasonable drawings of objects they cannot identify. A double dissociation can sometimes be shown between these two forms of deficit—failure to organise a coherent percept on the one hand, and failure to endow an adequately organised percept with meaning. In many patients, however, the features of both apperceptive and associative agnosia occur together, suggesting that the two may form a continuum (Jankowiak & Albert 1994).

Bay (1953, 1965) and others were sceptical of gnostic activity generally, and suggested that visual forms of agnosia were attributable to impaired primary perception combined in most cases with generalised impairment of intellect. They drew attention not only to the visual field defects which were commonly present, but also to other subtle deficits of primary visual perception in the intact parts of the field. Ettlinger (1956), however, argued against such an interpretation, and pointed to the frequency of patients with severe sensory disorders compared to the rarity of agnosia.

Nevertheless, all agree that clear-cut cases of visual object agnosia are rare. Lesions in the posterior parts of the cerebral hemispheres, involving the occipital, parietal and posterior temporal regions are almost invariably responsible. Warrington (1985) suggests that following basic sensory analysis, input to the right hemisphere achieves perceptual categorisation and input to the left hemisphere semantic (meaning) categorisation. Accordingly apperceptive agnosic deficits can occasionally be seen in unusually clear form with right hemisphere lesions and associative agnosia with left hemisphere lesions. Jankowiak and Albert's (1994) careful review makes it clear, however, that bilateral pathology can be detected in the great majority of cases, even though PET activation studies suggest that object identification takes place predominantly in the left posterior hemisphere. Apperceptive agnosia tends to be associated with diffuse or multifocal lesions, whereas associative agnosia may occur with more focal pathology within the territories of the posterior cerebral arteries. It is noteworthy that the three cases of apperceptive agnosia studied by Grossman et al. (1996) showed bilateral occipitotemporal hypoperfusion on PET scanning, even though the MRI appearances had been unremarkable in two.

Prosopagnosia

Inability to recognise familiar faces has been described as a distinct and separate defect, which may or may not be combined with visual object agnosia and is certainly much commoner than the latter (Hécaen & Angelergues 1962). In extreme form the patient cannot recognise his own face in a mirror. The defect has been reported to be commoner with right than with left hemisphere lesions

but in most cases there is probably bilateral involvement (Walsh 1994). This was strongly supported by Damasio et al. (1982b) in their analysis of postmortem and CT scan data; bilateral lesions of the central visual system, situated specifically in the medial occipitotemporal regions, proved to be crucial for the development of prosopagnosia.

The precise nature of the defect remains uncertain, and it seems likely that prosopagnosia is not a unitary disorder. Warrington and James (1967a) showed a distinction between impaired recognition of a previously well-known face, which depends on long-term storage of visual information, and impaired recognition of a previously unknown face from short-term memory. The former tended to be associated with right temporal lesions, and the latter with right parietal lesions. De Renzi et al. (1991) propose a division into 'apperceptive' forms, in which a disorder in processing shape information prevents a sufficiently clear representation of the face to activate memory for it, and 'associative' forms in which the memory itself is defective. McNeil and Warrington (1991) discuss the continuing controversies in this area.

Damasio et al. (1982b) have argued that a primary factor in the development of the condition may be the requirement to evoke the specific context of a given visual stimulus. They suggest, indeed, that the defect may not be specific to human faces, but may be prone to emerge in relation to any visual stimulus provided that it is sufficiently ambiguous and that its recognition depends on recall of the specific context in which it has previously been perceived. In some instances, however, the condition must be regarded as a 'face-specific disorder', as in the interesting example reported by McNeil and Warrington (1993); here a patient with severe and persistent prosopagnosia for human faces was still able to identify individual members of his flock of sheep from pictures of their faces alone! Neurophysiological recording from the human right temporal lobe has confirmed that there are discrete populations of neurones which are related to the perception and comparison of faces (Ojemann et al. 1992). Recent PET scan studies have also indicated foci of activation which are specifically associated with the processing of face identity (Sergent 1994).

The processing of facial expression, as opposed to facial identity, has also been studied by PET with interesting results. Morris et al. (1996) carried out PET scans while subjects viewed photographs of happy or fearful faces, which varied systematically in the intensity of the emotional expressions. The neuronal response in the left amygdala was significantly greater to fearful as opposed to happy expressions; and it increased with increasing intensity of fearfulness and decreased with increasing intensity of happiness. This emerged, moreover, without a requirement for explicit processing of the facial expressions; the subjects were merely asked to judge whether each face was male or female.

Colour agnosia

Patients with colour agnosia show defective appreciation of the differences between colours, and fail to relate colours to objects correctly, even though their primary colour vision is intact as shown by normal performance on the Ishihara chart. Thus they have difficulty in sorting objects according to colour, ordering them in series or matching colours one with another. A dominant occipital lobe lesion is usually responsible and a right homonymous hemianopia is frequently present.

A closely associated though separable defect consists of 'colour anomia', in which the subject is unable to name colours or to point appropriately to named colours, in the absence of any impairment of colour sense. Thus he may use the word 'blue' when shown a picture of a banana, yet be capable of placing the correctly coloured chip next to it. Such problems may be unaccompanied by any other form of language difficulty, representing an unusually clear example of disruption of neural systems which mediate between specific concepts and their corresponding word forms (Damasio & Damasio 1992). The lesion in such cases appears to lie in the temporal segment of the left lingual gyrus.

In 'achromatopsia' there is a more profound loss of colour sense, extending even to an inability to imagine colours. The concept of colour itself is abolished and the world around, though perceived normally in form and depth, is seen in shades of grey. Damage in such cases is situated in the occipital and subcalcarine portions of the lingual gyri bilaterally (Damasio & Damasio 1992).

Simultanagnosia

Classically the patient fails to recognise the meaning of a complex picture while details are correctly appreciated. However, this is not attributable to difficulty in forming meaningful concepts, since with auditory information there is prompt understanding. Moreover, if plenty of time is given, or every individual feature of the picture is pointed out, the patient ultimately comprehends the meaning. In a similar way, words cannot be read except by spelling out individual letters.

The key problem appears to be with the perception of more than a limited number of units or configurations at a time. Thus tachistoscopic studies have shown that such patients have normal thresholds for the perception of single shapes and letters, but greatly elevated thresholds when more than one stimulus is presented at a time

(Kinsbourne & Warrington 1962a, 1963). Luria *et al.* (1963) described an impairment of the eye movements involved in visual scanning in simultanagnosia, but this is probably a secondary effect resulting from restriction of visual attention.

Coslett and Saffran (1991), in a detailed analysis of a case, suggest that the fundamental difficulty lay in the integration between object identity and information concerning spatial location when multiple items of visual information needed to be processed. They point out that the processing of multiple targets in an array must be carried out serially beyond a certain level, with storage both of the products of identification and their positions as the 'spotlight on visual attention' moves from one location to another. The inability to maintain appropriate linkages during the process of visual search appeared to account for their patient's failure.

Posterior lesions of the dominant lobe have been implicated in patients who display the complete syndrome.

Visuospatial defects

The abstract conception of space is derived from the spatial relations which are observed to exist between objects. As Brain (1965) pointed out this must be learned primarily in relation to the position of our own bodies, with compensation for the apparent movement of objects when it is our own eyes or body which move. After cerebral lesions a number of defects of visuospatial perception may be demonstrated. It has proved difficult, however, to reach agreement about their classification and the precise nature of the defects involved, since many tests require at the same time perception, construction and even visual memory. It remains, for example, uncertain whether failure to reproduce simple models and drawings depends on dyspraxic difficulties or failure of visuospatial analysis, likewise how far inability to draw from memory may further depend on defective visual imagery. Classic visuospatial agnosia is indeed widely regarded as broadly synonymous with constructional apraxia, as will be discussed below. Nevertheless, certain syndromes of localising value can be recognised as follows.

Visuospatial agnosia is identified by failure on tasks which demand explicit analysis of the spatial properties of a visual display. This is most readily tested by asking the patient to reproduce simple designs under visual control— the copying of drawings or the construction of patterns with bricks or sticks. The Block Design and Object Assembly subtests of the Wechsler Adult Intelligence Scale will most readily indicate minor degrees of such a defect.

Usually the patient has no difficulty in finding his way about, though an itinerary on a map cannot be indicated and towns cannot be correctly located. In the most severe examples a loss of topographical memory (p. 63) may be present as well. An interesting fact, often noted, is that patients with marked visuospatial defects rarely make specific complaints about them. Thus visuospatial agnosia easily eludes routine examination and special tests are needed for its detection.

Visuospatial agnosia results from lesions in the parietal lobe, and appears to be considerably more common and severe with lesions of the right lobe than the left. Piercy (1964), De Renzi and Faglioni (1967) and Warrington (1970) discuss this evidence, also the indications that the defects may be qualitatively different when produced by left- or right-sided lesions.

The former appear to depend more on executive difficulties and the latter on perceptual components in the task. Thus drawings made by patients with left parietal lesions tend to be coherent but simplified versions of the model, with omission of details but with relative preservation of spatial relationships. Performance is notably improved when the patient is provided with a model to copy. Frequent associated defects are aphasia, apraxia or components of the Gerstmann syndrome such as right–left disorientation. Patients with right parietal lesions produce more elaborate drawings, but made hastily and without care, and the result is typically scattered and fragmented. Disorientation on the page is marked, the left side of the page is relatively neglected, and the drawings are often asymmetrical and show gross disorganisation of spatial relationships. The presence of a model is of little extra help.

Some therefore prefer to retain the term constructional apraxia when the disorder results from dominant hemisphere lesions, and visuospatial agnosia when it is due to non-dominant lesions, though the distinctions between the two are by no means universally acknowledged.

Strong evidence has come from studies of patients after section of the corpus callosum to uphold the greater importance of the non-dominant hemisphere in tasks demanding visuospatial analysis. After the operation, which effectively disconnects the hemispheres from each other, patients show better ability to copy geometrical figures with the left hand than the right, even though the right hand had been superior before the commissure section. The ability to assemble complex object puzzles, or to reconstruct from a model standard geometrical patterns of the Kohs' block design test, are also better performed with the left hand than the right (Bogen & Gazzaniga 1965).

Evidence from LeDoux *et al.* (1977) suggests, however, that these findings in split-brain patients may owe more to difficulties on the part of the right hemisphere in carrying out 'manipulo-spatial tasks' than in perceiving spatial relationships *per se*. Thus when no manual construction was required, and the patient was merely asked to match or select drawings exposed to the right

hemisphere, their patient performed well. Specifically, LeDoux *et al.* suggest that the right hemisphere is specially equipped for mapping spatial context onto the perceptual and motor activities of the hands.

Visual disorientation. A further defect of visuospatial ability consists of difficulty in localising objects in space by vision alone. As a result the patient cannot point accurately to an object or estimate its distance. Such difficulty can occur in either half-field of vision alone, contralateral to the side of a lesion, or involve the whole visual field with bilateral lesions. When involving the whole field of vision the patient has difficulty in finding his way around objects or in learning the topography of a room.

Visual disorientation is usually seen in conjunction with impairment on more complex visuospatial tasks, and the lesions are situated posteriorly within the hemispheres. Warrington and James (1967b) suggest that there may be areas within the occipital lobes which contribute to the absolute localisation in space of a single object, whereas the integration of several spatial stimuli necessary for the appreciation of spatial relations between two or more objects is impaired by unilateral lesions within the right parietal area. De Renzi *et al.* (1971) reported a test of spatial judgement which appeared to demonstrate complete dominance for the post-Rolandic region of the right hemisphere. This involved the moving of a hinged rod into the same position as a model; patients with right posterior lesions were found to perform much more poorly than patients with lesions in any other location, and this applied whether visual or tactile forms of the test were used. De Renzi *et al.* suggest that the test measures spatial perception at a very basic and simple level, thus accounting for the more complete right hemisphere dominance than is found with more complex tasks such as the copying of drawings.

Visual neglect. Unilateral visual neglect (or unilateral spatial agnosia) may be seen in spontaneous drawings, copies, description of pictures, or use of paper when writing. When eating the patient may ignore food on the left side of the plate. It may also lead the patient to fail to take turnings to the left and consequently he may lose his way on familiar routes. A hemianopia may or may not be present. This is an agnosia for space as such, not merely an agnosia for spatial relations between visual objects. It may be seen in many degrees of severity. It is well confirmed that neglect of the left half of space is very much more common than right, and depends upon a right temporoparietal lesion (Heilman *et al.* 1985).

In an interesting report Halligan and Marshall (1991) have described a patient who showed severe visuospatial neglect for near ('peripersonal') space but not for extrapersonal space. Following a right middle cerebral infarction he showed left visuospatial neglect, a left hemiparesis and an inferior homonymous quadrantanopia. On standard line bisection tests, performed with the paper immediately before him, he showed marked displacements to the right, but was able accurately to indicate the midpoint of lines and to direct darts accordingly when these were some 2.5 m away. There is evidence from animal experimental work that visual inattention and neglect can be differentially affected for far and near space by lesions in different parts of the frontal cortex.

Loss of topographical memory. Patients with visual object agnosia or visuospatial agnosia may sometimes still be able to visualise familiar scenes or describe familiar routes. Loss of topographical memory may, however, occur, again in conjunction with lesions in the parietal lobes.

Hécaen (1962) studied the clinical evidence of loss of topographical memory for a previously familiar environment, and found that in most cases the parietal lesions were bilateral, though more of the unilateral cases involved the right than the left hemisphere.

Topographical disorientation. Semmes *et al.* (1955) showed that on tasks of following routes from maps, patients with parietal lesions did worse than patients with lesions elsewhere. Neither parietal lobe emerged as especially important in this regard. The difficulties occurred irrespective of whether visual or tactile maps were employed, suggesting a defect of appreciation of extrapersonal space which was not modality specific.

Ratcliff and Newcombe (1973) produced especially interesting findings from a study of men with penetrating missile wounds of the brain. Two tests were employed—a visually guided stylus maze task, and a locomotor map-reading task in which the subject was required to trace out a designated route on foot. These were designed to tap visuospatial agnosia and topographical disorientation, respectively. Patients with lesions in the posterior part of the right hemisphere were significantly worse than those with left posterior lesions on the maze-learning test, but a significant deficit on the map-reading test emerged only in those with bilateral posterior lesions. A clear dissociation between the two tasks could sometimes be observed. Ratcliff and Newcombe were led to conclude that while the right hemisphere has a special role in the perception of space, it does not bear an exclusive responsibility for the maintenance of spatial orientation. Bilateral lesions appeared to be necessary before route finding was impaired, perhaps because this involves a constant reorientation to stimuli as the subject moves around and alters his frames of reference. Further experiments on the topic are described by De Renzi (1982), along with a detailed discussion of the various deficits which may contribute to topographical disorientation.

Other visual perceptual defects

Other disorders of visual perception and of visuospatial analysis, which fall short of complete agnosia by any definition, have also proved to show interesting associations with the site of brain pathology. In particular, they are more frequent and more marked with right hemisphere lesions than left.

Patients with right temporal lesions have been shown to do worse than other groups with focal brain damage on tasks of rapid visual identification, picture comprehension and picture arrangement. These deficits are reflected for example in their scores on the Picture Completion and Picture Arrangement subtests of the Wechsler Adult Intelligence Scale, or on the McGill Picture Anomalies test in which the patient is required to identify incongruous features in a series of sketchily drawn pictures (Milner 1958; Ettlinger 1960; McFie 1960). Right temporal lobectomy has been found to lead to greater difficulty than left in the learning and recall of material such as nonsense figures which are not susceptible to verbal mediation (Kimura 1963). Warrington and James (1967c) similarly found that patients with right hemisphere lesions are specially impaired on the recognition of incomplete drawings, but in this a parietal rather than a temporal lesion was found to be crucial, suggesting that difficulties with spatial perception may have made a decisive contribution.

Thus it appears from these various findings that the non-dominant hemisphere plays some special part in the processing of visual sensory data, and is to a considerable extent specialised in visual matters. In this it complements the dominant hemisphere's specialisation for language. Within the non-dominant hemisphere it is probable that the temporal lobe is especially important for pattern recognition, and more posterior regions in the parietal lobe for the appreciation of spatial relationships. Such a distinction was in general upheld by Newcombe's (1969) analysis of the long-term effects of missile wounds of the brain.

Auditory agnosia and auditory perceptual defects

In auditory agnosia hearing is unimpaired, as tested by pure tone thresholds, but the patient fails to recognise or distinguish the sounds that he hears. Thus in everyday life he may give the appearance of being 'deaf'. Typically the onset is with severe dysphasia, which then clears substantially to leave the auditory problem in evidence. The patient is unable to recognise speech, as in pure word-deafness (p. 49), but in addition cannot recognise non-speech sounds such as the pouring of water, crumpling of paper or jingling of keys. Usually there is also failure to recognise musical sounds. These three defects—word-deafness, auditory agnosia and 'sensory amusia'—can occur together with varying degrees of severity.

The disorder is extremely rare and few convincing examples have been reported. Vignolo (1969) provides a detailed review, both of the phenomena observed and of their relationships to dysphasia. Most examples have been associated with bilateral lesions of the posterior parts of the temporal lobes.

Less complete difficulty with the processing of auditory information may be demonstrated in some patients with brain lesions. Vignolo (1969) showed that patients with right hemisphere lesions fail relatively on tests of discriminating meaningless sounds, whereas patients with left-sided lesions have greater difficulty in identifying sounds to which meaning can be attached. This indicates that the auditory-receiving areas of the two hemispheres are to some extent specialised, that of the right being specifically concerned with grasping the acoustic structure of the auditory input (i.e. subtle perceptual discrimination) and that of the left with endowing the input with meaning by virtue of semantic associative links (i.e. semantic decoding). A double dissociation was demonstrated in the patients with right and left hemisphere lesions between these two aspects of the 'understanding' of the auditory inputs. Thus where non-verbal sounds are concerned, it appears likely that there are two types of 'agnosia' depending on the hemisphere involved; the left hemisphere defect is essentially one of semantic identification of the perceived sound and is closely linked with dysphasic defects, whereas the right hemisphere defect is qualitatively different and essentially of a perceptual discriminative nature. Analogous differences between the hemispheres have more recently been shown for tactile recognition as well (p. 65).

With regard to music, the right temporal lobe appears overall to be more important than the left. Right temporal lobectomy has been found to impair performance on tests of musical aptitude, whereas left temporal lobectomy does not (Kimura 1961; Milner 1962). Shankweiler (1966) played extracts of familiar songs to patients who had had temporal lobectomies, and found that the left lesion group had greater difficulty in recalling the titles or words, whereas the right lesion group had greater difficulty in reproducing or recognising the melody. Dichotic listening tasks, in which different information is fed simultaneously to the two ears, have supported these findings in normal subjects; words fed to the right ear (and proceeding thence by crossed pathways predominantly to the left hemisphere) are reported better than words fed to the left ear, whereas with fragments of melodies the situation is reversed (Kimura 1961, 1964). Moreover, when dichotic tests are given to lobectomised patients it is found that left temporal lobectomy produces a more severe decrement in the contralateral ear where words are concerned, and right temporal lobectomy for the recognition of musical passages (Shankweiler 1966).

Gordon and Bogen (1974) also reported interesting effects when patients were asked to sing familiar songs during the course of unilateral intracarotid amytal injections. When the left hemisphere was sedated with the drug the words of the song were severely affected while the melody continued well; by contrast when the right hemisphere was sedated the words remained relatively intact whereas the pitch and melodic line were severely disrupted.

It seems clear therefore that the right hemisphere is superior to the left in most people for the perception of 'structured' musical passages, i.e. of sounds built up into tuneful, melodic and harmonious combinations (Wyke 1977). The right temporal lobe is particularly important in this regard, though right frontal lesions may also disrupt the perception of pitch, rhythm and phrasing (Shapiro *et al.* 1981). Measurements of changes in cerebral blood flow using PET scans have confirmed activation of the right temporal cortex during the perceptual analysis of melodies, and of the right frontal cortex during pitch comparisons (Zatorre *et al.* 1994).

However, detailed analysis of various components of musical perception—pitch, timbre, discrimination and rhythm—have often given conflicting results, suggesting that neither hemisphere alone is specialised for all aspects of musical cognition. Lezak (1995) reviews the more recent clinical and experimental evidence, indicating that while the right hemisphere is in general the more important in melodic recognition and chord analysis, the left tends to predominate in the processing of sequential and discrete tonal components of music.

Interesting differences have emerged, moreover, between musically naïve and musically trained subjects. Thus in trained musicians the left hemisphere may be found to predominate for melodic recognition, as well as for tone discrimination which tends to be less lateralised in untrained persons. It is unclear how far this may reflect the effects of learning processes on cerebral organisation, or pre-existing differences which have conferred musical ability. A recent study using MRI has shown that musicians with 'perfect pitch' have greater asymmetry of the planum temporale than non-musicians, with stronger anatomical biases towards the left (Schlaug *et al.* 1995).

Amusia may be defined as an impairment or loss of musical function deriving from acquired disease of the brain (Henson 1985). Amusia without aphasia has proved to be rare, but examples have been described following right temporal or right frontal lesions. In such examples the deficit usually involves loss of capacity to sing or hum a tune ('oral-expressive amusia'). Henson (1985) reviews the scattered literature on other amusia syndromes—musical agraphia, musical alexia and musical amnesia, and 'receptive amusia' in which there is failure to discriminate pitch, intensity, timbre and rhythm. This latter disturbance is usually seen only as part of a more widespread auditory agnosia.

Finally, under the heading of 'auditory affective agnosia', Heilman *et al.* (1975) have drawn attention to deficits in the appreciation of the affective tone of speech in patients with right hemisphere lesions. After listening to tape-recorded sentences patients were asked to judge either the content or the emotional tone in which each sentence had been spoken (happy, sad, angry or indifferent). Six patients had right temporoparietal lesions (with left unilateral neglect) and six had left temporoparietal lesions (with fluent aphasia). The responses were made by selection from a series of line-drawn pictures appropriate to the sentences and emotions concerned. All subjects achieved perfect scores with respect to content, but those with right hemisphere lesions were significantly impaired in judging affective tone.

Tactile perceptual defects

In tactile agnosia the patient is unable to recognise an object by touch, even though the sensory functions of the hand being tested are normal. The same object is immediately recognised by other means, for example by touching it with the opposite hand or by vision.

There is uncertainty surrounding the distinction between tactile agnosia and the 'astereognosis' of cortical sensory loss, in which there is equally failure of tactile recognition. Some, however, claim that in tactile agnosia the patient can still distinguish the size, shape and texture of the object even though the object cannot be recognised, whereas in astereognosis the appreciation of these sensory elements is impaired as well.

Commonly tactile agnosia is restricted to one hand, and results from a lesion in the opposite parietal lobe. The supramarginal gyrus has been especially incriminated. Bilateral tactile agnosia is said to follow damage in this region in the dominant hemisphere, and it is possible that in such cases callosal fibres to the opposite lobe have also been destroyed by the lesion.

In an interesting experiment Bottini *et al.* (1995) have shown a double dissociation between the nature of the tactile recognition disorders produced by right and left hemisphere lesions. Tasks were devised for examining tactile recognition either of meaningless shapes or of meaningful objects. In each case a stimulus object was first explored manually, then a matching object had to be selected by palpation from a choice of four. Patients with right hemisphere damage were impaired on the first task ('apperceptive recognition') but not the second ('associative recognition'). Patients with left hemisphere damage showed the reverse. The results thus provide an analogy in the tactile domain for those previously described for the processing of auditory information (p. 64).

'Gerstmann's syndrome'

The concept of a 'Gerstmann syndrome' resulting from dominant parietal lobe lesions has become firmly entrenched in the neurological and psychological literature. It consists of finger agnosia, right–left disorientation, dyscalculia and dysgraphia. As such it remains a useful venue for the discussion of these disorders, and yields a useful group of simple clinical tests when one is looking for subtle signs of a lesion in the dominant hemisphere. The essential clustering together of the defects has, however, been seriously questioned, and it is now clear that they barely constitute a 'syndrome' in the accepted sense of the word.

It is known that the four components are not always found together, one or more being often absent when the others can be demonstrated clearly. Similarly, one or more components can occur along with other disorders of cognitive function—dysphasia, dyslexia, constructional apraxia, visual disorientation or generalised intellectual impairment. Benton (1961) examined the intercorrelations on tests of the four Gerstmann symptoms and of three other functions related to the parietal lobes (constructional ability, reading and visual memory) in a large unselected series of brain-damaged subjects; it emerged that the correlations of the Gerstmann abilities with each other was no higher than with the three abilities not included in the syndrome. In a separate analysis of patients with damage restricted to the left parietal lobe, the Gerstmann defects again failed to cluster together. Heimburger *et al.* (1964) in a similar study found that as the number of Gerstmann components increased the lesions tended to be larger in size. When all four defects did appear together they were usually accompanied by severe impairment of many other functions.

Nevertheless Roeltgen *et al.* (1983) have been able to report a patient with the 'pure' Gerstmann syndrome, all four defects occurring together and without other symptoms or signs. This followed a discrete area of infarction in the left parietal lobe, including the superior part of the angular gyrus and the adjacent part of the supramarginal gyrus. Undoubtedly, however, such cases are very rare.

It has not seemed possible to establish a common fundamental disturbance underlying each of the four defects, which can indeed result individually from more than one kind of functional loss. For example, finger agnosia and right–left disorientation may be due to limited forms of body image disturbance or result from comprehension defects, dyscalculia may exist in many forms as described below, and dysgraphia may represent a disturbance of language function or result primarily from dyspraxia. Warrington (1970) has suggested, however, that if the concept were re-examined, taking into account a more restricted definition of each of the elements, the status of the syndrome might be further clarified.

Dysgraphia has already been dealt with briefly on pp. 50 and 53, and the remaining three components are considered below.

Finger agnosia

Finger agnosia is shown by loss of ability to recognise, name, identify, indicate or select individual fingers, either on the patient's own body or on that of another person. Traditionally the patient is asked to point to named fingers or to name an individual finger, but the presence of dysphasia may confound this simple procedure. Kinsbourne and Warrington (1962b) advocated a test in which two fingers are simultaneously touched by the examiner and the patient is asked to state the number of fingers between those touched, first in practice sessions with the eyes open and then with the eyes closed.

The disorder appears bilaterally. The patient does not report it spontaneously, and thus like constructional apraxia it is a defect usually only revealed by specific testing. A lesion in the left parieto-occipital area appears to be critical for its appearance, but it is possible that it can occur very occasionally with right hemisphere lesions. The angular gyrus and the second occipital convolution have been especially incriminated.

Gerstmann (1958) himself proposed that finger agnosia may represent a minimal form of whole body autotopagnosia, in other words a defect of recognition of the body or appreciation of the interrelations of body parts (see p. 71). He suggested that complete autotopagnosia is very rarely seen because those lesions sufficient to produce it also result in concomitant defects which obscure the picture, whereas in the restricted form of finger agnosia it can be recognised as a clear-cut entity. Kinsbourne and Warrington (1964) viewed it instead as a difficulty in classifying fingers in terms of their relative positions, and saw this as part of an underlying disorder in the processing of information in terms of a spatiotemporal sequence. Thus they found a particular type of spelling error in association with finger agnosia, namely errors relating to the ordering of the letters in a word. Frederiks (1969, 1985) considers the defect to be polymorphous in origin, though usually closely bound to language disorder as the fundamental disturbance of function. He points out that no other part of the body is verbally differentiated to so great a degree as the hand, and that despite its extensive cerebral representation we habitually disregard the hand when in use. Thus the physiological representation of the hand is in many ways different from that of other body parts, which may account, whatever the exact pathogenesis, for the special vulnerability which emerges in finger agnosia.

Right–left disorientation

This defect shows as inability to carry out instructions which involve an appreciation of right and left. The patient fails to point on command to objects on his right and his left, to indicate parts of his body on the right and the left, or to perform more complex instructions in which these directions form an integral part of the task. It undoubtedly can reflect several complex disorders of function. Gerstmann (1958) suggested that like finger agnosia it represented a restricted form of body image disturbance. Benton (1959) on the other hand stressed that language is likely to be intrinsically concerned with many forms of the disorder. Sauget et al. (1971) investigated the relationship between sensory dysphasia and various forms of disturbance including right–left disorientation and finger agnosia, using both verbal and non-verbal tests. They concluded that these disturbances are closely linked to impairment of language comprehension, but that in addition impairment of somatosensory functions is necessary for their appearance. Frederiks (1985) suggests that visual aspects of the body schema, and the relation between corporeal and extracorporeal space, are likely to be fundamentally involved.

Right–left disorientation can in general be accepted as a sign of left hemisphere dysfunction, but is of little value for more precise localisation within the hemisphere. Occasionally, moreover, it may emerge with right hemisphere dysfunction (Benton & Sivan 1993).

Dyscalculia

Dyscalculia is an impairment of the capacity for calculation in persons who have hitherto shown no disorder of their arithmetical faculties. The complex problems in this field are reviewed by Grewel (1969), Boller and Grafman (1985) and Grafman (1988). It is clear that detailed analysis of the nature of the calculation defect is necessary if the symptom is to have any localising value since there are many possible sources of failure. Arithmetical ability can be disturbed independently of language functions and general intelligence, but pure cases of this nature are rare. Secondary dyscalculia can result from defects of short-term memory, perseveration or simple impairment of concentration.

Boller and Grafman (1985) subdivide primary dyscalculia into four varieties. First, there may be loss of ability to appreciate the names and significance of numbers or to combine them syntactically to produce a meaningful digit notation. Second, there may be problems with the spatial organisation required in numerical operations. Third, there may be difficulties in carrying out the basic computational aspects of addition, subtraction, multiplication and division ('anarithmetica'). This last may be subdivided into two sources of failure—inability to retrieve mathematical facts which are normally stored in memory (such as $5+4=9$), or inability to engage in mathematical thinking and reasoning and to understand the procedural rules that underlie mathematical operations.

Such a distinction was clarified by Warrington (1982) in a study of a physician with a left parietal subdural haematoma. Simple calculations were performed laboriously and inaccurately, and on introspection he found that the processes of addition and subtraction could no longer be performed 'automatically'. He could define the concepts of addition, subtraction, multiplication and division quite well and his understanding of such operations was unimpaired. What he lacked was direct access to the semantic memories of arithmetical facts so that he had to revert to the slow counting processes observed in children. Other anarithmetic patients differ from this in that they lack all concept of the mathematical operations, or are unable to comprehend the significance of individual numbers or number facts (e.g. that there are 100 pence in a pound, or that 12 is greater than 11).

Dyscalculia has been found in one form or another with lesions of the frontal, temporal, parietal or occipital lobes of the brain, but the parietal lobes have been most frequently involved and the left lobe more often than the right. Hécaen (1969) suggested that dyscalculia due to alexia or anarithmetica was commoner with left-sided lesions than right, whereas dyscalculia due to problems with visuospatial organisation was commoner with right-sided lesions than left. It appears, however, that even this last form of difficulty is also more prone to emerge with left-sided lesions (Grafman et al. 1982).

Warrington (1970) concluded that in general, when a patient is unable to do simple mechanical additions and subtractions, without sufficient dysphasia or generalised intellectual impairment to explain it, a focal lesion may be suspected in the left parietal cortex. This was supported by Grafman et al.'s (1982) study, in which patients with focal damage to either hemisphere performed significantly worse than controls, but the left posterior brain-damaged group was particularly impaired; and this was largely independent of such additional factors as dysphasia or visuoconstructive difficulties.

Disorders of body image

The body image, or 'body schema' may be regarded as a subjective model of the body against which changes in its posture, in the disposition of its parts, and in its soundness or integrity can be appreciated. As such the body image is not static, but changes constantly under the influence of internal and external sensory impressions. Moreover, it invariably includes important unconscious as well as conscious components, so cannot be viewed as a mere picture in the mind. Normally it exists on the fringe of awareness, but aspects can be brought into consciousness when subjective attention is focused upon them.

The body image is thus an abstract conception, acquired during development and compounded of physiological and psychological elements. Schilder (1935) extended the concept and in particular stressed that data from a wide range of sources must be incorporated into any notion of the body image, including aspects of personality, emotion and social interaction. For him the postural model proposed by Head (1920) represented only a low level of body image organisation, whilst higher levels are built out of instinctual needs and personal interactions.

Clearly, therefore, the body image occupies a central place among the problems of brain–mind relationships, and not unnaturally its disorders must often be considered in relation to both cerebral pathology and individual psychopathology. Disorders of the body image are implicit in a wide range of puzzling and often bizarre clinical states, around which a good deal of controversy exists. Some disturbances represent the influence of structural or physiological changes in the brain, as seen for example in the presence of cerebral disease or in the effects of drugs such as cannabis or lysergic acid diethylamide (LSD). Other disturbances may accompany severe sensory deprivation or psychiatric illnesses such as depression or schizophrenia, and then may appear to be mainly psychological in origin. In some particularly puzzling disorders, such as anosognosia, it is probably necessary to invoke both organic and psychogenic factors in an attempt at a complete explanation. The concept of body image disturbance is thus involved in many different areas of study. Frederiks (1969) suggests that we must strive at least to keep clear whether we use it in a neurological or a psychopathological sense. In the former the aim is to find data which can contribute to topographical diagnosis of brain disease, whereas in the latter the interest is in relationships which are understandable in psychological terms.

The body image disturbances which follow brain lesions are themselves very incompletely understood. Sometimes they have been regarded as based on primary perceptual disturbances of kinaesthetic or proprioceptive inflow and sometimes as purely agnosic defects. At least a partial contribution may result from deficits in language comprehension, spatial analysis or ability to analyse a whole in terms of its parts, as will be discussed in connection with individual disturbances below. In some manifestations of body image disturbance hallucinatory experiences appear also to be directly involved. Precise analysis is often hampered by some degree of impairment of consciousness or generalised intellectual impairment which frequently accompany the more severe disorders.

Here the body image disorders most closely tied to brain pathology will be considered first and in most detail, then those encountered in non-organic psychiatric illness will be briefly reviewed. It must be appreciated, however, that the dividing line where pathogenesis is concerned is sometimes far from clear-cut.

Body image disturbances associated with brain lesions can be broadly divided into those affecting half of the body only, and those which involve bilateral disturbances. Unilateral body image disturbances are commoner with right hemisphere lesions than left, and the left side of the body is therefore most often affected. They include unilateral inattention, neglect, feelings and beliefs that the left limbs are missing (hemisomatognosia), and lack of awareness or denial of disability (anosognosia). Bilateral body image disturbances are commoner with left cerebral lesions than right. They are usually restricted to finger agnosia (p. 66) or right–left disorientation (p. 66), but very occasionally there is difficulty in naming or pointing to any body part (autotopagnosia). Complex illusions of bodily transformation or displacement are less closely tied to lesions in known locations and seem to be more intimately involved with non-organic psychopathology.

Unilateral unawareness and neglect

This represents perhaps the best known and most frequently encountered change in the body image. For reasons incompletely understood the disorder affects the left limbs in the great majority of cases, and appears to derive particularly from lesions in the neighbourhood of the supramarginal and angular gyri of the right parietal lobe. A spectrum of disturbances is seen, ranging from inattention and unawareness to neglect.

The range and interrelationships of these phenomena were excellently described by Critchley (1953). A minor degree of inattention to the left limbs may require special techniques of examination to reveal it, such as double simultaneous stimulation of both sides of the body together (p. 18). In unawareness the disorder is more obtrusive, the patient failing to utilise the left hand in bimanual activities, or overlooking the left foot when putting on his slippers. When attention is specifically drawn to the left limbs, however, they are used with normal efficiency, or if a degree of paresis exists the patient admits his difficulties. It is as though the limbs of this side were 'occupying a lower level in a hierarchy of personal awareness' (Critchley 1953).

The disorder may involve no more than this, or may include the more elaborate symptoms of neglect. The limbs may be ignored in washing or dressing, one half of the face may be left unshaven or the hair uncombed. This is more likely in the presence of confusion or other impairment of intellect. Sometimes unawareness or neglect accompany the development of a hemiparesis, and when this is present the more florid features of anosognosia may be added (p. 69).

Such disorders are seen more commonly after acute brain lesions, and particularly after cerebrovascular accidents. The degree of unawareness or neglect appears to be related to the abruptness of the lesion, the clarity of consciousness and whether or not motor weakness is present. Usually these are transient phenomena, and changeable from time to time during clinical examination, but occasionally the disability persists in some form as an enduring defect.

While a special association has been noted with parietal, and especially right parietal, lesions, typical syndromes of neglect have been reported following damage in other locations. Damasio *et al.* (1980) reported five examples of contralateral inattention and neglect, coupled with limb akinesia, after lesions in the frontal lobes or basal ganglia. Surprisingly the frontal lesions were in the left hemisphere, leading to neglect on the right side of the body. Damasio *et al.* suggest that the various structures involved may belong to an anatomically interconnected system subserving selective attention. Right thalamic infarcts have also been noted to lead to contralateral neglect of hemiparetic or akinetic limbs, along with anosognosia, marked emotional flattening and visuospatial difficulties (Watson & Heilman 1979; Watson *et al.* 1981).

Hemisomatognosia (hemiasomatognosia, hemidepersonalisation)

In this much rarer phenomenon the patient feels as though the limbs on one side are missing, sometimes episodically but sometimes as a continuous subjective state. It may feature as part of an aura in a focal epileptic attack.

The disorder is accompanied by various degrees of loss of insight. The limbs may feel absent though the patient knows this is not so, or he may say they are absent but can be corrected in his belief, or he may have a fixed delusion that they are absent which cannot be corrected. When consciousness is clear the patient usually retains insight into the illusory nature of the condition, even though it may feel very vivid, and can reassure himself as to the presence of the limbs by feeling or looking at them. In the presence of confusion, however, he may proclaim that the limbs are missing, look for them under the bed, or accuse others of taking them away.

Fredericks (1985) distinguishes conscious and non-conscious forms of the disorder. In the former the patient spontaneously reports the experience of having lost the perception of one half of the body. This is usually a transient or a paroxysmal phenomenon, may affect either half of the body, and is possibly based on subcortical blocking of somaesthetic input from one body half. Non-conscious hemisomatognosia, by contrast, is manifest only as a disorder of behaviour—the patient has no conscious awareness of the loss but behaves as though the body half were missing. He ignores and neglects it and fails to move it on command. This may be an enduring state, lasting for days or even weeks. It affects the left limbs much more commonly than the right, and tends to be associated with hemiplegia, anosognosia and unilateral spatial agnosia. The condition is typically due to a parietal lobe lesion of the minor hemisphere, and essentially corresponds to the syndrome of unilateral unawareness and neglect described just above.

Anosognosia

Anosognosia implies lack of awareness of disease, and is most commonly shown for left hemiplegic limbs. It may occur along with unilateral neglect, hemisomatognosia or with the illusions of transformation and displacement which are considered below.

In its mildest form the patient merely shows a lack of normal concern for his disability, attaching little importance to it and not grasping its implications. Or when confronted by the disability and obliged to admit it, he belittles the problem and shows an inappropriately flat or facetious reaction ('anosodiaphoria'). In true anosognosia, however, the patient appears to be completely unaware of the hemiplegia, makes no complaints about it and ignores the inconvenience it causes.

Commonly, anosognosia is merely a transient state in the early days after acute hemiplegia has developed, and recedes along with the initial clouding of consciousness. It may, however, persist and become more floridly developed with obstinate denial or bizarre elaboration on a delusional basis. When attention is firmly drawn to the

hemiplegia, the patient makes some shallow rationalisation for not performing the task, perhaps explaining that he has been ill recently or that he is too tired. In more bizarre cases he insists that the paralysed limbs do not belong to him or attributes them to some neighbouring person ('somatoparaphrenia'). He may claim that the limbs are some mechanical object, or talk to them and fondle them as though they had an existence of their own ('personification'). Feelings of anger or hatred may be expressed towards them ('misoplegia').

A woman of 39 with left hemiplegia, hemianaesthesia and hemianopia, was garrulous and confused. She denied that she was paralysed and insisted that her left arm and leg belonged to her daughter Ann, who she said had been sharing her bed for the past week. When the patient's wedding ring was pointed out to her she said that Ann had borrowed it to wear. The patient was encouraged to talk to Ann and to tell her to move her arm—she then became confused and talked vaguely about Ann being asleep and not to be disturbed. When asked to indicate her own left limbs she turned her head and searched in a bemused way over her left shoulder.

The left arm of a patient with a right parietal lesion kept wandering about in the blind homonymous half-field of vision. When the patient wrote, the left hand would wander across and butt in and rest on the right hand. Not recognising this as his own he would exclaim: 'Let go my hand!' He would swear at it in exasperation: 'You bloody bastard! It's lost its soul, this bloody thing. It follows me around and gets in the way when I read'.

(Critchley 1964)

Such highly colourful reactions are rare, and it is doubtful whether they occur in the absence of clouding of consciousness or generalised intellectual impairment. They can usually be understood most readily in terms of psychogenic elaboration of some partially perceived defect, sometimes illustrating in unusually clear form the common psychological mechanisms of defence.

Anosognosia is also used as a generic term for imperception of deficits other than hemiplegia. Here again it may range in degree from lack of concern and attention to explicit verbal denial, and again it is often uncertain how far the disturbance is intrinsically related to cerebral disorder alone or how far it reflects superadded psychogenic mechanisms. It is perhaps most commonly seen in relation to dysphasic symptoms, classically with primary sensory dysphasia when the patient seems not to appreciate his mistakes. Unawareness or denial of amnesic defects is common as part of Korsakoff's syndrome. Blindness, especially when due to lesions of the optic radiations or striate cortices may be denied, the patient attempting to behave as though he can see and describing purely imaginary visual experiences when tested ('Anton's syndrome'). Deafness due to cerebral lesions may more rarely be denied. Unawareness of painful stimuli ('pain asymbolia') is another incompletely understood example, in which the patient may perceive a painful stimulus but fails to recognise it as unpleasant, so that little or no defensive reaction is produced. This rare disorder can result from an acquired cerebral lesion, usually in the dominant hemisphere, while other aspects of sensation are unaffected (Frederiks 1985). It has been regarded as a failure to integrate the awareness of pain with awareness of the body image, or alternatively as a gross denial in the psychogenic sense of painful experience.

Anosognosia for hemiplegia has been more closely studied than these other forms of the disorder. Nevertheless the mechanisms involved remain unclear and are the subject of controversy. In the majority of cases there are sensory as well as motor deficits in the limbs concerned, but the condition is not explainable in terms of perceptual deficit alone, since occasionally hemiplegia is denied while the patient remains fully aware of the existence of the limbs. Frederiks (1969, 1985) puts forward the interesting suggestion that sometimes kinaesthetic hallucinations of movement may occur in the paralysed limbs, explaining at least those cases where verbal denial of paralysis is the main feature rather than neglect. The role of general intellectual disturbance is also disputed. Some claim that anosognosia can occur in the presence of strictly focal brain damage and when the patient is mentally clear, while others deny its localising significance and find it only with evidence of some degree of clouding of consciousness. Still others emphasise the psychogenic component, and see anosognosia essentially as a motivated desire to repress the unpleasant facts of a disability. Such primitive defensive behaviour may admittedly be brought to the fore by the presence of cerebral disease.

Weinstein and Kahn (1950, 1955) stressed this last point of view in their survey of a large population of brain-injured patients. In addition to denial of the defects already mentioned they noted denial of incontinence and impotence, and patients totally confined to bed might occasionally insist that they had recently returned from a walk. Some degree of mental confusion could always be detected in their patients when specially sought out, though it was often of a subtle nature. Moreover when the signs of anosognosia disappeared, intravenous sodium amytal could cause them to return by lowering the level of consciousness. Generalised brain damage appeared to be the cause in the great majority of cases.

Weinstein and Cole (1963) continued these observations in a later study restricted to anosognosia for hemiplegia. Half of their patients showed explicit verbal denial of paralysis while the others showed neglect. Those with denial disclaimed other aspects of the illness such as vomiting, incontinence or recent craniotomy, and all showed either disorientation for time and place, reduplicative delusions, other delusions and confabulations, or paraphasic misnaming. Frequently some degree of awareness of the defect was betrayed, and medication or operation was accepted without demur. Those with neglect alone showed less evidence of mental confusion but some degree could still be detected in every case. Mood changes were more striking in this second group, with depression, euphoria or paranoid developments.

Common mental mechanisms for defence against anxiety could be seen to operate. The premorbid personalities of the patients had often shown strong perfectionistic traits, tendencies to deny illness, and to view health as important for their self-esteem. Where verbal anosognosia was concerned this often appeared to be an artefact of the interview situation, and the attitudes of observers and of the patient's relatives were important in determining the degree and duration of the denial.

Such observations have led some authorities to argue against the implication of focal brain damage in anosognosia, or indeed against any special relationship to body image disorder. However, there remains the rather obstinate fact that anosognosia, like uncomplicated unilateral neglect, has usually been found to be very much commoner for the left than for the right side of the body. In Starkstein et al.'s (1992) series of stroke patients, 38% with left-sided signs showed anosognosia compared with 11% of those with right-sided signs. Moreover the lesion, when focal, appears to implicate the temporoparietal region rather than the pre-Rolandic cortex or lower levels of motor organisation. Those upholding strict localisation point even to the supramarginal and angular gyri of the parietal lobe. Hence it is often suggested that anosognosia represents a special example of focal derangement of the body schema, dependent on subtle deficits of sensory experience and higher order defects of conceptualisation. In this view any concurrent diffuse cerebral disorder acts only to actualise the defect or allow its elaboration by lowering the patient's overall grasp and alertness.

Ullman et al. (1960) in an unusually clear review, attempted a synthesis of both physiological and psychodynamic factors leading to anosognosia. In the more florid examples of denial they suggest that the patient's initial subjective experiences have come to mesh and synchronise with his defensive mechanisms. Thus, for example, his first experience may be of an arm without feeling lying across his chest. This is not experienced as his own, and the feeling of separateness may be heightened when spontaneous movements are noted in it as on yawning. The initial fright and puzzlement can then be immediately relieved by disowning the limb or even identifying it as belonging to someone else. Early 'potential' anosognosic responses could be identified in a high proportion of patients with hemiplegia ('I didn't feel like I had an arm'; 'It seemed like something attached to me that wasn't mine'), but this did not progress to further elaboration in the absence of diffuse brain damage with accompanying mental changes. With a shift to concrete modes of thinking, however, and when the total social context could not be grasped, the patient might begin to utilise cues in a selective fashion to support and substantiate delusional beliefs.

The elaboration of explicit verbal denial could thus reflect the operation of various sets of factors. It could sometimes be primarily related to motivational factors embedded in the personality as Weinstein and Kahn suggest, but in others one might be witnessing a degree of sensory change or functional loss great enough to prevent the patient from making the necessary compensatory judgements. Social and interpersonal aspects of the immediate situation could then be closely implicated, in addition to the role of brain damage itself.

The rarity of anosognosia and related defects in the right limbs is very hard to explain by any theory. It has been suggested that since the left limbs are normally subordinate to the right, cerebral lesions merely exaggerate this tendency, or alternatively that with lesions of the dominant hemisphere intellectual deficits and dysphasia readily swamp these more subtle manifestations. Others have attempted to resolve the dilemma by proposing that the non-dominant hemisphere is prepotent where the body image is concerned, or at least that it contains special mechanisms for the recognition of unilateral inequalities. More complex formulations include the suggestion that the dominant hemisphere is principally concerned with the body image proper, but the non-dominant with the adequate recording of bodily alteration or disablement upon the body schema (Gerstmann 1958). Cutting's (1978a) study renders many of these arguments less necessary, in that a high incidence of anosognosia and associated 'anosognosic phenomena' was detectable in patients with right as well as with left hemiplegia:

Cutting took care to interview patients within a few days of onset of the hemiplegia, and to divide the right hemiplegics into those who were adequately testable (i.e. free from dysphasia) and those who were not. Fifty-eight per cent of the left hemiplegics showed explicit verbal denial in this early stage, and another 29% showed phenomena such as minimising the defect, adopting unusual attitudes to the limbs, or feeling that the limbs did not belong. Of the testable right hemiplegics 14% showed explicit denial and 41% showed the related phenomena. Clear examples of non-belonging and of 'misoplegia' could be detected among the latter. If the presumption was made that the dysphasic right hemiplegics might also harbour unusual attitudes to their disability, then the incidence of anosognosia from left and right brain lesions might not be very dissimilar. Some findings, nevertheless, lent support to the idea that different factors might be responsible in each hemisphere; left hemiplegics, for instance, could develop anosognosia or the related phenomena in the absence of disorientation or impairment of memory, whereas virtually all right hemiplegics with abnormal attitudes showed obvious cognitive impairment.

Autotopagnosia

Autotopagnosia refers to an inability to recognise, name or point on command to various parts of the body both on the right and on the left. The defect may apply to other people's bodies as well as to the subject's own, yet other external objects are dealt with normally.

Autotopagnosia in any extensive sense is extremely rare. However, restricted forms are seen in conjunction with many other types of body image disorder, in that a tendency may occur to misidentify certain body parts. Such a defect confined to one body half is seen in patients with unilateral neglect or anosognosia. Finger agnosia (p. 66) is sometimes regarded as a minimal degree of whole body autotopagnosia, and to represent the only clear-cut example which cannot be better explained in terms of other defects.

Most examples which implicate the body bilaterally are explainable in terms of apraxia, agnosia, dysphasia or disorder of spatial perception. De Renzi and Scotti (1970) described a case which perhaps illustrates essential mechanisms of another type. The patient, who had a tumour of the left parietal lobe, failed to point to body parts, but by contrast could promptly name all parts pointed to by the examiner. He could also correctly monitor the accuracy or otherwise of another person's pointing. The same dissociation between pointing himself and naming could be seen for parts of objects other than the human body, for example for parts of a bicycle. The defect thus appeared to be a part of a more general disturbance of failure to analyse a whole into parts, in other words a difficulty in conjuring up clear mental images of how individual parts were related to one another and to the whole. The patient's errors were noted to be concentrated on body parts which lacked definite boundaries, such as the wrists, cheeks, ankles and chin.

Autotopagnosia is usually seen in conjunction with diffuse bilateral lesions of the brain. Lesions of the left hemisphere alone can produce it, but must always involve the parieto-occipitotemporal region (Frederiks 1985).

Illusions of transformation displacement or reduplication

A great variety of body image disturbances may be loosely grouped together under this heading. They are relatively uncommon, and little is understood about the mechanisms underlying their appearance. It seems, however, that both physiogenic and psychogenic factors can be responsible. They are seen in many clinical settings. Some of the less dramatic, such as feelings of heaviness or enlargement of a limb, may occur in healthy subjects in states of extreme exhaustion, sensory deprivation or in the course of falling asleep. Others, like feelings of distortion or free floating of the body, occur with generalised cerebral disorder as in delirium or under the influence of drugs such as LSD. Many unilateral examples are seen with focal brain disturbance, particularly as part of an epileptic aura, and some of the most bizarre instances, including autoscopy, can occur in the course of migrainous attacks. A further group appear in association with static lesions, particularly those which have led to left hemiplegia and anosognosia, but here again the phenomena are usually short lived even if recurrent. Psychiatric illness without evidence of brain damage also contributes to such disorders as discussed in the section on p. 74.

This group therefore depends sometimes on neuropathological and sometimes on psychopathological mechanisms, and probably often on an inextricable mixture of the two. Strictly focal brain damage can sometimes be incriminated in the more basic examples, but in the more elaborate such an origin remains hypothetical.

Macrosomatognosia and microsomatognosia consist of feelings of abnormal largeness or smallness of parts, or of half or even the whole of the body. Most commonly a single limb or a hand is affected alone. Such changes may be accompanied by sensations of heaviness, distortion or displacement of the part concerned, or features such as these may constitute the sole abnormality. Feelings of swelling, elongation, shortening or twisting may be experienced, rather than a change which preserves the normal proportions of the part. Rarely the experience may be of physical separation of the part from the rest of the body. The following examples are reported by Lukianowicz (1967):

An epileptic girl sometimes had a somatic sensory aura during which she felt that '. . . my whole body grows very rapidly almost to the point of bursting. After a few seconds it collapses, like a deflated balloon, and then I lose consciousness and have a turn.'

A lorry driver discovered to have epilepsy had attacks 'when everything seems to run away from me, and then I get the feeling in my eyes that they tear out of their sockets, and rush out from the cabin, till they touch the people and the houses and the lampposts along the road . . . Then everything rushes towards me again and my eyeballs hurry back into their sockets. At other times I might feel that my hands and arms grow long very rapidly, till they seem to reach miles ahead. A moment later they begin to shrink until they come back to their normal size. I may have such a feeling several times in a minute or two.'

A woman with migraine complained: 'Before the ache I see coloured zig-zag stripes appearing always from the left side. After a while I begin to feel that my head shrinks until it becomes not bigger than a small orange. At that time it always occurs to me that my head must look like the small dried up heads of the

head-hunters in Borneo, which I had once seen on TV. This sensation lasts about 1 minute and then my head at once comes back to its normal size. This feeling of my head shrinking and expanding goes on for some time, until I get my splitting headache.'

An epileptic girl had attacks ushered in by the feeling of spinning round on her own axis: 'This speed is so terrific that my body can't stand its centrifugal force: at first my head falls to pieces, and then the rest of my body, its parts flying apart like sparks. In a second or two my whole body falls apart, disintegrates, ceases to exist, is reduced to a formless splash on the spot where I was standing just a minute ago. And then I lose consciousness and fall down.'

The patient almost always retains insight into the alien nature of the experiences, describing the abnormality in 'as if' terms. A truly delusional or hallucinatory experience is rare in the absence of marked impairment of consciousness or psychotic illness. It is of course hard to discern, in cases such as those just quoted, how far the abnormal experience is due to a primary disturbance of the body schema, or how far it represents an imaginative elaboration of simple kinaesthetic and vestibular sensory changes. Derangements of either right or left hemisphere function may lead to such phenomena, and when a focal lesion is responsible the parietotemporo-occipital region is said to be usually involved.

Reduplicative phenomena usually involve the limbs, and most often the hand or fingers alone. Such phantoms are usually transient, appearing with darkness and drowsiness. Many cases occur with anosognosia for left hemiplegia, and may lead to illusions of movement in the paralysed limbs. Insight is again usually preserved in large degree, and when the patient looks at the actual limbs the phantom promptly disappears. Occasional cases are reported, however, in which enduring phantoms prove an embarrassment and inconvenience, and the patient feels obliged to make the real limb coincide in position with the phantom. More dramatic instances of reduplication may involve the whole body image, as in the following case:

A student with migraine had severe splitting headache 'and after a while I suddenly would have the feeling that I have two bodies and two heads. It is like this: for a second or two I sort of "lose" myself and then it's there: I feel all doubled, I have two heads, two right hands and two left hands, I have four legs instead of two. Often I wonder how I am going to walk and to move about. I feel like a centipede, but her movements are perfectly synchronised and coordinated, while I feel awkward, like a dismembered doll or a rubber toy. I don't know which of my two right hands or legs to use—the "real" one, or so to say, the "imaginary" one. After a while I become confused and again "lose" myself. And then it is all over: my headache at once disappears and I feel my old "single" self again.'

(Lukianowicz 1967)

Weinstein *et al.* (1954) have reported a few patients with reduplicative phenomena all with cerebral lesions of rapid onset and producing some degree of generalised confusion. One patient with a left hemiplegia claimed to have an extra left hand, one with a left hemiparesis and a fracture of the right leg stated that he had four legs, and one with a severe head injury who had previously had an eye removed claimed to have several eyes. Another patient with a cerebellar astrocytoma and meningitis said that he had three heads and four bodies, one of each with him and the remainder upstairs in a closet. In all four cases the reduplications were accompanied by other forms of reduplication for time, place or person. The 'body image' disturbance therefore appeared to be but one manifestation of a general pattern of reduplicative delusions. As in the case of anosognosia these authors viewed the reduplication of body parts as symbolic mechanisms to express some personal motivation, particularly denial of illness.

In autoscopy (the Doppelgänger phenomenon) there is 'a complex psychosensorial hallucinatory perception of one's own body image projected into external visual space' (Lukianowicz 1958). Usually the image is in front of the patient at a certain distance, mostly fleetingly but very occasionally lasting for days at a time. It may be transparent, or coloured and definite, or show expressive movements. It may consist of the whole or a part only of the body, but the face is usually included. Cases have been described in which the image occurs to one side of the midline in a hemianopic field of vision. The experience may be extremely realistic but is almost always recognised by the subject to be a pathological event. The emotional reaction may be of anxiety or quiet surprise, depending on the patient's mental state.

Usually the experience is visual, as the name implies, but sometimes the body image is experienced as projected into outside space by senses other than vision.

A draughtsman of 34 reported: 'Often during an attack of migraine, or towards the end of it, I feel as if my head would split into two parts, right in the middle. Then a miniature image of myself emerges from the fissure. It rapidly expands to the size of my real body, and then for a moment I have two separate bodies. They are both "me" or "I". They are about 1 foot apart, the "new" body being always on the right side. It seems that I could touch him, i.e. "the other me". Yet, I have never seen him with my eyes, though I feel his presence very intensely. He mostly appears towards the end of a splitting headache and soon after he emerges from my head the headache ceases. Then this "other me" also disappears.'
(Lukianowicz 1967)

A number of subdivisions of this striking phenomenon are recognised as discussed by Brugger *et al.* (1996):

With *'autoscopic hallucinations'* only the visual part of the body image is split off, usually being perceived as a lifeless though multicoloured image of the patient's own person. In *'heautoscopy'* somaesthetic elements are additionally projected into peripersonal space so that the subject both sees and feels awareness of the presence of his double. The image is then experienced as a living being. The patient may indeed have difficulty in deciding whether he should refer to the phenomenon as 'seeing' or 'being' his double. In an *'out-of-the-body experience'* the core subjective experience is the illusion of being separated from one's body, and visual elements may play a minor role. *'Feeling of presence'* occurs without visual elements, the person having the illusion of being accompanied by an invisible being. Typical features include a distinct localisation for the 'presence', as a rule at a specific distance from the subject's own body, also a conviction that the invisible being is real. It is endowed with an intense sense of familiarity and affinity, and sometimes it dawns on the subject that the presence is in fact a replica of himself. Heautoscopy and 'feeling of presence' can occur in close temporal conjunction with one another in certain organic states.

The distinctions between these various phenomena can be hard to discern, as in the patient cited above, and are not always clearly observed in the literature. They may occur episodically with attacks of epilepsy or migraine, or in association with a variety of organic psychoses and intoxications. Classic examples are sometimes encountered in the course of depressive or schizophrenic psychoses. In addition 'feeling of presence' is not uncommonly reported by healthy persons under conditions of isolation and exhaustion, as with mountaineers, lone sailors and explorers. Autoscopic hallucinations are sometimes experienced habitually by persons without cerebral disease, especially while falling asleep. Nevertheless Frederiks (1985) makes the important practical point that autoscopy can very occasionally be the first manifestation of brain disorder and always warrants careful neurological examination.

Brugger *et al.* (1996) suggest that autoscopic hallucinations owe most to occipitotemporal lesions and heautoscopy proper to temporoparietal lesions. 'Feeling of presence' may be closely associated with parietal lobe impairment and is often seen along with a sensory hemisyndrome or hemispatial neglect. Commonly, however, the associated cerebral pathology is diffuse. With regard to laterality, Brugger *et al.* suggest that the visual Doppelgängers (autoscopic hallucinations and heautoscopy) occur more often with right hemisphere lesions than left, whereas out-of-the-body experiences are projected more often towards the right and presumably reflect left hemisphere dysfunction. In their analysis of 31 cases of 'feeling of presence', Brugger *et al.* found that the presence was typically confined to one hemispace and was rather more often lateralised to the right than the left; of 12 cases with unilateral brain lesions eight were in the left hemisphere and four in the right.

The phantom limb which occurs after amputation or peripheral lesions of the nervous system has a basis quite distinct from the supernumerary phantom that occurs with cerebral disease. It is nonetheless in some ways the most decisive proof of the existence of the body schema. Phantom limbs are seen most commonly after amputation, but similar phenomena may follow severe nerve plexus lesions or lesions of the brain stem and thalamus. Equivalent phantom phenomena have also been reported after removal of the breast, the genitalia or the eye.

Frederiks (1969) provides a comprehensive review, and distinguishes between the perception of the missing limb itself, including its spatial characteristics, and the perception of phantom limb sensations such as paraesthesiae, heaviness, cold, cramp and pain. If the phantom is to develop it usually does so immediately after the operation, persisting sometimes for several months and sometimes for the rest of the patient's life. It has a markedly realistic character, can usually be 'moved' at will, and may assume a relaxed or a cramped position. In the course of time it may appear only sporadically, or it may gradually telescope, the distal portion ultimately approaching the stump and disappearing into it.

Pain in the phantom limb can be distressing and intractable. It is typically paroxysmal, burning or shooting in character, sometimes occurring alone and sometimes with paraesthesiae. As with other phantom limb sensations the pain may be markedly affected by influences such as a change in the weather, use of a prosthesis, use of the contralateral limb, pain elsewhere in the body or firm efforts at mental concentration. Morganstern (1964) has shown the efficacy of frequently repeating a task of sensory distraction in diminishing awareness of the phantom and lessening pain. The current emotional state may likewise have a profound effect, depression contributing to such an extent that ECT has sometimes been found to abolish phantom limb pain. Stengel (1965) mentions a man whose phantom limb pain was markedly increased whenever he watched scenes of violence on television.

A psychogenic component thus undoubtedly exists, and has been interpreted in terms of loss of bodily integrity and reaction to disablement. Psychotherapy and hypnosis have accordingly sometimes met with success in treatment. However, a physiological component is also indicated by the efficacy, short lived though it may be, of surgical procedures. Relief may follow the excision of a stump neuroma, chordotomy, or lesions in the thalamic radiation or sensory cortex. Both peripheral and central nervous mechanisms thus appear to contribute to its

genesis, in addition to psychological factors in certain cases. It has been suggested that unpatterned somaesthetic sensory input acts in some way to stimulate and sensitise the central structures involved with the body image for the missing part.

Body image disturbances in non-organic psychiatric illness

The majority of the body image disturbances so far considered have been associated with cerebral pathology or pathophysiology. With some forms, however, psychogenic mechanisms also have to be taken into account, and seem to be strongly implicated for example with anosognosia, phantom limb phenomena and some of the more bizarre illusions of transformation and reduplication.

It is therefore interesting to view the range of body image disturbances that may accompany psychiatric illnesses devoid of known brain pathology. It is, of course, often hard to clarify the phenomenology when other mental disturbances are present as well. Many examples appear on close acquaintance not to represent true disturbance of the body schema, but rather to be based primarily on pathological changes in bodily experience. In neuroses, for example, minor bodily sensations may become exaggerated by anxiety or hypochondriacal concern, and in psychoses kinaesthetic hallucinations may become the subject of delusional elaboration. The area has rarely been examined systematically, and Lukianowicz's (1967) survey provides a valuable set of observations.

Among 200 consecutive admissions to a mental hospital, 31 patients complained spontaneously of unusual sensations and experiences in various parts of their bodies, and a further 21 answered affirmatively when questioned about such phenomena. Excluding the patients with epilepsy or migraine, 38 patients (19% of the total) were considered to show some body image disturbance, 23 in the presence of schizophrenia, 12 with depressive illness and three with anxiety neurosis. In the latter the disturbances were manifest only in the drowsy hypnagogic state.

Experiences of depersonalisation were not included in the survey. The remainder were classified entirely on phenomenological grounds in order to avoid the aetiological implications of the terms which are usually employed. Experience of change of shape was the commonest abnormality, followed by change of position in space, reduplication or splitting, change of size and change of mass. The schizophrenic patients tended more often than the others to experience changes of shape, and the depressed patients change of mass.

Disturbances of the shape of the body image took many forms. In schizophrenic patients there were examples of feelings of change of shape to that of another animal, the hands feeling shrunken like crab's claws or the whole body feeling as though transformed into a dog. Such changes appeared to be based essentially on misinterpreted bodily sensations, combined often with hallucinations of the sense of smell. Insight into the unreality of the experiences was commonly retained, though sometimes incompletely expressed. In some cases complex sensory experiences appeared to underlie feelings that the body was changing into that of the opposite sex, likewise in some examples of transformation into Christ or other figures. Care was taken to distinguish as far as possible between mechanisms such as these, in which there was a discernible relationship to corresponding bodily sensations and hallucinations, and the more usual situation in which a delusional belief in a new identity or sex was purely ideational.

Feelings of change of position in space included levitation, floating and falling, sometimes as hypnagogic phenomena but sometimes occurring in the full waking state. In epileptic patients equivalent sensations were sometimes observed as a kinaesthetic aura preceding an epileptic attack.

Feelings of reduplication and splitting occurred in schizophrenia and in depression.

A schizophrenic student had the feeling of 'two bodies, one outside the other, only a bit larger than my actual body. I feel that the "inner" body is the real one, and the "outer" is more like something artificial, a sort of shell over a hermit crab although it has the shape and the appearance of my "real" body.'

A woman when depressed had a feeling 'as if my body was split into two halves, like a stem of a tree struck by lightning. They both feel a few inches apart and there is nothing between them, but a black, empty hole; black and empty and dead.'

Again, in epileptic patients such experiences could herald an attack. Experiences of autoscopic doubling were also seen in patients with schizophrenia and depression.

Feelings of additional body parts occurred in several bizarre forms, sometimes inviting a psychodynamic formulation which would see them as symbolically representing displaced sexual organs:

A man whose potency was dwindling as a result of spinal injury developed recurrent depressive episodes. In one there were visual and haptic hallucinations of spurs and horns growing from his ankles, in another of a ball sticking out of his thigh, and in another of big screws growing from his abdomen and thighs. He retained insight into their unreal nature, and ECT was effective in banishing the phenomena along with the depression.

Change of size sometimes affected the whole body, and sometimes parts only, such as the ears, nose or limbs. Again, displaced sexual symbolism sometimes provided the most ready explanation, though analogous examples occurring in the course of epileptic and migrainous attacks may have rested primarily on disturbed cortical function. Lilliputian experiences were rare in comparison to feelings of enlargement, but one depressed woman had distressing hypnagogic experiences in which she felt her body shrink rapidly to the size of her little finger.

Changes in mass were usually manifest as feelings of emptiness and hollowness of body parts, particularly of the head. They were confined to patients with depressive illness or neurotic disorder, and often came close to nihilistic delusions. The following case illustrates the possible distinction.

A man with anxiety neurosis described a recurrent hypnopompic experience as follows: 'Just after I wake up, but before I move, I have a terrifying feeling that my whole body consists of skin with nothing inside, like an empty blown up balloon, or an empty shell, only pretending to be a human body. It is a very frightening feeling, which lasts only a few seconds and disappears immediately when I move any part of my body.'

In general these various disturbances in psychiatric patients seemed to be an integral part of their mental illnesses, along with the more common hallucinations and related psychotic symptoms. Misinterpretation of normal bodily sensations, or of hallucinations, appeared to be mainly responsible, rather than changes originating in the body schema itself. The initial sensations seemed often to be complex, mainly of visceral, kinaesthetic or labyrinthine origin, and then to become secondarily elaborated in terms of change in shape, position, size or mass. In schizophrenic patients the end result was frequently bizarre, in keeping with their tendencies towards bodily preoccupation, weakening of ego functions and autistic modes of thinking. In depressive illness the body image disturbances were often consonant with hypochondriacal and nihilistic developments. Successful treatment of the psychiatric illness invariably resulted in resolution of the body image disturbances.

Cutting (1989) has more recently analysed body image disturbances in a series of 100 schizophrenic patients. Rather surprisingly almost half had experienced some form of disorder, the predominant subjective change being alterations in structure, weight or shape. Other abnormalities included tactile hallucinations, feelings of additions to the body, or belief in the presence of localised devices within the body. As expected many of these changes were highly bizarre. Consonant with Cutting's (1985, 1990) view that right hemisphere dysfunction is important in the pathogenesis of schizophrenia, 13 of the

14 instances in which the disorder was lateralised concerned the left side of the body.

Non-cognitive disturbances and regional brain dysfunction

The forms of disability discussed above have all been more or less closely tied to cognitive or perceptual deficits, even though these have sometimes been of a rather subtle nature. There remain, however, certain abnormalities of emotion, behaviour and 'personality' which appear to be related to regional brain dysfunction yet do not necessarily have cognitive disturbance at the core. These are clearly of special interest to the psychiatrist. Certain examples will be selected for discussion.

The 'frontal lobe syndrome' will be considered first because of its classic position in the psychiatric literature. Aggressive behaviour will then be examined in relation to focal brain disturbances. Finally, the evidence linking schizophrenia-like illnesses to regional brain dysfunction and brain pathology will be outlined.

With all of these examples the task of elucidating the nature of the ties between clinical symptoms and brain dysfunction has been considerable. Abnormalities of emotion and personality cannot be assessed with anything like the precision that is usually possible for cognitive defects. It has already been seen how much uncertainty surrounds our understanding of such measurable disorders as memory impairment, and such testable defects as dysphasia or apraxia. With the body image disturbances there was an uncertain admixture of physiogenic and psychogenic mechanisms to be considered. Such problems are greatly extended in any analysis of disordered emotion or abnormalities of personality and social behaviour. A large element of subjectivity is involved in attempts at classifying or quantifying the phenomena concerned, and in trying to separate the abnormal from what must be judged as normal variation; the abnormalities are more variable from one situation to another than are cognitive defects and more protean in their manifestations; and their determinants will include factors which have nothing to do with damage to the brain — matters of genetic constitution, interpersonal relationships and current environmental circumstances. It is inherently likely, moreover, that the 'higher order' the function concerned the more complex will be the interplay between the different cerebral systems subserving it.

Despite such difficulties important leads have been obtained, and interesting clinicopathological correlations have emerged in the examples discussed below.

Frontal lobe syndrome

Certain clinical features emerge with especial frequency after damage to the frontal lobes. They are not unique to frontal lobe pathology, but are seen more regularly and perhaps more strikingly than after damage to other cerebral regions. A good deal of debate has surrounded this issue of localisation, likewise the question of the range of symptoms to be included and the means by which they come about. Detailed reviews are provided by Teuber (1964), Hécaen and Albert (1975) and Benson and Stuss (1989).

Clinical picture

In the typical case, the personality of the patient is more profoundly and obviously affected than his cognitive functions. The striking changes in well-marked examples are in the areas of volitional and psychomotor activity, habitual mood and social awareness and behaviour.

Lack of initiative and spontaneity is usually coupled with a general diminution of motor activity. Responses are sluggish, tasks are left unfinished and new initiatives rarely undertaken. In consequence the capacity to function independently in daily life can be profoundly affected. Yet when vigorously urged, or constrained by a structured situation, the patient may function quite well. He may achieve virtually normal performance in situations where the examiner provides the impetus, and thus show little or no difficulty over formal tests of intelligence. How far the impairment of initiative represents a true loss of interest, or an apparent loss due to impaired volition, is often hard to discern. Occasional patients tend to be restless and hyperactive rather than sluggish, but again are likely to display a lack of purposive goal-directed behaviour.

The mood is often mildly euphoric and out of keeping with the patient's situation. Rather empty high spirits may be accompanied by a boisterous over-familiarity of manner. Such changes are rarely sustained, however, and when left to himself the patient becomes inert and apathetic. Outbursts of irritability are also common and a child-like petulance may be seen. True depression is rare though the picture of asthenia and inertia may mimic it closely. The euphoria is sometimes elaborated into a tendency to joke or pun, to make facetious remarks or indulge in pranks ('Witzelsücht'). Very occasionally it extends to a state of excitement approaching hypomania ('moria').

Serious changes are observed in social awareness and behaviour. Typically the patient is less concerned with the consequences of his acts than formerly. Loss of 'finer feelings' and social graces form part of a general coarsening of the personality. In interpersonal relationships there is a lack of the normal adult tact and restraints, and a diminished appreciation of the impact of his behaviour upon others. Disinhibition is sometimes apparent in the sexual sphere with lewd remarks, promiscuity or the emergence of perverse tendencies.

Judgement may be markedly impaired in the conduct of affairs. The patient shows little concern about his personal future, and fails to plan ahead or carry through ideas. Inability to forejudge the consequences of actions can lead to foolish or irresponsible behaviour. Social and ethical controls may be weakened and have issue in antisocial conduct.

Psychometry, as already stressed, may show little by way of impairment on formal tests of intellectual ability, even when behaviour is markedly abnormal. Special test procedures, however, may show loss of abstracting ability and incapacity to shift between different frames of reference as discussed below. Inattention may also be marked, and memory may appear to be faulty. The latter, in particular, can be very hard to evaluate; it may sometimes seem that failures over recall represent a lack of initiative in memory rather than a true forgetting of material, in that given time and encouragement the answers are ultimately forthcoming.

Such changes are seen in varying degree, sometimes merely as a blunting of a previously sophisticated personality, but sometimes as a radical change of personality which is grossly disabling. The patient himself usually has little insight into the changes that have occurred. The component symptoms may be seen in different combinations, but with sufficient similarity from one patient to another to convey a definitive stamp to the picture.

The evidence concerning the 'frontal lobe syndrome' has come from studies of patients with various forms of brain pathology. That derived from head-injured patients is described in Chapter 5 (p. 180) and observations on patients with frontal lobe tumours in Chapter 6 (p. 223). Evidence has also accumulated from studies of patients after surgical excisions of frontal lobe lesions (Rylander 1939, 1943) and of patients who were exposed to the earlier extensive frontal leucotomies (Partridge 1950; Tow 1955; Greenblatt & Solomon 1958). The consensus of evidence suggests that lesions of the convex lateral surface are especially prone to produce aspontaneity and slowing, while lesions of the orbital undersurface are liable to have adverse effects on personality and social behaviour (Blumer & Benson 1975). Bifrontal lesions are especially hazardous in this regard.

Possible mechanisms

A number of intriguing suggestions have been put forward in attempts at explaining why such symptoms should arise. Detailed neuropsychological studies have produced a wealth of information both in animals and man, but it remains difficult to draw these strands together to form a satisfactory theory. This is scarcely surprising in view of the elusive nature of frontal lobe function in the intact brain.

Nevertheless, detailed analysis of failure on problem-solving and perceptual tasks has allowed tentative explanatory hypotheses to be put forward. The obvious deficits in man are in matters of personality and social behaviour rather than in cognitive and perceptual processes, yet experiments dealing with these more basic functions have sometimes seemed to illuminate the behavioural deficits observed.

Goldman-Rakic (1987) traces the development of experimental work on primates from the classic studies of Jacobsen onwards. Jacobsen (1935) showed that monkeys with frontal lobe lesions were selectively impaired on a delayed choice reaction task, in which they had to select which of two cups contained a food reward after witnessing the baiting of the cups some time before. Subsequent experiments have shown that this is not simply due to failure of memory or spatial perception, but rather to disturbance of complex aspects of the monkey's attention and response at the time of baiting one or other cup. Further work has shown that monkeys with frontal lesions have severe difficulty in learning to reverse a discrimination problem, despite normal ability to master the problem initially. Similar difficulty is seen in shifting back and forth between other related problems due to perseverative interference from previous responses. Yet paradoxically they also are unduly ready to select novel cues when these are progressively introduced into the experimental situation. The perseveration of set is thus combined with an enhancement of the normal tendency to be attracted to what is novel in the environment. In other words the monkeys show unusual difficulty in overcoming a preferred mode of response, whether spontaneous or experimentally induced, and despite the lack of reward for errors. They cannot suppress responses that naturally prevail in a given situation, and they appear to be little affected by the immediate consequences of their actions. Even in monkeys, therefore, detailed analysis of problem-solving behaviour turns out to reveal complex abnormalities of motivation and behavioural control.

Milner (1963, 1964) examined performance on certain psychometric tests which are particularly susceptible to frontal lobe damage in man. Again, careful analysis of sources of failure produced interesting results. On the Wisconsin Card Sorting Test (described in Chapter 3, p. 118), patients with frontal lesions show difficulty in shifting from one mode of response to another, which reveals itself as a strong perseverative tendency. In particular they fail to abandon a particular sorting strategy after being repeatedly told that it is wrong. This appears not to be due to lack of motivation, since the patients often work carefully and are manifestly distressed by their poor performance. They also seem capable of grasping the principle of the test in prior discussion. Yet they may continue to sort erroneously while themselves saying 'right' or 'wrong' as they place the cards. Thus the essential deficit emerges as persistence of inappropriate sets in the face of mounting errors, coupled perhaps with inability to modify behaviour in accordance with verbal signals. The failure to suppress an on-going tendency, despite growing proof of its inadequacy, has similarities with the concept of disinhibition invoked to account for the behavioural changes observed clinically.

Similarly on a stylus maze test, Milner (1964) reported a special type of frontal deficit—the patients fail to heed instructions, break rules and make repetitive errors much more than other groups. They seem unable to restrain themselves from impulsive mistakes which impair their learning curves. Milner points out that these tests, and others, demonstrate that patients with frontal lesions cannot maintain a constantly shifting response to meet changing environmental demands. Normal behaviour depends on simultaneous functioning of many complex 'sets', one of which can become prepotent when appropriate signals arise from the environment. Frontal lobe damage appears to disturb this modulating function, which may explain the coexistence in such patients of inadequate social behaviour and lack of initiative in many everyday situations, despite good achievement on standard tests of intelligence.

Teuber's (1964) contribution was more far reaching. He and his co-workers showed specific frontal deficits on several tasks which at first sight seem unrelated. Patients with frontal lesions were able to set a vertical midline correctly under normal conditions, but not when their bodies were tilted to one or other side. They failed in visual searching tasks and in certain aspects of the perception of reversible figures. And they had special difficulty with orienting tasks in relation to their own bodies when asked to transpose from front to back view. Teuber proffered a unitary interpretation in terms of a defect of 'corollary discharges' which allow the subject to predict, and thereby prepare for, incoming sensory stimuli. Such a defect would stand to impair the proper maintenance of

the perceived upright during changes of posture, and the proper direction of voluntary gaze; it could alter the facility of 'assumptive shifts' of the viewer's position on inspecting ambiguous figures, or the required reversals of standpoint when dealing with mirror images of the body.

Arguing further, Teuber pointed out that 'will' involves anticipation of the future course of events coupled with an awareness of the role of the self in bringing these events about. The patient with frontal lobe pathology is not altogether devoid of capacity to anticipate a course of events, but lacks the ability to picture himself as a potential agent in relation to those events. From such changes could follow lack of initiative, fixity of set, oscillation of action and impulsiveness. Thus the seemingly lower-level sensorimotor defects revealed in the experiments might be the conditions that give rise, in more severe forms of frontal lobe dysfunction, to pervasive changes of behaviour.

Luria's conclusions were not so very dissimilar to the above, involving a consideration of feedback processes and self-regulating systems in the control of behaviour (Luria & Homskaya 1964; Luria 1966; Luria et al. 1966). Luria pointed out that the organism not only reacts to stimuli, but can anticipate future events and prepare for them by constructing appropriate series of actions. In man such programmes become enormously complex as a result of social development, and are formed with the assistance of language which achieves an important role in the regulation of behaviour. During on-going activity there are not only 'action plans', but also a complex process of matching the effects achieved against the initial intentions. Frontal lobe damage has a disruptive effect on the programming of complicated activities and on this 'psychological control of action'. Behaviour in consequence loses its selective character and easily falls under the influence of outside associations.

Using a simple bulb-pressing task, Luria and Homskaya (1964) showed that patients with large frontal lesions were unable to translate verbal instructions accurately into motor behaviour. The instructions were understood and remembered but appeared to have lost their signalling function. With less severe frontal lesions similar deficits could be shown on more complex bulb-pressing tasks—when told to press twice for a single stimulus and once for a double, for example, behaviour soon gave way to a simple mirroring of the properties of the stimuli. The disturbed verbal regulation of function was shown in that errors persisted even when the patient was asked to repeat the instructions every time the signal appeared, and despite his running commentary which showed he knew what was required.

Disordered programming and feedback control have

also been shown in the domain of complex perceptual processes, especially those requiring a preliminary planned approach (Luria *et al.* 1966). Eye movements were monitored while patients with frontal lesions were invited to study a picture and answer questions about it. The eye movements were found to be disorganised and random, with failure to concentrate on important and significant details. Instead of singling out and correlating the most informative features, the patients would perceive a single detail and come up with an immediate impulsive idea of what the picture represented. Moreover eye movement records showed a stereotyped form of scanning no matter what question was asked about the picture, in sharp contrast to the situation in normal subjects. Thus patients with frontal damage lack the organised visual scanning needed to seek out cues relevant to solving a task, to compare them and to match them with several hypotheses.

Both of Luria's experiments reveal disturbed regulation of activity and disordered feedback and correction of errors. In everyday life such deficits would stand to impair many aspects of behaviour. Disordered regulation of activity, i.e. the loss of the controlling function of intentions upon behaviour, may underlie the apathy and aspontaneity of patients with frontal lesions and their lack of goal-orientated behaviour. Impaired feedback may account for their lack of critical attitudes towards the results of their own behaviour, their failure to modify it and their satisfaction with actions regardless of whether or not they are effective.

Further ambitious attempts at theoretical formulations of frontal lobe function have been put forward by Stuss and Benson (1986) and Fuster (1989). Both stress the superordinate control of the prefrontal cortex over the activities of more posterior brain functional systems. Stuss and Benson distinguish frontal systems concerned with sequencing, i.e. the ability to order multiple items of information into proper serial order, and those concerned with drive, i.e. the capacity to activate and actualise behaviours. Hierarchically superior to these are a number of 'executive' functions dealing with such matters as anticipation, goal selection, planning and the initiation and monitoring of novel responses.

Fuster (1989) places central emphasis on the critical role of the prefrontal cortex in the *temporal* organisation of behaviour, i.e. with the integration of sensory information and motor acts into novel and purposive behavioural sequences. He points out that the tasks most consistently disrupted by frontal lesions in primates are those which contain temporal or spatial discontinuities in the information used to guide behaviour. In man the most typical manifestation is inability to organise cognitive and behav-

ioural acts in the time domain, i.e. a failure to organise new and deliberate sequential activities. This in turn can be traced to problems with the short-term storage of information, planning and the control of interference. The temporal structuring of behaviour achieved by the prefrontal cortex enables behaviour to be adaptive to changing demands, and allows the proper ordering of events in temporal sequence towards a goal.

Finally, two sets of 'experimental' observations on patients with frontal lobe lesions have also been informative in revealing something of the mechanisms that may be at fault. Lhermitte's demonstration of imitation and utilisation behaviour (described on p. 106) was extended in remarkable fashion when he observed patients in complex everyday life situations, i.e. without the constraints normally imposed during clinical assessment (Lhermitte 1986):

Thus when taken into a room containing a buffet, his patient laid out the glasses and offered him food, spontaneously behaving like a hostess. Confronted with make up she used it immediately, and seeing wool and knitting needles began to knit. Another patient, when taken into a bedroom with the sheet turned back, got undressed, went to bed and prepared to go to sleep. On hearing the word 'museum' while in an apartment he began methodically to examine the paintings on the wall, and walked from room to room inspecting various objects.

In commenting on these behaviours Lhermitte (1986) proposes that they reflect a lack of personal autonomy, coupled with an excessive dependence on the social and physical environment ('environmental dependency syndrome'). The decisions concerning the patients' actions were not made for themselves, but the behaviours were called forth by surrounding external stimuli: 'for the patient, the social and physical environments issue the order to use them, even though the patient "himself" or "herself" has neither the idea nor the intention to do so'. Lhermitte suggests that the shift in the balance between personal autonomy and environmental influences reflects decreased control by frontal systems over the parietal sensorimotor systems which link the individual to the world around. From this may follow such classic features as disinhibited behaviour, distractibility, loss of flexibility of action and loss of self criticism. Similar environmental dependency has been described following the disinhibition of frontal systems secondary to focal thalamic infarction (Eslinger *et al.* 1991).

Damasio *et al.*'s (1990) investigation was more directly aimed at exploring the possible origin of sociopathic behaviour after orbitofrontal lesions. Specifically they studied autonomic responses to socially meaningful stimuli. Electrodermal skin conductance responses (SCRs) were measured while subjects viewed neutral or 'target' pictures exposed upon a screen. The latter depicted such matters as social disaster, mutilation or nudity, of a nature expected to elicit strong SCRs. Patients with orbitofrontal lesions and severe defects in social conduct were compared with non-frontal brain-damaged controls and normal subjects.

While viewing the pictures the frontally damaged patients failed to show the marked increase in SCRs which were elicited by the target pictures in the control groups. Moreover, on subsequent debriefing it was clear that the emotionally powerful stimuli had not provoked the appropriate feeling responses.

Damasio *et al.* interpret such results as support for their theory that patients with orbitofrontal damage fail to activate autonomic 'somatic states' linked to punishment and reward, which normally serve as a guide to the anticipated outcomes of behaviour. Such 'markers' have previously been learned in association with numerous social situations, signalling deleterious or advantageous outcomes of alternative forms of response and helping to defer immediate gratification for longer-term reward. Without such markers the frontally damaged patient cannot automatically and instantaneously distinguish advantageous from disadvantageous actions in the context of social rules and contingencies, despite the preservation of formal aspects of intelligence. The orbitomedial frontal cortex is the only known source of projections from frontal regions towards the central structures involved in autonomic control. Damage to such regions therefore stands to disable the immediate autonomic response which signals appropriate social behaviour in a variety of situations.

Disordered control of aggression

The emotional disturbances classically associated with brain damage include emotional lability and loss of control over emotional expression. In the former the prevailing mood shifts rapidly on little provocation and is ill sustained. In the latter, which in severe form is termed 'emotional incontinence', there are outbursts of crying or laughing in response to minimal stimuli and sometimes with little or no affective change subjectively.

Increasingly, however, attention has been focused on the specific question of impaired control of aggressive behaviour and its possible cerebral correlates. In extreme form this may be manifest as outbursts of uncontrollable violence. In some instances such disturbance is clearly attributable to focal cerebral pathology—in relation to epilepsy, certain cerebral tumours and other forms of brain disease. But the argument has been extended to suggest that in some habitually aggressive individuals, not

showing overt signs of cerebral disorder, there may be abnormalities of the neural apparatus subserving aggressive responses. Attention has been directed particularly at possible dysfunction of the 'limbic brain', and especially of the amygdaloid nuclei within the temporal lobes. This remains a contentious area, not least because of the frequent difficulty in apportioning blame between pathophysiological and psychosocial influences in clinical situations, as discussed below (p. 83).

In seeking correlates between aggressive behaviour and brain pathology one is handicapped by the difficulty of defining in what circumstances and to what degree aggression must be displayed before it is regarded as 'abnormal'. A variety of motivations may be involved, and many aspects of aggression are biologically valuable in man as in other animals. Its determinants include environmental, social, cultural and intrapsychic factors, also learned components, any of which can emerge as crucial in individual instances. But there appear to be persons who are subject to recurring and harmful outbursts of aggressive behaviour, sometimes on little or no provocation, and certain aggressive offenders whose episodes remain inexplicable in terms of personality, social adjustment and the situation at the time. Here it would seem that there may be important cerebral determinants of this pattern of behaviour—an abnormal triggering of aggressive responses based in disturbed cerebral functioning.

Neural substrate for aggressive responses

A neural substrate for the elaboration and display of aggression has been amply demonstrated both in animals and man. A large literature exists to show that in animals aggressive behaviour can be facilitated, decreased or abolished by cerebral lesions, mostly situated in or near the limbic system and hypothalamus. Bard (1928), for example, showed the importance of the caudal half of the hypothalamus for the elaboration of 'sham rage' in decorticate cats, and Klüver and Bucy (1939) demonstrated an abnormal absence of anger and fear after bitemporal lesions in monkeys. Downer (1962) elegantly showed how removal of the amygdaloid nucleus from a single temporal lobe would, after section of the cerebral commissures, allow the monkey to display normally aggressive behaviour when stimuli were fed to the sound hemisphere but unnatural tameness when fed to the lesioned side.

Delgado's work was particularly impressive in illustrating the need to take into account both intracerebral mechanisms and socioenvironmental factors in the understanding of aggressive behaviour in animals (Delgado 1969). Radio-stimulation via implanted electrodes in the amygdala, hypothalamus, septum and reticular formation, allowed discrete areas of the brain to be stimulated while monkeys and chimpanzees were free-ranging and interacting with their fellows. Certain areas when stimulated produced a threatening display or social conflict, but this depended on the hierarchical position of the animal in the group; such responses could be observed when a submissive monkey was at hand as a target, but were inhibited in the presence of a dominant animal. Moreover, elicited behaviour which might be interpreted as aggressive by the experimenter was apparently not always perceived as such by the other animals in the colony.

In different species of animals similar brain regions have emerged repeatedly as important in connection with 'aggressive' behaviour. Nonetheless considerable inter-species differences exist, and applicability of the results to man is a far from straightforward matter. Observations in man are necessarily limited in scope, and rely principally on indirect methods of study in a variety of pathological situations.

Clinical evidence

Some of the principal evidence has come from studies of patients with epilepsy. This is set out in Chapter 7, where the question of a special association between temporal lobe epilepsy and aggressive behaviour is discussed (p. 266 et seq.). A proportion of patients with temporal lobe epilepsy appear to show explosive aggressive tendencies, not only in relation to attacks but as an enduring trait of their personalities. Temporal lobectomy carried out for the relief of epilepsy may be followed by pronounced improvement in the control of such disorder (p. 270). The lesions in these patients commonly consist of sclerosis in the limbic structures on the medial aspects of the temporal lobes.

Patients with cerebral tumours have occasionally been observed to show abnormal outbursts of rage and destructive behaviour. Poeck (1969) reviews the literature, showing the frequent involvement in such cases of the hypothalamus, septal regions and medial temporal structures including the hippocampus and amygdaloid nucleus. Some patients have described their condition as a feeling of rage building up in spite of themselves, others as waiting tensely for the first opportunity to release their accumulated aggression. Poeck stresses, however, that the relation between symptoms and lesions is by no means strict and constant. Important additional factors derive from the premorbid emotional make up, and the presence or absence of diffuse brain damage.

A patient reported by Sweet et al. (1969) showed in

very striking fashion the possible relationship between a circumscribed tumour and the wildly aggressive behaviour that ultimately ensued. The case also illustrates the complex nature of 'aggressive' behaviour in man, and the hazards of attempting a simplistic formulation of the nature of the link between such behaviour and cerebral pathology:

In August 1966 a young man murdered his mother and wife in their apartments, then ascended the University of Texas tower, stepped on to the parapet and killed by gunfire 14 people, wounding 24 others. In his personal diaries he had recorded over several months that something peculiar was happening to him, which he did not understand but which he was noting down in the hope that its mention would help others to do so. Five months before the mass murder he had consulted a psychiatrist, stating early in the interview that sometimes he became so mad he could 'go up to the top of that University tower and start shooting at people'. Autopsy disclosed a glioblastoma multiforme; the damage to the brain from the gunshot wounds which terminated his barrage led to uncertainty about the precise location of the walnut-sized tumour, but it was considered to be probably in the medial part of one of the temporal lobes.

Other examples of an association between a lowered threshold for aggression and brain pathology include patients who become seriously disturbed as a result of birth trauma, head injury and intracerebral infections. However, in such situations clinicopathological correlations are rarely exact enough to allow firm conclusions to be drawn about the role of circumscribed as opposed to diffuse brain damage. Moreover there will often be intervening variables by way of affective disorder or paranoid psychosis, especially when serious violence is involved (Gunn 1993). Tonkonogy (1991) performed CT and MRI scans in a mixed group of patients with organic psychosyndromes who had shown repetitive violent behaviour; in five of the 14 patients, focal lesions were observed in the anterior temporal lobe structures close to the amygdala, most often attributable to head injury. The question of impaired control of aggression after head injury is further discussed in Chapter 5 (p. 188), and of antisocial conduct after encephalitis lethargica in Chapter 8 (p. 353).

Opportunities for assessing the effects of stimulating discrete brain structures in man have occasionally appeared to yield direct evidence for the role of limbic structures in elaborating emotional responses, including short-lived feelings of rage. Heath et al. (1955) stimulated the amygdaloid nucleus via implanted electrodes in a chronic schizophrenic patient, resulting in a sudden rage response when the current reached a certain intensity. She was perfectly aware of her feelings and was able to discuss them objectively between stimulations. The result was unstable, however, and later stimulation of the same point produced feelings of fear in place of rage. Delgado et *al.* (1968) found that stimulation of the amygdala and hippocampus in patients with temporal lobe epilepsy produced a variety of effects including pleasant sensations, elation, deep thoughtful concentration, relaxation and colour visions. However, in one patient with postencephalitic brain damage and epilepsy, stimulation of the right amygdala led to episodes of assaultive behaviour reminiscent of her spontaneous outbursts of anger. Seven seconds after the stimulation she interrupted her activities, threw herself against the wall in a fit of rage, then paced around the room for several minutes before resuming her normal behaviour. During the elicited rage attack no seizure activity was evident on depth recording. The observation proved to be of crucial importance for selecting the appropriate site for a destructive lesion within the temporal lobe. Fenwick (1986) reviews other early studies of this nature.

Psychosurgery for aggression

It thus seems fair to conclude that pathological derangements affecting the limbic areas, and perhaps especially the amygdaloid nuclei, are capable of leading to abnormal tendencies towards aggressive behaviour in man. The conclusion has led to attempts at modifying such behaviour by a variety of psychosurgical procedures. Unilateral temporal lobectomy can meet with success in patients with temporal lobe epilepsy, as already mentioned, but bilateral operations are contraindicated by the severe memory deficits that follow. Turner (1969, 1972), however, reported success with bilateral division of tracts within the temporal lobes and with posterior cingulectomy, mostly in patients with temporal lobe epilepsy but also in some abnormally aggressive patients who had never had seizures.

Attention has also been directed at stereotactic operations on the amygdaloid nuclei in patients with temporal lobe epilepsy and violent behaviour (Hitchcock *et al.* 1972; Mark *et al.* 1972). The results were reported as often markedly successful, and without disabling side effects. Narabayashi performed amygdalectomies on one or both sides in a large population of patients, some with epilepsy and some with 'severe behaviour disorders and hyperexcitability' (Narabayashi *et al.* 1963; Narabayashi & Uno 1966). Nearly all were mentally subnormal. Of 60 patients aged 5–35 years, 51 were said to show marked reduction in emotional excitability and 'normalisation of social behaviour'. The improvements were described in terms of increased obedience, calmness, a diminution of labile mood and a decreased tendency to attack persons and destroy objects. Of 40 patients followed 3–6 years later, 27 continued to show a satisfactory outcome,

though older patients who had been markedly aggressive fared less well than younger patients who had shown hyperactivity and 'unsteady moods'.

It is hard in these reports to discern how specific were the effects on aggressive behaviour, and how far the improvements may have been related to improved control of epilepsy. Sweet *et al.* (1969) reviewed the discrepant results obtained by different workers. In a patient of their own they found that stimulation of the medial part of the amygdala led to feelings of imminent loss of control, whereas stimulation just 4 mm lateral to the same point produced feelings of relaxation. The variable results of operation may thus be attributable to subdivisions of function within the relatively large complex of nuclei that constitute the amygdala.

Other reports have shown improvement in aggressive psychotic patients after amygdalectomy and basofrontal tractotomy (Vaernet & Madsen 1970), and in aggressive epileptic children and young adults after surgical lesions in the posteromedial hypothalamus (Sano *et al.* 1966, 1972). All such operations, needless to say, soon became the focus of considerable social controversy, especially when applied to minors and to persons held in custody on account of offences.

Habitually aggressive offenders

It remains to consider the situation in individuals who display persistently aggressive behaviour yet who lack overt evidence of brain pathology. These are the persons traditionally labelled as 'aggressive psychopaths' or as having an 'explosive personality disorder'. Their outbursts of violence are usually merely a part of wide-ranging personality and social maladjustments. They are notoriously resistant to efforts at therapeutic intervention, yet many seem to outgrow their aggressive propensities in middle years. It is obviously a matter of importance to attempt to clarify whether in some such persons there are definable abnormalities of the neural apparatus subserving aggressive responses, and to what degree such abnormalities are inherited or acquired.

A high proportion of persons with disturbed personalities are known to have abnormal EEGs, especially those who show aggressive antisocial behaviour. The evidence is discussed in Chapter 3 (p. 128). Such EEG abnormalities involve the temporal lobes particularly, are often of a type suggesting cerebral immaturity, and tend to decrease with age in parallel with improvements in behaviour. Hill (1944) found that the abnormalities in aggressive psychopaths were often bilateral, synchronous, and postcentral in location, suggesting dysfunction in subcortical centres or the deep temporal grey matter.

An important study by Williams (1969) reinforced the importance of earlier findings:

In a review of EEGs carried out on 333 men convicted of violent crimes he divided the population into two groups—206 who had a history of habitual aggression or explosive rage, and 127 who had committed an isolated act of aggression. In the first group the aggression appeared to be largely endogenous and related to personality factors, and in the second to be provoked by unusually stressful environmental situations. Sixty-five per cent of the habitually aggressive offenders had abnormal EEGs compared with only 24% of the remainder. Eighty per cent of both groups showed dysrhythmias known to be associated with temporal lobe dysfunction.

When persons with disabilities suggesting structural brain damage were excluded (i.e. those who were mentally subnormal, had epilepsy, or with a history of major head injury) 57% of the remaining habitual aggressives showed EEG abnormalities, whereas the figure for solitary aggressives had fallen to 12% (which was equivalent to the general population). It thus seemed reasonable to conclude that in the former, the EEG abnormalities were directly related to the disturbed behaviour and were not attributable to otherwise unrelated structural brain disease. Williams considered the disturbed behaviour and the EEG findings in the habitually aggressive men to be 'constitutional' in origin and to reflect a disturbance of cerebral physiology. They appeared to derive from dysfunction of diencephalic and limbic mechanisms, as judged by the features and distribution of the EEG abnormalities.

A study by Krynicki (1978) in repetitively assaultative adolescents, though based on very small numbers, produced essentially similar findings. Volkow *et al.* (1995) have recently produced preliminary evidence of cerebral dysfunction by FDG-PET (p. 144) in a group of eight psychiatric patients with a history of repetitive violent behaviour. Three had a diagnosis of schizophrenia or schizoaffective disorder, the remainder meeting DSM-III-R criteria for intermittent explosive disorder or antisocial personality disorder. In comparison with controls they showed significantly lower metabolism in the medial temporal and prefrontal cortices bilaterally.

The question has been argued further by certain observers who have elaborated the concept of a syndrome of *'episodic dyscontrol'* (Mark & Ervin 1970; Bach-y-Rita *et al.* 1971; Maletzky 1973). The term 'intermittent explosive disorder' is currently more widely used in the USA. The suggestion is that after excluding patients who have demonstrable epilepsy, brain damage or psychotic illness as a basis for their aggressive acts (also those pursuing a motivated career of premeditated crime for gain), one is left with a large number of persons who are victims of their disturbed cerebral physiology. The essence of the claim is that violent behaviour can, in effect, be the only overt symptom of brain disorder.

The great majority of such persons are male, from seriously disturbed family backgrounds, and with a history of repeated outbursts of violent behaviour dating back to adolescence or even childhood. Provocation for such outbursts has often been minimal. Evidence of minor neurological dysfunction is not uncommon, and there is a high frequency of abnormal EEGs, often involving the temporal lobes and sometimes quasi-epileptic in nature. Many have symptoms reminiscent of epileptic phenomena, even when not suffering from seizures; in particular the outbursts may be preceded or followed by features akin to those seen with temporal lobe epilepsy. The clinical picture is further described in Chapter 7 (pp. 297–8).

The implication is that such persons have functional abnormalities of the neural systems subserving aggressive responses, which set the threshold for the elicitation of outbursts at an unusually low level. There is then a complex interaction between such brain dysfunction, social disorganisation and significant psychopathological experiences in the individual concerned.

Such a 'syndrome' appears to stand at the borderland between what is conventionally regarded as psychopathic personality, and what with more definite clinical evidence might be included as temporal lobe epilepsy. Clear definition of the syndrome, and estimates of its frequency, are rendered difficult by the elusive nature of the ancillary evidence of cerebral dysfunction, and the ever-present confounding evidence of social and interpersonal stresses in the group.

The status, and indeed the existence, of the syndrome remains a matter of controversy. Some regard the concept as useful in clinical practice while recognising that it cuts across traditional diagnostic boundaries (Elliott 1992). Others regard it as serving no useful purpose. Lucas (1994) presents a detailed review of the evolution of the concept and concludes that its nosological status is invalid. He stresses that it lacks clear demarcation from allied forms of disordered behaviour, and suggests that it represents one extreme of a continuum rather than a distinct nosological category. Lucas advocates a multiaxial classification of patients who show repeated outbursts of anger or violence, encompassing the presence or absence of general psychiatric syndromes, developmental disorders, concomitant physical conditions and psychosocial difficulties.

Schizophrenia

Schizophrenia has gradually proved to be a fruitful arena for neuropsychiatric research. An organic contribution to the disorder has been suspected from Kraepelin's time onwards, but until recent decades has remained remarkably elusive. Now, however, there is evidence that 'symptomatic schizophrenias' associated with known brain lesions show affinities with certain brain locations; neuroimaging and autopsy studies show that aspects of brain structure and function are not uncommonly abnormal in the condition; and unusual patterns of cerebral lateralisation and interhemispheric organisation have been increasingly documented. Attention has therefore turned towards the possibility that definable aspects of brain malfunction may render genetic propensities to the disorder overt, or perhaps reflect abnormal neurodevelopmental processes which have conferred vulnerability to the disorder. It is possible, furthermore, that such neurodevelopmental anomalies may themselves be genetically determined.

In working toward such formulations there have been many false starts, not least because of the problems of defining schizophrenia and separating it from its surrounding territories. Improved diagnostic criteria, presented for example by Feighner *et al.* (1972) and Spitzer *et al.* (1975), and objective methods for rating key aspects of symptomatology such as the Present State Examination (Wing *et al.* 1967, 1974) have been important in allowing groups of well-defined patients to be assembled and studied with confidence. It has also become evident that the schizophrenias associated with obvious brain pathology or toxic influences can often be identical phenomenologically with 'idiopathic' forms. Valid attempts are therefore increasingly underway to seek a cerebral substrate for this common and extraordinarily puzzling illness.

Associations with regional brain pathology

Evidence has accumulated to suggest that schizophrenia, when associated with brain lesions, is commoner with pathology in certain brain areas. The subject is comprehensively reviewed in detailed analyses of the literature by Davison and Bagley (1969) and Davison (1983). There are clearly difficulties in resolving the nosological problems inherent in such an exercise, and particularly when dealing with data reported by others. Moreover, having identified a reasonably acceptable group of cases the problem remains how far any association with brain damage is fortuitous, or due to the unmasking of a genetic liability to the disorder, or more directly related by way of a causal influence of the brain lesion upon the development of the schizophrenia. These questions too were tackled by Davison and Bagley and their views are presented at many points in the chapters that follow.

The conclusion which emerges repeatedly is that lesions, particularly of the temporal lobes and diencephalon, appear to carry a small but definite risk of

increasing the likelihood that a schizophrenia-like illness will develop. This hazard appears to exceed what would be expected in view of the known genetic propensities in the populations concerned. Thus, at least where some forms of brain lesion are concerned, there appears to be a causal link between the disturbance of cerebral function engendered by the lesion and the appearance of the psychosis. The nature of such a link remains uncertain, but if the observations are accepted as valid a pathophysiology of some sort must be postulated. Certain speculations with regard to the mechanisms underlying the psychoses seen with epilepsy are described on pp. 282–4.

It has not yet been clarified whether such schizophrenias are identical in every respect with the naturally occurring idiopathic disorder, in particular with regard to the course that is followed. Phenomenologically, however, they appear to be indistinguishable from schizophrenias occurring in the absence of brain disease. The current impression is that paranoid forms are very much commoner than catatonic or hebephrenic varieties, as applies with schizophrenia generally, but the relative frequency of positive and negative symptoms remains to be properly explored.

Irrespective of such nosological refinements, the striking fact appears to be that psychotic illnesses with the major features of schizophrenia may coexist with cerebral lesions and may be generated in some fashion by them. The acute and chronic organic reactions described in Chapter 1 are by no means the exclusive hallmarks of mental disorder occasioned by cerebral dysfunction. The corollary implication is that, while in the great majority of schizophrenias no clear-cut brain lesion will be revealed by routine investigation, in some patients there may be identifiable pathology which warrants careful appraisal.

The evidence incriminating the temporal lobes and diencephalon has come from diverse forms of cerebral pathology. That concerning head injuries is described in Chapter 5 (p. 191), cerebral tumours are discussed in Chapter 6 (p. 225) and epilepsy in Chapter 7 (pp. 281–2). While far from satisfactory or entirely conclusive, for the reasons discussed above, the sum total of evidence begins to look impressive.

Other clinical evidence has pointed to disease of the basal ganglia as having a special relationship with schizophrenia-like illnesses, for example in Huntington's disease (p. 470), Wilson's disease (p. 665) and the rare syndrome of idiopathic calcification of the basal ganglia (p. 756). Bowman and Lewis (1980) reinforced this association in their analysis of the site of major pathology in a large variety of cerebral disorders liable to show aspects of schizophrenic symptomatology.

It remains puzzling that frontal lesions have rarely been

incriminated, with the exception of occasional disorders such as metachromatic leucodystrophy (p. 758). However, functional brain imaging in the naturally occurring illness strongly suggests that frontal systems may be specially at fault, as described on p. 87. Occasional anecdotal reports of schizophrenia following frontal damage are therefore of interest, as in the patient described by Pang and Lewis (1996):

A young man with a family history of depression suffered several episodes of bipolar affective illness over a 2-year period. He then sustained a head injury leading to a left frontal haematoma which necessitated a left frontal lobectomy. Nine months later he developed a classic schizophrenic illness which pursued a chronic course during 6 years' follow-up. A spike-discharging focus was detected 3 years after the injury when he developed epileptic seizures. The authors suggest that the transformation from bipolar affective disorder to schizophrenia, in a patient genetically predisposed to the former, was due to the unusual combination of damage to the left frontal lobe and an excitatory lesion in the left temporal lobe.

Structural brain imaging

Interest was renewed in the possibility of structural brain changes in schizophrenia by the demonstration of ventricular enlargement on CT scans, sometimes with sulcal widening, as described on p. 140. This has emerged repeatedly in controlled comparisons, though not in all studies to date. Particularly compelling were early reports that among sibships and monozygotic twin pairs discordant for schizophrenia the affected member virtually always had the larger ventricles (Weinberger et al. 1981; Reveley et al. 1982).

The implications of such findings have been the subject of numerous reviews (Lishman 1983a; Weinberger et al. 1983; Reveley 1985; Lewis 1990). The CT changes show a number of associations — with poor performance on neuropsychological tests, with the presence of tardive dyskinesia, and possibly with a preponderance of negative symptoms, poor response to neuroleptics and poor premorbid adjustment. More controversial are claims that they are commoner in patients who lack a family history of major psychiatric illness (Reveley et al. 1984; Jones et al. 1993) or in those with a history of obstetric complications at birth (Schulsinger et al. 1984; Owen et al. 1988). It seems clear that the changes are unrelated to the duration of illness or length of hospitalisation, and they have been detected in patients soon after the schizophrenia is declared (Weinberger et al. 1982; Turner et al. 1986). Several studies have confirmed that they do not progress during follow-up (Nasrallah 1990; Jaskiw et al. 1994). The consensus is therefore that such CT findings represent static brain changes, possibly reflecting early neurodevelopmental anomalies. Consistent with this is Lewis's (1990) report of unexpected focal abnormalities in a small percentage of scans—areas of low attenuation and calcification—also occasional anomalies of brain development such as septal cysts, aqueduct stenosis, agenesis of the corpus callosum and cavum septum pellucidum.

Magnetic resonance imaging has in the main confirmed the CT findings and added a good deal more. Andreasen et al. (1986) found evidence of smaller frontal lobe size in schizophrenic patients, not replicated in a better-controlled study (Andreasen et al. 1990) but emerging again with three-dimensional reconstructions (Andreasen et al. 1994b). Andreasen et al. (1994a) have also reported decreased thalamic size in the disorder. Others have reported smaller temporal lobes, most markedly on the left (Johnstone et al. 1989; DeLisi et al. 1991). Suddath et al. (1989) found a 67% enlargement of the ventricles in chronic patients, and reductions in temporal lobe grey matter by 20%, most markedly in areas corresponding to the amygdala and anterior hippocampus. Bogerts et al. (1990a) confirmed reductions in hippocampal tissue in first-episode schizophrenic patients, apparently restricted to the left side and to males. In a comparison of 15 monozygotic twin pairs discordant for schizophrenia, Suddath et al. (1990) reported enlargement of the lateral and third ventricles and virtually consistent bilateral reductions in hippocampal volume in the affected co-twins.

Several studies have attempted to explore the clinical associations of the reduction in temporal lobe structures in small groups of schizophrenic patients. Nestor et al. (1993) found modest but significant relationships between the volume of the parahippocampal and posterior superior temporal gyri and impairment on tests of verbal memory, abstraction and categorisation. More strikingly, associations have been found between reduced volume in the left superior temporal gyrus and the severity of auditory hallucinations (Barta et al. 1990), and between reductions in its posterior part and the severity of thought disorder (Shenton et al. 1992; Menon et al. 1995). Menon et al. (1995) found a significant *positive* correlation between the volume of the left posterior superior temporal gyrus and scores reflecting the presence of delusions.

In contrast to regional effects of this nature, Zipursky et al. (1992) have reported significant reductions in grey matter volumes in *most* parts of the cerebral cortex, including the prefrontal, frontal, temporoparietal and parieto-occipital regions, a result broadly confirmed by Harvey et al. (1993). This was not apparent in manic-depressive patients examined by similar procedures (Harvey et al. 1994). Such widespread cortical involvement could perhaps account for the pleomorphic features of the disease and its variability of expression in different patients. Significant reductions in subcortical grey matter volumes were also apparent in Zipursky et al.'s patients.

Other findings of interest include significant reductions in corpus callosum size on MRI, particularly of the anterior and central parts which connect the frontal and temporal regions (Woodruff et al. 1993, 1995). A number of preliminary findings from magnetic resonance spectroscopy in schizophrenia are mentioned on p. 143.

It appears, therefore, that the more closely one looks with modern neuroimaging methods, the more evidence one obtains of widespread neurodevelopmental anomalies in schizophrenia. Some, but not all, of these findings are mirrored in the autopsy investigations discussed immediately below.

Neuropathology

Neuropathological studies of schizophrenia appeared until recently to have run into an impasse. The Vogts, for example, had seemingly spent a life-time examining the brains of schizophrenics (Vogt & Vogt 1952), with results that failed to gain wide acceptance. Plum (1972) was led to make the memorable remark that 'schizophrenia is the graveyard of neuropathologists'. Now there has been an upsurge of interest again, fuelled in part by the findings from neuroimaging but also by advances in techniques such as quantitative morphometry and histochemistry. Important reviews are presented by Lantos (1988) and Roberts and Bruton (1990). Lantos cautions particularly that many of the more recent findings have yet to be shown convincingly to be specific for schizophrenia.

Stevens (1982), in a thorough investigation, found evidence of periventricular and periaqueductal gliosis, with appearances suggestive of previous low-grade inflammation. Not dissimilar observations had previously been made by Nieto and Escobar (1972) and Fisman (1975). Most others, however, have stressed that gliosis is rare, and ascribe the observed abnormalities to early embryonic insult or early prenatal developmental anomalies, since foetal brain tissues show a glial response only in the last trimester of gestation. (Roberts et al. 1987; Roberts & Crow 1987). In Bruton et al.'s (1990) carefully controlled investigation the excess gliosis disappeared after excluding patients with Alzheimer changes, cerebrovascular disease and focal pathologies.

Bogerts et al. (1985) found no evidence of gliosis in a re-examination of the Vogts' collection of brains, gathered before the era of neuroleptics and insulin treatment, but showed reductions in size of the globus pallidus and several limbic structures. Shrinkage of the hippocampal

formation was sometimes obvious macroscopically. Such findings were confirmed in a separate series, particularly among the males (Bogerts et al. 1990b). Corsellis's group measured a large sample from Runwell Hospital, showing pronounced enlargement of the temporal horns and thinning of the parahippocampal cortex (particularly on the left) in comparison with patients with affective disorder (Brown et al. 1986). Crow et al. (1989) showed enlargement principally restricted to the left temporal horn, i.e. to that part of the brain in which anatomical asymmetries are normally present. Jakob and Beckmann (1989) described abnormalities in the gyral pattern over the temporal lobe, most markedly on the left, again suggestive of early developmental disturbance. Falkai et al. (1992) noted reductions in the length of the left Sylvian fissure, perhaps indicative of early impairment of cerebral lateralisation.

Bruton et al. (1990) compared a series of 56 carefully diagnosed and prospectively gathered schizophrenic patients with normal controls matched for age and sex. Fixed brain weights were significantly reduced by 4.5%, with concomitant increases in ventricular size. Similar reductions were found in mean brain length, both measures being related to indices of poor premorbid adjustment. Arnold et al. (1991) concentrated attention on the entorhinal cortex, which forms the anterior part of the parahippocampal gyrus and contains important communications between the neocortex and the hippocampus. All six brains examined by Arnold et al. showed abnormalities by way of aberrant invaginations of the surface, disruption of cortical layers and heterotopic displacement of neurones indicative of disturbed neurodevelopment.

Benes and co-workers have made detailed neuronal counts in various brain regions with the help of sophisticated morphometric techniques (Benes et al. 1986, 1991a, 1991b; Benes & Bird 1987). The numbers of small interneurones were reduced in cingulate and prefrontal areas, without increased gliosis, likewise pyramidal neuronal counts in some parts of the hippocampus. The latter has been confirmed in some studies (Falkai & Bogerts 1986; Jeste & Lohr 1989) but not in others (Heckers et al. 1991). It is, however, supported by magnetic resonance spectroscopy (Maier et al. 1995). Scheibel's group noted alterations in pyramidal cell orientation in the hippocampus, with disorderly alignments and corresponding disorganisation of their dendritic arrays (Kovelman & Scheibel 1984; Conrad & Scheibel 1987; Conrad et al. 1991). In some areas the proportion of cells rotated by 30 degrees or more was increased seven or eightfold in comparison with controls, and the severity of the effect seemed to be related to the severity of the antemortem clinical picture.

Such changes appeared to be the product of disturbed migration of neurones into the primordial hippocampus during the second trimester of pregnancy. Again, however, there has not been universal agreement on the finding (Christison *et al.* 1989; Benes *et al.* 1991b).

Finally, recent studies by Akbarian and co-workers are interesting in providing more definitive evidence of disturbed migration of neurones during foetal development (Akbarian *et al.* 1993a, 1993b). Neurochemical techniques were used to identify a particular population of neurones in the grey matter and subjacent white matter ('NADPH-d neurones'). Having migrated towards the cortex these are normally found in greatest numbers immediately deep to layer VI of the cortex. In schizophrenic brains, however, their distribution was shifted significantly inwards and they were found in deeper layers of the white matter. Such findings applied to the medial and lateral temporal lobe structures, also to the dorsolateral prefrontal cortex which has emerged as dysfunctional in cerebral blood flow studies (see below).

In brief, therefore, neuropathological investigations have pointed most clearly to temporal lobe abnormalities, possibly because this region of the brain has been examined most carefully. Structural brain imaging, by contrast, has indicated more widespread cortical involvement (e.g. Zipursky *et al.* 1992; *vide supra*) and it is therefore interesting that pathological changes at a histological level are now reported in frontal regions as well. An important consensus from the more recent pathological studies is that the abnormalities observed are likely to be neurodevelopmental in origin.

Functional brain imaging

Functional imaging studies effectively took origin from Ingvar and Franzen's (1974) demonstration of diminished cerebral blood flow to frontal regions in older chronic schizophrenic patients. Such 'hypofrontality' was supported by Buchsbaum *et al.* (1982) who showed lowered uptake of glucose in frontal regions by FDG-PET, and particularly in the central grey matter of the left side of the brain. Subsequent PET studies have given variable results, as reviewed by Bench *et al.* (1990) and Buchsbaum (1990), seemingly due to variations in technique and differences in the populations investigated. Nevertheless, most reports have shown lower metabolism in the frontal and temporal regions and basal ganglia than in posterior brain areas. With further experience, however, such hypometabolism appears to lack specificity in that it may also be seen in some degree in patients with depressive illness (p. 145).

Single photon emission computerised tomography (SPECT) has given variable findings when carried out in schizophrenic patients at rest (Ebmeier *et al.* 1995). More consistent results are obtained when 'activation' techniques are employed. Thus Weinberger *et al.* (1986, 1988b) measured cerebral blood flow by xenon inhalation, first while the patient performed a simple number-matching task, then while engaged in a sorting task of the type normally expected to activate the prefrontal cortex (Plate 3). Activation of blood flow was found to be strikingly reduced over the dorsolateral prefrontal cortex (DLPFC), the patients' performance on the task being correlated with the degree of prefrontal activation. In a study of 10 pairs of monozygotic twins discordant for schizophrenia, the affected co-twin invariably showed less prefrontal activation than the healthy member of the pair (Berman *et al.* 1992). The phenomenon has appeared to be specific to schizophrenia, to the extent that patients with Huntington's disease, who also performed badly on the task, increased their frontal blood flows normally (Weinberger *et al.* 1988a). Patients with severe depression and with Down's syndrome also activated the DLPFC normally (Weinberger *et al.* 1991a). By contrast, during performance on an automated version of Raven's matrices schizophrenic patients were found to activate posterior parieto-occipital areas in a normal fashion (Berman *et al.* 1988).

Not dissimilarly, Warkentin *et al.* (1989) showed with xenon inhalation and a verbal fluency task that schizophrenic patients produced considerably less prefrontal activation in the left hemisphere than normal controls. Daniel *et al.* (1990) used SPECT to show that dextroamphetamine could restore left frontal activation in response to card sorting in a group of chronic schizophrenics, along with improvement in performance. Weinberger *et al.* (1991a) conclude that in all studies which have used cognitive tasks demanding prefrontal activation, schizophrenic patients have tended to show a 'hypofrontal' pattern as measured by cerebral blood flow or glucose utilisation. This provides a tempting explanation for such common symptoms as affective blunting and impaired volition.

In a more ambitious development, Liddle *et al.* (1992) have explored ^{15}O-PET indices of resting regional cerebral blood flow (rCBF) in cohorts of chronic schizophrenic patients with contrasting patterns of symptomatology. Patients classified as having the *'psychomotor poverty syndrome'* (i.e. poverty of speech, flattened affect and decreased spontaneous movement) showed decreased rCBF in the left prefrontal and parietal cortex, along with increases in the caudate nuclei. The area of left prefrontal hypoperfusion coincided with that shown by Frith *et al.* (1991) to be activated by the internal generation of willed as compared with routine actions. Patients with the *'disorganisation syndrome'* (disordered thought and inappropriate affect) showed increased resting rCBF most markedly in the anterior cingulate region. This coincides with the area maximally activated during performance of the Stroop test in which competing responses must be suppressed (p. 118); hence it may reflect a struggle in such patients to suppress inappropriate mental activity. Patients with the *'reality distortion syndrome'* (delusions and hallucinations) showed increases in rCBF most prominently in the left parahippocampal gyrus and contiguous areas. In each syndrome the detailed patterns of blood flow indicated that distributed neuronal networks rather than specific loci were implicated in the underlying abnormalities of brain function.

Kaplan *et al.* (1993) have broadly confirmed Liddle's clinical groupings and the associated sites of brain abnormality, using FDG-PET in untreated acute schizophrenic patients. An interesting difference lay, however, in the finding of *hyper*metabolism rather than hypometabolism in left prefrontal and parietal cortex in acute patients with the psychomotor poverty syndrome; this may conceivably reflect different stages of a compensatory or degenerative process which had proceeded further in Liddle's chronic patients.

Frith (1995) reviews further associations emerging from PET studies. He points out, for example, that 'self monitoring' depends on a tight correspondence between anterior brain regions concerned with voluntary motor output and posterior regions concerned with the relevant sensory inputs. When normal subjects generate words there is an increase in blood flow to the DLPFC and an associated decrease in the superior temporal cortex. In schizophrenic patients performing the same task the DLPFC increase was not associated with decreases in the left superior temporal cortex, implying a lack of connectivity between these two brain areas.

Interesting attempts have also been made to explore differences on neuroimaging between schizophrenic patients with and without persistent auditory hallucinations. Cleghorn *et al.* (1990) compared such groups using FDG-PET. No one region showed significant differences, but there were patterns of correlation between Broca's area and other brain areas (e.g. anterior cingulate and left superior temporal) in those who hallucinated but not in the others. McGuire *et al.* (1993) obtained more clear-cut results by arranging for each patient to serve as his own control, carrying out HMPAO-SPECT scans (p. 148) first in the presence of on-going auditory verbal hallucinations then again some weeks later when these had largely resolved. On each occasion the patient was asked to signal the presence or absence of hallucinations immediately prior to the injection of HMPAO. Increased blood flow was demonstrated in Broca's area during the occurrence of hallucinations, i.e. the area that has been implicated in the subvocal rehearsal of inner speech (Paulesu *et al.* 1993). Such a finding supports the idea that hallucinations arise from the patient's failure to monitor his own

thoughts and 'inner speech', which is therefore regarded as alien and perceived as emanating from others.

In a further study, schizophrenic patients *liable* to auditory verbal hallucinations were compared with those who were not, even though hallucinations were not occurring at the time of testing (McGuire *et al.* 1995b). ^{15}O-PET scans were carried out while the subject imagined sentences being spoken in another person's voice. In normal subjects this task is associated with increased activity in such areas as the left inferior frontal gyrus, the supplementary motor area and the left temporal cortex (McGuire *et al.* 1996). Patients prone to hallucinations showed the expected increase in frontal activity, but reductions rather than increases in the supplementary motor area and left temporal regions. Thus it appeared that a predisposition to auditory verbal hallucinations was reflected in aberrant connectivity between the areas concerned with the generation and monitoring of inner speech.

Functional MRI (p. 143) has also been used to explore the cerebral correlates of auditory verbal hallucinations (David *et al.* 1996). Images were obtained during periods of auditory stimulation (speech) and visual stimulation (flashing lights), both when the patient was hallucinating and when he was not. As can be seen from Plate 4, activation to visual stimulation occurred in the visual cortex irrespective of the presence or absence of auditory hallucinations, whereas temporal lobe activation to auditory stimulation was almost completely suppressed while hallucinations were in progress. David *et al.* interpret this as reflecting physiological competition for a common neural substrate, normally activated by speech, by the on-going verbal hallucinations.

Functional brain imaging has additionally made use of radiolabelled ligands, in particular to explore possibilities of dopamine overactivity in the striatum in drug-naïve schizophrenic patients. Early attempts using PET gave contradictory results, Wong *et al.* (1986) reporting a marked elevation in striatal D_2 receptor density but others finding no difference from controls (Farde *et al.* 1987; Martinot *et al.* 1990). Crawley *et al.* (1986) using SPECT found an increase, but Pilowsky *et al.* (1994) did not. The latter study, however, produced evidence of significant asymmetry in D_2 binding among male schizophrenics, the levels being higher in the left striatum than the right. Farde *et al.* (1995) have reported a similar asymmetry with PET. Martinot *et al.* (1994) further showed a significant correlation between PET indices of reduced striatal D_2 receptor density and certain negative symptoms such as poverty of speech and blunted affect.

Further clarification may need to await studies using ligands capable of identifying specific subtypes of dopamine receptors. Advances in PET technology may also permit the monitoring of dopamine receptors in relevant extrastriatal brain structures such as the hippocampus, nucleus accumbens and frontal limbic cortex (Farde *et al.* 1995). To date this has scarcely been possible because of limits on scanner resolution and the low concentrations of dopamine in brain areas other than the striatum.

Hemispheric differences

A separate but perhaps complementary strand to the picture concerns evidence that aspects of cerebral dominance may bear a special relationship to schizophrenia. As described on p. 282, the schizophrenia-like psychoses seen with epilepsy tend to be associated with foci in the left hemisphere. Furthermore, neuropathological investigations have drawn particular attention to changes in the left temporal lobe in the generality of schizophrenias (p. 86).

Other observations can be marshalled in support of left hemisphere dysfunction in the disease. For comprehensive reviews of cerebral laterality in relation to various forms of psychopathology Flor-Henry (1983) should be consulted, also the compilations of reports by Gruzelier and Flor-Henry (1979) and Flor-Henry and Gruzelier (1983). Brief reviews are presented by Merrin (1981), Gruzelier (1981) and Taylor (1987).

Dominant lobe dysfunction in schizophrenia has been inferred from asymmetries in skin conductance responses (Gruzelier & Venables 1974), patterns of functioning on dichotic and tachistoscopic tests (Colbourn & Lishman 1979; Gruzelier 1979; Connolly *et al.* 1983; Bruder *et al.* 1995), psychometric testing (Flor-Henry & Yeudall 1979; Flor-Henry *et al.* 1983; Taylor & Abrams 1987), electroencephalographic data (Abrams & Taylor 1979, 1980), and data from visual and auditory evoked responses (Buchsbaum *et al.* 1979; Shagass *et al.* 1979, 1983). In many of these respects depressive illness can be shown to be associated, on similar evidence, with dysfunction of the right side of the brain (Kronfol *et al.* 1978; Yozawitz *et al.* 1979; Von Knorring 1983; Taylor & Abrams 1987). In a direct comparison between patients with schizophrenia and affective disorder, David and Cutting (1992) found that the schizophrenic group failed to show the expected left hemisphere advantage on a tachistoscopic test of visual semantic judgements; however, both patient groups showed a normal right hemisphere advantage on an equivalent task involving visual imagery.

As might be expected, however, different avenues of investigation are not always in agreement with one another, all being indirect indices of hemispheric dysfunction. Such is the fragility of much of the evidence, that Cutting (1985, 1990, 1992, 1994) has been able to amass arguments in favour of quite the reverse, namely of *right* hemisphere dysfunction in schizophrenia. More specifically he suggests that diminution in the activity of the right hemisphere results in hemispheric imbalance, the left coming to be unusually prepotent over the right.

In reaching this conclusion Cutting draws both on clinical observations and certain test procedures. He points out, for example, that certain phenomena exhibited by patients with damage to the right hemisphere come close to resembling those seen in schizophrenia. Delusional misidentification, for example, is commoner with right hemisphere lesions than left, and feelings of dissolution of body boundaries may be observed following acute right hemisphere strokes. Flattening of affect is reminiscent of the aprosody seen with right hemisphere damage, similarly loss of figurative/metaphorical meaning in language and impaired proverb interpretation.

Certain neuropsychological tests with high specificity for right hemisphere dysfunction have emerged as impaired in schizophrenic subjects, for example judgements of facial expression (Gessler *et al.* 1989) and tests of ability to comprehend and express emotional prosody in speech (Murphy & Cutting 1990). Cutting and Murphy (1990) found that schizophrenic patients tended to select non-figurative rather than metaphorical pairings of words, as occurs with right but not left hemisphere lesions. David and Cutting (1990) demonstrated loss of the normal left hemifacial bias for judgements of facial expression on a chimeric faces test. Left-sided tactual extinction has been found to be common, particularly in chronic forms of schizophrenia (Scarone *et al.* 1987); and a tendency to exhibit an excess of right-directed eye movements during mental activity has been interpreted as a consequence of increased left hemisphere activity in compensation for a primary right hemisphere deficit (Schweitzer 1982).

Again, however, much of the evidence pointing to right rather than left hemisphere dysfunction is inferential.

Patterns of hand preference have been extensively studied in schizophrenia but with results that have varied markedly (Taylor *et al.* 1982a, 1982b; Manoach *et al.* 1988; Green *et al.* 1989; Nelson *et al.* 1993). Claims have included an excess of left-handedness, mixed handedness or even pure right-handedness, often with male patients diverging more than females from controls. Despite attempts to refine the subgroupings of patients according to chronicity or different forms of illness the conclusions to be drawn remain ambiguous.

Nevertheless, interest in left- and right-handedness has paved the way to important findings concerning cerebral anatomical asymmetry. As described on p. 41, Le May (1976, 1977) showed that the brain is normally asymmetrical, the frontal lobe being wider on the right and the occipital lobe on the left. Such asymmetries, evident on CT scans, were sometimes reversed in left-handers. Luchins *et al.* (1979, 1982) then showed that a subgroup of right-handed schizophrenics displayed the reversed left-handed pattern, a finding variably confirmed or refuted in subsequent studies.

Bullmore *et al.* (1995) have recently produced impressive evidence that this is a valid finding, by analysis of a large group of schizophrenics and controls. The strength of their study, derived from MRI images, relies on the measurement of a large number of brain slices obtained in the coronal plane from the frontal and temporal lobes. The reversed asymmetry was found, however, to apply only to male schizophrenics:

Bullmore et al. used sophisticated image analysis to delineate the boundaries between the cortex and subcortex in up to 19 coronal slices per subject. The 'radius of gyration' (Rg) was then measured on each slice, representing the mean dispersion of points organised radially about the centre of gravity of the residual images obtained. In right-handed controls the Rg for right brain boundaries was significantly greater than that for left brain boundaries, indicating larger anterior brain volumes on the right than the left. In left-handed controls the reverse obtained, with larger Rg on the left than the right. Right-handed male schizophrenics, however, were distinguished by reversal of the right-handed control pattern, due to a highly significant global reduction of Rg measures for right brain boundaries. This showed nearly significant associations with ratings of negative symptoms, and with categorisations according to outcome.

Biochemical observations on postmortem brain tissue have sometimes revealed unusual asymmetries in schizophrenic patients, for example increased dopamine in the left amygdaloid nucleus (Reynolds 1983, 1988). Decreased binding to kainate and quisqualate glutamate receptors has been demonstrated in the left hippocampus (Kerwin et al. 1988; Kerwin 1990), likewise a predominantly left-sided reduction in gamma aminobutyric acid (GABA) uptake in certain temporal lobe structures (Deakin et al. 1990; Reynolds & Czudek 1990). Biochemical studies thus tend to confirm a predominantly left-sided pathology, though it remains uncertain how far such findings may be the consequence of drug effects.

A particularly intriguing finding was reported by Bracha (1987) in seven unmedicated and three never-medicated schizophrenic patients who were observed during 8-hour periods while wearing a 'rotameter'. This portable device records the turns made to the left or the right while subjects pursue their daily activities. Normal controls registered an equivalent number of left and right turns (% right turns 49.9), whereas the schizophrenic patients made significantly more left turns than right (% right turns 30.7). All 10 patients turned more often to the left than the right. The possible relevance of the finding to dopamine asymmetry in the brain is suggested by analogous animal experiments; animals with unilateral striatal dopamine deficiency rotate more often towards the side which is depleted.

A further set of observations suggests a *disturbance of functional interrelationships between the two hemispheres* in the disease. Green (1978) and Carr (1980) showed impairment of transfer of information from one hand to the other in schizophrenic patients, and Dimond et al. (1980) found impairments in pointing with one hand to areas touched lightly on the other. In a test of naming objects by palpation, significantly more errors were made with the left hand than the right (Dimond et al. 1979). Such early studies combined to suggest inefficient transfer across channels of communication between the hemispheres.

Further striking evidence pointing to callosal dysfunction has come from David's (1987) tachistoscopic tests of colour naming and matching. Schizophrenic patients were found to make significantly more errors than controls in naming colours presented to the left visual field (i.e. to the right hemisphere), whereas performance to right visual field exposures was normal. Matching of colours exposed simultaneously across the two half-fields was also significantly impaired, whereas matching within a given half-field was unaffected.

In a second experiment, David (1993) examined the Stroop effect (p. 118), in which subjects were asked to name the colour of a vertical strip alongside which was printed a vertical colour word:

Presentations were made tachistoscopically and all responses were timed. In 'congruent' pairings the colour and the word were the same, in 'incongruent' pairings they differed from one another. The difference in reaction times between the two, reflecting the combined effects of interference and facilitation, was labelled the 'combined Stroop effect'. Schizophrenic patients, compared to controls, showed a larger combined Stroop effect when the colour patch and the colour word were separated across the midline and thus fed to different hemispheres. Pairings presented within the same half-field showed results no different from controls. There was in fact a double dissociation, schizophrenics showing greater combined Stroop effects in the interhemispheric than the intrahemispheric condition, and controls showing the reverse.

Such results could be interpreted either as evidence for increased interference between the hemispheres for incongruent stimuli, or increased facilitation for congruent stimuli—in both cases implying unusual callosal function in schizophrenia. A particular strength of David's two experiments is that patients with affective disorder as well as normal subjects served as controls.

Other interesting observations have been reported by Green and associates (Green & Kotenko 1980; Green et al. 1983). In normal subjects the monaural comprehension of short prose passages can be shown to be equivalent whether the input is to the left or right ear; however, simultaneous input to the two ears yields slightly improved scores. Schizophrenics, by contrast, tend to perform better through one ear than the other, the right usually being superior. And, rather strikingly, binaural inputs yield poorer scores than monaural input to the better of the two ears. The suggested explanation is that the right–left monaural differences reflect abnormal callosal transfer; and the impairment in binaural scores may also result from abnormal callosal function which prevents the smooth processing and integration of information when this is fed simultaneously to the two hemispheres. Abnormal information transfer across the corpus callosum may in effect lead to competition between the hemispheres, with consequent impairment of comprehension.

It is tempting to speculate that certain schizophrenic symptoms could arise on such a basis. Thought disorder, for example, might be the product, at least in part, of inefficient callosal transfer and complex interactions between rival systems in the two cerebral hemispheres.

Thus in addition to a role for focal brain pathology in relation to schizophrenia, it appears that dominance relationships between the hemispheres, and certain aspects of interhemispheric collaboration, may have a bearing on the disorder. Many of these findings must be regarded as provisional, but nevertheless they emerge, in sum, as impressive.

Neurodevelopmental and virogene models

Any attempt to unite these various strands of evidence to form a coherent theory meets with very considerable difficulties, especially since several are as yet insubstantial in themselves. Moreover, a convincing account of a cerebral basis to schizophrenia must try to encompass a number of clinical observations—genetic liability to the disorder, a tendency to appear in adolescence or early adult life, response to certain medications, and distinct associations in certain cases with pathology affecting the temporal lobes and limbic areas. Other findings almost as firm need also to be taken into account (Lishman 1995)—'season of birth effects' with an excess during the late winter and early spring months (Bradbury & Miller 1985; Hare 1987, 1988), vulnerability to life events and to 'expressed emotion' (Brown & Birley 1968; Vaughn & Leff 1976), the presence of antecedent impairments from childhood onwards (Jones et al. 1994), and a host of tantalising relationships with aspects of cerebral laterality.

Neurodevelopmental theory

The neurodevelopmental theory of schizophrenia has gained prominence in the field and is argued persuasively by a number of authorities (Weinberger 1987, 1995; Murray et al. 1988; Murray 1994). It encompasses both genetic and environmental factors as having a causal relationship to the disease. Though not applicable in every case the theory claims to account for a sizeable proportion of patients, particularly those with early onset of the illness and prominent negative symptoms.

It is suggested that many schizophrenic subjects harbour 'brain lesions', especially in the limbic system and frontal cortex, which have originated very early in life extending back even to the intrauterine period. Such lesions, which are of a subtle nature, predispose the affected person to develop schizophrenia later. They may be the product of genetic influences controlling early brain growth, of infection, immune disorder, complications of pregnancy or, the now favoured view, of abnormal patterns of neuronal migration. These last may be occasioned by damage to the foetus during pregnancy or may themselves be inherited directly. Important variables with respect to the risk of developing schizophrenia are likely to include the site and timing of the disturbances, and the presence or absence of a genetic predisposition to the disorder.

The environmental influences concerned are likely to be heterogeneous, varying from one individual to another. The question of maternal infection during pregnancy has been explored in some detail, as a possible explanation for the observation that schizophrenic patients are more likely to be born in the late winter or early spring months as mentioned above. The issue has become closely focused on influenza, with a number of studies showing an excess of schizophrenic births during the months following epidemics. The detailed evidence is reviewed by Murray (1994) and Sham (1995) and contested by Crow and Done (1992) and Cooper (1992). Among studies supporting the association the timing of the increase has been fairly consistent, following some 3–5 months after epidemics. It is clear, however, that influenza could be the causative agent in only a minority of schizophrenic births.

Lewis (1989) reviews the increasing evidence of a link with obstetric complications. Moreover, a recent analysis of a large cohort of patients from Scotland, compared with closely matched controls, has shown a significant excess of complications both of pregnancy and delivery as antecedents to schizophrenia, in particular an excess of pre-eclampsia and of infants detained in hospital for neonatal care (Kendell et al. 1996). In some surveys a history of obstetric complications has been found to be predictive of increased ventricular size once the illness is declared (e.g. Owen et al. 1988).

An additional study has highlighted the possible role of malnutrition during the first trimester of pregnancy. Susser and Lin (1992) investigated the risk of schizophrenia in cohorts of persons born to mothers who had endured severe starvation during the Nazi blockade of western Holland in the winter of 1944–45. In comparison with controls such persons showed a substantial increase in hospitalisations for schizophrenia during 1978–89, though applying only to females.

The brain abnormalities, however engendered, may have issue in a variety of impairments from childhood onwards. The child at risk for developing schizophrenia in adult life has been found to have a lower IQ than his sibs and peers (Aylward et al. 1984), and to show early social, cognitive and motor impairments (Fish 1977; Fish et al. 1992; Walker 1993; Jones et al. 1994). But it is suggested that the lesions declare themselves fully only 15–20 years later, because they need to interact with normal brain maturational processes before their true impact is revealed. This is the distinctive aspect of the 'schizophrenic brain lesion'—that it involves systems that have yet to mature functionally. Or putting it another way, the lesion remains largely dormant until further brain maturation calls the damaged neuronal systems into operation.

There are precedents for such a situation both in animal experimental work and in man (Weinberger 1987). Thus a lesion of the dorsolateral prefrontal cortex does not markedly affect the infant monkey's behaviour, but disrupts performance on delayed response tasks in adulthood. Similarly, perinatal hypoxia may lead to cerebral palsy in infancy but to athetosis and epilepsy some years later.

A good deal of theorising has centred on the mechanisms whereby the early lesion may come to be 'actualised' in later years. Murray *et al.* (1988) and Lewis (1989) discuss the possibility that immature circuitry is laid bare by synaptic pruning, a process which in some brain areas continues until after puberty. The developing brain has a large excess of neurones and axons which thin out during early development, serving to eliminate early errors of connection and to strengthen those that are useful. Early injury can prevent such processes from occurring, resulting in the perpetuation of anomalous patterns. These will eventually become operational, resulting, it is suggested, in the appearance of the disease.

Brain myelination is also known to continue well into postnatal life, particularly in areas such as the corpus callosum and the prefrontal cortex. Weinberger (1987) stresses that the dorsolateral prefrontal cortex is one of the last brain areas to myelinate, this continuing well into the second and third decades of life. In his model the declaration of symptoms may depend on the maturing of cortical–subcortical relationships:

In animals lesions of the dorsolateral prefrontal cortex can disturb the relationship between cortical and subcortical dopamine metabolism. In the rat a lesion of the dopamine afferents within the medial prefrontal cortex results in dopamine overactivity in subcortical sites, apparently through the operation of feedback control (Pycock *et al.* 1980). Thus a lesion in such a situation could account both for the negative symptoms of schizophrenia (low dopamine prefrontally) and for the positive symptoms (high dopamine subcortically). Evidence for such feedback control is, however, lacking to date in man.

Brain dopamine is known to be important in relation to stress, rising in frontal and subcortical sites in response to limb shock in rats, but in the frontal cortex alone when the rat is re-exposed to the environment where the shocks had occurred ('experiential stress') (Herman *et al.* 1982). This aspect could be relevant to schizophrenia in that stress could tax a faulty system. Adolescence is notably a time of stress, i.e. precisely when augmenta-

tion of prefrontal dopamine levels may be needed. The failure to increase prefrontal dopamine, and the failure of a feedback loop to come into operation, would cause subcortical dopamine levels to rise higher still, with issue in schizophrenic symptomatology.

Sex differences with regard to schizophrenia can be accommodated within the neurodevelopmental model. There is evidence that the onset of the illness is earlier in males than females, and that males show poorer premorbid adjustment and tend to have a poorer outcome (Castle & Murray 1991). This accords with the evidence from neuroimaging and neuropathology that the male schizophrenic brain is more often abnormal than the female (*vide supra*). Moreover, neurodevelopmental disorders are in general commoner in boys than girls, as with developmental dyslexia and autism, perhaps as a result of slower maturation or greater lateralisation of function which renders compensation for damage less successful.

Virogene theory

The viral theory of schizophrenia has been argued in similar detail and can account for certain observations. It originated from the finding of Tyrrell *et al.* (1979) and Crow *et al.* (1979) that the cerebrospinal fluid from a proportion of acute schizophrenic patients exerted cytopathic effects on fibroblast tissue cultures, similar to those induced by viruses. The responsible agent could not be identified, nor could it be propagated satisfactorily. Nevertheless the observation led to the hypothesis that viral infection might sometimes be localised to systems of the brain concerned with higher mental functions, resulting in mental disorder without accompanying neurological features. The idea was supported by the occasional development of schizophrenia-like pictures in the course of encephalitis due to conventional viruses (p. 347), also the finding of raised gamma globulin in the cerebrospinal fluid of certain acute psychotic patients (p. 355).

Crow (1983a) suggested that the putative virus might set in train the neurochemical disturbances underlying schizophrenia by its affinity for certain receptors, thus rendering the patient's genetic predisposition overt. Indirect evidence in support of an infective aetiology included the seasonal incidence of birth and presentations, and certain family data that could not be explained on a genetic basis alone (Crow 1983b). For example, concordance for schizophrenia is higher between same sex than opposite sex dizygotic twins and siblings, and higher in same sex dizygotic twins than same sex sibs, all suggesting that physical proximity, and thereby infection, may bring additional hazards to genetically predisposed persons.

As evidence of neurodevelopmental and hemispheric abnormalities in the condition accumulated, Crow (1984,

1986, 1987a) modified the hypothesis to suggest that a retrovirus (or 'retrotransposon') might be responsible, sometimes inherited from a parent or sometimes acquired at a critical stage of embryonic development. By integration into the host's genetic complement it would also contribute in part to vertical transmission of the disorder. The ingenious additional suggestion was made that the retrovirus might be integrated at a site close to the genes responsible for cerebral dominance and/or growth factors determining differential hemisphere development. In this way it would be possible to account for disturbed cerebral laterality in the disease and the special accent of pathology in the left temporal lobe. The anomalous cerebral development would often be manifest in behavioural abnormalities from childhood onwards, the gene then remaining latent until adolescence or adulthood. It might then be expressed as viral particles during episodes of illness. Models exist with certain animal diseases to support such a possibility.

In further papers Crow (1987b, 1987c, 1990) discusses how a retrovirus of this nature could account for the survival of the gene and the persistence of psychosis in the community despite lowered fertility among affected individuals. An interaction of the virus with the cerebral dominance gene could be advantageous to survival by promoting brain areas involved with the lateralisation of language. And since lateralisation is typically more pronounced in males than in females, an anomaly in the genes which determine it might explain the earlier onset of schizophrenia and the more pronounced brain morphological changes in the male. High rates of mutation, as a function of environmental temperature, could help to account for season of birth effects.

The models discussed above are undoubtedly premature given the present state of knowledge and may need substantial revision as new findings emerge. Nevertheless they already account for a surprising amount of what has quite recently been discovered about schizophrenia, and they provide an important framework for further research. Most importantly they have synthesised a great deal of disparate information into views about aetiology. The challenge remains to unravel the detailed pathophysiological processes which may account for the curious manifestations of the disorder.

Chapter 3: Clinical Assessment

The assessment of patients with organic psychiatric disorder follows the time-honoured principles of clinical practice generally. It is sometimes a time-consuming process, requiring a good deal of patience and persistence. A careful history is essential, the mental state must be systematically examined, and a thorough physical examination will be required as well. The picture will then often remain incomplete without evaluation by a clinical psychologist and the undertaking of certain ancillary investigations. A period of observation in hospital can do much to clarify the situation when the diagnosis is unclear, and may prove more valuable than a great number of visits to the out-patient clinic. In many cases, therefore, the initial contact with the patient will merely serve to establish the major probabilities in diagnosis and allow more detailed planning for further enquiries.

No attempt will be made in the present chapter to outline a comprehensive schema for psychiatric history taking or examination. This is dealt with in textbooks of general psychiatry and is summarised in the publication by the Departmental Teaching Committee of the Institute of Psychiatry (Notes on Eliciting and Recording Clinical Information 1987). The purpose here will be to focus on those aspects of clinical enquiry which assume particular importance when one suspects an organic disease process in the genesis of the patient's mental symptoms. The value of certain psychometric tests and other investigatory procedures will also be discussed.

History taking

Where the great majority of organic psychiatric illnesses are concerned the stage is clearly set by the history, certainly when the relatives have been interviewed. Or if the history is equivocal, certain features on examination usually soon indicate that there is likely to be an organic basis for the disturbance. The main task thereafter is to refine the diagnosis by seeking to determine the nature of the pathological process. It is only in a minority of patients, albeit a vitally important group, that the presentation may be misleading—in the very early case or in cases with an abundance of 'functional' psychiatric features.

Time spent in obtaining a detailed history is almost always rewarded, and may yield more important leads to the correct diagnosis than a host of investigations. Certainly it will indicate what investigations, if any, need to be pursued. Moreover, the patient's account and his behaviour during interview will provide a wealth of information about his mental state and the intactness or otherwise of cognitive functions.

The patient's own account will usually need to be supplemented by information from others. Statements derived from the patient alone frequently prove misleading, both with regard to the gravity of the symptoms and the time course of their evolution. This is clearly so when the patient is confused or suffering from obvious memory impairment, but can be equally important in other situations. The changes occasioned by brain damage can be hard for the patient to evaluate subjectively, even when insight is largely retained. Certainly, when asked to judge whether memory or other difficulties are worsening or improving, he will often seize on some recent instance which may have more to do with chance and circumstance than with the course of the clinical condition. In many cases there will be genuine loss of insight, and sometimes a desire to conceal from himself and from others that intellectual functions are failing. Sometimes, too, the early changes will be of a type more obvious to outsiders than to the patient himself—changes in mood, enthusiasms, habitual activities and attitudes. Such matters obviously require the detailed testimony of someone who has known the patient intimately throughout the evolution of the disorder.

Abnormalities are likely to include such matters as disordered behaviour, and disturbances of mood, memory and subjective experience. Physical symptoms will also often figure prominently. The full range of complaints and apparent defects of functioning must be carefully explored, with readiness to search beneath the immediately presenting picture. Physical symptoms may have come to serve as the focus of attention for the patient and his relatives, and the true extent of mental abnormalities may only be revealed by specific enquiry. On the other hand the physical components should not be lightly brushed aside; in particular complaints of headache, malaise or generalised weakness must not be underestimated. When there is a problem of differential diagnosis between organic and non-organic mental illness it will be necessary to preserve a delicate balance in the enquiries until information begins to tip the balance in one direction or the other (Lishman 1992).

Particular attention must always be paid to the mode of onset of the disorder, the duration of symptoms and the way they have progressed. Where developments have been insidious the onset is often dated very imprecisely, even by relatives, with some striking incident serving as a screen for much that went before. Systematic enquiry about the level of functioning prior to the alleged onset can then be useful—behaviour on a previous holiday or at Christmas time for example—and serve to remind informants of the earlier evidence of disorder.

Enquiry should always be made for fluctuations in behaviour or changes which have been observed from one situation to another. Nocturnal worsening is an important indicator of minor degrees of clouding of consciousness. Behaviour which is relatively intact in the restricted field of domestic activities may be dramatically changed when new experiences need to be confronted. Episodic abnormal behaviour of sudden onset and ending will raise the suspicion of an epileptic component.

Other salient matters which deserve specific enquiry are outlined in Chapter 4 where differential diagnosis is discussed. These include not only features among the presenting symptoms, but also antecedent conditions such as head injury, alcoholism or drug abuse. Tactful and careful enquiry may need to be made about sexual practices if any suspicion of AIDS arises. Any recent physical illness must be noted, or medications recently prescribed, or conditions predisposing to anoxia such as cardiac failure, respiratory inadequacy or the recent administration of an anaesthetic. Any history of dysphasia, paresis, fits or other transitory neurological disturbances must be ascertained.

It is perhaps worth emphasising that the formal psychiatric history remains important even when the presenting complaints have a markedly organic flavour. Where the question arises of a differential diagnosis between organic and non-organic mental illness, all parts of the standard psychiatric enquiry will need to be completed. Previous reactions to stress, and symptoms observed during previous episodes of ill health, may help to clarify the significance of the present clinical features. Of course when there is abundant evidence of a cerebral pathological process some parts of the formal psychiatric history will be redundant. But there is still a need to know about premorbid patterns of functioning, special vulnerabilities and details of the patient's social and family setting. Such information may throw light upon the content of the illness and on special factors which will need to be borne in mind in management. Knowledge of the level achieved in education and at work can similarly be valuable in assessing present evidence of intellectual decline.

Physical examination

The more one suspects an organic basis for the patient's mental condition, the more important will be the physical examination. Often it is the latter which yields decisive information about the precise aetiology and the treatment required. In practice the dichotomy between the physical and the mental examination can tend to melt away, with each providing essential leads to the other. This is particularly evident in the examination of higher mental functions where the neurological examination overlaps with the detailed assessment of cognitive status.

Special attention will usually need to be devoted to the neurological system, but other systems can be just as crucially important. Johnson (1968) found that among 250 consecutive admissions to a psychiatric hospital, 12% had some physical illness which was an important aetiological factor in the presenting mental disorder. The majority were diagnosable by routine physical examination and had been missed prior to admission. Among his examples were cases of myxoedema, neurosyphilis, cerebral anoxia due to cardiac failure, chest infections, anaemia, liver failure, carcinoma and cerebral vascular disease. In addition many other physical disorders were discovered which did not contribute directly to the presenting clinical picture. Among 534 elderly patients admitted to psychiatric receiving wards, Simon and Cahan (1963) found that 13% had an acute and reversible physical cause for their symptoms, and another 30% had an acute component added to their senile or vascular dementia. Cardiac failure, malnutrition and recent cerebrovascular accidents made up most of the latter group. More recently Koran et al. (1989), in a thorough evaluation of patients in the Californian mental health system, identified an important physical disease in almost 40% of cases. This was judged to be causal in 6% and to exacerbate the mental disorder in 9%. Relevant conditions included organic brain syndrome, epilepsy, migraine, head injury, diabetes and thyroid and parathyroid disorders. A sixth of the causal illnesses had been overlooked, also more than half of those which were exacerbating the picture. Some of the principal physical signs which must be sought out with care are described on pp. 152 and 154.

It is important, especially in the neurological examination, to interpret abnormal findings in relation to the total clinical picture. Among the elderly in particular, isolated neurological abnormalities can be without significance (Critchley 1931; Prakash & Stern 1973). Absent vibration sense, mild tremors, sluggish and irregular pupils, isolated abnormalities of tendon reflexes or a doubtfully positive plantar response may lack diagnostic significance, or be related to minor pathology without relevance to the present problem. On the other hand, when viewed against the total picture these can be just the features which lead eventually to the true diagnosis.

Gross neurological abnormalities will rarely be encountered in patients with diffuse cerebral impairment, but certain less striking features should be carefully observed. Some of these are not widely appreciated, and can be important in raising suspicion of a degenerative brain process. Lack of manual precision, motor impersistence and perseveration of motor acts may emerge clearly in the course of neurological testing. A clumsy graceless walk or minor unsteadiness may betray cerebral pathology, even in the absence of definite pyramidal, extrapyramidal or cerebellar signs (Allison 1962). This may be striking once attention has been directed towards it. In patients suspected of cerebral vascular disease, special attention should be paid to swallowing, speech and the jaw jerk as indicators of early pseudobulbar palsy. A wide-based gait has been stressed as an early indicator of normal-pressure hydrocephalus (p. 745). Minor parkinsonian features, such as a stooping posture or lack of associated arm movements on walking, may also be noticed in diffuse cerebral disease.

Paulson (1971) describes certain reflex abnormalities which can occasionally precede definite evidence of intellectual impairment in cortical disease processes. Reflex grasping movements of the hand may occur on stroking the palm, or sucking or pouting movements of the mouth on tapping the lips ('snout reflex'). Both are linked especially to frontal lobe disease. The 'palmomental reflex' consists of unilateral contraction of the muscles of the chin producing a wince-like movement when the thenar eminence of the ipsilateral hand is stroked briskly. The 'corneomandibular reflex' consists of a movement of the opposite side of the chin in addition to blinking when a cotton-tip is applied to the cornea. The 'glabella-tap reflex' is elicited by repeated tapping of the forehead above the root of the nose—this produces blinking in response to each tap which fails to habituate rapidly as it does in normal persons.

Keshavan et al. (1979) illustrate the limitations of such 'primitive' reflexes as an aid to diagnosis; the palmomental reflex, for example, was found to be positive in as high a proportion of patients with affective disorder or schizophrenia as in patients with organic brain disease. Jacobs and Gossman (1980) found that the palmomental reflex was present in over 20% of healthy subjects in their thirties and forties, and a snout reflex in almost a third of those over 60. Both increased in incidence with advancing age, as did the corneomandibular reflex. Koller et al. (1982) found that the snout reflex failed to distinguish between demented and age-matched healthy elderly subjects. The glabella-tap reflex did so but showed no correlation with the presence of cerebral atrophy or the results of psychometry.

The mental state

The evaluation of the mental state provides the cross-sectional view which supplements the longitudinal view of the illness derived from the history. It also adds decisive information of its own. It is essential to realise that key features such as memory impairment may have to be sought after diligently if they are to be properly displayed.

There are obviously certain aspects of the mental state which are of especial importance in organic psychiatric disease, and these will be described in some detail below. In particular the correct evaluation of cognitive functions is often central to the identification of cerebral pathology. However, too early or exclusive a preoccupation with the assessment of cognitive functions can be a mistake, and stands to leave much valuable information uncharted. Short cuts should be avoided, the aim being always towards a systematic and comprehensive examination of the full range of mental phenomena. Often, for example, it is uncertain how much of the picture may be explained on the basis of non-organic rather than organic mental disturbance, and such a differentiation requires careful assessment of all aspects of the mental state. Even when cerebral pathology is abundantly obvious it is still necessary to be thoroughly aware of the patient's affective state, the nature of his interpersonal reactions and the content of his subjective experiences. The emphasis below on certain aspects should therefore not be taken to imply that other areas are necessarily of minor importance.

The mental state observed at interview must be evaluated against background information from others who have observed the patient in real-life situations. The interview has its own importance in allowing a systematic exploration of relevant areas of function, but is necessarily restricted in scope and is in many ways an artificial situation. For this reason admission to hospital for a period of observation often adds greatly to the assessment. Nurses' reports of behaviour in the ward, interactions with others and variability during the day can yield crucial information. Occupational therapy can provide the best setting of all when it comes to observing the detailed nature of the patient's difficulties over everyday tasks.

Appearance and general behaviour

Certain features obvious at a glance may raise suspicion of an organic basis for mental symptoms. Any evidence of physical ill health should be noted—pallor, loss of weight or indications of physical weakness. The facies can be very important: a certain laxness of the muscles of the lower face and lack of emotional play about the features can suggest a cerebral degenerative process in the absence of depression. Movements may be slow, sparse or tremulous. The appearance may be older than expected for the patient's age, or standards of self care and general tidiness may be poor. A lapse of standards which cannot readily be explained on the basis of severe emotional disturbance can be a sensitive pointer to cerebral pathology.

Features which should be noted in the course of conversation include slowness, hesitancy, perseverative tendencies and defective uptake or grasp. This is the time to note whether the patient is alert and responsive or dull and apathetic, whether he is friendly and cooperative or distant and reserved. The adequacy with which attention can be held, diverted or shifted from one topic to another may be seen to be abnormal. Impulsiveness, disinhibition or blunted sensitivity to social interaction are other relevant features which may emerge during the interview. The patient may be noted to tire unusually quickly with mental effort.

Behaviour in the ward can also be revealing. The patient may prove to be indifferent to events and out of contact with his surroundings, sometimes with variability from one part of the day to another. Impaired awareness of the environment may be manifest in a puzzled expression, aimless wandering, restlessness or repetitive stereotyped behaviour. Responses to various requirements and situations may reveal defects not previously suspected. He may lose his way, misidentify people or betray serious lapses of memory. Interactions with those around may reveal paranoid tendencies, or he may be observed to react to hallucinatory experiences not previously disclosed. Competence over dressing, undressing and matters of hygiene can be assessed. Disordered feeding habits can occasionally reveal the inroads of dementia in a patient with an otherwise well-preserved social manner. Any episode of incontinence will of course be noted, along with the patient's reaction towards it.

Mood

A variety of abnormalities of mood can occur with organic cerebral dysfunction, depending partly on the nature of the cerebral pathology and partly on the premorbid personality. Some forms of reaction are particularly common and immediately raise suspicion.

Clouding of consciousness is often accompanied by an inappropriate placidity and lack of concern, coupled with some degree of disinhibition. The florid hostile or fearful moods of delirium are also characteristic, often changing rapidly from one moment to another. In early dementia a quiet wondering perplexity is often the predominant mood, or emotional lability in which signs of distress resolve as abruptly as they appear.

An empty shallow quality to the emotional display should always raise suspicion of organic cerebral disease, likewise apathy in which there is little discernible emotion, and euphoria in which a mild elevation of mood is unbacked by a true sense of happy elation. Emotional blunting and flattening are other characteristic signs. These classic forms are not invariable, however. Some patients with organic brain damage show heightened and sustained anxiety or marked depressive reactions.

Characteristic emotional responses may emerge when the patient is faced with problems which tax his ability. He may over-react in an anxious aggressive manner, or alternatively become quiet, sullen and withdrawn. Goldstein (1942) described the catastrophic reaction ('katastrophenreaktion') which can be observed in such circumstances, occasionally without warning but usually heralded by increasing anxiety and tension. The patient looks dazed and starts to fumble. Whereas a moment before he was calm and amiable he now shows an intense affective response, varying from irritability and temper to outbursts of crying and despair. Autonomic disturbance is seen in the form of flushing, sweating or trembling. He may become evasive where further questions are concerned, or show a sudden aimless restlessness.

Talk and content of thought

The patient's talk, both spontaneously and in response to questions, provides a wealth of important clues. Discursive tendencies may be noted, or minor incoherence, or perseverative and paraphasic errors. Perseveration is a sign of great importance in indicating cerebral pathology; having given a response the patient repeats this inappropriately to subsequent questions, in consequence of difficulty with shifting his attention. Perseveration must be distinguished from reiteration, in which the patient continually repeats some word, phrase or question without intervention by the examiner. The formal examination for dysphasic disturbances is considered below (p. 102 *et seq.*).

There may be pressure of talk which serves as a screen to cover defects. The patient may employ denials or evasions when pressed for details about his history, or try to explain away failures with facile rationalisations. It can be important to push gently beneath a well-preserved social façade in order to determine the true extent of the inroads made by cerebral pathology.

Observation of the content of talk is the chief means of access to the patient's thought processes. A surprising poverty of thought may be revealed, or preoccupation with restricted themes. Associations may be found to be impoverished and reasoning power impaired.

Time should be spent in attempts to get as complete a picture as possible of any pathological ideas, experiences or attitudes which may be present. Paranoid tendencies are common in the presence of intellectual deterioration and ideas of reference may be marked. Delusional ideas may be stamped with certain characteristic features, as already described on pp. 11 and 15.

Perceptual distortions, illusions and hallucinations must be noted. In organic psychiatric disorders these occur chiefly in the visual modality; they tend to be commoner when sensory cues diminish towards nightfall, and may be fleeting and changeable. Feelings of familiarity or unfamiliarity may be intrusive, with depersonalisation, derealisation or *déjà vu*. Body image disorders will merit careful assessment.

The patient's attitude to his illness should always be ascertained. He may fail to recognise that he is unwell, deny any disability or take a surprisingly lighthearted view of his case. At the same time he may prove to be fully compliant over examination or admission to hospital. His own explanations for his symptoms should be determined. This alone can give important indications concerning his capacity for making realistic judgements.

Assessment of the cognitive state

The cognitive state examination can be crucial for producing evidence of an organic component in a mental illness. The number of tests and procedures available for assessing cognitive functions is rather bewildering, and it is therefore helpful to acquire a standard routine. This also has value in building up the clinician's experience of the different tests and the meaning to be put on failure in various situations. He can then formulate subjective judgements in cases where the evidence is not clear-cut; such judgements in turn are essential when deciding whether more detailed investigations should be undertaken.

Most of the brief shorthand tests employed by the psychiatrist lack adequate standardisation and validation. Indeed when their value has been tested they have often, taken individually, proved to be remarkably inefficient in distinguishing between organic and non-organic psy-

chiatric illness (Shapiro *et al.* 1956; Hinton & Withers 1971). Many prove to be closely related to the patient's educational level and general intelligence, some are markedly affected by increasing age and others by emotional disturbance. Some of the more detailed psychometric procedures elaborated by psychologists are clearly superior for the task of identifying organic psychiatric disorder, but are too cumbersome for use in every patient.

Nevertheless, the routine tests available to the clinician have a value of their own. They have the important virtue of throwing a wide net and touching upon a number of facets of cognitive function in a reasonably concise manner. In the course of administering them the examiner also obtains numerous indirect clues; the patient's behaviour while attempting the tests, and the nature of his approach, provide important information in themselves. Thus when taken in conjunction with observations gleaned during the interview there is a substantial chance that cerebral impairment will be suspected when it exists. Such suspicions can then be followed up by more decisive means.

The fact that patients with non-organic psychiatric conditions sometimes show impaired performance on the tests is paradoxically of value as well. It is important, for example, to gauge how severely concentration is impaired in depressive illness, or to observe how little impact outside events have made in a patient with severe and sustained anxiety. The routine use of the tests in every patient is therefore seldom a waste of time.

The important matter is to recognise the limitations of the tests, and to have a clear strategy for knowing how far to press the cognitive status examination in a given situation. A brief examination is described below for use in every psychiatric patient, and then a more extended battery for use when organic cerebral disease is definitely suspected.

Routine cognitive state examination*

Orientation

Orientation for time is assessed by asking the patient to name the day of the week, date, month and year. Minor degrees of temporal disorientation may be identified by asking the patient to estimate the time of day, or to estimate how much time has elapsed since the interview was started. *Impaired appreciation of the flow of time* is sometimes surprisingly revealed.   Orientation

---

* Much of the material in the sections which follow up to p. 108 has previously appeared in condensed form in the publication produced by the Departmental Teaching Committee of the Institute of Psychiatry (Notes on Eliciting and Recording Clinical Information 1973, 1987) published by Oxford University Press.

for place is assessed by asking the patient to name his present whereabouts and to give the address. Orientation for person is tested simply by asking the patient his name.

Common sense must obviously be used in administering these simple questions. It will usually have become apparent in the course of history taking if the patient is correctly orientated for place and person and these questions can therefore often be omitted. Orientation for time is worth testing in all patients, however, since this is commonly the first area to suffer in the course of mild impairment of consciousness or intellectual impairment. Latitude will obviously be required in interpreting errors with respect to date; Brotchie *et al.* (1985) showed that errors of a day or more occurred in 29% of healthy elderly subjects when orientation was accurate in other respects.

Attention and concentration

Marked difficulties with attention and concentration will usually have become apparent in the course of history taking and examination. When so it is important to *record qualitative observations in full.*

Note deficiencies in the way in which attention is *aroused* or *sustained*, whether the patient is readily *distracted* by extraneous or internal stimuli, and whether *attention fluctuates* from one moment to another. There may be difficulty in *shifting attention* from one topic or frame of reference to another, or attention may be *diffuse* so that it cannot be directed to a particular purpose. Note impairment of ability to *concentrate upon a coherent line of thought or reasoning*, or undue readiness with which powers of concentration become *fatigued*.

Brief tests which can be used to record attention and concentration include asking the patient to give the days of the week or months of the year in reverse order; recording and timing his efforts to subtract serial sevens from 100; or asking him to perform other simple tests of mental arithmetic appropriate to his level of intelligence.

The ability to repeat digits forwards and backwards provides another useful yardstick ('digit span'). The digits must be delivered in an even tone and at a rate of one per second if accurate comparisons are to be made. A start will usually be made with two or three digits forwards, increasing by one each time until the patient's limit is reached.

Memory

The ability to register, retain and retrieve information should be assessed by two or three simple tests. The patient's capacity for current memorising (new learning) has the most important clinical implications and warrants close attention.

Ask the patient to listen carefully while you tell him a name and address, then ask for its immediate reproduction. Record his answer verbatim, and repeat if necessary when the first response

is unsatisfactory. Test retrieval 3–5 minutes later after interposing other cognitive tests, and again record the answer verbatim.

Test ability to repeat a sentence immediately after a single hearing. The sentence should be appropriate to the patient's intellectual level as in the following examples from the Stanford–Binet series. Year 13: 'The aeroplane made a careful landing in the space which had been prepared for it'. Average adult: 'The red-headed woodpeckers made a terrible fuss as they tried to drive the young away from the nest'. Superior adult: 'At the end of the week the newspaper published a complete account of the experiences of the great explorer'.

If suspicion of impairment has arisen test the number of repetitions necessary for the accurate reproduction of one of Babcock's (1930) sentences: 'One thing a nation must have to become rich and great is a large secure supply of wood'. Or 'The clouds hung low in the valley and the wind howled among the trees as the men went on through the rain'. Or 'As the great red sun came over the hills the Indians broke camp and prepared for another hard day's work'. Three repetitions of one of these sentences should allow word perfect reproduction in a patient of average intelligence.

A technique similar to that of Irving *et al.* (1970) (p. 114) may be useful with patients of limited ability or when it is hard to be sure of cooperation, as follows. The patient is told he will be given the name of a flower and asked to repeat it ('The flower is—a daffodil —please repeat daffodil'), then a colour ('The colour is—blue— please repeat blue'), then a town ('The town is—Brighton'), etc. The list may continue with makes of car, days of week, etc., until some six or 10 items have been given according to the patient's ability. Recall is tested 3–5 minutes later, first without prompting then if necessary after giving each category name. This provides the opportunity for testing free recall and cued recall separately, and will sometimes demonstrate good learning ability when other techniques have failed. Perseveration is sometimes clearly displayed on the test, likewise confabulatory tendencies.

Other aspects of memory assessment are necessarily largely subjective. Discrepancies may already have emerged between the patient's account of his illness and that given by informants. *Pay special attention to memory for recent happenings and in particular for the temporal sequence of recent events.* The circumstances surrounding the patient's admission to hospital and happenings in the ward thereafter should be briefly reviewed, since these are matters about which the examiner will have independent knowledge.

Retrieval from the remote past is more difficult to evaluate, but an attempt should be made to judge the adequacy of the patient's account of his earlier life, and to examine this for evidence of gaps or inconsistencies. Care must be taken in doubtful cases to frame questions in such a way that memory for the past its truly tested. Williams (1968) points out that many of the questions which patients are asked about their earlier life can be answered in very general terms. Thus the question 'How old were you when you started school?' can produce an easy habitual response and secure a correct reply, whereas 'Can you describe your first day at school?' requires the mobilisation of actual memories.

Record any *selective impairments of memory* which become apparent in the interview for *special incidents, periods or themes* in the patient's life. *Retrograde and anterograde amnesia* must be specified in detail in relation to head injury or epileptic phenomena. Describe any evidence of *confabulation* or *false memories. Note the patient's attitude to any memory difficulties which he displays.*

General information

A brief estimate should be made of the patient's knowledge of current events, and of his ability to handle material from his long-term memory store ('utilisation of old knowledge').

Ask about recent items of interest in the news, political, sporting or otherwise, in accordance with the patient's known interests and activities. Ask him to name key personalities—members of the Royal Family, Prime Ministers, members of the cabinet or well-known television performers. (Clearly such questions will only need to be pursued when reason has emerged to doubt the patient's competence.) In patients who disclaim any interest in political or sporting events, television soap operas can provide a useful vehicle for assessment, providing of course that the examiner is adequately informed about them! Surprisingly detailed knowledge may be forthcoming in patients who have seemed to be severely impaired.

Ask for the dates of the first and second world wars, and test for knowledge of capitals and countries. In the face of poor responses pursue the patient's general knowledge further by asking for names of cities in England, rivers, etc.

If reason has emerged to suspect a disturbance of abstract thinking ask the patient to explain the difference between concepts such as 'child' and 'dwarf', 'poverty' and 'misery', 'river' and 'canal', 'lie' and 'mistake', and test ability to give the meaning behind well-known proverbs.

Intelligence

The patient's educational and occupational history, taken in conjunction with his own interests and activities, should allow a rough estimate to be made of the expected level of intelligence. *Any aspects of performance during testing which are at variance with this should be carefully noted.* Patients in hospital can usually be asked to complete the Mill Hill Vocabulary Test and Raven's Progressive Matrices (p. 112) and these may provide further evidence to uphold a suspicion of deterioration.

The above battery of tests can often be abbreviated when responses are clear and accurate from the start. It is important, however, to gain a clear understanding of the patient's capacities under each of these headings whatever form the presenting illness may take. Much will have been learned about the patient's grasp and efficiency, and about his reactions and approach to problems. Covert organic disorders may be revealed, and obvious cerebral impairment will have been charted in a preliminary and valuable way.

The headings employed are not, of course, mutually exclusive. Orientation for time and place is closely bound up with current memorising ability and with clarity and coherence of thought. The tests of orientation as described above are nevertheless very useful, and have repeatedly emerged as among the most discriminating features in the mental state examination for distinguishing between organic and non-organic psychiatric disorders (Shapiro *et al.* 1956; Hinton & Withers 1971). Sometimes they have even been found to compare favourably with more elaborate and time-consuming psychometric procedures (Irving *et al.* 1970).

Attention is not a clearly defined concept and overlaps with functions described as alertness, awareness and responsiveness (Klein & Mayer-Gross 1957). It is nonetheless widely accepted as a clinically useful concept, with particular relevance to general mental acuity and minor impairment of consciousness. Concentration is a similarly imprecise term, referring to capacity for focusing and sustaining mental activity on the task in hand. Both stand to be markedly affected by preoccupations or abnormalities of mood, and can therefore be disturbed in many forms of psychiatric illness. Equally, however, they can give important indications of clouding of consciousness or general intellectual impairment.

It will be noted that simple tests of arithmetic form an integral part of the tests for attention and concentration, and this in itself can be valuable in revealing marked defects in numerical ability. The digit repetition test is included in this section, rather than in the assessment of memory, since it is well established that the immediate memory span is usually normal in amnesic subjects (Zangwill 1946; Milner 1966).

The assessment of memory is of the utmost importance, since memory failure is a particularly sensitive indicator of cerebral dysfunction. It is here that the most decisive evidence of an organic component in the illness will often be obtained. Fortunately for clinical practice, the aspect of memory that is most amenable to careful testing is also the aspect most vulnerable to cerebral dysfunction, namely the capacity for acquiring and retaining new information.

The section on general information extends the evaluation of memory, and at the same time brings added information against which to judge the likelihood of generalised intellectual impairment.

Extended cognitive state examination

The examination described above is adequate for routine psychiatric practice. The abnormalities which emerge will need to be evaluated against the total picture presented by the patient—sometimes they will raise the possibility of organic cerebral disorder, but quite often they will be attributable to factors such as low intelligence, emotional disturbance or psychotic thought disorder. More latitude will then be allowed for failure. When, however, they raise a strong suspicion of organic psychiatric illness more thoroughgoing evaluation will be required as described below.

In certain situations this will be undertaken from the outset—when, for example, there is doubt from the beginning over the differentiation between organic and non-organic psychiatric disorder, or when the clinical presentation immediately suggests the presence of cerebral dysfunction. The approach must then be more systematic and comprehensive. In particular it must embrace the possibilities of circumscribed defects of higher mental function due to focal brain pathology.

Some points of caution must be observed before embarking on the extended cognitive state examination. The examination can be lengthy and fatigue may produce misleading results; the procedures should not be hurried, and several brief sessions are usually preferable to a single long drawn-out examination. Secondly, the examiner must remain sensitive to the patient's reactions to failure. A particular test must sometimes be set aside for a while in the interests of sustaining cooperation; tests which are pressed too firmly may provoke 'catastrophic reactions' or bewilder the patient to the point where useful information is no longer obtained. Thirdly, the tests must be adapted to the patient's intelligence and educational level, and to his particular difficulties. Finally, it is essential to remain aware that one disability may have repercussions upon performance at other tasks. Defective comprehension, for example, will cloud the issue when it comes to testing for dyspraxia. Allowance will need to be made for this in the selection of the tests, the order of their administration and the assessment of results.

Consequently, it is helpful to have a simple routine at the outset which allows the key area of function to be assessed in an abbreviated fashion, before proceeding to lengthier parts of the examination:

First, take careful note of the patient's *level of cooperation*. His willingness to apply himself to the test procedures will be fundamental to the amount of reliable information that can be obtained.

Make a preliminary assessment of the *level of conscious awareness*. This must have an early priority since performance on all other tests may be affected by minor degrees of clouding of consciousness.

Next assess *language functions*. Much of what follows will depend upon the accuracy of verbal communication. In addition to noting verbal ability during conversation and history taking, ask the patient to name a series of objects and to perform a series of simple commands.

Memory functions, if not already tested, should be briefly examined as already described.

Visuospatial ability should always be screened because non-verbal deficits of this nature may otherwise remain concealed. Ask the patient to copy simple designs such as those illustrated on p. 104.

Test the integrity of *volitional movements* and at the same time of *right–left orientation* by asking the patient to point to various parts of the body. Ask him for example to 'Touch your left ear with your left hand', 'Touch your left knee with your right hand', etc.

This overture to the detailed examination will often save a good deal of time and avoid confusion later. It will chart important areas of disability and go some way towards exonerating others. The significance of failures during later more detailed testing will then be more readily appreciated.

Thereafter, individual areas of cognitive function must be systematically explored, with the aim of covering each of the sections described below. Some areas will need to be dealt with in detail and others more briefly. Those which require most careful assessment in the particular patient will by now be apparent—attention will have been directed towards them by the history, the neurological examination and the cognitive deficits already displayed.

Level of conscious awareness

Impairment of consciousness is obvious when there is frank drowsiness or somnolence during examination. It is over the detection of minor degrees that difficulties are encountered. There are no pathognomonic signs or tests for minor impairment of consciousness, and its detection is largely a matter for subjective clinical judgement based on a variety of clues:

Record any obvious impairment in the form of drowsiness or diminished awareness of the environment. Note fluctuations during examination, and question relatives or nursing staff about changes which occur from time to time during the day. Impairment may only become obvious towards nightfall or when the patient is fatigued.

Minor impairment will be suspected when the patient is dull, inert and uncertain in behaviour even though he is not drowsy, or when responses to external events are diminished. There may be a vagueness and hesitancy about the manner of speaking. Once the examiner suspects a reduction of the level of consciousness it can be helpful to repeat questions concerning dates and names of places, with the object of seeing whether consistent answers are given. Tests of orientation, attention, concentration and memory may be poorly performed, often with variability from one occasion to another. Judgement of the passage of time will often be markedly inaccurate. Attention will usually be ill sustained and ill focused, and the patient may tend to lose the thread in conversation. Lucid intervals may emerge from time to time and form a marked contrast to the general tenor of behaviour. Even when seemingly alert it may be discovered that the patient has failed to register on-going experiences, including those of the interview itself.

Simple procedures may be employed in order to assess capacity for sustained attention or 'vigilance' over a period of time. The patient may be asked, for example, to raise his hand whenever an 'A' is spoken, and a series of letters are then delivered in an even tone and at a constant rate. A more difficult version will consist in raising the hand whenever any vowel is spoken, or whenever two vowels succeed one another. A written form of the test can easily be made by asking the patient to cancel all letters of a designated type on a printed sheet or in a passage of prose material.

If somnolent, can the patient be roused to full or only partial awareness? If his attention cannot be sustained does he drift back towards sleep or does his attention wander onto other topics? When consciousness is severely impaired describe the nature of the stimulus required to evoke a response (for example conversation, firm commands, commands following arousal by shaking, painful stimuli) and the character of the response produced (for example a correct verbal reply or motor act, an incorrect and muddled response, failure to respond to commands but accurate localisation of a painful stimulus, ill-coordinated and ineffectual motor movements). The Glasgow Coma Scale (p. 167) will prove of value for monitoring progress in patients with seriously impaired consciousness.

Evidence for 'delirium', 'stupor' or 'coma' should be specified in detail.

Language functions

Language functions are conveniently examined under the six headings described below. Thorough examination of dysphasic disturbances can take a considerable time, but in the non-dysphasic subject screening need take only a few minutes.

At the onset it is important to *note whether the patient is predominantly right- or left-handed,* otherwise this important item of information may come to be overlooked.

Motor aspects of speech

Note the quality of spontaneous speech and that in reply to questions. Minor expressive speech defects may only emerge when the patient is pressed to engage in conversation, to describe his work, his house, or some event in his life.

Is there any disturbance of articulation (dysarthria)? When slight dysarthria is suspected test ability to pronounce a phrase such as 'West Register Street'.

Is there slowness or hesitancy with speech production and is the output sparse? Or conversely, is the output excessive with a definite pressure of speech (logorrhoea)?

Does he use wrong words, words which are nearly but not exactly correct, or words that do not exist? *Paraphasic errors* may be defined as 'substitutions within language' (Benson & Geschwind 1971) and exist in several forms; they may involve the substitution of one correct word for another, the distortion of one syllable within a word, or the production of a group of sounds with no specific meaning (neologisms).

Note whether words are omitted and sentences abbreviated (telegram style). Are there inaccuracies of grammatical construction (paragrammatisms)? Is the normal rhythm and inflexion of speech disturbed (dysprosody)? Is speech totally disorganised and incomprehensible (jargon aphasia)?

Observe carefully for perseverative errors of speech (p. 97). Also for reiteration of phrases just spoken (echolalia), of single words (pallilalia) or of a terminal syllable (logoclonia).

When defects are found test whether automatic speech or the naming of serials is better preserved than conversational speech — ask him to repeat a well-known nursery rhyme or prayer, to count to 20, or to give the days of the week. Are emotional utterances or ejaculations preserved when formal speech is defective?

From the phenomenological point of view, Benson and Geschwind (1971) recommend a basic division into *fluent and non-fluent forms of dysphasic speech,* the former characterising posterior lesions and the latter anterior lesions. Fluent dysphasias in general show clear articulation, the words are produced without effort, output is normal or excessive, paraphasic errors are frequent, phrase length is not curtailed, and normal rhythm and inflexion are preserved. Non-fluent dysphasias show poor articulation, the speech is produced with obvious difficulty, output is sparse but nonetheless the content is meaningful when this can be discerned, phrase length is reduced to one or two words, and the rhythm and inflexion are disturbed.

Comprehension of speech

The understanding of speech must be separately assessed, whether or not production is defective. Even when the patient is mute or his utterances totally incomprehensible it is still necessary to determine whether he can understand what is said to him.

Can he point correctly on command to objects around him? Can he carry out simple orders on request, for example pick up an object, show his tongue? Failure can be misleading since it may be due to dyspraxia; thus if commands are not carried out test whether he can signal his response to simple 'yes–no' questions.

Can he respond to more complex instructions, for example walk over to the door and come back again, or take his spectacles from his pocket and put them on the table. Can he follow a series of commands sequentially, for example go to the window, tap it twice, turn around, then come back again.

Marie's Three Paper Test is widely employed for the rapid assessment of mild comprehension defects. Three pieces of paper of different sizes are put before the patient. He is told to take the largest and hand it to the examiner, take the smallest and throw it to the ground, and take the middle-sized piece and put it in his pocket.

The understanding of prepositional and syntactic aspects of speech can be a sensitive indicator of minor comprehension difficulties. It is readily tested by providing the patient with three objects such as a book, pen and coin, then issuing increasingly complex instructions as follows: 'Put the coin on the book; put the coin and the pen under the book; tap the book and then the coin with the pen; put the book between the pen and the coin; place the book over the coin then put the pen inside it', etc.

If comprehension of spoken speech is defective, test whether understanding of written words and instructions is better preserved. *Test whether other hearing functions are intact*, for example the startle response to sudden noise. Test for *auditory agnosia* by noting whether the patient can recognise non-verbal noises—clapping hands, snapping fingers, jingling money—or copy the production of such sounds when they are made outside the field of vision.

Repetition of speech

Can the patient repeat digits, words, short phrases or sentences exactly as you give them? The classic phrase for testing repetition is 'No ifs, ands or buts'. Successful repetition involves both motor and sensory parts of the speech apparatus and also the connections between the two. Failure in repetition may occur despite adequate spontaneous articulation and good comprehension. Paraphasic errors often emerge most clearly in the testing of repetition.

Word finding

Does the patient have difficulty in finding words during conversation, or use circumlocutions? Test specifically for nominal dysphasia by asking him to name both common and uncommon objects (for example the parts of a wrist watch, and other objects in the room). Include an examination of his ability to name colours.

Nominal dysphasia may be the only language disturbance in patients with cerebral damage and must therefore always be tested with care. Newcombe *et al.* (1965) have shown that the ease of word finding is inversely related to the frequency of occurrence of the word in the language, and that the detection of slight nominal dysphasia requires testing with objects whose names occur at a frequency of less than one per 100 000 words. The latter include words such as 'buckle', 'pointer' or 'dial', but not 'watch' or 'strap'; 'lapel' or 'knuckle', but not 'button' or 'finger'; 'radiator' or 'linoleum', but not 'picture' or 'carpet' (Thorndike & Lorge 1944).

Reading

Present the patient with the written names of objects in the room and ask him to point to them. If this is performed correctly present him with written instructions to perform specific actions.

Test his ability to read aloud, and determine whether he understands what he has read. If the patient fails to read aloud it is still necessary to assess whether he has read, since some dysphasics comprehend well even though they fail to read aloud.

Table 1 Performance on tests of language function in different varieties of dysphasia (after Benson & Geschwind 1971).

	Spontaneous speech	Comprehension	Repetition	Naming	Reading	Writing
Pure word-deafness	F	−	−	+	+	+ (not to dictation)
Pure word-blindness (alexia without agraphia)	F	+	+	+	−	+
Pure word-dumbness	NF	+	−	±	+	+
Pure agraphia (agraphia without alexia)	F	+	+	+	+	−
Primary sensory (Wernicke's) dysphasia	F	−	−	±	−	−
Primary motor (Broca's) dysphasia	NF	±	−	±	Aloud − Compr ±	−
Nominal dysphasia	F	+	+	−	±	±
Conduction dysphasia	F	+	−	±	Aloud − Compr +	−
Isolation syndrome	NF	−	+	−	−	−
Transcortical motor dysphasia	NF	+	±	−	Aloud − Compr +	−
Transcortical sensory dysphasia	F	−	+	−	−	−
Alexia with agraphia (visual asymbolia)	F	+	+	+	−	−

Compr, comprehension; F, fluent speech productions; NF, non-fluent speech productions.

Writing

Test ability to write spontaneously and to dictation. Examine written productions for substitutions, perseverations, spelling errors and letter reversals. Is copying better preserved than writing to dictation? Is spelling out loud better preserved than spelling on paper? Is the writing of habitual material (signature, address) relatively intact? Are numbers written more accurately than words or letters?

The main syndromes of language impairment can be distinguished by the pattern of breakdown in the above examination. Table 1 on p. 103 summarises performance on the different tests of language function in relation to the syndromes of dysphasia described in Chapter 2.

Verbal fluency

Verbal fluency must be separately assessed, even when there is no other form of language disturbance, since fluency is characteristically impaired with frontal lesions (Benton 1968; Perret 1974; Lezak 1995).

A simple technique is to ask the patient to give as many words as he can think of beginning with a certain letter of the alphabet, for example 1 minute for words beginning with F, then 1 minute for A and 1 minute for S. The total achieved on this 'FAS test' should be in excess of 30. Norms are available in relation to the patient's age and educational level (see Lezak 1995). Alternatively, the patient may be asked to give the names of animals or the names of objects found in a kitchen.

The number of words accomplished will often be strikingly low even though there is no evidence of dysphasia. This accords with the impoverishment of spontaneous speech which may be observed with frontal lesions. It can be necessary to allow the patient a full minute over his attempts at each category, since words may be rapidly produced initially then tail off in noteworthy fashion. The effect is more pronounced with left frontal lesions than right. Corresponding deficits can also be demonstrated on a 'design fluency test', but in this case the task is more affected by right frontal lesions than left (Jones-Gotman & Milner 1977).

Number functions

Test the patient's ability to perform simple arithmetical operations—addition, subtraction, multiplication, division—in relation to his educational and occupational background. Assess his ability to handle money correctly.

Can he count objects and make a rough estimate of the number of matches laid before him? Can he give the average size and weight of a man? Can he estimate the size of various objects in the room?

Test his ability to read and write numbers of two and more digits.

Memory

Full examination of memory will always be required along the lines already set out on p. 99. Special attention should be directed at recent memory and new learning ability.

A convenient and sensitive method for supplementing the assessment of new learning ability consists of testing the patient's capacity for learning supra-span lists of digits (Drachman & Arbit 1966; Warrington 1970). The normal digit span is first determined (as on p. 99), then ability to extend the list by one or two items is assessed by repeated presentations. Amnesic subjects can perform adequately on the straightforward digit span test, but show a dramatic breakdown in performance as soon as this is exceeded.

Simple paired-associate learning may also be tested, using for example the pairs described by Isaacs and Walkey (1964), as outlined on p. 114.

Non-verbal memory should be tested in addition to verbal memory by asking the patient to reproduce simple geometrical figures (such as those shown below) after an interval of 5 minutes.

Visuospatial and constructional difficulties

Patients with visuospatial agnosia may make no complaints, thus failing to direct attention towards the problem. It is important, therefore, to include tests which betray such difficulties when a cerebral lesion is suspected.

Test the patient's ability to judge the relation between objects in space—to estimate distances, to say which of two objects is nearer to him, and which is larger. Can he with eyes closed indicate the spatial order of objects in the room around him?

Visuospatial agnosia is often associated with constructional dyspraxia and the distinction between the two defects is usually far from clear-cut (see pp. 61–2). Constructional dyspraxia is tested as follows.

Test ability to connect two dots by a straight line, and to find the middle of a straight line and of a circle. Test ability to draw simple figures such as a square, circle and triangle. Ask the patient to copy a series of line drawings of increasing complexity such as those shown below.

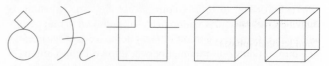

The test may be made more difficult by removing the model and asking the patient to draw the figure from immediate memory.

Ask him to draw a house, a bicycle, a clock face and set the hands, and to indicate the principal towns on a rough map of England. Note particularly whether he shows neglect of one half of visual space or crowds material into one part of the paper.

Test ability to construct simple figures when presented with sticks or matches. Can he construct a triangle and a square, or copy more complex designs?

Can the patient assemble a simple jig-saw puzzle, or reassemble a piece of paper which has been cut into several fragments?

If available test the patient's ability to reproduce patterns with Kohs' blocks.

The copying of a range of geometrical figures has the virtue of being graded in difficulty and of providing a permanent record. Most normal subjects will succeed in copying at least the first four of the figures illustrated above. Free drawing of a house or bicycle has the advantage of being more natural and also more difficult. It often reveals more subtle forms of defect, but can be hard to interpret since normal individuals vary considerably in drawing skill. Sometimes highly characteristic defects may emerge, as when windows are placed in the roof or outside the main body of the building. The drawing of a clock is particularly useful in showing how accurately the figures can be spaced around the dial, or in revealing unilateral neglect of space by the omission of figures from one half of the dial. The use of sticks and other materials for constructional tasks gives the opportunity to observe the patient's capacity to improve his performance and to alter mistakes.

Other agnosic disturbances

Other forms of agnosia are very rare. Before concluding that agnosia is present it is essential to try to exclude impairments of primary perception as the cause of failure on a test (such as impaired visual acuity, field defects or deafness). Firm indications of an agnosic problem will often be obtained by finding that an object which cannot be identified through one sensory modality is immediately identified through another.

Can the patient describe what he sees and identify objects and persons? Ask him to name a particular object in a group exposed to view and to describe its use, or if dysphasic, to indicate its use (*visual object agnosia*). If he fails, test whether he can identify the object by other senses such as touch. Ask him to name the colours of objects, to indicate their colour on a chart and to group objects according to their colour (*colour agnosia*). Ask him to describe a meaningful situation in a picture shown to him (*simultanagnosia*). Is his recognition of faces defective (*prosopagnosia*)? Ask him to point out a named person known to him among a group or to name photographs of relatives or of well-known public figures.

Auditory agnosia will already have been assessed (see under comprehension of speech, p. 103).

Tactile agnosia is tested by asking the patient to identify objects by touch with the eyes closed. Each hand must be tested separately. Care must be taken that other sensory information (such as the rattle of money) does not give the necessary clue for identification. Ask him to name the objects and to describe their shape, texture and use. In the event of failure, test whether the objects can then be identified by vision. If dysphasic, his responses must be assessed by testing selection from a group of objects exposed to view.

Dyspraxia and related disturbances

Before diagnosing dyspraxia it is essential to make sure that the patient's difficulties cannot be explained on the basis of muscular weakness, incoordination or profound sensory disturbance. Many dyspraxic patients are also dysphasic, so care must be taken to check whether instructions are understood. To prove the existence of dyspraxia it is necessary to show that a movement not made under one set of conditions (e.g. on command) can be performed under others (e.g. spontaneously), or that movements of equal or greater complexity can be made under other circumstances. It is also necessary to exclude simple unwillingness to cooperate. Because of the complexities of this area of dysfunction it is advisable in all cases to make a careful note of what the patient does, how he does it and what he fails to do (Critchley 1953). The examination should test the integrity of learned movements both to command and to imitation. It must also encompass the capacity for making familiar gestures, and for using objects in pantomime and in reality.

Test the patient's ability to carry out purposeful movements to command, such as holding out the arms, crossing legs, showing teeth, screwing up eyes or nodding the head. Test each hand separately for making a fist, opposition of thumb and little finger, pronation and supination ('ideomotor dyspraxia').

Test ability to rise from a chair on command and to turn around ('whole body dyspraxia').

Test ability to imitate postures of the hand and arm demonstrated by the examiner, and to adopt with one limb the posture imposed on the other.

Test expressive and make-believe movements such as knocking at a door or waving goodbye. Ask the patient to demonstrate how he would brush his teeth, use a hammer or kick a ball.

Test the patient's ability to carry out complex coordinated sequences of movements, such as taking a match from a box and striking it, winding a watch, cutting with scissors, or folding a piece of paper and putting it in an envelope ('ideational dyspraxia').

Does the patient show undue difficulty with dressing and undressing, get muddled when inserting limbs into clothing, or try to put garments on the wrong way round ('dressing dyspraxia')?

Tests of frontal lobe function

When frontal damage is suspected certain tests are specially indicated. Many of these tap 'executive functions', in that they examine the initiation, planning and regulation of goal-directed behaviours. Others assess capacities for abstract thinking, categorisation or judgement. Only some are suitable for bedside examination, which will therefore often need to be supplemented by neuropsychological tests as described on p. 118 *et seq*.

Verbal fluency should be assessed as on p. 104.

Luria's motor tests reflect the dynamic organisation of the motor act (Luria 1966). The most suitable are those which require the subject to perform a simple series of movements whose components follow in a connected alternating sequence. These are particularly disturbed by premotor frontal lesions:

Reciprocal coordination of the hands is tested by asking the patient to place both hands before him, one with the fist clenched and the other with the fingers extended. He is then asked to change the position of both hands simultaneously, extending the first and clenching the other. The smoothness and speed of the alternating actions is observed; he may break the task down and perform each movement separately, or perform similar movements with both hands so that reciprocal coordination is lost.

Alternating tapping is tested by asking the patient to alternately tap twice with the right hand and once with the left hand in an on-going alternating sequence.

A single limb may be tested by asking the patient alternately to make a fist and a ring with the fingers of the hand.

Alternating written sequences may be tested by asking the patient to draw a design composed of two alternating components, for example: x o x o x o x o x o, or in cursive script: u n u n u n u n u n.

An alternating choice task has similarly been shown to be sensitive to frontal lesions (Stevenson 1967). A simple version consists of asking the patient to predict in which of the examiner's hands a coin is hidden, when this is alternated R L R L R L or R R L L R R L L.

Capacity for abstract thinking should be tested by asking for the meaning of well-known proverbs, and for differences between concepts as described on p. 100.

The Cognitive Estimates Test (p. 119) assesses the patient's capacity for making realistic practical judgements of size and number:

Ask, for example: What is the largest object normally found in a house? What is the best paid job in Britain today? How fast do race horses gallop? How tall is the average English woman?

'Imitation and utilization behaviour' have been described in patients with frontal lesions, particularly those involving orbital parts of one or both lobes (Lhermitte 1983; Lhermitte *et al.* 1986). Both reflect pathological dependence on environmental stimuli:

With imitation behaviour the patient imitates the examiner's gestures and activities without being told to do so. On questioning he states that he thought he had to imitate the examiner, but may continue to do so after being told that it is unnecessary. Note, for example whether the patient copies gestures (bending the head and resting the chin on the hand, tapping the leg with the hand, crossing the legs, saluting) or simple activities (folding a sheet of paper, putting on spectacles, smelling a flower).

Utilization behaviour reflects a more severe disturbance, extending to objects in the physical environment. Everyday objects are presented visually or tactually to the patient, without speaking, and his response observed. In the presence of a frontal lesion the patient may seem compelled to grasp and use the objects. When presented with a paper and pen, for example, the patient takes the pen and writes; when given spectacles he puts them on; when a jug of water and a glass are advanced towards him he pours the water and drinks it. Once started the patient may continue using objects presented to him in this manner, persisting even after being told that this is not required.

Behavioural observations can be equally important in pointing to frontal dysfunction. Note whether the patient is apathetic, disinhibited, unkempt or lacking in normal social graces.

Topographical sense and right–left orientation

Does the patient have difficulty in finding his way about the ward (topographical disorientation)? Does he confuse his bed with other people's? Can he describe the relations between parts of the ward or of his own house? Can he describe the route from home to hospital? If necessary test his ability to follow a simple route in the ward or hospital.

Can the patient point on command to objects around him on the right and on the left? Ask him to move on command right and left parts of the body, and to point to individual parts on the right and left side of his own body, and of the examiner sitting opposite him. Can he perform complex instructions like 'touch your right ear with your left hand', 'pick up the left hand coin with your left hand and place it in my right hand'?

Body image disturbances

Body image disturbances will often be revealed by the patient's behaviour or his own subjective complaints, but sometimes special tests or questions will be required to elicit them. Asking the patient to make a rough drawing of a man will sometimes give the first indication of body image disorder (Cohn 1960).

Test for *finger agnosia*. Ask the patient to move on command or point to individual fingers—his own and the examiner's. Kinsbourne and Warrington (1962b) describe various tests which have proved to be more sensitive indicators of finger agnosia than the conventional tests. In one such, two of the patient's fingers are touched simultaneously and he is asked to state how many fingers lie between them.

Test for disturbance of identification of other body parts (*autotopagnosia*). Ask the patient to move on command and to name various parts of his body, to point to them and to parts of the examiner's body.

Note any evidence of *unilateral unawareness or neglect* of the body. When present this will usually involve the left side. Does the patient utilize the left hand normally in bimanual activities? Is the left side of the body relatively neglected in washing, combing or dressing? When attention is drawn to such defects does he recognise them and correct them?

Determine whether he has unusual subjective sensations or beliefs about the limbs of one half of the body. Do they feel as though absent or changed, either intermittently or continuously (*hemisomatognosia*)?

Does the patient ignore or show lack of concern about an injured or functionally defective part of the body, for example a left hemiparesis or hemianopic field defect (*anosognosia*)? He may verbally deny the defect or deny ownership of the affected body part.

Other general indications of organic cerebral disorder

Note the ability of the patient to *sustain attention* during the above test procedures. Did he *fatigue unduly easily*? Was he able to *shift attention* readily from one task to another? Did he show *perseveration* in the use of words or in response to commands (p. 97)? Note and describe any evidence of *lability of mood* or *euphoria*. Were emotional responses *exaggerated, flattened or lacking*? When confronted with a task beyond his ability did he show evidence of a *catastrophic reaction* (p. 97)? Did he show *impulsiveness, disinhibition or over-familiarity* at any point during the testing? Did the patient *appreciate his failings* and show *appropriate concern*? Did he use *evasions* or *excuses* to cover up his deficits?

Examination of the mute or apparently inaccessible patient

States of mutism, 'stupor' and apparent inaccessibility may be due to organic brain disease or to psychiatric disorders such as depression, catatonic schizophrenia or conversion hysteria. In all cases it is necessary to carry out a *detailed neurological examination* and to assess the apparent *level of conscious awareness* (as outlined on pp. 101–2) before considering other aspects of the problem.

The differential diagnosis of stupor is considered on p. 155 *et seq*. In addition to the intracerebral causes it is essential to bear in mind the possibilities of physical illness such as uraemia, hypoglycaemia or myxoedema, and to examine for physical complications of stupor such as hypotension or retention of urine. It is also important to remember that in stupors due to non-organic psychiatric illness the patient's comprehension of remarks made in his presence may be intact despite appearances to the contrary.

Stupor, semicoma and hypersomnia

The definitions of these terms are not sufficiently precise to be used as the sole description of the phenomena they comprise. The following features should therefore be described separately:

To what extent does the patient dress, feed himself or co-operate with feeding, and attend to matters of hygiene and elimination?

Are the eyes open or shut? If open, are they apparently watchful and do they follow moving objects? If shut, do they open in response to stimulation, and is there resistance to passive opening?

Assess the patient's response to graded stimulation as outlined on p. 102. When aroused does he become briefly alert and verbally responsive?

Is the physical posture comfortable, constrained, awkward, bizarre, or in any way indicative of possible delusional beliefs? Does the patient resume a previous posture if moved or when placed in an awkward position? Do movements display special meaning, for example on a possible delusional basis or in response to hallucinatory experiences?

Is the facial expression constant or varying, alert or vacant, blank or meaningful? Is it secretive, withdrawn, indicative of sadness, hopelessness or ecstasy; does it betray attention to hallucinatory experiences?

Is there any physical or emotional reaction to what is said or done to the patient or within his hearing? Does he show an emotional response when sensitive subjects are discussed? Does he show signs of irritation or annoyance when moved against his wishes?

Examine the state of the musculature. Is it relaxed or rigid? Is rigidity increased by passive movements? Examine for negativism, flexibilitas cerea, automatic obedience and echopraxia. Note evidence of resistiveness, irritability or defensive movements during examination.

In the neurological examination pay special attention to evidence of raised intracranial pressure or of diencephalic or upper brain stem disturbance: thus examine for papilloedema, observe equality and reactivity of pupils, note quality of respiration, look for evidence of long tract deficit in the limbs, and test for conjugate reflex eye movements on passive head rotation.

After recovery, examine for memory of events occurring during the abnormal phase and for fantasies or other subjective experiences occurring at the time.

Mutism

'Mutism' is a condition in which the person does not speak and makes no attempt at spoken communication despite preservation of an adequate level of consciousness. It may sometimes be the only abnormality in otherwise normal behaviour.

Is it elective, confined to some situations, or in relation to some persons but not others? Is the patient disturbed by it as shown by gesticulations or evidence of distress? Does he attempt to communicate by signs? When offered paper and pen does he communicate in writing?

Distinguish mutism from severe motor dysphasia, dysarthria, aphonia, poverty of speech or severe psychomotor retardation. Is partial vocalisation preserved, are emotional ejaculations possible, can simple 'yes–no' answers be given? Test separately for ability to articulate (to whisper or make the lip movements of speech) and ability to phonate (to produce coarse vocalisations or to hum). Can he cough? Does he speak very occasionally and briefly on restricted themes? Does he reply or signal responses to some questions but only after a long delay? In the distinction from dysphasia it is important to remember that the most profoundly dysphasic patient is never mute; he is always able to make some speech sounds, even if these are restricted to crude syllabic stereotypies or repeated expletives (Benson 1973).

A careful history from informants may sometimes enable distinctions to be made more readily than from examination alone.

Psychometric assessment

The clinical value of psychological testing in the field of organic psychiatry has been much debated. Overenthusiastic claims have sometimes followed the introduction of new tests and procedures for the identification of cerebral dysfunction, and have had to be tempered later in the light of experience. But even when the claims themselves have been modest the psychiatrist has often misunderstood the situation, and has expected a degree of exactitude from psychometric testing that is unrealistic. The experience of the present author has been that collaboration with clinical psychologists is extremely helpful, both in diagnosis and in management, provided a jointly balanced view is taken of the situation. In the diagnosis of brain damage the psychiatrist's and the psychologist's approach are both in their own ways fallible, but each may usefully supplement the other.

The limitations of psychometric tests must be appreciated. There appears to be no single test that will differentiate brain-damaged patients from others without some degree of overlap, and even the most skilful selection of groups of tests will occasionally produce misleading results. Accordingly, test results should only be interpreted in conjunction with all other sources of information relevant to the issue in question. The worst service to psychometry, and to the patient, is likely to come from attempts to rely on test scores viewed in isolation. Similar disappointment would be expected to follow if any clinical diagnostic procedure were singled out and given unique importance. It is essential, therefore, to retain a 'general clinical impression' as a back-up to the detailed findings.

Advantages

As diagnostic instruments, psychological tests have certain definite advantages over the ordinary procedures of clinical assessment. The tests can be given in strictly standardised form and the results are usually scored numerically. Hence they can be validated on large groups of patients, so that norms can be established and the extent of individual variation gauged with some precision. In these respects they represent a marked advance on the psychiatrist's assessment of the mental state. With their aid one can talk meaningfully in terms of *probabilities* where the presence or absence of brain damage is concerned, and the level of probability is often crucial in deciding what action to pursue. Similarly, the measures can be repeated on more than one occasion, permitting accurate comparisons over an interval of time. This can be invaluable when equivocal findings have emerged at the first consultation; after establishing a baseline the patient's progress can be charted with some accuracy, and any evidence of decline will be highlighted.

Psychological testing can also concentrate in detail on an individual area of functioning which has come under suspicion. Minor degrees of memory impairment or verbal disability, for example, can be pursued with much more thoroughness by psychometric tests than in the clinical interview. The structure of such deficits can also be explored in greater detail. It is here that the psychologist must sometimes be prepared to sacrifice the rigid standardisation of his approach in order to follow the leads that emerge. Piercy (1959) has argued cogently that some kinds of evidence are better assessed by an experienced human observer than by a standardised procedure; the nature of the failure can be important and this is not always obvious from the score alone. In other words, the advantages of the standardised approach must not be allowed to become an unduly restrictive influence or valuable information will sometimes be lost.

Limitations

Some fundamental difficulties concerning tests for brain damage are discussed by Yates (1954, 1966), Smith (1962) and Lezak (1995). Modern tests represent a distinct advance on their forerunners, but certain in-built difficulties remain.

Typically a test is standardised on groups of subjects known to be suffering from brain damage, and groups in whom this is known to be absent by independent criteria. A highly satisfactory level of discrimination is frequently achieved, and the test is then further validated on a separate population. However, the efficiency of the test has still emerged only where clear-cut cases are concerned. In clinical use the test will often be applied to borderline problems in which other evidence of brain damage is equivocal, and here it will not yet have established its credentials. The indications that it gives about the presence or absence of brain damage must still be viewed with caution, and may be no more valid than the clinical evidence which led to the patient being referred for testing. For this reason expectations must not be unrealistic. The difficulty in establishing the sensitivity of the test in equivocal cases lies in the problem of obtaining a final arbiter of brain damage. Follow up of disputed cases can help by displaying the *predictive* value of the test, but such studies have not been carried out extensively.

A separate problem arises from the fact that all tests require a certain level of attention and cooperation. Consequently they are vulnerable to emotional disturbance and other influences which have nothing to do with brain damage. Tests which distinguish well between brain-damaged and healthy subjects may, therefore, give misleading results when applied to certain psychiatric patients. Depression, for example, may disrupt performance on sensitive tests of memory, and schizophrenic thought disorder may lead to poor performance on tests of abstract thinking. Thus any test which is to be usefully employed for differential diagnosis between organic and non-organic psychiatric illness must first be standardised on patients suffering from a wide range of mental disorders. It is at this point that many excellent tests fail to uphold their promise.

Common misconceptions have also concerned the nature of brain damage itself, and the constancy of its relationship to the behavioural deficits that follow. Tests have sometimes relied heavily on unitary theories of cerebral dysfunction, and many of those put forward as global indicators of 'brain damage' pay little regard to what is known of regional cerebral organisation. The aim has often been to identify a fundamental disturbance of function which would emerge in every case, no matter what the extent, location or nature of the responsible brain damage. But no one defect or set of deficits can be expected to emerge in all brain-injured individuals. Thus tests which sample a restricted aspect of cognitive activity may fail to identify cerebral lesions which are sufficiently circumscribed to leave that particular function intact. Purely verbal tests, for example, may fail to detect visuo-spatial difficulties resulting from a restricted lesion of the non-dominant hemisphere. Even with diffuse brain damage the behavioural effects that follow may vary at different levels of functional disorganisation, so that tests which tap one hierarchical level of behaviour may fail entirely to tap another. Many of the differences between

one validation study and another would appear to arise from difficulties of this type. The greater the number of functions sampled by the test, the greater will be its usefulness as a general screening device, though a price will then usually be paid in that it will be less sensitive at detecting minor degrees of dysfunction in restricted areas of cognitive activity.

In some circumstances, the identification of patterns of impairment on different tests can be of more value than indicators of brain damage generally. McFie (1960) pointed out that psychologists had been rather slow to proceed from neurological knowledge and examine whether disturbances of higher cortical function, as revealed by tests, could be used as a guide to local cerebral injury. His own survey of cases from the National Hospital, Queen Square, gave indications that this was a fruitful line of enquiry. Left parietal lesions, for example, were associated with special difficulty with arithmetic, digit span and sentence learning; right parietal lesions with picture arrangement and memory for designs. On tests of learning and retention the impairment depended to a considerable extent on the nature of the material to be learned—verbal material was mainly affected by left-sided lesions (especially left temporal) and visual material by right-sided lesions (particularly right parietal). When the material to be retained was neither verbal nor visual, as in the estimation of the passage of time, the impairments appeared to have general rather than focal associations. Such regional associations have since been explored further, as described at many points in Chapter 2. Their importance in the present context is to stress that psychometric testing can occasionally be useful in viewing the patient's performance, not so much in terms of deviation from statistical normality, as in terms of conformity with a recognised syndrome of cognitive deficits (Piercy 1959). In such an exercise the identification of brain damage will depend much less on carefully validated norms, but will closely follow the strategies of clinical enquiry generally.

Applications

From the foregoing it will be clear that the questions asked of the psychologist must be realistic, and should reflect some knowledge both of the limitations and special advantages of the psychometric procedures available. It will usually be helpful to discuss the patient fully beforehand in order to focus on the problems to be solved. Requests that the psychologist should 'exclude the possibility of brain damage' or 'localise the lesion' will not yield unequivocal answers, but to ask for collaboration in assessing the *likelihood* of brain damage, focal or diffuse, may bring valuable evidence to add to that already available.

A faint suspicion of early dementia may be greatly sharpened by failure on sensitive tests of learning ability, even when the physician's examination has yielded doubtful results. In the absence of depression or other emotional disturbance such findings may be crucial in indicating that further investigations should be pursued. Minimal dysphasia or perceptual difficulties may likewise be exposed. Conversely, excellent performance on a reasonably wide range of cognitive tests can be greatly reassuring. And even when test results are less than clear-cut in one direction or another an important baseline will have been established for reference later on.

Apart from diagnosis, psychometry can also be valuable where rehabilitation is concerned. Areas of relatively intact function can be identified, and problems highlighted on which re-education should be concentrated. Progress can be monitored with a fair degree of accuracy, enabling ultimate goals to be discerned.

In the sections which follow some of the available tests are briefly described. Some provide essentially qualitative information, though the great majority yield numerical scores. Some rely on profiles of comparison between different functional capacities, or help to demonstrate the fall from estimated levels of premorbid intelligence (e.g. the National Adult Reading Test). Others concentrate on certain areas alone, such as perception, language or memory, though obviously considerable overlap will often occur. The Halstead–Reitan battery is briefly described as it was used extensively in earlier studies in the USA. Some recent developments in computerised testing are then outlined.

Mention is also made of certain aptitude tests, often initially designed for healthy individuals, but also useful as a guide to the rehabilitation and resettlement of brain-damaged patients. Questionnaires and rating scales which have been employed with severely brain-damaged subjects are also discussed.

The tests themselves vary widely in the extent to which they have been validated and the adequacy with which norms have been established. This is not the place to attempt a thorough review of their respective credentials, but rather to give an outline of their aims and procedures. Details can be found in the compilations produced by Crawford *et al.* (1992c) and Lezak (1995).

Intelligence tests

Wechsler Adult Intelligence Scale (WAIS)

The WAIS is an extensively standardised instrument for the measurement of intelligence, providing separate scores for 'verbal' and 'performance' abilities. Possible deterioration from estimated or established premorbid levels can be assessed, and this alone can yield important information about the likelihood of brain damage. Qualitative interpretation of different subtest scores may indicate areas of special cognitive difficulty.

Eleven subtests are involved. In the 1981 revision of the test (WAIS-R) they are as follows (Wechsler 1981):

Verbal subtests (untimed except for arithmetic)

1 Information: 29 questions covering a wide variety of information and arranged in order of difficulty.
2 Comprehension: 16 items in which the subject must explain what should be done in certain circumstances, the meaning of proverbs, etc. This aims at measuring practical judgement and common sense.
3 Arithmetic: 14 mental arithmetic problems set in the context of everyday activities.
4 Similarities: 14 items in which the subject must say in what way two things are alike.
5 Digit span: lists of 3–9 digits to be reproduced forwards and 2–8 digits to be reproduced backwards.
6 Vocabulary: 35 words graded in difficulty for which the subject must give the meaning.

Performance subtests (all timed)

1 Digit symbol: the subject must follow a simple code in matching symbols to digits, as quickly as he can.
2 Picture completion: the subject is shown 20 pictures of human features, familiar objects or scenes, and must say what important part is missing from each.
3 Block design: this is similar to the Kohs' Block Design Test. The subject must reproduce designs with red and white blocks.
4 Picture arrangement: 10 sets of cartoon pictures must be arranged in sequence so as to tell a sensible story.
5 Object assembly: four jigsaw-like puzzles of familiar objects must be assembled from their parts.

The raw score on each subtest is transmuted into a standard score (scaled score), which represents the individual's distance from the mean in terms of the distribution for that particular subtest. By this procedure all subtest scores are expressed in units which can be compared one with another. Abbreviated forms of the test are commonly used in clinical practice and have been shown to be reasonably valid (Crawford *et al.* 1992a).

Difficulties arise when comparing performance on the WAIS-R with earlier performance on the WAIS. Crawford *et al.* (1990a) have shown on a UK sample that the WAIS-R yields significantly lower full scale, verbal and performance IQs than with the WAIS, with mean differences of 7.5, 6.4 and 7.9 IQ points, respectively. Slightly smaller differences have been noted in the USA.

In addition to yielding an intelligence quotient, various

diagnostic uses have been proposed for the WAIS. Wechsler himself proposed such functions for the test (Wechsler 1958), including its use for the identification of brain damage. Others have carried these possibilities further, seeking to identify patterns characteristic of various illness processes. All such procedures involve comparisons between the individual's performance on different subtests. Some measure the amount of overall scatter, while others involve the computation of 'indices of deterioration'. However, all have come under criticism and have generally emerged as inferior to other psychometric tests for brain damage.

At the simplest level brain damage may be reflected in discrepancies between the verbal and performance IQs. The functions measured by the performance subtests usually prove to be more vulnerable than those measured by verbal subtests, though this is by no means invariable. Damage restricted to the dominant hemisphere may, for example, severely impair ability on the comprehension, arithmetic and vocabulary subtests of the verbal scale, while leaving performance abilities relatively intact. Moreover, significant discrepancies emerge in some normal subjects and in some patients suffering from non-organic mental illness. In very general terms verbal subtests will tend to be impaired by lesions in the dominant hemisphere, and those involving visuospatial functions by lesions in the non-dominant hemisphere. Verbal–performance discrepancies cannot, however, be used as a reliable guide to laterality of brain damage. Diffuse brain damage, moreover, tends to lower performance IQ disproportionately.

'Deterioration indices' involve comparisons between other contrasting groups of subtests. 'Hold' tests are identified which are found to be relatively impervious to the effects of brain damage, whereas 'Don't hold' tests show early decline. The former include subtests which reflect the use of old knowledge (vocabulary, information, object assembly, picture completion), whereas the latter require speed or the perception of new relations in verbal or spatial content (digit symbol, digit span, similarities, block design). Several such indices have been elaborated, but are open to the objection that they fail to allow for the diversity of the effects of brain damage in different locations. In practice they have sometimes shown a close correlation with severity of diffuse brain damage (McFie 1960; Gonen 1970), but equally they have often proved disappointing in differentiating organic from non-organic psychiatric disorders (Watson 1965; Bolton et al. 1966; Bersoff 1970).

Factor analysis has also been applied to WAIS-R data as a more robust way of looking at test results. A three-factor model yields factors reflecting 'verbal comprehension'

(information, vocabulary, comprehension and similarities), 'perceptual organisation' (block design, object assembly, picture completion and picture arrangement) and 'freedom from distractibility' (digit span, arithmetic and digit symbol). This last is more prominent in neurologically impaired subjects (Burgess et al. 1992).

The application of the WAIS as a diagnostic instrument has been widely criticised on theoretical grounds, in that the reliability of subtests taken individually is not sufficiently high to allow a confident interpretation of any but the largest differences between them. Scatter can result not only from pathological processes, but also from differences in educational, occupational and cultural factors. Nevertheless, qualitative interpretation of subtest scores may still on occasion provide useful clinical information, yielding important pointers for verification by more detailed testing.

National Adult Reading Test (NART)

A simple technique for yielding an approximate estimate of general intelligence consists in administering a series of words to be read aloud (Nelson 1982; Nelson & Willison 1991). Nelson and McKenna (1975) introduced this rapid method using words from the Schonell Graded Word Reading Test, and Nelson and O'Connell (1978) then modified it by drawing up a list of words which are spelled in an irregular manner. The level of word reading ability achieved by an adult has been shown to correlate highly with intelligence, and being well practiced and over-learned, it proves to be relatively resistant to influences which impair other aspects of cognitive function.

It is this last aspect which makes the test especially useful. The authors showed that even in patients with dementia the ability to read words declined little if at all, at least in the patients used in the samples they examined. Thus subjects without evidence of brain disorder gave results closely comparable to patients with cerebral atrophy, even though in the latter the WAIS IQ had deteriorated considerably. It was possible to show that estimates of premorbid intelligence derived from the NART were more stable even than those derived from the vocabulary subtest of the WAIS. The validity of the test in this regard has since been confirmed in further studies (Crawford et al. 1990b). The test has, however, come under criticism, with evidence that in patients with dementia of moderate severity it may yield an underestimate of premorbid competence (O'Carroll et al. 1995b).

The irregularly spelled words of the NART have proved more suitable for estimating premorbid intelligence than the words of the Schonell Test. Since their spelling does not conform to rules (e.g. ache, bouquet, naïve, sidereal) they depend for correct pronunciation on long familiarity and cannot be pronounced by guesses based on their alphabetic structure. Moreover the words available in the list extend the ceiling of the test, allowing estimation of IQs in the bright normal and superior range.

After administering the NART, regression equations are used to obtain an estimate of 'minimum premorbid intelligence', and discrepancies between this and current WAIS IQ can then be observed. With the latest revision of the NART, predicted IQs can be given in terms of the WAIS-R rather than the WAIS (Nelson & Willison 1991). It may also be used to estimate premorbid levels of verbal fluency (Crawford *et al.* 1992b). The test has obvious limitations, however, especially for subjects who were always poor readers, or who have acquired reading difficulties or dysarthria.

Raven's Progressive Matrices

Raven (1958a, 1982; Raven *et al.* 1992) developed a test of non-verbal intelligence which requires the perception of relations among abstract items. Coloured forms are available for use with children and adults (Raven 1965; Raven *et al.* 1984).

The test consists of a series of printed designs, from each of which a part has been removed. The subject must choose the missing portion from among a series of alternatives, in a manner which tests his ability at discrimination, analogy, permutation and alternation of patterns, and other logical relationships. Factor analysis has shown the test to be heavily loaded with a factor common to most intelligence tests, but to be influenced also by spatial aptitude, inductive reasoning, perceptual accuracy and other factors.

(Anastasi 1982)

The test is widely used as a rapid device for estimating performance IQ, often in association with the Mill Hill Vocabulary Test which provides a similarly rapid estimate of verbal ability (Raven 1958b). Surprisingly for an intelligence test it has sometimes compared well with other psychometric tests for differentiating between psychiatric patients with and without diffuse brain damage (Kendrick & Post 1967; Irving *et al.* 1970). The coloured form of the test has been especially commended in this regard. Some authors have found it to be more affected by right-sided lesions than left (Piercy & Smyth 1962), whereas others have found it to be equally impaired by damage to either hemisphere (Costa & Vaughan 1962; De Renzi & Faglioni 1965).

Tests of perception

Bender–Gestalt Test (Bender Visual Motor Gestalt Test)

Bender (1938, 1946) produced what is primarily a copying test, independent of memory and learning ability, though it can be varied to examine reproduction from memory after a lapse of time if required.

Nine simple designs are presented to the subject, one at a time, and he is asked to copy them. The type and frequency of errors are noted, and serve as the basis for identifying neurotic, psychotic and brain-damaged subjects. Interpretation relies to a large extent on subjective intuitive procedures, but attempts have been made to standardise it for certain purposes.

It has been widely used as a rapid screening test, but the overlap between groups reduces its value when applied to the individual subject. Nevertheless its efficiency at detecting brain damage has sometimes received surprisingly strong support when compared with other long-established psychometric tests (Shapiro *et al.* 1956; Brilliant & Gynther 1963). Lezak (1995) reviews the now extensive literature of this simple test and the sometimes elaborate scoring procedures employed.

Visual Object and Space Perception Battery

Warrington and James (1991) have introduced a nine-test battery for exploring visual perception which can be given in parts or as a whole. Minimal motor response is required from the patient so that any praxic element is eliminated.

The first test screens for visual impairment which might preclude proceeding further. A series of cards is shown with an all-over pattern and the patient must say which of them contain a degraded 'X'.

The next four tests show views of letters, animals or objects which have been rendered puzzling in various ways. In 'Incomplete Letters' the subject has to identify a series of randomly degraded letters. 'Silhouettes' requires the subject to identify animals and inanimate objects depicted as black silhouettes and rotated through various degrees. In 'Object Decision' the subject has to choose which of a group of silhouettes, again rotated, represents a real as opposed to an imaginary object. In 'Progressive Silhouettes' the subject sees two series of silhouettes, each representing a single object, presented at a series of angles which gradually approach normality.

The final four tests deal with aspects of space perception. 'Dot Counting' requires the subject to count the number of dots in a small array. In 'Position Discrimination' the subject must decide which of two squares, presented side by side, has the dot exactly in the centre. 'Number Location' consists of two squares one above the other; in the lower display there is a single dot, and the subject must say which number in the square above corresponds to its position. 'Cube Analysis' requires the subject to count the number of cubes depicted in line drawings of three-dimensional displays.

Patients with right hemisphere lesions have been shown to perform less well than patients with left hemisphere lesions on all of these subtests.

Behavioural Inattention Test

This battery of tests is designed to examine unilateral visual neglect (Wilson *et al.* 1987). The first six subtests are traditional procedures for examining for neglect, and the next nine 'behavioural tests' aim to identify everyday problems likely to be faced by patients, thereby serving as a guide to rehabilitation.

The traditional tests include line crossing, letter cancellation, star cancellation, figure- and shape-copying tests, line bisection tests and free drawing of a clock, a man or woman and a butterfly.

The behavioural tests examine picture scanning, telephone dialling, menu reading, article reading, telling and setting the time on a clock face, coin sorting, address and sentence copying, map navigation and card sorting.

Halligan *et al.* (1991) have shown excellent test–retest reliabilities for the battery, and good correlations on each of the two subsets with occupational therapists' reports and measures of activities of daily living.

Language tests

Boston Naming Test

This consists of 60 line drawings of objects which the patient must name (Kaplan *et al.* 1983). The items range in difficulty from common objects such as a tree or pencil, to more difficult ones like a sphinx or a trellis. When the subject cannot name the picture he is given cues, first a stimulus cue (e.g. 'it's something to eat'), then a phonemic cue (i.e. the opening sound of the word). These help to identify whether the subject knew the word at all. The number of cues needed is noted.

Normative data on the test are provided by Van Gorp *et al.* (1986). It effectively elicits naming impairments in patients with aphasia, but is also sensitive to the language difficulties of patients with dementia (Margolin *et al.* 1990). Edith Kaplan (quoted in Lezak 1995) has noted that patients with right hemisphere damage, especially right frontal damage, may show responses indicative of perceptual fragmentation, for example identifying the mouth-piece of a harmonica as the line of windows on a bus.

Graded Naming Test

The subject is presented with 30 line drawings of items and asked to name them (McKenna & Warrington 1983). These vary with regard to frequency of usage and consequently in naming difficulty. It is possible to judge whether naming ability is in line with reading ability, as estimated by the NART or the Schonell Graded Word Reading Test, or with vocabulary scores as measured on the WAIS.

Token Test

De Renzi and Vignolo (1962) introduced a test especially sensitive to minor degrees of impairment of language comprehension. This can be of considerable value since routine examination often fails to detect slight receptive language disorder. Moreover a patient with dysphasia may seem to have difficulties which are limited to verbal expression alone, and it can then be difficult to explore the more subtle aspects of language comprehension without taxing other cognitive functions as well.

The test uses a number of simple 'tokens' which are manipulated by the subject. He is given a series of verbal commands expressed in progressively more complex messages, in response to which he must perform simple manual tasks such as picking up, moving or touching the tokens. The tokens used are of two different shapes (circles and rectangles), two different sizes and five different colours. It is first necessary to ensure that the subject appreciates the meaning of circle and rectangle and that colour recognition is intact.

In the first part of the test the large circles and rectangles are displayed and the patient is asked to pick up each in turn by telling him to 'pick up the yellow rectangle', 'pick up the white circle', etc. Subsequent parts proceed in graded stages by introducing the small as well as the large tokens, by asking the subject to pick up two at a time, and by introducing more complex instructions which involve new grammatical elements. In the final part of the test, prepositions, conjunctions and adverbs are introduced so as to radically change the meaning of the action which the subject is required to perform. Thus: 'put the red circle on the green rectangle', 'touch the blue circle with the red rectangle', 'pick up all the rectangles except the yellow one', 'put the red circle between the yellow rectangle and the green rectangle', 'after picking up the green rectangle touch the white circle', etc.

Thus the test consists of messages which are conceptually elementary and short and easy to remember, but which make two kinds of demand on comprehension—the token must be identified by three independent features, and the subject must grasp the semantic complications which are later introduced. Deficits often become obvious only in the later stages of the test, and can then emerge clearly even among dysphasics who have shown no evidence of difficulty with comprehension during normal conversation.

Boller and Vignolo (1966) found that the test was more impaired in aphasics than non-aphasics, as expected, but also that among non-aphasics it was more impaired by left-sided brain damage than right. The 'latent sensory aphasia' thus identified was independent of non-language impairments as measured by Raven's Progressive Matrices, and appeared not merely to be a consequence of impaired general intelligence. The test was shown to be more sensitive for the detection of mild comprehension deficits than Marie's Three Paper Test which has been widely employed for this purpose (p. 102).

Benton (1967) has described a more extensive battery of tests for the detailed investigation of language functions, which incorporates the Token Test as one of many components. Other parts assess visual and tactile naming, sentence repetition, sentence construction, word fluency and several aspects of reading and writing. Profiles of language dysfunction can be drawn up and help to identify areas of relative difficulty and to assess progress during recovery.

Speed and Capacity of Language Processing Test

In the first part, the *Speed of Comprehension Test*, the rate of processing of language is measured (Baddeley *et al.* 1992). The subject is required to read a number of statements which vary in content and syntactic structure, putting a tick against those which are true or sensible and a cross if they are false or silly. The subject must work as quickly as possible through the series.

The second part, the *Spot-the-Word Test*, is introduced to control for poor verbal skills *per se*, rather than slowed information processing. In this test the subject is presented with 60 pairs of items, each consisting of a word and an invented non-word, and must indicate which of the pair is real. The extent to which the subject's speed of comprehension falls behind performance on the Spot-the-Word Test indicates how far language comprehension skills have been impaired.

The Spot-the-Word Test may have another value in itself, in that it has proved to be a potentially useful method for estimating premorbid intelligence. Thus it has been shown to correlate highly with verbal intelligence as estimated by Mill Hill Vocabulary scores or performance on the NART, and performance seems not to decline with age even in the presence of intellectual impairment (Baddeley *et al.* 1993). In performing the task a number of parallel routes are available for making the lexical decisions—the meaning of the word, its orthographic appearance, its sound, or a general feeling of familiarity—and this may be what makes it relatively resistant to brain damage.

Memory tests

Paired associate learning tests

Paired associate learning involves the mastery of the appropriate response when the first member of a pair of words is presented. Inglis (1959) elaborated such a test, designed to be sensitive to memory impairment in the elderly and as independent as possible of the patient's general level of intellectual functioning:

Three simple paired associates must be learned by repeated auditory presentation. In one form of the test, for example, the pairs are 'cabbage–pen', 'knife–chimney', and 'sponge–trumpet'. The examiner reads the list after telling the subject to remember the pairs that go together. The stimulus words are then given alone in random order, and repeated with appropriate corrections for errors until the subject achieves three consecutive correct responses on every one of the three different stimulus words. Any given stimulus word is dropped out as soon as its own criterion is reached. The score is the sum of the times the stimulus words must be presented before the total criterion is reached.

The test has proved to be a sensitive indicator of memory disorder in the elderly and to be independent of the patient's verbal intelligence. It is useful for measuring impairment in the acquisition phase of memory, but abnormally poor scores may be obtained in severely depressed and perplexed elderly subjects without evidence of brain damage (Post 1965). The test has been shown to correlate highly with the Modified Word Learning Test and the Synonym Learning Test (Kendrick *et al.* 1965; Bolton *et al.* 1967).

Isaacs and Walkey (1964) have prepared a simpler and shorter form which is less fatiguing and can be administered along with the clinical interview:

Three easy paired associates are given, and tested three times only in random order ('knife–fork', 'east–west', 'hand–foot'). The procedure is then repeated with three rather harder associates ('cup–plate', 'cat–milk', 'gold–lead'), and the result is simply scored in terms of the number of errors from 0 to 18. Normal scores were judged to be in the range of 0–2, moderate impairment 3–9, and severe impairment 10–18.

The range of functions covered includes attention, registration, short-term recall and, to some extent, verbal learning. Motivational factors are clearly involved as well. Priest *et al.* (1969) found significant differences between organic and non-organic psychiatric patients with Isaacs and Walkey's test, but many misclassifications occurred as would be expected from such an abbreviated procedure. However, it may be useful as a screening device provided its limitations are recognised.

Irving *et al.* (1970) have assessed a similar simplified test in which the appropriate response must be learned for each of 12 items. For example, in response to 'colour' the subject must learn 'purple', for 'country'—'Portugal', for 'flower'—'daisy' and so on. Repeated trials are given if necessary, and the number of correct responses charted. This was found to discriminate as efficiently as several more complicated procedures when a battery of tests were administered to depressed and demented patients.

Goldstein *et al.* (1988) investigated paired associate learning in patients who had undergone unilateral temporal lobectomy. A verbal paired associate task differentiated between left and right lobectomies better than did a test involving paired associate learning of designs, but when used together the two tests provided optimal discrimination between the two groups of patients.

Synonym Learning Test

Kendrick *et al.* (1965) introduced this as a modification of the more cumbersome Walton–Black Modified Word Learning Test (Walton & Black 1957) for use in elderly depressed subjects when the question of dementia had arisen.

Ten words unfamiliar to the subject are identified by administering a vocabulary test of ascending difficulty (the Mill Hill Vocabulary Test) until 10 consecutive words cannot be defined. Learning of the meanings of these words is then assessed by repeated administration, exactly the same definitions being used for each presentation. The fact that the test is based on failures in the initial vocabulary test, rather than on an arbitrary selection of unknown words, ensures that the subject is only required to learn at a level consistent with his own intellectual ability.

No overlap was found between normal and brain-damaged subjects, but 16% of depressed elderly patients were still found to obtain scores in the brain-damaged range. The misclassifications tended to occur in depressed patients with low intelligence, severe affective disturbance, complaints of perplexity and confusion, and poor knowledge of recent general events (Kendrick & Post 1967).

Kendrick (1967) later showed that the combination of the Synonym Learning Test with a simple test designed to measure the speed of copying digits (Digit Copying Test) could distinguish even more effectively between elderly demented patients and elderly depressed patients who gave a semblance of being demented.

Object Learning Test

Kendrick *et al.* (1979) have described an Object Learning Test which has proved more acceptable and less stressful to elderly patients than the Synonym Learning Test. This is again used in conjunction with the Digit Copying Test for aiding the distinction between the depressed and the demented elderly. The new 'battery' can be administered in approximately 10 minutes, and its reliability and validity have been examined on large samples of patients and controls.

Four cards are divided into 25 equal sections within which there are drawings of familiar objects (for example a comb, a teapot, etc.). The first card contains 10 items, the second 15, the third 20 and the fourth 25. Six of the items are repeated across all four cards and are always in the same position. Some items form a category across the cards. The cards are exposed to the subject for a standard length of time, and the score represents the total number of correct items recalled.

List learning tests

Tests examining the learning of word lists have a number of advantages. They provide information about the immediate memory span, the shape of the learning curve and the nature of the learning strategies employed (or their absence). In addition they give evidence of such matters as proactive interference and confabulation. Lezak (1995) reviews the two tests most widely used at present—the Rey Auditory Verbal Learning Test and the California Verbal Learning Test.

The *Rey Auditory Verbal Learning Test* consists of five presentations of a 15-word list, after each of which the subject must recall as many words as he can. A second 15-word list is then presented and tested for recall. The subject is then immediately asked to recall as much as he can of the first list, and retention is examined 30 minutes (or even 24 hours) later.

After each presentation the examiner writes down the words exactly as they are recalled. Scores are made of total words correctly recalled, of intrusions from one list to the other, and of errors made (i.e. words not on the lists). The shape of the learning curve over the repeated presentations of the first list can be examined, also retention after the period of delay. 'Primacy' and 'recency' effects (better recall of words towards the beginning and end of the list) are usually shown by normal subjects, but the primacy effect is often lacking when learning ability is defective. Extensive normative data is available for the test.

The *California Verbal Learning Test* is similar to the above, but includes 16 words which belong to four defined categories. This allows the subjects' learning strategies to be examined more closely. Category-cued recall is tested as well as free recall, and a recognition trial is included.

Recognition memory tests

Warrington (1974, 1984) has described a simple technique for separately assessing verbal and non-verbal memory by means of an easily administered recognition memory task. A recognition paradigm is used in preference to free recall, since recognition tasks appear to be less vulnerable to anxiety and depression. Moreover, identical procedures can be followed for the verbal and non-verbal material, allowing direct comparisons between the two.

The material consists of 50 high frequency words, each printed on a card, and 50 photographs of unknown faces. The words are presented to the subject at 3-second intervals, and he is asked to respond 'yes' or 'no' each time according to whether he judges the word to be pleasant or not pleasant. This strategy is adopted to ensure attention to the words. Recognition is tested immediately the presentation is complete by showing pairs of words, one of which is new and one of which has already been shown. A choice must be made each time between the two items.

The 50 photographs of faces are then shown at 3-second intervals, again with the requirement that the subject decides at each presentation whether the face is pleasant or unpleasant. Recognition is again tested as soon as presentation is complete by a similar forced-choice technique.

Benton Visual Retention Test

This visual recall test requires the reproduction of a series of geometrical figures shortly after their inspection (Benton 1955, 1963; Sivan 1992).

The subject must draw the designs from memory after each card has been exposed for 10 seconds and then removed. The test can be varied by giving shorter exposures, or by imposing delays before reproduction is required. Copying of the designs while the card is in front of the subject allows separation of memory difficulties from visuoperceptual difficulties. Performance is scored in terms of the number of designs correctly reproduced and the number of errors made. Additional qualitative information may be derived from inspection of the type of errors committed — distortions, omissions, perseverations, rotations, misplacements and errors of size. Three parallel forms of the test are available.

Performance correlates highly with intelligence and chronological age, but normative data are available to make allowance for this. The value of the test in differentiating brain-damaged and non-brain-damaged groups has been repeatedly upheld, and it has proved to be sensitive to early cognitive decline (Lezak 1995). This is probably because the test involves so many different capacities — spatial perception, visual and verbal conceptualisation, short-term retention and recall, and visuoconstructive abilities. It is sensitive to left brain damage as well as right since many of the designs can be conceptualised verbally.

Graham–Kendall Memory for Designs Test

Graham and Kendall's (1960) test again involves the copying of a series of simple geometrical figures from immediate memory, after exposure to the subject for 5 seconds at a time. In evolving the test a specific effort was made, not to measure some function of theoretical significance, but rather to crystallise in the scoring system the differences in response which served to distinguish defined groups of patients. Raw scores in terms of the number and kind of errors can be transmuted into scores that control for the effects of age and intellectual development as reflected in the patient's vocabulary level.

The test has been extensively validated. Poor performance has been found to indicate a high probability of brain damage, though good performance does not necessarily indicate an intact brain. Patients with damage to the left and right sides of the brain are equally affected. The test has been commended in comparison with others (Yates 1966), and the ease of its administration adds considerably to its popularity. Unfortunately, patients with non-organic psychiatric disorder show a good deal of overlap with brain-damaged subjects, and healthy elderly subjects have sometimes been found to score within the brain-damaged range. A significant correlation has also emerged between performance on the test and estimates of premorbid intelligence (Turland & Steinhard 1969).

Rey–Osterrieth Test

This involves the copying of a single geometrical figure of complex design, then testing reproduction from memory some time later (Rey 1941; Osterrieth 1944).

The figure is too complex to be adequately verbalised, hence the test is of visual, non-verbal memory. The subject is first asked to copy the design as accurately as he can with the original before him. Forty minutes later and without previous warning he is asked to draw the figure again, but this time from memory. The initial copying reflects any drawing disability or disorder of spatial perception, but the recall score reflects in addition any visual memory impairment.

The test usefully complements those which measure verbal memory functions. Patients with temporal lobe damage in the hemisphere dominant for speech tend to show little impairment with the Rey–Osterrieth Test, in contrast to their difficulties with verbal memory tests. Right temporal lobectomy, however, leads to a slight but significant defect on copying the figure, and a pronounced and disproportionate impairment when tested for delayed recall (Teuber et al. 1968; Teuber & Milner 1968; Milner 1969). Lezak (1995) reviews the extensive literature on the patterns of deficit seen with different brain lesions. Patients with parietal lobe lesions appear to show relatively stable retention despite having difficulty in copying the figure initially.

Wechsler Memory Scale (WMS-R)

Wechsler's battery of memory tests aims at measuring several different aspects of memory by rapid standardised procedures. With the original battery the raw scores could be translated into a 'memory quotient' which could be directly compared with the subject's IQ (Wechsler 1945; Wechsler & Stone 1945). The new revision of the scale (Wechsler 1987) discards this provision (which being a unitary score was not very informative), but includes norms stratified at nine age levels. Atkinson (1991) provides a table of the differences required between the various WMS-R indices and the WAIS-R full scale IQ before such discrepancies can be regarded as statistically significant.

Improvements with the revised scale include the more thorough assessment of visual/non-verbal memory and the introduction of measures of delayed recall. Unfortunately, the revision is presented in only one form, so practice effects cannot be avoided if testing is repeated.

The first subtest consists of *information and orientation questions*, included for the detection of dementia or severe disturbances of memory. The results are not used in formal scoring.

Next is a test of '*mental control*', aimed at detecting minor brain damage which might not emerge in tests of memory alone. It includes counting backwards from 20 to 1, repeating the alphabet and counting in 3s.

Figural memory involves the recognition of abstract patterns and their identification from an array of similar designs.

Logical memory examines the immediate recall of two short stories, each containing 25 scoring units.

Visual paired associates requires the subject to learn six couplings of abstract line drawings with different coloured squares; at recall he must name the colour when shown the design.

Verbal paired associates requires the learning of eight pairs of words, four being easy to associate and four having no obvious semantic connections.

Visual reproduction involves the immediate recall of four geometrical figures. The subject must draw what he remembers after seeing each card for 10 seconds.

Digit span is measured forwards and backwards.

Visual memory span is assessed forwards and backwards by asking the subject to touch a series of coloured squares in a predetermined order, which is first demonstrated by the examiner.

Delayed recall is tested after 30 minutes for the logical memory passages, the visual paired associates, the verbal paired associates and the visual reproduction items.

Adult Memory and Information Processing Battery

This brief battery of memory tests has British norms, stratified for age, and a parallel form is available (Coughlan & Hollows 1985). There are four memory subtests and two information-processing tests.

Short story recall: recall is tested immediately after presentation and again after a 30-minute delay.

Figure copy and recall: a complex two-dimensional figure is copied and recall is tested immediately and after a 30-minute delay.

List learning: a list of 15 words is presented in the same order for a maximum of five trials. A distracter trial is then presented, for which recall is tested, and then delayed recall of the original list is tested. The test assesses rote learning and susceptibility to interference.

Design learning: an abstract design must be learned, with up to five presentations. Recall of a distraction design is then followed by delayed recall of the original design. This again assesses rote learning and susceptibility to interference.

Information processing is tested by number cancellation and digit cancellation tasks.

Rivermead Behavioural Memory Test

This battery of tests was designed to be more 'ecologically valid' than most formal memory tests in that it emphasises skills needed in real-life situations (Wilson 1987; Wilson *et al.* 1991). It assesses memory impairment in terms of everyday memory functioning, thus bridging the gap between laboratory-based and naturalistic measures of memory. Four parallel forms of the test are available to allow repeat assessments during the course of rehabilitation. Good levels of correlation with standardised memory tests show that the battery is a valid indicator of memory functioning. Norms are available for adults and separately for elderly patients, and it may be adapted for use with children. A shortened form for use with aphasic patients has been shown to be sensitive to memory deficits rather than to the effects of language impairment (Cockburn *et al.* 1990). The several subtests include the following:

Orientation is tested for time and place and knowledge of the date.

Remembering a name: the subject is told the first and second name that goes with a photograph, and recall of these is tested when the photograph is re-presented later in the session.

Picture recognition: 10 line drawings of common objects are shown for 5 seconds each, and after a short delay the subject is asked to identify them from a set of 20.

Face recognition: five photographs of faces seen a few minutes earlier must be identified out of a group of 10.

Story recall: a short story similar to a newspaper item is read to the subject who is asked to repeat it immediately and again some 15 minutes later.

Route memory: a short route around the room is demonstrated and copied immediately by the subject. Recall is required some 15 minutes later.

Prospective memory: three innovative methods are used to test the subject's capacity to remember to do something:

1 At the start of the session an object (such as a comb or a key) is borrowed from the subject and hidden while the subject looks on; he must ask for it and remember where it was hidden at the end in response to a specific cue (e.g. 'We have now finished this test.').

2 When an alarm rings the subject must remember to ask a specific question, told to him when the alarm was set 20 minutes earlier (e.g. about the next appointment).

3 He must remember an errand, e.g. to leave an envelope at a specific location along the route around the room.

Frontal lobe ('executive function') tests

Verbal fluency tests

A large number of tests can be used for assessing the reduction in verbal fluency associated with frontal brain lesions, especially left frontal lesions. These are reviewed by Lezak (1995). The 'FAS' test is briefly described on p. 104. Tests which require word generation in response to an initial letter are often most revealing, in that the subject must develop his own strategies in guiding the search for words. Those asking for lists of animals, food articles, etc. are easier in that they provide some of the required structure for the patient. Even so there is room for the development of subcategories (farm animals, domestic animals, etc.) in the organisation of recall. Newcombe (1969) used a variant in which subjects were asked to *alternate* in naming birds and colours, thus adding a requirement for continual changes of set. Written tests of word fluency have been devised, also tests of 'design fluency' which are somewhat more affected by right frontal damage than left (p. 104).

Wisconsin Card Sorting Test

This complex sorting test has proved to be particularly sensitive to frontal lobe damage (Milner 1963, 1964, 1969). It has accordingly achieved considerable importance in neuropsychological testing, since frontal lesions may sometimes be difficult to detect by other psychometric procedures.

The material consists of 64 cards, each containing from one to four geometrical figures. These consist of any one of four shapes (triangles, stars, crosses and circles) in any one of four colours. Four stimulus cards are set out before the subject who must sort the remainder beneath them. His task is to discover by trial and error whether he is required to sort according to colour, form or number, the clue being the examiner's remark of 'right' or 'wrong' after each response is made. In administering the test the subject is required to sort first of all by colour, all other responses being called wrong, then when he has achieved 10 consecutive correct responses to colour the required sorting principle shifts *without warning* to form. Later it shifts to number, then back again to colour, and so on. The test thus combines the requirement for shifting frames of reference with a need for empirical discovery of categories. A total score can be obtained, also scores for perseverative and non-perseverative types of error.

Nelson (1976) has reported a simplified and improved version of the test (*Modified Wisconsin Card Sorting Test*) in which those cards which share more than one attribute with a stimulus card have been eliminated. Possible ambiguities for the patient are thereby reduced and the time of administration considerably shortened. The total number of cards to be sorted in the modified test is reduced from 64 to 24.

Milner (1963) obtained clear evidence that impairment was closely related to lesions of the frontal lobes of either hemisphere, with no comparable effects from lesions in other areas of the brain. The impairment was chiefly seen with lesions of the dorsolateral convexities of the frontal lobe, rather than with inferior and orbital lesions. Moreover, the errors in the patients with frontal lobe lesions were chiefly of the perseverative type. These results were obtained in patients with focal cortical excisions for epilepsy. They were broadly confirmed by Drewe (1974) in a heterogeneous group of brain-damaged patients. Certain qualitative differences were found between the nature of the errors with left and right frontal lesions, and the former produced the greater overall impairment. Grafman *et al.* (1990a) confirmed an excess of perseverative errors in veterans with left dorsolateral frontal and left anterior temporal lobe penetrating head injuries.

The precise nature of the deficits revealed by the test is uncertain. Motivational defects or primary disturbances of abstract thinking may contribute to failure, but do not appear adequate as a complete explanation. By analogy with observations on monkeys with frontal lesions it seems that there may be especial difficulty in overcoming a preferred mode of response, so that the immediate consequences of actions have less influence in modifying ongoing behaviour. Luria and Homskaya (1964) have stressed impairment in the verbal regulation of behaviour after frontal lobe lesions (p. 78), and this may also contribute to failure on the test.

Stroop tests

A variety of tests derive from Stroop's (1935) work on the interference which can arise between word reading and colour naming. Lezak (1995) reviews the several formats available. All are based on the observation that it takes longer to read printed colour names when they are printed in (and/or surrounded by) coloured ink different from the name of the colour word. This may be due to a variety of factors—response conflict, failure of response inhibition, or failure of selective attention. Studies have shown that the technique is sensitive to the effects of closed head injury, and that patients with left frontal lesions perform especially badly.

Pardo *et al.* (1990) carried out positron emission tomography (PET) scans during performance on the test, to reveal the brain areas involved in resolution of the interference effect. Images made during the reading of congruent material were subtracted from those made during incongruent readings. An extensive distributed network of regions was shown to be involved (left premotor, left post central, left putamen, supplementary motor area, right superior temporal gyrus and bilateral peristriate cortex), but the most robust responses were observed in the anterior cingulate region.

Tests vary in the number of words and colours employed, and whether the requirement is to read out the colour names or to report the colour in which each word is printed. Scoring may be by time, number of errors made, or number of items correctly performed within a designated time period. The *Stroop Neuropsychological Screening Test* (Trenerry *et al.* 1989) is as follows:

Columns of four colour names are presented (red, blue, green and tan), all being printed in colours incongruent with the colour name. The subject must first read the colour names aloud as quickly as possible. In the second, crucial, condition there are similar columns of colour names but this time the subject must say what colour ink the word is printed in. Thus, for example, if the word RED is printed in blue the subject must say 'blue'. The number completed correctly in 120 seconds is compared with two age bands of norms.

Cognitive Estimates Test

Shallice and Evans (1978) noted that a patient with selective frontal lobe damage showed gross inability to produce simple cognitive estimates despite having an IQ at the same level as prior to injury. When asked, for example, to estimate the height of the tallest building in London, or to name the best paid occupation in Britain, he gave remarkably inaccurate replies and seemed not to realise that the answers were bizarre. This appeared to reflect failures of judgement in dealing with novel situations, even though lower level cognitive skills were retained. In effect the patient was unable to select the appropriate cognitive plan for answering the question and failed to check the putative answer.

The value of the procedure was checked on groups of patients with anterior and posterior cerebral lesions, by devising a series of questions such that the appropriate plan for answering them was not immediately apparent, yet requiring no specialist knowledge. Scoring systems for the accuracy or bizarreness of the replies were established. The frontal lesion patients performed significantly worse than the posterior group, independently of the hemisphere involved. This persisted on partialling out scores on Raven's Matrices, indicating that the differences were not simply due to defects of reasoning or general intelligence. Examples of the questions used in the test are as follows:

How tall is the average English woman?

What is the best paid job in Britain today?
What is the largest object normally found in a house?
How fast do racehorses gallop?
What is the height of the Post Office Tower?
What is the age of the oldest person in Britain today?
What is the length of an average man's spine?

Strategy application tests

Some patients with known frontal damage can be observed to perform surprisingly well on tests of frontal lobe function yet show marked organisational difficulties in everyday life. Shallice and Burgess (1991) suggested that this might be due to the constraints incorporated in clinic-based tests where the subject has an explicit problem to be tackled, usually under guidance from the examiner. In most routine tests the patient rarely needs to organise and plan his behaviour over substantial periods of time, set a range of goals or deal with interleaving priorities. Yet 'executive' abilities of this nature are required in everyday activities.

Consequently two tests of 'strategy application' were devised to assess the capacity to exercise such functions by scheduling and carrying out a number of fairly simple activities:

The *Six Elements Test* requires the subject to carry out a group of open-ended tasks in a fixed period of time (15 minutes) so as to maximise the overall score obtained. The tasks are divided into two sets of three—dictating details of a route to and from the hospital, carrying out arithmetical problems of increasing difficulty, and writing down the names of pictures of objects. Detailed written instructions are presented concerning rules to be followed in carrying out the tasks. Basically, the test involves devising a simple plan, scheduling the tasks efficiently and keeping a check on time. The number of subtasks tackled and the time spent on each is recorded.

The *Multiple Errands Test* is more complex, requiring the subject to complete a number of tasks away from the hospital in an unfamiliar shopping precinct. Thus it involves the dovetailing of multiple activities in a real-life situation where minor unforeseen events can occur. Again detailed 'rules' must be followed and the subject's behaviour is observed throughout.

The tasks principally involve buying specified items, but one requires more ingenuity and social judgement, namely to write on a card the name of the shop likely to contain the most expensive item on sale in the precinct, the price of a pound of tomatoes, the name of the coldest place in Britain and the rate of exchange of the French franc on the previous day. Thus a range of goals must be defined, actions planned, outcomes evaluated and appropriate adaptations made. Scores are made in terms of efficiency, rule breaks, misinterpretations and task failures. Qualitative aspects of performance are also charted.

Shallice and Burgess were able to show impaired performance on both tests in three patients with frontal brain injuries, even though two of them performed normally on an extensive battery of standardised frontal lobe tests. Goldstein *et al.* (1993) have reported impaired performance on the Multiple Errands Test in a patient with a circumscribed excision on the left frontal lobe, who showed preserved intelligence and memory and normal performance on other tests of frontal lobe function. The planning difficulties elicited by the test mirrored those that the patient experienced in everyday life.

Tower of London Test

Shallice (1982) introduced this test, derived from the Tower of Hanoi oriental puzzle.

The subject must move a number of coloured beads placed on three upright poles so as to reproduce a pattern set by the examiner. It is a test of planning, in that the subject must look ahead and divide the task into a series of subtasks, and carry these out in the correct sequence in order to obtain the desired solution. Different grades of difficulty can be presented in terms of the minimum number of moves allowed to reproduce the pattern.

Shallice (1982) found that patients with left frontal lesions performed significantly worse than patients with brain lesions in other locations.

Trail Making Test

The Trail Making Test consists of 25 circles distributed over a sheet of paper. In the first part the circles are numbered, and the subject must draw a line connecting them in numerical sequence as quickly as possible. In the second part the circles contain both numbers and letters and the subject must alternate between numbers and letters as he proceeds in ascending sequence. The score is the time taken over the task. Errors must be corrected and are thus incorporated in the time scores.

Performance on the test requires spatial analysis, motor control, alertness, concentration and ability to shift attention between alternatives. In consequence, it is likely to be affected by brain damage in many locations. When the subject takes disproportionately longer to complete the second part than the first ('Trail B'), there are likely to be difficulties with complex conceptual tracking or with flexibly changing sets during on-going activity. For this reason the test is sometimes employed when frontal damage is suspected. Impulsive errors may be noted, and perseverations revealed.

More generally, Reitan (1958) demonstrated excellent differentiation between brain-damaged and nonbrain-damaged subjects, and this has since been repeatedly confirmed. However, both age and education have significant effects on performance, and depression has been shown to interact with the slowing produced by ageing (Lezak 1995).

Goldstein–Sheerer tests

Tests developed by Goldstein and Sheerer (1941) were formerly extensively employed for investigating capacity for abstract thinking and categorisation, but are now little used. Various tests in the group explore ability to abstract common properties of objects, to break up a whole into parts, and to shift from one frame of reference to another. Accordingly they can be particularly vulnerable to frontal lobe lesions.

This type of test relies heavily on qualitative observations, being concerned with the methods employed by the subject as well as with the end-point achieved, and it is difficult to obtain objective methods of scoring.

The *Goldstein–Sheerer Cube Test* consists of cubes with sides of different colours, which must be assembled to match printed designs. The *Gelb–Goldstein Colour Sorting Test* consists of woollen skeins of different colours and shades which must be selected by colour or brightness to go with chosen samples. The *Gelb–Goldstein–Weigl–Sheerer Object Sorting Test* consists of a miscellaneous group of objects which must be sorted into designated groups (according to form, colour, use, etc.). The *Colour Form Sorting Test* utilises circles, squares and triangles in different colours which must be sorted according to one common property and then another. The *Goldstein–Sheerer Stick Test* requires the subject to copy geometrical designs with a number of sticks of different lengths.

Vigilance tests

A number of tests aim to measure the subject's capacity for the continuous monitoring of stimuli over relatively long periods of time. Such 'vigilance tests' come closer than most other procedures to measuring ability for sustained attention and concentration. They have been shown to be sensitive to brain damage, and can have special advantages for detecting minor degrees of clouding of consciousness.

In routine clinical practice the simple procedures outlined on p. 102 will often suffice for obtaining an estimate of sustained attention. More complex information processing tests, such as the *Paced Auditory Serial Addition Test* (PASAT), described on p. 198, may be employed in patients who can cooperate with the procedure.

A further series of tests requires the subject to react rapidly in response to signals which arrive in a preset random manner. Efficient performance requires the prolonged maintenance of a high level of attention, and rapid activation of perceptual and motor mechanisms. Their disadvantage is that special apparatus is required.

The simple estimation of *reaction times* has often shown good differentiation between brain-damaged subjects and controls (Blackburn & Benton 1955; Benton & Joynt 1959). De Renzi and

Faglioni (1965) showed that measures of the reaction time to visual stimuli were more efficient than Raven's Matrices in discriminating between normal subjects and patients with focal cerebral lesions. However, Benton *et al.* (1959) found that reaction times were also significantly slowed in schizophrenic patients.

Rosvold *et al.* (1956) explored the value of a *Continuous Performance Test* in which letters were exposed by a revolving drum at 1-second intervals for periods of up to 10 minutes. The subject was required to press a button whenever the letter 'x' appeared, or in a more difficult version whenever an 'x' was preceded by an 'a'. Brain-damaged adults and children were shown to be significantly poorer at the test than normal controls.

The *Continuous Choice Reaction Test* used by De Renzi and Faglioni (1965) involved a screen on which various combinations of circles or squares in black or white could be briefly illuminated. The combinations were made to follow one another in irregular sequences, a new combination appearing every 1.5 seconds. The task was to press a button every time the combination 'black circle–white square' appeared, all other combinations being ignored. The test was again superior to Raven's Matrices in distinguishing between normal subjects and patients with focal brain damage. Performance was equally impaired by right and left hemisphere lesions in non-dysphasic patients, but was especially impaired in the presence of dysphasia, presumably because internal verbalisation was utilised during performance of the task.

Halstead–Reitan Battery

This extensive battery of tests represents one of the most ambitious attempts to produce a comprehensive battery for the investigation of brain damage. Reitan (1966) and Russell *et al.* (1970) describe its evolution and the attempts made to explore its diagnostic usefulness. The aim has been not only to detect brain damage, but to indicate whether this is likely to be focal or diffuse, lateralised to the right or left hemisphere, and whether acute and progressive or relatively static. Individual components of the battery are frequently used alone. Some of the principal tests involved are as follows:

Halstead's Category Test consists of groups of pictures displayed on a screen, in response to which the subject must press one of four levers. The lever required at each exposure is determined by certain unifying concepts among the group of pictures, and the subject must discover the rules by repeated trial and error. It is thus a relatively complex concept formation test which requires the subject to note similarities and differences, to set up hypotheses and to test and modify them.

The *Critical Flicker Frequency Test* measures the speed of flicker required before repeated brief exposures of light become fused.

The *Tactual Performance Test* requires the subject to fit blocks into their spaces on a board while blindfolded and later to draw the board from memory. It requires tactile form discrimination, manual dexterity and coordination, and the visualisation of spatial configurations.

The *Rhythm Test* requires the subject to differentiate between several pairs of rhythmic beats, and assesses alertness, ability for sustained attention and ability to perceive differing rhythmic sequences.

The *Speech Sounds Perception Test* consists of a series of tape-recorded nonsense words which the subject must identify by selection from printed alternatives.

The *Finger Tapping Test* is a simple measure of motor speed.

The *Time Sense Test* requires the subject to observe the time taken for a hand to rotate around a dial, then after several practice trials to estimate the time from memory.

The *Halstead–Wepman Aphasia Screening Test* contains items for testing ability to name objects, spell, identify single numbers and letters, read, write, calculate, name body parts and distinguish right from left.

The *Trail Making Test* already described on p. 120 is added as a further part of the battery.

Other tests include detailed assessments of the accuracy of sensory perception on each side of the body, and tests of finger recognition, graphaesthesia and stereognosis.

Computerised psychological tests

Tests which can be administered by microcomputer have an obvious attraction for certain purposes, either to economise with the time of a psychologist when large numbers of patients need to be examined in research, or to allow very detailed exploration of specific psychological functions. In both contexts they have special advantages in permitting accurate recording of response times in addition to examining levels of performance. Two such batteries will be briefly described.

Bexley Maudsley Automated Psychological Screening and Bexley Maudsley Category Sorting Test

These early automated tests were introduced in the context of research into alcoholic brain damage (Acker & Acker 1982; Acker *et al.* 1984). They were designed to be administered by non-psychologists on a Commodore microcomputer (and later an Apple) as a screening procedure which could be followed when necessary by orthodox testing. After the programme is loaded the testing proceeds largely autonomously and requires minimal supervision, the patient using a keyboard cover which is specially designed to facilitate ease of response. The tests proved to be acceptable to patients, and to identify impairments in alcoholics with an efficiency comparable to that of traditional testing methods. Typical results are described by Acker *et al.* (1984) and Acker (1985, 1986). The several components are derived from orthodox test procedures:

Visuospatial ability: a mannikin is displayed on the computer screen, either facing or with his back to the subject and sometimes upside down. The task is to decide whether an object is in his left or right hand.

Symbol digit coding: the subject must use a code to match digits to symbols appearing on the screen, working as quickly as he can.

Visual perceptual analysis: the subject must detect graduated differences in three matrix patterns appearing on the screen, one of which differs from the other two at each trial.

Verbal recognition memory: 36 high frequency nouns are presented serially in the first part of the test. In the second part, recognition memory is tested by forced choices between alternatives.

Visual spatial recognition memory: a pattern is exposed briefly on the screen and the subject must select it from alternatives after delays of 1, 5 or 10 seconds.

Category sorting test: this proceeds in a manner analogous to the Wisconsin Card Sorting Test (p. 118), with pictures of the material to be sorted appearing on the screen.

Cambridge Neuropsychological Test Automated Battery (CANTAB)

An ingenious and sensitive group of automated tests was developed in the context of exploring deficits in patients with Alzheimer's dementia and Parkinson's disease (Morris *et al.* 1987, 1988; Sahakian *et al.* 1988; Sahakian & Owen 1992; Robbins *et al.* 1994). They require a BBC microcomputer fitted with a touch-sensitive screen which is used to record the patient's responses. Component tests include the following, some of which are based on paradigms derived from animal work:

Motor screening test: the finger is placed on a flashing cross which moves to a new location after 6 seconds. The finger must follow the move. This serves to train the subject to point correctly, and also provides a measure of response speed.

Pattern recognition: a series of 12 abstract patterns appears on the screen, each for 3 seconds. After a short delay each must be identified by forced choices between alternatives.

Visual search task: a central box on the screen is surrounded by eight white boxes. On depressing a switch pad these 'open' to reveal patterns; the subject must locate the pattern at the periphery which matches that at the centre, responding as quickly as he can.

Spatial recognition: a sequence of squares is shown at five different positions on the screen, each square being presented for 3 seconds. After a short delay two squares are shown, one of which is in a location previously used and the other is not. The subject must point to the former.

Delayed matching to sample: a target pattern must be matched with one of four sample patterns which are presented after increasing delays.

Block span test: white squares turn blue in a preset order, each remaining blue for 1.5 seconds before returning to white again. The subject has to touch the squares in the same order as they were highlighted. Sequences of increasing length are presented.

Working memory test: an array of red squares, termed 'boxes', is presented on the screen. When a box is touched it 'opens' to show what is 'inside'. The subject must search through the boxes until a 'counter' is revealed, and having found one he must transfer it to a box at the side of the screen. He then continues searching for another counter. Errors can be made by returning to a box from which a counter has already been removed, or by returning to a box which has already been explored during the same search.

Tower of London test: this is a computerised adaptation of the test described on p. 120. The 'beads' are represented by coloured rectangular blocks superimposed one upon another; these must be moved by first touching the block itself and then the required destination.

Conditional visuospatial associative learning test: the subject must learn a set of pattern–location associations of increasing length. 'Boxes' around the margins of the screen 'open' successively for 3 seconds in random order to show their contents, these consisting of various patterns. Immediately after the last box has opened and closed a pattern is shown in the centre of the screen, and the subject must point to the box in which it had previously appeared. In later stages two, three, six and eight patterns must be located.

Aptitude tests

Tests are available for providing information concerning ability and aptitude for different kinds of task. These have mostly been introduced for educational and vocational guidance and have accordingly been standardised on healthy subjects. Nevertheless they sometimes find a useful place in the management of brain-damaged subjects. During rehabilitation they may indicate which functions require most attention, and when it comes to resettlement at work they can be valuable in indicating which forms of employment may be particularly suitable or unsuitable.

The *Differential Aptitude Test* yields scores on verbal reasoning, numerical ability, abstract reasoning, clerical speed and accuracy, mechanical reasoning, spatial relations, spelling and grammar. The *Primary Mental Abilities Test* produces similar scores on a more restricted range of functions. The *General Aptitude Test Battery* includes in addition scores for motor coordination, finger dexterity and manual dexterity, which may of course be crucial factors in the resettlement of a brain-damaged patient. Details are provided by Anastasi (1982).

Dementia questionnaires and rating scales

A number of questionnaires are available for making an approximate assessment of functions which tend to be impaired in dementing illnesses. These are not psychometric tests in the ordinary sense, but questionnaires filled in by doctors, nurses or relatives who have observed the patient closely. They often include questions relevant to social and emotional functioning in addition to observations about the patient's cognitive status.

Standardisation is often incomplete, but the questionnaires can give useful information in certain settings. Some have especial value in quantifying the degree of impairment when patients are too severely incapacitated to yield scores on formal psychometric tests. Others are useful for research purposes in allowing the separation of groups according to overall severity of disability. In clinical practice they can serve as an approximate screening device, or they can be repeated after an interval of time to gauge the rate of the patient's decline or improvement.

However, some of the more ambitious developments in the field approximate to a full clinical assessment of the patient (e.g. AGECAT and CAMDEX as described on p. 124), yielding a range of differential diagnoses and specifying the type of dementia encountered. These are proving to be invaluable in epidemiological research and other large-scale studies.

Gresham Ward Questionnaire

The Gresham Ward Questionnaire for use with elderly patients was described by Post (1965) and is set out in detail in Notes on Eliciting and Recording Clinical Information in Psychiatric Patients (1987).

Different sections contain questions relevant to orientation in time and place, memory for past personal events, memory for recent personal events, general information, and topographical orientation within the ward—each being scored separately. Uneven performance, or a total score of less than 35 points, should serve as a basis for more intensive enquiry about the possibility of brain damage.

Blessed's Dementia Scale

Blessed et al. (1968) used a standard 'dementia scale' in their study of the relationship between impairments of function and severity of neuropathological changes in the brains of old people (p. 436).

The questionnaire is administered to a close relative or friend, who must answer the questions on the basis of the patient's level of performance during the preceding 6 months. One group of questions contains items concerning competence in personal, domestic and social activities, such as ability to perform household tasks, to cope with small sums of money, to find the way in familiar surroundings and to recall recent outings and visits. The next group concerns changes of habits, such as impairment of eating, dressing and sphincter control. The third is relevant to change in personality, interest and drive, such as increased rigidity, egocentricity, coarsening of affect, impaired emotional control or the abandonment of habitual interests.

Information–Memory–Concentration Test

The Information–Memory–Concentration Test was also introduced by Blessed et al. (1968), after finding that many demented subjects could not complete more formal psychometric procedures. The test contains simple questions and tests which can usually be attempted even by severely demented subjects, thus yielding numerical scores across all grades of severity.

Information is tested by questions about name, age, time, date, place and recognition of persons. Memory is assessed by questions about past personal events and certain non-personal matters, and by testing 5-minute recall of a name and address. Concentration is tested by asking the patient to count forwards and backwards from 20, and to give the months in reverse order.

Mini-Mental State Examination (MMSE)

The MMSE was elaborated by Folstein et al. (1975) as a simplified form of the routine cognitive status examination. It has the virtue of brevity, taking only 5–10 minutes to administer, yet test–retest reliability is high and it has been shown to discriminate well between patients with dementia and delirium (Anthony et al. 1982).

The first section covers orientation, memory and attention. Memory is tested by noting the number of trials required to learn three object names, then testing recall later. Attention is assessed by the serial subtraction of 7s or by spelling a word backwards. The second section tests ability to name common objects, follow verbal and written commands, write a sentence spontaneously and copy a simple figure. The total score obtainable is 30, scores of less than 24 usually being indicative of cognitive impairment.

Geriatric Mental State Schedule (GMS)

The GMS is not simply a questionnaire but a standardised, semistructured interview for examining and recording the patient's mental state. It takes 30–40 minutes to administer and covers the period of a month prior to examination (Copeland et al. 1976).

Items are drawn from the 8th edition of the Present State Examination (Wing et al. 1967) and the Present Status Schedule (Spitzer et al. 1964) with extra sections dealing with disorientation and other cognitive abnormalities. The patient is required, for example, to spell his name, learn and recall the name of the interviewer, give his own age and date of birth, the present day and year, etc., and to recognise common objects and their functions. The cognitive sections are interspersed with less stressful questions of a more general nature. Most ratings are on a 5 point scale, with each point carefully defined. The examiner is allowed to cross-examine the patient with additional questions if he is not clear how an item should be rated.

The GMS allows classification of elderly patients by symptom profile and can demonstrate changes in the profile over time. Good reliability between raters has been shown both for individual items and for diagnoses made on the basis of the schedule (Copeland *et al.* 1976). In a correlational procedure 21 factors were produced, including three dealing with cognitive impairment ('impaired memory', 'cortical dysfunction' and 'disorientation') and others concerned with depression, anxiety, somatic concerns, etc. The ability of these factors to discriminate between organic and non-organic disorders of the elderly has been demonstrated (Gurland *et al.* 1976).

The related *Comprehensive Assessment and Referral Evaluation Schedule* (CARE) (Gurland *et al.* 1977) contains psychiatric components largely derived from the GMS, along with questions covering medical disorders, social functioning and capacity to undertake activities of daily living. Henderson *et al.* (1983) have combined parts of both instruments to produce an interview for use in community surveys.

Further developments with the GMS have involved computerisation of the data to yield diagnostic information (Copeland *et al.* 1986). The system, known as AGECAT, summates symptom components and arrives at levels of confidence with which diagnoses of organic brain syndrome, schizophrenia, depression, etc. can be made. GMS-AGECAT diagnoses of dementia and depression have been shown to agree well with diagnoses made according to DSM-III criteria (Copeland *et al.* 1990). The addition of data from an informant interview (the *History and Aetiology Schedule*, HAS) allows further refinement and subdivision of diagnoses (HAS-AGECAT), including subdivision of dementia into senile dementia of the Alzheimer type, multi-infarct dementia and alcohol-related dementia. HAS-AGECAT is being used in on-going studies of the prevalence and incidence of dementia in the elderly (Copeland *et al.* 1992).

Cambridge Examination for Mental Disorders of the Elderly (CAMDEX)

The CAMDEX was published in 1988 and has become widely influential (Roth *et al.* 1988). Its aim is to incorporate within a single standardised instrument all components needed to identify dementia in the elderly, even in the early stages. This is graded according to severity and subdivided into its main subcategories (senile dementia of Alzheimer type, vascular dementia, mixed forms, and dementia secondary to other causes). Items relevant to other confounding diagnoses are also included—delirium, depression, paranoid or paraphrenic illness, and anxiety and phobic disorders.

The schedule begins with a structured patient interview, incorporating questions regarding the present mental state, the previous personal and medical history and the family history. A standardised assessment is made of a broad range of cognitive functions, also of other aspects of the mental state, appearance and demeanour. A brief physical and neurological examination is recorded along with the results of investigations. Finally, observations and information from a relative or other informant are systematically recorded. The administration involves approximately 60 minutes with the patient and a further 20 minutes with the informant. The items of information obtained from these multiple approaches are then assembled to produce diagnostic categories according to operational diagnostic criteria. It is also possible to arrive at diagnoses in terms of ICD-10 and DSM-III-R criteria.

The subsection dealing with the cognitive examination (the CAMCOG) is particularly useful, being specially engineered to be 'user friendly' for non-psychologists. It incorporates tests of orientation, memory, language, perceptual abilities, praxis, attention and abstract thinking. Items contained within it comprise the MMSE (p. 123) but the CAMCOG is more thorough in its assessment. It can stand alone for certain purposes as a valuable brief means of performing a neuropsychological examination.

An earlier version of the CAMDEX was shown to be acceptable to patients, with a high inter-rater reliability (Roth *et al.* 1986). Detailed comparisons have been carried out between the CAMCOG and other instruments for the detection of dementia, including the AGECAT computer program outlined above (Blessed *et al.* 1991). High levels of agreement have been demonstrated, AGECAT being rather more conservative in its diagnoses. Using a cut-off point of between 69 and 70 for CAMCOG scores, high levels of sensitivity and specificity have been demonstrated.

Crichton Geriatric Behaviour Rating Scale

This is a group nursing assessment applied retrospectively on impressions gained during the preceding week (Robinson 1961, 1977). The 10 items involved convey a vignette of behaviour and functional capacities which can be drawn up rapidly and with reasonable reliability.

The areas covered were selected specifically for use with brain-damaged elderly patients: mobility, orientation, communication, cooperation, restlessness, dressing, feeding, continence, sleep and mood. Each is rated on a 5-point scale, 1 representing normality and 5 severe failure on the function concerned. Points on the scale are verbally described and the level most appropriate to the patient must be checked. In scoring 'communication', for example, the scale is as follows: Always clear and retains information (1); can indicate needs, can understand verbal directions, can deal with simple information (2); understands simple verbal and non-verbal information but does not indicate needs (3); cannot understand simple verbal or non-verbal information but retains some expressive ability (4); no effective contact (5).

Clifton Assessment Schedule

This is a brief assessment procedure for use with psychogeriatric patients. Twelve items are scored by nurses covering aspects of information, orientation and such mental abilities as counting, reading, writing and repeating the alphabet. The Gibson Spiral Maze is used in addition as a brief test of psychomotor performance. Scores derived from the schedule have been shown to have good predictive validity in terms of outcome at follow-up, and in the distinction between organic and non-organic psychiatric disorders in the elderly (Pattie & Gilleard 1975, 1976, 1978).

Stockton Geriatric Rating Scale

The Stockton Geriatric Rating Scale was introduced by Meer and Baker (1966) as a 33-item scale for assessing both physical disability and behaviour in elderly patients. It has been modified for British use and shortened to 18 items by Gilleard and Pattie (1977). Each item is rated by nurses on a simple 3-point scale and summated to yield four subscores: physical disability, apathy, communication difficulties and social disturbance. Their validity in terms of outcome and diagnostic groupings has been examined as for the Clifton Assessment Schedule (Pattie & Gilleard 1975, 1978).

Present Behavioural Examination (PBE)

The PBE aims to chart disturbed behaviours in detail in patients with dementia (Hope & Fairburn 1992). It is administered by interview with the carers of patients, covering behaviour over the preceding 4 weeks. This period was selected to be long enough for ratings to be little affected by day-to-day fluctuations and to pick up relatively rare but important aspects of behaviour. Questioning is by specified probes, followed by further detailed questioning where necessary. Eight main sections deal with mental health, walking (including wandering and hyperactivity), eating, diurnal rhythm, aggressive behaviour, sexual behaviour, incontinence and a number of individual behavioural abnormalities. Wherever possible ratings are made of the frequency of occurrence of the behaviour in question so that the measures will be sensitive to change, other items being rated in terms of sever-

ity. Test–retest and inter-rater reliabilities have emerged as satisfactory. With suitable adaptation it should be amenable for use with other disorders such as head injury, stroke and mental handicap.

Manchester and Oxford Universities Scale for the Psychopathological Assessment of Dementia (MOUSEPAD)

This scale, recently described by Allen et al. (1996), similarly charts psychopathological and behavioural changes in dementia, and like the PBE is administered by interviewing the carers of patients. Though briefer than the PBE it contains more items relevant to delusions and hallucinations. The questions refer to the entire duration of the dementia syndrome, but supplementary questions allow focusing on the past month alone.

Performance Test of Activities of Daily Living (PADL)

This is a simple and rapidly administered test for assessing capacity for self care. It is unaffected by lack of insight and has the special advantage of requiring the minimum of verbal communication. The patient is required to demonstrate his ability to perform 16 tasks which are essential for functional independence, such as drinking, dressing, etc. He is then assigned to a category of 'independent', 'moderately independent' or 'dependent' according to the proportion of tasks correctly performed. Kuriansky et al. (1976) have shown that the results obtained agree closely with an informant's assessment of the patient's self-care capacity, but not with the patient's own assessment. An objective test of this nature is thus preferable to a questionnaire administered to the patient himself. The test has been shown to discriminate well between elderly patients with organic and non-organic disorders and to correlate well with short-term outcome of hospitalisation.

Vineland Social Maturity Scale

The Vineland Social Maturity Scale (Doll 1947) has been mainly used for studies in child development and mental retardation, but can also be useful in providing a measure of social functioning in brain-damaged adults. Repeat administration after an interval of time can reveal gains or losses in the social field, usefully supplementing measures of intellectual ability.

The scale consists of 117 items which sample various aspects of social ability—capacity for self care, social independence in personal activities and social responsibility. The items are scored by interviewing someone closely acquainted with the patient. The chief categories of function measured by the scale are as follows: 'self help general' (for example 'cares for self at toilet', 'tells time to quarter hour'); 'self help eating' (for example 'drinks from cup or glass unaided', 'uses table knife for spreading'); 'self help dressing' ('dresses self except for tying', 'bathes self assisted', 'bathes self unaided'); 'self direction' ('makes minor purchases', 'uses money providently'); 'occupation' ('uses tools or utensils', 'does simple creative work'); 'communication' ('prints simple words', 'makes telephone calls', 'follows current events'); 'locomotion' ('goes about neighbourhood unattended', 'goes about home freely', 'goes to distant places alone'); and 'socialisation' ('plays simple table games', 'assumes responsibilities beyond own needs', 'shares community responsibility').

Ancillary investigations

Further investigations will often be required when an organic basis is suspected for psychiatric disorder. Certain routine tests should ideally be performed on all psychiatric in-patients, including estimation of haemoglobin, erythrocyte sedimentation rate, serological tests for syphilis, chest X-ray and routine urine examination. The patient's temperature should always be taken, with 4-hourly recording if minor rises are suspected. These serve as screening tests for coincidental as well as causally related physical disorders. Other investigations will be indicated on the basis of the history and clinical examination when specific disorders are suspected. An important principle is that investigations should always be planned to give the maximum of required information with the minimum of inconvenience to the patient. Investigations which are without discomfort or risk will obviously be more readily undertaken than those which carry the possibility of pain or complications. Skull X-ray, electroencephalography and computerised tomography (CT) scanning, for example, will sometimes be performed even when the level or suspicion of organic involvement is low, whereas lumbar puncture and other invasive procedures will be reserved until very specific and important questions need to be answered.

Some indication of the relative use made of different investigatory procedures was provided by Macfie (1972) who reviewed the diagnostic practices on a number of general psychiatric units at the Maudsley Hospital. Among 136 consecutive new admissions, the investigations shown in Table 2 were carried out.

It can be seen that the yield of abnormal results was low where many of the commoner investigations were concerned, but these were procedures which caused little discomfort to the patient. Some investigations such as serum protein bound iodine, B$_{12}$ and folate, and estimation of urinary porphyrins gave uniformly negative results, yet were each undertaken in approximately 10% of the patients. Here a very low level of suspicion clearly dictated the investigations because of the importance of detecting abnormalities when they exist. Lumbar puncture, by con-

Table 2 Ancillary investigations among 136 consecutive psychiatric in-patients (after Macfie 1972).

	% patients examined	% abnormal of those examined
Routine haematology	89	7
Serological tests for syphilis	75	1
Chest X-ray	75	12
Electroencephalogram	42	14
Serum electrolytes	33	9
Skull X-ray	29	5
Drugs in urine	24	3
Serum proteins and liver function tests	18	28
Serum protein bound iodine	14	0
Psychological tests for brain damage	13	65
Serum B$_{12}$	11	0
Urinary porphyrins	9	0
Serum folate	7	0
Lumbar puncture	7	20

trast, was used with considerable discrimination and yielded a high proportion of abnormal findings.

The requests for an EEG may be contrasted in Table 2 with requests for psychological investigation for brain damage. EEGs were requested three times as often as psychological tests yet the yield of abnormal results was very much lower. Here it would seem that common practice has been to use the EEG in a less discriminating manner, perhaps even as a screening test, whereas psychometry was undertaken only after full consultation between psychiatrist and psychologist.

This study was, of course, carried out before the introduction of CT scanning. The yield of abnormal CT scan results in psychiatric patients from various series is described by Roberts and Lishman (1984).

Examination of the blood will usually include estimation of haemoglobin, erythrocyte sedimentation rate, and white blood count and differential. In the presence of anaemia full haematological studies will be needed. Serological tests for syphilis remain extremely important. The serum B$_{12}$ and folate will sometimes be estimated even in the absence of anaemia (pp. 589 and 592). Biochemical investigations may include estimation of urea and electrolytes (including on occasion calcium and phosphorus), serum proteins, liver function tests, blood sugar studies, serum lipids and serum caeruloplasmin. The serum T$_3$ and T$_4$ may give indications of thyroid disorder. The blood alcohol level or other drug levels may need to be investigated. Very occasionally immunological tests will be required, including the search for antinuclear antibodies.

Examination of the urine will include routine tests for sugar, albumin and specific gravity, and sometimes microscopy and culture. Examination for drugs will sometimes be indicated, and more rarely for porphyrins, catecholamines or steroids. Very occasionally a search will be made for heavy metals in the urine or the blood.

Chest X-ray is important for the evaluation of cardiac and pulmonary status, and in particular for the detection of carcinoma of the lung or tuberculosis. Electrocardiography may provide evidence of dysrhythmia, cardiac ischaemia or recent coronary thrombosis, and can occasionally provide evidence of serum potassium abnormalities.

The indications for these and other investigations are detailed in the relevant chapters later in the book. The special investigations required in connection with some of the rarer causes of dementia are outlined on p. 496. Certain other investigations of particular relevance to cerebral dysfunction will be discussed in detail below.

Electroencephalography

The EEG has the important advantage over many other procedures that it is safe and without discomfort to the patient. It is accordingly used extensively when organic psychiatric disorders are suspected. It remains, furthermore, the major non-invasive means of determining the physiological or functional state of the brain, as opposed to its anatomical status. However, certain marked limitations in its diagnostic usefulness must be borne in mind.

Characteristics

EEG rhythms are conventionally classified into four components according to their frequencies — delta rhythms at less than 4 Hz, theta at 4–7 Hz, alpha at 8–13 Hz, and beta in excess of 13 Hz (Terminology Committee, Storm van Leeuwen *et al.* 1966). The normal EEG has a well-developed alpha rhythm, maximal in the occipital and parietal regions, which attenuates on opening the eyes and reappears when they are closed again. It similarly attenuates when the patient engages in mental activity such as simple mental arithmetic. The average voltage of the alpha rhythm is 30–50 μV with spindle-shaped modulations. Small amounts of other rhythms are allowable provided the alpha activity is well developed. Beta activity is seen mainly in the precentral regions, and low-voltage theta becomes more obvious with relaxation and drowsiness. Delta activity is normally seen only in very young children and during sleep.

Lambda waves are saw-toothed in form and characteristically situated over the occiput. They reflect small eyeball movements. Mu rhythm has a characteristic wave form and a frequency within the alpha range; it is commonly present in the Rolandic area and is diminished by

contralateral limb movement (Toone 1984). K complexes are brief bursts of high-voltage slow waves which may emerge during non-REM (rapid eye movement) sleep.

Abnormal EEG elements which can be important in diagnosis include the following:

'Spikes' are high peaked discharges which rise and fall abruptly and stand out above the general amplitude of the other waves. 'Sharp waves' rise steeply then fall more slowly, and may occupy the alpha, theta or delta range. Composite elements may consist of spikes alternating with delta waves ('spike and wave' or 'wave and spike' discharges) or slow waves preceded by several spikes ('poly-spike and wave'). Wave and spike discharges occurring at a rhythm of 3 Hz constitute the classic EEG feature of simple absence attacks; those faster and slower than this may be referred to as 'wave and spike variants'. Abnormal rhythms and other elements can be generalised, unilateral or focal, and may be described as synchronous or asynchronous depending on the coincidence of their appearance in different leads.

Various activating procedures may be used to clarify marginal abnormalities, or to bring out those which are concealed in the resting record. Hyperventilation is used to increase the excitability of cortical cells, probably mainly as a result of hypocapnic constriction of cerebral vessels leading to cerebral hypoxia (Meyer & Gotoh 1960). Epileptic foci and other disturbances may emerge more clearly. Photic stimulation consists of repetitive light flashes of varying frequency. Within certain ranges of flash frequency (especially 8–15 Hz) the occipital alpha rhythm adjusts itself to the flash rate (occipital 'driving'), and paroxysmal abnormalities may emerge in the form of high-voltage complex elements spreading to the frontal and temporal regions. Seizure patterns may emerge, and a generalised seizure may even be provoked. Sleep may be induced by barbiturates if it does not occur naturally. This can be useful in activating the spike or sharp wave discharges of epilepsy, especially those arising within the temporal lobes. Thiopentone may be given intravenously, and typically induces beta activity, often in the form of discrete runs or spindles. The induced beta activity is commonly less well developed at the electrodes over the site of damage in the affected temporal lobe. Other drugs which may occasionally be employed for the activation of seizure patterns are chlorpromazine or injections of metrazole. The latter must be reserved for use under skilled supervision in specialised centres, since fits are liable to be provoked.

In addition to the normal electrode placements over the scalp, sphenoidal, nasopharyngeal or foramen ovale electrodes can be valuable for locating discharges from the antero-inferior portions of the temporal lobes. These are chiefly used when assessing the suitability of epileptic patients for temporal lobectomy. Much may also be gained from depth electrode studies, or by recording directly from the exposed cortex at operation ('electrocorticography'). These procedures can obviously be undertaken only in special centres.

Limitations

In many ways the EEG has failed to satisfy early expectations as a diagnostic aid for reasons discussed by Kiloh *et al.* (1981). Accordingly it must only be interpreted with its limitations clearly in mind. Moreover much of its traditional advantage in being non-invasive has now been eroded by the introduction of modern brain imaging techniques (Toone 1984).

In the first place the EEG can be normal in patients with obvious cerebral dysfunction, certainly if reliance is put upon a single recording. It is probably true to say that a normal EEG never excludes any clinical condition, but can merely serve to diminish the probability of its existence. Conversely, a certain proportion of healthy individuals will show abnormal EEGs. The EEG is particularly sensitive to such physiological variables as level of awareness, acid–base equilibrium and blood sugar level. Such physiological changes in the record are indistinguishable from those associated with many pathological states, and can readily be misinterpreted as evidence of disease.

Again, with rare exceptions, the patterns obtained have little diagnostic specificity, and the EEG should only be used as an additional source of information to add to the evidence of the history and clinical examination. It can be a valuable aid in localisation but is of little help in pathological diagnosis. Even with regard to localisation it is known that a focal lesion can occasionally be associated with disturbance some distance away, or alternatively give rise to generalised EEG abnormalities. For these reasons the most useful help will be obtained from the investigation when the person interpreting the record is fully acquainted with all relevant clinical information about the patient's illness.

There can be added difficulties in psychiatric patients, in that mental disorders of apparently non-organic origin are known to be associated with an increased incidence of abnormalities in the EEG. This can sometimes cloud the issue when it comes to the differential diagnosis between organic and non-organic psychiatric conditions. The large and often confusing literature on the subject has been reviewed by Ellingson (1954), Hill (1963a) and Fenton (1974). Whereas perhaps 10–15% of normal subjects show some abnormality on the EEG, this figure has sometimes been found to be higher among patients with neurotic disorders. The abnormalities in such patients commonly lie just outside the normal range, with an excess of generalised theta or beta rhythms of rather low amplitude. Patients with manic depressive disorder have been reported to show marginally abnormal records in up to 20% of cases, though again the finding is far from consistently upheld. Schizophrenia is sometimes associated with more definite abnormalities, in perhaps a quarter of cases (Abenson 1970). Abrams and Taylor (1980) found abnormal records in a quarter of patients suffering from affective disorder or schizophrenia, with significantly more abnormalities in the latter. Correlations were noted between left-sided abnormalities and both thought disorder and emotional blunting. Catatonic schizophrenia shows abnormal records more commonly than other varieties. No particular pattern is characteristic, but Hill (1957a) reported epileptiform activity in a high proportion of schizophrenic patients, usually of low amplitude. This may consist of grouped spikes, fast spikes and waves, or paroxysmal slow waves with the spike components minimally in evidence. In catatonic stupor normal rhythms tend to be replaced by low-amplitude slow activity, sometimes extending to the delta range. However, these changes are not constant, failing to appear in some patients and sometimes varying from one attack to another in the same patient.

In patients with disorders of behaviour and personality the incidence of abnormalities is perhaps highest of all. Hill and Watterson (1942) found that 48% of patients diagnosed as psychopathic had abnormal EEGs compared with 15% of controls, and among aggressive psychopaths the proportion rose to 65%. A 70% incidence of EEG abnormalities in prisoners convicted of apparently motiveless murders has been observed (Stafford-Clark & Taylor 1949; Okasha *et al.* 1975). The majority of the abnormalities in patients with personality disorder appear to reflect cerebral immaturity, and are of a type which would be accepted as normal in a very much younger age group. Hill (1952) listed the abnormalities as bilateral rhythmic theta activity in central and temporal regions, alpha variants, and posterior temporal slow wave foci which were usually episodic. Personality disorder with antisocial conduct was especially liable to be associated with focal abnormality in the temporal lobes and particularly the posterior temporal areas. Sometimes the so-called immaturity may be the result of past cerebral insults, even of birth injury, but the great majority appear merely to be associated with delayed maturation. Thus the abnormalities tend to decrease with age, and this may be accompanied by a parallel improvement in behaviour.

Another difficulty with psychiatric patients can be the result of treatments currently or recently given. Many of the widely prescribed drugs affect the EEG, and in some individuals to a marked extent. Fenton (1974) and Kiloh *et al.* (1981) review the main changes that occur. Barbiturates and other sedatives increase fast activity and sometimes produce a small amount of diffuse theta or even delta activity. Most sedatives also tend to aggravate epileptic discharges. Anticonvulsants other than barbiturates, on the other hand, have little effect on the EEG. Chlorpromazine in low dosage may disturb alpha activity, with the occasional appearance of slow frequencies. In high dosage it may produce generalised delta waves or hypersynchronous high-voltage discharges. Chlorpromazine also potentiates epileptic discharges. Similar changes are produced by other phenothiazines, butyrophenones, tricyclic antidepressants and lithium. Chlordiazepoxide and diazepam are usually associated with increased fast activity.

Electroconvulsive therapy can render the EEG hard to interpret for a time. Each fit is followed by generalised theta and delta activity which becomes more persistent as successive treatments are given. After three or four treatments spaced at intervals of 2–3 days the abnormal rhythms may persist in the intervals between, often with frontal preponderance. As the course of treatment proceeds the disturbance becomes more widespread and of higher voltage, and alpha activity may disappear. Individual patients differ in the severity of these effects and in the time taken for return to normality. Shagass (1965) reported that most patients regained a normal pattern 1–3 months after the termination of a course of 6–12 treatments given thrice weekly.

Uses

This brief description of some of the difficulties surrounding the interpretation of the EEG is necessary before discussing situations where it can serve a useful purpose. In general terms, suspicions of abnormality of brain structure or function are confirmed by the EEG in 60% of cases (Kugler 1964); hence it can bring added information in psychiatric patients when the question of an organic basis for the illness has arisen. In diagnostically obscure cases one can look for clues which may indicate the need for further investigation. A single focus of abnormally fast or slow activity will always suggest the presence of a cerebral lesion and must be followed up further, likewise gross asymmetries of normal or abnormal activity between the hemispheres. The EEG also plays a part in the differentiation between organic and non-organic psychiatric illness, though caution must be observed. A normal record will be of little help in the distinction, but it will certainly be less easy to maintain a diagnosis of a purely psychogenic disturbance in the presence of a grossly abnormal record.

The disturbances seen in *epileptic subjects* are considered in detail in Chapter 7. Characteristic epileptic discharges consist of spikes, sharp waves or wave and spike complexes. When recurrent these are very strong evidence in favour of an epileptic process. In primary generalised epilepsy wave and spike complexes may consist of runs of classic three per second spike and wave, but in the presence of grand mal attacks they are commonly somewhat faster or consist of variants with polyspike and wave. Other abnormalities common in epileptics, but without the same degree of specificity, include paroxysms of symmetrical delta activity, bursts of theta, or a diffuse excess of delta and theta. Epilepsy which originates within the cortex shows a spike and sharp wave focus, or local spike discharges either singly or in groups. These often betray the point of origin of the seizures, though sometimes they are transmitted widely to other areas. Temporal lobe epilepsy often shows spike discharges over the temporal region, but occasionally the record can be normal until sleep is induced and sphenoidal or nasopharyngeal electrodes are employed.

The principal value of the EEG in epilepsy is to distinguish patients with a discharging cortical focus from those with primary generalised epilepsy. In patients without an aura to their grand mal attacks there may be no other means of making the distinction. The EEG can often localise the cortical lesion, and indicate whether it is circumscribed in extent, unilateral or bilateral. This becomes very important when deciding how far to explore the responsible pathology, and when the question of surgery for the relief of epilepsy is likely to arise.

On the broader question of the diagnosis of epilepsy, the EEG can be useful but is not an infallible guide. Epileptiform discharges are found in occasional normal persons, in many degenerative brain disorders and in some patients with psychosis or personality disorder. Conversely, in some 20–30% of patients with epilepsy, a single routine EEG will be normal. In exceptional cases the record can remain normal even during an attack, as in some cases of Jacksonian and psychomotor epilepsy when the foci are so discrete, and of such low voltage, that they fail to reach the surface electrodes. The recognition of the epileptic nature of a group of symptoms must therefore remain primarily a clinical task, but one which obtains firm confirmation from the EEG in the majority of cases. Where the clinical features are dubious this confirmation can have a decisive influence on the diagnosis and future management. Classic spike and wave discharges, for example, may resolve doubts when an adequate witnessed account of attacks is not forthcoming. And in temporal lobe epilepsy, the EEG can sometimes point directly to the diagnosis in patients who have hitherto been considered to suffer from 'hysteria', anxiety attacks or short-lived psychotic reactions.

Space-occupying lesions are revealed by the EEG in a high proportion of cases. A focal delta wave focus will constitute strong presumptive evidence of a cerebral tumour, especially when combined with the other features outlined in Chapter 6 (p. 232). Alternatively it may give the first indication of a developing cerebral abscess when this arises as a complication of a generalised infection. A subdural haematoma in the elderly sometimes presents with a psychiatric picture, and the EEG can be the factor which alerts one to the diagnosis. Typically there is diminished amplitude or suppression of cerebral rhythms over the affected hemisphere, and some irregular slow activity on the affected side, though the contralateral hemisphere may be affected as well (p. 412).

Positive findings are therefore of value, but negative findings must not be interpreted as excluding possible pathology. In approximately 20% of tumours a normal record may be obtained, particularly with slow-growing varieties which carry the best prognosis. The EEG may fail to reveal evidence of a subdural haematoma in a similar proportion of cases. One must also beware of the occasional cases with well-defined but utterly misleading foci, even sometimes locating the tumour or haematoma to the wrong side of the head.

With *cerebral infarctions* the EEG can be of help in gauging prognosis. Patients with minimal changes during the acute episode can in general be expected to make a good recovery, also patients in whom the EEG changes resolve steadily from an early date. An EEG which becomes normal while neurological deficits persist, however, will suggest that little further clinical improvement can be expected.

After *head injury* the EEG may again sometimes help in gauging prognosis (p. 165), or in pointing to an organic component in disturbances which have seemed to be purely psychological in origin. EEG changes may occasionally foreshadow the development of post-traumatic epilepsy, but the interseizure record remains normal in a high proportion of patients even when fits have already become established.

In *encephalitis* the EEG, together with examination of the cerebrospinal fluid (CSF), can be a valuable means of following progress. Abnormalities consist of diffuse irregular slow waves and scattered sharp waves, with slowing or reduction in alpha activity. Seizure patterns are not uncommon in the acute stage. There may be a warning of complications and of permanent brain damage when slow waves persist. The appearance of new spikes or spike and wave complexes raises the possibility that secondary epilepsy will develop. In subacute sclerosing panencephalitis the EEG changes described on p. 362 have high diagnostic value.

In *metabolic disorders* the EEG is a sensitive indicator of cerebral insufficiency, and can reflect worsening or improvement of the clinical condition with a fair degree of accuracy. The changes lack specificity for the various metabolic disorders, being for example similar in hypoglycaemia, anoxia, hypokalaemia, carbon dioxide retention or vitamin B_{12} deficiency. Nevertheless, they can provide important information in patients who present with indefinite features in the mental state. They may help to confirm the organic basis for paranoid syndromes or disturbances of behaviour in patients who are only minimally confused. Or when organic features are well developed the EEG may help in the sometimes difficult distinction between reversible causes and progressive brain pathology. Obrecht *et al.* (1979) have demonstrated the value of the EEG in patients with acute confusional states in general hospital practice, in particular in helping to distinguish metabolic and other systemic disorders from intracranial pathologies.

The earliest changes are slowing of the alpha rhythm along with diminution of voltage. Later there is progressive slowing and disorganisation, with runs of theta which come to replace all other activity. Finally, in metabolic coma regular high-voltage delta activity appears, sometimes bilaterally synchronous and sometimes more random in distribution. In deep coma, when the patient is quite unresponsive, the amplitude of the EEG diminishes and ultimately the record becomes flat and featureless.

Engel and Romano (1959) re-emphasised earlier findings about the importance of the EEG in the diagnosis of delirium and in the detection of minor degrees of impairment of consciousness. A close correlation was demonstrated between the degree of slowing of the EEG, and the degree of disturbance of consciousness as reflected in impairment of functions such as awareness, attention, memory and comprehension (Romano & Engel 1944). Moreover, when the effects of hypoxia, hypoglycaemia and alcohol were observed in the same individuals, an equivalent degree of cognitive disturbance was obtained for comparable degrees of slowing of the EEG, even though more personal aspects of behaviour, affect and thought content could be very different (Engel *et al.* 1945).

With very mild affections, when cognitive difficulty can be hard to detect on clinical examination, the EEG has already begun to slow. This can be shown by serial recordings, and can occasionally be useful in the retrospective diagnosis of minimal degrees of clouding of consciousness. The absolute frequency of the dominant rhythm is less important than the degree of slowing. Thus 8–9 Hz may be abnormal if it has replaced alpha of a higher frequency. This explains why patients with clouding of consciousness can have an apparently normal EEG. When slowing has reached 5–6 Hz the characteristic disruption of activity on eye opening no longer occurs, representing the physiological correlate of the reduced impact of perceptions derived from the environment. Fluctuations in the severity of delirium, as reflected in outward behaviour, prove not to be related to changes in the underlying metabolic disturbance as reflected in the EEG, but to be more closely tied to psychological and environmental factors.

How widely Engel and Romano's findings may be applied to all causes of delirium is unknown. Kiloh *et al.* (1981) suggest that there is often a direct relationship between level of consciousness and degree of EEG abnormality but that this is not invariable. Delirium tremens is an obvious exception, in that during profound delirium the EEG may be normal or show fast activity of low to moderate voltage rather than slowing of rhythms. Lipowski (1990) suggests that slowing of the EEG is characteristic of delirium which presents with reduced alertness and wakefulness, whereas in hyperactive delirium fast activity may be superimposed on this, sometimes with features resembling those of REM sleep.

The EEG can be of some diagnostic help in comatose patients. Comas due to metabolic disturbance will show diffuse high-voltage delta activity as described above, whereas in barbiturate overdosage there will be augmented amplitude and an increase in fast frequencies. Space-occupying lesions may be indicated by focal abnormalities, or epileptic activity may be revealed.

In the *presenile and senile dementias* the degree of EEG abnormality appears to be more closely related to the rate of progression of the disorder than to the degree of intellectual impairment at a given point in time. The changes are described along with the individual diseases in Chapter 10. Briefly, in senile dementia of the Alzheimer type the commonest abnormality is accentuation of the normal EEG changes with ageing, and may therefore be difficult to diagnose with confidence. Alpha activity is slowed in frequency and reduced in quantity, and diffuse theta or delta rhythms tend to appear. The vascular dementias show a similar picture, though often with focal features where local cerebral infarctions have occurred. Presenile Alzheimer's disease is associated with a particularly high incidence of abnormalities. Alpha activity tends to disappear, and is replaced with irregular theta upon which runs of delta activity may be superimposed. Pronounced flattening of the record will raise the possibility

of Huntington's chorea, whereas repetitive spike discharges or characteristic triphasic sharp wave complexes may be indicative of Creutzfeldt–Jakob disease.

In all of these conditions the EEG abnormalities may fail to develop in a significant proportion of mild to moderate cases, and even advanced dementia can occasionally exist alongside a normal EEG. Moreover, with some exceptions, the changes that occur lack specificity for the illnesses in question. Nevertheless an EEG can be helpful in early and uncertain cases of dementia. A normal EEG in such circumstances will make Alzheimer's disease unlikely, but will not exclude other varieties of dementia. The EEG may also help in the distinction between diffuse and focal lesions.

Finally, in elderly patients the EEG may aid in the differentiation between depressive pseudodementia and degenerative brain disease. A normal EEG in a patient who has been diagnosed as suffering from Alzheimer's disease or vascular dementia, and who shows features of depression, will at least suggest that the diagnosis should be reconsidered (Kiloh *et al.* 1981).

Event-related potentials (evoked potentials, ERPs, EPs)

Incoming sensory stimuli are associated with brief changes in brain potentials, and these can be detected when suitable averaging methods are used to demarcate them from the background EEG activity. Successive epochs of EEG are summated and averaged by computer while repeated visual, auditory or somatosensory stimuli are presented to the subject. The value of such techniques lies in their non-invasive nature, and the minimal requirement for cooperation from the subject. Moreover certain late components of ERPs, when coupled with minimal task demands, have proved to reflect psychological processes such as expectation and motivation, and to be abnormal in some psychiatric conditions.

The early components, generated within 20 ms or so from stimulus presentation, reflect neuronal activity in the sensory end organs and afferent pathways, and can be sensitive indicators of pathology in the auditory apparatus, optic pathways and brain stem. The value of visual pattern evoked responses, brain stem auditory evoked responses and somatosensory responses in the diagnosis of multiple sclerosis is described on p. 689. Wright *et al.* (1984) found that while pattern evoked responses were normal in dementia, the major positive component (P_2) to flash was considerably delayed, presumably because this is generated in association cortex rather than primary visual cortex.

The principal interest for psychiatry, however, centres

on the late components of ERPs elicited while the subject is engaged in some simple task ('cognitive ERPs'). Grey Walter *et al.* (1964) described the 'contingent negative variation' (CNV), observed when a subject was told to press a button in response to a flash of light which occurred 3 seconds after hearing a warning click. During the period of expectation a negative potential could be recorded from the scalp which increased steadily in amplitude until the button press was performed. Sutton *et al.* (1965) then showed that certain late potentials were a function of the uncertainty experienced by the subject during simple test procedures, in particular the development of a large late positive potential some 300 ms after stimulus presentation ('P_{300} response'). In a typical test paradigm the subject listens to a series of auditory tones, most of which are identical in pitch, but with the random appearance of rarer stimuli at another pitch ('odd-ball paradigm'). The subject must attend carefully, and respond with a button press or make a mental count of the abnormal target stimuli. These then induce a series of late potentials—a negative deflection at approximately 100 ms (N_1 or N_{100}), a positive potential at 200 ms (P_2), followed by N_2 then P_{300} potentials at 300 ms. This last component has been extensively studied in relation to dementia and schizophrenia.

The P_{300} is significantly delayed in a majority of patients with dementia, and in proportion to the severity of the dementia (Gordon *et al.* 1986; Neshige *et al.* 1988). There are indications, moreover, that differences can be discerned in different varieties of dementia. Goodin and Aminoff (1986) showed that patients with 'subcortical dementia' (Parkinson's and Huntington's disease) showed more severe delays in the P_{300} than Alzheimer patients, also longer delays in the earlier N_1 and P_2 components. The Parkinson and the Huntington patients differed from one another by greater P_2 delay in the latter group. Observations have also been made in Parkinson patients during 'on' and 'off' phases, with significant decreases in P_{300} latency while motor ability is improved (Starkstein *et al.* 1989). Goodin *et al.* (1990) found delayed latencies in all four components in patients with AIDS dementia, and to a lesser extent in many HIV-positive men who were clinically asymptomatic and with normal EEGs. It remains to be determined how far this may indicate subclinical brain infection and be of prognostic significance.

P_{300} findings in schizophrenia are more variable, but a majority of investigators have found diminished amplitudes of response, with or without abnormal latencies. Blackwood and Muir (1990) summarise studies showing differences between schizophrenic and depressed patients, and which may hold promise for circumscribing

the boundaries of schizophrenia more closely. The P_{300} changes appear to be largely independent of the state of relapse or remission, and have been detected in asymptomatic relatives of schizophrenic patients, McConaghy *et al.* (1993) have demonstrated a relationship between P_{300} amplitude and measures of schizophrenic thought disorder, also with measures of 'allusive thinking' in normal subjects. In a combined ERP and magnetic resonance imaging (MRI) study of schizophrenic patients, McCarley *et al.* (1993) found that reductions in P_{300} amplitude were significantly related to reductions of grey matter in the left posterior superior temporal gyrus (including Heschl's gyrus and the planum temporale), suggesting that these structures may play a major role in generating the auditory P_{300} response. Asymmetries between left and right P_{300} responses went in hand with the asymmetries in temporal volume reductions.

Brain electrical activity mapping (BEAM)

Brain electrical activity mapping represents an attempt to gain maximal information from EEG and evoked potential data, by displaying regional brain activity in the form of visual topographic maps. Several systems are now in use, the common aim being to extract visual information relevant to electrophysiological abnormality as a complement to structural and metabolic methods of brain imaging.

Duffy *et al.* (1979) introduced BEAM, using 24 scalp electrodes to record EEG and visual evoked responses. The EEG data were subjected to spectral analysis, and runs containing spike discharges were digitised. Extremely brief epochs of the evoked responses were displayed in quick succession. The spatiotemporal information obtained in this manner was displayed as colour-coded maps, interpolated values being calculated for points between electrode placements. Buchsbaum *et al.* (1982) developed an analogous system. Morihisa (1989) describes the strengths and limitations of such techniques, and the findings that have emerged in relation to schizophrenia and developmental dyslexia. The value of BEAM in diagnosis has been largely superseded by the other brain imaging techniques described on p. 137 *et seq.*

Fractal analysis

Bullmore *et al.* (1992, 1994) have recently described a promising development in 'fractal analysis' of EEG patterns, which substantially reduces the volume of EEG data without loss of diagnostically important information.

The fractal dimensions of consecutive 10-second epochs of digitised EEG data were estimated and shown to be sensitive in detecting ictal events.

Magnetoencephalography (MEG)

Magnetoencephalography has been developed during the past two decades as a method for studying brain electrical activity which is complementary to the EEG. It aims to measure, not the electrical activity directly, but the minute magnetic fields which are a by-product of that activity. These are charted over extremely brief epochs of time, measured in milliseconds. The fundamentals of the technique are described by Reeve et al. (1989), Fagaly (1990) and Andrews (1996).

The advantage of charting magnetic fields is that they are not attenuated and distorted by passage through the brain tissue, skull and scalp as are the electrical currents which make up the EEG. Consequently localisation, whether superficial or deep, stands to be enhanced. And since the EEG is partly derived from radially orientated current sources and MEG from tangential sources, the simultaneous recording of both together can provide complementary information with regard to the intracranial origin of electrical activity.

In recording the magnetoencephalogram a detection coil is placed in close proximity to the head surface and feeds information to a SQUID sensor (superconducting quantum interference device). Both the detection coil and the SQUID must be kept at superconducting temperatures, either by enclosing them in liquid helium in a vacuum-insulated chamber or by using closed-cycle refrigeration. This 'magnetometer' is capable of measuring extremely small variations in magnetic flux. The resulting information is fed through appropriate electronics to a data acquisition system. Since the SQUID must be protected from major changes in environmental magnetic fields it is usually necessary to carry out the recordings in a magnetically shielded room. Multichannel detection systems with up to 100 detector units are now available in certain research centres.

Though still largely a research technique, MEG has shown its potential for answering both fundamental and clinical problems. A principal virtue is its capacity to localise the source of electrical signals, whether in the form of epileptic discharges or during studies of sensory evoked potentials. Sutherling and Barth (1990) outline the benefits likely to accrue in the localisation of epileptic foci without the need for depth electrodes, and in revealing the patterns of propagation of spike discharges. Fenwick (1990a) describes the potential for monitoring deep discharges from the limbic system in patients with schizophrenia or behavioural disorder. Reite (1990) has studied the magnetic evoked response to auditory stimulation (M_{50}), finding that schizophrenic patients show less asymmetry than normal subjects, possibly reflecting anatomical differences in the left planum temporale.

Considerable technical problems remain to be resolved before MEG becomes widely available as a clinical or research instrument. Not least is the problem of developing valid models for localisation deep within the brain in the presence of multiple dipole sources with differing orientations. It is likely, however, that the technique will contribute importantly to the understanding of the genesis of signals related to perception, cognition and behavioural responses, and it possibly stands to clarify the site of major electrophysiological disturbances associated with psychiatric disorders. It could ultimately find a valuable place in the clinical investigation of patients with epilepsy.

Lumbar puncture

Examination of the CSF can give valuable information in many clinical situations. It is usually a safe procedure but should never be undertaken lightly. The principal hazard is in patients with raised intracranial pressure and particularly when an intracranial tumour is present. The abrupt reduction of pressure due to withdrawal of fluid can bring about tentorial herniation or a medullary pressure cone with fatal results. Even when the needle is quickly removed there may be continued leakage from the puncture hole in the dura mater so that complications can follow some time later. Lumbar puncture is therefore strictly contraindicated in the presence of papilloedema or when there are symptoms suggestive of raised intracranial pressure, except under skilled supervision and when neurosurgical help is immediately to hand.

In the absence of raised intracranial pressure the risk attached to lumbar puncture is small. Conversely the risk of withholding it can be high. In psychiatric practice it will sometimes be indicated in patients who show disturbance of consciousness or unexplained change of behaviour, even in the absence of definite neurological signs. It can be a dangerous mistake to postpone the investigation on account of the severity of illness or uncooperative behaviour, though it will often be wise to delay in such circumstances until a CT scan and a neurological opinion have been obtained.

Walton (1993a) reviews the information to be obtained from lumbar puncture. The pressure is raised in the presence of tumour, haematoma, abscess or cerebral oedema.

A moderate rise may be seen in patients with severe arterial hypertension. The pressure may also be raised in certain rare disorders such as lead poisoning or hypoparathyroidism.

A pleocytosis implies inflammatory changes in the meninges, either primary as in meningitis, or secondary to cerebral infection as in encephalitis or cerebral abscess. Polymorphonuclear leucocytes predominate with pyogenic infections, and may number many thousands per cubic millimetre rendering the fluid turbid. Virus encephalitis shows mainly lymphocytes, though with some varieties there may be polymorphs in the early stages. The number of cells is normally rather low. When present the pleocytosis can be an essential observation for confirming the diagnosis. A moderate cellular reaction can similarly be important in the diagnosis of cerebral abscess, usually with 20–200 cells/mm^3, most of which are polymorphs. In untreated general paresis, 5–50 lymphocytes/mm^3 are usual, and as described on p. 343 the monitoring of the cellular content of the CSF is essential for judging the adequacy of treatment and for the early detection of relapse. A slight pleocytosis, nearly always of lymphocytes, may be present in other conditions including primary and secondary cerebral tumours, cerebral infarctions or multiple sclerosis.

Blood is found in the CSF after subarachnoid haemorrhage or when a primary intracerebral haemorrhage has extended to the subarachnoid space. Xanthochromia may persist as a yellow discoloration for several weeks thereafter. Xanthochromia in the absence of frank blood is also sometimes found with subdural haematomas.

An increased protein content is common to many conditions and can be difficult to interpret. The protein rises with meningitic infections and this can persist for some time after the pleocytosis has resolved. A moderate increase to 1.0 g/l (100 mg/100 ml) or a little more may occur with encephalitis, cerebral abscess, cerebral infarction, neurosyphilis, cerebral tumours and multiple sclerosis. Similar levels can be seen with cervical spondylosis or with myxoedema. In the latter situation it can be particularly misleading. With certain tumours such as meningiomas or acoustic neuromas the level is often considerably higher. Very high levels of up to 10 g/l (1000 mg/100 ml) without an accompanying cellular reaction is characteristic of the polyneuropathy of the Guillain–Barré syndrome, also of spinal blockage from any cause.

The globulin fraction is raised in relation to the albumin in many inflammatory conditions. The gamma globulins are abnormally high, with a selective increase in the immunoglobulin G (IgG) fraction in the majority of cases of multiple sclerosis. The colloidal gold (Lange) curve, which probably reflects selective changes in the protein content of the fluid, can give additional information. The 'paretic' first zone curve is characteristic of general paresis (e.g. 5544322110), the 'luetic' early mid-zone curve is seen with tabes dorsalis (0123322100), and the 'meningitic' late mid-zone curve with meningitis of various kinds (0001223210). The technique has, however, been largely superseded by modern quantitative methods for estimating the major immunoglobulins (IgG, IgA and IgM), such as radioimmunoassay, immunoelectrophoresis and isoelectric focusing. 'Oligoclonal banding' reflects the typical pattern of such changes in multiple sclerosis, but is also found in various forms of meningoencephalitis, subacute sclerosing panencephalitis and the Guillain–Barré syndrome. Thus it is indicative of an immunological response rather than being diagnostic of a particular condition (Walton 1993a). Immunoassay for protein 14-3-3 appears to be highly specific for Creutzfeldt–Jakob disease (p. 478).

The sugar content of the fluid is greatly lowered or abolished in pyogenic meningitis. A moderate fall is found in tuberculous meningitis and can be a valuable pointer in differentiating this from the various forms of aseptic meningitis due to viral infection. The chloride content is also low in tuberculous meningitis.

Examination of films and culture of the fluid are important for determining the responsible organism when infection is present. Virological studies can be useful, but usually only in retrospect since a considerable time is required before the results become available. However, the development of polymerase chain reaction techniques for the detection of viral DNA in the CSF holds promise of yielding an immediate and specific diagnosis with some infections. Examination of films may also reveal neoplastic cells, especially in carcinomatosis and the medulloblastomas of childhood. Serological tests for syphilis are important since sometimes they are negative in the serum in active cases of general paresis.

Thus in many situations examination of the CSF gives important information which contributes to the diagnosis. In some conditions such as encephalitis, general paresis and cerebral abscess it may be crucial in alerting one to the diagnosis. A normal CSF does not, however, mean that a pathological process within the central nervous system can be excluded. The degenerative processes responsible for the presenile and senile dementias do not as a rule show changes, and a completely normal fluid may be found in occasional cases of encephalitis. Moreover many pathological processes responsible for enduring brain damage and neuropsychiatric disturbance will have subsided by the time the patient is examined, and will have left a normal fluid in their wake.

Radiography of the skull

The chief indication for skull X-ray is usually suspicion of a cerebral tumour. There may be erosion or bony overgrowth over the vault due to a meningioma, or abnormal vascular markings indicative of a tumour or angioma. Special views may show erosion of the internal auditory meatus due to an acoustic neuroma. Osteolytic bone lesions may give the first indication of carcinomatosis or multiple myeloma. General thickening or 'woolliness' may indicate Paget's disease.

The next main focus of interest is the sella turcica. Decalcification or erosion of the posterior clinoid processes is an important indication of raised intracranial pressure, or the fossa may be enlarged due to a pituitary or suprasellar lesion.

Intracranial calcification provides other clues. The pineal is calcified in approximately 50% of adults and may display shifts of the midline structures. The choroid plexuses and the falx cerebri may occasionally be calcified as well. Calcification within the body of a tumour can be of direct localising value, similarly calcification within the walls of a large cerebral aneurysm. Other rare conditions include calcification within the basal ganglia in hypoparathyroidism, calcification within the nodules in tuberose sclerosis or in the cysts of cysticercosis.

The value of skull X-ray in psychiatric practice was indicated by Kraft et al. (1965) who found abnormalities in 2.5% of patients when a chronic psychiatric population was screened routinely. Rubin and Rubin (1966) found relevant positive findings in 3% of a younger and more acutely ill psychiatric population, even though all cerebral tumours had been excluded by careful pre-admission screening.

Echoencephalography (ultrasound)

Echoencephalography is used as a simple screening test for detecting displacement of midline structures within the skull. It is a rapid procedure, entirely without discomfort or risk to the patient. When necessary it can be carried out at out-patient consultation, though considerable expertise is needed in order to achieve reliable results.

A beam of ultrasound is passed transversely through the skull and waves are reflected back when they meet surfaces with different physical properties. They are transduced into electrical energy so that the resulting impulses can be displayed to view. Midline displacements are readily detected, and more recent refined techniques can display ventricular shifts as well.

The technique has been largely supplanted by CT scanning, but where such facilities are not available echoen-

cephalography can form a useful preliminary to decisions regarding contrast radiography.

Radioisotope scan (radionuclide scan, gamma encephalography)

Radioisotope scanning can be a valuable technique for the investigation of cerebral tumours and some cerebral infarctions. However, its use has declined very markedly since the introduction of CT and other scan procedures though it still finds an important place where access to these is limited.

An isotope preparation such as technetium-99 (^{99}Tc) is injected intravenously in a dose according to body weight. This is picked up by vascular tissue, especially neovascular tissue, and the gamma radiation may be detected by a 'scan' of the skull with radioactive counting equipment. Remarkably precise localisation can be achieved. Readings are usually taken 15–30 minutes after injection or at 2–4 hours when a tumour is suspected. Rapid readings may be taken immediately after injection in suspected cerebrovascular disease.

The clinical usefulness of the procedure is reviewed by Heck et al. (1971). Diagnostic accuracy is high for vascular tumours though with others it may fail. Lesions which are cystic or necrotic in the centre, such as astrocytomas or abscesses, may show a characteristic 'doughnut' sign. Multiple metastases are well displayed. In general, however, resolution is poor in comparison to CT scanning.

Cerebral infarctions are revealed if the timing is correct. The conversion of a normal scan to abnormal in the distribution of one of the major cerebral vessels, within a few days of a suspected cerebrovascular accident, allows the diagnosis to be made with a high degree of confidence. A distinction cannot always be made from a tumour on a single examination, but repetition of the study can be valuable in aiding the differentiation.

A subdural haematoma may show as a crescent-shaped defect over the hemisphere. Here the results can be very helpful towards the diagnosis, particularly in haematomas which have become isodense with brain tissue on the CT scan (p. 412).

Isotope cisternography (isotope encephalography)

Isotope cisternography provides a means of obtaining a dynamic picture of the CSF circulation. It found its main clinical application in conjunction with air encephalography in the investigation of patients with communicating hydrocephalus, but since the advent of CT scanning its usefulness has declined. When it is thought necessary to visualise the morphology and the dynamics of the CSF circulation it is now generally preferable to employ an intrathecal injection of metrizamide in conjunction with a CT scan (Isherwood 1983).

In performing a scan, isotope-labelled material (^{99m}Tc-EDTA or indium-113m) is injected intrathecally by lumbar puncture, and serial scintillation scans of the head are made at intervals ranging from 2 hours to several days. In normal subjects the radioactivity appears in the basal cisterns within 1–3 hours, and by 24 hours is well disseminated over the hemispheres and along the superior longitudinal sinus with little remaining at the base of the brain. Activity fades rapidly after 48 hours, and at no stage does the scan show activity within the ventricular system.

Distinctive findings were demonstrated in patients with normal-pressure hydrocephalus (Bannister 1970; Benson *et al.* 1970). The dilated ventricles show early filling, and come to contain a high concentration of the isotope which persists throughout the series. Moreover the radioactive material fails to circulate over the hemispheres and does not appear in the sagittal area. A delay may be seen with degenerative diseases such as primary presenile dementia, but within 48 hours these ultimately show adequate saggital activity. When little or no radioactivity has appeared in the sagittal area after 48–72 hours, normal-pressure hydrocephalus is strongly suggested.

The procedure is safe, with little or no discomfort to the patient afterwards. CT scanning and techniques for continuous intracranial pressure monitoring have now, however, emerged as the favoured diagnostic procedures when hydrocephalus requires investigation (p. 746).

Cerebral angiography

Cerebral angiography consists of taking X-ray films in rapid succession after an injection of contrast medium into the cerebral circulation. Injection of the common carotid artery displays the internal carotid and its area of supply by way of the anterior and middle cerebral arteries, and sometimes the posterior cerebral arteries also. Vertebral arteriography is more hazardous, but can be used to outline the vertebral, basilar and posterior cerebral arteries.

Angiography is in the main without serious risk, but can be dangerous in the presence of cerebrovascular disease or severe hypertension. The injected vessel may go into spasm, or a clot may be dislodged leading to cerebral infarction; or damage to the wall may be slow to heal and form a focus for thrombosis later. For this reason arteriography by means of a catheter inserted into the femoral or radial artery is often preferred to direct puncture.

Vascular lesions are usually clearly demonstrated, including intracranial aneurysms, arteriovenous malformations, or stenosis or obstruction of the internal carotid arteries. A subdural haematoma may show as an avascular area beneath the vault of the skull in the anteroposterior view. Space-occupying lesions of the cerebral hemispheres are often well localised, including tumours, abscesses or haematomas. The nature of the tumour may be indicated by its degree of vascularity, and meningiomas often produce a characteristic 'blush' in the venous phase of the angiogram. Vertebral arteriography may help in the diagnosis of tumours of the posterior fossa, and is of value in patients suspected of having vascular abnormalities of the hindbrain circulation.

Angiography carries small but definite hazards, so has now been supplanted by CT scanning (p. 137) as a screening procedure for tumours. It is still required, however, for the demonstration of most aneurysms and angiomas, and is still sometimes employed to confirm that a tumour is a meningioma. The precise delineation of vascular anomalies and occlusive vascular disease seem likely to remain essential roles for the procedure.

Air encephalography (pneumoencephalography)

Before CT scanning became available air encephalography was a technique of great importance for visualising intracranial pathology. It was the only means available for demonstrating cortical atrophy or yielding reasonable estimates of ventricular size. Space-occupying lesions were shown by displacements of the ventricular system. In virtually all respects, however, it has now been superseded by CT scanning, which is a great deal safer and without discomfort for the patient.

For a while a place remained for the technique in a small minority of patients, chiefly for visualising small basal tumours near the optic or auditory nerves or in the brain stem, and for clarifying obstructions in the aqueductal region. Such areas are relatively inaccessible on the CT scan but are now well visualised by magnetic resonance imaging. MRI has also displaced the use of air encephalography for the investigation of patients with temporal lobe epilepsy, since coronal views allow detailed visualisation of the temporal horns of the lateral ventricles. A knowledge of the uses of air encephalography nevertheless remains important, since in many parts of the world the new imaging techniques are not available.

Lumbar air encephalography involved the introduction of air into the subarachnoid space by lumbar puncture, and allowing it to ascend to outline the ventricular system and basal cisterns of the brain. Earlier techniques which utilised large quantities of air gave way to more refined procedures which employed no more than 20–40 cm³ of air, but nonetheless considerable discomfort usually resulted. Headache could be severe, and could persist for 48 hours or longer, with nausea and meningeal irritation.

The decision to perform air encephalography therefore always required the most careful consideration of the benefits which might result. In addition to discomfort there is a considerable element of risk in certain situations. When the intracranial pressure is raised the alteration of cerebral hydrodynamics following the introduction of air may lead to the development of tentorial herniation or a medullary pressure cone, and patients with degenerative brain disease may be worsened at least temporarily after the procedure.

A chief indication was to explore the possibility of cerebral atrophy due to degenerative or other brain diseases. Ventricular dilatation was shown more clearly by air studies than by angiography or isotope cisternography. Cortical atrophy could also be revealed by the pooling of air in dilated sulci over the convexity of the brain or around the cerebellar hemispheres. Air encephalography could therefore bring important confirmatory evidence in patients suffering from presenile dementia, and could be indicated in borderline cases to add to the other evidence available.

In normal-pressure hydrocephalus the findings on air encephalography were virtually diagnostic, showing massive symmetrical dilatation of the lateral ventricles but complete absence of air over the cortical surface. Space-occupying lesions were revealed by shift of the midline structures and local deformities of the ventricular system. However, air encephalography should never be carried out when the intracranial pressure is known to be raised, and when a tumour is suspected it should be withheld unless full neurosurgical facilities are to hand.

Computerised axial tomography (CAT scan, CT scan, EMI scan)

Computerised axial tomography probably represents the most significant advance in the use of X-rays for diagnosis since their discovery, and has quickly established itself as invaluable in the diagnosis of cerebral disorder. Very significantly, wherever facilities for CT scanning have been established, the requirements for earlier neuroradiological procedures have dropped abruptly. In particular it has come to replace the air encephalogram except in a tiny minority of cases, and these are now adequately dealt with by MRI (see below).

Descriptions of the technique and early reports of its value in clinical practice are provided by Hounsfield (1973), Ambrose (1973, 1974), Gawler et al. (1974), Paxton and Ambrose (1974) and Kazner et al. (1975). It is essentially a procedure in which X-ray transmission readings are taken through the head at a multitude of angles by means of a narrow collimated beam of X-rays; from these data, absorption values of the material contained within the head are calculated by computer, and presented as a series of pictures of transverse slices of the cranial contents. The system is approximately 100 times more sensitive than conventional X-ray systems, yet exposes the patient to no greater radiation dosage than a standard series of ordinary skull X-rays. There is no need for anaesthesia or any form of invasive procedure, rendering it entirely safe for patients who might be unfit for contrast neuroradiology.

Gawler et al. (1975) describe the findings in the normal brain and the range of structures identified. The ventricular system is clearly shown along with certain of the basal cisterns. The cortical sulci are often detectable, and readily so when enlarged. Within the cerebral substance variations in soft tissues of nearly similar absorption density may be displayed; thus the thalami and heads of the caudate nuclei are generally identifiable as discrete structures, also the internal capsule and optic radiations. The cortical grey matter mantle is visible over the surface of the cerebral hemispheres. Progressive refinements incorporated into the more recent scan machines have considerably increased the amount of detail displayed.

In investigating cerebral pathology the scan may show displacements of normal intracranial contents, but in addition many focal pathological processes produce changes in brain absorption density which enable lesions to be displayed directly. Space-occupying lesions are readily shown, including tumours, abscesses and haematomas. Local cerebral oedema is demonstrated, and infarction is revealed as a region of low absorption density.

The nature as well as the location of a tumour can often be demonstrated—whether benign or malignant, solid or cystic—as well as the degree to which surrounding oedema infiltrates brain tissue. A diffuse increase in absorption density is seen with meningiomas, colloid cysts and pituitary adenomas, whereas gliomas and metastases may be hyper- or hypodense. A special advantage is the capacity to distinguish tumours from infarctions at an early stage, and in cases where angiography might well have been contraindicated. Intravenous injections of sodium iothalamate (Conray) can be used in doubtful cases to enhance the contrast between the tumour and surrounding brain tissue. A high level of efficiency in diagnosis has been found, though certain tumours near the base of the skull can be difficult to visualise (Kendall 1980). Scanning after the introduction of intrathecal metrizamide can improve the detection of small brain stem, suprasellar and cerebellopontine tumours.

In the management of strokes the differentiation between infarction and haemorrhage is relatively simple. This can be especially important if the patient is taking or due to take anticoagulants (Sandercock *et al.* 1985). The location, size and direction of propagation of intracerebral haematomas can be defined. After head injuries various important forms of cerebral pathology are displayed (p. 165). In the acute stage of injury, scanning can be invaluable in demonstrating intracranial haematomas before the patient's deterioration makes them obvious to the surgeon.

Cerebral atrophy shows as enlargement of the ventricles, broadening of the Sylvian and interhemispheric fissures, and widening of the cerebral sulci, much as after air encephalography. Enlarged sulci are best seen from a high slice near the vertex. CT has entirely replaced air contrast studies in the investigation of the dementias (p. 495). Gawler *et al.* (1975, 1976) found it to be as accurate as earlier neuroradiological methods for revealing cerebral atrophy or hydrocephalus. Metrizamide studies can add important information in the investigation of communicating hydrocephalus (p. 136).

Areas of relative translucency may be shown in the cerebral white matter in demyelinating disorders such as multiple sclerosis (p. 690) and Schilder's disease (p. 700). White matter changes may also be found in a proportion of demented patients and even sometimes in the healthy elderly ('leukoaraiosis'), as discussed on p. 495 *et seq.*

Some of the potentials which CT scanning has opened up for research into psychiatric disorders are briefly indicated on p. 140. For the reliable detection of differences between groups, which may often be of a relatively minor nature, objective methods of scan analysis must be used. Those commonly employed vary in sophistication, from simple threshold methods for determination of the brain–CSF margins (Penn *et al.* 1978; Reveley *et al.* 1984) to methods which use techniques for detecting edges or following boundaries (Walser & Ackerman 1977; Keller *et al.* 1981). Computer-assisted automated methods hold special value in yielding greater objectivity and permitting adjustments for 'partial volume artefact' in regions which lie at the brain–CSF interface (Jernigan *et al.* 1979; Baldy *et al.* 1986).

A further development, largely confined to research, involves the direct estimation of brain absorption density values as a guide to more subtle changes in the brain parenchyma, for example in patients with dementia (see below). Findings of some interest have emerged in alcoholic patients as discussed on p. 606. In schizophrenia there have been rather tenuous indications of reduced absorption densities in the left hemisphere

(Golden *et al.* 1981; Largen *et al.* 1983) and increased absorption densities in the thalamic and caudate nuclei (Dewan *et al.* 1983). Reveley *et al.*'s (1987) study is the most impressive to date and appears to uphold left hemisphere hypodensity.

Computerised tomography densitometry is, however, vulnerable to numerous sources of artefact, including beam-hardening effects due to differing skull thickness and size, systematic drifts in scanner stability, and problems with the consistency of sampling of regions of interest (Jacobson *et al.* 1985). Few studies to date have addressed such issues adequately. It is, moreover, likely that this extension of CT scanning will be overtaken by developments in MRI spectroscopy (p. 142) and the various forms of functional brain imaging discussed on p. 143 *et seq.*

Xenon-enhanced CT uses the inhalation of xenon gas in conjunction with CT scanning for the non-invasive imaging of regional cerebral blood flow (Yonas *et al.* 1987; Meyer *et al.* 1988). Colour-coded maps representing local brain–blood partition coefficients are formatted onto CT images for correlation with brain anatomy and structural pathology. An application in the field of alcoholism is described on p. 606.

Significance of cerebral atrophy

Sometimes neuroimaging shows changes which are hard to interpret, particularly where cerebral atrophy is concerned. It is often easier to assess distortion by a space-occupying lesion than to decide on the significance of minor ventricular enlargement. Occasionally, moreover, the ventricles may prove to be enlarged or the sulci prominent in patients who show no evidence of cerebral disorder. Such examples raise obvious diagnostic difficulties, and are a reminder that a range of normal variation must be allowed where the appearances of the brain are concerned.

Attempts were made to establish criteria of normality on the air encephalogram, but for obvious reasons it was impossible to study unselected groups of healthy individuals. Indications were obtained that the ventricles increase in size with age, at least over the age of 60, though even this was far from firmly established (Willanger *et al.* 1968). CT scanning has allowed more reliable assessments to be made. It is now clear that ventricular size increases with age even in healthy persons, and particularly so in the later decades of life (Barron *et al.* 1976; Gyldensted 1977; Haug 1977; Jacobs *et al.* 1978). Barron *et al.* (1976), for example, examined 135 normal volunteers by CT scan, demonstrating a gradual increase from the first to the sixth decades followed by a dramatic increase from the age of 70 onwards. The range encountered in ventricular size also became wider among the elderly subjects.

With regard to dementia there is usually an obvious

association with evidence of atrophy, though this is not absolute in every case. Younger demented patients are more likely to show decisively abnormal findings, in comparison with their peers, whereas in the elderly there may be considerable overlap with healthy persons of equivalent age.

Gosling (1955) reviewed the air encephalograms of a large group of patients suspected of dementia, mostly in the presenile age range, and found that 85% showed cerebral atrophy. Among those who did not, the features indicative of dementia had usually been slight and follow-up often showed a lack of progression. During the same period, and in the same department, 19% of air studies on non-demented patients had shown atrophy, sometimes with an obvious cause but in 11% without. Many of the latter patients were suffering from epilepsy of late onset. The features particularly associated with dementia were cortical sulci wider than 0.5 cm, air trapped in the insular regions, and enlargement of the lateral ventricles most markedly in the trigone area.

Among elderly demented patients, CT studies have shown greater sulcal and ventricular size than in age-matched healthy controls, though the overlap tends to be considerable (Jacoby & Levy 1980a; Gado et al. 1982). Jacoby and Levy found on discriminant function analysis that CT scan measurements produced a correct prediction in 83% of elderly subjects, cortical atrophy being a rather better discriminator than ventricular size. Interestingly, however, patients over the age of 80 were significantly less likely to have large ventricles when compared with those a decade or so younger, perhaps reflecting the more benign course of dementia in the very elderly. Hubbard and Anderson (1981) were able to show by detailed autopsy measurements that the ventricles were of normal size for age in approximately 40% of patients with senile dementia.

The severity of cognitive impairment in dementia has proved to be closely related to the degree of cerebral atrophy, both in air encephalographic and CT scan studies, and in the elderly as well as the middle aged (Kiev et al. 1962; Willanger et al. 1968; Roberts & Caird 1976; De Leon et al. 1979; Jacoby & Levy 1980a). Most agree that the relationship with cognitive impairment is closer for ventricular enlargement than for widening of the sulci. Burns and Pearlson (1994) review the many CT studies in this area, showing that significant correlations with cognition have emerged twice as often for ventricular as for cortical measurements. There are indications, too, that the progression of cognitive deterioration on follow-up is paralleled by further ventricular enlargement (Naguib & Levy 1982b). In Burns et al.'s (1991) study of elderly Alzheimer patients, both ventricular and cortical atrophy

worsened significantly over a 12-month period, the increase in ventricular size being associated with further deterioration of memory.

Interest in the CT scan in dementia has also centred on the absorption density to X-rays in various brain regions. White matter absorption density appears to decrease gradually with age among healthy volunteers (Zatz et al. 1982), but in both presenile and senile Alzheimer's disease further reductions are seen (Naeser et al. 1980; Bondareff et al. 1981a). As mentioned on p. 433, there is some evidence that decreased absorption density in the parietal region may be associated with shorter survival. How far measurements such as these may prove of value in refining diagnostic accuracy in dementia remains to be determined.

Certain MRI features relevant to the brain parenchyma have also attracted interest. Besson et al. (1985) found that T_1 relaxation times were increased in elderly patients with Alzheimer's disease, especially in parietal and frontal regions, and that this was significantly related to the severity of dementia. Christie et al. (1988) showed in presenile Alzeimer's disease that frontal T_1 values increased with progression of the disorder in individual patients. Elevated values emerged in a small group of patients with multi-infarct dementia, though the variability was too high to make this a reliable differentiating feature. Bondareff et al. (1990) quantified T_2 white matter lesions in Alzheimer's disease, showing significant correlations with certain dementia scores.

In general, therefore, clinical evidence of dementia is accompanied by evidence of atrophy, and this tends to be more severe the more advanced the dementia. In occasional early cases, however, no abnormality will emerge, and in the elderly it may be hard to judge the significance of the findings. It is extremely important, as stressed on p. 495, that the results of brain imaging should only be interpreted in conjunction with the overall clinical picture, and that the diagnosis of a dementing illness should not be allowed to hinge on such findings alone.

This point gains a special importance in that indications of cerebral atrophy are found in a considerable number of persons without dementia. Among institutionalised epileptic patients, for example, Larsby and Lindgren (1940) found abnormalities on air encephalography in over two-thirds of cases. CT and MRI studies have shown abnormalities in a high percentage of epileptics (p. 289), focal or generalised atrophy being by far the commonest finding. Alcoholic subjects are similarly prone to show cortical shrinkage and ventricular dilatation, sometimes quite marked in degree and not necessarily accompanied by obvious cognitive change. The findings in this area are discussed in some detail on pp. 605–6. Finally, chronic psychiatric illness of many varieties has been found, when investigated, to be associated with a considerable prevalence of radiographic changes as described immediately below.

Haug (1962) carried out a large air encephalographic

survey on 278 long-stay patients in a mental hospital, and reported 'definite cerebral atrophy' in 60% of patients. This usually consisted of ventricular enlargement, but cortical atrophy was shown in many cases where filling over the cortical surface had been achieved. Among patients with organic mental disorders abnormalities were found in 72%, in those with schizophrenia 61%, and in those with other 'functional' illnesses 49%. The latter consisted of a variety of paranoid, affective and neurotic conditions, all of which had been long lasting and rather resistant to treatment. Haug suggested that earlier brain damage may have contributed to the genesis of these illnesses by lowering resistance to stress. Among the patients with organic mental syndromes the atrophy was usually diffuse, whereas half of the non-organic group showed purely focal abnormalities, often of a single temporal horn. The majority appeared to be non-progressive on follow-up, but mortality was increased in patients with abnormal air encephalograms.

Hunter *et al.* (1968b) attempted a similar study in patients who had been continuously in hospital for more than 40 years. Twenty-seven patients were examined, all previously diagnosed as schizophrenic. More than half showed abnormal air encephalograms, usually with unilateral ventricular enlargement. The suggestion again was that some underlying condition, of uncertain nature, may have caused structural damage as reflected both in the air encephalogram and in the patient's mental illness.

The findings in schizophrenia were the subject of several air encephalographic studies, notably Huber's (1957) investigation of 190 patients. Those with the more severe defects in social competence showed the most marked changes on air encephalography. Broadening of the third ventricle went step by step with the severity of personality deterioration when the effects of age were controlled, and frontal atrophy was associated with illnesses of long duration. In a prolonged follow-up of many of these patients it emerged that ventricular enlargement was associated with a poor outcome (Huber *et al.* 1975). Many similar indications of atrophy in chronic schizophrenia are scattered through the air encephalographic literature as reviewed by Storey (1966). However, negative reports emerged as well (Peltonen 1962; Storey 1966) and much of the evidence tended to be contradictory. The availability of CT scanning has, however, brought more clarity to the picture.

Starting with a small study by Johnstone *et al.* (1976, 1978) several CT scan surveys have been carried out on carefully diagnosed schizophrenic patients, the non-invasive nature of the scan permitting relatively unselected groups to be examined (for example Weinberger *et al.* 1979a, 1979b; Andreasen *et al.* 1982; Nasrallah *et al.*

1982a). Comparison with age-matched controls has repeatedly shown mild but definite ventricular enlargement in a considerable proportion, this varying by up to 60% from one study to another. Minor degrees of sulcal enlargement have also been detected (Pfefferbaum *et al.* 1988), and atrophy of the vermis of the cerebellum can sometimes be shown (Weinberger *et al.* 1979c; Lippmann *et al.* 1982). The implications of such findings are discussed on p. 85 *et seq.* In brief the sum total of evidence suggests that such atrophy antedates the development of the schizophrenic illness, but may be a significant factor in helping to determine it and shape its manifestations. Adverse influences operating very early in life, even intrauterine life, are perhaps chiefly to be held responsible. On present evidence there is little to support a causative role for neuroleptic medication in leading to the changes, or to suggest that a specific pathological process is at work.

Not dissimilar findings have begun to emerge in patients with affective disorder, where ventricular enlargement and cerebellar vermis atrophy have also been reported (Pearlson & Veroff 1981; Lippmann *et al.* 1982). Both patients with mania and patients with major depressive illness have sometimes shown significantly larger ventricles than controls (Nasrallah *et al.* 1982b; Scott *et al.* 1983). Elderly patients with first-onset depression have been found to have larger ventricles than age-matched healthy volunteers (Jacoby & Levy 1980b), and there are indications that this is predictive of increased mortality at follow-up (Jacoby *et al.* 1981).

Dolan *et al.* (1985, 1986) investigated 101 patients with a clear-cut history of depression in the recent past. In comparison to healthy controls they had significantly larger ventricles, the differences being more marked in the middle-aged and elderly and scarcely apparent in those under 40. Bipolar and unipolar groups were equivalently affected, likewise those with or without a family history of depression. Again the findings appeared to have antedated the onset of the illness, in that there was no relationship to illness duration or treatment parameters. Sulcal widening was also commoner in patients than controls, particularly over the frontal and temporal regions. Those who had received electroconvulsive treatment showed more sulcal changes than those who had not, but a causal relationship seemed unlikely since there was no relationship to the number of treatments given.

Computerised tomography and MRI studies are thus increasing our appreciation that a degree of cerebral disorder may play some part in contributing to a considerable range of mental illness. The degree of cerebral change encountered on CT scanning will only rarely lead to difficulties with diagnosis, but on occasion it will be sufficient to call for detailed re-evaluation of the patient's illness. The cortical shrinkage and ventricular dilatation accompanying severe alcohol abuse will quite often be perplexing when the drinking history is unknown, likewise the appearances of atrophy that may accompany steroid administration (Bentson *et al.* 1978; Lagenstein *et al.* 1979). The latter appears to be largely reversible on discontinuation of the steroids. Minor reversible changes have also been reported in patients with anorexia nervosa (Enzmann & Lane 1977; Heinz *et al.* 1977; Palazidou *et al.* 1990).

Studies dating from the air encephalographic era have confirmed that unexpected cerebral atrophy need not imply progressive cerebral disorder or necessarily impair response to treatment for the associated psychiatric condition. Eitinger (1959) followed 46 psychiatric patients with cerebral atrophy of unknown origin and found that 11 improved in social functioning over the years that followed. He concluded that it must often represent a static condition, perhaps dating from early life, thus altering the patient's reaction pattern and increasing his vulnerability to psychological trauma. The important conclusion was that the discovery of atrophy should not lead to therapeutic pessimism, and that treatment should be given in the normal manner for the psychiatric symptoms present.

Mann (1972, 1973) followed a consecutive group of 49 patients from the Maudsley Hospital who showed significant generalised atrophy, with both ventricular dilatation and widening of sulci over the cortex. Some were suffering from obvious dementia but others had presented with non-organic psychiatric syndromes. Follow-up 5–10 years later allowed 16 survivors to be traced and 15 were available for re-examination. The majority of those who had died had shown clear evidence of dementia prior to death, but among the survivors there was no suggestion of progressive organic disease. Most were still under out-patient psychiatric supervision, but half were leading an active social life and many of them were working. Others were functioning at a reduced social level which appeared to be static, with a good deal of depression or anxiety and sometimes with complaints of subjective memory impairment. Seven had originally presented with depression, six with epilepsy, two with paranoid states and one with suspected dementia, but in all there had been sufficient clinical indication of brain damage at the time to warrant air encephalography. Detailed comparisons of the radiographic findings in those who had dementia and those who had not, surprisingly showed no difference in the amount of air over the cortical surface. Significant differences emerged, however, in ventricular measurements which were larger in those who deteriorated later.

Studies using CT and MRI obviously stand to clarify this situation further. The readiness with which large samples of patients can be examined without risk of discomfort, and the facility with which the scan can be repeated after an interval of time, should ultimately allow an increased understanding of the significance of cerebral atrophy in a variety of psychiatric settings.

Magnetic resonance imaging (nuclear magnetic resonance, MRI scan, NMR scan)

Magnetic resonance imaging is a more recent technique for non-invasive imaging of the brain. It competes strongly with CT as a neurodiagnostic procedure, yielding greatly superior anatomical and pathological information, though the high costs involved tend to limit its application. Unlike CT scanning it involves no X-irradiation, but makes use of the magnetic properties of nuclei and their capacity to be excited by radiofrequency pulses. Early reviews of the procedure and its clinical applications are found in Bydder and Steiner (1982) and Young *et al.* (1982). Besson (1990) provides a comprehensive outline of its use in neuropsychiatric disorders.

Most routine magnetic resonance imaging utilises the hydrogen nuclei of the tissues. In essence these are made to 'resonate' in response to rapidly changing magnetic fields around them, and the signals they emit are then processed to yield a visual image based on their distribution and physicochemical state.

The patient is placed in a static magnetic field, varying in different machines from 0.5 to 2.5 Tesla in strength. This produces a net alignment of the magnetic moments of the hydrogen nuclei in the tissues. Under such circumstances the nuclei 'precess' in a circular course about this axis, much as a spinning top will wobble. Brief bursts of radiofrequency pulses, applied at the appropriate frequency from a surrounding coil, augment the precession, and when the excitation pulse ends the nuclei return to their lower energy state. The electrical signals emitted from the tissues in the course of such energy changes can be detected and analysed by computer to reveal the distribution of the hydrogen nuclei involved. Techniques are used to 'scan' the tissues systematically, yielding visual images much as with the CT scan.

A variety of scanning 'sequences' can be selected in order to optimise the particular parameters used in image reconstruction. 'Repeated free induction decay' or 'saturation recovery' (RFID or SR) produce images that reflect proton density (PD). 'Inversion-recovery' (IR) sequences reflect the 'longitudinal' or 'spin-lattice' relaxation time (T_1) of the protons as they return to their previous equilibrium in line with the axis of the static magnetic field. 'Spin-echo' (SE) sequences are differently derived to display the 'transverse' or 'spin-spin' relaxation time (T_2), during which the spinning protons are relaxing in phase with one another but interacting with the spins of other nuclei. These different scanning sequences are each suited to different purposes in visual imaging. In T_1 images the CSF appears dark in relation to brain tissue; in T_2 images the CSF is light, with grey matter also light and the white matter dark, as illustrated in Plate 5.

An outstanding feature of MRI is the high level of soft tissue contrast obtained by scanning in the IR sequence

('T$_1$-weighted images'). Grey and white matter are strongly differentiated, yielding fine anatomical detail. The cortical grey matter is shown clearly and the thalami and basal ganglia are demarcated from the surrounding white matter and ventricular system. Sagittal scans show the corpus callosum, the columns of the fornix and the brain stem. In the posterior fossa the substantia nigra and the middle cerebral peduncles can be discerned. Cerebral and cerebellar atrophy are of course well displayed. IR sequences also show infarcts, and can reveal plaques of multiple sclerosis in a manner superior to CT scanning (p. 690). SE sequences (T$_2$-weighted images), by contrast, produce little grey–white differentiation, but have proved to be a sensitive indicator of pathological change (Bailes *et al.* 1982). Infarctions, haemorrhages and tumours are well displayed, likewise tissue changes caused by cerebral oedema and encephalitis. Repeated free induction decay (RFID) is of less value in routine diagnosis but has the special advantage of revealing blood flow and thus outlining major vessels.

MRI scanning holds several pronounced advantages over CT. Improved detection of small demyelinating lesions is coupled with excellent visualisation of the posterior fossa and pituitary regions, since there is little or no bone artefact to intrude on the images obtained. The various scanning sequences available give versatility of choice; and the slices to be viewed are readily switched from transverse to coronal or sagittal planes without disturbing or moving the patient.

Its superiority over CT scanning has emerged in many clinical settings—in the detection of cerebral tumours (p. 232), small infarcts and other vascular disease of the brain (pp. 377 and 421), and in revealing the lesions responsible for epilepsy (p. 289). It is very much better at showing the residua of cerebral trauma (p. 166), and in the detection of cerebral infections including those due to AIDS (p. 325). The value of MRI in relation to the dementias and other neurodegenerative disorders is described in the appropriate sections of the book. Routine examination may be supplemented by the intravenous administration of a paramagnetic contrast agent (gadolinium bound to a chelating agent, diethylene triaminepenta-acetic acid—Gd-DTPA) which yields additional information about derangements of the blood–brain barrier in the vicinity of lesions (Hawkins *et al.* 1990). This can be valuable in the context of vascular disease and in distinguishing a tumour from the oedema that surrounds it. Developments in magnetic resonance angiography can be used for imaging the larger intracranial arteries and veins (Bradley 1992).

In all of these settings MRI has the added advantage that repeat examinations are possible without hazard from radiation exposure. Indeed no adverse effects have been encountered to date, provided that patients with intracranial metallic foreign bodies, including aneurysmal clips, are excluded, likewise patients with cochlear implants or cardiac pacemakers. Other potential exclusion criteria are discussed by Moseley (1994). Budinger (1981) reviews the evidence concerning safe levels for exposure to the static and changing magnetic fields, the principal risk being the induction of heating in large metal objects such as skull prostheses. There is a theoretical risk of producing cardiac fibrillation or cerebral dysrhythmia from the currents induced by the rapid field changes, and on this account persons with heart disease, epilepsy or pregnancy must be excluded in volunteer procedures. Apart from feelings of claustrophobia and a certain amount of noise while in the machine, which some patients find very distressing, the examination is without discomfort, though with the strong magnetic fields and rapid switching employed in echoplanar imaging (see below) patients may sometimes complain of sensations ranging from tickling to actual pain (Stehling *et al.* 1991).

As a research tool the virtues of MRI over CT scanning include additionally the capacity to delineate very fine anatomical detail in whatever plane may be required. Coronal sections may be used for the examination of medial temporal lobe structures in a manner not previously possible during life. The interesting results which are emerging in relation to schizophrenia are described on p. 85, and work on amnesic patients on p. 27. Computer-assisted methods have been developed for the accurate measurement and comparison of discrete brain structures, also for the reconstruction of remarkably faithful three-dimensional models of the brain (Andreasen *et al.* 1993) (Plate 6). The more recent developments in MRI spectroscopy and echoplanar imaging (see below) hold particular promise for advancing research in the field of neuropsychiatry since they permit investigation of brain function as well as structure.

Magnetic resonance spectroscopy

Magnetic resonance spectroscopy (MRS) is an important extension of MRI, in effect yielding information about certain chemical constituents of tissues. It depends on the principle that in a given magnetic field each distinct nuclear species spins at a unique frequency (Larmor frequency) which is altered slightly according to the chemical compound containing the element. This effect is called the 'chemical shift'. When tissue within a static magnetic field is exposed to another competing field, by applying a radiofrequency pulse tuned to the Larmor frequency of the element in question, a spectrum can be obtained which reflects the various compounds in which the element is incorporated. By examining the spectrum the relative ratios of these components one to another can be calculated. The biochemical information is necessarily obtained at the expense of spatial information, though techniques are available which seek a compromise between the two.

Technical details are described by Bottomley (1989), Lock *et al.* (1990), Guze (1991), Keshavan (1993) and Maier (1995), including applications of relevance for neuropsychiatry. In essence the patient is placed in an MRI scanner of strong magnetic capability (1.5 Tesla or above) and a radiofrequency coil is centred over the area of the head to be sampled. By appropriate tuning of the coil spectra can be obtained which reflect the hydrogen nucleus (^{1}H) or the phosphorous nucleus (^{31}P). A range of other nuclei are also accessible (^{19}F, ^{13}C, ^{23}Na, ^{7}Li), but for technical reasons have been less explored to date.

Hydrogen-1 MRS yields spectra representing the tissue content of water, choline, creatine, lactate and *N*-acetyl aspartate (NAA), also smaller peaks derived from amino acids such as glutamate and aspartate. The water peak must be suppressed by appropriate techniques to prevent it from overriding the others. ^{1}H MRS thus gives information about the metabolic status of amino acids, neurotransmitters and their derivatives. In addition, it has potential for investigating histological change, in that NAA appears to be located entirely within neurones and their processes. Van der Knaap *et al.* (1992) have shown that in cerebral degenerative conditions the ratio of NAA to creatine falls as the severity of neuronal damage increases, this sometimes being evident before structural change is demonstrable. With astrocytosis the relative concentrations of choline and creatine are increased, while creatine falls with membrane breakdown. ^{1}H MRS has been studied in relation to multiple sclerosis, epilepsy, inborn errors of metabolism and cerebrovascular disorders. In schizophrenia, Maier *et al.* (1995) have shown significant reductions of NAA, creatine and choline in the left hippocampus, with smaller losses on the right. Buckley *et al.* (1994) have detected decreases in NAA in the frontal cortex in schizophrenia patients. Decreases in glutamate and aspartate have also been found in the dorsolateral prefrontal cortex, indicative of early neuronal degeneration (Stanley *et al.* 1992, 1993).

Phosphorus-31 MRS yields spectra of particular relevance to impaired energy metabolism, showing peaks for adenosine triphosphate (ATP), phosphocreatine (PCr) and inorganic phosphate (Pi). Ratios of ATP and PCr to Pi provide a measure of tissue health, varying with ischaemia, metabolic disorders and drug therapy (Bottomley *et al.* 1983). ^{31}P resonances can also reflect membrane metabolism by revealing peaks for phosphomonoesters and diesters. ^{31}P MRS has been employed to study brain anoxia, trauma and demyelination, as well as Alzheimer's disease (Pettegrew *et al.* 1988; Brown *et al.*

1989) and AIDS dementia (Bottomley *et al.* 1989). In schizophrenia evidence has been obtained of metabolic hypoactivity and disturbed membrane phospholipid metabolism in the dorsolateral prefrontal cortex (Keshavan *et al.* 1991b; Pettegrew *et al.* 1991, 1993; Stanley *et al.* 1993).

Other promising areas for neuropsychiatric research include the use of ^{19}F MRS for the study of fluorine-containing antipsychotics such as trifluoperazine and fluphenazine, and ^{7}Li MRS for following the pharmacokinetics of lithium (Keshavan *et al.* 1991a). The labelling of glucose with ^{13}C has potential for brain metabolic investigations, and ^{23}Na MRS for differentiating the intracellular and extracellular pools of sodium.

Functional magnetic resonance imaging (fMRI)

This still more recent development consists of ultrafast imaging, whereby minute changes in regional cerebral blood flow can be detected and related to physiological activity occurring locally in the cortex. Brain changes can be charted in response to sensorimotor or cognitive activities, and it is possible even to capture alterations occurring with subjective events such as hallucinatory experiences (see below). Thus fMRI is a technique which can integrate structure with function by providing high resolution mapping of the brain areas involved in discrete tasks and activities. As such it holds particular promise for neuropsychiatry.

The technique and some of its principal achievements to date are summarised by David *et al.* (1994) and Binder and Rao (1994). Two main methods are used—fast low-angle shot (FLASH) and echoplanar imaging (EPI). FLASH depends on extremely brief intervals between successive radiofrequency pulses (5–15 ms), coupled with narrow 'flip angles' so that the proton nuclei return quickly towards their previous state of equilibrium. The resulting free induction decay images reveal any transient alterations of blood flow that occur. The echoplanar technique involves the encoding of free induction decay following a single radiofrequency excitation pulse, while a rapidly oscillating gradient is applied to generate a train of closely spaced signals from the tissue ('gradient echoes').

Earlier studies used gadolinium enhancement which increases the decay rate of the MRI signal (Belliveau *et al.* 1991), but Kwong *et al.* (1992) showed that it was possible to exploit the changed magnetic properties of haemoglobin when it changes from the oxy- to the deoxy- state ('blood oxygenation-level-dependent contrast imaging' or BOLD) (Ogawa *et al.* 1992). Changes in the relative proportions of oxy- and deoxyhaemoglobin, in response to local neuronal activity and the ensuing increased local blood flow, increases the relaxation time leading to a brightening of the magnetic resonance image in active regions. This completely non-invasive method of imaging transient changes in blood flow has obvious advantages over its precursors.

Neuropsychological studies summarised by David *et al.* (1994) include the demonstration of calcarine cortex activation in response to photic stimulation or checkerboard presentations; activation of contralateral and to some extent ipsilateral sensorimotor cortex on touching fingers to thumb; and activation of areas similar to those found with PET scanning on repetition of nouns and generation of verbs (p. 45). Passive word listening activates the superior temporal gyri, especially on the left, and pattern recognition memory activates areas within the medial temporal and frontal lobes. Symptom provocation in patients with obsessive compulsive disorder has been shown to activate orbitofrontal and lateral frontal cortex and related limbic and paralimbic areas (Breiter *et al.* 1996). An application of the technique to study the cerebral correlates of auditory hallucinations in schizophrenia is described on p. 88 and illustrated in Plate 4.

Certain advantages are evident for fMRI over PET as an avenue for further studies, notably much higher resolution with fine localisation, and the ability to track cortical responses which are as brief as 1 second or less. The non-invasiveness of the procedure and its lack of radiation exposure readily permit repeat examinations. A main disadvantage is the difficulty of adapting task paradigms to the restricted space available while the patient lies within the scanner.

Positron emission tomography (PET scan, ECAT scan)

PET is restricted to special centres, since a cyclotron must be close at hand for the manufacture of the short-lived isotopes involved. In essence the PET scan produces a cross-sectional image of brain radioactivity after the injection of a suitably labelled compound, yielding information about the site and rate of dynamic processes such as cerebral blood flow and metabolism. The principal value of the technique is its ability to reveal aspects of regional brain metabolism which are not otherwise accessible to study.

The principles involved are outlined by Oldendorf (1980), Bench *et al.* (1990) and Watson (1991). Compounds labelled with short-lived isotopes, for example ^{18}F or ^{15}O, are injected or inhaled and allowed to reach a steady state in the tissues. The excess of protons over neutrons in such isotopes confers instability, leading to the emission of positrons (positively charged electrons). With the discharge of a positron one of the protons in the nucleus becomes a neutron and stability is achieved again.

An emitted positron has a range of only a few millimetres in the tissues before it encounters an ordinary electron and the two then annihilate each other. Their mass is converted into two gamma rays, which originate simultaneously and propagate in almost precisely opposite directions. This allows their point of origin to be determined by 'coincidence counting' with suitably placed detectors, and this point of origin will be very close to the point where the positron was released.

Hence paired detectors arranged around the head can be used to compute the distribution of the isotope with a fair degree of accuracy. Algorithms similar to those used in CT scanning can yield a visual image of its location within the brain. Resolution of the order of 5 mm can be obtained with the most modern scanners. With appropriate calibration the absolute tissue concentrations of the labelled tracers can be determined, reliable quantitative figures being obtained from cubes with a volume of approximately 2 ml. And by using a stereotaxic head holder, it is possible when required to collect both MRI (or CT) and PET scan data, allowing integration of structural and functional information. Special image-analysis software is now available to permit accurate 'co-registration' of PET and MRI images (Watson *et al.* 1993). More simply Pellizari *et al.* (1989) have described a 'surface matching' technique; or each PET scan may be specially fitted to a standard template derived from an anatomical atlas (Friston *et al.* 1989).

The analysis of PET scan data for purposes of research can be immensely complex, requiring numerous comparisons and the generation of extensive statistical data. In the identification of regional changes in blood flow, for example, regional shifts must be 'normalised' against global reductions elsewhere. Where activation paradigms are employed, to assess changes in metabolism or blood flow consequent upon cognitive or other activity, special care must be taken in this regard. 'Subtraction' techniques have proved to be extremely valuable, whereby images generated in a given subject are compared while at rest and when engaged in some specific activity—task-state minus control-state subtractions then reveal the regional changes associated with the activity in question (e.g. in the studies of linguistic processing described on p. 45). Similar methods have been developed for comparisons between different groups of subjects; the subtraction of common activity again allows display of an image which represents statistically significant differences on a pixel-by-pixel basis ('statistical parametric maps') (Fox *et al.* 1988; Friston *et al.* 1991).

The isotopes chiefly used are ^{15}O, ^{13}N, ^{11}C and ^{18}F which have half-lives of approximately 2, 10, 20 and 110 minutes, respectively. ^{15}O may be inhaled and the arterial blood sampled, to yield quantitative measurements of regional cerebral blood flow and regional cerebral oxygen utilisation (Frackowiak *et al.* 1980). Alternatively, a bolus of ^{15}O-labelled water may be injected intravenously to obtain brief repeated images of cerebral blood flow which serve as a marker of neuronal activity (Raichle *et al.* 1983). ^{18}F may be incorporated into 2-deoxy-D-glucose (^{18}FDG) which is injected to measure local glucose metabolic rates (Phelps *et al.* 1979). The compound enters the brain as though it were glucose, but cannot be degraded and remains trapped within the cells for several hours. Estimates of regional glucose utilization can therefore be made by repeated venous sampling in conjunction with the scan. ^{11}C may be incorporated into deoxyglucose for similar purposes.

The important PET studies carried out in relation to ageing and dementia are described in Chapter 10 (p. 434). They have revealed differing patterns of regional brain hypometabolism in different varieties of dementia, such changes often predating evidence of atrophy on CT scans. In Huntington's disease, in particular, caudate hypometabolism can be an early indicator of the developing disorder, and may have some predictive value in disclosing susceptibility to the disease (pp. 470–1). Interesting information has been obtained concerning brain metabolic failure in regions remote from areas of focal infarction (p. 377), and with regard to patterns of brain adaptation and recovery in response to injury (p. 378). In consequence we have achieved a more comprehensive view of brain functional organisation. Studies in Parkinson's disease and epilepsy are described on pp. 655 and 289. The burgeoning field of PET scan studies in schizophrenia is outlined in Chapter 2. Here certain findings in relation to depression and other psychiatric disorders will be briefly outlined.

Whole brain hypometabolism has been reported in bipolar depressed patients, with a return towards normal following changes to euthymic or hypomanic states (Baxter et al. 1985). In a further study, depression was associated with impaired glucose metabolism in the dorsal anterolateral prefrontal cortex, particularly on the left (Baxter et al. 1989). Ratings of the severity of depression correlated with the degree of left prefrontal hypometabolism, and parallel improvements were observed on recovery with medication. Post et al. (1987) found temporal rather than frontal hypometabolism in their patients. Using more sophisticated methods for comparison, Bench et al. (1992) have confirmed decreased regional cerebral blood flow in the left dorsolateral frontal cortex and also in the left anterior cingulate region; furthermore patients with depression-related cognitive impairments showed decreases in the left medial frontal gyrus along with increased blood flow in the cerebellar vermis.

PET scans in patients suffering from DSM-III panic disorder have shown asymmetries of blood flow and oxygen metabolism in a discrete region of the limbic system, namely the parahippocampal gyri (Reiman et al. 1984, 1986). This applied only in those patients whose panic attacks were reproducible by lactate infusions. In a further investigation Reiman et al. (1989) studied patients who were actively experiencing panic attacks, demonstrating significant increases in blood flow in the temporal poles, insular cortex and claustrum/lateral putamen.

Obsessive–compulsive disorder has attracted considerable attention. Baxter et al. (1987, 1988) showed significant increases in metabolism in the left orbital gyrus and both caudate nuclei, in comparison to normal controls and to patients with depression. The caudate/hemisphere metabolic ratios increased significantly with symptom improvement after drug treatment, but

remained unchanged in those who did not respond. Further PET studies are reviewed by McGuire (1995) and McGuire et al. (1995a), including their own investigation of patients during the elicitation of obsessive–compulsive symptoms; a graded relationship was observed between symptom intensity and increased blood flow to inferior prefrontal, cingulate and striate areas. The implication of basal ganglia dysfunction in obsessive–compulsive disorder is interesting in view of the tendency for such symptoms to emerge with encephalitis lethargica and Tourette's syndrome. Possible findings of striatal dysfunction in Tourette's syndrome are described on p. 685. Baxter et al. (1987) hypothesise that in patients suffering from obsessive–compulsive symptoms there is a mismatch between orbitofrontal and caudate activity; in effect cortical activity is elevated beyond the capacity of the caudate to maintain its integrative role.

PET studies with cerebral activation

'Activation' paradigms may be employed with PET to provide further insights into cerebral organisation and function. The subject is scanned at rest and again when engaged in some specific perceptual, motor or cognitive activity. By subtraction of one image from the other, areas of discrete activation are revealed. The use of ^{15}O with its short half-life has proved especially valuable; scans may be repeated at intervals of 12–15 minutes, allowing several tasks to be investigated in a single session without head repositioning.

Reviews are provided by Phelps and Mazziotta (1985), Haxby et al. (1991) and Chertkow and Bub (1994). A motor task of sequential finger movement, for example, activates the contralateral motor strip and supplementary motor cortex. Studies of the visual system have shown differing patterns of activation during tasks of object recognition and spatial localisation; both activate the lateral visual cortex, but the former additionally involves more anterior occipitotemporal regions and the latter activates regions in the superior parietal cortex. Colour processing selectively activates the lingual and fusiform gyri in the ventromedial occipital and temporal cortex, while the perception of movement activates a small region at the junction of the temporoparieto-occipital cortex (Zeki et al. 1991). Such fine differentiation greatly exceeds what could have accrued from lesion studies.

Studies in the auditory system have shown differing patterns of activation according to the nature of the stimulus received, and even to some extent the strategy used by the subject to solve a related task (Phelps & Mazziotta 1985). Verbal stimuli are associated with increased left hemisphere metabolism, whereas musical chords activate primarily the right. When comparing sequences of notes, subjects who used visual imagery activated left posterior temporal regions, while those who mentally 're-signed' the notes activated inferior parietal and temporo-occipital regions on the right. Subjects who were asked to recall specific aspects of auditory stimuli showed activations in medial temporal lobe structures, which were not seen during auditory perceptions which made no demands on memory.

Attentional mechanisms have also been dissected. Selective attention to colour, shape and velocity modulates activity in relevant extrastriate regions—in occipital, temporal and inferior parietal cortex, respectively. But tasks which make heavy demands on attention activate frontal and subcortical regions as well. A particular frontal region, the anterior cingulate cortex, is activated by both the Stroop colour–word interference task (Pardo *et al.* 1990) and a semantic verbal association task (Petersen *et al.* 1988), and may be critical for 'attention for action'.

PET studies which have attempted to display thinking and imagery in the absence of any sensory input or motor output are discussed by Haxby *et al.* (1991). In general, widespread bilateral prefrontal activation is accompanied by activation in the sensory association regions appropriate to the task involved. Imagined route finding, for example, activates inferior temporal and posterosuperior parietal areas bilaterally, and mental subtraction activates the region of the angular gyrus. With regard to 'frontal lobe tests', analogues of card sorting have been shown to activate the dorsolateral prefrontal cortex bilaterally, and verbal fluency tasks the left only, as reviewed by Chertkow and Bub (1994). PET studies in relation to memory are described on p. 28, and those dealing with language on p. 45.

In addition to exploring neuropsychological paradigms, activation studies can be used to increase the specificity and sensitivity of PET in clinical situations. Studies in relation to schizophrenia are outlined on p. 88. Activation studies have also been used to explore fundamental theories about the nature of psychosis as described by Joyce (1992). Thus Frith (1987) has proposed that the phenomena of schizophrenia are secondary to a disturbance of the perception and initiation of willed action; positive features such as hallucinations and delusions represent failures of systems which register that an act has been willed, while negative features such as poverty of speech and flatness of affect result from inability to generate intentions *per se*. PET activation studies in normal subjects have indicated that the monitoring of intended movements is particularly associated with activity in the left hippocampus, whereas the willed initiation of behaviour depends on dorsolateral prefrontal cortex and anterior cingulate cortex. It is therefore intriguing that in Liddle's (1987) subcategorisation of schizophrenia, patients with 'reality distortion syndrome' (i.e. hallucinations and delusions) have shown focal changes in cerebral blood flow in the former region, and patients with 'psychomotor poverty syndrome' in the latter (pp. 87–8). Furthermore, correlational analysis has shown that psychomotor retardation in depressed patients is likewise significantly related to decreased blood flow in the dorsolateral prefrontal

cortex, suggesting that this reflects a fundamental psychological–cerebral association rather than an attribute of a specific disease process.

Radioligands and psychopharmacology

In addition to studies of brain metabolism and blood flow, PET scanning has opened up windows to other biochemical processes in the brain. A large number of compounds can be labelled with appropriate radioisotopes to reveal, for example, aspects of neurotransmitter function and the fate of pharmacological agents.

The technique, where neurotransmitters are concerned, is to find a 'ligand' (i.e. a substance which binds to a class of receptor sites) and label it with a positron-emitting isotope. After testing for its specificity and sensitivity in the laboratory it can then be used to reveal the distribution of receptor sites within the brain. In some cases detailed quantitative measures can be obtained of the density of such receptors, and of the extent to which they are free or already occupied by drugs or the natural neurotransmitters of the brain. The technical complexities inherent in such studies are outlined by Dolan *et al.* (1990) and Pilowsky (1996).

Most interest has centred on the dopaminergic system, in relation for example to movement disorders and schizophrenia as described in Chapters 14 and 2. Postsynaptic D_2 receptors can be studied using raclopride labelled with ^{11}C. Presynaptic function is examined with ^{18}F-dopa which detects dopamine stores in nerve terminals, and with ^{11}C-nomifensine which labels presynaptic re-uptake sites.

Other radiolabelled ligands include ^{11}C-flumazenil for central benzodiazepine receptors, ^{11}C-carfentanil for opiate receptors, ^{11}C-dexetimide for muscarinic cholinergic receptors, and ^{11}C-deprenyl for monoamine oxidase B. ^{11}C-N-methylspiperone binds to both D_2 and S_2 receptors, but the reversibility of its binding in the cortex can provide an index of serotonergic function there. Complex tracer kinetic models are utilised in certain studies to reveal subtle changes in receptor numbers and affinity, especially in the investigation of psychiatric disorders.

Pharmacological studies are summarised by Dolan *et al.* (1990) and Pilowsky (1996). PET can be used to examine the influx of drugs into brain tissue and assess their interaction with receptors, to monitor receptor blockade in relation to clinical effect, or to observe responsivity of distinct neurochemical pathways to pharmacological agonists and antagonists. This last may be combined with simultaneous cognitive activation in order to reveal more clearly the differences between patients and controls. Some drugs may be labelled directly, such as the neuroleptics pimozide and clozapine, and the anticonvulsants valproate and diphenylhydantoin. After injection in tracer amounts their distribution within the brain can be studied directly, also their affinities at specific receptor sites.

Studies in relation to the neuroleptic treatment of schizophrenia are reviewed by List and Cleghorn (1993). PET has been used to show the rapidity of D_2-receptor blockade in the striatum on commencing neuroleptics, and the time course of reversal of the blockade when they are discontinued. Dose-dependent relationships have been demonstrated between serum levels of neuroleptics and the degree of inhibition of striatal D_2 binding, and attempts have been made to detect differences in patients who are resistant to neuroleptic effect.

Another approach has been to examine the effects of neuroleptics on regional brain metabolism and blood flow, since it is clear that striatal receptor blockade occurs within hours whereas clinical improvement follows only gradually over several days or weeks. It has been shown that the metabolic rate of the basal ganglia is increased by long-term neuroleptic treatment, whereas the ratio of frontal to parietal cortical metabolism falls. The determination of which of these changes may correlate with the time course of symptom improvement could serve as a guide towards the cerebral mechanisms of neuroleptic effect. The relationship of cerebral changes to drug-induced side effects will similarly warrant clarification.

Other molecules which may be labelled include amino acids, fatty acids, alcohols and sugars. A considerable variety of active metabolic processes are thus accessible to study.

Single photon emission computerised tomography (SPECT scanning, SPET scanning)

SPECT scanning has come into prominence more recently than PET, though in some respects its origins go back further. It is essentially an elaboration of radioisotope scanning (p. 135), brought about by the harnessing of computer technology analogous to that used in CT for reconstructing images of the brain. This, coupled with improved radiotracer biochemistry has brought the technique to a high degree of sophistication. It may also be seen as an elaboration of the xenon-133 planar blood flow studies introduced by Ingvar and Lassen (1961) which lacked the capacity for exploring deeper regions of the brain.

Though considerably less accurate than PET scanning, and a good deal less amenable to quantitation, the images obtained with the most modern machines can be of remarkable quality (Plate 7). Since the radioisotopes employed have much longer half-lives than those used for PET scanning there is no requirement to have a cyclotron close at hand. This accounts in large measure

for the increasing attention devoted to the technique. SPECT scanning can be available at any hospital where a nuclear medicine facility is available; and its greatly reduced cost in comparison with PET means that larger samples may be investigated and that it can be applied more readily in a clinical context. The range of normal variation encountered is, however, considerable, rendering the technique in general more suitable for group comparisons than for precise diagnosis in the individual patient.

The procedure involves the administration of radiopharmaceuticals which emit, not positrons, but gamma rays (photons) directly. The tracers are taken up into the brain, and their regional concentration detected by focused collimators arranged around the head or by a rotating gamma camera. At each point the detector samples a cone of brain tissue, brain images then being obtained by summation according to the standard tomographic technique. Costa and Ell (1991) describe the evolution of progressively more sophisticated equipment and the methods available for data analysis. Since the gamma rays are emitted directly from the radiotracers employed, there is no annihilation process as with PET. 'Coincidence counting' is therefore precluded and the points of origin of the gamma rays are simply determined from their trajectories, consequently with less precision. Nevertheless, resolution approaches 8–12 mm with the most recent systems.

The tracers most used to date are markers of cerebral blood flow. Glucose and oxygen uptake cannot be revealed directly by SPECT, but will normally be closely coupled to blood flow in the situations where SPECT is employed. With the continued development of tracer biochemistry methods are also available for imaging a variety of neurotransmitters and their receptor sites as described below.

Xenon-133 (with a half-life of 5.3 days) may be administered by inhalation or injection for cerebral blood flow studies. Xenon is inert and freely diffusible, with a short retention time in the brain, hence uptake and clearance must be measured throughout the procedure. Its chief virtues are the brief scanning time required and the capacity to measure regional blood flow in absolute units, but resolution is relatively poor. Isopropylamphetamine (IMP) labelled with ^{123}I is simpler to use. It has a half-life of 13 hours, and being lipophylic it penetrates brain tissue and becomes trapped within it, revealing patterns of distribution of blood flow which remain stable over a substantial period of time. Scanning is carried out after a single intravenous injection; higher resolution is obtained than with xenon but at the expense of longer scanning times. IMP has now been superseded by hexamethylpropyleneamineoxine (HMPAO) labelled with tech-netium-99 molybdenum (^{99m}Tc) which is similarly lipophylic, but having a shorter half-life (6 hours) it can be given in higher dosage yielding improved definition and shorter scanning times. ^{99m}Tc is routinely available and can be obtained from a 'generator' which has a shelf life of 67 hours. The HMPAO is taken up in the brain in proportion to blood flow within a few minutes, yielding a 'frozen image' which remains stable for several hours. Scanning is normally undertaken some 20–30 minutes after injection.

In general xenon is used in studies which seek to inves-tigate dynamic changes in blood flow, as in activation pro-cedures, and HMPAO when the requirement is for a static and more detailed picture. Split-dose techniques are, however, applicable with HMPAO; a portion of the tracer is injected for imaging at rest, then the remainder after some cognitive or other activation procedure has been performed by the subject (Shedlack *et al.* 1991).

The typical picture obtained with xenon consists of low flows at the periphery, representing skin, scalp and bone; a ring of higher flows which reflect cortical grey matter, either continuous or broken in the posterior temporal region; then lower flows centrally over the white matter and ventricles. The highest flows are usually observed in the visual cortex and cerebellum. HMPAO scans show sharper definition between grey and white matter and are greatly superior in revealing regional cortical deficits and the presence of brain pathology. The heads of the caudate nuclei, the putamen/globus pallidus, thalamus and cere-bellum can often be clearly displayed (Plate 7).

SPECT scans have proved of clinical value in relation to strokes, and for the investigation of blood flow during migraine attacks (pp. 377 and 402). In the dementias they can reveal the reductions of uptake in the temporopari-etal regions typical of Alzheimer's disease (p. 434), and have been used to demarcate the contrasting group of 'frontal lobe dementias' (p. 463 *et seq.*). Multi-infarct dementia may be indicated by scattered focal deficits (p. 457). In Huntington's disease changes may be detected in the heads of the caudate nuclei (Smith *et al.* 1988; Gemmell *et al.* 1989). Applications in the field of epilepsy and alcoholism are described on pp. 289 and 606.

In a retrospective evaluation of 20 neuropsychiatric patients suf-fering from dementia, amnesic states, depression and personality disorder, Trzepacz *et al.* (1992) have shown the value of IMP SPECT in revealing clinically relevant brain abnormalities. They concluded, somewhat surprisingly, that it was possibly superior to CT or even MRI in this regard. In particular it appeared to be better than structural imaging in the differential diagnosis of the dementias and in yielding improved understanding of amnesic disorders.

Studies in schizophrenic patients have revealed hypoperfu-sion frontally (p. 87), much as in PET scan studies, and decreased blood flow has been reported in depression with significant increases on recovery (Rush *et al.* 1982; Sackheim *et al.* 1990). Musalek *et al.* (1989) have reported distinctive patterns in patients with auditory and tactile hallucinations. McGuire *et al.*'s (1993) investigation of auditory verbal hallucinations is outlined on p. 88.

Investigations have also revealed redistributions of flow during the performance of perceptual and cognitive activities which, though modest in comparison with PET, allow the devel-opment of activation paradigms. Thus the visual cortex can be shown to increase its uptake during visual stimulation (Devous 1989). Attempts have likewise been made to reveal blood flow changes associated with various thinking and imagery tasks (Roland & Friberg 1985; Goldenberg *et al.* 1989a, 1989b) and during card sorting and verbal fluency tests (Devous *et al.* 1985; Shedlack *et al.* 1991).

Neurotransmitter imaging

With further developments in radiotracer chemistry it has proved possible to image certain neurotransmitter recep-tors. Most success has been achieved to date with the dopamine system, Crawley *et al.* (1986) used bromo-spiperone-77, and Pilowsky *et al.* (1994) iodobenzamide (IBZM) labelled with ^{123}I to explore D_2-receptor binding in a semiquantitative manner. Quinuclidinyl-4-iodo-benzilate (QNB) labelled with ^{123}I may be used to detect muscarinic acetylcholine receptors, a decrease being re-vealed in the posterior temporal cortex in patients with Alzheimer's dementia (Holman *et al.* 1985; Weinberger *et al.* 1991b). Other potential ligands include raclopride for D_2 receptors, IBZP for D_1 receptors and flumazenil for benzodiazepine receptors, all labelled with ^{123}I.

Chapter 4: Differential Diagnosis

The correct appraisal of patients with organic psychiatric disorders is a test both of psychiatric and general medical skills. The detailed differential diagnosis of individual conditions will be considered in the appropriate sections elsewhere, but here certain general principles will be outlined.

Of first importance is the ability to distinguish between organic and non-organic psychiatric illness, in other words to recognise when identifiable brain disorder is the root cause of the presenting clinical picture. The nature of the cerebral disorder must then be determined by a process of enquiry which proceeds logically in accordance with reasonable expectations. A distinction between acute and chronic organic reactions is often helpful in deciding on probabilities, as is the distinction between diffuse or focal cerebral disorder. Thereafter the range of possible causes remains wide, and will also be briefly discussed below.

Differentiation from non-organic conditions

There can be little difficulty in deciding on an organic aetiology when impairment of consciousness or of cognitive processes is marked, when there are epileptic fits, or when psychiatric symptoms are accompanied by obvious neurological symptoms and signs. But this is not always the case. Some organic disorders can present with hallucinations, affective change or schizophrenia-like symptomatology and lack clear organic accompaniments throughout their course. Others unfold very gradually, with indefinite organic features and with symptomatology suggestive of virtually any form of psychiatric illness. Special predisposition to neurotic forms of reaction, or to psychotic illness, may confer distinctive features which for some time obscure the true situation.

The converse is also true, since patients with non-organic psychiatric illness may show features which raise the possibility of cerebral disease. For example, disorientation and minor impairment of consciousness may be detected at the onset of acute schizophrenia, also some-

times in mania and agitated depression, yet without evidence of identifiable brain malfunction either at the time or subsequently. Similarly, cognitive impairment, including difficulty with recent memory, may accompany purely affective disorders particularly in later life, as discussed on p. 485 *et seq*. Features resembling delirium, including characteristic disturbances of thought processes and even hallucinations, can follow psychological stress, as in sensory deprivation (Zuckerman 1964) or sleep deprivation (Morris & Singer 1966). It is probable that subtle perturbations of brain function underlie all such examples, though these are not identifiable by clinical investigation; moreover the possibility of their presence has little practical implication for treatment.

Thus it is clear that the line of demarcation between organic and non-organic psychiatric disorders is not hard and fast. It remains valid and useful in practice for the great majority of cases, but in a substantial number there can be continuing uncertainty. The margin for error is reduced when special investigations are undertaken, but even so is not removed completely. The electroencephalogram can yield equivocal results. Psychometric testing can occasionally be misleading. Radiographic procedures may reveal findings of uncertain significance, likewise functional brain imaging techniques. Clinical examination therefore remains of the first importance, and is in any case the chief guideline which determines whether or not special investigations should be undertaken. Examples of patients in whom unusual problems in the differentiation between organic and non-organic disorder have arisen, often with surprising results, have been described by the present author (Lishman 1992).

Neurotic disorder may be simulated in the early stages of cerebral disease by virtue of diffuse complaints of anxiety, depression, irritability and insomnia. The patient may himself complain of forgetfulness and difficulty in concentration, but these tend to be discounted because of the multitude of other vague somatic symptoms. Phobic and obsessional symptomatology is not uncommon at the onset, and may remain a prominent feature for some considerable time. The need to differentiate between the 'worried well' and patients in the earliest stages of HIV brain infection has drawn particular attention to problems in this area. It is also well known that one must be wary of neurotic developments beginning only in middle life and when the previous mental constitution was good, also to seek for clear evidence of adequate immediate causes for their appearance.

Sometimes the clue may lie in the patient's attitude towards his symptoms. The organic patient will often tend to play down his deficits so that a graver picture is obtained from relatives than from the patient himself. The neurotic patient, by contrast, presses home his symptoms and actively seeks a remedy for them. The patient's evasiveness may raise suspicion, or when pressed he may display abrupt 'catastrophic' reactions of distress or anger. Typically also the organic patient's symptomatology lacks the richness and diversity seen in purely neurotic disorders.

Hysterical forms of reaction may also be simulated. Acute organic reactions tend to fluctuate with periods of lucidity, and symptoms may thus be fleeting. A shallow affective quality and a tendency to make light of symptoms may suggest the 'belle indifference' of hysteria. In mild delirium the cardinal features of impairment of consciousness and subtle deficits of attention may sometimes be hard to determine, and behaviour may be seemingly motivated for display. Thus it may be necessary to watch closely for signs of perseveration, slight dysarthria and other minimal features which betray the organic basis of the disorder.

Episodes of bizarre behaviour in hypoglycaemic attacks, or of paralysis in porphyria, provide well-known diagnostic hazards in which hysteria comes to be suspected. Similar difficulty is sometimes found with periods of long-continued abnormal behaviour following encephalitis. Frank conversion symptoms may, of course, occur with chronic brain disease and be mistaken for the primary disorder. It is unclear how far these reflect in some way the direct effects of cerebral damage, or how far they merely represent a psychogenic response to the patient's partial awareness of his deficits. Again, it is axiomatic to view with grave suspicion hysterical symptoms which make their first appearance only in middle life. The problem of the differential diagnosis of hysterical pseudodementia is discussed on p. 484.

Schizophrenic symptoms in association with cerebral disease can readily be misleading. A preponderance of visual over auditory hallucinations should raise suspicion of an organic disorder, similarly an empty or shallow affective colouring to delusional beliefs and passivity phenomena. Delusions in both acute and chronic organic reactions may take any form which is seen in schizophrenia, but paranoid delusions are by far the most common. Certain qualities of the delusions strongly suggest an organic basis, namely those which are vague, poorly systematised, incoherent, fleeting and changeable, or restricted and stereotyped in content. Nevertheless schizophrenic illnesses which are typical in every respect occasionally prove ultimately to be founded on identifiable cerebral disease.

Depressive symptoms can also give rise to difficulty. Ordinary affective disorder can be associated with marked slowness of thinking, difficulty with concentration and uncertainty with memory. There may be considerable doubt about the correct evaluation of such features, and psychometric testing may give equivocal results. The difficulties are increased when electroconvulsive treatments have already been given.

Features which may help in distinguishing primary depressive illness from organic psychiatric disorder include the careful appraisal of the setting in which disturbances of concentration and memory occur. In depressive illness it can often be observed that lack of interest or excessive anxiety prevent the focusing of attention on the matter in hand, rather than any pervasive difficulty with the organisation of thought and memory. Preoccupation with morbid thoughts may operate similarly. Typically the patient with uncomplicated depression is able to give a more coherent account of his discomforts and a more accurate chronology of his illness than would be possible in the presence of cerebral disease. These important aspects of differential diagnosis are considered more fully in the section on depressive pseudodementia (pp. 487–9).

Personality disorder is especially liable to be suspected where frontal lobe dysfunction is concerned, for example following injury or in the early stages of a frontal dementia. Irresponsible behaviour or lapses of social conduct may be attributed to pre-existing personality factors, particularly when there has been some recent stress or problem in the patient's life. Here the essential clue will lie in a careful history from an informant which reveals the change that has occurred. Other avenues to the differential diagnosis are less reliable. Thus the patient may fail to display the classic features of frontal lobe disturbance at interview. And psychometric testing cannot always be relied upon in making the distinction; cognitive ability may be well preserved, and even tests specially devised to reveal frontal deficits can occasionally be misleading (p. 119). Examples of frontal tumours or general paresis presenting with change of disposition and behaviour are described on pp. 223 and 340. An example where functional neuroimaging finally disclosed the presence of a frontal lobe dementia is described on p. 464. Special difficulty will of course arise in patients whose personality has always been abnormal.

Differentiation between acute and chronic organic reactions

In practice this distinction is most directly made from the history of the mode of onset of the disorder. A short history and firm knowledge of an acute onset will make a chronic organic reaction unlikely. Onset in association with a physical illness rather strongly suggests an acute organic reaction. But when such leads are lacking close attention to phenomenology may be necessary.

Acute organic reactions are characterised by impairment of consciousness in some degree, as revealed by careful observation of the patient's alertness, wakefulness, and ability to focus and sustain attention. In chronic organic reactions, by contrast, the patient is fully in touch, and attempts to cooperate despite cognitive difficulties. Fluctuation from time to time is also an observation of importance in pointing to acute disorders. Nocturnal worsening may be apparent, or a picture which changes rapidly from one occasion to another. When stimulated the patient may become lucid for a while, and one can then determine that intellectual processes are basically intact. Moreover during lucid periods he may demonstrate adequate recall of events immediately preceding the development of the illness, confirming that until very recently mental functioning had been normal.

Acute rather than chronic cerebral disorder is suggested when there are severe perceptual disturbances and distortions, with prominent illusions and hallucinations in the visual modality. Defective appreciation of reality may lead to rich and intrusive fantasies, in contrast to the emptiness and impoverishment of thought characteristic of chronic organic reactions. Similarly in the presence of florid behaviour disturbance this will be seen to be dictated by disturbed thought processes of a more sophisticated kind in acute than in chronic cerebral disorder. Roth and Myers (1969) describe this difference well: 'Psychic life in clouding is full, sometimes extravagantly so, but distorted: the patient lives in a private world of shifting experiences richly supplied with detail from the resources of a brain which is essentially intact. . . . His statements about his experiences and misconstrued orientations are positive and sometimes detailed. In dementia, by contrast, the patient lives in the actual world but does so deficiently. His disorientation results from ignorance, and when asked about his experiences, he is likely querulously to dismiss the question as unimportant, or proffer feeble inventions or readily accept suggestions, however, absurd.'

The affective state of the patient may also help with the distinction. In acute organic reactions the emotional disturbances are typically of a positive kind—fear or terror, perplexity and agitation—whereas the demented patient may be flat, apathetic and emotionally unresponsive (Roth 1981). Emotional rapport can usually be established in patients showing clouding of consciousness, but tends to be poor in dementia.

This said, it must be recognised that in practice the differentiation between acute and chronic organic reactions can sometimes be very difficult. Despite careful observation the distinction may come to be revealed only by the time course that is followed. For example, a prolonged subacute delirious state due to anoxia, uraemia or hepatic disorder can simulate dementia very closely. Or the patient may be admitted to hospital without a history to point to the acute and recent onset of the disorder. Perhaps most difficulty is encountered with elderly patients who show postoperative disturbances, due to metabolic derangements or anoxia, and in whom the mental state was incompletely evaluated beforehand. The electroencephalogram may provide some guidance in such examples (p. 130).

Acute disturbance of cerebral function may, of course, give way gradually to irreversible structural pathology with a corresponding admixture of features appropriate to both. The two may also coexist when a chronic dementing process is complicated by superadded anoxia, infection or some other concurrent disease, or when fresh progressions occur in the course of a vascular dementia. Not uncommonly it is such a transient phase of acute disorder which first draws attention to chronic brain disease which has hitherto gone unrecognised.

Differentiation between diffuse and focal lesions

Symptoms and signs of localising significance must be carefully sought out in all organic psychiatric disorders, and when discovered must not be ignored. Local disturbances of cerebral function can, of course, occur with progressive cortical disease before it is sufficiently extensive to produce a global dementia; well-known examples are a circumscribed amnesic syndrome in the early stages of Alzheimer's disease, or a frontal lobe syndrome in Pick's disease. Evidence of focal brain damage may also emerge later in the course of such disorders when the pathological changes become especially advanced in certain regions of the brain. Signs of focal damage must therefore be carefully assessed in relation to the clinical picture as a whole, but will usually dictate that further investigations should be undertaken. The important problem is to distinguish the essentially focal lesion from diffuse brain damage, because a remediable cause may then come to light.

Neurological signs are of first importance in this connection. Every attempt must be made to exclude the possibility of raised intracranial pressure, and to examine for cranial nerve palsies, visual field defects or unilateral motor and sensory disturbances. Physical signs in the presenile and senile dementias are rarely strictly unilateral or even markedly asymmetrical, and dense motor and sensory disturbances will always be strongly suggestive of cerebrovascular disease, cerebral tumour or cerebral syphilis. Unilateral anosmia or optic atrophy are important signs which may betray a frontal tumour. Finally the neurological examination should always be supplemented by careful enquiry and observation for epileptic disturbances of focal origin.

Psychological symptoms of possible localising value include amnesia out of proportion to other cognitive deficits, dysphasia, somnolence, and the several aspects of parietal lobe symptomatology that have been discussed (pp. 17–18). It is necessary to beware especially of an amnesic syndrome which masquerades as generalised dementia. The relative preservation of other cognitive functions must be carefully assessed, and due attention paid to any marked discrepancy between memory for remote and recent events or the presence of a circumscribed retrograde gap. Although the patient with Korsakoff's syndrome is anergic and apathetic, he shows better preservation of intellect in general conversation than the patient with dementia. In the latter it often proves difficult to determine the relative contributions of impaired memory and impairment of other cognitive functions to the total disability.

Mild dysphasia due to focal cerebral disease may also be mistaken for early dementia, when the patient's account is hesitant and incoherent, or when he is anxious and depressed as a result of his disability. Careful observation usually shows, however, that behaviour not involving language remains substantially intact. Dysphasic difficulties, and especially nominal dysphasia, may be seen with diffuse cerebral disorder, but then insight into the defect is less likely to be well preserved. Indeed the demented patient is often oblivious of his disability, and untroubled by failures rather than distressed and struggling. The greatest difficulty in differentiation is therefore likely to arise with primary sensory or conduction dysphasia (pp. 51 and 53). A clinical point that is said to be helpful in the distinction is that dysphasic patients with focal lesions have as much difficulty in naming objects from sight as in recalling names from memory, whereas patients with diffuse brain disease perform better when the object can be seen or handled.

Agnosic and apraxic deficits, disturbances of the body image and of spatial orientation, likewise raise suspicion of focal cerebral disorder when severe and out of all proportion to other cognitive difficulties. Such deficits are, however, relatively common in acute organic reactions or consciousness is impaired to a significant extent, and when chronic diffuse brain disease has progressed beyond the early stages.

Special investigatory procedures, as outlined in Chapter 3 are the most reliable arbiters in the distinction between focal and diffuse brain damage, and will often need to be undertaken before a firm differentiation is achieved.

Causes of acute and chronic organic reactions

The specific cause in the majority of cases will readily become apparent in the course of history taking and examination. In many it is self-evident from the outset. Sometimes, however, the cause may be elusive and it is then essential to consider systematically a wide range of possibilities. These are shown in Tables 3 and 4.

It is helpful in approaching a given case to consider first the possible causes arising within the central nervous system itself, then derangements of cerebral function consequent upon disorders in other systems of the body. This division is reflected approximately in the ordering of causes in Tables 3 and 4. Even some of the very rare conditions are remediable, and enquiry must therefore be extensive when the solution is not soon forthcoming.

The antecedent history will give important clues, and it is essential that a relative or close acquaintance should be seen. The time and mode of onset must always be carefully established. The classic presenile and senile dementias usually begin insidiously and their history commonly extends over several months, whereas remediable illnesses often have an abrupt and relatively recent onset. Careful enquiry should always be made for a history of head injury, fits, alcoholism, drug abuse, recent illness or anaesthesia. Even in the absence of known head injury the possibility of subdural haematoma should be kept in mind, since this may follow trivial injury in arteriosclerotic subjects or be forgotten in alcoholics. It may be followed by a latent interval, and be accompanied by minimal neurological signs. A known epileptic tendency may suggest that the present disturbance is an unusually prolonged complex partial seizure or post-ictal state. Fits of recent onset may indicate a space-occupying lesion, or some acute cerebrovascular accident or injury which has left a residual focus of brain damage. A history of alcoholism or drug abuse may be long concealed in some cases, even on occasion by relatives as well as by the patient. Suspicion may only be raised by indirect evidence

Table 3 Causes of acute organic reactions.

1	Degenerative	Presenile or senile dementias complicated by infection, anoxia, etc. Episode in Lewy body dementia
2	Space-occupying lesions	Cerebral tumour, subdural haematoma, cerebral abscess
3	Trauma	'Acute post-traumatic psychosis'
4	Infection	Encephalitis, meningitis, HIV infection, subacute meningovascular syphilis Exanthemata, streptococcal infection, septicaemia, pneumonia, influenza, typhoid, typhus, cerebral malaria, trypanosomiasis, rheumatic chorea
5	Vascular	Acute cerebral thrombosis or embolism, episode in multi-infarct dementia, transient cerebral ischaemic attack, subarachnoid haemorrhage, hypertensive encephalopathy, systemic lupus erythematosus
6	Epileptic	Complex partial seizures, petit mal status, post-ictal states
7	Metabolic	Uraemia, liver disorder, electrolyte disturbances, alkalosis, acidosis, hypercapnia, remote effects of carcinoma, porphyria
8	Endocrine	Hyperthyroid crises, myxoedema, Addisonian crises, hypopituitarism, hypo- and hyperparathyroidism, diabetic precoma, hypoglycaemia
9	Toxic	Alcohol—Wernicke's encephalopathy, delirium tremens Drugs—benzodiazepines and other sedatives (including withdrawal), salicylate intoxication, cannabis, LSD, prescribed medications (antiparkinsonian drugs, scopolamine, tricyclic and MAOI antidepressants, etc.) Others—lead, arsenic, organic mercury compounds, carbon disulphide
10	Anoxic	Bronchopneumonia, congestive cardiac failure, cardiac dysrhythmias, silent coronary infarction, silent gastrointestinal bleeding, carbon monoxide poisoning, postanaesthetic
11	Vitamin lack	Thiamine (Wernicke's encephalopathy), nicotinic acid (pellagra, acute nicotinic acid deficiency encephalopathy), B_{12} and folic acid deficiency

LSD, lysergic acid diethylamide; MAOI, monoamine oxidase inhibitor.

Table 4 Causes of chronic organic reactions.

1	Degenerative	Senile and presenile Alzheimer's disease, multi-infarct dementia, Lewy body dementia, frontal lobe dementia, Pick's, Huntington's and Creutzfeldt–Jakob diseases, normal-pressure hydrocephalus, multiple sclerosis, Parkinson's, Schilder's and Wilson's diseases, progressive supranuclear palsy, progressive multifocal leucoencephalopathy, progressive myoclonic epilepsy, metachromatic leucodystrophy, neuroacanthocytosis, Kufs' disease, mitochondrial myopathy, etc.
2	Space-occupying lesions	Cerebral tumour, subdural haematoma
3	Trauma	Post-traumatic dementia
4	Infection	HIV-associated dementia, general paresis, chronic meningovascular syphilis, subacute and chronic encephalitis
5	Vascular	Cerebral vascular disease, 'état lacunaire'
6	Epileptic	'Epileptic dementia'
7	Metabolic	Uraemia, liver disorder, remote effects of carcinoma
8	Endocrine	Myxoedema, Addison's disease, hypopituitarism, hypo- and hyperparathyroidism, hypoglycaemia
9	Toxic	Korsakoff's syndrome, 'alcoholic dementia', chronic intoxication with sedative drugs, manganese, carbon disulphide
10	Anoxic	Anaemia, congestive cardiac failure, chronic pulmonary disease, postanaesthetic, post-carbon-monoxide poisoning, post cardiac arrest
11	Vitamin lack	Lack of thiamine, nicotinic acid, B_{12}, folic acid

from the patient's attitude to enquiry or unwillingness for hospitalisation. A history of repeated episodes over a considerable period of time may strongly suggest that drug abuse is responsible.

Apart from self-administered drugs it is always important to enquire about medication recently prescribed. This may have contributed by way of toxic effects, idiosyncratic reactions or the lowering of blood pressure. Diuretics given without proper supervision may have led to electrolyte depletion. If the patient is a known diabetic enquiry must be made about previous hypoglycaemic reactions, the current dose of insulin and the current diet.

A history of recent illness and operation should be noted, also the quality of recovery from any recent anaesthetic. Previous episodes of dysphasia, paralysis or other neurological deficit will be suggestive of cerebral arterial disease. Any indications that the patient may be at risk of HIV infection should be noted, also a family history of illness such as Huntington's disease.

In patients with acute organic reactions it is important still to enquire for an antecedent history of failing memory or intellect over some period of time, since an incipient chronic dementia may be being aggravated by intercurrent disease. The adequacy of diet should be assessed in elderly patients, especially when living alone, or in patients of low intelligence and low economic means. Vitamin depletion is, indeed, not excluded in patients suffering from presenile or senile dementing illnesses and may be adding to the disability. Finally, in the more immediate history, specific enquiry should always be made for headache, vomiting or visual disturbance indicative of raised intracranial pressure, and in elderly patients for breathlessness, ankle swelling or substernal pain which may indicate recent cardiac decompensation.

On examination one must pay attention to any appearance of physical ill health which may betoken metabolic disorder, carcinoma or an infective process. The general appearance of the patient may indicate anaemia, or an endocrine disorder such as myxoedema which is otherwise easily missed. Dehydration may suggest uraemia or diabetic precoma. Muscular twitching suggests uraemia, electrolyte disturbance or hypoglycaemia. There may be skin lesions diagnostic of exanthemata or indicative of vitamin deficiency. It may be necessary to search closely, by 4-hourly temperature recording, for evidence of low-grade intermittent pyrexia indicating, for example, encephalitis or cerebral abscess. Finally, very careful general observation may sometimes reveal the choreiform movements diagnostic of early Huntington's chorea.

Examination of the central nervous system must pay careful attention to the optic fundi for signs of raised intracranial pressure, to abnormalities of pupil size or reactions indicative of syphilis, or nystagmus which may suggest drug intoxication. Transient disorders of external ocular movement may be the essential sign for confirming a diagnosis of Wernicke's encephalopathy. Evidence of focal neurological defects in motor or sensory systems (including unsuspected visual field defects) will suggest a space-occupying lesion or cerebrovascular disease. Neck stiffness may indicate subarachnoid haemorrhage or meningitis, and evidence of recent ear infection will raise the possibility of cerebral abscess.

Signs of arteriosclerosis should be noted both at the periphery and in the optic fundi. The patency of the carotid arteries should be tested by palpation and auscultation in the neck. Hypertension must be assessed, likewise evidence of cardiac failure, heart block or recent coronary infarction. Respiratory infection or inadequacy must also be noted as possible causes of cerebral anoxia. Even in the absence of hepatic or splenic enlargement it may be necessary to examine for liver flap, spider naevi or foetor hepaticus. It can be important to examine for prostatic enlargement. Carcinoma with secondary cerebral deposits, or secondary 'remote' effects upon the central nervous system, may need to be excluded by palpation of breasts, neck, axillae, and rectal and vaginal examinations. A chest X-ray will be obligatory for exclusion of carcinoma of the lung.

Particular features in the mental state will only rarely help in the differential diagnosis of causes. The ceaseless overactivity of delirium tremens may sometimes be virtually diagnostic of this disorder when coupled with evidence of marked autonomic disturbance and vivid visual and tactile hallucinations. In general, hallucinations appear to be commoner in acute organic reactions due to drugs or metabolic derangements than after trauma or anoxia. The myxoedematous patient is typically dull and underactive, likewise the patient with uraemia who will probably also be somnolent. Episodes of euphoria and foolish jocularity may suggest hepatic disorder, while expansiveness is still sometimes seen with general paresis.

Investigations in every case should include haematology, erythrocyte sedimentation rate, serological tests for syphilis, urine examination and chest X-ray, no matter what may appear to be the cause. Skull X-ray and electroencephalography may be required, and a computerised tomography (CT) or magnetic resonance imaging (MRI) scan will quite often be undertaken. It may be necessary to proceed with estimation of blood urea, serum electrolytes and proteins, liver function tests, serum thyroxine, estimation of blood sugar, serum B_{12} and folate, or urinary examination for drugs or evidence of porphyria. An electrocardiogram may be indicated if silent myocardial infarction or Stokes–Adams attacks are suspected. The problems surrounding HIV testing and the need to obtain informed consent beforehand are discussed on p. 333. Lumbar puncture will sometimes be required when the diagnosis remains in doubt, and in particular to confirm suspicions of intracranial infection. Further investigations such as a radioisotope scan or angiography will sometimes be indicated, though CT and MRI scanning have greatly reduced the need for these.

Causes of stupor

Mention may be made of the differential diagnosis of stupor. The causes may be organic or non-organic, and the differential diagnosis must embrace schizophrenia, depression and hysteria in addition to organic brain dysfunction.

Joyston-Bechal (1966) examined the records of 100 cases of stupor diagnosed at the Bethlem Royal and Maudsley Hospitals in order to obtain an indication of the frequency of different causes. The results are shown in Table 5. In this setting organic causes are seen to have been relatively uncommon. The essential features of the stupor were closely similar in the organic and non-organic cases, but in the majority a firm diagnosis could ultimately be made. The 14 cases where the cause remained uncertain had, however, led to great diagnostic difficulty. Sometimes the true situation was unclear at the time of the patient's presentation, but was revealed in retrospect when the stupor had resolved.

Knowledge of the antecedent psychiatric history is often invaluable in suggesting the cause, and a careful neurological examination is always essential with special attention to signs which may indicate a diencephalic or upper brain stem lesion (p. 107). Patients with stupor due to non-organic psychiatric illness are more likely to show some partial preservation of ability to help with feeding or eliminative functions, though this is by no means invariable. The facial expression and posture is also more likely to be meaningful or show some emotional reaction to what is said or done. On recovery, patients with non-organic stupors often prove to have retained awareness of what transpired during the episode, whereas in organic stupor the level of awareness as well as the level of responsiveness is usually severely diminished.

Schizophrenic stupor is mainly a catatonic phenomenon, and is usually seen along with other catatonic features such as negativism, echopraxia, posturing or flexibilitas cerea. The patient's posture is often fixed and bizarre, and may have symbolic meaning in connection with his delusions. When disturbed the special posture is often resumed. The facial expression may be secretive or withdrawn, and may betray attention to hallucinatory experiences. Some schizophrenic stupors appear to represent withdrawal into a world of delusional fantasies, whereas in others it seems that nothing at all is experienced by the patient. The latter may represent a prolongation in severe form of schizophrenic blocking of thought and of willed action.

Depressive stupor may occasionally be just as profound as the above, and the differentiation can be difficult if the antecedent psychiatric history is unknown. Usually it can be seen to develop out of severe psychomotor retardation, which increases until there is universal motor inhibition. The posture and expression are sometimes indicative of sadness and hopelessness, and silent tears may be shed. Sometimes, however, the expression is apathetic and vacant. Conscious awareness is usually fully retained and the patient can later relate most of what was said and done to him.

Manic stupor is usually described as uncommon. The expression may be of elation or ecstasy, and the patient may later report that his mind was filled with teeming ideas to the extent that he was unable to react to anything around him. Surprisingly, in Abrams and Taylor's (1976) prospective study of catatonic patients mania emerged as the commonest diagnosis, applying also to the subgroup who had shown stupor.

Hysterical and psychogenic stupors usually occur in a situation of stress, and manifest superficial motives can often be discerned. Signs of conversion hysteria are commonly in evidence. The condition is more likely than others to wax and wane, and there may be a marked emotional reaction when sensitive subjects are discussed. Completely passive dependence on others for feeding and toilet functions is rare, and the patient may show signs

Table 5 Causes of stupor (after Joyston-Bechal 1966).

All causes		Organic causes	
Schizophrenia	31	Presenile or senile dementia	7
Depressive illness	25	'Confusional state'	4
Organic disease	20	Cerebral tumour or cyst	3
Neurosis and hysteria	10	Neurosyphilis	3
Uncertain	14	Postencephalitic disturbance	2
		Post epileptic	1
Total	100	Total	20

of irritability and annoyance when moved against his wishes.

Organic stupor has many causes, the most urgent of which is raised intracranial pressure producing a medullary or midbrain pressure cone. Focal pathologies in the region of the posterior diencephalon or upper midbrain include tumours (especially craniopharyngiomas), infarctions, meningitis (especially tuberculous meningitis), neurosyphilis and formerly encephalitis lethargica. Senile or presenile dementias may lead to stupor late in their course, likewise HIV-associated dementia. Complex partial seizures may take this form, or alternatively stupor may follow briefly in the wake of an epileptic seizure.

When a brain lesion is responsible for stupor the site will commonly lie in the upper brain stem or mesencephalon. Sometimes, however, it is due to involvement of the anteromedial frontal lobes and adjacent septal area (Segarra 1970). With stupors of brain stem origin the patient tends to be apathetic and somnolent most of the time and will frequently show pareses of external ocular movement. Patients with frontal stupor are more likely to appear alert, ready to be roused and with seeming vigilant gaze ('hyperpathic akinetic mutism').

Extracerebral causes which must be considered include a number of the conditions listed in Table 3 (p. 153). Pictures typical of stupor may occasionally be seen with uraemia, hypoglycaemia or liver disorder, or postoperatively with electrolyte disturbance or water intoxication. Endocrine disorders include myxoedema, Cushing's disease, Addison's disease, hypopituitarism and hyperparathyroidism. Stupor may also emerge with severe alcoholic intoxication, other intoxications, nicotinic acid deficiency encephalopathy, or terminally with certain infections such as typhus fever. It is important to remember that it can occasionally be seen as an adverse reaction to psychotropic medication; in Johnson's (1982) series of 25 cases, two were due to intoxication with lithium and one to excessive medication with flupenthixol.

Fortunately, with the great majority of organic causes there will be evidence of neurological dysfunction or systemic disturbance. In equivocal cases the electroencephalogram will often be helpful in deciding between a psychiatric or a neurological aetiology. When psychogenic causes are suspected, an interview under sodium amytal may confirm the situation, while in schizophrenic and depressive stupors the response to electroconvulsive therapy can be dramatic.

In Joyston-Bechal's (1966) series almost half of the stupors resolved within a week, and only one-fifth lasted more than a month. The six patients who remained in stupor for more than 6 months were all severely brain damaged.

Causes of mutism

Mutism is rarely an isolated phenomenon, often occurring along with catatonic signs such as negativism, stereotypy, posturing or stupor. It may therefore be associated with the several psychiatric conditions discussed above. Important organic causes include head injury, encephalitis, frontal lobe lesions, the post-ictal phase of epilepsy, and endocrine disorders including hyperparathyroidism, myxoedema, diabetic ketoacidosis and Addison's disease. Behrman (1972) drew attention to an important group of patients who developed mutism shortly after starting treatment with neuroleptics.

Mutism without catatonic features may also be due to organic or non-organic causes. Dissociative states are among the commoner associated conditions, though here it is essential that severe dysphasia is excluded as outlined on p. 108.

Altshuler et al. (1986) drew together collected series of patients presenting with mutism and attempted to assess the frequency of various causes. The pooled results showed that some 40% were likely to have affective disorder, 30% schizophrenia, 9% personality disorder and 17% an organic cerebral cause. In the remainder the responsible factors were uncertain. The diagnoses in their own series of 22 patients presenting over a 2-year period are shown in Table 6. Fourteen of these had shown additional catatonic signs but eight had presented with mutism alone. Not uncommonly organic causes had been overlooked initially, for example in a patient with stroke who was first diagnosed as having hysterical aphonia, and a patient with herpes encephalitis who was first thought to have catatonic schizophrenia. This emphasises the importance of careful neurological examination in every case.

Features stressed by Altshuler et al. as important in pointing to a neurological cause include irregular respiration, abnormal pupil responses, roving eye movements, facial weakness and an exaggerated jaw jerk. A psychiatric cause is suggested in patients who resist eye opening.

Table 6 Causes of mutism (after Altshuler et al. 1986).

All causes		Organic causes	
Schizophrenia	6	Stroke	4
Schizoaffective disorder	2	Postencephalitic disturbance	2
Other psychosis	1	Organic affective disorder	2
Affective disorder	3	Organic delusion syndrome	1
Organic disease	10	Phencyclidine psychosis	1
Total	22	Total	10

Occasionally patients with a primary psychiatric disorder may be induced to whisper or communicate in writing, though the latter may also occur with infarctions leading to pure word-dumbness as described on p. 50. The presence of accompanying catatonic phenomena cannot be relied upon as aiding the distinction between organic and non-organic causes. Again, however, interview under sodium amytal can often be informative.

PART 2
SPECIFIC DISORDERS

PART 2
SPECIFIC DISORDERS

Chapter 5: Head Injury

The size of the problem presented by head injuries to medical services and to the economy generally is immense. In the UK Lewin (1966) found that some 100 000 patients with head injuries were admitted to hospital yearly, and London (1967) calculated that such injuries produced 1000 severely disabled people every year. Moreover, more than half of the hospital admissions are of persons under the age of 20 (Field 1976). In 1980 the economic cost in the USA was put at almost 4 billion dollars per year (Kalsbeek *et al.* 1980). It has been estimated more recently that in the UK a million patients attend accident and emergency departments with head injuries yearly, leaving 5000 dead and 1500 with permanent brain damage (Jennett 1986). In the USA over a million persons per year sustain head injuries severe enough to require hospitalisation, and from these 30 000–50 000 persons have such serious intellectual and behavioural dysfunction that they are unable to return to normal life (National Head Injury Foundation 1992).

Early mortality has been considerably improved as a result of advances in the management of the early acute stages. The chronic sequelae remain, however, as a serious challenge to medical care and communal resources, and this can only be reflected very approximately in statistics. Quite apart from the physical sequelae, the psychiatric consequences and their social repercussions may be judged to be significant in upwards of a quarter of patients who survive. Precise figures are hard to obtain because it is clear that many patients, even with severe incapacities, do not present themselves for continuing medical attention. But what is virtually certain is that the mental sequelae outstrip the physical as a cause of difficulty with rehabilitation, hardship at work and social incapacity generally, and in terms of the strain thrown on the families to whom the head-injured patients return.

Fahy *et al.*'s (1967) follow-up of a small group of very severe civilian head injuries vividly illustrated the amount of disturbance enduring 6 years later. Only five of 22 patients were free from psychiatric sequelae, and psy-chiatric disturbance was a prominent cause of incapacity for work. Problems in the home included affective outbursts, chronic irritability, epileptiform and hallucinatory episodes and paranoid developments, in addition to impairment of intellectual processes. Yet only two of the patients had been referred for psychiatric advice during the follow-up period. It appears therefore that the psychiatrist sees only a small proportion of the problem.

The greater part of the present chapter will be devoted to the long-term mental sequelae of head injury, since this is the sphere in which the psychiatrist is most frequently engaged. The acute phases are primarily the province of the casualty officer, neurologist or neurosurgeon. Nevertheless, the psychiatrist must also have a proper understanding of acute effects, since these have important bearings on the correct evaluation of the mechanisms which underlie the longer-term disturbances.

Pathology and pathophysiology

The pathological changes following head injury have been carefully documented. Such investigations have illuminated some of the principal mechanisms by which clinical symptoms follow head injury, and indicate in general terms what sort of pathology may be expected to follow from different types of trauma. This information must be taken into account when considering matters of prognosis, or when marshalling evidence for the relationship likely to obtain between the injury and symptoms which persist long afterwards.

Unfortunately there must remain a margin of conjecture, particularly in milder injuries where opportunities for pathological study are rare. Yet these are the changes about which we need most understanding for routine clinical practice. In particular we lack a satisfactory experimental paradigm in animals, where the margin is extremely narrow between the blow which barely concusses and the blow which kills the animal outright. The more recent development of pathophysiological studies during life is, therefore, to be welcomed and may ultimately help to answer some of the outstanding questions.

Pathology of concussion

Most elusive of all has been firm evidence concerning the basis for the brief loss of consciousness which follows all but the mildest blow to the head. Cerebral ischaemia was at first thought to be the cause, either from temporary paralysis of the vasomotor regulating centres, or from arrest of the cerebral circulation due to the abrupt rise of intracranial pressure at the moment of injury.

Support for the ischaemic hypothesis was slight, however, and direct traumatic paresis of nervous functions was proposed instead. But the most notable advance has come from the conception of rotational sheer stresses within the brain. Denny-Brown and Russell (1941) showed that in anaesthetised animals uncomplicated concussion, as observed by loss of brain stem reflexes, could be produced only if the head was free to move when struck, that is when forces of acceleration or deceleration acted upon the brain within the cranium. Holbourn (1943) experimented with gelatin models of the brain, and Pudenz and Shelden (1946) directly observed the brains of monkeys after replacing their skull caps with transparent material; swirling movements of brain tissue could be witnessed after acceleration injury, both at the point of impact and elsewhere. This, then, may explain why concussion is common when the head is in motion at the time of injury, but relatively rare in static crushing injuries (Russell & Schiller 1949).

An additional problem is whether concussion depends on diffuse or focal damage to brain tissue. Swirling movements within the rigid skull stand to produce diffuse effects throughout the brain, yet the cardinal symptoms of concussion point to a major involvement of brain stem centres. In addition to loss of consciousness there is respiratory arrest, generalised vasoconstriction, loss of corneal reflexes and paralysis of deglutition. Neurophysiological studies (reviewed by Ward 1966) have certainly emphasised disturbance of brain stem structures; experimental concussion in monkeys produces surprisingly little effect on cortical EEG rhythms and far more disturbance in the medial reticular formation.

Histological studies can provide only indirect evidence on the issue, especially since mild examples may represent loss of function without structural alteration. Neuronal changes have been shown in the brain stem of animals in proportion to the strength of the blows inflicted (Windle *et al.* 1944; Groat & Simmons 1950), but these may be secondary to cervical cord damage occasioned by bending and stretching of the neck (Friede 1961). Brain stem damage has also been implicated in penetrating injuries, due to a 'plunger effect' of the brain stem within the foramen magnum (Webster & Gurdjian 1943). However, the possibility remains that similar damage may exist throughout the brain, and that hemisphere lesions may play a contributory or even primary role in the genesis of concussion. The magnetic resonance imaging (MRI) evidence discussed on p. 166 serves to reinstate the importance of hemisphere damage, with brain stem mechanisms suffering secondarily.

Biochemical evidence concerning the basis of concussion is outlined on p. 164.

Pathology of amnesia

The pathological basis for the amnesic defects which accompany concussion is also uncertain. These too may depend on focal or diffuse brain changes.

The fact that registration and recall are affected together would suggest that the specialised neural mechanisms in the hippocampus and/or diencephalon have been temporarily put out of action. The temporal lobes are tightly encased within a bony framework, and the medial temporal lobe structures may be liable to disproportionate damage when the brain is set in sudden motion. However, in closed head injuries the length of post-traumatic amnesia is intimately associated with measures of the overall severity of injury, suggesting that it may be founded in diffuse rather than focal disturbance of cerebral function. Moreover, substantial amnesia is much less common in crushing or penetrating injuries where shearing stresses are unlikely to occur throughout the brain.

It is probable that both diffuse and focal effects contribute in different degrees from one case to another. The hippocampal or diencephalic mechanisms may be especially affected in cases with long and persistent retrograde amnesias, whereas a generalised effect on the brain may produce the more common situation in which the retrograde amnesia is brief (and compatible with the time required for registration) no matter how long the post-traumatic amnesia. Certainly in the occasional patient who is left with permanent memory difficulties, but without gross disturbance of other intellectual functions, it is reasonable to assume that focal damage has been caused to the parts of the brain especially concerned with memorising.

General pathology of head injury

The more severe injuries which come to postmortem examination show a variety of pathological changes. Some are the result of direct physical damage to the brain parenchyma, and some the result of complicating factors such as vascular disturbances, cerebral oedema and anoxia. In penetrating injuries infection may be superadded.

Direct physical damage will vary in important respects according to the type of trauma inflicted. Closed head injury is by far the commonest form in civilian life, and here important factors are the direction of the blow, its force and velocity, and whether or not the head was free to move at impact. Contusion and laceration tend to be marked at the site of impact, at the opposite pole ('contre-coup') and at the poles of the hemispheres generally. When the head is at rest at the time of injury, as in assault, the lesion will be maximal at the site of impact, but when in motion, as in falls or traffic accidents, the contrecoup effect is likely to be the most pronounced (Bloomquist & Courville 1947; Löken 1959). Contrecoup effects are often particularly marked in the temporal and orbital regions. Such lesions lead to loss of neurones locally and, ultimately, to areas of subcortical demyelination.

Acceleration injuries, as in the impact of a car with the head, or deceleration injuries, as when a motorcyclist hits a wall after flying through the air, cause swirling movements throughout the brain as already described. The resulting rotational and linear stresses tear and damage nerve fibres throughout the brain. First reported in patients dying after very severe brain injuries, there is now little doubt that a distinctive diffuse pathology can result from such a mechanism in mild closed injuries as well (Strich 1956, 1969; Teasdale & Mendelow 1984). Widespread interruption and degeneration of nerve fibres can be detected, with breakdown and resorption of myelin and the formation of retraction balls. The changes are mainly confined to the central white matter of the hemispheres, the corpus callosum and the long tracts in the brain stem. The distribution of lesions is often asymmetrical. A striking aspect is that severely affected tracts of fibres may be seen near normal areas, with a sharp boundary between the two, suggesting selective sparing or involvement by virtue of fibre tract direction. Such pathology can exist with only moderate cerebral atrophy, and only limited dilatation of the ventricles. Studies by Adams *et al.* (1977) have emphasised that diffuse white matter damage of this nature can occur from the moment of injury, and is probably the most important single factor governing outcome in closed head injuries. In patients remaining in a 'persistent vegetative state' until death (p. 183) this was the typical finding, rather than any special accent of pathology on the brain stem.

Experimental models of injury have allowed careful study to be made of the changes following minor blows to the head (Povlishock & Coburn 1989). Electron microscopy reveals highly focal areas of axonal damage, without contusions or glial reactivity in the neighbourhood. Damaged axons can be seen lying adjacent to intact fibres, and rather than being torn they appear to have been subjected to stretching and compression. The resulting impairment of axoplasmic transport sets in train changes which continue over several hours—axonal swelling, lobulation, segmentation, and ultimately separation of the distal segment from that still attached to the cell body. The latter forms the classic 'retraction ball'. Over the ensuing weeks and months attempts at regrowth and regeneration can be observed, with sprouting from the proximal segment.

Vascular lesions include scattered punctate haemorrhages throughout the brain, along with large and small infarcts. Sometimes the whole or part of the territory of a major cerebral artery may become necrotic. Such vascular lesions probably result from a combination of factors—reduced cerebral blood flow immediately after the injury, hypotension, embolism, pre-existing atheroma, rise of intracranial pressure sufficient to occlude the arteries, and spasm of vessels due to mechanical strain at the junction of brain and vessel (Strich 1969; Graham & Adams 1971).

Extensive bleeding may occur into the subarachnoid space, with the appearance of blood in the cerebrospinal fluid. Subdural haematomas may collect and become organised over the cerebral hemispheres. Blood collecting in the basal cisterns or over the surface of the brain may later lead to organised adhesions which obstruct the flow of cerebrospinal fluid and lead to hydrocephalus. Bleeding into the brain tissue itself may result in an intracerebral haematoma.

Cerebral oedema may develop in the acute stages and further complicate the picture. It is especially liable to occur in the region of contusions, lacerations, infarcts and haematomas. The raised intracranial pressure which results can have serious consequences in terms of herniation of brain tissue through the tentorium and under the falx cerebri. If severe, such 'coning' may be fatal. Less severe cases can be followed by focal necrosis and haemorrhage in the medial temporal lobe structures and brain stem.

Cerebral anoxia accounts for other pathological findings, such as cortical necrosis in the depths of the cortical sulci, lesions in Ammon's horn and the basal ganglia, and the disappearance of Purkinje cells from the cerebellum. Cases studied early after injury show widespread chromatolysis in neurones both in the brain stem and throughout the cortex. The anoxia will derive not only from cerebral oedema and other local changes, but also from hypotension, blood loss, disturbances of regulation of the cerebral circulation, and ventilatory insufficiency in the acute stages. The importance of early metabolic and neurochemical derangements in leading to brain damage is also increasingly recognised (see below).

Resolution of such acute changes will be followed by variable gliosis and cerebral atrophy, often with considerable distortion of brain tissue, cyst formation, enlargement of the ventricles or the development of ventricular diverticula. Where prolonged coma has followed injury a special emphasis of pathology may be expected in the central part of the upper brain stem, chiefly as a result of the mechanical and vascular sequelae of raised intracranial pressure (Jellinger & Seitelberger 1969).

In *open head injuries* the skull and dural coverings are perforated. Laceration of brain tissue is present at the site of impact but contrecoup is slight or even absent. This is probably explained by the limited and direct effect of the trauma which expends its energy locally, together with the resilience of fractured bones which act as a buffer to prevent the propagation of the force (Löken 1959). Extensive local laceration may lead to large cystic cavities and ventricular dilatations. Haemorrhage may occur locally, and infection is an ever-present risk. Small fractures in the neighbourhood of the nasal sinuses may pave the way for meningitis or local abscess formation.

Any inflammatory process provokes a connective tissue reaction from the vascular adventitia, and results in a fibroglial scar in which infection may linger. This tends to be adherent to the dura, and ultimately retracts with distortion and traction on the brain. Such a lesion brings special hazards for the later development of epilepsy.

Biochemical and physiological changes

In addition to the structural changes following head injury, alterations occur in biochemical, circulatory and electrical aspects of brain function. These too will play a part in determining the clinical picture, and after mild trauma may be unaccompanied by structural pathology. Recent evidence has focused increasingly on the damaging effects of ionic changes within the cells, and on alterations in central neurotransmitters. Possibilities of 'excitotoxic' brain damage from glutamate release have commanded especial attention, by analogy with the substantial body of evidence which incriminates glutamate in hypoxic and hypoglycaemic brain damage.

Marshall (1990) reviews the changes occurring within cells during the first few hours after trauma. Much of the damage appears to depend on sudden calcium entry into the cell consequent upon altered permeability of the cell membrane. Once inside the cell, calcium activates a variety of proteases which destroy cell constituents, also phospholipases which increase the formation of free radicals. Chains of harmful chemical processes are thereby set in motion. A fall in intracellular magnesium also appears to be important and has been shown

to correlate with outcome in experimental models of injury.

Among neurotransmitters, acetylcholine was the first to be clearly implicated. Free acetylcholine appears in the cerebrospinal fluid after injury and may persist for days or even weeks. The amount roughly parallels the degree of unconsciousness and the severity of EEG changes, and the level gradually falls with clinical improvement. The acetylcholine is probably released from neural membranes as a direct result of the trauma or the massive neuronal discharge at the time of impact. It has been suggested that this may constitute a biochemical basis for concussion by the blocking of neural transmission in the reticular formation (Ward 1966). Alternatively, Hayes *et al.* (1989) suggest that the phenomena of concussion may result from transient activation of an inhibitory cholinergic system in the rostral pons. Thus the turnover of acetylcholine in the pons is increased after experimental concussion, and pretreatment with scopolamine can attenuate the length of coma. Some of the longer-term sequelae may also be attributable to excessive release of acetylcholine, resulting in abnormal agonist–receptor interactions which contribute to persisting changes in cell function.

The concept of damaging 'excitotoxicity' has recently been greatly expanded in relation to the glutamate/aspartate system (Choi & Rothman 1990; Meldrum & Garthwaite 1990; Sauer *et al.* 1992). These excitatory amino acids were shown in experimental animals to be capable of inducing postsynaptic changes in neurones and dendrites, including cell death, of a nature identical to that following cerebral ischaemia or status epilepticus. Moreover, microdialysis experiments have demonstrated that cerebral ischaemia is accompanied by a large increase in extracellular glutamate and aspartate; and antagonists, principally those which block N-methyl-D-aspartate (NMDA) glutamate receptors, have been shown to ameliorate the effects of ischaemic brain damage and to reduce calcium entry into the cell.

More directly in relation to traumatic injury, Faden *et al.* (1989) have demonstrated a marked rise in extracellular glutamate and aspartate adjacent to the site of trauma in experimentally injured animals, the degree of elevation being related to the severity of the injury. Treatment with the NMDA antagonist dextrorphan, even 30 minutes after the trauma, was shown to limit the extent of neurological dysfunction, indicating that excitatory amino acids contribute to delayed as well as to immediate tissue damage after head injury.

The mechanisms underlying such secondary effects are complex and as yet incompletely understood. The acute release of extracellular glutamate and aspartate clearly sets in motion a cascade of self-propagating biochemical changes within the cells—ionic imbalances, with increase in calcium and sodium and a fall in free magnesium, the accumulation of lactic acid, changes in lipid metabolism with accumulation of free fatty acids, protein degradation, reduction in high energy phosphates, activation of nitric oxide synthetase, and the production of highly reactive free radicals. Precisely which of these components are chiefly responsible for cellular injury remains to be determined.

Endogenous opioids may also be involved in some components of brain damage following trauma, exerting a protective effect (Hayes *et al.* 1990). Beta-endorphins are increased in the cerebrospinal fluid in patients after head injury, and pretreatment of animals with an opioid antagonist (naloxone) has been shown to exacerbate the deficits associated with injury.

The importance of these discoveries lies in the promise they offer for the development of 'neuroprotective agents', in relation to both stroke and head trauma. In particular a 'window of opportunity' would appear to exist, during which appropriate interventions might ameliorate the cascade of changes leading to irreversible brain damage. Strategies under appraisal include the use of NMDA antagonists such as MK 801, calcium channel blockers, opiate antagonists and free radical scavengers. Mahadik (1992) reviews the use of exogenous gangliosides, which act to maintain and restore plasma membrane structure and function. Hall (1992a, 1992b) describes the development of novel compounds (21-amino steroids, 'lazaroids') which aim to replicate the effects of synthetic glucocorticoids, such as methylprednisolone, in inhibiting the lipid peroxidation in cell membranes induced by free radicals.

Cerebral circulatory changes are also important in the development of delayed or 'secondary' brain changes. Overgaard and Tweed (1974) demonstrated wide variability in resting cerebral blood flow after severe head injuries. Commonly, normal or low flow rates in the first 24 hours were succeeded by relative hyperaemia ('luxury perfusion') which persisted into the second or third week and then subsided. Either ischaemia or hyperaemia in the acute stage appeared to be related to a poor clinical outcome. Distinct regional changes in cerebral blood flow, either ischaemic or hyperaemic in type, were also observed, chiefly in relation to focal lesions such as haematomas or lacerations.

Electroencephalogram after head injury

Bickford and Klass (1966) review the EEG alterations seen after head injury. One of the most sensitive changes is local suppression of alpha rhythm in the region of a localised blow or in the contrecoup area. This can occur with trivial injuries and can be helpful in indicating

unsuspected damage, especially in a region which is clinically 'silent'. With greater severity the suppression may extend bilaterally and occasional slow waves appear. With severe injury delta waves at 1–3 Hz appear and may persist for several weeks or months. During recovery there is a gradual trend towards increase of frequency and normality over the weeks and months that follow. The development and persistence of spike discharges indicate that gliosis has occurred.

The EEG can be helpful in the differential diagnosis of the unconscious patient, chiefly by pointing to causes other than head injury which might be overlooked. Fast activity may suggest drug overdosage, marked localised delta activity will point to a primary intracerebral lesion, and spike and wave bursts will indicate an epileptic process. The EEG can also draw attention to complications following head injury. With a subdural haematoma there may be increasing slow activity over one hemisphere, or the development of unilateral alpha wave suppression. A delta focus of increasing magnitude after open head injury suggests the development of a cerebral abscess.

With regard to prognosis, less can be said with certainty. The degree of overall EEG abnormality is not a firm guide, and must always be taken in conjunction with other clinical data. Serial recordings may, however, be helpful, especially in revealing the organic component in cases thought to be due entirely to psychogenic factors. The EEG is unreliable as a guide to the later development of epilepsy, some 50% of patients who develop post-traumatic epilepsy having normal or only minimally abnormal EEGs initially. Jennett (1975) found no consistent correlation between EEG abnormalities during the first year after injury and the development of late epilepsy. However, the appearance of focal discharges which spread and intensify can be taken as a strong indication that pathology is developing which will ultimately lead to seizures.

Neuroimaging and head injury

Computerised tomography (CT) scanning has proved to be invaluable in displaying the neuropathological effects of head injury and in serving as a guide to surgical intervention. Acute mass effects are revealed by shift of the midline structures or compression of the midbrain cisterns, also areas of contusion and oedema. Coup and contrecoup lesions may be demonstrated. Extradural, subdural and intracerebral haematomas are shown. In the later stages ventricular enlargement may become apparent, along with focal or generalised atrophy. With severe injuries only some 5% will yield scans that can be considered normal in all respects (Eisenberg & Levin 1989).

MRI is more sensitive at revealing brain pathology, but is less suited to the investigation of patients in the acute stages, especially when on life support equipment. Moreover the superiority of MRI does not lie in matters likely to influence acute surgical management. Nonetheless, the yield from MRI greatly exceeds that from CT scanning. Small areas of haemorrhage and oedema are shown that would be missed by CT, likewise very small subdural haematomas. Jenkins *et al.* (1986) were able to visualise cortical contusions even when there had been no loss of consciousness, and deep white matter lesions could occasionally be seen after losses as brief as 5 minutes. In the chronic stages MRI is superior to CT in the detection of white matter changes consequent upon diffuse axonal injury (Kelly *et al.* 1988).

Certain clinicopathological correlations have emerged from this improved visualisation of lesions. Severity of injury, as judged by degree and duration of consciousness, is related both to the number and the location of MRI lesions (Jenkins *et al.* 1986). Their depth from the cortical surface was found to increase with severity, reinforcing the view that the brain is injured concentrically inwards from the surface in closed head injury. Only one of 50 patients showed a brain stem lesion, compared with 46 showing hemisphere damage, suggesting that white matter hemisphere lesions may be the primary event in traumatic loss of consciousness, the brain stem arousal mechanisms then being suppressed secondarily.

Levin *et al.* (1987a) noted the frequency of MRI lesions in the frontal and temporal regions, both being areas which are often neurologically silent. Deficits on neuropsychological testing in the acute stage were related to size and location of such abnormalities, for example perseveration with frontal involvement, and memory difficulties with temporal lesions. At follow-up, MRI scans in individual patients could be informative, for example in a patient whose left frontal haematoma and diminished verbal fluency were observed to resolve together.

Wilson *et al.* (1988) examined the relationship between MRI lesions and outcome. Patients were scanned in the acute stages and then at follow-up 5–18 months later. Measures of neuropsychological outcome showed a strong correlation with the abnormalities that persisted, especially those in the deeper brain regions. Ventricular enlargement on follow-up correlated strongly with residual neuropsychological disability.

Single photon emission computerised tomography (SPECT) scanning has been shown to complement the information obtained with CT or MRI, and indeed to reveal additional areas of cerebral damage which correlate with clinical signs (Newton *et al.* 1992). Nineteen patients undergoing rehabilitation between 3 months and 3 years after injury were subjected to all three investigations. A total of 43 perfusion deficits were shown by SPECT, compared with 21 focal lesions on MRI and 13 on CT. Of these 43 lesions, 31 were not apparent on either CT or MRI. The highest number of SPECT lesions, presumed to reflect areas of contusion or ischaemia, were seen in the most disabled patients, and their frequency correlated significantly with the Glasgow Outcome Score. Measures of global cerebral blood flow also correlated with the functional status of the patient.

An important aspect of the study was that lesions shown by SPECT, but not apparent on CT or MRI, sometimes revealed important clinical correlations. One patient, for example, was left with reading difficulties 5 months after injury, and SPECT showed a perfusion defect in the left posterior parietal region. No such lesion was apparent on CT or MRI. Another severely injured patient showed defects in the right parietal region, unique to SPECT, which correlated with a left hemi-neglect syndrome.

Postitron emission tomography (PET) scanning may also provide additional information. Langfitt *et al.* (1986) showed that all lesions demonstrated by CT or MRI, other than tiny haemorrhages, were accompanied by FDG-PET changes in the corresponding regions. The areas of hypometabolism often extended beyond the structural abnormalities and new regions could be revealed. Anterior temporal lobe dysfunction was particularly common.

A student was unconscious for 20 minutes after a fall, and MRI examination showed right frontal and temporal lobe contusions. CT showed the right frontal contusion only. PET scanning 17 days later, when he was alert but slowed, demonstrated impaired glucose metabolism in the frontal poles and orbital cortex of *both* hemispheres and in both anterior temporal lobe regions. Six months later the right frontal and temporal damage was still evident on structural scans; metabolism had improved in both frontal lobes but the right was still impaired. The left but not the right temporal abnormality had recovered. At this stage he still complained of difficulty with concentration, and though performing well on IQ tests he was inattentive and slowed in conversation.

Ruff *et al.* (1989) attempted to show the value of PET scanning when neuropsychological deficits persisted in the presence of normal CT and MRI scans. Six such patients were scanned 3–5 years after injury, and anterior frontal hypometabolism was shown in five. It will be important to determine how much reliance can be placed on such findings, especially in view of their medicolegal implications. Some of Ruff *et al.*'s patients had had minimal injuries and the significance of the hypometabolism in such cases should perhaps be viewed with caution.

Acute effects of head injury

The most constant of the acute effects of head injury is impairment of consciousness, ranging from momentary dazing to prolonged coma. This is usually succeeded during recovery by a variable period of confusion, and the whole episode proves later to be surrounded by characteristic amnesic defects. These three features form the cardinal symptoms of the early effects of head injury. They provide important information about the severity of brain damage that is likely to have occurred, and must therefore be taken carefully into account when assessing prognosis. In addition, of course, there may be added effects due to damage to specific parts of the brain, and as a result of the various complications outlined above.

Impairment of consciousness

A good deal of debate has surrounded the definition of 'concussion'. That given by Caveness and Walker (1966) is reproduced here: '. . . a clinical syndrome characterised by immediate and transient impairment of neural function, such as alteration of consciousness, disturbances of vision, equilibrium, etcetera, due to mechanical forces'.

Impairment of consciousness, however transient, follows all but the mildest blow in closed head injuries, and especially when the head is free to move at impact. After penetrating head injuries it is considerably less common, also in static crushing injuries as already discussed. In occasional cases there may be no detectable impairment of consciousness, but merely transient dizziness or blurring of vision; or there may be no outward sign of impairment of consciousness to onlookers, yet the patient has no recollection of the injury, showing that registration was failing to occur at the time.

In the typical case loss of consciousness is complete. The patient falls to the ground, displays no response to stimuli, and for a moment shows arrest of respiration, profound fall of blood pressure, pallor, dilated pupils, loss of corneal reflexes and paralysis of deglutition. Mass contraction of the limbs may be followed by flaccid paralysis and loss of tendon reflexes. With recovery shallow sighing respiration is resumed and the circulatory state gradually returns to normal. Consciousness returns after a variable interval depending on the severity of injury. Usually this is followed by a period of confusion, drowsiness and headache, and sometimes by vomiting and dizziness. The duration of complete unconsciousness is often overestimated by the patient, because of the confusion which follows and the post-traumatic amnesia which may greatly outlast the resumption of outwardly normal behaviour. Conversely, the patient may sometimes underestimate the period of unconsciousness or in rare cases deny any knowledge of it.

Periods of unconsciousness lasting several hours are compatible with uneventful and complete recovery. The longer its duration, however, and the deeper the level of coma, the more probable it is that permanent brain damage will have been sustained. It is no longer fashionable on clinical grounds to attempt to distinguish between simple concussion, contusion and laceration of the brain, but prolonged unconsciousness is more likely to be accompanied by evidence of brain damage on neurological examination, by evidence of raised intracranial pressure and by the presence of blood in the cerebrospinal fluid. It is also more likely to be followed by a considerable period of post-traumatic confusion and by both physical and mental long-term sequelae.

In severe cases unconsciousness may persist for weeks or even months, and here permanent after-effects are to be expected. Lewin (1959) assessed the quality of recovery in 102 patients who had remained unconscious for over a month. Thirty-nine died, 15 were left very severely disabled, 29 made partial recoveries and 19 were ultimately well enough to return to their former work. If a good recovery was to be made then some improvement was usually seen within the first month after injury— not necessarily return of consciousness but certainly increased responsiveness to pain or diminution of spasticity. Thomsen (1984) followed 40 survivors with post-traumatic amnesias exceeding a month; 10–15 years later impairments were still severe in many cases, especially incoordination, dysarthria and memory problems, and two-thirds showed change of personality.

The Glasgow Coma Scale (Teasdale & Jennett 1974) is now in routine use in many countries in units caring for acutely head-injured patients. It has proved to be of considerable predictive value in pointing to long-term outcome, in terms of both survival and ultimate levels of disability (Jennett et al. 1975, 1977). The patient's clinical state is charted regularly on a number of graded parameters: motor responsiveness (no response, extensor response to pain, flexor response, localising response, obeying commands), verbal performance (nil, without recognisable words, no sustained exchange possible, confused conversation, orientated for person, place and time) and eye opening (nil, in response to pain, in response to speech, spontaneously). Numerical scores are summated for the best responses obtained under each category at a defined point in time. In this way useful predictions can be made, often within 24 hours of injury and more certainly within the first week.

The prolonged post-traumatic coma may be profound from the outset, or may deepen rapidly in the early stages due to intracerebral or subarachnoid bleeding. Decerebrate rigidity is common, with tonic fits, stertorous breathing, tachycardia and hyperpyrexia. Anoxia is a special hazard, resulting from obstruction of the airways or damage to the respiratory and vasomotor centres in the brain stem. Ominous signs of brain stem compression include muscular flaccidity, failing respiration, falling blood pressure and fixed dilated pupils. Skilled nursing and watchful medical supervision are therefore essential, with readiness to operate for extradural, subdural and intracerebral haematomas. Artificial aids to sustain respiration may be required for considerable periods of time, and electrolyte imbalance or anaemia due to blood loss may need correction.

Acute post-traumatic psychosis (post-traumatic acute organic reaction, post-traumatic confusional state)

As unconsciousness recedes the patient passes through a phase of disorientation and impaired cognitive ability before the ultimate level of recovery is attained. This stage shows much variation, depending on the severity of the injury and its complications, and coloured also by aspects of the patient's personality and present surroundings. The term 'acute post-traumatic psychosis' thus covers a wide range of different clinical pictures.

After momentary concussion a return to normal may be expected within a few minutes. After unconsciousness lasting several hours the ensuing disturbance may last for some days or weeks. In the most severe injuries, where permanent disablement is to follow, the phase of acute confusion may last for many months and ultimately shade into the picture of post-traumatic dementia. Thus there exists a fairly close relationship between severity of injury and the duration of disorientation, which may be used in the early stages as an approximate guide to prognosis (Moore & Ruesch 1944). Exceptions are seen, however, since the severity of the acute traumatic psychosis also often depends on complicating factors such as anoxia, electrolyte disturbance, systemic infection or severe blood loss which need not lead to enduring brain damage. The disturbance is usually more prolonged and severe in the elderly, the arteriosclerotic and the alcoholic.

The form which the disturbance takes is also variable, ranging from apathetic withdrawal, through restless irritability, to pictures of florid 'post-traumatic delirium'. The determinants of the clinical picture will include not only the nature of the brain damage and complicating factors, but also the pretraumatic personality of the patient. Some may react by marked depression, others by boisterous

noisy disturbance. Hysterical or paranoid traits may be released, and sometimes a schizophrenic colouring is evident.

In many cases outward behaviour is little disturbed beyond obvious lethargy and failure of cognitive function. Perplexity is common, and there may be initial restlessness and irritability. Thereafter progress usually follows a torpid apathetic course until consciousness is fully regained. On the other hand, some patients pass through an excitable and overactive phase with florid disturbance of behaviour which can be long continued and pose serious problems of management. Sometimes this is attributable to the abnormal experiences and delusional misinterpretations of a post-traumatic delirium, but sometimes it proves to foreshadow enduring changes of temperament and behaviour occasioned by the injury. The patient may be abusive, aggressive and markedly uncooperative. Very occasionally crimes of violence are committed at the height of such disturbance, and afterwards the patient has no knowledge of their occurrence.

In this stage there is always some degree of residual impairment of consciousness and failure to retain new information. Accordingly, the period of acute traumatic psychosis comes to be incorporated within the post-traumatic amnesic gap. Impairment of consciousness is usually clinically obvious, though occasionally the patient may seem to be fully alert and capable of a high degree of motivated behaviour. The subsequent amnesic gap is then important evidence that the brain was still in an abnormal state at the time.

Disorientation for time and place, and sometimes even for personal identity, is marked at first. Later during recovery a bizarre state of double orientation may be maintained, as described on p. 11. Confabulation is sometimes much in evidence. Cognitive dysfunction is also shown in difficulty with simple mental tests and obvious inability to concentrate or sustain mental effort.

Misinterpretation of surroundings and misidentification of people are common. Sometimes these are described only upon recovery. There may be suspicious disbelief of the role and purpose of those around, such that nurses and other patients are thought to be spies or gaolers. More openly expressed delusions often originate in sensory falsifications and poverty of grasp. They are usually highly charged with emotion, changeable and unsystematised, and paranoid in content.

Very occasionally the circumstances of the injury are recalled in a confused and muddled manner, and become woven into a delusional system. This can have important medicolegal repercussions. Russell (1935) reported a patient who had a motorcycle accident and subsequently ascribed his injuries to an attack by the dog which had caused it. He later elaborated this by maintaining that the dog's owner had attacked him directly. In this case the delusions were short lived and cleared as the post-traumatic confusion receded. A similar case was cited in which a doctor took home a boy who had fallen off his bicycle and was later accused by the boy of having run him down.

Weston and Whitlock (1971) describe another example in which delusions apparently stemmed from a vivid hallucinatory experience occurring as part of the early post-traumatic delirium. The patient related an episode in which he believed he saw his parents being shot by Chinese communists. Thereafter when his family visited him he believed them to be impostors who had assumed their exact appearance in order to trick him (Capgras' syndrome, p. 15). The profound memory disturbance from which the patient was suffering at the time had prevented him from realising that the head injury had occurred, or from reintegrating his vivid fantasy into normal daily experience.

With resolution of the acute post-traumatic psychosis the patient may recover completely or be left with defects of intellect or change of temperament. These may yet improve slowly over time or remain as permanent sequelae.

Amnesic defects surrounding injury

On recovery of consciousness, and whether or not an acute post-traumatic psychosis has followed, events often fail to be recorded in memory for a time. The injury is therefore followed by a post-traumatic amnesic gap. In addition, events immediately preceding the injury are sometimes no longer available for recall so that a retrograde amnesic gap exists as well. The correct evaluation of these amnesic phenomena is of considerable clinical importance, particularly in relation to prognosis.

Post-traumatic amnesia

The length of the post-traumatic amnesia (PTA) may be defined as *the time from the moment of injury to the time of resumption of normal continuous memory*. It therefore ends at the time from which the patient can later give a clear and consecutive account of what was happening around him. It includes any period of unconsciousness or overt confusion, and often, in addition, a further period thereafter during which outward behaviour has appeared to return to normal.

Characteristically the termination is abrupt, except in those very severe injuries where enduring memory difficulties are to supervene. The amnesic phase may have lasted from several minutes to several weeks, yet finally ends sharply with the return of normal continuous

memory. It is for this reason that the majority of patients can retrospectively give a firm end-point to their PTA, usually though not invariably with some highlighted experience of a pleasurable, painful or surprising nature. In some cases brief islands of memory at first emerge, vaguely recalled and jumbled in temporal sequence, before the continuity of memory is restored, but this is exceptional.

Detailed studies of patients during the course of the PTA have only rarely been undertaken, but Levin and co-workers have made a number of interesting observations. Tests of remote memory for autobiographical information, carried out by administering a structured interview of life events to patients during their PTA, have revealed a marked temporal gradient (Levin et al. 1985). Events from primary school days were, for example, better remembered than events from young adult life. The same technique applied to patients after resolution of the PTA showed no such gradient, but demonstrated equivalent levels of recall for all life periods.

A study of orientation during PTA showed that the usual sequence of recovery was for person, then place, then time (Levin 1989). The date was characteristically displaced backwards, for up to 5 years in severe injuries, then the discrepancy diminished as orientation improved. Such changes mirror, in effect, the receding retrograde gap.

In a study of rates of forgetting using the Huppert–Piercy technique (p. 38), patients tested during PTA required longer periods of exposure of the material for adequate initial acquisition; and thereafter they showed accelerated forgetting over 32 hours compared to normal controls or to patients recovered from PTA (Levin et al. 1988).

Ewert et al. (1989) made an interesting comparison between procedural and declarative (episodic) memory during the course of the PTA. A group of patients were tested on three consecutive days during their PTAs, then again when the PTA had terminated. On procedural tasks (mirror reading, maze learning and a pursuit–rotor task) performance improved across sessions, and showed transfer with further gains when tested after resolution of the PTA. By contrast, tests of declarative memory (tests of recognition of the words used in mirror reading, and a questionnaire concerning details of the previous session) showed stable impairments throughout. Thus it is clear that patients can acquire and retain new *skills* during the PTA, while remaining disorientated and amnesic for on-going events.

Behaviour during the PTA gap may vary from apparent normality to obvious difficulty with memory and mental confusion. Some degree of temporal disorientation is almost always in evidence if opportunities arise to test for it with care. The general tenor of behaviour may, however, be surprisingly intact so that observers are easily misled into thinking that full recovery has occurred. Even questions designed to test short-term memory may sometimes be answered adequately, since memory functions may have recovered sufficiently for this but not yet enough to lay down a permanent record. It is thus only in retrospect that the true duration of the post-traumatic gap can be determined with certainty. Commonly, the patient appears to be unaware himself of the abnormality of memory functions at the time, and gives superficial explanations or confabulations for the deficits which are discovered.

False memories, which at first sight are convincing enough, have sometimes been found to centre on a previous injury:

A dispatch rider was concussed in a motorcycle accident. Following a period of complete unconsciousness he was confused and drowsy for 2–3 days, and after treatment at a local hospital was transferred to a special head injury unit 10 days later. When seen at that time he gave details of the accident, including its locale and the incident leading up to it, and recounted his journey from the first hospital. He gave his name and army number correctly, but persistently underestimated his age by 2 years. At clinical examination he appeared to be rational and fully orientated. It finally transpired, however, that he was giving details of an accident he had had before joining the army some 2 years previously, and that the description of his journey to the second hospital was also a false reminiscence. His final PTA was assessed as 12 days. It involved the period of false reminiscence and the first 2 days of his stay in the second hospital.

(Whitty & Zangwill 1966)

In the majority of cases, as already indicated, the purely amnesic phase follows upon the clearing of overt signs of confusion and impairment of consciousness, but occasionally it follows immediately upon the injury and is the sole defect. The classic example is that of the schoolboy struck during a game of football but not rendered unconscious. He may then continue to play, but later proves to have no recollection of the part of the game which immediately followed the injury (post-traumatic automatism). Similar examples are sometimes seen in boxers. Usually performance is noted to be substandard during the continuation of activity.

Occasionally, but rarely, the amnesic period is delayed by a few moments after the blow. Some brief isolated experiences are recalled immediately after the injury, usually in an inaccurate and confused way, and thereafter the dense amnesic period begins.

A boy of 18 skidded in a car and hit a telegraph pole, sustaining a fractured skull and broken leg. He clearly recalled switching off the engine and forcing open the jammed car door, both of which were subsequently corroborated. Thereafter he could recall nothing until he came round in hospital some 48 hours later.

(Whitty & Zangwill 1966)

A more delayed onset to the amnesic phase may of course be seen when complications such as extradural haemorrhage lead to a second period of unconsciousness after full recovery has been attained; here events may be recalled from the lucid interval preceding the haemorrhage, and this may be of several hours' duration.

Retrograde amnesia

The duration of the retrograde amnesia (RA) is measured as *the time between the moment of injury and the last clear memory from before the injury which the patient can recall*. The patient can often indicate with fair precision the last event which he can clearly recollect. In road accidents the journey is typically recalled up to a certain point, and this allows an estimate to be made of the extent of the retrograde gap.

The RA is usually dense, including events of high emotional significance and, of course, involving details of the accident itself. Usually the RA is much shorter than the PTA, though in rare exceptions the reverse is seen. Indeed the great majority of RAs are surprisingly uniform in extent, occupying only a few seconds or up to 1 minute in time, which may be regarded as the period required for the processes of consolidation of the original perceptions. Longer retrograde gaps are generally seen only with more severe injuries, and these may be of many days' or weeks' duration. Conversely, examples of mild injury are seen in which no RA occurs whatever, and full details of the injury can be recalled up to the moment of loss of consciousness.

The organic basis for the very long RA has come under suspicion, and certainly those which follow mild head injury have often proved to be psychogenic in origin. Here the emotional shock of the accident is principally to be blamed. Nevertheless, long RAs may be seen with other forms of organic brain damage, and experienced observers have agreed that after severe head injury a long RA may sometimes be directly attributable to organic factors. Symonds (1962a), for example, reported a permanent RA of 1 year for which there was no indication that other than organic factors were at work. Russell and Nathan (1946) investigated the effect of thiopentone narcosis on the duration of amnesias, and found a reduction in only 12 of 40 cases investigated. The reductions were mostly trivial in amount, and did not include material likely to have been repressed by psychological mechanisms. Moreover the recovered material always bordered the fringes of the amnesic gap, suggesting again that it was substantially organic in origin.

With long RAs it is usual to find that the amnesia is most dense for events shortly preceding the injury, with only patchy loss for the more remote periods. Dislocation from correct temporal sequence is also characteristic for events recalled from within the retrograde gap.

The RA as determined shortly after injury may prove to

be misleading. At first it may be very long, then shrink in the days or weeks that follow as normal orientation is regained. The final estimate should therefore not be made until the patient has emerged from the period of the PTA and the fullest possible recovery of cerebral function has occurred. The shrinkage of the RA is itself a phenomenon of some interest, as described on pp. 30 and 36.

Amnesia in relation to severity of injury

The importance of the duration of amnesia as a guide to the severity of injury and prognosis for recovery was first clearly shown by Russell (1932). This has now become a well-attested part of clinical practice, hence the importance of striving to record in every case the precise details of the retrograde and post-traumatic gaps.

The PTA has proved to be more valid and useful than the RA in this regard. In general the RA tends to increase in length with the PTA (Russell & Nathan 1946), but since the great majority of RAs are extremely brief they are less valuable as a guide to severity. The PTA shows all gradations of length and is highly variable from case to case, thus allowing it to be used as an index of severity. It also emerges as more valid for this purpose than the duration of unconsciousness or overt confusion, probably because the latter depend more closely on secondary complications. The PTA is, moreover, a permanent index of severity, and available to the clinician who enquires long after the injury.

Viewed first in the most general terms, the duration of the PTA in closed head injuries is related to the time which is likely to elapse before the patient returns to work (Symonds & Russell 1943; Steadman & Graham 1970). Within broad limits it may be predicted that a patient with a PTA of less than an hour will usually return to work within a month, with a PTA of less than a day within 2 months, and with a PTA of less than a week within 4 months. PTAs exceeding 1 week will often be followed by invalidism extending over the greater part of a year.

More specifically, the duration of PTA shows close correlations with objective evidence of damage to brain tissue, as reflected in neurological residua such as motor disorder, dysphasia or anosmia, or enduring defects of memory and calculation (Russell & Smith 1961; Smith 1961). Psychiatric disablement likewise shows an important relationship to the duration of PTA, particularly where organic mental disabilities such as intellectual impairment, euphoria, disinhibition or aspects of the 'frontal lobe syndrome' are concerned (Lishman 1968). In Steadman and Graham's (1970) series the mean duration of PTA was significantly increased in patients who showed post-traumatic change of personality.

An important, though not over-riding qualification to the above, concerns the situation in open as opposed to closed head injuries. In penetrating injuries, particularly those due to high velocity missiles, there is a tendency for the PTA to be very short or even absent in up to 50% of cases (Russell 1951). Similarly, in crushing injuries, where the brain is not subject to the forces of acceleration, loss of consciousness is relatively rare (Russell & Schiller 1949). Nevertheless, Table 7 shows that even among penetrating head injuries a close relationship exists between the length of PTA and the amount of psychiatric disability or intellectual impairment as assessed in general terms 1–5 years later.

Chronic sequelae of head injury

With recovery from the acute stages, a mild head injury is quite compatible with return to full efficiency, both physically and mentally. This important fact is not always appreciated by the patient and his relatives for whom the very term 'concussion' can have ominous overtones. Nevertheless, head injury does account for a great deal of chronic disability. Common physical defects include cranial nerve lesions such as anosmia, oculomotor pareses, visual field defects and motor disorders resulting from cortical or brain stem lesions. Peripheral sensory

Table 7 Duration of post-traumatic amnesia in relation to psychiatric disability and generalised intellectual impairment (after Lishman 1968). (Figures in italics represent percentages calculated on the equivalent totals shown at the bottom of each column.)

Length of post-traumatic amnesia	Psychiatric disability			Intellectual impairment		
	Nil	Mild	Severe	Nil	Mild	Severe
<1 hour	62 *67*	226 *52*	41 *28*	116 *65*	208 *45*	5 *16*
<7 days	17 *18*	83 *19*	31 *22*	32 *18*	95 *21*	4 *12*
>7 days	14 *15*	124 *29*	72 *50*	31 *17*	156 *34*	23 *72*
Total cases	93	433	144	179	459	32

defects are seen less frequently. In penetrating injuries, or after complications due to intracranial bleeding, such focal neurological defects will be more common. They are fully described in textbooks of neurology and neurosurgery and will not be dealt with further here.

Only the mental sequelae will be considered in detail. These are extremely important in clinical practice, and furthermore provide valuable material for academic study —both in demonstrating the complex interplay of many factors in the genesis of psychiatric disorder and in increasing our understanding of the cerebral basis of behaviour.

The clinical importance of the mental aftermaths cannot be overstressed. Observers are uniformly agreed that problems such as cognitive incapacity or change of personality far outstrip the physical sequelae as obstacles in rehabilitation and as a source of long-term disability (Bond 1976; Field 1976; Jennett *et al.* 1981). Decline in employment is more likely to be associated with mental than physical factors (Roberts 1976; Brooks *et al.* 1987c), likewise the strain imposed on families and those responsible for care (Thomsen 1974; McKinlay *et al.* 1981; Florian *et al.* 1989).

The range of mental sequelae is very great and embraces most that can be found in psychiatric symptomatology. It is therefore most unlikely that all will share a common aetiology, even though all will appear to have originated from a common event, namely the blow to the head. At one extreme there are enduring defects of cognitive function which can confidently be ascribed to the brain damage sustained. At the other extreme there are certain groups of symptoms—phobias, anxiety states and depression—which sometimes follow the most trivial injuries and commonly occur in a setting of environmental and interpersonal difficulties consequent upon the injury. They may also be closely tied to the frightening experiences of the accident itself, especially when threat to life has been involved. These often differ little if at all from the general run of neurotic and affective disturbances, and appear to owe little to the brain damage which may have been sustained. In between there exists a range of phenomena in which the relative contribution of organic and psychogenic factors can be hard to disentangle, such as enduring difficulty with concentration, persistent headache, undue irritability and other subtle changes of temperament. Schizophrenic and affective psychoses may also follow head injury, and have likewise been the subject of controversy where aetiological mechanisms are concerned.

Thus it has steadily become apparent that over and above any obvious brain damage there are a multitude of factors, constitutional and environmental, which can decisively shape the psychiatric picture in the individual. Such a situation is, of course, common in psychiatric illness, and head-injured patients illustrate particularly well the interplay of many contributory factors rebounding each upon the other. Confronted with an individual case the clinician must nevertheless try to decide which are the causal factors presently operating, and the relative weights to be given to each, before he can hope to tackle the problem effectively or make a reasoned estimate at prognosis. It will therefore be useful first to review the range of aetiological factors which may contribute to post-traumatic psychiatric disability before describing the common clinical pictures that result.

Aetiology of psychiatric disability after head injury

The aetiological factors shown in Table 8 have all been demonstrated to operate significantly in contributing to the mental after-effects of head injury. The case in which any one of them operates alone will be rare, and in particular one cannot expect a firm dichotomy between physiogenic and psychogenic causes. Most often the two will be found to be inextricably combined. However, each aetiological factor will first be considered individually since this is the process that clinical enquiry must follow in seeking to clarify the determinants of disability in an individual case.

Some factors, such as the influence of environmental difficulties, have been readily shown to exert a powerful effect; others, including the effects of brain damage itself, have been more difficult to demonstrate, certainly where symptoms other than cognitive deficits are concerned. But it is important to avoid the fallacy of concluding that where aetiological factors are easy to demonstrate they are necessarily most potent in action. In particular it is difficult to demonstrate minor degrees of brain damage during life, and one must therefore be wary of dismissing

Table 8 Aetiological factors contributing to psychiatric disturbance after head injury.

Mental constitution
Premorbid personality
Emotional impact of injury
Circumstances, setting and repercussions of injury
Iatrogenic factors
Environmental factors
Compensation and litigation
Response to intellectual impairments
Development of epilepsy
Amount of brain damage incurred
Location of brain damage incurred

the physiogenic contribution. On the other hand, we must not cling to the possibility that 'subclinical' brain damage is responsible in the face of overwhelming evidence that psychogenesis leads the field.

In the discussion that follows it is equally important to remember that even very large series of head-injured patients are liable to special selection because of the settings in which they are studied and the populations from which they are drawn. Most civilian series consist predominantly of closed head injuries due to road traffic accidents, whereas soldiers wounded in combat suffer mainly from penetrating missile wounds. Series derived from acute sources will differ substantially from patients referred later for treatment in rehabilitation units. Patients seen solely in connection with claims for compensation will be different again. All such factors may strongly bias interpretations concerning causal factors.

Mental constitution

Reliable assessments of premorbid mental constitution are hard to make and it is therefore not surprising that different studies have placed differing emphasis on its importance. Among soldiers invalided after head injury, a family or personal history of mental disorder has been found to increase the likelihood of chronic incapacity (Symonds & Russell 1943). A history of character deviations, mental retardation and psychosis in near relatives has likewise emerged as important in both soldiers and civilians (Adler 1945; Kozol 1945; Hillbom 1960).

Several studies have directly assessed the importance of constitutional factors by comparing head-injured patients with non-head-injured neurotics. Lewis (1942), studying soldiers in an army neurosis centre, found a remarkable degree of similarity in constitutional background between the two, and concluded that the 'long-lasting relatively intractable post-concussional syndrome is apt to occur in much the same person as develops a psychiatric syndrome anyway'. Ruesch and Bowman (1945) showed that head-injured patients with neurotic symptoms but who lacked obvious signs of brain damage resembled non-head-injured neurotics very closely, both in the range and diffuseness of their complaints and in profiles from the Minnesota Multiphasic Personality Inventory. In particular, it appeared that the longer the disability persisted the less likely was it to be the expression of brain damage.

An alternative approach has been to compare head-injured twins with their non-head-injured controls. Dencker (1958, 1960) collected 37 monozygotic pairs and 81 dizygotic pairs in which only one of the twins had been injured. The head-injured twins were inferior to their controls on a variety of tests of intellectual function, though the deficits were usually subtle and unobtrusive in everyday life. No significant differences were found where emotional and other psychiatric symptoms were concerned, nor in rates of admission to mental hospitals in the years that followed injury. The monozygotic pairs were more concordant than the dizygotic where certain post-traumatic symptoms were concerned—headache, dizziness, impaired memory, sensitivity to noise and decreased alcohol tolerance—suggesting that these at least were founded in genetic constitution rather than in any brain damage that had occurred. Several patients were found to have undergone a 'change of personality' since the injury, with increased tension, fatiguability or lessened ability to work, but where monozygotic partners were available for comparison they proved to be closely similar for the traits concerned. Among the dizygotic pairs the 'new' personality traits were often found to have caused divergence from the partner before the head injury occurred.

Dencker's investigation was carried out with scrupulous attention to detail and underlines the misleading impression which can be obtained from a cursory psychiatric history; constitutional factors emerged as crucial in many areas of disability which would otherwise have been readily ascribed to the head injury itself. It is important to note, however, that the patients were examined on average 10 years after injury, by which time many of the more specific consequences had probably become submerged. It seems, therefore, to be long-continued psychiatric disability which relies most heavily on constitutional factors rather than on the specific consequences of brain damage.

Slater's (1943) classic study of 2000 neurotic soldiers also showed the importance of constitutional factors, but here a contribution due to brain damage also emerged. In this investigation acute conditions were under scrutiny. A quantitative relationship was demonstrated between the degree of stress antedating breakdown and the degree of constitutional vulnerability in the soldiers concerned. But it was clearly shown that soldiers who had sustained brain damage scored lower than average on most items of constitutional vulnerability, just as did the soldiers who had undergone maximal military stress before breakdown. Head injury, in effect, appeared to contribute something additional to disturb the overall balance which could be discerned between stress and predisposition in the genesis of neurotic symptoms. A similar conclusion emerged from Guttmann's (1946) investigation of service patients.

The development of psychotic illness after head injury appears to rely heavily on constitutional predisposition, and it is only recently that more specific factors related to brain damage have come under serious suspicion. This is considered in some detail on pp. 191–2.

Age at time of injury. Finally under the heading of constitution it is important to note that many aspects of post-traumatic disability, and especially cognitive impairments, increase with age at the time of injury. This is probably due to the rising incidence of complicating factors such as cerebral vascular disease, the diminishing reserve of neurones, and the general loss of resilience and adaptability among older persons. Mortality also rises sharply. In Kerr *et al.*'s (1971) series of civilian head injuries a steady rise in mortality occurred after the age of 50, this appearing to be due to age-related factors such as medical complications or pre-existing disease. Pentland *et al.* (1986) showed that patients over 65 admitted to the head injury unit in Edinburgh with severe injuries were twice as likely to die (77%) as younger patients with the same severity of injury (39%). The elderly with moderately severe injuries were more than twice as likely to remain severely disabled or in a vegetative state (35% compared to 14%).

In Heiskanen and Sipponen's (1970) group of severe brain injuries less than 30% of the survivors aged 50 or over were able to return to their former work, whereas more than 70% of those under 20 were able to do so. Russell (1932) found that memory difficulties increased regularly with age and were three times as common among patients over 40 as in younger patients. Adler (1945) found that neurotic symptoms, mainly anxieties and fears, were more frequent as age at time of injury advanced, and attributed this to the increased problems of occupational and financial adjustment which had to be faced by older people.

Premorbid personality

Head injury is liable to accentuate special vulnerabilities of personality, and to call upon personality resources during the difficult stages of convalescence. Thus it is not surprising that more psychiatric disability is likely to follow when premorbid traits of instability or inadequacy have been in evidence (Adler 1945). Further than this, however, it has proved difficult to specify what special aspects of personality are important. Classification into personality types such as psychopathic or neurotic does not add much additional information (Kozol 1945, 1946), though studies with the Minnesota Multiphasic Personality Inventory have indicated that high scores on the hysterical, depressive and hypochondriacal scales are associated with the long persistence of neurotic complaints (Walker & Erculei 1969). In general, however, analysis of individual personality traits allows only broad generalisations to be made:

'The patient who was altrocentric rather than egocentric, social minded and endowed with a high sense of responsibility was most likely to escape substantial sequelae, despite the fact that such a person might be heavily endowed with neurotic traits' (Kozol 1946). '. . . people who pity themselves instead of making attempts at more rational and active behaviour in conditions of stress do so also after head injuries and consequently are prone to meet with later difficulties in the course of rehabilitation' (Gruvstad *et al.* 1958). Such generalisations are of course of little help in assessing the individual case.

It is likely that specific personality features will tend to influence the form that post-traumatic disability takes. Patients with neurotic traits have been shown to be especially liable to fatigue, insomnia, headache and dizziness (Kozol 1946). It has also been suggested that disinhibition after frontal lesions tends to involve those aspects of personality where inhibition had previously been marked (Jarvie 1954). Such evidence is, however, impressionistic and hampered by lack of opportunity for objective assessments before the injury occurred. Aspects of personality will, of course, also contribute to the way in which the psychogenic factors, discussed immediately below, come to shape the pattern of disability after head injury.

Emotional impact of injury

The purely emotional shock occasioned by the injury can be an important determinant of the psychiatric disturbances that follow. Early reactions will be particularly coloured in this fashion, but persistent states of chronic anxiety may also be set in train. This has been recognised in the concept of post-traumatic stress disorder (PTSD) as described on p. 194. The circumstances of the accident may recur vividly in dreams, or be re-experienced as 'flashbacks' with realistic intensity. In other individuals the details of the accident become the focus for obsessional ruminations or conversion hysteria. Psychotic disorder may be precipitated in predisposed persons.

Neurotic disabilities appear to be related especially closely to emotional shock, also the so-called post-traumatic syndrome (p. 196). These are found more commonly when emotional reactions have been marked immediately after injury (Brenner *et al.* 1944), or when the injury has occurred in an emotionally loaded setting (Guttmann 1946). A striking finding is that neurotic disabilities have sometimes proved to be most frequent after minor injuries, and sometimes to be particularly common when there has been no PTA to obliterate the memory of the accident and its immediate consequences (Denny-Brown 1945; Miller 1961).

The head holds an especially important place in the body image, and is widely regarded as the seat of the soul or of sanity. The lay attitude to 'concussion' is one of unusual alarm, and unconsciousness and confusion are always deeply impressive symptoms. There may be lurking fears of insanity, or an inner conviction that one can never be quite the same again. Psychoanalysts have stressed the part which barely conscious factors may play, and have described the trauma situation in terms of a threat to the patient's integrity and a blow to his ego-security (Ferenczi *et al.* 1921).

Circumstances, setting and repercussions of injury

The circumstances of the accident can also be important, as when a reckless driver has injured his family or a workman has been forced against his will to use faulty equipment. The setting may have been peculiarly conducive to fear, anger or resentment as in the following case:

A man aged 48 was coshed on the way to bank his firm's takings and rendered briefly unconscious. For 12 months thereafter he showed enduring symptoms of anxiety and depression despite full physical and intellectual recovery. His ability to function at work appeared to be unaccountably impaired. It ultimately emerged that after a series of frustrating setbacks he had come to be employed in a humble capacity by his successful younger brother who ran a flourishing business. Years of suppressed resentment and hostility were now focused on the injury, and the full significance to him of being attacked while banking the firm's profits immediately became apparent.   (Lishman 1973)

Pilowsky (1985) describes other examples in which exploration of the details surrounding the accident can be rewarding in revealing circumstances of special significance. And even ignoring individual determinants of this nature, it is possible to show that disability tends to differ from one broad category of accident to another—whether on the roads, at work or in the home (Brain 1942; Adler 1945; Miller 1966a).

The emotional repercussions of the accident may also be more influential than was at first sight supposed. Time spent in detailed enquiry here can sometimes be rewarding, especially in intractable neurotic states or long-continued affective reactions. Such enquiry is particularly indicated when psychiatric disability is disproportionate to the likely severity of brain damage incurred, or when it outstrips expectations derived from a knowledge of previous mental stability:

A woman of 45 was disabled for many months by a number of neurotic complaints after surviving intact from a car crash. The head injury had been mild but her vision had been threatened for a time. Her persistent neurotic reaction was surprising in view of her excellent previous mental health and stability. She eventually confessed to a long-standing secret liaison with the

husband of a friend, in whose company the accident had occurred. She had made a fervent resolve to end the relationship by way of atonement if her sight should be spared, and this she was now striving to do. Here the injury served as a focus for long-standing conflict and guilt, in addition to providing on-going emotional distress of a deeply disturbing kind.   (Lishman 1973)

In such a case the true nature of the conflict underlying the symptoms needed to be revealed before treatment could begin to be effective.

Iatrogenic factors

Iatrogenic factors can sometimes assume major importance. In the early stages after injury the patient is vulnerable and often highly suggestible. In particular he may be strongly influenced by what he hears from fellow patients, the treatment received and how much is or is not explained to him. Protracted investigations can sometimes stir up enduring anxiety:

A policewoman of 22 sustained a minor blow on the head when travelling on duty in a car. Continuing headache led to skull X-ray which showed some increased convolutional markings. A CT scan was therefore undertaken in case a pre-existing hydrocephalus had been exacerbated. This was normal but the foramen magnum seemed enlarged. A myelogram was therefore in turn carried out to exclude any possibility of abnormality at the craniocervical junction and was also normal. Throughout the 6 weeks of investigation her headaches steadily worsened— and were still troublesome some 3 years later when she was referred for a second opinion. Her attention had indeed been firmly focused on her early symptoms.   (Lishman 1988)

Environmental factors

Environmental difficulties encountered during convalescence and thereafter must always be carefully evaluated, along with the general social setting of the patient. In practice such aspects are extremely important since environmental problems may be accessible to remediation.

Careful management during convalescence and a healthy home environment have been found to be factors of great prognostic importance (Aita 1948). In less severe injuries these features become of correspondingly greater significance in determining progress. Threats to family or personal security and occupational difficulties frequently assume crucial importance, especially if physical or intellectual deficits require new adaptation on the part of the patient. Fear of returning to a dangerous occupation where the accident has occurred can have a powerful influence in determining prolonged invalidism. An unstable domestic background will often stand to impede progress, likewise oversolicitude on the part of the family.

Tarsh and Royston (1985) have documented the influence of changes within the family in contributing to prolongation of disability, especially overprotection from family members and changes in the normal family hierarchies and roles.

It is necessary to consider not only the new problems accruing from the injury, but also environmental and interpersonal difficulties which may have been present long before. Sometimes prolonged disability turns out to be motivated by problems which have antedated the head injury, and the latter then serves as a tangible focus or 'scapegoat' on which they can be blamed (Ruesch & Bowman 1945). Frustrations which have previously been tolerated may now be released in full force. Patients who have long feared economic disaster may focus their anxiety on the reality of the injury; others may be seen to utilize it as an escape from some unbearable situation. With the injury in the forefront of his mind the patient now has a reason around which to crystallize his discomforts—to become outspokenly irritable or to find his work exhausting.

It is also important to recognize that disturbing life events may have shortly antedated the accident. Selzer et al. (1968) were able to show an excess of personal conflicts and stresses in the lives of drivers causing fatal accidents during the 12 months preceding these events, many of which were still affecting the driver at the time. No less than 20% had had an acutely disturbing experience during the preceding 6 hours. Whitlock et al. (1977) similarly found an excess of such items as moving house, marital separations, serious discord or changes of work in the recent lives of victims of accidental injury. Among 45 consecutive admissions with minor head injury, Fenton et al. (1993) found that adverse life events were twice as frequent as among controls—mainly ill health and changes in job, school and personal relationships during the preceding 12 months. Thus accidents seem prone to occur just when the person already has to cope with other sources of conflict or upheaval. Detailed exploration of the life situation antedating as well as following the injury is therefore often indicated.

Compensation and litigation

The important medicolegal aspects of head injury are dealt with on pp. 207–11. Here it will suffice to note that impending litigation can strongly motivate the aggravation and prolongation of disability. Especially after industrial accidents, powerful social influences are often brought to bear on the patient and lead him to hope for financial reward. Advice is received from many sources,

and tempting examples of other similar cases are often much discussed.

That the compensation issue, like other conflicts, can operate at many levels of consciousness should be no cause for surprise. In some, probably rare cases, there will be entirely conscious simulation for gain, but in the great majority the compensation issue colours the picture in more subtle ways. Once the possibility of compensation is raised the patient finds himself in complex legal dealings; there are frustrations due to delay, anxieties due to conflicting advice and often capital outlay. In effect the injured person is invited to complain and, having done so, finds he must complain repeatedly, often over years to a number of specialists (Cole 1970). Repeated questioning from lawyers and doctors not only focuses the patient's attention on early symptoms which perhaps were due to recede, but in addition reinforces the prospect of their continuance or of worse to come. Nor is it surprising that conflict over compensation should dictate neurotic forms of disability; it is in the nature of conflict, both conscious and subconscious, to provoke subjective forms of disability which lack external and objective cues to keep it in proportion.

Where patients have been selected to optimise the chance of revealing the compensation issue, as in series seen especially for the courts, it is sometimes found to outweigh all other factors in the prolongation of disability. But just how common or important it may be in the generality of head-injured patients is hard to determine, because we lack comprehensive investigations of parallel series of cases in which compensation is and is not a possible consequence. Miller (1961, 1966a) estimated that the compensation issue contributes to disability in one-quarter to one-third of all patients when the accident has fulfilled two criteria—when someone else is at fault in the patient's view, and when payment of financial compensation is at least a possibility. In reviewing 200 patients seen for medicolegal assessment after head injury he found that gross psychoneurotic complaints or the postconcussional syndrome were the outstanding disabilities in more than a third. Patients of low social status, unskilled or semiskilled, were particularly affected, and men were implicated twice as often as women. Neurotic disability was twice as common after industrial accidents as after road traffic accidents, and employees of large organisations or nationalised concerns were affected more commonly than those of small intimate firms. The alarming nature of the accident was not clearly related to neurotic disability in this group, and the actual severity of the injury to the head was inversely related to such developments. Additional evidence of the importance of litigation has been deduced from the fact that postconcussional symptoms are rare after injuries at sport or in the home where compensation is not payable (Miller 1969).

With regard to outcome it is clear that prolonged legal negotiations often aggravate the situation. It is also sometimes reported that disability continues until the compensation issue is settled, then clears abruptly whether or not financial reward has been forthcoming. These oft-quoted instances show the tenacity with which the compensation motive can sometimes operate. Even so, improvement on settlement need not imply that the patient has been 'manufacturing' his symptoms—genuine uncertainty and worry have been decisively removed (Merskey & Woodforde 1972).

Examples of abrupt resolution on settlement are, in fact, much rarer than is commonly supposed. Steadman and Graham (1970) found that patients whose claims were rejected took a long time to recover or return to work, and 'neurotic resentment' seemed a possible explanation for this. Kelly and Smith (1981) traced 43 of 100 patients to determine the long-term outcome of the post-traumatic syndrome when the compensation issue was at stake; of 26 who had failed to return to work by the settlement date, only one was at work 18 months later, yet all but four had considered the settlement adequate.

In a review of the literature Mendelson (1982) has underlined such findings, obtaining little support for the view that many patients become symptom-free on settlement; in some series up to two-thirds of those injured in compensatible accidents had failed to return to work during the next year or two. With regard to postconcussional symptoms, Rutherford (1989) has strikingly illustrated their tendency to persist, by following 44 consecutive patients referred for medicolegal reports. At the time of writing the reports 57% had symptoms, but this had fallen to 39% at the time of settlement; there was little further fall in the proportion still complaining (34%) when followed up 1 year later.

Response to intellectual impairments

Intellectual impairment after head injury is important not only for its cognitive effects, but also for the role that subtle impairments may play in dictating emotional and behavioural changes. Goldstein (1942, 1952) made an important contribution here in stressing how the various psychological results of brain injury can have repercussions one upon another.

After brain injury some symptoms are the direct result of loss of brain tissue, while others represent the necessary modification of related functions consequent upon this.

Furthermore, in Goldstein's view, a large number of symptoms and alterations of behaviour are in no direct sense a result of damage to a part of the brain, but must be viewed holistically as 'the expression of the struggle of the changed organism to cope with the (primary) defect and to meet the demands of the milieu with which it is no longer equipped to deal'. Some symptoms reflect the struggle, and some the tendency to build up substitute performances. In this way Goldstein saw the origin of such symptoms as anxiety, restlessness, overorderliness, social withdrawal and the catastrophic reaction (pp. 14 and 97).

The disabilities which Goldstein thought to be fundamental lay chiefly within the intellectual sphere. These may be of a subtle nature and not obvious until special testing is carried out. He emphasised disturbances in conceptual thinking, such as difficulty with abstract as opposed to concrete matters, and difficulty in singling out important features from the general background of perceptions. Such disturbances have found ample confirmation in the hands of subsequent workers. In the twin studies of Dencker (pp. 173 and 184) these were the outstanding post-traumatic defects which distinguished the injured twin from his partner.

Goldstein perhaps overstated his case in contending that so large a spectrum of secondary disabilities followed in the wake of intellectual disturbance, but he drew attention to possibilities which had previously been neglected. Goldstein's point of view is implicit in Hillbom's (1960) explanation for the special frequency of severe neuroses after mild head injuries, namely that 'contradictions with the environment originate more easily when invalidity is not easily visible and the requirement is too high'; also in Guttmann's (1946) suggestion that attempted denial of mild intellectual impairment is often the basis for neurotic reactions after head injury. It is therefore essential when considering psychiatric disturbance after head injury to explore in detail for minor intellectual deficits. Clinical impressions must be adequately backed by psychometric testing.

Development of epilepsy

Post-traumatic epilepsy is known to develop in about 5% of closed head injuries and in over 30% when the dura mater has been penetrated. The general question of post-traumatic epilepsy is considered on pp. 244–5.

The development of seizures represents a serious complication, and is regarded by Jennett (1962) as next in frequency to organic psychological deficits as the cause of enduring occupational difficulty. It certainly stands to aggravate the psychiatric disability ensuing from the injury. First there is the socially disruptive effect of the epilepsy which increases self concern, hinders rehabilitation and brings special problems in readaptation to daily life. The fits may make their appearance when the patient is on the point of regaining confidence, and represent an added hurdle to be overcome. In addition, the physiological disturbance underlying the epilepsy may add to the effects of brain damage already present. After closed head injury temporal lobe epilepsy is the commonest form (Jennett 1962), and this is the type most frequently incriminated in leading to psychiatric disturbance.

Lishman (1968) found that epilepsy occurred during the ensuing 5 years in 45% of patients with penetrating injuries, and there was a highly significant relationship between its development and the degree of overall psychiatric disability. Epilepsy of early rather than late onset was mainly responsible for the association, especially that developing during the first year after injury. The relationship remained significant after controlling for the differing amounts of brain damage sustained among the epileptic and non-epileptic patients.

Amount of brain damage incurred

The main difficulty in estimating the contribution of brain damage to different forms of post-traumatic psychiatric disability lies in the problem of detecting minor degrees of damage while the patient is alive. The available techniques of neuroimaging, electroencephalography and psychometry cannot be expected always to reflect small amounts of neuronal loss or focal brain dysfunction. When positive findings do emerge it can be difficult to assess their causal relationship to different aspects of the clinical picture. Intellectual impairment after head injury is readily attributed to brain damage, but there is a less clear answer where emotional and behavioural disorders are concerned. Some common somatic symptoms, such as headache and dizziness, have sometimes been attributed to brain damage and sometimes not.

The divergences of opinion in the literature are very striking. Mapother (1937) was led to include psychasthenia among the organic consequences of head injury. This was defined as 'the persistence of ultimate incapacity for employment by mental disabilities which are not gross or obvious'. Similarly many clinicians have been impressed with the stereotyped nature of post-traumatic headache and associated nervous symptoms, and have urged that these too must have some constant basis in minor neuronal damage, perhaps even at the subcellular level. Doubt has now been cast on such clinical impressions and has grown with a more sensitive appreciation of the role of psychogenic factors of the type outlined above.

A common approach has been to examine the nature and severity of post-traumatic symptoms against clinical indices known to reflect severity of brain damage, such as length of coma, length of PTA, and other clinical features seen shortly after injury. Personality change has been found to be commoner after the more severe injuries, also the average severity of overall psychiatric disability (Kremer 1943; Aita 1948; Steadman & Graham 1970). In Walker and Jablon's (1959) large series the severity of injury appeared to bear some relation to many aspects of psychiatric disorder—impaired judgement, mentation, memory, alterations of personality and even the post-traumatic syndrome. Norrman and Svahn (1961), however, in injuries studied more than 2 years later, found that severity correlated only with impairment of intellectual functions and very little, if at all, with emotional instability or post-traumatic headache and dizziness.

Lishman's (1968) investigation of 670 soldiers with penetrating injuries used objective measures from X-ray data and surgeons' operating notes, to allow a direct estimation of the extent of brain tissue destruction. This material was chosen to optimise the chance of obtaining reliable measures of brain damage and of demonstrating their relationship to symptoms. All cases had been followed up irrespective of the development of mental sequelae, and thus served as their own controls when the clinical picture was reviewed 1–5 years later. A wide spectrum of psychiatric disabilities was investigated, including intellectual, affective and behavioural changes, also persistent somatic complaints for which no physical basis could be discovered. From this a global measure of psychiatric disability was obtained and graded according to severity.

It was readily shown that simple measures of the amount of brain damage incurred were related to the amount of psychiatric disorder encountered 1–5 years later. A close and regular relationship was found, for example, between the depth of penetration of brain tissue at initial wounding and the severity of the ensuing psychiatric disability, and this relationship was broadly maintained when allowance was made for effects due solely to intellectual impairment. In a similar manner, PTA was used as an index of diffuse as opposed to focal brain damage, and again regular correlations were seen with the severity of eventual psychiatric disability (Table 7, p. 171). Statistical analyses of the data strongly upheld the significance of these results.

Analysis of individual symptoms and symptom groups allowed some estimate to be made of which components of psychiatric disability were particularly closely tied to the indices of brain damage. These included generalised intellectual impairment and dysphasia, as might be expected, but also apathy, euphoria, and behavioural disorders such as disinhibition, facile or childish behaviour and lack of judgement and consideration for others. Among symptoms which had apparently contributed little if at all to the relationships with brain damage were difficulty in concentration, depression, anxiety, irritability, and somatic complaints such as headache, dizziness, fatigue and sensitivity to noise. Difficulty with memory occupied an intermediate position suggesting a more variable aetiology—some patients suffering principally from organic disturbance of memory and some from psychogenic elaboration of minimal defects.

Brain damage thus emerged as undeniably important in contributing to the long-term psychiatric sequelae of head injury, and appeared to be operative where several different types of disability were concerned. Nevertheless, the correlations between brain damage and psychiatric disability, while highly significant statistically, were relatively small (the correlation coefficients being in the region of 0.25). In other words, brain damage could be shown to contribute little more than one-fifteenth part of the total causation of psychiatric disability in the material, and other unmeasured aetiological factors had also clearly been at work.

The availability of sensitive brain-imaging techniques for assessing and quantifying brain damage holds considerable promise for refining such observations further. Studies to date which have sought to relate MRI findings to clinical parameters are outlined on p. 166.

Finally, the special hazard of brain damage when blood alcohol levels are elevated must be emphasised. Waller (1968), investigating road deaths in California, found that 58% of drivers, 47% of passengers and 36% of pedestrians had alcohol in the blood, most with levels exceeding the legal maximum for drivers. Moreover, 75% of the drivers could be classified as problem drinkers. In the UK it has been estimated that a quarter of all road accident deaths are associated with alcohol (Raffle 1989). The effects of acute alcohol intake in increasing the extent of brain injury, and of chronic intake in delaying reparative processes within the nervous system, are now appreciated from laboratory experimental studies (Flamm et al. 1977; West et al. 1982; Albin & Bunegin 1986). There is also evidence that the prevalence of head injury in alcoholic subjects is some 2–4 times that of the general population (Hillbom & Holm 1986).

Despite earlier negative reports (e.g. Nath et al. 1986), there is now some clinical evidence that alcohol consumption at the time of injury worsens the outcome of head injury. Brooks et al. (1989) found that alcohol intake at injury was a significant predictor of the severity of

memory impairment 2–6 years later. Moreover, there was an interaction between the severity of the injury and amount of alcohol consumed on the size of the memory deficit; to have a short PTA and to have drunk heavily led to a worse outcome than occurred in patients with a considerably longer PTA who had drunk lightly or not at all.

In Brooks et al.'s study the deleterious effects of drinking at the time of the accident emerged more clearly than the effects of habitual consumption, though the two were strongly interrelated. Recently, however, Rönty et al. (1993) have shown the effects of habitual excessive consumption on CT measures of brain damage. Fifty-six consecutive patients with mild or moderate injury included 15 alcohol abusers and 41 non-alcoholics. The groups were comparable in terms of age and severity of injury. The alcoholics showed markedly larger initial volumes of brain injury on CT, and longer cerebral circulation times at the site of injury when compared to the contralateral side. On rescanning 6 months and 1 year later the alcoholics had developed more local brain atrophy, and greater ventricular and sulcal enlargement, despite equivalence on these measures with the non-alcoholic group at the time of injury. Only 40% of the alcoholics returned to work after the injury compared with 73% of the remainder.

Location of brain damage incurred

Many investigations have sought to determine how far psychiatric disability depends on the location of damage within the brain. Here the difficulties inherent in attempting to measure brain damage during life are further increased by the problem of estimating its location with reasonable accuracy.

Efforts in this direction have formed a substantial part of the general endeavour to seek correlations between disturbed mental function and regional brain disorder. Head-injury material is in some ways particularly suitable for such investigation. Seen in the stationary state, post-traumatic brain lesions are in the main non-progressive and uncomplicated by changes in intracranial pressure. The principal disadvantage is the uncertainty which often exists about the site of focal pathology, and the degree to which it is truly circumscribed. Moreover, focal deficits are often overlaid by the generalised effects of brain damage. Penetrating injuries are more suitable for analysis than closed head injuries in these regards, and have been studied in more detail, though even here it must be recognised that damage may exist where it is unsuspected.

Focal syndromes of cognitive defect may certainly result from head injury, and it is likely that several aspects of emotional and behavioural disorder may similarly depend on circumscribed pathology. Dysphasia remains the prime example in the cognitive sphere, and frontal lobe symptoms in the behavioural sphere. Both may stand out against the background effects of coexisting diffuse brain damage.

After each world war extensive series of head-injured patients were investigated from this point of view. Unfortunately many early studies relied heavily on impressionistic statements, and were interpreted in terms of an outmoded psychopathology. The quest for a unifying theme or a 'fundamental disturbance of function' produced concepts which were vague, hard to confirm and hard to translate into the language of another psychiatric school (for example 'Antriebstörung'—disturbance of vital force or drive, and 'Hirnleistungsschwäche'—general weakness of brain capacity or performance). In consequence the valuable clinical material of early studies is nowadays hard to assess and to compare with more recent investigations.

The frontal lobes were soon the site of special interest, and Phelps' (1898) investigation has historical importance. In a series of head-injured patients he investigated the site of laceration of the brain at autopsy and compared this with the presence or absence of mental abnormalities immediately before death. Opportunities for observation were limited since most cases died within a few days of injury, but among 225 autopsies mental change had existed in only four cases where lacerations had spared the left frontal lobe. Furthermore, among 28 cases with frontal lobe laceration abnormalities had been noted only when the left lobe was damaged. Phelps concluded that there 'seems to be a general law of relationship between a very limited region of the brain and the manifestation of the higher psychical phenomena'. This was supported by his analysis of 110 pistol shot wounds of the brain culled from the English and American literature of the period.

Some of the first detailed reports from war-injured patients were produced by Röper (1917), Forster (1919) and Feuchtwanger (1923). Feuchtwanger compared 200 frontal gunshot wounds with 200 cases where bullets had penetrated other parts of the skull. The outstanding changes in the frontal group included euphoria, facetiousness, irritability, apathy and defects of attention. There was often an incapacity for planning ahead, tactlessness and moral defects. Where intellect was disturbed this seemed usually to be secondary to disorders of emotion and volition. Much of this, of course, was later well substantiated from observation on leucotomised patients.

Kleist (1934) in a similar study added loss of initiative, aspontaneity of motor activity, lack of ideation and mutism as characteristic of frontal injuries. The special psychiatric hazard of bifrontal injuries was noted (Heygster 1949), also the liability of frontal lesions to produce changes of character which led to criminality (Lindenberg 1951; Mutschler 1956).

Differences have been described between wounds of the convex lateral surface and wounds of the orbital parts of the lobe, the former producing mainly intellectual and motor changes while the latter had more serious effects on the personality (Kleist 1934; Faust 1955, 1960; Walch 1956). Walch found that with convexity lesions the disturbance was mainly lack of drive (Antriebstörung) or disinhibition, though many patients showed no psychic changes whatever. By contrast, few among the patients with orbital lesions were without striking psychological symptoms, and a high proportion showed changes in 'the more highly developed qualities of personality'. Faust similarly stressed the lack of productive thinking, indifference and incapacity for decisions with convexity lesions. Patients with orbital lesions often failed to show defects on formal intelligence testing, but were prone to develop marked personality changes. They failed to maintain satisfactory relationships, lacked perseverance and were sometimes demanding, disinhibited and aggressive. Sexual behaviour was often marked by increased libido and potency, coupled with disregard for the partner. Criminality was especially common in the orbital group and often took the form of sexual offences.

Injury to the basal parts of the brain also attracted special attention. Kretschmer (1949, 1956) described a 'basal syndrome' which found wide support in the German literature. This results from lesions of the midbrain, hypothalamus and orbital frontal cortex. It is characterised by sluggishness and apathy along with fluctuations of mood and sudden outbursts of irritability, typically coupled with disturbance of fundamental drives and instincts—appetite, thirst and sleep rhythm—and varied sexual pathologies. Hoheisel and Walch (1952) described five patients with marked bipolar fluctuations of mood persisting for a long time after head injury; one such case had a shell splinter in the hypothalamus and the other four showed clinical signs which indicated diencephalic injury.

In contrast to the above, remarkably little has been written of distinctive psychiatric pictures after injury to other parts of the brain. Teuber (1959, 1962) and co-workers investigated cognitive and perceptual defects in a large series of penetrating injuries with regional brain damage. Patients with left parietotemporal lesions showed significant losses on the Army General Classification Test (AGCT) of general intelligence when pre- and post-traumatic scores were compared. No such losses were found after lesions elsewhere. The differences persisted after excluding patients with dysphasia, and the left parietotemporal cases also showed maximal impairment on a non-verbal task (a visual conditional reaction). The evidence, therefore, suggested that lesions of this region of the brain may be especially associated with intellectual deficits and, to a considerable extent, independently of language loss.

Temporal lobe injuries appear to show a special frequency of personality disorder, both in their own right and by virtue of the temporal lobe epilepsy which may accompany them (Ajuriaguerra & Hécaen 1960). Hillbom (1951, 1960) also noted a preponderance of atypical psychoses after temporal lobe injury, especially schizophrenia-like psychoses.

Hillbom's (1960) important investigation surveyed a large number of wartime head injuries, of which 415 were randomly selected for special study. Amongst unilateral wounds the left were associated with more psychiatric disturbance than the right, particularly where dementias and psychoses were concerned. Bilateral and midline wounds appeared to cause a great excess of dementias. Frontal injuries were associated with a significant excess of psychiatric disturbance, especially changes of character, and particularly when disordered behaviour was prominent. By contrast, patients with parietal, occipital and cerebellar lesions were relatively free from psychiatric disturbance.

The study described on p. 178 (Lishman 1968) paid special attention to the site of known brain damage in a subsample of 345 cases of penetrating head injury. Left hemisphere lesions again proved to be more closely associated with overall psychiatric disability than right hemisphere lesions. Temporal lobe wounds had led to significantly more psychiatric disability than frontal, parietal or occipital lobe wounds, and this was very largely due to injuries of the left temporal lobe.

Some neurological defects appearing immediately after injury were also used as a guide to the location of cerebral

Table 9 Symptoms and symptom groups seen 1–5 years after penetrating injury in relation to the location of brain damage (after Lishman 1968).

	Number of cases (total = 345)	Hemisphere		Lobe(s) (R, L or both)			
		Left	Right	Frontal	Parietal	Temporal	Occipital
Any intellectual disorder	117	*			*	*	?*
General intellectual impairment	32	*				*	?*
Dysphasia	24	*			*	*	
Impairment of memory	50	*			*		*
Difficulty in concentration	87		*				*
Any affective disorder	113		*	*			
Depression	58		*	*	*		
Anxiety	40						*
Irritability	72		*	*	*		
Aggression	10			*			
Apathy	35		*				
Euphoria	10			*			
Any behavioural disorder	40		*	*			
Crime or misdemeanours	5			*			
Sexual disturbance	8			*			
Lack of judgement, etc.	20			*			
Facile or childish behaviour	17		*	*			
Disinhibition	13			*			
Somatic complaints	71		*	*			
Headache or dizziness	62			*			
Fatigue	16				*		
Sensitivity to noise	24			*			
'Frontal lobe syndrome'	32		*	*			

* Indicates strong evidence of special association.

damage, and showed certain associations with psychiatric disability. In effect damage to different 'functional systems' within the brain could be shown to carry special hazards for psychiatric disability, in addition to damage to specific anatomical areas. Thus sensorimotor defects originating within the left hemisphere, but not those originating within the right, were associated with a significant excess of psychiatric disability. Similarly, visual field defects were closely associated with psychiatric disability when they originated in the left parietal or temporal lobes, but not when caused by occipital lobe lesions.

The number of cases available did not allow confident conclusions to be drawn about special regional associations for different types of psychiatric disability. However, intellectual disorders were found more commonly after left hemisphere damage, while affective disorders, behavioural disorders and somatic complaints were more frequent after right hemisphere damage (Table 9, p. 181). Intellectual disorders were especially associated with damage to the parietal and temporal lobes, and were in fact less frequent after damage to the frontal lobe than after damage to other parts of the brain. Affective disorders, behavioural disorders and somatic complaints were more frequent after frontal lobe damage than after damage elsewhere. All component symptoms among the group of behavioural disorders showed this special frontal association. Sexual disturbances were seen only after frontal wounds, and with one exception this was also true of criminal behaviour. The 'frontal lobe syndrome' (recorded for patients who showed euphoria, lack of judgement, facile or childish behaviour or disinhibition) was especially common after frontal wounds, but nine of the 32 examples were found after wounds which did not apparently involve the frontal lobes at all.

MRI investigations have upheld the importance of frontal and temporal lesions in relation to defined neuropsychological deficits, as discussed on p. 166. PET scan studies appear to hold special promise in revealing cerebral dysfunction extending beyond areas of structural abnormality. The application of such techniques in conjunction with thorough psychiatric and psychological assessments will doubtless increase our understanding of brain–behaviour correlations very considerably.

It has therefore steadily become apparent that psychiatric disability after head injury may vary according to the location of damage within the brain. Taken together, the various studies quoted above provide considerable support for the broad generalisation that lesions in some areas provide a greater psychiatric hazard than others, and that this involves emotional and behavioural disturbances as well as cognitive defects.

Categories of post-traumatic psychiatric disorder

The many different forms of post-traumatic psychiatric disablement cannot be rigidly classified, and complex admixtures of symptoms are frequently seen. For example, changes of temperament may occur along with intellectual impairment, or paranoid developments may arise in association with neurotic disability. Quite often, however, specific features or a combination of related features are outstanding, or even seen in relative isolation. For this reason the four main categories of psychiatric disturbance will be examined separately below—cognitive impairment, change of personality, psychosis and neurosis. The problem of the so-called 'post-traumatic syndrome' will be dealt with separately because of the special difficulties surrounding its nosological status.

The relative frequency of these changes may be gauged from the analysis of two large series of patients in which these broad divisions have been observed. Hillbom's (1960) follow up of 3552 wartime injuries, of which 1505 were penetrating, showed cognitive impairment in 2%, changes of character in 18%, psychoses in 8% and severe neuroses in 11%. Ota's (1969) large series of 1168 closed head injuries among Japanese civilians showed cognitive impairment in 3%, changes of character in 6%, psychoses in 5% and neuroses in 22%. The differences between the two reflect matters of definition, selection, and type of injury, but both agree in finding that changes of character and neurotic manifestations are the most common, and enduring cognitive defects the least common among psychiatric sequelae. The frequency of the post-traumatic syndrome is difficult to judge because of the many different ways in which the syndrome is defined (p. 196), though often this is reported to rank as the commonest after-effect of all.

Under each heading below the clinical pictures will be described, along with comments on the aetiology, course and differential diagnosis.

Cognitive impairment

Cognitive impairment is, of course, the direct result of the damage to brain tissue which has occurred. Minor injuries are compatible with full intellectual recovery, even when indubitable loss of consciousness has occurred, in the sense that the patient feels himself to be unimpaired and psychometric tests reveal no deficits in performance. Levin et al. (1987c) followed a group of patients with minor head injury (defined as loss of consciousness for 20 minutes or less and absence of neurological deficits) and tested them serially along with controls. Patients with a previous history of alcohol or drug abuse, previous head injury or a history of neurological or psychiatric disorder were excluded. Tests of memory, attention and information processing showed impairments at 1 week, but these generally resolved during the next 3 months. Somatic complaints and affective symptoms also diminished but cleared less completely. It was concluded that a single uncomplicated minor head injury produces no permanent neurobehavioural sequelae in the great majority of patients, provided they have been free from pre-existing neuropsychiatric disorder. It is arguable nevertheless that subtle changes too minor to be detected may still exist. The observations of Gronwall and Wrightson (1975) on the cumulative effect of a second minor concussion, discussed on p. 204, are relevant here.

More severe head injuries are likely to be followed by persisting cognitive impairment of a degree proportional to the amount of brain damage incurred. In closed head injuries a PTA of 24 hours may be taken as a very approximate clinical guide; below this complete intellectual recovery may be expected in a fair proportion of cases, but with durations in excess of 24 hours the patient will be fortunate to escape without some intellectual impairment. With penetrating injuries due to missiles or with depressed skull fractures, however, the length of PTA is a somewhat less reliable guide. Concussion and amnesia may then be brief or absent, yet focal cognitive defects can be severe, especially if haemorrhage or infection have occurred. Any such complicating factors must be taken carefully into account in assessing the prognosis. With increasing age the chance of intellectual impairment is increased (p. 174) and, in general, damage to the dominant hemisphere will produce more severe effects on intellectual function than damage to the non-dominant hemisphere (Teuber 1959, 1962; Piercy 1964).

Generalised intellectual impairment

After closed head injury the impairment of intellect is usually global, affecting a wide range of cognitive functions together. Marked post-traumatic dementia is usually accompanied by hemiparesis, quadriparesis or other striking neurological disablement. In the most severe cases the patient remains mute and immobile on recovery from coma, persisting thus until death supervenes, usually within a year. This is the 'persistent vegetative state' which represents the most severe form of disability compatible with survival (Jennett & Plum 1972; Jennett & Bond 1975). The sleep–waking cycle is preserved, indicating that the patient is no longer comatose, but all mental function appears to be lost. The eyes may be open and blink to menace or follow moving objects, but they are not attentive. Liquids placed in the mouth may be swallowed. Beyond this, however, responsiveness is usually limited to primitive postural and reflex movements of the limbs. Such a condition represents essentially a state of wakefulness without awareness. The similarity to akinetic mutism (p. 229) is obvious, though in the latter the potential for responding may be considerably greater. The management of such patients, including the difficult ethical and legal problems surrounding the point at which life-sustaining treatment might possibly be withdrawn, is discussed by Howard and Miller (1995). The responsible lesions may lie in the cortex, subcortex or brain stem, diffuse white matter damage being universal at autopsy.

Short of this the patient is profoundly slow and apathetic, frequently with incontinence and gross dysarthria. All intellectual processes are severely affected and even recognition of relatives may be long delayed. Further recovery often brings evidence of emotional lability, with episodes of uncontrolled weeping or laughing, or more rarely with outbursts of poorly coordinated aggressive behaviour. The 'catastrophic reaction' may be called forth when the patient is confronted with a task beyond his ability—sudden flushing, restless overactivity and either explosive anger or weeping.

Slow improvement over many months or sometimes years may be expected in all but the most severe examples. The final level of incapacity is characterised by mental slowing, sluggishness of response, impairment of memory and blunting of affect. Apathy or empty euphoria may remain as persistent features. Logical and abstract thinking will be most markedly affected as in other forms of dementia. Loss of libido is the rule, and paranoid developments are not uncommon.

All gradations are seen between such pictures of established post-traumatic dementia and minimal degrees of intellectual impairment which may come to light only when the patient returns to work. Such minor degrees of impairment present the most difficulty for clinical evaluation. Complaints of forgetfulness and difficulty with concentration can be particularly hard to assess, especially when persisting after minor injuries or occurring along with features suggestive of neurotic disturbance. Both may represent organic changes of slight degree, but both are also met with frequently in nonorganic psychiatric disorder. After head injury they may therefore sometimes be attributable entirely to depression, preoccupation or anxiety. Careful psychometric examination will often, but not invariably, resolve the dilemma; follow-up over time and close attention to other concomitant symptoms will sometimes be necessary to clarify the picture.

With regard to psychometry, tests should explore the subtler aspects of cognitive function in addition to the orthodox tests of memory and intelligence. Dencker and Löfving (1958) made careful psychometric comparisons between head-injured twins and their identical uninjured partners, and found that while the groups were almost identical in general intelligence and capacity for new learning, the probands were significantly inferior in ability for abstraction (sorting tests), tests of figure–ground discrimination and ability to shift frames of reference.

More recent studies have focused on deficits in selective attention, vigilance and speed of information processing (Van Zomeren et al. 1984; Gronwall 1987, 1989; Stuss et al. 1989). Simple reaction time tests usually show maximal recovery within a year and are unrelated to severity of injury; the more sensitive choice reaction time tests prove to be related to severity, and can show continuing recovery more than 2 years after injury. The Paced Auditory Serial Addition Test (PASAT) (p. 198) reveals speed of information processing and correlates with the duration of PTA. Reduced capacity for information processing presents as slowness over tasks, inattention due to overload, and distractibility due to lack of spare capacity for the monitoring of irrelevant stimuli. Problems in such areas appear to be common after even minor injury and may contribute to the genesis of quasi-neurotic symptomatology.

In an interesting study Barth et al. (1989) investigated very mild head injuries (loss of consciousness less than 2 minutes) among university football players, comparing PASAT scores at 24 hours and thereafter with pre-injury performance. Players with mild orthopaedic injuries served as controls. When tested at 24 hours after head injury, the PASAT scores failed to improve as they did in controls due to practice effect. Thereafter, serial testing showed resolution of the impairment. Symbol–digit decoding revealed a similar pattern of transient deficits. Symptom scores for headache, dizziness, nausea, weakness and difficulty with memory were also increased at 24 hours, and then subsided to normal by 10 days. Thus a single very mild head injury caused cognitive/information-processing deficits which could be documented at 24 hours, and which were accompanied and followed by subjective complaints.

Focal cognitive impairment

A focal emphasis of brain pathology may result in focal cognitive deficits, which either stand out against a background of general intellectual impairment or on occasion appear in highly circumscribed form. Strictly focal deficits are more likely after penetrating injuries than closed head injuries, but nonetheless the search for focal emphasis in disorder must always be pursued. A dysphasic or an amnesic syndrome can readily come to be mistaken for global dementia. And areas of relatively intact cognitive function must always be demarcated so that they can be used to the full in rehabilitation.

Newcombe (1983) and Brooks (1984a) provide valuable reviews of the range of deficits encountered and the problems involved in charting and quantifying them by psychometric tests. Disorders of memory, language and visuospatial competence will often require appraisal. Deficits in sustained attention and mental speed may emerge when carefully sought out and will sometimes prove most handicapping of all.

Selective impairment of memory may persist despite excellent restitution of other intellectual functions. This may be sufficiently marked to constitute a 'post-traumatic Korsakoff syndrome', and presumably depends upon circumscribed damage to structures in the diencephalon or medial temporal lobe structures.

Dominant hemisphere damage is associated with language difficulties, manifested variously as difficulty with comprehension, speech production, reading, writing or spelling. Short of overt dysphasia, subtle impairments of verbal function may be revealed by special testing— deficits in verbal learning or verbal retention. Impairment of verbal fluency may owe much to frontal involvement. Arithmetical functions may also be specifically impaired. Dyspraxic difficulties rarely persist in relative isolation, but again characterise dominant hemisphere lesions.

Non-dominant hemisphere damage tends to be associated with special difficulties with visual and spatial functions, including visuospatial agnosic defects and disturbances of topographical orientation. Disturbances of body image, dressing dyspraxia and anosognosia may be marked in the early stages, but rarely persist in the absence of gross generalised impairment of cognitive function.

It is unfortunately true that when focal deficits are very marked and persistent, the likelihood of impairment in other areas of intellectual function is also increased, but this is not invariably so. Newcombe (1969), studying men with focal injuries due to high-velocity missiles, was able to demonstrate highly selective impairments in language, visual perception and spatial orientation persisting 20 years after injury, yet without any evidence of generalised intellectual deterioration.

Recovery of intellectual function

A surprising finding is the relative rarity of profound enduring dementia even after injuries of considerable severity. It is known that some patients, possibly those with severe brain stem injuries, show little improvement over time, also that many partially demented patients survive precariously in their own homes and escape medical attention (Fahy *et al.* 1967). Nevertheless, the fact remains that others improve slowly to an extent that would probably not have been predicted. Certainly experience teaches that in all but the most extreme cases a firm prognosis should not be attempted until 2 or 3 years have elapsed from the time of injury.

Several studies have attempted to chart the pattern and speed of recovery in patients followed prospectively. All agree that the major gains are usually made during the first post-injury year, the most substantial improvement occurring in the first 6 months. During subsequent years continuing improvement can certainly be encountered, but much of this can be seen as adaptation and adjustment to the deficits which persist.

The Glasgow workers (Bond & Brooks 1976; Jennett *et al.* 1977, 1981) have used broad categories of social outcome rather than focusing on cognitive defects alone; using the Glasgow Outcome Scale, patients were classified in terms of remaining dependent on daily support, being able to travel and work in sheltered environments, or resuming normal life even in the face of minor continuing deficits (Jennett & Bond 1975). Only a minority of severely injured patients proved to change from one major grade of social outcome to another after the first post-injury year, though further gains insufficient for reclassification could clearly continue after that period.

Psychometric testing has shown that different components of cognitive function tend to plateau at different periods. Thus Mandleberg and Brooks (1975) found that scores on verbal subtests of the Wechsler Adult Intelligence Scale (WAIS) tended to approach those of a non-injured control group after 1 year, whereas recovery on performance subtests continued for about 3 years. The slower restitution on performance items no doubt depends on their complex nature, requiring a synthesis of numerous capacities such as perception, attention, learning and psychomotor speed. The recovery of memory functions has been investigated similarly (Brooks 1976; Parker & Serrats 1976), again with indications that most of the improvement takes place during the first year.

Surprising examples of apparent long-continued cognitive improvement can, however, be seen. This was underlined by Miller and Stern's (1965) follow up of 92 patients injured on average 11 years earlier. Despite the severity of the initial injuries, with a mean PTA of 13 days, only 10 patients showed persistent cognitive impairment and of these only five were unemployed. Half had escaped any loss of occupational status. Of 38 in whom an initial report, made on average 3 years after the injury, had expressed serious doubts whether they would ever work again, 28 were employed and 16 without loss of status. Spastic paresis likewise showed an unexpected degree of recovery, persisting in only four out of 25 cases.

These observations obtain support from clinical experience and call for some attempt at explanation. They challenge the simple idea that clinical impressions of the severity of dementia always match the extent of brain pathology. It would seem unlikely that long-continued improvement over a number of years could be due to those aspects of brain pathology which are reversible. The time course is more in keeping with the re-education of intact brain tissue to take over new functions, and such capacities in the adult brain may be greater than is generally recognised. But an additional explanation is perhaps that a part of the dementia seen in the early phase of recovery is more apparent than real, and that from the outset there has been less brain damage than one was led to infer from the clinical picture. Two situations may have been responsible for this; first, that the patient was suffering from coincident affective disorder, and second that motivational defects have been particularly marked and have then slowly yielded to the process of rehabilitation.

Affective disorder may easily be missed in the early months of convalescence when the patient is already slowed, anergic and withdrawn. It is important to remember that the typical patient with severe dementia after gross brain injury shows a bland, even euphoric disposition, in spite of his disabilities; a complicating depressive reaction is therefore to be suspected if the patient remains agitated or profoundly apathetic, or if anorexic or sleeping badly. Antidepressant medication may sometimes produce dramatic improvement and electroconvulsive therapy is not absolutely contraindicated.

With regard to motivational defects, these may lead to spuriously low performance on tests of intellectual capacity, and the general sluggishness of the patient may increase the clinical impression of the severity of dementia. It is therefore perhaps in the areas of motivation and drive that we should sometimes seek an explanation for the progressive improvement over very long periods of time which may occur. Little is known about the neural basis of motivation, but it is possible that motivational defects are themselves based in cerebral pathology, at least in the early post-traumatic phase. Certain evidence suggests that dopaminergic underactivity may be involved, and treatment with dopamine agonists has occasionally met with success (p. 214). Later in recovery, psychological processes of readjustment and adaptation will play back powerfully to improve motivation, and personality resources are likely to contribute increasingly.

Psychological means are therefore necessary to combat such deficits, and it is for this reason that graded and stimulating programmes of rehabilitation can often meet with conspicuous success when instituted early and pursued with constant encouragement.

Complicating factors

In rather rare instances a degree of dementia persists which is out of keeping with the severity of the injury that has occurred. This should raise the possibility of subdural haematoma, of normal-pressure hydrocephalus or of a coincident presenile or senile dementing illness.

Subdural haematoma (p. 411) is a particular hazard in the arteriosclerotic and the elderly, and should be especially suspected when the degree of intellectual impairment appears to fluctuate from time to time. Normal-pressure hydrocephalus (p. 744) is a rare but important complication which must also be considered, especially when intellectual failure sets in or worsens some time after the injury. The patient reported by Christie Brown (1975), in whom profound mental impairment persisted for 1–2 years after injury then spontaneously and progressively resolved, would appear to represent a rare example of normal-pressure hydrocephalus which underwent spontaneous resolution.

The rare cases of post-traumatic dementia in which subsequent histological examination of the brain reveals changes typical of a primary presenile dementia have been discussed by Corsellis and Brierley (1959) and Strich (1969). Here it remains possible that trauma has precipitated or at least accelerated the degenerative process, but for this there is no proof. In the great majority of instances it would seem more likely that the patient was already suffering from a dementing illness to which attention has been drawn by the injury. Roberts (1976, 1979) focused particular attention on the question of late dementia in his follow up of 291 survivors from very severe injuries. Careful enquiry 10–25 years later yielded evidence of worsening in 31 patients, and in 10 the possibility was raised of a progressive dementia. On taking all associated factors into account, however, such as age, alcoholism, epilepsy and hydrocephalus, there was little to support the notion that a single head injury could set in train a progressive dementing process. Some patients may have had Alzheimer's disease unrelated to the injury, but a more general explanation seemed to lie with the natural processes of ageing affecting a brain already depleted of its functional reserves.

Nonetheless, the evidence that there may be a statistical link between Alzheimer's disease and earlier head trauma remains intriguing, as is the recent finding of increased beta-amyloid deposition in the cortex in the wake of trauma. These matters are discussed on p. 438. Occasional patients have been reported who have demented exceptionally early, for example the man described by Rudelli *et al.* (1982) who had a severe head injury at 22, began to dement at 30, and died of Alzheimer's disease at 38 years. With regard to accelerated decline with ageing, in consequence of depleted neuronal reserves, rather striking evidence has come from Corkin *et al.*'s studies of soldiers surviving from World War II:

Corkin *et al.* (1989) traced 84 soldiers who had had penetrating head injuries and compared them with 27 controls who had suffered peripheral nerve injuries. The groups were matched for age, education and premorbid intelligence. All subjects had already undergone extensive neuropsychological investigation 30 years earlier, and changes in performance on these same tests could now be accurately assessed.

Head injury had led to accelerated decline on total scores from the AGCT, and on its arithmetic subtest, when head-injured and non-head-injured subjects were compared. Means were in the same direction for the vocabulary and the block-counting subscales, and on a hidden figures test. Exacerbated decline was greatest among older subjects, and was common rather than restricted to a small subsample, affecting for example some 75% of persons where the AGCT total scores were concerned.

Regional effects of the initial brain damage were also evident. Those who had had left parietal lobe injuries showed significantly greater decline on the vocabulary and arithmetic subscales, whereas right parietal lobe injuries were associated with significantly greater decline on the hidden figures test.

Although the head-injured patients were not demented, these results point to the possibility that decreased neuronal reserves, consequent upon injury, lead to accelerated decline with ageing. Additional possibilities include the reaction of the brain to the extra stress placed on it by needing to function in a compromised state during the many years following injury. The important clinical point made by Corkin *et al.* is that before diagnosing dementia in a patient with a history of head trauma, one should consider the possibility that exacerbated cognitive decline is the responsible factor rather than a new pathological process.

These findings from detailed psychometry support the impressionistic report from Walker and Blummer (1989) that mental deterioration appeared to affect a quarter of the head-injured soldiers they followed up after World War II, starting at around 25 years after injury. The changes were often not recognised by the subjects themselves but were apparent to their wives and friends—in the form of forgetfulness, inattention, mental fatigue and confusion. These men had all suffered from post-traumatic epilepsy, but the tendency to deteriorate did not correlate with the persistence of any type of seizure. In contrast to Corkin *et al.*'s (1989) findings, however, Newcombe (1996) has been unable to find evidence of accelerated cognitive decline from her extensive survey of British soldiers sustaining focal brain injuries in World War II.

The special situation with regard to repeated mild head

injuries, as sustained during boxing, is discussed on p. 204 *et seq.*

Change of personality

'Change of personality' implies an alteration in the patient's habitual attitudes and patterns of behaviour, so that his reactions to events and to people are different from what they were before. This may occur as a persistent sequel of head injury and is undoubtedly one of the most distressing after effects for the families of the victims. The patient may be aware of the change in himself, though quite often he is completely oblivious of it. Sometimes the alterations are gross and obvious, or sometimes detectable only to those who knew him well beforehand.

Alexander (1982a) points out that head injury is particularly prone to damage the neocortical portions of the limbic system—the frontopolar, orbitofrontal and anterior temporal regions; few other pathologies routinely damage such areas in a symmetrical fashion while largely sparing the rest of the neocortex. This may explain why behavioural problems are often greatly out of proportion to the severity of neurological defects, and why profound changes in behaviour, affect and emotion can occur even when there is little by way of long-term cognitive impairment.

The term is used to cover a wide variety of disturbances which can be hard to evaluate or to classify with precision. Accordingly, this area of post-traumatic change is particularly difficult to interpret. Different aspects tend to be singled out for discussion by different observers, and the mechanisms responsible are often unclear. Sometimes the changes will be determined by brain damage, sometimes by psychogenic factors and sometimes by a combination of the two together. Aspects of the pretraumatic personality will usually be found to colour the picture, and many of the changes will represent intensification of traits that were present all along. But sometimes, as with frontal lobe damage, there will be elements of change which are new and broadly similar in all individuals affected. Where brain damage is insubstantial, the stress of the accident and its subsequent repercussions will often be found to be the factors mainly responsible, acting on special vulnerabilities in the person concerned.

A broad division may therefore be made into personality changes consequent upon brain damage and those in which it appears to play little or no part.

Personality change with brain damage

Here the personality change will often be but one aspect of the global dementia which follows injury, and cognitive deficits of some degree will be in evidence. With minor degrees of intellectual loss the change may be understandable in terms of the patient's reaction to awareness of impairment. In other cases, however, circumscribed brain damage may operate more directly by disruption of cerebral systems upon which the synthesis of the personality depends. The latter situation is compatible with excellent preservation of intellect to formal testing, yet the personality change is nonetheless 'organic' in origin.

The changes which accompany intellectual impairment may be no more than a loss of refinement or lessened vitality of behaviour, sometimes seen only as transient disturbances which gradually recede over the months that follow. Even so these may combine with adverse circumstances in marriage or at work to set in train severe problems for the patient and his family. Minor degrees of cognitive impairment may also call forth anxiety and depression, especially when the previous personality has been marked by traits of insecurity or feelings of personal inadequacy. Much will depend on the demands made by the environment, and on the handling which the patient receives during the early post-traumatic phase.

With more severe dementia there will be slowing, impairment of motivation, loss of libido and withdrawal of interest in surrounding events and people. Emotional changes include blunting, instability, apathy or euphoria. Irritability and explosive anger occur in some cases and paranoid developments in others. A passive and childish dependence may develop, with petulant behaviour and egocentricity. In very severe examples the essential individuality of the person may be to a large extent obscured.

Frontal lobe lesions remain the best known example of the effects of regional cerebral damage on personality. These have already been described on pp. 76–7. Centrally there are changes which it is difficult to quantify or demonstrate objectively—lack of foresight, tact and concern, inability to plan ahead or judge the consequences of actions, and a facile euphoric disposition. This may lead to antisocial conduct and conflict with the law. Disinhibition is often marked, emerging in social interactions and in some cases in sexual behaviour. Amorous advances may be made from soon after recovery, conversation is interlarded with sexual innuendos, perverse sexual tendencies may emerge, or interest may come to be focused on pornographic material. The patient typically has little insight into the changes which occur.

The alterations are seen in varying degree, sometimes representing little more than coarsening of a previously sophisticated personality or sometimes appearing with gross and disabling severity. Different components of the picture may be prominent, depending perhaps on attributes of the previous personality and on the precise location of damage within the brain. As indicated on p. 180, bilateral frontal lesions, particularly of the orbital parts of the lobes, appear to lead to the most severe examples, often with markedly irresponsible and antisocial conduct. While not entirely the prerogative of frontal lesions, changes of this nature are seen more commonly with frontal damage than with damage restricted to other parts of the brain.

In Roberts' (1976, 1979) survey of the long-term outcome of severe head injuries, the commonest pattern of personality change had a distinctly frontal character. This he termed 'fronto-limbic dementia'—a combination of disabling euphoria, disinhibition or anergia, associated in the majority of cases with intense irritability. Outbursts of ungovernable rage had in some cases led to commitment to institutions. Marked examples were seen only after very severe injuries. Memory was usually also very defective. Less commonly the frontal personality change was present without undue irritability. Occasional patients indeed could be said to have shown *improvement* in personality, in that they were now less prone to worry and were more outgoing and sociable.

A point of great clinical importance is that frontal lobe personality change can occur without evidence of impairment on formal tests of cognitive ability, though of course the two may also be seen together.

A 34-year-old man was referred for psychiatric rehabilitation 7 years after head injury. A fall at work had resulted in fractures of the frontal bones of the skull and these had opened up pathways of infection from the frontal sinuses to the brain. Despite careful neurosurgical care over the ensuing years extensive chronic abscess formation had caused much brain destruction in both frontal lobes. Prior to the accident he had been a stable thoughtful man, happily married and interested in his family. Now he was talkative, restless and grossly disinhibited. His wife had divorced him on account of his preoccupation with pornographic material and his irresponsibility generally. Twelve thousand pounds awarded to him by way of compensation had been spent within a few months, partly on extravagant presents for relatives and acquaintances, and partly on the reckless purchase of a business which soon went bankrupt. He showed no concern or insight into his disabilities, and made jocular comments about the troubles which had befallen him. Full psychometric testing showed a level of intelligence within the average range and consistent with his previous education and work record. No memory or learning deficits could be detected.   (Lishman 1973)

A 24-year-old guardsman shot himself through both frontal lobes while playing 'Russian roulette'. He was in coma for 10 days, and mute, incontinent and profoundly anergic for many months thereafter. When seen 3 years later he was permanently hospitalised and appeared to have reached a plateau where improvement was concerned. Apart from dysarthria there were no neurological abnormalities. He was polite and friendly, and on first acquaintance there was little abnormal to detect. Conversation revealed a rather off-hand manner with some degree of euphoria, but he was reasonably well-informed about current events. In his daily life, however, he was profoundly lacking in initiative and needed supervision to care for his appearance. When left to his own devices he preferred to lie in bed for most of the day. He was inclined to indulge in childish pranks, and to buy pin-up magazines and talk of women though libido was totally lacking. He was extremely easily led into mischief and had twice been convicted for breaking and entering while on leave from hospital. The only change he recognised in himself was that nothing worried him any more. He showed no remorse about the recent convictions and no concern about his future. When asked about the game of 'Russian roulette' he replied that it had been 'a bit silly, I suppose'. Psychological testing showed intelligence in the average to superior range with no disturbance of memory. But perseverative tendencies were marked and there was considerable difficulty in shifting attention from one task to another.

The picture just described has obtained recognition on account of the uniformity of the changes seen from case to case. Frontal lobe personality change bears a definitive stamp which in large measure cuts across differences in premorbid personality. Little is known in comparison about specific personality changes which may follow circumscribed lesions of other parts of the brain, though such may yet remain to be discovered. The characteristic picture claimed for *hypothalamic and basal brain injuries* has already been outlined (p. 180). *Temporal lobe injury* might also be expected to confer distinctive features, by analogy with what is known of personality disturbance in temporal lobe epilepsy, though these have not yet been defined in any detail.

The symptom of reduced control over aggression deserves special consideration. This is seen with sufficient frequency after head injury, and often enough in relative isolation, to suggest that it may sometimes be founded in focal cerebral pathology. Typically the patient is subject, under minor provocation, to sudden explosions of violent behaviour which sometimes bring him repeatedly before the courts. Hooper *et al.* (1945) described 12 such cases. They stressed that the condition was very different from the more common symptom of post-traumatic irritability, especially in its explosive quality. It could, moreover, occur without evidence of irritability between attacks. In general the problem was found to follow severe head injury, though in a few cases the blow had been quite mild.

These cases do not form a homogeneous group. Sometimes the outbursts of aggression may merely represent an exaggeration of personality traits which were previously well in evidence. Careful enquiry may show, indeed, that aggressive outbursts have characterised the individual from childhood and adolescence onwards, and that the head injury is merely being blamed for a pre-existing condition; a recent interpersonal crisis or impending court action for violent behaviour may have led to the patient presenting his complaint at this particular point in time (Lishman 1978).

Other habitually aggressive persons may, however, show true worsening. The more severe the injury, the more likely it will be that brain damage is responsible. Frontal lobe damage may be particularly significant on account of its disinhibiting effects on the personality. One must remain alert, nonetheless, to the possibility that current life stresses or affective disorder are the factors principally operating to aggravate the situation. Paranoid developments may be important, including conspicuous jealousy within the marital context.

Alcohol will often prove to be a significant factor. Consumption may have increased since the injury, or brain damage may have conferred sensitivity to the intake of normal amounts. The so-called 'pathological intoxication' or 'manie à potu' has been ascribed to head injury, as discussed on p. 595. Drug abuse may similarly be responsible.

In other cases no such associated conditions will be found. The explosive diathesis will have emerged as a new disorder, out of character for the individual and relevant directly to the injury. Occasionally it may represent an epileptic phenomenon. Short of this, EEG studies may reveal focal temporal lobe disturbance, and on theoretical grounds suspicion falls heavily on brain damage implicating the periamygdaloid region within the temporal lobes. Sweet et al. (1969) have discussed the evidence linking violent behaviour with diverse forms of pathology within the medial temporal lobe structures.

Clearly every case must be carefully assessed on its merits. The setting of the outbursts, their character and concomitants, the degree of provocation, and the persons against whom aggression is habitually displayed, may all provide essential clues for the origins of the disorder. Sometimes psychogenic factors may emerge in the end as playing the most important part:

A man of 21 had shown repeated episodes of markedly aggressive behaviour, chiefly directed towards the police, since a road traffic accident 2.5 years earlier. These had led to repeated convictions and several brief periods of imprisonment. He had previously been a police cadet and there was ample evidence that his conduct prior to the injury had been entirely satisfactory. Detailed investigations failed to show any evidence of brain damage; full EEG studies revealed no abnormality, psychological testing indicated good intelligence without evidence of intellectual impairment, and prolonged fasting showed no evidence of hypoglycaemia. The injury itself had been mild, without neurological sequelae and with a PTA of only 20 minutes.

The great majority of aggressive outbursts occurred after excessive drinking, and when the patient felt that he had been provoked in some degree. Excessive drinking had set in during a phase of severe depression following the loss of a friend in the accident, and continued as the patient became progressively embittered and disgruntled at his failure to find a new career. He now found himself in a vicious circle as a result of repeated convictions, and much of his aggressive behaviour could be seen as bravado in attempts to regain his self esteem. His hatred of the police force was overt, and he felt their rejection keenly. When drunk, encounters with the police led immediately to the release of explosive outbursts of violence.

Personality change without brain damage

Changes of temperament less likely to be based on brain pathology include fluctuating depression, morbid anxiety, obsessional traits and persistent irritability. All are common, and frequently come to be included under the rubric of personality change. Often they represent an intensification of previous personality traits and will have emerged on other occasions under different conditions of stress. They may emerge as responses to physical defects or minor cognitive impairments, certainly in the early stages of convalesence, but when persistent they can more commonly be traced to stresses consequent upon the injury. They are, in fact, often more accurately to be regarded as neurotic reactions than as changes of personality. In some cases detailed enquiry will show that they conform to the picture of post-traumatic stress disorder (PTSD), with intrusive thoughts concerning the accident and avoidance of situations related to it. PTSD can be long lasting as a source of chronic disability, with reports of it persisting even several decades after wartime stresses (p. 195). Such patients may readily come to be labelled as suffering from personality change.

It must be allowed, however, that the stress of a head injury and its attendant disruptions can sometimes have profound effects on patterns of life adaptation, and thus come to engender true changes of personality even though brain damage has not occurred. A head injury may have profound sequelae in terms of career, marriage and life-style, and in certain persons even minor injuries may be invested with great significance. Individuals who are narcissistic, insecure or who prize their bodily integrity and activity, may develop far-reaching changes in habitual attitudes and behaviour. Those who must cope with physical incapacity or disfigurement will be especially likely to do so.

Here, as so often with the psychological consequences of head injury, the time course has to be taken into account—the longer the changes persist in the absence of evidence of organic defect, the more confidently can they be ascribed to psychogenic rather than physiogenic mechanisms.

Psychoses

The acute post-traumatic psychoses of organic origin have already been described (p. 168). Psychotic episodes may develop later in association with post-traumatic epilepsy, and here also an organic basis can be discerned. The problem is more complex when schizophrenic, paranoid or affective psychoses develop in a patient whose head has been injured. The causal role of the injury may then be far from clear, especially if some considerable time has elapsed between the trauma and the onset of the illness. Frequently the patient or his relatives will seize upon the injury in retrospect as an acceptable and understandable cause, and the issue may become a matter of medicolegal importance.

Various possibilities exist. Brain disturbance may itself contribute directly to such developments; or it may act merely as a precipitant in someone already predisposed; or cerebral damage may create a proneness to psychotic disorder by altering the subject's patterns of reaction to stresses and difficulties. Alternatively, organic factors may be unimportant in themselves: the injury or its psychological repercussions may have acted as a non-specific stress to precipitate the psychosis, or psychogenic causes may lie in the changes wrought in the patient's life or the special difficulties he has to face. Finally, of course, the possibility of simple coincidence must also be considered.

These matters have not been disentangled to a satisfactory extent. Large numbers of cases are hard to assemble, and comparisons between different series raise special difficulties, not least with regard to diagnostic criteria. In general the longer the lapse of time between the injury and the onset of the psychosis, the more likely it will be that the relationship is coincidental. But even with a lapse of many years it can be very difficult to discount the injury entirely as a contributory factor, especially if there is clear evidence of persisting brain damage with symptoms derived therefrom in the interim. Both organic disturbances and psychological aftermaths can sometimes be expected to operate over long periods of time in contributing to psychotic developments, vide the long interval characteristically observed between the onset of epilepsy and the onset of the schizophrenia-like psychoses related to it (p. 279).

Nevertheless, the generally accepted view is that a constitutional predisposition to the psychosis is a major factor in most cases of schizophrenia or affective psychosis following head injury. Early observations such as those of Tennent (1937) showed that evidence of special vulnera-

bility could usually be found, even in cases where the psychotic illness followed directly on the head injury and became manifest as soon as the acute confusional stage subsided. In five such cases of schizophrenia Tennent found that all had shown evidence of schizoid traits in the premorbid personality, and the illnesses followed the course of ordinary schizophrenia. Among four depressive psychoses three had been treated previously for similar affective disorder. The injuries therefore appeared to have made manifest, at a particular point in time, what would in all probability have followed other stressful situations in that particular person. Since then, however, other studies have combined to suggest more specific factors at work, at least where schizophrenia and hypomania are concerned.

Schizophrenia

All forms of schizophrenia have been reported after head injury—hebephrenic, paranoid and catatonic. Cases indistinguishable from the naturally occurring illness may be seen, also certain variants and atypical forms. Davison and Bagley (1969) review the extensive literature on the subject. Paranoid forms are reported to be especially common, also schizophrenia-like hallucinoses in which affect is preserved and thought disorder is not intrusive. Definite information appears to be lacking about the course of schizophrenia following head injury (Davison & Bagley 1969). Gradual progression to a state of organic deficits has been reported, and factors of adverse prognostic significance have included a latent interval before the onset of the illness, but such matters are far from well established.

Achté et al. (1967, 1969) produced one of the most comprehensive studies of psychotic illness after head injury by following 3552 Finnish soldiers from World War II for 22–26 years. During this period 92 patients (2.6%) developed psychoses resembling schizophrenia, which is well above the incidence to be expected in the general population. However, only 0.84% developed 'primary or malignant' schizophrenia, the remainder being schizophreniform or borderline states. These findings are strikingly similar to the earlier survey of Feuchtwanger and Mayer-Gross (1938), who found no excess of 'process' schizophrenia in brain-injured subjects when compared to the general population, but a considerable excess of schizophrenia-like states. Clearly these somewhat tantalising results reflect the difficulties encountered in achieving precise diagnostic criteria for schizophrenia.

Achté et al. found that patients with mild injuries developed schizophrenia more frequently than those with severe injuries, and suggested that factors independent of the injury usually played a decisive role. Detailed analysis of the location of brain damage failed to highlight any region as having special importance. Other investigations, however, have produced rather different findings, suggesting that brain damage may be important in itself, and especially damage to the temporal lobes.

Shapiro (1939), for example, reported 21 patients in whom schizophrenia had followed within a few hours to 3 months after injury. Ten showed no enduring evidence of injury to the brain but all had had evidence of a constitutional predisposition to schizophrenia; 11 did show evidence of brain damage, and in this group only two had positive family histories and seven had had well-integrated premorbid personalities. Thus in the former group the trauma appeared to have precipitated a latent tendency towards schizophrenia, whereas in the latter group brain injury would seem to have played a more direct role in the genesis of the disorder. Hillbom (1951) further supported an organic contribution by noting that 17 of his 20 patients with schizophrenia-like symptoms after head injury had sustained damage to the temporal lobes of the brain. Finally, Davison and Bagley (1969) have made an extensive and detailed review of evidence from many sources, including a re-analysis of data from several of the largest and most comprehensively reported series of patients in the literature. Their conclusions, which cannot be bettered to date, are that the incidence of schizophrenia-like psychoses after head injury is certainly greater than chance expectation, and that the trauma may often be of direct aetiological significance rather than merely a precipitating factor. The total evidence of genetic or personality predisposition was found to be less than in the naturally occurring disease, the early onset of the psychosis was related to severity of diffuse brain injury, and a possible special association with temporal lobe damage was upheld.

Paranoid psychoses

Paranoid developments may be the cause of much distress and disturbance after head injury. They not uncommonly colour the picture of post-traumatic dementia, or emerge as one facet of personality disturbance. Ideas of persecution or of marital infidelity often figure prominently. Frank paranoid psychoses occurring independently of schizophrenia were seen in 77 patients (2.1%) in Achté et al.'s (1967) series, and represented the second largest group of psychotic developments. The onset of the psychosis was often long delayed and typically occurred in middle age. No relationship was shown to severity of injury, and no particular site of brain damage could be especially incriminated. Evidence of premorbid instability

and early deprivation was common, and the development of the psychosis appeared often to be related to serious difficulties in life and to marital conflicts. Conspicuous jealousy was manifest in half of the cases. Almost a quarter were impotent and this proportion was significantly higher than in the series as a whole.

Affective psychoses

Affective psychoses may emerge in all degrees of severity, both in the presence and in the absence of objective signs of brain injury. Marked examples may be seen after minimal trauma. Here the idea of precipitation in the predisposed person has until recently gone largely unchallenged, though there are now some indications that factors related to brain injury may be operative in both major depression and mania.

Early suggestions in this direction include the two patients with depressive psychosis reported by Symonds (1937), in whom the symptoms developed before they had recovered from their acute post-traumatic confusion. Symonds proposed that as the patients could not appreciate the effects of the injury at the time, this was evidence favouring the view that the illness was the direct result of organic brain disturbance. Hoheisel and Walch (1952) suggested that hypothalamic damage might play a part, reporting five patients with lasting bipolar affective disorder after injuries implicating this part of the brain. But organic features were also present in the mental state, and the pictures were atypical in that the fluctuations of mood were rapid, lasting only hours or days. More suggestive was the patient reported by Parker (1957), in whom marked swings of mood developed within 10 weeks of a severe closed head injury, and continued over the next 10 years with repeated attacks of depression and hypomania. There was no previous history or family history of such disorder.

Recently Jorge et al. (1993) have produced evidence that major depression seen shortly after head injury may owe something to lesion location, and thus may be partly based in biological responses of the injured brain. Later-onset depression, by contrast, was more closely tied to psychosocial factors:

Of 66 consecutive patients admitted to hospital with closed head injury, 17 (26%) met DSM-III criteria for major depression at examination 1 month later. When compared to non-depressed patients they showed an increased past history of psychiatric disorder and a higher frequency of alcohol or drug abuse. Severity of injury was not significantly different, but analysis of lesion location from CT scans showed an excess of left anterior brain damage in the depressed group. Follow-up of 41 of the non-depressed group at 3 months, 6 months and 1 year revealed the later onset of major depression in 11 (27%). Again these showed an excess of previous psychiatric disorder, but lesion location was not a significant factor. Direct comparisons between early and later-onset depression groups confirmed the importance of lesion location in the former (frequency of subcortical involvement) and of poorer social functioning in the latter.

Manic psychoses after head injury have come under fresh appraisal following a number of scattered case reports. Bracken (1987) found 20 cases in the literature and reported a striking example of his own as follows:

A 48-year-old woman fell from a trapeze sustaining multiple injuries. She lost consciousness for 10 minutes and had a PTA of approximately 3 days. On recovery from her physical injuries she was confused and disorientated, and over the next few days became overactive and grandiose. This was 3 weeks after her fall. The CT scan was normal. On transfer to a psychiatric unit she was fully orientated but with marked pressure of speech and flight of ideas. She reported feeling very happy and 'very strong' and said she was writing a book which would be a best seller. There was no previous personal or family history of psychiatric disorder.

With chlorpromazine and haloperidol she gradually settled over the next 8 weeks. She then developed a depressive episode which responded to mianserin. Psychological tests suggested possible residual deficits in visual and verbal memory, and there was persistent diplopia due to fourth cranial nerve palsies. She was well again 3 months after the accident.

Clark and Davison (1987) reported two further cases, one setting in 2 months after closed head injury and the other 6 months after operation for post-traumatic subdural haematomas. Shukla *et al.* (1987) assembled 20 cases, the mania following closed head injury by a mean of 2.8 years (range 0–12 years). No patient had a family history of bipolar illness, though six had one or more relatives with histories of depression. Epilepsy had developed in half of the patients and appeared to be a predisposing factor. Among phenomenological features, Shukla *et al.* stressed that irritable moods were commoner than euphoria and that assaultive behaviour was common. Fourteen patients experienced recurrent mania without depression, and the sample as a whole showed an excess of manic over depressive episodes.

A study of 12 patients who developed mania after a variety of brain lesions—tumours, strokes and head injuries—was presented by Starkstein *et al.* (1988). None had had a previous history of affective disorder. In the group as a whole right hemisphere lesions were commoner than left, and involvement of structures functionally connected to the orbitofrontal cortex seemed to be strongly associated with the development of mania. Of the two head injuries in the series, one developed repeated manic episodes after an interval of 18 months,

and the other became manic 2 years after frontal injury associated with marked change of personality.

Manic psychosis after injury is nevertheless very much less common than major depression. Achté *et al.* (1967) found 47 cases of affective disorder (1.3% of their series) which could be described as 'psychotic' in intensity. Only three were typically manic–depressive, the rest showing depressive illnesses without manic phases.

Other psychoses

Other forms of psychosis considered by Achté *et al.* (1967) included epileptic psychoses, episodes of delirium, and rarer forms such as hysterical psychoses, hypochondriacal psychoses and hallucinoses. The epileptic psychoses consisted of confusional states associated with seizures, and were the next most frequent after schizophrenic and paranoid psychoses. States of delirium were due to abuse of alcohol or drugs. 'Hysterical' (or reactive psychogenic) psychoses were diagnosed when the disorder, though undoubtedly psychotic, could be seen as a reaction to difficulties, and were characterised by demonstrative behaviour and hysterical conversion symptoms. Hypochondriacal psychoses and simple hallucinoses were very rare.

Suicide

Death by suicide is very considerably increased among head-injured patients, accounting for up to 14% of all deaths (Vauhkonen 1959; Achté & Anttinen 1963). In Vauhkonen's series of 3700 soldiers injured in World War II, no less than 1% had committed suicide by 1957. In many there had been financial difficulties or family disputes arising from the disability, or the patient had been depressed on account of inability to adjust to a new occupation. The lesions were commonly in the frontal and temporal lobes of the brain. Achté and Anttinen (1963) found a tendency for the frequency of suicide to increase with the length of time elapsed since injury, reaching a maximum after 15–19 years. In the majority of cases the injuries had been severe, but the predominance of frontal or temporal lesions could not be confirmed. Most of the patients had had marital problems or other difficulties in personal relationships, and excessive drinking had often made these worse. Over half had been psychotic at some stage in the past, and it seemed that a change of personality had taken place in over 40%. Hillbom (1960) found that change of personality made the largest single contribution to the suicides in his series, occurring in approximately a third. In Achté *et al.*'s (1967) series, 41% of suicides had taken place during a depressive psychosis.

Neurotic disability

The post-traumatic neuroses represent the commonest of the psychiatric sequelae of head injury, in some series outnumbering all other forms of disability together (Ota 1969). Included here are a number of emotional disorders —minor depression; states of tension and anxiety, often with phobic symptomatology; neurasthenic reactions with fatigue, irritability and sensitivity to noise; cases of conversion hysteria and of obsessional neurosis; and most common of all, a variety of somatic complaints including headaches and dizziness, which may be the subject of anxious introspection and hypochondriacal concern. Patients suffering from post-traumatic stress disorder (PTSD) have been increasingly recognised among the victims of accidents, and careful enquiry will reveal the distinctive picture in a considerable number of cases, as described on pp. 194–5.

Neurotic symptomatology may be found in any and every combination, and patients will sometimes show different components from one time to another. Sometimes they occur as mild and transient disturbances during convalescence, but sometimes as severe and persistent disabilities which can present formidable therapeutic problems. They can also provide protracted difficulty with diagnosis:

A 50-year-old man was referred for assessment 6 years after an injury which had occurred when his lorry was involved in an accident. He had not been rendered unconscious at the time, and indeed the likelihood of trauma to the head had been very slight indeed. He had, however, been exposed to severe emotional shock. During the early months after the accident he had been extremely depressed and lacking in confidence, afraid to meet people and afraid to leave the house. He had attended regularly at a psychiatric day centre and was found to be grossly slowed and lacking in initiative or spontaneity. Psychological testing at this time had shown intelligence within the average range but certain memory tests raised the possibility of organic brain damage.

During the second year after injury he continued to be severely disabled with depression, insomnia and inability to concentrate. His wife described episodes at night in which he would wet the bed, wander from the house, or wake in fear claiming that spiders, frogs and snakes were biting him in bed. He was able to wash and dress himself but his wife had to shave him. She was noted to be excessively overprotective and to smother him with affection. At a medical interview in connection with a claim of compensation it was reported that he appeared to be largely unaware of his surroundings, and that it was virtually impossible to get coherent statements from him The clinical impression at this time was of 'a fairly rapid dementing process'.

During the third and fourth years after injury he continued to deteriorate, becoming increasingly retarded and vague, with incoherent speech and flattened affect, although the florid nocturnal features were no longer in evidence. He was unemploy-

able at the day centre and unable to take part in group activities. The diagnosis remained that of 'a steadily progressive cerebral degenerative process of uncertain cause'.

When examined 5 years after injury it was reported that he could not answer simple questions regarding his name, age or address. He exhibited a gross tremor of the hands, however, and his general demeanour now suggested an element of psychogenic elaboration.

Six years after injury he was referred anew for full evaluation, and for the first time was hospitalised at a considerable distance from his home. At first he was hesitant, anxious and incoherent, and the general picture strongly suggested an organic dementing process. Gradually, however, he improved with encouragement, and was observed at times to perform efficiently and well in occupational therapy. At times he would converse normally, display full orientation and reasonable memory for the events of the past 6 years. During his wife's visits, however, he relapsed into his earlier vague manner, became childishly dependent and expressed irrational fears about being abandoned or subjected to unnecessary operations.

By the end of his 4 weeks' stay in hospital it was obvious that he was capable of functioning at a normal level, and comprehensive investigations, including full psychometric testing, failed to reveal any evidence of brain damage. He remained somewhat tense but there was no evidence of depression. He expressed a desire to return to work, and appeared quite genuine in his statement that he wished to have nothing further to do with proceedings for compensation. He viewed the previous 6 years as 'blown out of all proportion' and 'being caught up in a network of problems'. Unfortunately his wife insisted on removing him from hospital before definitive steps could be taken to secure his return to work.

In this case the appearance of severe and progressive dementia proved ultimately to be due to a severe neurotic reaction in response to the psychological trauma of the accident. This had then become intensified and prolonged by the pathological degree of dependence which he had formed in relation to his wife. There was abundant evidence that his wife had colluded and reinforced this aspect of the situation, and in many ways the compensation motive appeared to be more active where his wife was concerned than with the patient himself.

(Lishman 1973)

Clearly these are the areas in which psychogenic factors come into their own, and can often be seen to operate exclusively. Severe neurosis is chiefly found in subjects prone to neurotic reactions generally, and post-traumatic neurotics, when compared to non-organic neurotics, have shown much the same range of complaints and a similar degree of vulnerability as judged by family and personal history (p. 173).

The important question arises, however, whether subtle aspects of brain damage may sometimes operate in addition as further contributory factors. Such matters are hard to disentangle and require comparisons among large numbers of subjects. Slater's (1943) study of soldiers subject to breakdown in war has already been described

(p. 173), and appeared to indicate that organic factors did play some part. But Slater was dealing essentially with acute neurotic breakdowns. In psychiatric practice it is chiefly the long-lasting post-traumatic neuroses which present for attention, and here in the great majority there is little to suggest that organic factors continue over the years to play a part. There is, for example, a conspicuous lack of relationship between severity of injury and severity of enduring neurotic disability, and neurotic symptoms are rare in the presence of marked intellectual or neurological disabilities. It would appear, indeed, that when the consequences of injury are not immediately obvious to external view, the patient with neurotic potential is more than ever liable to manifest subjective forms of complaint. Thus, in general, it seems fair to conclude with Ruesch and Bowman (1945) that the longer neurotic symptoms persist, the less likely they are to be the expression of brain damage.

Depression in this context shows the features conventionally regarded as characteristic of 'neurotic depression'. Anorexia, insomnia and early morning waking are rarely marked. The depression often fluctuates in severity, and may be responsive to change of activity and surroundings. Sometimes it proves to be no more than a readiness to be cast down by the troubles of daily life, and sometimes it is more accurately described as a state of gloomy and morose preoccupation.

Complaints of difficulty with concentration, lack of normal interest and minor forgetfulness may be marked, and will, of course, require careful investigation to exclude the coexistence of minor intellectual deficits. Paranoid features may sometimes be prominent. Hypochondriasis may be intrusive, with overconcern about real or imagined disabilities. Headache often fluctuates with the prevailing mood.

Anxiety may coexist with depression or stand alone. Persistent states of anxiety and tension tend to be seen after accidents of an especially frightening nature. In a survey of 188 consecutive victims of road traffic accidents Mayou *et al.* (1993) found that one-fifth suffered from an *acute stress syndrome* as an aftermath, with mood disturbance and horrific memories of the accident. At follow-up 3 months and 1 year later one-tenth of the series showed persisting mood disorder with anxiety as the major component. The acute stress syndrome was significantly related to neuroticism in the premorbid personality; continuing emotional distress was also especially likely in those who were psychologically and socially vulnerable, but was additionally strongly associated with chronic medical disability and social, financial and work problems.

The patient may dwell on the circumstances of the injury or relive it in terrifying dreams. There may be marked startle responses and phobic avoidance of situations which bring the accident to mind. These are the typical symptoms of *post-traumatic stress disorder*, which has attracted increasing attention since its inclusion as a distinct clinical syndrome in DSM-III (American Psychiatric Association 1980, 1987). It is now clear that the cardinal features of the syndrome must sometimes be sought out with care, in that patients may not always vouchsafe them directly. The disturbance can be long lasting and disabling, and in chronic form the patient may merely present with non-specific complaints of irritability, insomnia, depression and general inability to cope.

Three major groups of symptoms are characteristic (Gersons & Carlier 1992). The first consists of reliving the trauma, with nightmares, intrusive daytime recollections and sudden 'flashbacks' in which the traumatic event is re-experienced with realistic intensity. Rainey *et al.* (1987) have demonstrated that such flashbacks can be provoked by lactate infusions, much as panic attacks may be provoked in patients with panic disorder. Re-experiencing acute distress may be cued when the individual finds himself in a situation analogous to that of the accident. Anniversary reactions have also been described, for example at the anniversary of the event or on the birthday of a person who has died.

The second group of symptoms comprise avoidance behaviours in relation to anything likely to remind the patient of the trauma. Phobic avoidance is shown towards situations or activities that bring the traumatic event to mind, and there may be striking inability to remember key aspects of the experience. In an interesting experiment McNally *et al.* (1990) used a modified Stroop test to show that PTSD patients exhibited enhanced interference when dealing with words related to their traumatic experiences. Closely related to avoidance there may be emotional numbing and detachment, incapacity to express affection and a decrease in habitual interests. Painful guilt feelings are common.

The third group includes symptoms indicative of heightened arousal, such as sleep disturbance, startle responses, irritability and outbursts of anger, often accompanied by difficulties with memory and concentration.

It is still to some extent disputed how far PTSD may be delimited from other related disorders such as generalised anxiety disorder, panic disorder and simple phobias. McNally (1992) reviews the evidence which increasingly supports its validity as a distinct nosological entity, though it frequently coexists with other anxiety syndromes, also with depression and alcohol misuse.

The origin of the concept derives from studies of combat stress, and studies of surviving prisoners of war and victims of large-scale disasters in civilian life. Attention has more recently been turned to examples occurring in individuals after exposure to traumas such as rape, assault and road traffic accidents. Mayou *et al.* (1993) suggest that the last may prove to be the commonest cause of the syndrome in the general population. An important common denominator is not only exposure to a terrifying experience but also the risk, real or perceived, of coming close to death. Additional features likely to produce the disorder are when the individual had little or no control over the event, or if it was unanticipated and unpreventable (Raphael 1981).

A key issue is the primacy given to the acutely distressing event as the principal aetiological factor, unlike other stress reactions whose persistence often owes much to personal vulnerability and continuing adverse circumstances. With PTSD a dose–response effect has often been shown, with the probability of developing the disorder increasing as a function of the severity of the trauma experienced. Though widely accepted, the overriding importance of this 'stressor criterion' has not gone entirely unchallenged. After an Australian bush fire disaster, McFarlane (1989) found that premorbid personality factors were a better predictor of morbidity than were degree of exposure or losses sustained. Feinstein and Dolan (1991) have also emphasised individual variability in ability to cope with the stressful situation, independently of the severity of the traumatic situation itself.

Remarkably prolonged examples of PTSD have been reported in veterans from Vietnam and World War II, with persistence or recrudescence of symptoms even 40 years later (Kluznik *et al.* 1986; Speed *et al.* 1989). In such examples vulnerability factors appear to have been of less importance than the overwhelming nature of the trauma. It is well recognised that delays of many months, sometimes years, can elapse before symptoms are declared, the pictures then being indistinguishable from those of immediate onset (Watson *et al.* 1988).

Treatment consists of appropriate pharmacotherapy with tricyclic or other antidepressants, combined with cognitive–behavioural therapy (Davidson 1992). The phobias that develop may require additional specific treatment in their own right.

In Mayou *et al.*'s (1993) survey of road traffic accidents, one-tenth of the victims were judged to meet criteria for PTSD during the subsequent year. Overlap was seen with a rather larger group who suffered phobic anxiety in relation to driving or travelling generally, often with marked limitation of work, social and leisure activities. The development of PTSD was not associated with premorbid neuroticism or a history of previous psychological problems; the principal and very strong predictor was the rating of 'horrific' memories of the accident at interview shortly after it occurred. Predictors of phobic travel anxiety were similar. PTSD did not occur in subjects who had been unconscious and were amnesic for the accident. Similarly, Warden *et al.* (1997) were unable to find patients who met the full criteria for PTSD among head-injured veterans who had sustained substantial PTA.

It seems clear, nonetheless, that aspects of the typical picture can sometimes develop when the patient has lost consciousness after head injury, and in the presence of post-traumatic amnesia. Several of Warden *et al.*'s patients met the avoidance and arousal criteria for PTSD while lacking the re-experiencing criteria. The following case is also instructive:

A girl of 18 sustained a severe head injury in a road traffic accident and was unconscious for 3 or 4 days. She initially had a mild right hemiparesis, dysphasia, euphoria and poor memory, and spent 3 months in a rehabilitation unit. The duration of PTA was about 6 weeks. After 7 months she returned to her job as a bank clerk.

Fourteen months after the accident she was referred with symptoms of fatigue, poor concentration, dizziness, headache and difficulty in coping at work. There was a good deal of evidence of depression. Other symptoms, however, were not consistent with low mood or a postconcussional syndrome. She had intrusive thoughts several times a day about her friend who had died in the accident, and could not prevent these from entering her mind. They were triggered by situations where the two might conceivably have met, such as in the local supermarket. In addition she showed cognitive and physical avoidance of reminders of the accident, including hospitals in general. The thought of entering the rehabilitation unit where she had been treated was particularly anxiety-provoking. She did not talk about the accident to anyone, and continually postponed visiting the grave of her friend. She suffered from continual and irrational guilt, believing that she had somehow caused or failed to prevent the accident. Treatment involved cognitive–behavioural exposure techniques and resulted in marked improvement.

(McMillan 1991)

Other settings in which anxiety may figure prominently after head injury have been described by Roberts (1979). He found two characteristic patterns among long-term survivors of severe head injury, each rarely associated with more than minimal evidence of residual brain damage.

'Dysmnesic inadequacy' appeared as a neurotic response to memory or other less obvious cognitive defects; 'phobic imbalance' had emerged in response to various forms of vestibular damage. The anxiety was commonly manifest as reluctance to leave the home and could remain severely disabling over the course of several years. An example of the latter syndrome was as follows:

A man of 30 was seen 18 months after a head injury occasioned by a falling ladder. He had been only briefly concussed, but immediately afterwards became dizzy and vomited several times. Thereafter he experienced vertigo and nausea on sudden head movement, persisting on occasion 1 month later. During this time he became acutely phobic of enclosed spaces and travelling and gave in his notice at work.

The dizziness subsided but the phobias persisted and intensified. He began drinking heavily and quarrelled with his wife, who left him. Detailed examination showed no evidence of brain damage, and it was strongly argued by the defendants that his present neurotic condition owed much to alcohol and little, if anything, to the injury. The genuineness of the phobias themselves was called into question.

Examination, however, revealed two striking signs. On tilting him backwards to a horizontal position with the head to one side he developed bursts of nystagmus, indicative of labyrinthine damage. And on persuading him to enter the hospital lift he developed obvious signs of autonomic distress, with the pulse rate rising from 84 to 120 per minute. Subsequent neuro-ootological examination showed that the right labyrinth was completely non-functioning. Crucial evidence was thus available to demonstrate labyrinthine damage accruing from the injury, and to confirm the genuine nature of his phobias.

(Lishman 1978)

A *neurasthenic reaction* may incapacitate the patient for months or even years after injury. The patient complains that he is always tired, feels weak and is lacking in energy. Fatigue, both mental and physical, is readily precipitated by effort and there is marked curtailment of activity. A good deal of hypochondriacal concern typically comes to centre around such disability.

Irritability is among the most common of the emotional consequences of injury. The patient is more short-tempered than usual, more inclined to be snappy and stricter in matters of discipline. All grades are seen, extending to the serious loss of control of aggression already considered on pp. 188–9. It can be difficult to decide how far this represents an affective disturbance, or alternatively a personality change due to brain damage. Among patients with severe irritability persisting more than a year after injury, Lishman (1968) found little evidence to suggest that brain damage was an important factor in the group as a whole. Moreover it showed strong associations with other non-organic symptoms such as depression, anxiety and post-traumatic headache.

Hysterical symptoms have figured prominently in some series of head-injured patients, perhaps especially those admitted to army neurosis centres during times of war (Anderson 1942). The usual range of dissociative states may occur—fits, fugues, amnesias, Ganser states, motor paralyses, anaesthesias, and disturbances of speech, sight or hearing. The onset is usually soon after the injury, though later developments may occur in association with depression or when complex neurotic states emerge in relation to compensation issues.

Whitlock (1967a) compared 56 patients admitted to psychiatric units with hysterical conversion symptoms, with a group of controls matched for age and sex but suffering from depressive or anxiety states. Almost two-thirds of the patients with hysterical disorders had suffered significant preceding or coexisting brain disorder, compared with only 5% of the controls. Head injury had preceded the onset of hysterical phenomena within 6 months in 21% of the hysterical patients but in none of the controls. It would seem, therefore, that head injury may be a more frequent antecedent of the clinical picture of hysteria than is commonly supposed.

Obsessive–compulsive symptoms may emerge in susceptible individuals, usually as a colouring to pictures of depression or anxiety. Typically the patient is tense and ruminative, focusing his doubt, indecision and compulsive preoccupation on the injured head (Anderson 1942). Frank obsessional neuroses are rarely mentioned in the literature, with the exception of Hillbom (1960) who reported 14 examples among 415 cases (3.4%). Several also had depersonalisation symptoms, and epilepsy occurred in almost two-thirds which was three times the prevalence among the patients generally. Unlike the most common neuroses, Hillbom found that compulsive disorders tended to occur after reasonably severe rather than mild injuries. They appeared to be associated with lesions which had caused a noticeable but not very severe disability; in other words just those circumstances where the patient was still able to struggle against his disability in attempts to preserve his former standing.

More recently McKeon *et al.* (1984) have reported four patients with severe obsessive–compulsive disorders following directly on head injuries of moderate severity. Three were from a consecutive series of 25 patients suffering from obsessive–compulsive neurosis, the fourth from a pair of monozygotic twins discordant for the disorder. The prompt onset of symptoms, usually within 24 hours of injury, and the absence of premorbid obsessional traits in all but one case suggested that the brain trauma may have contributed directly to the neurosis by some physiogenic mechanism rather than acting as a non-specific stress.

Headache and dizziness are considered in detail immediately below.

Post-traumatic syndrome
('postconcussional syndrome')

The so-called 'post-traumatic syndrome' is the area around which most controversy has existed. The term is unsatisfactory, chiefly because it has come to be used in a somewhat capricious way. The syndrome is rarely clearly defined and different authors include different symptoms under the heading. Central to most definitions are headache and dizziness, but to these may be added fatigue, intolerance of noise and light, irritability, emotional instability, insomnia, difficulty with memory, difficulty with concentration or simply 'mental symptoms'. Minor degrees of overt intellectual impairment or of change in personality have sometimes also been included, which complicates the picture further. It is not surprising that the concept lacks clarity, and that its aetiology has remained in doubt. Lewis (1942) referred to it as 'that common dubious psychopathic condition—the bugbear of the clear-minded doctor and lawyer'.

Headache and dizziness are two of the most common

post-traumatic symptoms in this category. Their correct evaluation is of the utmost importance since both can be due to organic causes which may continue to operate for long periods of time. Such causes can be easily overlooked. On the other hand, both are also frequent concomitants of psychological stress.

Jones (1974), in a follow-up of 3500 patients discharged from emergency room practice after slight head injuries, illustrated the natural history of such complaints. Forty-two per cent of the patients became asymptomatic within 3 weeks of injury, another 57% continuing with headache, dizziness or both for at least 2 months. These too had become asymptomatic by the 1-year follow-up. Of the remaining 1% (36 patients), 30 were still symptomatic at 1 year and had continued to seek medical advice. Twenty of these had been hospitalised for re-examination but nothing abnormal was discovered. Four patients had developed haematomas or hydrocephalus, and two had died from non-related causes.

Persistent headache must raise the possibility of subdural haematoma (p. 411) and requires full and careful neurological examination, supplemented by electroencephalography and where possible CT scanning. It may derive from pathology in the upper cervical spine, especially after whiplash injuries. Examination may reveal focal areas of tenderness in the occipital muscles or in relation to healed scalp lacerations. Abnormal vasospastic responses of the arteries of the scalp, or tension headache due to muscle contraction, must also be considered. Friedman (1969) reviewed the numerous theories about the pathogenesis of chronic post-traumatic headache and concluded that there was no specific type. He suggested that it may mimic almost any form of chronic recurring headache, which supports the idea that no single mechanism is responsible.

Commonly, however, and particularly when headache has persisted for many months after injury, no demonstrable physical basis will be discovered. Headache which is diffuse, vaguely described and unremitting throughout the day, immediately raises the possibility of a psychogenic basis. The lack of clear precipitants which cause it to worsen, and resistance to analgesics, also bias the diagnosis in this direction. Frequently post-traumatic headache is found along with other components of neurotic disability, and may be noted to fluctuate in severity along with tension or depression.

Walker and Erculei (1969) analysed the features of post-traumatic headache seen in men 14–17 years after injury. The onset and termination of episodes was usually gradual, the headache was commonly bilateral and referred to frontal regions. Precipitants in order of frequency included noise, nervousness, work, eye strain and lack of sleep. Aggravating factors in order of frequency were noise, movement, light, coughing or sneezing, and breathing. The descriptions used by the patients were of dull ache, throbbing, pressure, sharp pain or scalp soreness. The headaches were occasionally coupled with nausea and visual disturbances, possibly representing migraine.

Dizziness must likewise be carefully distinguished from true vertigo, and in borderline cases testing of labyrinthine and vestibular function will be necessary by caloric and other tests, including where possible electronystagmography. Toglia (1969) showed the value of comprehensive tests of vestibular function in doubtful cases. Harrison (1956) stressed the frequency after head injury of positional nystagmus of the benign paroxysmal type. Seventeen of 108 post-traumatic subjects, most of whom complained of dizziness, showed characteristic nystagmus after rotation of the head to the right or left, then hyperextension of the neck so that the head is almost upside down and turned to one side. However, most of these patients reported a true rotational component to their dizziness, and they were seen within 2 weeks of injury. Care must also be taken to exclude orthostatic hypotension which may lead to feelings of syncope.

Dizziness which persists for many months will, like headache, often be found to have no demonstrable physical basis. Careful enquiry often shows that it is no more than uncertainty of balance, light headedness or subjective unsteadiness of gait. It is frequently associated with headache, likewise with other neurotic complaints. The syndrome of 'phobic imbalance' which may be traceable to early vestibular damage but then persists as a disabling neurosis, is described on p. 195.

When easily demonstrable causes cannot be found we are again left uncertain how much is physiogenic and how much psychogenic with regard to post-traumatic symptoms such as these. Some see them as founded in subtle cerebral pathology, while others argue that their roots lie in conflict and anxiety. Much may depend on whether the symptoms are under observation early or late after injury (Lishman 1988).

Thus in Lidvall *et al.*'s (1974) prospective study there was a marked and continuing decline in the percentage of patients displaying one or more postconcussional symptom, from 73% at 2 days to 24% at 3 months, the fall being particularly marked during the first post-injury week. In the longer term such changes doubtless continue. Jones (1974), in the follow-up cited above, found that only 1% of patients were still symptomatic after a year. It is therefore important to realise that very different populations of patients with postconcussional symptoms will be encountered according to whether they are studied weeks or years after the injury has occurred. The sum total of evidence, as reviewed elsewhere (Lishman 1988), suggests that organic influences may be operative in the early stages, but that psychogenic mechanisms may often be prepotent when the symptoms are long-lasting.

Organic contributions to the picture are suggested by the frequency of the 'clustered symptom complex' early after injury, with headache, dizziness and fatigue in the forefront of the picture. Some 50% of patients can be expected to experience such symptoms, even though in the majority they will subside with time. McMillan and Glucksman (1987), moreover, found that headache, dizziness, fatigue and sensitivity to noise and light were commoner after minor head injury than after injury to the limbs. Support for a physiogenic basis has also been forthcoming from investigations performed early after the injury. Taylor and Bell (1966) found prolongation of the cerebral circulation time, in comparison to controls, with recovery to normal sometimes coinciding with resolution of the symptoms. Brain stem auditory evoked responses have been found to be delayed (Rowe & Carlson 1980; Noseworthy *et al.* 1981; Montgomery *et al.* 1984, 1991), and lowered thresholds for tolerance to light and sound have been shown during the first few weeks (Waddell & Gronwall 1984).

Gronwall and Wrightson (1974) demonstrated slowed information processing on the PASAT test, with impairments at 1–2 months which progressively resolved thereafter. The task was to listen to digits presented continuously at a standard rate, and to add each digit to the one immediately preceding it. Patients with postconcussional symptoms showed diminished accuracy compared to those without, and took longer to achieve scores in the normal range. Moreover, symptoms could often be observed to recede in step as the patients' scores improved. MacFlynn *et al.* (1984) found similar delays on a four-choice reaction-time test at 24 hours and 6 weeks after injury, but without relationship to the presence or absence of postconcussional complaints.

In clinical terms, Rutherford *et al.* (1977) were able to show an association between the prevalence of symptoms at 6 weeks and the presence of diplopia, anosmia or other neurological abnormalities during the first 24 hours after injury. Some, though certainly not all, investigations have found a positive association with indices of severity of injury, such as duration of PTA or evidence of intellectual impairment (e.g. Keshavan *et al.* 1981). In these last respects, however, different studies have given remarkably diverse results.

Such observations support the notion of some alteration of cerebral function shortly after injury, which may well dictate the symptomatology in large degree. Even

then, however, non-organic factors appear to be operative. Rutherford *et al.* (1977) found that the symptom rate was significantly higher at 6 weeks in those who blamed their employers for their accidents than in those who blamed themselves, and Keshavan *et al.* (1981) showed that premorbid 'neuroticism' scores were influential at 3 months. Lidvall *et al.* (1974) found that patients with postconcussional symptoms during the early months had had more anxiety about the accident from the earliest stages, more worries about other ailments and more fears that they had sustained serious and possibly permanent brain damage.

Non-organic contributions become much easier to discern when patients are still complaining of symptoms after the first few months have gone by. At 3–6 months after injury, Kay *et al.* (1971) found that psychosocial factors were influential in distinguishing between patients with postconcussional symptoms and those without—marital status, social class, type of accident and previous history of psychiatric illness. No measure of severity of injury did so. Interestingly, however, as in Rutherford's study, disturbances of vision and anosmia persisting after the acute stages were commoner in the group with postconcussional symptoms. At 6 months also, Bohnen *et al.* (1991) have shown that patients with such symptoms have decreased tolerance to light and sound when compared with those without.

When persisting beyond a year, the evidence becomes overwhelming that such *long-lasting* postconcussional symptoms rest principally on psychogenic mechanisms. The component symptoms lack demonstrable relationship to extent or severity of brain damage (Norrman & Svahn 1961; Lishman 1968), show close concordance between injured and non-injured twin pairs (Dencker 1958, 1960) and figure with great frequency among litigants for compensation. They may indeed sometimes set in only after a latent interval following injury, and sometimes the fully-fledged syndrome follows an injury in which there has been no physical trauma to the head but merely severe emotional shock (Walshe 1958). Finally, such symptoms are remarkably rare, as long-continued and disabling features, in the presence of marked intellectual impairment or neurological disability.

With certain techniques it is sometimes claimed that disturbed brain function can be demonstrated even some years after minor head injury. Ewing *et al.* (1980), for example, showed impairment on tests of memory and vigilance under conditions of hypoxic stress 1–3 years later; even so there was no suggestion that this was related to the presence or absence of postconcussional symptoms. Rather more convincing in relation to post-concussional symptoms was Watson *et al.*'s (1995) follow-up of a sample of young mildly injured patients. Residual psychiatric morbidity at 12 months, as reflected in Present State Examination scores, was associated with delays in brain stem auditory evoked responses at 24 hours and with delayed recovery of left temporal EEG rhythms over the course of the first 6 weeks. These associations, however, failed to reach statistical significance.

Thus it may be concluded that the 'post-traumatic syndrome' has a complex aetiology in which numerous factors come to play a part. A model is proposed (Lishman 1988) whereby the cerebral dysfunction engendered by head injury, even mild head injury, commonly yields a nuclear group of symptoms, headache, dizziness and fatigue being prominent among them. At the outset these are largely organic in origin, but they are destined to recede by a natural process of healing towards the status quo. If the patient is able to feel untroubled by them, and if left undisturbed by his environment, recuperation will in favourable cases be complete.

However, obstacles to their resolution may arise, and it seems likely that these are mainly of a psychological nature. They may lie in the patient's tendency to worry unduly and to build anxiety around the symptoms, in the handling he receives from those around and the attention he is encouraged to focus on them. Obstacles may arise from other sources of distress—domestic difficulties, resentment about the accident, the need to cope too early or to face an uncongenial job. He may become significantly depressed, and there may be conflict over compensation.

Secondary neurotic developments, founded on anxiety, are then sometimes destined to become long lasting. What has initially been based in physiogenic disturbance readily thereafter becomes prolonged, and nonetheless disabling, by virtue of a complicated interplay of psychogenic factors.

Such a model is broadly confirmed by the evidence presently available, and would appear to apply to the great majority of patients. Doubtless, however, exceptional instances occur, and detailed clinical appraisal of all factors is essential whether the patient presents for attention early or late after injury.

Jacobson (1995) presents a more complex model which attempts to avoid a rigid distinction between physiological disorder and psychological disturbance in the genesis and maintenance of symptoms. Cognitive–behavioural factors, including social stresses, personal resources and coping processes are seen as influential over the entire time course of the syndrome, much also depending on individual differences in sensory sensitivity and psychophysiological reactivity. Analogies are drawn with the large range of factors known to be important in relation,

for example, to persistent pain. Again the model serves as an important focus around which to explore treatment options in the individual patient.

Whiplash injuries

Whiplash injury results from a sudden unexpected jolt to the body while the head is free to move at the time of impact. The common cause is a road accident collision. Since the normal protective reflexes which splint the neck cannot come into operation it is subjected to abrupt hyperextension/flexion or rotational stresses. The result is damage and bruising to the ligaments and other soft tissues of the neck. By any strict definition bony injuries, dislocations or disc protrusions of the spine are excluded, likewise direct trauma to the head.

The condition has attracted a great deal of attention on account of the sometimes prolonged sequelae, which include local pain and stiffness along with considerable invalidism due to headache and nervous complaints. Characteristically such patients become more disabled, and handicapped for longer periods of time, than would be anticipated from the mild character of their accidents (Gay & Abbott 1953). Many such patients are soon involved in litigation, and it is often a matter of dispute whether enduring symptoms are determined by organic or psychological factors. When complaints of difficulty with concentration and memory are prominent it may further be suggested that brain damage has been sustained, despite the lack of any direct trauma to the head.

Typically the victim's car is struck from behind, often while stationary. The result is acute shock and bewilderment, and there may be momentary dazing and confusion. 'Concussion' has been reported in 20–60% of cases—momentary loss of consciousness followed by feeling stunned and out of contact with surroundings. In many cases, however, it will be hard to judge whether this represents a true impairment of consciousness or a transient episode of dissociation occasioned by stress. Pain and stiffness in the neck, often with headache, develop within minutes or hours, but may be delayed until the following day. In an analysis of 190 acute cases Balla and Iansek (1988) reported neck ache in 90%, headache in 75% and limitation of neck movement in 50%. As in most series they found a female preponderance, unlike the usual male preponderance in other types of accident. Tenderness and spasm of the neck muscles is often severe, with pain spreading to the shoulders and back and into the occipital region. Sharp radicular pain may radiate to the lower jaw, arms and upper anterior chest.

Treatment with rest, analgesics and temporary immobilization in a soft collar allows resolution of symptoms over the following weeks in favourable cases. The remain-der, varying in different reports from 25 to 50%, progress to develop the *'late whiplash syndrome'*, in which neck and head pain persist for many months along with symptoms reminiscent of the post-traumatic syndrome (p. 196). Balla and Iansek (1988) reported 300 patients with symp-toms persisting beyond 6 months: 98% continued to com-plain of neck ache, 97% of headache, 85% of neck stiffness and 39% of arm ache. Other symptoms included anxiety in 63%, irritability in 57%, depression in 50%, insomnia in 47%, poor concentration in 23% and loss of libido in 7%. Not dissimilar figures were reported by Radanov *et al.* (1994).

The headache is mainly occipital but can be generalised or frontal. It may be dull, sharp or throbbing, and is often accompanied by dizziness. Additional symptoms include prominent fatigue and decreased tolerance to light and sound. Difficulty with sleeping may be due to distressing dreams of the accident. The disability engendered is often remarkably severe, with inability to work and curtailment of social life. In unfavourable cases the syndrome may persist for several years.

The genesis of this chronic syndrome is open to much uncertainty. *Organic components* may lie in pain referred from strains to the ligaments and the small apophysial joints of the spine, aggravated no doubt by spasm of the cervical muscles. Disinclination on the part of the patient to attempt gradual mobilisation may lead to a vicious circle of continuing tension from efforts to guard and splint the spine. Much of the psychological distress may stem from the pain and disability engendered in this manner.

The possibility that *brain damage of a subtle nature* may sometimes make a contribution is hard to rule out with certainty. The sudden bending and stretching of the neck may conceivably cause brain stem contusion, and sheer stresses set up within the brain may have led to neuronal damage. For this, however, there has been little direct evi-dence in human cases.

Experiments by Ommaya *et al.* (1968) in lightly anaesthetized monkeys have, by contrast, shown that brain contusions can result from purely whiplash injuries. Nineteen of 50 rhesus monkeys showed evidence of concussion, by way of temporary loss of responses to stimuli and abolition of the corneal reflexes. Fifteen of these had macroscopic evidence of brain damage in the form of haemorrhages and contusions over the brain. The main sites involved were the parasagittal parietal regions, over the medial supracallosal surfaces of the hemispheres, the tempo-ral and frontal poles, the inferior orbital-temporal regions, and the brain stem and upper cervical cord. Moreover such contu-sions were unaccompanied by obvious neurological deficits, pro-viding a possible analogy with human cases. Gennarelli *et al.* (1982) have described diffuse axonal injury within the hemi-

spheres, cerebellum and upper brain stem in monkeys subjected to sudden angular head rotation, but only in those which were rendered unconscious for considerable periods of time.

Possibilities of brain damage are also raised by reports of momentary 'concussion' in a proportion of cases, as already described. An example of amnesia lasting for 72 hours was reported by Fisher (1982a):

A woman of 67 was struck from behind while a passenger in a stationary car, sustaining a whiplash injury but no direct trauma to the head. When asked immediately if she was hurt she replied 'What am I doing here?', and proved to be muddled and to have no idea of the purpose of the journey. She was nevertheless fully alert. When examined 2.5 and 10 hours later she was still disori-entated and unable to retain any new information. She could not recall anything of the past 4 days and showed faulty recall of the previous weeks and months. She repeatedly asked where she was and what time it was. There was horizontal nystagmus to the left but no other neurological abnormality. Seventy-two hours after the accident her memory had returned to normal. She could finally recall the car being struck but remained amnesic for the 48 hours that followed. Suggested explanations included sheer stresses in the brain, or alternatively interference with circulation in the vertebral arteries.

Neuropsychological testing has occasionally appeared to uphold the presence of mild brain damage. Bohnen *et al.* (1993) reported two patients complaining of cognitive difficulties some 2 years after their injuries; both showed impairment of information processing and clear dysfunc-tion on tests of memory, despite well-preserved intelli-gence and normal perceptual and motor functions. Both also showed otoneurological dysfunction by way of gaze nystagmus. There has been little else, however, to support the presence of brain damage in the generality of whiplash patients. Electroencephalography has shown abnormalities in some studies but not in others (Torres & Schapiro 1961; Jacome 1987). MRI scans were normal in the four patients examined by Maimaris (1989).

Psychogenic factors are strongly suspected of making an important contribution in many of the prolonged cases. In the first place, symptoms often worsen steadily over several weeks after the accident which seems inconsistent with organic pathological factors (Gotten 1956). More-over, the development of essentially neurotic disability is understandable in terms of the sudden shock attaching to the acute experience, especially since consciousness is usually fully retained throughout. Further apprehension is generated when disturbing symptoms begin without warning some time later, often on the succeeding day (Gay & Abbott 1953). Thus elements of post-traumatic stress disorder (p. 194) may be discerned in the high inci-dence of anxiety and in insomnia with recurrent dreams. The spasm and tension in the neck muscles may them-selves owe much to emotional tension.

The resulting disability may sometimes be seen to solve interpersonal problems, focus attention on the patient, provide an escape from work or fulfil some other psychological need. Certainly once symptoms have developed fully they tend to persist for many months and to be refractory to reassurance and other treatments. The pictures of 'neurosis' that result are strikingly similar to those of the post-traumatic syndrome as discussed on p. 196 *et seq.*, and a similar range of determinants may often apply. Mayou *et al.* (1993) found a strong relationship between emotional disorder 1 year after whiplash injury and scores of neuroticism in the premorbid personality.

The role of litigation will often be thought to be important, and surveys of litigants have highlighted psychological factors in the maintenance and prolongation of symptoms. Among patients seen for medicolegal assessment, Pearce (1989) reported spurious weakness of grip in over half and non-anatomical sensory loss in one-third. He concluded rather cryptically that 'unusually severe or protracted complaints may demand explanations which lie outside the fields of organic and psychiatric illness'. It is clear, however, that some patients remain symptomatic after settlement of all compensation issues (Gotten 1956; Maimaris *et al.* 1988; Newman 1990), also that the chronic syndrome can be seen when litigation has not been at issue.

Few studies have attempted to explore the relative importance of organic and non-organic factors in the aftermath of whiplash injuries. An exception is the report from Radanov *et al.* (1994), who followed 117 patients prospectively over a 12-month period. Generalisation from their findings is, however, difficult since the Swiss system of accident insurance meant that none of the subjects was engaged in litigation. At all follow-up examinations (3 months, 6 months and 12 months), the outcome was strongly related to the severity of the neck injury, as reflected in initial symptoms of radicular irritation and intensity of neck pain. These proved in effect to be the most reliable indicators of recovery. Other predictors of poor outcome at 6 and 12 months were indicative of the initial reaction to the injury, namely severity of sleep disturbance and scores of 'nervousness', both of which may have been attributable to pain. By contrast no relationship could be found to aspects of psychosocial stress at any phase of recovery, and 'neuroticism' as measured by a personality inventory showed a negative correlation with recovery at 6 and 12 months.

These results therefore serve to play down the importance of non-organic factors, at least in non-litigants. The authors accept that additional factors developing during follow-up could yet be important, for example anxiety and depression consequent upon the frustrations imposed by the disability. They suggest that a dynamic relationship obtains between damage to cervical structures and problems in adjusting to damage-related symptoms, i.e. that progress is determined by a complex interplay between severity of injury and the reaction induced by the trauma.

Head injury in childhood

The after-effects of head injury in children differ from those in adults in certain important respects. The reasons are to be sought in several different factors. On the one hand the neural apparatus as a whole appears to be more resilient to damage in childhood. Yet conversely certain functions are particularly vulnerable when they are damaged during the course of their development. The issues involved, and the complex balance between advantageous and disadvantageous effects when the brain is damaged before maturity, are discussed by Rutter (1993). The social setting of the child is also different to the adult's and will have important influences—the compensation motive is likely to be absent, whereas the cognitive and emotional aftermaths of injury are likely to hamper school work and call forth interactions with the parents which may have important effects.

There is general agreement that the overall incidence of sequelae is lower in children than adults (Black *et al.* 1969). In physical terms this can partly be attributed to the greater pliability of the skull and intracranial structures in childhood. The pressure effects of the blow will be better absorbed, vessels less readily ruptured and transient rises of intracranial pressure more easily accommodated. The powers of restitution and compensation also seem to be greater in the young nervous system; Teuber and Rudel (1962) review evidence indicating that animals are less disabled from brain lesions sustained early in life than in maturity, at least where elementary sensorimotor functions are concerned. Thus severe head injury in childhood may be followed by grave neurological defects, but these quite often regress rapidly; similarly early psychiatric symptoms can sometimes be observed to resolve remarkably well (Hjern & Nylander 1962).

Valid comparisons between groups of child and adult patients are, however, difficult. In particular it is hard to use the usual criteria of severity of injury when comparing cases. The length of PTA cannot be measured accurately in young children, and it is uncertain that it carries the same implications for severity as in adults. Duration of unconsciousness or disorientation can also be hard to assess—immediately after injury the child may be apathetic, fretful and morose, this later clearing abruptly, suggesting that emotional disturbance has been the principal manifestation of impairment of consciousness (Guttmann & Horder 1943).

The form which residual disturbances take is also rather different in children as described below. Cognitive disturbances will be influenced by the stage of development which has been reached. Whilst in adults somatic symptoms such as headache and dizziness are the most frequent and long-lasting effects, these are rarely disabling in children. Instead certain serious disorders of behaviour may be much in evidence, and tend to take distinctive forms as described below.

Cognitive defects have different implications compared to adults, since mental skills are in the process of development. The child stands not only to lose what has already been acquired, but also to prejudice chances of future intellectual growth.

In practice profound intellectual disablement appears to be distinctly rare as a result of head injuries sustained other than at birth. This is probably because injuries of the necessary severity are not often compatible with survival. However, occasional examples of severe dementia do occur in children, usually in association with spasticity and other marked neurological defects.

More commonly the child is observed to be set back only temporarily, and to make good in the months that follow. Recently acquired abilities to walk or talk may be lost, or school work is found to be impaired for a time in relation to his fellows. For a while he may appear to be more backward than is truly the case, as a result of ill-sustained attention, sluggishness or ready mental fatigue. While they persist, however, such factors can hamper education to a serious degree. Behavioural changes are sometimes even more disruptive of progress at school, leading to persistent under-achievement even when no intellectual loss can be identified.

Chadwick *et al.* (1981) have reported one of the few prospective studies of the cognitive sequelae of head injury in school-age children. A group of 29 children with 'mild' injuries (PTA less than 7 days) and 31 with 'severe' injuries (PTA more than 7 days) were followed with repeat testing for up to 27 months. Twenty-eight non-head-injured children served as controls. When the PTA had been less than 24 hours in duration there was no convincing evidence of intellectual impairment, even transient in nature. Deficits were common, however, when the PTA had exceeded 3 weeks and in some cases could still be detected at the final follow-up examination. Transient impairments, resolving completely, seemed to characterise those in the intermediate PTA range. In general visuospatial and visuomotor skills tended to be more severely affected than verbal skills. Substantial recoveries in intellectual function could be charted during the

follow-up period; improvement was most rapid during the early months, but further gains were observed for a year and sometimes continued into the second post-injury year as well. A definitely adverse effect upon school performance was observed only in children with the most severe injuries, where the PTA had exceeded 3 weeks in duration.

Klonoff *et al.* (1977), in a 5-year prospective study of a large cohort of head-injured children, were able to demonstrate the long time-scale of the improvements that could occur. Serial testing, carried out along with matched non-injured controls, showed that recovery sometimes extended over the whole 5-year period, with significant gains still occurring between the fourth and fifth year follow-up examinations.

The precise effects of childhood injury on intellectual function are incompletely understood. Teuber and Rudel (1962) illustrated the complex relationships which may obtain between brain injury in childhood and performance on different types of task. Performance on one of the perceptual tasks which they examined was lowered by injury at any age, another revealed the effects only up to the age of 11 but then diminished as the child grew older, whereas a third task revealed no impairment while the child was young but from 11 onwards the deficits became increasingly apparent. Clearly the dynamics of cerebral organisation change during the course of development, so that functions which are crucial at one stage can later be supplemented by others, or deficits which at first remain latent may later be revealed.

Among focal defects, dysphasia has been most closely investigated. A change in cerebral dominance is possible after unilateral brain injury in early life, and this plasticity appears to persist in some degree in later childhood (p. 40). Complex relationships obtain, however, with respect to the reorganisation of language and other cognitive functions, as shown by Varga-Khadem and Polkey's (1992) review of the effects of hemi-decortication in childhood. A particular feature of childhood dysphasia is often the quantitative reduction of spoken and written language, extending even to gesture activities (Alajouanine & Lhermitte 1965). Spontaneous speech is sparse, and the child must be strongly encouraged to get him to reply to questions. Loss of acquired language is sometimes less striking than subsequent slowing of speech maturation, especially in very young children who are still in the process of learning to talk. Comprehension difficulties may only become obvious when the child must sustain attention for long periods as at school, or difficulties in learning to read or spell may later emerge even when spoken speech has made a good recovery. Thus even though the prognosis is better than in adults, Alajouanine and Lhermitte found that continuing difficulties were still to be found in a large proportion of children.

Behaviour disturbances are repeatedly stressed as the commonest and most disruptive of the sequelae of head injury in children (Dillon & Leopold 1961; Black *et al.* 1969). Commonly they consist of restless overactivity ('hyperkinesis'), impulsive disobedience at home and at school, and explosive outbursts of anger and irritability. Marked delinquency may appear by way of stealing, cruelty and destructiveness. Black *et al.* (1969) followed up an unselected cohort of 105 children injured between the ages of 2 and 14 years and showed the incidence of such changes. At 1 year after injury approximately 20% of the children showed behaviour disorders which had not been present before. The most disruptive effects on adjustment were produced by hyperkinesis (present in 32% and appearing as a new phenomenon in 15%) and problems with anger control (present in 20% and a new development in 13%). Both represented a very definite increase in incidence compared to the pretraumatic state. Problems of discipline such as lying, stealing or destructiveness were a major problem in 10%, and excessive lethargy or passivity had persisted since the accident in 8%. Sleep disturbances and problems with appetite were also occasionally observed. Hyperkinesis was commoner in younger than older children, and behaviour disturbance generally was more frequent in boys than girls.

Brown *et al.*'s (1981) careful prospective study of 50 school-age children demonstrated that the development of new behavioural disorder was related to severity of injury. The group with PTAs of less than 1 week showed a raised level of *pre*-accident psychiatric disturbance compared to controls, but no increase following injury. By contrast approximately half of those with PTAs exceeding 1 week developed new behavioural disorders, this being commoner the more severe the injury. In general there was little that was specific about the forms of psychiatric disturbance encountered in this study, the sole exception being a tendency to disinhibition and socially inappropriate behaviour reminiscent of the adult frontal lobe syndrome. Hyperkinesis in particular did not emerge in this sample as strongly related to brain damage.

Both organic and non-organic factors can be discerned in the development of post-injury behavioural disturbances and it can be difficult to apportion the blame. The combination of restless hyperactivity, impulsiveness and resistance to discipline is reminiscent of that seen after encephalitis lethargica (p. 353), and has long been regarded as a distinctive result of brain damage in childhood (Strecker & Ebaugh 1924; Blau 1936). The child appears to be dominated by instinctual and emotional impulses, as though he has lost the inhibiting and restraining influences normally acquired during development. As with postencephalitic children, and unlike delinquents generally, these children are said to know that what they do is wrong and to realise that they lack the ability to control their misbehaviour. In these respects an organic origin is strongly suggested.

There is evidence, however, that other factors contribute as well. Brown *et al.* (1981) were able to demonstrate the influence of the child's pre-accident behaviour, his cognitive level and his psychosocial circumstances in leading to behaviour disorder, in addition to the effects of brain damage. Harrington and Letemendia (1958) compared a group of head-injured children attending a child guidance clinic with a group who were not under psychiatric care. The latter, as expected, showed less psychiatric disorder, but proved to have had the more severe injuries. In general terms the pretraumatic personality and family setting of the child emerged as more important for the psychiatric outcome than the nature and severity of the injury. A favourable outcome was possible even after severe injuries provided the child had previously been well adjusted; and the families of children who presented with chronic behaviour disturbance showed a high incidence of emotional and psychiatric disorder among immediate relatives. The authors were further led to challenge the specificity of the pictures so often described after head injury. The range of disturbances in their material was similar to that encountered in non-organic child psychiatry generally, with aggression, tics, tension habits and hyperactive behaviour heading the list.

Clearly, as with head injuries in adults, the environment of the child and his premorbid constitution will have important effects, particularly where later progress is concerned. But it would seem unwise to discount the organic contribution entirely. The observations already outlined imply a definite organic stamp in the more severe examples, and in Black *et al.*'s (1969) series the incidence of new behavioural disorders was identical in the groups with and without evidence of premorbid behavioural difficulties.

Whatever its origin, post-traumatic behaviour disturbance can have serious consequences in terms of school achievement, which may be markedly impaired despite good preservation of intellect to formal testing. In the presence of severe hyperkinesis and impulsivity schooling may be completely disrupted. Minor degrees of disturbance are sometimes tolerated for several years before psychiatric help is sought, and the apparent worsening may then be due to the manifestations becoming more marked as the child's behavioural repertoire expands. Sometimes self control is gradually re-established as the child matures, and hyperkinesis appears usually to wane as the child grows older. Hill (1989) discusses the serious impact which personality changes after severe head injury can have on schooling and social development; blunting of emotional responsiveness may make continuing social education extremely difficult, and loss of tact and judgement may lead to social isolation, particularly in adolescents. Considerable adverse effects on personality may accrue from changes in self appraisal and self identity during a vulnerable phase of development.

Neurotic disturbances are by contrast rare in head-injured children. Nightmares, tension habits and hysterical features are said to be uncommon as enduring features unless the child has shown obvious maladjustment beforehand. Headache may be present in the early post-traumatic phase, but is rarely prolonged and usually has negligible effects on the child's adjustment. It becomes more pronounced and frequent as age at time of injury increases, and in older children may approach the adult pattern with psychological and social features which account for its continuation (Guttmann & Horder 1943; Black *et al.* 1969). Dizziness is likewise very rare after injuries early in life.

Head injuries due to boxing

The question of 'chronic traumatic encephalopathy' in boxers is of special interest, because here serious sequelae appear to follow repeated mild head injuries, each in itself leading to no more than brief concussion. The mechanisms underlying such a cumulative effect are unknown, though the finding of beta-amyloid deposition in the brain may be a pointer towards the pathophysiological process (p. 207). It is interesting, moreover, that Gronwall and Wrightson (1975) have been able to show that even a single concussion renders the brain slower to recover from a subsequent episode. Using a sensitive psychological test procedure (p. 198), they demonstrated that rates of information processing were slower after a second mild head injury than after a single injury of equivalent severity, despite a mean of 4.5 years between the two. The time taken to recover to normal levels of functioning was also significantly delayed.

The whole subject has been a matter of dispute for many years. The picture of 'punch-drunkenness' in retired boxers is widely recognised, but the supporters of boxing have sought to attribute it to coincidental neurological disease or alcoholism, rather than blaming the patient's boxing career. Several series of cases have combined to suggest a syndrome with highly characteristic features, but have been open to criticism on the grounds of special selection (Martland 1928; Critchley 1957; Spillane 1962; Mawdsley & Ferguson 1963). Roberts'

(1969) extensive survey, described below, was therefore particularly important in establishing the syndrome as a valid entity, and in providing clear indications that the boxing career had been responsible.

In its fully developed form the syndrome consists of cerebellar, pyramidal and extrapyramidal features, along with a varying degree of intellectual deterioration. This unusual combination of neurological features provides a characteristic picture, and suggests that a distinctive pathological process is responsible. Severe examples date mostly from boxing careers pursued before World War II when medical control over boxing was less rigorous than at present. Fairground booth boxing appears to have been especially hazardous. However, there are indications, especially from CT scan and neuropsychological studies, that present safeguards are still inadequate to prevent brain injury, as will be discussed below. Kaste *et al.* (1982) suggest, indeed, that modern medical controls create a dangerous illusion of safety.

Neurological features

In mild examples there is dysarthria, facial immobility and poverty and slowness of movement. Unsteadiness of gait may not be present, but evidence of asymmetrical pyramidal lesions is common from an early stage. At its most severe there is disabling ataxia, disequilibrium, a festinant gait, tremor of the hands and head, and spasticity or rigidity of the limbs. All grades of cerebellar, pyramidal and extrapyramidal disorder may be seen between these extremes. The disabilities usually set in towards the end of the boxing career while the patient is still relatively young. Sometimes the onset is acute and can be traced to a series of particularly hard fights, thereafter dictating retirement.

Roberts (1969) carefully traced a random sample of professional boxers who had held a professional licence for at least 3 years between 1929 and 1955. Of the 250 boxers chosen for study, 224 were available for examination. Thirty-seven (17% of the total) showed evidence of the characteristic syndrome, while 11 more had other neurological lesions which could not be attributed to boxing. Approximately one-third of the 37 were judged to be affected severely enough to be recognisable by a layman as 'punch drunk'. The clinical picture, while varying in degree, was remarkably constant from one case to another, and appeared distinct from other common neurological diseases. Moreover the prevalence of the syndrome increased with increasing exposure to boxing as judged from the history, again strongly upholding a causal relationship. A number of other isolated symptoms such as vertigo and impairment of vision also increased with the length of exposure, but epilepsy occurred no more frequently than in the general population.

Progression of the disablement has been described as characteristic, but Roberts found that the majority of cases remained static once boxing was discontinued. Occasionally the condition had become more obvious with advancing age, but it was hard to distinguish this from the changes associated with ageing generally. However, undoubted progression was seen in four cases, three with extrapyramidal disturbance and one with cerebellar symptoms and dementia, at an age and with a rapidity that was clearly independent of ageing. In a few cases there had been undoubted improvement after retirement from the ring.

Psychiatric features

Almost half of Roberts' 37 cases showed intellectual and personality changes indicative of dementia in addition to their neurological disablement. This occurred with all degrees of severity. Nine had severe memory impairment, often in conjunction with apathy, irritability or marked disinhibition. In five others thinking was profoundly slowed. Two were demented to a degree which required permanent hospitalisation. In the series as a whole subjective difficulty with memory increased in proportion to the length of the boxing career.

The incidence of personality change was hard to assess, but the boxers' wives often described irritability, progressive apathy and liability to outbursts of temper. Severe paranoid illness appeared to be common, particularly in subjects who showed intellectual deterioration.

Johnson (1969) paid special attention to the psychiatric features in 17 ex-boxers with chronic traumatic encephalopathy. The neurological features had usually appeared before the psychological manifestations, and each could then follow an independent course. Four main areas of psychiatric disturbance were apparent.

A *chronic amnesic state* was present in 11 patients, chiefly affecting recent memory and without any tendency to confabulate. Progression was uncommon, and apart from social embarrassment the memory deficit caused little concern. *Progressive dementia* with disorganisation of intellect and personality occurred in three cases, and paralleled progressive neurological disablement in two. *Morbid jealousy* had led to the primary psychiatric referral in five cases, with persistent accusations and sometimes frank delusions concerning the wives' infidelity. All showed evidence of brain damage, and some degree of impotence appeared to be an important determining factor. *Rage reactions*, with uncontrolled outbursts of anger and violence, were prominent in three patients. All had shown impul-

sive aggressive behaviour as a life-long trait, and the worsening after boxing was attributed by the patients to decreased alcohol tolerance. In addition five had shown evidence of psychotic illness; one a chronic paranoid state associated with organic memory disturbance, two with transient paranoid–hallucinatory states, one with endogenous depression, and one with acute catatonic schizophrenia which developed after a fight and was followed by gradual intellectual and social deterioration.

More recent investigations

More recent studies have concentrated on 'modern era' boxers who have fought under present medical controls. The debate now centres on whether such controls have rendered boxing safe, and the answer would appear to be in the negative. The consensus of recent evidence from brain imaging and psychometry is that chronic as well as acute brain damage is still prone to occur, even in comparatively young boxers who are pursuing successful careers. Cerebral atrophy, as revealed by CT scans, has been found to antedate the development of overt signs of brain damage; and sometimes to show association with the number of bouts fought rather than with the number of knock-outs sustained, suggesting a cumulative effect of multiple subconcussive blows to the head (Casson *et al.* 1982, 1984; Ross *et al.* 1983). In the field of amateur as opposed to professional boxing the evidence is less straightforward, with negative as well as positive findings as described below.

Earlier studies, while giving grounds for concern, suffered from lack of control comparisons. Casson *et al.* (1982) reported mild to moderate cerebral atrophy on CT in five of 10 active professional boxers aged 20–31 years. None of the five showed mental or neurological abnormalities. Atrophy was detected in three of six professionals and one of eight amateurs by Kaste *et al.* (1982), the mean age of the group being 31. Ross *et al.* (1983) found a significant relationship between the number of bouts fought and both ventricular enlargement and EEG changes in a group of 40 ex-boxers, the presence of CT abnormalities being associated with more frequent neurological symptoms and signs.

Casson *et al.*'s second study focused on boxers with no known medical, neurological or psychiatric illness, and without histories of drug or alcohol abuse (Casson *et al.* 1984). All 18 had been active only since the Second World War, and 15 since 1960. Thirteen were professionals and five were amateurs. Eight were found to have atrophy on the CT scan, three also showing a cavum septum pellucidum. Seven of the 13 had abnormal EEGs. Neuropsychological testing revealed deficits in several areas of functioning, performance being particularly poor on tests of short-term memory. Neuropsychological impairment, like cerebral atrophy, showed a significant relationship to the number of bouts fought, and was significantly more common in those with CT or EEG abnormalities. Three of the older subjects had a clinically obvious organic mental syndrome manifest by disorientation, confusion and memory loss.

McLatchie et al. (1987) restricted attention to active amateur boxers, aged 18–49 years. Seven of the 20 showed minor neurological abnormalities such as up-going plantar responses or a degree of manual incoordination, eight were judged to have abnormal EEGs, and nine of 15 were impaired on tests of verbal and non-verbal learning. Only one, however, showed an abnormal CT scan with ventricular dilatation. The presence of abnormalities on neurological examination correlated significantly with the number of bouts fought. Again, however, controls were lacking, so it remains possible that the abnormalities detected antedated involvement with boxing. Jordan and Zimmerman (1988) found no abnormalities on MRI scanning in nine amateurs who had been suspended after knock-outs or excessive head blows. By contrast seven of 21 amateurs and professionals referred for examination showed white matter changes and focal contusions on CT and MRI (Jordan & Zimmerman 1990).

More thorough-going investigations have used carefully selected controls, usually sportsmen from other fields or prospective boxers in training who have not yet been involved in bouts. Here the evidence has sometimes been conflicting. Drew et al. (1986) examined a group of young professionals, aged 18–25, and compared them with control athletes. They were significantly inferior on a memory test and on several subtests from the Halstead–Reitan battery. The deficits were highly correlated with the number of bouts fought, also with the number of losses and draws sustained. By contrast, Levin et al. (1987b) found little difference on psychometry between 13 young professionals early in their careers and matched controls involved with other sports. Brooks et al. (1987b) similarly found essentially negative results on psychological tests in a group of active amateur boxers; it could be significant, however, that in this study less than half of those invited took part in testing, and those refusing may have been subjectively aware of impairments.

A thorough investigation of former amateur boxers has been reported from Sweden, where professional boxing has been prohibited for many years (Haglund & Bergstrand 1990; Haglund & Persson 1990; Murelius & Haglund 1991). Fifty were randomly selected from the boxing register and compared with soccer players and track and field athletes. No differences were found on CT and MRI indices, and indeed a cavum septum pellucidum was found rather more often in the controls than the boxers (at 8% and 4%, respectively). Findings on electroencephalography were similar in both groups. On psychometric testing no definite intellectual impairment was revealed, the sole difference from controls being on a test of finger tapping which correlated significantly with the length of the boxing career and the number of bouts fought.

Kemp et al. (1991, 1995) have recently investigated the situation using functional imaging, arguing that by the time CT scans are abnormal the brain damage is likely to be irreversible. Thirty-four amateur boxers were compared with 34 controls using HMPAO-SPECT, all scans being compared with an 'atlas of normality'. The boxers showed a significantly greater number of perfusion abnormalities than the controls.

Thus, with certain exceptions, surveys to date would appear to suggest that amateur, as opposed to professional boxing, is relatively safe with respect to the risk of long-term brain damage. Some findings, however, still raise concern, and further comprehensive studies are clearly needed. The British Medical Association continues to campaign actively for the abolition of both professional and amateur boxing, and has presented its views in two influential reports (Report of the Board of Science and Education Working Party 1984; British Medical Association 1993). It remains to be seen whether the recent introduction of new safety measures by the British Boxing Board of Control, including tighter medical checks, will serve to diminish the current level of concern (Carnall & Warden 1995).

Pathology

Cerebral atrophy is commonly revealed on CT scanning, with dilatation of the ventricles, sulcal shrinkage and sometimes obvious cerebellar atrophy. A characteristic finding is perforation of the septum pellucidum (cavum septum pellucidum) which is rarely seen in other conditions. It is thought to be a direct result of rupture of the walls of the septum consequent upon recurrent abrupt rises of intracerebral pressure.

The EEG may be abnormal with flattening of the record, diminution of the alpha rhythm or diffuse slow waves. However, Roberts (1969) found no reliable differences between boxers and a healthy control group, nor within his sample in relation to the clinical condition or the degree of exposure. Single EEG records are therefore of little use in establishing or refuting a diagnosis of traumatic encephalopathy, and cannot be used to detect early changes which might indicate that retirement is advisable.

At autopsy cerebral atrophy and ventricular enlargement are often obvious to the naked eye, and ragged holes may be seen in the septum pellucidum. The detailed neuropathological findings have been clarified by the thorough studies carried out by Corsellis and colleagues (Corsellis *et al.* 1973; Corsellis 1989). The most obvious abnormalities are in the deep midline structures, with tearing of the septal region and atrophy of the fornices. On microscopy, severe gliosis is seen in such regions, also in the thalamus and hypothalamus. The cerebellum is affected, with gliosis and loss of Purkinje cells. In the substantia nigra there is loss of pigmented neurones similar to that seen in Parkinson's disease.

The cerebral cortex shows extensive loss of neurones, many of those surviving showing neurofibrillary degeneration of the Alzheimer type. Such changes are particularly obvious in the temporal grey matter. The 'senile plaques' typical of Alzheimer's disease do not, however, occur.

This varied combination of histological abnormalities forms a pattern not described in other conditions and apparently unique to the effects of boxing. Additional findings include tearing of axons in the white matter and distorted axonal swellings, attributable to swirling of the brain within the skull (Lampert & Hardman 1984), also evidence of previous perivascular, meningeal and subpial haemorrhages (Adams & Bruton 1989).

Johnson (1969) suggests that the clinical features are probably related to damage to two main areas of the brain —the upper brain stem and the hippocampal–limbic system, accounting for the fact that the neurological and psychiatric features may progress independently of each other. Dysarthria, ataxia, parkinsonism and pyramidal disorder are consistent with lesions in the midbrain. These probably derive from the repeated rotational stresses to which the brain stem is subjected in the blows of boxing. The memory difficulties probably depend on hippocampal or mamillothalamic lesions. Corsellis *et al.* (1973) ascribe them to the intense neurofibrillary changes which may be seen in the hippocampi and related parts of the limbic grey matter, and perhaps also to the atrophic state of the fornix bundles which are often displaced by the septal damage. Johnson suggests that impotence may also be due to lesions within the limbic system or in the neighbourhood of the third ventricle. With regard to the accentuation of rage reactions, this may depend on limbic lesions or even directly on structural changes in the septal area.

In the occasional cases of severe and progressive dementia it is hard to discount the possibility of coincident Alzheimer's disease. In cases coming to necropsy a picture typical of this condition has been reported. It remains possible, of course, that repeated head trauma may precipitate the disease, in line with the link between Alzheimer's dementia and head injury generally (p. 438), but for this there is no decisive clinical evidence to date.

Recent laboratory findings by Roberts *et al.* (1990a) are, however, of considerable interest. In a re-examination of the material reported by Corsellis *et al.*, using immunocytochemical methods, it was shown that though congophilic plaques were absent there was an accumulation of beta protein in the brain. All cases with substantial neurofibrillary tangle formation showed extensive immunoreactive deposits of beta protein, not congregated in plaques as in Alzheimer's disease but distributed more diffusely. Such deposits may represent plaques at an early stage of formation. Roberts (1988) had previously used antisera to demonstrate that the neurofibrillary tangles in the brains of boxers were immunologically indistinguishable from those of Alzheimer's disease, so the parallels in pathology are close.

With regard to mechanism, it is possible that frequent disruptions of the blood–brain barrier may allow leakage of beta-protein precursors from the serum into the brain. Brayne *et al.* (1982) obtained evidence of such disruptions by measuring the levels of creatinine kinase BB before and after fights; greater rises occurred in boxers than in cyclists after a track race, and the rise in levels correlated significantly with the number of blows received to the head.

Medicolegal considerations

In peace-time the great majority of head injuries result either from road traffic accidents or accidents at work, and therefore frequently become an issue before the courts. Motor insurance covers road traffic accidents, and personal accident insurance covers many accidents which occur in other settings. Legal problems may involve the proof of prime responsibility or of negligence. With industrial injuries the employee will need to show that the employer was negligent or in breach of a statutory duty.

The system operative in New Zealand has attracted considerable interest, in that injured persons have no need to take legal action. An Accident Compensation Corporation exists as a statutory body, with responsibility for compensation, rehabilitation and accident prevention, being funded from a levy on all employers, from general taxation and from vehicle licence fees (Smith 1982a, 1982b).

In such a system there is no requirement to prove that anyone was at fault; problems can hinge, nonetheless, on defining what may properly be deemed an 'accident'. A not dissimilar 'no fault' scheme is operative in Sweden for work-related injuries.

Whatever the setting of the accident a medical report usually comes to form an important part of the proceedings, and few neurologists or psychiatrists are in practice for long without being required to furnish such evidence. In complicated or disputed cases attendance at court may be obligatory.

Facilities for legal aid in the UK allow patients of modest means to obtain legal representation after satisfying a panel of lawyers that their claim has a reasonable chance of success. In industrial accidents the patient will normally consult his trade union where applicable, and the union's lawyers will act on his behalf. Formerly it was usual for solicitors to call in chosen medical experts to intercede on the patient's behalf and to argue his case in return for a special fee, but present practice is increasingly to contact the consultant under whose care the patient has always been treated.

The defendant in the case, usually an insurance company, will often wish to seek an independent opinion and may call upon doctors specially retained for such a function. In some instances the doctors from the two sides meet and agree on a report for the court, but this is not always the happy solution. It is then that clashes of medical opinion may arise and legal proceedings become burdensome and prolonged. Nevertheless in the interests of justice to all parties the situation must be accepted, and a proper skill in the presentation of evidence must be acquired.

The court will need to make its decision on three main aspects of the situation where the medical evidence is concerned: first on the nature and degree of disablement which has followed the injury; second, on the likely duration and future course of such disablement, and the impact it will make on the quality of the patient's life; third, and fundamental to all the rest, the causative relationship between the disability and the injury which preceded it. All three can in some circumstances be the subject of uncertainty and open to argument.

Nature and degree of disablement

The nature of the disablement and its severity are decided from clinical examination, supplemented wherever possible by objective test procedures. With many areas, however, it is necessary to depend largely on the patient's own account, that of his friends and relatives and sometimes that of his employers. Evidence from observation in hospital or rehabilitation units is invaluable, since the other sources can hardly be expected to be free from bias once litigation is under way. Very important information can often be obtained from records from the patient's general practitioner, particularly where premorbid levels of functioning are concerned.

All too often it is necessary to accept unsubstantiated evidence and to make a reasoned interpretation of its reliability. Evidence of altered disposition or of emotional instability, for example, must often be derived from accounts of behaviour furnished by others. The situation can be particularly difficult when subjective complaints form the main burden of the patient's disability, as with persistent headache, dizziness, fatigue or inability to concentrate.

The impression made at interview, and equally that made before the court, can be misleading in both directions. The patient with intellectual impairment or frontal lobe damage may cheerfully disclaim any symptoms whatever, and the likely impact of the injury on his life may be revealed only by skilled examination and psychological testing. Conversely, the patient may greatly exaggerate his symptoms, and claim unfitness for work or inability for enjoyment when objective evidence of disability is slight. The circumstances of the clinical interview do not permit a wealth of suspicious cross-questioning and the follow-up of every lead for verification, but the patient's permission for access to important informants should always be sought when there is room for doubt.

A diagnosis of deliberate simulation must be made with extreme caution. The distinction from hysteria will sometimes be difficult if not impossible, though the criteria outlined on p. 485 may help in arriving at a reasonably valid conclusion. The parties contesting the claim for compensation will nowadays sometimes arrange for covert surveillance of the claimant in order to determine his true level of functioning; this is scarcely appropriate in the context of clinical evaluation, but it is well to be aware that such evidence may be produced at the eventual trial proceedings. Miller and Cartlidge (1972) rather brusquely criticise the unwillingness of doctors to consider simulation, and report a vivid example as follows:

A 30-year-old labourer had sustained a mild head injury without loss of consciousness. During the ensuing months he developed anxiety, depression and stammering, unrelieved by psychotropic drugs, and after a course of electroconvulsive therapy he became totally mute. At the time of examination he had not been heard to utter for nearly 2 years. Numerous referrals had led to a multitude of diagnoses, but 11 psychiatric reports had failed to mention the possibility of malingering.

'As can be imagined, examination presented considerable difficulty. The case was well-documented and the patient's wife most informative. His own contribution consisted in grimly nodding his head in affirmation or negation of questions and of written notes passed across the table. This he accomplished fluently and accurately. In this manner he registered complaints of frequent headaches, dizziness on change of posture, forgetfulness, and intermittent severe depression . . . From the beginning of this remarkable consultation it was difficult to escape the impression that the patient was malingering. He was tense, evasive, suspicious and defensive—and his wife's attitude was very similar. The examiner's conviction that the patient was endeavouring to deceive was so strong that he telephoned a colleague and arranged for him to accompany the claimant unobserved on his mainline train back to the Midlands. The patient exchanged his first remarks with his wife as the train drew out of Newcastle station, and by the time his companion left the train at Durham the whole compartment was engaged in uninhibited and cheerful conversation on matters of the day.'

(Miller & Cartlidge 1972)

Careful note should be made of the patient's attitude to detailed history taking, and of any striking inconsistencies which emerge. For example, the vigour with which he pursues the claim and the detail with which he recounts events connected with it may be at variance with his complaints of torpor, failing memory or difficulty in sustaining concentration. His appearance may belie complaints of insomnia or constant headache. Or the clinical features of the latter may raise suspicion, especially when it is said to be unremitting over very long periods of time and totally unresponsive to analgesics. The medical advice that the patient has sought in the interim, and the regularity with which he has attended and followed the treatment prescribed, may also give important indications of the true extent of his suffering. It is fair and just to tell him on occasion of conflicts in his evidence, and to reassess this further in the light of his response and explanations.

Estimate of prognosis

The question of prognosis will certainly be considered by the court. Here it is usually possible to do no more than give a reasoned expectation and to be frank about the measure of uncertainty which surrounds it. It could be argued that after head injury of any severity the patient's condition is never likely to reach stability, and that full justice could only be met by a life-time's follow-up (Miller 1969). In practice, however, a compromise must be accepted, since compensation is likely to be paid as a lump sum on the basis of shorter term assessment together with prediction of the likely future course. Steadman and Graham's (1970) review of a series of civilian head injuries in the UK showed that in one-third the compensation issue was settled within 1 year, in one-third within 2 years, and in all by 5 years. However, in particularly complex cases much longer periods can ensue.

Follow-up studies of patients coming before the courts are remarkably few, and opinions expressed by eminent practitioners in the literature are not uncommonly at variance with one another. Such a situation is grist to the mill of contending counsel. The frustrating delays which so commonly attend legal proceedings can here sometimes prove to be an indirect advantage, especially when the patient has remained under regular surveillance and when repeated detailed examinations have been carried out. Even severe post-traumatic dementias are known to be compatible with improvement over long periods of time (p. 185), and serial testing may already have indicated the course that is likely to be followed in the present instance. Moreover a truly confident prognosis can sometimes only be given when the patient has returned to work. Examination may have failed to reveal much in the way of intellectual loss, yet impaired judgement and irresponsibility may later prove to make him totally unsuitable for his former occupation.

On the other hand, where the compensation motive is suspected to be active it may be felt that until litigation is ended the future course will remain uncertain. If the compensation issue is thought to play a part in determining the prolongation of symptoms this should be clearly stated in the report. If a substantial element of simulation has been confidently detected the likely resolution of the disorder after settlement may likewise be predicted. Otherwise it is sometimes better not to venture too firm a forecast but merely to state the uncertainties which surround the patient's future course. It is the decision of the court which will be operative, and where present medical knowledge is insufficient to help in this decision it must not be allowed to bias it unfairly.

The question of post-traumatic epilepsy should be considered in every case, and when epilepsy has not already occurred the possibility of its future development should be kept in mind. The court should be reminded of the possibility of onset even some years after injury, otherwise final settlement may deprive the patient of adequate compensation for what is later to prove his most substantial handicap. Other possible late effects of head injury—post-traumatic parkinsonism or the development of multiple sclerosis or Alzheimer's disease—are too rare and too controversial to warrant mention unless they have already made an appearance.

In all questions of prognosis, and particularly where mental symptoms are concerned, the patient's age, general physical and mental health, and the intelligence which he may bring to bear on adjusting to his disability should be fully considered. His social setting must also be carefully evaluated. A patient of restricted ability or resources is likely to experience greater continuing hardship in response to new disabilities than one who is better endowed. On the other hand, the patient who relies on his intellect for pursuing his career may be especially handicapped by even slight disturbance of cognitive function. A professional man, for example, is likely to be more handicapped in his occupation than a labourer when the injury is followed by some degree of loss of verbal fluency. Since the court will strive to make a just award on the basis of the *impairment of the quality of life to be followed*, rather than on the actual severity of individual symptoms, these important background factors will need to be appropriately evaluated and stressed.

Relationship to injury

With regard to the causative relationship between the injury and the disability that follows, we are liable to find that the further we move away from purely physical disabilities, the more is causation likely to be open to question. Cosmetic, orthopaedic and neurological defects can usually be directly blamed upon the injury, but psychiatric sequelae with their multifactorial aetiologies can raise very special problems.

The physician must not always expect to find a strict concordance between what is accepted as causal medically and what is viewed as causal in the legal sense of the term (Spielmeyer 1969; Zülch 1969; Trimble 1981a). The medical definition of causation is based on 'natural' correlations and deduced from knowledge of the interplay of factors, external and internal to the patient, in leading to medical disorder. It embraces all the things which have contributed to the result, not only the proximate events but also pre-existing conditions such as special vulnerability in the individual. Its primary concern is with finding some means of treatment. The juridical definition of causation, on the other hand, depends on artificial correlations set up by man through regulations and laws, and modified through accumulated experience as reflected in case law. The interest here is almost wholly absorbed in whether some specified event, in this case an injury, can be shown to have contributed to the result. Consequently the law cannot always be expected to recognise the niceties of the interplay of factors which are propounded in the medical view of the problem.

When predisposing factors have existed it is logical to argue that liability should not be limited, even though these were previously undetected. Arteriosclerotic brain disease, for example, may have led to a more severe deficit from head injury than would have been found with a healthy brain. In just the same way a neurotic constitution, special vulnerabilities of personality, or a genetic loading for psychotic illness may have predisposed the patient to suffer prolonged disability from an injury which in the 'normal' person would not have called forth such a reaction. In general nowadays the courts prove sympathetic to such an argument when abundant evidence of special vulnerability can be presented. On the other hand, compensation may not be awarded if the court decides that a similar result could have occurred with a high probability at any time or in other circumstances, no matter how closely associated with the injury it may happen to be. Thus a patient long subject to recurring neurotic disability may receive scant sympathy from the court when injury is seen to lead once more to a situation which has often occurred before. The correctness or otherwise of such views could be the subject of long debate. Again, it is the legal decision which carries force, and the duty of the medical referee is to place before the court the sum total of evidence in the individual case.

When complicating factors follow injury the court will similarly need to decide what weight to put upon them. Sometimes the injury will be seen to have set in motion a whole chain of circumstances which contribute towards the psychiatric disability. Thus the break up of a marriage or the loss of a career may be traceable directly to the injury, and may be factors of great importance in prolonging affective disorder or neurotic forms of reaction. The injury itself may have been mild, even when repercussions have been severe.

It is therefore essential for the physician to formulate all aetiological factors which have a clear bearing on the case, in addition to the restricted role of the trauma itself. Unfortunately, in the determination of psychiatric sequelae some of the contributory factors will be idiosyncratic to the individual concerned, and it will be more difficult to demonstrate their operation than to display aspects of causation which have universal application.

Finally, when the clinical picture agrees closely with what would have been expected from the severity or location of known brain damage, this concordance should be stressed. For example, egocentricity, irresponsibility or coarseness of personality will be more readily attributed to head injury when damage has involved the frontal lobes, even if the premorbid personality was poorly integrated beforehand. Similarly the auras of post-traumatic epileptic attacks may conform to the site of penetrating injury, and confirm that a new disorder has been produced even though the patient has experienced epilepsy before.

The court report

A first essential in undertaking examinations for the courts is to obtain the patient's written permission for access to any additional sources of information, and his consent for the report to be sent to the solicitors who request it. Adequate time should be devoted to the interview and examination, or to a series of examinations if these are indicated. Full notes must be kept of all the information obtained since medical documents may be called before the court. Bell (1992) gives detailed advice about the evidence to be gathered and the preparation of the report.

Time should be spent in obtaining *the fullest possible information about details of the injury itself,* from which to judge the likely severity and distribution of brain damage. The duration of unconsciousness, confusion, RA and PTA should be carefully assessed, along with the extent of early neurological defects. Complications such as skull fracture, raised intracranial pressure, blood in the cerebrospinal fluid, haematomas or intracranial infection should be noted, also early episodes of fainting or other transient disorders which may prove to be the prelude to post-traumatic epilepsy. Due regard must also be paid to features of the initial injury which may specially predispose to epilepsy developing later (p. 244).

Any deficiency in investigations which come to light should be remedied. Skull X-ray, CT scan, electroencephalography and careful psychometric testing are the minimum of investigations which should be to hand. The last three should be repeated if a considerable time has elapsed since they were previously carried out. It is rarely possible to compare the results of psychological testing with results obtained before the injury occurred, but valuable interpretations can often be made when results are judged against previous educational and occupational attainments. The results of psychological testing should not be given unbacked by the general clinical impression of severity of impairment, since dementia may be manifest in behaviour and personality deterioration as well as in cognitive dysfunction. When there are substantial cognitive deficits, or when the question of impairment is in serious doubt, MRI scanning may be a useful supplement to CT.

The report should embody the date and place of examination and specify the length of contact with the patient and his illness. Additional sources of information which have contributed to the material in the report should be listed—reports from informants, general practitioners and other hospitals, and the results of special investigations performed. The patient's symptoms and all objective evidence of deficits should be described in detail, and only thereafter should any tentative opinion be expressed about the reliability or otherwise with which the patient's complaints can be taken to represent the true state of his disability. In other words, full descriptive evidence should always be presented before matters of interpretation.

The question of prognosis should be handled with caution, and expressed in probabilities rather than certainties. Writing in 1938 about the problem of dementia Lewis said: 'The subtleties of modern psychiatric classification and prognosis are unfamiliar, and perhaps unwelcome, to the legal mind; clear-cut diseases, simple labels and firm statements are likely to obtain readier hearing'. This is probably less true today than formerly, but nevertheless the temptation to oversimplify the situation must be avoided. Whatever guidance can be given regarding the future course of events should be spelled out in full, remembering that it is the reflection of disability on the quality of future life, rather than the symptoms and deficits themselves, that will be of most interest to the courts. In this the problems peculiar to the case in question—matters of age, intelligence, general health and social setting—will need to be described.

Finally, the formulation of aetiology will embrace the likely role of trauma in relation to the individual picture presented by the patient, together with such constitutional and other antecedent circumstances which may have conferred special vulnerability. Where causal chains of circumstances have followed in the wake of injury and added to the disability, these should also be clearly and simply explained. Full supporting data must always be given to help define the contribution due to injury and that due to other additional factors. Evaluations which merely state opinions or conclusions do not help the lawyers to present the case or to argue it in a satisfactory manner.

The report should be as concise as possible and should avoid technical jargon, or where this is inevitable a simple explanation may need to be included. It is sometimes necessary to bear in mind that the patient may himself have access to the report, though this should not be allowed to dictate any alteration in material content. Finally, it is perhaps worth mentioning that in the interests of justice it behoves the doctor to re-read his report with scrupulous attention to the overall impression that it makes. His evidence will have a powerful influence, even though the final decision regarding compensation will be made by others. It is all too easy for the doctor to identify with the patient's wish for compensation, especially when this is to be forthcoming from a large impersonal body, or when the patient is already well known to him. Conversely, when the patient has been importunate, dilatory or difficult to treat, a careful re-reading of the report may indicate that the writer has come to be unfairly biased against him.

Treatment

The treatment of the acute stages and early complications of head injury will not be dealt with here, since this is rarely the province of the psychiatrist. However, with commencing recovery the proper psychological management of the patient becomes of great importance, and can do much to reduce prolonged and disabling sequelae.

Early management

Rehabilitation should be planned and supervised with care from the early stages of recovery. Fortunately the majority of patients with mild injuries make satisfactory progress without a great deal of specialised attention, but every effort should be made to identify those who are specially at risk, because of personality factors or environmental difficulties, before confidence is lost and invalidism established.

The initial convalescent period is usually undertaken in hospital, and ideally in an atmosphere as free from stress as possible. Demands upon the intellect should at first be at a minimum since ready mental fatigue is likely to be evident. Physical activities, on the other hand, are beneficial, provided certain limits are imposed, and the value of early mobilisation has come to be generally recognised (Lewin 1966, 1968). Graduated exercises and games help to restore the patient's physical self confidence, and morale is improved by opportunities for social interaction. Simple advice should be given to avoid sudden bending or stooping if headache and dizziness are troublesome. At a later stage the patient should be encouraged to seek fresh air and avoid oppressive surroundings.

Usually little is needed by way of psychotherapy in any formal sense, but the value of the doctor–patient relationship should not be overlooked. It is essential that the patient should know that a full assessment has been made of any possible damage to his brain, and feel confident that the advice he is given is soundly based. Time devoted to exploration of anxieties is always well spent, and fears should not be lightly brushed aside however unfounded they may seem. The patient is often in a highly suggestible state, and lurking fears can easily take root. Explanation should be given about residual symptoms at an early date —fatigue, mental slowing, headache, dizziness—but difficulties not already present should not be implanted in the patient's mind.

An appropriate period of time away from work will need to be advised, after taking into account the severity of the injury, its complications, and the patient's personality and the stresses of the work to which he will return. Too early a return is liable to provoke a second wave of anxieties if powers of concentration are still deficient; on the other hand a long period of enforced idleness can engender morbid preoccupation and pave the way for neurotic developments. The general practitioner who is well acquainted with the patient is often well placed to

know what suits his temperament best. Patients of striving and conscientious disposition must sometimes be held back from premature attempts, while others may need encouragement to try.

More detailed and specialised care is required by patients who have sustained substantial brain damage with neurological sequelae and intellectual impairment, also by patients with minor injuries where psychiatric complications have become pronounced. The treatment programme will then need careful planning and must often be pursued over a long period of time.

From what has gone before it will be apparent that the first step must always be the systematic evaluation of residual disabilities and assessment of the causes operating in the individual case. In general it is less important to place the patient in a firm diagnostic category than to aim at a comprehensive understanding of his individual problems, personality and environment. Treatment will often need to follow a many-sided approach involving medical and allied workers from several different disciplines. The key question of the patient's motivation will almost always require attention, with special efforts to maintain or augment it.

Neurological sequelae

The main areas which require evaluation are locomotion, upper extremity function and impairment of communication. Visual acuity and visual field defects must also be assessed. Hemiparesis requires physiotherapy when more than mild and transient, similarly paraparesis or ataxia of gait. Occupational therapy has a special place in restoring useful function to the upper limbs, and speech therapy in helping the resolution of dysphasia or dysarthria. When treatment is undertaken in hospital or in rehabilitation units the nursing staff can contribute usefully in these areas, likewise the relatives when patients are treated on an out-patient basis.

Intellectual impairment

The rehabilitation of cognitive functions presents a special therapeutic challenge, and is a field where further research is badly needed (Newcombe *et al.* 1980). Full psychometric assessment is a first essential, and serves both to highlight areas of deficit and areas of preserved function on which to capitalise. Memory functions are of crucial importance and should be comprehensively evaluated from the outset. Verbal ability, comprehension, visuospatial ability, manual dexterity and capacity for sustained attention also require careful assessment.

Some general principles which should underlie the

planning of the therapeutic programme can be stated. First the confidence, and where possible the full cooperation, of the patient must be secured. The relatives also must be kept informed of aims, progress and necessary limitations. Second, an optimistic and positive approach is required in order to instil enthusiasm, with ready allowance for fatigue and tolerance of shortcomings. The personalities of the therapists can therefore be of great importance. Third, the programme must be graded, with goals at any stage that are realisable, rational and acceptable to the patient (Jousse *et al.* 1969). Self esteem is bolstered by the setting of tasks which can be mastered, however simple these may need to be at first. Success then serves as a catalyst which encourages and maintains endeavour. The tasks must also be suited to the patient's needs and inclinations. Simple repetitive craft work has a place only with the most severely disabled, or when planned specifically as remedial exercises for the restoration of manual skills. Assembly or packing work is more realistic for the factory worker, or domestic activities for the housewife. Simple clerical tasks find a special place in those better orientated towards mental than physical occupations. Finally, throughout the course of rehabilitation careful attention must be paid to basic matters such as the maintenance of optimal physical health. It is vital to detect depression, and to make due allowance for matters of personality change as well as intellectual impairment.

Zangwill (1947) stressed the emphasis that should be placed on *re-education, compensation* and *substitution* in rehabilitation. Re-education involves a direct attempt to retrain the patient in skills and accomplishments which have been impaired. For intellectual deficits, simple exercises of an ordinary scholastic kind are often of definite benefit and prove to be surprisingly well accepted. However, compensatory functions must be systematically trained if improvement of a primary function is not noted over time, since the rehabilitation aim must be to augment remaining functions rather than to exercise faculties which are destroyed (Gerstenbrand 1969). Compensation may take place spontaneously, but can often be helped further. Obvious examples are the use of props to memory, or compensatory methods of expression in severe motor dysphasia. Again the speeding of recovery through such means can have a powerful effect on the patient's morale and thus influence progress in other spheres. Substitution is required when a function is damaged irreparably, and a new method of approach must then be sought to replace it. Zangwill describes a patient who lost all ability to recognise printed symbols, until he was taught to rapidly trace the form of the letters with his forefinger. Lip-reading for the deaf is another

obvious example, or methods of seeking to alleviate the difficulties of dyscalculia (see Slade & Russell 1971).

Newcombe (1983) reviews the various strategies being developed to assist with cognitive retraining. An important requirement is to separate primary defects, attributable directly to brain injury, from the coping mechanisms adopted by the patient. The latter may be successful and deserving of encouragement, but in some cases may be counterproductive. In the retraining of memory it can be valuable to teach the use of visual imagery, verbal coding or other systems of mnemonics as outlined on p. 391.

Retraining in attentional mechanisms can be of particular importance since deficits in such areas tend to be pervasive in their effects. Wood (1984b) reviews the strategies available. Sohlberg and Mateer (1987) have described successful results with a 5–10-week course of 'attention training'. In this a variety of tasks, including specially designed computer programs, were used to concentrate on five aspects of attention—focused, sustained and selective attention, also alternating attention as needed for mental flexibility, and divided attention which is required for simultaneous responses to multiple tasks. Impressive aspects of the results were the capacity of patients to respond long after injury, the persistence of improvement after training had ceased, and the apparently beneficial effects in terms of regaining independence and gainful employment.

Personality change and behavioural disorder

Personality changes following brain damage are notoriously difficult to modify. There is relatively little that can be done by way of specific treatment, though much may be achieved by broader lines of management.

A period spent in hospital or a rehabilitation unit is often valuable for assessing the full extent of the patient's difficulties and limitations, and may help towards the elimination of socially disruptive behaviour.

Psychotherapy at a relatively superficial level can be of considerable benefit if a working relationship can be established. It should aim at helping the patient to achieve some insight when this is lacking, at least into the more disturbing aspects of his behaviour. A measure of control may sometimes be achieved in such matters as disinhibition, impulsiveness or emotional outbursts, though progress is usually limited. Discussion can also usefully centre on problems which arise day-to-day in consequence of the patient's altered disposition, and here group therapy can be particularly effective.

A valuable development is the application of behavioural modification techniques to brain-injured persons, with the aim of reducing disruptive behaviour and encouraging more constructive involvement in the rehabilitation process. Such methods have been tried mainly with severely injured persons, usually in special units, but could perhaps find wider application. Hollon (1973) reported success with a form of operant therapy in a rehabilitation unit, whereby cooperative self-helping behaviour was systematically rewarded, while belligerent or manipulative behaviour was ignored. By such means disruptive patients could become accessible to therapy when this had not been possible before.

Wood and Eames (1981) and Wood (1984a) have described their extensive experience with behaviour modification in St Andrew's Hospital, Northampton. They point out that maladaptive patterns of behaviour have often been acquired by a process of learning, then become positively reinforced by the attention they evoke. Programmes were devised to control such matters as temper outbursts or antisocial behaviour, while at the same time shaping and encouraging more constructive responses. A token economy regime is fundamental in the treatment, being carefully adapted to the circumstances of each individual patient. Tokens are earned or forfeited in relation to key aspects of the day's behaviour, then exchanged for privileges within the unit. Imposed periods of social isolation ('time out') may also be required, or abrupt 'on the spot' withdrawal of staff attention, all against a background of positive reinforcement when things are going well. More intensive conditioning sessions may further help in the elimination of particularly resistant matters such as repetitive spitting, striking or stereotyped nonsensical utterances. In favourable cases such programmes can apparently meet with considerable and lasting success, bringing the patient closer into contact and allowing further adaptive behaviours to be progressively encouraged (Eames & Wood 1985).

Short of such decisive intervention much may still be required by way of clinical surveillance. When irresponsibility is a marked feature close supervision may be needed over matters of finance, and the patient's family must be brought fully into the picture. Indeed post-traumatic personality change is often the area in which the relatives most require advice, explanation and support. On-going contact with a social worker or 'case manager' can prove invaluable in helping to avoid domestic, financial and occupational crises. Placement in work requires careful choice, sometimes with full discussion with the employer.

Tranquillising drugs such as diazepam may help with tension and anxiety, and antidepressants should be tried if an element of depression is thought to colour the picture. The author has observed benefit from low dose chlorpromazine in patients with frontal lobe damage where euphoria and disinhibited prankish behaviour were disturbing in degree. Barrett (1991) has reported considerable success with dopamine agonists such as bromocriptine or lisuride in patients with severe passivity and anergia ('abulia') after brain damage of varied aetiologies, and these may find a useful role in treatment in certain patients. There may also be a place, under carefully supervised conditions, for a cautious trial of stimulating agents such as methylphenidate (Ritalin) or amphetamine in patients whose sluggishness and anergia derive from hypothalamic damage. Anticonvulsants are of doubtful value in preventing outbursts of aggression unless these are clearly related to epileptic activity, though phenytoin or other agents may warrant a trial in certain cases (p. 298).

Psychotic illness

Psychoses which develop after head injury require, in general, the same psychiatric management as the equivalent illnesses which occur in other settings. Schizophrenia and affective disorder may need appropriate medication along with attention to psychosocial aspects of the patient's situation. Electroconvulsive therapy is not contraindicated when other measures have failed, and can occasionally be dramatically effective in cases of severe depression or prolonged stupor following head injury (Silverman 1964).

Neurotic sequelae

Neurotic complications call for careful evaluation especially when long continued after injury, with readiness to explore the detailed factors operating in the individual case. The situation of the patient, including his family setting, must be comprehensively reviewed; where litigation is in progress liaison with the lawyers representing the case can be helpful.

Once the possibility of brain damage has been fully assessed, further physical investigations are best kept to a minimum. Repeated questioning about symptoms can also delay the patient's progress, and in cases of litigation it may be advisable to tell the lawyers that this is considered to be the case.

Antidepressant medication and the minor tranquillisers are valuable aids, but the mainstay of treatment lies usually in psychotherapy and in attention to the social problems that exist. Psychotherapy may need to consist of little more than on-going support, reassurance and the ventilation of anxieties. But as the patient's confidence is gained more detailed problems may emerge, as in the cases outlined on p. 175. Post-traumatic stress disorder may require a cognitive–behavioural approach, and phobic conditions will often respond well to behaviour therapy.

Speedy resolution of litigation is in general to be desired, certainly in cases where brain damage does not play an identifiable part. Return to work should also be secured at the earliest possible opportunity. In very severe and protracted examples removal from the home environment can be valuable in clarifying the issues at stake, either by admission to hospital or to a rehabilitation unit. Indeed severe neurotic sequelae, no less than intellectual impairments, may need the full range of rehabilitation facilities for the restoration of morale and preparation for taking up the normal course of life again.

Post-traumatic headache

Long continued and disabling post-traumatic headache can come to pose a difficult therapeutic problem. Frequently, a number of simple remedies will have been tried without success, and the headache will be found to be inextricably intertwined with a variety of neurotic complaints. Evaluation and treatment must give full attention to both organic and psychological factors. The range of organic causes which need to be considered has already been outlined on p. 197.

Friedman (1969) provides a useful review of treatment. Short-term psychotherapy can be surprisingly helpful, and must aim at understanding the role the symptoms play in relation to the patient's personality and environment. Anxieties, frustrations and in particular resentments, must often be ventilated in full.

Non-addictive analgesics have a place, also tranquillisers such as diazepam. The latter is especially indicated when tension headache is the cause. Ergotamine preparations may be tried when episodic headache is suspected to have a vascular basis. Antidepressants can sometimes produce dramatic results:

A man of 60 was somewhat depressed and tense 2 years after a second mild head injury to the left parietal region. He felt that he was failing at his work, and complained of severe persistent headache and odd indefinable sensations in the left side of the head. After 1 week on amitriptyline he was surprised to find that the headache and other sensations had abruptly disappeared. The depression yielded more slowly but ultimately he made an excellent recovery.

Physical treatments which will often have been tried include local heat, and procaine injections to tender sites and to the upper cervical spine. These have a useful place, but when overemployed they carry the danger of focusing attention exclusively on one aspect of the problem alone.

Post-traumatic epilepsy

This important complication needs to be managed along the same lines as epilepsy due to other causes, as outlined on p. 298 *et seq*. There may be a place, in carefully selected cases, for operative removal of an epileptogenic scar. Prophylactic medication is reserved for those forms of head injury which carry special risk (pp. 244–5).

Rehabilitation units: resettlement at work

From the range of treatments required, and the many special problems encountered, it is clearly advantageous to have centres for the rehabilitation of the more severely disabled patients. This need is widely recognised, but facilities are not equally widely available. Recent reports from the Royal College of Physicians (1986), the Medical Disability Society (1988) and the Royal College of Psychiatrists (Working Group of the Research Committee of Royal College of Psychiatrists 1991) have emphasised the size of the problem and the requirement for a coordinated national strategy in the UK.

Head-injured patients often present a combination of physical handicap with disturbances of intellect, mood and behaviour. They are therefore liable to fall between the two stools of adequate provision for physical therapy and adequate facilities for psychiatric supervision (Lishman 1983b). Properly organised rehabilitation units allow a multidisciplinary approach, both in evaluation and in the supervision of treatment, with neurologists, psychiatrists and specialists in physical medicine and orthopaedics working together. Moreover, the patient can receive the prolonged attention of other skilled personnel whose services can be coordinated—physiotherapists, psychologists, occupational therapists, speech therapists and social workers. Social aspects of rehabilitation are also facilitated when large numbers of patients can be treated together. However, where special units are not available rehabilitation must often be managed on an *ad hoc* basis within the hospital or out-patient department.

An essential part of rehabilitation lies in the help and guidance offered when the time comes for preparation for return to work. The ideal of return to the original occupation may have to be changed on account of persistent physical or mental handicaps. In practice the chief hindrances usually prove to be of a psychological kind—inadequacy of memory, weakness of attention, early fatigue, lowered vitality, slowness, or persistent depression (Schmid 1969). Dresser *et al.* (1973), in a study of Korean war veterans in the USA, showed the importance of *pre*morbid mental capacity, as well as severity of injury, in predicting return to work. A period of retraining may be necessary, or entry to a sheltered workshop or day centre, for those who are unable to manage under ordinary working conditions.

Short of this a full assessment must be made to guide the patient towards a suitable form of intermediate or final employment. Conditions usually to be avoided include shift or night work, noisy or oppressive conditions, high frequency vibration, working at heights or with moving machinery, or work which must be carried out under pressure of time. The patient may require sympathetic help when compromises are to be made. The patient's family may also need support at this important stage, especially in adjusting to the social and financial implications of a change in occupational status.

Rusk *et al.* (1969) followed the results of rehabilitation from the New York Institute of Rehabilitation Medicine with interesting results. Female patients more often needed to be institutionalised than males, perhaps because a wife can more easily assume the major care of a disabled husband than vice versa. Patients adequately ambulant at discharge maintained their progress, whereas those only partially ambulant frequently regressed. Similar findings emerged with regard to dressing, feeding and toilet care, the principal cause of failure being lack of adequate time to perform the functions unaided, rather than loss of basic skills. Two factors of importance in the patients' continuing welfare proved to be the presence or absence of depression, and the continuity of care after discharge. Those who lived near to the centre, or maintained contact with an interested doctor or social worker, were more likely to maintain or even improve their gains. Conversely, isolation from professional advisers was markedly evident in those who relapsed.

A more recent study from New Hampshire has shown the success that can often be achieved by intensive rehabilitation, even among severely injured and behaviourly disturbed patients who would normally be considered to have a poor prognosis (Burke *et al.* 1988). Most were young victims of road traffic accidents, the majority having been unconscious for over 6 weeks and showing evidence of diffuse or frontal brain damage. Almost 90% had been referred because of emotional and behavioural problems, and a third were admitted directly from secure psychiatric settings. In-patient rehabilitation included cognitive therapy, social skills training, vocational rehabilitation and techniques designed to decrease the frequency of maladaptive behaviours. Follow-up 3–12 months later showed that half were living independently, and half were maintaining successful employment, albeit often in supported settings. Discharge to independent living arrangements or group homes appeared to be more successful than return to the care of the family which often encouraged prolonged dependence. The assignment of a case manager to serve as an advocate appeared to be an important factor in aiding reintegration into the community.

McMillan *et al.* (1988) argue for the benefits of intro-

ducing case management for severely head-injured patients in the UK. Surveys have indicated that only a small proportion of such patients receive the full range of rehabilitation they require after discharge from hospital (Murphy *et al.* 1990). Moreover many lose contact with specialist services after post-acute rehabilitation, whereas problems and disabilities can continue for many years. Patients can easily fall through the net of service provision, or lack guidance over where to seek help in specific situations. A designated case manager should be in a position to establish a continuous link among the various service providers, build up knowledge of what is available locally, and coordinate input to the patient and the family. A recent attempt at evaluating the usefulness of such a role in the UK has given inconclusive results, largely it seems because of difficulties in augmenting contact with the scarce rehabilitation services available (Greenwood *et al.* 1994).

Social adaptation and effects upon the family

Consideration of the sequelae of head injury is incomplete without mention of the broad effects on the quality of the patient's life and that of his family. Valuable reviews are presented by Oddy (1984), Brooks (1984b) and Florian *et al.* (1989). It is abundantly clear that leisure and social activities are often profoundly disrupted, sometimes in the long-term view, quite apart from the consequences in terms of employment and finance. Family relationships can come under considerable strain. In all these respects the mental aftermaths, and particularly changes in personality, can prove more disruptive than purely physical disabilities.

Jennett *et al.* (1981) discuss various aspects of living relevant to 'quality of life'. First are the 'activities of daily living' most related to dependence on others—capacity to feed, dress, move and cope with toilet requirements. Next is the question of mobility beyond the patient's immediate surroundings, which can be as severely hampered by mental as physical handicaps. Social relationships require quite separate assessment, much depending on the patient's capacities for initiative and response. Work and leisure activities, present satisfaction and future prospects must also be borne in mind. Finally there is the question of the burden borne by the persons with whom the patient lives.

It was apparent in Thomsen's (1974) follow-up of severely head-injured patients that loss of social contact featured prominently among their problems. Most had lost touch with previous friends, and possibilities for making new acquaintances were few. Intellectual deficits, but even more so changes in personality, created the major problems in daily living. A prospective follow-up by Oddy and Humphrey (1980) reinforced these findings— leisure activities were still impaired 2 years after injury in half of their patients, this rarely being due to physical problems alone. Weddell *et al.* (1980) demonstrated marked changes in the social milieu of young adults followed 2 years later, in terms of changes in work, leisure activities, contact with friends and family life. Working capacity was affected by neurophysical status, memory difficulties and personality problems; it was the last, however, which contributed most to loss of friendships and dependence on the family.

Florian *et al.* (1989) contrast the obstacles to adjustment in head-injured patients with those who suffer from purely physical disabilities. Normally adjustment to loss or disablement is helped by continuity between the past and the present in the lives of the person and his family, but in the brain-damaged patient this stands to be disrupted. Another prerequisite is acceptance of the reality of the deficits that exist, and this too is often compromised. Internal resources needed for the process of adaptation are frequently curtailed, likewise necessary elements of judgement and flexibility. Added to this, the combined effects of cognitive, emotional and behavioural dysfunction are often greater than their individual parts, and can have more deleterious effects than physical disability alone.

With respect to family dynamics, Florian *et al.* (1989) emphasise difficulties often unique to head injury. Lack of comprehension of the patient's behaviour and its origins can lead to unhelpful responses on the part of those around. Anger may arise from a suspicion that the patient is not making proper effort, or guilt that disappointing progress reflects the carer's own inadequacy. This circle of anger and guilt can lead to emotional distancing. Denial by parents or spouses of the severity of the impact of the injury may persist for many years, along with unrealistic expectations of progress; and with eventual disappointment this can turn to anger directed at those responsible for rehabilitation.

With the passage of time, as a physical condition stabilises, the family's social contacts generally begin to improve. By contrast, after head injury, the family often suffers gradual social withdrawal. Conflict and tension among family members tend to increase in consequence. The wives of victims are liable to suffer particularly; they will often need to adjust to regressive, childlike behaviour, to altered sexual behaviour, and to facing the burden of child care alone. Such issues are reinforced by Lezak's (1978) account of working with the families of head-injured patients; guidelines are presented for goals in counselling and in dealing with the common family problems that arise.

Direct assessment of the relatives of head-injured persons has shown the extent of their difficulties, and has consistently related this to the mental rather than the physical aftermaths. Oddy *et al.* (1978) interviewed relatives at intervals over a year, finding that scores for depression were related not to severity of injury but to factors reflecting the patient's social adjustment. Two aspects emerged as particularly distressing: first the patient's forgetfulness and disorientation; second his 'verbal expansiveness' which referred to talking too long, too loudly and with poor logical continuity.

McKinlay *et al.* (1981) in a similar study found that the problems most frequently encountered by the family concerned the patient's slowness, irritability, poor memory and emotional changes. Physical disability was less commonly a problem. Thomsen (1974) stressed the burden of aspontaneity, irritability, restlessness and stubbornness. Emotional lability and outbursts of pathological laughter were especially embarrassing features.

Very strikingly, Rosenbaum and Najenson (1976) compared the wives of 10 patients suffering from severe head injury with those of paraplegic controls who had sustained no loss of cognitive function. At 1 year follow-up the wives of the head-injured patients were significantly more depressed, had experienced greater changes in their lives and had suffered greater social restriction.

For reasons such as these the National Head Injuries Association ('Headway') has been established as a voluntary charitable trust, with the aim of providing counselling, support and social activities for patients handicapped in the long-term view and for their families.

Chapter 6: Cerebral Tumours

Cerebral tumours commonly present with symptoms of raised intracranial pressure, focal neurological signs or epileptic fits which lead the patient directly to the neurologist or neurosurgeon. Some, however, develop such evidence only late in the evolution of the tumour, and the earliest manifestations may consist of mental symptoms alone. When mental disturbance is the most prominent feature the patient may come first to the attention of the psychiatrist, and thereby run the risk of delayed or even missed diagnosis.

It is, of course, comparatively rare for the psychiatrist to find a cerebral tumour in a patient with mental disorder. Parry's (1968) finding of one per 200 patients admitted to a psychiatric unit is probably higher than average. The converse, however, is extremely common and many patients with cerebral tumours show pronounced mental symptoms at some time in their course. The frequency has been reported variously from 10% to virtually 100% of cases, depending on the care with which psychological symptoms are sought out and recorded, and the stage of evolution of the tumour at the time the observations are made. Two of the larger series of tumour patients studied personally by the authors, and with psychological symptoms in mind, were those of Keschner *et al.* (1938) and Hécaen and Ajuriaguerra (1956). Keschner *et al.* reported mental symptoms in 78% of 530 cases, Hécaen and Ajuriaguerra in 52% of 439 cases.

From the clinical point of view, mental symptoms are in general of little use as a guide to the location or the nature of the tumour. Neurological signs are greatly superior in this regard, and neuroimaging has diminished the importance even of those mental symptoms which might have been of value. Tumour material has also proved disappointing for the study of the cerebral basis of mental phenomena. It is often hard to disentangle the effects of the lesion itself from remote pressure effects, circulatory disturbances or the generalised effects of raised intracranial pressure. Nevertheless the psychological effects of cerebral tumours show many features of interest, and can on occasion be of crucial clinical importance.

General characteristics of mental symptoms

Changes may be seen in any aspect of psychological function. Sometimes certain areas are affected alone, for example the level of consciousness, aspects of cognitive function or the affective state, though usually several areas are affected together. The interaction and synthesis of several functions may be disturbed in a manner which emerges as 'change of personality'. Complex psychological symptoms such as hallucinations and delusions may also appear, and the picture can be complicated by paroxysmal disorders consequent upon an epileptogenic focus. Occasionally frank psychotic illnesses are seen, or more frequently neurotic disturbances occasioned by the make-up of the individual.

In very general terms it may be said that slow-growing tumours tend to produce changes of personality, and allow premorbid tendencies to manifest themselves; more rapid tumours lead to cognitive defects; whereas the most rapid lead to acute organic reactions with obvious impairment of consciousness.

Cognitive changes

Disturbance of cognitive function is the most commonly noted psychological change. In minor degree it shows as diminished capacity to attend and concentrate, faulty memory and ready mental fatigue. These rather subtle changes may be the first manifestation of the lesion, and sometimes provide the sole indication of disease for long periods of time.

More severe cognitive impairment may present in the form of dementia, with slowed and concrete thinking, impoverished associations, defective judgement and obvious difficulty with memory. Perseveration is sometimes marked. Speech may be slowed and incoherent, even in the absence of dysphasia and even with tumours of the non-dominant hemisphere. Such changes can be steadily progressive, but more characteristically tend to fluctuate in severity from one occasion to another.

Focal cognitive changes are commoner than generalised dementia as befits the focal nature of the lesion. Or a focal emphasis may be detected even when global deterioration is present. A circumscribed amnesic syndrome may appear while other functions remain well preserved, with markedly defective memory for recent events, disorientation and even confabulation. All varieties of dysphasia can be seen, also apraxia, visuospatial defects, topographical disorientation and components of the Gerstmann syndrome. These will be important pointers to the focal nature of the disorder and serve as a guide to its location. Certain cognitive disturbances characteristic of tumours in special locations will be considered further below.

Disturbance in the level of consciousness will add to the cognitive changes, again tending to fluctuate with periods of relative lucidity. Later, drowsiness and somnolence appear, and as the lesion extends the level of consciousness declines progressively, ending, if untreated, in coma.

Affective changes

Affective changes rarely occur in isolation, but frequently accompany other mental manifestations. With intellectual impairment there tends to be emotional dullness, apathy and aspontaneity; or euphoria may stand in striking contrast to what would be expected in view of the patient's physical defects and disabilities. However, depression and anxiety are also common with cerebral tumours, sometimes as understandable reactions and sometimes pathological in degree. Irritability can be a prominent feature, or emotional lability with marked and evanescent swings of mood. Sustained elation is rarely seen. Henry (1932) attempted to outline the usual sequence of mood changes during the evolution of cerebral tumours. He found that irritability in the early stages typically gave way to growing anxiety and depression. Suicidal tendencies were estimated to occur in 10% of cases. Up to this point the emotional reactions were largely determined by inherent tendencies in the patient, but thereafter the disease process itself appeared more important, leading to indifference, apathy, euphoria or emotional lability.

Hallucinations

Hallucinations may occur in any modality, commonly as part of an epileptic disturbance but also without evidence of paroxysmal activity. The nature of the hallucinations will depend on the location of the tumour. Occipital tumours are associated with simple visual hallucinations; temporal lobe tumours with more complex formed visual and auditory hallucinations, also gustatory and olfactory hallucinations; and parietal lobe tumours with localised tactile and kinaesthetic hallucinations. The distinctions are not, however, absolute. Circumscribed frontal lobe tumours may sometimes produce visual, auditory or even gustatory hallucinations, presumably through effects on the neighbouring temporal lobe. Medial frontal lesions can also discharge directly to the temporal lobe and produce hallucinations and other phenomena by this means. Subtentorial tumours may be accompanied by visual hallucinations, presumably by pressure effects on the adjacent occipital lobe (Keschner *et al.* 1937).

Psychotic and neurotic phenomena

Any form of psychotic illness may accompany cerebral tumour, either early or late in its evolution. Depressive, schizophrenic, paranoid and hypomanic illnesses have all been reported, usually but not always in association with evidence of organic brain dysfunction. Delusions when they occur may have a characteristic organic colouring, being poorly elaborated, shallow or fleeting. A wide variety of neurotic manifestations also occur, especially in the early stages, and may likewise be misleading (as discussed on p. 235).

Such disorders are obviously more common in those cerebral tumours which come the way of the psychiatrist. Minski's (1933) report of psychiatric symptomatology among patients from the Maudsley Hospital is typical: 25 out of 58 patients with cerebral tumour showed 'functional' mental illness, and in almost half of these physical signs were absent. Fourteen patients displayed severe depression, seven excitement, and one each showed schizophrenia, an anxiety state, an obsessional disorder and hysteria.

Factors governing symptom formation

The mental disturbances accompanying cerebral tumours have, as is usual with psychiatric symptomatology, several sources of origin. Some of these are common to all patients affected, while others are largely idiosyncratic to the individual.

Raised intracranial pressure

Raised intracranial pressure accounts for a good deal of the mental symptomatology. When the pressure is lowered by decompression or by dexamethasone, dramatic changes in mental state can follow, with resolution of confusion, drowsiness, apathy or even coma.

Fluctuations in the level of consciousness probably depend principally upon fluctuations in the dynamics of the cerebrospinal fluid (CSF) circulation. Other symptoms—difficulties with thinking, perception and memory, also emotional dullness and apathy—may often be similarly ascribed to impaired cerebral function due to raised intracranial pressure. The pathophysiology of these effects may lie largely with disturbance of the brain stem reticular formation and its rostral projections to the cortex, or with direct compression of brain tissue, impeded circulation, and impaired flow of CSF. After long-continued elevation of pressure there may be extensive parenchymal damage resulting from such factors, and the mental impairments will then remain even after the pressure is lowered.

Focal effects in the region of the tumour may also be aggravated by increased pressure, as seen for example when dysphasic symptoms recede as the pressure is lowered. But much psychiatric symptomatology appears to have little connection with intracranial pressure. Busch (1940) contrasted the overall prevalence of psychiatric disturbance and raised intracranial pressure in a large unselected series of tumour patients. Temporal lobe tumours showed mental symptoms in 50% of cases, whilst intracranial pressure was raised in only 25%; infratentorial tumours by contrast showed mental symptoms in 10% but raised intracranial pressure in 99%. The studies of Keschner et al. (1938) and Hécaen and Ajuriaguerra (1956) have confirmed this distinction in tumours arising above and below the tentorium. Thus even when intracranial pressure is raised, there are likely to be other important factors at work which lead to the appearance of mental symptoms. Of these, localized cerebral oedema in the neighbourhood of the tumour is clearly of special importance.

Nature of the tumour

The nature of the tumour and the rapidity of its growth appear to be important factors determining the incidence and severity of mental symptoms. Keschner et al. (1938) found that tumours which produced no mental symptoms whatsoever were mainly of the slow-growing type. Busch (1940) found that symptoms were more frequent with malignant tumours than benign.

Gliomas have repeatedly been found to produce a higher incidence of mental disturbance than meningiomas. In Hécaen and Ajuriaguerra's (1956) series, for example, mental disturbances were noted in 61% of gliomas as compared to 43% of meningiomas. Further-

more, within the group of gliomas, rapidity of growth appears to be important. Busch (1940) found, among left hemisphere tumours, that 25% of astrocytomas had mental symptoms compared to 70% of glioblastomas; the corresponding figures for right hemisphere tumours were 35% and 80%, respectively. It is important, however, to distinguish these general associations from the relative diagnostic hazards of slow- and fast-growing tumours. Rapid growth is associated with more severe mental disturbance, but slow-growing tumours are more liable to present with mental symptoms alone so that they may more easily be missed.

The greater frequency of mental disturbances among malignant as compared to benign cerebral tumours is probably due to the greater prevalence of raised intracranial pressure in the former group. Malignant tumours also invade the brain more widely. It is perhaps for the latter reason that metastatic tumours with several deposits scattered throughout the brain have proved to be associated with a higher prevalence of mental disturbance than any variety of primary intracerebral tumour (Keschner et al. 1938).

Location of the tumour

The importance of tumour location in relation to mental symptoms has been much debated. Many observations concerning special regional effects can be offset by negative findings. There are, of course, considerable difficulties in amassing large and unselected series of tumour patients in a setting which allows for careful appraisal and comparison of psychiatric features. Most tumours are progressive and present changing mental pictures during their evolution. Moreover there may be effects which derive from cerebral involvement at a distance, due to distortions of the brain, compression against the skull and dural openings, or obstruction to free arterial supply and venous drainage. The patient's awareness of the illness will profoundly influence his response, and this in turn will depend on many features of his personality and situation. Thus any direct contribution made by the location of the lesion can be hard to disentangle from other factors.

Bleuler (1951a), reviewing 600 unselected tumours from the Zurich neurosurgical clinic, suggested that the psychopathological picture was, in fact, very uniform. Eighty-three per cent of his patients showed mental symptoms, but there were no significant differences according to the site of the tumour. Only two mental syndromes could be reliably differentiated—clouding of consciousness in the acute stage and a 'chronic amnesic syndrome' in the chronic stage. The latter embraced much more than memory defects alone, including also widespread cognitive disturbances, emotional instability and impairment of personality.

Bleuler's results, however, run counter to most other findings in the literature, and special association between site of tumour and certain aspects of psychiatric disturbance have frequently emerged. This will be discussed further in the sections that follow, but here we may note that focal cognitive defects may appear with parietal tumours, and focal amnesic syndromes with tumours of the diencephalon. Hallucinations also clearly derive from focal lesions of the brain.

When considering more than such relatively elementary symptoms, it becomes harder to demonstrate the role of focal cerebral disorder in the pictures that result. Thus disturbances of affect and personality cannot be tied convincingly to tumours in specific parts of the brain, and psychotic illness appears to be largely determined by other factors. The evidence indicating special characteristics of personality disturbance in association with frontal lobe tumours is outlined on p. 223, and that linking schizophrenia-like psychoses with temporal lobe tumours is discussed on p. 225. In these areas, however, the evidence which can be derived from tumour material remains relatively slender.

Table 10 shows the overall frequency of mental symptoms with tumours in different locations, as reported by Keschner et al. (1938) and Hécaen and Ajuriaguerra (1956). These are two of the largest series investigated by observers whose primary interest was to evaluate mental symptoms against a constant set of criteria. A fair degree of agreement is seen between the two, even though Hécaen and Ajuriaguerra's criteria for recording symptoms were clearly stricter than those of Keschner et al. Supratentorial tumours show a greatly increased frequency of mental disturbances when compared to infratentorial tumours, and this is especially marked when attention is restricted to symptoms appearing at the onset or early in the illness. This is particularly noteworthy since raised intracranial pressure was considerably less frequent among the supratentorial than the infratentorial tumours in both series of cases. Frontal and temporal lobe tumours show a somewhat higher frequency of mental disturbance than do tumours in the parietal or occipital lobes. Parry (1968), commenting on Hécaen and Ajuriaguerra's series, points out that the high frequency of cases with mental symptoms at onset in the temporal and occipital groups is entirely due to paroxysmal disturbances; if one considers only those with enduring mental symptoms the frontal preponderance is statistically significant, and all other locations are approximately equivalent with one another. However, in Keschner et al.'s series, where patients with paroxysmal disturbances were excluded, temporal lobe tumours still retain their lead.

Individual constitution and response

Finally the individual response to a cerebral tumour will play a part in determining the mental symptoms. The importance of this probably emerges less forcibly in most published studies than its true influence would warrant.

In patients with special genetic predisposition to mental disorder the tumour may act as little more than a precipitating factor in the psychiatric disturbance that develops. This is likely to be especially so where neurotic disorders or psychotic developments are concerned. Much emotional disturbance will also be an understandable response to physical impairments such as paralysis, fits or visual symptoms, or to the threat presented by the illness. In all of this the patient's response will be largely shaped by his premorbid personality and will reflect his habitual

Table 10 Prevalence of mental symptoms with cerebral tumours.

Location of tumour	Study 1 (Keschner et al. 1938)*			Study 2 (Hécaen & Ajuriaguerra 1956)†		
	Number of cases	% with mental symptoms	% with 'early' mental symptoms	Number of cases	% with mental symptoms	% onset with mental symptoms
All tumours	530	78	15	439	52	18
All supratentorial	401	87	18	354	56	19
All infratentorial	129	47	5	85	40	12
Frontal	68	85	25	80	68	20
Temporal	56	93	29	75	68	28
Parietal	32	81	19	75	52	16
Occipital	11	82	9	25	52	32

* Excluding paroxysmal disturbances.
† Including paroxysmal disturbances.

modes of reaction to stress. It will also be modified to a very considerable extent by the handling the patient receives from medical and nursing personnel.

Such highly individual factors may be expected to modify the psychological effects of a cerebral lesion wherever it is situated. It is not surprising therefore that precise evidence about aetiological factors becomes harder to obtain as one deals with the more complex aspects of psychiatric disorder in the presence of cerebral tumours.

Mental symptoms with tumours in different locations

Despite the complexities outlined above, a large literature has accumulated describing characteristic mental pictures for tumours in different parts of the brain. A good deal is contradictory from one report to another, but certain aspects emerge repeatedly. These deserve emphasis since they can be of diagnostic importance. Much of what follows has been drawn from the detailed monograph by Hécaen and Ajuriaguerra (1956).

Frontal lobe tumours

Frontal lobe tumours are notorious for their liability to present under guises which may lead to a mistaken diagnosis of a primary dementing illness. This is due partly to the paucity of striking neurological signs which accompany frontal lesions, and in part to the frequency with which mental disturbances appear from an early stage.

Impairment of consciousness and intellectual deterioration were found more frequently with frontal tumours than with tumours in any other location in Hécaen and Ajuriaguerra's own series. Sachs (1950), in a large series of patients with meningiomas, found eight who presented with dementia before any symptoms indicative of tumour had appeared, and in six the tumours were frontal in location. Sometimes dramatically successful results can follow the removal of such a tumour:

A woman of 64 was admitted to hospital in a deteriorated state and unable to give an account of herself. Her husband stated that the illness had begun 2 years previously when she became excessively preoccupied with the ills of her pet dog. For 3 months there had been episodes of trembling all over, worse in the morning, but not associated with any loss of consciousness. She had gradually become forgetful and muddled and had lost all initiative. For 3 weeks she had been confined to bed and was too confused to dress herself. She was doubly incontinent. There had been no headache, fits or vomiting.

On examination she showed a profound dementia with disorientation in time and place. She lay inert in bed but was not difficult to rouse. There was no dysphasia or apraxia, but she could

not cooperate over detailed tests of intellectual function. The only neurological signs were a persistent tremor of the outstretched hands and an equivocal left plantar response. The sense of smell was intact.

The EEG showed evidence of a lesion in the left frontotemporal region, and skull X-ray showed erosion of the posterior clinoid processes. At operation a left frontal parasagittal meningioma was removed.

Two months postoperatively her mental state was judged to be entirely normal and she said she felt better than for several years. She recalled little of her preoperative condition except that she had been distressed over her incontinence.   (Sachs 1950)

A woman developed grand mal epileptic fits at the age of 40, and at 53 was admitted to a psychiatric hospital because she had become apathetic, inert, incontinent and bedridden. She was aggressive when approached and deteriorated in habits. A skull X-ray was interpreted as showing hyperostosis frontalis interna. After 12 years in hospital she remained severely demented, was somnolent and showed little response to questions. She sat with the tongue protruded to the right, and making purposeless repetitive movements of the right arm and leg. She was anosmic, could only just distinguish between light and dark, and showed a left-sided facial weakness. There was no obvious weakness of the limbs but she could neither stand nor walk.

Investigations revealed a massive bifrontal meningioma, probably attached above the crista galli. After its removal she made a remarkable improvement, regained some degree of spontaneity, speech and sight and was able to get about. She recognised and talked with relatives for the first time in 12 years. She had a dense amnesia for the 15–20 years before the operation and misjudged events and ages accordingly.   (Hunter et al. 1968a)

Chee et al. (1985) have charted improvement in six patients with frontal meningiomas who presented with dementia, sometimes with recovery postoperatively to normal intellectual function as confirmed by psychometry.

Tumours of the left frontal lobe appear to be associated with greater cognitive disturbance than tumours of the right. Smith's (1966b) careful analysis of psychometric test results showed greater losses in both verbal and performance abilities with left compared to right frontal tumours, the difference still persisting when aphasic patients were excluded. Bilateral involvement, as with tumours originating in the midline, produce more disturbance than when a single lobe is implicated alone (Strauss & Keschner 1935).

Generalised dementia is the most frequent picture, but disturbance of memory can occasionally be seen in relative isolation. Hécaen and Ajuriaguerra found that 10 of their 80 cases presented with mental disturbances in which amnésie de fixation was prominent. In one case there was a typical Korsakoff syndrome together with confabulation. Often, however, the apparent memory failure occurs in a setting of profound apathy and indifference which makes it hard to decide whether the patient is trying to remember or to give the answer.

Other special characteristics of cognitive disturbance include aspontaneity, slowing and inertia. The slowing of mental and physical activities may be striking, with long periods during which virtually all activity comes to a halt. Speech may be extremely slow and laboured, even when the tumour is in the non-dominant lobe and evidence of dysphasia is lacking. Akinetic states have been described in which the patient is mute and immobile, yet when forcibly roused proves to be normally orientated. In other cases somnolence may be extreme, usually but not invariably in association with raised intracranial pressure.

The disturbances of affect most characteristic of frontal lobe tumours appear to be irritability, depression, euphoria and apathy. Irritability is repeatedly stressed and may sometimes occur as a presenting symptom. Some of Direkze et al.'s (1971) patients had initially been admitted to psychiatric units on account of depression, which then proved unresponsive to electroconvulsive therapy. Euphoria and apathy generally occur along with intellectual enfeeblement, or in conjunction with other organically determined changes of personality.

Frontal lobe tumours may present with changes of disposition and behaviour, even in the absence of intellectual deficits or neurological signs. This appears to be particularly characteristic of slow-growing meningiomas. In Strauss and Keschner's (1935) series of frontal tumours, for example, change of personality was one of the earliest manifestations in almost a quarter of patients. Eleven of 25 patients reported by Direkze et al. (1971) presented with subtle personality alterations. A 53-year-old clergyman began outlining rather smutty jokes, a greengrocer was charged on five occasions for speeding, all within 3 weeks, and a pharmacist became forgetful, easily provoked and asked his wife to play cowboys and indians with him. All proved to have frontal astrocytomas.

Irresponsibility, childishness and lack of reserve are the changes stressed most frequently, and can sometimes occur before there is any evidence of intellectual deterioration. A tendency towards facetiousness and indifference to those around may combine to give a particular stamp to the clinical picture. Disinhibition sometimes leads to striking social lapses or minor misdemeanours as the first obvious sign of change; sexual excitation and erotic behaviour very occasionally occur.

A man of 58 presented with a 12-month history of extravagance, boastfulness, excessive drinking, marital discord, unrealistic planning and several changes of job. He had previously held a responsible job in a senior position. He showed a happy confi-dent manner and believed he was rich, but was self neglectful and severely lacking in insight. The plantar reflexes were upgoing and there was papilloedema on the left with reduced visual acuity. A left olfactory groove meningioma was discovered.
                                                    (Avery 1971)

Frontal lobe tumours are not unique in their capacity to engender such personality changes, and it has even been questioned whether they show them more frequently than tumours elsewhere in the cortex. Keschner et al. (1936) found little difference between frontal and temporal lobe tumours in this regard. Most are agreed, however, that bifrontal tumours show such changes with especial frequency and severity. Tumours arising from the small sphenoidal wing, which marks the transition between the frontal and temporal lobes, have also been noted to show a very high frequency of mental changes (David & Askenasy 1937).

Lack of insight is characteristically marked, and in part may represent a lack of feedback from environmental cues. Frequently the patient is completely indifferent about his illness and situation, even when intellect is well preserved. In a paradoxical fashion denial of illness may coexist with placid compliance and calm acceptance of treatment.

Severe urgency, frequency and incontinence are often present early in the course of a frontal tumour, and can occur in the absence of dementia, indifference or lack of social concern (Andrew & Nathan 1964; Maurice-Williams 1974). The ability to inhibit the micturition reflex appears to be impaired, likewise ability to stop the flow once it has begun. A similar disorder of defaecation may develop, though less often and less severely. Contrary to common teaching the patients are usually upset and embarrassed by their incontinence at this stage, though later on it may emerge in the context of general indifference and self neglect.

The neurological signs which may betray frontal lesions are outlined on p. 17. In addition, hallucinations may derive from the neighbouring temporal lobe (p. 219), and hypothalamic damage due to pressure or distortion may occasionally lead to obesity, stupor or narcoleptic attacks (Hunter et al. 1968a).

Corpus callosum tumours

Tumours originating within the corpus callosum are notorious for the severity of the mental disturbances that follow. They are said, moreover, to present with mental symptoms more frequently than tumours elsewhere. A large series was reported by Schlesinger (1950), who found mental changes in 92% when the rostrum was involved, in 57% with mid-callosal tumours and in 89%

with tumours of the splenium. Selecki (1964) in a small consecutive series confirmed the special frequency of mental symptoms with anterior and posterior tumours when compared with those arising from the middle portion. Anterior tumours in particular tended to lead to rapid mental deterioration before the appearance of neurological signs, headache or other evidence of raised intracranial pressure. Rudge and Warrington (1991) have drawn attention to the special tendency for tumours of the splenium to present with marked deficits of memory and visual perception, sometimes while other aspects of intellectual function are relatively well preserved.

The usual picture is of a rapidly progressive impairment of cognitive functions, beginning with marked memory difficulties. Sometimes there is striking blocking of thought and action which may resemble that seen with catatonic schizophrenia. Alpers (1936) thought that the clinical picture was often sufficiently characteristic for the diagnosis to be made directly:

A man of 64 had a 4-week history of behaving strangely at work, seeming oblivious of questions and unable to focus his attention. At home he would sit in the same place for hours at a time, once wound a clock for 3 hours on end and once lathered his face for 2 hours. On examination there was bilateral spasticity but no papilloedema. He sat staring ahead oblivious of his surroundings, or with his eyes closed picking aimlessly at the bed clothes. Sometimes he lay for long periods tapping his head with his hand. It was hard to make contact with him, and most questions met with no response. He was disoriented, but at times seemed to recognise people. Perseveration was extremely marked. He proved to have a glioblastoma practically confined to the genu of the corpus callosum.   (Alpers 1936)

Personality change may also be an early feature, similar in all respects to that seen with frontal lobe tumours. Florid psychotic symptoms have also been reported. Elliott (1969), in his comprehensive review, suggests that the combination of delusions and stupor can come to resemble schizophrenia closely.

A large part of the mental disturbance is probably due to the tendency for tumours of the corpus callosum to involve adjacent structures. Those of the anterior portion rapidly extend into the frontal lobes bilaterally, and those of the splenium invade the thalamus and midbrain posteriorly. Almost all involve the third ventricle and diencephalon at some stage, which probably accounts for the somnolence, akinesis and stupor which ultimately appear. However, the lesion of the corpus callosum is also likely to be important in itself by leading to disturbance of interhemispheric communication, also the disruption of fibres in the neighbouring cingulum bundle which connects important association areas ipsilaterally (Schlesinger 1950).

Temporal lobe tumours

As noted in Table 10 (p. 221), temporal lobe tumours produce perhaps the highest frequency of mental disturbances. In part this may be ascribed to the paroxysmal phenomena occasioned by temporal lobe epilepsy, though temporal tumours retain their lead over other groups in Keschner et al.'s series where disturbances due to epilepsy were excluded.

Apart from features particular to temporal lobe epilepsy, there does not seem to be any form of mental disturbance specific enough to be of localising value. The early onset and rapid progression of dementia has been said to be characteristic, though this impression may be largely due to the marked dysphasic disturbances which accompany tumours on the dominant side. Certainly non-dominant temporal lobe tumours can be clinically silent until they are very large.

Bingley (1958) reported one of the largest series of temporal lobe tumours—253 temporal lobe gliomas—and concluded that tumours on the dominant side produced the greater impairment of intellect. This appeared to apply to both verbal and non-verbal functions. Moreover the excess of intellectual disturbance with dominant tumours was even more pronounced when attention was restricted to cases without papilloedema. Bingley also found that among the dominant lobe tumours those with dysphasia did not have a higher incidence of other mental changes than those without. These findings, however, do not go unchallenged, and tumour material is in many ways unsatisfactory for exploring the complex interrelationships between language and non-language impairments after cerebral lesions.

The slowing and aspontaneity of speech and movement seen with frontal lobe tumours has also been reported with temporal lobe tumours. Keschner et al. (1936) compared frontal and temporal tumours in this regard and could find no substantial difference between them. Sixty-three per cent of temporal cases showed dullness, apathy or torpor; some showed no spontaneous speech whatever, yet when roused spoke slowly and deliberately without evidence of dysphasia. Indifference to surroundings may also be seen with temporal as with frontal lobe tumours; memory disturbances may likewise feature prominently, including occasional cases which present with a florid Korsakoff syndrome.

Affective disturbances appear to be common. In Hécaen and Ajuriaguerra's (1956) series, frontal, frontotemporal and temporal tumours taken together showed double the frequency of affective changes seen with tumours in other locations. Euphoria is probably as common with temporal as with frontal tumours (Keschner et al. 1936; Schlesinger

1950), and again occurs mainly in the presence of intellectual impairment. Paroxysms of anxiety or anger have been described, and occasional cases have presented with mania or hypomania. Depression, anxiety and irritability are all common, perhaps particularly with tumours on the dominant side and in association with dysphasia (Keschner *et al.* 1936). Bingley (1958) found that emotional changes generally were more frequent with dominant than non-dominant tumours, especially where blunting and flattening of affect were concerned.

There does not appear to be a form of personality change specific for temporal lobe tumours. A change towards facetiousness, foolish joking and childish behaviour may be indistinguishable from that seen with frontal lesions, and has been reported to be just as common. Strobos (1953) observed marked personality alterations in seven of 62 patients with temporal lobe tumours, including psychopathic and paranoid trends, hypochondriasis and extreme irritability. Three of these patients were without papilloedema. Most examples seemed to represent a reaction to the disease or to the epileptic attacks which occurred, and to reflect aspects of the premorbid personality. An accentuation of neurotic traits has also been stressed, with dramatisation of complaints, unjustified fears and preoccupation with troubles remote from the present situation (Hécaen & Ajuriaguerra 1956).

Occasionally patients with temporal lobe tumours develop psychotic illnesses resembling schizophrenia. This may sometimes be the initial manifestation. Such cases are rare, but were drawn together in a review of the literature by Davison and Bagley (1969). The location of the tumour in 77 cases of 'schizophrenia' from 42 published reports was compared with two large unselected series of tumours. A significantly higher proportion of temporal lobe tumours and pituitary tumours were present in the schizophrenic group. There was insufficient information to indicate whether such patients had been genetically predisposed to schizophrenia, or whether the temporal lobe pathology might play a more direct aetiological role.

Some isolated clinical examples rather strongly suggest that the temporal lobe pathology may itself be responsible:

A 53-year-old woman was admitted to hospital after attacking her husband with a knife. She had recently been behaving bizarrely, accusing her family of trying to poison her and refusing to eat in self defence. She believed they were spraying the house with poison gas in an attempt to harm her, and that her son was turning her into a dog. She also complained of severe headache and pains in the chest and stomach. Her previous personality

had been that of a sociable, quick tempered and outspoken woman.

On examination there were no abnormal neurological signs. Speech was incoherent but she was mostly unresponsive to questioning. She showed bizarre facial mannerisms and sudden unexpected actions from time to time, for example rolling of the eyes or abrupt attempts at undressing. After 3 weeks in hospital she became stuporose and died. A glioblastoma was found in the right temporal lobe.   (Haberland 1965)

In a case seen personally, a woman of 51 developed florid schizophrenic symptomatology in association with a possible local recurrence of a temporal lobe tumour which had been removed 2 years previously. There was no family history of schizophrenia, and her premorbid personality had shown no schizoid traits.

She had presented originally with a 15-year history of attacks of visual disturbance in the right field of vision, and a 1-year history of grand mal epilepsy. A slow-growing astrocytoma of the left temporal lobe was discovered and partially removed. She made an excellent recovery, but 2 years later became depressed for several weeks after her husband had a stroke. As the depression receded she gradually developed a number of strange ideas —she believed that strangers could read her thoughts and communicate with her, became distressed when she saw the colour red, and felt that words had special significance for her if they contained 'a' as the second letter. With this she developed occasional hallucinations in the right half-field of vision—of an eye, of a man standing in a room or by a car, or of a sepia-coloured scene.

These disturbances increased over several months until she was admitted to hospital. She then showed many of the first rank symptoms of schizophrenia. She believed that her thoughts were read by some radio mechanism, and that others betrayed this by gestures; she believed that her husband could alter the train of her thoughts and cause them to block, and that he had taken over control of the limbs on the left of her body; she felt that other patients were talking about her and looking at her in a special way, and that when she put on her spectacles a neighbouring patient and her doctor could both see more clearly. She felt that she was caught up in some ill-defined plan involving many people.

Her speech was somewhat circumstantial with loosening of associations, tangential thinking and occasional thought block. However, her affect remained warm and her personality intact, and she preserved a certain measure of insight into the abnormal nature of her beliefs and experiences.

Examination revealed a new upper quadrantic visual field defect, a return of her dysphasia, some defect of recent memory and slight dropping away of the outstretched right arm. The EEG showed an increase in slow activity in the left frontotemporal region. A local extension of the tumour was suspected but angiography failed to give definite evidence of this.

She was started on chlorpromazine and over the next 2 weeks the schizophrenia-like symptoms began to recede. Coincidentally her dysphasia and right arm weakness also began to resolve, and the EEG improved to its baseline state. Within 2 months all psychotic symptoms had disappeared and she had regained full insight. She remained well when followed up 6 months later, apart from occasional grand mal and minor epileptic attacks and a persistent mild deficit of recent memory. Residual dysphasic symptoms were again evident, especially when she was tired.

One year later she was re-admitted with increasing dysphasia and frequent attacks of falling. She developed increasing drowsiness and a right hemiparesis, and died after 3 weeks in hospital. At autopsy recurrence of the tumour was found in the left frontotemporal region.

In addition to patients who present with schizophrenic symptomatology, the complex hallucinations of temporal lobe tumours may lead to diagnostic confusion. Fifteen of 110 cases reported by Keschner *et al.* (1936) showed hallucinations independently of epileptic phenomena. Visual and auditory hallucinations can be either simple or complex, the latter being especially liable to lead to a mistaken diagnosis of psychotic illness. Visual hallucinations occurring within a hemianopic field of vision are particularly characteristic of temporal lobe disturbance. Olfactory and gustatory hallucinations may arise from the uncinate region. Typically, the patient accepts such hallucinatory experiences as real at the time of their occurrence, but thereafter rapidly regains insight into their abnormal nature, unlike the situation with schizophrenia.

Epilepsy occurs in approximately 50% of patients with temporal lobe tumours, which is commoner than with tumours in other locations (Paillas & Tamalet 1950; Strobos 1953). In addition to hallucinatory experiences, the epileptic auras may contain a variety of abnormal subjective experiences which lead to diagnostic difficulty — unreality, *déjà vu*, dreamy states, forced thoughts, overwhelming fears and other sudden emotional changes (pp. 250–2). Automatisms and other complex psychomotor seizures may occur, though these are probably less common with tumours than with temporal lobe epilepsy

arising from other causes (Hécaen & Ajuriaguerra 1956; Bingley 1958).

Parietal tumours

Tumours of the parietal lobe appear to be distinctly less likely than frontal or temporal lobe tumours to produce psychological changes. Table 11 shows this where several different areas of mental disturbance are concerned. They are also prone to lead to early neurological signs in motor and sensory systems, so that an erroneous diagnosis of primary psychiatric disorder is less likely to be made.

With regard to affective changes, depression has been noted with considerable frequency (Hécaen & Ajuriaguerra 1956). Personality disturbances appear to be relatively uncommon. Hallucinatory disturbances consist of tactile or kinaesthetic hallucinations confined to the opposite half of the body, also 'tactile perseveration' as when the patient continues to perceive a contact long after the stimulus has been removed.

The principal psychiatric interest attaching to parietal lobe tumours lies in the complex and fascinating cognitive disturbances that may occur. It is here that care must be taken, since the clinical picture may at first sight be mistaken for dementia or hysteria. Dominant lobe tumours may produce dysphasia, more rarely ideomotor or ideational dyspraxia. Components of the Gerstmann syndrome—finger agnosia, dyscalculia, dysgraphia and right–left disorientation—may be found in relative isolation or may stand out among more generalised cognitive disturbances. Tumours of the non-dominant lobe are associated with disorders of visuospatial perception, dressing difficulty and topographical disorientation,

Table 11 Prevalence of forms of mental disturbance with cerebral tumours.

| | Study 1 (Keschner *et al.* 1938) | | | | | Study 2 (Hécaen & Ajuriaguerra 1956) | | |
Location of tumour	Number of cases	% with disturbance of consciousness	% with change of intellect	% with disturbance of memory and orientation	% with disturbance of affect	Number of cases	% with intellectual disturbance	% with affective and personality disturbance
Frontal	68	65	47	50	59	80	60	38
Temporal	56	75	50	57	61	75	43	24
Parietal	32	69	38	25	38	75	35	19
Occipital	11	64	36	45	45	25	24	20
Mesodiencephalic	—	—	—	—	—	61	26	21
All supratentorial	401	69	44	45	54	—	—	—
All infratentorial	129	37	12	8	23	85	22	12

which again can sometimes occur in relative isolation. Any of these disorders, when accompanied by marked indifference or social withdrawal, may easily lead to an erroneous diagnosis of dementia. However, with careful examination it can often be established that other cognitive functions remain intact.

Non-dominant tumours are also liable to be associated with complex disturbances of the body image. Best known are the phenomena of unilateral inattention or neglect, and anosognosia in which the patient appears to be unaware of a left hemiplegia or denies the disability when this is pointed out to him. A range of disturbances is seen, extending even to denial of ownership of the affected limbs, or attribution of the limbs to another person (p. 69 *et seq.*). Though less common with tumours than with vascular parietal lesions, these elaborate disturbances may at first sight strongly suggest hysteria. Fortunately such a diagnostic error is unlikely to be made after even a cursory neurological examination. Critchley (1964) stressed other similarities between hysteria and parietal disease: difficulties with communication may make it hard to secure the patient's attention or cooperation, and performance may show marked inconsistencies such that he succeeds in a task which a moment before had appeared to be beyond him.

Finally, the epileptic manifestations which accompany parietal lobe tumours, and which may antedate the appearance of neurological signs, sometimes consist of transient disturbances of the body image. These again may be sufficiently bizarre to suggest a non-organic psychiatric disorder. Examples reported by Hécaen and Ajuriaguerra (1956) included the spasmodic feeling of someone standing close by, absence or displacement of a part of the body, transformation of a limb into a mechanical object, and the phantom appearance of a third limb.

Occipital tumours

In the early literature, occipital tumours were sometimes reported to show a particularly high frequency of mental disturbances. This may have been a result of their tendency to produce early and pronounced elevation of intracranial pressure. Allen (1930), for example, stressed the frequency of neurotic manifestations early in the course of 40 such patients, and noted pronounced defects of attention and memory in almost a third.

However, detailed comparisons between patients with tumours in different locations have failed to reveal an excess of mental symptoms with occipital tumours (Table 11). Amnesic difficulties and dementia can occasionally be striking, but affective disturbances and personality changes seem to occur with rather less frequency than with tumours elsewhere.

Visual agnosic defects and other features which may be of localising value are outlined on p. 19.

Diencephalic tumours

Tumours originating in the deep midline structures of the diencephalon (i.e. the thalamus, hypothalamus and other structures in the neighbourhood of the third ventricle) are not remarkable for the overall frequency with which they produce mental symptoms, as shown in Table 11. However, the disturbances that do occur are often striking and some have important localising significance.

Marked amnesic difficulties are well established as typical of tumours in the neighbourhood of the third ventricle (Delay *et al.* 1964). Hécaen and Ajuriaguerra (1956) regarded this as one of the few psychiatric syndromes of practical importance to the neurosurgeon. The picture is of marked inability to fixate current events, impairment of new learning and distortion of the recent past, while remote memory and other cognitive functions remain substantially intact. Confabulation may be much in evidence. Sprofkin and Sciarra (1952) reported three patients in whom the clinical picture was that of a Korsakoff syndrome but alcoholism had been excluded. All had tumours limited to the region of the hypothalamus and third ventricle. Previously, coincidence had been held to account for examples of Korsakoff's syndrome with third ventricle tumours, and a history of alcoholism was said to be usually present.

Williams and Pennybacker (1954) provided further evidence from a systematic study of 180 patients with cerebral tumours, all of whom were given psychological tests to assess memory function. In 26 impairment of memory was the outstanding cognitive deficit, and more than half of these had tumours involving the region of the third ventricle. Four patients had a classic amnesic–confabulatory syndrome, and all four had localised lesions directly involving the floor or walls of the third ventricle. Pursuing the question of localisation further, Williams and Pennybacker reviewed 32 patients with craniopharyngiomas implicating the diencephalon and third ventricle, and compared them with patients with posterior fossa tumours to control for the effects of raised intracranial pressure. The craniopharyngiomas showed a clear excess of cases with characteristic memory defects, especially when the more posterior parts of the hypothalamus and third ventricle had been involved.

One of Williams and Pennybacker's patients illustrates the distinction which can at times be made between the general mental changes of raised intracranial pressure and the specific memory changes related to the focal lesion:

A young man of 22 was found to have a craniopharyngioma involving the floor of the third ventricle. It had interrupted the circulation of the CSF and caused a marked rise of intracranial pressure, producing some local brain stem signs, severe confusion, drowsiness and intermittent coma. Ventricular tapping relieved these symptoms and he became alert and cooperative. However, a marked memory deficit for recent events then emerged, with elaborate and detailed confabulation. Part of the tumour was cystic and was directly tapped, thereby reducing local pressure on the hypothalamus. Following this he became fully orientated and his confabulation ceased. As the cyst again filled up the amnesic–confabulatory syndrome reappeared. As the CSF circulation was again interrupted and general intracranial tension rose, so drowsiness and mental confusion supervened. These sequences were repeated on several occasions.

A patient reported by Burkle and Lipowski (1978) is also instructive in that memory deficits were accompanied by such prominent psychiatric disorder that the organic nature of her troubles was at first overlooked. The lesion, a colloid cyst of the third ventricle, was eventually removed with excellent results:

A woman of 24 complained of increasing depression, sleepiness, loss of interest and recurrent memory lapses. Her depression had been coming on gradually over several months. On examination she was disoriented for the day of the week, showed poor recall of objects, but had no neurological abnormalities. She was apathetic, spoke slowly and stared impassively. A diagnosis was made of severe depression.

Further examination confirmed marked impairment of judgement and recent memory, and she was considered to be affectively flat rather than depressed. The possibility was raised of hysteria or an organic brain syndrome. Skull X-ray surprisingly showed evidence of raised intracranial pressure, and a computerised tomography (CT) scan showed dilated lateral ventricles and a spherical mass in the third ventricle. A colloid cyst was removed and she ultimately made a full recovery.

(Burkle & Lipowski 1978)

Steadily progressive intellectual impairment with tumours of the diencephalon are usually the result of cortical atrophy consequent upon chronic obstruction to the CSF circulation. Thus even simple cysts of the third ventricle may present with progressive dementia. Russell and Pennybacker (1961) showed that craniopharyngiomas, when coming to light only in middle or old age, may present with clinical pictures dominated by failing intellect and memory and that obvious neurological signs could be absent. Visual symptoms were common but not universal. These tumours are strategically situated to compress the optic chiasma, but the demented patient was sometimes unaware of field defects even when these

could be demonstrated. The clue in such diencephalic dementias may lie in marked somnolence or the other symptoms of hypothalamic disturbance considered below, but these are not obvious in every case.

Thalamic tumours have been reported to show early and severe dementia which may run a rapid course. Smyth and Stern (1938) reported six such cases. In two, severe dementia coexisted with little evidence of raised intracranial pressure or ventricular dilatation, and at postmortem examination the tumour had not extended widely into the surrounding white matter. The focal lesion may therefore be significant in itself in causing intellectual disturbance, perhaps by virtue of the important connections between medial thalamic structures and the cerebral cortex. Again neurological signs need not be an early feature; disturbances of pupillary reflexes were common in Smyth and Stern's cases, but sensory and motor focal signs were sometimes late in appearance or even completely absent.

Somnolence and hypersomnia are frequent with diencephalic tumours. They are symptoms of localising importance, and can alert one to the diencephalic origin of disturbances of memory or intellect. Fulton and Bailey (1929) stressed that it is necessary to distinguish true hypersomnia from the impairment of consciousness that results from raised intracranial pressure. The hypersomnia due to diencephalic lesions is essentially an excess of normal sleep, and when roused the patient awakens normally and fully; patients with torpor due to raised intracranial pressure may similarly be roused, but usually then display a muddled awareness and obvious intellectual impairment. With some diencephalic lesions there may be a history of transient attacks of hypersomnia for several years during the evolution of the tumour, and well before the intracranial pressure has risen. Very rarely attacks virtually indistinguishable from idiopathic narcolepsy are said to occur, with uncontrollable drowsiness and sometimes also with episodes of weakness of the limbs. These may be provoked by laughter or other sudden emotional reactions.

Such disorders of sleep are due to lesions which impinge upon the hypothalamus, especially in its posterior part, and the contiguous regions of the upper midbrain. The tumour may originate within the hypothalamus itself, but more commonly compresses it from above as with third ventricular tumours, or from below as with craniopharyngiomas or pituitary tumours. Frequently, but not invariably, the sleep disturbances are accompanied by other evidence of hypothalamic disorder —amenorrhoea, impotence, diabetes insipidus with polydipsia and polyuria, or a voracious appetite. Disturbances of thermoregulation may cause pyrexia and lead to a mistaken diagnosis of an infective process. Tumours affecting the hypothalamus or third ventricular region in childhood, such as craniopharyngiomas or pinealomas, can lead to delayed sexual development or occasionally to precocious puberty. These varied disturbances may, of course, also occur in the absence of somnolence and provide their own clues to the diencephalic origin of disturbances of memory and intellect.

'Akinetic mutism' is another striking syndrome seen with lesions of the posterior diencephalon or upper midbrain. It was first clearly described by Cairns *et al.* (1941) in a patient with an epidermoid cyst of the third ventricle:

'The patient sleeps more than normally, but he is easily roused. In the fully developed state he makes no sound and lies inert, except that his eyes regard the observer steadily, or follow the movements of objects, and they may be diverted by sound. Despite his steady gaze, which seems to give promise of speech, the patient is quite mute or he answers only in whispered monosyllables. Oft-repeated commands may be carried out in a feeble, slow and incomplete manner, but usually there are no movements of a voluntary character; no restless movements, struggling or evidence of negativism. Emotional movement also is almost in abeyance. A painful stimulus produces reflex withdrawal of the limb and, if the stimulus is sustained, slow feeble voluntary movements of the limbs may occur in an attempt to remove the source of stimulation, but usually without tears, noise or other manifestations of pain or displeasure. The patient swallows readily, but has to be fed. Food seen may be recognised as such, but there is evidently little appreciation of its taste and other characteristics: objects normally chewed or sucked may be swallowed whole. There is total incontinence of urine and faeces.

Fluctuations may occur in the intensity of this state. In its incomplete manifestations the patient may respond at times, though slowly and imperfectly, by speech and voluntary movement. Voluntary movement may be accompanied by a coarse tremor of the limbs. Incontinence persists, and there is little or no trace of spontaneous activity or speech. The onset of the condition is gradual. In certain circumstances there may be slow spontaneous recovery; but if the state is caused by pressure of a tumour it may be followed by coma. The condition is sometimes, though not always, associated with decorticate rigidity.'

When caused by a cystic tumour which can be aspirated the syndrome is found to be potentially reversible. A dense amnesic gap is then left for the duration of the episode. The syndrome is thus clearly not due to the general effects of raised intracranial pressure, but attributable to focal disturbance of particular diencephalic mechanisms. It may very occasionally need to be distinguished from depressive or catatonic stupor (pp. 155–6).

Affective disturbances with diencephalic tumours have been much discussed, but mainly in anecdotal form. Marked swings of mood have been described, from severe depression to exuberant gaiety, or defective emotional control leading to sudden outbursts of temper on minor provocation (Alpers 1940). Reeves and Plum (1969) reported a patient whose dementia was accompanied by outbursts of rage and marked hyperphagia; at autopsy a circumscribed hamartoma was found in the hypothalamus. Transient manic reactions have occasionally been observed during the course of operations on hypothalamic tumours, also in the postoperative phase. Other patients have presented from the outset with psychotic depression of marked degree. In the presence of dementia, a euphoric or grandiose colouring has led to a mistaken impression of general paresis.

Complex disturbances of personality have also been reported in occasional cases of hypothalamic tumour:

A patient of 39 was found at postmortem to have a teratoma of the third ventricle which had destroyed the hypothalamus, but without evidence of hydrocephalus or cortical damage. For a year before signs of the tumour developed he had become irritable, hypersensitive, aggressive, unreasonable and stubborn, in contrast to his previous personality. He had shown periods of great excitement, and frequently flew into a rage over trivial matters. Meanwhile his business judgement had become impaired and he had become careless of responsibilities. Ultimately he exhibited severe loss of memory.   (Alpers 1937)

Other patients are described with features suggestive of frontal lobe disturbance—carelessness, fatuous serenity, disinhibition and lack of concern for those around. Indifference to the gravity of the condition may be striking, with affirmation of well-being and denial of illness.

Pituitary tumours

Tumours arising from the pituitary gland commonly present with raised intracranial pressure, pituitary dysfunction or visual failure. Other tumours in the region of the sella turcica, such as suprasellar meningiomas and craniopharyngiomas, may show similar symptoms. All, however, may also produce mental changes at an early stage and well before these other features are marked.

With some forms of pituitary tumour the psychiatric picture may in part be attributable to the endocrine disturbances which result, for example when Cushing's disease develops with basophil tumours (p. 515) or acromegaly with acidophil tumours (p. 521). The common prolactin-secreting adenoma may be accompanied by marked depression which resolves when the prolactin levels are corrected (pp. 522–3). It is therefore often hard to apportion the blame between the effects of hormonal changes and the effects of the lesion of the nervous system, but there is general agreement that much of the psychiatric disturbance is due directly to extensions of the tumour beyond the sella turcica. Upward extension occurs in the direction of the third ventricle, and will cause the mental symptoms typical of diencephalic tumours. Forward extension may occur between the frontal lobes, or laterally into the temporal lobe, all of which will contribute to the picture that ensues. Clearly pituitary tumours are prone to involve some of the regions where damage is especially likely to lead to psychiatric disturbance. They are also well situated to cause obstruction to the circulation of the CSF, with additional effects on the mental state due to raised intracranial pressure.

It is therefore not surprising that the literature on pituitary tumours reports a high incidence of mental changes. Accurate comparison with other groups of tumours is difficult since strictly comparable series are not available, but reviews by White and Cobb (1955) and Jefferson (1955) indicated the range of disturbances seen—hypothalamic disturbances with somnolence, polyuria and obesity, circumscribed amnesic states, deterioration of personality, and epilepsy including the uncinate fits of temporal lobe epilepsy.

Dullness, apathy and passivity appear to be particularly characteristic, with mental slowing out of proportion to changes in intracranial pressure. Lack of concern may be striking, even in face of progressive blindness. Emotional instability is also stressed, with liability to episodes of irritability and sudden rage.

A tendency towards paranoid developments seems to be common, and Davison and Bagley's (1969) data (p. 225) have suggested a particular association between pituitary tumours and schizophrenia.

Apart from the amnesic syndrome and the disturbances of hypothalamic regulatory function, it is difficult to apportion these psychological changes between diencephalic, frontal and temporal effects. Even so it is important to pay attention to early mental changes, since they are likely to represent extensions of the tumour beyond the sella turcica which may render the tumour inoperable.

Subtentorial tumours (posterior fossa tumours)

Under this heading are included tumours of the cerebellum, cerebellopontine angle and brain stem. As already seen, tumours originating below the tentorium cerebelli have a considerably lower incidence of mental symptoms than those originating above (Table 10, p. 221) despite the fact that raised intracranial pressure is much commoner and tends to occur earlier in the former. This distinction is one of the firmer strands of evidence in favour of the view that tumour location plays a part in determining the severity of mental sequelae.

Table 11 (p. 226) shows that cognitive, affective and personality disturbances are all less frequent with subtentorial tumours when compared to tumours elsewhere. Moreover Keschner et al. (1937) found that the mental disturbances that did occur were usually mild, were rarely persistent and tended to arise late in the disease.

Cognitive disturbances appear to be very closely tied to evidence of raised intracranial pressure. The intellectual impairment is usually global, and amnesic defects or other focal cognitive deficits rarely appear in isolation. The impairments usually develop insidiously, and parallel the development of internal hydrocephalus caused by obstruction to the flow of CSF. Very slow-growing subtentorial tumours sometimes result in profound ventricular dilatation before they present for attention, and by then dementia may be severe.

It is important, however, to allow for exceptional instances. Wilson and Rupp (1946) reported a group of 21 patients with posterior fossa tumours, of whom five had initially been admitted to psychiatric units with symptoms of memory disturbance, confusion, retardation of thinking and emotional instability; in these cases evidence of raised intracranial pressure was sometimes absent at the time of their presentation. A patient reported by Whitty (1956) is also instructive in this regard:

A woman of 59 with no previous or family history of mental disorder became increasingly depressed and unable to manage her housework following the unexpected death of her mother. Her family noted marked memory impairment. She would put household utensils and money carefully away and then forget where they were, which upset her greatly. When first examined there were no abnormal physical signs and her symptoms were considered to be a psychological reaction to the death of her mother 2 months before.

Over the next 6 months she developed occasional incontinence of urine and some ill-defined difficulty with walking. She was now euphoric and showed emotional lability. There was a marked memory deficit for recent events, some nominal dysphasia and a suggestion of constructional apraxia. Neurological examination showed a fine tremor of the outstretched hands, brisk tendon reflexes and a shuffling gait, but no papilloedema or other abnormal signs. The CSF protein was 90 mg/100 ml but under normal pressure.

She was considered to have an early organic dementia, but in view of the high CSF protein ventriculograms were carried out. A posterior fossa tumour was revealed, and at operation a haemangioblastoma of the right cerebellar lobe was successfully removed. Over the next 3 months she improved rapidly and steadily, and on discharge was fully orientated with normal memory to formal testing. She returned to full household duties and social life, and had maintained the improvement when followed up 3 years later.

Disturbances of affect include euphoria and emotional lability in association with intellectual impairments, and sometimes a marked degree of depression, apprehension or irritability. The latter are probably chiefly reactions to the neurological deficits resulting from cerebellar, brain stem or cranial nerve lesions. Bristow's (1991) two patients with tumours of the brain stem had reacted to dizziness, loss of balance and other minor symptoms by becoming depressed and anxious, and had initially been diagnosed as neurotic. Change of personality appears to occur mainly as part of the general dementing process, though sometimes frontal lobe disturbance is prominent in consequence of internal hydrocephalus.

The mental symptoms that can emerge with acoustic neuromas have attracted attention. Shepherd and Wadia (1956) reported six patients in whom chronic hydrocephalus produced confusion, impaired memory, change of personality, apathy and lack of insight. In two the mental changes were the presenting feature. Woodcock (1967) found mental changes in seven of 31 cases— personality deterioration, impairment of memory and intellect, confusion, depression, euphoria and neurotic traits—and concluded that these were attributable to vascular disturbances consequent upon brain stem distortion. Psychotic developments have been reported both preoperatively and postoperatively in a surprising number of cases, chiefly depressive or paranoid psychoses occurring in clear consciousness (Dobrokhotova & Faller 1969; Scott 1970).

In children posterior fossa tumours appear to lead rather often to early and pronounced changes of behaviour. In Hécaen and Ajuriaguerra's (1956) series there were four cases of cerebellar tumour in children which had produced anxiety, withdrawal, deterioration in school work, hyperactivity and problems of control. Pontine tumours may present similarly in childhood. Cairns (1950) reported three children with astrocytomas of the pons in whom the initial symptoms included irritability, fretfulness, cruelty and obstinacy. In two these were sufficiently pronounced to constitute a complete change of character, and in all three they antedated the appearance of headache or the development of physical signs. Cairns suggested that the inhibitory functions of the cortex over the lower centres were perhaps less well developed in children, allowing emotional and behavioural disorders to declare themselves more promptly in the presence of a subtentorial lesion.

Visual hallucinations may occur with subtentorial tumours, presumably via pressure effects transmitted through the tentorium to the adjacent occipital cortex.

Investigations

When there are grounds for seriously suspecting the existence of a tumour, neurological or neurosurgical help should be obtained without delay. But in doubtful cases certain preliminary investigations may be undertaken by the psychiatrist himself, so a brief survey may not be inappropriate here.

The value of different investigatory procedures is usefully outlined by Sumner (1969) and Mendelow (1993). Kendall (1980) has reviewed the changed situation since CT scans became available, and Armstrong and Keevil (1991) outline the advantages of magnetic resonance imaging (MRI). A detailed neurological examination is the first essential, and here the importance of false localising signs must be remembered. Oculomotor and other cranial nerve palsies may result from secondary distortion of the brain stem, the stretching of cranial nerves or compression of the cerebral peduncles against the tentorium. An extensor plantar response may be obtained on the side ipsilateral to the tumour for similar reasons.

Full medical examination and chest X-ray are essential in case the tumour should be a secondary deposit from primary neoplasia elsewhere. The erythrocyte sedimentation rate is more commonly raised in secondary than primary intracerebral tumours. Serological tests for syphilis should be carried out while any uncertainty persists.

Skull X-ray may be expected to outline the pineal gland in approximately 50% of adults and a lateral shift may be revealed. Evidence of raised intracranial pressure may be seen in erosion of the dorsum sellae or posterior clinoid processes, or the situation of the tumour may be indicated by bone destruction, new bone formation or enlarged vascular channels in the overlying skull. Sometimes there may be calcification within the tumour itself when this is very slow growing. With many pituitary tumours the pituitary fossa shows expansion; and special views may reveal widening or erosion of the internal auditory meatus with acoustic neuromas.

The *electroencephalogram* is discussed by Kiloh *et al.* (1981). In approximately 20% of cases a normal record is obtained, so the investigation cannot be relied upon to exclude the possibility of a tumour. Occasionally it may point to the lesion when other methods short of contrast radiography or CT scanning fail, being particularly valuable with tumours situated in 'silent' areas such as the frontal regions. Malignant tumours produce more abnormalities than benign, and meningiomas may occasionally yield abnormal tracings only several years after the onset of clinical symptoms.

Focal evidence consists usually of a delta wave focus, irregular in form and amplitude, often with faster waves in the vicinity. Local spikes or spike and wave complexes may be seen, especially if the patient has symptomatic epilepsy. Diffuse changes may consist of less well developed alpha activity or an increase of slow waves on the side of the tumour. Distant signs may also be produced by mass displacements and cerebral circulatory disturbances; focal evidence of a tumour may therefore sometimes be misleading as to site. A single recording will often fail to distinguish between a tumour and an infarct, though serial recordings can be of value, with worsening indicating the former and improvement the latter.

Brain imaging is now essential in the investigation of suspected tumours. CT and MRI can be expected to give firm indications as to site, and the nature of the tumour may also be disclosed. The capacity to distinguish tumours from infarctions at an early stage is particularly useful, and in cases of doubt repetition after an interval of 2–3 weeks will usually clarify the issue.

In addition to direct visualisation of the tumour mass, important information is obtained from brain displacements, surrounding oedema and changes in the overlying bone. With CT scanning a meningioma shows as an area of increased density, whereas gliomas and metastases may be either hypo- or hyperdense. Calcification or bleeding within the tumour may be detected. Contrast enhancement is essential before concluding that a CT examination is negative. Abnormal enhancement occurs with vascular tumours, and cystic or necrotic areas may be clearly displayed.

MRI holds several advantages over CT scanning and is the investigation of choice whenever facilities are available (Armstrong & Keevil 1991). Its increased sensitivity allows the detection of very small lesions, the images are not degraded by artefact from overlying bone, and the capacity to image in multiple planes can yield extra information about tumour size, shape and position. These emerge as marked advantages in, for example, the detection of metastases in asymptomatic patients. MRI frequently shows that the tumour and its associated brain response is more extensive than suspected on CT, and gadolinium enhancement helps delineate the tumour margins from surrounding oedema. CT remains superior, however, in the detection of calcification, for example in meningiomas.

MRI is of special value in the investigation of pituitary and posterior fossa tumours. Microadenomas of the pituitary less than 1 cm in diameter are well displayed (Naheedy *et al.* 1987; Levy & Lightman 1994), likewise the upward and lateral extension of large lesions in relation to the optic tract, third ventricle and cavernous sinuses. Early lesions of the brain stem, such as tiny acoustic neuromas which are below the threshold for CT scanning, are shown by appropriate sequences.

A puzzling syndrome which not infrequently gives rise to suspicion of a cerebral tumour is *'benign intracranial hypertension'* ('pseudotumour cerebri'). This consists of a sustained rise of intracranial pressure in the absence of a space-occupying lesion, the ventricles usually being normal or even reduced in size (Mendelow 1993). The patient presents with headache, and papilloedema is discovered on examination. Diplopia and unsteadiness of gait may be present and vomiting may occur, but there are no progressive neurological signs.

The condition may follow infections or head injury, or result from intracranial venous sinus thrombosis secondary to middle ear disease ('otitic hydrocephalus'). In many patients, however, there are no identifiable antecedents, this most commonly occurring in obese women in their third or fourth decades. Certain drugs have also been incriminated, notably corticosteroids, tetracycline, isotretinoin given for acne, and excessive administration of vitamin A (Gibberd 1991). Among drugs used in psychiatric practice lithium and phenytoin have occasionally been blamed.

The *echoencephalogram* was formerly of value as a noninvasive procedure. It may demonstrate a shift of the midline structures in cases where the pineal is not calcified, but provides little information about the nature of the lesion. It has the advantage of occupying only a few minutes of time, though both false positives and false negatives are sometimes seen. At best it is therefore no more than a screening test.

The *radioisotope scan* (p. 135) is also entirely safe but has considerably lower resolution than CT. It demonstrates vascular tumours such as glioblastomas, many meningiomas and multiple secondary deposits. Failure is more likely with slow-growing avascular tumours such as certain astrocytomas, oligodendrogliomas and pituitary tumours, and with tumours smaller than 2 cm in diameter.

Lumbar puncture is best avoided when a cerebral tumour is suspected, and certainly when there are indications of raised intracranial pressure. Abnormalities in the CSF are not, moreover, universal. Warning signs of increased pressure include headache and papilloedema, though even the latter is not invariably present. Thus if a cerebral tumour is remotely suspected lumbar puncture must always be deferred until a CT scan and neurological opinion have been obtained.

Lumbar air encephalography should likewise be avoided in anyone suspected of having tumour, certainly unless full neurosurgical cover is immediately to hand. CT and

MRI scanning have now rendered air studies obsolete in this context. Ventriculography is similarly very rarely required.

Angiography is comparatively safe in the presence of raised intracranial pressure. It is unlikely to show a tumour when the CT scan is negative, but is still needed for differentiation from aneurysms and angiomas. It can also be valuable in confirming that a tumour is a meningioma by revealing the capillary circulation supplied by a meningeal artery. Angiography, however, is no longer acceptable as the primary screening procedure for tumours.

Clearly these different investigations can find a place where facilities for neuroimaging are not easily to hand. However, several carry definite hazards, so expert guidance is essential in deciding upon priorities in the individual patient.

Problems of misdiagnosis

The possibility of the psychiatrist overlooking a cerebral tumour in a patient under his care is small in numerical terms, but nevertheless of great importance. Kraft *et al.* (1963) performed routine skull X-rays on 1000 new admissions to a psychiatric hospital and found 14 unsuspected tumours, 11 of which were pituitary adenomas. Extending their investigation to 1200 chronic schizophrenic in-patients three more cerebral tumours came to light, plus 14 more pituitary adenomas (Kraft *et al.* 1965).

Surveys of autopsy material from psychiatric hospitals have given cause for concern. Patton and Sheppard (1956) suggested that the chance of finding a cerebral tumour at autopsy was significantly greater among patients dying in state mental hospitals in North America than in non-mental hospitals (3.7% compared to 2.4%). Moreover this difference was particularly great for benign meningiomas, which constituted 33% of the tumours in mental hospitals but only 14% in non-mental hospitals. Such statistics have been disputed, but obtain support from several quarters. Klotz (1957) could not confirm a higher overall incidence of tumours in psychiatric hospital autopsies, but agreed that meningiomas were over-represented. Klotz also agreed that approximately half of the tumours had been unsuspected during life.

It is hard to estimate what proportion of such tumours may have been incidental to the presenting mental illness. Certainly the pituitary tumours mentioned above could have been without pathological effects. But Remington and Rubert (1962) reported 34 patients discharged from a psychiatric hospital over a 30-year period with a diagnosis of cerebral tumour, all of whom had been admitted initially with disturbances of behaviour or cog-

nition, but in only 10 of whom the tumour was diagnosed on admission. Where opportunities for careful screening are sparse, such patients may easily remain undiagnosed. Andersson's (1970) findings from the state mental hospitals of Denmark are also relevant. A tumour frequency of 3% was found at autopsy and two-thirds had been missed during life; moreover the great majority of these patients had been hospitalised for less than 6 months prior to death, so presumably the tumour had been present at the time of admission. In some, at least, the tumours are likely to have been directly responsible for the symptoms which led to hospitalisation.

The distribution of tumour types is important, since as seen above benign meningiomas appear to be especially common in psychiatric patients. Raskin's (1956) series from the Boston State Hospital is typical—86 tumours were discovered in 2430 consecutive autopsies on psychiatric patients (3.5%), with the distribution of tumour types shown in Table 12. Comparison is made in the table with two large series from neurological units as reported by Sumner (1969). Meningiomas are clearly over-represented and gliomas under-represented among the psychiatric patients. Dumas-Duport (1970), in a detailed survey of the literature, makes the further interesting point that when tumour types are studied in a living psychiatric population the frequencies approach much more closely those of the general population; it is only when autopsy psychiatric material is studied that the proportion of meningiomas rises and the proportion of gliomas falls so markedly. This is probably because autopsy surveys deal mostly with chronically hospitalised patients, and meningiomas tend to produce chronic pictures of mental disorder and therefore tend to be missed.

Some of the principal misdiagnoses met with in psychiatric practice include the following:

Presenile or senile dementia is all too readily diagnosed when a patient comes before the psychiatrist with features of organic brain dysfunction. In particular the

Table 12 Comparison of tumour types between psychiatric (Raskin 1956) and neurological (Sumner 1969) patients with cerebral tumours.

	Psychiatric patients (%)	Neurological patients (%)
Meningiomas	30	15
Gliomas	20	45
Metastatic tumours	18	5*
Pituitary tumours	13	10
Others	19	25

* 40% considered more realistic today by Sumner.

predilection of meningiomas for the anterior basal parts of the skull often allows them to grow large without clinical findings other than progressive failure of intellect. Hunter *et al.* (1968a) were able to report three patients with frontal meningiomas who had been mentally ill for 3, 25 and 43 years, respectively, before the correct diagnosis was made. Focal neurological signs of great importance may easily be missed owing to the intellectual enfeeblement of the patient; in particular it is difficult to assess visual fields or unilateral anosmia without the patient's full cooperation.

The misdiagnosis of dementia is, of course, a special hazard among the elderly. Deterioration of intellect and personality is readily ascribed to Alzheimer's disease, and in addition the subarachnoid space becomes more capacious with increasing age so that symptoms of raised intracranial pressure are especially liable to be late (McMenemey 1941).

Cerebral arteriosclerosis is likewise among the common misdiagnoses, and in Raskin's (1956) series accounted for all 10 of the meningiomas which had been missed during life. Evidence of arteriosclerosis on clinical examination, or a past history of focal cerebrovascular accidents, may lead the examiner to undervalue the significance of focal symptoms and signs even when these exist. In addition some tumours first declare themselves with an episode of infarction, and further investigation may then not be pursued.

Alcoholism may also be misleading. When a clear history of alcohol abuse is obtained, persistent amnesic difficulties will often be ascribed to this. Similarly, episodes of confusion in the early stages of a tumour may be mistaken for intoxication. In the following patient the diagnosis was only made because of the patient's request for a CT scan:

A man of 34 was referred because of his concern over impaired concentration and memory. He had been a severe alcoholic until 2 years previously, but since then had abstained completely. Problems with memory had been marked when drinking and had improved considerably since he stopped, but this improvement had reached a plateau. He was also aware of ready mental fatigue, and was eager to know whether brain damage due to alcoholism had persisted. His only other complaint was of episodes of vertigo and nausea for the past 3 months, ascribed by his general practitioner to labyrinthitis. Examination showed positional nystagmus but no other neurological signs. There was no evidence of cognitive impairment on examining his mental state.

He was strongly reassured that there was little likelihood of alcohol-induced brain damage, and it was thought that he was presenting now because of concern about his past alcoholic history. Psychometric testing reinforced this conclusion, showing superior intelligence and intact memory functions.

By way of further reassurance his request for a CT scan was granted. A large cystic lesion was revealed in the cerebellum, compressing the fourth ventricle and causing dilatation of the third and lateral ventricles. By the time of the scan examination, 1 month after presentation, he had developed ataxia of gait and papilloedema was apparent. This had not been present before. At operation a low-grade cystic astrocytoma was removed and he made an excellent recovery.

Epileptic fits may be misinterpreted as due to idiopathic epilepsy. Approximately 20% of tumours are estimated to present with epilepsy, mostly of a focal nature. In psychiatric practice temporal lobe epilepsy will present a special hazard, since even the epileptic nature of the phenomena may be missed. Malamud (1967) reviewed the case histories of 18 patients coming to autopsy in psychiatric hospitals with tumours of the limbic areas of the brain; all had been diagnosed as suffering from non-organic psychiatric illnesses, though much of the symptomatology appeared to have been based in temporal lobe epilepsy which had been overlooked.

Psychoses, both schizophrenic and affective, can be particularly misleading. Symptoms of psychosis in association with tumours usually coexist with evidence of organic deficits, but occasionally present alone as the sole aspect of the clinical picture. It is then only with further progression of the tumour that the true situation is revealed.

As described on p. 225, Davison and Bagley (1969) collected the evidence regarding schizophrenia in several large series of tumour patients. They concluded that the association between cerebral tumour and schizophrenia exceeded chance expectation, though the question of special genetic predisposition could not be resolved. Epilepsy did not seem to be the significant factor linking tumour to psychosis. There was no evidence for a special association with different pathological types of tumour, but a significant association emerged with tumours of the temporal lobe and hypophyseal region. Such conclusions could of course only be tentative in view of the large number of uncontrolled variables.

Major depressive illness may occasionally be the presenting feature, as in the patient with a craniopharyngioma reported by Spence *et al.* (1995). Here the clues to the presence of the tumour lay in hypersomnia and hyperphagia, in contrast to the insomnia and anorexia which had characterised previous bouts of depression. Another feature, always deserving of note, was the failure of the present episode to respond to antidepressant medication. Maurice-Williams and Dunwoody (1988) further stress the importance of distinguishing between true depression and the apathy and indifference which characterise frontal lobe tumours.

In the remarkable patient reported by Maurice-Williams and Sinar (1984) an intractable depressive illness had responded to bifrontal leucotomy 23 years before her left frontal meningioma was diagnosed. It seemed probable, moreover, that the tumour had caused or precipitated the depression since its onset coincided with the development of focal seizures involving the right arm and face. An EEG carried out prior to the leucotomy had shown a left frontotemporal focus, but inexplicably was ignored. The depression remained in abeyance following the leucotomy, though the seizures had continued. At the time of her depression the patient had been obsessed that her fits were due to a brain tumour!

Mania appears to be rare, though occasional patients have been reported to present in this way. Starkstein *et al.* (1988) have described six patients with tumours who developed mania either before or after surgical removal; all but one were frontal or temporal in location and there appeared to be a special relationship with right hemisphere involvement.

Neurotic symptoms can be an early feature and are sometimes severe enough to dominate the picture. Minor degrees of depression, irritability and anxiety are extremely common, representing an exaggeration of premorbid traits and probably often occurring in response to subjective awareness of subtle changes in intellectual function. Symptoms of dizziness and subjective unsteadiness with posterior fossa lesions also readily provoke psychological distress (Bristow 1991). Occasionally, elaborate neurotic developments emerge, with obsessional, hypochondriacal and hysterical features, before the focal signs of the tumour have declared themselves.

A special source of error is the readiness with which the patient's family, and his physician, are liable to interpret such early symptoms in terms of current stresses in the life situation. Minski (1933) found that 19 of 58 patients with cerebral tumours admitted to the Maudsley Hospital had a clear history of stress antedating admission in the form of recent accidents, bereavements or occupational difficulties. Sometimes the stress may have served to focus attention on early symptoms, or sometimes the patient's attempt to cope with the problem may have unmasked his reduced adaptability.

A man of 37 was referred by a neurologist for psychiatric treatment on account of depression and irritability of recent onset, together with panicky feelings when travelling. He had developed epilepsy 4 years earlier, after a mild head injury, but this remained well controlled by anticonvulsant medication. He also complained of intermittent headache and difficulty in concentrating on his job, but in fact was coping well and had recently been promoted. Neurological examination was entirely normal.

He had always been of an anxious, pedantic disposition and prone to take his responsibilities very seriously. His wife was now expecting the birth of a second child and they were due to face considerable financial difficulties. He was treated with minor tranquillisers and supportive psychotherapy for 6 months, and showed a measure of improvement. Suddenly, however, he developed a hemianopia and a sixth nerve palsy, and was admitted to hospital in semicoma. A slow-growing astrocytoma in the non-dominant temporal lobe was discovered.

The principal safeguard in such difficult examples is to be especially cautious in accepting as 'neurotic' someone whose previous adjustment has been good, and in whom precipitating causes seem insufficient. These highly subjective assessments must of course be backed up by careful neurological examination and a readiness to investigate whenever there is room for doubt.

Hysteria is a well known source of error. Neurological signs of a puzzling or unconvincing nature readily invite this label, especially in patients with an unstable background. Certain symptoms, such as somnolence, may be viewed with suspicion when they are unbacked by physical findings. The patient who has displayed conversion symptoms in the past is especially at risk:

A 'kept woman' was finding it hard to maintain influence over the man who supported her as she grew older. On several occasions she had shown evidence of conversion hysteria, once going blind temporarily when he refused to take her on a customary spring trip to Florida. Again he declined to take her on this trip, and she became too weak on the left side to care for herself. She was admitted to hospital with the diagnosis of 'major hysteria'. The left plantar response was found to be up-going and the abdominal reflexes were absent on the left. A right temporal lobe glioma was eventually discovered.   (Chambers 1955)

Factors contributing to misdiagnosis

It is useful to look at some of the principal reasons why tumours appear to have been overlooked in psychiatric patients, as listed by workers who have made a retrospective analysis of the situation (McIntyre & McIntyre 1942; Olin & Weisman 1964; Hunter *et al.* 1968a; Dumas-Duport 1970).

A lack of 'brain tumour consciousness' in the mind of the examiner is repeatedly stressed. Such a lack is perhaps not surprising in view of the rarity of cerebral tumours even in busy psychiatric practice. But a greater awareness, and readiness to investigate, could undoubtedly reduce the errors that occur.

It is likely that the doctor often allows himself to be influenced by explanations furnished by the patient or his family, and too readily views the early symptoms in terms of current psychosocial stresses. The problem can be seen as part of the general tendency for psychiatrists to underrate physical causes as a possible basis for mental symptoms, at least until the physical disorder becomes obtrusive.

The psychiatrist's preoccupation with the mental picture may further lead him to disregard important details of the history or symptomatology. Olin and Weisman (1964), for example, reported a patient whose episodes of severe anxiety, and a manipulative manner, allowed the physician to overlook his clear report of inter-mittent attacks of an unpleasant taste sensation. Ulti-mately a temporal lobe tumour was revealed. Again, with psychiatric troubles in the foreground an adequate neuro-logical examination may fail to be performed, or there may be considerable practical difficulties in carrying this out. Not only does the intensity of psychiatric disorder make a primary psychiatric diagnosis more plausible but it also makes the neurological diagnosis more difficult. It may be hard to get an adequate description of symptoms in the mentally disturbed patient, or to secure co-operation for a comprehensive neurological examination.

Other sources of error include failure to realise that headache, vomiting and papilloedema are frequently absent in the early stages of tumours. It is particularly noteworthy that it is the slow-growing and potentially remediable tumours which are apt to be late in declaring themselves by evidence of raised intracranial pressure. False assurance is also sometimes derived from a normal skull X-ray or EEG.

Finally, one must contend with the relative lack of specificity in the psychiatric symptomatology of cerebral tumours, and especially with the risk attaching to the term 'dementia'. When such a label has been applied it sometimes discourages attempts at further refinement of the diagnosis. Unfortunately in many psychiatric hospi-tals the situation is aggravated by a lack of facilities readily at hand for suitable investigations.

Chapter 7: Epilepsy

The manifestations of epilepsy include facets of equal importance to the psychiatrist and the neurologist. Some aspects indeed stand firmly at the junction between the two disciplines. The seizure itself may take the form of the classic motor convulsion or consist instead of complex abnormalities of behaviour and subjective experience. Associated disorders may sometimes include cognitive difficulties, personality disturbances or psychotic illnesses of various types and durations. In all these respects the study of patients with epilepsy has played an important part in advancing our knowledge of brain function and dysfunction, and in indicating something of the pathophysiological basis for certain forms of psychological disorder.

The accent in the present chapter will be on those aspects most relevant to the work of the psychiatrist. It is now clear that the great majority of people with epilepsy suffer little or no mental disturbance, but those who do can present difficult and complicated problems. Psychosocial and organic factors are often inextricably mixed in causation, and the assessment of all the evidence available in the individual patient can be a complex and time-consuming matter.

At a theoretical level epilepsy presents considerable problems of terminology and classification and these must often be met by compromise solutions. Such difficulties become compounded when seeking to explore the psychiatric concomitants of seizures, and many areas remain in which our understanding is remarkably incomplete.

Varieties of epilepsy

Brain (1955) defined epilepsy as 'a paroxysmal and transitory disturbance of the functions of the brain which develops suddenly, ceases spontaneously and exhibits a conspicuous tendency to recurrence'. It is important, however, to bring electrophysiological events into the definition to separate the above from, for example, migraine or syncope. Chadwick (1993) recommends defining an *epileptic seizure* as 'an intermittent, stereo-typed, disturbance of consciousness, behaviour, emotion, motor function or sensation that on clinical grounds is believed to result from cortical neuronal discharge'. *Epilepsy* can then be defined as a condition in which seizures recur, usually spontaneously.

Epilepsy may be subdivided according to observed content of attacks, presumed aetiology and pathology, electroencephalographic manifestations or presumed site of origin of the abnormal activity within the brain. No single classification is entirely satisfactory and attempts at any comprehensive subdivision soon become unwieldy. A broad classification which is useful for clinical purposes is shown in Table 13. It is derived from proposals put forward at a meeting of the International League Against Epilepsy for an international classification of the epilepsies and epileptic seizures (Gastaut 1970; Merlis 1970).

Generalised epilepsies

Generalised epileptic attacks derive from hyperexcitability in thalamocortical connecting pathways. Competing hypotheses have proposed that the primary abnormality lies in the cortex or in the subcortical 'centrencephalic' system (i.e. the brain stem reticular formation and the nuclei of the diffuse thalamic projection system) and the debate has not been resolved decisively. In either event the resulting discharges spread immediately to involve all areas of the cortex at virtually the same moment. The resulting seizures are bilaterally symmetrical and consciousness is impaired from the outset. An aura is lacking and there is no evidence whatever of a local onset. Usually there is no warning at all, though very occasionally the patient may experience ill-defined malaise for a few seconds immediately before the seizure.

Such attacks may be generalised from the outset (primary generalised epilepsy, primary subcortical epilepsy, centrencephalic epilepsy), or they may develop in consequence of a focal cortical seizure which then spreads to involve the thalamocortical pathways (secondary generalised epilepsy, secondary subcortical epilepsy). In some

Table 13 Varieties of epilepsy.

1 Generalised epilepsies:
   (a) primary generalised epilepsy (petit mal, grand mal)
   (b) secondary generalised epilepsy

2 Focal epilepsies ('partial' or 'local' epilepsies):
   (a) with elementary (simple) symptomatology
   (b) with complex symptomatology

3 Unclassifiable and mixed forms

of the latter, especially those originating in the basal frontal cortex, the spread to generalisation may be extremely rapid; the clinical manifestations are then identical to primary generalised epilepsy and the differentiation is essentially made by electroencephalography.

The generalised epilepsies are divided into two sharply differing forms, petit mal and grand mal, as described below.

Petit mal is the term formerly used to refer to the triad of absence, akinetic and myoclonic attacks. It is now used less frequently than formerly, but is retained at this point for ease of reference to the literature. In the revised classification of epileptic seizures put forward in 1981 the term petit mal was abandoned, and a division was made into absence seizures (typical or atypical), atonic seizures and myoclonic seizures (Commission on Classification and Terminology of the International League Against Epilepsy 1981).

The commonest and most clear-cut form is the *simple (typical) absence attack*. This is always of primary generalised origin and it is virtually always without evidence of any gross brain lesion. It is sometimes termed 'pyknolepsy' when, as is usual, it sets in in childhood and clears at adolescence. Occasionally simple absence and grand mal seizures are seen together, and the prognosis is then less favourable.

Without warning the patient loses contact with the environment, usually for 4 or 5 seconds but occasionally for as long as half a minute. To the onlooker he appears momentarily dazed, stops speaking and becomes immobile. The face is pale, the eyes assume a fixed glazed appearance and the pupils may be observed to be fixed and dilated. Posture and balance are usually well maintained, though muscular relaxation may allow the head to slump forward. Brief muscular twitches may be seen around the eyes, occasionally extending to brief myoclonic jerks of the limbs. Such movements are always bilateral and symmetrical. Consciousness is typically deeply impaired during the attack, though in rare cases the subject may remain dimly aware of what is happening around him.

In 'absence with automatism' there may be lip smacking, chewing, mouthing or fumbling movements, even brief aimless walking, and vocalisations may occur. Such automatisms can present difficulty over clinical differentiation from brief temporal lobe seizures, particularly when the latter are partially controlled by drugs. Close observation of the content of the attacks and the EEG picture usually serve to make the distinction, but sometimes even the latter will yield inconclusive results. In such circumstances one may ultimately be forced to a trial of different medications (Marsden & Reynolds 1982).

There are usually no after-effects whatever. The patient may later be aware of the attack as a momentary break in the continuity of events, but quite often does not know it has occurred and continues immediately with the word or activity that was interrupted. While each attack is brief, runs of attacks sometimes occur in rapid succession. The frequency of episodes is commonly 5–10 per day, but sometimes hundreds may be noted in the course of a single day. Lennox (1960) suggests that if attacks do not occur daily the diagnosis should be questioned.

Atypical (complex) absences show more protean manifestations, yet are accompanied in the main by the EEG features of simple absences. The duration of attacks is likely to be longer, and they are often accompanied by prominent increases or decreases in muscle tone (Holmes *et al.* 1987). They are more likely to occur in patients with developmental delay and additional seizure types, and the inter-ictal EEG is more frequently abnormal. However, typical and atypical absences seem not to be discrete entities, but rather to form parts of a continuum.

The second main variety consists of *atonic seizures (akinetic seizures)*. These primarily involve the mechanisms governing posture, resulting in precipitate muscular relaxation so that the patient nods abruptly, slumps in the chair or falls to the ground. Attacks again occur without warning and last for only a few seconds. After-effects, other than those due to bruising or emotional shock, do not occur. Such attacks may be seen along with typical or atypical absences. Quite often, however, drop attacks of this nature occur in patients with grand mal epilepsy and represent unusually brief and abortive forms of major seizure discharges.

The third form consists of *myoclonic seizures* – sudden shock-like movements lasting for only a fraction of a second and mainly affecting the neck, arms and shoulders. Objects which are held may be dropped or flung violently. If the trunk or legs are affected the patient may be flung off balance. It is uncertain whether consciousness is lost or retained, since the seizures last for so very short a time. Single myoclonic jerks of this nature frequently occur in subjects suffering from absences or atonic seizures. Myoclonic jerks may, however, also be seen as an occasional manifestation in normal persons when falling asleep, or in association with grand mal epilepsy or several serious brain diseases. They are characteristic of subacute encephalitis, the cerebral lipoidoses and Creutzfeldt–Jakob disease. Rare progressive forms of myoclonic epilepsy, which may be associated with increasing ataxia or dementia, include Unverricht–Lundborg disease, Lafora-body disease and the Ramsay Hunt syndrome (p. 242).

These three main forms of attack may be displayed by a single patient on different occasions, and they show certain EEG features in common.

The EEG picture in simple absences is striking and very characteristic. During attacks the record is suddenly interrupted by bilaterally synchronous spike and slow wave complexes of high amplitude, occurring at approximately three per second and seen synchronously (simultaneously) throughout all scalp leads but with a frontal emphasis. With atypical absences the picture is more heterogeneous, with irregular spike and slow wave complexes and other paroxysmal activity. Akinetic seizures usually show slower two per second wave and spike formations or polyspike and wave. Myoclonic jerks may sometimes be accompanied by a single wave and spike complex, by multiple spikes or by polyspike and wave.

The interseizure record may display brief bursts of similar activity unaccompanied by overt attacks, or symmetrical spike and wave variants without the strict three per second regularity. These subclinical manifestations are usually less well organised and of lower amplitude than in the actual attack, but are always widespread, bilaterally synchronous and more or less symmetrical. Their incidence is considerably increased by overbreathing. The runs are unaccompanied by obvious clinical phenomena, but it has been shown that during wave and spike discharges there is slowing of response times and an increase in errors on simple psychological tests (p. 262).

Grand mal seizures of the primary generalised type occur without immediate warning and consciousness is lost abruptly. Thus there is no preceding aura. Some subjects, however, may be aware that a fit is imminent on account of ill-defined prodromata which build up for hours or days, such as malaise, tension, nausea or headache. In subjects liable to myoclonic jerks these may increase in frequency for some hours before the grand mal attack. The seizure consists of tonic and clonic phases which involve all parts of the body symmetrically and from the same moment. The fit is usually followed by a deep sleep which may then be succeeded by nausea, vomiting and headache. If sleep does not occur a period of confusion is usually seen before full consciousness is regained. During this period the patient is disorientated, often restless, rambling and incoherent, and sometimes unaware of his personal identity. On recovery there is total amnesia for the content of the attack and frequently for a period of several seconds extending in a retrograde direction.

The EEG pattern during the attack is characteristic. For a few seconds before the fit there is a crescendo of low voltage fast activity. With the tonic phase this gives way to a generalised synchronous discharge of high amplitude spikes at 8–12 per second. After some 15–30 seconds the spikes become grouped and separated by slow waves as the clonic phase begins. When the fit is over low amplitude delta waves predominate throughout the record, often as slow as one per second and without focal preponderance. Thereafter the record gradually resumes its usual appearance, though the slow activity sometimes persists for several hours. After status epilepticus random diffuse slow activity can persist for several days.

In approximately 20–30% of cases the interseizure EEG is normal on a single routine record (Kiloh *et al.* 1981). Forty per cent show non-specific abnormalities in the form of paroxysms of symmetrical delta, bursts of theta, or a diffuse excess of slow rhythms. The remainder show *formes frustes* of seizure discharges with wave and spike or polyspike and wave complexes. As with petit mal absences these are always widespread and more or less symmetrical. Patients with grand mal alone can show paroxysms of three per second wave and spike, but faster variants at 3.5–4.5 per second are more typical.

Focal epilepsies

In focal epilepsy the seizure discharge begins in some part of the cortex. This always implies the presence of a localised brain lesion, even though techniques presently available may fail to reveal its nature. Focal symptoms in the form of an aura therefore usually usher in the seizure, the precise symptomatology depending on the area of the brain in which the discharge originates and the direction of its subsequent spread. The main varieties of aura and their significance for localisation are discussed on p. 249 *et seq.*

All varieties of focal epilepsy are liable to lead on to a generalised convulsion, but this is not an invariable sequel. Some attacks may consist of no more than the focal manifestations of the epileptic process. They may be very brief indeed, consisting only of the opening phases of the aura. Such 'minor' attacks are more common when the patient is already on medication. Even extended attacks may fail to generalise to the rest of the brain, in which case the seizure consists only of the focal disturbance while consciousness is wholly or partially retained. In Jacksonian epilepsy, for example, the motor 'march' may sometimes spread along a limb and then recede, while the subject retains full awareness throughout. Consciousness is also usually retained in 'epilepsia partialis continua', in which clonic motor spasms remain confined to the part of the body where they originate, sometimes continuing for hours or even days with little or no inter-mission. The grand mal convulsions which do occur are often asymmetrical in distribution, and may be followed by longer lasting focal functional defects such as dysphasia or transient weakness of the affected limb (Todd's paralysis).

Sometimes, and particularly in temporal lobe epilepsy, the focal discharge spreads to the limbic system rather than to the centrencephalic system, and remains confined there throughout the attack. In such cases consciousness is profoundly impaired during the seizure, yet complex behaviour can still be carried out (complex partial seizure, psychomotor attack). Whether or not a grand mal convulsion eventually ensues will depend upon the degree of generalisation of the seizure discharge, i.e. whether there is ultimate involvement of the thalamocortical pathways.

The classification and terminology used for the focal epilepsies has undergone repeated revisions. The terms 'focal' and 'partial' are in general used interchangeably. Thereafter such epilepsies are most readily classified according to their predominant type of seizure as shown in Table 14. A first division is made into simple and complex partial seizures according to whether or not consciousness is impaired. This criterion must not, however, be regarded as absolute. In some simple partial seizures, as with the example of Jacksonian epilepsy described above, it is clear that consciousness is well preserved throughout, whereas in others this may be difficult to determine with certainty. Partial seizures which display 'psychic' symptomatology can be particularly hard to classify in this regard. In some cases the simple partial seizure represents essentially the aural component of an attack which would

Table 14 Classification of focal seizures (after Commission on Classification and Terminology of the International League Against Epilepsy 1981).

1 Simple partial seizures (consciousness not impaired):
  (a) with motor symptoms
  (b) with somatosensory or special sensory symptoms
  (c) with autonomic symptoms
  (d) with psychic symptoms

2 Complex partial seizures (with impairment of consciousness):
  (a) beginning as simple partial seizures then progressing to impairment of consciousness
  (b) with impairment of consciousness at onset:
    (i) with impairment of consciousness only
    (ii) with automatism, fugues or 'twilight states'

3 Partial seizures evolving to secondarily generalised seizures:
  (a) simple partial evolving to generalised seizures
  (b) complex partial evolving to generalised seizures
  (c) simple partial evolving to complex partial evolving to generalised seizures

have progressed further if the subject had not been on antiepileptic medication, as discussed on p. 249.

Simple motor attacks may be tonic–clonic, involving a part of the body, or merely tonic in form, the latter often with dystonic posturing of the limbs and adversion of the head and eyes. Negative motor phenomena classically include speech arrest during which comprehension remains unimpaired. Simple sensory attacks can involve paraesthesias and numbness, or more rarely pain. Olfactory and gustatory symptoms are common; visual and auditory experiences are usually relatively primitive in type. Autonomic and psychic symptoms are mostly associated with temporal lobe epilepsy, and include the wealth of visceral, cognitive, perceptual and emotional changes outlined on p. 250 *et seq*.

Complex partial seizures are by definition accompanied by impairment of consciousness. They may, however, start with a simple partial seizure or an aura, succeeded by a brief period of arrested motion and staring before more complicated activity develops. The great majority, though not all, are temporal lobe in origin. As with simple partial seizures they may sometimes end with a grand mal fit due to secondary generalisation. The various pictures encountered are described on p. 252 *et seq*.

During attacks of focal epilepsy the EEG may show a variety of abnormal electrical discharges. There may be rhythmic spikes, sharp waves, spikes and slow waves or rhythmical runs of theta and delta. The abnormal activity may remain strictly localised or may be spread widely over one or both hemispheres. In occasional cases the record may remain normal during an attack, as in some cases of Jacksonian epilepsy when the focus is very discrete and of insufficient voltage to reach the surface electrodes. Once the attack has ceased normal rhythms may return at once or after a period of random low voltage slow activity.

During automatisms (pp. 253–4) bilaterally synchronous theta or delta discharges are usually seen, most marked in the frontotemporal regions and sometimes interspersed with slow waves or spikes. Other pictures may occur, however, such as generalised fast activity, 'normalisation' of the record with disappearance of inter-ictal discharges, or no change whatever. (The EEG during automatisms and other psychomotor attacks is discussed further on p. 258.) After the attack focal slow activity may persist in the affected temporal lobe for hours or days.

In the interseizure record the commonest evidence of a cortical epileptogenic lesion is a spike and sharp wave focus. Alternatively there may be local spikes, singly or in groups, spikes and slow waves or paroxysmal theta or delta. The underlying lesion may produce electrical disturbance itself, usually in the form of focal slow waves. The abnormal discharges commonly betray the point of origin of the attacks though sometimes they are transmitted widely to other areas. There may even be a 'mirror' focus over the homologous area of the contralateral hemisphere. Such distant foci can be seriously misleading, but it is usual for them to be less consistent than the primary focus from one recording to another.

The inter-ictal record in temporal lobe epilepsy typically shows spikes or sharp waves at the temporal electrodes, but the record can be normal until sleep activation is employed. Sphenoidal or foramen ovale electrodes may be necessary to detect discharges originating in the medial temporal lobe structures. Light thiopentone anaesthesia is also useful for inducing beta activity, which may be less well developed at the electrodes over the site of damage in the affected temporal lobe.

Unclassifiable and mixed forms of epilepsy

In some patients the most careful investigation will fail to clarify the source of origin of the attacks, or alternatively there may be diffuse and scattered lesions leading to multiple foci both in cortical and subcortical structures. Some of the more severe and intractable cases of epilepsy fall into this latter category. Clinical manifestations may include a mixture of focal seizures, grand mal and myoclonic attacks. There are likely to be abnormal neurological findings. Progressive dementia may sometimes occur.

In patients with mixed forms of epilepsy the EEG is more continuously abnormal than in other groups. It can occasionally be difficult to find normal stretches of record. Multiple independent foci may be seen, with groups of spikes, sharp waves or spike and slow waves. Slow waves may be widespread over the hemispheres and are often irregular in form.

Other special forms of epilepsy

Other forms of epilepsy which occur more rarely but can produce puzzling clinical pictures will be mentioned briefly.

'*Reflex epilepsy*' is the term used for attacks which are liable to occur in response to some specific precipitating stimulus. Detailed reviews of the many varieties are provided by Daube (1965), Merlis (1974) and Fenwick (1981a). In some patients fits result from sensory stimulation of discrete regions of the body. Music is the precipitating stimulus in 'musicogenic epilepsy', sometimes music with special emotional significance for the patient (Critchley 1937; Shaw & Hill 1947; Daly & Barry 1957). In 'television epilepsy' the photic stimulation from the flickering of the television screen is the precipitant (Mawdsley 1961; Pallis & Louis 1961; Jeavons & Harding 1970). An interesting variety, also due to photic stimulation, has been reported in children who pass their hand repeatedly in front of their eyes while staring at the sky, or jump up and down in front of venetian blinds, and perhaps derive satisfaction from the minor seizures that result (Robertson 1954; Sherwood 1962). Other patients have been reported with attacks precipitated by reading (Bickford *et al.* 1956; Critchley *et al.* 1959; Antebi & Bird 1992) or by

sudden voluntary movement of the limbs (Lishman *et al.* 1962; Whitty *et al.* 1964).

The chief importance of reflex epilepsy for the psychiatrist is that attacks may easily be suspected of being psychogenic in origin until their reflex epileptic basis is recognised. The existence of such clear-cut examples is also a reminder of the importance of searching for possible precipitating factors in other epileptic patients (as discussed on p. 309).

'*Tonic seizures*' consist of sustained spasm, usually affecting the whole musculature but often asymmetrically so that slow twisting, writhing movements are produced. Groping and grasping of a limb may occur. There is no clonic phase, the attacks are usually brief and after-effects are slight. The bizarre nature of the attacks may again suggest a purely psychogenic disorder. Such seizures have been thought to originate in the basal ganglia, and have been variously termed extrapyramidal, striatal or subcortical epilepsy (Lennox 1960). Most are now thought to originate in the frontal lobes (pp. 249–50). 'Tonic postural fits' represent a more severe variety, with sustained rigidity of the antigravity muscles resulting in opisthotonos, extension of the neck and legs, and flexion of the arms as in decerebrate rigidity. Such attacks have been presumed to have a focal origin in the lower midbrain or upper pons. They may sometimes be seen with cerebellar tumours by virtue of pressure effects on the neighbouring brain stem (cerebellar fits). It is likely that many examples are in fact not epilepsy at all but represent transient attacks of decerebrate rigidity.

'*Gelastic epilepsy*' is a term occasionally used for seizures preceded or accompanied by uncontrollable laughter. A child, for example, may suddenly bend his head and giggle for no apparent reason. Such attacks may be regarded as a curious habit, and not be recognised as epileptic in origin for a considerable time until more definitive features appear. The laughter may occasionally be accompanied by a subjective experience of mirth, but is most typically without affect and of a hollow quality. It may be evoked by the emotional content of a brief temporal lobe aura or occur as part of an automatism. Gloor (1991) has drawn attention to cases associated with hypothalamic hamartomas, often in the presence of mental retardation.

'*Diencephalic*' or '*autonomic epilepsy*' is characterised by autonomic symptoms which predominate during attacks. It is likely that most reported examples represent partial seizures arising from the medial temporal lobe. Fox *et al.* (1973) reported a patient whose attacks consisted of episodic flushing and sweating, lasting 10–20 minutes, followed by feeling cold and shivering. Slight confusion could sometimes ensue. The rectal temperature fell during attacks and was recorded as low as 34°C. In other cases seizures may take the form of a sudden desire to urinate, to defaecate, sensations of heat or cold, flushing, hyperpnoea, difficulty with breathing, salivation, lachrymation or abnormal gastric sensations. It may be hard to distinguish such symptoms from those of an anxiety state, though the sudden onset and ending and the regular stereotyped nature of the attacks may give the clue.

West syndrome consists of the triad of infantile spasms, arrest of psychomotor development and the characteristic EEG finding of *hypsarrhythmia*. The latter consists of almost continuously abnormal electrical activity, with irregularly recurring spikes and slow waves of high amplitude in all leads. The typical spasms consist of brief repeated flexor, or more rarely extensor, spasms of the trunk and limbs. 'Salaam attacks' with bowing of the head and trunk are a common but not a constant manifestation.

The onset peaks at 4–7 months of age and almost all cases present during the first year of life. Boys are affected more often than girls. In the majority the condition represents a non-specific response to a variety of cerebral disorders—metabolic disorders, birth hypoxia or the presence of tuberous sclerosis — and developmental abnormality has been obvious since birth (symptomatic group). In a smaller proportion the spasms set in after normal development, but thereafter psychomotor progress may be halted or reversed (idiopathic group). The prognosis is in general grave, particularly in symptomatic cases. The spasms rarely persist beyond 3 years of age, but other seizures continue in some 50% of children, particularly in the form of the Lennox–Gastaut syndrome (see below). Mental retardation is observed in approximately 85% of cases (Aicardi 1986). Antiepileptic treatment is often without effect, though vigabatrin may be helpful (Duncan 1994). Adrenocorticotrophic hormone (ACTH) or steroids can be successful in suppressing the spasms and the EEG abnormalities. In idiopathic cases such treatment may sometimes effect a cure of the condition.

Lennox–Gastaut syndrome, like the above, is age-related and non-specific in aetiology and often associated with intellectual failure. The onset is typically between 1 and 8 years of age and mainly in preschool children. Some 60% show evidence of pre-existing brain damage with delay in mental development before the onset.

The seizures are frequent, severe and hard to control, consisting of mixed seizure types—tonic attacks occurring particularly during sleep and affecting the axial musculature, atonic and myoclonic attacks and atypical absences (Neville 1993). Episodes of non-convulsive status are frequent. In consequence much of the child's waking life may be spent in an obtunded state. The seizures com-

monly persist into adult life, and less than 10% of cases make a full recovery. Continuing intellectual impairment is common. The EEG typically shows abnormal background activity, slow spike waves and often multifocal abnormalities. Bursts of fast rhythms may occur during sleep. The abnormalities are sometimes unilateral, and such cases may be amenable to surgery. Lamotrigine has recently been found to help considerably in a proportion of cases (Wallace 1994).

Landau–Kleffner syndrome (acquired epileptic aphasia) is a rare childhood disorder which may present either with seizures or aphasia. In some 20% of cases obvious seizures remain in abeyance, though close inspection may reveal minor episodes. The child loses comprehension of speech after seemingly normal development, and rapidly ceases to use speech to communicate. The cognitive deficits may sometimes extend beyond auditory comprehension, and behaviour disorder may develop. Seizures are usually mild and infrequent, consisting mostly of grand mal or partial motor attacks. EEG abnormalities consist of spikes or spike wave complexes, usually bilaterally in the temporal and parietal regions. The seizures usually remit before the age of 15, but language difficulties may persist even into adult life. The cause of the condition is unknown.

Ramsay Hunt syndrome (dyssynergia cerebellaris myoclonica) is a heterogeneous syndrome which overlaps with other progressive myoclonic epilepsies of childhood. Some cases are associated with mitochondrial myopathy (p. 761), showing abnormalities of lactate and pyruvate metabolism. The onset is usually between 6 and 20 years of age, presenting either with myoclonus or grand mal seizures. Action and intention myoclonus are accompanied by cerebellar ataxia, and there may be gradual mental deterioration. The EEG shows normal background activity, with generalised spikes, spike waves and polyspike waves, often with marked photosensitivity. During rapid eye movement (REM) sleep rapid polyspikes appear over the central and vertex regions (Commission on Classification and Terminology of the International League Against Epilepsy 1989).

Prevalence and aetiology

General practice surveys have indicated that in England and Wales some 4–6 persons per 1000 are currently suffering from epilepsy, and that approximately 5% of the population will have a fit of some sort during their lifetime (College of General Practitioners Report 1960; Pond *et al.* 1960). The overall incidence is about the same in males and females. Age of onset shows the highest rate in the first year of life, a considerably lower incidence during childhood and adolescence, and a lower level still during adulthood. In Pond *et al.*'s (1960) survey almost a quarter of cases had begun before the age of 5, another quarter during schooldays (5–14 years), one-tenth during adolescence (15–19 years), and the remaining 40% after 20 years. Of the different types of epilepsy the great majority appearing in the first 20 years of life are generalised grand mal attacks, while after this age the proportion of focal epilepsies rapidly increases.

With regard to aetiology, epilepsy must be viewed as a symptom and not as a disease in itself. A great variety of causes may underlie the occurrence of the fits and need to be carefully investigated. When this is done, however, a considerable proportion of cases remains in which no cause is discernible, either during life or on eventual histological examination of the brain. It is therefore necessary to make a first division into epilepsy of unknown aetiology and epilepsy of known aetiology. The latter is often referred to as 'secondary' or 'symptomatic' epilepsy.

Epilepsy of unknown aetiology

This simply represents those cases in which no evidence can be found in the history or on examination for an adequate underlying cause. The older term 'idiopathic' epilepsy has fallen into disfavour because it carries the implication that the group represents a distinct clinical entity and this is far from clearly established. Other terms are 'cryptogenic' epilepsy, suggesting that some brain lesion is responsible but evades detection, or 'functional' or 'metabolic' epilepsy suggesting that the fits result from disordered metabolism or other faults of cerebral function rather than any structural abnormality. For obvious reasons all of these terms can be misleading, and the group is most accurately termed 'epilepsy of unknown aetiology'.

The proportion of such cases was remarkably constant in earlier surveys, representing approximately two-thirds of patients in several large populations (Alstrom 1950; Juul-Jensen 1964; Gudmundsson 1966). The proportion was somewhat higher (75%) in Pond *et al.*'s (1960) survey, but here there was no first-hand opportunity for investigating causes. It is now clear, however, that the proportion of such cases will fall as modern neuroimaging techniques are systematically applied to patients with epilepsy. The discovery of subtle forms of cortical dysgenesis by high resolution magnetic resonance imaging (MRI), and the detection of small hamartomas and neoplastic lesions in resected brain specimens, serve gradually to erode the territory of 'idiopathic' or 'cryptogenic' epilepsy. Recent advances in this area are described on p. 244.

The great majority of epilepsies of unknown aetiology are generalised from the start, being either simple absences or grand mal without warning. Indeed the classic simple absence proves virtually always to be without demonstrable cause. A focal component to the seizures will strongly indicate that some form of structural brain lesion is present, but of course this will not invariably be demonstrated. In a small proportion of cases with focal seizures no cause will be found even at autopsy, and here it must be presumed that the 'idiopathic discharge' simply happens to arise in some particular area other than the usual midline structures. In most epilepsies of unknown aetiology no neurological abnormality will be found between attacks. The incidence of psychiatric disabilities is also lower than in other groups; Alstrom (1950) found mental disturbance in 21% of cases of unknown aetiology, in 37% where a probable cause could be discerned, and in 58% where the epilepsy was clearly secondary to a structural lesion.

The precise mechanisms underlying the electrical abnormality responsible for the seizures are unknown, but appear to be based on biochemical changes in neurones and synapses leading to prolonged depolarising shifts in resting membrane potentials (Chadwick 1993). Neurotransmitters, especially gamma aminobutyric acid (GABA) and glutamate, are closely involved. An hereditary basis almost certainly plays some part (as discussed on p. 247) and a family history is found more commonly than for epilepsies secondary to known to brain lesions.

Epilepsy due to birth injury or congenital malformations

Complications of pregnancy and delivery may damage the brain and lead to epilepsy. Most often the seizures will be declared in infancy or date from very early in childhood. Anoxia is an important cause of damage, likewise direct trauma leading to cerebral haemorrhage. In the early neonatal period similar brain damage may result from cardiorespiratory disorders, infections or metabolic disturbances. A large proportion of children with spasticity, infantile hemiplegia or severe mental defect will accordingly suffer from seizures. Covert brain injury without such gross defects is likely to account for fits in many more.

Congenital disorders and developmental defects may likewise be found in epilepsies of early onset, and are increasingly demonstrated in cases of adult onset as well. The types of pathology responsible are legion, including porencephaly, tuberous sclerosis and arteriovenous malformations (Sturge–Weber and Lindau's diseases). Particular attention has recently been focused on various forms of *cortical dysgenesis* which appear to owe their origin to abnormalities in the orderly migration of neurones from the germinal matrix to the cortical plate during the course of foetal development. The most common forms probably derive from insults to the brain—ischaemia, infections or exposure to drugs—during the third and fourth months of gestation when neuronal migration is at its peak.

Raymond *et al.* (1994a, 1995) discuss the various forms of cortical dysgenesis now recognised, though terminology and classification remain incompletely standardised. High-resolution MRI, using thin-section volume acquisition techniques and multiplanar reformatting, has enabled some of the principal forms to be detected by neuroimaging, though more subtle varieties still depend on histological examination. In a survey of 100 adults with chronic epilepsy from the National Hospital, cortical dysgenesis emerged as the second most common cause of epilepsy after hippocampal sclerosis, accounting for 24% of the cases. In a further study of 100 adults with refractory epilepsy due to cortical dysgenesis the median age at onset was 10 years but in 30 patients the onset was in adulthood. The great majority of these patients had previously been labelled as suffering from 'cryptogenic' epilepsy. In three-quarters the dysgenesis was established by MRI, and in the remainder by histological examination of surgical or postmortem material.

The largest group was made up of *gyral abnormalities*, particularly focal macrogyria (pachygyria) or polymicrogyria. Diffuse agyria (lissencephaly) occurred more rarely. A second major group consisted of *grey matter heterotopias*, showing as nodular areas of grey matter where the migrating neurones had become arrested in the course of traversing the white matter. These were often found along the lateral margins of the ventricles. Diffuse band-like heterotopias were less common. Rarer abnormalities, recognised only on histological examination, included areas of *focal cortical dysplasia* and *microdysgenesis*, in which the normal laminar architecture of the cortex was disrupted and the clusters of heterotopic neurones were too small to be identified as heterotopic grey matter lesions. Formes frustes of *tuberous sclerosis* made up a further group, all of which could be seen in conjunction with one another and with or without abnormalities of gyral formation.

Dysembrioplastic neuroepithelial tumours represent another form of lesion, recently recognised, and emerging as one of the commonest types of tumour in epileptic patients (Daumas-Duport *et al.* 1988; Raymond *et al.* 1994c). It is uncertain at present how far this too should be included among the forms of cortical dysgenesis or whether it is to be regarded as a type of low-grade neoplasm. Its frequent association with cortical dysplasia, and the uniformly early onset of the epilepsy, favour the former view. The lesions are predominantly intracortical, usually involving the temporal lobe, and the MRI picture is sometimes sufficiently distinctive to be diagnostic. Characteristics of the tumour include a multinodular architecture, calcification, and cellular polymorphism with an admixture of glial cells, neuronal cells and sometimes germinal matrix components. The prognosis for control of epilepsy after resection appears to be considerably better than for other forms of cortical dysgenesis.

Post-traumatic epilepsy

Head injury is a common cause of secondary epilepsy in young adults. The underlying pathology may be a small cicatrix due to organisation of a circumscribed and superficial haemorrhage, or a more extensive glial reaction with focal atrophy and distortion of brain tissue demonstrable on neuroimaging.

The development of post-traumatic epilepsy can be profoundly disabling and has important medicolegal implications. Guidance towards the likelihood of its appearance in the individual case is therefore important. Jennett (1975) showed that the overall incidence after closed head injury was 5% after excluding cases with fits only in the first week after injury. More than half of the cases had their first fit within 1 year of injury, and three-quarters within 3 years; this means, however, that the risk of developing post-traumatic epilepsy is by no means over when the third year has gone by. Indeed almost one-fifth made their first appearance only 4 years after injury; and these late-onset fits were more likely to occur frequently and less likely to remit. Temporal lobe epilepsy accounted for almost 20% of cases in Jennett's (1975) series, again underlining the seriousness of this possible complication.

Certain features can be identified which substantially increase the risk (Lewin 1970; Jennett 1975). About 1% of patients are likely to develop epilepsy when there has been no fit within 1 week after injury, and when there has been no haematoma or depressed skull fracture. Irrespective of the severity of injury, a fit occurring within the first week raises the incidence to 25%. The occurrence of a depressed skull fracture raises the incidence to 15%, and an intracranial haematoma to 31%. A depressed fracture associated with a post-traumatic amnesia in excess of 24 hours leads to an incidence of 32%. If in addition these features are associated with a fit within the first week the incidence is 57%.

There is reason to regard fits which develop within the first week after injury rather differently from those which develop in subsequent weeks or later. Thus Jennett (1969, 1975) showed that the prognosis was better with a lessened tendency for the epilepsy to persist (even though as described above, subsequent epilepsy is still much commoner than in those who do not have such an early fit). Fits within the first week are commonly focal motor attacks, in contrast to epilepsies which develop later, but temporal lobe seizures are rare.

Penetrating injuries carry a much higher incidence of post-traumatic epilepsy, reported as being 30–50% (Russell & Whitty 1952; Walker & Jablon 1961). In Russell and Whitty's series the highest incidence was from wounds in the central regions of the brain (parietal 65%, motor and premotor cortex 55%), with a diminished incidence towards the poles (prefrontal 39%, temporal 38%, occipital 38%).

Caveness *et al.* (1979), reviewing studies from World Wars I and II and the Korean and Vietnam wars, showed that the incidence of post-traumatic epilepsy had remained substantially the same despite marked improvements in the management of acute head injuries. With regard to prognosis, experience from the Korean campaign showed that approximately half of the patients with seizures had ceased to have them within 5–10 years, and that in half of the remainder (here 8%) the fits proved to be intractable.

Postinfective epilepsy

Infections of the brain and its meningeal coverings may lead to fits in the acute stage, or produce scarring which becomes the source of seizures some considerable time later. Encephalitis is more likely to be followed by epilepsy than meningitis, likewise cerebral abscess or venous sinus thrombosis. The incidence of epilepsy due to covert brain involvement during the course of mumps, whooping cough and other infectious diseases of childhood is impossible to determine. Neurosyphilis must not be overlooked as a cause of late-onset epilepsy. Parasitic cysts within the brain are an important cause of fits in certain parts of the world (p. 370).

The common 'febrile convulsions' of childhood are distinct from the above. Any systemic infection may be responsible, presumably by virtue of a lowered threshold for seizures induced by the effect of toxins or pyrexia on the brain. A genetic predisposition is found to be operative, siblings of affected children being also more likely to respond to pyrexia with convulsions, but nonetheless the predisposition appears to fade rapidly after the age of 3 or 4 years and the great majority of cases do not develop persistent epilepsy. Febrile convulsions nevertheless warrant careful management. When severe they may be responsible for the genesis of the anoxic brain lesions which underlie temporal lobe epilepsy in later years (p. 246).

Epilepsy due to cerebrovascular disease

Cerebral arteriosclerosis and episodes of hypertensive encephalopathy are important causes of epilepsy in later adult life. A cerebral embolus is more likely to lead to a fit than a thrombosis or haemorrhage, but any cerebral infarct may leave behind a focal source for epileptic seizures. Sometimes the acute cerebrovascular episode may have gone undiagnosed at the time.

Epilepsy due to cerebral tumour

A space-occupying lesion may first declare itself by fits and must be given special consideration in late-onset epilepsy. Tumours in the so-called silent regions of the brain naturally present a special hazard in this regard. Approximately 40% of patients with fits due to tumour will have seizures as the first symptom (Chadwick 1993). Both primary and secondary tumours can be responsible.

Epilepsy due to degenerative disorders

Epilepsy may be caused by demyelinating and degenerative disorders both in childhood and later life. In childhood, lipoidoses or tuberous sclerosis may be responsible. In adult life, multiple sclerosis or one of the presenile or senile dementias may be complicated in this fashion. Romanelli *et al.* (1990) found that advanced Alzheimer's disease was an important risk factor for new-onset epilepsy in the elderly; on following a group of patients over several years they found that 15% had at least one documented seizure by the time they had progressed to severe dementia.

Epilepsy due to drugs and toxins

Alcohol and drug withdrawal are important causes of seizures, as described in Chapter 13. The abuse of sedative drugs can easily be overlooked as a cause of epilepsy beginning only in adult life. The administration of certain drugs such as amphetamines, ergot alkaloids or steroids may provoke seizures, also certain psychotropic medications such as phenothiazines or tricyclic antidepressants (Toone & Fenton 1977). Intoxication with substances such as lead, or the chlorinated hydrocarbons found in insecticides, may be responsible.

Metabolic causes

In infancy seizures may be associated with specific metabolic disorders such as galactosaemia or pyridoxine deficiency. Uraemia or hypocalcaemia may be responsible at any age. Electrolyte disturbances are important, particularly in eclampsia and perhaps in occasional seizures which occur premenstrually. Hypoglycaemia due to islet cell tumours of the pancreas may very occasionally emerge as the cause for seemingly idiopathic epilepsies of later onset. Porphyria may declare itself similarly.

The relative likelihood of these different aetiological factors will vary according to the nature of the population studied. The most representative sample to date has been reported by Sander *et al.* (1990) from the National General Practice Study of Epilepsy. This was a prospective survey of newly diagnosed patients with epilepsy reported from 275 general practices in the UK. Over a 3-year period some 1000 patients were incepted, 564 with definite epileptic seizures, 228 with possible seizures and 220 with febrile seizures. Of the definite group 61% were idiopathic/cryptogenic, 15% due to vascular causes, 6% attributable to alcohol, 6% due to tumour, 3% posttraumatic, 2% postinfective and 7% due to other causes. A quarter were younger than 15 years and a similar proportion aged 60 or over, and the relative incidence of causes differed according to the age group studied. A vascular aetiology accounted for almost half of those aged 60 or over; alcohol was responsible for 27% of those aged 30–39; and cerebral tumours varied from 1% in those under 30 to 19% in patients aged 50–59 and 11% in those over 60.

Aetiology of temporal lobe epilepsy

A good deal of interest has centred on the pathological substrate of temporal lobe epilepsy, since this may be examined in resected brain tissue obtained at temporal lobectomy. A variety of lesions are found—scars, infarcts, small benign tumours of developmental origin (hamartomas) or 'mesial temporal lobe sclerosis'. The latter is by far the commonest lesion found at operation, occurring in some 50% of cases, and appears to be the commonest single finding in any epileptic patient who dies a natural death (Falconer & Taylor 1968). The pathogenesis of mesial temporal lobe sclerosis is thus a subject of considerable importance.

The sclerosis consists of dense glial infiltration of Ammon's horn and adjacent structures such as the amygdala and uncus in the medial part of the temporal lobe. It is usually unilateral. The associated epilepsy commonly sets in during the first decade of life, is frequently severe and responds particularly well to surgical resection of the lesion. Initially it was thought to result from birth injury, either through generalised hypoxia or as a result of herniation and compression of the posterior cerebral arteries against the tentorial opening. Careful studies, however, suggest that this is not so (Ounsted *et al.* 1966; Falconer & Taylor 1968; Falconer 1974). Neither high birth weight nor prematurity predispose to temporal lobe epilepsy, and the incidence of birth injury in patients with medial temporal lobe sclerosis has usually been found to be no higher than in other groups with temporal lobe epilepsy. Nonetheless Bruton (1988), in a recent analysis of a large material of resected temporal lobe specimens, found a weakly significant relationship between the presence of

the lesion and a history of birth injury, suggesting that the latter may be operative in a small proportion of cases.

A factor which has clearly emerged as especially common is a history of febrile convulsions, often with status epilepticus, occurring in early childhood. This was confirmed in Bruton's study. It is suggested that the anoxia deriving from such episodes, if sufficiently prolonged at this vulnerable period, may cause irreversible damage to the medial temporal lobe structures and result in due course in the sclerotic epileptogenic lesion. A similar lesion can be produced experimentally in adolescent baboons by inducing serial epileptic attacks or status epilepticus, and as in man the resulting lesion is usually unilateral (Meldrum *et al.* 1973, 1974).

The availability of high-resolution MRI has allowed this hypothesis to be explored in more detail (Kuks *et al.* 1993). Among 107 patients with drug-resistant epilepsy, 45 showed evidence of focal or diffuse hippocampal damage and 20 had a history of childhood febrile seizures. The two were highly significantly associated, especially where diffuse hippocampal lesions were concerned. Furthermore the severity of hippocampal damage was greater in those with such a history. This finding confirmed Sagar and Oxbury's (1987) observation that severe and diffuse loss of neurones in resected temporal lobe specimens was closely associated with a history of prolonged childhood convulsions.

Kuks *et al.* (1993) suggest three possible explanations for this relationship. The patients may have been born with normal brains and the febrile seizures then produced the diffuse hippocampal damage; or they may have been born with focal hippocampal abnormalities which were then converted to diffuse sclerosis by the seizures; or they may have been born with diffuse sclerosis which put them at increased risk of developing febrile seizures. In favour of the last two possibilities is the observation that some 15% of patients with hippocampal sclerosis had additional MRI or histological evidence of cortical dysgenesis, suggesting that the two may sometimes have shared a common aetiology by way of abnormal embryogenesis (Kuzniecky 1994; Raymond *et al.* 1994b). Scheibel (1991) marshalls further arguments in support of this view.

Factors other than febrile convulsions must clearly be incriminated in many cases. Two-thirds of Kuks *et al.*'s patients showed MRI evidence of the lesion in the absence of such a history. Developmental abnormalities may then be responsible, or other causes of anoxia may have operated to produce the pathological changes. Perinatal or postnatal trauma may sometimes have contributed to the lesion—perhaps not directly, but by setting up some other epileptogenic focus which eventually leads, by way of anoxic episodes during seizures, to the mesial temporal lobe sclerosis.

Genetics of epilepsy

Genetic aspects of epilepsy have been extensively studied

but have met with a good deal of difficulty. An hereditary contribution has usually emerged in large-scale studies, but clear-cut patterns have seldom been observed. Mendelian patterns of inheritance have been established in relation to a few specific forms of epilepsy, as discussed below, but in the vast majority of cases genetic counselling is dependent on empirical risks estimated from family studies.

This should not be surprising since the epilepsies are a heterogeneous group of disorders. No satisfactory genetic hypothesis could be expected to fit the facts when the epileptic symptom may result from so many different forms of cerebral disorder, some inherited and some acquired. Moreover the capacity to have an epileptic attack is apparently universal in the population provided precipitating factors are sufficient; it is possible therefore that separate genetic mechanisms may govern such matters as aptitude for convulsions (convulsive threshold) even though the subject has not experienced a seizure, and the specific epileptic predisposition which may not always be paralleled by lowering of the threshold (Radermecker & Dumon 1969). Basic research further shows how many different mechanisms can lead to seizures, any of which may be influenced by genetic factors — hypersensitivity of neurones, inactivation of excitatory neurotransmitters, or control of spread of discharges (Anderson & Hauser 1993).

Nevertheless twin studies have shown much greater concordance for epilepsy among monozygotic than dizygotic twin pairs, especially when attention is restricted to epilepsies without identifiable cause. Large-scale family studies have also long supported a genetic factor. Conrad's surveys from German hospitals and institutions in the 1930s showed, for example, that when patients were classified into those showing 'idiopathic', 'intermediate' and 'symptomatic' clinical types, the incidence of epilepsy in their children was 6.0, 2.7 and 1.6%, respectively (Slater & Cowie 1971). It is also clear that family concentrations are more marked with certain types of epilepsy, especially those with generalised epilepsy showing inter-ictal spike and wave discharges, whether grand mal or petit mal, and in relation to febrile seizures. Anderson and Hauser (1993) provide a detailed review of the literature:

Taking 1% as the baseline risk, and summarizing data from Metrakos and Metrakos (1961, 1970) and Doose *et al.* (1973, 1984), Anderson and Hauser estimate that the risk to siblings is increased some 3–5-fold when onset in the proband has been below the age of 15, and 2–3-fold when after this age. A 5–6-fold increased risk is associated with EEGs showing generalised spike and wave discharges in the proband, this rising to 15-fold when the sibling in question also has such an EEG pattern.

Children with febrile seizures have a 3–6-fold increased risk of developing epilepsy later. The risk to siblings is increased both for febrile convulsions and for epilepsy, risk of the former rising to 20% when one parent has also had febrile convulsions and to 55% when both parents have been affected (Hauser *et al.* 1985). In a small subgroup of children with three or more febrile convulsions such episodes may follow an autosomal dominant pattern (Rich *et al.* 1987).

With partial epilepsies sibling risk is lower, being estimated variously from no increase to 5- or 6-fold. Focal epilepsy involving paroxysmal sharp waves or spikes in the mid-temporal regions tends, however, to show a familial incidence (Bray & Wiser 1965).

It is much harder to obtain data for risk to the offspring of probands with epilepsy, though in general this seems to be higher or the same as that to siblings. Anderson and Hauser conclude that the risk to offspring is increased when the parent has had idiopathic epilepsy, when this developed at a young age, and when the mother rather than the father has been affected (8.7% compared with 2.4%). The risk is also higher for children who themselves show a specific EEG abnormality.

In contrast to the above approximations, some epilepsies, perhaps 1–2%, are associated with diagnosable Mendelian traits or chromosomal abnormalities. Examples include the epilepsy associated with tuberous sclerosis which is inherited as an autosomal dominant, and progressive myoclonic epilepsy of the Unverricht–Lundborg type which follows a recessive pattern. An autosomal dominant form of nocturnal frontal lobe epilepsy has recently been identified (Scheffer *et al.* 1995). Certain rare chromosomal abnormalities such as ring chromosome 14, ring chromosome 20, an extra inverted chromosome 15, and fragile X syndrome are closely associated with seizures. Finally, genetic loci have been mapped for three epileptic syndromes—on chromosome 20 for benign familial neonatal convulsions, on chromosome 6 for juvenile myoclonic epilepsy, and on chromosome 21 for progressive myoclonic epilepsy in Finnish families. Further molecular genetic studies may be expected to expand this list.

It seems therefore that there may be a number of genes in circulation which produce clinically recognisable forms of epilepsy. These, however, must still be regarded as exceptional instances, even when attention is restricted to special varieties of epilepsy. For most of the remainder, polygenic inheritance is likely to play a considerable role, acting in conjunction with important environmental influences.

The important point for genetic counselling is that the chance of an epileptic patient having an epileptic child appears to be not very greatly increased provided the partner is unaffected. Hill (1963b) recommends that as a prelude to any advice with regard to procreation, a full personal and family history should be obtained from both partners of the marriage with special reference to the occurrence of epilepsy in both families, also comprehensive EEG examinations of both partners. 'If the partner's EEG is normal and the family history is negative, and the patient's epilepsy is clearly of acquired origin (focal corti-cal EEG), the chances that a child of the relationship will be epileptic are probably not more than one in 40. The risk of epileptic progeny increases from this, depending on the evidence that the patient's epilepsy is dependent upon a genetic factor (e.g. family history positive, EEG showing subcortical three per second spike and wave dis-charges) to the opposed extreme position in which both partners are epileptic and both show this type of seizure discharge in their EEGs.'

Aggravating and precipitating factors in epilepsy

Whatever the underlying cause of the seizures, certain factors may operate to facilitate attacks. Some are largely idiosyncratic to the individual concerned, as seen in extreme degree in reflex epilepsy (p. 241). Some may be responsible for a single attack in an otherwise unaffected person whose threshold for an epileptic seizure merely happens to be relatively low.

Lowering of physical health from any cause may increase the chance of attacks. Sleep deprivation or extreme fatigue are sometimes found to be important. Starvation or even mild degrees of hypoglycaemia can be responsible for attacks in some patients, similarly tran-sient states of anoxia. In women, attacks sometimes increase in the premenstrual phase, probably by virtue of shifts in water and electrolyte balance. Drugs which increase the likelihood of attacks have already been men-tioned (p. 245).

Frequently noted precipitants include emotional dis-turbances, startle, shock or surprise (Daube 1965). Inter-personal stresses and tensions are widely recognised to increase the frequency and severity of attacks; accord-ingly the emotional stability of the patient may be a factor of considerable importance in securing optimal control. Servit et al. (1963) made an analysis of activating situa-tions in 895 epileptics, and found that more than a third had an increase of seizures in relation to factors in the external environment. Conflict situations were reported to aggravate seizures in 23%, and mental or physical activity in 6%. Eighteen per cent of the patients claimed that their first seizure had followed immediately upon an emotional trauma, mostly an episode of alarm or an expe-rience of horror or fear. Mattson (1991) and Antebi and Bird (1992) review further evidence that tension, anxiety and depression increase the frequency of seizures in a substantial proportion of patients.

Stevens (1959), in an interesting experiment, found that an emotionally stressful interview could have a markedly adverse effect on the stability of EEG patterns in a large proportion of epileptics, but was without effect in normal controls. More specifically, Barker and Wolf (1947) illustrated the highly individual triggering which could occur in relation to certain conflict situations. They presented a detailed psychological study of a patient whose epileptic attacks appeared to be related to occa-sions when his anger broke through customary inhibitory restraints. When interviewed under sodium amytal he expressed mounting rage against his mother, culminating in a fit with coincident epileptic discharges on the EEG.

Fenwick distinguishes between 'evoked' and 'psy-chogenic' seizures (Fenwick 1981a; Fenwick & Brown 1989). The former depend on a specific external precipi-tant and correspond to 'reflex epilepsy' as discussed on p. 241. Psychogenic seizures, in the correct sense of the term, are generated by an act of will or by specific func-tions of the mind *without* any external stimulus. Fenwick estimates that evoked seizures probably account for 5–6% of all cases of epilepsy, whereas the psychogenic variety may be three times as common. Some patients, for example, find that an act of attention, dwelling on a par-ticular emotion, or some mental function such as think-ing, calculating or searching for a word increases the likelihood of seizures. A patient described by Cirignotta et al. (1980a) had attacks when playing cards or draughts or solving mathematical puzzles, but rarely in other situa-tions, suggesting that the precipitant was a specific pattern of 'strategic thinking'. He was unable to learn chess because efforts to concentrate on it were frustrated by attacks. Forster et al. (1975) described a not dissimilar patient in whom the precipitant appeared to be complex decision making in a sequential fashion. In other patients a direct act of will may be involved, such as making the mind blank, attending closely to a particular point in the visual field or concentrating on an emotion of sadness or guilt. In such cases the particular mental function which serves as a precipitant may not always be vouchsafed readily.

By contrast some patients find that they can arrest or abort a seizure after it has begun by some form of mental or bodily activity. Symonds (1959) recorded such a situa-tion in 53 of 1000 cases seen consecutively. Twenty-five stated that they could cut short attacks by some kind of mental effort, usually described as 'pulling themselves together' or making an 'effort of concentration'. Eight patients volunteered that a deliberate switch of mental attention could be successful, for example away from the contents of the aura. Twelve could arrest focal seizures by local stimulation of some part of the body. Such inhibitory manoeuvres may be discovered spontaneously by the patient. Failing this, it may be possible to direct his atten-tion towards them and to utilise the process in therapy, as discussed on p. 308 *et seq.*

Auras of epilepsy

The auras which precede focal epileptic attacks are of great clinical importance. They represent the initial focal onset of the attack, and in conjunction with the EEG findings can give essential information about the site of origin of the epileptic disturbance within the brain. In essence the aura is that portion of the seizure which occurs before consciousness is lost and for which memory is retained afterwards (Commission on Classification and Terminology of the International League Against Epilepsy 1981). It is thus a retrospective term, applying to what the patient can describe after the seizure has ended. Auras may sometimes arise without further progression, as in simple partial seizures (p. 240). This is especially likely early in the evolution of a lesion or when the epilepsy is partially controlled by drugs. They will then produce irregularly recurrent symptoms whose significance may easily be overlooked or misinterpreted.

The detailed content of auras can range from simple discrete sensations to complex abnormalities of ideation and emotion as described below. The pattern shows a fair degree of specificity for the brain region in which the epileptic discharge originates, and in a given patient is usually constant from one attack to another. The symptoms appear abruptly, and in the majority of cases are experienced passively as foreign intrusions on the stream of awareness. They probably rarely occupy more than a few seconds or perhaps a minute, though subjectively the time course may seem much longer (Pond 1957). With recovery of consciousness the aura is usually recalled but not invariably so. At the time the patient may have indicated his aura by a frightened look, an exclamation or by moving to safety, yet afterwards can remember nothing of it. Or he may distinctly recall having had some warning by way of a definite sensation or experience which now cannot be described.

Auras must be distinguished from prodromata. The latter do not appear abruptly, but build up slowly for hours or days before the attacks occur. Prodromata are commoner in children than adults, and probably commoner in temporal lobe epilepsy than other forms. Typically they consist of psychological manifestations—mounting irritability, apprehension, sullenness, apathy or periods of mental dullness. Rarely the patient may have a feeling of well being and show increased energy during the prodromal period. Changes in appetite may occur, or autonomic changes such as pallor, flushing or dyspepsia. Such prodromata are incompletely understood and lack the clinical significance of the well-defined aura. Nevertheless, they may be of value in occasional patients in warning that attacks are to be expected.

Frontal seizures

Seizures arising within the frontal lobes are remarkable for the variety of pictures produced and their sometimes bizarre manifestations (Riggio & Harner 1992; Chauvel *et al.* 1995; Williamson 1995). Moreover their origin is frequently difficult to detect on the scalp EEG. Stores *et al.* (1991) have described the diagnostic difficulties that may arise in children.

The spread of discharge is often so rapid that no aura is experienced, leading to sudden loss of consciousness and a grand mal seizure resembling primary generalised epilepsy. The rare cases of frontal lobe absence can present like petit mal with arrest of speech and inhibition of movement. Discharges originating in the more posterior part of the lobe may implicate the frontal eye fields, with an 'adversive aura' in which the head and eyes turn towards the opposite side. Ipsilateral deviation has also been described. Implication of the pre-Rolandic motor cortex can lead to the classic Jacksonian motor 'march', consisting of involuntary rhythmic clonic movements commencing in some part of the opposite limb or side of the face or tongue, and spreading thence to involve contiguous regions until the major convulsion results. Alternatively the Jacksonian seizure may die away without progressing to generalised convulsions, and in this case consciousness may be fully retained throughout. Speech arrest may similarly occur with fully preserved consciousness, and can be found with discharges originating in either hemisphere.

Involvement of the supplementary motor cortex leads to the sudden, even explosive assumption of an asymmetrical tonic posture. The characteristic picture is of dystonic abduction and flexion of the contralateral arm and turning of the head towards the upraised hand. The contralateral leg is usually extended. Such posturing may be accompanied by speech arrest or repeated utterance of a single syllable word, but awareness is usually strikingly retained.

Sensory aural symptoms may include dizziness, light headedness and feelings of constriction or oppression in the head, also vague sensations of heat or shivering in the trunk and limbs. Autonomic symptoms consist of piloerection and flushing, often accompanied by a frightened facial expression, palpitations or a sudden desire to urinate. Chauvel *et al.* (1995) also describe forced thinking, with obsessive intrusion of thoughts, and 'gaze attraction' to some object in the environment. In addition the discharges may sometimes come to implicate the temporal lobes, with the production of auras indistinguishable from those of temporal lobe epilepsy (see below).

The most dramatic and often puzzling manifestations

consist of frontal lobe automatisms, mostly arising from the anterior and medial parts of the lobe. Their bizarre manifestations not infrequently lead to a mistaken diagnosis of pseudoseizures. Some are identical to the automatisms of temporal lobe epilepsy (p. 253), but distinguishing features include their brevity and the rapid resumption of consciousness. They characteristically include perseverative motor phenomena of a florid and idiosyncratic nature – arm flailing, rubbing, rolling, kicking or bicycling movements of the legs. If standing the patient may hop, jump or run in circles. Sexual automatisms may consist of pelvic thrusting and genital manipulation. Tonic posturing may accompany the motor activity, also vocalisations in the form of shouting, screaming, moaning or howling. Intracranial recording has shown that in many such patients the seizure discharges remain confined to the frontal lobes (Williamson *et al.* 1985). In others there has clearly been spread to the medial temporal lobe structures.

Parietal seizures

Parietal lobe seizures may commence with a 'sensory Jacksonian march' consisting of paraesthesiae, numbness, tingling or feelings of heat and cold, which begin focally and spread to contiguous areas of the body as the sensory cortex becomes progressively involved. The parts most frequently affected are those with the most extensive cortical representation, namely the hand, arm and face. Visual phenomena include complex hallucinations or disturbances of shape or size. Paracentral involvement may lead to lateralised genital sensations. Seizures beginning more posteriorly can lead to pronounced disorders of the body image. A limb or even half of the entire body may appear to be heavier, larger, smaller, missing or separated from the rest of the body. The limb may feel to be displaced, extended or contracted into the body, even though the patient can see for himself that it is normal. Very occasionally a phantom limb may be felt to be present. Some of the bizarre forms which such auras can take are illustrated in the examples described in Chapter 2 (p. 72).

Medial surface seizures

Seizures arising from the medial surface and superior border of the hemisphere show several interesting features (Kennedy 1959b). Involvement of the supplementary motor area, just anterior to the Rolandic fissure, may produce tonic postural movements as described above (p. 249). Epigastric sensations indistinguishable from those of temporal lobe epilepsy may occur, also speech arrest

and confusion. More posterior lesions are associated with paraesthesiae in the contralateral foot and leg, rectal sensations and sometimes genital sensations including feelings of orgasm.

Erickson (1945) reported a woman who for 16 years had suffered attacks of feeling 'hot all over' as if she were having coitus, associated with a marked increase of libido. Although the feeling in the genitalia was a pleasurable sensation, resembling ordinary intercourse, it was limited to the contralateral side of the vagina. Nevertheless she had twice been hospitalised with a diagnosis of nymphomania. Later the sensory experience was followed by Jacksonian seizures and finally by progressive paraplegia. A haemangioma was ultimately removed from the upper end of the right Rolandic sulcus on the medial surface of the hemisphere, with prompt cessation of the sexual disturbance.

Occipital seizures

These commence with visual disturbances, well localised within the opposite half-field of vision. A scotoma or hemianopic field defect may occur, or more commonly simple visual hallucinations consisting of flashes of light, colours, zigzags or radiating spectra. Complex formed hallucinations with meaningful content may occur with discharges involving the temporoparieto-occipital junction.

Temporal lobe seizures

Temporal lobe seizures produce the most varied and complex auras of all. They are of great importance to the psychiatrist since they often contain elements which may raise a suspicion of neurotic or psychotic disorder. This is particularly likely when the auras arise repeatedly without an ensuing motor convulsion. Isolated auras with prominent psychological content such as hallucinations, depersonalisation or other subjective experiences are sometimes referred to as 'psychic seizures'.

A variety of *autonomic effects and visceral sensations* figure prominently in temporal lobe auras. The 'epigastric aura' is perhaps the most common, consisting of ill-defined sensations rising from the epigastrium upwards towards the throat, typically described as churning in the stomach, fear in the stomach or even pain. Also frequent are inexplicable odd feelings in the head. Other autonomic effects include salivation, borborygmi, flushing, pallor, tachycardia, praecordial pain, cough and apnoea. Subjective dizziness is common, or true vertigo accompanied by tinnitus and changes in auditory perception.

Altered perceptual experiences include both distortions of real perceptions and spontaneous hallucinations. Sounds may seem suddenly remote or intensely loud, objects may seem larger or smaller, nearer or further away. The evaluation attached to percepts may change, so that objects, sounds or events suddenly acquire a peculiar vivid significance. Alternatively, the subject may feel remote from the environment and out of meaningful contact with things around him. Feelings of derealisation and depersonalisation may be marked. The essential quality of recognition may change, with strong feelings of familiarity or unfamiliarity which lead to *déjà vu* and *jamais vu*. Stimulation studies carried out on the temporal lobes exposed at operation have suggested that visual hallucinations, interpretive illusions (such as objects seeming nearer or further away) and illusions of familiarity derive more commonly from the right temporal lobe than the left (Mullan & Penfield 1959; Penfield & Perot 1963).

Visual hallucinations may consist of the simple elements described for occipital seizures, but also complex formed hallucinations of scenes, faces or visions of past experiences. 'Lilliputian hallucinations', in which hallucinated visual material appears very small, must be distinguished from micropsia in which actual objects look to be smaller than normal. Auditory hallucinations stemming from the region of the superior lateral temporal gyrus may also be simple or complex — ringing and buzzing or organised experiences of music or voices.

Hallucinations of taste and smell derive from the medial temporal lobe structures, particularly the uncinate region, and are of great significance for the diagnosis of temporal lobe epilepsy. They may be accompanied by a characteristic smacking or pursing of the lips, or chewing, tasting and swallowing movements. Olfactory and gustatory sensations may occur alone or in conjunction with a peculiar alteration of consciousness composed of depersonalisation, *déjà vu* and dream-like reminiscence — the classic 'dreamy state' or 'uncinate crisis' of earlier writers.

Cognitive abnormalities include disturbances of speech, thought and memory. Transient dysphasia may occur, or sudden ejaculations, or a press of incorrect and inappropriate speech. Dysphasia as part of an aura indicates a left temporal lobe focus, whereas speech automatisms (recurrent, irrelevant or emotionally toned utterances) are strongly related to a right temporal lobe focus (Serafetinides & Falconer 1963).

The purely subjective disorders of thinking and memory constitute some of the most striking manifestations of temporal lobe auras. The patient may become abruptly aware of difficulty in thinking coherently, of mixing things up, or of great confusion and turmoil in his mind. There may be a compulsion to think on certain restricted topics such as eternity, suicide or death ('forced thinking'). Or there may be intrusion of thoughts or of stereotyped words or phrases against the subject's will ('evocation of thoughts'). A sudden cessation in the stream of thought may occur and later be described in a manner indistinguishable from schizophrenic 'blocking'.

Disturbances of memory range from sudden difficulty with recall to compulsive reminiscence on topics, scenes or events from the past. Many of the phenomena of *déjà vu* or *jamais vu* should perhaps be interpreted as distortions of the memory process. In the rare 'panoramic memory' the patient feels that whole episodes from his past life are lived through again in a brief period of time as complex organised experiences. Indeed distortion of time sense is often an integral part of the experience of the aura, time appearing to rush by precipitately or alternatively to stand quite still. Amidst all of these experiences the patient usually retains a hold on reality to some degree, so that subsequently he can relate that he was aware of himself experiencing the abnormal phenomena.

Finally, strong *affective experiences* frequently appear in temporal lobe auras. The most common are fear and intense anxiety, which well up suddenly without provocation. Other unpleasant affects include depression, guilt and anger, all of which may reach extreme degree. Pleasurable affects of joy, elation or ecstasy occur more rarely, though Cirignotta *et al.* (1980b) have documented a patient with a well-marked ecstatic content to the attacks (so-called 'Dostoevsky epilepsy'). Williams (1956) showed that fear was experienced when the epileptic discharge involved the anterior half of either temporal lobe and occurred in 70% of patients with foci in this region. Depression was associated with lesions anywhere in the temporal part of the brain. Non-specific pleasant and unpleasant affects were mainly associated with posterior temporal lesions. Hermann *et al.* (1992) showed that in 13 of 15 patients with ictal fear the origin of the seizures was in the right (non-dominant) lobe.

These affective experiences must be accepted as an intrinsic part of the attack, and not merely a reaction to other aspects of the aura. Thus the affect aroused is usually stereotyped and crude, and lacks the subtlety of normal emotions. It tends to be constant both in quality and in time of occurrence during the attack, though it may sometimes change sequentially over time in a given patient. The emotional content of the aura may nevertheless colour hallucinatory experiences or occasionally have issue in disturbed behaviour.

These manifold aspects of the auras can occur in any and every combination. There is often a characteristic 'march', passing for example from an initial epigastric sensation to gustatory hallucinations to forced thinking, or from intense *déjà vu* to an overwhelming sense of fear. Sometimes various aspects of the aura appear to occur simultaneously, or the content is so rich and strange that the patient lacks the vocabulary to describe his experiences. Many are extremely bizarre, particularly those which involve disturbance of appreciation of reality and of the self. Williams (1966) pointed out that the temporal lobes perform the function of integrating sensations of all kinds, and in addition probably contain the neural substrates for emotion itself: 'It is the integration of the whole of exteroceptive and proprioceptive sensations with emotions and moods which culminates in the ultimate sense of "I am", so that it is not at all surprising that disintegration of this organisation, with retention of sensation, leads to so many of the bizarre disturbances of self which disturb the patient with temporal lobe epilepsy.'

The precise content of the auras may sometimes change with the passage of time, and scrutiny of the patient's notes may reveal well-documented phenomena earlier in the illness of which the patient now has no recollection. This tendency can sometimes increase the risk of the patient being regarded as suffering from a psychogenic disorder.

Special interest attaches to the possible psychopathological significance of some temporal lobe auras. The perceptual–ideational content may prove to be related to an early traumatic situation which is perhaps only partially, if at all, accessible to recall in the normal state. But when activated by the epileptic process the claim of the material to occupy the field of consciousness becomes irresistible and overwhelming:

A man of 39 had fits from the age of 10. The aura consisted of nausea, raising a hand above the face and saying 'Don't hit me dad, please don't hit me'. The patient described a visual scene of his father threatening him with a poker. An informant stated that the father had actually struck the patient with a poker just before the first fit.
(Hill & Mitchell 1953)

A patient's aura consisted of vertigo, a bell ringing and the subjective compulsion to think of 'number two' before losing consciousness. The patient had been faecally incontinent until the age of 6, and had at that time called faeces 'number two'.
(Hill & Mitchell 1953)

A patient had her first epileptic attack in an anxious situation after living in a desolate war environment. The aura consisted of a scene of a city in ruins accompanied by strong *déjà vu*. Even many years later it was possible to provoke a characteristic dysrhythmia in the EEG by inviting the visual evocation of the symbolic scene of the city in ruins.
(Krapf 1957)

Hill and Mitchell (1953) discuss the gradations which may be seen in such auras, between the complete re-enactment of organised experience from the past as in the first example, to more abbreviated forms in which merely a word or two, or a simple forced thought, intrude into consciousness. These may be devoid of meaning to the patient, yet, as in the second example, have a possible relation to emotionally significant past events. Hill and Mitchell found cases in which the ideational content of the aura had changed over time from complete memories to the more abbreviated and hidden forms. These then resembled 'screen memories', and had apparently undergone the psychological processes of repression, condensation or symbol formation. In some cases the process had gone still further: the patient merely experienced strong *déjà vu* and felt that some important memory was about to be recalled but lost consciousness before it arrived. Or he might later say that an important memory was recalled just before the fit but was now forgotten again.

The mechanisms underlying these changes over time are unknown. They may rest on physiological mechanisms, whereby the neuronal circuits responsible for the activation into awareness of the content of the aura become destroyed or by-passed, or on psychological mechanisms of defence by which the significant event is barred increasingly from access to consciousness. The two, of course, may in the last analysis be synonymous.

Complex partial seizures ('psychomotor seizures')

Complex partial seizures are notable for the striking clinical phenomena which may be displayed or experienced. In particular the fit proper may be replaced as the ictal manifestation of the epileptic attack. The clinical pictures involved range from periods of disturbed motor behaviour, sometimes of a complex and semipurposeful nature, to periods of abnormal subjective experience of varying duration. All have in common impairment of consciousness of some degree, an abrupt onset and a more or less abrupt termination, and all are accompanied by alteration of the electrical activity of the brain throughout the time they are taking place. In essence these are *the complex behavioural and experiential manifestations of on-going epileptic discharge*.

They are frequently preceded by aural manifestations of the type which usher in more conventional motor seizures. They may displace the grand mal convulsion entirely and constitute the sole manifestation of the seizure, or give way later to grand mal which then terminates the episode. When of long duration they may occasionally be interrupted by one or more convulsions which punctuate their course.

A bewildering number of names have been used for such episodes—'psychomotor seizures', 'epileptic equivalents', 'psychic variants', 'automatisms,' 'fugues' and 'twilight states'. Such terms have often been used without clear definition, or even interchangeably, which has led to very considerable confusion in the literature. 'Epileptic equivalent' had long usage as a generic term but cannot be commended; these attacks are not the 'equivalents' of epilepsy in any exact sense of the word. 'Psychomotor seizure' comes nearer to indicating the content of the attacks. Its chief disadvantage is that 'psychomotor epilepsy' is sometimes regarded as synonymous with 'temporal lobe epilepsy', namely as referring to seizures arising within the anatomical boundaries of the temporal lobes. Complex partial seizures certainly have a special association with epilepsy originating in the medial temporal lobe structures, but this association is by no means exclusive. It is accepted that some 20% of complex partial seizures derive from lesions elsewhere in the brain, and will fail to show a temporal focus on repeated EEG examination, while 20% of patients with temporal lobe epilepsy suffer from grand mal seizures alone (Stevens 1966b). Using depth electrodes, Williamson and Spencer (1986) found that 30% of complex partial seizures were of extratemporal origin.

An additional complication is that clinically similar but physiologically distinct phenomena may ensue upon a grand mal convulsion. They are then not manifestations of the ictus itself, but of the disturbance of cerebral activity which follows upon the ictus. The close similarity of content between complex partial seizures and some of these post-ictal disorders is discussed on p. 258.

In what follows an attempt will be made to describe the various manifestations of complex partial seizures under headings which reach some measure of agreement in the literature, while recognizing that the distinctions between them are often far from clear-cut and that a good deal of overlap must be expected to occur.

Epileptic automatisms

An epileptic automatism may be defined as 'a state of clouding of consciousness which occurs during or immediately after a seizure, and during which the individual retains control of posture and muscle tone but performs simple or complex movements and actions without being aware of what is happening' (Fenton 1972). It is accompanied by continuous electrical disturbance in the EEG.

Commonly an ictal automatism is preceded by aural manifestations, usually those typical of temporal lobe epilepsy. Eighty per cent of Feindel and Penfield's (1954) patients had warnings of their attacks, chiefly in the form of epigastric sensations, confusion or difficulty with memory, feelings of strangeness or unreality, lightness or dizziness in the head, or masticatory movements with salivation. Occasionally, though not very frequently, the automatism terminates with a grand mal convulsion. The majority of patients with automatisms also suffer from other forms of seizure, especially grand mal attacks, though occasionally they occur as the sole manifestation of the epilepsy.

The great majority are brief, lasting from a few seconds to several minutes, though occasional examples have lasted for up to an hour. Knox (1968) found that 80% occupied less than 5 minutes, and another 12% less than 15 minutes. The detailed patterns of behaviour are variable, sometimes even in the same individual on different occasions. The subject may merely continue with what he was doing, a dazed expression and sudden inaccessibility being the only indications of the seizure. Or there may be no more than some regular stereotyped manoeuvre such as pulling at the clothes, passing a hand over the face or fumbling with objects near at hand. Brief automatisms can in fact pass unnoticed by onlookers. In more extended attacks the patient performs a whole sequence of related actions—walking about the room, searching in drawers, moving objects or attempting to remove his clothing. The actions tend to be repetitive, fumbling and clumsy, but are sometimes reasonably well coordinated. The apparent purposiveness behind the movements also varies considerably. Intentions are usually poorly conceived and executed, but are sometimes successfully carried through even though inappropriate to the situation.

The following examples described by Lennox (1960) are typical:

A woman abruptly ceased her conversation, assumed a strained worried expression and walked away. Led into an adjoining room, she walked quickly from place to place saying 'I must get my coat'. After 5 minutes she consented to sit down and converse, asking what she should do about her affairs, but seemingly not satisfied with the answers because her questions would be repeated again and again. She had no recollection of this seizure or of the post-ictal conversation nor, in fact, of anything until after she awoke the next day.

While in a physician's office a patient suddenly stopped talking and stared into space. He slumped in his chair for a brief moment, then sat up and began to rub his abdomen with both hands. A flashlight was shone into his eyes and he turned away. He began to rummage about the desk as if looking for something. When questioned as to what he wanted he said 'I wanna, I wanna'. At this point he took a cigarette from his packet, lit it and started to smoke. He then got up from his chair, walked out of the office and wandered down the hall opening all the doors and saying 'I want a toilet'. Next, he walked down the hall but could not be distracted by any outside contact. He then lay on the bed and appeared to regain contact gradually.

A policeman directing traffic walked to a waiting car, opened the door, opened and examined the contents of the woman driver's handbag, then returned the bag and went back to his post. The woman reported the occurrence and the policeman denied knowledge of it. Subsequent seizures were predominantly convulsive.

Environmental cues may to some extent determine the detailed patterns of behaviour, accounting perhaps for the variations seen from one attack to another in the individual patient (Forster & Liske 1963). Patterns of cognitive function in train at the time no doubt also help to shape behaviour. Thus the content may be in accord with the current environment, as in patients who continue with on-going behaviour during the attack — performing household tasks, or even continuing to drive and obeying regulations with subsequent dense amnesia for what has transpired. Sometimes, however, behaviour is in direct opposition with environmental cues. One patient, for example, developed an attack while playing the organ for a carol service — he interrupted the carol to render jazz music for 3 minutes, thereafter returning to the exact bar of the hymn when the seizure was over (Forster & Liske 1963).

To the onlooker the subject is clearly out of touch with his surroundings in the great majority of automatisms. Typically he looks somewhat dazed and vacant, and often anxious and tense. When spoken to there may be no response, or he may mumble incoherently or answer quite irrelevantly. Attempts at distraction are likely to be resisted, and interference may meet with opposition amounting on rare occasions to combative behaviour. Only very rarely are patients reported in whom judgement and awareness were seemingly maintained during attacks. Hughlings Jackson (1889) recorded the case of a physician who apparently persisted with reasonably competent behaviour during some of his automatisms—in one he continued to write a prescription though the details of dosage were incorrect, and in another he correctly diagnosed a case of pneumonia during an episode for which he was afterwards completely amnesic. Such examples are exceptional and should perhaps be accepted with reserve. It is now widely agreed that behaviour is unlikely ever to be entirely normal, or conversation rational, while the attack is in progress (Jasper 1964; Fenton 1972). Even when complex coordinated activities are maintained these are usually inappropriate in some respects to the immediate situation, and judgement will be seen to have been impaired.

Subjectively the essential and constant feature noted by the patient himself is amnesia for the period of the automatism, and sometimes for a period after its termination as well. The amnesia is usually total, though a vague and muddled awareness of some parts may very occasionally be retained. Failure to lay down a durable record of experience is often clinically important in allowing automatisms to be recognised even in retrospect.

The commonest source of origin of automatisms is epilepsy arising within the medial temporal lobe structures. This evidence comes from the study of traumatic epilepsy after brain wounds of known location, from the EEG and especially from the study of responses to stimulation of the brain at neurosurgical exploration. Feindel and Penfield (1954) found that 78 of 155 patients undergoing temporal lobectomies for epilepsy had a history of automatisms at one time or another. Such attacks were usually accompanied by spontaneous epileptic discharges in the medial and inferior temporal regions, contemporaneous with the duration of the seizure; in such cases electrical stimulation within a fairly discrete region around the amygdaloid nucleus and deep in the uncus could reproduce the automatism. In a very much smaller group automatisms were found to depend on discharges originating in the frontal grey matter and spreading thence to involve subcortical structures. It is now increasingly apparent that automatisms deriving from frontal lobe discharges may show certain distinctive features, as described on p. 250. Moreover, when in such form there is evidence that the seizure discharges can remain confined within the frontal lobes (Williamson et al. 1985).

Fugues

Epileptic fugues are much less common than automatisms and their physiological basis is less completely understood. They consist of longer lasting disturbances of behaviour associated with a tendency to wander away. The distinction between automatisms and fugues can thus be partly a matter of degree; consciousness is said to be less severely impaired in fugues and the abnormal behaviour more complex, extended and integrated.

A confident differentiation between epileptic fugues and those which rest on an hysterical or depressive basis (pp. 296–7) is often difficult, since detailed observation, including EEG recording, has rarely been possible during the occurrence of the abnormal state. Some experienced observers are even inclined to doubt whether epileptic fugues constitute a valid clinical entity, and view all examples as essentially psychogenic in origin. Organic and psychogenic factors may often, of course, be inextricably mixed, with epileptic clouding helping to release dissociative mechanisms. Thus in some cases an initial brief automatism may become greatly prolonged thereafter as an episode of hysterical dissociation.

In general the longer lasting the fugue the more wary one will be of accepting a basis in cerebral dysrhythmia alone. Considerable doubt also surrounds the 'orderly' fugue in which purposive extended behaviour is carried through, and especially when antisocial acts have been performed. A history of grand mal epilepsy or of typical brief automatisms will certainly bias the diagnosis towards an epileptic aetiology, also EEG findings which are strongly indicative of seizures arising within the temporal lobes.

Epileptic fugues are described as lasting for many hours or even days. The patient may wander far from home and later recover spontaneously in a strange setting not knowing how he has got there. Or he may be discovered while still in the abnormal state, appearing vague, perplexed and incoherent. These are some of the patients who are picked up by the police not knowing their personal identity. The patient may have walked long distances, made purchases or travelled by public transport. A limited amount of conversation may sometimes have taken place, though none of this is subsequently remembered. During most periods when the subject is under observation, however, his behaviour is clearly abnormal. Actions are usually seen to be erratic and he may appear to be drowsy or intoxicated. His appearance is often untidy and his demeanour absent minded. Money will usually have been spent carelessly, and the wanderings will rarely have had any clear aim or purpose. Upon recovery amnesia is typically complete for all events which have occurred while the fugue was in progress.

A man of 48 set out for his work in Oxford at the normal time one morning and remembered nothing more until he found himself on the sea-front at Bournemouth. This was some 10 hours later. He had apparently travelled by train, changing twice, and had eaten a meal and paid for it normally. During this period he had lost his hat and coat. The patient was known to have had occasional grand mal epilepsy. Further investigation showed that he had an epileptic focus in the left temporal region. His wife recalled previous episodes of brief confused behaviour of which he himself had been unaware.

(Whitty, Stores & Lishman 1977)

Epileptic fugues lasting for several weeks have occasionally been reported, as in the case described by Spratling (1902) where a travelling salesman undertook his normal circuit of work, recording events in his diary including convulsive seizures from which he was known to suffer. The total period covered was 28 days, for all of which there was no recollection afterwards. The purely epileptic nature of such a case must, however, remain very doubtful.

As with automatisms the epileptic focus will usually be sited in the inferomedial temporal lobe structures. Fugues and automatisms will quite often be found to occur at different times in the same individual.

Twilight states

The term 'twilight state' has been applied to many forms of abnormal episode in epileptic subjects, ranging from automatisms and fugues, as described above, to brief discrete periods of schizophrenia-like disorder. Sometimes it has been used as a generic term for all episodes short of grand mal convulsions in which the level of consciousness is temporarily reduced. Its most useful application in connection with epilepsy, however, would seem to be to separate off those episodes which are distinguished by the occurrence of abnormal subjective experience, rather than by objective motor manifestations.

Twilight states of this nature commonly last from one to several hours, though sometimes they may be prolonged for a week or more. Consciousness is always impaired but this varies greatly in degree from one example to another. It may show only as dream-like absent-minded behaviour or as some slowness of reaction and muddling of comprehension, while at the other extreme there may be complete unawareness of the environment with lack of all response to external stimuli. Psychomotor retardation is commonly profound throughout the attack with marked perseveration in speech and action.

The outstanding phenomena are in the realms of affective and perceptual experience. Abnormal affective states figure prominently in most attacks — panic, terror, anger or ecstasy being the most frequent. Affective storms of great intensity occasionally break up the otherwise passive and apathetic picture which is observed externally. Hallucinations may occupy a large part of the twilight attack, and often contribute directly to the patient's reactions of fear or ecstasy. They are usually visual and typically vivid and highly coloured, perhaps involving whole complex scenes which unfold before the mind's eye. Delusions may be extensively elaborated. A paranoid colouring is often marked and may have issue in the behaviour displayed.

The patient often sits quietly throughout the attack and only tells of his experiences afterwards, or he may show spells of sudden overactivity including aggressive and destructive behaviour. There is sometimes great irritability and sensitivity to minor stimuli, and attempts at interference can precipitate outbursts of primitive rage.

Twilight states usually run their course and end spontaneously, but are said to terminate with a grand mal convulsion rather more commonly than do automatisms. Indeed electroconvulsive therapy can meet with considerable success in terminating twilight states of long duration. Memory for the content of the attack is usually incomplete and fragmentary, though sometimes a remarkably detailed account can be given. In particular a vivid recollection of the hallucinations may be retained. What the patient tells of his experiences can frequently be supplemented by what has been inferred from observation of his expression and reactions at the time.

It is clear that a great variety of abnormal mental states are subsumed under the heading of twilight states, even when the term is restricted in the manner described. Some appear to be characterised by cognitive, some by affective and some by complex 'psychotic' experiences. The precise classification of these varied manifestations and their electrophysiological correlates must await further clarification. All are accompanied by profound disturbance of the electrical activity of the brain, and again the source of origin of the epilepsy is most commonly within the medial temporal lobe structures.

Other forms of automatism

Absence status (petit mal status)

A rather longer lasting form of automatism has been found to depend essentially on generalised runs of three per second spike and wave discharges in the EEG. The discharges may sometimes be discontinuous, but the periods of normality which separate them are too brief for the resumption of complete awareness. It is essentially the EEG pattern which distinguishes this variety of automatism from those initiated from within the temporal lobes (Lennox 1960).

The features of the disorder are summarised by Fenton (1978) and Toone (1981). In most cases the patient will already have experienced absence attacks, or more rarely grand mal, though occasionally absence status appears without a prior history of epilepsy. It occurs before the age of 20 in three-quarters of cases but can appear for the first time in middle age. With late-onset cases there will frequently be some underlying toxic or metabolic disturbance which serves as a precipitant.

The episodes usually start and stop abruptly, occasionally finishing with sleep or a grand mal convulsion. They may last from several minutes to several hours or even days, during which the subject is markedly confused, uncoordinated, slowed and perseverative. The degree of clouding of consciousness varies: at its slightest there is simply slowing of ideation and expression, but more commonly there is marked disorientation, impaired grasp and automatic behaviour. The patient may be virtually stuporose, remaining motionless and apathetic, but if partially aroused is usually capable of limited voluntary action and may sometimes even respond to simple commands. Fluttering of the eyelids and myoclonus of the arms and face are common. Sometimes environmental stimulation will interrupt the condition, both in its clinical and EEG manifestations (Landolt 1958). Subsequently there is complete amnesia for the episode or only a blurred and fragmentary memory.

Niedermeyer and Khalifeh (1965) reported similar examples, but preferred the term 'spike and wave stupor' since regular three per second spike and wave discharges were seen less commonly than atypical spike wave complexes, slow spike wave variants and intermingled multiple spikes. In some of their cases the level of awareness was not markedly lowered, and relatively light arousing stimuli could immediately block the paroxysmal activity.

Abnormal mental states other than clouding are very uncommon, but psychotic pictures have been reported in late-onset cases with paranoid delusional ideation, thought blocking and visual and auditory hallucinations (Toone 1981). Presentation as a depressive psychosis in middle age has been described. Schwartz and Scott (1971) reported an important group of four cases presenting *de novo* with acute confusion in middle age, in whom the provisional diagnoses had included subdural haematoma, acute psychosis and acute confusional state. Without an EEG the correct diagnosis would almost certainly have been missed. When the acute episode was over three of the four patients had no further attacks and required no further treatment.

The course of absence status is essentially benign. Episodes can usually be successfully terminated with intravenous diazepam.

Temporal lobe status (psychomotor status)

Psychomotor status has been much less commonly reported than the above, perhaps surprisingly in view of the frequency of temporal lobe epilepsy. In part this may be due to the difficulty in recognising it on clinical or EEG grounds and of differentiating it from absence status (Toone 1981).

The episodes last for hours or days, and can be ushered in or terminated by a grand mal seizure. The patient is confused, withdrawn and retarded, sometimes with continuous movements of the hands, lip smacking and picking at the clothes. Recurrent automatisms can be interspersed with long periods when the patient is withdrawn but able to respond to simple stimulation. Hallucinations may figure prominently during the course of attacks. There may be psychotic features with a paranoid flavour, including paranoid delusions, but the presence of confusion and disorientation usually makes the organic nature of the disorder apparent (Fenwick 1987a).

The EEG shows unifocal, predominantly medial temporal lobe discharges, spreading bilaterally to involve the prefrontal and lateral temporal regions at times of unresponsiveness. Periods of relatively normal EEG may be interspersed between such episodes. Markand *et al.* (1978) have reported a typical example with EEG recording during two attacks. Intravenous diazepam promptly terminated both the abnormal behaviour and the ictal discharges on the EEG.

Post-ictal disorders

Post-ictal disorders are conveniently considered along with complex partial seizures, since some of their manifestations are similar or indeed indistinguishable if the preceding convulsion has gone unrecognised. The majority of grand mal convulsions are followed by a period of sleep or by transient malaise, headache and nausea. Sometimes, however, post-ictal manifestations are more complex and a period of confusion or disturbed behaviour ensues directly upon recovery from the fit itself. Post-ictal confusional states may sometimes last for hours or even days, and on rare occasions for as long as 1 or 2 weeks (Fenwick 1987a).

The recovery of full consciousness may lag behind the resumption of motor activity, resulting in an episode of *post-ictal automatic behaviour*. Particularly in temporal lobe epilepsy, the actual epileptic attack may be brief and trivial in comparison to the post-ictal automatism which follows. The majority of such episodes are brief, lasting no more than a minute or two, but post-ictal automatisms are rather more likely to be prolonged than ictal automatisms, and more likely to involve complex behaviour which may be semipurposive in nature.

The patient is usually very obviously confused and his movements clumsy and incoordinated, but the degree of organisation of behaviour will vary with the severity of disturbance of consciousness. Pond (1957) pointed out that psychogenic factors may on occasion play a considerable part in determining behaviour, since emotionally charged impulses are more likely to gain control while higher level functions are impaired. Agitation and irritability are sometimes prominent features, and paranoid thought content may be much in evidence. In a small minority of patients, usually those with gross brain damage, dangerously aggressive behaviour may occur. This is the 'epileptic furore' in which the subject becomes wildly overactive for several minutes after the fit, and may indulge in seriously destructive behaviour including physical attacks on people. In all post-ictal automatisms complete amnesia for what transpires is the rule.

Post-ictal 'twilight states' often last considerably longer, sometimes for several hours or even days. As with the ictal twilight states already described they are characterised by psychomotor retardation, vivid hallucinations and marked abnormalities of affective experience. In the patients reported by Landolt (1958) post-ictal twilight states were often accompanied by marked resistance and restlessness, and violent reactions could sometimes be released by even light touch stimuli.

'Post-ictal psychoses' are indistinctly demarcated from the above, but tend to last considerably longer and are characteristically separated from the seizures by a lucid interval. A large group of such cases was included among the patients with 'epileptic clouded states' reported by Levin (1952). Most cleared spontaneously in less than a week, but some lasted for a month or more. The detailed features of such psychoses have only recently come under systematic observation. Logsdail and Toone (1988) have reported 14 examples, most by retrospective review:

The criteria for inclusion were that an episode of confusion or psychosis was manifest immediately after a seizure or emerged within a week of the return of apparently normal mental function; that the episode had a minimum duration of 24 hours and a maximum of 3 months; that the mental state showed clouding or delirium, delusions and hallucinations in clear consciousness, or a mixture of the two together; and that there was no evidence of anticonvulsant toxicity, EEG evidence of petit mal status, a previous history of inter-ictal psychosis, or a recent history of head injury or alcohol or drug abuse.

Five patients had experienced a single episode, six had experienced two to four episodes and three over 10 episodes, all in the wake of seizures. The time from the onset of epilepsy to the first episode ranged from 3 to 33 years with a mean of 15.5 years. Three patients suffered from primary generalised epilepsy and 11 from complex partial seizures with intermittent secondary generalisation. There had typically been an increase in seizure frequency prior to the onset of the psychosis, usually as a cluster of two or three attacks. Eleven of the 14 patients had had a lucid interval with complete recovery from the seizure and the immediate post-ictal confusional phase before the psychosis began, usually lasting 1–2 days but sometimes as long as 6 days in duration.

The pictures encountered were pleomorphic rather than manifesting as discrete easily recognised syndromes. Clouding of consciousness was not invariably present. Nine patients were confused at the onset, this persisting throughout the episode in five. Three showed no evidence of confusion at any time, and two could not cooperate sufficently to clarify the level of consciousness. Mood abnormalities were marked in nine, either elation, depression or both. Six reported paranoid delusions, six visual hallucinations, six auditory hallucinations and two somatic hallucinations. Three initially showed a period of stupor. Diagnoses according to the Present State Examination or Syndrome Check List were schizophrenia (four cases), paranoid psychosis (four), manic or mixed affective psychosis (three) and other psychosis (three). These diagnostic classes were obtained both in patients who were confused and in those who were not. The psychosis lasted 1–2 days in four cases, 4–7 days in four, 8–21 days in four, and 1 month and 3 months in the other two. Six patients were seriously behaviourally disturbed, two were physically aggressive and one made a suicide attempt. Six experienced further generalised seizures while psychotic, usually followed by worsening of the mental symptoms. Where repeat EEG examination was possible during the episode this commonly showed an increase in slow wave abnormalities and in spikes and/or sharp waves.

Factors in common with inter-ictal psychoses (p. 279 *et seq.*) included the lack of a family history of psychotic illness, the over-representation of complex partial seizures, and a similar interval between the age of onset of epilepsy and of the psychosis. Moreover, follow-up showed that three patients later developed a chronic inter-ictal psychosis, usually after several years.

The frequency of affective changes in Logsdail and Toone's patients is mirrored in occasional reports of hypomania following complex partial seizures. Barczak *et al.* (1988) described three such patients, all without evidence of impaired consciousness, two with repeated attacks. Four further cases were reported by Humphries and Dickinson (1988), Morphew (1988) and Byrne (1988). Rather strikingly six of these seven patients had a right-sided focus of origin for their seizures, congruent with the excess of right hemisphere lesions in the patients with mania reported by Starkstein *et al.* (1988) (p. 192).

Interrelations between automatisms, twilight states and post-ictal disturbances

From the descriptions already given it will be obvious that complex partial seizures and post-ictal disturbances embrace a wide variety of clinical phenomena which are hard to classify with precision. All share an intimate relationship with disturbances of the electrical rhythms of the brain, but our understanding of such relationships awaits clarification in many important respects. A step in this direction was reported by Dongier (1959) who presented a synthesis of the experience of several contributors to a colloquium in Marseilles on 'acute psychotic episodes' in epileptics.

Five hundred and thirty-six episodes were considered in 516 epileptics. The several series of patients involved were often highly selected, so even with this large material the findings may not have wholly general application. The episodes were classified purely on their symptomatic content, and viewed in relation to the type of epilepsy from which the patient was suffering, the timing of the episodes in relation to overt seizures, and the EEG disturbances observed during the course of the abnormal

behaviour. Twenty-five per cent of the episodes were preceded by seizures, 10% ended in seizures, and in the remainder the relationship was questionable or lacking entirely.

Those episodes characterised mainly by confusion and disturbance of consciousness showed two types of EEG abnormality during attacks — either continuous bisynchronous spike and wave discharges or diffuse delta dysrhythmia. The former clearly corresponded to the 'absence status' type of automatism, were commoner in children than adults, and showed exclusively simple confusion without marked affective change, agitation or delusions. Most were brief, and none lasted for more than a few hours. They rarely either began or ended with a grand mal convulsion. The confusional states accompanied by diffuse delta dysrhythmia often followed a grand mal convulsion, and thus corresponded mainly to post-ictal automatisms. These were also mostly brief and similarly showed impairment of consciousness as the predominant feature, but here agitated behaviour was more often in evidence. Dongier suggested that agitation and aggression may more readily appear in post-ictal states because the impairment of consciousness is less profound than during episodes of absence status.

In this material confusional episodes were commoner among generalised than focal epilepsies, but this may have been because examples of absence status were over-represented. When confusion was accompanied by marked agitation or visual hallucinations, however, focal epilepsy originating in the temporal lobes was much commoner than other forms of epilepsy. Aggressive behaviour was also somewhat more common in the temporal lobe epilepsies than in other groups. It was suggested that in post-ictal confusional states associated with temporal lobe epilepsy the aggression might be due to exclusion of cortical function by virtue of the diffuse delta dysrhythmia, which then permitted emotionally charged impulses originating within the temporal lobes to be directly expressed in behaviour.

In general the episodes seen in conjunction with temporal lobe epilepsy stood in considerable contrast to those seen with the generalised epilepsies. The accent tended to be less on impairment of consciousness and a great deal more on affective changes, delusions and schizophreniform disturbances. These episodes were sometimes long, even days or weeks in duration, and often occurred without relation to grand mal convulsions. Some no doubt corresponded to twilight states or post-ictal psychoses as described above, and others to the transient psychotic developments discussed on p. 284. The EEG in such episodes often showed reinforcement of the focal temporal lobe discharges, but sometimes no change from the inter-ictal state and sometimes disappearance of all abnormal rhythms ('normalisation'). Thus the majority of episodes in the temporal lobe group were best conceived as pre-ictal or sub-ictal, with their manifestations representing the direct on-going effects of focal disturbance of brain function. Ultimately, in some cases, the prolonged increase in focal or perifocal excitation might exceed the threshold for generalisation to the rest of the brain, accounting for the occasional cases in which the episode terminated with a grand mal convulsion.

Dongier's review stressed, however, that a good deal of overlap occurred between the varieties of epilepsy, the type of episode produced, and to a lesser extent the nature of the accompanying electrical disturbance in the brain. The neurophysiological mechanisms hypothesised for the genesis of these complex disturbances must therefore be regarded as no more than provisional approximations.

Psychiatric disability among persons with epilepsy

It is difficult to form an accurate estimate of the prevalence of psychiatric disturbance among persons with epilepsy. The general problem is compounded when attempts are made to compare the frequency of disabilities in patients with different types of epilepsy, and here a special controversy has centred over the question of temporal lobe epilepsy. Yet these are matters of both practical and theoretical importance — for the proper planning of services and for the understanding which might follow concerning brain–behaviour relationships.

Surveys have often produced conflicting results, largely because most are based on highly selected populations of epileptic subjects. Clearly, patients coming before a psychiatrist, or requiring institutional care, will have a higher frequency of psychiatric and social problems than epileptics in general. Equally, patients under supervision in hospital out-patient departments will be unrepresentative of epileptics as a whole. Edeh *et al.* (1990) showed that they had higher psychiatric morbidity than clinic non-attenders, and were more likely to suffer from complex partial seizures and poor seizure control. The College of General Practitioners Report (1960) indicated that hospital consultants probably saw no more than 75% of the epileptics in the community.

Perhaps the most accurate estimates are to be found in general practice surveys, or better still in surveys of the general population. The College of General Practitioners (1960) collected information about 1209 chronic epileptics from 67 practices in England and Wales, and found that 17% had significant social problems. Eight per cent of those of employable age were out of work or incapable of

work because of their epilepsy, and a further 12% were capable only of restricted employment. Pond and Bidwell (1960) made a more detailed survey of 245 cases from 14 practices in South East England, and found that 10% were unemployable, most on account of mental impairment and the remainder because of marked behaviour disturbance. No case was found in which the fits alone were adequate to account for unemployability. Altogether, however, over 50% of the men had experienced serious job difficulties, being presently downgraded or having had long periods out of work in the past. The difficulties in retaining satisfactory employment were principally due to the occurrence of fits, and next most frequently to behaviour disorder. Job difficulties were markedly more frequent in patients with psychiatric symptoms.

Other data demonstrated the hardships imposed by epilepsy (Pond *et al.* 1960). Compared to the normal population there was an excess of single over married persons, and social class as measured by occupation was much reduced. These differences were especially marked in the younger age groups, and particularly among the males.

With regard to psychiatric disability, Pond and Bidwell (1960) found that 29% showed conspicuous mental problems and this was felt to be an underestimate. The figure rose to over 50% among patients with temporal lobe epilepsy. At the time of the survey 7% of the total had already had psychiatric in-patient care, which was twice the rate to be expected in the general population. The special hazards of temporal lobe epilepsy were again indicated — the proportion of patients with temporal lobe epilepsy who had already been in psychiatric hospitals was three times that of the total epileptic population.

The commonest problem throughout was neurotic disability and this appeared to be reactive to environmental difficulties. Some 15% of the patients were affected in this way, which may not be substantially higher than in the population as a whole. Rather less common were those psychiatric disturbances—intellectual deficits and personality disorders—which could more directly be attributed to the epileptic process itself or to associated brain damage.

Edeh and Toone (1987) carried out a not dissimilar community survey of 88 patients with epilepsy gathered from general practices in south London. Though smaller in size, this had the advantage of using a standardised rating instrument for psychiatric assessment (the Clinical Interview Schedule) and of investigating each patient thoroughly before categorisation of the epilepsy. Thirty-one per cent had a history of psychiatric referral, a figure close to the 29% of Pond and Bidwell's study who showed 'conspicuous mental problems'. On scores from the interview schedule 48% of patients emerged as psychiatric 'cases', the great majority representing minor affective disturbance of an anxious or depressive nature. Both in terms of previous psychiatric referral and in Interview Schedule scores the patients with focal epilepsy showed significantly more disturbance than those with primary generalised epilepsy, despite equivalence in sex, age and duration of epilepsy. Possible reasons for this difference lay with greater brain damage in the focal epilepsy group, as confirmed by computerised tomography (CT) scans, or their relatively poorer seizure control and the wider range of drugs they were receiving. Few differences emerged, however, between the group with temporal lobe epilepsy and the patients with other focal seizures, though depression and anxiety were commoner among the temporal lobe epileptics.

Fiordelli et al. (1993) used the same Clinical Interview Schedule to assess 100 out-patients with epilepsy but found a much lower prevalence of 'caseness' at 19%, this differing little from controls attending hospital for minor surgical procedures. Again depression and anxiety were the commonest problems. The lower prevalence of psychiatric disturbance compared with Edeh and Toone's survey may have reflected the exclusion of patients with IQs below 80, also those with evidence of brain lesions responsible for their epilepsy. To the extent that the latter explains the difference, it would suggest that much of the psychiatric disability encountered in epileptic patients is attributable to brain damage rather than to the epilepsy per se. Most patients were on monotherapy, usually with carbamazepine, and it was possible to show that polypharmacy carried increased risk of psychiatric disorder. Altogether Fiordelli et al.'s results indicate that patients with cryptogenic epilepsy and normal intelligence, managed by modern means, may be at no greater risk of psychiatric disorder than a non-neurological control population.

Graham and Rutter's (1968) survey dealt with school children between the ages of 5 and 14 on the Isle of Wight, and showed a high prevalence of psychiatric disturbance. The entire population of children on the island was screened and 85 cases of epilepsy were discovered (7.2 per 1000). Twenty-nine per cent of those with epilepsy, but no other evidence of a brain lesion ('uncomplicated epilepsy'), showed some psychiatric disorder; when in addition to epilepsy there was other independent evidence of brain damage the figure rose to 58%. Children with temporal lobe epilepsy showed significantly more disturbance than children with other types. These figures could be compared with the prevalence of psychiatric disorder among the rest of the school children of the island which emerged at 6.8%.

The type of psychiatric disorder shown by the children with 'uncomplicated epilepsy' was closely similar to that seen in other disturbed children—mainly neurotic disorders or antisocial conduct. Teachers' ratings showed that they were more restless and fidgety and more inclined to fight than the generality of school children, but again these characteristics applied to disturbed children even in the absence of epilepsy.

In a careful analysis of causes it was shown that lowered intelligence was unlikely to be a factor. The uncomplicated epileptic group showed a normal distribution of intelligence, likewise the subgroup with temporal lobe epilepsy. The on-going handicap of epilepsy alone was unlikely to be responsible, since less than 12% of children with other chronic handicaps (asthma, heart disease, diabetes) showed psychiatric disorder, and in any case many of the children with epilepsy were little incapacitated by it. Widespread community prejudice against epilepsy was thought to be an adverse factor in the epileptic child's development, though many of the sample had nocturnal seizures only and psychiatric disability was not especially frequent in children whose teachers knew of their condition.

Thus by exclusion it seemed that an important factor was probably the dysfunction occurring specifically within the brain. In addition the influence of parental handling appeared to be important; an adverse family background, measured in terms of the mother's emotional stability, was significantly more common among the epileptic children with psychiatric disability than in those without.

Thus, while in the majority of persons epilepsy is compatible with normal mental health, psychiatric disturbance appears to be far from uncommon and to outstrip that found in the general population. That it is found from a very early age and is accompanied by a good deal of chronic social disability, underlines the importance with which it must be viewed. The genesis of such disability is clearly a complex matter, partly psychological, partly social and partly pathophysiological in origin. In the sections that follow an attempt will be made to explore in further detail the forms which psychiatric disability may take, its aetiology and its association with different varieties of epilepsy.

Cognitive function

The earlier gloomy view that epileptic patients were characterised by low intelligence has been corrected over the years. Vislie and Henriksen (1958) reviewed numerous studies which showed that while intellectual impairment was common in institutionalised epileptics, the range of intelligence was almost normal when out-patient populations were investigated. In the Isle of Wight survey, described above, the epileptic children without other evidence of brain damage showed a normal distribution of intelligence. Similarly, twin studies have indicated that epilepsy rarely lowers the genetic endowment for intelligence unless there is additional evidence of a gross brain lesion (Lennox 1960). In general therefore there is little reason to fear that epilepsy, in the absence of overt brain damage, will lead to a sustained lowering of cognitive ability.

Nevertheless a proportion of epileptics show obvious impairment of intellect, and in rare cases even progressive intellectual deterioration. The factors which contribute to such difficulties are incompletely understood. They are likely to include the effects of hereditary endowment and psychosocial influences as with intelligence generally; also the effects of brain damage, the effects of the epileptic process itself and the effects of anticonvulsant drugs.

Psychosocial effects. Environmental influences during childhood doubtless affect the degree to which the epileptic child can achieve his intellectual potential. Parental attitudes and the child's own reaction to his epilepsy may have an adverse effect, determining his stability, his receptivity and the degree to which he will be exposed to normal formative influences. Schooling may be disrupted and the normal processes of play curtailed. A vicious circle is likely to develop in which emotional disturbance, consequent upon poor attainment, leads to further difficulties with education. The high level of psychiatric disability noted by Graham and Rutter (1968) was particularly marked in children of low intelligence and when reading was severely retarded in relation to the child's potential.

Effects of brain damage. It is widely agreed that the brain damage responsible for the fits is chiefly to be blamed when intelligence is substantially reduced. Thus simple absences, in which there is no evidence of structural brain damage, are very rarely associated with lowered intelligence, even when attacks are very frequent indeed (Metrakos & Metrakos 1960). Conversely, marked mental retardation is almost invariably accompanied by evidence of severe and extensive cerebral lesions.

The location of the cerebral damage is a factor of importance. Patients with grand mal tend to have lower intelligence than patients with simple absences, but when grand mal and psychomotor seizures occur together intelligence is lowest of all (Vislie & Henriksen 1958). Thus temporal lobe epilepsy appears to carry the greatest hazard for impaired intellectual function, and almost certainly by virtue of the location of brain damage responsible for the seizures. In Ounsted *et al.*'s (1966) series of children with temporal lobe epilepsy, retardation was restricted to those who had suffered acute cerebral insults in the form of perinatal damage, head injury or infection, or who had experienced status epilepticus at an early age.

In the remainder there was no evidence whatever of intellectual loss.

Stores (1978) carried out a series of careful studies on epileptic children attending ordinary schools. Children with generalised epilepsy were matched with those showing temporal lobe discharges, and compared with non-epileptic children in the same school class. Reading attainment (when viewed against age and IQ) was significantly impaired among the temporal lobe epileptics, but only in those who showed foci in the left temporal lobe. Children with generalised epilepsy or right temporal lobe epilepsy performed as well as their controls. When subdivided according to sex it was only the boys who showed retarded reading skills, girls appearing unaffected irrespective of type of epilepsy. On ratings and measures of inattentiveness the epileptic boys again fared worse than the girls, likewise on ratings of behaviour disorder and hyperactivity. Gender effects, in addition to location of brain paroxysmal activity, thus appeared to be operative in determining the relationship between epilepsy and disturbed performance at school.

Among adults, subtle forms of cognitive defect have been discerned when patients with temporal lobe epilepsy are compared with patients suffering from generalised grand mal, even after controlling for full scale intelligence. Quadfasel and Pruyser (1955) showed a high frequency of deficits on tests of verbal ability and on efficiency of retention and recall. Many temporal lobe patients were aware of their difficulties in verbal usage, though the deficits were not constant or gross enough to be labelled as dysphasia. Guerrant *et al.* (1962) similarly found that temporal lobe epileptics had an especially high frequency of psychological impairments indicative of brain damage — memory difficulties, slowed speech and impaired concentration and attention.

Detailed comparisons of patients with lateralised foci have shown that the patterns of deficit may vary with the side of the lesion. Even prior to lobectomy, patients with epileptogenic foci in the dominant temporal lobe tend to be impaired on verbal as compared to non-verbal tasks, and patients with foci in the non-dominant lobe show the reverse (Milner 1958, 1962; Dennerll 1964). With regard to memory, Delaney *et al.* (1980) have shown impairment of verbal memory in patients with left temporal lobe foci when compared with patients with right temporal or frontal foci or controls; and impairment of memory for non-verbal visual material in patients with right temporal foci when compared with these other groups. Similar differential effects on memory and learning tasks have been demonstrated in children with temporal lobe epilepsy (Feido & Mirsky 1969), and will clearly have implications for processes of education. These special problems in temporal lobe epilepsy may partly be due to the location of the fixed brain damage in the temporal lobes, and partly to on-going subclinical epileptic disturbances as discussed below.

Effects of seizures and abnormal electrical activity. The seizures themselves can provide an educational handicap by disruption of schooling and lessening of concentration when attacks are frequent. In addition, however, it is possible that intelligence may sometimes be adversely affected by the pathological and pathophysiological disturbances occasioned by seizures, or by inter-ictal subclinical discharges.

Grand mal seizures may contribute to further brain damage as a result of cerebral anoxia, especially if prolonged and particularly when status epilepticus occurs. It is possible that this is a special hazard in childhood, and may account for Taylor and Falconer's (1968) finding that patients with temporal lobe epilepsy showed lower intelligence the earlier the onset of epilepsy.

Secondly, epileptic activity may intensify the extent to which existing brain damage interferes with cerebral function, particularly when frequent attacks and their associated dysrhythmia disrupt the activity of normal parts of the brain (Pond 1961). In addition to the overt disturbance which is manifest as seizures one must take account of the continuing 'subclinical' disturbance of electrical activity which persists during inter-ictal periods. Chaudhry and Pond (1961) found that the adequacy of control of attacks was a significant factor distinguishing between a group of 'deteriorating' epileptic children and a group of non-deteriorating brain-damaged epileptic controls. Such deterioration could occasionally be reversed when attacks came under control once more (Pond 1961). Certainly in animals it has been shown that discharging lesions in the amygdaloid region can have a profoundly disturbing effect on learning, and that there is a marked improvement after excision of the discharging lesion (Morrell *et al.* 1956).

Several experimental observations have demonstrated the short-lived effects of seizures on on-going intellectual activity. Jus and Jus (1962) carried out tests of continuous registration while recording the EEG in patients subject to frequent absence attacks. During absence attacks or myoclonic jerks there was lack of registration of material as expected, but also a variable retrograde amnesia, usually 4–15 seconds in length, for events preceding the seizure. Ounsted *et al.* (1963) showed similar deficits during episodes of spike wave discharge induced by stroboscopic stimulation. Goode *et al.* (1970) employed a pursuit–rotor task, requiring continuing vigilance over eye–hand coordination, while recording the EEG in patients with absence attacks. A strong relationship was observed between the incidence of errors in performance and the presence of spike wave bursts lasting for more than 3 seconds at a time. Hutt *et al.* (1977) showed impair-

ments in reaction time on a continuous choice response task. Such observations suggest that generalised spike wave activity functions as 'neural noise', thereby reducing the child's information-processing capacity.

Tizard and Margerison (1964) studied adults subject to frequent bursts of generalised synchronous wave spike discharges, and demonstrated that cognitive efficiency was lowered during runs of EEG abnormality even though no overt clinical seizures occurred. Tasks were performed more slowly and inaccurately during periods of discharge than between them; even discharges lasting as little as 0.5–1.5 seconds were accompanied by significantly slower response times.

The advent of computerised tests for continuous assessment of cognitive performance has allowed more sensitive studies to be performed. Using such a technique, Aarts *et al.* (1984) have documented cognitive deficits even during brief focal discharges, and have shown an interaction between lateralisation of discharge and the nature of the task performed. Focal discharges on the left affected a verbal task more consistently than a spatial task, and focal right-sided discharges the reverse. With regard to the impact of subclinical discharges on day-to-day tasks, Kasteleijn-Nolst Trenité *et al.* (1988) examined reading performance among children under continuous EEG and video monitoring; both during and immediately after subclinical discharges there was a significant increase in the rate of errors observed.

Finally, direct comparisons have been made between children with temporal lobe epilepsy and children with generalised centrencephalic epilepsy on various tasks of memory and sustained attention (Lansdell & Mirsky 1964; Feido & Mirsky 1969). The centrencephalic children lacked the focal deficits of memory and learning which characterised the temporal lobe children, but performed more poorly when selective attention was required over a period of time. It seemed that this was not solely due to subclinical absence attacks, since poor performance could be observed in the absence of concurrent EEG abnormality. The task of sustained attention thus possibly revealed some permanent disturbance of central subcortical structures. Such deficits, which would otherwise be likely to pass unnoticed, would stand to have an adverse effect on the natural processes of learning.

A remarkable example of the effects of controlling subclinical epileptic discharges on memory was obtained in a 54-year-old man who had suffered an apparent attack of encephalitis 6 months earlier (Goldstein *et al.* 1992). Some weeks after the illness he had developed marked memory difficulties, fluctuating in severity from day to day, sometimes to the extent that they were suspected of being hysterical in nature. On one occasion, for example, he appeared to have forgotten that his father was dead but at subsequent interview was quite clear on the issue. Sometimes he could not recall his telephone number nor his daughter's age or remember anything of previous hospital admissions. It was considered likely, nevertheless, that his memory had been damaged by the encephalitis, even though CT and MRI scans showed no abnormalities.

There had been a possible epileptic seizure soon after the onset of the illness, and when transferred to the Maudsley Hospital for reassessment 6 months later two further brief attacks were witnessed. He also showed occasional myoclonic jerks. The EEG revealed epileptiform activity in the right temporal region, with more widespread sharp waves extending over both hemispheres during sleep. It was therefore decided to start him on anticonvulsants while monitoring his memory closely, in order to see whether subclinical epileptic discharges may have been interfering with memory functioning.

A small battery of ward-based memory tests was administered on a day-to-day basis, both before and after starting anticonvulsants. Measurable improvements were charted after treatment commenced, with further gains once all myoclonic seizures had come under control. Improved memory functioning was confirmed by repeat administration of the Rivermead Behavioural Test battery. His ability to recognise and name members of staff had improved dramatically. He remained greatly improved on discharge home and when followed-up 12 months later.

Effects of anticonvulsant drugs. High dosage of drugs can undoubtedly impair concentration and lead to intellectual slowing. Folic acid deficiency due to anticonvulsants may also have an adverse effect on mental function, as discussed in Chapter 12 (p. 592). Trimble *et al.* (1980) showed that epileptic children in a hospital school who experienced a fall in IQ had significantly lower serum folates than the remainder. With well conducted regimens, however, it has generally been held that drug effects are rarely important as a cause of lowered cognitive performance, and careful studies in children and in adults seemed initially to support this conclusion (Loveland *et al.* 1957; Chaudhry & Pond 1961).

Later more critical studies have, however, suggested that the chronic administration of anticonvulsants has been underestimated as a cause of impairment (Trimble & Reynolds 1976, 1984). There are indications, moreover, that intellectual impairment may sometimes occur even when conventional signs of toxicity are absent. Reynolds and Travers (1974) surveyed 57 patients taking phenobarbitone and phenytoin, and showed that the serum levels of each drug were considerably higher in patients with certain mental symptoms than in those without. Psychomotor slowing and intellectual deterioration both appeared to be related to high serum levels of the drugs, even after excluding patients with clear clinical evidence of drug toxicity.

Psychometric investigations have confirmed such effects. Guey *et al.* (1967) tested 25 children before and after adding ethosuximide to their regimens, and observed a negative influence on intellectual efficiency. Slowing, perseveration and memory troubles emerged, particularly in the older (adolescent) child. Tchicaloff and Gaillard (1970) examined 20 patients of normal intelligence who were taking varied doses of phenobarbitone and phenytoin, and found significant correlations between the dosages employed and impaired performance on certain tests. Phenobarbitone was associated with impairment on the object assembly and comprehension subtests of the Wechsler Adult Intelligence Scale, and phenytoin with impaired digit repetition. The cumulative effects of the two medications given together were revealed on tests of visuospatial ability which had failed to show correlations with the dose of either drug alone.

In prospective studies, Thompson and Trimble (1982, 1983) have explored the effects of alterations of dosage or reduction of polypharmacy on psychometric performance, testing control groups in parallel in whom there had been no change of drug. Significant improvements could be observed on measures of concentration, memory and motor speed when serum levels were reduced or the number of drugs diminished. An important finding was that several months sometimes elapsed before the beneficial effects became evident. A change to carbamazepine led to particularly clear improvements and these were more quickly apparent.

Even in patients on monotherapy, however, impairments can be detected, and these tend to affect different aspects of performance according to the drug employed. Gillham *et al.* (1990) tested 35 patients on carbamazepine, 19 on phenytoin and 30 on sodium valproate, comparing the results with those of untreated epileptics and non-epileptic controls. None of the patients had specifically complained about cognitive side effects. Nevertheless, patients taking carbamazepine showed poorer performance on tests of speed of perception and/or movement when compared with both control groups and with patients taking valproate; and those taking phenytoin scored less well on memory tests than the non-epileptics and those on valproate. Andrewes *et al.* (1986) similarly found that phenytoin had adverse effects on memory, this time in comparison with untreated patients and those on carbamazepine. Thus important, albeit subtle, differences appear to exist in the effects of these first-line drugs on cognitive function, even when given singly and with adequate serum monitoring. Sodium valproate, though less comprehensively studied than the others, appears to influence cognitive function relatively little, and only at high concentrations (Smith 1991).

Over and above any such general effects it is important to be alert to idiosyncratic reactions in certain individuals and to adjust their medication accordingly. Phenobarbitone is perhaps most often responsible for such adverse reactions. Hutt *et al.* (1968) demonstrated that in therapeutic dosage it could sometimes affect capacity for sustained attention very considerably. Rosen (1968) reported decreased intellectual performance attributable to pheny-toin in therapeutic dosage as a rare but important idiosyn-cratic reaction; 20 epileptic patients were found in whom IQ and school or work performance improved markedly after stopping the drug, even though there had been no obvious signs of sedation or lethargy beforehand. Stores (1981) describes more recent evidence of problems with learning and behaviour in children attributable to pheno-barbitone or phenytoin.

In the converse direction, of course, the administration of anticonvulsants can sometimes dramatically improve intellectual function when fits are brought under improved control.

Epileptic 'dementia'

Most large series of epileptic patients include a small pro-portion who undergo a decline in intellectual ability, with progressive impairment of memory, concentration and judgement. This may set in after many years of function-ing at a reasonably adequate level. Usually it is coupled with severe personality deterioration, and sometimes with marked behaviour disorder in the form of impulsiv-ity, irritability and outbursts of rage. Neuroimaging may demonstrate cerebral atrophy. Such cases appear to be commoner when the epilepsy is secondary to a known brain lesion and when the epilepsy has been severe and of long duration.

As a group these conditions have attracted remarkably little attention and the responsible factors are far from clear. Betts (1982) suggests that the concept of epileptic dementia requires critical examination, and that it is still uncertain whether epilepsy itself can be responsible for a progressive dementing process.

In children it is clear that prolonged febrile status can result in brain damage, also that rare conditions such as West syndrome (p. 242) and Lennox–Gastaut syndrome (p. 242) can be associated with profound mental impair-ment, including failure of subsequent development and perhaps even cognitive decline. Often, however, these syndromes can be attributed to some underlying 'encephalopathy' which is responsible for both the epilepsy and the cognitive deficits. The question therefore remains whether repeated fits can of themselves lead directly to fixed impairment or deterioration.

Besag (1988) discusses the situation in children in some detail and reviews his experience at Lingfield Hospital School (now St Piers, Lingfield). A close examination of eight children who had apparently deteriorated, and for whom sequential IQ results were available, revealed that they had undergone intellectual arrest rather than decline; because the mental age had hardly increased over several years the IQ appeared to have fallen pro-

gressively. While recognizing the need for further systematic prospective studies, Besag concludes that a small subgroup of children with epilepsy do deteriorate intellectually, some with recognised pre-existing brain damage and some without. Risk factors appear to include early age of onset, frequent and pro-longed seizures, mixed epilepsy with several seizure types occur-ring together, and pre-existing brain damage. Additionally, status epilepticus can undoubtedly cause intellectual and neuro-logical deterioration when not treated promptly, and it is possible that phenytoin sometimes causes a chronic encephalopathy with cognitive deterioration.

In adults the aetiology in those who appear to dement probably differs from one case to another. A progressive cerebral pathology may sometimes be present, such as a tumour or degenerative process; it is therefore always important to search anew for an underlying cause which may be responsible at one and the same time for the fits and the intellectual decline (Williams 1963). Recurrent head injuries may make a contribution.

Brown and Vaughan (1988) have attempted to clarify other factors which may be involved. A sample of 12 patients was col-lected from the Maudsley and King's College Hospitals who showed evidence of intellectual deterioration, based on knowl-edge of previous attainments and repeat psychometric testing. They showed a tendency to have more than one seizure type, and to have had very large numbers of seizures, often in excess of 50, during the year before the deterioration was first noted. Five had abnormal CT scans with focal or generalised atrophy. Some showed neurotic or psychotic symptomatology in addition to their cognitive problems. In two the decline was apparently reversed following a change of medication.

More systematic studies from the David Lewis Centre, which caters for people with very severe epilepsy, allowed Brown and Vaughan to examine 10 males and 10 females with clear evi-dence of deterioration. Patients were excluded if aged 50 or over, when the predicted IQ was below 75, or when there was a record of severe head injury in adult life or of alcohol abuse. The deteri-oration from predicted IQ levels (derived from the National Adult Reading Test) averaged 24 points in the males and 20 points in the females. Such deterioration appeared to affect both vocabulary and block design scores in five subjects, the former alone in six and the latter alone in eight, indicating that a selec-tive impairment of cognitive function was perhaps commoner than global decline. Frontotemporal dysfunction, as judged from psychometric testing, also seemed to make a contribution in several cases.

In later years it is quite likely that epileptics with sub-stantial brain damage may dement earlier than the general population, since their neuronal reserves are reduced even though the brain damage underlying the epilepsy remains static. Studies to examine such a possi-bility, analogous to those of Corkin et al. (1989) in head-injured subjects (outlined on p. 186), appear not to have been carried out in epileptic patients.

In all cases the anticonvulsant regimen will need

careful reappraisal, including the estimation of serum levels, since the patient may be suffering from unsuspected toxic effects or abnormal metabolic responses to certain drug combinations (p. 263).

Sometimes the dementia will be found to be more apparent than real, representing mainly a neurotic withdrawal or the effects of institutionalisation (Pond 1957). In others it may represent the chronic end-state of a schizophrenia-like psychosis (p. 279), a depressive disorder, or progressive worsening of personality traits which have long been present.

Personality

Among the prejudices that have surrounded epilepsy and coloured public attitudes towards it, is the old established idea that the sufferer is in some fundamental way changed by the disorder. Guerrant *et al.* (1962) summarised the changing views on the personality of epileptics, starting with the previous century when 'deterioration' was thought to be the rule and a consequence of the seizures. Early in the present century personality changes were still regarded as common, but ascribed to an hereditary 'degenerative stigma' of which the epilepsy was one manifestation and certain personality attributes another. Gradually, however, the idea of a specific epileptic personality has been rejected, and most epileptics are now recognised as substantially normal in this regard. When personality problems are present they can take many forms and can be ascribed to a variety of factors including brain damage, uncontrolled seizures and psychosocial influences. The most recent debate centres on the possibility that temporal lobe epilepsy carries special hazards where personality function is concerned, and this will be further discussed below.

The older concept of an 'epileptic personality' is now seen as an artefact derived from close observation and selective reporting of patients long confined to an institutional life.

The epileptic was said to be untrustworthy, sly and disruptive in the community. He was prone to curry favour, but beneath his subservience lay resentment and strong paranoid feelings. He was liable to sudden explosions of affect, sometimes with dangerously aggressive behaviour as a result. In general he tended to be egocentric, importunate, irritable and needed tactful handling. Religiosity of an obtrusive and sentimental kind was particularly common. He was ponderous, slow and perseverative, and his thinking tended to be stereotyped and concrete. In both thought and emotions he was described as 'adhesive', 'sticky' or 'viscous'.

In the above, some traits can be discerned which were probably a direct result of institutionalisation, and others which are characteristic of patients with substantial brain damage from any

cause. The widespread use of bromides at toxic levels no doubt added a further contribution. It is also worth noting that the majority of patients in psychiatric hospitals, from whom the above picture was largely derived, were likely to be suffering from temporal lobe epilepsy rather than other forms (Liddell 1953; Margerison & Liddell 1961).

It is now clear from the community surveys already mentioned that only a small proportion of patients with epilepsy suffer from personality difficulties of any great degree. It seems equally clear that those that occur do not conform to any broad pattern which is distinctive for epilepsy generally. Certain traits may characterise certain types of epilepsy, but even this is still a matter for controversy. What is certain is the seriousness in terms of social adjustment and overall prognosis of those personality problems that do occur. They markedly interfere with the ability to hold employment, as shown by surveys in general practice and in neurological and psychiatric clinics (Gordon & Russell 1958; Kennedy & Seccombe 1959; Pond & Bidwell 1960). The emotional disturbances they engender can render the control of fits difficult and they are themselves very hard to remedy. Personality difficulties are therefore an extremely important aspect of epilepsy, and their origins and associations deserve careful study.

Association with varieties of epilepsy

It is commonly held that personality disturbance is more frequent with epilepsy of known than unknown aetiology (Alstrom 1950), commoner in grand mal than with absence attacks, and commonest of all in temporal lobe epilepsy (Gudmundsson 1966). Such assertions are found repeatedly in the literature, but rest principally on clinical impressions or on comparisons between groups of cases which are small and specially selected. Satisfactory surveys are hard to find and contradictory results have frequently emerged.

Disturbance of personality appears to be rarely obtrusive with absence attacks. Pond (1952a) reviewed 150 epileptic children seen at the Maudsley Hospital and described those with petit mal absences as generally passive and 'nice mannered'. They had been referred for treatment on account of neurotic symptoms rather than disorders of conduct. By contrast the brain-injured epileptic children in the same population were often aggressive, explosive and unpredictable, and suffered from many varieties of grand mal and focal epilepsy but never from petit mal alone. Children with temporal lobe epilepsy showed behaviour disturbance to the most marked degree.

Nuffield (1961) pursued the question in detail by

analysing neurotic symptoms (fears, timidity, nightmares) and manifestations of aggression (temper tantrums, violence, cruelty) in 233 Maudsley epileptic children. Classification both by fit pattern and EEG showed highly significant differences between those with petit mal absences and those with temporal lobe epilepsy. The petit mal child showed more neurotic symptoms and less aggression than other groups, and the temporal lobe epileptic child a great deal more aggression and less neurotic disorder. These differences demarcated the two groups clearly from a neutral sample of cases with non-temporal cortical foci.

Such contrasting personality patterns in children may, however, depend partly or even wholly on their different home backgrounds. Pond had already noted that the petit mal child usually came from a gentle but anxious family, whereas the brain-injured child often had a family history of instability and emotional disturbance. The differences therefore, while marked, cannot be definitely attributed to the type of epilepsy suffered and its electrophysiological correlates.

The important symptom of hyperkinesis has also shown certain relationships to the type of epilepsy suffered in childhood. Ounsted (1955) found that petit mal children were not liable to the disorder, whereas all other forms of generalised and focal seizures were represented in his material. Most if not all of the children with hyperkinesis had considerable brain damage, and half had IQs below 70. Boys were affected much more commonly than girls. The special vulnerability of epileptic boys also emerged in Stores' (1978) investigations of school-age children referred to on p. 261. On ratings of conduct disorder, overactivity, inattentiveness and social isolation boys fared particularly badly, those with left temporal lobe epilepsy being the worst affected of all.

In adult life the patient with temporal lobe epilepsy has been singled out repeatedly as being especially prone to personality disturbance. Gibbs (1951) reported the prevalence of psychiatric disturbance in 275 patients with restricted seizure discharges on electroencephalography; 'severe personality disorder' was found considerably more frequently with temporal lobe discharges than with discharges elsewhere—it occurred in 32% of cases with anterior temporal foci, 13% with mid-temporal foci, 10% with occipital foci and 5% with frontal foci. Hill (1953) estimated that some 50% of patients with temporal lobe epilepsy showed severe personality disorder, and Gibbs and Gibbs (1964) estimated that 44–58% had moderate to severe psychopathology compared to less than 10% of patients with other types of seizure. Left temporal lobe foci possibly carry a greater hazard than right. Lindsay et al.'s (1979a) follow-up of temporal lobe epileptic children

into adult life showed that only 12% of left focus children achieved full independence, compared with 43% of those with foci on the other side.

Aggressiveness of an explosive and immature kind has been regarded as especially characteristic of patients with temporal lobe epilepsy, occurring as a predominant symptom in about a third of the patients who present for temporal lobectomy (Falconer & Taylor 1970). Outbursts are described as typically sudden, extreme, inexplicable and without remorse. In such patients aggression appears to be associated with early onset of seizures, male sex, low IQ, social class and a focus in the dominant temporal lobe (Serafetinides 1965; Taylor 1969a; Sherwin 1980). Considerable doubt has, however, been raised over whether patients with temporal lobe epilepsy as a group show an excess of aggressive behaviour when compared to patients with other seizure types (Stevens & Hermann 1981).

Herrington (1969) has reviewed other personality characteristics seen in temporal lobe epileptics—impulsiveness which can lead to antisocial conduct, sensitive suspiciousness, frankly paranoid attitudes, moodiness, anxiety, depression and hysterical manifestations. The 'ixophrenic syndrome' of slowness, perseveration and 'viscosity' of thought has been said to be particularly common.

Unfortunately there is a lack of well-controlled studies to support or refute these strong clinical impressions. Pond and Bidwell's (1960) community survey found an increased frequency of psychiatric disturbance among temporal lobe epileptics compared to patients with other forms of seizure, and this often consisted essentially of personality disorder. But the numbers were too small and the personality assessments too approximate to allow definite and detailed conclusions to be drawn. Similar criticisms apply to several studies which have sought to refute the special frequency of personality disorder in temporal lobe epileptics (Small et al. 1962, 1966; Stevens 1966b). Guerrant et al.'s (1962) study involved especially careful comparisons between matched groups of patients with temporal lobe epilepsy and generalised grand mal epilepsy, but the numbers involved were again relatively small (32 and 26 patients, respectively). The total psychiatric disturbance was similar in both, but the predominant forms differed—the temporal lobe epileptics had a higher prevalence of organic brain symptoms, and the grand mal group a higher prevalence of personality disorder.

In an important refinement and extension of the argument, Dodrill and Batzel (1986) point out that patients with temporal lobe epilepsy often have more than one type of seizure, and review evidence that this could be significant in relation to maladjustment. When patients with generalised tonic–clonic seizures alone were compared with those having partial seizures alone (mostly complex partial), no differences emerged on the Minnesota Multiphasic Personality Inventory. However, patients exhibiting both types of seizure showed elevated scores on several indices and exceeded the normal cut-off points on the 'depression' and 'schizophrenia' scales. It thus seems possible that the number of seizure types experienced may be more relevant to personality and psychiatric problems than the particular form of seizures that occur.

Reynolds (1983) emphasises the numerous confounding variables that are often at work in contributing to psychopathology in epilepsy, probably accounting in large measure for this continuing controversy. It could be relevant, for example, that temporal lobe seizures are often hard to control, especially when associated with brain damage, so that the patients experience more frequent attacks, take more drugs and suffer more psychosocial stresses than patients with generalised epilepsy. The association between temporal lobe epilepsy and aggression may similarly depend on factors which are not always readily apparent (Kligman & Goldberg 1975; Fenton 1981; Stevens & Hermann 1981). In addition to matters of special selection in the groups reported to date, socioeconomic factors have rarely been given due consideration: clusters of adverse environmental factors such as poor parenting, neglect and impaired general health, may have themselves conspired to produce the seeming correlations with irritability and violent behaviour.

There is, of course, abundant evidence from animal experimental work to support the notion that disturbance within the limbic system should be particularly closely associated with aggressive behaviour (Fenwick 1986). Stimulation in the region of the amygdaloid nucleus in human subjects has also been shown to lead to a range of aggressive responses, from coherent verbal threats to uncontrolled swearing and physically destructive behaviour (Heath *et al.* 1955; Delgado *et al.* 1968; Hitchcock & Cairns 1973).

Treffert (1963) showed that EEG disturbance within the temporal lobes, whether or not it was associated with clear evidence of epilepsy, was closely associated with aggressive behaviour in psychiatric patients. Patients with clinically obvious temporal lobe epilepsy, and patients with temporal lobe spiking on the EEG but without temporal lobe epilepsy, were carefully matched with a variety of controls. The temporal lobe patients, with and without fits, were remarkably like one another in terms of presenting behaviour and in the historical evolution of the disorder. Aggressive behaviour, including episodic rage, assault and impulsive acting out, had led to their admission more often than in the control subjects.

Further indirect evidence in support of the association between temporal lobe epilepsy and aggression comes from the marked improvement in personality which may follow temporal lobectomy as discussed below (p. 270).

Thus in the present state of knowledge we can only conclude that there is a good deal of presumptive evidence for a special relationship between temporal lobe epilepsy and some aspects of personality disorder, but that as yet this lacks a firm scientific foundation. Any simplistic view about the mechanisms underlying such an association is almost certain to be erroneous, since multiple determinants will usually be at work.

'Temporal lobe syndrome'. A recent approach to the problem has sought to side step the question of categories of personality or psychiatric disorder, and to concentrate instead on defining clusters of behavioural traits in epileptic patients. In this manner a 'syndrome' characteristic of the inter-ictal behaviour of temporal lobe epileptic patients has been proposed. The concept, however, has not proved to be without difficulties.

Bear and Fedio (1977) selected a number of traits previously highlighted in the literature as being characteristic of patients with temporal lobe foci. Dewhurst and Beard (1970), for example, had noted a tendency towards mystical experiences and sudden religious conversions in a number of patients who were psychotic ('religiosity'). Waxman and Geschwind (1974, 1975) had reported a group who showed unusually detailed and copious writings, of a degree out of proportion to their educational background ('hypergraphia'). These often centred on moral, philosophical or religious issues ('hypermoralism'). The deepened emotionality, the hyposexuality and the excessive tendency to adhere to each thought and action ('viscosity') could be viewed in certain respects as the converse of features noted in the Klüver–Bucy syndrome (p. 23) following extirpations of the temporal lobes. These, along with a number of other traits (elation, anger, aggression, guilt, obsessionality, circumstantiality, sense of personal significance, dependence, humourlessness and paranoia), were incorporated in a detailed questionnaire filled in by temporal lobe epileptics and also by observers who knew them well. Fifteen patients with right temporal lobe foci and 12 with left were compared with normal controls and with patients with neuromuscular disorders.

The great majority of the chosen traits differentiated the epileptic patients from the controls to a significant extent. Particularly striking differences were seen with humourlessness, circumstantiality, dependence, sense of personal destiny and preoccupation with philosophical concerns. A possible unifying mechanism behind the cluster seemed to centre on enhanced affective associations to previously neutral stimuli, events or concepts; by this means even the smallest acts might come to be endowed with emotional importance, and affective coloration would tend to encourage a mystically religious outlook on the world.

The profiles of traits tended to differ according to the hemisphere primarily involved. Patients with right temporal foci showed an excess of overt emotional traits (deepened emotionality, sadness, hypermoralism), whereas those with left temporal foci showed ruminative intellectual tendencies (religiosity, philosophical interests, humourlessness, sense of personal destiny). Each hemisphere thus appeared to have responded to the enhanced affective coloration of experience in a manner reflecting its own particular style.

Further studies, however, have thrown doubt upon many of these associations, in particular detracting from their unique association with temporal lobe disorder. Bear and Fedio's initial study failed to include patients with other forms of epilepsy, nor did it control for the presence or absence of psychiatric disorder. Hermann and Riel (1981) compared patients with temporal lobe epilepsy and patients with primary generalised epilepsy, and found that only four of the traits differentiated them significantly (sense of personal destiny, philosophical interests, dependence and paranoia). Mungas (1982) found that no trait discriminated between patients with temporal lobe epilepsy and patients with psychiatric disorder; indeed when tested on a separate group of patients a large proportion of the variance in the trait scores seemed attributable to the presence or absence of psychiatric illness. Master *et al.* (1984), in a thorough study, compared patients with temporal lobe epilepsy, other forms of epilepsy, psychiatric disorder and normal volunteers. The results again underlined the prominent effect of psychiatric disturbance. Temporal lobe epilepsy made no discernible contribution of its own, and no differences in trait scores were observed between patients with right or left temporal lobe foci.

Sensky *et al.* (1984), after excluding patients with a history of psychiatric illness, found that religious beliefs and practices were similar in patients with temporal lobe epilepsy and generalised epilepsy, and corresponded to norms for the general population. No special association could be discerned between mystical experiences and temporal lobe attacks.

Thus the temporal lobe syndrome as first proposed does not appear to hold up or have general application. In effect it meets with the same doubts as did earlier concepts of distinctive personality categories. However, the possibility remains that a subgroup of patients with temporal lobe epilepsy may display significant clusterings of some components of the syndrome, perhaps especially in the presence of psychiatric disorder. The search for clearly definable traits, and their detailed associations, still has much to commend it. Considerable interest still attaches, moreover, to phenomena such as hypergraphia. This continues to be reported in association with temporal lobe epilepsy, with some indications that it may be particularly common in patients with right-sided epileptic foci (Roberts *et al.* 1982). However, a recent study discounts such laterality bias and stresses instead associations with emotional maladjustment, brain damage and a history of psychiatric illness (Okamura *et al.* 1993).

Aetiology of personality disorders in epilepsy

When epileptic patients show personality disorders, a multifactorial aetiology must usually be recognised. The interplay of factors will often be complex, especially when the epilepsy has dated from the formative period of life. As in the section on cognitive function it will be convenient to consider separately the contributions of psychosocial influences, the effects of brain damage, the effects of the epileptic process itself and the effects of anticonvulsant drugs.

Psychosocial effects. Psychosocial contributions will often be evident. The epileptic child reacts keenly to his emo-

tional background, and behaviour disturbance in epileptic children is closely tied to adverse factors in the family environment (Grunberg & Pond 1957; Graham & Rutter 1968). Thus, as with any child, the early environment may contribute to enduring problems of personality.

But in addition, the epileptic child is liable to be the object of anxious concern and over-protection, to excite parental anxiety or to become the focus of conflict between the parents. He will almost certainly be treated differently from his siblings. Others may be encouraged to protect him and make allowances for him, and many play activities may be debarred. His own reaction to the fits themselves may contribute to fundamental aspects of self evaluation. Feelings of isolation and estrangement are likely to result, and the foundations may be laid for attitudes of dependency, egocentricity or hypochondriasis in the personality.

At adolescence further problems must be faced in relation to sexual identity and choice of career. In adult life frustrations must be tolerated in many spheres, particularly in work and in the attitudes of others to the disorder. Taylor and Falconer (1968) showed that in temporal lobe epileptics the frequency of fits affected social adjustment, mainly in those situations where the patient had to relate to others outside the family; thus work and non-family relationships were adversely associated with fit frequency, and family relationships less so.

Williams (1963) has vividly described the problems which the epileptic patient has to face in adult life:

'To have epilepsy is to be different from one's fellows as the result of a persistent, intangible and recalcitrant disorder which even in the most enlightened society carries with it the stigma of the unusual. The epileptic nearly always feels different from his contemporaries; the more intelligent and enlightened he is, and the more understanding and enlightened his contemporaries, the bigger the problem he has to face, for it is greater trauma to have to be consciously treated as normal than to be naturally accepted as different. This hurtful dilemma, in all its degrees ranging from sentencious and embarrassing over-understanding to miserable restriction and loneliness, pervades his life at home, at school, at work and sometimes into marriage . . .

. . . At work the adult pattern of the problem asserts itself first with limitation of choice of vocation, secondly with lowering of levels and ambition either through limitations of choice or through acquired disturbance of attitude. A career having been started there is often insecurity of tenure, limitation of activities, and the faulty attitudes of ill-informed equals or defensive and self-protective seniors, including the insurance companies responsible for his future security.

In marriage the mate's attitude is usually ideal, which is one reason why the marriage took place, and one's impression is that marriage to an epileptic is usually a secure one. Nevertheless, the epileptic subject now has the attitude of two families and a new circle of friends to contend with. He may be less privileged than they in his work, is less secure, and for the first time begins to feel guilty rather than bitter about his afflictions . . .

. . . There are as many causes for disorders of feeling and behaviour in the epileptic subject whether brain damaged or not as in the ordinary population, but his stresses are more continuous, usually more intense, and many are peculiar to him.'

Caveness *et al.* (1969) demonstrated the steady improvement in social attitudes to epilepsy in the USA during the previous 20 years by repeated Gallup poll analyses. Nevertheless in 1969, 9% of the population still answered that they would object to their children associating in school or at play with persons who had seizures, and 12% still thought that epileptics should not be employed. In the UK attitudes were less favourable than in the USA, the respective figures being 15% and 23% (Burden 1969). The epileptic patient even then was clearly obliged to face strong social prejudices which are only slowly yielding to more enlightened attitudes. It is easy to see how traits of sensitivity or insecurity may become implanted or enhanced.

If the patient carries the added burden of low intelligence, poor genetic background or poor social status the impact of adverse psychosocial factors will stand to be increased. Taylor and Falconer (1968) were able to demonstrate that broad measures of social adjustment were related to such features — being significantly worse in the presence of low intelligence, a family history of mental illness and difficulties with schooling. The effect of intelligence was particularly marked. When epilepsy had been of early onset social adjustment was poorer, and psychopathic traits were more likely to be evident.

Effects of brain damage. Many of the personality problems seen in epilepsy are similar to those seen with brain damage due to any cause. There may be nothing specific to epilepsy about mental slowing, ponderousness and perseveration, nor in the 'stickiness' or 'viscosity' of thoughts and emotions which has been labelled the 'ixophrenic syndrome'. Irritability, impulsiveness and emotional lability are similarly the hallmarks of many forms of brain damage. The majority of abnormal personality attributes which cannot be attributed to psychosocial causes are therefore likely to be due to the brain damage underlying the epilepsy.

This probably accounts for the rarity of behaviour disorder or personality problems with absence attacks, even when attacks are very frequent. The high frequency of psychiatric disturbance in epilepsy secondary to known brain damage will also rest on such a basis, and the special associations claimed between temporal lobe epilepsy and personality disorder is likely to be due to the strategic location of the brain damage in the limbic system of the brain.

Effects of seizures and abnormal electrical activity. In addition to the effects of structural brain pathology, a further contribution to personality disorder may come from the disorganisation of cerebral functioning occasioned by epileptic discharges. Pathophysiological effects due to abnormal electrical activity may spread widely in neural systems beyond the area of the structural lesion. Moreover it is clear that in addition to overt attacks, a good deal of background subclinical discharge may continue in the inter-ictal periods. Electrocorticography at operation has shown that prolonged and widespread discharges can often be recorded without any accompanying clinical phenomena (Pampiglione & Falconer 1960). The question arises how far these special aspects of the epileptogenic lesion may affect personality functioning, over and above the effects due to any structural brain damage present.

A particularly intriguing suggestion has concerned the possible pathophysiology underlying certain behavioural changes in patients with temporal lobe epilepsy, occasioned by the frequent spike discharges arising within the limbic structures (Waxman & Geschwind 1975; Bear & Fedio 1977; Bear 1979; Geschwind 1979). It is proposed that such discharges lead in time to a 'hyperconnection' between neocortical and limbic systems ('sensory–limbic hyperconnection') with far-reaching effects on the patient's behaviour and experience. Such an alteration of limbic reactivity to environmental stimuli, it is suggested, could result in the suffusion of experience with affective coloration and a deepening of the patient's emotional life. The features considered to derive from this — religiosity, mystical and philosophical tendencies, and an enhanced sense of personal significance — are discussed in some detail on p. 267.

In more general support one may note that some patients show increasing disturbance of behaviour for hours or days prior to a fit, with moodiness, tension or irritability which are relieved when the convulsion occurs. Conversely, some habitually disturbed patients show marked improvement after a fit, becoming calmer and easier to manage for some time afterwards. Here one may hypothesise the gradual build up of subclinical discharges, or the post-ictal diminution of such discharges, to account for the behavioural changes seen.

Brady (1964) studied these phenomena in a group of hospitalised epileptic patients, most of whom were suffering from marked personality disturbance. Fit frequency was recorded each month, along with a checklist to monitor disturbed behaviour. Among patients with temporal lobe epilepsy both varied in the same direction, disturbed behaviour increasing when seizures were frequent. Among non-temporal lobe epileptics the converse tended to occur, disturbance of behaviour being significantly less common when fit frequency was elevated. Thus among the temporal lobe epileptics it could be argued that the disturbed behaviour and the seizures were both manifestations of a common pathophysiological disturbance, which waxed and waned over considerable periods of time. In the non-temporal lobe epileptics the disturbed behaviour and the seizures appeared to be alternative manifestations, representing different facets of the pathophysiological background. Brady stressed, however, that explanations on a physiological basis might yet be faulty. The relationships between fits and behaviour could also be mediated by psychological or social mechanisms, especially in a hospitalised population where fits would call forth both positive and negative reactions from other patients and staff.

Direct recording of electrophysiological disturbance within the brain would obviously be necessary to clarify the situation. It is interesting therefore that Ervin *et al.* (1969) noted electrophysiological correlates of aggression by depth recording from the limbic system in patients. Aggressive behaviour could be elicited by stimulation of appropriately placed electrodes, occurring independently of traditional seizures. The stimulation was followed by focal electrophysiological changes which preceded the disturbed behaviour. Such focal discharges, usually in the amygdaloid region, could also be seen to occur in response to appropriate environmental stimuli as a prelude to the alterations in behaviour.

It is a common observation that difficult traits in the personality may improve when fit frequency is reduced by appropriate medication. Evidence has also accumulated to suggest that when epileptogenic brain tissue is removed at operation personality disorder may improve dramatically along with abolition of the seizures. Wilson (1970) reported such effects in a high proportion of children undergoing hemispherectomy for intractable epilepsy associated with infantile hemiplegia—behaviour disorder could sometimes improve remarkably, with abolition of violent rages, explosive tantrums, hyperactivity and negativism.

The effects of temporal lobectomy on personality have attracted especial attention. Between a half and two-thirds of disturbed temporal lobe epileptics are reported to show significant improvement in psychiatric status postoperatively (Hill *et al.* 1957; James 1960; Taylor & Falconer 1968). In part this may depend on the psychological effect of improved fit control, since the most marked benefits follow when fits are greatly reduced (Jensen & Larsen 1979a). The latter is not, however, always essential, and the improvement is often striking enough to suggest that removal of the discharging focus has had a more direct effect.

Most striking is the reduction in aggressiveness in patients who have previously shown a liability to unpredictable explosive outbursts. After operation tolerance of frustration is increased, irritability subsides and there is no longer the constant risk of provoking displays of anger. In this group improvement has proved to be very closely related to fit control. It has been particularly gratifying in

patients with mesial temporal lobe sclerosis (Falconer 1973; Bruton 1988).

A considerable proportion have shown depressive episodes during the first year or two after operation despite the excellent result in other respects. Such episodes are frequently severe, with retardation and delusion formation, but respond well to electroconvulsive therapy and tend not to recur after the first 18 months. It has been suggested that the substitution of depression for aggression is physiologically based, a new equilibrium being required between aggression which is turned outwards and that which is turned inwards upon the self (James 1960). Alternative explanations have, however, been put forward in psychodynamic terms (Ferguson & Rayport 1965; Horowitz *et al.* 1970). The depression may reflect the need for psychological readjustments — learning to live without the help of an accustomed handicap or being suddenly 'burdened' with normality. When seizures are abolished the family may begin to express their negative feelings more openly, and become more critical of behaviour previously excused. In effect the patient now has to establish his identity as a person without conspicuous disability.

Improvement in sexual adjustment is a second area in which gratifying results have been reported after temporal lobectomy. Increased drive and potency, and replacement of perverse tendencies by normal libidinal interest have been observed. In Taylor's (1969b) series of 100 consecutive cases, of whom two-thirds had had significant sexual difficulties, almost a quarter showed improved adjustment after surgery. This is further considered on p. 271 *et seq.*

Thirdly, Hill *et al.* (1957) reported increased warmth in social relationships after temporal lobectomy. This could be striking from the early months onwards, with lessened egotism, more friendliness and concern for the feelings of others, and a more 'extroverted' attitude towards life.

Such changes after surgery strongly suggest that the previously discharging lesion may have exerted a continuing effect on certain aspects of personality functioning. They also add to the evidence discussed on p. 266 that special personality attributes may be connected with this particular type of epilepsy. The fact that in some cases personality improvement can follow resection, not of diffuse but of highly discrete focal lesions within the temporal lobe, underlines the importance of regional cerebral damage in contributing to personality difficulties.

Effects of anticonvulsant drugs. Finally, it remains to consider the effect that anticonvulsant medication may have on personality functioning. Improved control of fits by medication is often followed by improved emotional stability, but the converse can also be seen. Sometimes as fits are reduced disturbances of behaviour increase. Very occasionally, in very disturbed patients, a balance must be struck between the control of fits and control of behaviour, but such cases are relatively rare. The dilemma can usually be resolved by the addition of psychotropic drugs to the anticonvulsant regimen.

Over and above the effects of fit control, it is important to know whether anticonvulsant drugs can have an aggravating or beneficial effect on personality attributes. The situation is unclear and has rarely been tested by controlled comparisons. Reynolds and Travers (1974) produced evidence that several aspects of mental disturbance, including personality change, could be related to increased serum levels of phenobarbitone or phenytoin, even while these remain within the therapeutic range. It remains uncertain, however, how common such effects may be in clinical practice. Trimble and Reynolds (1984) review anecdotal reports of depression as a side effect of phenobarbitone and phenytoin, personality change following primidone and hysterical reactions seen with phenytoin. Conversely, drugs such as carbamazepine or diazepam are reported to have beneficial effects on behaviour, as discussed in the section on treatment, though here it is far from clear whether their action is by way of a direct psychotropic effect or improved control of seizures.

In certain situations drugs are widely recognised to have adverse effects. In children sedative and stimulating drugs can have a paradoxical action (Pond 1961); phenobarbitone may make epileptic children restless and irritable, whereas amphetamines can improve behaviour and reduce hyperkinesis (Ounsted 1955). Phenobarbitone may also increase the irritability of adult patients with temporal lobe epilepsy, and a change to an alternative anticonvulsant may then have a markedly beneficial effect. This may in part underlie the reputation which newer drugs come to acquire for helping the personality difficulties of patients with temporal lobe epilepsy.

The observations of Reynolds (1967a) and others on the disturbances of folate metabolism which may be associated with anticonvulsant medication are also relevant. Disturbances of mood and behaviour, in addition to intellectual retardation, have sometimes appeared to be due to the lowering of folate levels and to improve when this is remedied. However, the situation is complex and to some extent controversial as discussed in Chapter 12 (p. 592). In Edeh and Toone's (1985, 1987) community survey of epileptic subjects (p. 259), significantly lower folate levels were obtained in patients with psychiatric disorder, particularly in those with depression.

Sexual disorder in epilepsy

Sexual disorder attracted little attention in epileptic patients until relatively recently. Several reports, however, now stress the frequency of sexual disturbance in patients with temporal lobe epilepsy. Hyposexuality has emerged as the commonest abnormality, with perversions of sexual interest and outlet occurring in a much smaller number.

Gastaut and Collomb (1954) were the first to draw attention to hyposexuality after specific enquiry in 36 patients with temporal lobe epilepsy. More than two-thirds showed marked diminution or absence of interest, appetite or sexual activity. Other forms of focal and generalised epilepsy appeared to be unassociated with such problems. There was often a remarkable lack of sexual curiosity, fantasies or erotic dreams, yet little to suggest inhibition since the patients talked easily and without reserve about such matters. Indeed they appeared to be quite indifferent about the subject.

Gastaut and Collomb's patients were resident in a psychiatric hospital and none were living in a normal environment. Hierons and Saunders (1966), however, reported impotence in 15 patients with temporal lobe lesions, all of whom were living at home. Twelve were suffering from temporal lobe epileptic attacks. In contrast to Gastaut and Collomb's patients libido appeared to be normal, and in four patients the impotence improved when the epilepsy was brought under control with drugs.

Taylor (1969b) found poor sexual adjustment in two-thirds of 100 consecutive cases referred for temporal lobectomy. The commonest problem was again lack of sexual drive and a bland denial of interest in sex. Masturbation was rare, and marital problems were attributable to lack of interest in sex rather than actual impotence. Blumer (1970) found hyposexuality in 29 of 50 patients with temporal lobe epilepsy, and observed improvement in a third of those who underwent temporal lobectomy, especially when seizures were substantially relieved.

Shukla et al. (1979) have upheld the special association between temporal lobe epilepsy and hyposexuality in a controlled study. Seventy patients with temporal lobe epilepsy were compared with 70 patients with generalised epilepsy attending the same clinic in India. The groups were similar in age, duration of illness, seizure frequency and marital history. By detailed interviews it was established that 41% of the male temporal lobe epileptics were hyposexual, compared to 8% of the males with generalised epilepsy. The corresponding figures for females were 38% and 5%, respectively. On restricting attention to patients over the age of 15 and where adequate information was available these differences were accentuated, reaching statistically significant levels. Among the males the disorder was manifest as a global lack of interest, failure of erections and nocturnal emissions, and absence of fantasies or dreams of a sexual nature. The females remained totally passive in sexual relations and failed to reach orgasm. When the temporal lobe epilepsy had set in during childhood the patients had commonly failed to develop any interest in sexual matters; when it was of late onset there had been a decline in interest and activity. The lack of concern evidenced by the patients, and their failure to make complaints, probably accounted for the problem having attracted so little attention in the past. Toone *et al.* (1989) found that temporal lobe epileptics and other focal epileptics recruited from general practice were equivalently impaired, both more often lacking sexual interest and activity than patients with primary generalised epilepsy.

Lindsay *et al.*'s (1979b) follow-up into adult life of 100 children with temporal lobe epilepsy showed the striking importance of time of remission of seizures where sexual maturing was concerned. Of those men who were marriageable, 17 had married and 24 were unmarried, the two groups being comparable in terms of age, intelligence and frequency and severity of seizures. The distinguishing factor was whether or not their seizures had remitted before the age of 12. Twelve of the 15 early remitters had married, compared with only five of the 26 non-remitters, a statistically significant difference. Furthermore, at least 14 of the 24 single men showed no interest in sexual matters and only one of these had been an early remitter. It thus appeared that continuing epileptic disruption of temporolimbic functions during the normal period of sexual maturing often resulted in a lack of interest in sex; conversely remission before puberty allowed relatively normal sexual development.

Male hormone metabolism also appears to be often disturbed in epileptic patients. Following a report by Christiansen *et al.* (1975) of reduced androgen excretion in male epileptics, Toone *et al.* (1983, 1984, 1989) carried out hormonal studies in several groups of patients. Free testosterone levels were found to be significantly reduced in a mixed group of male epileptics resident in the David Lewis Centre, in male epileptics attending an out-patient clinic and in those recruited from general practice. Luteinising hormone, follicle-stimulating hormone and sex-hormone-binding globulin were by contrast significantly raised. When the resident patients were divided into low and high sex drive categories on a number of measures, the free testosterone levels were shown to be significantly lower in the former than in the latter. The hormonal abnormalities seemed likely to be the product of metabolic changes consequent upon anticonvulsant medication. Thus in addition to impaired maturation of sexual interest, male hyposexuality may also derive in part from hormonal derangements.

Hypersexuality, by contrast, appears to be rare. Taylor (1969b) and Shukla *et al.* (1979) each found only one example, but Blumer (1970) found seven who showed distinct episodes of increased sexual drive. This occurred post-ictally, but in one patient accompanied the actual seizures. Two hyposexual patients showed hypersexuality as a transient postoperative reversal, severe in degree. One patient experienced increased desire when the seizures were controlled by medication.

Fifteen per cent of Taylor's (1969b) patients showed perverse tendencies in the form of masochism or exhibitionism. None showed transvestism or fetishism though several other reports have drawn attention to examples. Kolarsky *et al.*'s (1967) patients showed a wide range of sexual deviations — sadomasochism, exhibitionism and fetishism—the disorders often appearing to be associated with temporal lobe damage dating from very early in life.

The relationship of abnormal sexual activity to the epileptic process has sometimes emerged as very close indeed:

Hunter *et al.* (1963) reported a patient with transvestism and fetishism of 30 years' duration and temporal lobe attacks for 10 years. The abnormal sexual impulses diminished as the epilepsy was controlled by drugs and were later abolished completely by temporal lobectomy. The onset of the perversion 20 years before the epilepsy was considered to be compatible with the natural history of the temporal lobe gliosis found at operation.

Of particular interest are cases in which transvestism has appeared in association with temporal lobe epilepsy well after the attainment of a normal adult sexual orientation:

Davies and Morganstern (1960) reported a patient of 36 who had developed grand mal epilepsy 12 years previously. This proved to be due to cerebral cysticercosis. For 7 years the auras to attacks had included features typical of temporal lobe epilepsy, and for some 3 years had consisted of epigastric and jaw sensations. The epigastric auras were followed by an episodic desire to transvest. Initially this was exclusively in relation to the epigastric and jaw sensations, but for 2 years the desire to transvest had increased and become independent of any epileptic phenomena.

Mitchell *et al.* (1954) reported a striking example of fetishism in association with temporal lobe epilepsy which deserves to be described in detail:

A man of 38 had enjoyed what he described as 'thought satisfaction' for as long as he could remember when looking at a safety pin. This was highly pleasurable to him but even as a child he felt that it was an odd and potentially embarrassing habit. Between the ages of 8 and 11 the 'thought satisfaction' began to be followed by a blank period, but since the phenomenon was kept secret no such attacks were observed until after his marriage.

Attacks were first accidentally observed by his wife when he was 23. She reported that he would stare at a pin for a minute, then become glassy eyed, make a humming noise and sucking movements of the lips. This was followed by a 2-minute period in which he would be immobile and unresponsive. Just before some of his attacks his right pupil would dilate. By 31 the period of immobility was regularly succeeded by a brief motor automatism in which he would mark time and later march backwards while his right hand plucked at his left sleeve. Brief post-ictal confusion was evident during which he occasionally dressed himself in his wife's clothing.

Such seizures occurred only after staring at a safety pin or after fantasies of doing so. A 'bright shiny' whole pin was essential and often several of them were more effective than one. Two or three attacks occurred every 7–10 days. The desire to look at a pin arose mostly during sexual stimulation or in anxiety-provoking situations. During sexual intercourse or masturbation he occasionally had a seizure if he thought about the fetish. He had become increasingly impotent during the past 5 years. There had been three episodes of florid but short-lived paranoid psychosis in the past 12 months.

A left-sided temporal lobe focus was found on EEG. This was exacerbated by exhibiting pins, followed after some 30 seconds by a clinical seizure. Air encephalography showed focal dilatation of the left temporal horn. At operation the left temporal lobe was resected, and showed slight atrophy and gliosis but no other abnormality.

Postoperatively there were no further fits, and at follow-up 16 months later he reported that he had had no further desire to look at a safety pin. He had become as potent as in early marriage. The EEG was now normal and the exhibition of a safety pin did not affect it.

The mechanisms which may underlie the association of such abnormal sexual behaviour with temporal lobe epilepsy are far from clear. Epstein (1961) suggested that the limbic system may subserve mechanisms concerned with such functions as imitation, identification and sexual arousal; dysfunction within this neural system may prevent the proper subordination and integration of such features during sexual development, so that the 'symbol and sign' aspects of sex are allowed to become dominant. This may then have issue in fetishism or transvestism, in both of which sign and symbol serve not only as stimulus but also as object of consummation. Hunter et al. (1963) suggested that rather than a direct pathophysiological link the disorders may arise by purely psychological means. Sexual ideas may occur as an integral part of dreamy states or déjà vu experiences, and by repeatedly reviving memories of childhood scenes and fantasies may keep alive early autistic forms of sexual activity. Neither theory, however, would explain the onset in adult life of transvestism in Davies and Morganstern's (1960) patient after many years of apparently normal sexual behaviour.

Such theories are of course no more than speculation. It remains possible that in the great majority of cases there is no direct causal link with the temporal lobe dysfunction, but that the disturbed sexuality is merely the outcome of distorted relationships during vulnerable phases of development and the limitations imposed on opportunities for experimentation and choice.

Occasional cases have been reported in which sexual sensations or activity accompany or follow epileptic discharges. Freemon and Nevis (1969) described a woman who experienced auras of genital sexual stimulation followed by automatisms of sexual statements and actions, sometimes proceeding thereafter to grand mal convulsions. Currier et al. (1971) reported a woman with temporal lobe epilepsy who carried out the activities of sexual intercourse in the course of psychomotor attacks, and another who masturbated briefly during an attack while an EEG examination was in progress. Both were regarded as showing unconscious release or lack of inhibition in relation to post-ictal confusion.

A sexual content to automatisms appears to be especially common in those which derive from the anterior and medial parts of the frontal lobe (p. 250). Spencer et al. (1983) found that ictal automatisms such as pelvic thrusting or masturbatory activity occurred only with frontal foci as confirmed by depth EEG studies, even though anterior temporal lobe spiking was sometimes observed on scalp recordings. Sexual emotions as part of an aura could, however, be temporal lobe in origin, and somatosensory genital sensations could derive from parietal lobe foci.

Other disturbances of sexual function may occur, and appear to be reported mainly in temporal lobe epilepsy. In Taylor's (1969b) series one woman claimed that her fits always followed the excitement of sexual intercourse. Two men reported that they could only have intercourse mechanically and unemotionally lest fits should be precipitated. Another woman only experienced desire postictally. Hunter et al. (1963) mention a woman with temporal lobe epilepsy whose frigidity was threatening her marriage. When her husband approached her she experienced such strong déjà vu that she could not sustain interest in present reality. It emerged that she had in fact experienced an incestuous assault in her teens. Finally, Hooshmand and Brawley (1969) report two patients initially thought to be exhibitionists when they had undressed in public during the course of a temporal lobe automatism. One of them had never been known to have a grand mal seizure.

Crime and epilepsy

Early writers such as Lombroso (1911) came to view

epilepsy and criminality as intimately related. Though not all epileptics were criminals, most criminals were thought to have an 'epileptoid' constitution. 'If fully developed epileptic fits are often lacking in the born criminal, this is because they remain latent, and only show themselves later under the influence of the causes assigned (anger, alcoholism), which bring them to the surface.' Violent crimes such as murder, arson, rape and theft were thought to be particularly characteristic of epileptic subjects. Maudsley (1873, 1906) emphasised that epilepsy should always be considered in aggressive crimes, and felt that crimes committed suddenly and in a 'blind fury' were often due to some form of epileptic process.

These views were decisively altered when careful surveys were carried out. Alstrom (1950) found no excess of criminal records compared to the population generally in 897 epileptics attending a Swedish clinic, provided they were not mentally affected. Those with psychiatric complications did show a significant excess, though even so the figure was not strikingly high (12% compared to 5%). Major aggression was not observed in the sample, and the acts of violence that had occurred were usually trivial and closely connected with abuse of alcohol. Juul-Jensen's (1964) large Danish survey of 1020 adult epileptics substantially confirmed these findings. Both surveys, however, were largely confined to patients attending hospitals and clinics, and many epileptics in institutions and in the community were doubtless omitted. Gudmundsson's (1966) attempt to survey all epileptics resident in Iceland (987 patients) produced rather different results—the male epileptics had been convicted three times as often as the male population generally.

Gunn approached the problem by an extensive survey of the prevalence of epilepsy among the prison and borstal populations of England and Wales (Gunn 1969; Gunn & Fenton 1971). At a conservative estimate seven to eight prisoners per 1000 were found to be suffering from epilepsy, which is considerably higher than the prevalence of epilepsy in the general population. Young prisoners in particular were much more likely to be suffering from epilepsy than persons of a similar age in the community. It seems, therefore, that epileptics do have a higher probability of being committed to prison than other members of the population.

A representative sample of epileptic prisoners was then examined to see whether the types of crime committed differed from those of matched controls (Gunn & Bonn 1971). The great majority had been convicted for non-violent larceny, as with prisoners generally. There was no suggestion that epileptics were more prone to any particular form of offence, and no support for the view that

they were especially liable to crimes of violence. Whitman *et al.* (1984) confirmed these findings in a survey of men entering the Illinois prison system; the prevalence of epilepsy was again raised, but there was no excess of more serious or violent crimes.

The number of homicides committed in Gunn's survey was too small for testing an earlier suggestion that there may be some special relationship between epilepsy and murder. Stafford-Clark and Taylor (1949) reported a remarkable association between EEG abnormality and type of crime among 64 prisoners facing charges of murder. Where the killing had been incidental to some other crime or in self defence 9% of EEGs were abnormal; where there was a clear motive for killing 25% were abnormal; where the crime was apparently motiveless 73% were abnormal; and among those found unfit to plead or guilty but insane 86% were abnormal. Hill and Pond (1952) extended this series to 105 murderers and reinforced the findings; accidental murderers appeared to have no greater incidence of EEG abnormality than the general population, clearly motivated murderers were intermediate, and motiveless murderers had an extremely high proportion of abnormal EEGs. Eighteen of the 105 subjects had definite evidence of epilepsy, which was more than 30 times the incidence of epilepsy in the population generally. Even allowing for matters of special selection, in that referral for EEG meant that epilepsy or brain disease had already been suspected, Hill and Pond (1952) concluded that there was undoubtedly some relationship between murder and epilepsy.

The question arises whether murder, or more minor crimes of violence, often occur during seizures or post-ictal 'automatisms'. Most now agree that although this can occur it must be very rare indeed. Hill and Pond (1952), for example, could not find a case in their material where they were satisfied that a seizure had preceded the murder. Gunn and Fenton (1971), in a survey of 158 prisoners with epilepsy, found five who had fits just after committing a crime, four who had fits just before committing a crime, and four others in whom a possible association with automatism could be considered. However, when the detailed evidence was reviewed none showed convincing evidence of 'automatic' criminal behaviour. Subsequently, however, further evidence came forward to suggest that one of these prisoners probably killed his wife in the course of an epileptic attack or its immediate sequelae (Gunn 1978). Moreover, among 32 epileptics committed to Broadmoor Hospital, Gunn and Fenton (1971) found two who had probably committed their crimes during a post-ictal confusional state as in the following example:

A 32-year-old patient in Broadmoor had developed convulsions at the age of 18. Two and a half years later he had a generalised convulsion early in the morning while getting ready for work. On recovery 20 minutes later his speech was slurred and his eyes seemed 'vacant'. He violently attacked an elderly man who lived in the house, striking him with a spade and kicking him. (The man died as a result of severe head injuries 6 days later.) He then attacked his girl friend and the victim's wife, smashed some panes of glass and cycled aimlessly away with blood on his arms. One and a half miles from the house he fell off the cycle, and on admission to hospital was mentally confused and amnesic for all events following the seizure.

In Broadmoor he continued to have major seizures every 1–2 years without aura. Each was followed by confusion for up to an hour during which he would appear perplexed and frightened, and if restrained in any way he would become dangerously aggressive. His behaviour at all other times was impeccable. The EEG showed spike and wave discharges of subcortical origin, but no evidence of a focal lesion.

Dangerous behaviour during ictal automatisms is also occasionally reported. The patient may continue with an act in progress at the time and do harm by virtue of a confused state of mind. A patient mentioned by Macdonald (1969) was filling a kettle with a view to placing it on the fire when her seizure commenced, and she placed her baby on the fire instead. Such situations are, however, exceedingly rare, and acts of violence have emerged as distinctly unusual in reviews of patients subject to automatisms (Knox 1968). Delgado-Escueta *et al.* (1981) reviewed videotaped recordings of 33 seizures in 19 patients, selected from over 5000 as showing possible aggressive behaviour. Only seven were rated as showing substantial aggression, usually in the form of struggling when restrained or kicking out in fear, but three showed elements of physical attack with spitting, shouting or scratching and three attempted to destroy property. Five of these seven had histories of inter-ictal personality disturbance or psychiatric disorder, including aggressive behaviour unassociated with seizures. Videotaped seizures witnessed in a laboratory are probably considerably less likely to reveal aggression than those taking place in the community when the patient is interacting with those around; nevertheless Roth's (1968) conclusion would seem to be valid — that insofar as there is any increased risk of violent or antisocial conduct among epileptics, it is unlikely to arise from the attacks themselves but rather from the psychiatric complications of the epilepsy.

It can be important in medicolegal work to have guidelines for assessing the probability that a crime may have been committed during an episode of ictal or post-ictal confusion. Walker (1961), Knox (1968) and Fenton (1972) have discussed a series of criteria which may be applied:

First of all the patient should have a past history of unequivocal epileptic attacks. In the majority of cases it is likely that a history of grand mal attacks or other partial epileptic attacks will be elicited, as well as the alleged automatic behaviour. A story of vague perceptual disturbances, such as *déjà vu* sensations or feelings of depersonalization, should not be accepted as indicating temporal lobe epilepsy in the absence of other distinctive features, since these are frequently experienced by neurotic patients and can sometimes be elicited on enquiry from perfectly healthy people. There need not necessarily be a previous history of automatism as such, though clearly when this is elicited it will strengthen the confidence with which the present example is so diagnosed. The diagnosis must always be made on clinical grounds, for epilepsy can occur in the presence of a normal EEG, and, conversely, abnormal records may be obtained in patients who have never had a clinical attack. Nevertheless an EEG compatible with the type of clinical disorder presumed to be present will constitute important additional evidence.

With regard to the circumstances of the crime itself, this will always have been sudden, obvious motives will be lacking and there should be no evidence of planning or premeditation. The crime will appear to be senseless, there will typically have been little or no attempt at concealment and often no attempt at escape. The abnormal behaviour will usually have been of short duration, lasting minutes rather than hours, and will never have been entirely appropriate to the circumstances. Witnesses may have noted evidence of impairment of awareness, for example inappropriate actions or gestures, stereotyped movements, unresponsiveness or irrelevant replies to questions, aimless wandering around, or a dazed and vacant expression. These features may not, however, be readily apparent to the untrained eye. Amnesia for the crime is the rule, but there should be no continuing anterograde amnesia for events following the resumption of conscious awareness. The more that these criteria are not fulfilled, the more will an epileptic basis for the act be regarded with suspicion.

Neurosis

The more florid psychiatric disturbances in epilepsy are greatly outnumbered by neurotic forms of disability. This has emerged in all the community surveys outlined on pp. 259–60, and it is uncertain to what degree the prevalence exceeds that in the population generally. Nevertheless, those epileptics who are subject to neurotic disturbance warrant close attention, since emotional stability is likely to be an important factor in contributing to adequacy of fit control. States of heightened anxiety, in particular, may come to be self reinforcing in leading to an increase of seizures.

The forms that the neurotic disability takes have little that is distinctive for epilepsy. Pond (1957) concluded that the characteristics of the neurotic reaction depended principally on patterns of premorbid personality and family relationships, as with neurosis generally, and owed little to the epileptic phenomena themselves. The epileptic has, of course, more than his share of psychosocial difficulties to account for such developments. In Shukla and Katiyar's (1980) series of 62 temporal lobe epileptics neurosis was significantly more common in those with a right temporal lobe focus, but such laterality effects do not appear to have been reported by others.

States of depression and anxiety are the most frequent and can usually be related to current environmental problems. Many epileptic patients pass through a difficult period of adjustment when first given the diagnosis; others react adversely to the social and personal problems occasioned by the disorder (Betts 1981). Surveys of epileptics attending neurological clinics have repeatedly highlighted the frequency of depressive mood and anxiety symptoms, even among patients unknown to psychiatric agencies (Currie *et al.* 1971; Standage & Fenton 1975; Kogeorgos *et al.* 1982). The relationships between affective disorder and epilepsy are discussed in more detail on p. 285.

Hysterical forms of reaction can often be traced to stresses operating on the vulnerable personality. These occur chiefly in patients of low intelligence or with marked personality disorder, but this is not always so. Sometimes the association between hysterical symptoms and epilepsy may be determined, in part at least, by organic brain dysfunction as implied by Slater and Roth (1969) — 'It is probably true that, as with many chronic organic conditions, the long persistence of an epilepsy can encourage the changes on which a hysterical alteration of personality, and an enhanced susceptibility to hysterical symptoms, can arise.' There has been some suggestion that 'hysteria', as measured by the Crown–Crisp Experiential Index self-rating questionnaire, may be more prominent among generalised as compared to focal epilepsies (Kogeorgos *et al.* 1982), but as yet there is no firm evidence to link hysterical symptoms with specific forms of epilepsy or with any particular locus of cerebral disorder. The important matter of the differential diagnosis between hysterical and epileptic seizures is discussed on p. 292 *et seq.*

Obsessive–compulsive disorders do not appear to be unusually common among epileptics. Phobic states sometimes centre around the dread of having an attack, and it is perhaps surprising that this is not encountered more frequently. Occasionally agoraphobia develops to an incapacitating degree, sometimes immediately after a fit which has occurred in a particularly dangerous situation. Pinto (1972) has described the successful treatment of a

patient by behaviour therapy, with parallel improvement in seizure frequency.

An unusual case of agoraphobia, which also illustrates pitfalls in the diagnosis of epilepsy, was as follows:

A woman of 34 had attended an epileptic clinic for many years on account of nocturnal attacks. These commenced at the age of 8, but increased greatly in severity at the age of 23 when she first presented at the clinic. They had shown temporary responses to various medications but were still occurring several times per week although she was on phenobarbitone, phenytoin and primidone.

For several years there had been a progressive restriction of activities and increasing dependence on her husband. For 2 years she had been unable to leave the house on her own. She complained of many strange symptoms—a feeling of walking on air, of internal shaking and of being dragged down from behind. On this account she was referred for psychiatric opinion.

She was clearly terrified of her 'epilepsy' and it was the dread of a daytime attack that prevented her from going out on her own. She described a striking family history; her father had had attacks during childhood and adolescence, two cousins had had epilepsy, one of whom had died in bed as a result, and her brother, 3 years her junior, had had nocturnal fits and had died in bed at the age of 20. At inquest his death was attributed to smothering during an epileptic fit.

Her own attacks were exclusively nocturnal. She was woken with abdominal cramps followed by a shooting pain passing from the right cheek to the left temple. She did not lose consciousness but felt an uncontrollable urge to bury her head in the pillow, and was obliged to struggle against this for up to 10 minutes. There had been no tongue biting or incontinence. Her husband confirmed that he would find her groaning, flushed, staring and anxious, attempting to talk and sometimes crying 'Hold me!'. She was stiff but there was no twitching or jerking. He had known of her attacks and of the family history since marrying her 8 years previously but the subject of epilepsy was taboo within the family.

The attacks were clearly most unusual for epilepsy and the EEG showed only mild and non-specific abnormalities. After much persuasion she allowed her father and his sister to be interviewed in order to clarify the family history.

It transpired that she had kept all knowledge of her own attacks from her father and her aunt in view of the tragedy which had befallen her brother. Her father was vague about his own youthful attacks, but his sister said that they had been diagnosed as hysterical in nature. Of the cousins with epilepsy, one had merely been examined by EEG after an episode of fainting, and the other had had no history of epilepsy but had died in bed from a brain haemorrhage following a cycle accident. It was only the patient's brother who had truly suffered from epilepsy, and he indeed died from smothering as the patient described. It also emerged that the father's mother had achieved notoriety in the national press in 1907 when her doctor had prescribed strychnine in mistake for some stomach medicine; she had died in convulsions, witnessed by her children including the patient's father when he was 5 years old.

It was decided that in all probability the patient's attacks were psychogenic in origin, as possibly her father's had been in his youth. She appeared, indeed, to represent the second generation of psychogenic attacks, deriving perhaps from the incident in 1907. Her fear of epilepsy was clearly intense and had led her to misinterpret and distort the family history. This fear was greatly aggravated by her brother's death, and it was shortly after this, when the patient was 23, that she had first presented herself at the epileptic clinic.

She was admitted to hospital for withdrawal of anticonvulsants after full explanation that no evidence for epilepsy could be found. Withdrawal was accomplished over several weeks, though the period was stormy with intense anxiety and many obviously psychogenic nocturnal attacks. Gradually, however, they subsided, along with her daytime odd sensations. After 2 months she had recovered her confidence in going out alone, and the following year she obtained employment as a travelling saleswoman. She felt better than for many years previously and accepted that she did not suffer from epilepsy. When followed up 18 months later there were still occasional disturbances at night, presumed to be hypnagogic in origin, but these no longer occasioned her much concern.

Another unusual patient was for a long time suspected of a psychogenic disorder, but in this case her complex phobias proved to be accompanied by post-ictal electro-physiological disturbance within the brain. The patient has already been briefly reported by Marks (1969):

A woman of 51 developed attacks suggestive of temporal lobe epilepsy from the age of 29. Prior to this she had seemed a stable and healthy person, surviving the loss of her husband and bringing up her daughter alone. Every 1–2 months she experienced brief attacks of feeling light-headed together with numbness bilaterally in the face. These were sometimes accompanied by a strange smell or taste, or incontinence of a few drops of urine, but she did not lose consciousness. For several days after each attack she felt depressed and generally unwell. The EEG showed no definite abnormalities.

At 38 she remarried and encountered great domestic disharmony. Her attacks increased to runs of three or four at a time, and she began to show marked hysterical features. There were three episodes of blindness lasting several minutes, and an episode of loss of speech for an hour. She made several suicidal gestures, and often collapsed motionless to the floor after arguments with her husband. The epileptic basis of her previous seizures began to be questioned and EEGs continued to show no abnormalities.

In 1958, at the age of 41 she had two of her usual seizures in quick succession, and was in her usual post-ictal phase of feeling 'washed out' and nervous when a furious argument developed with her husband. He became violent and she sought refuge by locking herself in a room. From this point onwards the post-ictal phase of all attacks became characterised by intense and unreasonable fears of men and of the dark. The invariable pattern was now for attacks to be followed by a period of 7–10 days during which these phobias were incapacitating, while in the interim they did not trouble her at all. Two years later she separated from her husband and resumed work as a telephonist, but the pattern of attacks continued unaltered.

The extent of the phobias was remarkable. Her fear of the dark led her to keep the light on all night, and she would take a bucket into her room since she was unable to go to the lavatory downstairs. Her fear of men made it difficult or impossible to travel to work lest a man should come close in the street or on public transport. The phobias always ran a characteristic course, setting in 12–24 hours after the seizure, remaining at their peak for several days, then gradually waning over 3 or 4 days thereafter.

In 1966 Dr R.T.C. Pratt obtained an opportunity to perform an EEG shortly after an attack and while the phobias were present. A marked abnormality, consisting of theta and delta waves together with some sharp elements, was seen in the right frontotemporal region. Sphenoidal leads confirmed focal sharp waves in the right anterior temporal region. The findings were confirmed after another attack and followed by repeat examinations; the right temporal abnormalities were marked immediately after the fit, and waned over 10 days as the phobias subsided.

The seizures changed somewhat in character at about this time, though she was an unreliable witness and gave different descriptions at different times. In place of the olfactory warning she noted a feeling as of water trickling over her back, epigastric sensations and mild confusion of thought. In some attacks she would slump in her chair and pick at her left cheek, and occasionally she lost consciousness and frothed at the mouth. After some attacks she claimed total amnesia for the events of several days preceding the seizure. The only constant and invariable feature continued to be the post-ictal phobias.

During 1968–69 she was admitted to the Maudsley Hospital on several occasions following attacks, and the focal right temporal disturbance on the EEG was repeatedly confirmed during phobic periods. In addition Dr Isaac Marks was able to obtain physiological confirmation of the post-ictal phobias — fantasies of the phobic situations led to marked physiological fear responses on the polygraph, whereas fantasies of neutral situations produced no such response. In between attacks, fantasies of the phobic situations were without effect. Physiological measures thus confirmed that selective phobic anxiety was present post-ictally but absent inter-ictally.

It thus seemed indubitable that the patient suffered from genuine and disabling phobias, uniquely during a 10-day period following each of her temporal lobe seizures, and accompanied by contemporaneous electrical disturbance within the right temporal lobe of the brain. The apparent onset of the phobic disorder in 1958, dating from an emotionally traumatic experience shortly after a seizure, was a striking feature in the history. It would appear that she may have been unusually vulnerable to the acquisition of a new 'neurotic' pattern of disability during the period immediately following her attacks, perhaps by virtue of temporal lobe dysfunction occurring at such times.

Psychoses

The proper understanding and classification of the epileptic psychoses is beset with difficulties. A bewildering variety of pictures may be encountered, ranging from transient self-limiting episodes to chronic illnesses which persist for many years. Some are immediately related to the fits themselves, or to identifiable alterations in the electrical activity of the brain, while others appear to arise independently of any seizure manifestations. The clinical content is similarly variable, some disturbances being dominated by organic features in the mental state, while others show affective or schizophreniform symptomatology with no evidence of clouding of consciousness. The well-known difficulty of detecting minor degrees of clouding adds to the problems of understanding and classifying such phenomena.

The epileptic psychoses are of great theoretical interest for obvious reasons. They provide an unusual opportunity for exploring relationships between cerebral dysfunction and mental disorder, both of organic and 'functional' types. It is unfortunate therefore that the literature concerning the forms they may take and their electrophysiological associations has often been far from clear. The selection of patients for report is open to many influences, terminology is often confused and phenomenology inadequately described. Our present state of knowledge is therefore likely to prove no more than an approximation to the true state of affairs.

A simple division may be made into (i) psychoses in which confusion and impairment of consciousness are the outstanding features while affective or schizophreniform elements are absent or unobtrusive; (ii) psychoses which contain an admixture of 'organic' and 'functional' manifestations; and (iii) psychoses which occur in a setting of clear consciousness and take a form characteristic of schizophrenia or affective disorder.

As might be expected the first and most decisively organic group shows the most regular and definite relationship with the cerebral dysrhythmias of epilepsy. Indeed such episodes prove mostly to reflect either ictal or immediately post-ictal disturbances of cerebral function. As such they are transient phenomena, lasting for minutes, hours or occasionally days but rarely longer. The great majority of these disturbances represent ictal automatisms, absence status or post-ictal confusional states, as already described in the sections on complex partial seizures and post-ictal disorders (p. 252 *et seq.* and p. 257).

The intermediate group, showing both impairment of consciousness and 'functional' psychotic features, tends likewise to be tied to on-going electrical disturbances within the brain, though perhaps less commonly in direct apposition to seizures. Temporal lobe epilepsy appears to be particularly associated with such manifestations (see discussion on p. 258). A common picture is the combination of marked confusion, visual and auditory hallucinations, paranoid delusions and depression sometimes amounting to stupor. The impairment of consciousness may be obvious at the time, or revealed only subsequently by evidence of patchy or complete amnesia for the episode. Such disorders may be many days or weeks in duration, but again are almost always self limiting. The post-ictal psychoses described on p. 257 represent the clearest delineation of this group, with pleomorphic pictures in which mood abnormalities, hallucinations and delusions are commonly but not always accompanied by clouding of consciousness. Here it is interesting that a lucid interval of one to several days may intervene between the seizure and the psychosis that follows. Others within this intermediate group will overlap with the 'twilight states' described on p. 255.

The psychotic illnesses which present regularly in clear consciousness may occur either as transient self-limiting episodes, or alternatively as chronic and severely disabling illnesses. They may be affective, schizoaffective or schizophrenic in form. It is this group, and particularly the schizophrenia-like psychoses within it, which has been clarified in several respects in recent years and which accordingly warrants more extended discussion.

Schizophrenia and epilepsy

The study of the relationship between schizophrenia and epilepsy has had a curious history as reviewed, for example, by Flor-Henry (1969), Wolf and Trimble (1985) and Trimble (1991). The relationship has been extensively investigated from two different points of view—the occurrence of epileptic manifestations in schizophrenic patients, and the development of schizophrenia in established epileptics.

With regard to the former, Hill (1948, 1957a) illustrated the unusual frequency of epileptic wave forms in the EEGs of schizophrenics. These were found in up to 25% of young acute cases and particularly in catatonic schizophrenia. Typical paroxysmal phenomena with three per second spike and wave activity may be seen. Among such patients convulsions were sometimes observed during the course of insulin coma therapy, or occurred spontaneously shortly after recovery. Variations could sometimes be demonstrated in the photometrazol threshold during periods of catatonic stupor, or in the ease of provoking spike and wave discharges by induced hypoglycaemia.

With regard to the prevalence of schizophrenia in known epileptics, directly contradictory conclusions arose from different investigations in the past. Thus some suggested an affinity between the two disorders, such that they occurred together in the same patient more often than chance expectation. Others, however, found quite the reverse, with a lowered prevalence of schizophrenia in epileptics. The idea of a fundamental antagonism between the two disorders was strengthened by reports of patients in whom epileptic and schizophrenic manifestations appeared to alternate, periods of psychosis developing when seizures were in abeyance and periods of sanity accompanying the return of convulsions. The latter viewpoint led to Meduna's introduction of convulsive therapy for the management of schizophrenia in 1937.

Gradually the situation has become clearer. It now appears that chronic paranoid–hallucinatory psychoses closely similar to schizophrenia, and phenomenologically often indistinguishable from it, do occur more often than chance expectation in epileptic patients, and show a particularly close relationship to epilepsy arising within the temporal lobes. The work of Slater et al. (1963), described below, was of central importance in arriving at this conclusion. It furthermore seems probable that a distinct subgroup of schizophrenia-like psychoses may warrant separate recognition from the above; in these the psychotic episodes are transient and self limiting, often setting in when fits are diminishing in frequency and tending to subside when fits return. These are discussed further on p. 284.

Thus both the 'affinity' and the 'antagonism' hypotheses appear to have had their roots in valid clinical observations, but in different groups of patients. A given series of patients will sometimes have contained a preponderance of one type of schizophrenia-like psychosis, sometimes of the other, accounting for the divergent views expressed in the literature. It is also likely that the distinctions are not absolute but that a variety of intermediate forms occur.

Mendez et al. (1993) have recently produced an unusually clear illustration of the excess occurrence of schizophrenia with epilepsy. Among attenders at a neurology clinic in Minnesota, inter-ictal schizophrenic disorders had been documented in 9.25% of 1611 epileptic patients compared with only 1.06% of 2167 migraine patients. In a comparison of matched subgroups with and without schizophrenia, the group with schizophrenia contained more epileptics with complex partial seizures and fewer with generalised epilepsy; and compared with non-epileptic schizophrenics they were less likely to have a family history of psychosis. Though limited by the retrospective nature of the study these results confirm much that has come to be suspected from other investigations as detailed below.

Chronic schizophrenia-like psychoses

The occurrence of chronic paranoid–hallucinatory states in patients with temporal lobe epilepsy was reported by Hill (1953, 1957b) and Pond (1957). These were described as resembling schizophrenia very closely

indeed. Delusions were often systematised and coupled with ideas of influence and auditory hallucinations. Frank thought disorder could appear, with neologisms, condensed words and inconsequential sentences. In contrast to ordinary schizophrenia, however, the affect tended to remain warm and appropriate, and typical hebephrenic deterioration was not seen. In the patients described by Hill and Pond the psychoses tended to begin at a time when fit frequency was declining, either spontaneously or as a result of medication.

Slater et al. (1963) tackled the problem by systematically collecting patients who had unequivocal evidence of epilepsy and who had subsequently developed an illness diagnosed as schizophrenia. Sixty-nine patients, 36 male and 33 female, were collected from the Maudsley Hospital and the National Hospital, Queen Square over a 10-year period. Care was taken to include only those in whom there was good clinical evidence for the diagnosis of schizophrenia, and in whom the psychosis had persisted for several weeks or months. Cases were excluded where psychotic symptoms had been confined to episodes in which alteration of consciousness could have played some part.

The clinical features were as follows. The mean age of onset was 30 years, after a mean duration of epilepsy of 14 years. The range extended, however, from 12 to 59 years, and the duration of epilepsy prior to onset from several months to 48 years. In the great majority (80%) the onset had been insidious with the gradual development of delusions as the first manifestation. In a smaller proportion there was an acute or subacute onset which then progressed to a more lasting psychosis. Sometimes there had been a number of acute episodes, perhaps in association with confusional states, before the chronic condition supervened. In the series as a whole there was no clear relationship between onset and alteration of fit frequency, but in a small number there was a suggestion of diminishing frequency before the psychosis appeared.

The following case from Slater et al. (1963) is typical:

The patient had had epilepsy since the age of 10. At 38, when he was having one major attack a month, he began to complain of depression. He told the psychiatrist he did not know whether he was coming or going. Someone had told him he was being a 'Billy Muggins'. For 6 months he had had the idea he was being followed; people had followed him around who looked like foreigners. At a tea bar the man who served him had said 'thank you very much, your Majesty'; and he was only a plain mister—as far as he knew. These vague ideas in course of time became systematised into the delusion that he was a scion of a noble family and could expect a vast sum from a will. He became auditorily hallucinated and heard voices in his head which said 'Duke of York', 'Duke of Cambridge' (the names of pubs in his neighbourhood), 'Duke of Salisbury' and 'Squire'. The voices knew everything he had done, and they must have recordings of his entire life. There was a pick-up in his body, 'a pin in my body to pick up the nerve vibrations', which transmitted thoughts from the brain, and also made the brain receive.

Sometimes the psychosis became manifest as a gradual change of personality as in the following example:

The patient had had screaming attacks as a little girl, and grand mal attacks without aura or focal signs since 13. Her attacks practically ceased at the age of 32. From this time on there was a progressive personality change. From being normally affectionate and active, she became unaffectionate, sulky and aggressive and lost all her interests. When admitted to hospital at the age of 38 she was becoming more and more difficult, refusing her food and her tablets, and refusing to get out of bed or to wash herself. In hospital she showed thought blocking, incongruities of thought and affect, grimacing and fragmentary delusional ideas. This state persisted even when the possibility of drug intoxication, which had first been considered, had been eliminated. She was then found to be also auditorily hallucinated.

The established psychoses were in the main chronic paranoid illnesses typical of paranoid schizophrenia. A small number, some 10%, showed the picture of hebephrenic schizophrenia. Delusions occurred in almost every case, frequently of a religious or mystical nature. Some clearly took origin from primary delusional experiences, others apparently arose from feelings of depersonalisation or derealisation. Passivity feelings of being controlled or influenced were prominent, and were more closely connected with systematised ideas of persecution. Bizarre features characteristic of schizophrenia often entered into these delusions—rays, electronic wires, magnetic powers, thought reading and hypnosis. Special powers were often claimed, special significance was attached to commonplace events and happenings fell into a special pattern.

Hallucinations were chiefly in the auditory modality (46% of cases), though visual, somatic, olfactory and gustatory hallucinations occurred as well. Persecutory voices were particularly common, commenting on the patient's actions, repeating his thoughts, discussing him in the third person or telling him what to do. Visual hallucinations (16% of cases) were often complex and full of meaning, and often of a mystical nature. Almost always they were accompanied by auditory hallucinations as well.

Almost half of the patients showed thought disorder of schizophrenic type, with answering beside the point, neologisms, thought blocking and occasional incoherence amounting to word salad. Several patients felt that their thoughts were read or interrupted, or that thoughts could be put into their minds. Manneristic behaviour was sometimes observed, and impaired volition or initiative could

be marked. Gross catatonic phenomena were rare, but occasional patients showed negativism of the classic type, statuesque postures, sudden impulsive acts or repetitive stereotyped movements.

The commonest emotional disturbances were irritability, aggressiveness and short-lived severe depression. Exaltation or ecstasy were usually associated with some semi-mystical experience. Occasional patients described intense fear, bewilderment or loneliness. Flatness of affect was shown, at least at times, by rather less than half of the patients, and some showed silly or inappropriate emotional responses.

In summary, therefore, all of the cardinal symptoms of schizophrenia were exhibited at some time or another by this large group of patients. Slater et al. (1963) stressed that it would not be possible to diagnose them, on psychiatric symptomatology alone, as suffering from anything other than a schizophrenic psychosis. They noted, however, that the combination of symptoms shown by individual patients differed slightly from the usual schizophrenic patterns. Thus catatonic phenomena of gross degree were rare, and loss of affective response did not occur so early or become so marked as in the usual run of schizophrenias. By and large the patients were friendlier, more cooperative and less suspicious towards hospital staff. Moreover, at the time of observation a very high proportion (80%) showed what Slater et al. (1963) interpreted as 'organic' personality changes in addition to their schizophrenia-like symptoms—lack of spontaneity, dullness and retardation, concrete and circumstantial thinking and impairments of memory.

Slater et al.'s observations concerning phenomenology rested essentially on clinical judgements. More recent studies have attempted direct control comparisons between smaller groups of epileptic and non-epileptic psychotic patients, in an attempt to define the clinical symptomatology more precisely. Toone et al. (1982b), in a retrospective review using the Syndrome Check List, confirmed that catatonic syndromes were less common in epileptic schizophrenics than in their non-epileptic counterparts. Paranoid delusions and delusions of reference were significantly more common. Affective flattening and grandiose and religious delusions did not, however, differentiate the groups. Perez et al. (1985) used the Present State Examination to identify 'nuclear schizophrenias', and compared 11 temporal lobe epileptics with non-epileptic controls. The profiles of symptoms proved to be virtually identical in the two groups. IQs were in the main within the normal range, and there was little to suggest impairments of an organic nature.

The course in Slater et al.'s series was usually a tendency to chronicity once the psychosis had been declared. This was the course followed by almost half of the patients. When the onset had been acute the prognosis was better, sometimes with improvement even to the point of recovery. Those with an episodic onset sometimes pursued a fluctuating course thereafter. Follow-up at a mean interval of 8 years from the onset showed that a third had achieved remission, and a further third had improved with regard to psychotic manifestations. The epilepsy had also tended to become less troublesome with time. Many patients, however, showed psycho-organic sequelae in the form of perseveration, retardation or impairment of memory, half being substantially handicapped on account of such problems. It seemed that the chronic schizophrenia-like illness had often merely been one phase in the total course of the illness, with later development towards a picture more characteristic of organic cerebral disorder.

This last point has not been confirmed in other series to date. Toone et al. (1982b) found evidence of organic deterioration in only six of a mixed group of 68 psychotic epileptics. Perez et al. (1985) found that most patients with a clear diagnosis of temporal lobe epilepsy and schizophrenia showed little to indicate deterioration of intellect; indeed they comment that most patients within this category managed to avoid institutionalisation and to live reasonably well within the community, perhaps by virtue of preserved affect and family relationships.

The epilepsy from which Slater et al.'s 69 patients suffered was most frequently temporal lobe in origin. Two-thirds had clinical evidence, and rather more had EEG evidence of such a focus. The few patients with centrencephalic epilepsy (seven of the 69) showed predominantly hebephrenic rather than paranoid–hallucinatory pictures, and their age of onset was considerably earlier than the average. Chance association may well have been operative in this small subgroup. Perez et al. (1985) found that when the Present State Examination was used to define 'nuclear schizophrenia' this was entirely confined to the temporal lobe epileptics in their series.

A high proportion of Slater et al.'s patients appeared to have a lesional basis for their epilepsy, in that some definable cause could be detected in the history—birth injury, middle ear infection or encephalitis. Kristensen and Sindrup (1978a) confirmed this impression in a controlled study. Ninety-six temporal lobe epileptics with paranoid–hallucinatory psychoses were matched with non-psychotic patients with the same type of epilepsy, age of onset and present age. The former contained a greater proportion with histories indicative of brain damage as a basis for their epilepsy, also a significantly greater number of left-handers which may similarly have reflected brain insult. Slater et al. found that air encephalography

demonstrated cerebral atrophy in two-thirds of cases; Toone et al. (1982a), however, found CT scan abnormalities to be no more common in epileptics with schizophrenia than in those with other psychoses or psychiatric disorders, the frequency being approximately 50% in all subgroups.

Using MRI, Conlon et al. (1990) found no differences between psychotic and non-psychotic epileptics, either on visual inspection or measurement of T_1 relaxation times, though within the psychotic group those who experienced hallucinations showed significantly higher T_1 values in the left temporal lobe. Positron emission tomography (PET) scanning in a small series has shown indications of reduced metabolism, especially in frontal, temporal and basal ganglia regions (Gallhofer et al. 1985). Marshall et al. (1993), in a small pilot study, obtained evidence from single photon emission computerised tomography (SPECT) of lowered cerebral blood flow in the left medial temporal region in psychotic epileptic patients, and also, surprisingly, in both thalami. In a larger SPECT investigation Mellers et al. (1996) observed a significant decrease in blood flow in the left superior temporal gyrus during verbal activation, in contrast to non-psychotic epileptics and non-epileptic schizophrenic controls.

An additional curious finding is that where patients with schizophrenia-like psychoses have come to temporal lobectomy, mesial temporal lobe sclerosis has seemed less common than in temporal lobe epileptics generally, and small cryptic tumours (hamartomas) have been particularly common (Taylor 1972; Falconer 1973). Taylor (1975) compared 47 patients whose resected specimens showed 'alien tissue' (small tumours, hamartomas and focal dysplasia) with 41 showing mesial sclerosis; 23% of the former but only 5% of the latter had been psychotic. A marked effect of left-handedness was also seen in Taylor's material, seven of the 13 psychotic patients being left-handed compared with only 11 of the 75 non-psychotic patients. In the alien tissue group females, and particularly left-handed females, were especially likely to have developed a schizophrenia-like psychosis. By contrast, Roberts et al. (1990b) in a further analysis of the material, found that mesial sclerosis was not uncommon in the presence of a schizophrenia-like psychosis, affecting the left hemisphere more often than the right. A second form of pathology – alien tissue ganglioglioma – was significantly above chance expectation in those who developed psychoses postoperatively. Both of these pathologies arise early in foetal or neonatal life and were associated with a particularly early onset of seizures. Where lesions were found in the resected specimens from patients with schizophrenia-like psychoses they always involved the medial temporal lobe structures (amygdala, hippocampus and parahippocampal gyrus), the lateral parts of the lobe being rarely affected.

The significance to be attached to these observations remains unknown, but they combine to suggest that the development of psychosis in temporal lobe epilepsy is more than a random matter. The indications of a special association with left-sided temporal lobe foci, discussed below, is further evidence in this regard.

The idea of a special association with temporal lobe epilepsy has been criticised by Small et al. (1966) and Stevens (1966b, 1991). It is not known, for example, how large a proportion of non-psychotic epileptic patients of equivalent age would show discharges arising within the temporal lobes. There is also the problem that a substantial proportion of patients with complex partial seizures have an epileptic focus in extratemporal sites (p. 253), and these will not have been detected in surveys which lack detailed EEG studies (Mace 1993). The matter will be hard to resolve conclusively until further large series of psychotic and non-psychotic epileptics can be accumulated, in a manner which avoids special selection and permits careful categorisation of both the psychoses and the epilepsy. Nevertheless, McKenna et al. (1985) and Trimble (1991) support the special association from their detailed reviews of the literature.

Moreover, Flor-Henry (1969) has produced further evidence in favour of special regional associations, by demonstrating that among psychotic temporal lobe epileptics the schizophrenias were strongly associated with foci in the dominant rather than the non-dominant lobe. This important finding has been both confirmed (Gregoriadis et al. 1971; Taylor 1975; Lindsay et al. 1979c; Sherwin 1981; Perez et al. 1985) and refuted (Kristensen & Sindrup 1978b; Jensen & Larsen 1979b), though the balance of evidence appears to support Flor-Henry's initial observation. Perez et al. (1985) present a summation of reports from the literature concerning 180 patients with schizophrenia-like psychoses and temporal lobe epilepsy, yielding a total of 62% with left, 15% with right and 23% with bilateral foci. They point out that the link with left-sided foci has emerged most consistently when Schneiderian criteria have been employed in the diagnosis of the schizophrenia.

The mechanisms behind the association between epilepsy and chronic schizophrenia-like psychoses have been considered in some detail (Pond 1962; Symonds 1962b; Slater et al. 1963; Davison and Bagley 1969; Flor-Henry 1969). Chance association may be operative, or precipitation in individuals already predisposed to schizophrenia. Or there may be more direct links of a psychological or physiological nature.

A merely chance association appears to be unlikely. Statistical reasoning from the known frequencies of epilepsy and of schizophrenia in the general population makes it improbable that 69 examples could have been collected by Slater et al. (1963) from two hospitals over a relatively short period of time. Moreover the 'schizophrenia' was mainly of a particular type (paranoid) and the epilepsy of a particular type (temporal lobe epilepsy), whereas chance association should have led to a more normal representation of all varieties. The psychoses also had some features unusual for schizophrenia, such as relatively good preservation of affective response. The special associations with alien tissue lesions and with left-sided foci, as discussed above, also argue for more than a chance association.

Precipitation in individuals predisposed to schizophrenia similarly appears unlikely. A family history of schizophrenia was very rare in first-degree relatives in Slater et al.'s material, occurring no more often than in the general population and certainly less often than in ordinary schizophrenia. Nor did the premorbid personalities of the patients contain an undue frequency of schizoid traits. Both of these points were confirmed by Flor-Henry (1969). In a direct comparison between epileptic and non-epileptic schizophrenics, Toone et al. (1982b) again found that abnormalities of premorbid personality had been less common in the epileptics.

Thus one is led to infer more direct aetiological links between the epilepsy (or its attendant brain dysfunction) and the psychosis. The latter may be viewed as a 'symptomatic schizophrenia' analogous to that emerging with other brain lesions (p. 84) or with amphetamine abuse. Taking a more conservative view, some have argued that the psychoses observed are not, strictly speaking, schizophrenias at all, but are more properly to be regarded as epileptic psychoses of a special kind ('paranoid–hallucinatory psychoses'). Though taking on the appearances of schizophrenia, and resembling it very closely indeed, they differ markedly from 'endogenous' examples of the disease in their associations. To some extent the argument is tautologous; but whatever the precise nosological position may be the pathogenesis of such disorders is clearly a matter of considerable interest.

The aetiological link with the epilepsy could be via the seizures themselves, or alternatively by way of the basic disorder of cerebral functioning which manifests itself as epilepsy. In favour of the view that the fits themselves might be responsible is the finding that they have usually been occurring for many years before the psychosis supervenes, also that they tend to be of a certain clinical type. Temporal lobe seizures commonly involve recurrent abnormal experiences, often of a compelling and disquieting kind—sudden affects of fear, anxiety or ecstasy unconnected with external reality, or abnormal perceptual experiences in the form of hallucinations, *déjà vu* or de-realisation. Symonds (1962b) suggests that there is hardly one of the characteristic symptoms of schizophrenia, of a positive kind, which may not be experienced at some time or another in the auras of temporal lobe epilepsy. The psychotic patients in Slater *et al.*'s series had often experienced such aural symptoms, and a number explained them in a delusional way; the symptoms in fact came to enter into the content of the delusional psychoses. Epileptic twilight states may also contain material of a mystical or religious nature which is later recollected, and some patients remain convinced of the reality of such experiences. Years of attacks of clouding of consciousness may accordingly lead to a confusion between reality on the one hand and autistic thinking and experience on the other. Thus Pond (1962) advanced the view that there may sometimes be a causal relationship of a psychological kind between the fits and the psychosis, the latter depending essentially on abnormal emotional experiences, physically caused, which then become integrated into the totality of psychic life as a psychodynamic process.

There are difficulties, however, in accepting such a mechanism as a general explanation. Slater *et al.* (1963) were unable to find evidence that the frequency or severity of attacks was related to the development of psychosis. More decisively, Flor-Henry (1969) compared psychotic and non-psychotic temporal lobe epileptics and found that the former had had significantly fewer seizures than the latter, in particular fewer seizures of a psychomotor or psychosensory character. Kristensen and Sindrup (1978a), in a similar comparison, showed that psychotic patients experienced fewer 'psychical' seizures involving disturbance of interpretive functions such as derealisation or hallucinations. Furthermore, a psychological explanation might be plausible for the derivation of delusional symptoms, but it would be hard to account for thought disorder or volitional disturbance on such a basis.

A physiogenic formulation of the link was put forward by Symonds (1962b). In this view, both the epilepsy and the psychosis are manifestations of the same basic disorder of cerebral function within the temporal lobes, the epilepsy being an earlier and intermittent manifestation, and the psychosis a later product. Symonds postulated that this abnormality might consist not so much of the static lesion responsible for the epilepsy, but rather of the disordered electrophysiological activity which spreads within the temporolimbic system. At peaks of such disorder seizures are likely to occur, but the background disturbance may persist in between attacks with far-reaching effects on psychological function. In effect Symonds sug-

gested that 'the temporal lobe includes within its boundaries circuits concerned with the physiological basis of the psychological disorder we call schizophrenia . . . it is not the loss of neurones in the temporal lobe that is responsible for the psychosis, but the disorderly activity of those that remain'.

A not dissimilar formulation, in more modern terms, has been put forward by Stevens (1992). Brain damage is known to provoke regenerative sprouting of axons and synaptic proliferation, even in adults, and resected specimens from patients with temporal lobe epilepsy have shown sprouting of cells in the dentate gyrus and expansion of postsynaptic receptor sites in the parahippocampal gyrus. The functional consequences of such changes are largely unknown, but reorganisation of this nature, as a consequence of insults from seizures, could be associated with the onset of schizophrenia.

A pathogenesis of this nature is supported by the high correlation observed in Slater *et al.*'s material between the ages of onset of epilepsy and of psychosis, suggesting an autonomous developmental tendency liable to produce fits at one stage and psychosis at another. Slater *et al.* suggested that it might be cells in the process of dying which contribute largely to the psychosis, rather than cells which are dead, as indicated by the eventual tendency for the psychosis to subside and its occasional progression to a syndrome of organic deficit.

Further support for a physiogenic link comes from the increasing evidence that site of focus may be significant in relation to liability to psychosis. The indications of a preponderance of left-sided foci have already been discussed (p. 282), this association emerging most clearly when the psychoses resemble classic schizophrenia closely. Kristensen and Sindrup (1978a, 1978b) have emphasised dysfunction deep within the temporal lobes as an important aetiological factor, as revealed by spike foci in the mediobasal temporal regions on sphenoidal recordings. The interesting suggestion has been made that a process akin to 'kindling' (p. 598) might be involved, with progressive and spreading changes occurring within the limbic system as a result of repeated inter-ictal discharges continuing over the years (Livingston 1977). This could be relevant to the long time interval commonly observed between the onset of the epilepsy and of the psychosis.

The relative claims of psychological and physiological explanations remain unresolved in what is clearly a complex pathogenesis. In the meantime the essential conclusions put forward by Slater *et al.* in 1963 should perhaps be allowed to stand—that there is an 'aetiological relationship between the epilepsy, or a pathological process causing epilepsy, and the psychosis. . . . The evidence is however ambiguous in value and insufficient to let us decide on the nature of the relationship, whether the epileptic fits themselves tend to cause the psychosis, or whether the cause of the epilepsy tends to cause the psychosis. . . . Our final conclusion then must be a somewhat inconclusive one. Both the modes of explanation suggested by Pond and by Symonds have evidence in their favour and seem likely to account for at least a part of the observations. Our own tendency is to think the physiogenic causation of the psychosis the more important factor . . .'.

Transient schizophrenia-like episodes

In addition to the chronic psychoses described above, certain transient self-limiting schizophrenia-like episodes may also arise in epileptic patients. It is possible that these may rest on a different pathophysiological basis, and that they should be viewed as a distinct subgroup (Davison & Bagley 1969). It remains to be determined, however, how far such distinctions are valid: overlap may occur, with transitional forms and several subvarieties.

The justification for regarding transient episodes as physiologically distinct lies largely with the work of Landolt, who drew attention to the phenomenon of 'forced normalisation' of the EEG during certain epileptic disturbances. In reporting 107 examples of 'epileptic twilight states and psychotic episodes', he included 47 patients in whom the EEG showed reduction of paroxysmal foci or other epileptic activity during the episode, with subsequent reappearance of the abnormal electrical activity when the psychosis subsided (Landolt 1958). The EEG abnormalities were usually absent altogether while the psychotic manifestations were in evidence. The clinical features witnessed in such episodes were polymorphous, but some examples apparently showed pictures virtually indistinguishable from schizophrenia.

The patients were often restless, noisy and overactive, though some remained composed and seemed only slightly tense. Hallucinations and delusions were prominent. Orientation was normal, or when abnormal this appeared to be due to autistic preoccupation rather than impairment of consciousness. Most remained entirely lucid and with normal clarity of thought processes, though with little awareness of the morbid change within themselves. Some episodes were followed by amnesia, but with others there was normal recollection of the content. They typically lasted for several days or weeks, and fits remained in abeyance throughout the psychotic period. The onset had often followed the institution of anticonvulsant treatment, and cautious discontinuation of medication could frequently be seen to have a beneficial effect. Sometimes the psychotic episode was terminated by an induced fit (electroconvulsive therapy). The

majority of patients had focal temporal lobe epilepsy, but similar pictures could also be observed with other focal seizures or with generalised epilepsy.

Landolt reviewed evidence from other series which supported his observations, and sought to extend his thesis into schizophrenias occurring in non-epileptics. Thus among 42 schizophrenics, spontaneous relapses were often accompanied by normalisation of the EEG, by way of reduction of generalised or focal dysrhythmias which had existed in non-psychotic phases. Remissions of schizophrenia were similarly associated with a return of abnormal rhythms.

Davison and Bagley (1969) referred to other examples of schizophrenia-like psychoses in epileptics which may reflect a process analogous to this – episodes arising shortly after starting a new anticonvulsant drug and subsiding when this was discontinued. Dongier (1959) found an association between paranoid episodes and normalisation of temporal lobe discharges. Others, however, failed to confirm such findings. Glaser et al. (1963) could rarely discern distinct time relationships between EEG changes and psychotic developments, and when present there was usually an increase rather than a decrease in paroxysmal activity.

More recently there has been a revival of interest in the subject, often under the term 'alternative psychosis'. Trimble (1991) describes scattered examples and small recent series from the literature (Pakalnis et al. 1987; Sander et al. 1991). Most cases appear to have set in after recent changes in medication and may reflect the greater effectiveness of the newer anticonvulsants available. Many have occurred in patients suffering from complex partial seizures, but others in patients with primary generalised epilepsy including petit mal (Fischer et al. 1965; Roger et al. 1968; Wolf 1991). Ethosuximide has been implicated in a considerable number of cases.

The possibility that some schizophrenia-like psychoses may bear an antithetical relationship to fit frequency and EEG disturbance could have important implications for treatment. As discussed on p. 279, the existence of this class of disturbance might stand to reconcile the conflicting views about the affinity or antagonism existing between epilepsy and schizophrenia. Certainly it may explain some of the divergent findings in the literature concerning fit frequency prior to the onset of schizophrenia-like psychoses; Pond (1957) and Kristensen and Sindrup (1978a) specifically mention diminished fit frequency in relation to such developments, whereas in Slater et al.'s (1963) large series no clear associations of this nature were observed. Here it may have been significant that the great majority of Slater's cases did not pursue an episodic course.

Reynolds (1967b, 1968) has discussed the possibility that there may be a biochemical contribution to the aetiology of schizophrenia-like psychoses in epileptics. Disturbance of folate or B_{12} metabolism was proposed as playing a part in precipitating such disorders, and it is perhaps in the type of psychosis just discussed that this warrants most careful exploration.

Affective disorder

Affective disorder, and particularly affective psychoses, have been less comprehensively studied in epileptic patients than the schizophrenia-like psychoses discussed above. Disturbance of affect is common in epileptics, but chiefly takes the form of neurotic disorder with fluctuating depression and anxiety. Others show periodic 'dysphoria', in the form of episodes of irritability and aggressiveness (Lorentz de Haas & Magnus 1958). A clear distinction is not always made between such pictures and depressive psychosis, so the prevalence of the latter is uncertain. Furthermore short-lived depressive or hypomanic episodes may be labelled as manic–depressive when in fact they represent post-ictal confusional states or automatisms with only minor disturbance of consciousness.

Nevertheless, clear-cut examples of affective psychosis do occur, depressive episodes being commoner than hypomania. Among 72 epileptic patients admitted to psychiatric hospitals Betts (1974) found that almost a third were suffering primarily from depressive illnesses, 12 being endogenous in type and 10 being reactive in nature. Moreover, a significant relationship was observed between decline in fit frequency prior to admission and the onset of endogenous depression.

Apart from the possible relationship to declining fit frequency, few special associations or unique characteristics have been described for affective disorder. Betts (1981) reported a clinical impression that the onset and remission of depression both tend to be sudden in epileptic patients, also that the mood disorder may fluctuate quite markedly while present. Serafetinides and Falconer (1962b) suggested that paranoid features were often found in association with psychotic depression, sometimes with an alternation between the paranoid and affective manifestations. As yet, however, firm evidence for such distinctive features has not been forthcoming.

Robertson has provided a detailed account of 66 patients referred to hospital with diagnoses of both epilepsy and depression (Robertson 1983, 1985; Robertson & Trimble 1983). The depression was judged to be endogenous in type in 40%, and 13 of the 66 were 'psychotic' as defined by the presence of mood-congruent hallucinations or delusions. Characteristics of the depression included high scores on anxiety, neuroticism, hostility and feelings of depersonalisation as reflected in questionnaire responses, and there was a suggestion that the duration of epilepsy correlated with the severity of the depression. More than half of the patients had a family history of psychiatric illness, mainly depressive in nature. Patients receiving phenobarbitone were significantly more depressed than the remainder, while those receiving carbamazepine were less so. The serum and red cell folate levels were significantly lower than in a control population. No clear relationship emerged, however, between depression and age of onset of epilepsy, seizure type or frequency, or site of focus on the EEG. The overall results thus combined to suggest that the depression was not directly interlinked with epileptic variables themselves, but was more likely to be the outcome of multiple factors operating in genetically predisposed individuals.

Toone *et al.* (1982b), in a retrospective survey, again found little support for a special relationship between affective psychoses and epilepsy. Nineteen patients who had received the combined diagnoses were compared with non-epileptic manic–depressive controls. The epileptic depressives often lacked convincing psychotic features, and objective scoring procedures (Catego diagnoses derived from the Syndrome Check List) indicated that half had probably been improperly labelled. Electroconvulsive therapy and lithium had rarely been prescribed, and only three of the 19 epileptics had shown bipolar illnesses. In this material the conjunction of affective psychosis and epilepsy was therefore judged to represent no more than a chance association.

In clinical practice affective and schizoaffective psychoses may be considerably more common than purely schizophrenic disorders (Fenton 1978). This seems rarely to be reflected in published reports, perhaps because many affective episodes are fleeting and relatively mild in degree. In Dongier's (1959) large series of transient psychotic episodes 30% showed change of affect as the predominant feature, compared to 56% with predominant change of consciousness and 10% with schizophrenia-like features. Depressive episodes were more closely related to temporal lobe epilepsy than to other varieties. Among patients who come to temporal lobectomy, affective psychoses have again been rather commoner than schizophrenia-like psychoses, though here the selection of cases may have contributed to the result (James 1960; Serafetinides & Falconer 1962b). Hypomanic and manic psychoses rarely appear to be reported in epileptic patients. Wolf (1982) reviews the cases in the literature and reports six additional patients, five of them suffering from temporal lobe epilepsy. The more recent reports of hypomania developing in the wake of seizures are described on p. 258.

Flor-Henry (1969) presented a detailed comparison between affective and other forms of psychosis in a series of 50 patients with temporal lobe epilepsy. These comprised all the cases admitted to the Maudsley Hospital over a 15-year period with a combined diagnosis of temporal lobe epilepsy and psychosis. Nine were diagnosed as manic–depressive, on the basis of elation or depression which exhibited periodicity and left the personality intact between phases; 11 were schizoaffective, showing features of both schizophrenia and affective disturbance; 21 showed schizophrenia-like psychoses; and nine showed an organic picture dominated by disorientation and clouding of consciousness. The manic–depressive and schizoaffective psychoses lasted on average several months, compared to several years for the schizophrenia-like psychoses and several weeks for the confusional psychoses. The patients with manic–depressive psychoses showed more stable previous personalities and better marital and occupational adjustment than the other groups. They also tended to have less frequent seizures than the others, and the fits that occurred were usually grand mal rather than psychomotor in type. Manic–depressive and schizoaffective patients showed a lower incidence of structural brain damage than those with schizophrenic or confusional psychoses.

A potentially interesting finding in Flor-Henry's series was that the manic–depressive patients showed a preponderance of foci in the right temporal lobe, whereas the schizophrenia-like and confusional groups had an excess of left temporal lobe involvement. There was a suggestion that the schizoaffective group might be transitional in this regard. However, while the association between schizophrenia-like psychoses and left-sided foci has received substantial support (p. 282), affective psychoses have emerged in other series as independent of laterality (Robertson 1983, 1985; Perez et al. 1985). Gregoriadis et al. (1971) seem to be alone in confirming a predominantly right-sided pathology among psychotic epileptics with affective symptomatology.

Suicide and epilepsy

Several studies have indicated that the suicide rate is higher among epileptics than in the general population. Prudhomme (1941) gathered data on an estimated 75 000 epileptic patients by contacting physicians and institutions in the USA. Sixty-seven deaths had occurred by suicide, which was considered greatly in excess of expectation. At one colony in New York it was estimated that the incidence was twice that of the general population,

or five times greater when the figures were corrected for age.

Henriksen et al. (1970) produced a more definitive study from Denmark. A representative sample of all adult epileptics discharged from four neurological clinics was traced, and the cause of death ascertained from death certificates. One hundred and sixty-four deaths had occurred among 2763 patients, which was 2.5–3 times the number to be expected. The mortality was higher among the mentally abnormal epileptics than the remainder. After excluding patients with other diseases likely to have reduced life expectancy, 20% of the deaths were due to suicide, representing three times the number that could have been predicted.

White et al. (1979) produced further striking figures. Some 2000 patients admitted to the Chalfont Centre for Epilepsy between 1931 and 1971 were followed up to the end of 1977, and their mortality rates compared with expected values from English life tables. Of 425 deaths, 21 were due to suicide, compared to an expected value of less than four. Reviewing this and other studies Barraclough (1981) concluded that the risk of suicide is increased approximately fivefold among epileptic patients; moreover four investigations relevant to temporal lobe epilepsy concurred in showing the highest risk of all, with suicide some 25 times above expectation.

Suicide attempts, as opposed to successful suicide, also appear to be especially common. Delay et al. (1957) found that almost a third of a large series of epileptics, either hospitalised for treatment or detained on criminal charges, had made suicide attempts. In more than half of the cases there had been multiple attempts. Gunn (1973), comparing epileptic prisoners with matched controls from the prison population, found a higher frequency of suicide attempts in the previous history, and a higher prevalence of suicidal feelings at interview.

In studies of patients presenting with self poisoning or self injury, Mackay (1979) in Glasgow and Hawton et al. (1980) in Oxford both found that epileptic patients were over-represented some 5–7-fold when viewed against the prevalence of epilepsy in the community. Both observed, moreover, that repeated attempts were more common than in non-epileptic patients. Mackay found that two-thirds of the epileptics used their current antiepileptic medication in the suicide attempts. In Hawton et al.'s series the attempted suicide rate was twice as high in epileptic men as in women, perhaps reflecting special psychosocial handicaps imposed by epilepsy in men.

Investigation and differential diagnosis

In the majority of cases a carefully taken history leaves

little doubt about the epileptic nature of attacks, especially when an adequate account is available from witnesses. Enquiry must always be made into the circumstances of attacks, the details of their commencement, the subjective sensations felt by the patient and the disturbed behaviour witnessed by others. Seizures of petit mal or grand mal type are usually readily identified, though more difficulty is likely to be encountered with complex partial seizures. In the presence of undoubted epilepsy the aims must be to reach conclusions concerning the type of epilepsy and its focus of origin within the brain, and to elucidate possible causes for the seizures. This will almost always require the undertaking of certain ancillary investigations as described below.

It is only in a minority of patients that diagnostic difficulties arise, but it may then be necessary to embrace a wide range of possibilities other than epilepsy itself. Indeed Slater and Roth (1969) suggest that the differential diagnosis of epilepsy can be one of the most complex problems in medicine. Problems of diagnosis are likely to be particularly great among patients who come before the psychiatrist, since very often they will have been referred to him because the attacks are of an unusual type, or because a disturbed mental state has raised the question of a psychogenic component to the seizures. Here, again, ancillary investigations may be indispensable, but as in many other areas of psychiatry the cornerstone for differential diagnosis will usually rest on a full and detailed history, coupled with careful clinical examination and close observation of behaviour. Observation may need to be prolonged and on an in-patient basis, especially when differentiation is required from hysteria, personality disorder or other psychiatric conditions.

Investigation of known epileptic attacks

It must be re-emphasised that epilepsy is to be regarded as a symptom and not as a disease entity on its own. Consequently every effort must be made to determine the underlying cause. In some patients this will remain elusive, but in others a structural or biochemical basis may be revealed. Obviously the extent to which investigations are pursued in the individual case will depend on the likelihood in the mind of the physician that a responsible pathology is to be discovered. Increased age at the time of the first attack will increase the chance that a cerebral lesion may be responsible. Associated symptoms, such as headache, or associated neurological signs or evidence of systemic disturbance will similarly dictate more rigorous investigation.

Another important factor in guiding the extent of investigation is the type of epileptic attack that occurs. In cases of simple absence attacks it will rarely be necessary to pursue a search for structural pathology; with grand mal one will need to be more cautious, and most careful of all with focal attacks. In making these distinctions the information provided by the EEG can be invaluable when viewed in conjunction with evidence from other sources.

The type of epilepsy from which the patient suffers also has implications for treatment (p. 300 *et seq.*). Particular care must be taken to distinguish between absence attacks and brief automatisms of temporal lobe origin, since each will respond to different anticonvulsant medication.

Falconer and Taylor (1970) particularly stress the importance of recognizing temporal lobe attacks in children. If diagnosed as petit mal absences, ethosuximide would be ineffective, and if diagnosed as grand mal and treated with phenobarbitone the associated behavioural abnormalities could be worsened. Here the history and observation of attacks may sometimes be the sole basis for the correct diagnosis, since the EEG may show little to support the temporal lobe origin until many years later. Young children will often fail to verbalise their auras, but may produce giveaway signs such as clutching the abdomen and flexing the hips in pain (epigastric aura), flying to their mother (fear), or show obvious borborigmi, drooling, pallor or flushing.

Some patients who suffer from generalised convulsions will prove to have a focal discharge limited to one temporal lobe, raising the possibility of surgical treatment. Conversely the EEG may reveal multiple foci of origin, effectively precluding surgery even though medication has achieved only poor control.

In searching for the cause of the epilepsy, the *clinical history* will usually be of first importance. Genetic factors may be obvious from the family history. Enquiry must be made for known difficulties surrounding the patient's birth, a history of febrile convulsions in childhood or illnesses suggestive of encephalitis. Any history of head injury must be carefully evaluated with regard to severity and timing in relation to the onset of the epilepsy. Enquiry must always be made for headache or other possible indications of cerebral tumour. Abuse of alcohol or drugs will sometimes be suspected. In older patients a history of even minor cerebral infarction may be relevant, or indications may be obtained of cerebral degenerative disease.

In the *clinical examination* attention will be directed primarily towards the central nervous system, with a search for focal neurological signs or indications of raised intracranial pressure. Slight inequalities in the size of limbs or hands may provide the clue to brain damage dating from early life. General medical assessment is essential, particularly when metabolic disease is suspected. In older patients the possibility of secondary cerebral malignancy must be borne in mind.

Investigations will usually include the routines of blood

count, erythrocyte sedimentation rate, serological tests for syphilis, urine examination and chest X-ray. The possibilities of hypoglycaemia, uraemia, hypocalcaemia and drug abuse may occasionally require appropriate exploration. In all cases a skull X-ray and EEG will normally be performed. A CT or MRI scan will be carried out where facilities are available, and will be specially indicated in certain situations as described below. Prolonged EEG recording by telemetry or ambulatory monitoring can give valuable information in specially selected patients (see below).

The *skull X-ray* may show displacement of the pineal body or calcification within a glial hamartoma or angioma. In temporal lobe epilepsy it may be of lateralising value, showing a slightly smaller middle cranial fossa on the affected side when the lesion dates from early life.

The *electroencephalogram* is often indispensable for determining the type of epilepsy and its source of origin within the brain. Its value can be paramount in the following situations (Parsonage 1973) — when seizures are habitually generalised and there is no indication of their site of origin; when they have no lateralising features as in many temporal lobe attacks; if there is more than one source of seizure discharge; and when the clinical description of the seizures does not permit accurate or reliable localisation. It can be of practical value in management, as mentioned above, in distinguishing absence attacks from brief temporal lobe seizures. In addition, the EEG may show abnormalities of background activity which indicate something of the underlying cause. A structural lesion such as a tumour will be suspected when there is a local decrease in background activity or a delta wave focus, and metabolic derangements may be indicated by slowing of the dominant rhythm or generalised disorganisation with runs of theta activity.

These should be regarded as the principal uses of the EEG in epilepsy. It may also help towards deciding whether or not epilepsy is present, but as discussed in Chapter 3 (p. 129) its value here is limited in certain important ways. A normal EEG can never be accepted as excluding epilepsy or a causative lesion, and the recognition of epilepsy remains essentially a clinical matter whatever the EEG may or may not show.

Clinical studies have not supported the common assumption that records obtained while the patient is on anticonvulsants are less liable to disclose epileptic activity (Marsan & Zivin 1970). It is therefore not necessary routinely to discontinue medication prior to the recording, although in cases where the EEG is normal and the diagnosis still in doubt it may sometimes be reasonable to reduce or gradually stop anticonvulsants before repeating the examination (Gibberd 1973). Activating techniques can be of considerable value, light sleep for example revealing a temporal lobe focus when the waking EEG has been within normal limits. Sphenoidal or foramen ovale recordings may be indicated for more precise localisation of discharges originating in the medial temporal lobe structures. More invasive explorations such as depth electrode recording or even electrocorticography may be required if surgical treatment is envisaged.

EEG telemetry has established itself as especially useful in the investigation of bizarre or unusual attacks, enabling a more reliable differentiation between epileptic and non-epileptic seizures (Binnie *et al.* 1981; Fenwick 1981b; Cull *et al.* 1982). In patients with refractory epilepsy it can yield more precise information about seizure type, thus permitting improved pharmacological control (Sutula *et al.* 1981). Other advantages are in increasing the detection rate of inter-ictal seizure discharges, in locating a possible focus, in monitoring the effects of anticonvulsant treatment or in identifying possible factors which trigger attacks.

A variety of systems are in use, predominantly in special centres. For recordings over the course of some hours or even days the patient occupies a special room or suite of rooms, the EEG being transmitted to the recording apparatus by a light flexible cable or radio transmission. The former is less prone to artefacts. Closed-circuit television or video monitoring of the patient's behaviour allows any change or ictus to be viewed in relation to the accompanying EEG pattern by split-screen display. The patient or the observer can be equipped with a button to allow storage of epochs of special significance.

Even when artefacts obscure the EEG during the course of an actual seizure, review of the record may reveal spiking immediately preceding it or slowing or asymmetry of the record as an aftermath. Conversely, the presence of well-marked alpha rhythm in an apparently unconscious patient following a substantial seizure will strongly suggest that this was an hysterical or simulated attack. Overnight studies, using an infrared camera, may clarify the distinction between nocturnal seizures, nightmares and night terrors.

For more prolonged recordings in the patient's home or in special situations a portable cassette recorder can be used. The EEG and other physiological parameters can then be monitored while the patient is fully ambulant and engaged in normal activities. An event marker is used by the patient to draw attention to periods of special significance. Such a system lacks the advantage of simultaneous video monitoring and the number of channels is limited, but it has proved useful in searching for epileptic activity over prolonged periods of time and in differing situations. With petit mal, particularly, it may allow precise monitoring of the effects of different treatment regimens.

Neuroimaging has proved invaluable in the detection of structural cerebral abnormalities in patients with epilepsy. CT or MRI are obviously indicated whenever a space-occupying lesion is remotely suspected, and should ideally be carried out in all patients when there is clinical or EEG evidence of a focal onset to the attacks. Beyond this, where access to scanning is limited, patients will be selected when the epilepsy has begun only in late adolescence or adult life, or when patients are being considered for surgery.

Surveys have demonstrated the yield and range of abnormalities likely to be encountered by CT scanning in various groups of patients (Gastaut 1976; Gastaut & Gastaut 1976). Those with primary generalised epilepsy, whether grand mal or petit mal, show the lowest incidence of changes at some 10% or less; primary and secondary generalised grand mal seizures considered together show abnormalities in 39–63% of cases from one series to another; and patients with focal (partial) seizures show the highest incidence of all, often in excess of 60%. Altogether, abnormalities may be expected in approximately a third to a half of any large series of epileptic patients.

Rather more than half of the abnormal findings will be atrophic changes, and some 10% space-occupying lesions. In Gastaut and Gastaut's (1976) series the incidence of tumours rose from 11% overall, to 16% when the epilepsy had begun after the age of 20, to 23% in partial epilepsies with complex symptomatology, and to 49% in partial epilepsies with elementary symptomatology. In 80% of cases the tumours had previously been unsuspected, and 11% had been missed on skull X-ray. Bauer *et al.* (1980) confined attention to focal epilepsies after excluding patients with known space-occupying lesions or progressive neurological disease; 5% were found to have slow-growing tumours and some 50% other lesions, mainly the residue of perinatal, post-traumatic or postinfective brain damage. The correspondence between CT and EEG evidence of focal disorder was in general high but by no means complete, an important number of EEG foci lacking a CT scan counterpart and vice versa.

CT scanning may occasionally show small well-demarcated enhancing cortical lesions shortly after ictal activity, which disappear spontaneously or in response to treatment of the seizures. Typically the abnormality disappears within several weeks or months. This has been reported with remarkable frequency in India, where the balance of evidence has suggested cysticercosis as the cause (Wadia *et al.* 1987; Bansal *et al.* 1989; Rajshekhar & Abraham 1990). Isolated tuberculomas are another possibility. Kennedy and Schon (1991) have reported four similar cases from the UK, all with negative investigations for infection in the blood and cerebrospinal fluid. Feinstein *et al.* (1990) describe two further patients in whom the scan abnormality was associated with psychiatric disturbance. In some examples, detected shortly after seizures, local brain changes due to hypoxia and/or oedema may be responsible. This seemed to be the mechanism in the examples reported by Goulatia *et al.* (1987) in patients with no evidence of cysticercosis or tuberculoma; the maximal radiological change lay in the area of maximal epileptic discharge and sometimes reappeared with recurrence of the ictus.

The superior definition afforded by MRI gives many advantages over CT (Lesser *et al.* 1986; Kuzniecky *et al.* 1987; Andermann 1994). The yield of lesions responsible for epilepsy is higher, including small tumours and areas of cortical dysplasia too small to be visualised otherwise. Focal areas of cortical atrophy on CT may prove to represent tumour tissue, and this may be more extensive than was previously apparent. In temporal lobe epilepsy, coronal MRI images yield extra information, allowing close comparison of temporal horn asymmetries and often visualizing hippocampal shrinkage directly. In mesial temporal lobe sclerosis T_1 images show the loss of grey matter in the hippocampal formation, while T_2 sequences display increased signal activity due to reactive gliosis (Berkovic *et al.* 1994). Cook *et al.* (1992) have described a method for estimating three-dimensional hippocampal volume from MRI scans, permitting accurate comparison between the two sides and assessment of focal involvement of the hippocampus throughout its length.

PET and SPECT scanning can add additional information. Inter-ictal hypometabolic areas shown by FDG-PET correlate well with the epileptic focus as revealed by EEG or histological examination of resected material, though often exceeding the area of anatomical abnormality (Engel *et al.* 1982a, 1982b). Greater precision may be obtained by ligand studies of benzodiazepine binding as a marker of GABA receptor sites, this being reduced in the area of the epileptic focus (Savic *et al.* 1988). SPECT scans can also be of value (Costa & Ell 1991). In Ryding *et al.*'s (1988) survey, hexamethylpropyleneamineoxine (HMPAO)-SPECT was almost as sensitive as the EEG in detecting epileptic foci, and significantly better than CT or MRI. Low uptake areas were seen inter-ictally, and hyper-perfused areas during ictal studies. Duncan *et al.* (1990) confirmed the value of SPECT as an adjunct to other investigations in determining the laterality of temporal lobe foci. Ictal SPECT studies seem to be particularly useful in this regard, and the simplicity of the procedure makes its use for such purposes a realistic possibility (Lancet 1989). HMPAO, for example, can be injected when the patient has a seizure, and the scan performed later to show where the increased uptake has been fixed within the brain. It is likely that such functional imaging techniques will contribute increasingly in the selection of patients for surgical treatment, and may obviate the need for depth electrode studies in many cases.

Neuroimaging techniques and the EEG thus complement each other in the investigation of epilepsy. The former may reveal the location and often the nature of associated cerebral lesions, whereas the latter remains the only technique for demonstrating the epileptic character of the disorder. Since the advent of neuroimaging other investigative procedures have receded greatly in importance. If no abnormality is shown on plain skull X-ray or neuroimaging it is unlikely that further radiological studies will reveal significant findings in patients with well-controlled epilepsy and no other symptoms. *Angiography* may, nevertheless, be indicated in special situations, as when a vascular malformation is suspected. *Lumbar puncture* is rarely employed in the investigation of epilepsy, but may occasionally be helpful in excluding conditions such as encephalitis or neurosyphilis.

Psychometry is often helpful as a further guide to localisation, and in particular for confirming the laterality of a temporal lobe focus. Assessment of the patient's intellectual capabilities will help in judging possibilities for employment or rehabilitation, and serve as a general guide to management. Establishing a reliable baseline of intellectual performance will be particularly important in any patient who is suspected of gradual intellectual decline.

The investigations described above may need to be repeated from time to time when the initial evaluation has given negative results. The need to reopen enquiry will be indicated particularly when seizures increase in frequency or severity at a later stage, or if signs of intellectual or personality deterioration set in.

Finally, *serum prolactin estimations* will often prove of value when uncertainty surrounds the genuinely epileptic nature of attacks. After generalised tonic–clonic seizures the serum prolactin rises sharply to a peak at 20 minutes, returning to baseline levels after approximately 1 hour. No such effect was observed in a group of patients with hysteria whose major attacks had previously been diagnosed as epilepsy (Trimble 1978). With partial seizures the rise is less pronounced, particularly in the case of simple partial seizures where the estimation is unlikely to be of value.

Dana-Haeri *et al.* (1983) recommend taking blood for prolactin estimation 20 minutes after an attack, then again at 1 hour to check that baseline levels had been within the normal range (100–360 mU/l). After generalised tonic–clonic seizures they observed a rise at 20 minutes to more than 1000 mU/l in 60% of patients, and to more than 500 mU/l in 96% of patients. Rises in excess of 500 mU/l after supposedly complex partial seizures can be regarded as highly suggestive that the attack was epileptic. The phenomenon appears to be related to central stimulation of the hypothalamic–pituitary axis

during the epileptic seizure; equivalent rises are seen in non-epileptic patients following electroconvulsive therapy carried out with full muscular relaxation under anaesthesia. Rao *et al.* (1989) have demonstrated similar transient elevation of other pituitary hormones and of cortisol.

Diagnostic possibilities other than epilepsy

A number of conditions which lead to intermittent disturbance of cerebral function may be mistaken for epilepsy—for example syncope, hypoglycaemia, transient cerebral ischaemia and occasionally migraine. Various psychiatric disorders can also resemble certain epileptic manifestations and vice versa. Here hysteria takes pride of place, but diagnostic difficulties can also be encountered with anxiety attacks, certain schizophrenic manifestations and short-lived acute organic reactions. Special problems may surround the diagnosis of epileptic automatisms, in particular their distinction from outbursts of violence in patients of unstable personality. These and related matters are discussed below.

Paroxysmal disorders of cerebral function resembling epilepsy

The classic *vasovagal attack* or *syncope* is usually readily distinguished from epilepsy by its setting. The subject is typically standing or has just risen to his feet when fainting occurs. In some instances an acutely upsetting experience may be the precipitant, or pain or an injection. The onset tends to be more gradual than with epilepsy, with a feeling of faintness, dizziness or darkening of vision leading directly into loss of consciousness. Unconsciousness is accompanied by pallor, a slow pulse and general flaccidity. When cerebral hypoperfusion is prolonged there may be stiffening or twitching movements which are hard to distinguish from seizures, but they lack the typical tonic–clonic sequence (Riley 1982). Incontinence or tongue biting are very rare indeed. Recovery is prompt after a minute or two, whereas after a fit there may be sleep or gradual recovery through a phase of confusion. Memory is intact up to the point where consciousness was lost, whereas an epileptic fit may be followed by a brief period of retrograde amnesia.

Diagnostic difficulty is more likely to be encountered with so-called 'micturition syncope', in which the patient gets out of bed to void urine, faints due to postural hypotension and is then incontinent due to fullness of the bladder. Very occasionally, moreover, the cerebral ischaemia responsible for syncope may trigger a true convulsive attack.

EEG studies have discounted any pathophysiological relationship between syncope and epilepsy (Gastaut & Fischer-Williams 1957). The loss of consciousness in syncope is accompanied by slow activity in the EEG, or in longer attacks by a period of electrical silence which resolves when consciousness is regained. Thus, while in epilepsy the cortex is functionally active, in syncope it is electrically silent. On recovery there is none of the generalised slow activity in the EEG that may persist for several hours after resolution of a grand mal attack.

Hyperventilation (p. 562), common in states of anxiety or stress, can actually precipitate a seizure. Short of this the induced tetany may cause spasms or shaking in the extremities, and this can be sudden in onset resembling an epileptic attack. Focal paraesthesias, dizziness and feelings of unreality may likewise mimic seizures. Riley (1982) suggests that syncope and hyperventilation are probably the most common episodic disorders of consciousness to be confused with epilepsy. Differentiation can on occasion only be made by witnessing or provoking a characteristic attack.

Stokes–Adams attacks may lead to repeated episodes of impaired consciousness, with or without convulsions. These can be hard to diagnose because the change in cardiac rhythm may be abrupt and transient. Usually, however, the electrocardiogram will reveal conduction defects or abnormal rhythms even between attacks. Schott *et al.* (1977) have reported 10 patients referred to hospital as possible cases of idiopathic epilepsy whose symptoms appeared to derive largely from various cardiac dysrhythmias. Many were relatively young, and the dysrhythmias were sometimes only apparent after prolonged electrocardiogram monitoring. *Aortic stenosis* may similarly lead to sudden episodes of unconsciousness.

Hypoglycaemic attacks can simulate epilepsy closely. The periods of confused and abnormal behaviour are easily mistaken for epileptic automatisms. Characteristic features of faintness, sweating, palpitations, tremor or dizziness should immediately raise suspicion. Occasionally true petit mal, grand mal or focal seizures may be provoked.

Transient cerebral ischaemic attacks, when brief, can produce symptoms very similar to focal epilepsy (Gibberd 1973). Attacks may start suddenly, develop, and then regress over a period of several minutes or sometimes hours. Usually, however, motor symptoms are of a positive kind in epilepsy, whereas in transient cerebral ischaemia paralysis is the rule. Considerable uncertainty may arise when motor weakness persists after a focal epileptic attack (Todd's paralysis). Usually this lasts for only a few hours; when persisting longer it is likely to have resulted from cerebral ischaemia or a localised structural lesion.

Migraine leads to positive symptoms as in epilepsy, usually in the form of visual disturbance of a highly characteristic kind. Other sensory phenomena may, however, be encountered and lead to a suspicion of epilepsy. The associated headache usually allows a distinction, but in some attacks this may be lacking. Syncopal manifestations may occasionally occur. Even so the history will usually be decisive in revealing typical migraine at other times. Special difficulty can arise with occipital seizures when auras consist of elementary visual hallucinations. However, the hallucinations of epilepsy are usually brief (less than 3 minutes) and are predominantly multi-coloured with spherical patterns, wheras those of migraine seldom last less than 3 minutes and are mainly black and white with linear or zigzag patterns (Panayiotopoulos *et al.* 1997). Difficulty may also be encountered in the rare migrainous attacks associated with amnesia, lasting sometimes for several hours then clearing gradually (Moersch 1924; Nielsen 1958). These can arise during attacks of visual disturbance and headache, or as a variant of classic attacks (p. 406). Brief automatisms are also said to occur in certain migrainous attacks (p. 407).

Musical hallucinations can occur as part of an epileptic aura, but in Keshavan *et al.*'s (1992) review this appeared to be an uncommon cause. The commonest associated feature was deafness, usually of long standing and sensorineural in origin (26 cases), while other patients had coarse brain lesions (22 cases) or a primary psychiatric illness (11 cases). It emerged that the hallucinations did not represent a unitary phenomenon, two or more of the three risk factors quite often existing together.

Typically the onset was abrupt, with the patient hearing songs or instrumental music for varying periods of time, ranging from repetitive short musical phrases to virtually constant elaborate musical hallucinations. Females preponderated and most patients were middle aged or elderly. Interestingly, a considerable proportion heard songs or music dating from early childhood. Many could alter the tempo or change the tune at will, but none could abolish the hallucinations voluntarily.

Paroxysmal choreoathetosis is a rare condition, sometimes familial, which appears to incorporate features both of convulsive disorder and extrapyramidal dyskinesia. Opinion is divided over whether it should be regarded as a form of reflex epilepsy (Lishman *et al.* 1962; Lishman & Whitty 1965; Stevens 1966a) or whether it is essentially a disorder of the extrapyramidal motor system (Rosen 1964). Alexander (1982b) and Fahn (1994a) have drawn together the literature on this interesting condition.

Short paroxysms of tonic posturing or choreiform and athetoid movements are provoked by sudden movement, as when the patient rises quickly from a chair or abruptly accelerates his pace while walking or running. Attacks last no more than a minute or two and may be unilateral or generalised, involving the limbs, trunk and face. Sudden startle or surprise may often induce the paroxysms. In a subgroup similar attacks occur spontaneously, then tending to be more prolonged and less frequent. A vague sensory aura, or a feeling of tightness in the limb of origin, may precede attacks. Many episodes are commonly aborted by slackening the pace or standing still. Awareness of the environment is generally fully retained throughout.

In most examples the condition is idiopathic or familial, setting in during childhood or adolescence, affecting males predominantly and proving to be a significant social embarrassment. Gradual amelioration is usually seen as the patient gets older. A good response to anticonvulsants, particularly to phenytoin, has been observed in the majority of cases described, even though the EEG may show little by way of paroxysmal features. Occasional examples are symptomatic, following multiple sclerosis or head injury, or occurring in the context of idiopathic hypoparathyroidism (Fahn 1994a).

Hyperekplexia ('startle disease') is another rare condition, often familial, though sporadic cases are also reported. Andermann *et al.* (1980) describe three examples and review accounts of the disorder. Matsumoto and Hallett (1994) describe the more recent literature. In essence it represents a greatly exaggerated response to startle, even to minor stimuli, to the extent that the patient loses his balance and falls. It is now apparent that many cases result from dominant mutations in the α_1 subunit of the glycine receptor gene on chromosome 5 (Andrew & Owen 1997). A recessive mutation in the same gene has been described in a sporadic example.

There is no associated loss of consciousness but self injury is common. The patient freezes as he falls, with the arms held stiffly at the sides, and thus cannot protect himself. The minor form shows the startle response alone. In the major form there are a number of associated features: hyperreflexia, repetitive jerking of the limbs, chiefly at night, and a peculiar insecure gait. In addition the major form often carries a history of generalised hypertonia in infancy, in response to handling or awakening, which gradually recedes during the first year of life. From the time of learning to walk the child then tends to fall on account of momentary periods of generalised muscular stiffness in response to noise or startle.

The course thereafter is variable, some patients gradually improving while others tend to worsen. The drugs of choice in treatment appear to be clonazepam and sodium valproate (Andermann *et al.* 1990). Clonazepam can greatly reduce the falling attacks and jerking though the startle response may not return to normal. Moreover, the patient may be left with secondary handicaps by way of depression, or anxiety (including agoraphobia) due to fear of falling (Andrew & Owen 1997).

The EEG between attacks is essentially normal, but a distinctive response is seen to startle. An initial spike is recorded from the centroparieto-occipital regions, followed by a brief train of slow waves, then desynchronised background activity lasting for 2–3 seconds.

Many cases are liable to be diagnosed as epileptic when first encountered, especially since a family history of epilepsy is not uncommon. Others are regarded as suffering from states of heightened anxiety. However, there is little to suggest an epileptic basis for the condition. The essential pathophysiology would seem to lie with a disorder of motor control, perhaps by way of impaired maturation of higher inhibitory centres over lower motor mechanisms.

Epilepsy versus 'pseudoseizures'

The recognition of hysteria as a cause of seizures resembling epilepsy has a long history, as outlined by Trimble (1986). Hysterical seizures and 'hysteroepilepsy' were the focus of intense interest by Charcot and his school at the Salpêtrière during the 19th century, and became influential in the elaboration of theories about hypnosis. In typical cases so-called 'stigmata' were often in evidence—areas of anaesthesia, narrowing of the visual fields or monocular polyopia.

Nowadays hysterical manifestations which take the form of major convulsions appear to be less common than formerly. Problems of differentiation between the two disorders centre more often on episodes of simple loss of consciousness, or episodes of disturbed behaviour followed by amnesia. The classic stigmata are more rarely elicited, and the hysterical basis of such attacks is often called into question. Some seem to be based primarily on anxiety, and others to represent aspects of abnormal illness behaviour with a variety of complex determinants. The term 'hysteria' has therefore gradually been replaced in favour of 'pseudoseizures', 'psychogenic seizures' or 'non-epileptic attack disorder'. This last is the label preferred by Betts who divides such attacks into several subvarieties (Betts 1990, 1993; Betts & Boden 1992):

Those accompanied by falling with apparent unconsciousness and convulsions may be due to hysteria or more rarely simulation. The vigorous body movements represent the lay concept of epilepsy and rarely look like tonic–clonic seizures. More often there is rigid extension of the limbs and incoordinated thrashing movements which may transport the patient across the room. Breathing is not suspended and is often noisy and gasping. With true hysteria there may be hemianaesthesia or other classic signs.

'Abreactive attacks' represent another convulsive form. After a period of overbreathing the body stiffens, then becomes involved in incoordinated jerking, characteristically with arching of the back and pelvic thrusting. The picture may closely resemble the movements of sexual intercourse. Attacks of this nature occurred in over 20% of the patients with non-epileptic attack disorder in Betts' series, and seemed often to occur in women who had previously suffered sexual abuse.

A third variety consists of 'tantrums', leading to sudden collapse with convulsions. This often starts noisily with a scream. The patient then throws himself to the ground with kicking or screaming and may bite himself or others. Such attacks tend to occur in the mentally or socially handicapped and resemble a childhood tantrum. They are typically the result of feeling frustrated or angry, and represent a form of 'acting out behaviour'.

Among non-convulsive attacks there are emotionally induced syncope, hyperventilation accompanying panic attacks leading sometimes to loss of consciousness, and the classic 'swoon'. In this last the patient abruptly withdraws from reality, closes the eyes and sinks to the floor, lying passively inert, often with a characteristic flickering of the eyelids. Such attacks may be long lasting, with the patient unrousable to vigorous stimulation. They represent 'cutting off behaviour'. Usually they are not consciously motivated, but serve as escape from environmental stress or unpleasant obtrusive thoughts.

In very rare cases attacks may be seen as part of Munchausen's syndrome. Savard et al. (1988) report a young woman who had been admitted to over 25 hospitals on account of seizures or status epilepticus, eventually admitting that she had mimicked her epilepsy by copying a school mate and reading medical texts.

A major difficulty in clinical assessment is that pseudoseizures and epilepsy do not preclude each other; there will sometimes be an admixture of the two, with psychogenic disturbances appearing against a background of cerebral disease. In consequence it is important to follow very carefully any patient whose attacks do not appear at first sight to have an organic basis.

It is estimated, indeed, that some 5% of genuinely epileptic patients are also liable to develop pseudoseizures at some point in their course (Scott 1982a). Occasionally it will appear that improved control of the epilepsy by medication provokes the appearance of classic pseudoseizures, the balance reverting again once the drugs are decreased (Trimble 1982). This paradoxical effect may reflect the patient's need to maintain his dependence on the family, or alternatively a liability to psychogenic reactions may have been exacerbated by some degree of intoxication with the anticonvulsant drugs.

It is unlikely, moreover, that in the last analysis the distinction between epileptic seizures and pseudoseizures is always absolute. Physiogenic or psychogenic influences will be seen to operate exclusively in a large proportion of cases, but in some the two will be inextricably combined.

Krapf (1957) has traced the recent history of our conceptions in this area. In the 1920s the differentiation between epilepsy and hysteria seemed to offer no difficulty. Epilepsy was the term for attacks which had an elementary or strictly 'neurological' character, and hysteria the term for attacks which contained elaborate and psychologically meaningful symptomatology. Even at that time some problem cases were noted, but the basic notion persisted that epilepsy and hysteria were different diseases between which no transition could exist. In part this attitude was born out of opposition to Charcot's concept of 'hysteroepilepsy'.

The EEG, however, failed to corroborate so firm a distinction, and correlations between type of attack and abnormalities of record were soon found to be imperfect. The recognition of psychomotor seizures did still more to dispel so clear-cut a view. Seizures clearly related to neuronal discharges were found to go far beyond what could clinically be considered as elementary and 'epileptic'. Pronounced instability of personality was found to characterise some patients with clearly organic seizures, and the role of psychologically disturbing situations in provoking epileptic attacks became recognised increasingly.

Krapf suggested that all 'epileptiform' seizures should be regarded as the outcome of an interplay between stress and predisposition, in which both of these factors were of a multifactorial nature. The predisposition could lie in the pathophysiology of the brain or in psychological immaturity, or in a combination of the two together. The nature of the seizures themselves might then be determined by the level of 'physiogenic or psychogenic regression' which prevailed in different cases.

Such a view can be useful in the understanding of borderline cases, though one would hesitate to follow Krapf further in seeing a fundamental parallel between the genesis of psychological and physiological immaturity, and in interpreting epileptiform dysrhythmias as sometimes reflecting functional immaturity of the brain.

The features which lead one to suspect a psychogenic component in a motor convulsion, are as follows. The pseudoseizure usually fails to conform to any recognised type of epilepsy, and may be bizarre in pattern or variable from one occasion to another. A typical tonic–clonic phase will normally be absent and movements will often have an organised pattern. An element of display may be noted, with movements obviously expressive in nature. Convulsions may increase if restraint is imposed.

Cyanosis or pallor accompany most epileptic attacks but are rarely seen with pseudoseizures. Reflexes are unaltered during or immediately after the attack, whereas in grand mal convulsions up-going plantars and wide fixed pupils may be observed for a time. The loss or preservation of corneal reflexes is rather less clear-cut as a differentiating sign. Incontinence and self injury are rare, though exceptions are occasionally seen. Severe self injury may indeed be skilfully avoided. Tongue biting is uncommon in pseudoseizures, but the inner mouth or lips may be abraided. Henry and Woodruff (1978) have described a positive sign which they regard as strongly indicative of feigned or hysterical unconsciousness: when the patient is turned from one side to another the eyes deviate each time towards the ground, in a manner not seen with organic coma.

The presence or absence of diminished awareness during the attack can be difficult to determine. Moreover some epileptic attacks, especially those of focal cortical origin, are compatible with preservation of consciousness throughout their course. Nevertheless, the demonstration of retained awareness of the environment while bilateral whole body convulsions are in progress will strongly suggest that the attack was not epileptic in origin. A marked emotional display when the attack is over is suggestive but by no means conclusive of pseudoseizures. Precipitation by shock, surprise or distress must also be interpreted with caution, since such factors may trigger epileptic attacks in susceptible individuals. Moreover overbreathing, ensuing on mental distress, may ultimately precipitate a genuine epileptic fit.

The taking of a detailed history can often be informative. Painstaking appraisal of the total situation must always be attempted, with evaluation of current stresses and premorbid modes of functioning. Roy (1979) identified several factors which were significantly more common in patients with pseudoseizures than in epileptic controls: a past history or family history of psychiatric disorder, a history of attempted suicide, and the presence of sexual maladjustment or of a current affective disorder. The mode of evolution of the attacks must also be considered. Sudden loss of control in an established epileptic, for example, may indicate the development of non-epileptic seizures, particularly when anticonvulsant levels have remained stable and recent stresses can be identified (Trimble 1983). When a history of obvious pseudoseizures is of long duration it can be important to obtain full details of the earliest attacks, since these may represent the genuine epilepsy upon which pseudoseizures have come to be superimposed. When repeated episodes occur their habitual setting can be of value in diagnosis: pseudoseizures almost invariably take place where they can be witnessed, particularly in the home and in the presence of the family.

Admission to hospital is indicated when uncertainty persists, though sometimes even close observation by skilled personnel can fail to resolve the issue. Estimation of serum prolactin levels shortly after attacks can give important and sometimes decisive information as described on p. 290. The EEG can also prove invaluable.

The interseizure record may give a lead, in that it would be rare for this to show no abnormalities in a patient experiencing several epileptic attacks per day. The converse, however, can be misleading, since many patients with pseudoseizures will also be liable to genuine attacks and will then show epileptiform abnormalities in the EEG. A record taken during or shortly after an attack provides the firmest evidence of all (Scott 1982a, 1982b). Consistent absence of seizure discharges, or of the slow activity that commonly succeeds a grand mal fit, will strongly suggest a non-organic seizure. Epilepsy will be indicated by spiking and other discharges which are seen to commence locally and spread widely, or in the post-ictal period by flattening of background elements and localised or generalised slow activity persisting for many minutes or even hours. Rare examples exist, nonetheless, in which definite epileptic seizures, particularly partial seizures, are witnessed by the clinician without EEG concomitants. Where facilities exist for prolonged EEG monitoring (p. 288) the chances of clarifying the diagnosis will be considerably increased.

The mistake of interpreting epilepsy as hysteria is probably much commoner than the converse situation. Special difficulty is likely to be encountered with temporal lobe epilepsy, where attacks may be bizarre in character and accompanied by pronounced emotional disturbance. The EEG may fail to reveal abnormalities until activating techniques are employed. Complex partial seizures which are unaccompanied by grand mal convulsions are especially liable to be mistaken for non-organic disturbances, particularly when consciousness is not very obviously altered. Complex partial seizures of frontal lobe origin can give rise to especial difficulty. Abnormalities of behaviour are more likely to be epileptic in origin when they are sudden in onset, short lived, irregularly recurrent and out of character for the individual concerned (Falconer & Taylor 1970). The problems of diagnosis raised by automatisms and fugues are further considered below.

Epilepsy versus other psychiatric disorders

Epilepsy may not only be associated with a wide range of neurotic and psychotic manifestations but can also be mistaken for them. These difficulties in diagnosis again centre principally on temporal lobe epilepsy.

Episodic attacks of anxiety may be difficult to distinguish from temporal lobe epilepsy, especially when panic wells up suddenly accompanied by marked depersonalisation. Harper and Roth (1962) illustrated this clearly in their comparison between 30 patients with temporal lobe epilepsy and 30 patients suffering from the 'phobic anxiety depersonalisation syndrome'. In both conditions there were episodic bouts of fear, depersonalisation, *déjà vu* and distortions of perception. In rare cases the neurotic patients also reported hallucinations. Occasionally they had fainted at the height of their attacks, even voiding urine if the bladder was full. Disturbance of conscious awareness was sometimes observed at the peaks of emotional disturbance.

Important differences lay in the tendency for severe psychiatric symptoms to persist between episodes in the anxious patients, and for their attacks to have more clear-cut emotional precipitation. Attacks began abruptly in both groups, but tended to end gradually in the neurotics and abruptly in temporal lobe epilepsy. There was often a characteristic 'march' in the evolution of symptoms in the epileptics, and complete loss of consciousness typically dominated the clinical picture. Episodic disturbances of speech and automatic behaviour were also largely confined to the epileptics. Other differences, of more value in distinguishing groups than individuals, lay in the greater neurotic background of the anxious patients, with more prominent traits of immaturity or overdependence in the personality. The patients with temporal lobe epilepsy frequently had a history of some disease leading to cerebral damage, and they alone had abnormalities of a specifically epileptic nature in the EEG.

Occasionally the true diagnosis can remain in doubt even after detailed clinical enquiry and a period of observation. The majority of such patients were considered by Harper and Roth to suffer from neurotic disturbance. They suggested that only specifically epileptic abnormalities in the EEG should be allowed to decide the issue in favour of epilepsy when the problem could not be resolved by other means.

Schizophrenia and temporal lobe epilepsy may sometimes be confused with one another. Karagulla and Robertson (1955) drew attention to several psychopathological phenomena which may be seen both in schizophrenia and in the auras of temporal lobe epilepsy—the evocation of thoughts, either indefinite or formulated and including thoughts which entered the mind unbidden, the hearing of voices both within and without the head, and visual hallucinations. To these may be added thought block, perceptual distortions of space, time and the body image, sudden experiences of unreality and perplexity, and the autochthonous welling up of emotions such as dread, anxiety and ecstasy.

It may therefore happen, when grand mal is absent or infrequent, that such auras will be interpreted as evidence of schizophrenia. Special difficulties are likely to be encountered in patients with markedly schizoid personalities who experience complex auras including hallucina-

tions and thought disorders (Pond 1957). The clue will usually lie in the episodic nature of attacks in temporal lobe epilepsy and in the evidence of impairment of consciousness at the time. Epileptic hallucinations are typically fleeting and sometimes tantalisingly difficult, if not impossible, to recall. Those of schizophrenia are usually longer lasting, can be described in more detail and are less stereotyped and restricted in content. Schizophrenic disorders of thought and affect also persist in between such episodes. Post-ictal confusion may similarly be mistaken for schizophrenia when hallucinations and paranoid ideas are prominent.

Conversely, epilepsy may be suspected in patients with typical schizophrenic illnesses who are discovered to have temporal lobe spiking on the EEG (Treffert 1963), or when a grand mal convulsion is precipitated in a schizophrenic patient on phenothiazine medication. Catatonic schizophrenics are especially liable to show epileptic phenomena during relapses, either in the EEG or in the form of myoclonic jerks or grand mal convulsions. When such illnesses have been of relatively short duration it may be questioned whether the psychotic episode has been in fact a prolonged psychomotor attack or 'twilight state'. Usually the dullness and retardation of the epileptic twilight state is distinctive, and the hallucinations are more massive, complex and chiefly in the visual sphere. Short recurrences of abnormal experience are also usual in twilight states, with intervening lucid periods during which no gross abnormality or loss of affect can be detected (Slater & Roth 1969).

Episodic visual hallucinations may occasionally raise the suspicion of an epileptic disorder, for example in the so-called 'Charles Bonnet syndrome' of the elderly. Here extremely vivid and well-formed visual hallucinations occur with great profusion, sometimes episodically and compellingly. Typically they are experienced in clear consciousness, and insight is either retained or very quickly attained into the unreal nature of the phenomena. In these respects the similarity to formed visual hallucinations of epileptic auras can sometimes be striking.

.The Charles Bonnet syndrome is reviewed by Damas-Mora *et al.* (1982) and Berrios and Brook (1982). It appears to represent a heterogeneous collection of patients and the usefulness of the eponym is doubtful. Defining characteristics have included the occurrence of visual hallucinations in the elderly, the preservation of intellectual competence, the absence of impairment of consciousness and the preservation of insight. Peripheral ocular pathology may be present or absent. The quality of the hallucinations is commonly vivid, elaborate and well organised, persisting for seconds or hours at a time. The scenes may change continuously, and richness of themes is the rule—trees, flowers, buildings or persons appear in considerable array. The patient sometimes greets such phenomena with surprise, curiosity or delight. They may disappear or persist when the eyes are closed.

The cause is unknown and other psychiatric disorder is commonly absent. Ball (1991) reviews the evidence that midbrain arterial disease may be responsible, with peripheral ocular pathology facilitating the development of the syndrome by diminishing the normal flow of afferents to the visual cortex.

Finally, epileptic disturbances may sometimes be diagnosed as *acute organic reactions due to some other cause*. On rare occasions ictal or post-ictal disturbances can last for a week or more, and a history of epilepsy may not be forthcoming. The abruptness of onset of the condition is usually the feature which suggests an epileptic basis. Absence status may similarly be misleading until the highly characteristic disturbance in the EEG is discovered.

Differential diagnosis of automatisms

Epileptic automatisms can raise special diagnostic problems, particularly when, as is commonly the case, they are unaccompanied by a grand mal convulsion. In the majority of cases the diagnosis rests primarily on clinical assessment of the pattern of behaviour manifest during attacks, so eye-witness accounts should be obtained whenever possible. Particular enquiry should be made about the occurrence of other types of epileptic seizure, either in the past or present. Where the possibility of hysteria has arisen it is essential to be conversant with the patient's current life situation, personality and previous history, and to corroborate this from someone who knows him well. In working towards the correct diagnosis full medical evaluation will usually be required, together with careful EEG and other investigations.

Possible misdiagnoses in this area are discussed by Fenton (1972). The episode may be attributed to *intoxication with alcohol or drugs*. Or the subsequent amnesia may be attributed to *hysteria* or *simulation*, especially when the personality is abnormal or antisocial behaviour has occurred. In the converse direction epileptic automatism may be diagnosed in mistake for attacks of *hypoglycaemia*, due to an islet cell tumour or overdosage with insulin in diabetic subjects. Clouding of consciousness due to other conditions such as *encephalitis* or *cerebral ischaemia* may need to be excluded. Automatic behaviour can occasionally occur with cerebral degenerative conditions such as *Alzheimer's disease*. However, episodes of confusion due to toxic, metabolic, infective or structural causes are usually more prolonged, lasting days or weeks, and are not necessarily recurrent events.

Very occasionally the posturing and stereotyped movements seen in brief episodes of *catatonic schizophrenia* may be mistaken for epileptic automatisms. Episodes of *transient global amnesia* (p. 413) can resemble automatisms in being of sudden onset, lasting a few minutes then recovering spontaneously, and in sometimes being recurrent.

However, the patient's 'confusion' is restricted to difficulties with memory—during the amnesic episode he usually acts quite normally, movements are perfectly coordinated, and he responds to questions appropriately apart from his obvious memory defects. There is no clouding of consciousness and the personality remains intact.

Ictal automatisms confined to sleep may be confused with *somnambulism* (p. 735). However, sleep-walking episodes are usually of longer duration, the behaviour is better integrated, and the sleep walker may mumble or answer monosyllabically if spoken to. During epileptic automatisms the patient is usually inaccessible, and stereotyped automatic behaviour is more likely to be prominent. Pedley and Guilleminault (1977) described an interesting group of six patients who presented with unusual sleep-walking episodes but in whom the balance of evidence favoured an atypical form of epilepsy. Attacks commonly occurred in the early morning hours, were characterised by screaming, unintelligible vocalisations and complex automatisms, and in several the EEGs showed epileptiform abnormalities. Treatment with phenytoin or carbamazepine led to cessation of the abnormal behaviour. A striking example was as follows:

A previously healthy 18-year-old man began having episodes lasting 2–10 minutes between 2 and 6 a.m. He would jump suddenly from the bed, climb onto a chair and begin leaping from one piece of furniture to another. The movements were violent, and occasionally punctuated by screaming or hitting his head against the wall. Each episode characteristically ended by his diving onto the bed where he would grab semi-purposefully at his sleeping partner then fall deeply asleep. If awakened a few minutes later he was amnesic for what had transpired. During the episode he was unresponsive to questions, admonitions or stimuli. At other times he would sit up, shout, then stare for 30–40 seconds before falling back asleep; or mumble incoherently and appear frightened. Initially attacks occurred once every 6 months, but 2 years later they were happening five nights out of seven. An active epileptic focus was present in the right temporal region, and phenytoin abolished the disorder within 2 weeks.   (Pedley & Guilleminault 1977)

In older patients, and particularly in the presence of cerebral disease, the syndrome of '*REM sleep behaviour disorder*' in which patients seemingly act out dreams with aggressive content, should be explored by polysomnographic studies (p. 737).

Hysterical dissociation with amnesia is a particularly common source of uncertainty. This, however, usually occurs at a time of crisis in the patient's life, and the behaviour will often be purposeful and directed at removing him from a situation of stress. The features typical of psychogenic amnesia (p. 33) may be evident when the patient presents for attention. Moreover the amnesic gap may last for hours, days or weeks, in contrast to the brief duration of most automatisms. The behaviour displayed during the episode itself will usually reveal little firm evidence of loss of awareness of the environment.

Longer-lasting epileptic fugue states, in which the patient wanders away, may raise similar problems of diagnosis. An hysterical basis is strongly suggested in fugues which have lasted for several days or more, when there is no clear history of conventional epileptic attacks, and when the patient has been observed during the course of the episode to show well-integrated behaviour. At the end of the fugue, the hysterical patient is usually well preserved—has eaten and cared for himself quite normally—whereas in the case suggesting epilepsy he is often dirty, dishevelled and neglected. In hysterical fugues, personal emotional factors will usually be found to be operative. Sometimes the patient may return to some place which has special meaning for him, as in the example described on p. 416, whereas in epileptic fugues he will have wandered quite aimlessly.

Stengel (1941, 1943a), however, emphasised the areas of overlap which occur between fugue states of hysterical and epileptic origin, and concluded that there was little fundamental difference between them. His survey also showed the importance of a depressive component in the great majority of fugues, whether or not epileptic tendencies were present. Often a suicidal impulse appeared to have been transformed into an impulse to wander. Clearly the possibility of an affective disorder needs to be carefully borne in mind in the management of such patients.

Simulation rather than hysterical dissociation may sometimes be suspected. Amnesia may occasionally be feigned by the patient to protect himself from the legal consequences of an act or in attempts to maintain self esteem. Detailed investigation of the circumstances surrounding the behaviour concerned will usually reveal discrepancies and inconsistencies in the patient's story. The criteria which may usefully be applied in assessing whether or not an epileptic automatism was likely to be in progress when a crime was committed are discussed on p. 275.

Aggressive outbursts in patients with unstable personalities can raise the possibility of epileptic automatism, especially when the disturbed behaviour is of an impulsive and paroxysmal nature. The distinction can on occasion be difficult; a high proportion of patients with aggressive personality disorders show temporal lobe abnormalities on the EEG, and problems in the control of aggression are found in a number of patients with epilepsy. Yet the distinction has important implications for treatment, and can be crucial in medicolegal proceedings.

Clinical assessment of the details of the attacks is of first importance. Epileptic automatisms usually begin abruptly, whereas in simple outbursts of aggression there is often a gradual build up of anger and tension before the peak of disturbance is reached. Automatisms also usually end abruptly, with spontaneous resumption of the patient's normal personality. The abnormal behaviour during automatisms is typically purposeless and unmotivated, whereas aggression is directed against specific targets in most outbursts of anger. Motor coordination in automatism will often be faulty, and the patient's expression may clearly reveal that consciousness is clouded. Subsequent amnesia cannot, however, always be taken as firm evidence of epilepsy, since memory can be blurred during phases of intense emotion, and an element of dissociation may have occurred at the peak of an outburst of anger.

The circumstances in which attacks occur must be taken into account—outbursts which are regularly precipitated by external circumstances are most unlikely to represent epileptic automatisms. Careful enquiry into the patient's life situation may reveal specific stresses which dictate his behaviour. Sometimes the aggressive tendencies will have extended far back into childhood or adolescence, but occasionally they will have appeared only recently in relation to definable marital or other difficulties. In some patients the personality may prove to be inhibited rather than habitually aggressive, with difficulty in the expression of feelings until a threshold of provocation or frustration has been exceeded.

The existence of specific epileptic abnormalities in the EEG, and the appearance of epileptic fits in intimate relationship to outbursts, will of course bias the diagnosis towards epilepsy. In recurrent cases, where the diagnosis remains in doubt, a trial of anticonvulsant medication is usually indicated and may help to resolve the dilemma.

In occasional cases, however, assessment of all the available information will leave one undecided whether organic or psychogenic factors are mainly to be blamed. This is well illustrated by the so-called *syndrome of episodic dyscontrol* (p. 83). The term is used for patients characterised by uncontrollable storms of aggression, sometimes on minimal or no provocation and sometimes associated with phenomena of a quasi-epileptic nature.

Maletzky (1973) in a study of 22 such patients suggested that 'episodic dyscontrol' might represent a fairly distinct clinical entity. Patients were excluded from consideration if their outbursts had occurred in the context of pathological intoxication, acute drug reactions or schizophrenia, or if they showed evidence of undoubted temporal lobe epilepsy. All were men in their twenties or thirties from lower socioeconomic groups, and with a history of episodes of violence increasing in frequency and severity from adolescence onwards. Sometimes isolated episodes could be traced back to childhood. Two-thirds had seriously injured their victims at some time or another, and five had committed homicide. The outbursts were usually provoked but the stimuli were typically minimal. The frequency varied from one episode per day to several per year, the average being one per week. In most cases the anger had habitually been directed against a close family member. There was a high frequency of a history of violence among the male relatives of patients, and also of epilepsy. The patients' personal situations were mostly chaotic, with frequent histories of divorce, arrest and repeated dismissal from work.

Attacks were similar to epilepsy in a number of ways. There were often auras preceding attacks in the form of hyperacusis, visual illusions, numbness of the extremities or nausea. Headache and drowsiness often followed the outbursts. More than half of the patients had episodes of altered consciousness without associated aggression, usually in the form of brief staring spells. Some claimed amnesia for the attacks or even for a period just preceding them. Extreme remorse was prominent, and the majority viewed the episodes as foreign and distasteful. Many showed mild recent memory impairments, or 'soft' neurological signs in the form of minor ataxia, incoordination or some degree of left–right uncertainty. Fourteen had abnormal EEGs, six with temporal lobe spiking and the remainder with non-specific abnormalities which, however, always involved the temporal lobe.

Liability to attacks was notably worsened by alcohol and sometimes also by attempts at treatment with chlordiazepoxide. In an uncontrolled trial phenytoin was found to have a markedly beneficial effect—19 of the 22 patients achieved a good response, with an approximately 75% reduction in the frequency and severity of attacks. Stein (1993) has, however, stressed the magnitude of the placebo response which may explain such a result. Carbamazepine by contrast has been shown to be effective in controlled trials (Gardner & Cowdry 1986). Other reports have indicated possible benefit from lithium (Sheard 1971; Tupin *et al.* 1973) or propanolol (Williams *et al.* 1982).

In such patients it can clearly be difficult to decide how far epileptic or non-epileptic factors are operative. Maletzky suggests that it is reasonable to assume that in the majority there are functional abnormalities of the limbic (or amygdaloid) regions of the brain. Such abnormalities may set the threshold for episodes of uncontrollable anger at an unusually low level. Nevertheless the problem appears to become less disabling with age, since it is rare to encounter similar examples in older patients. The uncertain nosological status of the syndrome is discussed on p. 83.

The legal situation regarding automatisms has become illogical, at least in England and Wales, as a result of a series of court decisions (d'Orbán 1989; Fenwick 1990b, 1993). Whereas medical usage of the term is largely restricted to epilepsy and defined as on p. 253, the legal definition transcends medical causation and merely implies 'unconscious involuntary action' in which 'the mind does not go with what is being done'. Thus it involves complete absence of *mens rea* (i.e. of intention, recklessness or guilty knowledge).

The legal definition is very wide, extending from simple reflex action such as an intuitive defensive gesture, through inattentiveness due to preoccupation (for example driving through red traffic lights), to confusional states in which consciousness is absent. Automatisms in the legal sense can arise from epilepsy, somnambulism, hypo- or hyperglycaemia, concussion, brain disease, hysterical dissociation or the effects of drugs (except those taken voluntarily such as alcohol or drugs of addiction). All can give rise to a state of mind which is incompatible with *mens rea*.

Two types of automatism are then recognised legally—'sane' and 'insane' automatisms, the former resulting in acquittal and the latter until recently requiring mandatory detention in hospital. This could be for an indefinite period. Since the Criminal Procedure (Insanity and Unfitness to Plead) Act of 1991, there is no longer an absolute requirement for admission to hospital and the judge can decide on disposal as he sees fit. Nevertheless the distinction between sane and insane automatism is of immense importance, since the former leads to instant acquittal. Such distinction made on legal grounds can be medically indefensible.

The principle behind current decisions appears to be that sane automatism ('automatism simpliciter') occurs when the mind is disordered by an external factor and the automatism is therefore unlikely to recur. Insane automatism occurs when the mind is disordered due to an intrinsic factor (i.e. malfunctioning due to 'disease'), leading to a situation that is prone to recur and that may conceivably result in violence. Thus a blow to the head resulting in concussion, or an injection of insulin causing hypoglycaemia, result in sane automatism; cerebral arteriosclerosis leading to a confusional state can produce insane automatism.

Nonsensical instances arise, however. Hypoglycaemia can be due to an internal factor such as insulinoma, which might therefore be legally judged to lead to 'insane automatism' even though the manifestations will be the same as those produced by injected insulin; and a defence of somnambulism, which having an internal physiological cause might be regarded as 'insane automatism', has until recently always led to acquittal. In the case of R. vs Charlson the patient was acquitted ('sane automatism') on the grounds of probably having a cerebral tumour which was not regarded as a 'disease of the mind'.

Automatisms due to epilepsy are regarded on all grounds legally as insane automatisms.

Treatment

The management of patients with epilepsy requires appropriate investigation as already discussed, with diagnosis of type of attack and definition of the cause as far as possible. Anticonvulsant drugs then form the mainstay of treatment and are accordingly given pride of place below. Drug treatment, however, is but one part of the care required by the majority of epileptics—psychological and social aspects warrant attention to some degree in virtually every patient who is subject to recurring attacks. In those who come before the psychiatrist these aspects can be of overriding importance, and are often decisive in determining the level of overall success achieved.

Anticonvulsant drugs

Many drugs are available, some of which have stood the test of time. Other more recent acquisitions can prove efficacious but may have serious side effects which limit their usefulness. The field is large and is usefully reviewed by Fenton (1983) and Richens and Perucca (1993). Reynolds (1982) outlines the special considerations which may govern the drugs of choice in patients with psychological disorder.

Whenever possible drugs should be used singly or at most in small-sized combinations. The temptation to add several drugs in sequence must be resisted; unfavourable interactions can lead to disturbances in drug metabolism, either increasing the serum concentrations to toxic levels or lowering them so that seizure control is impaired. The feasibility of monotherapy for a high proportion of patients, and the benefits which result when polypharmacy is carefully rationalised to one or two drugs, have been amply demonstrated (Shorvon & Reynolds 1979; Reynolds & Shorvon 1982). A start should be made with drugs which are well established for the type of epilepsy in question, and in general once started a drug should not be discarded until it has been increased to tolerance.

Nevertheless several drugs may need to be tried in rotation in difficult cases. Sometimes the administration of two or even three together will be indicated in order to obtain their additive effects, but this must only be tried when the first drugs have been used to full efficiency. The various classes of drugs are known to act by different mechanisms — probably none have a significant effect in suppressing the focus itself, but some appear to block the spread of the seizure discharge by suppressing post-tetanic potentiation, and others may modify the levels of neurotransmitters or affect ionic transport within the brain.

The aim is complete abolition of seizures, but this must not be at the expense of side effects which handicap the patient. It is better to tolerate occasional fits than to leave the patient permanently drowsy or muddled. Sometimes complete control may lead to severe disturbances of mood, with recurring tension states or even the appearance of epileptic psychoses. Thus drug treatment is a highly individual matter which needs to be carefully adjusted to the patient's particular needs and responses.

The monitoring of therapy by estimation of blood levels has shown its value, since the relationship between the dose ingested and the plasma levels obtained can vary considerably from one patient to another. With some drugs, moreover, the difference between therapeutic and toxic levels is narrow, and when several drugs are used together there can be complex interactions. Serum monitoring is of especial importance in any patient whose seizures are poorly controlled, when toxic reactions are suspected, during pregnancy, or in the presence of hepatic or renal disease which can markedly affect blood levels. Ranges can now be defined within which most patients will be expected to obtain substantial benefit, and above which toxic effects are likely to be encountered: phenytoin 10–20 µg/ml (40–80 µmol/l); phenobarbitone 15–40 µg/ml (65–170 µmol/l); carbamazepine 5–10 µg/ml (20–40 µmol/l); sodium valproate 50–100 µg/ml (350–700 µmol/l); ethosuximide 50–100 µg/ml (350–700 µmol/l). Primidone is monitored in terms of its major metabolite, phenobarbitone. These ranges may not be required by all patients, but they should always be achieved on a single drug before contemplating the addition of a second.

When difficulties of control arise it will often be necessary to look beyond the details of medication. Before automatically increasing the dose one must be alert to psychological conflicts or emotional disturbances which may have temporarily aggravated the situation and which obviously require first attention. It is also important to bear in mind that deteriorating seizure control may sometimes indicate the need for reduction rather than increase of medication, since toxic levels, particularly of phenytoin or phenobarbitone, can increase seizures.

The question of stopping drugs may arise when the patient has been free from seizures for 2–3 years, since there is evidence that some 70% of patients with epilepsy eventually enter a prolonged remission (Drug & Therapeutics Bulletin 1989). The risk of recurrence must then be balanced against the disadvantages of continuation on an individual basis. Cessation will be deferred if having a seizure stands to imperil the patient's well being, for example if loss of a driving licence will cause special difficulties. The problems surrounding the decision are discussed by Chadwick and Reynolds (1985). Partial epilepsy carries more risk of relapse than primary generalised epilepsy, also seizures symptomatic of pre-existing cerebral disease. The duration of the epilepsy, the frequency of seizures and the presence of continuing abnormalities on the EEG must also be taken into account.

The special problems that arise with pregnancy are discussed by Brodie (1989a) and O'Brien and Gilmour-White (1993). The most important is the increased risk of congenital abnormalities among babies born to women taking antiepileptic drugs. Pre-pregnancy counselling is therefore important, and if the patient has been seizure-free for more than 2 years and has no evidence of an anatomical lesion, withdrawal of medication should be offered before pregnancy is contemplated. Otherwise monotherapy should be employed whenever possible, and in the smallest practicable dose. No drug has been exonerated completely from teratogenic effects, but it is clear that the number of drugs taken together increases the risk of foetal abnormality — from double the natural risk in women taking two antiepileptic drugs to almost 10 times the risk in those taking four. The present consensus of opinion is that carbamazepine is the safest anticonvulsant during pregnancy. Newer drugs such as vigabatrin and lamotrigine should be avoided since there is as yet insufficient information about their safety.

The commonest malformations resulting are cleft lip and palate and congenital heart disease. Phenytoin has been particularly implicated in these, and is also associated with minor craniofacial and digital anomalies — the so-called 'foetal hydantoin syndrome'. Valproate, and to a lesser extent carbamazepine, carry a risk of leading to neural tube defects. Nevertheless in patients who have achieved good control with valproate, it may be judged safer to continue with this than to expose the foetus to the risk of hypoxia occasioned during maternal seizures.

All women taking antiepileptic drugs should receive folic acid supplements, ideally starting before pregnancy since neural tube defects develop during the first 28 days of gestation. Alpha-fetoprotein concentrations should be measured at 18 weeks, and high-definition ultrasound should be performed for the detection of neural tube defects and cardiac malformations. Regular monitoring of serum anticonvulsant levels is important since they tend to fall as pregnancy progresses. Vitamin K_1 should be given for at least 1 week before delivery, and to the baby immediately after birth, to reduce the risk of perinatal bleeding.

Choice of drugs

The drug of first choice is determined by the type of seizures and EEG findings. Within a given category of epilepsy there is often little to choose in terms of anticonvulsant effect, and liability to side effects will be the important consideration.

Generalised tonic–clonic seizures respond best to phenytoin or carbamazepine, which seem to be largely equivalent in efficacy. Experience increasingly favours the latter on account of its fewer side effects and the wider margin between therapeutic and toxic levels. Sodium valproate is also regarded as a drug of first choice and is probably equally effective. In resistant cases two of these drugs may be needed together. If control is not achieved it will nowadays be usual to try one of the newer antiepileptics such as vigabatrin or lamotrigine, or very occasionally to resort to primidone or phenobarbitone which are considerably more sedative.

Partial seizures tend to respond to the same drugs as generalised grand mal seizures but the drug may need to be taken in higher dosage towards the top of the therapeutic range. Temporal lobe epilepsy can be particularly difficult to control. Carbamazepine is consequently now regarded as the drug of choice for this form of epilepsy, since it can be given in high dosage with less risk of confusion or sedation. It may also have psychotropic properties as discussed below.

For petit mal absences ethosuximide has until recently been the drug of choice, but sodium valproate is probably equally effective. The latter has the advantage of also helping any grand mal seizures which may be present. Atypical absences and myoclonic seizures can be hard to control, and here sodium valproate and clonazepam have proved particularly helpful. Sodium valproate is preferable because clonazepam is often markedly sedative. A combination of the two should be avoided since this can lead to stupor. Among the newer antiepileptics lamotrigine has proved to be particularly effective.

Most of these drugs will be given twice per day to ensure stable serum levels, though phenobarbitone, primidone and phenytoin can be given once per day, at night. Sodium valproate may need to be given three times per day on account of its short half-life.

While the above represents a consensus of opinion concerning drugs of first choice, individual differences in response exist. Other drugs must therefore be tried when the first drug gives incomplete control, and sometimes the additional drugs mentioned below will prove their worth.

Drugs of first choice

Carbamazepine

Carbamazepine (Tegretol) was formerly principally employed in the treatment of trigeminal neuralgia. However it has now established itself as a highly effective anticonvulsant for use with grand mal and partial seizures, though not with petit mal. In general it emerges as equivalent to phenytoin and phenobarbitone in antiepileptic potency, but may be preferred to these on account of its relative lack of sedation and side effects. As mentioned above it is now widely regarded as the drug of choice for temporal lobe epilepsy, particularly in the presence of complex partial seizures.

Carbamazepine almost certainly has less adverse effects on cognitive functioning than phenobarbitone, phenytoin or primidone. This makes it particularly useful in patients who are already impaired. In both children and adults improvements in alertness and personality have been noted on changing to the drug (Bower 1978; Reynolds 1982). Thompson et al. (1980), in studies on normal volunteers, showed that while phenytoin produced a dose-related impairment in cognitive processes, this was insignificant with carbamazepine. Dodrill and Troupin (1977) compared epileptic patients on monotherapy with phenytoin or carbamazepine in a cross-over study, and showed fewer errors on tasks requiring attention and problem-solving with the latter.

Several reports have raised the further possibility that carbamazepine may have a positive psychotropic influence in improving mood and behaviour, though it remains uncertain whether this is a primary effect or the result of withdrawal of more sedative medications. Dalby (1971) described the improvements in psychiatric status which could be seen among patients with temporal lobe epilepsy. The most marked effect emerged in patients with phasic psychiatric disturbances, especially phasic depression, though benefit was also observed in patients with emotional instability and 'hysterical elaboration'. These psychotropic effects were largely related to improved control of seizures, but were also attributed to the disappearance of the debilitating side effects caused by previous medication. Sillanpää (1981) reviews other studies in which a psychotropic effect is emphasised. Andrewes et al. (1986), in a study of patients on monotherapy, found significant inverse correlations between serum levels of carbamazepine and ratings of anxiety, depression and fatigue. It could be relevant that carbamazepine has a tricyclic structure similar to that of imipramine, and (along with its derivative oxcarbazepine) is the only tricyclic anticonvulsant in clinical use.

The starting dose is 100 mg twice daily, increased when necessary up to 1800 mg per day. Serious side effects are rare. If the dose is increased too rapidly the patient may experience tiredness, drowsiness, dizziness, headache, nausea and unsteadiness of gait, though these disappear with time. Diplopia and blurring of vision may also occur. A rash develops in some 4% of cases. Hyponatraemia may occur, probably through altered regulation of antidiuretic hormone. Anticoagulant levels may be lowered as a result of increased hepatic clearance, and the efficacy of oral contraceptives may be reduced. In chronic use agranulocytosis and aplastic anaemia have very occasionally been encountered, also osteomalacia.

Phenytoin sodium

Phenytoin sodium (Epanutin, Dilantin) vies with carbamazepine as the drug of first choice in grand mal seizures. Some use it first for all forms of seizure other than petit mal. Its highly effective antiepileptic properties are, however, combined with disadvantages in terms of long-term side effects.

The margin between therapeutic and toxic levels is rather low and the therapeutic level varies from patient to patient. The plasma level is also markedly affected by interaction with other drugs, including phenothiazines and antidepressants. Serum monitoring is therefore especially important when using phenytoin, particularly when control of seizures is poor or if toxic symptoms have appeared. The pharmacokinetics are moreover distinctive in that phenytoin undergoes 'saturable metabolism'. This means that as the dosage increases the plasma levels can rise to a greater degree than would be expected. Increases in dosage should therefore not exceed 25 mg when the therapeutic range is approached.

The chief toxic effects are ataxia, with dysarthria, nystagmus and incoordination. Such symptoms may set in abruptly and to such an extent that a cerebellar lesion is suspected, either early in treatment or after many years on the drug. The syndrome almost invariably subsides rapidly on withdrawal, though the development of permanent cerebellar deficits appears to be a rare possibility (Reynolds 1975). Diplopia, blurring of vision and headache may occur, or occasionally confusional states. After prolonged use acne and gum hypertrophy are common, and hirsutism may be a distressing side effect in females. The general coarsening of facial features which may ultimately emerge was strikingly demonstrated by Falconer and Davidson (1973) in comparisons of twins. Hypocalcaemia, with rickets or osteomalacia, may develop. Hepatic enzyme induction may reduce the efficacy of oral anticoagulants or oral contraceptives.

Experience has shown that even in the absence of overt toxic symptoms phenytoin can have subtle effects on concentration, memory and psychomotor performance. This 'subacute encephalopathy' can easily pass unnoticed as a cause of mental deterioration, especially since serum levels are not always elevated beyond the therapeutic range (Reynolds 1981, 1982). Brain-damaged and retarded patients appear to be especially susceptible. Another hazard in psychiatric practice is toxicity from the combination of lithium with phenytoin; serum lithium levels may become unreliable when the drugs are given together.

The dosage of phenytoin is 100 mg twice per day, up to 600 mg per day in adults. A combined tablet containing 50 mg phenobarbitone with 100 mg phenytoin is available (Garoin); while combined medications are in general undesirable this may simplify treatment for patients who are unreliable or of limited intelligence.

Sodium valproate

Sodium valproate (Epilim) has a particularly wide spectrum of action, controlling both partial and generalised seizures including petit mal absences and myoclonic attacks (Davis *et al.* 1994). This commends its use when both grand mal and petit mal occur together.

It is regarded as equal, if not superior, to ethosuximide in the treatment of simple absences. Atypical absences and myoclonic seizures also stand to be controlled and it is of special value with the latter. The mode of action of sodium valproate appears to be different from that of the other antiepileptics above in that it increases the level of GABA in the brain.

Side effects are in general slight, though weight gain, ankle oedema, tremor and drowsiness may occur. Cognitive impairment appears to be rare, though the combination of sodium valproate and phenobarbitone is liable to lead to additive sedative effects. Temporary gastrointestinal irritation and nausea can develop at the start. Hair thinning can be troublesome and alopecia may occasionally develop. Liver disorder has proved to be a rare complication, and liver function should be monitored during the first few months of therapy and at intervals thereafter. Platelet disturbance is indicated by the appearance of bruising or petechiae. A 'valproate encephalopathy' has occasionally been reported, with profound impairment of cognitive processes leading to semi-stuporose states and dystonic posturing. This is reversible on withdrawal of the drug.

Treatment should be started with 200 mg twice daily, increasing up to 2000–3000 mg per day. In adults the short half-life of sodium valproate may lead to large fluctuations in blood levels, requiring it to be given three times per day.

Ethosuximide

Ethosuximide (Zarontin) has been regarded as the drug of first choice in patients with simple absences alone, though sodium valproate now appears to be equally effective. It has a marked and almost specific effect on simple absences accompanied by characteristic three per second wave and spike discharges, but is unlikely to be of use in other forms of epilepsy. For the control of atypical absences it usually needs to be combined with sodium valproate.

Ethosuximide has few side effects. The chief problems that arise are gastric disturbances and nausea, also dizziness, headache and drowsiness. It may occasionally precipitate a grand mal convulsion but this appears to be rare. In adults brief psychotic episodes have sometimes been reported, with visual and auditory hallucinations, depression and slight impairment of consciousness (Fischer *et al.* 1965). Lupus-like reactions have been reported in chil-dren. The adult dose is 250 mg twice daily, up to 1500 mg per day.

Clonazepam

Clonazepam (Rivotril), a benzodiazepine, was initially reported to be successful against a wide variety of seizures (Lund & Trolle 1973; Mikkelsen & Birket-Smith 1973). However, its chief value has proved to lie with myoclonic seizures as an alternative to sodium valproate. The two should not be given together.

The main drawback of clonazepam is its sedative effect in therapeutic doses. A tendency to aggravate behaviour disorder has also been reported. Tolerance gradually develops to the drowsiness induced, but adaptation to the anticonvulsant effect may occur along with this. In children it is usually too sedative for use, but in the myoclonic epilepsies of infancy and adulthood it can be given as a single dose at night. Sometimes this sedative effect is of value with other types of seizure when anxiety levels are high. Clonazepam is also important as an alternative to diazepam for the treatment of status epilepticus (*vide infra*). The dosage in routine treatment is 0.5–1.0 mg, very gradually increasing to a maximum of 10 mg per day.

Newer antiepileptics

Vigabatrin

Vigabatrin (Sabril) was introduced in 1989. It was designed specifically as a structural analogue of GABA, the inhibitory neurotransmitter. By binding irreversibly to GABA transaminase, the enzyme responsible for its breakdown, it increases GABA concentrations at synapses in a dose-dependent manner (Brodie 1992). The drug has proved its value in relation to complex partial seizures, with or without secondary generalisation, and is also effective with primary generalised grand mal though perhaps less impressively so. Petit mal does not respond, and myoclonic seizures may be worsened. Vigabatrin is used at present when epilepsy has proved resistant to first-line drugs such as carbamazepine or phenytoin.

Its elimination half-life is relatively short, but since it acts by binding to a target enzyme the duration of action exceeds 24 hours. Serum monitoring of drug levels is without value since the efficacy is unrelated to the amount circulating in the blood. It does not cause liver enzyme induction, but results in a fall of some 20% in serum phenytoin concentrations through unknown mechanisms. These should therefore be monitored when the two drugs are given together.

The chief side effects are weight gain and sedation. Tolerance usually develops to the latter, but drowsiness can occasionally be severe and necessitate discontinuation. Headache and ataxia are mostly short lived. Visual field constriction has recently come under suspicion as a rare complication (Wilson & Brodie 1997; Wong *et al.* 1997). Paradoxical excitement and agitation may be seen in children, as with phenobarbitone.

The most troublesome side effects, however, are in relation to psychiatric complications, including depression, confusion and psychosis. Some 5–10% of patients develop behavioural changes, often progressing to psychotic illness. Typical features are irritability, confusion and aggression, eventually with auditory and visual hallucinations and paranoid ideation. Sander *et al.* (1991) have described both schizophrenia-like pictures in clear consciousness and, more rarely, organic psychoses. In eight of their 15 cases the psychosis followed a change in the habitual pattern of seizure activity—sometimes after cessation of seizures for several weeks, with a degree of EEG normalisation, and sometimes after a period of freedom followed by a cluster of attacks. Such psychoses are reversible with discontinuation of the drug or perhaps with reduction of dosage. Small doses of haloperidol are effective in treatment. Similar psychotic pictures can also follow abrupt withdrawal, so this must always proceed very slowly over several weeks. On account of the mental complications the drug is usually contraindicated in the presence of major psychiatric illness and must be used with care when there is a history of such. In certain animal species widespread microvacuolation has been detected in the cerebral white matter, but no such changes have been reported with clinically used doses in humans (Duncan 1994).

The starting dose is 500–1000 mg per day, increasing by 500 mg every 1–2 weeks. Some patients respond optimally to doses as low as 1 g per day, but the standard dosage is 2–3 g per day given as a single or divided dose. Lower doses should be used in patients with renal impairment. When substantial improvement occurs, other medication can be withdrawn over a number of months if sedation is proving troublesome.

Lamotrigine

Lamotrigine (Lamictal) is another new drug which has shown considerable promise in patients with refractory seizures. It acts by quite different mechanisms, blocking voltage-sensitive sodium channels to stabilise neuronal membranes and inhibiting the release of glutamate. Trials have shown its effectiveness, both as add-on treatment and monotherapy. The spectrum of action has emerged as wide, with good effects in partial seizures with or without secondary generalisation, primary generalised seizures, myoclonic seizures, and particularly with typical and atypical absences. It is chiefly metabolised in the liver, with a mean plasma elimination half-life of 30 hours (Drug & Therapeutics Bulletin 1992c).

In general lamotrigine is well tolerated, the commonest side effect being an allergic skin rash in 5–10% of patients, appearing within 4 weeks and clearing when the drug is stopped. Other unwanted effects include diplopia, blurred vision, headache, drowsiness, asthenia, dizziness, irritability and nausea. Angioedema and Stevens–Johnson syndrome are rare complications. It is in general free from neuropsychiatric side effects but aggressive reactions have been observed.

Very occasional deaths have been reported following a rapidly progressive illness with status epilepticus, multiorgan dysfunction and disseminated intravascular coagulation. Close monitoring is therefore essential in any patient who suddenly develops an unexplained rash, fever, flu-like symptoms, drowsiness or worsening of seizure control, especially within the first month of treatment, and must include the estimation of hepatic, renal and clotting parameters. Other abrupt unexplained deaths have occurred in patients on the drug but lamotrigine has not been incriminated directly in these. It is contraindicated in patients with hepatic or renal disease.

Gradual introduction is important, and the dosage depends on the other medication being prescribed. Drugs which induce liver enzymes (carbamazepine, phenytoin and primidone) can halve the half-life of lamotrigine, whereas valproate can double it. Patients already taking the former drugs should start on 50 mg per day for 2 weeks, with a gradual increase to 100–200 mg twice per day. Those taking valproate should start with 25 mg every alternate day for 2 weeks, increasing gradually to 100–200 mg given once per day. Lamotrigine inhibits epoxide hydrolase, thus increasing serum concentrations of an active metabolite of carbamazepine, and may therefore precipitate carbamazepine toxicity with dizziness and diplopia. When given as monotherapy the initial dose is 25 mg per day for 2 weeks, increasing to 100–200 mg given once per day.

Oxcarbazepine

Oxcarbazepine (Trileptal) has been developed by manipulation of the structure of carbamazepine with the aim of decreasing its allergenic and other side effects. Experience with its use over the past 10 years suggests that this has been successful and that it may now be regarded as a drug of first choice (Sabers & Gram 1994). Though chemically similar to carbamazepine it follows different metabolic pathways, without the formation of carbamazepine epoxide which appears to be responsible for many of the neurotoxic side effects. In consequence the dosage can be titrated upwards to therapeutic levels more quickly. Moreover, it causes minimal hepatic induction, and the elimination of its principal derivative (mono-hydroxy derivate, MHD) is unaffected by the presence of other anticonvulsants; hence there are fewer troublesome drug interactions than when using carbamazepine itself.

In double-blind cross-over studies it has shown comparable anticonvulsant action to carbamazepine and against a similar range of seizure types. In some studies on patients taking several drugs it has emerged as superior to carbamazepine, but this result may be attributable to rises in serum levels of other medication as a result of lessened hepatic enzyme induction.

With monotherapy, trials have confirmed a significant reduction in side effects compared to carbamazepine. The nature of neurotoxic effects is similar (tiredness, dizziness, headache and ataxia) but they occur less frequently. Allergic skin rashes are considerably less common. Hyponatraemia is, however, more frequently encountered, though it is usually mild and reversible. As with carbamazepine, the efficacy of oral contraceptives may be reduced, with breakthrough bleeding as a result. The metabolism of warfarin appears to be unaffected.

The starting dose is 600 mg per day, rising to 900–3000 mg per day given in two or three divided doses. Dosage can be increased more rapidly than with carbamazepine, which is an added advantage. In monotherapy, carbamazepine can be abruptly replaced by oxcarbazepine and vice versa, 300 mg of oxcarbazepine corresponding to 200 mg of carbamazepine. With polytherapy, however, the changeover must be more gradual and accompanied by serum monitoring, since the reduced enzyme induction on oxcarbazepine will lead to an abrupt rise in serum levels of other antiepileptics.

Gabapentin

Gabapentin (Neurontin) was designed as a GABA agonist and is structurally similar to GABA, but does not appear to act via the GABA system. Its mechanism of action remains obscure, but probably depends on alterations in the metabolism of brain amino acids (Taylor 1994). It is effective as add-on therapy for partial seizures with or without secondary generalisation, in patients who have not achieved satisfactory control with standard anticonvulsants (Ramsay 1994). It is ineffective with absence

seizures and may cause their exacerbation. Trials of monotherapy are under way. It is not metabolised, does not induce liver enzymes and is excreted unchanged in the urine. A chief virtue is the lack of significant interactions with standard antiepileptic medications, which can be important in patients who require polytherapy.

Gabapentin is in general well tolerated, though transient adverse effects are common when used in conjunction with other anticonvulsants. The most frequent are somnolence, dizziness, ataxia, nystagmus, headache, diplopia, rhinitis and nausea or vomiting. These rarely dictate withdrawal. Less commonly patients may experience pharyngitis, weight gain and dyspepsia.

Dosage begins at 300 mg per day, increasing to 300 mg three times per day over several days. This may be increased to 1200–2400 mg per day, given in three divided doses.

Other new antiepileptics

Other new antiepileptics include tiagabine, topiramate and zionisamide. A recent review of randomised placebo-controlled trials concluded that all are effective as add-on treatment in patients with refractory partial seizures, but that there was no evidence pointing to the superiority of any one of them, nor of vigabatrin, lamotrigine or gabapentin (Marson et al. 1996).

Other drugs

Phenobarbitone

Phenobarbitone (Gardenal, Luminal) held sway in the treatment of epilepsy for many decades after its introduction in 1912, but has gradually yielded pride of place to the above medications. It has a wide margin of safety, is cheap in relation to other anticonvulsants and serious side effects other than sedation are rare. Unfortunately, however, it is now apparent that it produces an unacceptable degree of cognitive impairment in many patients.

It is probably equal in anticonvulsant effect to carbamazepine or phenytoin for generalised grand mal, also for focal motor and sensory seizures. It is often less satisfactory in temporal lobe epilepsy, and may indeed aggravate attacks or lead to an increase in aggressive behaviour. Young children can react paradoxically to phenobarbitone, becoming restless, hyperactive and with worsened behaviour.

The chief drawback of phenobarbitone in routine practice is a tendency to produce oversedation. Occasional patients are particularly sensitive in this respect, developing mental dullness, drowsiness and lethargy. Impotence, blurred vision, headache and muscular incoordination may also be troublesome. Depression can become severe and should be watched for carefully. Phenobarbitone also shares with phenytoin and primidone the liability to disturb folate metabolism, with the possible psychological effects discussed in Chapter 12 (p. 592). *Methyl phenobarbitone* (Prominal) was introduced in attempts to overcome the sedative actions of phenobarbitone but has proved to be less effective as an anticonvulsant.

The dose of phenobarbitone is 30 mg at night, increased usually to no more than 120 mg per day on account of sedation.

Primidone

Primidone (Mysoline) may be tried when other drugs have proved ineffective. It is often used in place of phenobarbitone while phenytoin is continued, though it remains uncertain whether this combination is superior. There is little point in using phenobarbitone and primidone together, since the latter is largely metabolised to phenobarbitone in the liver. In the past primidone was regarded as the drug of choice for temporal lobe epilepsy, although there has been no controlled evidence to support this opinion.

The chief side effect is sedation with drowsiness, dizziness and confusion, but this usually soon subsides. Slowing of mental performance may, however, persist. Ataxia and dysarthria may occur, or less commonly nausea, anorexia and skin rashes.

It is important to start primidone gradually, in a dose of 125 mg each night, because of initial intolerance. Up to 1500 mg per day may ultimately be required.

Clobazam

Clobazam (Frisium), a benzodiazepine, possesses strong anticonvulsant properties, but adaptation to its effects tends to occur. It is nevertheless regarded as one of the first among the second-line drugs. Dellaportas *et al.* (1984) reported sustained benefit in a group of patients with poorly controlled generalised and partial seizures when the drug was added to existing regimens. This was maintained over a 6-month trial period.

Since effective doses can be employed from the outset, clobazam can be particularly useful as a short-term addition to existing regimens in patients whose attacks occur in clusters. A single dose of 20–30 mg can be taken immediately after the first seizure of a group and continued for several days (Feely 1989). It can similarly be used to provide 'cover' for special events in patients with refractory epilepsy. The chief side effects are sedation and drowsiness. Withdrawal seizures are particularly prone to occur when the drug is discontinued after long-term administration.

Sulthiame

Sulthiame (Ospolot) is of relatively little value as a primary antiepileptic agent, but can occasionally be useful as an adjunct to other medication in the treatment of generalised grand mal and focal seizures. Its success probably largely depended on inhibiting the metabolism of phenytoin, phenobarbitone or primidone given concurrently, thereby raising their blood levels. It is now less used than formerly.

Sulthiame enjoyed a vogue in the treatment of temporal lobe epilepsy, also for ameliorating disturbed behaviour. Improvements in conduct, social adjustment and emotional stability were occasionally reported, particularly among mentally handicapped epileptics (Liu 1966), and even among such patients who did not suffer from epilepsy (Moffatt *et al.* 1970).

Toxic symptoms may appear at high dosage—headache, drowsiness, paraesthesiae, weight loss, and hyperpnoea. Phenytoin intoxication can be induced. It must therefore be used cautiously in relatively low dosage, 200 mg twice per day up to 600 mg per day.

Troxidone

Troxidone (Tridione) was formerly extensively used for petit mal absences, but its popularity has declined in favour of newer medications. It can aggravate concurrent grand mal seizures and have serious toxic effects on the bone marrow or kidney. Regular blood counts are essential while patients are on treatment. Skin rashes may occur, or photophobia and 'glare' due to the increased time required for adaptation to changes in illumination. The dose is 300 mg twice per day, to a maximum of 1200 mg in adults. The related drug *paramethadione* (Paradione) is rather less toxic than troxidone but also less potent.

Diazepam

Diazepam (Valium) has a potent initial anticonvulsant effect, coupled with low toxicity, which makes it extremely effective in status epilepticus. It has proved of little use in the treatment of chronic epilepsy, however, because tolerance develops and the anticonvulsant effect declines. Nevertheless it can be given as an adjunct to other anticonvulsants, and here its action as a tranquillising agent may be its principal value. Among hospitalised epileptic patients it has sometimes been shown to have a favourable effect on seizure frequency and to control excitement, hostility and possibly paranoia (Lehmann & Ban 1968; Goddard & Lokare 1970).

Nitrazepam

Nitrazepam (Mogadon) can be of value in the myoclonic epilepsies of infancy, childhood and adolescence, combined when necessary with sodium valproate.

Dextroamphetamine sulphate

Dextroamphetamine sulphate (Dexedrine), 5–10 mg mane, occasionally produces good results in children with simple absences, also in epileptic children who show hyperkinesis or other behaviour disorders.

Acetazolamide

Acetazolamide (Diamox) can sometimes produce improvement but its usefulness is limited by the rapid development of tolerance.

Status epilepticus

Status epilepticus is a grave medical emergency in which speed of control is of the utmost importance. Cerebral anoxia may lead to permanent physical or mental handicaps, and there is a significant mortality with long-continued attacks.

An adequate airway must be ensured from the outset and oxygen administered where possible. Blood should ideally be withdrawn at an early stage to measure serum anticonvulsant levels, blood glucose, urea, electrolytes, calcium, haemoglobin and blood gases. Commonly, however, this will be deferred until emergency drug treatment has been administered.

Intravenous diazepam is regarded as the treatment of choice when veins are readily accessible, up to a maximum of 20 mg. The first 10 mg should be injected quickly, then the rest in 2 mg boluses over the next minute or two. Rectal diazepam is worth trying if venous access is a problem (Brodie 1989b). This should be followed immediately by phenytoin intravenously at a rate no greater than 50 mg per minute, to a total of 15 mg per kilogram body weight to prevent recurrence. An alternative is paraldehyde, 10 ml intramuscularly, with not more than 5 ml being injected at one intramuscular site. Although unpleasant, paraldehyde remains an effective drug. When intravenous diazepam is not available the latter drugs may be used alone, or 200–300 mg of pheno-

barbitone may be given intramuscularly. Clonazepam (Rivotril) has also been shown to be effective, sometimes even when intravenous diazepam has failed (Gastaut et al. 1971). The dose is 1 mg by slow intravenous infusion.

If these measures do not suffice an intravenous drip is likely to be required. An infusion of a 0.8% solution of chlormethiazole is commonly employed, giving 40–100 ml over a period of 5–10 minutes then reducing to a maintenance dose of 1 ml per minute if convulsions persist. Care must be taken to watch for overhydration, respiratory depression or hypotension. Alternatively 10 ml of paraldehyde may be diluted in 100 ml normal saline and administered over 10–15 minutes or until fitting ceases. A further infusion of diazepam can also be effective – 40 mg diluted in 500 ml of 5% dextrose and administered at 100 ml per hour. However, when large doses of diazepam have been infused coma may persist for some considerable time after the status has been controlled.

If status still continues thiopentone anaesthesia will be necessary, with muscle relaxants and positive-pressure ventilation together with continuous monitoring of EEG activity. This may very occasionally be required for several days along with the administration of anticonvulsants and chlormethiazole.

When status has been controlled it is important to assess the factors that have led to it. The anticonvulsant regimen may need reappraisal, infection may be present or a progressive cerebral lesion may require investigation.

Absence status (p. 256) is a benign self-limiting disorder, but when necessary can usually be abruptly terminated by a small amount of intravenous diazepam.

Psychological and social aspects of management

As already emphasised, drug treatment is rarely the sole aspect of management that needs to be considered. A liability to seizures, at unpredictable intervals and often with serious or embarrassing consequences, is bound to be a deeply unsettling disability. Social repercussions may add profoundly to the patient's difficulties of adjustment, particularly in the fields of education, employment and personal relationships. Time must therefore be devoted to understanding the patient and his current situation in some detail if he is to receive optimum help.

On-going surveillance will always be required, with periodic reviews even when things are going well. Much can be achieved by sympathetic support over long periods of time, with discussion of difficulties as they arise. The doctor–patient relationship is of particular importance and must sometimes be fostered with more than the average degree of skill. Some patients seek to ignore their epilepsy and are careless about medication; others become markedly frustrated by the problems they encounter, develop paranoid attitudes or seek fresh consultations and frequent changes of doctor. Thus a good deal of tolerance and understanding may be required if continuity of care is to be achieved. Patients who are handicapped by low intelligence or difficulties of personality will pose special problems in this regard, and will, of course, be particularly common among those who come before the psychiatrist.

The nature of the disorder should be explained frankly and realistically to the patient and the relatives. Any necessary limitation of activities must be discussed, and the need for regular medication emphasised. Where the patient appears to be unreliable, medication may need to be entrusted to a parent or spouse. Exploration of attitudes to the disorder will often prove helpful, particularly in correcting misconceptions and prejudices which can otherwise become deeply ingrained. Young patients must be helped to regard themselves in as normal a light as possible. Parents should be encouraged to allow every possible freedom, to use normal discipline and to integrate the child into ordinary family life if social and emotional growth is to be fostered.

Beyond this, psychotherapy at any intensive level is rarely indicated. It may indeed be harmful, with aggravation of seizures if too much anxiety is engendered. The occasional patient, however, will warrant a more detailed approach, particularly when passing through vulnerable periods of development such as adolescence, or when special emotional or interpersonal difficulties need to be resolved. Claims have occasionally been made for the efficacy of analytically orientated psychotherapy as a direct aid to the alleviation of seizures, by revealing their dynamic origin and symbolic significance (Sperling 1953), but here the credentials of psychotherapy are not impressive.

Obviously some restrictions on the patient's life will be necessary as long as a liability to seizures persists. Those that are indicated are dictated largely by common sense. Climbing or cycling should be forbidden in children. Swimming should be undertaken only in company. Other athletic pursuits are usually to be encouraged. With regard to employment, the patient must not be in a position to injure himself or others if a seizure should occur. Thus working at heights or in proximity to fire will be unsuitable, likewise driving or work involving dangerous machinery. Certain professional activities are best avoided if it is considered that even an occasional attack could have seriously adverse consequences.

With regard to driving, a person who has had epileptic seizures will not be issued with a driving licence unless the licensing authority (in the UK the Driving and Vehicle Licensing Agency) is satisfied that he is unlikely to be a source of danger to the public. Until recently it was necessary for the applicant to have been free from attacks for a minimum of 2 years, but this requirement has been reduced to 1 year since August 1994 (Shorvon 1995). In persons whose attacks occur only during sleep this pattern must have existed for at least 3 years. The regulations apply whether or not the person is receiving anticonvulsants, and there is thus no incentive to try going without medication in order to qualify more surely for a licence. In effect the regulations recognise the existence of the fully controlled epileptic, and the person who consistently has attacks only while sleeping. 'Provoked seizures', which are precipitated by exceptional and non-recurring circumstances, are not considered to warrant a diagnosis of epilepsy, and driving is usually allowed once the provoking factor has been successfully treated or removed. Seizures related to alcohol or illicit drugs do not qualify in this sense as provoked.

It is important, of course, that if medication is subsequently withdrawn the patient should cease driving for at least 6 months, during which it can be ensured that seizures remain in abeyance. Driving should also be suspended during changes in drug treatment, although this is not covered by legislation. Should an attack occur during change of treatment the regulations will of course immediately apply and the licence will be withdrawn.

The above applies to the issuing of ordinary licences. Stricter conditions surround the granting of vocational (Group 2) licences, for which there must have been complete freedom from attacks for a minimum of 10 years. The person must have taken no antiepileptic medication throughout this period, and there must not be a continuing liability to seizures by way of a potentially epileptogenic brain lesion.

Fitness for marriage or procreation are among the more emotionally loaded social problems which the epileptic must face. If advice is requested this can only be given on an individual basis. Psychological fitness for marriage or parenthood will often be a more important deciding factor than the occasional fit that occurs, yet the latter may have weighed unduly in the patient's mind. Qualities in the spouse will need to be considered, and the degree of the patient's disablement in economic terms. The advice which can be offered on the question of heredity is discussed on pp. 247–8.

Valuable assistance can be given in the epileptic clinic by a social worker experienced in the problems encountered by epileptics. Most patients tend to be confronted with difficulties in making an adequate social adjustment, and may face considerable rejection from time to time. Counselling of relatives can often usefully be extended to school teachers, employers and wardens of hostels. The patient may be put in touch with fellow sufferers through branches of the British Epilepsy Association, which also provide advice and information on a wide range of social and employment problems.

A hard core of patients will require very considerable help on account of refractory epilepsy, personality difficulties and severe social problems. A multidisciplinary team may then be essential for proper guidance, with collaboration among physicians, social workers, occupational therapists and nurses. A period away from home will often help where deteriorating family relationships are concerned, and a stay in hospital or a rehabilitation centre can provide new support by way of a disciplined yet understanding environment. Employment problems typically loom large in such patients, and a comprehensive evaluation may be required of the patient's assets and liabilities, motivation for work and social competence in interpersonal relationships. Fortunately it is only a small minority of patients who defeat all efforts at rehabilitation and prove ultimately to require long-term sheltered care.

Other aspects of treatment

Certain relatively simple matters deserve attention, particularly in patients who have shown a disappointing response to medication. Daily life should be as well ordered as possible, with regular sleep, regular meals and the avoidance of sudden changes in routine. Prolonged physical exertion should be discouraged, also sudden excitement or situations predisposing to tension or emotional stress. Alcohol intake should be strictly limited. Careful consideration of factors such as these may indicate why seizures have occurred on some occasions but not on others. Sometimes highly specific precipitants will be discovered as already discussed (p. 241).

Behavioural treatment

The conditioned inhibition or arrest of seizures may occasionally be possible as in the interesting example reported by Efron (1957):

The patient had a complex aura to her seizures, beginning with depersonalisation then leading on to forced thinking, olfactory hallucinations, auditory hallucinations and adversive head movements preceding the grand mal climax. The march of the aura, and thereby the grand mal convulsion, was found to be averted by the application of a strong unpleasant odour at a sufficiently early point in the development of the aura. This was assumed to be due to the activation of a widespread inhibitory system by the unpleasant olfactory stimulus. Later it was shown that repeated couplings of the odour with a visual stimulus (a silver bracelet) allowed the latter alone to become effective in terminating attacks. By looking at the bracelet the patient could inhibit impending attacks. In other words it had become a conditioned stimulus. Later, merely thinking intensely about the bracelet could arrest the seizures without the necessity of looking at it — a second order conditioning situation had been achieved.

Systematic deconditioning may also be effective when a specific precipitating situation can be identified. Forster and colleagues reported success with a number of types of sensory-evoked seizures (Forster *et al.* 1965; Forster 1969). In patients with photosensitive seizures repeated stroboscopic stimulation was employed, at first in a brightly lit room so that the stroboscope was barely perceptible, then gradually proceeding to stimulation in darkness. Or a start could be made with monocular presentations, or presentations outside the flash frequency to which the patient was sensitive. Pattern-provoked epilepsies were deconditioned by starting with presentations in dim light or out of focus, then gradually moving to clear presentation of the noxious patterns. Somatosensory seizures were treated by tapping outside the sensitive area of the body, then moving into it; or starting with very light taps and gradually increasing their intensity. In startle epilepsies the provoking stimulus was delivered with gradually increasing intensity, starting well below the level which evoked a seizure.

An interesting example of deconditioning to musicogenic epilepsy involved a patient in whom psychomotor attacks were provoked by a particular piece of music when presented in an orchestrated version but not when rendered on the piano or organ (Forster *et al.* 1965). The availability of many commercial variants allowed deconditioning to be achieved by proceeding carefully along a gradient from innocuous to noxious forms of the music; generalisation was ultimately achieved, extending to other noxious music not directly implicated in the deconditioning process. In other cases a simpler method was employed, utilizing the refractory period after a seizure — the music was continuously replayed during the ictal and post-ictal period until it lost its ability to provoke dysrhythmia.

Adams (1976) reviewed other methods employed to decondition patients to special precipitants in reflex epilepsy. In startle epilepsy to sound, for example, ambient background noise can be progressively decreased while the patient is trained to relax. For reading-induced seizures the patient may be trained in competing responses, such as tapping the knee whenever selected letters occur in the text. With all such deconditioning procedures the beneficial outcome often tends to be temporary, and reinforcement may be necessary on a day-to-day basis. Sometimes a 'second signal system' can be elaborated, for instance by coupling auditory clicks with flashes of light during the process of deconditioning photosensitive patients, thereby enabling the clicks to acquire protective properties.

A range of psychological manoeuvres may warrant a trial even in patients whose seizures do not have an obvious precipitant. These are discussed by Powell (1981), Brown and Fenwick (1989) and Fenwick (1991). Goldstein (1990) provides a critical review. It may be possible to identify emotional triggers to the fits, and desensitise the patient to these by frequent rehearsal or systematic desensitisation; or to train the patient in relaxation while he imagines situations in which fits are likely to occur or while he relives the prodromata to his usual seizures. Such relaxation may be coupled to a cue word such as 'relax' or 'stop', or to some activity such as clenching the fist. These can then be employed when fits are felt to be imminent. Case reports have shown the value of such procedures in reducing seizures in suitably motivated individuals. Often, however, the precise elements in the training which are most beneficial remain uncertain. Some patients appear to benefit from cue-controlled relaxation at the threshold of seizure onset, others from abrupt induced arousal.

Operant management techniques have also been employed with some success, most notably in patients in an institutional setting. These may involve positive reinforcement, as in token economy regimes, or the withdrawal of reinforcement by ignoring seizures, shifting attention away from them or imposing periods of 'time out' immediately after a fit. This last must obviously be applied only with care and sensitivity. Lavender (1981) used a token economy regime for reinforcing seizure-free periods among children in a residential hospital school. The patients were first helped to develop methods for interrupting their seizures, then rewarded systematically to motivate their use. Success from such methods will obviously stand to be greater in patients with self-induced seizures or pseudoseizures, but appear sometimes to be effective more generally.

The application of abrupt external stimulation has long been known to cut short seizures in certain patients, and this has been exploited systematically by Carasso *et al.* (1992). They report that the induction of pain, by dorsiflexion of the palm, can be highly effective in terminating seizures, whether focal or generalised in nature. The pressure must be continually applied until the convulsive frequency is visibly reduced. The technique may be temporarily effective even in status epilepticus. Coincident EEG recording in several cases has shown abrupt cessation of dysrhythmic activity following application of the noxious stimulation. An advantage of such a relatively simple technique is that it can be taught to family members. Experience of using it

in some 120 patients is claimed to have resulted in successful termination of attacks in 90% of instances, usually within 30–60 seconds.

A controversial area, of still unproved value, concerns biofeedback training to augment specific EEG rhythms. This is based on the premise that epileptiform discharges are incompatible with certain frequency bands in the EEG. The studies carried out with such methods are reviewed by Fischer-Williams *et al.* (1981), Kogeorgos and Scott (1981) and Fenwick (1981a, 1991). It has proved possible, for example, to train patients to enhance their occipital alpha rhythm, to suppress low frequency activity in the neighbourhood of a focus, or to augment low voltage fast activity. Training in the augmentation of the 12–14 Hz 'sensorimotor rhythm' (SMR) has attracted considerable interest. Reports of success have not, however, been uniformly upheld and powerful placebo effects are often likely to be at work. The biofeedback setting is conducive to relaxation which may be beneficial in itself. Further careful studies may define the true value of such approaches.

Treatment of psychiatric complications

Where patients show the various complications of epilepsy already outlined, every effort must be made in the first place to reduce seizures to a minimum. There will often be a corresponding improvement in personality disorder, emotional instability or intellectual deterioration. Unfortunately, however, this is not always so. Some patients may show an antithetical relationship between frequency of seizures and mental disturbance; moodiness and irritability may increase when seizures are few in number and improve when fits occur, or psychotic episodes may make an appearance shortly after seizures are brought under strict control (pp. 269 and 284). In such patients an uneasy compromise may need to be established, in which occasional seizures are tolerated for the sake of improved overall adjustment.

An important step in any patient showing psychiatric disorder is to review the antiepileptic medication currently being given. Subtle toxic effects may otherwise readily escape detection. The benefits observed when polypharmacy is reduced, and those sometimes strikingly achieved when patients are transferred to carbamazepine, are outlined on pp. 263 and 299.

The management of personality problems proceeds along the lines applicable to personality disorders generally. Supportive psychotherapy may need to be combined with appropriate psychotropic medication. Phenothiazines and butyrophenones can be a considerable aid in patients who are markedly aggressive or paranoid, but must be used with caution on account of their liability to increase seizures. Anticonvulsant medication may need to be adjusted accordingly. Benzodiazepines may be indicated for tension or apprehension, though care must be taken that irritability and aggression are not worsened coincidentally.

Problems can be encountered in the treatment of depression in that most antidepressants, including tricyclics, monoamine oxidase inhibitors and 5-hydroxytryptamine reuptake inhibitors, lower the seizure threshold. Drugs particularly incriminated in this regard include imipramine, amitriptyline and mianserin. Nomifensine was an exception though this has been withdrawn in the UK on account of toxic effects. In a double-blind comparison, Robertson (1985) showed that nomifensine was significantly more effective than amitriptyline in relieving depression in epileptic patients. The same trial demonstrated, however, that response to a placebo was common in the early phases of treatment, so it may be worth withholding antidepressants for a while when the depression is not severe. The rationalisation of polypharmacy can usefully be undertaken in the interim, perhaps with the substitution of carbamazepine for other anticonvulsants. In severe depressive illnesses with substantial risk of suicide, electroconvulsive therapy is not contraindicated.

Medication will play an important part in the management of many epileptic psychoses. For transient psychotic states occurring in close relationship to seizures it may be possible to avoid major tranquillisers, with their risk of aggravating seizures, and to sedate the patient with benzodiazepines or chlormethiazole instead (Trimble 1981b). Stronger neuroleptics will usually be required, however, for inter-ictal psychoses with schizophrenic or paranoid features. Haloperidol or pimozide are probably least liable to provoke seizures, and sulpiride is a useful alternative (Trimble 1991). For longer-term management flupenthixol decanoate may be required intramuscularly. Close monitoring of serum anticonvulsant levels will always be indicated once neuroleptic treatment is commenced. When dealing with a first episode of psychotic illness, the antipsychotic drugs will warrant withdrawal once the symptoms are controlled and the mental state is stable. Relapse will then indicate the need for maintenance therapy, but the possibilities of spontaneous remission must still be kept in mind — attempts to withdraw medication should in principle be deferred rather than abandoned altogether (Toone 1981). In addition, chronically disabled patients with a schizophrenia-like psychosis will require management as for schizophrenia generally, with every effort at rehabilitation towards life within the community.

The majority of acute organic psychoses resolve spontaneously, either with or without a convulsion occurring. Prolonged twilight states and post-ictal disorders are best treated conservatively initially, or at least as long as the patient is no danger to himself or others. A first step should be the estimation of serum anticonvulsant levels since medication may have been omitted by the patient. Hospitalisation will obviously be indicated for long-continued episodes, and nursing observation must be close. Anticonvulsants are rarely effective in terminating such episodes, but treatment as for status epilepticus may occasionally be required if the patient becomes dangerously overactive. When antipsychotic medication is indicated haloperidol or pimozide are again the drugs of choice. Electroconvulsive therapy can bring an abrupt resolution and should not be long withheld if the patient is in danger of becoming exhausted. Such treatment is said to be particularly effective in episodes accompanied by marked abnormalities of mood or florid delusions and hallucinations (Slater & Roth 1969). The presence of confusion and clouding of consciousness is no contraindication, provided the epileptic basis of the disorder is well established and other intracranial causes have been excluded.

Here it may be noted that electroconvulsive therapy has very occasionally found a place in the management of epileptic patients who show no psychotic phenomena. It is an old observation that a major convulsion may resolve a phase of mood or behaviour disturbance in epileptic subjects, and a case can sometimes be made for trying the effect of a single induced convulsion in such a situation.

Electroconvulsive treatment has also been used as a temporary protection against spontaneous fits. Kalinowsky and Kennedy (1943) showed that after such treatment the threshold for convulsions was temporarily raised, and in two patients with regularly recurring seizures they were able to avert spontaneous attacks for several months by its judicious use. With modern anticonvulsant medication, however, there will rarely be occasion to attempt such a therapeutic approach.

Surgical treatment

Surgical approaches to epilepsy can be extremely successful in properly selected patients. Two main approaches can be distinguished — the excision of damaged brain tissue responsible for focal seizures and the interruption of tracts which propagate seizure discharges to other parts of the brain. The former is by far the most common, especially temporal lobectomy. Hemispherectomy has special indications in childhood. Among lesional approaches, division of the corpus callosum can be effective with non-focal seizures, and multiple subpial transection finds a place in sensitive areas such as the motor cortex.

Reviewing the effects of over 6000 operations carried out worldwide between 1986 and 1990, Engel (1993) reported that almost 60% of patients were rendered fit-free and a further 29% were improved. Descriptions of the surgical procedures commonly employed, and their indications and complications, are provided by Oxbury and Adams (1989) and Polkey and Binnie (1993), with special emphasis on experience gained at the Maudsley Hospital and at Oxford.

Pre-requisites for surgery are that the patient should have true epileptic seizures, as determined by a careful clinical history and where possible observation of attacks, along with good evidence that the seizures are occurring at an unacceptable frequency despite anticonvulsant medication. A frequency of at least one seizure per week will usually be required, despite adequate trials of three standard anticonvulsants for at least 2 years. Surgery may, however, be offered earlier than this when definite focal pathology is demonstrated in an operable site. Age must usually be less than 55 years. A full scale IQ of less than 70 will sometimes be a bar to operation, since with intelligence less than this it is more probable that diffuse brain damage is responsible for the seizures; however, low intelligence is not a contraindication in all situations, particularly when a structural lesion can be shown.

A history of psychiatric disturbance is encountered in a considerable proportion of patients referred for operation, and in the main is not a contraindication. It is important, however, to distinguish aspects associated with the epilepsy from those that are unrelated to it, and to be confident that the patient can cope with the procedure and subsequent rehabilitation. Where resective surgery is concerned it will be necessary to show that the fits originate in one part of the brain, preferably with evidence of a structural lesion, also that the rest of the brain is normal. Hence the need for thorough investigation in every case before deciding that the operation and its attendant risks are justified (see below).

Temporal lobectomy

Temporal lobectomy is the commonest procedure carried out both in the UK and North America. Some form of unilateral temporal lobe resection accounts for two-thirds of operations worldwide (Engel 1993). The operation in the UK consists of a tailored *en bloc* removal of some 4.5–6.5 cm of the temporal neocortex as measured from the pole, along with an equivalent portion (usually 2–3 cm) of the hippocampus and the amygdala (Falconer 1969, 1971). The precise extent of the removal may be determined by electrocorticography carried out at operation, and will normally be more restricted when in the hemisphere dominant for language. The outcome is more likely to be successful when the amygdala and at least part of the hippocampus is included in the excision, even when the primary pathology (for example an indolent glioma) does not involve these structures.

A more *selective amygdalohippocampectomy* may be the operation of choice when depth recordings show consistent seizure onset from within the hippocampus and/or amygdala of one side. This involves resection of the medial temporal structures alone. It probably results in less adverse consequences on cognitive function (Goldstein & Polkey 1993), and may be particularly indicated in operations on the hemisphere dominant for language or when amytal tests have shown significant disruption of memory on the side to be resected.

The selection of patients for operation requires great care. In addition to the general indications outlined above, investigations must be performed to clarify the site and extent of likely pathology. The better the concordance between the various indices of localisation, the more confidently will surgery be undertaken. Scalp EEGs are of limited value in confirming unilateral pathology, but it is reassuring when EEG data, during waking and sleep, is entirely concordant with all other sources of information. It is known, however, that bilateral foci on scalp recordings may sometimes exist with unilateral pathology, these secondary foci usually regressing after surgery. Foramen ovale electrodes can be valuable in indicating foci originating in the medial temporal lobe structures, and are now regarded as superior to sphenoidal lead recordings. In cases of uncertainty, and especially when a frontal lobe focus is suspected, it may be necessary to proceed to subdural electrodes or depth recordings before a decision over operation is reached. Binnie *et al.* (1994) have demonstrated the value of such procedures in a large series of patients. Telemetry may enable ictal activity to be recorded in successive attacks, confirming a constant site of origin for the ictal discharge.

Neuroimaging is essential, the gold standard being good quality MRI, or failing that CT orientated along the axis of the temporal lobe. The former is better at detecting small discrete lesions or temporal lobe asymmetries as described on p. 289, and may yield direct evidence of mesial temporal sclerosis. FDG-PET or SPECT may occasionally be employed to confirm unilaterality, the latter allowing peri-ictal blood flow changes to be charted in a clinical setting (p. 289).

Neuropsychological testing adds further information, revealing evidence of localised malfunction and helping to predict the likely effects of the proposed resection. A useful review of neuropsychological testing in this context is provided by Goldstein (1991). An important component consists of the Wada intracarotid amytal test (p. 40), during which language dominance and the memory capacity of each hemisphere can be assessed. Powell *et al.* (1987) describe the procedures involved and the results in a series of patients. Ideally the test should demonstrate preservation of speech and memory during inactivation of the hemisphere to be operated upon, and abolition of these functions when the contralateral hemisphere is anaesthetised. Often, however, incomplete lateralisation is revealed in epileptic patients.

Bilateral pathology contradicting operation is suggested by absence of a clear unilateral preponderance of spikes at the foramen ovale or sphenoidal electrodes, neuroradiological evidence of bilateral temporal lobe atrophy or atrophy opposite to the predominant EEG focus, or the combination of verbal with non-verbal memory deficits on neuropsychological assessment.

The mortality from temporal lobe resections is less than 0.5%, though some 1–2% of patients may be left with dysphasia or hemiparesis. An asymptomatic upper quadratic homonymous visual field defect results in most cases. Outcome in terms of seizure relief is usually excellent, with more than 50% of patients being rendered fit-free and less than 20% being unimproved. In successful cases anticonvulsant medication can usually be withdrawn. In a small proportion seizures may ultimately recur on long-term follow-up, this occurring in 15% of the Maudsley series after a fit-free period of 2–10 years. The nature of the pathology discovered is strongly related to a successful outcome: benign lesions such as indolent tumours are associated with a seizure relief rate of 80%, mesial temporal sclerosis 60%, and non-specific pathology only 15% (Polkey & Binnie 1993). In a reanalysis of Falconer's cases, Bruton (1988) showed that the best results in terms of social adjustment in addition to fit control were obtained when the resected specimen showed mesial sclerosis.

The effects on cognitive function are variable, some patients improving along with seizure control. Others, however, may be aware of mild memory difficulties, particularly with excisions from the dominant hemisphere. Older patients, especially, are liable to acquire material-specific memory deficits which are demonstrable on neuropsychological testing — for verbal material after dominant lobectomy and for non-verbal material after non-dominant lobectomy (Goldstein *et al.* 1988). Quantitative MRI has shown that the severity of such deficits is related to the extent of removal of medial temporal lobe brain tissue (Katz *et al.* 1989). Impairments of this nature are rarely severe enough to handicap the patient in everyday life, but self-report questionnaires show that both the patients and their relatives are often aware of some degree of memory difficulty (Goldstein & Polkey 1992). After left-sided dominant operations patients tended to complain of 'tip-of-the-tongue' phenomena, forgetting names and details of books they had read; right-sided operations were associated with poor memory for faces and difficulty with placing a previously seen face.

Where the epilepsy is relieved or lessened social adaptation is often markedly improved, with reduction of behaviour and personality disturbances (Taylor & Falconer 1968; Falconer 1973). However, such problems are not a prime reason for the operation and do not stand to improve with surgery if the epilepsy is already well controlled. The particular benefit that may be seen with aggression has already been discussed (p. 270), likewise improvement in psychosexual adjustment (p. 270). Inadequate or hysterical traits are not benefited and may contraindicate operation (Hill 1958).

There are concerns that depression may be increased above expectation after lobectomy. Depressive episodes in the first year or two after surgery (p. 270) may extend to a depressive psychosis, and an excess of suicides has been suspected. Taylor and Marsh (1977) reviewed the deaths in Falconer's series. Of 193 patients operated on before 1970 and with a minimum of 5 years' follow-up, 37 had died, nine from suicide and six in 'unclear' circumstances. Half of the patients who died from suicide had been fit-free since operation. When suicidal deaths were combined with probable suicides from the 'unclear' group, the total suicide risk rose to 50 times that expected for the British population. Right-sided lobectomy appears to be especially prone to be followed by depression, this being reported in up to a third of Polkey's patients (Polkey & Binnie 1993).

Jensen and Larsen (1979a, 1979b) found that surgery had no discernible effect on psychoses that were present preoperatively, and concluded that the presence of psychosis was not useful as a criterion either for or against operation. Of 74 patients followed up 1–10 years later, 11 had had a schizophrenia-like or schizoaffective psychosis before operation, and nine others developed psychoses during the follow-up period. Trimble (1991, 1992) reviews a number of reports where schizophrenia-like or paranoid psychoses have arisen as a new development postoperatively, noting an apparent excess after right- as opposed to left-sided lobectomy. A curious effect seems apparent from close inspection of the literature, whereby left lobectomy may be effective in sometimes terminating a psychosis of this nature, whereas right lobectomy is followed by its development, often many years later. These impressions have not yet been checked by comprehensive prospective studies. It was striking, nonetheless, that among six consecutive referrals of lobectomised patients to a psychiatric service Mace and Trimble (1991) found that the operation had been right-sided in all cases. The interval since operation varied from 1 month to 9 years; four patients were schizophrenic, one showed a delusional depression and one a Capgras' syndrome with depression. Manchanda *et al.* (1993) have reported four patients in whom post-ictal psychoses developed for the first time after surgery, all following right-sided lobectomy. Stevens (1990) suggests that aberrant reinnervation in projection sites related to the damaged or removed medial temporal structures may contribute to such developments. The phenomenon of 'forced normalisation' (p. 284) may also be relevant in some cases (Trimble 1992).

Other cortical resections

Other cortical resections vary from the removal of small discrete areas of cerebral cortex to ablation of a large part of a lobe. Guidance from electrocorticography at operation can be particularly important. With frontal lobectomy it is essential to preserve the frontal operculum of the Sylvian fissure on the side dominant for speech. Occipital lobectomy will inevitably result in a hemianopia, and parietal excisions may leave motor and sensory deficits. However, the patient may decide that such disability is worthwhile for relief from intractable seizures.

Hemispherectomy

Hemispherectomy has proved to be highly successful in patients with infantile hemiplegia, relieving the epilepsy and concurrently improving behaviour disorder (Beardsworth & Adams 1988). There may also be some lessening of spasticity. Interestingly, intelligence does not deteriorate postoperatively, and with the passage of time there may be considerable gains. Hemispherectomy has also been successful in children with Rasmussen's disease or 'chronic progressive encephalitis' (Rasmussen *et al.* 1958). This little-understood condition presents with intractable focal seizures and progressive neurological deterioration (Honovar *et al.* 1992).

Earlier attempts at the operation were abandoned when it became clear that there was a high incidence of delayed haemorrhagic complications, often many years later, with the development of obstructive hydrocephalus, haemosiderosis and intracranial haematomas.

However, a number of technical modifications have overcome such problems and the operation now yields excellent long-term results. Adams' (1983) operation creates a large extradural space and insulates the ventricular system from the remaining subdural cavity. Various techniques of 'functional hemispherectomy' and 'hemispherotomy' aim to isolate the hemisphere by severance of major tracts while leaving most of the hemisphere intact along with its blood supply (Delalande *et al.* 1993; Villemure *et al.* 1993; Schramm *et al.* 1995).

Section of the corpus callosum

Section of the corpus callosum was introduced as a means of preventing the spread of ictal discharges from one hemisphere to the other, and thereby the recruitment of abnormal discharges which culminates in the major seizure (Van Wagenen & Herren 1940). The operation was revived by Bogen and Vogel (1962), and more recently by Wilson *et al.* (1982) using a two-stage microsurgical technique. Roberts (1991) describes the operative procedures employed. It can prove beneficial with intractable generalised seizures, particularly akinetic seizures, or in patients with unilateral hemisphere disease which is not severe enough for hemispherectomy. Partial seizures are less responsive.

After section of the corpus callosum and other midline commissures, patients are often remarkably free from subjective psychological difficulties, despite the fact that appropriate testing procedures show that each hemisphere now processes information largely independently of the other (p. 41). The postoperative psychological studies carried out on these patients have clarified understanding of many aspects of brain organisation and function, particularly with regard to cerebral dominance for language and visuospatial functions (Gazzaniga *et al.* 1965; Sperry & Gazzaniga 1967; Bogen 1969). Some of the neuropsychological and psychiatric implications of the findings were summarised by Lishman (1969, 1971) and are discussed more recently by Gazzaniga (1985), Holtzman (1985), Sidtis (1985) and Volpe (1985). It has become clear, however, that occasional patients experience long-lasting deficits postoperatively in relation to language, attention and memory, and that there may sometimes be evidence of hemisphere competition in everyday activities (Ferguson *et al.* 1985).

Reeves (1991) reports that in the early postoperative period the non-dominant hand will often act in an antagonistic manner to the other, leading to difficulties with bimanual tasks such as eating, washing or opening and closing doors. Cooperation is ultimately established in most cases for well-learned bimanual tasks though new ones may be difficult to acquire. In a very small proportion 'interhemispheric antagonism' remains as a chronic problem. In one remarkable patient Reeves reports that the left and right arms abuse each other, potentially causing physical injury; and that the dominant left hemisphere sometimes verbally expresses hostility towards the left arm and leg, considering them to be another hostile person, altogether creating a disability which outweighs the excellent result in terms of seizure control.

Other disconnection procedures

These include temporal lobotomy and multiple subpial transection. Temporal lobotomy involves division of tracts lying above the anterior parts of the temporal horns but without removal of tissue (Turner 1969). Unlike lobectomy it can be carried out bilaterally without risk of damaging memory when there are independent epileptogenic foci in both temporal lobes. In Turner's hands it was frequently combined with lesions made in other parts of the brain. Outbursts of rage were said to be uniformly improved and seizures abolished in 65% of cases.

Multiple subpial transection consists of division of tangential intracortical fibres in blocks of cerebral cortex while vertical fibre connections are spared, so preserving function in sensitive areas such as the cortex subserving speech or motor function (Morrell *et al.* 1989). The technique has been employed in the Landau–Kleffner syndrome (p. 242).

Various stereotactic ablation procedures have also been devised, including ablation of the amygdaloid nucleus (Vaernet 1972). Hitchcock and Cairns (1973) have reported the benefit of amygdalotomy in diminishing aggressive behaviour, mood changes and suspiciousness, in addition to improving seizures.

Recently chronic intermittent stimulation of the vagus nerve has been shown to reduce the number of seizures in patients with medically refractory epilepsy, and may be an effective alternative for subjects who are not optimal candidates for surgery (Vagus Nerve Stimulation Study Group 1995).

Chapter 8: Intracranial Infections

Intracranial infections are usually the province of the neurologist or general physician but must occasionally be considered in the differential diagnosis of psychiatric patients. AIDS is of particular importance, likewise cerebral syphilis which, though rare, has crucial treatment implications. These will be dealt with in some detail, also certain encephalitic illnesses in which diagnostic confusion can arise. More space will be devoted to encephalitis lethargica than its present-day incidence warrants, because of the important lessons which were learned for psychiatry during outbreaks of the disease. Meningitis, cerebral abscess and other nervous system infections will be dealt with very briefly.

Acquired immune deficiency syndrome
(AIDS, human immunodeficiency virus (HIV) disease)

The appearance of AIDS on the medical and social scene in the early 1980s has been followed by worldwide spread of the disease and escalating numbers of persons affected. While rife in the USA and Europe, its impact is far greater in sub-Saharan Africa and other developing countries. Forecasts suggest that by the year 2000 there could be over 20 million people who are HIV positive or with AIDS; a cumulative total of 30–40 million people will have been infected, 90% of whom live in developing countries; the total of deaths could have exceeded 8 million and over 5 million children will have been orphaned (Communicable Disease Report 1994a).

Over 10 000 cases of AIDS were reported in the UK between 1982, when reporting began, and the end of 1994, 8.6% affecting females (Communicable Disease Report 1995). Seven thousand of these patients (68%) are known to have died. Infections with the HIV-1 virus have exceeded 23 000 since reporting began in 1984 (14% in females). Figures from the USA are many times in excess of this, a cumulative total of some 440 000 cases having been reported since 1981 (Morbidity & Mortality Weekly Report 1995). Altogether it is estimated that by 1994 there were 10 million infected adults in sub-Saharan Africa, 2.5 million in South and South East Asia, 2 million in Latin America and the Caribbean, and 1.5 million in North America and Western Europe (Communicable Disease Report 1994a).

Problems associated with the disease include not only its devastating clinical manifestations and their economic cost, but also the cultural and social problems that must be tackled in attempts to limit its spread. For the first time in a worldwide epidemic it has been necessary to try to change fundamental aspects of human behaviour by education and the dissemination of information. This, moreover, centres on topics as sensitive as sexual practices and the control of risk-taking behaviour among persons addicted to drugs. A particularly disturbing aspect concerns the risk of transmission to children born to infected women; the proportion of females has slowly risen and is particularly high, approaching 50%, in Africa.

Added difficulties arise from the stigma attaching to the disease and the fear engendered among populations at special risk, particularly the male homosexual community. This is fuelled by the ever-present risk of transmission from infected but asymptomatic individuals. Social difficulties in terms of employment, insurance and disruption of family relationships exacerbate the problems associated with the disease. In many respects, therefore, AIDS represents a new and unique threat to individuals and to society, and raises public health issues of a remarkably difficult nature.

Discussion of the evolution of the present epidemic and groups at special risk will be followed by an outline of the systemic manifestations of the disease. The impact on the nervous system will be described in some detail. Thereafter the question of subtle impairments in patients during the asymptomatic stage will be considered, also the range of other psychiatric disturbances that may present for attention, including the problem of the 'worried well'. Finally, certain treatment options will be reviewed as they exist at present.

Epidemiology and groups at risk

The disease was first recognised in 1981 when cases of *Pneumocystis carinii* pneumonia and Kaposi's sarcoma were reported from California and New York in men who were both homosexual and immunocompromised. The first UK cases were recognised soon afterwards. With hindsight, however, the disease had existed in the USA since at least 1978, and stored serum samples have indicated that the virus was entering the drug-injecting population in the mid-1970s (Des Jarlais *et al.* 1989). The disease is thought to have originated in Zaïre, travelling thence via Haiti to the USA and UK. Spread has been especially devastating among the countries of sub-Saharan Africa which are now the most severely affected of all, accounting for more than two-thirds of the estimated cases of AIDS worldwide and over 90% of the cases in women and children (Johnson & De Cock 1994). India and Thailand are also heavily affected with numbers of cases escalating alarmingly. One hundred and fifty-eight countries are now known to harbour the disease.

The subgroups of the population mainly affected differ with geographical location. In Western Europe, North America and Australasia homosexual and bisexual men are predominantly affected, followed by injecting drug users and heterosexual contacts with infected persons. On the west coast of America about 90% of HIV-infected persons are homosexual men, whereas on the east coast 40% are intravenous drug users. More than half of the estimated 200 000 drug injectors in New York are infected with HIV, and appear there to be the principal source of heterosexual and perinatal transmission (Des Jarlais *et al.* 1989). In the UK the prevalence varies among drug users,

from 10% in London to 55% in Edinburgh (Adler 1987). In Italy and Spain drug injection accounts for over two-thirds of the cases of AIDS; whereas in sub-Saharan Africa the commonest mode of transmission is heterosexual intercourse (Communicable Disease Report 1994a).

Table 15 shows the presumed routes of infection among cases reported during 1994 in the USA and the UK. Male homosexual transmission is clearly the commonest route. A large proportion of infections through heterosexual intercourse in the UK is thought to derive from infections acquired abroad, particularly from African countries. Transmissions via contaminated blood products were recognised from 1983, largely stemming from contaminated pooled factors VIII and IX given to haemophiliac patients. Mother to infant transmissions in the UK may be due in large part to mothers who acquired the infection in Africa.

The largest focus of infection in the UK is in London (Communicable Disease Report Review 1993), with the four Thames regions accounting for 70% of all cases. Homosexual transmission is the commonest route in all areas except Scotland, where it is exceeded by injecting drug use (29% and 48% of cases, respectively) (Communicable Disease Report 1994b). It seems possible that the steady upward trend among male homosexuals may be nearing its end in the UK, though this is disputed, and there are clear indications that the epidemic among drug addicts showed a decline towards the end of the 1980s (Working Group Report 1993). This is almost certainly due to education in safer injection practices and needle exchange schemes. Such hopeful signs are, however, offset by the increase in heterosexual transmission (Table 15).

Table 15 Exposure category in relation to AIDS and HIV-1 infection, January to December 1994 (after Communicable Disease Report 1995; Morbidity & Mortality Weekly Report 1995).

	AIDS (USA)	AIDS (UK)	HIV-1 infection (UK)
Total cases	80 691*	1789	2411
(% female)	(18%)	(12%)	(19%)
Possible mode of acquisition			
1 Sexual intercourse between men	43%	64%	56%
2 Heterosexual intercourse	10%	18%	28%†
3 Injecting drug use	27%	8%	7.5%
1 or 3	5%	1.5%	1%
4 Contaminated blood products	1.5%	4.5%	1%
5 Mother to infant	1%	2.5%	2%
6 Other/undetermined	12%	1%	4.5%

* Approximately half reflecting expanded definition of AIDS to include reduced CD_4 counts (p. 319).
† Compared with 17% since reporting began in 1984.

The HIV virus

The virus responsible for AIDS was isolated in 1983. It was at first named lymphadenopathy-associated virus (LAV) in France, and human T-cell lymphotropic virus type III (HTLV-III) in the USA, but by common consent is now termed the human immunodeficiency virus (HIV). The overwhelming majority of cases worldwide are caused by HIV-1, though the related HIV-2 virus (LAV-2, HTLV-IV) has proved to be responsible for a similar AIDS syndrome, principally among West Africans. HTLV-I virus is responsible for epidemics of tropical spastic paraparesis which may be transmitted sexually.

Related viruses in animals include visna virus in sheep and caprine arthritis encephalitis virus in goats, which lead to neurodegenerative disorders. Of particular interest is the simian immunodeficiency virus (SIV), which is closely related to HIV-2 and induces a disease similar in many respects to AIDS in macaque monkeys, providing a valuable animal model (Gravell 1988; Clements et al. 1994).

These are 'lentiviruses' (i.e. slow to replicate and produce pathological effects) from the general class of 'retroviruses'. Retroviruses have the unique characteristic of replicating by entering host cells, then using the enzyme reverse transcriptase to integrate their own genetic material into the DNA of the host cell nucleus. This then continues to manufacture the virus until the cell dies, resulting in persistent infection. The HIV virus infects cells which bear the CD_4 surface receptor, using a glycoprotein on its surface (gp 120) for the initial interaction. CD_4 receptors are found on monocytes, macrophages and a subset of T-helper lymphocytes (T_4 cells). Once inside the cell, reverse transcriptase carried in the genome of the virus catalyses the production of a DNA copy of the single-stranded viral RNA. This migrates to the nucleus of the cell and becomes integrated into its genome. The integrated DNA copy is called a 'provirus'. Thereafter it may exist in latent form without pathogenic effect, reproducing along with the cell, or it may change to become productive and cytopathic. Such change involves the production of new viral RNA, the assembly of viral proteins which are toxic to the cell, and the budding of new virus from the surface of the cell to infect others. The mechanisms underlying such change are poorly understood.

The hallmark of active HIV infection is the gradual depletion of T_4-helper lymphocytes in the blood, with correspondingly disastrous impairment of the body's immunological competence. Infection of macrophages and microglia leads to a further range of complications involving the nervous system directly as described below.

Natural history and clinical signs of HIV infection

Infection with HIV-1 follows a characteristic course, though with wide variation in the timing of the various stages (Communicable Disease Report Review 1994).

An acute 'seroconversion' illness affects 50–90% of people, setting in 2–6 weeks after exposure and probably reflecting direct invasion by the virus. Symptoms often take the form of a mild glandular fever-like illness with fever, myalgia, sore throat, lymphadenopathy and a maculopapular rash, generally subsiding within 1–2 weeks. More severe manifestations include mucocutaneous ulceration, or reflect nervous system invasion with aseptic meningitis, myelopathy or neuropathy, or a transient acute confusional state sometimes with seizures (Carne et al. 1985).

Early during this period, virus nucleic acid can be detected in the blood, the cerebrospinal fluid and most organs of the body. A transient lymphopaenia affects both CD_4 and CD_8 lymphocytes (T-helper and cytotoxic cells, respectively), followed a week or two later by lymphocytosis. Towards the end of this stage HIV-1 antibodies begin to appear in the serum, conventional antibody tests becoming positive after 2–6 weeks or occasionally after a delay of several months.

An asymptomatic phase then follows and may last for many years, during which the person is nonetheless infective. Viral levels remain low in the blood, but high levels of activity are maintained in the lymphoid system. The semen, blood and possibly the cervical secretions are particularly infective. There is no documented evidence of spread by saliva, ingestion or droplet inhalation, nor by casual or social contact. Health care workers must, however, beware of needle-stick injuries.

Generalised lymphadenopathy persists in up to a third of patients after seroconversion, and minor skin complaints may be troublesome, but otherwise the person remains well. Thrombocytopaenia of severe degree occasionally occurs. Throughout this period CD_4 counts remain in the normal range (450–1500/μl in women; 350–1440/μl in men), but tend to decline slowly with time. The duration of the asymptomatic phase varies widely, most persons progressing to further stages within 2–10 years but some remaining well for considerably longer. Recent cohort studies of homosexual and bisexual men have shown that up to half remain free from AIDS 10 years after initial infection and that 8% remain clinically normal after 10–15 years (Buchbinder et al. 1994; Rutherford 1994). Moreover some 5% appear to have nonprogressive infection in that they do not show declining CD_4 counts. A recent estimate of survival in a cohort of haemophiliac men, based on extrapolations of changes in CD_4 counts, suggests that as many as a quarter may remain free from AIDS for 20 years (Phillips *et al.* 1994).

Prolonged survival may owe much to treatment interventions with zidovudine (p. 335) and the use of prophylactic antibiotics and vaccines to prevent the more common opportunistic infections. Much may also depend on the robustness of the host's immunological response, and perhaps on characteristics of the viral strain involved. The study of long-term survivors has become important in efforts to determine the factors which may be protective (Baltimore 1995).

Early symptomatic infection begins to appear as the proportion of infected lymphocytes increases. Cell-mediated immunity falls, and recurrent viral infections such as herpes or warts make an appearance. Infections may also result from common bacterial pathogens such as *Pneumococcus*, *Haemophilus* and *Salmonella*. Recurrent vaginal candidiasis may occur in women.

Late symptomatic infection includes a constellation of symptoms which predict the progression to AIDS. Oral candidiasis and hairy leucoplakia of the tongue and cheek are usually of serious import. 'Constitutional symptoms' include low-grade pyrexia, night sweats, weight loss, fatigue and diarrhoea. The most valuable laboratory marker of disease progression is the declining trend in CD_4 counts, which correlates with progression to AIDS. Serum markers reflecting immune activation — β_2 microglobulin and serum neopterin — yield additional information for assessing prognosis. The clinical indicators described above are, however, the most valuable means for estimating progression of the disease; the risk of progression to AIDS within 2 years is approximately 40% in the presence of oral candidiasis or hairy leucoplakia, and virtually 100% when constitutional symptoms have appeared.

AIDS-defining illnesses finally make their appearance as definitive indications of severely compromised immunological function. By this stage viral replication is increasing rapidly and the CD_4 count has generally fallen below 200/μl. The three principal groups of illnesses are opportunistic infections, certain neoplastic conditions and the results of direct involvement of the nervous system by the HIV virus. This last may antedate evidence of immunodeficiency.

Opportunistic infections are legion, affecting the lungs, gastrointestinal tract and nervous system as low-grade organisms which have previously been tolerated gain hold. Pneumonia results from *Pneumocystis carinii*, cytomegalovirus, herpes simplex, *Cryptococcus* and atypical mycobacteria. Tuberculosis has increased very substantially in HIV-infected patients in Africa where it may

now be the most common opportunistic problem (Lucas *et al.* 1993). Severe diarrhoea may be caused by the protozoa cryptosporidium, *Isospora belli* and microsporidium, also *Candida*, cytomegalovirus and *Mycobacterium avium intracellulare*. The range of infections affecting the central nervous system is discussed in detail on p. 320 *et seq*.

Neoplasia characteristically consists of Kaposi's sarcoma of the skin or other organs, lymphomas, or more rarely squamous carcinoma of the mouth or anorectum.

Direct HIV infection of the nervous system is described on p. 322 *et seq*. Other conditions may mark the later stages of infection, including lymphoid interstitial pneumonitis, granulomatous hepatitis and recurrent salmonella septicaemia.

The commonest presenting symptoms in the UK between 1989 and 1992 were *Pneumocystis carinii* pneumonia (41% of cases), Kaposi's sarcoma (14%), oesophageal candidiasis (13%) and lymphomas (4%) (Communicable Disease Report Review 1994). However, the incidence of these manifestations varies in different groups of subjects at risk. European women rarely develop Kaposi's sarcoma, likewise patients with haemophilia, and injecting drug users in the USA have an unusually high frequency of pneumococcal pneumonia, pulmonary tuberculosis and bacterial sepsis. Changes are also occurring over time. *Pneumocystis carinii* pneumonia, though still very common, has fallen in frequency as the first AIDS-defining illness, probably due to effective prophylaxis with co-trimoxazole or pentamidine. Presentations with Kaposi's skin sarcoma have also fallen, though with improved length of survival patients more frequently progress to pulmonary or visceral forms of the neoplasm. By contrast, the incidence of non-Hodgkin's lymphoma and primary cerebral lymphoma is thought to be increasing.

Classification of HIV-related illness

Increasing awareness of the diversity of HIV-related manifestations has led to an evolving nomenclature which has been at times confusing.

Three categories of disorder were early recognised following upon the asymptomatic carrier stage — persistent generalised lymphadenopathy (PGL), AIDS-related complex (ARC) and the acquired immune deficiency syndrome (AIDS).

PGL is identified by enlargement of lymph nodes, 1 cm or more in diameter, in at least two extrainguinal sites and persisting for at least 3 months. A third of such cases show associated splenomegaly. PGL is largely symptomless, and is often thought to carry a relatively good prognosis with respect to early further progression. A proportion of such patients, however, show peripheral nerve disorder, and subjective memory difficulty and affective disorder appear to be commoner than in controls (Janssen *et al.*

1988). Neuropsychological evaluation may confirm mild cognitive impairment.

ARC is defined as a category of chronic disease which fails to fulfil the criteria for AIDS in that there is no clear evidence of opportunistic infection or neoplasia. The diagnosis usually requires two or more of the following, persisting for at least 3 months: low-grade pyrexia, weight loss exceeding 10% of body weight, PGL as defined above, oral candidiasis, diarrhoea, night sweats or fatigue interfering with work. One or more laboratory abnormalities such as decreased CD_4 lymphocyte counts are sometimes required in addition.

AIDS was originally diagnosed only when there was reliable evidence of a disease at least moderately indicative of underlying cellular immune deficiency, for example Kaposi's sarcoma (in a person under 60) or some opportunistic infection. Other causes of cellular immune deficiency or of reduced resistance to infection had also to be excluded.

With further experience of the range of disorders encountered, and armed with reliable serological tests, this cumbersome terminology has now been revised (Centers for Disease Control 1986). The new terminology allows, for example, for neurological disorder consequent upon invasion of the nervous system by the HIV virus, even when cellular immune deficiency has not been declared by systemic disease. Four categories of infection are recognised, the last being subdivided:

Group I (acute infection) represents transient symptoms occurring at the time of or shortly after seroconversion.

Group II (asymptomatic infection) is self explanatory.

Group III (persistent generalised lymphadenopathy) is defined as above (also known as lymphadenopathy syndrome or LAS).

Group IV (other disease) in effect incorporates both ARC and AIDS. It is subdivided into: (a) *constitutional disease*, consisting of one or more of fever for over a month, diarrhoea for over a month or weight loss exceeding 10% of body weight; (b) *neurological disease*, including dementia, myelopathy and peripheral neuropathy; (c) *secondary infectious disease*s; (d) *secondary cancers*; and (e) *other conditions*. The last includes, for example, patients with constitutional symptoms not meeting the criteria for subgroup IV(a), infections not listed in IV(c) or neoplasms not specified in IV(d).

The diagnosis of AIDS is confined to patients infected with the HIV virus when they develop certain defined opportunistic infections or malignancies for the first time, for example *Pneumocystis carinii* pneumonia, Kaposi's sarcoma or other specified conditions including HIV-related encephalopathy (Centers for Disease Control 1992). In addition, the USA surveillance case definition of AIDS has been expanded to include HIV-positive persons whose CD_4 lymphocyte count is less than 200/μl (or CD_4 percentage is less than 14%), but this is not included in case definition in Europe. An analogous classification system has been introduced for HIV infection in children under 13 years of age (Centers for Disease Control 1987).

Neuropsychiatric manifestations

HIV disease has proved to be of immense importance to neurology and psychiatry. Early reports by Snider *et al.* (1983) and Levy *et al.* (1985) drew attention to the range of neurological problems encountered and set the stage for their elaboration. It was also soon evident that the psychosocial consequences of infection could lead to profound emotional disturbance, even among those who were physically well or had sustained no more than a risk of exposure to the virus. Vulnerable persons, in groups at special risk, could display neurotic and sometimes psychotic symptomatology which needed to be distinguished from the effects of brain pathology. In this manner neurology and psychiatry have been drawn closer together in seeking to disentangle the impact of the disorder. In the sections which follow those disorders reflecting identifiable pathology will be considered first, then those which may be viewed as 'reactions' to knowledge of being infected.

Both the central and the peripheral nervous system are involved in a high proportion of cases, variously estimated at between 30% and 60% (McArthur *et al.* 1994). Special importance attaches to the resulting manifestations in that they can be the presenting feature in some 10% of cases (Levy *et al.* 1988). It has become clear that the nervous system is an early target in HIV disease, with abnormalities developing in the cerebrospinal fluid in a large proportion of asymptomatic HIV-positive individuals (Marshall *et al.* 1988). In a prospective study of homosexual men, McArthur *et al.* (1988) were able to demonstrate cerebrospinal fluid abnormalities, and sometimes to isolate the virus from the fluid, within 6–24 months of seroconversion. Ho *et al.* (1985) detected the virus in the cerebrospinal fluid of a patient suffering from aseptic meningitis at the actual time of seroconversion. Gray *et al.* (1996) review neuropathological reports of HIV-positive individuals who have died accidentally during the asymptomatic period, often showing vascular inflammation and gliosis in the white matter along with early myelin pallor. By the time patients with AIDS come to autopsy, neuropathological changes have been demonstrated in over 90% of cases, even in patients who have shown no relevant neurological symptomatology during life (Budka *et al.* 1987).

Multiple pathologies occur together in about a third of cases (Levy *et al.* 1988). The pictures observed are therefore pleomorphic and can present considerable problems for diagnosis. Three main forms of involvement are recognised — opportunistic infections, neoplastic change and direct invasion of the nervous system by the HIV virus. Evidence for the last has been increasingly forthcoming, both from laboratory studies and from the clinical observation that nervous system involvement can sometimes antedate impaired immunological competence. The change in terminology for HIV-related illness (p. 319) was largely prompted by this realisation. Thus neurological involvement can span the entire spectrum of HIV infection, from the time of seroconversion to its most advanced manifestations.

Additional pathology in the central nervous system results from vascular disorders, such as infarction, haemorrhage and vasculitis. The brain is also vulnerable to hypoxia and metabolic derangements due to pulmonary, hepatic and renal failure, and to the toxic effects of systemic infections or drugs. In the peripheral nervous system the relative importance of HIV infection and metabolic factors remains uncertain, with the added complication that autoimmune mechanisms appear often to be involved.

A very approximate guide to the relative frequency of the different forms of pathology is given by Petito *et al.*'s (1986) review of neuropathological findings in 153 patients dying from HIV disease. Twenty-eight per cent showed evidence of HIV encephalitis (presumed due to HIV viral invasion, p. 324), 26% of encephalomyelitis due to cytomegalovirus, 10% toxoplasmosis, 6% central nervous system lymphoma and 29% vacuomyelopathy of the cord. Different risk groups of patients may, however, be differently affected. Lantos *et al.* (1989) showed that haemophiliacs were less likely to develop HIV encephalitis while vascular lesions were common. Children are unlikely to develop opportunistic infections or lymphomas, but mainly show the picture of HIV encephalitis.

Opportunistic infections of the central nervous system

Viral, fungal and parasitic infections of the central nervous system are common, while bacterial invasion is rare. The manifestations are broadly similar to those occurring in other settings except that they are more florid in the immunocompromised state. This may also be due in some instances to co-infection with the HIV virus which serves to exacerbate the tissue destruction.

Such infections occur in about a third of patients (De la Monte *et al.* 1987) and multiple infections are common (Gray *et al.* 1988). The incidence of the different organisms varies geographically, toxoplasmosis for example

occurring especially frequently in France and cryptococcal meningitis more often in New Jersey than California (Everall & Lantos 1991).

The principal infections encountered are toxoplasmosis, viral infection with cytomegalovirus, herpes simplex and herpes zoster, also the papova virus leading to progressive multifocal leukoencephalopathy. Fungal infections include *Cryptococcus*, *Candida albicans* or more rarely aspergillosis and coccidioidomycosis. The tubercle bacillus is occasionally involved, also other mycobacteria, *Escherichia coli*, *Listeria*, *Histoplasma* and *Treponema pallidum*. The detailed pictures are described by Levy *et al.* (1988) and will be presented in summary form.

Toxoplasmosis results from reactivation of latent infection with the intracellular protozoon, *Toxoplasma gondii*. It appears to be especially frequent among patients from Haiti and Florida and also from France. The infection leads to an acute focal or diffuse meningoencephalitis, presenting usually with headache, fever and altered consciousness, and focal neurological signs such as hemiparesis, aphasia or cerebellar ataxia. These may be preceded for several days or weeks by lethargy, confusion or weakness. Koppel *et al.* (1985) found that patients with focal neurological features usually proved to have toxoplasmosis, similarly patients with mass lesions on computerised tomography (CT) scans (Levy *et al.* 1986). Seizures occur in some 15% of cases. Raised intracranial pressure is rare.

The pathology consists of scattered focal areas of abscess formation, varying in size according to the patient's immunological response. Each has a necrotic core surrounded by granuloma formation consisting of an intense mononuclear reaction. Encysted *Toxoplasma gondii* and tachyzoites can usually be detected. Thrombosis of blood vessels may lead to large areas of necrosis, producing mass lesions in the brain.

The CT scan shows a characteristic picture of ring-enhancing lesions in cortical and subcortical regions, which when large may be mistaken for lymphoma (p. 321). Early diagnosis can lead to a dramatic response to antibiotic treatment (p. 334). Lumbar puncture often reveals a pleocytosis and elevation of protein.

Cytomegalovirus typically leads to a subacute encephalitis with fever, confusion and ataxia. Associated features which may be of diagnostic importance are mentioned on p. 326. The pathology varies in severity from scattered microglial nodules to multiple necrotising lesions (Everall & Lantos 1991). The ventricular lining is frequently involved, likewise the choroid plexus. Microglia and macrophages contain intranuclear inclusions indicative of the presence of the virus. Concurrent retinitis is common and is the most frequent cause of loss of vision in AIDS.

Herpes simplex produces a severe haemorrhagic

encephalitis, typically limited to the temporofrontal regions (p. 356), presenting with headache, fever, seizures, aphasia and other focal neurological deficits. Necrosis and softening affect both the grey and white matter, and eosinophilic nuclear inclusions are seen in neurones and glial cells. Occasional cases present as an ascending myelitis.

Herpes zoster may involve the peripheral or central nervous system, the latter leading to diffuse encephalitis with multiple necrotic lesions similar to those of progressive multifocal leukoencephalopathy. Small eosinophilic inclusions in neurones and glial cells contain the virus.

Progressive multifocal leukoencephalopathy results from infection with the JC papova virus. It usually presents with the subacute development of mental impairment accompanied by varied neurological deficits as described on p. 751. Dementia, blindness, dysphasia, hemiparesis and ataxia are among the classic features. The CT scan may show characteristic low density lesions in the white matter with a 'scalloped' appearance to their margins, without mass effect, enhancement or associated oedema. Magnetic resonance imaging (MRI) may show that the grey matter is involved as well, possibly reflecting a more aggressive form of the disease in the presence of AIDS (Mark & Atlas 1989).

The lesions consist essentially of areas of demyelination with sparing of axis cylinders and often with necrosis. The papova virus can be detected in the bizarre glial cells around their margins which are the hallmark of the disorder—enlarged astrocytes with distorted nuclei and oligodendrocytes containing eosinophilic inclusions. The condition carries a grave prognosis, with survival rarely extending beyond a few months. Antemortem diagnosis is made by biopsy. No treatment is currently effective.

Cryptococcus is the commonest fungal infection of the central nervous system, typically leading to a subacute granulomatous meningitis producing a gelatinous exudate at the base of the brain. Headache and malaise may be the sole complaints, perhaps because of the minimal inflammatory response. In other patients progressive headache, photophobia and nuchal rigidity are accompanied by confused and altered behaviour. Sometimes there is additional cyst and granuloma formation within the brain, such patients presenting with focal neurological signs. Raised intracranial pressure may develop in consequence of hydrocephalus. The diagnosis is confirmed by lumbar puncture. Cells may be absent and the protein and glucose normal, but indian ink staining reveals the fungus in a high proportion of cases. Detection of the cryptococcal antigen in the cerebrospinal fluid is a more reliable procedure.

Candida albicans rarely involves the brain despite the frequency of this infection elsewhere in the body in HIV disease. When it does invade the central nervous system this takes the form of meningitis or multiple brain abscesses with focal neurological signs.

Coccidioidomycosis may produce a chronic relapsing meningitis, which is occasionally fulminant with microabscess formation in the brain.

Tuberculous infection can present either with a mass lesion or as tuberculous meningitis as described on p. 366.

Treponema pallidum may lead to neurosyphilis after an unusually brief latent interval, and sometimes despite previous adequate therapy for the initial syphilitic infection (Nieman 1991). In the immunocompromised state the manifestations of meningovascular syphilis may be especially florid, leading to unusual acute neurological syndromes. Serological tests for syphilis may also be altered, becoming positive in the cerebrospinal fluid only after repeated serial testing.

Neoplasia of the central nervous system

The commonest central nervous system neoplasm is a primary non-Hodgkin's malignant lymphoma, occurring in some 2–6% of patients. This is a B-cell lymphoma, usually unifocal but sometimes multifocal and extensive, involving the cerebral hemispheres, cerebellum and brain stem. The presentation is usually with focal neurological deficits, similar to those seen with toxoplasmosis or progressive multifocal leukoencephalopathy, but with more gradual onset (Stern & Marder 1991). Sometimes, however, the picture is surprisingly non-specific with lethargy, confusion and memory impairment (Rosenblum *et al.* 1988). Headache and evidence of raised intracranial pressure may be lacking and unexplained fever may occur. Seizures develop in a third of cases.

The pictures on brain imaging may also be hard to distinguish from toxoplasmosis or progressive multifocal leukoencephalopathy. The space-occupying lesions show ill-defined margins with surrounding oedema, and may enhance irregularly (Sze *et al.* 1987). They lie mainly in the basal ganglia, thalamus, corpus callosum and cerebellum. Biopsy is usually needed for definitive diagnosis, or the distinction may ultimately be made by the rapid initial response to radiation. The long-term effects of treatment are poor.

Pathological examination shows lymphoid cells invading vascular walls and brain tissue, along with a marked astrocytic response. The Epstein–Barr virus is implicated in a high proportion of cases and may be identified by *in situ* hybridisation (Hamilton-Dutoit *et al.* 1991).

Secondary brain involvement from lymphoma elsewhere in the body occurs more rarely, also metastatic deposits from Kaposi's sarcoma. Plasmocytomas and lymphoid granulomatosis may also occur.

Primary HIV infection of the central nervous system

As described above (p. 319) it has become clear that the nervous system is a prime target for the HIV virus in addition to its predilection for the immunological system. This was not at first apparent, but has now been fully proven by electron microscopy, immunocytochemistry and *in situ* hybridisation. Shaw *et al.* (1985) were the first to identify the virus in five of 15 brains from AIDS patients with dementia, and Koenig *et al.* (1986) showed that the cell type harbouring the virus was the macrophage and the multinucleated giant cells deriving from it (Plates 8 and 9). Such cells often contain enormous quantities of the virus. The microglia are also involved. It is possible that oligodendrocytes and vascular epithelial cells may be infected, but astrocytes and neurones do not appear to be implicated directly (Price 1994). Evidence has accumulated to suggest that the nervous system is infected at an early stage of the disease (p. 319), even though pronounced clinical sequelae may take a considerable time to appear.

It seems, furthermore, that the virus in the brain represents a distinct strain, differing in certain respects from that occurring elsewhere. 'Neurotropic' (or more accurately 'macrophage tropic') variants isolated from the nervous system differ from those from peripheral blood in their ability to infect and destroy certain cell lines, and in their patterns of sensitivity to serum neutralisation (Cheng-Mayer & Levy 1988). Thus they show preferential replication in macrophages rather than lymphocytes, in contrast to isolates from the blood. They are also less genetically heterogeneous than those from organs such as the spleen (O'Brien 1994b).

A major characteristic of the HIV virus is its genetic variability, such that an inoculum quickly gives rise to a population of 'quasi-species' with differing antigenic and biological properties. This is in consequence of the poor fidelity of transcription during the replication of the virus. Thus the viruses which invade the nervous system probably represent a subset generated from the original infecting dose, and this selection appears to involve a limited subset only.

The precise mode of entry into the nervous system remains uncertain. The 'Trojan horse theory' proposes that HIV-infected macrophages and microglia carry the virus into the brain. There is also evidence that activated T-lymphocytes can enter the central nervous system. Alternatively the virus may enter and replicate in the vascular endothelium, or via the choroid plexus and cerebrospinal fluid. Entrance by way of peripheral nerves has also been considered.

The consequences of such invasion have been clarified to some extent at the level of tissue pathology, with the delineation of several more or less distinct patterns of neuropathological change. Their clinical counterparts are, however, as yet unclear, and classification in terms of presenting clinical features remains incomplete. The major clinical syndromes which appear to be due to primary brain infection are the so-called 'AIDS–dementia complex' or 'HIV-associated dementia', and the progressive encephalopathy which occurs in children. Aseptic meningitis is almost certainly so caused. Vacuolar myelopathy of the spinal cord may be due to direct infection, also certain affections of the peripheral nervous system and muscle. Here, however, the evidence is less convincing.

The clinical uncertainties are due to a lack of long-term prospective studies from which clinicopathological correlations may be drawn, also to the coincident operation of opportunistic infections and other pathologies in many cases. The pathological changes associated with HIV infection will therefore be briefly reviewed before consideration of the clinical pictures encountered.

HIV-associated pathology of the central nervous system

Budka *et al.* (1991) have produced a consensus report for the classification of HIV-associated neuropathologies as listed below. Everall and Lantos (1991) provide a concise description of the several categories. With some pathologies, namely HIV encephalitis and HIV leukoencephalopathy, there is clear evidence that the lesion is caused by the HIV virus itself, these forms not occurring in other settings of immunosuppression. In the others the pathogenic role of direct HIV infection is less completely established. Though the classification is provisional it serves as a framework for further studies. By far the most common are HIV encephalitis, HIV leukoencephalopathy and vacuolar myelopathy.

HIV encephalitis refers to the picture of multiple foci of inflammatory change throughout the cortex and white matter, also involving the basal ganglia and brain stem. The cortex may be spared relative to deeper parts of the brain, and the globus pallidus is often particularly severely affected. The foci consist of aggregations of macrophages, microglia and multinucleated giant cells, these last being the hallmark of the condition and probably deriving from macrophages (Plates 8 and 9). The glycoprotein gp 41 on the surface of the HIV virus mediates cell fusion and may be responsible for the formation of these characteristic cell syncytia. The HIV virus can be detected in all three types of cell. In addition there may be foci of microglial nodules and sometimes damage to myelinated fibres.

HIV leukoencephalopathy is characterised by diffuse and

usually symmetrical white matter damage, particularly in deep areas of the centrum semiovale, involving loss of myelin, reactive astrocytosis and the accumulation of macrophages and multinucleated giant cells. Such indications of inflammatory change are accompanied by alterations in small blood vessel walls and possible damage to the blood–brain barrier. A degree of overlap with HIV encephalitis is sometimes obvious and the validity of the distinction between the two is not firmly established. It is possible that they represent the same pathological process, but with accent on the white matter in HIV leukoencephalopathy.

It must be distinguished from the so-called 'myelin pallor' frequently observed in the deep white matter with myelin stains. This is an extremely common finding in patients with HIV disease and may be the sole brain abnormality at autopsy. The myelin sheaths are preserved, and the appearances may be mainly due to increased interstitial water or represent an artefact of staining techniques.

Vacuolar myelopathy is a distinctive finding confined to the spinal cord, chiefly in the cervical and high thoracic regions and mainly affecting the posterior and lateral columns. It is often a late development. Multiple areas show vacuolar myelin swellings, similar to the lesions seen in subacute combined degeneration due to vitamin B_{12} deficiency. The early lesions show scattered vacuoles due to swellings within the myelin sheaths and occasional lipid-laden macrophages; with severe cases there is secondary axonal degeneration (Petito *et al.* 1985; Petito 1988).

Virological studies have not implicated the HIV virus conclusively. The virus can be cultured from the cord, but has not been demonstrated in the areas with vacuolar change. Other viruses could be responsible, or nutritional and metabolic factors could play a part.

Vacuolar leukoencephalopathy shows a not dissimilar picture affecting the white matter of the cerebral hemispheres, cerebellum, basal ganglia and brain stem. It may accompany HIV leukoencephalopathy.

Diffuse poliodystrophy consists of diffuse astrocytosis, gliosis and microglial activation in the grey matter of the cerebral cortex, basal ganglia and brain stem nuclei. This is the only category in Budka *et al.*'s (1991) classification which recognises the possibility of the neuronal loss discussed below. The validity of diffuse poliodystrophy as a separate entity is uncertain, since gliosis is so commonly found in patients dying from HIV disease.

Cerebral vasculitis including granulomatous angiitis consists of infiltration of the walls of cerebral blood vessels with lymphocytes and multinucleated giant cells. There may be accompanying areas of necrosis.

Lymphocytic meningitis usually occurs soon after HIV infection as a self-limiting condition, but may recur or appear for the first time later in the asymptomatic or early symptomatic phases. The usual pathogens responsible for meningitis cannot be isolated, but in many cases HIV virus can be identified in the cerebrospinal fluid.

Neuronal loss with HIV infection

An important development has been the demonstration of substantial neuronal loss in the cerebral cortex of patients with HIV disease. This has recently attracted increasing attention.

Everall *et al.* (1991) made counts in the frontal cortex of 11 patients with HIV disease, all without opportunistic brain infection or neoplastic change, and demonstrated a 38% depletion of neurones. Such loss was equivalently severe in the five with obvious HIV encephalitis and the six who showed only minimal pathology by way of slight astrocytosis and perivascular accumulations of mononuclear cells. Neuronal loss has since been established more widely in the occipital, parietal and superior temporal areas (Wiley *et al.* 1991; Everall *et al.* 1993a), also in the substantia nigra and cerebellar nuclei (Abe *et al.* 1993; Everall *et al.* 1993b). The frontal losses have, however, emerged as the most severe. A significant association has been observed between such losses and the presence of dementia (Asare *et al.* 1995).

The mechanisms responsible are unclear. It seems that the presence of HIV encephalitis with multinucleated giant cells is not an accurate marker for neuronal loss, which can occur in the presence of minimal or absent inflammatory change (Everall *et al.* 1993b). Thus dual pathogenic processes may be at work, the one an inflammatory response and the other damaging neurones by mechanisms that wait to be clarified. Since neurones seem not to be infected directly one must postulate some 'toxic' effect on neuronal viability. On theoretical grounds there are reasons to implicate the release of cytokines or other damaging factors from infected macrophages and microglia, or to blame the glycoprotein gp 120 in the envelope of the virus. This has been shown to be neurotoxic *in vitro* by an effect on calcium channels analogous to that of glutamate-mediated excitotoxicity.

Dendritic morphology has also been found to be altered in the HIV-infected brain, with shortened, vacuolated and tortuous dendrites and a marked decrease in the number of dendritic spines (Wiley *et al.* 1991; Masliah *et al.* 1994). Synaptic density has been shown to be reduced in the frontal cortex. These observations have been made in brains with concurrent evidence of HIV encephalitis, so they, at least, may be a product of the inflammatory process.

HIV-associated dementia (AIDS–dementia complex,
HIV-related encephalopathy, AIDS encephalopathy,
HIV-associated cognitive/motor complex,
HIV encephalitis, subacute encephalitis)

Clinical pictures of central nervous system impairment
occur against the pathological backgrounds described
above and take a variety of forms. Prominent among
them is a syndrome of progressive cognitive impairment,
referred to by the bewildering variety of labels just listed,
and carrying in general a poor prognosis. This is regarded
as the commonest of all central nervous system complications of HIV disease. Evidence increasingly suggests that it
results in large part from direct brain invasion by the HIV
virus, but beyond that it has proved difficult to relate it to
defined aspects of brain pathology.

This problem pervades other aspects of HIV-associated neurological disorder as well. When the opportunistic brain infections
and neoplasias have been set aside, it is remarkably difficult to
relate clinical syndromes to different aspects of pathological
change. Cognitive impairment can be ascribed to changes within
the cerebrum, and motor disorder probably owes much to vacuolar myelopathy in the cord. Focal neurological deficits are
likely to be associated with cerebral vasculitis. Other than this,
however, little has been established with confidence.

The reasons are not far to seek. Attempts at clinicopathological
correlations have mostly been derived from retrospective case
note surveys or from the pooling of several smaller series of
patients. Clinical evaluations have rarely made use of carefully
defined criteria, and the pathology observed has often been
varied and overlapping in type. Moreover, patients have commonly been found to suffer from multiple pathologies, some
derived from HIV infection and some from opportunistic infections and neoplastic changes.

Terminology and definition

In early descriptions the condition was labelled 'subacute
encephalitis' and thought to be due to opportunistic brain
infection, probably with cytomegalovirus (Snider *et al.*
1983; Levy *et al.* 1985). It was rechristened 'AIDS–dementia complex' by Navia *et al.* (1986a, 1986b), 'complex'
being added because motor and behavioural components
were often prominent in addition to the cognitive failure.
The Working Group of the American Academy of Neurology proposed the term 'HIV-1-associated cognitive/motor
complex', with subcategories referring to patients with
behavioural or motor manifestations in addition to their
cognitive impairment (Report of a Working Group of the
American Academy of Neurology AIDS Task Force 1991).
All appear to refer to a broadly similar clinical syndrome
which for present purposes will be termed 'HIV-associated
dementia'.

The WHO Consultation Committee (World Health Organization
1990a) has recommended the use of operationally defined criteria for the condition, which are essentially modifications of the
ICD-10 reseach criteria for dementia generally (p. 7):

Thus there must be evidence of decline in memory, objectively
verified, also of decline in other cognitive abilities and in the processing of information. Clouding of consciousness must be
absent. Deterioration in emotional control or motivation, or a
change in social behaviour, are also required.

The modifications of ICD-10 suggested for AIDS-associated
dementia are:
1 Decline in memory may not be severe enough to impair activities of daily living.
2 Decline in motor functions may be present, but should not be
entirely caused by myelopathy of the cord, peripheral neuropathy or other physical illness.
3 The minimum duration of symptoms required is 1 month
(instead of 6 months as with ICD-10).
4 Aphasia, agnosia and apraxia are recognised as unusual.

Additionally there must be laboratory evidence of systemic
HIV-1 infection, and other processes such as tumours or opportunistic central nervous system infections should be ruled out by
neuroimaging and lumbar puncture.

Such a firm definition should refine understanding of
the disorder and aid its demarcation from other clinical
syndromes. Catalan (1991) points out that in many
surveys of HIV-positive patients dementia has been used
as an umbrella term, encompassing syndromes of cognitive decline, sometimes without impairment of memory,
also acute brain syndromes, motor syndromes and possibly conditions characterised chiefly by depression and
other psychiatric disorders.

Prevalence

HIV-associated dementia has emerged as the commonest
central nervous system manifestation in patients with
HIV disease. Brew *et al.* (1988) reported that over 60% of
patients dying of HIV disease in New York exhibited some
degree of dementia prior to death. Catalan (1991) reviews
various estimates of its prevalence, ranging from 8% to
almost 40%, much probably depending on matters of
patient selection and the criteria adopted for diagnosis.
Prospective surveys in the UK have shown prevalences of
7–16% when other causes of chronic organic reactions,
such as opportunistic infections, have been excluded.

Clinical features

The principal features emphasised in early descriptions
were cognitive impairment, accompanied by behavioural
change and often motor deficits (Snider *et al.* 1983; Levy
et al. 1985). Behavioural manifestations included lethargy
and social withdrawal, also marked psychomotor slowing

which could at first be mistaken for depression. A confusional state could mark the outset and malaise was frequently profound.

Navia *et al.* (1986a, 1986b) gave the first full description of the syndrome and its pathological background. They found it in 38% of 121 patients coming to autopsy, or almost two-thirds in the absence of opportunistic brain infection or neoplasia. In a quarter it appeared to antedate other manifestations of AIDS. Some cases, indeed, failed to show systemic features of AIDS right up to the time of death (Navia & Price 1987). Further experience has indicated, however, that this is rare. Dementia can occur relatively early in the evolution of HIV disease, and occasionally in the face of minimal or no systemic manifestations, but mostly it occurs in a setting of profound immunosuppression (Price 1994). McArthur *et al.* (1994) suggest that only 3% of patients present with dementia, and Manji and Connolly (1992) suggest that all will have reduced CD_4 counts.

The onset was sometimes insidious and sometimes fairly abrupt in Navia *et al.*'s cases. Impairment of memory and loss of concentration were the commonest early symptoms, but when these were mild they could easily be attributed to systemic illness or depression. Mental slowing was prominent, and confusion often present. Approximately half presented with cognitive change, while in the remainder motor or behavioural changes predominated.

Motor dysfunction took the form of imbalance, ataxia or leg weakness, sometimes for several months before cognitive deficits appeared. Loss of fine hand coordination and deterioration of handwriting was frequently observed.

Of the behavioural changes apathy and social withdrawal were most frequent, irritability and emotional lability less so. Such changes were the opening feature in almost a quarter of patients. The typical picture was of becoming subdued, with loss of interest and loss of emotional responsiveness. Frank dysphoria was, however, infrequent. A subgroup showed agitation with hyperactivity.

Less common symptoms included headache, seizures and episodes of speech disturbance. Some patients showed psychotic episodes with delusions and hallucinations. Perry and Jacobsen (1986) described several patients who presented with acute psychoses resembling schizophrenia, acute paranoid disorder, mania or psychotic depression.

This clinical picture has been broadly confirmed in subsequent reports. On examination there may be little to find neurologically in the early stages, though rapid eye and limb movements may be impaired along with diffuse hyperreflexia. Later there is often ataxia of gait, leg weakness and clonus. Frontal release signs may be prominent, especially the snout reflex. Some patients show tremors and dysarthria, and evidence of peripheral neuropathy is common.

Course

The course is typically steadily progressive though punctuated at times by abrupt accelerations. Half of Navia *et al.*'s patients progressed to severe global impairment within 2 months, but some 20% followed a more protracted course. McArthur (1987) found that of 20 patients seen initially in the early stages nine progressed to advanced dementia within a few months, while six remained stable and failed to deteriorate over 3–13 months. Once severely demented the mean survival time was less than 3 months. In 18 patients who died with dementia, the average interval from the first symptom of cognitive dysfunction to death was 5.5 months.

Insight is often relatively preserved until late in the disorder. The delayed appearance of focal cognitive symptoms such as apraxia or agnosia is in keeping with the predominantly subcortical nature of the dementia. The final stages are marked by severe global dementia, akinetic mutism, incontinence, paraplegia and sometimes myoclonus. Even in the terminal stages, however, the level of consciousness is unimpaired.

Investigations

The EEG is often normal initially, with diffuse slowing later. Neuroimaging usually shows variable cortical atrophy and ventricular dilatation, but the absence of atrophy does not countermand the diagnosis. White matter rarefaction is common, and MRI may show areas of increased T_2 signal in the white matter which becomes more diffuse as the dementia progresses (Levy *et al.* 1986; Olsen *et al.* 1988). However, the essential role of neuroimaging is to exclude features indicative of treatable conditions such as opportunistic infections or lymphomas. Positron emission tomography (PET) has demonstrated subcortical hypermetabolism in the thalamus and basal ganglia in the early stages, with progression to cortical and subcortical hypometabolism later (Rottenberg *et al.* 1987). Single photon emission computerised tomography (SPECT) may show perfusion deficits despite the absence of gross brain lesions (Costa *et al.* 1988), and MRI proton spectroscopy has shown reduced levels of *N*-acetyl aspartate indicative of neuronal loss, even in areas apparently normal on structural scans (Menon *et al.* 1990).

Examination of the cerebrospinal fluid is essential to exclude opportunistic infections. It may be normal, but elevation of protein and a mild lymphocytic pleocytosis can occur. This, however, is non-specific and can be found in asymptomatic persons. Oligoclonal bands are sometimes detected. Levels of β_2-microglobulin appear to correlate highly with the severity of the dementia (Brew *et al.* 1992), and this can be a pointer to the diagnosis in the absence of opportunistic infections. HIV virus may be isolated from the fluid.

Differential diagnosis

The diagnosis of HIV-associated dementia during life is essentially one of exclusion. In mild examples differentiation will be required from anxiety or depression, also from fatigue and the effects of systemic illness. Metabolic causes of encephalopathy should be excluded, also the effects of psychotropic medication to which AIDS patients may be sensitive. When psychotic features are present it is important to consider the possibility of an independent schizophrenia or paranoid state.

With more severe dementia the essential differentiation is from opportunistic brain infections or neoplasia. Infections such as cytomegalovirus, toxoplasmosis, neurosyphilis and cryptococcal or tuberculous meningitis must be carefully excluded since they lead to therapeutic options. Distinguishing features characteristic of cytomegalovirus encephalitis include coexisting retinitis or colitis, electrolyte abnormalities reflecting adrenalitis, or periventricular abnormalities on MRI indicative of periventriculitis (McArthur *et al.* 1994). Other causes of dementia must clearly be considered, particularly in the middle aged or elderly.

Pathology

The pathological substrate of HIV-associated dementia remains unclear for the reasons outlined on p. 324. Price (1994) summarises the attempts made to relate the severity of cognitive impairment to the extent and nature of brain pathology (Price *et al.* 1988, 1991), but such correlations are far from exact. Severe dementia is often associated with the prominent development of multinucleated HIV encephalitis, and mild forms tend to show little more than white matter pallor and gliosis. Sometimes, however, the neuropathology can be remarkably bland even in the presence of severe dementia. Much may then depend on more subtle changes such as cortical neuronal loss, as discussed on p. 323. McArthur *et al.* (1994) report that only a quarter of cases show multinucleated giant

cells, and half show neither these nor white matter pallor, suggesting that correlations must be sought elsewhere to explain the clinical picture. Some 25% of cases show an associated vacuolar myelopathy of the spinal cord.

Successive stages of severity of dementia tend to arise in the context of increasing levels of systemic immunosuppression, raising the possibility that the virus both creates the opportunity for infection and then exploits it by infecting the central nervous system (Price 1994). However, there is much variability here as well, some patients failing to develop dementia despite repeated episodes of systemic opportunistic infection, while occasional patients develop severe dementia as the sole feature of the illness.

Vacuolar myelopathy of the spinal cord

Vacuolar myelopathy affects some 20–30% of patients, commonly in the context of HIV-associated dementia. Dementia had been present in 70% of the cases identified at autopsy by Petito *et al.* (1985). Moreover the severity of the pathological lesions correlates not only with clinical evidence of cord damage but also with the presence of dementia (Petito 1988). Sometimes, however, the motor deficit predominates over evidence of cognitive dysfunction, and worsens progressively while mentation is relatively preserved.

The picture typically evolves over weeks or months as a spastic–ataxic paraparesis, with slowness of gait, clumsiness of leg movements, sensory ataxia and eventual weakness. It may be accompanied by incontinence of the bladder and bowels and by complaints of paraesthesia or vague discomfort in the legs. Sensation is relatively spared except for loss of vibratory and position sense unless peripheral neuropathy is also present. However, the frequent co-occurrence of the latter may render precise attribution of symptoms difficult.

Examination of the cerebrospinal fluid may show non-specific abnormalities, including raised protein and a mononuclear pleocytosis. Differential diagnoses must include cord damage due to herpes simplex, herpes zoster and cytomegalovirus as well as lymphoma in the epidural space. The pathology is described on p. 323.

HIV-associated progressive encephalopathy of childhood

Many children born to HIV-infected mothers develop cognitive and motor disabilities, usually presenting during the first 2 years of life but with wide variability from 2 months to 5 years. Epstein *et al.* (1988) estimate that a progressive encephalopathy develops in 30–50% of children so infected, with a poor prognosis and almost invariably a fatal outcome. In other cases the deficits appear to be relatively static. The infection is usually acquired *in utero* or possibly during birth. In occasional cases it may have been transmitted postnatally through breast feeding. Exposure to contaminated blood products accounts for a small proportion of cases, especially those in older children.

Belman (1994) describes the pictures that can result, with considerable variability in clinical manifestations and modes of progression. Much is likely to be influenced by the timing of the maternal–foetal transmission and the stage of maturity of the brain when it becomes infected. Common manifestations are developmental delays, cognitive impairment, poor brain growth leading to acquired microcephaly, and corticospinal tract signs. Progressive cognitive impairment is sometimes in the forefront of the picture, whereas other children develop disabling motor involvement while cognitive function remains relatively stable.

The most severe syndrome takes the form of increasing spasticity, impaired brain growth and loss of previously acquired milestones. The progression of decline is usually slow but can be rapid over several weeks. Plateau periods occasionally occur, lasting for several months. The typical result is spastic quadriparesis, sometimes with rigidity, dystonia and tremor, along with progressive apathy and loss of interest in the environment. The characteristic facial appearance is of an alert, wide-eyed child with diminished blinking and a mask-like face.

Most children show a more indolent course, which can be mild with long periods during which progression is halted. Cognitive impairment becomes manifest as a decline in the rate of mental development, but previously acquired milestones are preserved. Motor involvement is again common, with paraparesis or disturbance of gait.

A stable/static form is also recognised in children with histories of developmental delay or non-progressive motor deficits. Intelligence is low but remains relatively stable and neurological deficits do not worsen. Motor dysfunction shows as poor coordination, hyperreflexia and increased tone in the legs. The role of HIV infection is less clear in these cases, but has probably served to compromise normal development.

Neuroimaging in the more severe varieties shows cerebral atrophy which can be observed to progress. White matter hypodensity is often apparent, but the characteristic finding is calcification in the basal ganglia and sometimes also in the frontal white matter.

Pathology

Autopsy may show the characteristic features of HIV encephalitis, with foci of microglia, macrophages and multinucleated giant cells. However, this is found less frequently than in adults. Characteristically the basal ganglia show calcification, chiefly in relation to blood vessels and the adjacent neuropil, and sometimes in the absence of inflammatory change elsewhere. White matter leukoencephalopathy may be present in the cerebral hemispheres. The spinal cord shows myelin pallor, often restricted in distribution to the corticospinal tracts. Vacuolar myelopathy is infrequent and usually found only in older children.

Opportunistic infections and neoplasms of the brain occasionally occur in childhood but are rare.

Aseptic meningitis

HIV-positive subjects not infrequently show a lymphocytic pleocytosis in the cerebrospinal fluid during the asymptomatic stage (Marshall *et al.* 1988). Some, however, present with symptoms of meningitis, usually early after infection and while still relatively immunocompetent. Obvious pathogens cannot be isolated, hence the term 'aseptic', but in several cases the HIV virus has been recovered directly from the fluid.

The condition appears to be clinically heterogeneous. In an important group the meningitis develops acutely after infection at the time of seroconversion, presenting with fever, headache, photophobia and meningism (Ho *et al.* 1985). This is typically a mild and self-limiting disorder, lasting for 1–4 weeks, though cranial nerve palsies are occasionally seen. Similar examples may occur later in the asymptomatic phase, or shortly after defining features of AIDS have appeared. Hollander and Stringari (1987) describe two patterns of presentation. One resembles the above, sometimes with recurrent bouts of acute meningeal infection. The other presents with chronic headache in the absence of meningeal signs and may run a protracted course over several months. This appears to represent a more indolent infection, with less marked abnormalities in cell count and protein in the cerebrospinal fluid.

Peripheral nerve and muscle disorders

Peripheral nerve disorders can complicate all stages of HIV infection and appear to be attributable to a variety of mechanisms. They are reviewed by Parry (1988), Dalakas and Pezeshkpour (1988) and Griffin *et al.* (1994). Direct infection by the HIV virus has not been established with certainty.

Acute and chronic inflammatory demyelinating polyneuropathies are commonest early in the disease and can be the presenting manifestation. The acute form (Guillain–Barré syndrome) can occur at the time of seroconversion.

There is profound motor impairment with loss of tendon reflexes, variable degrees of sensory loss and often radicular pains in the back and legs. The cerebrospinal fluid protein is characteristically elevated. The pathogenesis almost certainly reflects a disorder of immune regulation. Treatment by plasmapheresis or intravenous immunoglobulin can be of benefit. Steroids must only be used with caution and with close monitoring of immune function because they may reduce resistance to opportunistic infections.

Sensory ganglioneuritis and acute cranial nerve palsies may also occur in the early asymptomatic phase of infection.

Predominantly sensory neuropathy (PSN) (also known as distal symmetrical polyneuropathy or DSPN) is the main form in the later stages of HIV disease, rivalling HIV dementia in prevalence. The two frequently occur together. It may develop acutely or gradually, presenting usually with burning pain and hyperalgesia in the feet. Intense neuropathic pain may lead to considerable disablement. Mild distal motor involvement can often be found when carefully sought out, by way of muscle atrophy or weakness. Tendon reflexes are diminished at the ankles and vibratory thresholds are elevated. Occasionally the disaesthesias may begin in the hands. The pathogenic factors at work are unclear, and may involve infectious, toxic or nutritional processes. Some cases may be due to the side effects of drugs.

Other neuropathies take the form of polyradiculopathies, consisting of rapidly evolving flaccid paralysis and pain in the back and legs, or sometimes present as a cauda equina lesion. Multiple mononeuropathy (mononeuritis multiplex) appears often to be due to cytomegalovirus infections, and partial response may be obtained with gancyclovir. Herpes simplex is sometimes implicated. The role of direct infection with HIV virus is suspected, and the virus can sometimes be isolated from the peripheral nerves.

Myopathy may present at any stage with slowly progressive proximal muscle weakness of the limbs, myalgia and excessive fatiguability. Creatine phosphokinase levels are elevated in the serum, and cautious treatment with steroids can be beneficial. The relative roles of immunological factors and infection with the HIV virus are uncertain. Other affections of muscle include necrotising myopathy, necrotising vasculitis, nemaline rod myopathy and mitochondrial myopathy. An acute self-limiting

myopathic process may also be observed at the time of seroconversion.

Impairment in asymptomatic HIV-positive subjects

In view of the known early invasion of the nervous system by the HIV virus, the question arises whether impairments of a subtle nature may be detectable during the asymptomatic phase. The issue is important for both theoretical and practical reasons. If impairments commonly exist while asymptomatic persons are active at work and in social life this could be relevant to their competence and reliability. In particular, impairment of judgement or change of behaviour could increase their risks of spreading the infection. Early therapeutic intervention might be indicated.

Despite several surveys, some on large numbers of subjects, the matter remains *sub judice*. Stern and Marder (1991) and Grant *et al.* (1992) discuss the pitfalls inherent in attempting to document impairments when these are minor in nature—problems in the sampling of persons to be tested, the selection of appropriate neuropsychological tests and the need to allow for variables such as past head injury or alcohol and drug abuse. The selection of controls raises problems of its own; the most suitable are HIV-negative persons from similar sections of the population, but those who volunteer may be biased towards well-motivated and better educated members of the group.

The controversy began with a preliminary study by Grant *et al.* (1987), who found indications that the frequency of neuropsychological impairment increased across small groups of homosexual men divided into those who were HIV negative, those who were HIV positive but asymptomatic, or those with ARC and AIDS. The results, though slender, raised the possibility that HIV-positive asymptomatic persons might have 'incipient central nervous system impairment'. Some of these persons were not in fact entirely asymptomatic, though their symptoms were too mild to meet the criteria for ARC or AIDS (Grant *et al.* 1988). The results were reinforced by the finding of white matter hyperintensities on MRI in three of four asymptomatic patients (Grant *et al.* 1992).

The findings were supported by Wilkie *et al.* (1990), who examined a rather larger group and found significant slowing on tests of information processing, possibly relevant to subcortical pathology, and on tests of delayed recall. Some of these subjects had persistent lymphadenopathy. Stern *et al.* (1991) found slight but significant impairment on certain tests of verbal memory, language and executive function in a group of 49 asymptomatic patients. Marder *et al.* (1992) studied a cohort of intravenous drug users in New York, including 33 who were HIV positive but completely asymptomatic; no differences emerged in neuropsychological performance, but in comparison with HIV-negative controls they showed more extrapyramidal disorder and frontal release signs. These differences persisted on controlling for age, education, current drug use and history of head injury.

A number of negative reports must be set against such findings. The strongest evidence against early impairment comes from the Multicenter AIDS Cohort Study, which recruited large numbers of homosexual and bisexual men from cities in the USA for prospective examinations. In a cross-sectional comparison of 270 HIV-positive asymptomatic subjects and 193 HIV negatives no differences could be discerned in the prevalence of neuropsychiatric symptoms or on screening tests of neuropsychological performance (McArthur *et al.* 1989). More detailed examination was made of 75 HIV positives and 44 HIV negatives who had shown possible abnormalities, and again no differences emerged on detailed neurological and psychological examinations. White matter hyperintensities on MRI were equally frequent in the two groups and showed no association with neurological or neuropsychological impairments. The majority of the abnormalities which did emerge could be attributed to other factors such as alcohol or concurrent psychiatric disorder.

A further survey, using the screening test battery on very large numbers from the Multicenter AIDS Cohort Study (727 HIV-positive asymptomatics and 769 HIV negatives) upheld these negative findings (Miller *et al.* 1990). Furthermore, no significant relationships could be discerned between cognitive performance in the asymptomatic subjects and duration of HIV infection or level of immune functioning. Negative results have also been reported from cross-sectional studies by Janssen *et al.* (1989), Goethe *et al.* (1989) and Riccio *et al.* (1993). Sinforiani *et al.* (1991) found some mild impairment on verbal memory tests, but this did not progress over 18 months' follow-up, suggesting that it was due to pre-existing factors rather than HIV infection *per se*.

Selnes *et al.* (1990) carried out a longitudinal follow-up of 238 HIV-positive asymptomatic subjects and 170 uninfected controls from the Multicentre AIDS Cohort Study. One hundred and thirty-two individuals from each group could be compared at 18 months, and there was no evidence of decline over time. Selnes *et al.* (1992) similarly followed a large cohort of intravenous drug users for 12 months, and found no differences in cognitive performance according to serostatus group. Burgess *et al.* (1994) found no differences initially or at the 12-month follow-up where mean test scores were concerned, but performance at follow-up was significantly poorer in the HIV-positive group than would have been predicted on the basis of baseline performance and other variables. The significance of this more sophisticated approach to analysis is uncertain, and has not yet been adopted in a more substantial series of subjects.

Altogether some 56 research reports have now addressed the issue, 26 with negative findings and 30 reporting evidence, variable in quality, pointing to mild cognitive deficits (Burgess *et al.* 1994). Results have been conflicting even among studies employing similar test procedures. This is perhaps not surprising in view of the heterogeneity of the samples studied—in terms of degree of immunocompetence, time from seroconversion and the influence of factors such as head trauma, alcohol and drug abuse. Added difficulties arise from the effects of depression and anxiety on the sensitive test procedures employed.

Certain important conclusions can nevertheless be drawn. Cognitive impairment in infected but asymptomatic persons appears to be neither widespread nor severe in degree. It may, however, affect a minority of individuals, and it can then be hard to apportion the blame between HIV infection and other confounding factors. The impairments identified seem to be without effect in terms of day-to-day functioning, and on balance seem not to be the harbinger of incipient HIV-associated dementia. A decisive answer will need to await longer term prospective studies and control of the numerous sources of artefact already known to bias results.

Other psychiatric disorders

In addition to the neuropsychiatric disorders described above, HIV-infected patients are vulnerable to a variety of psychiatric disturbances, many of which may owe little or nothing to primary brain pathology. The range is wide, from states of acute distress on becoming aware of HIV positivity to profound depression and psychotic illnesses. These latter may sometimes show an admixture of organic psychiatric symptoms, since mood disorder and psychoses can be early manifestations of brain disease. A separate group of patients consists of the 'worried well'—persons who are not infected but develop an intense fear, or even a protracted conviction of harbouring the disease, which may be hard to dispel. Accounts of these various manifestations are presented by Fenton (1987), Maj (1990) and King (1993).

Other factors have been noted as contributing to psychiatric morbidity over and above the threats inherent in an unpleasant and life-threatening disorder. Surveys have stressed the vulnerability of the populations from which

HIV-infected persons tend to be drawn, and the powerful role of psychosocial influences in determining adverse reactions (Dilley *et al.* 1985; Faulstich 1987). A degree of isolation is common among homosexual and drug-injecting persons, and their social supports may be tenuous or lacking. The acquisition of infection can increase feelings of stigma or guilt, and provoke intense concern about others to whom the disease may have been transmitted. An additional stress is the uncertainty, extending sometimes over many years, about the course the disease will take, occurring often against a background of illness and losses among close friends and partners. In consequence it is scarcely surprising that a high prevalence of psychiatric disorder is reported both in physically asymptomatic and symptomatic persons. Such rates have been variable from one survey to another, much undoubtedly depending on the support available to subjects from medical and lay organisations.

Acute psychological reactions

Acute stress reactions are most commonly observed at the time of notification of a positive serological test result. Confirmation of the diagnosis brings the realisation of fears which may have long been present, also the need to tell others, including homosexual and heterosexual partners. Life styles which have previously been concealed may be exposed to parents and colleagues for the first time. Later in the illness, patients may undergo further cycles of crisis as new symptoms make an appearance.

The principal manifestations are acute shock, bewilderment and anxiety, typically lasting for several weeks. Major depression may be precipitated, with depersonalisation, insomnia and suicidal ideation. A preoccupation may develop with bodily symptoms thought to be indicative of commencing disease. Other reactions include anger, despair, guilt, increased use of alcohol or drugs, social withdrawal or denial. This last may lead to a dangerous disregard of medical advice and failure to take precautions against infecting others.

The incidence of acute psychological reactions at the time of testing has varied widely in different reports, perhaps reflecting the adequacy of pre- and post-test counselling. Perry *et al.* (1990g) found that psychological distress had diminished in most cases by 10 weeks after notification. Jadresic *et al.* (1994) found that the reduction in anxiety among a group of homosexual men at 6 months was greater in seropositive than seronegative subjects, this possibly reflecting the extensive support they received.

Longer-term psychiatric disorder

Longer-lasting psychiatric disorder may emerge during the asymptomatic or symptomatic stages of infection, but it is uncertain whether this is commoner than in patients with other serious medical conditions (King 1989, 1993). A particularly high prevalence has sometimes been noted in patients with ARC when compared with those with AIDS, perhaps reflecting the renewed uncertainties reawakened during this phase (Miller & Riccio 1990).

Adjustment disorders make up a substantial proportion of the problems encountered. These are diagnosed when distress is judged to exceed what might be expected in the circumstances, either in duration or intensity, or when it results in significant impairment in social or occupational functioning (DSM-IV 1994). Such disorders may last for many months, or result in chronic symptomatology when in response to continuing medical disability. Principal determinants have been found to include a previous history of psychiatric disorder, lack of social acceptance and lack of support. Three forms of adjustment disorder have been described, dominated respectively by anxiety, depression and obsessional symptoms.

Anxiety often centres on the uncertainties surrounding the long-term outcome, the availability of care in the future and the loss of physical and financial independence. The risk of infecting others, or of being identified as homosexual or a drug abuser, may be at the forefront of concerns. Somatic symptoms of anxiety are sometimes interpreted as evidence of progression to further stages of the disorder, giving rise to an escalating vicious circle. Alcohol or drugs may be abused in attempts to self medicate the symptoms of anxiety.

Depression has varied in prevalence from 6% to more than 30% of patients in different surveys (Perry 1994). It has proved to be strongly associated with a previous history of depressive illness, the presence of personality disorder and low perceived social support. Rather surprisingly the severity of physical symptoms of HIV disease seems to be no more than a moderate predictor. Depression and withdrawal can significantly interfere with ability to cope with the procedures required for the management of the illness (Ostrow 1990).

Perry (1994) makes the important point that depressive disorders are the exception rather than the rule in HIV-infected persons; severe depressive symptoms should not be assumed to be understandable and justified, and must always receive full evaluation and treatment. The problems which may arise in distinguishing between depression and the early stages of HIV-associated dementia are discussed on p. 325. Difficulty may also be encountered with ARC when this presents with fatigue, insomnia, weight loss and loss of libido.

Obsessive–compulsive disorder can occur with or without depressed mood, commonly involving repeated bodily scrutiny for evidence of progression of disease. Obsessive ruminations may centre on death and dying, or endeavours to recollect past sexual partners to whom the infection may have been transmitted.

Suicide presents a considerable risk both in the early and late stages of the disorder. Perry *et al.* (1990f) found that suicidal ideation was common, affecting almost 30% of individuals at the time of serological testing, but falling significantly within 2 months of notification. Suicide attempts tend to cluster in the first 6 months after diagnosis, underlining the importance of pre- and post-test counselling (World Health Organization 1990b).

Later, with symptomatic AIDS, completed suicide is considerably increased. Rates among New York residents were estimated to be some 36-fold above expectation in one retrospective review, but such a very large excess has yet to be confirmed (Marzuk *et al.* 1988; Marzuk 1991). Factors apparently associated with increased risk include social stigma, withdrawal of family support, loss of friends and partners, long-term dependency and the prospect of an inexorable terminal illness. Additional factors which increase the risk include previous psychiatric illness and the presence of alcohol and drug abuse.

An important consideration is the extent to which suicide in the later stages may be considered to be 'rational' in view of the poor outcome to be expected. Against this is the close association between suicide and psychiatric illness, inappropriate guilt, and erroneous perceptions about the development of the illness and methods available to relieve suffering (Glass 1988; King 1993).

Marzuk (1991) discusses other AIDS-related suicides, including persons grieving for loss of friends and family members, psychotic patients who were deluded that they suffered from AIDS, and a small group of people, mainly homosexual, who had deliberately sought to contract AIDS as a means of ending their lives.

Psychoses appear to be not infrequent, though the scattered reports of small numbers of cases make any estimate of prevalence uncertain. Many pictures have been reported, some seemingly typical of psychoses occurring in other settings, while others have shown special features. Major affective disorders, both depressive and manic, occur, as well as schizophrenia and paranoid states.

A considerable proportion develop in the context of cognitive impairment or clouding of consciousness, sometimes of a subtle or evanescent nature. In others, evidence of cognitive impairment emerges only later when the more florid manifestations have been brought under control. Sometimes, however, organic symptomatology remains absent throughout the illness which presents as a purely 'functional' psychosis (Halstead *et al.* 1988).

Many cases arise in patients who already show physical manifestations of ARC or AIDS, but even then the psychosis may first draw attention to the disease. In other examples an acute psychosis presents as the sole manifestation and the patient is only later found to be HIV positive. Maj (1990) reviews the mechanisms that may be responsible—chance association, reactions to the threat of the disorder, precipitation in predisposed persons or a response to drugs used or abused. Alternatively the psychosis may reflect HIV brain infection, especially in patients with no previous history of psychiatric illness or drug abuse and who are unaware of their seropositivity (Buhrich *et al.* 1988). The predilection of the virus for the limbic regions of the brain could be relevant in this regard.

The variety of pictures encountered is illustrated by several reports and reviews (Thomas & Szabadi 1987; Buhrich *et al.* 1988; Halstead *et al.* 1988; Vogel-Scibilia *et al.* 1988; Harris *et al.* 1991). Delusions, hallucinations, bizarre behaviour, thought disorder, lability of mood and major affective disorder may feature prominently, with or without organic accompaniments in the mental state. Among the 31 cases reviewed by Harris *et al.* (1991), after excluding those due to substance abuse or delirium, the psychosis was the presenting feature in 12. CT scans were abnormal in half and the cerebrospinal fluid in a quarter, these patients tending to decline rapidly in physical and cognitive status.

It seems unlikely that a specific 'HIV psychosis' exists, but it appears that mania may be especially common. Kieburtz *et al.* (1991) described eight such patients, all with evidence of cognitive impairment once the florid symptoms had subsided. Irritability was more prominent than elation, and all showed MRI abnormalities. King (1993) reported that all psychotic patients referred to his AIDS liaison psychiatry service exhibited major manic symptoms. Treisman *et al.* (1994) present data suggesting that when mania develops in patients with low genetic risk this tends to occur late in the disease and in the context of dementia; whereas in those with personal or family histories of affective disorder mania may occur at any stage and while cognitive function is well preserved.

The 'worried well' (AIDS phobia, pseudo-AIDS)

The intense public concern aroused by AIDS, and the amount of media attention devoted to it, have raised anxieties in many segments of the population. People at risk, particularly homosexual and bisexual men, may present themselves for testing in states of considerable alarm ('AIDS anxiety', 'AIDS panic'). Psychotic patients may incorporate AIDS into their delusions and become convinced that they are harbouring the disease (Mahorney & Cavenar 1988). Todd (1989) describes typical examples—patients presenting with anxiety or panic after casual affairs, especially in the face of mild physical symptoms, or with obsessional fears of touching people and compulsive hand washing, or with paranoid psychosis developing some time after an affair.

Distinct from these are a group of neurotic patients who focus on the condition as a vehicle for hypochondriacal concern. Such patients can absorb a great deal of attention in fruitless attempts at reassurance. These are the 'worried well'. They are remarkable not only for the persistence of their anxieties, which can fail to be allayed by repeated negative tests, but often for the remoteness of the chance that they have been exposed to risk of infection. An interesting constellation of influences appears to underlie this sometimes intractable disorder.

Miller *et al.* (1988) reported experience with 19 such patients. Of the 17 males six were heterosexual, eight homosexual and three bisexual. The mean age was 35 years. The uniform presentation was with an unshakable and anxiety-laden conviction that they had HIV infection or disease, as indicated by symptoms such as fatigue, dizziness, sweating, skin rashes, muscle pain, diarrhoea, sore throat, slight weight loss, minor mouth infections or slight lymphadenopathy. The misattribution of such features had often stemmed directly from media reports describing AIDS-related symptoms. Obsessional ruminations were almost universal, centring on thoughts of HIV disease and death, possible 'high-risk' sexual practices in the past and the dangers they may have presented to others. Repeated body checking for signs of the disease and palpation for enlarged lymph nodes were common, likewise questioning and scrutiny of spouses or partners for evidence of the disease. Three-quarters were depressed and over half suicidal. Two patients later progressed to a delusional conviction of supposed infection. Most of the patients had already made repeated attendances at clinics or general practice surgeries, often receiving several negative serological test results.

Background features included a fairly consistent picture of constrained and problematic sexual adaptation, including non-acceptance of homosexual tendencies, difficulties with sexual expression, or constricting religious or family influences on sexual behaviour. This had often resulted in episodes of covert sexual activity, either homosexual or heterosexual, with high levels of associated guilt. In most cases there was a history of no more than low-risk sexual experiences, and only two patients reported activities that could have led to infection within the previous 6 years. A past history of psychiatric disorder, mostly depression or anxiety, was common.

It would appear therefore that the disorder affects a group of people with vulnerable personalities and constrained sexual adjustment, in whom public anxiety about AIDS has served as a vehicle for expression of their sexual guilt and anxiety. The remarkable persistence of such anxieties has been stressed in most reports. Negative test results may be attributed by the patient to laboratory error, to the appearance of a 'new form' of the virus, or to their inability to form antibodies as other people do (Maj 1990). Miller *et al.* (1988) acknowledge the futility of repeated reassurance, which appears merely to maintain the problem. They recommend a cognitive–behavioural strategy based on cue exposure and response prevention, with attempts at the reinterpretation of symptoms in terms of their origin in anxiety. In occasional patients, however, the excessive fear of infection may prove to be part of a major depressive illness and be responsive to antidepressant medication (Jenike & Pato 1986).

Factitious/fraudulent AIDS

In contrast to the above group who have an unfounded fear of infection, occasional patients present with unfounded claims of having the disease. Some state that they are HIV positive to secure financial assistance, rehousing or social support (King 1993). Drug abusers may hope to ensure a supply of maintenance medication and obviate therapeutic attempts to promote withdrawal. Falsified documents and forged reports may be presented to these ends (Zumwalt *et al.* 1987).

More remarkable are those patients who attend hospitals and clinics with a complex history of HIV-related illness, including opportunistic infections and their treatment, all of which turns out to have been fabricated. Sometimes a similar story has been repeated during visits at several hospitals. These patients represent a variant of Munchausen's syndrome, the underlying motive being apparently to secure medical attention. Zuger and O'Dowd (1992) describe such a patient who had received in-patient and out-patient treatment at AIDS facilities for almost a year before the true situation was established. They review 14 more cases from the literature. The usual presentations were with acute neurological or psychiatric complaints, and most patients were members of groups at high risk for HIV infection. Only HIV testing, and where possible confirmation of the history, can protect against a false diagnosis.

Bereavement in AIDS

Fawzy et al. (1991) describe the multifaceted problems of bereavement in patients with AIDS, also in their families, friends and partners. In contrast with individuals suffering from other life-threatening diseases, the patient with AIDS will often have to deal with AIDS-related deaths among many associates and in unrelenting succession.

There is a high risk of the development of abnormal bereavement reactions for a number of reasons. There may be constraints on the public display of grief when homosexuality has previously been concealed; and in the case of drug abuse there is likely to be disapproval or even a punitive response from those around. The patient's ambivalent feelings about homosexuality or drug abuse may be brought to the surface, and may conspire against the development of new supportive relationships. There is the threat of progression to later stages of the disorder, also the risk of 'emotional exhaustion' as losses of friends are repeated. Family members may need to contend with the first awareness of their relative's sexual orientation or drug abuse, and may find themselves lying about the cause of death. Health care workers who treat patients with AIDS also carry a heavy burden in adjusting to the loss of their patients.

Investigation and treatment

HIV-related disease can require the attention of physicians, psychiatrists, psychologists, social workers and specially trained counsellors. The problems which arise are frequently complex, both in terms of medical diagnosis and psychosocial impact. It is therefore common practice, both in the UK and the USA, to establish specialised HIV and AIDS units or centres, where staff can gain particular expertise in matters of investigation and management. In such a context it is also possible to arrange for comprehensive education and support for the staff engaged in the care of patients.

Investigations during the symptomatic stages will often involve extensive laboratory and radiographic procedures. Some of the principal findings in patients with opportunistic infections and tumours of the nervous system have been mentioned above, also findings in relation to HIV-associated dementia. Space does not permit a comprehensive account where other organ systems are concerned, but reference may be made to Weller et al. (1996) for details of the investigations often required. However, the issue of serological testing will be considered in some detail in view of the problems encountered for psychiatric practice.

Serological testing

The technique routinely employed for detecting HIV infection relies on assessment of antibodies to the virus using enzyme immunoassay. When a positive result is obtained the test is first repeated, then checked with a more specific approach such as immunofluorescence, radioimmune precipitation or Western blotting (Dr Anton Pozniak, personal communication). Lymphocyte culture for isolation of the virus can be useful in paediatric practice, since HIV antibody testing can remain positive through passive maternal transfer for up to 18 months. Minute amounts of HIV nucleic acid can be detected by polymerase chain reaction, and this can yield a measurement of viral load.

The important issues surrounding testing are discussed by Catalan et al. (1989). Testing should only be carried out with the patient's informed and explicit consent except in very rare instances, and in the context of careful pre- and post-test counselling. A positive result carries not only implications for the patient's future health but also far-reaching social, financial and often legal consequences. The specific points to be covered in counselling have been set out in guidelines by the World Health Organization and the British Medical Association and are summarised by Bor et al. (1991).

There are, however, exceptional circumstances in which testing may need to be performed without explicit consent, namely where a test is imperative in order to secure the safety of persons other than the patient and where it is not possible for the prior consent of the patient to be obtained (General Medical Council 1988, 1993). In psychiatric practice other situations may also arise, for example when a patient is unable or unwilling to give consent by reason of psychiatric disorder such as severe affective illness, mental handicap or an organic brain syndrome. It is then necessary before proceeding to be clear that the result would be both of real diagnostic value and of likely benefit to the patient. In many instances there is no immediate and pressing need for a definitive diagnosis, and it may be possible to defer testing until the patient becomes well enough to reconsider giving consent in the normal way. The need to know urgently for the protection of staff or other patients is likely to apply only in patients showing aggressive or seriously uninhibited behaviour.

When performed without consent, it is important to record reasons for taking such action in the patient's notes, to discuss it with the psychiatric team and to obtain a second opinion from a psychiatrist or physician. It is wise also to inform the health authority's solicitor and the relevant medical defence body. In essence the test should be carried out with awareness that the decision may have to be defended in court.

Matters of confidentiality surrounding the test result can also be problematical (General Medical Council 1988, 1993; Catalan *et al.* 1989). Only those team members who need to know should be informed. The importance of telling the patient's general practitioner, who is likely to be involved in future care, should be discussed with the patient and consent obtained for this. But if after full discussion the patient refuses, his request for privacy should normally be respected. The exception is when failure of disclosure could put the health of any carer at serious risk. Similarly, disclosure to a spouse or partner without consent is warranted only when there is a serious and identifiable risk to a specific individual who, if not informed, would be exposed to infection.

Treatment

General aspects

General aspects of management include the need for support and counselling, not only for the infected person but often for the family, partners and friends as well. Even in the asymptomatic stage it is important to allow for full discussion of the disease and its significance, including the likelihood that there may be considerable delay before symptoms make an appearance. Detailed information is essential over methods to minimise the risk of infecting others, including 'safe' sexual practices and, in addicts, the strict avoidance of needle-sharing. The patient should be advised to inform the dentist before any dental procedure.

Prophylactic drug treatment is often undertaken to ward off opportunistic infections such as *Pneumocystis carinii*, tuberculosis and toxoplasmosis (Beiser 1997). Problems over employment and in coping with negative reactions from associates will often need attention. Many patients will benefit from regular follow-up, when weight and blood counts can be checked routinely and enquiry made about general health and fitness. Referral to local self-help organisations will usually be of very considerable assistance.

Psychological aspects

Psychological management assumes particular importance in patients suffering from adjustment reactions or sustained anxiety or depression. A behavioural–cognitive approach can prove effective, particularly in the management of anxiety. Depression will sometimes require pharmacotherapy, and careful attention must be given to the risk of suicide. Where alcohol abuse is a problem this may need to become a focus in treatment, because of disin-

hibiting which may lead to unsafe sexual encounters (King 1993).

Later, with ARC or AIDS, psychotropic medication must often be given with special care. Small starting doses may be required because of sensitivity to side effects such as sedation, confusion or postural hypotension. Medications with strong anticholinergic side effects run the risk of inducing delirium or drying mucous membranes. Patients with central nervous system involvement may be sensitive to the extrapyramidal side effects of major tranquillisers. Electroconvulsive therapy for major depression appears not to be contraindicated, except in the context of dementia when it is liable to increase confusion.

Treatment of opportunistic infections and neoplasms

This is a matter for specialist attention. The differential diagnosis is often wide, infections can be multiple and investigations may need to be extensive. *Pneumocystis carinii* pneumonia will often respond, at least early on, to co-trimoxazole, and Kaposi's sarcoma skin lesions to local radiotherapy or intralesional injections of vinblastine. Kaposi's sarcoma occurring elsewhere, such as the lungs or gastrointestinal tract, may be treated with intravenous chemotherapy. Oral candidiasis may be kept in check with nystatin suspension or amphotericin lozenges; oesophageal and severe oral infection will require ketoconazole. Details of treatment for these and other systemic infections are given in textbooks of medicine.

Many central nervous system pathogens can be treated similarly. *Toxoplasma* brain infection will often respond, both clinically and radiologically, to pyrimethamine and sulphadiazine, occasionally with complete resolution of symptoms and control of the disease. Improvement can be seen within 1–2 weeks, this sometimes being used empirically as a diagnostic test. If there is no response, biopsy is required to investigate for other treatable conditions such as lymphoma, tuberculosis or cytomegalovirus infection. Cryptococcal infection is usually treated with amphotericin B, with or without 5-flucytosine, followed by maintenance therapy with fluconazole (Manji & Connolly 1992). Herpes simplex requires acyclovir, and cytomegalovirus infection foscarnet or ganciclovir; the latter should not be combined with zidovudine because of severe myelosuppression. Cerebral lymphoma often responds initially to radiotherapy.

Inflammatory neuropathies are sometimes considered best treated with plasmapheresis because of the risks of steroid therapy in the immunocompromised patient. Others, however, use steroids on the basis that autoimmune mechanisms are at work. Distal sensory neuropathy may respond to zidovudine.

Anti-retroviral treatment

Zidovudine (3-azido-2,3-diethoxythymidine, AZT, Retrovir) has been used in treatment since 1987. It is a thymidine analogue which competes with thymidine for incorporation into the DNA produced by the virus, inhibiting viral reverse transcriptase and blocking formation of further proviral DNA. It can be shown to be highly active against the HIV virus *in vitro*, but is effective only against virus in the process of replication. Resistant strains may accordingly develop after several months of use. Other antiretroviral agents licensed for trials in the USA and the UK include dideoxyinosine (didanosine, DDI) and dideoxycytidine (zalcitabine, DDC) but these have been less comprehensively studied. Still others under investigation include lamivudine, stavudine, and the non-nucleoside reverse transcriptase inhibitors nevirapine and delavirdine. A group of protease enzyme inhibitors which prevent cleavage of proteins in newly formed virus particles also show promise, including saquinavir, ritonavir, indinavir and nelfinavir (Cohn 1997). These are now being assessed in various combinations on the basis that greater success may be achieved by targeting several aspects of the viral life cycle together (p. 336). However, zidovudine has been most comprehensively studied and is therefore considered in detail below.

The most frequent adverse effect of zidovudine is bone marrow suppression, resulting in anaemia or neutropenia, which may dictate reduction of dose or cessation of treatment. Regular monitoring of the blood picture is therefore essential during treatment. Other side effects include nausea, anorexia, abdominal pain, rashes, headache and insomnia, largely restricted to the early weeks of treatment. A reversible myopathy occasionally develops after long-continued use.

Early open studies reported improvements in peripheral neuropathy and early dementia, sometimes sustained for several months (Yarchoan *et al.* 1987, 1988). Children with HIV encephalopathy showed improvement in cognitive function, also in appetite, weight and CD_4 counts (Pizzo *et al.* 1988). The first major trial with placebo control was conducted on 282 patients with AIDS presenting as *Pneumocystis* pneumonia or with advanced ARC (Fischl *et al.* 1987). It was stopped after a median follow-up of 4 months because only one patient under treatment had died compared with 19 on placebo. Twenty-four patients on zidovudine compared with 45 on placebo developed opportunistic infections; weight increased significantly with treatment, patients reported improved well being, and CD_4 cell counts increased significantly. In the course of the trial Schmitt *et al.* (1988) were able to demonstrate improved cognitive functioning among those taking zidovudine on measures of attention, memory and psychomotor speed.

HIV-associated dementia also appears to respond to zidovudine in some degree. Sidtis *et al.* (1993) randomised 40 patients with mild to moderate dementia to placebo and treatment doses of 1000 or 2000 mg per day, and after 16 weeks observed significant improvement in the combined treatment groups on neurological and neuropsychological examination. The placebo group was then re-randomised to high or low treatment and showed significant gains after a further 16 weeks. The most decisive improvements were at the higher dosage.

It seems possible, furthermore, that treatment may prevent or at least delay progression to dementia if started early in the disorder. Portegies *et al.* (1989) carried out a retrospective review of patients with AIDS and neurological symptoms seen between 1982 and 1988. Dementia had been diagnosed in 36% of those never taking zidovudine compared with 2% of those who had had the drug. Moreover 26% of samples of cerebrospinal fluid from the former group were positive for HIV-1 p 24 antigen, compared with none of the latter, suggesting that the drug may inhibit viral replication in the central nervous system. In an extension of the study, Portegies *et al.* (1993) examined survival in the 40 patients who had developed dementia: mean survival had been 4 months in the 20 not given zidovudine, compared with 14.8 months in the 10 who started treatment after the dementia had developed. Three of these 10 had improved remarkably and two slightly under treatment. Only one patient had developed dementia while taking zidovudine, whereas nine developed it after discontinuation. Gray *et al.* (1991), in an autopsy survey, found significantly fewer multinucleated giant cells in the brains of patients who had been treated continuously until death, compared with those who had never had the drug or in whom it had been given only briefly.

The question therefore arises whether zidovudine and allied agents should be started early after infection on the grounds that they may exert a 'neuroprotective' effect. There is some evidence in favour of this. Hamilton *et al.* (1992) carried out a controlled trial of early versus late treatment with zidovudine in patients who were already symptomatic but not yet suffering from AIDS-defining illnesses. 'Late' treatment involved delaying zidovudine until CD_4 counts had fallen below 200/μl. Over the 2 years' follow-up 16% of patients in the early-treatment group progressed to AIDS, compared with 29% in the late-treatment group. Dementia developed in none of the patients who started treatment early, but in six of the 168 who started it late. High dosage may, however, be essential for protecting against dementia: the Nordic

Medical Research Council's HIV Therapy Group (1992) found a trend indicative of a dose–response effect—8% of patients taking 400 mg zidovudine per day progressed to dementia over 19 months, compared with 6% on 800 mg per day and 3% on 1200 mg per day.

A more difficult problem concerns possible long-term benefits from starting treatment in the asymptomatic stage of infection, when advantages may be outweighed by the early development of viral resistance (Drug & Therapeutics Bulletin 1991a). Volberding *et al.* (1990) randomised 1338 asymptomatic subjects to placebo or zidovudine, all with CD_4 counts below 500/μl. Analysis after a mean of 1 year showed that significantly fewer had progressed to AIDS when on active treatment (2.7% compared with 7.7%) and the trial was discontinued. Fischl *et al.* (1990) followed 711 mildly symptomatic patients for a median of 11 months, and found that 4.2% of those on treatment died or developed ARC or AIDS compared with 10.3% of those on placebo. In both trials zidovudine either prevented or delayed the fall in CD_4 counts seen over time in the control patients. Such encouraging results have, however, been criticised on a number of methodological grounds (Lancet 1990a). Moreover, they refer to gains over a relatively short period of time and could be interpreted as displaying no more than a transient effect in delaying progression.

The more recent Concorde trial extended the period of observation to a median of 3.3 years and has shown essentially negative results (Concorde Coordinating Committee 1994). One thousand seven hundred and forty-nine asymptomatic HIV-positive individuals were recruited from the UK, Ireland and France, and randomised to early or deferred treatment with 1000 mg zidovudine per day. The early treatment group was given zidovudine from the time of randomisation, while the deferred group was maintained on placebo until ARC or AIDS had developed or CD_4 counts became persistently low. No statistically significant differences in outcome emerged. The estimated 3-year probabilities of death were 8% and 6%, respectively, the 3-year progression rates to AIDS or death were 18% in both groups, and the 3-year progression rates to ARC, AIDS or death were 29% and 32%. CD_4 counts did, however, change significantly, median changes from baseline at 3 months being +20/μl in the early treatment group and −9/μl in the deferred group. These differences persisted for up to 3 years despite the lack of long-term gains in clinical outcome. The use of CD_4 counts as a surrogate end-point must therefore be questioned.

In discussing the Concorde results, and a meta-analysis of six other long-term trials, Egger *et al.* (1994) conclude that trials lasting less than 18 months appear to show some benefit from immediate treatment, while those lasting more than 2 years raise the possibility even of small adverse effects. The issue of early treatment in the absence of symptoms thus remains controversial.

In summary, therefore, zidovudine clearly prolongs survival and reduces opportunistic infections in symptomatic patients, and has proved capable of helping with dementia in some degree. However, it acts to slow rather than prevent viral replication, so delays rather than halts disease progression. The possible development of viral resistance, and the side effects encountered, make the virtues of starting treatment in the asymptomatic stage uncertain, but commencement soon after ARC or AIDS has developed appears to reduce the incidence of later dementia.

Current dosage schemes for zidovudine vary from 500 to 1800 mg or more per day. The optimal dosages to be employed at various stages of the disorder remain uncertain. Combined therapy with other agents currently being developed may hold the key to greater success, as witnessed by recent results from large-scale trials of combination therapy with zidovudine and didanosine or zidovudine and zalcitabine (Pinching 1996). These have shown significant benefit when compared with zidovudine alone in delaying disease progression, and it seems likely that such combinations will rapidly become standard practice. Other combinations under review include zidovudine, lamivudine and the protease enzyme inhibitor ritonavir; zidovudine, zalcitabine and saquinavir; and zidovudine, didanosine and nevirapine (Cohn 1997). Meanwhile efforts continue to discover vaccines effective against the initial viral infection.

Syphilis of the central nervous system

Syphilitic infections of the nervous system have shown a tremendous decrease during the present century and particularly since the introduction of penicillin. During 1936–39 there were 1629 deaths registered as due to general paresis or tabes in the UK, but by 1966–69 these had fallen to 224 (Wilkinson 1972).

Primary syphilitic infections had already shown a gradual decline from the time of World War I onwards. A new peak arose during World War II but this subsided rapidly in the years that followed. It was feared, however, that late manifestations would ultimately rise again, due to unwitting partial treatment in the early stages when penicillin was given for other conditions, but this has not occurred. What does seem to have happened is that partial but incomplete suppression of infection leads to neurosyphilis appearing later in atypical and attenuated forms, with consequent difficulty in diagnosis in many instances. This important problem is discussed on p. 342. There has also been a pronounced shift away from parenchymatous neurosyphilis (general paresis and tabes dorsalis) towards meningovascular syphilis which now accounts for most of the new cases encountered (Nieman 1991). Male homosexuals are particularly at risk and constitute a high proportion of patients, with particular problems when HIV and syphilitic infection occur together (p. 321).

Paradoxically the success of treatment brings its own particular risks, since as the disease becomes increasingly rare it runs the hazard of being more often overlooked. The psychiatrist must continue to bear it in mind, to check regularly with serological tests and look carefully for cardinal signs in the pupillary reactions and tendon reflexes. The 'classic presentation' of general paresis is nowadays rare, and syphilis of the central nervous system can present with virtually any form of psychiatric complaint.

Traditionally the effects of syphilis are divided into four stages: the primary stage with the appearance of the local lesion at the site of inoculation; the secondary stage with early generalised lesions, chiefly manifest as a variety of skin rashes which appear within 4–8 weeks; the tertiary stage with the appearance of late destructive lesions such as gummata, gummatous ulcers, glossitis and bone changes; and the quaternary stage of parenchymatous changes in the central nervous system leading to tabes dorsalis and general paresis. These divisions are empirical, and with the exception of the last not easily applied to the spectrum of changes which occur in the central nervous system. Meningovascular syphilis can appear in the secondary or tertiary stages; and even with primary infections the nervous system is sometimes involved without overt signs of disorder (early asymptomatic neurosyphilis).

Other affections which fall principally on the spinal cord — myelitis, cervical pachymeningitis and syphilitic amyotrophy—are the province of neurology and will not be dealt with here.

Early asymptomatic neurosyphilis

This term is used for cases with abnormalities in the cerebrospinal fluid but no symptoms or signs of central nervous system disorder. The cells or protein may be raised, the pressure increased or the cerebrospinal fluid immunological tests may give a positive result. Such findings emerge in approximately 10% of cases of primary syphilis and 30% of cases of secondary syphilis when the cerebrospinal fluid is examined routinely (Hahn & Clark 1946a).

Thus it appears that a meningeal reaction can set in very early in a surprising number of cases and without producing overt disorder. When adequate treatment is given the disturbance dies out within a year or two and proves to have been benign. In some cases the prognosis is favourable even when treatment has been inadequate (Hahn & Clark 1946b), though in others the changes probably have implications for the later development of quaternary neurosyphilis. It remains uncertain whether tissue immunity is the protective factor, or whether a neurotropic strain of spirochaete is responsible for those cases which progress to general paresis.

Acute syphilitic meningitis

In rare cases infection of the nervous system may be overwhelming with the production of an acute meningitis. This usually develops within the first 2 years, and can even accompany the secondary rash within a month or two of the primary infection. The illness is indistinguishable from other forms of acute meningitis until specific tests are performed.

There is a pyrexia of approximately 39°C (102°F) with headache, delirium, neck stiffness and somnolence. Lumbar puncture reveals fluid under pressure, containing upwards of 1000 cells/mm^3, of which a considerable proportion may be polymorphs. Specific tests for syphilis may be negative in the cerebrospinal fluid but are invariably positive in the blood. With prompt treatment there is usually good recovery, though some permanent intellectual impairment may result.

Subacute and chronic meningovascular syphilis

A variety of clinical pictures are subsumed under this heading and are most easily understood in terms of the underlying pathology. The disorders usually declare themselves within 1–5 years of the primary infection, though the range may extend from the first few months to 30 years or more.

Pathology

Changes affect both the meninges and the cerebral vasculature. In the meninges there is a diffuse inflammatory process with thickening, areas of necrosis and the formation of exudate which may become gelatinous and adherent ('gummatous leptomeningitis'). Changes are often most in evidence at the base of the brain, resulting in cranial nerve lesions or hydrocephalus due to obstruction of the flow of cerebrospinal fluid. Less commonly they are localised over the convexity, or extend to envelop the whole of a hemisphere in a thickened sheath. Similar changes may extend along the perivascular channels, with the formation of localised gummata within the brain or in relation to the overlying bones of the skull.

Vascular pathology forms an integral part of the reaction in the meninges but can also involve the cerebral vessels directly. The vessels at the base of the brain are chiefly affected, first the small and then the larger branches of the circle of Willis. There is both a periarteritis and an endarteritis, the latter producing great hypertrophy of the intimal layer and leading to thrombosis. Around affected vessels there is fibroblastic proliferation and necrosis, again sometimes proceeding to scattered gummata. The large isolated gumma leading to tumour-like symptoms is extremely rare.

Clinical features

Subacute forms of meningitis may progress rapidly once they are declared, though chronic forms are often insidious and intermittent with periods of several months between exacerbations of disease. Hence the delay which may be encountered in diagnosis.

Early generalised symptoms consist of intermittent headache, lethargy and malaise. The patient is usually slow and forgetful, with difficulty in concentration and faulty judgement. Emotional instability and irritability are common. Mental deterioration may progress to definite evidence of dementia, sometimes with fleeting delusions or episodes of excited overactivity. Alternatively there may be periods of clouding of consciousness or florid delirium separated by intervals of relative normality. The vague quality of the complaints, and the fleeting nature of the early disabilities, can lead to the organic nature of the disturbance being overlooked for some considerable time.

The focal evidence of basal meningitis consists chiefly of cranial nerve disturbances. Paresis of external ocular movements and abnormalities of pupil size and reaction are common, but the fully developed Argyll Robertson pupil (p. 341) is rarely seen. Papilloedema, optic atrophy and visual field defects from chiasmatic lesions also occur. Hypothalamic involvement may produce polyuria, obesity and somnolence. Convexity meningitis can result in focal fits, aphasia or hemiparesis. Headache is often sharply localised and the overlying skull may be tender.

When vascular pathology is predominant, minor arterial occlusions lead to episodes of transient neurological disorder—hemiparesis, hemianopia, aphasia or amnesia—while occlusion of major vessels can result in a completed stroke. The picture of 'pseudobulbar palsy' may develop with bilateral spasticity and emotional lability.

Unusual presentations include isolated ocular palsy and trigeminal neuralgia as well as meningitic symptoms (Nieman 1991). Meningovascular syphilis may also mimic encephalitis and even multiple sclerosis. It should be considered in any acute encephalopathy, and in any acute stroke in younger patients.

The cerebrospinal fluid shows a moderate cellular reaction with up to 200 cells/mm^3, mostly mononuclear leucocytes, and a moderate increase of protein. The pressure is usually normal. Serological tests are usually positive in the blood but may be negative in the cerebrospinal fluid.

With adequate treatment the prognosis is generally good provided extensive cerebral infarction has not occurred. Sometimes the patient is left with fits, hydrocephalus or permanent intellectual impairment.

Tabes dorsalis

Tabes dorsalis is seen in conjunction with approximately 20% of cases of general paresis. Its highly characteristic signs and symptoms may therefore alert the psychiatrist to the latter disease.

Onset is usually 8–12 years after primary infection, though a range of 3–20 years is seen. Males are affected much more frequently than females with a peak age of onset in the fifth decade (Orban 1957). The essential pathology consists of degeneration of the ascending fibres from the dorsal root ganglia, resulting in atrophy of the dorsal roots and shrinkage and demyelination in the posterior columns of the cord.

Characteristic symptoms include pain, paraesthesiae and a marked disturbance of gait. These usually develop insidiously. The lightning pains of tabes are extraordinarily severe, typically brief and stabbing in nature and sharply localised in the legs. Burning and tearing pains may also occur, or girdle pains around the trunk. Paraesthesiae are also most common in the legs and feet; the skin may be hyperaesthetic to touch or the patient may feel he is walking on cotton wool.

The ataxia is sensory in origin and due to loss of proprioceptive sensibility. The patient walks with a wide base or a typical 'high stepping gait', and finds more difficulty in the dark when visual control is reduced. Romberg's test is positive from an early stage.

'Tabetic crises' consist of episodic pain in the viscera. The gastric crisis is most common, with attacks of epigastric pain and vomiting. Laryngeal crises consist of dyspnoea, cough and stridor, rectal crises of tenesmus, and vesical crises of pain in the bladder and penis. Other manifestations are impotence and sphincter disturbances.

On examination sensory changes are found earliest in the legs. Loss of postural sense and vibration sense are marked, and compression of the Achilles tendon may fail to produce pain. Other characteristic sites of sensory loss, involving both touch and pain, are the side of the nose, the ulnar aspect of the arms, patchy loss over the trunk and the dorsum of the feet. The musculature is hypotonic and the tendon reflexes diminished or absent, particularly at the ankles. The pupils are abnormal in 90% of cases, though the full spectrum of the Argyll Robertson pupil (p. 341) tends to be a late development. Ptosis and optic atrophy are frequently seen.

Painless disorganisation of joints may result in gross deformity (Charcot's joints), most frequently at the knee or the hip. Perforating ulcers and other trophic skin changes may appear.

The cerebrospinal fluid is usually under increased pressure, with a moderate number of mononuclear cells and a slightly raised protein. The Lange colloidal gold curve is 'luetic' with increased precipitation in the middle zone. The Venereal Disease Research Laboratory test (VDRL) may be negative in both the blood and the cerebrospinal fluid in 20% of cases, and the fluorescent treponemal antibody absorption test (FTA-ABS) may be negative in the cerebrospinal fluid despite an excess of cells and protein (Wiles 1993b).

Without treatment the disease is slowly progressive. General paresis may appear after a lapse of many years, or even if it does not long-standing cases may develop psychotic illnesses of a paranoid or depressive nature (Wilson 1940).

General paresis (dementia paralytica, general paralysis of the insane, GPI)

Hare (1959) has traced the fascinating history of this disease. It was first clearly described in the early 19th century by physicians working in the mental hospitals of Paris. It appears to have assumed epidemic proportions in France soon after the Napoleonic wars, and thereafter the spread by venereal infection can be traced along the trade routes of Europe and to the New World. Hare adduces detailed evidence to suggest that general paresis may have arisen as a new disease by mutation of the syphilitic spirochaete.

The disease occupies a unique place in several respects in the history of psychiatry. The final proof of its aetiology was an important landmark, likewise the discovery of its response to treatment. A relationship between syphilis and insanity had long been recognised, but there was much controversy before a syphilitic aetiology became accepted for general paresis. Hereditary taint, alcohol consumption, mental strain and even sexual excess were all championed as causes by various authorities despite the increasing epidemiological evidence that syphilis was

responsible. The development of the Wassermann test in 1906 did not end the disputes, which persisted until Noguchi and Moore (1913) finally demonstrated the *Treponema pallidum* in the brain itself. Thus a clear aetiology was eventually established for a mental disorder which was then extremely common. Some few years later the same disease proved to be the first major mental illness to respond to medical treatment, and ultimately earned the Nobel prize for Wagner-Jauregg in 1927.

Pathology

General paresis is the only syphilitic disease in which spirochaetes can be demonstrated in the tissues of the brain, and the pathology is thought to be the direct result of their action there.

Macroscopically the dura mater is thickened and opaque, and chronic subdural haemorrhage may contribute to the formation of a thick membrane over the brain (pachymeningitis haemorrhagica). The pia mater is firmly adherent to the underlying cortex. The brain itself is small and atrophied with widening of the cerebral sulci and dilatation of the ventricles.

Microscopically there are inflammatory lesions throughout the cortex, consisting of dense perivascular collections of lymphocytes and plasma cells and attributable to the irritation produced by the spirochaetes. Equally prominent are degenerative changes, with cortical thinning and outfall of neurones, especially in the frontal and parietal regions. Neuroglial proliferation is marked, forming a dense feltwork below the meninges and beneath the ventricular walls, the latter giving a 'frosted' granular appearance to the naked eye. Enlarged microglial cells (rod cells) are characteristically arranged in rows, and stain with Prussian blue to show iron-containing pigments in their cytoplasm. This reaction is held to be pathognomonic for general paresis.

The spinal cord may show secondary degeneration of the pyramidal tracts, or a combination of paretic and tabetic pathology with degeneration of the posterior columns.

Clinical features

In essence general paresis is a dementing process of insidious onset, but often coloured at first by other features which tend to obscure the intellectual impairment. Changes in affect or personality are frequently the presenting abnormalities as with Pick's disease (p. 461); alternatively the dementing process may be concealed until some unexplained lapse of conduct brings the true situation abruptly to light. Thereafter the progress of the disorder is marked by certain characteristic features and by neurological disabilities which give the disease its name.

It is usual to describe several forms of general paresis according to salient aspects of the mental state. This remains useful in serving to underline the varied manifestations of the disease, although as indicated below the frequency of the different varieties has changed considerably and many atypical forms are now seen.

The disease affects males much more commonly than females, with a peak age of onset between 30 and 50 though the latitude is wide. Congenital general paresis can be declared in early childhood and cases are also seen in extreme old age. The time from infection is difficult to determine, but is usually quoted as being from 5 to 25 years with an average of 10–15 years.

Presenting features

In retrospect it is often discovered that the patient has experienced minor ill-defined symptoms such as headache, insomnia and lethargy for several months before more definite manifestations appear. Relatives commonly report an insidious change of temperament — moodiness, apathy or lessened emotional control. Other common early changes may suggest frontal lobe involvement by way of coarsening of behaviour and loss of refinement in the personality.

Episodic forgetfulness is usually the first cognitive change, followed by defective concentration, reduction of interests and mental and physical slowing in the manner typical of a dementing process. Difficulty with calculation is stressed as an early feature, also disturbances of speech and writing. Insight is impaired from an early stage.

In approximately 50% of patients the presentation is abrupt, with some striking incident which first brings the patient to medical attention (Dewhurst 1969). Sometimes it is a lapse of social conduct which reveals the true state of affairs — law breaking, an outburst of violence or an episode of indecent exposure. Foolish, eccentric or reckless behaviour may be the opening sign:

In one case the first whim was the purchase of a quantity of old silver for which payment could not be made; another patient rose in his stall at the theatre and threw sovereigns at a comedienne on the stage; a third ordered 700 hymn books for a hospital ward of 16 beds, and a ton of guano for the ward plants. Another wrote to the War Office demanding three Victoria Crosses which he considered he had won in fighting some 10 years before. At the outbreak of hostilities in August 1914, an incipient paralytic sent telegrams to all the crowned heads and rulers, proffering his services as peacemaker.   (Wilson 1940)

Alternatively some organic feature may be abruptly declared, such as an episode of amnesia, an epileptic fit or an acute delirious episode. In Dewhurst's (1969) series five out of 91 cases presented with attempted suicide.

Grandiose or expansive form

This was by far the most frequent type of general paresis when the condition was first described, and it has tended to remain the prototype of the disorder in medical teaching. But there is evidence that it had already become less common in Europe during the latter half of the 19th century and perhaps somewhat later in England (Hare 1959). Nowadays it is comparatively rare. In large series of cases from England, America and Norway it has represented only 10%, 18% and 7% of cases, respectively (Fröshaug & Ytrehus 1956; Hahn et al. 1959; Dewhurst 1969). How far the change over time has depended on alterations in the host, the infecting organism or cultural factors is unknown. In some countries the proportion apparently continued to be high, for example in India (Varma 1952) and China (Liu 1960), when it had already become rare elsewhere.

Florid examples are certainly impressive, which may lead to their being highlighted in reports of the disease. The hallmark is the patient's bombastic and expansive demeanour, with delusions of power, wealth or social position. The patient boasts of fantastic riches, exploits in battle, or tells of his athletic and sexual prowess. He may believe he is some eminent person from the past or present, yet at the same time accepts his stay in hospital without complaint.

The mood is euphoric and frequently condescending. The patient's recital may be amusing but his jocularity is rarely infectious, the underlying dementia imparting a shallowness to the prevailing affect. If his beliefs are questioned the mood may readily turn to petulance or anger.

With arrest of the disease the clinical picture can remain remarkably static over many years. Formerly the delusions tended to die out with progression of the disease, and expansiveness gave way to apathy, lethargy and indifference.

Simple dementing form

This appears over time to have gradually replaced the grandiose form and is now a great deal more common. It represented 20% in Dewhurst's series, 60% in Hahn et al.'s series and 48% in Fröshaug and Ytrehus' series.

The usual symptoms of generalised dementia are in evidence, with impairment of memory, slowed and laboured thinking and early loss of insight. Progress may be punctuated by transient episodes of impairment of consciousness during which behaviour becomes even more confused. The affect is shallow; a mild euphoria is common, though many patients are dull and apathetic from the start. As with other dementing illnesses the patient may develop fleeting and ill-systematised delusions, mostly of a persecutory nature. Generally, however, such patients are quiet, lethargic and amenable throughout the course of the disease.

Depressive form

This important variety appears also to have increased considerably at the expense of the grandiose form. It emerged as the commonest variety at 27% in Dewhurst's (1969) series.

The patient presents with classic symptoms of a depressive illness. If dementia is already advanced it may be noted that the affect is somewhat shallow, and that the patient is more readily lifted from his gloom than in primary affective disorders. Sometimes, however, no such distinction can be made. Delusions are of a typically melancholic kind; nihilistic and hypochondriacal delusions may be grotesque in degree, though again the mood may be noted to be disproportionately shallow.

Taboparetic form

In perhaps 20% of patients the pictures of general paresis and tabes dorsalis are combined. Along with dementia the classic tabetic symptoms and signs (p. 338) are observed. The mental symptoms are then often rather mild. True Argyll Robertson pupils and optic atrophy are seen more commonly in this variety than with general paresis alone.

Other forms

Other forms of the disorder are much less common. There may occasionally be a picture of true *manic elation* accompanied by flight of ideas, or a presentation with *schizophrenic features* which mask the true diagnosis. Paranoid delusions are then common, together with ideas of influence, passivity phenomena and auditory hallucinations of an abusing or threatening nature (*'paranoid' or 'paraphrenic' form*). In the *'neurasthenic form'* the outstanding features are weakness, fatigue, irritability and complaints of general ill health. Presentation with an *acute organic reaction* represents an active and rapidly progressive form of the disease. Very occasionally this follows a fulminating course with fever, fits and a picture simulating encephalitis. Cases have been reported which for some time preserve the appearance of *Korsakoff's psychosis* (Wilson 1940). An epileptic or apoplectic presentation occurred in 15% of Fröshaug and Ytrehus' (1956) series. In *Lissauer's*

type the patient presents with hemiparesis, aphasia or other evidence of focal brain disease as a result of massive localised brain destruction. The common presentation nowadays, with a markedly attenuated picture, is outlined on p. 342.

Juvenile general paresis

This has always been extremely rare and is now hardly ever seen. Infection is transmitted via the placenta and the disease is declared in childhood or adolescence. The usual age of onset is between 6 and 21 years. Onset in childhood leads to backwardness at school and results in symptoms of mental subnormality. Epileptic fits are common. Onset in adolescence leads usually to the simple dementing type of general paresis. The same neurological and cerebrospinal fluid abnormalities are seen as in the adult form of the disease.

Abnormalities on examination

The patient frequently shows evidence of poor physical health. In the mental state there will usually be evidence of some degree of dementia if full attention is paid to the assessment of recent memory and other cognitive functions. This may, however, require considerable persistence in the face of facile excuses and evasive behaviour.

Confirmatory signs may be found on neurological examination even in the absence of definite organic features in the mental state. Pupillary abnormalities, tremor and dysarthria head the list of abnormal findings.

The pupils show abnormalities in about two-thirds of cases. A variety of changes is seen—inequality, irregularity and sluggishness of reactions. The full syndrome of the Argyll Robertson pupil may be present, but not so commonly — a small pupil, irregular in outline and with atrophy of the iris, which reacts normally to convergence but not at all to light, and does not dilate fully under the influence of a mydriatic. Optic atrophy may be in evidence even when the patient has no complaint of visual impairment.

Tremor also occurs in about two-thirds of patients when first seen. It typically involves the face and hands particularly. Close attention may be required to detect it in the lips and around the mouth. Tremor of the hands and fingers contributes to the clumsiness which is seen on manual tasks.

Dysarthria is partly due to the tremor of the lips and tongue. Speech becomes slurred, hesitant and jerky, and the voice feeble and lacking in intonation. Dysphasic difficulties may also be found.

Reflex abnormalities consist of exaggeration of the knee

and ankle jerks, with clonus and spasticity in the lower limbs. With progression of the disease the plantar responses become extensor, and there is increasing weakness of the limbs leading eventually to severe spastic paralysis. By contrast tendon reflexes may be absent when tabes dorsalis is combined with general paresis.

Incoordination is seen in the clumsiness of the hands and the characteristic slouching, unsteady gait. In taboparesis it becomes a marked feature, with Rombergism and the classic high-stepping gait.

Further progress

In the absence of treatment the dementia increases steadily along with marked physical deterioration. Periods of arrest or even complete remission were occasionally seen, but usually only for a few weeks or months at a time. Incontinence of urine appears early. Delusions gradually fade away with the other more florid mental features, and the patient becomes quiet, incoherent and apathetic. The characteristic picture in the later stages was of a childish gentle personality, seldom aggressive and with much of the dementia concealed beneath good-tempered polite behaviour (Storm-Mathisen 1969). Spastic paralysis and ataxia increased until the patient was enfeebled and confined to bed. Epileptic attacks, both grand mal and psychomotor, occurred in approximately half of the cases, and the progression of neurological disabilities was often speeded by the appearance of 'congestive attacks'. These consist of sudden episodes of loss of consciousness, hemiplegia, monoplegia, aphasia or hemianopia, lasting a few days or weeks at a time but eventually leaving enduring deficits in their wake. The mechanism responsible remains uncertain but a vascular basis is probable. Death usually occurred within 4–5 years of presentation. This uniformly disastrous prognosis has, of course, been dramatically altered by present methods of treatment as described below.

Atypical present-day forms of neurosyphilis

In addition to the risk of overlooking the disease on account of its rarity, we nowadays face the additional problem that neurosyphilis can occur in atypical or attenuated forms. This may be due in large measure to unwitting partial suppression of the infection in the earlier stages by antibiotics given for other purposes.

Thus while fully developed examples of general paresis and tabes dorsalis have become rare, modified forms of neurosyphilis with atypical presentations and relatively minor symptomatology are increasingly encountered

(British Medical Journal 1978). In Hooshmand *et al.*'s (1972) series of 241 patients in the USA, almost half presented with unrelated symptoms, the diagnosis being made by routine investigation after suspicion had been aroused by neurological or ocular findings. In a quarter the presentation was with focal or generalised seizures. Twelve per cent presented with declining vision or other ophthalmological features, and 11% with confusion following a cerebrovascular accident. Only 5% had the full clinical picture of general paresis. Three-quarters, however, showed abnormal neurological signs, particularly absent tendon reflexes at the ankles, loss of posterior column sensation in the legs or pupillary changes. Uveitis and choroidoretinitis were common. Joyce-Clark and Molteno (1978) have reported similar experience from South Africa. Luxon *et al.* (1979) describe patients presenting with diplopia due to sixth nerve palsy, deterioration of vision due to optic neuritis, primary optic atrophy or choroidoretinitis, and otological symptoms such as sudden deafness or repeated vertigo.

In such atypical cases little may appear to be pathognomonic, either in the clinical picture or on cerebrospinal fluid examination. Hooshmand *et al.*'s (1972) criteria for the diagnosis of neurosyphilis are therefore important. They recommend a firm diagnosis (i) when the blood FTA-ABS test (see below) is positive and there are ocular or neurological findings suggestive of neurosyphilis; (ii) when the FTA-ABS test is positive in both blood and cerebrospinal fluid and the latter contains over 5 leucocytes/mm³ in the absence of bacterial or viral meningitis; or (iii) when the blood and cerebrospinal fluid FTA-ABS are positive in the presence of progressive neurological symptoms not otherwise explained. In the last category there must also be either a transient leucocytosis in the cerebrospinal fluid after administering penicillin, or the patient must improve clinically on penicillin. A positive FTA-ABS result in the blood and cerebrospinal fluid as the sole abnormal finding may not necessarily imply active neurosyphilis, since this can have persisted as a serological finding after adequate antibiotic treatment.

Investigations

Serological tests such as the Wassermann reaction (WR) or Veneral Disease Research Laboratory test (VDRL) are positive in the blood in 90% or more of untreated cases of general paresis, but this figure may be considerably lower if penicillin has been given for some other infection or if a previous course of treatment has been carried out. They may also be negative in patients with AIDS. False positives may be obtained in certain diseases, notably leprosy, disseminated lupus erythematosus, thyroiditis, haemolytic anaemia and some cases of rheumatoid arthritis. The tests may also be positive for a while after some virus infections, after vaccination, during pregnancy and in an appreciable proportion of drug addicts. The cardiolipin WR uses a purer antigen and gives fewer false positives in these situations. The Reiter protein complement fixation test (RPCF) operates on spirochaetal material from non-pathogenic treponemes, and is therefore negative in the above diseases but may be positive in other spirochaetal infections such as yaws.

Positive results from the WR or VDRL, along with a positive RPCF, means that the possibility of syphilitic infection is high. More certainty will be given in marginal cases by modern procedures such as the TPI, TPHA or FTA. The *Treponema* immobilisation test (TPI) is reasonably specific to *T. pallidum*, but is technically difficult to perform. The *Treponema pallidum* haemagglutination test (TPHA) uses an indirect haemagglutination technique, yielding a high degree of specificity and lending itself to automated methods. The development of the fluorescent treponemal antibody test (FTA) has marked an important advance, particularly in the form of an absorption test (FTA-ABS). This is in general very reliable, though false positives occasionally occur with sera containing antinuclear or rheumatoid factor, and true positive results are obtained with yaws. Negative results are occasionally seen in patients who are HIV positive. The FTA-ABS is fortunately almost invariably positive, both in the cerebrospinal fluid and the blood, in the modified forms of neurosyphilis encountered in present-day practice (Oates 1979).

The possibility of negative results with certain serological tests in the blood means that the cerebrospinal fluid must be examined in every case when the presence of neurosyphilis is even remotely suspected. Such tests are positive in the cerebrospinal fluid in almost every untreated case of general paresis, though the VDRL may be negative in a considerable proportion (Davis & Schmitt 1989). The pressure is often raised, there is a moderate lymphocytosis of 5–50 cells/mm^3, and the protein is also usually elevated (50–100 mg/100 ml). The globulin ratio is greatly increased, oligoclonal bands may be present, and Lange's colloidal gold curve typically shows the 'paretic' form with maximum change in the first five tubes (e.g. 5544322110). There is in general little correlation between the initial cerebrospinal fluid cell or protein levels and the severity of the clinical picture. A cerebrospinal fluid without raised cells or protein may be seen if there has been previous treatment.

The EEG is abnormal in the great majority of patients with general paresis, with an excess of theta and slower wave activity.

Differential diagnosis

The forms of neurosyphilis are so variable in presentation that serological tests should be carried out on the blood in all patients admitted to psychiatric units. In the outpatient clinic there must be a readiness to do such tests when the index of suspicion is high. Roberts and Emsley (1992) reported 21 patients admitted to acute psychiatric units with neurosyphilis, in only three of whom the diagnosis had been considered before the results of routine serology were known. The initial diagnoses had encompassed schizophrenia, depression, mania and hysteria, in addition to delirium and dementia. Cleare *et al.* (1993) found a continuing low prevalence of positive serology (at almost 4%) among psychogeriatric in-patients, this not infrequently reflecting active disease. Other recent examples where mistakes were averted are reported by Sirota *et al.* (1989) and Sivakumar and Okocha (1992). At the very minimum the pupil reactions and tendon reflexes should be examined at every new consultation. However, clinical examination without serology is not always enough to avoid errors in diagnosis; this was illustrated by Steel (1960) in patients in a psychiatric observation ward and by Joffe *et al.* (1968) in patients seen in a neurological clinic. The present-day frequency of attenuated forms and atypical presentations makes the application of routine serology very much more important.

A history of change of personality, impaired emotional control and intellectual decline will immediately suggest general paresis, and the presence of tremor, dysarthria or pupillary or reflex abnormalities will almost suffice to confirm the diagnosis. But such well-established cases are nowadays rare at the time of initial presentation. In Dewhurst's (1969) series only 24 out of 91 cases were diagnosed as having neurosyphilis from the outset. The most common initial diagnoses were of depressive illness, dementia, confusional states, schizophrenia, hypomania and epilepsy.

General paresis must obviously be considered in all patients who present with organic impairment of intellect, and no patient should be diagnosed as suffering from a primary senile or presenile dementia until syphilis has been excluded. Among older arteriopathic patients mistakes are particularly likely to be made, since tremor and dysarthria are then not entirely unexpected. Pupillary abnormalities are, however, rarely seen in cerebral arteriosclerosis or other dementing illnesses.

Affective psychoses appear to have been closely simulated in many of Dewhurst's patients. On occasion the clinical picture may also be typical of schizophrenia, to the extent that the cerebrospinal fluid findings come as a surprise (Fröshaug & Ytrehus 1956). Where routine serological testing is not possible the principal safeguard must lie in careful and systematic examination of the nervous system, and due attention to any organic mental impairments which emerge.

There is a special risk of overlooking the diagnosis in alcoholic patients. Emotional instability or expansiveness may be attributed to alcoholic deterioration, likewise social lapses, facile behaviour, tremulousness and dysarthria.

General paresis may be confused with cerebral tumour when headache is marked and the personality attributes of frontal lobe damage conspicuous. An anterior basal meningioma may mimic the disease closely when compression of the optic pathways leads to pupillary changes and optic atrophy.

General paresis must also be borne in mind in the differential diagnosis of epilepsy of late onset, and in all acute organic reactions when other causes are not immediately obvious.

Finally it is necessary to distinguish between general paresis and other neurosyphilitic diseases, in particular chronic meningovascular syphilis and asymptomatic neurosyphilis. In chronic meningovascular syphilis the prognosis is much better than in general paresis, though the cerebrospinal fluid may show similar changes including a paretic Lange curve. Meningovascular syphilis tends to occur earlier than general paresis, shows a more acute development, and fluctuations in its course are usually marked. Insight is generally better preserved, the personality less deteriorated and focal neurological signs somewhat more common. Some patients with asymptomatic neurosyphilis will tend to be diagnosed as having general paresis when in reality the problem is of coincidental cerebral arteriosclerosis, chronic alcoholism, mental retardation or functional psychotic illness. This group will, however, be small, and antisyphilitic treatment will still be indicated in full.

Treatment

Adequate treatment of syphilis in the primary stage prevents the development of general paresis later. Similarly energetic treatment must be pursued, essentially as for general paresis, in those cases of 'asymptomatic neurosyphilis' where lumbar puncture reveals abnormalities in the cerebrospinal fluid before any clinical signs or symptoms of nervous involvement have become apparent. For this reason routine lumbar puncture is often advocated in every case of primary syphilis, and yearly examination of the cerebrospinal fluid in those who show abnormalities in the early stages. In patients who are HIV positive it is generally agreed that treatment should be as for general paresis, even for those in the primary or secondary stages (Nieman 1991).

Penicillin therapy

For the treatment of established general paresis penicillin alone is generally agreed to be adequate, and can eliminate syphilitic infection in the brain in the great majority of cases. Benzylpenicillin G is the preparation of choice and must be given by intramuscular injection; as procaine penicillin G it can be given by daily injections. Benzathine penicillin, given as a single injection per week, will not, however, suffice. This regimen appears to be effective for the treatment of primary syphilis in patients who are likely to be uncooperative over daily attendance, but there is now evidence that it yields inadequate cerebrospinal fluid levels for the treatment of neurosyphilis (Mohr *et al.* 1976; Tramont 1976).

The minimum effective dose has not been established with certainty. In Hahn *et al.*'s (1959) series a total of 6 million units appeared to be sufficient, and was traditionally given as 600 000 units (600 mg) of procaine penicillin intramuscularly each day for 10 consecutive days. More recent recommendations are of considerably higher dosage — 2.4 million units daily intramuscularly for 14 days, along with probenecid 2 g orally (Simon 1985). Aqueous penicillin G, 12–24 million units intravenously daily for 10–15 days, is sometimes regarded as preferable (Greenwood 1996).

A Herxheimer reaction is liable to occur in 5–10% of cases within the first few days of treatment. On this account these days of treatment are best undertaken in hospital. The reaction may consist of malaise and fever alone or result in an exacerbation of symptoms, sometimes with seizures. Oral prednisone given the day before and during the first few days of treatment helps to prevent its occurrence. When sensitivity to penicillin precludes its use it may be necessary to substitute oxytetracycline or erythromycin 2 g daily for 15–20 days (Gilroy & Meyer 1969). Fortunately spirochaetal resistance to penicillin does not appear to have developed; all early syphilis continues to respond and it is unlikely that other antibiotics confer extra benefit.

Other treatment

Pyrexia therapy enjoyed a vogue, particularly in the form of malaria therapy after its introduction by Wagner-

Jauregg in 1917. Such treatments, along with arsenic, bismuth and iodides, are no longer used and appear to give no additional benefit over treatment with penicillin alone.

Neuroleptic drugs are indicated for the control of excitement, agitation or florid delusions or hallucinations as in any other psychotic illness, similarly antidepressant drugs for severe depressive symptoms. Anticonvulsants are required for the symptomatic treatment of epilepsy. It must be borne in mind that a small proportion of cases may represent a coincidence between asymptomatic neurosyphilis and an independent psychotic illness, and the latter will then warrant full psychiatric management in its own right.

There is some evidence to contraindicate the use of electroconvulsive therapy in general paresis, particularly in the presence of active disease as mirrored in the cerebrospinal fluid. Sudden worsening with focal signs of neurological defect has been reported to follow electroconvulsive therapy in such cases, and Dewhurst (1969) provides data which suggest the possibility of an impaired overall prognosis.

The complete care of the patient will include planned rehabilitation when deficits persist, in the knowledge that they may show continued slow improvement for up to 2 years following arrest of the disease. From the outset it is necessary to make every effort to test the blood serology of the patient's spouse and children. This is usually best arranged through the patient's general practitioner.

Follow-up and re-treatment

The cerebrospinal fluid should be re-examined 2 months after penicillin treatment is completed. If abnormalities in cells or protein persist a second course should be given immediately. Failure to show clinical improvement does not automatically warrant re-treatment if the cerebrospinal fluid has shown an entirely satisfactory response. In this situation the essential step is a re-evaluation of the diagnosis, since syphilitic infection may have been coincidental with other disease.

Thereafter lumbar puncture should be repeated at 6 months, 12 months, then ideally yearly for the next 5 years. The first sign of relapse is seen in the cell count of the cerebrospinal fluid, and if this rises above 5 cells/mm³ at any follow-up examination re-treatment is strongly indicated. A persistently elevated protein is not of the same significance, and can usually be disregarded if cell counts remain low and there is no clinical evidence of progression. Serological tests may remain positive in the blood and the cerebrospinal fluid for several years after resolution of all active infection. Rising titres in the blood

serology should cause concern, however, and may point to continuing activity or reinfection. This will always indicate the need for re-examination of the cerebrospinal fluid at any point during the follow-up period.

The patient must similarly remain under regular clinical observation for evidence of relapse during the 5 post-treatment years. Clinical evidence of progression of the disease will always raise the possibility of the need for re-treatment, especially when the initial response was good. Routine re-treatment, however, confers no additional benefit.

In summary, re-treatment is indicated when cell counts in excess of 5 cells/mm³ persist or reappear in the cerebrospinal fluid, or when temporary clinical improvement is followed by evidence of progression of the disease; also of course if it cannot be firmly established that an adequate course of penicillin was given in the first place. Re-treatment is not indicated by the absence of initial clinical improvement provided the cerebrospinal fluid response is satisfactory, nor by persistent abnormalities in the protein or serology of the fluid.

Outcome of treatment

The outcome that can be expected was comprehensively described by Hahn *et al.* (1959) from a multicentre follow-up study of 1086 patients in the USA. Their general conclusion is of great importance, namely that success depends essentially on early diagnosis and the prompt administration of a fully adequate course of treatment.

Eighty per cent of mild or early cases obtained a clinical remission and proved capable of resuming work. In this group there were hardly any deaths from paresis. The prognosis for ability to work and to live in the community was directly proportional to the severity of the illness and the duration of decreased work capacity at the time of treatment. However, even severely affected institutionalised patients were still capable of considerable benefit, and stood a one in three chance of improving sufficiently for rehabilitation and ultimate return to work. Certain symptoms were associated with a poor overall prognosis, including incontinence, inability to dress and neglect of personal hygiene. In patients over 60 remission or improvement became much less frequent, probably because of the presence of cerebrovascular changes.

Interesting correlations were found in relation to the cerebrospinal fluid abnormalities at the time of treatment. The more active the fluid in terms of cell count, the greater was the chance of a good clinical response; at the same time, however, the likelihood of clinical progression was then also increased in certain cases. This apparent paradox is explained by the fact that pleocytosis in the cerebrospinal fluid reflects an active and labile process, whereas an inactive fluid indicates a relatively static pathology. The latter is less susceptible to treatment but also less likely to result in clinical progression.

The quality of recovery extended to a wide range of organic mental symptoms and florid psychotic phenomena. At the 5-year follow-up the following symptoms and signs had resolved completely in over half of the patients who showed them: disorientation, convulsions, tremors, incontinence, euphoria and depression. In over a quarter there was resolution of impaired memory, judgement, insight, speech, calculation, delusions and hallucinations. Clearly there is considerable leeway for restoration of function in favourable cases, though with long-established disease one can hope merely to halt progression of the disorder.

The overall death rate 10 years after treatment was 31%: 9% being attributable to general paresis and a further 22% to other causes. Altogether this was almost four times the death rate to be expected for non-syphilitic patients of a similar age.

Wilner and Brody (1968), in a prolonged follow-up of 100 patients, showed that new neurological manifestations were liable to develop in some 30% of cases, consisting of grand mal epilepsy, paraplegia, hemiparesis, optic atrophy or oculomotor palsies. These occurred even among patients who had been treated with penicillin, the average interval between treatment and such developments being 12 years. It was uncertain, however, whether this always represented progression of the neurosyphilis rather than increased susceptibility to other neurological disease, and penicillin may often have been given in inadequate dosage.

Encephalitis

An encephalitic process can occasionally arise in pyogenic infections such as septicaemia, or develop by direct extension of the inflammatory reaction in diseases such as cerebral abscess or meningitis. But in the more restricted sense to be dealt with here, encephalitis refers to a primary disease in which inflammation of the brain is caused by viral agents. Meningoencephalitis is the more appropriate term when a marked element of meningeal irritation exists as well.

Virological studies have gone some way towards isolating and demonstrating the responsible organisms, especially in large epidemics, but a large number of cases remain in which a viral aetiology is merely presumed to operate on account of the general features of the illness. This applies particularly to sporadic cases where opportunities for extensive virological investigations may not

be available, but is also true of some large epidemics, notably the epidemics of encephalitis lethargica in which a specific agent was never conclusively demonstrated.

In some cases of known viral infection it is uncertain whether the virus actually gains access to the central nervous system, or whether the central nervous changes represent an autoimmune or hypersensitivity reaction to the presence of viral infection elsewhere in the body. The latter is thought to be the principal mechanism in many of the forms of encephalitis which follow upon childhood infectious diseases.

It is now also apparent that viruses play a part in some subacute degenerative diseases of the brain, for example the measles virus in subacute sclerosing panencephalitis (p. 362) and the JC papova virus in progressive multifocal leukoencephalopathy (p. 752). Direct infection of the brain with the HIV-1 virus appears to be central to the development of HIV-associated dementia (p. 324). The implication of 'slow viruses' in the development of Creutzfeldt–Jakob disease and other transmissible encephalopathies has now been clarified by the discovery of the role of prion protein in such disorders (p. 474).

A comprehensive classification of encephalitis is difficult but Table 16 delineates the main categories for discussion. The relative incidence of the different forms in the USA between 1969 and 1978 was as follows (Centers for Disease Control 1981): arbovirus infection 25%, enterovirus infection 2%, sporadic encephalitis 7% and childhood virus infection (generally para-infectious encephalitis) 13%. However, the cause remained uncertain in the remainder.

Kennard and Swash (1981) illustrated the principal varieties encountered in the UK by a retrospective review of 60 patients with encephalitis admitted to the London Hospital. Of the 12 where the causative virus was proven this was herpes simplex in six, infectious mononucleosis in three, mumps in two and influenza in one. In 29 with similar features to the above no specific virus could be incriminated. Of the 19 post-infectious cases, 15 followed upon upper respiratory tract infections or influenza-like illnesses, three followed acute exanthemata and one vaccination against smallpox.

The clinical picture in most forms of acute encephalitis is of a rapidly developing illness with headache, considerable prostration, and features of central nervous system involvement. Vomiting, irritability and photophobia are common. Some degree of neck stiffness is often detectable, and papilloedema may develop due to cerebral oedema. Pyrexia is variable, but may be low grade and easily overlooked.

The principal feature of cerebral involvement is disturbance of consciousness, ranging from mild somnolence to

Table 16 Varieties of encephalitis (after Robbins 1958).

Epidemic virus infections of the central nervous system
Arthropod borne (arboviruses)
   Eastern equine, Western equine, St Louis
   Japanese B
   Murray Valley
   Russian spring-summer
   Louping ill
Enteroviruses
   Poliomyelitis
   Coxsackie group
   Echo group
Encephalitis lethargica

Sporadic virus infections of the central nervous system
Herpes simplex
Mumps
Infectious mononucleosis
Herpes zoster
Adenoviruses
Infectious hepatitis
Rabies

Para-infectious encephalitis
Following upper respiratory tract infections
Influenza
Post-vaccination
Measles
Rubella
Chickenpox
Scarlet fever
Atypical pneumonia

Subacute and chronic encephalitis

coma. Delirium figures prominently in some varieties. Epileptic fits are common, especially in children, and can be the opening feature of the illness. Focal neurological signs vary greatly according to the site of major impact of the inflammatory process, and are sometimes remarkably slight or even totally absent. Among the most common are pupillary changes, ocular palsies, nystagmus, ataxia, or affection of the long tracts with alteration of tendon reflexes, up-going plantar responses and pareses of the limbs. Symptoms of temporal lobe involvement such as dysphasia strongly suggest herpes simplex infection. Sometimes the spinal cord is involved with retention of urine or paraparesis.

Special interest attaches to the occasional cases which present with psychiatric disorder. This was recognised in the early epidemics of encephalitis lethargica (p. 350) and examples still occur with other varieties. Sometimes impairment of consciousness and neurological signs are absent at the time of presentation, as in the three patients reported by Misra and Hay (1971) who were admitted to a psychiatric unit with a provisional diagnosis of schizophrenia. Virological studies were apparently not performed:

A boy of 18 was admitted with a 2-day history of odd behaviour. He was excited, overactive and aggressive, with thought disorder and catatonic features. Two days after admission one plantar response was equivocal, and 2 days later both plantars were extensor and the left abdominal reflexes diminished. Lumbar puncture revealed no abnormality. He became pyrexial and developed subacute delirium. The EEG showed a reduction of alpha rhythm and generalised slow activity. He was treated with corticotrophin. Subsequently he developed postencephalitic parkinsonism.

A woman of 45 was admitted with a 3-week history of depression and irritability and a 2-week history of paranoid delusions. On examination she admitted to thought withdrawal and auditory hallucinations. Three days after admission she became pyrexial and an extensor plantar response was elicited. Lumbar puncture was normal but the EEG showed a general excess of symmetrical fast activity. She developed auricular fibrillation and congestive heart failure. She was treated for encephalitis and myocarditis and eventually made a complete recovery.

(Misra & Hay 1971)

Wilson (1976) presented further striking cases of this nature, showing abrupt onset of psychological disturbance and little by way of neurological dysfunction in the early stages. Crow (1978) reviews other scattered examples which illustrate the potential overlap with schizophrenia. The majority probably represent cases of herpes simplex encephalitis (p. 356).

The course can vary greatly from one patient to another, and from time to time in a single patient no matter what the causative organism. Profound coma may improve dramatically after some days or weeks, or unexpected relapse may follow steady recovery. When the acute phase is over there is generally a long period of physical and mental recuperation which may continue for several months. Occasionally the acute phase is succeeded by a prolonged phase of disturbed behaviour which may outlast all evidence of active infection and closely simulate a psychogenic reaction.

There may be no residua, or these may vary from trivial neurological signs to profound brain damage.

Young children are especially at risk, and the contribution of encephalitis to childhood behaviour disturbance has probably been underestimated. Greenbaum and Lurie (1948) described 78 children referred on account of personality difficulties or behaviour disorder attributable to previous encephalitis, representing almost 3% of their total patients. Boys showed postencephalitic changes much more often than girls, and the psychiatric sequelae were worse the younger the patient at the time of the attack. Characteristically there was lack of inhibition, restlessness, impulsiveness and extreme distractibility; intellect was often well preserved, but the prognosis was poor in terms of social adjustment.

Rautonen *et al.* (1991) examined the outcome in 462 Finnish children aged between 1 month and 16 years who were admitted to hospital with acute encephalitis. Death occurred in 2.8%, and 6.7% were severely damaged to the extent that they needed continual care 3–6 months later. The remainder survived with minor or no sequelae. The risk of death or severe disability was increased fivefold among those less than 1 year old, and 25-fold when unconsciousness had preceded admission. Herpes simplex and *Mycoplasma pneumoniae* encephalitis carried an especially poor prognosis.

A recent follow-up of the large cohort of children admitted to the National Childhood Encephalopathy Study, all under 3 years of age, has further underlined the seriousness of encephalitis in the very young (Madge *et al.* 1993). Three hundred and ninety-three children had presented with various forms of encephalitis or encephalopathy, some 60% following measles or other infectious disease of childhood. Almost one-third died, mostly within a month of the onset. Follow-up 10 years later showed that over 40% had motor or educational dysfunction, 20% had epilepsy and a similar proportion had behavioural difficulties by way of hyperactivity or unsociable behaviour.

Further aspects of the clinical picture and after-effects will be described as the varieties of encephalitis are dealt with in turn.

Arthropod-borne encephalitis

This group contains illnesses broadly similar to one another. They occur in epidemics in different parts of the world and are transmitted to humans by the bite of an infected insect, chiefly the mosquito, though in some cases ticks and mites are involved. In the USA the main varieties are Eastern and Western encephalitis and St Louis encephalitis, distinguished mainly by their geographical locations. Louping ill is the only member of the group which is seen in England and this is very rare. It is derived from sheep via sheep ticks. Japanese B encephalitis became well known to the Western world by affecting troops in the Far East during the Second World War.

Recurrent epidemics are a feature of all the diseases listed, often with a seasonal incidence in the warm summer months, and varying somewhat in virulence from one epidemic to another. In some epidemics overt disease is rare in comparison to the number of abortive cases who are found to harbour the viruses without showing signs of illness. This naturally leads to considerable difficulty in reaching a satisfactory laboratory confirmation of the disease when sporadic cases arise, though rising titres of antibodies on repeat examination may help.

Pathological changes are similar in the different varieties. There is diffuse rather than focal cerebral involve-

ment, affecting the grey matter particularly. Microscopy shows infiltration of lymphocytes and polymorphs, congregated especially around the blood vessels ('perivascular cuffing'), scattered small focal haemorrhages, necrosis of neurones and areas of reactive astrocytosis (Booss & Esiri 1986). Demyelination is rarely seen, in contrast to the para-infectious encephalitides.

The clinical picture is similarly uniform, though varying in intensity and prognosis according to the virulence of the epidemic. There is usually a predilection with regard to age, the very young and the old being especially affected. The onset is with fever, headache and gastrointestinal disturbance, often with signs of meningeal irritation. Fits are common, likewise progression to coma or semicoma, but marked delirium is rarely a feature (Drachman & Adams 1962). Focal signs include cranial nerve palsies, especially of the oculomotor nerve, and pareses in the limbs of upper motor neurone type. Eastern equine encephalitis is among the most severe, with early onset of profound neurological deficits and death in approximately 70% of cases (Feemster 1957).

The blood usually shows a polymorphonuclear leucocytosis. The cerebrospinal fluid shows some increase of pressure, a moderate rise of protein, and 200–1000 cells/mm³ of which polymorphs predominate early and mononuclears later. The cerebrospinal fluid sugar is normal. Serological tests may allow the identification of the causative organism by evidence of rising antibody titres to a particular arbovirus; and in the acute phase it may be possible to demonstrate immune-specific immunoglobulin M in the serum or cerebrospinal fluid.

The frequency of enduring sequelae is related to the length of coma in the acute stage and to the age at which infection occurs. Follow-up of a large Californian series showed residual deficits in some 50% of infants under 1 year and in 20% of adults, the former being much the more severe and including mental subnormality, spastic paralysis, athetosis and fits (Finley 1958). Among adults, transient depression and exhaustion are common during convalescence but serious organic residua are rare. Occasionally some degree of intellectual impairment or personality change becomes apparent in the year that follows, and a very small number show ataxia, dysarthria or hemiparesis. Postencephalitic parkinsonism is vary rare indeed. Subjective complaints are much more frequent—depression, irritability, insomnia and nervousness—and can persist for a year or two in a manner which simulates neurosis. These may be accompanied by forgetfulness, difficulty in concentration, tremors or ataxia which suggest a basis in minor cerebral damage. Zeifert *et al.* (1962) found that the EEG findings on follow-up were often at variance with the objective evidence of neurological damage, and abnormal recordings proved to correlate more closely with emotional disturbances than with motor or intellectual deficits.

Enterovirus encephalitis

The enteroviruses are more prone to produce the picture of aseptic meningitis than encephalitis (p. 365). The poliomyelitis virus is distinguished by its effects on the spinal cord and the accompanying encephalitis is usually very slight in degree, but the related Coxsackie and echo viruses can occasionally produce definite encephalitic manifestations.

Outbreaks are commonest in summer and autumn. The Coxsackie and echo illnesses usually run a benign course, accompanied by other systemic symptoms characteristic of the virus concerned—maculopapular rashes, muscular pains or pleurodynia. The changes in the cerebrospinal fluid resemble those of poliomyelitis, with a moderate elevation of protein, normal sugar and 50–100 cells/mm^3 (polymorphs early and mononuclears later). The virus may be isolated from throat swabs or stool specimens, but is of more significance if found in the cerebrospinal fluid. A rise in serum antibodies may be demonstrated during the course of the disease by neutralisation or complement fixation tests, though many asymptomatic infections evoke the same response. Serological testing is also made difficult by the large number of antigenically distinct viruses in this group.

Children affected before 1 year of age may occasionally be left with neurological impairment and seizures (Sells *et al.* 1975). Otherwise serious sequelae are uncommon with Coxsackie and echo virus infections. Muscular weakness may be marked and persist for some time during convalescence, but true paralysis is rare. Poser *et al.* (1969) have reported the occasional development of post-encephalitic parkinsonism after such infections, but this is usually a transient and mild disability unlike that following encephalitis lethargica (p. 352).

Encephalitis lethargica ('epidemic encephalitis')

An earlier generation of neurologists and psychiatrists was much concerned with this disease on account of the devastating epidemics of 1918–20 and the chronic sequelae that occurred. From the 1930s onwards it largely disappeared, at least in its original form, though champions exist for the view that variants still occur sporadically and often go unrecognised (p. 354). Strangely no causative organism was isolated despite extensive researches, and laboratory proof has never been available to uphold the diagnosis in disputed cases.

Whether or not the disease may be relegated to history, it remains an exceptionally important disorder. The thousands of cases available for observation displayed a wealth of psychopathological phenomena which could be clearly ascribed to pathological changes in the brain. This had an important influence on psychiatric thinking at a time when psychodynamic explanations for mental pathology were gaining too much ground. Certainly it focused attention on the relation between mental symptoms and brain structure in a way which few affections of the nervous system had done before. The sequelae of the disease demonstrated that an organic basis could sometimes exist for 'functional' disturbances, including tics, psychotic developments, far-reaching disturbances of personality and, particularly, compulsions and other profound disturbances of will. Hendrick (1928) reviews the attempts which were made by psychiatrists of every school to capitalise on the lessons to be learned from encephalitis lethargica for understanding the neuroses and psychoses, and von Economo (1929) wrote '. . . just as we find it hard today to follow up the trend of thought of our scientific predecessors for whom bacteriology and the lore of brain localisation did not exist, future generations will hardly be able to appreciate our pre-encephalitic neurological and psychiatric conceptions, particularly with regard to so-called functional disturbances'. There is, of course, a danger that these important lessons will be forgotten with the passage of time. The clinical features of the disease will therefore be described in some detail.

Encephalitis lethargica was first reported by von Economo in 1917, after a small local epidemic had led to numerous patients being seen in the Vienna Psychiatric Clinic with strange symptoms that did not fit into any known diagnostic category. The shared features were slight influenza-like prodromata followed by a variety of nervous manifestations, marked lethargy, disturbance of sleep and disturbance of ocular movement. At autopsy the picture of microscopic foci of inflammation, particularly in the grey matter of the midbrain and basal ganglia, was sufficiently constant to suggest a common cause despite the variety of phenomena that occurred. Complete recognition followed in the great pandemic which started in London in 1918 and spread throughout Europe during the next 2 years, approximately coincident with the influenza pandemic of that time. The polymorphic forms of the disease continued to be a striking feature, fresh epidemics often running close to type and differing from those nearby both in the acute phases and in the incidence of sequelae.

There was a seasonal pattern with most epidemics beginning in early winter. The peak incidence was in early adult life from age 15 to 45 years, though no age group was spared. At one time a toxic agent was suspected, but the general pattern combined to suggest an airborne infective agent, gaining access via the nasopharynx and transferred by carriers or those in the presymptomatic stages of infection. The agent was shown to be filter-passable and the disease was transmissible to monkeys by injection of brain tissue from infected patients, but the virus itself continued to elude attempts at isolation. It was a matter of controversy whether the coincident influenza epidemics had predisposed the host to react abnormally to some relatively innocuous organism, and some evidence suggested that the herpes virus might itself be responsible. These questions were not decisively settled, but the great majority of epidemiological evidence suggested that an independent virus was responsible.

In retrospect it appeared that this was not entirely a new disease, and similar widespread epidemics could be traced in history. In England a second peak occurred in 1924, but thereafter there was a striking fall off of new cases throughout the 1930s, though sporadic cases continued to be seen and small local epidemics appeared from time to time.

The following description is largely taken from von Economo's (1929) classic account.

Acute clinical picture

A prodromal stage lasting several days consisted of malaise, mild pharyngitis, headache, lassitude and low pyrexia, all symptoms being slight and resembling the prodomata of influenza. A great variety of nervous symptoms then appeared, depending on the localisation of the virus within the central nervous system. The polymorphic forms of the disease were much documented at the time, varying somewhat between epidemics and to a rather lesser extent in different patients during the same epidemic. Often there was change from day to day in a given patient.

The 'basic' form, and that most usual in sporadic cases, was the *somnolent–ophthalmoplegic variety*. Somnolence developed after the prodromal phase, with slight signs of meningeal irritation. Initially there was merely a tendency to drowsiness from which the patient could easily be roused, sometimes with evidence of confusion or mild delirium. If recovery did not occur at this stage the disorder progressed further to more or less permanent sleep for weeks or sometimes months, often deepening to coma. On recovery disturbances of sleep function might persist for many months during convalescence.

Pareses of the cranial nerves set in early, especially of the third and sixth, with ptosis, paralysis of ocular movements and less commonly pupillary abnormalities or nystagmus. Such signs were usually persistent, but sometimes fugitive and fleeting. Facial palsy or bulbar palsy occasionally developed. In the limbs isolated pareses and reflex abnormalities were seen, with spasticity, hypotonia or ataxia. An admixture of other phenomena appeared in some cases — parkinsonism, chorea, athetosis and catatonic phenomena. Rarely there were fits, transient aphasias or cerebellar symptoms.

In other cases the picture was dominated after the prodromal stage by signs of motor unrest. This was the *hyperkinetic form*, with myoclonic twitches, severe jerking chorea, wild jactitations and anxious excited behaviour. Sometimes compulsive tic-like movements, torticollis and torsion spasm appeared. Oculomotor signs and epileptic fits were common. Delirium could be marked with constant unrest by day and night, sometimes closely resembling delirium tremens with anxiety amounting to terror in response to vivid hallucinations. Typically the acute disturbance lasted a few days only, but insomnia or reversal of sleep rhythm then usually persisted for weeks or months after recovery. Other cases passed on to the typical somnolent–ophthalmoplegic form or to the parkinsonian form.

The *parkinsonian form* was characterised by rigidity and akinesis from the outset. Movements were remarkably slowed and sparse, the patient lying still for hours at a time or responding with profound psychomotor retardation. Speech, like motor movements, was greatly delayed, yet the patient could be shown to be mentally intact despite the appearance of dementia. The limbs showed increased tone and often a coarse tremor. The gait was festinant, and salivation occurred as in paralysis agitans. Catatonic phenomena could be seen, including classic flexibilitas cerea. Along with these features somnolence, sleep inversion and oculomotor signs might be in evidence. Many progressed thereafter to the chronic parkinsonian phase of the disease.

The *psychotic forms* were rare, but presented with acute psychiatric disturbance as the initial feature. Here mistakes in diagnosis frequently occurred until neurological signs declared themselves. The usual picture was of an acute organic reaction, but stupor, depression, hypomania and catatonia were also reported. Sometimes impulsive and bizarre behaviour was the sole manifestation for several days, accompanied by bewildered and fearful affect. Or mental conflicts were brought to the fore, adding a psychogenic colouring to the presenting symptoms. Several examples were reported by Sands (1928):

A woman of 28 developed a sore throat lasting for a week. A few days later she became excited, rambling and impulsive and was diagnosed as suffering from manic–depressive psychosis. No neurological abnormalities were found. She became extremely fearful, asking whether she was about to die or if something terrible was going to happen to her family. She spoke irrelevantly and was very tense. The pupils were later found to be irregular with sluggish reactions, and the tendon reflexes were diminished. In the following week she developed choreiform and athetoid movements and a left facial weakness. She died a few days later after a period of disorientation, high pyrexia and noisy disturbed behaviour.

A woman of 32 suddenly became restless and noisy, sang and screamed, and claimed to be the daughter of Christ and impregnated by him. She lay in bed in a strained attitude, and was markedly deluded and uncooperative. The pupils were widely dilated and reacted sluggishly to light, and the tendon reflexes were diminished. She continued in a state of excitement for 3 days then became drowsy, with diplopia and irregularity of the pupils. Three weeks later she recovered completely.

A woman of 30 developed headache for 2 days then became excitable, restless and uncooperative. She was admitted to hospital with a diagnosis of manic–depressive psychosis. She proved to be deluded and occasionally hallucinated, and claimed at times to be a physician or a great singer. Her temperature was found to be 102°F, and the cerebrospinal fluid was under increased pressure with 6 cells/mm³. Many weeks later she developed ocular palsies and other neurological signs typical of encephalitis lethargica.

It was disputed whether some cases might run their course as a psychotic illness alone without somatic symptoms at any stage. This could neither be proved nor disproved owing to the lack of specific tests for the disease. But in 1924 the Board of Control in the UK reported that many patients had been admitted to mental hospitals with diagnoses of non-specific confusional, delusional and hallucinatory states, yet in later years proved to show the classic sequelae of encephalitis lethargica (Lancet 1966a). The psychiatric literature abounded with case reports, and arguments centred on whether the cases had been missed because the neurological signs had been mild and fleeting, or whether the disease could present as a 'cerebral' form without localised manifestations.

Other forms presented with acute bulbar palsy, or mono-symptomatically with intense chorea, persistent hiccough or neuritis. Abortive types were common in most epidemics, with symptoms capable of arousing suspicion during the epidemic but easily overlooked at other times. There might be little more than headache and sleeplessness, with perhaps diplopia as the suggestive feature. Hysterical symptoms or mild confusion might be all that was noted in the mental state.

During the acute phase there was usually rapid debility and loss of weight. Fever might accompany the prodromal phase or persist throughout, while other cases ran their whole course without pyrexia. A moderate leucocytosis was often present but was not invariable. Examination of the cerebrospinal fluid was not in any way decisive,

though most cases showed some abnormalities — moderate increase in pressure, 5–20 lymphocytes/mm³, a slight rise in protein or a weakly luetic Lange curve. In other well-marked cases, however, the fluid was entirely normal. Many abortive cases developed only the prodromata, while others recovered early after definite symptoms and signs had appeared. Some ran a fulminating course with death after a few days or weeks. Usually, however, the acute disturbances lasted for several weeks, with some months more before ocular palsies, lethargy and sleep disturbances resolved.

A protracted convalescence was not uncommon with repeated relapses and fresh exacerbations. Convalescence also brought prolonged asthenic states, incapacitating depressive illness and a variety of sleep disturbances — insomnia, sleep reversal and narcoleptic phenomena.

Upon recovery focal neurological abnormalities might persist. Paralysis of external ocular movements or of isolated eye muscles was frequently permanent, also pupillary abnormalities, difficulty with accommodation and inability to converge the eyes. Hemiparesis, aphasia or other focal cerebral symptoms might remain, likewise chorea, tics, torticollis, torsion spasm or epilepsy. Hypothalamic damage was seen in adiposity, menstrual disturbance, impotence or precocious puberty. The outstanding sequelae, however, were parkinsonism and changes of personality as considered below.

Altogether in clinically well-marked acute cases, some 40% ended fatally, 40% were left with residual deficits and 20% recovered completely. Approximately half of those with residual defects were permanently disabled from working, mostly on account of progressive parkinsonian symptoms (von Economo 1929).

Chronic sequelae

The most seriously disabling sequelae consisted of parkinsonian developments, change of personality and mental defect. Severe psychiatric illnesses were also seen. The incidence of each varied in different epidemics, but a definite relationship emerged with regard to the age at which the acute infection had occurred. Adults tended to develop parkinsonism, children personality disturbances, and infants were left with mental defect. Generalised dementia did not appear to occur when the mature brain had been affected.

Parkinsonism sometimes developed gradually out of the acute stage, or could set in unexpectedly after full recovery. In the interval the patient may have shown persistent symptoms such as headache, irritability and sleep disturbance but this was by no means invariable. Indeed as time went by it became apparent that sequelae could develop after many months or years of completely normal health. By contrast personality change and mental defect were usually evident immediately after the acute infection.

Sometimes typical sequelae were seen without any clear history of acute disturbance, perhaps because the latter had been exceptionally mild, or perhaps because the causative agent could produce chronic disturbance from the outset. Certainly the severity of sequelae was unrelated to the severity of the original attack. Interestingly the brain pathology accompanying chronic sequelae usually showed new foci of disease as well as the residua of the acute attack, suggesting that the inflammatory process had once again become reactivated.

Postencephalitic parkinsonism

This was the most common sequel and could develop even when parkinsonian symptoms had been absent during the acute phase. Its development was usually insidious, with weakness and slowing of movements or the gradual development of a stiff and unnatural posture. The ensuing picture closely resembled other forms of parkinsonism, with mask-like face, stooping posture, festinant gait and excessive salivation. Tremor was less common than in paralysis agitans; the typical pill-rolling tremor was rarely seen, but coarser tremor and violent shaking of the limbs occasionally occurred.

Paucity of movement was sometimes a striking sign even in the absence of paresis or marked rigidity. It appeared that in large degree this represented a *primary disturbance of willed movement*, such that the patient was unable to supply the volitional impulse in spite of a wish to perform. There might be much difficulty in passing from rest to activity, the patient remaining for minutes on end in a state of trance-like immobility. Or a movement once started might freeze half-way, as when raising a spoon to the mouth. Later typical rigidity developed, with extrapyramidal increase of tone that was obvious on examination. Characteristically the akinesis and the rigidity could vary markedly, improving at some stage during the day, or allowing some activities while preventing others which required exactly the same musculature. Speech became slurred, jerky and monotonous, and writing was often strikingly small and cramped (micrographia).

Other distinctive features were *repetitive motor phenomena* in the form of tics, blepharospasm, torticollis, spells of sighing and yawning, or complex respiratory spasms. Complicated motor stereotypies developed in advanced cases, for example stamping of the feet accompanied by

writhing movements of the head and neck. Speech might show marked repetitive phenomena — of a phrase (echolalia), word (pallilalia) or syllable (logoclonia).

A *compulsive element* was often very prominent indeed, and emerged in speech and thought as well as in motor behaviour. A repeated phrase or question might accompany the motor movements, or the latter might be 'subjectivated' in a characteristic fashion; the patient would state 'I have got to move my hand that way' rather than 'I have a twitch in my hand' as would be the case with ordinary tics. Compulsive thoughts and urges also appeared independently of the motor phenomena, with the patient ruminating endlessly on restricted themes or being driven to complex rituals. Compulsive urges sometimes led to trouble with the law, for example with repeated episodes of indecent exposure. Claude *et al.* (1927) reported patients with compulsions to tear their clothes, pull out teeth, tie themselves with bonds and to strangle cats; he stressed the abrupt appearance of the obsessions, their fixity over time and the patient's clear awareness of the absurdity of the acts.

It is of considerable theoretical interest that motor and psychological features of compulsion should so regularly have occurred together and in intimate association. Schilder (1938) considered that the compulsive phenomena could often be directly traced to motor sources. The encephalitic process liberated motor impulses, with a tendency towards impulsive actions of a sadistic nature, and when checked these led in turn to the compulsions. He believed that in ordinary obsessional neurosis a similar impulse disturbance on an organic basis might sometimes be at work, and estimated that a third of obsessional neurotics at that time showed slight organic signs similar to those found in chronic encephalitis lethargica.

Oculogyric crises were another characteristic feature, again often intimately associated with compulsive phenomena. For a few minutes, or rarely hours, the eyes would deviate upwards or to the side, perhaps with contortions of the head, neck and extremities. Flushing and other autonomic disturbances were common accompaniments. At the onset the patient might be beset by some compulsive thought or enact some complex compulsive ritual. The crisis was sometimes accompanied by a fugue-like mental state, with inability to speak and lack of response to commands, or by marked affective disturbance—surges of depression, anxiety or fear, ideas of reference or feelings of persecution. Schwab *et al.* (1951) mention a patient whose episodes of paranoia were localised to one side of her body during oculogyric crises— she felt that everything and everybody on her left were hostile and unfriendly, whereas the environment on her right was normal. When the attack was over her thinking returned to normal.

Suggestibility was sometimes found to be an important factor, oculogyric attacks being provoked by talking about them or terminating in response to a sharp command. Attacks could also be precipitated by annoyance, shock or grief, and could be contagious in a ward of patients similarly affected. Thus again we see the complex admixture of motor and psychological phenomena which characterised the disease.

The typical mental state in postencephalitic parkinsonism was of marked slowing (bradyphrenia) and lack of the normal fluidity of thought, though otherwise with good preservation of mental clarity. Depression was common, in the early stages at least, and suicide was frequent. Torpor, irritability and disinclination for activity usually accompanied the compulsive elements of the disease (psychasthenia). Later, apathy became the striking emotional feature, with marked difficulty in arousing an affective reaction and little evidence of subjective distress. As the parkinsonian features progressed the patients showed increasing emotional impoverishment, egocentric restriction and peevish hypochondriasis, no doubt aggravated by the institutionalised lives which many were obliged to lead.

The parkinsonism itself usually advanced steadily, sometimes with intermittent progressions, but sometimes came to a halt with fixed residual defect. The combination of physical and mental disabilities inevitably meant that a large number of victims were permanently incapacitated for work, and such patients came to form a substantial proportion of the chronic mental hospital population. Sacks (1973) has provided a striking account of the remarkable motor and behavioural abnormalities encountered in a group of very long-term institutionalised survivors in the USA, and of the effects of attempted treatment with levodopa (pp. 659–60).

Postencephalitic personality change

Children and young adolescents were mostly the victims of this serious development, but adults were not completely immune. It was estimated that approximately a third of patients below the age of 16 developed some form of mental change after encephalitis lethargica. Frequently it was accompanied by other sequelae such as parkinsonism, sleep disturbance, obesity or other evidence of hypothalamic damage.

The common change was towards overactivity and impulsive antisocial behaviour, as though the child now had lessened control over his instinctual drives. He became excited and restless, with inability to settle at school or remain occupied at any task for long. He was talkative, importunate and disinhibited, often indulging in stealing or sexual misbehaviour. Emotional lability was marked, with cheerful affectionate behaviour one moment and outbursts of anger the next. Moral and social senses were undermined, so that the child became destructive, abusive and hard to control. There was usually no primary intellectual deficit, though as time went by education suffered severely or became impossible. Frequently the child appeared to be aware of the change in himself, to apologise repeatedly, yet immediately afterwards be compelled to err again. The general picture could be seen as a primary excess of 'impetus' (in contrast to the akinesis of parkinsonian developments in adults), resulting from brain damage occurring at a time when personality development was gaining control over basic impulsive drives.

The subsequent course was often unfavourable, with worsening over the years leading eventually to institutionalisation. Fairweather's (1947) account of postencephalitic patients admitted to Rampton State Institution for patients of violent and dangerous propensities gives a vivid illustration of the pictures which could ensue, with repeated serious aggression, sexual perversions and self mutilation. Some of the most severe behaviour disorders in Fairweather's group were found in the small group of patients with a definite history of encephalitis lethargica but without parkinsonism or other gross physical residua.

At puberty improvement occurred in perhaps a third of cases. In later years some 50% developed parkinsonian changes, with ultimate benefit where the behaviour disorder was concerned (Slater & Roth 1969).

Postencephalitic psychoses

A variety of psychotic illnesses supervened in other patients upon recovery from the acute stages. Depression and hypomania were relatively common, also paranoid–hallucinatory states and a variety of illnesses resembling schizophrenia. Severe hypochondriasis of 'psychotic' severity was often reported.

Hall (1929) described 18 patients from among 113 cases of encephalitis lethargica, mostly with manic–depressive psychoses or schizophrenia. They differed from the generality of psychoses in that delusions were more transient and variable, and even relatively mild depression was accompanied by profound retardation and immobility. Fairweather (1947) noted that 25% of men and 12% of women admitted to Rampton after encephalitis lethargica were deluded, mainly in a paranoid fashion.

Davison and Bagley (1969) review the evidence concerning schizophrenia. Paranoid–hallucinatory psychoses were estimated to occur in 15–30% of postencephalitics, and psychoses indistinguishable from paraphrenia or dementia praecox in 10% of those admitted to mental hospitals. All reported patients were selected for psychiatric disorder so the true frequency is unknown, but clearly such developments were not uncommon. Hebephrenic forms of schizophrenia occurred, but paranoid types predominated. Catatonic motor symptoms were seen, sometimes even independently of psychotic mental phenomena. Some claimed that the illnesses were indistinguishable from other schizophrenias, but others noted better preservation of rapport and lack of personality deterioration. Davison and Bagley's analysis of 40 cases from the literature revealed only one with a schizoid premorbid personality and two with family histories of schizophrenia, discounting the view that there was usually a predisposition towards the disorder.

Pathology of encephalitis lethargica

In patients dying in the acute stage little macroscopic change was seen other than hyperaemia of brain tissue and perhaps scattered 'flea-bite' punctate haemorrhages. Microscopically, tiny foci of non-purulent 'inflammation' were seen throughout the brain, confined almost exclusively to grey matter and with a marked preponderance in the midbrain, diencephalon and basal ganglia. The distribution of lesions was extremely variable from case to case. Vessels were found to be engorged, sometimes with perivascular collars of chronic inflammatory cells. Toxic–degenerative changes occurred in neurones, with patchy outfall of cells. Glial overgrowth was seldom marked.

With recovery glial proliferation occurred in damaged areas, and the remaining neurones were often filled with fatty material. The latter was regarded as typical of the chronic disease. Scattered calcifications were seen in vessel walls and the brain parenchyma, and small acidophil inclusions were found in neurones.

In the chronic stages old scarred foci were often seen in conjunction with newly active lesions, suggesting that the inflammatory process had persisted during the latent interval and then become reactivated. Degeneration and disappearance of the pigmented cells of the substantia nigra was a striking feature. Neurofibrillary tangles were prominent in the nerve cells, not only of the pigmented nuclei of the brain stem but often scattered throughout the cortex and subcortical nuclear masses as well.

The exact pathological basis for the mental developments — compulsions, personality changes, etc., could

not be determined because the lesions were so very widespread.

Present-day encephalitis lethargica

It would be a matter of some importance if sporadic cases of the disease were still continuing to occur. There would be a substantial chance that the diagnosis would be overlooked, especially with mild affections, yet the sequelae might still dictate considerable psychiatric disability. The problem is difficult to resolve. The laboratory findings were variable even when the disease was common, and specific confirmatory tests were not achieved. During life the diagnosis must therefore rest on the clinical features alone yet these were always variable; and von Economo (1929) predicted that future examples would probably produce different pictures again.

Many authorities doubt whether new acute cases occur, and consider that the disease disappeared completely before the onset of the Second World War. Leigh (1946), however, reported two possible cases during an influenza epidemic, and thought that one if not both might be regarded as classic examples of the acute disease. Espir and Spalding (1956) reported three further examples, all with acute illnesses, two merging into parkinsonism and the third developing it some years after recovery:

A police cadet of 16 developed headache and later that afternoon was found unconscious in bed. An hour later he was confused and talked nonsense. In the evening he lost consciousness again and was admitted to the Radcliffe Infirmary at Oxford.

On examination he responded to painful stimulation but did not speak. There was a pyrexia of 100°F and some nasal discharge. Myoclonic twitching was observed around the mouth and in the limbs. The pupils were unresponsive to light and the right eye was deviated laterally. All limbs were flaccid with normal tendon reflexes but with bilateral extensor plantar responses.

The cerebrospinal fluid was under a pressure of 240 mm but showed normal constituents. The white blood count was normal. The EEG showed a generalised disturbance but no focal abnormalities.

The fever subsided next day but the level of consciousness fluctuated over the next 3 weeks. There were almost continuous involuntary movements of chewing, swallowing, yawning and writhing of the limbs. He was occasionally incontinent of urine. The pupils became unequally dilated, conjugate movements of the eyes were defective in vertical directions, and slight left facial weakness appeared.

Thereafter he slowly recovered and was discharged 2 months after the onset. He was still almost completely mute and apt to have crying spells, but within the next few weeks he was speaking normally and he returned to work a month or two later.

During the next 18 months he complained of undue sleepiness by day and was treated with dexamphetamine sulphate. In other respects he seemed to have recovered completely.

Subsequently, however, he committed a series of crimes, mainly of a violent and unpremeditated nature and with little attempt at concealment. Previously he had been of exemplary character. The legal proceedings which followed brought him under medical supervision some 4 years after the initial illness. He then described episodes lasting 15–20 minutes during which his eyes involuntarily turned upwards and to the right in a manner strongly suggestive of oculogyric crises. There was occasional titubation of the head, his facial expression was stiff and there was slight cogwheel rigidity of the upper limbs.

Espir and Spalding support their diagnosis of encephalitis lethargica by pointing out that such a picture is rarely produced by the many known types of present-day viral encephalitis. Ophthalmoplegia is rare with other varieties, and parkinsonism a distinctly uncommon complication. The prolonged sleep disturbance during convalescence was also typical.

Rail *et al.* (1981) reviewed eight further examples occurring during the preceding two decades, some presenting with prominent psychiatric features. Pathological examination of the brain in two patients showed extensive loss of neurones from the substantia nigra and locus caeruleus, along with widespread neurofibrillary changes elsewhere in the brain stem, dentate nuclei and corpus striatum. They stressed that the diagnosis still rested essentially on the clinical features, and suggested that the following criteria be applied: an encephalitic illness, parkinsonism developing acutely or after a delay of months or years, alteration in the sleep cycle, oculogyric crises which are not drug induced, ocular or pupillary changes, respiratory disturbances, involuntary movements, corticospinal tract signs and mental abnormalities. While these represent the specific features of encephalitis lethargica, it is clear that not all will be present in every case. More recently Johnson and Lucey (1987) have reported two suspected examples in young men, both presenting with severe catatonic stupor in the setting of depressive psychosis. One had a low-grade pyrexia and the other showed blepharospasm and complex compulsive rituals.

The debate concerning latter-day examples was extended by Hunter and Jones (1966), who argued that sporadic cases might be appearing in mild or attenuated form and with clinical pictures increasingly dominated by psychiatric manifestations. Consequently the neurological signs on which the diagnosis depends could readily be overshadowed. They reported six possible cases seen during a 3-month period in a psychiatric hospital. All had presented with psychiatric syndromes, and all had initially been seen at general hospitals where diagnoses of hypomania, depression and anxiety neurosis had been applied:

Two were admitted in a state of excitement and confusion, two after overdoses of sleeping pills, one in a catatonic state and one at his own request on account of feeling ill and 'nervous'. Most had a history of progressive personality change over the course of several months with irritability, emotionality, perplexed–paranoid developments and impaired memory and concentration. They complained of malaise, headache, lethargy, hypersomnia, insomnia, giddiness, blurred and double vision, and altered taste and smell. All had worsened in the week or two before admission, with increasing agitation and depression, paranoid and bizarre bodily delusions, and nocturnal excitement and hallucinosis.

On examination all showed some degree of mental confusion, three had mild pyrexia and all had some ocular abnormality — dilated or unequal pupils, absent accommodation reflexes, ptosis, nystagmus, or weakness of upward, downward or conjugate gaze. A variety of other neurological signs were present, often fluctuating from day to day. Four showed loss of associated arm movements on walking, indicative of early parkinsonism, and several showed tremor, sialorrhoea and typical vasomotor disturbances.

The authors suggested that the combination of cerebral, hypothalamic and midbrain involvement was strongly reminiscent of encephalitis lethargica, likewise the symptoms of lethargy, sleep disorder and visual disturbance, the rapid fluctuation of symptoms, the fugitive signs and the relapsing course.

It is extremely difficult to evaluate these examples, but Hunter and Jones made an important point in urging that encephalitic antecedents should more often be considered in the differential diagnosis of psychiatric patients. Hunter *et al.* (1969) pursued the question further by examining the cerebrospinal fluid in 256 patients admitted to a psychiatric unit. More than a quarter showed abnormalities, as defined by a total protein in excess of 60 mg/100 ml or a gamma globulin exceeding 10% of the total protein. More importantly, in a group subjected to serial lumbar punctures the cerebrospinal fluid showed a return to normality more often when the clinical condition improved than when it did not. The abnormal findings emerged in patients with affective, schizophrenic and paranoid syndromes. Among the younger patients there was sometimes evidence of extrapyramidal disturbances, and here at least the authors concluded that an encephalitic type of illness might have been responsible.

Finally, it is worth considering whether encephalitic processes may have contributed to the prevalence of 'catatonia' in earlier psychiatric practice Mahendra (1981) reviews the decline of 'catatonic schizophrenia' over the past 40 years, and suggests that many examples in the earlier literature may have owed much to a viral, and possibly an encephalitic, origin. Present-day catatonia, when it occurs, may be seen in association with an impressive range of physical conditions, ranging from brain lesions and infections to toxic and metabolic disorders (Gelenberg 1976). In the absence of clearly organic determinants it appears now to be associated with affective disorder very much more commonly than with schizophrenia (Abrams & Taylor 1976).

Herpes simplex encephalitis

Herpes simplex is regarded as one of the commonest single causes of severe sporadic encephalitis. It has been incriminated in up to 20% of cases in Britain and this may be an underestimate. The disease is severe with a high mortality, and shows certain special features including marked psychological disturbance both in the acute phase and as a major sequel.

The subject was controversial for many years since herpes simplex infection is very widely distributed with antibodies detectable in 80–90% of adults. It was also known that the virus could occasionally be cultured from random samples of cerebrospinal fluid. But the evidence that it truly caused encephalitis came from the finding of Cowdry type A inclusion bodies in the brains of affected persons, identical with those seen in cutaneous and visceral forms of the disease. Smith et al. (1941) were finally able to show a convincing association with acute encephalitis by isolating the virus from the brain of a case which showed this specific pathological feature.

It is now recognised that herpes simplex is responsible not only for cases of ordinary acute encephalitis, but also for many of the cases of 'acute inclusion body', 'acute necrotising' and 'haemorrhagic' encephalitis which had formerly been regarded as distinct entities (Drachman & Adams 1962). In acute necrotising encephalitis the characteristic inclusion bodies can sometimes be demonstrated in biopsy material from the brain, and the virus has been obtained on culture; inclusion bodies are not invariable, however, so the situation is not definite in all cases.

Pathology

Changes characteristic of other forms of encephalitis are seen—perivascular infiltration of lymphocytes and histiocytes in the cortex and adjacent white matter, proliferation of microglia and the formation of glial nodules. The cerebral cortex is mainly affected in adults, with less involvement of subcortical structures. A distinctive feature is the severity of the process. In areas of maximal involvement there is necrosis with softening, haemorrhage and loss of all nervous and glial elements. Such lesions tend to be asymmetrical between the hemispheres, and involve the medial temporal and orbital regions especially. They can be seen both grossly and

microscopically. Cowdry type A inclusion bodies are often detected in the neurones, astrocytes and oligodendrocytes, in the form of large eosinophilic intranuclear masses surrounded by a clear halo and displacing the nucleolus to the periphery (Drachman & Adams 1962; Kibrick & Gooding 1965). In biopsy material obtained early in the disease it may be possible to demonstrate herpes viral antigen by immunofluorescence or immunoperoxidase techniques, thus confirming the diagnosis (Booss & Esiri 1986).

Clinical features

The disease affects all age groups, occurring sporadically without seasonal incidence. It may be either a primary infection or a recrudescence of an established infection. Only a small proportion of patients give a history of recurrent herpes labialis (Leider et al. 1965; Gostling 1967).

Typically there is rapid onset with a severe illness in the acute stage. Pyrexia may be up to 39.5°C (103°F), fits are frequent in all age groups, meningeal irritation is common and drowsiness or global confusion are prominent. Focal neurological signs include reflex asymmetry, up-going plantar responses, cortical sensory loss and cogwheel rigidity in the limbs.

Sometimes the clinical picture can at first be misleading. In five of six cases reported by Drachman and Adams (1962) psychological symptoms were the most striking initial feature. At first these patients appeared only mildly unwell and it was aberrations of behaviour which called attention to the seriousness of the illness. One patient packed a case a week in advance of a short journey, one dressed at night to go to an imagined funeral, one failed to recognise his wife and another slept until four o'clock in the afternoon then suddenly rushed from the house without explanation.

Once the illness is declared a delirious phase is often prominent before the patient sinks into coma. Hallucinations can resemble those of delirium tremens in being vivid and colourful, and in provoking a marked emotional reaction. On recovery from coma behaviour disturbance may again be marked, with a phase of restless hyperactivity.

The prominence of psychiatric disturbance no doubt owes much to the characteristic accent of pathology on the temporal lobes and orbitofrontal structures. This may bring added focal symptoms such as anosmia, olfactory and gustatory hallucinations, or marked memory disturbance out of proportion to the impairment of intellect. Sometimes an area of focal necrosis becomes swollen to such a degree that the illness presents with features indicative of an acute intracranial mass, usually in the temporal lobe. This may be revealed by CT scan or angiography and lead to referral as a case of brain tumour or abscess (Adams & Jennett 1967; Potter 1969). Biopsy then reveals the changes characteristic of acute necrotising encephalitis.

Much more rarely cases present with aseptic meningitis and run a benign course (Leider *et al.* 1965; Olson *et al.* 1967). Very occasionally there may be recurrent episodes of organic psychosis, as in the interesting patient reported by Shearer and Finch (1964): a 9-year-old boy had 17 episodes in a 3-year period, lasting a little over a week at a time, and consisting of fever, headache, drowsiness, disorientation and grossly irrational behaviour. Each episode was accompanied by electroencephalographic abnormalities and an outbreak of herpes labialis.

Investigations

Examination of the cerebrospinal fluid should be carried out only if this is judged safe after performing a CT scan (Anderson 1993). Other infectious conditions can be excluded, and it may be possible to demonstrate intrathecal synthesis of antibody to the virus. The application of the polymerase chain reaction to detect viral DNA in the cerebrospinal fluid holds promise of yielding a definitive means for confirming the diagnosis. The EEG shows nonspecific slowing early on, with later localisation of periodic spike and slow wave activity to one or both temporal lobes (Kugler 1964; Smith *et al.* 1975). CT scanning can aid materially in excluding an abscess or tumour (Kaufman *et al.* 1979). The scan may be normal in the early stages, but later reveals characteristic low density areas in one or both temporal lobes, or evidence of mass effects along with contrast enhancement (Zimmerman *et al.* 1980). MRI is more sensitive in revealing early changes at a time when therapy is most likely to be useful. Currently brain biopsy is the only certain method for confirming the diagnosis. Type A inclusion bodies may be detected and the virus demonstrated in the tissue obtained. However, the procedure is not without risk and a negative result does not exclude the condition. Rising titres of antibodies in the blood may give supportive evidence, but can be useful only in retrospect.

Differential diagnosis

The disease is not infrequently puzzling. In addition to cases which present as possible tumours or abscesses, other conditions can be simulated. When pyrexia is low and neurological signs markedly asymmetrical, the picture may suggest subdural haematoma or head injury. Acute and fulminating examples may resemble meningi-

tis. The prominence of mental confusion with vivid hallucinations may lead to a diagnosis of delirium tremens, or an acute onset with drowsiness, confabulation and fits may suggest Wernicke's encephalopathy. The residual end-state can closely resemble Korsakoff's psychosis or raise the possibility of general paresis.

Treatment and outcome

Treatment is often a matter of urgency. Seizures should be controlled, and dexamethasone may be required to reduce cerebral oedema. The antiviral agent acyclovir has emerged as superior to vidarabine and other drugs employed in the past, and should be started as soon as possible (Sköldenberg *et al.* 1984; Whitley *et al.* 1986). Decompression of the brain is a useful adjunct in appropriate cases.

The outcome depends on the speed with which treatment is initiated. Before the advent of acyclovir approximately 70% of patients died and half of the survivors were left with sequelae which could be severe (Illis & Merry 1972). With acyclovir the prognosis has improved considerably, but when the temporal lobes have been damaged severely the consequences can still be grave. Mental retardation can ensue in children, or dementia in adults. Seizures, dysphasia, personality change and severe amnesic states have also been described (Oxbury & Mac-Callum 1973). Hierons *et al.* (1978) reported pictures ranging from relatively pure amnesic syndromes to severe dementia, often accompanied by bizarre behaviour reminiscent of the Klüver Bucy syndrome. The patients reported by Rose and Symonds (1960), in whom encephalitis was followed by a Korsakoff-like syndrome, were probably examples of herpes simplex encephalitis.

Even among patients who apparently make excellent recoveries after treatment with acyclovir, neuropsychological testing may reveal evidence of cognitive deficits. Gordon *et al.* (1990) followed four such patients for several years, and all showed deficits on language and memory tests. Some showed additional impairments in calculation, visuoconstructive ability and facial recognition, and none were able to function at their prior level of achievement. Such results underline the importance of careful follow-up evaluation and counselling in patients who have had the disease.

Herpes simplex infection and other psychiatric conditions

The predilection of the herpes virus for the temporolimbic areas has suggested that covert brain infection may be important in relation to certain psychiatric disorders.

Cleobury *et al.* (1971) found neutralising antibodies to herpes simplex type 1 more commonly in a group of aggressive psychopaths than in non-aggressive psychiatric patients or healthy controls. Titres to herpes type 2 and other viruses were within the normal range. They suggested that infection in childhood, unapparent or unrecognised at the time, may have damaged the temporal lobes and interfered with personality development.

Evidence of infection, from complement fixation and neutralising antibody titres, has been found to be common in psychiatric patients, particularly those with major depression (Rimon & Halonen 1969; Halonen *et al.* 1974). Here it could be relevant that disturbance of monoamine metabolism has been demonstrated after intracerebral infection with herpes simplex in animals. Lycke *et al.* (1974) have demonstrated an increased prevalence of infection with both herpes simplex and cytomegalovirus in patients with major depression when compared with other diagnostic groups and normal controls.

Type B herpes simplex encephalitis

The monkey form of herpes simplex produces an almost invariably fatal disease in humans, and is a hazard to workers in animal laboratories. It is transmitted by the bite of an infected monkey. A vesicle is produced at the site of entry, and along with encephalitis of severe degree there is often an ascending paraplegia. Widespread necrotic lesions are found in other organs as well as the brain.

Other sporadic viral encephalitides

In a great number of cases of sporadic encephalitis the cause is never identified, and the yield even with extensive virological studies remains rather low. The following known varieties are all relatively infrequent.

Mumps encephalitis

It appears that the mumps virus affects the nervous system more commonly than was previously supposed, even in the absence of parotitis or other typical evidence of the disease. This is probably the only common childhood infectious disease in which the virus itself can invade the central nervous system. The usual picture is an aseptic meningitis (p. 365), though an encephalitic illness is occasionally seen. When it occurs there is usually some degree of coincident meningitis and sometimes myelitis.

Symptoms appear some 2–10 days after the onset of parotitis, but can precede it or occur without any overt evidence of mumps elsewhere in the body. Meningeal symptoms are usually prominent with headache, vomiting, fever, neck stiffness and irritability. Drowsiness and delirium occur, sometimes with cranial nerve palsies, ataxia or pareses in the limbs. Fits are uncommon. In the acute myelitic form there is profound paresis and sensory changes in the limbs. The varied psychiatric and neurological pictures that may be seen are reviewed by Keddie (1965).

The cerebrospinal fluid shows a moderate pleocytosis, usually of mononuclears, from the outset. Serological tests are useful if a rise in titre of complement fixation or haemagglutination-inhibition antibodies can be demonstrated during convalescence. Permanent sequelae are common enough to suggest that the prognosis should be guarded (Lees 1970; Johnstone *et al.* 1972).

Infectious mononucleosis

The neurological complications of infectious mononucleosis occasionally include an encephalitic picture. This may be due to direct viral invasion of the nervous system, but sometimes it appears to represent an allergic encephalomyelitis similar to that following the acute exanthemata (p. 360). A benign lymphocytic meningitis (p. 365) can also occur.

Headache and meningism are frequently encountered in glandular fever, suggesting that minor involvement of the nervous system may be not uncommon (Gautier-Smith 1965). Diffuse electroencephalographic abnormalities have been reported in up to 30% of cases. Frank neurological complications are, however, rare. Gautier-Smith (1965) and Boughton (1970) have described patients with acute confusion progressing to stupor or coma, usually setting in abruptly within 5–9 days of the illness. Other cases present with seizures or focal cerebral disturbances such as hemiplegia. Syndromes of brain stem, cerebellar or cord dysfunction may also be seen. The cerebrospinal fluid shows a moderate rise of cells and protein. Complete recovery appears to be the rule.

Of considerable interest are patients who develop acute psychiatric disturbances in clear consciousness during the course of glandular fever. Raymond and Williams (1948) described a patient who became acutely psychotic within a few days of onset, settling over 3 weeks as the illness improved. Klaber and Lacey (1968) reported five of 76 cases presenting with severe psychiatric disorder during the course of an epidemic, only subsequently being diagnosed as suffering from glandular fever. Two showed pictures of acute schizophrenia and three acute depression. Here it seems likely that the patients were responding to the non-specific stress of the physical illness rather than to direct nervous system involvement.

A depressive aftermath has also been widely recognised, very occasional patients showing depression of psychotic intensity (White & Lewis 1987). Careful prospective studies by White *et al.* (1995a, 1995b) have shown that a fatigue syndrome similar phenomenologically to that described on p. 370 *et seq.* may develop in the 6 months following glandular fever, and that to a large extent it could be differentiated from depression. Whereas social adversity correlated significantly with the development of depression this had little association with the development of a fatigue syndrome or delayed physical recovery (Bruce-Jones *et al.* 1994).

An investigation by Hamblin *et al.* (1983) could be relevant in pointing to immunological dysfunction. Seventeen patients complaining of lethargy and inability to get back to work for a year or more after the illness were compared with a group making a full recovery. The ratio of T-helper to T-suppressor cells in the blood was significantly lower in the former than the latter, and lower than in controls who had not had the disease. Two patients were followed for several months, and the ratios rose as their complaints resolved. It is conceivable that long-lasting immunological abnormalities of this nature could serve in large measure to precipitate and maintain fatigue and/or depression during the convalescent period.

Herpes zoster encephalitis

Some degree of meningeal reaction is common in herpes zoster, with elevation of the protein and an excess of mononuclears in the cerebrospinal fluid. Features of meningitis are observed very occasionally and encephalitis more rarely still. Hall (1963) has reported a clear example of encephalitis following ophthalmic zoster and resulting in a chronic amnesic syndrome.

Adenoviruses

Adenovirus infections are discussed by Booss and Esiri (1986). The several varieties are associated with acute respiratory infections, conjunctivitis and pharyngitis. Adenovirus type 7 may lead to encephalitis in children with respiratory disease, sometimes in the form of small outbreaks.

Infectious hepatitis

Encephalitic or meningitic complications may accompany infectious hepatitis, sometimes antedating the onset of jaundice. Headache, photophobia, neck stiffness and

pyrexia progress to typical severe encephalitic manifestations. The condition must be distinguished from the encephalitis occasionally seen with leptospirosis (Weil's disease).

Rabies

Rabies is transmitted by infected animal saliva from dogs, bats or wolves. There is a long and variable incubation period, commonly 1–2 months, but with a wide latitude extending sometimes up to a year. The onset is then sudden, with a pyrexial illness, excitement, hydrophobia and violent muscular spasms involving the oesophagus and respiratory muscles. Crises are characterised by intense fury or profound terror, and in the intervals between the mind is clear. An ascending paralysis may occur. Death occurs during paroxysms, or in coma if the patient survives sufficiently long.

Rabies must be distinguished from tetanus and from hysteria when a patient has been bitten by a supposedly rabid dog. In hysteria true pharyngeal spasm does not occur, and the mental disturbance is amenable to sedatives and suggestion.

Influenza encephalitis

It appears that the influenza virus itself may be responsible for occasional cases of encephalitis. Small groups of cases have been reported during influenza outbreaks in many parts of the world, including the large epidemic of 'Asian' influenza which affected the British Isles in 1957–58 (Dubowitz 1958; McConkey & Daws 1958).

A variety of pictures is seen, some setting in at the height of the upper respiratory tract infection, others beginning towards the end of the attack, and others following some days later after a brief afebrile episode. The usual picture is of headache, vomiting, delirium and coma, with transient reflex abnormalities or weakness of the limbs. The cerebrospinal fluid may be normal or show a slight pleocytosis. The EEG is often diffusely abnormal. The illness usually resolves after several days and excellent recovery is said to be the rule.

In other varieties the patient shows no more than a period of mental confusion and headache, accompanied by electroencephalographic abnormalities and succeeded by complete amnesia for the episode (Bental 1958). Cases have been reported from Barbados with an unusual hallucinatory syndrome in which bizarre smells were experienced (Lloyd-Still 1958). Other forms include spinal and radicular syndromes, transverse myelopathy and ascending motor and sensory disturbances of the Guillain–Barré type (Flewett & Hoult 1958; Wells 1971a).

The nature of the causal relationship between these illnesses and the influenza virus remains uncertain. They are rare, even during extensive epidemics, and it is hard to exclude the possibility of coincident infection with another sporadic virus. Dunbar *et al.* (1958) estimated that their cases represented only one in 10 000 of the persons affected by the influenza epidemic in the area. Other possibilities are the activation of some associated neurotropic virus or the occasional development by mutation of a neurotropic strain of influenza virus. Kapila *et al.* (1958) were able to isolate influenza A virus from the brain substance of one fatal case, but such reports are few. Examples which occur at the height of an attack may sometimes be merely attributable to the cerebral anoxia and metabolic derangements consequent upon pneumonia. However, the evidence increasingly favours the view that the great majority represent an autoimmune or hypersensitivity response on the part of the brain, similar to that which occurs after other infective illnesses (see below), and precipitated by the presence of virus in the body but not necessarily within the brain (British Medical Journal 1971). The pathology in fatal cases often supports this view by showing perivascular demyelination similar to that of postinfectious encephalitis generally.

The broader question arises of the relationship between influenza and other psychiatric disturbances that follow it. Depression appears to be common and may sometimes be unusually refractory to treatment; this has been ascribed to invasion of the brain by the influenza virus but there is no direct evidence to support the view (British Medical Journal 1971). Hysterical reactions may also be seen, and are usually ascribed to the non-specific stress of the illness and the physically weakening effects of its aftermath.

Steinberg *et al.* (1972) re-opened this question by presenting a case which suggested a more direct pathophysiological relationship between the infection and a manic psychosis that followed:

The illness, in a woman of 21, began with a typical attack of influenza. After a brief remission she again became febrile, with headache, sore throat and an unproductive cough. She complained of paraesthesiae in the limbs and experienced a transient episode of blindness lasting for less than a minute. Over the next 2 weeks a typical manic illness developed, with evidence of confusion and disorientation during the first few days. The affective disturbance gradually subsided with treatment over the next few months.

Antibody titres to influenza A were abnormally high at the onset of the psychosis, and showed an unusually slow decline in comparison with other influenza patients while the manic illness was resolving.

Despite normal findings in the cerebrospinal fluid and EEG the authors postulated that a mild attack of influenza encephalitis had probably occurred, producing minimal brain damage which acted as an intervening factor and contributed to the subsequent affective disorder.

The evidence is clearly tenuous, but combined virological and psychiatric studies on a larger number of patients might illuminate the relationship further as Steinberg *et al.* suggest.

Other para-infectious encephalitides

The forms of encephalitis that occasionally follow the acute exanthemata account for a large proportion of the cases seen in childhood. The chief causes are measles, rubella, pertussis, chickenpox and scarlet fever, though similar developments may be seen after viral pneumonias and infectious mononucleosis. In Kennard and Swash's (1981) series the predominant antecedent was an upper respiratory tract infection of influenzal type. All share a common pathology and possibly a common pathogenesis. Closely similar illnesses may follow vaccination against smallpox or injections of serum, or sometimes they arise for no apparent reason. The brain may be involved alone or there may be more widespread affection throughout the neuraxis with brain stem or cord involvement. In such cases the term 'acute disseminated encephalomyelitis' is usually employed.

The pathological changes differ from those of the virus infections already described in certain definite respects, though some degree of overlap can be seen. The brain and cord show congestion, often with petechial haemorrhages. But the most striking changes are seen in the white matter, with discrete areas of acute perivenous demyelination, mononuclear perivascular infiltration and neuroglial proliferation. Similar though less severe changes may occur in the grey matter as well. There is no evidence of a direct attack upon the nerve cells themselves, and the cortical neurones are characteristically spared completely unless there has been a complicating factor such as hypoxia (Booss & Esiri 1986). In 'acute haemorrhagic leucoencephalitis' the changes are particularly severely developed, along with brain congestion and swelling and foci of perivascular necrosis.

The exact pathogenesis is unknown, but there is little to suggest direct invasion of the central nervous system by the viruses concerned. Allergic or autoimmune mechanisms are generally held to be the cause. The picture closely resembles that of experimental allergic encephalomyelitis, produced in animals by injection of brain tissue together with certain adjuvants, and a response may be seen to treatment with adrenocorticotrophic hormone or steroids.

The clinical picture consists of headache, drowsiness, photophobia and irritability, setting in some 3–14 days after the onset of the specific illness but with a wide latitude of timing. There is commonly an interval of normal health between the acute viral illness and the encephalopathic development. Convulsions are common and meningism is often prominent. Cranial nerve palsies may appear, or myoclonic and choreiform movements may be seen. Loss of abdominal reflexes and extensor plantar responses are usual findings. The brain stem may be principally involved with vertigo, vomiting, nystagmus and dysarthria, or in myelitic forms there may be paraparesis with retention of urine. Peripheral nerve involvement is common. The form which follows chickenpox is said to be characterised by ataxia.

The cerebrospinal fluid may be normal, but is often under increased pressure with a mild lymphocytic pleocytosis and a moderate elevation of protein. When infectious mononucleosis is the cause a high protein and the absence of cells are characteristic. CT or MRI may show multiple white matter abnormalities similar to those of multiple sclerosis, or more extensive symmetrical changes in the cerebral and cerebellar white matter and basal ganglia (Kesselring *et al.* 1990). Serial MRI can be useful in contributing to the distinction from multiple sclerosis in uncertain cases. Textbooks of neurology should be consulted for further details of the pictures seen with different infections.

If the patient does not succumb during the first week or two a remarkably complete recovery may be seen. The mortality is much higher in infants than in older children or adults. In some survivors there may be severe neurological sequelae with hemiparesis, paraparesis, epilepsy and impairment of intellect. In children behaviour disorders similar to those that follow encephalitis lethargica may occur.

Subacute and chronic encephalitis
(Dawson's subacute inclusion body encephalitis,
van Bogaert's subacute sclerosing leucoencephalitis,
subacute sclerosing panencephalitis)

Certain rare diseases, referred to by the above labels, have long been suspected on pathological grounds to represent subacute infection within the brain. Modern virological techniques now show that the measles virus is responsible. They commonly present with features of dementia, and it is in this context that problems of differential diagnosis usually arise. Sometimes, however, the possibility of other psychiatric illness is raised in the early stages.

Until fairly recently such illnesses were regarded as uniformly fatal, with a progressive course lasting several weeks or months, but occasional cases have now been reported with arrest or even improvement over long periods of time. The likelihood that mild and relatively benign examples may occur has accordingly brought new interest to the subject.

Cases were first described by Dawson in 1933 (subacute inclusion body encephalitis), by van Bogaert in 1945 (subacute sclerosing leucoencephalitis) and by Brain *et al.* in 1943 and 1948. These now appear to be essentially variants of the same disease process (Adams 1976). Dawson's cases occurred in infants and young children, and derived their name from the intranuclear inclusions which were seen in affected neurones. Van Bogaert's cases occurred in children and young adults but showed more evident sclerotic lesions in the white matter. However, it is now generally accepted that a sharp line of demarcation cannot be drawn; great variation occurs in the incidence of pathological changes in grey or white matter, and inclusion bodies have been reported in van Bogaert's as well as in Dawson's varieties of the disease. *Subacute sclerosing panencephalitis* (SSPE) is the term now generally used to refer to these diseases.

Pathology

Adams (1976) described the typical pathological picture. The brain may be normal macroscopically, or firm and shrunken with areas of focal necrosis. Microscopy shows evidence of subacute inflammation, usually in both the grey and the white matter. There is perivascular infiltration with lymphocytes and plasma cells, and proliferation of astrocytes and microglia. Slight meningeal infiltration may also occur. The white matter lesions are of particular interest in that they are closely similar to those seen in para-infectious encephalomyelitis and HIV-associated dementia (Poser 1990). In the grey matter neuronal degeneration is apparent, often with characteristic intranuclear inclusions, and in the white matter areas of demyelination are seen with fibrous gliosis. Considerable variation is met with from case to case, but the more rapidly progressive cases are more prone to show intranuclear inclusions and the more chronic cases greater demyelination and sclerosis of the white matter.

The typical 'type A' intranuclear inclusions are strongly acidophilic homogeneous bodies with a sharp outline, separated from the nuclear membrane by a clear halo. They are the feature which originally suggested a viral aetiology, and are similar to those which occur in herpes simplex encephalitis (p. 356). In severely degenerated cells the inclusions may fill the nucleus so that the surrounding cytoplasm is reduced to a vestige. Sometimes they are found in the cytoplasm itself, or in glial cells as well as neurones. Such changes may be focal in distribution, affecting particularly the parieto-occipital and temporal lobes or the hippocampus and subcortical nuclei. Inclusions have also been reported in the brain stem nuclei, especially the nuclei pontis, and in rare cases in the cells of the spinal cord. In some entirely typical cases they may be very hard to detect; a negative result from biopsy material must therefore be interpreted with caution since inclusion bodies can be found in the same case at autopsy very shortly afterwards (Kennedy 1968).

Evidence has accumulated to suggest that the measles paramyxovirus is responsible. Almost all patients have a history of measles, usually at an early age, or of measles immunisation. Very high antibody titres to the virus are found in the serum and cerebrospinal fluid, and specific immunofluorescence with measles antibody has been demonstrated in brain biopsy material (Connolly *et al.* 1967; Legg 1967). Electron microscopy has shown particles indistinguishable from paramyxovirus budding from cytoplasmic inclusions, and measles virus has been isolated from brain cell tissue cultures derived from patients with the disease (Horta-Barbosa *et al.* 1969). Finally, the disease has been transmitted to animals by intracerebral inoculation of brain tissue from patients with the disorder (Lehrich *et al.* 1970).

It remains unclear why such an illness should develop in a minute proportion of those who have suffered a primary measles infection. The virus probably gains access to the brain at the time of initial infection and develops into a less invasive and more persistent form which evades immune destruction (Anderson 1993). The original infection may have been with an unusual strain of virus. At some stage the latent infection then triggers an immune-mediated response which results in the widespread pathological changes in the brain. Possibilities of reactivation by subsequent infection, even by a different organism, have not been discounted.

Clinical features

The great majority of cases occur in children or adolescents, though occasional examples have been reported in middle age (Brierley *et al.* 1960; Himmelhoch *et al.* 1970) and are probably to be regarded as variants of the disease.

Classic examples present with insidious deterioration of intellect, such that the child begins to fail at school, becomes forgetful and inattentive, slowed and slovenly. Other early symptoms are nocturnal delirium with hallucinations, marked lethargy and difficult uncontrollable behaviour. The prodromal manifestations may occasionally occur alone for a period of several months, but neurological abnormalities generally develop early. Char-

acteristically the patient develops marked involuntary movements, including myoclonic jerks of the face, fingers and limbs, athetosis or rapid torsion spasms of the trunk which lead to sudden stumbles and falls. Myoclonia may be regularly periodic, occurring at fixed intervals of 5–10 seconds for hours or days at a time. The limbs develop bilateral extrapyramidal rigidity or progressive spasticity. Epileptic fits are common, and aphasia, apraxia or akinetic mutism may appear. A low-grade pyrexia may accompany the prodromal or later stages of the disorder, but this is not invariable.

Atypical presentations sometimes raise the possibility of non-organic psychiatric illness in the early stages. Koehler and Jakumeit (1976), for example, reported a woman of 20 who presented with an apparently hysterical blindness and gave Ganser responses of a classic nature. She showed a profound lack of initiative and spent much of the time asleep. Within a week of admission, however, the true disease was declared. In the 21-year-old patient described by Salib (1988), who presented with dysmorphophobic features, the diagnosis was delayed for several months and schizophrenia was suspected initially.

The EEG often shows highly characteristic features, though many variants occur. Typically there are high voltage slow wave complexes, synchronous in all leads, and occurring at fixed intervals of 5–10 seconds along with the myoclonic jerks. They may also appear in the absence of motor abnormalities and can sometimes be focal in the frontal or occipital regions. The cerebrospinal fluid may show a slight increase of cells, but the total protein is often normal. A feature of diagnostic importance is that the majority of cases show a raised immunoglobulin G in the cerebrospinal fluid and a paretic curve on Lange's colloidal gold test. The complement fixation titres for measles are high in the serum and the cerebrospinal fluid. CT or MRI may show white matter abnormalities and later atrophy of the cerebrum, cerebellum and brain stem (Jayakumar *et al.* 1988).

The first descriptions stressed that the disease had a hopeless prognosis, with rapidly progressive dementia over 6 weeks to 6 months and death after a period of coma and decerebrate rigidity. However, cases have since been reported with temporary arrest for months or even years in the middle stage of the disorder, and a very few have been described with partial recovery. Of Kennedy's (1968) five cases in children, two achieved remission and one returned to school after regaining much coherent speech and a diminution of myoclonic jerks. Resnick *et al.* (1968) followed a patient for 5 years who showed considerable sustained improvement despite the continued elevation of measles antibody in the serum and cerebrospinal fluid. Cobb and Morgan-Hughes (1968) mention other scattered examples in the literature and suggest that the following patient may have had the disease in a mild form:

A 21-year-old chemistry student was admitted with a 5-month history of falling attacks, momentary blank spells and recent difficulty with concentration. Neurological examination was normal apart from brisk reflexes, the EEG showed persistent slow waves in the left occipitotemporal region, and the cerebrospinal fluid showed a paretic Lange curve. He was readmitted 8 months later with impairment of memory and difficulty with reading, writing and calculation, which had come on over the preceding 2 months. He showed a severe global dementia with loss of recent memory, disorientation in time, agraphia, acalculia and profound constructional apraxia. The Wechsler Adult Intelligence Scale (WAIS) showed a verbal IQ of 79 and a performance IQ of less than 35. Affect was flattened and inappropriate. Neurological examination was still negative, but the EEG showed bilateral recurrent monophasic and biphasic slow wave complexes. A ventriculogram was normal, but right frontal biopsy showed changes consistent with subacute encephalitis of the Dawson or van Bogaert type. Inclusion bodies were not seen.

He was treated with prednisone in addition to anticonvulsants and slowly improved. By the following year he was working, though he had been dismissed from several jobs on account of general slowness and difficulty with reading and writing. Seven years later he was working as a gardener and had recently married. He was still mildly dysgraphic, with reading difficulties and profound constructional apraxia, but he was orientated in time and place and able to do simple calculations. Psychological testing showed a verbal IQ of 82 and a performance IQ of 40.

Risk *et al.* (1978) estimated that improvement could be expected in about 5% of cases, even after severe illnesses. Relapse may subsequently occur, however, after remissions lasting for several years. Their experience with 118 patients showed substantial long-term improvement in six. Two of these were still improving 4–5 years later, two were stable 4–6 years later, and two relapsed after 8 and 11 years, respectively. Remittent cases tended to have shown milder variants of the disease and to have been somewhat older than usual at onset.

Progressive rubella panencephalitis

A variant of subacute sclerosing panencephalitis has been described in which the rubella rather than the measles virus appears to be responsible (Townsend *et al.* 1975, 1976; Weil *et al.* 1975). This sets in, usually during the second decade, in children who have been affected by rubella *in utero*. Mental and motor deterioration develop as with subacute sclerosing panencephalitis, and the pathological changes in the brain are similar. The serum and cerebrospinal fluid show elevated titres of antibodies to the rubella virus and normal titres to measles. The

rubella virus has been isolated from the brain in such cases.

Other varieties of subacute encephalitis

Himmelhoch *et al.* (1970) reported an interesting group of eight cases, mostly in adults, some apparently representing variants of subacute sclerosing panencephalitis. Symptoms characteristic of functional psychiatric disorder were prominent in all, and seven had originally been diagnosed as suffering from depression, schizophrenia or hysteria.

In some the onset was acute, with sudden withdrawal and seclusiveness following a period of coryza, malaise and headache. Retardation was prominent and a psychogenic reaction was usually diagnosed at this stage. The patients then quickly developed disorientation and visual hallucinations and showed intellectual deterioration. In others the development was more protracted, with irritability, depression, phobias and ruminations over a period of several months. They then became mute and retarded and showed progressive intellectual impairment.

The bizarreness of behaviour had strongly biased the initial diagnoses, and neurological signs had often been ignored even when they were noted. Evidence of mild confusion, disorientation or visual hallucinations had sometimes been disregarded, changes of sleep and appetite had been ascribed to depression, and fugue-like states to catatonia or hysteria.

Characteristically there were rapid fluctuations, with impaired awareness and disorientation one day followed by complete lucidity the next. Periods of aggressiveness and sexual provocativeness were often followed by profuse apology, and the patients seemed bewildered by their behaviour. Bizarre behaviour became increasingly frequent as time went on. It was markedly unresponsive to pharmacotherapy. Hallucinations were mainly visual but occurred in other modalities, and clear-cut paranoid delusions were common. At times an isolated episode was hard to distinguish from schizophrenia.

There were no consistently helpful laboratory findings, but all patients showed abnormal electroencephalographic changes at some point in the disease. Some died within several weeks or months, some ran a protracted course with remissions, but three recovered to premorbid levels of intellectual functioning:

A housewife of 38 became deluded after a period of fever, coryza and headache. She was committed to hospital with a diagnosis of paranoid schizophrenia. She alternated between a delusional state, when she was boisterous, abusive and combative, and periods of complete lucidity. Neurological examination revealed nothing abnormal, and her behaviour was unresponsive to phenothiazines or electroconvulsive therapy. Her later course was stormy, with grand mal seizures and periods of coma. She required tracheostomy and intragastric feeding. Lumbar puncture and air encephalography revealed no abnormalities, and the EEG showed episodic synchronous high voltage slow waves alternating with periods of relative electrical suppression. Biopsy of the right temporal lobe showed the features of encephalitis but no inclusion bodies were found.

Over the next 3 months the patient made a partial recovery, but 6 months later she still had severe impairment of memory, with disorientation for time and place and occasional nocturnal seizures. Five years later her memory deficit had cleared markedly, but the seizures continued and she had developed progressive paraplegia. The measles antibody titre remained elevated in the serum.

A 35-year-old woman graduate with a stable previous history became abruptly combative, confused and 'animalistic'. The EEG was diffusely slowed, and the cerebrospinal fluid showed a mild pleocytosis. She became unkempt, cachectic and totally uncommunicative, and showed aggressive and sexually provocative behaviour. She was incontinent of urine and faeces and required tube feeding. Even so she had intermittent periods of complete lucidity.

One month later she began to improve, with lessening of memory deficit and improvement of intellectual functions. At the same time, however, her behaviour became increasingly difficult to control. She refused to attend group meetings, with biting, kicking or pulling up her dress when she was urged to attend. With her family she behaved rather better and ultimately she was discharged. Two further admissions were required in the next few months on account of disturbed behaviour, but thereafter she unexpectedly began to improve. At first she had to carry a note book to help with her memory, but after 18 months this became unnecessary. After 2 years she had recovered completely and continued to function normally.

(Himmelhoch *et al.* 1970)

Himmelhoch *et al.* suggested that the marked behavioural disturbance in their patients was probably due to an accent of the pathological process on the temporal lobes and limbic structures. Since three out of eight recovered they suggest that other examples of subacute encephalitis may be commoner than is realised, especially when the process is mild and the patient is referred for psychiatric treatment on account of disturbed behaviour. The measles antibody titre might give helpful information in suspected cases.

Brierley *et al.* (1960) reported another group of three patients, all with onset in the fifties and all of whom were diagnostic problems during life. One had been regarded as having presenile dementia, but in the others a low-grade pyrexia early in the illness had raised the possibility of a viral encephalitis. One presented as a severe depressive illness coloured by bizarre behaviour and later developed minor epileptic attacks, another began with depression following a respiratory infection, and the third began with

pains in the shoulders and arms then progressed to tiredness and depression over the course of several weeks. All developed progressive dementia and died in coma several months thereafter. Myoclonic jerks and other motor features characteristic of subacute sclerosing panencephalitis were not seen, but at postmortem all showed severe encephalitic changes concentrated to a notable degree on the medial temporal lobe structures. Inclusion bodies were not present.

Corsellis (1969a) notes that one of these cases suffered from bronchial carcinoma, though a causal connection was not suspected at the time. He adds three further cases of bronchial carcinoma with similar pathological changes in the limbic areas, all of whom had shown marked abnormalities of affect and striking disturbance of memory during life. Whether the process should be regarded as inflammatory or degenerative in these latter cases remains uncertain. The problem is discussed further in Chapter 15, pp. 743–4.

Differential diagnosis

Subacute encephalitis clearly gives rise to diagnostic confusion during life. It is a rare condition, so that the clinician is unlikely to see more than the very occasional case. Many examples are likely to be missed completely, especially when postmortem examination is lacking or on the rare occasions when spontaneous recovery occurs.

Difficulties with diagnosis are especially likely to arise in the prodromal period. In children the picture may suggest behaviour disorder or autism, and in adults other psychiatric disorder may be simulated as described above. Careful attention must be directed towards minor neurological abnormalities, sudden involuntary jerks, evidence of nocturnal delirium or intermittent low-grade pyrexia.

Presenile dementia is probably the commonest misdiagnosis in the later stages in adults. Disseminated sclerosis may be suggested by the combination of early neurological disability with a paretic Lange curve and negative reactions for syphilis in the cerebrospinal fluid. Herpes simplex encephalitis can show identical inclusion bodies in biopsy material, but the course is acute, and progressive dementia and myoclonic jerking are not seen.

Classic examples of subacute sclerosing panencephalitis usually declare themselves eventually when involuntary movements and typical electroencephalographic features appear. It now seems, however, that these developments are not inevitable. A paretic Lange curve in the cerebrospinal fluid should alert one to the possibility of the disorder, and a greatly elevated titre of measles antibody may be discovered in the serum and the cerebrospinal fluid. Brain biopsy can be crucial in demonstrating characteristic changes, though intranuclear inclusions will frequently be missed. Such investigations are often worth pursuing in view of the possibilities of treatment with corticotrophin or steroids.

Meningitis

Meningeal infection is less liable to lead to diagnostic problems than encephalitis. In most varieties pyrexia and neck stiffness are soon in evidence, headache is marked and lumbar puncture rapidly confirms the diagnosis. Tuberculous meningitis is the important exception, sometimes presenting with insidious and ill-defined mental changes as described below. Enduring sequelae are also less common after meningitis than encephalitis provided full and effective treatment has been instituted early.

Three varieties will be discussed—pyogenic meningitis, aseptic meningitis and tuberculous meningitis.

Pyogenic meningitis

The principal organisms responsible are the meningococcus, *Pneumococcus*, *Streptococcus*, *Staphylococcus*, *Haemophilus influenzae* and *Escherichia coli*. Among adults the meningococcus accounts for about three-quarters of cases and the *Pneumococcus* for most of the remainder (Grinker & Sahs 1966).

Headache is usually the presenting feature, with pyrexia and rapidly increasing evidence of general ill health. Vomiting, photophobia and irritability are common from an early stage. Fits are frequent in children but rare in adults. Mental disturbance takes the form of an acute organic reaction, with drowsiness extending to coma and sometimes hallucinations, excitement and other features of delirium. Neck stiffness and a positive Kernig's sign are important confirmatory features. Pupillary abnormalities and oculomotor palsies are common, slight incoordination or tremor may appear in the limbs and the tendon reflexes are sluggish. The plantar reflexes are sometimes up-going.

The cerebrospinal fluid is under increased pressure and is often cloudy or frankly purulent. Polymorphonuclear cells may number thousands per cubic millimetre, the protein is raised and Lange's colloidal gold curve is 'meningitic' with a peak in the mid-zone or to the right. The chloride content is slightly reduced and the sugar content greatly diminished or even abolished. The causative organisms may be cultured or demonstrated on films.

Formerly the mortality rate was high and neurological complications were seen in a large proportion of survivors —hydrocephalus, spastic paralysis, mental defect, blindness, deafness and epilepsy. Pneumococcal meningitis carried an especially poor prognosis. Change of personality was also reported in children with moroseness, irritability or moral deterioration similar to that seen after encephalitis lethargica (Pai 1945). Nowadays, however, complete recovery is the rule, provided the diagnosis has been promptly made and the causative organism has not proved resistant to antibiotics. Meningococcal meningitis in particular proves to have a good outcome in the great majority of cases, despite the severity of the illness which may be seen in the acute stage.

Nevertheless, Berg (1962) found that meningitis still accounted for 22 of 800 consecutive admissions of severely retarded children to the Fountain Hospital between 1949 and 1960 (2.8%). Half of these had had tuberculous meningitis and half purulent meningitis. All had received antibiotics and up-to-date management of the acute illness, but in many the diagnosis had been delayed. Altogether meningitis was second only to mongolism as an identifiable cause of severe mental defect, exceeding in frequency such syndromes as rhesus incompatibility and phenylketonuria.

In adults mild but prolonged depression is common during convalescence, no doubt partly as a reaction to the stress of the illness. A period of fatigue and inefficiency may precede full recovery, and loss of libido may last for several months. Pai (1945) investigated 51 adults after meningococcal meningitis, all of whom were seen in a neuropsychiatric unit. Sulphonamides had been used in the treatment of some but not all cases. Psychogenic reactions outnumbered syndromes of organic defect. Sixteen patients showed intellectual deterioration or organic change of personality, and these were the ones who had had severe meningitis with marked delirium. In the other 35 patients psychogenic factors seemed to predominate. Disorders of gait and hysterical paresis had often set in after complete recovery and could be related to external stress. Depression was almost universal. Evidence of premorbid instability could often be discerned, but not in every case. Four patients had developed obsessional disorders for the first time. Other symptoms such as headache, blackouts and temporary loss of memory were occasionally hard to apportion to psychogenic or physiogenic causes.

Aseptic meningitis (acute benign lymphocytic meningitis)

Aseptic meningitis is mainly due to viral infection. The echoviruses are most frequently incriminated, or the mumps virus even in the absence of obvious parotitis (Grist 1967). Other viruses include the Coxsackie group, the virus of acute lymphocytic choriomeningitis, infectious mononucleosis, preparalytic poliomyelitis and psittacosis. HIV infection must also be borne in mind (p. 327). Investigation of the precise cause is often inconclusive. Non-viral causes must also be considered, including the early stages of tuberculous meningitis, brain abscess, cerebral syphilis, leptospirosis and incompletely treated pyogenic meningitis.

Cases occur in small epidemics and also arise sporadically. Epidemics are commoner in the summer and autumn when the circulation of enteroviruses among the population reaches a peak. The onset is abrupt with symptoms similar to those of pyogenic meningitis, but most illnesses are mild, running a course of 2–10 days then subsiding spontaneously. General malaise may persist for several weeks thereafter. Occasionally the meningitic symptoms and the cerebrospinal fluid abnormalities persist much longer and tuberculous meningitis may then be diagnosed in error.

The cerebrospinal fluid is under increased pressure and contains 50–1000 cells/mm³ of which most are lymphocytes. The protein is elevated but the chloride and sugar content are usually normal.

Enduring sequelae are distinctly rare, except for the paralysis which follows poliomyelitis and some infections with the Coxsackie type A7 virus. Minor temporary debilities, on the other hand, are fairly common during convalescence. Muller et al. (1958) carried out a long-term follow-up of a large group of cases of aseptic meningitis and 'meningoencephalitis of unknown cause', and compared them with controls from the normal population. No major differences could be found with regard to mental symptoms, occupation, school performance or social adjustment. Out of 238 patients only four were definitely mentally disordered with impaired capacity for work, two had epilepsy, two had tonic pupils and two had endocrine disorder.

Tuberculous meningitis

This more than any other form of meningitis is liable to lead to diagnostic error. The onset is insidious, pyrexia is low grade and often considerably delayed, and neck stiffness can be very slight. Mental symptoms figure prominently from the outset, and evidence of an acute organic reaction can precede overt signs of meningeal infection.

The cerebral pathology is characteristic. A yellowish gelatinous exudate forms mainly at the base of the brain in the anterior basal cisterns and extending along the lateral sulci. Miliary tubercles are visible on the leptomeninges and along the principal cerebral arteries.

Microscopically the inflammatory reaction can be seen to involve the floor of the third ventricle but is usually nowhere pronounced. The neurones show degenerative changes and old caseous foci can often be found in the substance of the brain. Arteritis is prominent in large and small vessels at the base of the brain, and areas of infarction may occur. The basal exudate is often organised and adherent, obstructing the flow of cerebrospinal fluid and leading to internal hydrocephalus.

A prodromal phase of vague ill health is usual, lasting for 2–3 weeks or longer. Anorexia is marked, but headache may be transient or even absent at this stage. Mental changes form an integral part of the picture, typically apathy, irritability and insidious change of personality. As long ago as 1868, Trousseau stressed that 'sadness setting in unaccountably is a premonitory sign of great value in a child'. Williams and Smith (1954) found that the earliest mental changes in their cases were often so gradual that they were imperceptible except to those who knew the patient well beforehand. A change towards clouded awareness was usually the first definite sign, the patient lying quietly and without apprehension. In one case the presenting symptom was of subjective impairment of memory.

As the disease progresses headache intensifies and low-grade pyrexia develops. Focal signs appear in the form of ptosis, oculomotor palsies, coarse tremor of the limbs and reflex abnormalities. Hemiplegia or other gross neurological defects may occur. Papilloedema is a late development, but choroidal tubercles are seen in the retina in up to 20% of cases (Wiles 1993a). These are rounded or oval yellow patches, approximately half the size of the optic disc.

The cerebrospinal fluid is under increased pressure, with up to 500 cells/mm³, mostly lymphocytes. The protein is moderately increased to 100 mg/100 ml with a meningitic Lange curve, the sugar is reduced below 50 mg/100 ml and the chloride much reduced to 500 mg/100 ml or below. The diagnosis is confirmed when tubercle bacilli can be identified or cultured from the fluid, but this is not achieved in every case. The CT scan may show hydrocephalus, focal infarcts and exudate in basal brain cisterns (Rovira et al. 1980).

The mental abnormalities increase with drowsiness, confusion, disorientation and inability to sustain a rational conversation. Characteristically the patient sleeps when alone but becomes disturbed when roused, in contrast to the perpetual 'silent struggling delirium' of purulent meningitis. Occasionally the patient is hallucinated and wildly delirious. The terror may resemble that of delirium tremens, or Wernicke's encephalopathy may be simulated when the onset is abrupt and oculomotor palsies are present. Formerly typhoid was often suggested by the combination of headache, fever and delirium.

Without treatment progressive internal hydrocephalus develops, coma supervenes and the patient dies in a state of decerebrate rigidity. Nowadays, however, the 'confusional' stage evolves during treatment to an 'amnesic' stage which may last for many weeks. Williams and Smith (1954) have described the picture in detail. It is remarkably constant in kind though varying in degree, consisting essentially of a disproportionate disturbance of memory in relation to other cognitive deficits. The patient may appear reasonably alert, and copes fairly well with intellectual problems, but proves to have a grave defect in retaining new information for more than a few minutes. Confabulation may be much in evidence and memory for temporal sequences is severely disorganised. Memory is hazy for the events of the illness and those preceding it for several weeks or months, but beyond this is usually intact. This stage was sufficiently characteristic to betray a diagnostic error in one of Williams and Smith's cases:

A man with a recent extension of known pulmonary tuberculosis complained of headache, became irrational and aggressive, and later had a fit. The cerebrospinal fluid showed a pleocytosis with raised protein and reduced sugar. He developed a slight dysarthria but no other focal signs.

Tuberculous meningitis was diagnosed and treatment started. In spite of this he deteriorated, became euphoric and fatuous, and showed gross intellectual deterioration. He remained normally orientated, however, and memory functions were well preserved. The diagnosis was reconsidered, the Wassermann reaction was found to be positive in the blood and cerebrospinal fluid, and he proved to be suffering from general paresis.

(Williams & Smith 1954)

Throughout the amnesic phase the patient is usually euphoric and shows little concern about his memory difficulties. Some, however, are withdrawn, negativistic, paranoid or acutely depressed.

During recovery, memory continues to lag behind improvement in other intellectual faculties. Retention of current events improves gradually, or occasionally returns with dramatic suddenness. The period of retrograde amnesia meanwhile steadily contracts towards the time of onset of the illness.

With cure of the infection, as judged by the return of the cerebrospinal fluid to normal, there is usually a complete restitution of normal memory functions, though a persistent amnesic gap remains for the period of overt confusion and disorientation. Williams and Smith followed 19 cases for periods of up to 4 years; none showed measurable defects of intellect, personality or memorising ability, although four complained of subjective forgetfulness for minor day-to-day events. Three others complained of slight impairment of concentration or were said by their relatives to show a lessened sense of responsibility. All, however, were amnesic for the early weeks or months of the illness, even those who had seemed alert and rational throughout. Six had a persistent retrograde amnesia, sometimes extending for periods of months or years prior to the illness, with haziness for details, some complete gaps and inability to organise past events into the correct temporal sequence:

A young man of 22 developed severe tuberculous meningitis. He had a long and difficult illness requiring some 9 months of treatment. Three years later he was doing well in clerical work and had recently been promoted. His memorising of current experience was normal. However, he still had a substantial retrograde amnesia for events some 6 months before the clinical onset of his illness, and had entirely lost some specific skills such as typing acquired during this period. The amnesia extended also to the first 4 months of the illness itself.

With present-day management a full physical and mental recovery can usually be secured when diagnosis has been prompt. Williams and Smith (1954) found that the majority of patients returned gradually to their former efficiency. Headache or neurotic developments were conspicuous by their absence. However, when neurological complications have been grave at the height of the illness there may be residual hemiparesis, paraparesis, epilepsy or intellectual impairment in association with hydrocephalus. Blindness or visual defects may result from optic atrophy, and deafness occurs in a minority. Hypothalamic damage occasionally leads to diabetes insipidus, disturbance of sleep rhythm or precocious puberty in children.

Lorber (1961) followed the long-term results in 100 children who survived the acute illness. A large variety of sequelae were seen but the number of children seriously affected was surprisingly small. Seventy-seven had made a complete recovery, including some with very severe neurological abnormalities during the active phase of the illness. Twenty-three showed defects in the form of paresis, fits, deafness or blindness, sometimes with gratifying improvement over time. Fits persisted in only eight children despite their frequency in the acute stages. Six of the 23 were profoundly mentally retarded; all of these had been under 2 years of age and severely affected when first seen, and all had major neurological sequelae. In the remainder there was no evidence that intellect had been impaired. Among children of normal intellect there were six with disorders of character and behaviour, four in association with a physical handicap and two without apparent relation to the meningitis.

Details of treatment are fully described by Wiles (1993a).

Cerebral abscess

Cerebral abscesses can present with remarkably few definite signs and symptoms. Headache may be slight and intermittent, papilloedema is often late, focal cerebral signs can be minimal and pyrexia tends to be absent in the chronic stage. It is essential therefore to consider the diagnosis when change of temperament or mild confusion is accompanied by evidence of ill health for which no immediate cause is obvious. In a large series of metastatic brain abscesses Gates *et al.* (1950) found that psychiatric symptoms were present from the start in almost a quarter of cases, and were exceeded in frequency only by headache.

Cerebral abscess is rarely seen without a focus of infection elsewhere, though this may be well concealed. Important sources near the brain include infection of the middle ear and mastoid cells, and extension from the frontal and sphenoidal sinuses. Head injury may convey infection by direct penetration or may open up pathways from the sinuses or ear when the base of the skull is fractured. The principal extracranial source is chronic suppurative disease of the lungs and pleura — bronchiectasis, lung abscess and empyema. Less commonly the abscess results from a general pyaemic infection caused by pelvic or abdominal suppuration, osteomyelitis, boils, cellulitis or subacute bacterial endocarditis. Paradoxical embolism of infected material may occur via septal defects in patients with congenital heart disease. With extracranial sources the abscesses are often multiple.

The organisms chiefly responsible are the *Streptococcus*, *Staphylococcus*, *Pneumococcus* or *Escherichia coli*. The developing abscess arises from an area of suppurating encephalitis which becomes progressively walled off from the surrounding brain by a fibrous and glial reaction. Inflammation of the overlying meninges varies in severity with the activity of the lesion. The abscess may grow large with distortion and compression of surrounding brain structures, but intracranial pressure may be little disturbed because the process is so gradual.

Classic symptoms are headache, vomiting and mild delirium, but these may sometimes be submerged in the symptoms of the predisposing infection. Alternatively the abscess may remain quiescent at the time of the original infection, and a latent interval of many months may follow before symptoms are declared. In the interim the patient shows evidence of chronic ill health—intermittent headache, malaise, loss of appetite and weight, constipation, occasional chills, depression and irritability. Ultimately more definite signs appear, sometimes closely simulating cerebral tumour. Headache intensifies and may be paroxysmal, evidence of toxaemia increases, fits may occur and focal neurological signs are declared.

The common temporal lobe abscess is usually derived from middle ear infection. Motor signs are often very slight, and careful testing of the visual fields may be needed to display the quadrantic hemianopia. Dysphasic symptoms may be detected with abscesses of the dominant lobe. The alternative route from the middle ear is to the cerebellum. Signs can again be slight, with nystagmus, hypotonia and incoordination of the ipsilateral limbs, or cranial nerve pareses from involvement of the nearby brain stem. Frontal lobe abscesses arise from sinus infection or frontal fracture, and may lack all focal signs apart from unilateral anosmia. Concentration and memory may be markedly impaired and personality change much in evidence. In all such cases signs of raised intracranial pressure can be slight or absent, even with very large abscesses, and papilloedema may be late.

Some degree of aseptic meningitis may produce obvious neck stiffness on examination. Examination of the cerebrospinal fluid is valuable for diagnosis but can be hazardous. The pressure is often raised and the protein elevated. The cells are mostly lymphocytes and rarely exceed 100 cells/mm³ so long as the abscess remains walled off. The sugar and chloride are normal, and organisms are not obtained. With the advent of the CT scan lumbar puncture can usually be avoided. The abscess is revealed after scan enhancement and has a characteristic appearance—the capsule shows as a ring-shaped area of increased density surrounded by cerebral oedema. The MRI appearances are often specific enough for exact diagnosis, with the capsule forming a discrete isointense or hyperintense ring surrounding a central cavity (Sze & Zimmerman 1988). Nevertheless exploratory puncture may be necessary to determine the causative organism. A polymorphonuclear leucocytosis is usual in the blood. The EEG shows changes broadly similar to those of tumour.

With modern management the mortality has fallen progressively to around 10% (Alderson *et al.* 1981). Some degree of permanent incapacity may nonetheless persist, and epilepsy is liable to develop in up to 70% of patients. Anticonvulsants should therefore be prescribed routinely for at least 5 years.

Other infective processes

Acute organic reactions may accompany many systemic infections, especially at the extremes of life. An obvious example is the delirium sometimes seen with the acute exanthemata of childhood, likewise the impairment of consciousness or delirium which occur with pneumonia in the elderly. Slater and Roth (1969) discuss the various causes which may be operative. Cerebral anoxia often appears to be responsible, or the influence of toxins derived from the infecting micro-organisms. More complex metabolic disturbances or the accumulation of toxic intermediate products must sometimes be postulated. Fever itself may play a direct part.

In the infections considered below, however, there is more definite evidence of cerebral involvement by the disease process itself. The conditions will be dealt with briefly, and textbooks of general medicine should be consulted for further details.

Lyme disease

Lyme disease is caused by the spirochaete *Borrelia burgdorferi* which is transmitted to humans through tick bites. It occurs in several regions of the USA and Europe, and cases have recently been reported from the UK, especially from the New Forest area. It can lead to cutaneous, neurological, arthritic and cardiac manifestations, though the course is usually benign and self limiting. The clinical pictures encountered are described by Burgdorfer (1987), and British experience of the disease is summarised by Bateman and White (1990) and O'Connell (1995).

The tick bite is followed by a characteristic rash, 'erythema migrans', which develops after some days or weeks and is often the pointer to the diagnosis. This consists of a spreading annular erythema which extends slowly outwards, usually on the trunk or limbs. It may be accompanied by systemic disturbances such as fever, headache or backache.

Neurological manifestations develop in some 15% of cases during the ensuing weeks or months, or can be the presenting feature. Eight cases from the New Forest region were described by Bateman *et al.* (1988). Some show a chronic low-grade meningitis with persistent headache and dizziness, others intense burning radicular pains and/or lower motor neurone facial palsies (Bannwarth's syndrome). Focal neurological signs and seizures may indicate brain parenchymal involvement. Complete recovery is the rule, though cases of chronic progressive encephalomyelitis have been reported in Europe and a syndrome resembling multiple sclerosis in the USA. Occasional patients are left with chronic fatigue and sometimes mild neuropsychological impairments. Recurrent attacks of arthritis may affect both large and small joints, and a transient myocarditis may occur, but these have been rare in the UK.

When the diagnosis is suspected serological tests for antibodies to *B. burgdorferi* should be carried out (O'Connell 1995). False negatives and false positives can occur, but rising titres over several weeks may give definitive evidence of the infection. The results may be positive in the cerebrospinal fluid when the serum is negative, so lumbar puncture should be performed when there are neurological manifestations. The cerebrospinal fluid shows pleocytosis with raised protein levels and often oligoclonal bands. The presence of borrelial DNA may be detected by the polymerase chain reaction.

Treatment consists of penicillin or tetracycline and should be given promptly once the skin rash is detected. In the presence of neurological complications penicillin must be given parenterally, and cefotaxime may be required (Muhlemann 1992).

Typhus fever

Of the several varieties of typhus, that due to *Rickettsia prowazeki* is the most common. Epidemics are intimately associated with famines and wars and the infection is transmitted by the body louse. Mental and neurological manifestations are usually prominent, and there is abundant evidence that the causative organism invades the nervous system directly. The rickettsiae invade the endothelial cells of small blood vessels, producing foci of thrombosis and necrosis in various organs including the brain. Characteristic 'typhus nodules' consist of perivascular accumulations of glial, endothelial and phagocytic cells.

Symptoms consist of pyrexia, delirium, malaise, severe headache, cough and generalised aching. A characteristic rash appears on the fifth day of fever. More definite nervous system manifestations appear towards the end of the febrile period and are of serious import. Headache becomes continuous and periods of delirium alternate with stupor or coma. Focal signs appear in the form of hemiplegia, ataxia, bulbar dysfunction, deafness or optic neuritis. Meningeal irritation is common and the cerebrospinal fluid shows a lymphocytosis and increased globulin. Among survivors evidence of cerebral damage frequently persists.

Trypanosomiasis (sleeping sickness)

The South African forms of trypanosomiasis are due to the protozoa *Trypanosoma gambiense* and *T. rhodesiense*. They are transmitted by the bite of the tsetse fly. An initial febrile stage consists of bouts of pyrexia, asthenia, adenitis, rashes and hepatosplenomegaly. This merges into the sleeping sickness stage which is essentially a chronic meningoencephalitis with the organisms appearing in the cerebrospinal fluid. The patient develops tremors, fits, incoordination or hemiplegia. Mental disturbances are prominent with somnolence, apathy and eventually coma. Death usually occurs within a year if the disease is untreated.

Cerebral malaria

Delirium may be marked at the peaks of fever in any variety of malaria, but sometimes there is more acute and dramatic evidence of cerebral involvement. This is most common with infections due to *Plasmodium falciparum* (malignant tertian malaria). In fatal cases the brain is seen to be congested and oedematous, with numerous areas of haemorrhage and softening around vessels.

The cerebral capillaries are filled with parasites in various stages of development. The cerebral symptoms usually appear in the second or third week of the illness, but they may sometimes be the initial manifestation. They can be cataclysmic in onset. Severe delirium is accompanied by bursting headache and high pyrexia. The patient is often combative and excitable before coma supervenes. Fits can be the presenting feature and focal signs are common—hemiplegia, dysphasia, hemianopia or cerebellar ataxia. Retinal haemorrhages and papilloedema may occur.

The picture can simulate encephalitis, meningitis, cerebral tumour, epilepsy, cerebrovascular lesions or a variety of acute psychiatric disorders (Boshes 1947). Mistakes are particularly likely to be made in the rare examples when the patient is afebrile. Nadeem and Younis (1977) also stressed that clouding of consciousness may be absent initially. Of 39 patients admitted to a Sudanese psychiatric hospital with mental illness precipitated by physical disease, 17 proved to have malaria. Half of these showed psychiatric disturbances in clear consciousness. Thus where malaria is endemic it must be borne in mind in all patients with psychoses of acute onset, whether or not organic features are evident in the mental state.

Rapid treatment is vital, so examination of blood smears must not be delayed in suspected cases. Care must be taken to enquire about countries in which the patient may have lived or travelled whenever an acute organic reaction occurs without obvious cause. The number of cases reported in the UK has increased substantially over the years in consequence of visits by businessmen and back-packers to heavily infected regions (Wyatt 1992).

Cerebral cysticercosis

The cysticercus stage of the tapeworm, usually *Taenia solium*, may occur in humans. Common sites include the skeletal muscles and the brain. The infestation is extremely common in Mexico. McCormick *et al.* (1982) and Grisolia and Wiederholt (1982) describe the typical clinical pictures.

Multiple cysts are usually present within the brain and the main damage appears to occur when the larvae begin to die. There is then an intense inflammatory reaction in an attempt to wall off the irritating process. The circulation of the cerebrospinal fluid is often obstructed.

The usual presentation is with focal seizures, or with symptoms of raised intracranial pressure due to internal hydrocephalus. Localizing signs are relatively uncommon, though sudden neurological deficits can result from infarcts. Very occasionally dementia is the presenting feature. Retinal involvement may accompany the central nervous system disturbance.

The cerebrospinal fluid shows a pleocytosis including eosinophils, an increase in protein and a positive reaction to serological tests for cysticercosis. However, the latter may be negative in up to 40% of patients (McCormick *et al.* 1982). Calcification of the cysts may be seen on X-ray, both within the skull and in the skeletal muscles. Neuroimaging is valuable in revealing the lesions or the resulting hydrocephalus when the skull X-ray is negative.

Chronic fatigue syndrome (postviral fatigue syndrome, epidemic neuromyasthenia, myalgic encephalomyelitis, ME)

The variety of labels attaching to this debilitating condition betrays uncertainty about its aetiology and, indeed, whether it is a unitary entity. While many examples follow in the wake of viral infection this is not an invariable precursor; and the title of myalgic encephalomyelitis, applied to the outbreak at the Royal Free Hospital, London in 1955, presupposes an inflammatory central nervous system pathology for which the evidence is slender. 'Chronic fatigue syndrome' appears to be the most acceptable label in that it remains neutral about pathogenesis. Not dissimilar pictures in the past have been referred to as 'chronic neurasthenia', 'effort syndrome', 'neurocirculatory asthenia' and 'fibromyalgia'. White (1990) reviews the interrelationships between these conditions.

The chronic fatigue syndrome is not uncommon as a cause of severe, protracted disability, chiefly among young adults. Most cases arise sporadically, though from time to time there have been small epidemics in institutions or in restricted geographical locations with some hundreds of persons affected. It is nowadays one of the most controversial and emotive topics in medicine, with contending theories about its aetiology. There are those who argue strongly, even stridently, for an organic causation, while others account for it in terms of depression or neurosis. In many long-continued cases it is possible that both sets of factors are operative, an organic affliction becoming prolonged by virtue of secondary psychological developments, much as may occur with the post-traumatic syndrome (p. 199).

Clinical features

The symptoms have tended to vary somewhat in different series. The onset is typically abrupt with intense malaise, lassitude and dizziness, often with sore throat, headache or gastrointestinal disturbance. Pyrexia is slight or absent. Generalised pains occur in the limbs and back, and muscle pain and tenderness may be marked. There may be slight neck stiffness and some lymphadenopathy.

A variety of rather insubstantial neurological features may then appear—flaccid weakness of the limbs, intermittency of muscle contraction on effort, or paraesthesiae, hyperaesthesia and analgesia of irregular distribution. Cranial nerve palsies have very occasionally been reported. Psychological symptoms are usually prominent, especially depression or severe emotional lability, and an hysterical component may be grafted onto the neurological picture. The symptoms typically show considerable variation from day to day.

Objective neurological findings are rare (British Medical Journal 1970a). The tendon reflexes are usually normal, or only slightly increased or decreased, and sensory changes may be difficult to confirm by neurological examination.

In most recorded outbreaks the majority of patients recover completely as with ordinary viral infections. Some, however, enter a chronic stage with persistent fatiguability, weakness of the limbs and muscle pain. Such patients may be severely incapacitated for many months or even years. In the common sporadic examples of the disorder it is during the chronic stage that the patient will usually first come to medical attention, and in many such examples there has been no evidence whatever of a preceding infection.

The outstanding feature is then fatigue, leading to progressive restriction of activities. After attempted exercise there is delayed recovery and often postexertional malaise. Mental fatiguability may also be in evidence, short periods of concentration leading to feelings of physical exhaustion. The patient may gradually recover over several months, but some have continuing relapses or persistent symptoms for very prolonged periods. Depression is a common accompaniment, with irritability, forgetfulness and difficulty with concentration. Jenkins (1991) stresses that lability of mood is commoner than sustained depression, swings of mood being closely related to levels of physical energy and fatigue. The classic diurnal variation of depressive illness is rarely seen, patients often starting the day feeling reasonably well but quickly becoming depressed when fatigue sets in. The depression is often related to the frustration experienced at being unable to carry out habitual activities, while enjoyment of passive pursuits is largely retained. Patients rarely report feelings of guilt, unworthiness or self blame. Introspective and hypochondriacal attitudes are liable to become entrenched, and attempts at rehabilitation can be long and tedious with lowering of morale.

Kendell (1967) surveyed the widespread psychiatric disturbances which may be observed. He described two patients in detail who showed long-lasting and severe changes of mood and behaviour as an aftermath. One had recurrent depressions and frequent self-destructive outbursts, still present 5 years after the illness. The other developed temporal lobe epilepsy and similarly had recurrent bouts of depression for 8 years thereafter, with histrionic attention-seeking behaviour and numerous suicide attempts. Damage was postulated to have occurred in neural mechanisms underlying the control of mood and behaviour to account for such severe and prolonged disturbances.

Diagnostic criteria

In view of the pleomorphic features described in various series, Holmes et al. (1988) have proposed precise diagnostic criteria for the syndrome. The major criterion is the new onset of persistent or relapsing debilitating fatigue, or easy fatiguability, that does not resolve with bed rest and that is severe enough to reduce daily activity below 50% of premorbid levels for a period of at least 6 months. The second major criterion is that clinical conditions which produce similar symptoms must be excluded by thorough evaluation—for example malignancy, chronic infections with known organisms, endocrine and toxic disorders, abuse of drugs or alcohol, myasthenia gravis, chronic depression, schizophrenia or hysterical personality disorder. A certain number of minor criteria must also be satisfied, selected from the following—low-grade fever, sore throat, painful lymphadenopathy, generalised muscle weakness, myalgia, headache, arthralgia, sleep disturbance, complaints of depression, irritability, forgetfulness or inability to concentrate, and a history of the main symptom complex initially developing over a few hours or days. Sharpe et al. (1991) have refined these criteria further, and have separated out a subtype of 'postinfectious fatigue syndrome' when there is definite evidence of infection at onset or presentation. The revised definition presented by Fukuda et al. (1994) is broadly similar to that of Holmes et al. but recognises in addition unrefreshing sleep and postexertional malaise lasting for more than 24 hours.

Investigations

Investigations typically give negative or at most border-line results. The blood picture is in general unremarkable. Buchwald (1991) reviews studies which have variously revealed leucocytosis, leucopaenia and raised or lowered erythrocyte sedimentation rates (ESRs) in a proportion of patients, concluding that such findings have been diverse, conflicting, modest in degree and of unclear clinical importance. Studies of the lumbar cerebrospinal fluid have similarly sometimes shown modest elevations of cells or protein, though in the main no abnormalities are detected.

Minor EEG changes are quite commonly reported, but do not resemble the picture of acute encephalitis. Single fibre electromyograph recordings have, however, shown clear evidence of muscle abnormality (Jamal 1991). Muscle biopsy may reveal fibre atrophy and necrosis, also structural and functional abnormalities in the mitochondria (Edwards *et al.* 1991). Creatine kinase levels are normal. Brain imaging has in general been uninformative, as reviewed by Cope and David (1996). Costa *et al.* (1995) have reported brain stem hypoperfusion on HMPAO-SPECT, but the significance of such a finding remains uncertain.

Aetiology

With regard to aetiology, opposing views support a viral/immunological origin or a primarily psychological explanation for the syndrome. In support of a viral causation it is noteworthy that most outbreaks have occurred in the summer months and that medical and nursing staff have often been victims of the disorder. In some patients there is clear evidence of viral precipitation at the outset, but uncertainty persists about the role of viruses in relation to chronic continuing disability. Numerous virological studies have been conducted, both in the UK and the USA, with implication of enteroviruses (especially the Coxsackie virus) or the Epstein–Barr virus, respectively. Elevated levels of the corresponding antibodies have been reported in up to 30% of patients, with immunological evidence sometimes pointing to persistent continuing infection (Mowbray 1991). It is suggested that abnormalities in the host response may be crucial to the continuation of symptoms, also that interferon production may account for much of the fatigue and myalgia experienced. Where repeated relapses are accompanied by 'flu-like symptoms, this may represent fluctuations in interferon production during the course of a single chronic infection. Some evidence exists for the presence of enteroviral RNA in muscle fibres in the disorder (Gow *et al.* 1991), perhaps accounting in part for the myalgic symptoms. Evidence of viral infection within the central nervous system has not, however, been forthcoming.

The issue of a psychological explanation for the disorder became pivotal following McEvedy and Beard's re-evaluation of the 1955 outbreak at the Royal Free Hospital. McEvedy and Beard (1970a, 1970b, 1973) pointed out that the initial manifestations in the epidemic had consisted entirely of subjective complaints, and that those cases showing pharyngitis might have been due to a coincident outbreak of streptococcal sore throat in the hospital at the time. Pyrexia exceeding 37.8°C (100°F) occurred in only 4.5% of cases and the ESR was over 20 in only 1.5%. The sensory changes had been mostly of glove and stocking type, and the motor weaknesses were unbacked by reflex changes. An encephalitic process seemed unlikely in that prolonged disturbance of consciousness was never seen and changes were uniformly absent in the cerebrospinal fluid. They concluded that a case could be made for regarding the manifestations as 'the subjective complaints of a frightened and hysterical population'. Overbreathing may have been responsible for dizziness, paraesthesiae and minor tetanic spasms.

In a review of 15 recorded outbreaks of the disease, McEvedy and Beard (1970b) stressed that the attack rate was higher in females than males, and that relatively closed communities appeared to be especially susceptible. Eight of the outbreaks had occurred among hospital nurses, and sometimes there had been a worrying epidemic of poliomyelitis in the community at the time. In retrospect several of the outbreaks could be regarded as psychosocial phenomena, caused either by mass hysteria or altered 'medical perception' in the community. Thus medical attention had come to be concentrated on the central nervous system, and cases had probably often been included when they were not immediately diagnosable as having some other condition.

This challenging view provoked a good deal of controversy at the time (British Medical Journal 1970b; Ramsay 1973) and this continues to the present day. McEvedy and Beard's formulation of the acute phenomena is unlikely to apply to the many cases which arise sporadically, though it remains an open question how far the long-continued aftermaths may depend on psychological factors. The attention given to the disorder in the lay press, and the activity of several pressure groups, have brought the conflicting views about the nature of the condition strongly before public attention.

A central problem in evaluating research findings, both in the organic and psychiatric domains, is the uncertainty about how much is primary or secondary among the observed abnormalities. Thus depression may be the consequence of a prolonged and debilitating illness which is organic in origin; or impaired mitochondrial activity may be the result of disuse muscle atrophy. A further problem is that fatigue is common as shown by community surveys, and can have both physical and psychosocial determinants (Pawlikowska *et al.* 1994). In such surveys the experiencing of fatigue has proved to be highly correlated with emotional distress. Ratings show that it occurs as a continuum, much as with levels of blood pressure, and cut-off points for labelling it as pathological are hard to achieve. Not least, fatigue is largely a subjective phenomenon, strongly affected by individual perceptions of its severity and implications.

Thomas (1993) concludes that there can be no simple explanation for the chronic fatigue syndrome, and that it reflects an interaction between cerebral dysfunction, trigger factors and social attitudes, being then complicated by secondary symptoms. He concedes, however, that the setting of the neural mechanisms responsible for the sensation of fatigue may be altered in the disorder, and in this connection it is interesting that hypothalamic dysfunction of a subtle nature has been reported. Thus Bakheit *et al.* (1992), measuring serum prolactin levels after a buspirone challenge test, have obtained evidence of upregulation of hypothalamic 5-hydroxytryptamine receptors in patients with the syndrome, when compared with normal subjects and with patients suffering from primary depressive illness. Nevertheless with respect to prognosis psychological factors have often emerged as extremely important, Wilson *et al.* (1994) showing that illness attitudes and coping styles predict long-term outcome better than measures of immunological or other factors.

Treatment

Numerous specific treatments have been advocated for the chronic fatigue syndrome, including gamma globulin injections, antiviral remedies, antibiotics, mineral and vitamin supplements and high dosages of essential fatty acids. None have achieved widespread success, and the management of patients remains often a difficult exercise. Antidepressants can obviously have a role to play, likewise analgesics when muscle pain is severe. Wessely *et al.* (1989, 1991) and Sharpe *et al.* (1992) give detailed descriptions of a cognitive–behavioural approach which aims, *inter alia*, to break the vicious cycle of exercise avoidance leading to diminished exercise tolerance and the production of further symptoms. The encouragement of the patient to engage in graded activity by planned stages requires careful assessment of the capacities in each individual and full explanation of the aims of treatment. Bonner *et al.* (1994) obtained strong indications of the long-term success of such an approach in a follow-up of patients 4 years after completion of treatment. More

recently Sharpe *et al.* (1996) have reported a prospective controlled trial of cognitive–behavioural therapy, showing undoubted benefits both in terms of significant improvement of functioning and reduction of depression and perception of fatigue. At 12 months' follow-up almost three-quarters of patients who had received treatment had achieved normal daily functioning compared with only a quarter of controls.

Rheumatic fever and rheumatic chorea
(Sydenham's chorea)

The relationship between rheumatic fever and rheumatic chorea is incompletely understood, but chorea has sometimes been regarded as a form of rheumatic encephalitis (Lees 1970). The two may occur together, or chorea may be seen in the absence of joint, skin or heart manifestations. Fatal cases, however, almost always show evidence of rheumatic carditis. Nausieda *et al.* (1980) have documented the marked progressive decline in the number of cases of rheumatic chorea seen during the preceding 30 years. In their review of 240 patients a high familial incidence was noted, both for chorea (13% of cases) and for rheumatic fever (36%). As expected there was a strong association with antecedent group A streptococcal infection.

The literature concerning the possible cerebral effects of the diseases is inconclusive. Both rheumatic fever and chorea may occasionally be associated with psychotic illnesses, and behaviour disorder is recognised as extremely common in children after rheumatic chorea. Lewis (1956) pointed out that chorea exemplifies the interplay of hereditary, psychic and structural factors in the production of symptoms; it is more prone to occur in families with nervous disorder, the motor abnormalities can appear and disappear under emotional influences, and after-effects such as tics often seem to be conditioned by the original choreic disturbances of neuromuscular function.

Guttmann (1936) stressed the frequency of psychiatric disorder among the relatives of patients, and thought it likely that a particular type of person was prone to the disease. The persistence of personality disturbances and emotional disorder after the chorea had subsided could not therefore be confidently ascribed to cerebral pathological change. Bender (1942), however, found that the restless, irritable and undisciplined behaviour of choreic children could often improve spontaneously as the rheumatic process receded.

Uncertainty still surrounds the question of cerebral pathology. Bruetsch (1940) reported 'rheumatic' changes in the cerebral vessels, similar to those seen in the myocardium and elsewhere. Walton (1977) described oedema, neuronal degeneration and occasional perivascular infiltration in rheumatic chorea. Such changes are said to be most marked in the corpus striatum, substantia nigra and subthalamic nucleus, but localisation has not been well established.

The general picture in postchoreic children is of the gradual onset of restless hyperactivity, with inattention, fidgetiness and inability to sit still. Motility may be awkward, and tics and compulsive utterances may develop. Krauss (1946) described characteristic peculiarities of personality—patients became sensitive, suspicious and seclusive — also neurasthenic symptoms by way of headache, fatigue and insomnia. Nausieda *et al.* (1980) noted that dysarthria was common but that other neurological abnormalities were rare. Some 10% of their cases showed emotional lability, disorientation, confusion or more rarely delirium. Swedo *et al.* (1989) compared 23 children and adolescents with rheumatic chorea and 14 with rheumatic fever alone, following small outbreaks in the USA. The former showed significantly more obsessional thoughts and compulsive behaviour than the latter, suggesting that obsessional–compulsive disorder might be related to basal ganglia dysfunction.

Some children show more bizarre disturbances with vague hallucinations, fears and episodes of panic (Bender 1942). The abnormalities of motility occasionally showed catatonic as well as choreiform features, the picture resembling schizophrenia quite closely. Lewis and Minski (1935) similarly noted that in the more severe cases delusional ideas could accompany the fleeting phases of anger or terror.

Still more severe manifestations can develop in the rare cases of rheumatic chorea in young adults, typified by chorea gravidarum in pregnant women. Delirium may occur, with hallucinations, delusions of persecution, persistent insomnia and much excitement (maniacal chorea). One of Lewis and Minski's (1935) patients, a nurse of 18, showed a grave choreic illness accompanied by clouding of consciousness, disorientation, auditory hallucinations and ideas of reference which gradually improved over several months. For 2 days at the height of the illness she showed a right-sided flaccid paralysis, but the cerebrospinal fluid was normal.

The following is another example in which electroencephalographic evidence pointed clearly to an organic basis for the protracted and puzzling mental illness:

A woman of 36 was seen when her son was referred to hospital on account of truanting from school and delinquent behaviour. She showed an abnormal personality, with high anxiety, numerous panic attacks and bizarre beliefs of a quasi-psychotic nature. In her own previous history she had been hospitalised for over a year at the age of 17 with a diagnosis of 'rheumatic encephalitis associated with hysterical and schizophrenic features'.

She had been a delicate and imaginative child, extremely able at school but with a disturbed home background. At 10 she had suffered rheumatic fever. For some months prior to admission she had been depressed and listless with considerable loss of weight. Gradually she had become restless, with nervous tics of the hands and feet which were diagnosed first as hysterical and later as rheumatic chorea.

On admission there were numerous tic-like movements of the limbs, shrugging of the shoulders and occasional myoclonic-like jerks. No other abnormalities were discovered on physical examination. Her mood was labile, and she eventually revealed a delusional belief that she had an evil thing inside her which accounted for her sister's death 2 years before she herself was born. She was hallucinated, seeing animals and seeing everything blue from time to time. She insisted that she could feel an insect crawling around inside her skull.

The choreiform movements settled after several weeks, but her subsequent course in hospital was stormy, with unpredictable and impulsive behaviour, marked seclusiveness and difficulty in making any therapeutic contact. She habitually carried a teddy bear and a copy of Shelley to which she attributed magical qualities. From time to time she absconded from hospital or cut her left arm with glass or razor blades.

The EEG showed marked abnormalities, with frequent high voltage spikes and persistent evidence of a discharging focus in the right frontal region. After 6 months in hospital this improved progressively along with improvement in her behaviour and mental state. On follow-up during the next few years she remained manipulative and disturbed at home from time to time, and occasional choreiform movements appeared when under stress. The EEG still showed evidence of residual brain damage 3 years after the onset of the illness. When seen at the age of 36, however, the EEG was entirely normal.

Finally, certain affinities between rheumatic diseases and schizophrenia have attracted attention. Schizophrenia has been noted to be common in the family histories of choreics, and Guttmann (1936) found that a history of chorea was twice as common in patients with schizophrenia as in those with manic–depressive psychosis. Krauss (1957) reported six patients with schizophrenia-like illnesses following rheumatic fever with cerebral involvement. Further evidence was presented by Bruetsch (1940), who found progressive obliterating cerebral arteritis together with rheumatic heart disease in a small group of schizophrenics at autopsy. It is possible, however, that these may have been examples of systemic lupus erythematosus with psychosis, rather than rheumatic fever with cerebral involvement (Fessel & Solomon 1960).

Chapter 9: Cerebrovascular Disorders

Diseases of the vascular system contribute greatly to the sum total of psychiatric disability, chiefly in the elderly population and mainly as a result of stroke. Cerebrovascular accidents will therefore be considered first, with emphasis on their psychiatric sequelae and the problems encountered in rehabilitation. Hypertension and migraine illustrate in an important fashion the possible role of emotional factors in organic disease and will also be dealt with here.

The syndrome of 'transient global amnesia' appears sometimes to rest on a cerebrovascular basis and, like subdural haematoma, may occasionally lead to mistakes in psychiatric diagnosis. Finally, certain diseases of rather obscure aetiology, such as systemic lupus erythematosus and other forms of vasculitis will be described. The psychiatric components of such illnesses have gained increasing recognition and appear to be attributable in part to involvement of the cerebral vasculature.

Cerebrovascular accidents

Cerebrovascular accidents are the third commonest cause of death after heart disease and cancer in the Western world. In Great Britain they emerge as the most frequent cause of severe disability in the community (Harris *et al.* 1971). From a population of 250 000 (the basis for a district general hospital) it is estimated that some 500 strokes will occur per annum, of which 250 will need a lot of help and about 150 will be added to the accumulating number needing continued care (Hurwitz & Adams 1972). The Oxfordshire Community Stroke Project (Bamford *et al.* 1988) has confirmed such an incidence for first-ever strokes (two per 1000 population), the risk for males exceeding that for females by 26%. The burden to the community, and to health and rehabilitation services is clearly enormous. Moreover approximately a quarter of victims are affected under 65 years of age and are thus disabled during the productive years of their lives.

The principal causes—atherosclerosis and hypertension—slowly yield to greater understanding, though opportu-nities for taking preventive action remain limited to certain categories of patient. Factors susceptible to modification among predisposing causes include hypertension, heart disease, diabetes, raised serum lipids and smoking. There are also indications that severely threatening life events are commoner in stroke victims than controls throughout the year preceding the stroke (House *et al.* 1990a).

A new interest and vigour attaches to the problems of rehabilitating the survivors, though psychiatrists are often little involved in the process. This is disappointing, in that much of the disability resulting from strokes is mental rather than physical, and psychological influences can be paramount in determining what progress is made. The lack of psychiatric involvement would appear to be largely a consequence of the way services for patients are organised, with the burden of care falling chiefly on geriatricians, general physicians and specialists in physical rehabilitation.

In what follows the general background to cerebrovascular accidents will be briefly sketched before reviewing what is known of the psychological and psychiatric aftermaths.

Forms of cerebrovascular accident

Virtually all enduring effects of vascular disease on the brain can be reduced to two essential pathological processes — infarction and haemorrhage. The common denominator of both from the clinical point of view is the 'stroke', which has been defined by the World Health Organization as 'a rapidly developed clinical sign of a focal disturbance of cerebral function of presumed vascular origin and of more than 24 hours duration' (Marquardsen 1983).

Infarction is commoner than haemorrhage in a ratio of approximately 4 : 1. It is not only more frequent as an acute development but very much more so as a source of enduring disability. Thus approximately three-quarters of patients with infarctions survive, whereas almost two-thirds of patients with cerebral haemorrhage die within a year (Bamford *et al.* 1990). Infarction may result from thrombosis of vessels or from emboli which come to lodge within them. Haemorrhage may be primarily into the substance of the brain or into the subarachnoid space.

In addition to examples of 'completed stroke' one must recognise the multitude of patients with episodes, often recurrent, which depend upon brief and transient ischaemia of the brain. Such 'transient ischaemic attacks' have attracted increasing attention, and the understanding of their pathophysiological basis has led to important therapeutic advances.

Cerebral haemorrhage

Intracranial haemorrhage, representing some 15% of all strokes, may be divided into primary intracerebral haemorrhage and subarachnoid haemorrhage. The former is intimately associated with hypertension as the main aetiological factor, and the latter with rupture of an aneurysm or angioma. The differentiation is not always absolute, since bleeding may occur into brain tissue in the neighbourhood of a ruptured aneurysm, and blood may gain access to the ventricular system and subarachnoid space after primary intracerebral haemorrhage. The two disorders are, however, in the main distinct. Subarachnoid haemorrhage is dealt with separately on p. 392 *et seq.* because the sequelae have been studied especially closely from the psychiatric point of view.

Primary intracerebral haemorrhage is most common in patients between the ages of 60 and 80. For practical purposes it is almost always associated with hypertension. The precise mechanism whereby haemorrhage develops has been the subject of controversy, but it seems probable that bleeding is often initiated from microaneurysms situated along the course of small arteries. These appear to develop in relation to hypertension in older subjects, and their distribution accords well with sites where haemorrhage is common (Russell 1963).

The onset is often during exertion, and very rarely during sleep as with cerebral thrombosis. The patient is abruptly seized with an ill-defined sensation of something wrong within the head, and shortly thereafter develops hemiparesis, dysphasia or some other form of neurological deficit. Headache and vomiting frequently occur. As the paralysis worsens mental confusion gives way to rapid impairment of consciousness. The picture characteristically worsens over one or more hours, usually to deep coma with stertorous breathing and a slow bounding pulse. Neck stiffness is common and the cerebrospinal fluid is often bloodstained.

The most common site of haemorrhage is in the putamen and internal capsule, from rupture of the lenticulostriate artery. A dense contralateral hemiplegia may be accompanied by deviation of the head and eyes away from the side of the lesion. The formation of a large intracerebral haematoma can lead to secondary effects due to tentorial herniation and brain stem compression. Another site of predilection is the cerebellum, leading to a similar picture but with vertigo and ataxia during the early stages. With haemorrhage into the pons consciousness is usually lost rapidly, the pupils are unequal or pinpoint, hyperpyrexia may occur and quadriplegia is likely to be present.

Early mortality is high, and survivors are usually severely crippled. Mild examples with only brief loss of consciousness may, however, make a reasonably good recovery. Medical treatment during the acute stages rests primarily on excellent nursing care. Corticosteroids or manitol may be given to reduce cerebral swelling. Surgical evacuation of the clot has been undertaken in carefully selected cases but has proved in general to be of limited value. It is most likely to be of benefit when the haematoma is in the central white matter or the cerebellar hemisphere.

Cerebral infarction

Thrombosis is considerably more common than embolism as a cause of infarction. This has tended, however, to be used as the diagnostic category when no other cause is clinically evident for the stroke. The role of embolism has come to be recognised increasingly, and is now thought to account for about 30% of all strokes (Kannel & Wolf 1983).

Cerebral thrombosis is mostly seen in patients over 60, but appears to be increasing in frequency among the middle aged. It has emerged as a rare but serious complication in young women taking the contraceptive pill. The principal cause is atherosclerosis, namely that form of arteriosclerosis in which lipid material accumulates beneath the intima of affected vessels. Hypertension aggravates the process, and this, like diabetes mellitus, may be an important contributory factor in younger subjects. As the plaques thicken the lumen narrows and flow becomes reduced. The vessels chiefly involved are the larger arteries — the aorta, carotids, middle cerebrals and vertebrobasilar arteries. The size of the infarct eventually produced will depend on the vessels principally involved and also on the efficiency of the collateral circulation.

An important factor in precipitating thrombosis may often be a transient fall in blood pressure, further compromising the flow in vessels already critically affected. Thus an abrupt reduction of cardiac output, as after myocardial infarction or episodes of ventricular fibrillation, may present with cerebral symptoms. The reduction of blood pressure which occurs during sleep may sometimes be enough to tip the scales (Walton 1982).

Great importance attaches to the minute 'lacunar infarcts' which develop deep in the brain substance from occlusion of small penetrating arteries supplying the basal ganglia, thalamus, internal capsule, pons or convolutional white matter (Fisher 1982b; Weisberg 1982). Such infarcts may be multiple and almost microscopic in size. They have been found to outnumber all other strokes combined at autopsy. Hypertension is an associated finding in the great majority of cases, and the incidence of cerebral lacunes may possibly have declined with the introduction of antihypertensive therapy (Fisher 1982b).

The clinical picture in cerebral thrombosis usually develops abruptly, though less markedly so than with embolism. Occasionally the development is ingravescent, with the neurological deficit increasing over hours or days and progressing in a stepwise or saltatory fashion. Onset is often during sleep, with the patient waking to find paralysis, dysphasia, diplopia or other deficits. Headache may be present in the early stages but is often absent throughout. Some degree of mental confusion is common, but consciousness may be little if at all impaired. Much will depend on the size and location of the infarcted brain tissue. Large infarcts may be followed by swelling of the affected hemisphere, leading to coma and a picture closely resembling cerebral haemorrhage. An important differentiating feature may be a history of previous small episodes, rapidly clearing, and perhaps disregarded by the patient and his family at the time.

Cerebral embolism can in the majority of cases be traced to disease of the heart or great vessels. Fragments of thrombus are derived from atheromatous plaques in the aorta or carotids, or consist of newly formed platelet aggregates ('white emboli') which have formed in relation to abnormal areas of the vessel wall. A cardiac origin is probable when there is atrial fibrillation, mitral stenosis, subacute bacterial endocarditis or a recent myocardial infarction. Rare forms include paradoxical embolism, in which a congenital cardiac malformation allows material from the veins of the legs to reach the brain by bypassing the pulmonary circulation. Cerebral fat embolism is closely linked to trauma.

The clinical picture is usually extremely acute in onset, developing within seconds or a minute and usually during activity. The neurological deficit is typically maximal from the outset, often with rapid resolution over the first few hours thereafter. Headache is usually absent. Consciousness is often relatively preserved, or even retained completely.

Rare cases have been reported of multiple microembolism, in which a fluctuating acute confusional state is punctuated by transient episodes of dysphasia, multiple pareses and episodes of visual disturbance, pursuing a progressive downhill course to death (McDonald 1967). The source in the examples reported was an ulcerating atheromatous lesion in the aorta or internal carotid artery, the emboli consisting of multiple cholesterol crystals.

The prognosis for cerebral infarction is much better than for cerebral haemorrhage. Approximately 20% of patients die in the acute stage, 20% recover completely and 60% are left with residual disability. Recovery from emboli is in general much quicker and more complete than after thrombosis, since collateral channels will usually be more readily available. In both, however, much will depend on the size of the infarct produced.

Treatment in the acute stage includes not only nursing care and physiotherapy as appropriate, but also evaluation of the patient's cardiovascular status. Possible sources of emboli must be sought out with care. Anticoagulant therapy may be indicated where embolism is suspected, or operative intervention may be needed on a stenosed or atheromatous carotid artery, but these are matters for neurological assessment.

Magnetic resonance imaging (MRI) is more sensitive than computerised tomography (CT) for detecting infarcts at an early stage and for the visualisation of very small lacunar infarcts. CT scanning is, however, more capable of distinguishing between infarction and haemorrhage early on and is the investigation of choice when imaging is required during the first 48 hours after stroke (Armstrong & Keevil 1991). Ultimately, however, intracranial blood becomes isodense with brain tissue, so scanning must be carried out within the first 2 weeks if small haemorrhages are not to be missed.

Positron emission tomography (PET) and single photon emission computerised tomography (SPECT) will typically reveal considerably larger areas of disturbed brain function than is apparent on structural scans. These also have the unique advantage of displaying remote effects ('diaschisis') at a distance from the point of infarction (Baron 1987; Costa & Ell 1991). Thus it can be shown that thalamic infarcts lead to reduced blood flow and metabolism over a wide area of the ipsilateral cortical mantle, sometimes with corresponding neuropsychological deficits in the acute stage (Caselli *et al.* 1991). Crossed cerebellar hypometabolism results from large cortical infarcts, especially those in the frontal and parietal regions, also from subcortical infarctions in the internal capsule. PET scanning, moreover, can show the degree to which blood flow and cerebral metabolism remain coupled or dissociated from one another in the infarcted area, by measurement of the oxygen extraction ratio, this having implications for the potential viability of the damaged brain tissue (Wise *et al.* 1983a, 1983b).

Frackowiak and colleagues have also used PET scanning to investigate patterns of brain recovery and adaptation after stroke

(Chollet *et al.* 1991). Serial scans were undertaken during the inhalation of ^{15}O-labelled carbon dioxide, while at rest and during the performance of fine finger movements, in patients who had recovered from hemiplegic stroke. Finger movements on the unaffected side activated regional blood flow in the contralateral sensorimotor and premotor cortex and the ipsilateral cerebellar hemisphere. Small changes were also observed in the contralateral insula, striatum, inferior parietal and supplementary motor cortex. The same movements in the recovered hand produced more widespread activations, including significant increases *bilaterally* in sensorimotor and premotor cortex and both cerebellar hemispheres. Thus bilateral involvement of motor systems was seen when the recovered fingers were employed, indicating significant reorganisation and recruitment of ipsilateral motor pathways.

In a further study using the same experimental paradigm, Weiller *et al.* (1992) compared post-stroke patients with normal subjects and obtained evidence of further complex patterns of functional reorganisation, namely the recruitment of additional motor systems involving inferior parietal and anterior insular regions. Activations were also observed in cingulate and prefrontal areas which are not normally involved in finger movement but are known to be involved in selective attentional and intentional mechanisms, suggesting that these too may play an important part in the recovery process.

Individual patients were then studied in an attempt to discover how far individual patterns of reorganisation might relate to different sites of infarction (Weiller *et al.* 1993). Lesions in the posterior, but not the anterior, limb of the internal capsule were found to produce expansions of the hand field into the face area of the contralateral sensorimotor cortex. This may reflect the somatotopic organisation of pyramidal fibres in the internal capsule; those destined for the arm and leg lie posteriorly to those for the tongue and face, so expansions into the face territory may only be possible with more posteriorly situated lesions.

Cerebral arterial syndromes

The form which the neurological deficits take after thrombosis or embolism obviously depends on the vessels principally affected. It is now recognised, however, that much variation occurs from one individual to another, and that partial and incomplete syndromes are extremely common. The following can, however, be diagnosed with reasonable confidence.

Occlusion of the main trunk of the *middle cerebral artery* leads to a contralateral hemiparesis and sensory loss of cortical type, often with hemianopia due to involvement of the optic radiation. When the more distal parts of the artery are affected alone the weakness mainly involves the face, arm and hand. Dysphasia is common in dominant hemisphere lesions, and agnosic syndromes and body image disturbances with non-dominant hemisphere lesions. Infarction of the deep territory of the middle cerebral artery, which includes the posterior limb of the internal capsule, leads to a dense and global hemiplegia.

Mesulam *et al.* (1976) drew attention to the states of mental confusion which can follow middle cerebral infarctions on the right, sometimes leading to diagnostic difficulties in that focal signs may consist of little more than left-sided cortical sensory loss and visual inattention. A toxic or metabolic cause for the acute organic reaction had often been suspected in their patients. Salient features were inattentiveness to relevant stimuli and inability to maintain a coherent stream of thought or behaviour. Disorientation, anomia, incontinence, an abnormal gait and lack of concern for the illness were characteristic. An example was as follows:

A 61-year-old man was discovered in an incoherent agitated state, banging on doors and shouting in the night. He was disoriented in all spheres, very distractible, and with a severely diminished span of attention. His speech contained paraphasic errors and there were difficulties in naming objects. Gait was unsteady and he was incontinent and unkempt. Over the next few days the agitation gave way to an amiable placid state, but the incoherence and impaired attention span persisted for several weeks. Angiography showed occlusion of the right angular branch of the middle cerebral artery.   (Mesulam *et al.* 1976)

Infarctions in the distribution of the *anterior cerebral artery* lead to contralateral hemiparesis affecting the leg more severely than the arm. There may be a grasp reflex in the hand. Cortical sensory loss and motor dysphasia are often present as well. Mental changes may resemble those of a global dementia and incontinence may be a prominent feature. Residual personality changes of frontal lobe type may occur. Involvement of the penetrating branch which supplies the anterior limb of the internal capsule (Heubner's artery) leads to paralysis of the contralateral side of the face and arm, often with sensory loss of spinothalamic type in the contralateral limbs.

Occlusion of the *internal carotid artery* can be entirely asymptomatic, emerging as a chance finding at autopsy. If the circulation should fail, infarction occurs principally in the territory of the middle cerebral artery, though the distribution of the anterior cerebral artery may be involved as well. Much depends on the efficiency of the collateral circulation and the patency of the circle of Willis. The common 'watershed infarct' lies at the borderland of the major arterial territories—a sickle-shaped zone on the lateral surface of the hemisphere (Fisher 1968). The resulting clinical picture is often indistinguishable from that of middle cerebral infarction. A common tell-tale sign is monocular blindness, fleeting or permanent, in the eye contralateral to the hemiplegia, due to interruption of blood flow in the ophthalmic or retinal arteries. Evidence of the source of infarction may also be obtained by noting a bruit over the bifurcation of the common carotid, loss of pulsation unilaterally in the neck, or decreased retinal arterial pressure on the affected side. An ipsilateral Horner's syndrome may result from involvement of the sympathetic fibres in the carotid sheath.

Sometimes mental symptoms may predominate with general slowing, decreased spontaneous activity, dyspraxia and incontinence, all pointing to a frontal lobe deficit. If the abruptness of onset and fluctuation in the symptoms is not appreciated, the nature of the lesion may not be detected, as in the following example reported by Fisher (1968):

A man of 68 had shown a change of personality for some 4 months, consisting of selfishness, overeating and impoliteness, combined with clumsiness, falling, spilling food, episodic difficulty in speaking and urinary incontinence. On examination he stared vacantly into space, spoke in a quiet voice, forgot quickly and was clumsy in all his movements. There were elements of dysphasia, both hands were dyspraxic, and he broke spasmodically into tears. Angiography showed left carotid occlusion but this was felt to be irrelevant. He died suddenly, however, and autopsy revealed an extensive watershed infarct in the left hemisphere.

The main effect of *posterior cerebral artery* infarction is a contralateral hemianopia, sometimes with visual hallucinations, visual agnosias or spatial disorientation. Visual perseveration may consist of a train of objects repeating within the affected field, or persistence of an image in the centre of the field after the object is removed (Caplan 1980). Alexia without agraphia occurs when damage has affected the dominant occipital lobe along with the splenium of the corpus callosum (p. 50). Involvement of the perforating branches to the thalamus and brain stem may lead to a contralateral thalamic syndrome or mild contralateral hemiparesis and cerebellar ataxia. Bilateral infarctions may lead to cortical blindness, sometimes with conspicuous denial of disability (Anton's syndrome).

Adams and Hurwitz (1974) stressed that psychological disturbances are frequent with posterior cerebral infarctions. Transient mental confusion may be the only manifestation apart from a hemianopia which is difficult to demonstrate. Amnesic syndromes may also figure prominently when the hippocampus and other limbic structures are involved bilaterally on the inferomedial surfaces of the temporal lobes (Victor *et al.* 1961; Benson *et al.* 1974). The question of whether amnesia can occur after strictly unilateral infarctions in the posterior cerebral territory is reviewed by Benson *et al.* (1974), likewise the problem of whether amnesia can ever be the sole manifestation. Both are questions which cannot be answered decisively.

Strokes in the distribution of the *vertebrobasilar system* are extremely diverse in their manifestations. The vertebrals unite to form the basilar artery which in turn feeds the posterior cerebral arteries; from this system perforating branches supply the brain stem and cerebellum.

Total occlusion of the basilar artery is usually rapidly fatal with loss of consciousness, a decerebrate state and quadriplegia. Partial occlusions of the system, with infarctions in the territory of individual branches, can lead to a multitude of pictures. The hallmark is brain stem involvement, with bilateral or unilateral pyramidal signs and a variety of ipsilateral cranial nerve palsies. Ipsilateral cerebellar deficits may also be present. Common signs therefore include weakness or paralysis of one or all four limbs, long-tract sensory deficits which may be contralateral to the hemiparesis, diplopia, pupillary changes, Horner's syndrome, facial numbness, vertigo, unilateral or bilateral deafness, dysarthria, dysphagia, cerebellar ataxia and visual field defects. Major obstacles to recovery include disturbances of balance and persistent dizziness. Intellectual processes are usually little if at all affected.

The various pictures of coma, decerebration and akinetic mutism which may follow brain stem infarction are described by Plum and Posner (1972). One rare but striking picture is the so-called 'locked in' syndrome which follows a circumscribed infarction affecting the descending motor pathways in the ventral part of the pons. This is compatible with full wakefulness and alertness, despite aphonia and total paralysis of the limbs, trunk and lower cranial nerves. Such patients are responsive and sentient, although their repertoire of responses may be limited to blinking and jaw and eye movements. Feldman's (1971) patient was able to learn to employ blinks and eye movements, using Morse code, to communicate with those around her, displaying preserved memory and appropriate awareness of her environment.

Caplan (1980) reviews further striking pictures with prominent behavioural change following occlusion of the rostral branches of the basilar artery (the 'top of the basilar' syndrome). The result is infarction in the midbrain, thalamus and portions of the temporal and occipital lobes, producing an array of visual, oculomotor and behavioural abnormalities. Motor dysfunction can be minimal, leading to difficulties with diagnosis. The remarkable syndrome of *peduncular hallucinosis* (p. 388) consists of vivid, well-formed hallucinations, sometimes confined to a half-field of vision and occurring with or without visual field defects. The hallucinations are recognised by the patient as unreal despite their dramatic nature. Caplan's patient saw a parrot in beautiful plumage to the right, and pictures of a relative flashed on the wall to the left. Others have reported vivid hallucinations of animals, of children at play with toys, fleeting images of the head of a dog or intricate lines and colours lasting for an hour or two at a time. States of *bizarre disorientation* accompanied by somnolence may likewise reflect disturbance in the rostral portions of the brain stem reticular formation. In response to questions one patient said she was lying on a beach at Nice, another that she was speaking to friends on the telephone. Such answers, entirely divorced from the current reality, may appear as an extraordinary form of confabulation. Other patients may dream excessively, with inability to distinguish the dreams from reality. Oculomotor disturbances and pupillary abnormalities will usually betray the origins of such abnormal mental states.

Lacunar infarcts

The syndromes associated with lacunar infarcts are outlined by Fisher (1982b) and Gautier (1983). Very small lacunes may be asymptomatic, but those 0.5–1.5 cm in diameter are likely to produce deficits, especially when situated along the corticobulbar–spinal–motor system or long sensory tracts. Lacunes in the posterior limb of the internal capsule or pons may lead to a pure motor hemiparesis, those in the posterolateral thalamus to a pure sensory stroke. Others are associated with ataxia, dysarthria and a variety of cranial nerve palsies. The deficits resulting from lacunar infarcts are usually slight and recover rapidly, but the effects of successive small lesions may sometimes be cumulative, leading eventually to dementia and pseudobulbar palsy as described on pp. 384 and 454.

Transient cerebral ischaemic attacks

Vasospasm was formerly invoked to explain short-lived attacks of hemiparesis, dysphasia or other neurological disturbance, though clear evidence for such a basis was not forthcoming. Attacks of this nature were commonly recurrent, with complete recovery between episodes, yet leading ultimately in a proportion of cases to a full-blown stroke.

Such episodes are now designated transient ischaemic attacks (TIAs) and the mechanisms behind their occurrence are more clearly understood (Russell 1983). The feature common to all is a temporary reduction of the blood supply to a small area of the brain, long enough to cause manifest loss of function but not enough to lead to clinical signs of infarction. Nevertheless abnormalities by way of focal parenchymal changes are seen in up to a third of cases on CT scanning and in up to 80% with MRI (Perrone et al. 1979; Salgado et al. 1986). In some cases the reduction in blood supply is occasioned by temporary occlusion of vessels, and in others by reduction of flow while the patency remains unimpaired.

The occlusive variety appears mainly to be due to microemboli derived from extracranial sources in the heart or great vessels. Atheromatous plaques on the wall of the internal carotid artery itself are frequently the source. The emboli may consist of platelet aggregates, cholesterol or small fragments of thrombus which come to lodge in small end-arteries within the brain. In other cases haemodynamic factors are essentially responsible and emboli cannot be blamed. Thus a sudden fall in cardiac output, or systemic hypotension due to any cause, may compromise flow in vessels already critically narrowed by atherosclerosis. Occasionally the flow is reduced by kinking of the carotid artery on rotation of the head, or by compression of the vertebrals by osteophytes associated with cervical spondylosis. Sometimes the responsible lesion is an occlusive or stenotic lesion of the subclavian artery proximal to the origin of the vertebrals, leading to 'stealing' of blood from the vertebral distribution. The blood pressure is then found to be different in the two arms and a bruit may be detectable in the supraclavicular fossa. Anaemia or polycythaemia may be background factors facilitating the development of attacks.

Clearly a multitude of factors may be responsible and require careful investigation in every case. The tendency for the same vascular territory to be involved in successive attacks is explained in the haemodynamic group by the sites of maximal atheroma in cerebral vessels. In the embolic group the predilection for certain territories may rest on the fact that flow in vessels appears to adopt a uniform laminar pattern, so that emboli entering the circulation at a particular point will tend to follow the same route to their eventual destination.

TIAs are commonly very brief, most lasting less than an hour and some for a few minutes only. By definition the maximum period allowed is 24 hours. They may occur at frequent intervals over days, weeks or months, or alternatively as isolated and widely spaced attacks over many years. After a number of attacks complete resolution becomes less likely and increasing deficit is liable to develop. The symptoms produced are extremely variable depending on the territory of the brain which has been rendered ischaemic. A broad division may be made into those implicating the territory of the internal carotid and its branches, and those involving the areas of supply of the vertebrobasilar system.

TIAs in the carotid territory typically show contralateral pareses, paraesthesiae, hemianopias or dysphasia, sometimes with transient blurring or even episodes of total blindness in the ipsilateral eye (amaurosis fugax). Microemboli may actually be observed in the retinal arteries on ophthalmoscopy in such cases. Motor impairments may take the form of a brief monoparesis involving only part of a limb. Transient numbness of the face or arm is a common variety. Mental confusion may occasionally be marked, and in some cases the recurrent motor and sensory symptoms are merely the more dramatic part of a picture which contains other evidence of accumulating frontal and parietal lobe damage (Adams & Hurwitz 1974). Relatives may have noted signs of deterioration in intellect, memory and personality as the attacks continue. Alvarez (1966) similarly stressed the mental deterioration which could follow in the wake of 'little strokes', presenting numerous case vignettes of people who lost their efficiency and ability over the years, gradually becoming untidy, irascible and difficult to live with. Only a careful history could trace this change to a sudden point in time when some 'dizzy spell' or transient neurological deficit had been declared, often recurring thereafter as the deterioration progressed.

Vertebrobasilar TIAs present with a multitude of pictures. Spells of vertigo, tinnitus or diplopia are typical. Episodes of paresis or numbness may involve different sides of the body in successive attacks. Drop attacks are commonly attributable to such a cause in the elderly—the person falls abruptly to the ground without loss of consciousness then can rise immediately—as a result of acute and transient failure of the antigravity muscles. Sometimes a staggering ataxia may be combined with dysarthria and drowsiness, leading to an impression of drunkenness. Visual phenomena include blurred vision, altitudinal or homonymous hemianopias, or scintillation scotomata. Transient bilateral blindness may occur where both posterior cerebral arteries are implicated.

TIAs may at first be mistaken for epileptic seizures, migraine, simple faints, labyrinthine disease or the early symptoms of cerebral tumour. They may be so slight and transient as to be overlooked entirely. It is important, however, that the significance of the symptoms should be recognised as early as possible so that appropriate investigation and treatment can be started.

Follow-up of such patients has shown that they have an increased risk of developing a frank cerebral infarction or myocardial infarction (Russell 1983). The risk of stroke is particularly high in the first month after the first TIA, but remains markedly elevated throughout the following year. It then declines, but remains higher than in the normal population, perhaps indefinitely. The presence of an obstructive or ulcerative lesion in the carotid artery increases the risk considerably. There is some evidence that the prognosis is relatively benign when vertebrobasilar symptoms have been confined to vertigo, disturbed vision, diplopia or drop attacks (Marshall 1964).

Carotid endarterectomy has an important role in the prevention of later infarction when stenosis of the carotid is more than mild in degree. Auscultation may reveal a bruit over the artery but this is insufficient guidance of itself. Non-invasive methods such as Doppler ultrasound or MRI imaging are useful as screening tests, but angiography will usually be required before a decision is taken over operation. Intra-arterial digital subtraction angiography (IADSA) will often be preferred over conventional angiography. Vertebral angiography carries special hazards in this situation and is usually contraindicated. For patients not amenable to surgery anticoagulants may be indicated, or treatment with drugs such as aspirin to reduce platelet aggregation. The study by the SALT Collaborative Group (1991) showed the efficacy of 75 mg aspirin per day in reducing the risk of stroke or death after TIAs or minor stroke. Attention may need to be directed to hypertension, anaemia, polycythaemia, diabetes, episodes of cardiac dysrhythmia or other aspects of heart disease.

Sequelae of stroke

The disablement resulting from strokes is frequently an admixture of physical and mental problems. The latter may be attributable directly to the brain damage sustained, or largely represent the individual's reaction to the handicaps imposed upon him. In either event the patient's personality make-up and life situation can have a profound effect on overall adjustment to the disability, and the mental components of the picture will often be decisive in determining the level of success achieved in rehabilitation. It is therefore unfortunate that relatively little attention has been directed at the problem of the psychiatric aftermaths of strokes, and of the ways in which these interact with the physical disabilities. The studies of Adams and Hurwitz, discussed below, were important exceptions in this regard, and have highlighted the practical value of paying due regard to matters other than the purely physical sequelae (Adams & Hurwitz 1963, 1974; Adams 1967; Hurwitz & Adams 1972). The more recent findings concerning post-stroke depression and its associations are discussed on pp. 385–6.

In what follows an attempt will be made to review the principal components of psychiatric disability after stroke, but first the question of overall prognosis will be considered. The general picture of the incidence of defects and quality of survival provides the framework against which to view the range and extent of the problems encountered.

Overall prognosis

Marquardsen (1969) analysed the mortality and long-term morbidity of 769 patients admitted to hospital with acute cerebral infarcts and haemorrhages. The immediate mortality was high, almost half dying within the first 3 weeks. Of the 407 survivors 52% were restored to independence and self care, a further 15% were able to walk unaided but required some assistance with personal needs, and the remaining 33% failed to achieve independence in either walking or self care. Factors indicative of a poor prognosis for functional recovery were age over 70 years, extracerebral complications and indices of the extent of cerebral damage such as severe motor deficit, conjugate ocular deviation, prolonged impairment of consciousness, incontinence and persistent confusion or apathy.

Improvement in motor function usually continued for several months. Contrary to general belief, patients with right hemisphere lesions fared less well than patients with left-sided lesions in terms of recovery of independence; the accompanying visuospatial and allied difficulties appeared to provide a greater handicap to rehabilitation than dysphasia. Patients who survived after brain stem lesions did somewhat better than patients with hemisphere strokes, presumably because of the absence of cortical deficits.

At 1 year after the stroke two-thirds still had residual hemiplegia, a quarter had substantial mental impairment and 40% had other cerebral symptoms such as dysphasia, vertigo or cranial nerve palsies. Residual hemiplegia was the main problem in approximately half, a third were mainly handicapped by other cerebral symptoms including dementia, and in most of the remainder the clinical picture was dominated by cardiac disabilities such as angina or dyspnoea. Very few were entirely symptom-free.

Follow-up showed further cerebrovascular accidents in a third, occurring at a mean interval of 3 years after the primary stroke. Recurrent epileptic convulsions developed in 6%. Forty-six per cent had died within 3 years compared to an expected 12% for the general population. The principal causes of death were cardiac failure, bronchopneumonia, recurrent stroke, myocardial infarction, pulmonary infarction and uraemia.

Thus it appeared that the majority of strokes appeared merely as incidents in the progress of a generalised vascular disorder, either atherosclerotic or hypertensive vascular disease, the extent of which essentially determined the long-term prognosis. The realistic goal of rehabilitation was usually not re-employment but independence in self care and domestic resettlement. Of the younger patients in employment at the time of the stroke only a third were able to return to work.

Marquardsen's survey was based on patients admitted to hospital. Gresham *et al.* (1975) traced 123 survivors of cerebrovascular accidents from a large community-based study, and compared them with controls matched for age and sex. The mean age at which the strokes had occurred was 64, and the mean interval to re-examination 7 years. Eighty-four per cent of the stroke survivors were living at home, 80% were independent in mobility and 69% were rated as independent with regard to activities of daily living (compared to 97%, 95% and 92% of controls, respectively). Sixty-two per cent showed decreased socialisation compared to 31% of controls. Comparisons with controls showed in each case significantly greater disability than would be expected from age alone; but the differences were less than might have been anticipated on account of the widespread functional limitations accruing from other causes in the elderly population.

Cognitive impairments

Deficits in cognitive function are among the more serious of the sequelae of stroke, delaying and often gravely compromising attempts at rehabilitation. Such elements in the clinical picture may be less immediately obvious than the hemiplegia or other physical handicap, yet often prove to be the factors which are responsible for failure to regain independence. Thus among patients who become long-stay invalids, permanently confined to chair or bed, paralysis by itself rather seldom accounts for their incapacity and may even contribute little towards it (Adams & Hurwitz 1963, 1974).

In a review of 45 bedfast hemiplegics, Adams and Hurwitz (1963) showed that physical disability, such as dense paralysis or limited exercise tolerance, accounted for failure in less than half. In 18 patients severe residual paralysis and sensory defect were accompanied by varying degrees of generalised intellectual impairment and a correspondingly high rate of incontinence. Failure to respond to treatment seemed to derive from impaired comprehension, difficulties in communication, inattentiveness and lack of spontaneous effort. They were frustrated by perseveration and could not assimilate or retain instructions. Insight into their illnesses had been lacking in the critical early months. Most of these infarctions had occurred in the distribution of the middle cerebral artery of the dominant hemisphere. Ten further patients showed neglect of the affected limbs or even denied that they were in any way abnormal. Some disowned their hemiplegic limbs or complained of bizarre changes within them. The latter had at first given a superficial impression of alert and responsible behaviour, which was later belied by defective grasp, inattentive lapses and persistent incontinence. Seven were mainly incapacitated by postural imbalance which had often led to profound loss of confidence. Other patients showed severe receptive dysphasia, apraxia of gait or emotional disturbance with catastrophic reactions.

The mental impairment that may follow a single stroke usually proves to be focal in nature once the initial clouding of consciousness has cleared. For some time, however, global confusion and disorientation may be much in evidence, and can be slow to clear when the cerebral damage has been extensive. It may be aggravated by anoxia from congestive cardiac failure or respiratory infection, or be attributable in part to the patient's difficulty in coping with new-found barriers to communication with his environment. As the situation improves the true extent of cognitive dysfunction is revealed. The longer clouding of consciousness has persisted the more likely will it be that residual mental deficits are severe and extensive.

Considerable difficulty may be encountered in assessing the extent of global intellectual impairment, particularly if the patient is dysphasic or with marked constructional difficulties. Hurwitz and Adams (1972) suggest that sometimes the best early indication is an alert glint in the patient's eye, and the nurses' opinion that the patient is 'with it'. Agitation, depression or apathy in the early stages may give a false impression of dementia. Likewise behaviour resulting from visual disorientation or agnosic difficulties. A circumscribed amnesic syndrome due to posterior cerebral infarction may not at first be appreciated as such.

Much of our understanding of the classic focal cortical syndromes—the dysphasias, apraxias and body image disturbances—has come from studies of stroke survivors. The essentials of such disorders have been outlined in Chapter 2 and will not be recapitulated here. Disturbances of language accompany some two-thirds of right hemiplegias, or may be found without paralysis. They contribute a large added handicap and source of frustration, frequently outlasting recovery of motor function. Patients with expressive loss but good comprehension will in general make much better adjustment than when understanding is faulty. Apraxic disturbances may persist as a barrier to rehabilitation when motor paralysis has cleared, particularly an apraxia of gait. Thus occasional patients with dominant hemisphere infarction appear to make a quick recovery from hemiparesis, but fail to regain a normal pattern of walking and postural control; they shuffle shakily, tend to fall backwards and their feet seem to 'stick to the floor' (Adams 1967).

Disturbed awareness of the self or of space more commonly occurs after right hemisphere lesions than left. Neglect of the left half of external space may be accompanied by left sensory inattention, neglect or unawareness of body parts, or frank denial of disability. Occasionally, however, exceptions are found and such symptoms result from left hemisphere lesions leading to a complex admixture of deficits:

Welman (1969) for example reported a right-handed man who had a left parietotemporal infarction. This led to a right hemiplegia, aphasia for some hours, apraxia, hemisomatognosia and anosognosia for the right side of the body, left unilateral spatial agnosia, visual–constructive apraxia, left–right disorientation, loss of memory and finger agnosia in both hands.

The more florid aspects of anosognosia, involving verbal denial or disowning of paralysed limbs, usually subside over several weeks, but neglect and inattention may endure. After severe infarction in the non-dominant hemisphere a characteristic pattern may emerge, providing immense difficulties for effective rehabilitation—the patient has a dense hemianopia, hemiplegia and hemi-anaesthesia but lacks insight into his predicament, may admit to nothing wrong with the left limbs or disown the arm (Adams 1967). Sometimes this persists even after quite good recovery of power and the patient makes no constructive attempts to walk. Persistent incontinence is a common accompaniment, adding to the poor prognosis for recovery of independence and social functioning.

Improvement over time in specific cognitive and perceptual disabilities may be expected to follow the course of a decelerating learning curve, the percentage return of function gradually diminishing as time after stroke increases. In general most improvement can be expected within the first 6 months, but wide variation is seen. The influence of affective or motivational factors is often profound, delaying full recovery until several years have gone by.

A considerably longer period must usually be allowed for the optimal resolution of dysphasia and visuospatial or topographical defects than is allowed for physical disabilities such as hemiplegia. The ultimate level achieved will depend crucially on the amount of brain tissue destroyed, the number of separate deficits involved, and on the multitude of factors peculiar to the individual which dictate his adaptive capacity.

Dementia

Very occasionally dementia may follow a single strategically situated cerebrovascular accident (p. 453), but more usually it ensues on multiple strokes whose deficits combine together. Strokes within the dominant hemisphere, or which affect both hemispheres, are particularly liable to produce dementia, also those involving the thalamus (Ladurner et al. 1982). Where multiple strokes are involved each episode is accompanied by some further loss of mental ability, accruing over time in a step-like fashion to lead to a more or less global deterioration of memory, intellect and personality. This is the 'multi-infarct' form of dementia as described in Chapter 10. A careful history will usually make it evident that infarctions have occurred, from the tempo of events combined with episodes of neurological disorder. The latter, however, may be slight and transient, at least in the early stages, and the dementia will then emerge as the dominant symptom.

The *role of 'lacunar' infarcts* in producing dementia is discussed by Fisher (1965, 1968) and Cummings and Mahler (1991). The deficits resulting from each such minor stroke are often mild and recover rapidly, but as their number increases the effects may be cumulative leading to the so-called 'état lacunaire' with dementia and some degree of pseudobulbar palsy. The mental deterioration generally lags behind physical changes of weakness, slowness, dysarthria, dysphagia, a small-stepped gait and neurological evidence of bilateral pyramidal involvement. An associated normal-pressure hydrocephalus may contribute to the clinical picture (Fisher 1982b). Very occasionally, however, the dementia may emerge in a gradual fashion, resembling a primary degenerative dementia and without sudden infarcts to betray the minor strokes (Fisher 1968; Weisberg 1982). This is probably rare, though with increasingly sensitive brain imaging studies such patients are now being detected. If the history fails the neurological findings will usually be decisive. Weisberg (1982), however, has described a small group of patients with bilateral capsular lacunae and gradual mental deterioration who showed no neurological deficits whatsoever. Emotional lability with spasmodic laughing and crying also serves to make the differentiation from Alzheimer's disease, being rare in the latter but frequent in the lacunar state.

Dementia may result from *vascular lesions of the thalamus*, much as may occur with tumours in this location (p. 228). De Boucaud *et al.* (1968) reported an example with autopsy confirmation. The dementia was accompanied by disturbance of gait, but there were few clear neurological signs. Autopsy showed old haemorrhagic softenings in both thalami and the cortex was free from pathological changes.

Cases revealed by CT scanning were reported by Guberman and Stuss (1983) and Graf-Radford *et al.* (1984). Left thalamic infarction appears to cause more pervasive cognitive disturbance than right, and personality changes may be marked. Bilateral medial thalamic infarctions typically lead to a hypersomnolent apathetic state and vertical gaze disturbance, with dementia of the 'subcortical' type (p. 667). A Korsakoff-like amnesic state may also be seen.

The possible *role of caroticovertebral stenosis* in leading to dementia has also attracted attention. There have been hopes that surgical intervention on narrowed or occluded carotid arteries might help to remedy diminished blood flow to the brain, and thereby improve mental functioning, but results in general have been disappointing.

Thus Clarke and Harrison (1956), reviewing the cases of bilateral carotid occlusion in the literature, found that mental changes were encountered in almost a third, often taking the form of a progressive dementia. Neurological accompaniments such as hemiplegia or visual difficulties were frequent but often transient, and in the early stages neurological signs could be entirely absent. Fisher (1951, 1954) described examples of carotid occlusion associated with progressive cerebral deterioration, and cautiously proposed that sometimes this may have been the cause of the dementia rather than a coincidental finding.

Subsequent experience has shown that this is very unlikely. Stenosis or occlusion of the carotids is not uncommon in unselected series of autopsies of people past middle age (Schwartz & Mitchell 1961). And Corsellis and Evans (1965) demonstrated that when the entire vascular tree from the heart to the brain was examined, whether in demented or non-demented subjects, the cerebral and extracerebral vessels were usually found to be spared or to be involved in stenosis to roughly the same extent. Altogether there was little to suggest that structural interference with blood supply in the neck had any special or unique role to play in contributing to dementia. There also appeared to be little leeway for the re-establishment of improved cerebral circulation by operative procedures.

Present opinion is therefore that it is most unlikely that chronic marginal ischaemia from carotid stenosis can lead to a progressive deterioration resembling Alzheimer's senile dementia. When dementing symptoms are attributable to carotid occlusion infarctions will have occurred within the hemispheres, and there will almost invariably be motor and sensory signs to indicate the nature of the process (Fisher 1968).

Organic personality change

Personality changes attributable to brain damage are among the most troublesome of the sequelae of stroke, and may overshadow the intellectual deficits. Most are probably attributable to widespread vascular changes within the damaged brain, and as such they may progress even though the focal sequelae of the stroke improve. Usually they prove to be the prelude to a progressive dementing illness.

A woman of 69 had a very mild stroke affecting the left arm transiently. She seemed well for a while thereafter, but gradually changed, becoming irritable, hard to please and with vague complaints of headache and giddiness. She became anxious and did not want to be left alone. Loss of interests and slowing were accompanied by episodes of confusion and disorientation. On examination 15 months after the stroke she was not grossly demented, but showed some difficulty in understanding questions and had only a vague idea of the date. There was a residual left hemiparesis, a left homonymous hemianopia, some dyscalculia and a mild nominal dysphasia. Her affective state was, however, worse than her intellect — she was mostly apathetic and dull, though cheerful in a facile way at times. Eventually she needed long-term hospitalisation.   (Slater 1962)

Slater (1962) outlined the range of problems encountered. Typically one sees a 'reduction of margins'. The patient cannot adjust to new circumstances, and small matters make him anxious, irritable or depressed. Consciously or unconsciously he avoids new experiences and restricts himself to an unvarying routine. The barriers this can impose to rehabilitation are obvious. Confrontations with a task or with social demands carries the risk of provoking a catastrophic reaction. The patient may become irritable, abusive and uncooperative if asked to make any effort, yet be affable and obliging when left in peace.

Minor bodily ills are apt to be felt as oppressive, and hypochondriacal concern may centre around sleep or the bowels. The picture may bear a deceptively neurotic appearance until evidence of cognitive impairment is detected. Constitutional predispositions may also be revealed or accentuated: a previously lonely person may become suspicious or frankly paranoid, or cyclothymic tendencies may have issue in frank depression.

At a later stage the emotional state is recognisably abnormal, with dulled and flattened responsiveness, marked irritability and emotional reactions which are stereotyped and lacking in flexibility. The patient is unmoved by pleasure or dismay where the interests of others are concerned, but if his own security is threatened the emotional reaction is severe and prolonged. These changes may be in evidence for some time, hindering rehabilitation and providing a considerable burden for relatives, before more decisive evidence of failing memory and impoverishment of thought supervene.

Depression

It is scarcely surprising that depressive reactions should be common in survivors of strokes. Ullman (1962) vividly describes the subjective impact which the experience may have. The patient finds himself abruptly in the grip of something novel, frightening and ill understood. He may well not be in a position to evaluate the situation objectively, but may project the blame outwards or alternatively against himself. Even slight interference in free communication with those around will greatly intensify feelings of isolation, threat or loss.

When the acute stage is over there are a variety of factors around which depression may come to be organised — the frustrations of physical handicaps, uncertainty about the prospects of their resolution, the enforced dependency and imposition of the invalid role. In the longer term the patient may face loss of job and status, financial insecurity, a sense of uselessness or the prospect of permanent loss of independence. Robinson and Price (1982), in a survey of 103 patients attending a stroke clinic, found that one-third were depressed, the majority remaining so for at least 6 months. The peak incidence of depression was in the period 6 months to 2 years after the stroke had occurred. Considerably lower rates than this were reported by House et al. (1991) from an Oxfordshire community-based sample, where depression was only moderately increased in comparison to age-matched controls and the excess had largely disappeared by 12 months. The difference probably reflects lower rates of physical disability in the Oxfordshire sample and their relatively good socioeconomic status.

The reaction to the situation will also be strongly determined by aspects of the premorbid personality. Patients of striving and self-sufficient disposition may react more adversely to handicap than those with strong dependency needs. Those who have experienced anxiety and depressive reactions under previous stress will be at increased risk. Much will also depend on the family setting and relationships with which the patient is surrounded. Quite frequently, at the era of life in which most strokes occur, the patient is relatively unsupported — the spouse may have died or be infirm, and children will have moved away.

Others may experience depression of an 'endogenous' type, sometimes precipitated by strokes of a relatively minor nature and persisting after excellent recovery from the more immediate disabilities. Complaints of difficulty with memory and concentration, and inability to take up the threads of life again, may then give a false impression of the severity of residual brain damage. Insomnia, feelings of hopelessness and hypochondriacal concern over minor handicaps may greatly retard the resumption of normal activities.

Interesting evidence has now emerged to suggest that there may be a special relationship between strokes and depression, depending at least in part on the effects of the cerebral lesion itself. Thus stroke patients have been found to show a higher incidence of depression than orthopaedic controls or patients suffering from traumatic brain injuries, despite equivalent levels of disability in terms of 'activities of daily living' or cognitive dysfunction (Folstein et al. 1977; Robinson & Szetela 1981). Moreover the location of the infarction may be a significant factor. Left hemisphere strokes appear to result in significantly more depression than right hemisphere or brain stem strokes (Robinson & Price 1982; Robinson et al. 1984); and within the left hemisphere the proximity of the lesion to the frontal pole has proved to be an influential factor (Robinson & Szetela 1981; Lipsey *et al.* 1983; Robinson *et al.* 1984). This has been shown to apply both with cortical and basal ganglia lesions (Starkstein *et al.* 1987). In effect, left anterior brain lesions seem to produce more depression than lesions in any other location, at least in the early post-stroke phase.

It has been suggested that this may be related to the anatomical disposition of monoamine-containing pathways in the brain, which pass from subcortical centres through the frontal cortex *en route* to their diffuse projections elsewhere. Related animal experiments have demonstrated differential effects on brain biochemistry according to the laterality of the lesion. After right middle cerebral artery ligations noradrenaline concentrations fall in both cerebral hemispheres, whereas left middle cerebral ligations produce no such change (Robinson 1979; Robinson & Coyle 1980). This, however, would appear to run counter to the laterality effects observed with post-stroke depression in humans.

Evidence, employing ^{11}C-methylspiperone and PET to detect cortical S_2-serotonin receptor binding, is more persuasive in indicating differential effects between left and right hemisphere strokes. Right, but not left, hemisphere strokes were associated with an increase in 5-hydroxytryptamine (5-HT) receptor binding in uninjured regions, which may have served to prevent or ameliorate depression. With left hemisphere strokes this was not observed, and a relationship could be discerned between 5-HT levels and the severity of the depression encountered (Mayberg *et al.* 1988). In a single patient study, Mayberg *et al.* (1991) demonstrated a 25% increase in 5-HT binding in the left temporal cortex during the course of recovery from depression (without medication) following an infarction of the left basal ganglia.

The importance of lesion location in relation to depression has been supported in some though not all subsequent investigations. Proximity of the lesion to the left frontal pole was related to severity of depression in samples studied by Sinyor *et al.* (1986), Eastwood *et al.* (1989) and Morris *et al.* (1992), but no overall effect of laterality of lesion was observed. House *et al.* (1990b) found no strong relationships to location of lesion in the Oxfordshire community sample during the first year after stroke. Sharpe *et al.* (1990) showed that size but not location of the infarct was strongly related to depression in patients examined 3–5 years later. The other main determinants at this stage were female sex and levels of functional impairment, also greater age, residence in an institution and absence of close personal relationships (Sharpe *et al.* 1994). The importance of social support has been underlined by Morris *et al.* (1991).

Thus it appears that lesion location plays some part, among a complex set of other determinants, in contributing to depression after stroke. It seems, moreover, that it may be an especially important factor in the early months following the infarct. With the passage of time, social and interpersonal factors become increasingly important in determining the affective state and may then obscure the effects of lesion location *per se*. Possible reasons for the discrepancies among the different investigations to date are likely to include differing levels of physical and cognitive impairment, pre-existing brain damage and a host of psychosocial variables in the samples studied, in addition to the time elapsed since the stroke occurred.

The importance of recognising the depression need scarcely be stressed. On occasion this can be difficult, especially when the development has been insidious. Sometimes it is masked by stoical attitudes, or absorbed into habitual or automatic patterns of behaviour. It may lead to lack of cooperation or poor motivation for rehabilitation, and aggravate dysphasic and similar difficulties. In all such circumstances appropriate treatment can be quickly rewarding. It is important, however, to distinguish depressive disorder from simple loss of confidence, or from the emotional lability associated with intellectual impairment. It is also necessary to remain sensitively aware that sometimes, in severely disabled patients, feelings of resignation and futility are realistically based; some elderly patients really are so frail, and the odds so genuinely against them, that their wish 'not to bother' deserves to be treated with proper respect. Needless to say this is an aspect of differential 'diagnosis' which requires the utmost care.

Attention has recently been drawn to another aspect of differential diagnosis by Förstl and Sahakian (1991). Three patients were described who were admitted to hospital with supposed major depression, exhibiting severe psychomotor retardation, weight loss, exhaustion and self reproach. All had evidence of infarcts or atrophy in the left frontal lobe, and SPECT scanning in two showed left frontal hypoperfusion. The shared clinical feature was abrupt improvement under hospital care, with relapse to extreme lack of initiative and energy on discharge to the home environment. Such cycles were followed repeatedly, with the patients neglecting to eat or drink and spending most of their time at home in bed. It was suggested that this may represent a specific syndrome of extreme abulia (i.e. lack of will) consequent upon left frontal pathology. The profound disturbance of motivation induced by the brain damage appeared to respond to the structured hospital regime, but to relapse in the context of the more permissive home environment.

Pathological emotionalism

A heightened tendency to cry, often uncontrollably and with little warning, has traditionally been attributed to pseudobulbar palsy resulting from bilateral lesions of the corticobulbar tracts. In such a setting the crying may occur with little or no provocation. Recent studies, however, have shown that the disorder has broader connotations, and that it is not uncommon as an embarrassing and disabling aftermath of strokes.

House *et al.* (1989) followed up 128 patients who had suffered a first-ever stroke, and examined them specifically for heightened emotionalism. The criteria were that the patient should experience an increase in episodes of crying (or more rarely laughing), with little or no warning, and with an inability to control them. The term 'pathological emotionalism' was preferred to 'emotional lability' or 'emotional incontinence' as a more accurate description of the phenomenon.

At 6 months, 21% of patients reported such symptoms and at 12 months, 11%. All showed crying as the principal problem, but two had episodes of pathological laughter in addition. In most the disorder had set in during the 4–6 weeks following the stroke, with a tendency to ameliorate over the following year. In virtually all patients the episodes were provoked by emotional stimuli of a sad or sentimental nature—thoughts of illness or death, distressing pictures on television, visits from grandchildren or expressions of greeting or concern. In half the tearfulness was provoked at interview by enquiry about the symptom.

The patients as a group scored higher on indices of depression than the remainder, but they were also more intellectually impaired and showed more extensive lesions on CT scans. A special relationship appeared to obtain with lesions in the anterior left hemisphere, and patients with such lesions showed longer-lasting disorder. The observation that the emotionalism was usually appropriate to the patient's feelings and emotional context, while being associated with special characteristics of the lesion, suggested that it should be viewed as a form of disinhibition — a loss of ability to suppress a response at low levels of stimulation.

Allman (1991) reported an analysis of the phenomenon in 30 post-stroke patients. Complete lack of warning was uncommon, and the majority had some degree of control over the crying. The most common precipitants were thoughts about the family or the illness, expressions of sympathy or visitors arriving or departing. Five of the 30, however, reported episodes for which no precipitant could be identified. With regard to subjective mood, over half described feeling sad and miserable when crying, a quarter were unable to describe their mood and the remainder felt no change.

Drug treatment with antidepressants or levodopa can help with severe examples of the disorder as described on p. 392.

Psychoses

There are no figures against which to gauge the incidence of psychotic illness after cerebrovascular accidents. A depression of psychotic intensity may be provoked in susceptible subjects, as mentioned above. Hypomanic pictures have also been reported (van der Lugt & de Visser 1967), and from the data presented by Starkstein *et al.* (1988) may be expected to be commoner after right hemisphere strokes than left. They reported 12 cases of mania after a variety of brain lesions, seven being restricted to the right hemisphere, one to the left, and four with bilateral or midline damage. Of the four strokes in this series, two were in the right hemisphere, one in the left and one was a right thalamocapsular bleed. The episodes of mania often followed the strokes within days or weeks.

A remarkable example of bipolar affective disorder following thalamic infarction was described by McGilchrist *et al.* (1993):

A 43-year-old man with mild hypercholesterolaemia and indications of autoimmune dysfunction experienced an episode of transient loss of consciousness, followed by drowsiness and left-sided pyramidal signs for 24 hours. Thereafter he appeared to have undergone a marked change of personality, becoming apathetic, dulled and fatuous, and eating and sleeping excessively. At intervals of 3 weeks or so he would suddenly become alert, excitable and elated for about 36 hours, then relapse to his former condition. The picture was sufficiently bizarre to suggest at one time that he might be malingering.

When referred for a second opinion 18 months later he was histrionic and tearful, smiled incongruously and had poor self esteem. He was profoundly apathetic and self care was poor. He complained that he was like 'an engine that won't tick over'. CT scanning revealed bilateral thalamic infarcts, and a SPECT scan showed severe hypoperfusion of both frontal lobes. Psychological testing showed poor performance on a visual memory task and impaired frontal functioning on the Trail Making and the Cognitive Estimates tests. While in hospital he showed two episodes of elation lasting for several days, the second being frankly manic with pressure of speech, flight of ideas and possibly auditory hallucinations.

It was concluded that the thalamic infarctions had led by 'diaschisis' to metabolic hypofunction in the frontal lobes, resulting in the abrupt onset of cyclical mood disorder accompanied by features of frontal lobe dysfunction.

Davison and Bagley (1969) reviewed the evidence concerning the relationship between psychotic disorder and cerebrovascular disease. There was some suggestion that late-onset schizophrenia might be significantly associated with cerebral atheroma and its complications, but there was insufficient information on which to base firm conclusions. Davison and Bagley also mentioned reports of paranoid–hallucinatory syndromes developing shortly after cerebrovascular catastrophes. One such example, at first thought to be a 'functional' illness but later recognised as organic, was reported by Shapiro (1959) in association with carotid artery occlusion:

A woman of 60 developed a psychosis of acute onset, with hallucinations and delusions that people were saying she had married her husband for his money. She was hypertensive but showed no abnormal neurological signs. Improvement occurred with eight electroconvulsive treatments, and she became normal for a week, but then relapsed with confusion and a return of hallucinations. She developed a transient left hemiparesis, and angiography showed right carotid occlusion. Two days later she died, and at autopsy bilateral carotid occlusions were revealed.

Levine and Finklestein (1982) have noted an apparent relationship between cerebrovascular lesions of the right hemisphere, specifically of the right temporoparieto-occipital areas, and the development of psychotic illnesses some time later. Eight patients were described, with the psychoses appearing some weeks or years after the stroke. All but one had developed seizures in the interim which may have been a connecting factor. The psychoses developed acutely, with formed auditory and visual hallucinations; the majority of patients showed agitation, persecutory delusions and confusion, but in some the hallucinatory phenomena were relatively pure. All had constructional apraxia, and most showed a variety of other neurological residua. The right-sided location in every case may have reflected the freedom from dysphasia, allowing the psychoses to be revealed, or alternatively may have reflected the predisposing effects of spatial disabilities in leading to environmental misinterpretations. Rabins *et al.* (1991) have confirmed the importance of right hemisphere infarctions for the development of post-stroke psychoses in five further patients, also the likely role of seizures in their genesis. Pre-existing subcortical atrophy appeared to be an additional risk factor.

Hallucinosis, in which the patient retains insight into the unreal nature of the hallucinated material, has traditionally been related to lesions in the midbrain and pons—the 'peduncular hallucinosis' of Lhermitte (1922, 1932) described on p. 379. Such hallucinosis can occur in the visual or auditory modalities, is typically complex and vivid, and usually resolves within days or weeks. The midbrain lesion responsible has been demonstrated on MRI (Geller & Bellur 1987), and cases have been reported with lesions restricted to the reticular portion of the substantia nigra (McKee *et al.* 1990). Other patients have shown lesions in the thalamus (Feinberg & Rapcsak 1989;

Serra Catafau *et al.* 1992). Starkstein *et al.* (1992) suggest that hallucinosis of this nature is related to damage involving primary sensory pathways and the reticular activating system. Lhermitte (1922) stressed the similarity between the nature of the images perceived and those experienced during dream activity, and proposed that disturbances of the sleep–wake cycle might be important for their development.

Other psychiatric sequelae

Other significant developments include a variety of psychological reactions which may greatly impede convalescence and prove an enormous burden to relatives. An accentuation of paranoid traits is common. Some patients develop rebellious aggressive attitudes and unwillingness to conform to medical regimens and treatment, others become hostile, vindictive and spiteful (Rees 1961). The predominant factor will usually lie in the patient's response to his disabilities, often aggravated or brought to the fore by the brain damage that has occurred.

In a careful follow-up of patients, House *et al.* (1991) stressed the importance of persistent agoraphobia and social withdrawal in a small proportion of cases. Such developments were often associated with fear of looking conspicuous on account of disabilities, or fear of recurrence provoked by physical activity. Tension, worry and lack of energy were common complaints.

Two main channels into which irrational modes of adaptation may flow are unrealistic strivings for independence and unrealistic dependency (Ullman 1962). Thus the patient may attempt to deny his limitations and refuse the provision of simple aids. Or an overzealous, impatient attitude may interfere with progress. Others, by contrast, regress considerably and succumb to invalidism to an unnecessary degree. Here a profound loss of confidence may be the essential ingredient, or there may be elements of secondary gain. Manipulative tendencies may be effective within the family circle because of the feelings of guilt they arouse. In this way the patient may evade responsibilities and exploit his disabilities, perhaps protesting against dependence while renouncing many of the things he could do for himself.

Psychological problems can be severe when the life situation is profoundly altered as a consequence of the stroke. Many important sources of gratification, pleasure and interest may be lost both for the patient and other family members. There are often far-reaching domestic upheavals, particularly in younger patients—the wife may need to work and the husband adjust to a new domestic role. Marital problems may come to the fore, with rejection by the spouse. Sexual sequelae, commonly impotence in the face of continuing desire, can have highly distressing repercussions.

Many components will therefore enter into the success or failure of the adaptation which is made to the sequelae of stroke, and will combine to determine the change of life pattern that follows. Ullman (1962) provides case histories which illustrate the social, psychological and physical variables which can contribute to the final adaptive response on the part of the victim and his family.

Rehabilitation after stroke

The management of the acute phase of stroke is a matter for the medical and neurological team, an integral part being attention to differential diagnosis and the mounting of appropriate investigations. Thereafter skilled nursing care is of the utmost importance. Steroids may have a part to play in reducing cerebral oedema, but vasodilator drugs are of uncertain value (Hutchinson 1983). Decisions may be required over anticoagulants; these find little place in the management of completed stroke, but can be of prophylactic importance in transient ischaemic attacks or when sources of emboli are discovered in the heart and great vessels. The use of low dosage aspirin as a prophylactic has a good deal of evidence to commend it in reducing the chance of further vascular events and death (SALT Collaborative Group 1991; Underwood & More 1994).

Correct management of hypertension is of great importance, and has been shown to be effective in reducing recurrence (Beevers et al. 1973). Even so antihypertensive therapy must be carried out with care. When the evidence points to infarction rather than haemorrhage it will usually be prudent to defer any lowering of blood pressure at least until the acute phase of the stroke is over.

Operative intervention may be considered in certain circumstances. Carotid endarterectomy can play an important preventive role in carefully selected patients (p. 381), and extracranial–intracranial bypass operations have had enthusiastic advocates. Their value in preventing further ischaemic attacks or strokes, or in ameliorating existing deficits, requires on-going appraisal (Browse 1983).

Further details of medical management are summarised by Hutchinson (1983) and Wade et al. (1985). Here attention will be restricted to the longer-term problems of rehabilitation which must be tackled once the acute phase is over. Three stages can usually be envisaged in the process of recovery—2 weeks concerned with survival, 8–12 weeks of effort to restore activity and independence in standing, walking and self care, then often 2 years more before the full capacity of the patient to participate in normal social activities is realised (Hurwitz & Adams 1972).

The processes of recovery are largely spontaneous and usually slow. Rehabilitation implies efforts aimed at promoting recovery and the optimal utilisation of residual functions (Isaacs 1973). The mechanisms underlying such changes over time are undoubtedly complex and incompletely understood. In part there would appear to be transfer of lost functions to unaffected brain areas, reorganisation within the brain to allow other areas to contribute more (pp. 377–8), and perhaps removal of inhibitory influences from elements which are still intact. Key structures such as the anterior horn cells may improve in their ability to modify the influences playing upon them. Better utilisation of unaffected body parts will help with substitute performances.

Rehabilitation in any extensive sense requires a multidisciplinary team. It may proceed in the hospital, the home or specialised rehabilitation units, depending on circumstances and the severity of the problems involved. Proper liaison among the different persons in the team is essential for success, also adequate continuing care when the patient returns home.

Isaacs (1971) offers a useful practical guide to the planning of rehabilitation by classifying stroke disability into four principal categories—motor deficit alone, major disorder in communication, major perceptual disorder and major cognitive disturbance. Among 115 patients in his series, 23 showed a motor deficit alone, 43 a major disorder of communication with or without perceptual or cognitive disturbance, 31 major perceptual disorder without disturbance of communication, and 18 major cognitive disturbance without perceptual or communication deficits.

Motor deficits require physiotherapy from the earliest stages. Voluntary movements should be encouraged while the patient is still confined to bed, and a full range of passive movements will help to prevent contractures and joint immobility in the affected limbs. Exercises in standing and balancing from the early weeks aim to achieve a correct postural background for the walking exercises which follow. These must often be pursued over many months in an atmosphere of constant encouragement. Fundamental to success is the gradual restoration of the patient's self confidence, and hence his motivation to help himself further.

The occupational therapist will concentrate on matters of fine motor control, particularly in the upper limbs. Restoration of function after hemiplegia is commonly much less complete in the arm than the leg, so that patients with excellent mobility remain at risk of dependence on others. Re-training may be needed for activities of daily living—how to dress, feed, wash and cook despite the handicaps that persist. The provision of simple mechanical aids can be of immense help in restoring capabilities which would otherwise be lost. A graded occupational therapy programme is thus a further important boost to morale.

Sensory handicaps gravely complicate rehabilitation, particularly sensory impairments in paralysed limbs. Loss of position sense which persists after the early weeks carries a bad prognosis in hemiplegic patients, and may need special training under visual and tactile control. Constant emphasis is required on the existence and position in space of the limbs. Cortical sensory loss, with defective discrimination, adds to difficulties with fine manipulations of the fingers.

Hemianopic or quadrantic field defects tend to resolve with time, or the alert patient learns to compensate for them. In the early stages, however, or when there is mental impairment, care must be taken to approach the patient from the sound side, and to arrange the disposition of belongings and work materials accordingly. A tendency to ignore the left half of space may be a greater barrier, contributing to falls and mishaps and hindering mastery of a new environment.

Refractive errors or defective hearing must not be overlooked as remediable sources of additional difficulty.

Disturbed body awareness can provide a serious obstacle to progress when long continued. Persistent denial or disowning of hemiplegic limbs carries an especially poor prognosis for recovery of independence, and is often accompanied by prolonged incontinence. Neglect, disuse or seeming unawareness of paralysed limbs must therefore be countered by stimulation and exercises. Repeated testing of the limits of what can and cannot be done may help to rectify the situation, and the incontinence may respond to careful training regimes. Nevertheless, it would seem to be deficits such as these which make an important contribution to the poorer overall prognosis of right hemisphere strokes than left, even despite the absence of dysphasic difficulties.

Communication disorders warrant close and early attention. The dysphasic patient has lost not only the ability to speak but also his primary means of relating with those around. Once communication is re-established, however small in degree, the patient's frustration and fear begin to diminish.

In addition to inducing feelings of isolation language difficulties play a central role in impairing other aspects of progress. The patient may have lost the means of stabilising internally the events which are occurring around him, and will be at a grave disadvantage in relearning other patterns of behaviour and activities (Hagen 1969).

Without personal understanding of the requisite goals it will be hard for him to muster and sustain effort towards those goals.

A first aim must be to establish emotional contact with the patient, using whatever channels of communication are most intact. Pictures may be used with which he can indicate requests, even though he cannot read or speak. Cards with words or short phrases may be useful later on. Gestures or visual signs may be employed when verbal understanding is very poor, coupled with one or two concrete words but avoiding a confusing flow of speech. Later in recovery instructions must be carefully spaced, given slowly, and as far as possible in the same manner on each occasion. Thus a special approach is needed from all the staff. Every attempt must be made to avoid withdrawal after early failures, to keep the patient involved and active, and to stimulate a continuing desire to communicate.

Formal speech therapy has rarely been rigorously tested, which is surprising in view of the magnitude of the problem. Whether the final level achieved exceeds that which would have occurred spontaneously is uncertain, but few doubt the effects of retraining programmes on emotional adjustment and morale. Butfield and Zangwill (1946) obtained some evidence that training begun early was more effective than that begun late, and that predominantly expressive dysphasias did better than receptive or mixed dysphasias. Speech fared better than reading or writing, and mathematical ability did particularly badly. Darley (1982) and Enderby and Emerson (1996) review other attempts to gauge the efficacy of retraining programmes, sometimes with results suggesting that measurable gains are attributable to therapeutic intervention.

The role of the speech therapist is outlined by Leche (1972) and Wade *et al.* (1985). After establishing the range of the deficits, re-education must aim at maximising spontaneous recovery, sustaining incentives and preventing the development of undesirable speech habits. Throughout the process the patient is reassured to know that his difficulties are understood, and his own attention is focused constructively upon them. Later, group therapy can have an important part to play, also the counselling of relatives about optimal means of overcoming the communication problem.

Impairment of memory must be specially catered for with a more gradual programme, frequent rehearsals and the provision of props and supports by way of notes and written instructions. The relative preservation of old memories may initially produce a misleading impression until ability to acquire new knowledge is specifically tested.

Strategies for assisting in memory retraining include the use of mnemonic devices such as first-letter cueing, rhyming strategies, visual imagery, or 'motor coding' whereby a movement is associated to a name to be remembered. Where multiple items are to be remembered these may be 'pegged' to a standard list of words, or to standard loci such as body parts or rooms within a house. Embedding the items in a brief manufactured story can be particularly effective. Other more general techniques concentrate on organising the study of material to be learned, chunking information into subsets and breaking down new skills into a series of steps. Such matters are reviewed by Wilson and Moffat (1984), Wade *et al.* (1985) and Wilson (1982, 1987), including attempts to assess their efficacy in patients following stroke.

Other intellectual impairments are a serious barrier to progress when at all extensive. Ill-sustained attention, perseveration, fatiguability and failure to grasp instructions may combine to render attempts at rehabilitation fruitless. To maximise the chances of success, verbal instructions must be presented in simple language with deliberate methodical repetition. Practical demonstrations of what is expected may get the ideas across when other methods have failed. The pace will necessarily be slow, and allowance must be made for variability in performance from day to day.

Much ingenuity is obviously required in devising special methods of treatment to counteract these various obstacles to recovery. It is here that the studies of Hurwitz and Adams were particularly valuable in drawing attention to the 'mental barriers' which may impede progress and which can all too easily be overlooked. Defective comprehension, impaired memory, apraxia, loss of sensation and disturbed body awareness may not be appreciated as such, and the patient's failure is attributed simply to inadequate motivation or to generalised dementia. The patient seldom has the insight to appreciate or complain about such difficulties himself, so they must be sought out with care by systematic examination. Adams (1967) reported remarkably improved results in the rehabilitation of hemiplegics after routinely searching for barriers of this nature. Whereas 42% of an earlier series regained independence in self care and walking, 59% of a more recent series did so. Thirty-eight per cent of the former remained chronic invalids compared to 26% of the latter.

Motivation itself is, nevertheless, among the most crucial determinants of progress and every means must be taken to optimise and maintain it. The day-to-day enthusiasm and encouragement of the therapeutic team is an essential ingredient, and the patient's own awareness of progress then plays back to reinforce it. All through the programme, proper communication must be maintained so that he is aware of the plans and goals at every stage.

A watch must be kept for evidence of depression, which will commonly respond to appropriate medication. Tactful handling may be required in the face of discouragement, withdrawal or obstinacy. Clear guidelines must sometimes be drawn up, especially for patients with intellectual impairment who will benefit from a structured environment. By contrast, flexibility must be built into the programme to allow for patients with differing needs and personalities. Rigid conformity to set standards cannot always be expected, and in some persons will be counterproductive.

Attention must also be devoted to the relatives of the patient. They too will need full discussion of aims and procedures, and help in adjusting to the disabilities that are likely to remain. Careful physical rehabilitation may be doomed to failure if insufficient attention has been given to the family situation and to the impact of the problem on family members. Here the social worker has a vital part to play, and should be brought into the picture at an early stage. Much time may be needed to allay unrealistic expectations or needless anxieties and fears. The stroke and its repercussions may have had a far-reaching effect on many members of the household, disturbing the family equilibrium and requiring a reorganisation of roles. The range of the problems encountered, and the value of counselling in surmounting them, are illustrated by de la Mata *et al.* (1960), Collins (1961), Overs and Healy (1973) and Holbrook (1982).

Preparations for discharge must be made well in advance, on a practical as well as an emotional level. The patient's assets and liabilities must be carefully assessed, likewise the family and community resources available to help. Physical adaptations may be needed in the home by way of ramps or simple supports. Proper liaison will be required with local authority and voluntary services. Where work is being considered, extended evaluation and retraining will often be indicated. Sheltered employment may need to be found when the patient is too disabled to cope on the open market.

In older patients, and those severely disabled, attendance at a day centre or social centre may need to be organised. Transport problems in particular will need attention. For those who remain at home every effort must be made to combat feelings of loneliness and isolation, by building new contacts, encouraging a return to hobbies and mobilising community resources.

Sadly, some patients will need to remain in institutions, usually by virtue of extensive mental impairments in addition to their neurological defects. Others will have complicating pathologies, such as heart disease or arthritis, which have conspired to make effective rehabilitation impossible. Here nursing care and occupational therapy will be required long term in order to maintain a reasonable quality of life. Adequate stimulation must be ensured, with routines that are as varied and congenial as possible. Psychotropic medication will occasionally be required to combat anxiety and depression.

The effectiveness of antidepressants in relieving poststroke depression has been documented (Lipsey *et al.* 1984). Tricyclic antidepressants have also been shown to be remarkably effective in patients who develop 'emotional incontinence' with pathological laughing and crying, whether or not this is associated with other features of pseudobulbar palsy (Lawson & MacLeod 1969). Even in the absence of subjective depression such medication can apparently alleviate the disruptive and socially embarrassing effects of the disorder. Udaka *et al.* (1984) have reported similar success with levodopa. In patients with pathological emotionalism due to other causes, such as multiple sclerosis, these medications can also be effective (Wolf *et al.* 1979; Schiffer *et al.* 1985).

Subarachnoid haemorrhage

It is estimated that subarachnoid haemorrhage makes up some 5% of cerebrovascular catastrophes. It is particularly important in that it affects a younger age group than other strokes, and because correct management can substantially reduce mortality. Since the site of origin of the haemorrhage is often demonstrable on angiography, and the ensuing brain damage is commonly localised, the mental sequelae have attracted detailed attention. Moreover the pictures which are produced are less liable than with other strokes to be contaminated by the effects of diffuse cerebrovascular disease.

The usual cause is rupture of an intracranial aneurysm, estimated to account for some 60% of cases. A smaller group derive from ruptured angiomas (5–10%). In 15–20% no structural cause for the bleeding can be found, and it is in this group that hypertensive crises due to monoamine oxidase inhibitor drugs may occasionally be to blame. During a 2-year period Villiers (1966) found 16 patients who had developed subarachnoid haemorrhage while taking monoamine oxidase inhibitors. It was estimated that 3.3% of unexplained subarachnoid haemorrhages occurred in patients on such drugs, the ingestion of cheese or other tyramine-containing foods commonly being the precipitant. Rare additional causes include bleeds from intracranial and spinal tumours, blood dyscrasias or inflammatory conditions of the brain and meninges. Others represent primary intracerebral or cerebellar haemorrhages which have bled into the ventricular system and thereby reached the subarachnoid space.

Aneurysms arise from congenital defects in the media, usually at the forks of the cerebral arteries. The great majority arise close to the circle of Willis at the base of the brain. Common sites are on the anterior cerebral or anterior communicating arteries, at the point of division of the middle cerebral arteries, or where the posterior communicating artery arises from the upper end of the internal carotid artery. Another common site is on the intracavernous part of the internal carotid, but this more often leads to local pressure effects than to subarachnoid haemorrhage (p. 412). Rupture occurs spontaneously and suddenly, with bleeding directly into the subarachnoid space and often into the adjacent brain substance as well. Spasm of adjacent vessels may lead to infarction in their territories of supply.

Anterior communicating aneurysms lie between the frontal lobes and near to the anterior hypothalamus. Rupture is often unaccompanied by localising signs, but ischaemia can be extensive in one or both frontal lobes due to occlusion or spasm of the anterior cerebral arteries. Middle cerebral aneurysms lie in the Sylvian fissure or embedded in the frontal or temporal lobes nearby. Rupture is often accompanied by hemiparesis due to vascular spasm in the territory of the middle cerebral artery or by haematoma formation. Posterior communicating aneurysms lie medial to the uncus of the temporal lobe. They often bleed directly into the subarachnoid space, but infarction can be widespread in the territory of the middle cerebral arteries, and there may also be interference with the fine perforating vessels to the basal ganglia and hypothalamus.

Whatever the site of the bleed, vasospasm may develop focally or diffusely, involving vessels near to or distant from the site of rupture. Local vasospasm leads to evanescent symptoms, but widespread involvement carries a grave prognosis.

(Saito *et al.* 1977)

Acute clinical picture

The patient is usually between 40 and 60 though cases can be seen at an early age. The onset is abrupt with intense, often catastrophic pain in the head, mainly in the occipital region but radiating into the neck and later becoming generalised. Vomiting, photophobia and fits may occur. Consciousness may be lost from the outset though some patients retain full awareness throughout. Others are drowsy, confused and irritable. Sometimes the mental symptoms overshadow the headache to such an extent that the diagnosis is not immediately apparent. Walton (1956) mentioned three patients who had been accused of drunkenness at the onset, and two who were regarded as hysterical on first admission to hospital.

Neck stiffness generally becomes intense. The tendon

reflexes are diminished and the plantars extensor. Papilloedema may develop immediately or within a few days, and subhyaloid haemorrhages may be observed spreading from the edges of the optic discs. Focal ophthalmoplegias are common, and aphasia or hemiplegia may result from arterial spasm or intracerebral extension. Lumbar puncture shows uniformly bloodstained cerebrospinal fluid, usually under increased pressure, becoming xanthochromic after 36–45 hours. CT scanning performed within a week of the bleed may obviate the need for lumbar puncture by demonstrating the presence of blood in the cerebrospinal fluid directly (Moseley 1981). Any intracerebral bleeding is usually clearly shown. Small aneurysms will often escape detection on CT, but are better shown on MRI (Jenkins et al. 1988). MRI can be particularly valuable in the identification of arteriovenous malformations, and in this respect may render angiography unnecessary.

Immediate bed rest is mandatory with sedation and analgesics. Early treatment with nimodipine, a calcium channel blocker which acts preferentially on cerebral vessels, has been shown to decrease the important complication of delayed cerebral ischaemia with subsequent infarction (Drug & Therapeutics Bulletin 1992a). A recurrence of the bleed is particularly likely during the first 2 weeks and the risk diminishes considerably thereafter.

The delicate questions of timing of angiography and the relative virtues of early versus late operation are discussed by Maurice-Williams (1987). Untreated, 65–70% of patients may be expected to die within a year, 35–40% from rebleeding. Eighty per cent of rebleeds will occur within a month. Operative mortality with proper selection of patients has fallen over the past 30 years from 20–30% to 5–10%. The techniques available include occlusion of the neck of the aneurysm or the feeding vessels, reinforcement of the wall by muslin or acrylic compounds, or ligation of the common carotid artery in the neck. Complications such as intracerebral haematomas may need surgical treatment in their own right.

Coma persisting for more than 24 hours is a bad prognostic sign. With modern management some two-thirds of patients may be expected to survive a first bleed, though a third of survivors will be left with some major neurological disability. In patients with no aneurysm demonstrable on angiography the mortality and morbidity rates are considerably lower.

Psychiatric sequelae of subarachnoid haemorrhage

Mental symptoms in the wake of subarachnoid haemorrhage received remarkably scant attention until Walton (1952, 1956) emphasised their importance as a source of persistent disability. Among 120 survivors, examined 2–11 years later, he found that important residua included paresis in 10%, epilepsy in 13% and persistent headache in 23%; also organic mental symptoms in 9% and anxiety symptoms in 27%. The anxiety was occasionally severely disabling, resulting in chronic psychiatric invalidism.

Subsequently two large series of patients were reported with attention directed primarily at the psychiatric sequelae. Storey (1967, 1970, 1972) studied 261 patients who had had a subarachnoid haemorrhage 6 months to 6 years earlier, noting the site of the responsible aneurysm and correlating this with the psychiatric aftermaths. Eighty-one patients had bled from anterior communicating aneurysms, 71 from middle cerebral aneurysms, 72 from posterior communicating aneurysms and seven from multiple aneurysms, while in the remaining 30 no aneurysm could be detected. Logue et al. (1968) confined attention to 79 survivors of haemorrhages from anterior cerebral aneurysms, studied 6 months to 8.5 years later.

Both studies confirmed the high incidence of mental disablement among survivors, especially as a result of organic mental impairments and personality change attributable to brain damage. Rather surprisingly both also stressed that improvement in personality could occur in occasional survivors, mainly evident to relatives but sometimes also to the patients themselves.

Cognitive impairments

Severe confusion and states of akinetic mutism can be seen in the early stages of recovery. Most are transient, but when substantial brain damage has occurred there may be enduring cognitive sequelae. These range from mild difficulties with memory to gross and disabling dementia. Focal dysphasic symptoms may be prominent.

Storey (1967) found persistent intellectual difficulties in about 40% of patients as judged by simple clinical criteria. They were rated as moderate to severe in some 10% of cases, and occasional patients remained grossly demented and bedfast. Those with middle cerebral aneurysms fared considerably worse than other groups, while patients with no demonstrable aneurysms had the lowest morbidity of all. Logue et al.'s (1968) patients with anterior cerebral aneurysms showed 10% with global dementia but many more with minor persistent deficits. Forty per cent showed dysphasic errors on detailed testing. Memory was often more impaired than intelligence, perhaps by virtue of the close proximity of these anterior aneurysms to the base of the third ventricle.

Intellectual impairment when severe is usually associated with other evidence of residual brain damage by way of neurological deficits. Occasional examples may owe their origin to the development of normal-pressure hydrocephalus (p. 744), as a result of obstruction of the flow of cerebrospinal fluid by organisation of exudate at the base of the brain. Considerable improvement may then result from shunting procedures.

Amnesic syndromes

A picture resembling Korsakoff's syndrome may emerge shortly after the haemorrhage, with disorientation, confabulation and marked memory difficulties. Tarachow (1939) and Walton (1953) recorded several examples, often developing after a latent interval of several days or weeks. The disorder was temporary in all of their cases, usually recovering gradually over a few weeks, but occasionally with abrupt resolution overnight. It was hard to explain the syndrome on the basis of focal brain damage because of the frequent latent interval and the examples of abrupt recovery.

Theander and Granholm (1967), reviewing 56 survivors of subarachnoid haemorrhage, demonstrated communicating hydrocephalus in five, four of whom had had severe dysmnesic syndromes lasting months or years. Intraventricular pressure was normal, and three of the four improved remarkably on shunting. It is therefore possible that some of the earlier transient examples may have been due to similar mechanisms. The latent interval may have been attributable to the time required for the development of adhesive arachnoiditis, and the subsequent improvement to the eventual freeing of the cerebrospinal fluid circulation. In Theander and Granholm's cases, by contrast, the obstructions had become permanent and required operative intervention. The dramatic success achieved is indicated in the following example:

A 57-year-old woman had a subarachnoid haemorrhage, and on recovery of consciousness showed signs of severe cerebral injury with disorientation. She was transferred to a home for the chronically sick. At examination 3 years later she was bedridden with contractures of the hips and knees—lively, talkative, almost euphoric, but completely disoriented in time and place. She could not remember having fallen ill and was unaware of her disease. Air encephalography showed severe hydrocephalus due to obstruction of cerebrospinal fluid circulation in the basal cisterns. A shunt operation produced rapid improvement. She became fully orientated and her ability to add to her store of new memories became virtually normal. An amnesic gap persisted, however, for the 3 years between the bleeding and the shunt. Extensive orthopaedic treatment and rehabilitation eventually allowed her discharge home.   (Theander & Granholm 1967)

A distinct group would seem after all to owe their amnesia to focal brain damage, particularly after rupture of anterior communicating aneurysms. Transient confabulation was noted in almost a quarter of Logue et al.'s (1968) cases, and two striking examples of enduring memory difficulties have been reported after operative intervention on aneurysms in this location (Sweet et al. 1966; Talland et al. 1967):

Preoperatively both patients had been confused and apathetic, but immediately postoperatively they showed severe disorientation, nonsensical confabulation, some retrograde and virtually complete anterograde amnesia. The disorientation improved considerably within a few weeks, and at the same time their confabulation changed from fantastic fabrications to temporal misplacement of actual incidents. Over the next 3 years the memory disorder became chronic, together with impotence and lack of initiative. The lesions seen at operation had involved the posteromedial aspects of the orbital surface of both frontal lobes and the adjoining medial surface of the hemispheres—the so-called septal region in front of the lamina terminalis and anterior commissure. The crucial region was thought to lie in the septal region bilaterally.

Lindqvist and Norlén (1966) reported similar amnesic syndromes in 17 of 33 patients after operations on anterior communicating aneurysms. Eleven improved markedly within 6 months, but five appeared destined to be permanent. The memory disorder was accompanied by elevation of mood, indifference and apathy, and even in those which resolved there was sometimes persistent emotional shallowness.

It seems hard to escape the conclusion that operative intervention may play a part in the development of such changes, especially from some of the case histories presented by Lindqvist and Norlén. Gade (1982) has reported persistent amnesic syndromes very much more commonly after 'trapping' than after ligations confined to the neck of anterior communicating aneurysms. 'Trapping' involved ligatures placed on the anterior communicating artery on either side of the aneurysm, thus depriving blood supply to the fine perforating branches which supply structures along the anterior wall of the third ventricle — regions known to be implicated in memory functions.

Personality changes

Personality deterioration after subarachnoid haemorrhage usually has an obvious organic stamp and occurs in a setting of intellectual impairment. Prominent changes include loss of drive and vitality, decreased interest and initiative, withdrawal, irritability and easily provoked anxiety. Emotional lability and catastrophic tendencies may be marked. Storey (1970) described a picture of 'organic moodiness' with chronic shallow depression, often lifting in response to some new stimulus but rapidly falling back again with boredom, loss of interest and easy fatigue. Changes reminiscent of the frontal lobe syndrome may occur, with uninhibited selfish behaviour, tactlessness, elevation of mood and a decreased tendency to worry. Some of these latter aspects can be construed as improvements in personality as discussed below.

Personality impairment was rated as moderate or severe in 19% of Storey's patients, and mild in 22% more. It was most common after rupture of middle cerebral aneurysms, and in general the incidence paralleled that of intellectual impairment and neurological disability. The exception was a significant tendency for anterior communicating aneurysms to show relatively less intellectual impairment in the presence of personality deterioration. Descriptions of uninhibited behaviour, lessened worry and lessened irritability were commoner with anterior aneurysms than other groups, lending support to the classic idea of a frontal lobe syndrome. Logue et al. (1968), in a factor analysis of symptoms, similarly found a relatively independent component of elevation of mood and reduction of anxiety which could occasionally occur without anything by way of intellectual impairment.

Improvement in personality was noted by relatives in 13 of Storey's patients, eight after bleeds from anterior aneurysms. The same was seen in nine of Logue et al.'s patients. In both series, therefore, approximately 10% of patients with anterior bleeds showed a favourable outcome of this nature. Storey's patients were described as being more pleasant to live with, less sarcastic and irritable, less anxious and fussy, and often more affectionate and tolerant. Most were aware of increased well-being subjectively. The majority had previously been tense, perfectionistic or inhibited. Two who had been gloomy and readily fatigued became cheerful, vigorous and lost their tension headaches. Another lost compulsive rituals of long standing. Two of the 13 showed minor forgetfulness, but in the remainder there was no detectable intellectual impairment. None showed loss of drive or fall-off in work ability.

By contrast Logue et al. found that a price was usually paid for the improvements, in terms of memory impairment or an increase in irritability or outspokenness. The improvements consisted mainly of a decreased tendency to worry or get depressed. In three patients there was relief of a pre-existing endogenous depression, and another showed virtual relief of an obsessional neurosis.

Both Storey and Logue attributed the improvements to a 'leucotomy effect' consequent upon frontal lobe damage or ischaemia.

Anxiety and depression

Walton (1952) emphasised anxiety symptoms in 27% of his cases, half with premorbid neurotic tendencies and half without. The anxiety was often severe and incapacitating, centring largely on fear of recurrence of the haemorrhage. Some patients were afraid for months afterwards to leave the house, or retired to bed immediately they had a headache. In some instances the situation had been worsened by medical advice to avoid exertion.

Storey (1972) found symptoms of anxiety or depression in a quarter of patients, being moderate or severe in 14%. Such symptoms showed an association with indices of brain damage, but depression could also be severe when there was no evidence of brain damage whatever. The depressives without neurological signs had been more neurotic and prone to depression in their premorbid personalities, while those with brain damage had more often been energetic and were therefore perhaps reacting to their losses of function. The patients in whom aneurysms had not been detected appeared to form a special group, with a similar incidence of depression to the remainder despite considerably less evidence of intellectual impairment or neurological disability. Depression was commonest of all, and more liable to be severe and persistent, in patients with posterior communicating aneurysms, where rupture is known to interfere with the fine perforating vessels to the hypothalamus.

Other disturbances

'Neurasthenic' symptoms can occasionally be marked with fatigue, headache, dizziness and sensitivity to noise. These were persistent and incapacitating in seven of 56 patients followed by Theander and Granholm (1967), and present in mild degree in many more. Their origin was obscure and showed no relation to the duration of loss of consciousness. Walton (1952) commented on the general similarity between such symptoms after subarachnoid haemorrhage and after head injury.

Psychotic developments appear to be rare. Silverman (1949) reviewed occasional examples, and reported a patient of his own who became paranoid for several weeks despite normal orientation. Walton (1953) observed paranoid developments in two patients, one in association with a Korsakoff syndrome. Storey (1972), however, found no examples of psychosis among 261 patients who were studied closely from the psychiatric point of view. One of his patients developed schizophrenia a year later, but the illness seemed unrelated to the haemorrhage.

Emotional precipitation of subarachnoid haemorrhage

Occasional examples are reported of cerebrovascular accidents which show a striking temporal relationship to emotionally stressful events. The question has attracted some interest, since the development of a stroke at a given point in time may well depend on general circulatory as well as local occlusive processes. Ecker (1954) regarded a high proportion of his cases as having some special emotional stress immediately preceding their strokes. In Ullman's (1962) series there were occasional cases where the stroke was closely associated with an unusual and deeply disturbing life event, for example in a woman who had just returned from visiting her son who was being held on a charge of homicide, and in another on the night before being admitted to hospital for a mitral valvotomy which she dreaded. Adler *et al.* (1971), in a retrospective study, found that strokes typically occurred during a period of sustained or intermittent emotional disturbance which had been going on for weeks or months, and which sometimes had become intensified shortly before the stroke occurred.

The most dramatic instances, however, appear to involve patients with subarachnoid haemorrhage. Particularly striking examples have been recorded by Storey (1969, 1972) in which the haemorrhage followed immediately upon some emotionally traumatic event, presumably by virtue of the rise of blood pressure engendered. Thus a woman answered the door to a policeman who told her that the woman next door, her closest friend, had hanged herself—she said 'Oh, my God' and forthwith had her haemorrhage. Another woman was watching television when an aeroplane on a test flight was shown exploding in the air; she believed (erroneously as it turned out) that her son was on it, put her hands to her head and had the haemorrhage within seconds of the disaster. Another had a subarachnoid haemorrhage within a minute of being told by her husband that he knew of her adultery and was going to divorce her.

Altogether Storey found evidence of a striking emotional precipitant in four of his original 261 patients, and two further less dramatic examples. All were in women, although 43% of the series were male. Such precipitation appeared to be markedly more common in patients with no obvious source for the haemorrhage than in patients with aneurysms demonstrable on angiography. A history

of affective disorder antedating the haemorrhage was also more common in the non-aneurysm cases.

Exploring this further, Penrose and Storey (1970) carried out a blind prospective study by interviewing the relatives of 56 patients admitted with subarachnoid haemorrhage before the results of angiography were known. Significantly more emotional disturbance immediately antedating the haemorrhage was confirmed in the patients with normal angiograms. A standardised life events schedule also showed a significant increase in the number of upsetting life experiences during the 3 weeks prior to haemorrhage in patients without aneurysms (Penrose 1972).

The reason for a greater incidence of emotional precipitation in patients with normal angiograms is intriguing and not immediately clear. Part of the explanation may be that they are less often engaged in physical activity at the onset than are patients who bleed from aneurysms, or they may represent persons with unusually labile blood pressures and unusual reactivity to emotional traumas.

Mention must finally be made of two patients described by Engel (1972) in whom there was an astonishing conjunction between the timing of subarachnoid haemorrhage and antecedent events:

A 17-year-old boy collapsed and died at 6 a.m. from a ruptured aneurysm of the anterior communicating artery. Exactly 1 year earlier his brother had died at 5.12 a.m., a few hours after a car crash. The family had heard the boy stirring in his room around 5 a.m., earlier than he normally arose.

In the second case a man of 46 had his subarachnoid haemorrhage on the same date and in the same hospital as his father, who had died of a subarachnoid haemorrhage when 46 after a quarrel with the patient who was then a boy of 15. The patient had felt himself impelled to provoke a quarrel with his own teenage son on the day prior to his own subarachnoid haemorrhage.

Hypertension

Hypertension attracts psychiatric interest on several grounds. First, there is the intriguing possibility that essential hypertension may owe its aetiology, at least in part, to psychological factors. The question of a relationship to stress, or of an association between hypertension and certain personality attributes, has therefore received a good deal of attention. Secondly, the more discriminating assessment of common 'symptoms' of hypertension, such as headache and fatigue, has shown that they appear often to arise secondarily to knowledge of the disorder, rather than being attributable to elevation of the blood pressure *per se*. Thirdly, clinical syndromes such as hypertensive encephalopathy may develop in the course of the disorder and present with marked mental changes. All of this is additional to the important role of hypertension in contributing to cerebrovascular disease and stroke which has already been considered.

Psychological factors in causation

The pathogenesis of hypertension remains elusive in the great majority of cases. Rather less than 10% of patients show some specific causative pathology such as chronic renal disease, renal artery stenosis or, more rarely, a primary adrenal disorder. In the remainder, with so-called 'essential' hypertension, there is probably multifactorial causation involving genetic and environmental factors. A model frequently proposed envisages such persons as unusually susceptible to vasomotor reactions resulting from a stressful environment, by virtue of inherited traits, intrinsic emotional instability or a hyperreactive peripheral vasculature. The frequent excessive rises of blood pressure so provoked lead on to changes in small blood vessels, and thereby to secondary humoral mechanisms originating in the kidneys and elsewhere which maintain the blood pressure at sustained excessive levels. Claims for including essential hypertension among the 'psychosomatic disorders' in this way merit close examination, in view of its high incidence and associated mortality. Two facets warrant exploration here—the relationship to stress and the predisposition in terms of specific personality features.

There is a wealth of evidence that transient rises of blood pressure accompany psychological stimuli and stress, as reviewed by McGinn *et al.* (1964). The relationship has been shown to be extremely sensitive, with short-lived rises accompanying such matters as telling a lie, discussing life problems or dealing with material of threatening significance. The problem is whether lasting elevation of blood pressure may be related to stress, and here the evidence is necessarily indirect. Chronically stressed animals may develop hypertension which persists for several months after exposure to the stressful situation. In humans, Graham (1945) observed symptomless hypertension in 27% of soldiers resting after a year in active field operations, with diastolic pressures over 100 mmHg which lasted for several weeks or months. Following the severe explosion in Texas City in 1947, diastolic hypertension was present in more than half of the patients observed, often persisting for 1 or 2 weeks or even longer (Ruskin *et al.* 1948). Cruz-Coke (1960) drew attention to possible cultural stress influences, showing that blood pressure levels were significantly raised in a subsection of the population of Lima who were in rapid cultural transition from a primitive society to the stress of 'Western'-type civilization.

An interesting model for exploring the question was utilised by Heine *et al.* (1969). They argued that persons who had undergone the emotional disturbance of an agitated depressive illness, severe enough to warrant electroconvulsive therapy, might be expected to show an irreversible increase of blood pressure on recovery, and that the levels would be proportional to the duration of distress. Examining 25 such patients, they found a significant correlation between the blood pressure on recovery and both the duration and number of spells of illness, thus confirming their hypothesis. It seemed unlikely from the data that the results could be explained by common genetic determinants for depression and hypertension, or that pre-existing hypertension had predisposed to the depressive episodes. It should be noted, however, that the levels of hypertension observed were relatively low in comparison with those of patients seeking treatment for raised blood pressure.

Direct approaches to evaluating stress in the lives of established hypertensive patients have rarely been undertaken on any comprehensive scale. Reiser *et al.* (1951) reported an uncontrolled investigation of patients entering the malignant phase of hypertension, and felt that a close chronological correlation could be observed with emotionally charged life situations occurring at the time. Others, however, have found no difference between hypertensives and controls with regard to preceding life events, in particular when community-based samples have been studied (Wheatley *et al.* 1975). Stressful occupations have been examined, sometimes with highly suggestive findings. Cobb and Rose (1973), for example, found that the incidence of hypertension at annual physical examination was many times greater among air traffic controllers than among second-class airmen whose jobs were considerably less stressful. Moreover, those controllers working with high traffic densities showed more cases of hypertension than those working at low densities, and developed the disorder at an earlier age.

Thus the sum total of evidence rather strongly suggests that stress may be related to the development of sustained hypertension in certain situations. It is not inconceivable that stress may operate in this way in the hypertensive population generally. It is therefore necessary also to examine whether those who fall victim to hypertension are in any way unusual in their constitutional reactivity to environmental or interpersonal stresses. This has involved studies of vasomotor reactivity and of certain personality features in hypertensive patients.

Emotionally stressful situations have been shown to produce higher rises in blood pressure in hypertensive than normotensive persons, both in absolute terms and as a proportion of the original level (Robinson 1963). This, however, could be a feature secondary to the hypertensive process itself rather than reflecting an innate tendency. Thus it seems to apply equally in renal and essential hypertension (Ostfeld & Lebovits 1958). 'Neuroticism', as a feature in the personality, has often emerged as high in hypertensives, and has connotations for emotional lability, emotional over-responsiveness and perhaps vasomotor reactivity. Here, however, there has been difficulty in deciding how far the association is causal, coincidental or secondary to knowledge of having the disorder.

Sainsbury (1964) found that hypertensives attending an out-patient clinic obtained high neuroticism scores on the Maudsley Personality Inventory, being similar to 'psychosomatic' groups but scoring significantly higher than non-psychosomatic patients. Robinson (1963) found similar evidence among hospital attenders, but in a community survey found little relationship between neuroticism and the level of the blood pressure. He concluded that patients attending hospital were open to special selection, probably by their general practitioners. Cochrane (1969) compared the neuroticism scores of patients discovered to be hypertensive by general practitioners with those discovered to be normotensive in the same practices, and found no difference between them. The hypertensives had virtually normal neuroticism scores. He suggested that the results in Sainsbury's and Robinson's out-patient surveys may have been partly due to the use of rauwolfia at that time, which may have led to artificially elevated responses on the neuroticism scale. Kidson (1973) compared hypertensive clinic attenders with persons randomly selected from industry and found to have elevated or normal blood pressures. On a range of personality measures the hypertensive patients were strikingly different from the non-patient subjects, with higher neuroticism, more insecurity, more tension and higher total scores for somatic discomfort on the Cornell Medical Index. But among the non-patient groups, hypertensives and normotensives were in most respects similar on psychological variables. Thus the 'neurosis' of the hospital attenders appeared more likely to be a reaction to knowledge of the disease, or a by-product of treatment, rather than representing a psychological precursor of the hypertensive process.

The lack of any innate relationship between psychological factors and raised blood pressure was strongly confirmed in the course of a large treatment trial for mild to moderate hypertension (Mann 1977, 1981, 1984). Psychiatric morbidity was assessed by means of the General Health Questionnaire in over 2000 persons attending screening clinics, before the blood pressure was taken. No significant differences emerged between the scores of those subsequently found to be normotensive or hypertensive. Interestingly, moreover, when trial entrants were followed over the first year of treatment their level of psychiatric morbidity fell in relation to normotensive controls; the evidence suggested that this was attributable to the support derived from regular clinic attendance rather than to more specific factors such as the effects of medication or control of the hypertension.

A specific personality attribute claimed to characterise hypertensive patients is the chronic inhibition of aggressive, hostile impulses. Alexander (1939) suggested that a central feature was their inability to freely resolve either of two opposing tendencies—passive dependent needs on the one hand, and overcompensatory aggressive impulses on the other. Such conflict was often brought to the fore by the culturally determined complexities of present civilisation. Saul (1939) similarly reported intense, chronic and unexpressed hostility in his patients, along with marked inhibition and anxiety over heterosexuality. These, however, were uncontrolled observations in patients selected for psychoanalysis. Mann's (1977, 1984) study, referred to above, has indeed indicated a precisely opposite tendency, with hypertensive patients showing more overt hostility and reduced self criticism when compared with normotensive controls. Altogether the evidence in favour of specific predisposing personality patterns must be judged as very slender.

We are left therefore with highly suggestive findings that stress may be important in the aetiology of hypertension, but with rather little to support the notion that personality attributes make a definite contribution. The factors which select out the peripheral vasculature, and hence the blood pressure, as the system to be affected remain to be determined.

Symptoms

The repeated finding that hypertensives attending out-patient clinics score highly on indices of neurosis, whereas those discovered in the community do not, must call into question many of the symptoms which in the past have been attributed to elevation of blood pressure. Robinson (1963) pointed out that many of the so-called symptoms of hypertension are similar to those of emotional disorder — symptoms such as headache, dizziness, fatigue, palpitations, insomnia, depression and anxiety. Of the patients who are sent to hospital with complaints of this nature, those with elevated blood pressure will often tend to be directed to medical clinics and those without to psychiatric clinics, yet in both groups the symptoms may be founded equivalently in anxiety.

Stewart (1953) made a careful comparison between

two groups of patients with hypertension of comparable severity—those who were unaware and those who were aware of the elevation of their blood pressure. Only 16% of the former had headache and only 3% complained of this spontaneously, compared with 74% of those who had knowledge of their hypertension. Most of the latter described it in terms characteristic of anxiety. It was only in a very small group that headache appeared to be attributable directly to the elevation of blood pressure, and these headaches closely resembled migraine in character. Robinson (1969) compared groups of patients attending their general practitioners, noting whether or not the blood pressure had been measured and whether this was high or normal. Again little evidence emerged for linking headache, or any other symptom, to elevation of the blood pressure *per se*.

Thus the present consensus of opinion is that hypertension is essentially a symptomless disorder until complications occur. Frequently, however, there will be superadded anxiety with its attendant somatic complaints. The development of exceedingly high levels of blood pressure in the malignant phase is a different matter. Headache is then often severe, and may be associated with raised intracranial pressure and visual failure.

Hypertensive encephalopathy

This was never a common condition, and is now even rarer as a result of management of hypertension which prevents the malignant phase. When it does arise it is always a serious medical emergency. Very occasionally it may be the presenting manifestation of the hypertension.

Onset is acute with headache, drowsiness, apprehension and mental confusion. Epileptic fits frequently occur. The disorder evolves rapidly, often within the space of 24 hours, and if untreated progresses to coma with a fatal outcome in a high proportion of cases. The diastolic blood pressure is extremely high, often exceeding 140 mmHg. Vomiting may occur and papilloedema frequently develops. Differentiation from a tumour or abscess may be difficult if facilities for CT scanning are not to hand. The scan may show widespread white matter hypodensity which resolves when the blood pressure is brought under control (Rail & Perkin 1980). Advanced retinopathy is invariably present, and impending kidney or heart failure are common.

Focal signs such as nystagmus, cortical blindness or limb weakness are variable and tend to come and go. Usually, however, focal neurological signs are not a part of the picture. When present they imply complicating factors such as thrombosis, embolism or haemorrhage. Many focal syndromes previously labelled as hyperten-

sive encephalopathy were probably transient cerebral ischaemic attacks occurring in severely hypertensive patients.

Pathological examination may reveal a normal brain, but usually there is marked oedema or petechial haemorrhages and microinfarcts. Byrom (1954) showed in the rat that with hypertension of advanced degree there was intense segmental constriction of cerebral arterioles, attributable to attempts at autoregulation which fail when the pressure exceeds a certain limit. Dilatation occurs between the constricted segments and the vessel wall is damaged, leading to hyperperfusion and cerebral oedema which may be the essential factors underlying hypertensive encephalopathy (Skinhoj & Strandgaard 1973).

Migraine

Migraine is a common and sometimes severely incapacitating disorder, estimated to affect 5–10% of the population at some time or another. Comprehensive reviews of the condition are provided by Pearce (1969), Sacks (1970) and Lance (1993). Psychological factors can play an important role in the precipitation of attacks and psychiatric phenomena may feature prominently in the course of the attacks. Psychological aspects of management often prove to be of importance, especially in recalcitrant cases.

The syndrome is hard to delineate precisely since to some extent boundaries are blurred between this and other forms of vascular headache. Many variations occur and several subtypes have come to be established. The Research Group on Migraine and Headache of the World Federation of Neurology defined migraine as a familial disorder, characterised by recurrent attacks of headache widely variable in intensity, frequency and duration, commonly unilateral, usually associated with anorexia, nausea and vomiting, and sometimes preceded by or associated with neurological and mood disturbances (Critchley 1969). Others have chosen a more empirical approach to definition. Whitty *et al.* (1966), for example, used the criteria of recurrent throbbing headaches together with two of the following five features—unilateral headache, an association with nausea or vomiting, a visual or other sensory aura, a history of cyclical vomiting in childhood or a family history of migraine. More comprehensive criteria for use in research have been proposed by the Headache Classification Committee of the International Headache Society (1988).

Clinical features

The disorder is commoner in women than men in a ratio of 2–3 : 1. Onset is usually in childhood or early adult life, some 25% of cases beginning before the age of 10 and very few after 45. A childhood history of cyclical vomiting with abdominal pain can sometimes be traced as a precursor. Affected individuals show an increased frequency of allergic disorders such as asthma or hay fever, and very probably an increased frequency of epilepsy. A family history of migraine is reported in some two-thirds of cases.

Headache is the most constant element, lasting usually for 8–24 hours though occasionally several days, and varying from mild discomfort to pain of incapacitating violence. It is mostly unilateral at onset, though tending to become diffuse later in the attack. The chief focus may be temporal, supraorbital, retrobulbar or more rarely over the parietal or occipital regions. Throbbing is common, at least initially, with aggravation on coughing or jolting. Anorexia, nausea and vomiting usually develop, also photophobia and intolerance of noise. Autonomic changes may include pallor, facial oedema, conjunctival injection, abdominal distension or the passing of one or more loose stools. In attacks of any severity the patient is usually obliged to lie down until the episode has passed.

This variety is designated *common migraine*. Difficulty will be encountered in certain cases in distinguishing it from tension headache (p. 408). In perhaps a third of cases the headache is preceded by more dramatic phenomena in the form of a visual aura, the syndrome then being known as *classic migraine*. Here visual disturbance is the first indication of an impending attack, lasting some 10–60 minutes and subsiding as the headache sets in. Most typical are the well-known 'fortification spectra' (teichopsia), starting near the fixation point in one half-field and expanding to the periphery as a semicircle of shimmering highly coloured zigzag lights. Hare (1973) has drawn attention to the remarkably constant duration of 20 minutes for such classic spectra. Other forms consist of moving coils, curving lights or rippling sensations in the visual field. Not all are confined to one half-field of vision. A negative scotoma may follow in their wake, or constitute the whole of the aura in itself. Monocular scotoma can occur due to involvement of retinal vessels. Other disturbances include micropsia, macropsia, distortions of shape and position, 'zoom vision' and 'mosaic vision'. Occasionally there are hallucinations and distortion of taste, smell and hearing. Tactile paraesthesiae may coexist with the visual disturbances or occur alone. Problems with language may take the form of anomia or difficulty with speaking (Ardila & Sanchez 1988). Body image disturbances, though rare, can take fascinating forms, as discussed on pp. 406–7.

A not uncommon variant is *basilar artery migraine* (Bickerstaff 1961a, 1961b). The attacks begin with a visual aura, sometimes extending to both half-fields and obscuring vision, then proceeding to symptoms of brain stem dysfunction such as vertigo, dysarthria, ataxia, tinnitus, and sensory symptoms distally in the limbs and around the lips and tongue. After several minutes to three-quarters of an hour these give way to throbbing headache usually of occipital distribution. Loss of consciousness may be interposed between the brain stem symptoms and headache, lasting sometimes for up to half an hour and presumably due to ischaemia of the reticular formation. The impairment is gradual in onset, resembling deep sleep rather than syncope. Attacks of basilar migraine appear to be especially common in adolescent girls and to be associated with a strong family history of migraine. The episodes are usually infrequent and interspersed among classic attacks.

More marked neurological phenomena can occur in patients with so-called *'complicated migraine'*. With *hemiplegic migraine* unilateral motor (or sensory) disturbances in the limbs accompany or replace the visual aura, or may appear in the later stages of the attack. Dysphasia can accompany the paresis when the dominant side is affected, and consciousness is sometimes impaired (Whitty 1953; Bradshaw & Parsons 1965). The neurological signs may outlast other components of the attack, sometimes persisting for several days. In such cases there tends to be a strong family history of similar attacks. In *ophthalmoplegic migraine* attacks are accompanied by paresis of external ocular movement, again often outlasting the headache.

Other variants include *facial migraine (lower half headache)* in which episodes of unilateral facial pain are associated with typical migrainous phenomena, starting in the cheek or palate and spreading to the ear or neck. *Migrainous neuralgia (cluster headaches)* consists of severe unilateral head or face pain, usually periorbital, typically occurring in bouts over a period of several weeks and often appearing at exactly the same time each day. Attacks are accompanied by lachrymation and nasal blockage on the ipsilateral side, and sometimes by a Horner's syndrome. Some consider this to be a distinct entity rather than a variant of migraine.

A further variation consists of attacks in which components other than headache dominate the clinical picture (*migraine equivalents*). The headache may be mild or even totally absent, leading to considerable diagnostic difficulty if a history of more typical attacks is not forthcoming. Thus the visual aura or other neurological disturbance may occur alone, or there may be episodes of nausea and vomiting, abdominal pain or drowsiness. Some of the mental phenomena which may constitute equivalents are discussed below.

Course and outcome

Once established migraine is commonly a life-long complaint, though spells of relief may occur for years at a time. The frequency and severity of attacks vary greatly from one patient to another. Some are affected at fairly regular intervals, and a small number of women are especially susceptible around the time of their menstrual periods. Temporary relief during pregnancy is well attested in approximately 60% of cases. Improvement at the menopause may occur but is less regularly observed. A general indication of outcome is given by Whitty and Hockaday (1968) who reviewed a large group of patients 15–20 years after their first attendance at a clinic. Attacks had ceased in a third, improved over time in half and continued without improvement in the remainder. Changing patterns over time were not uncommon, as well as dissociation between the auras and the headaches so that either could occur alone.

Psychological precipitants (p. 404) are universally recognised and in some patients play a major role in determining the frequency and timing of attacks. Dietary factors may also be blamed, including alcohol, cheese and chocolate. Red wine appears to be an especially common precipitant. In some patients missing a meal or going without sleep appears regularly to precipitate attacks. Oral contraceptives have been found to exacerbate migraine, or indeed to induce its first appearance (Whitty et al. 1966; Bickerstaff & Holmes 1967).

Permanent sequelae to attacks are extremely uncommon and constitute clinical rarities. Nevertheless Davis-Jones et al. (1973) refer to 145 cases in the literature and add 14 more of their own. Most frequent are enduring visual field defects, attributable to retinal or cerebral lesions, also pareses, dysphasia, ophthalmoplegias and oculosympathetic lesions. Most owe their origin to migraine-related strokes which, though very rare, constitute a significant proportion of the strokes that occur among young people.

Dorfman et al. (1979) demonstrated infarctions by angiography or CT in four young adults with migraine, one representing a posterior cerebral artery occlusion and three infarctions in the middle cerebral territory. Titus et al. (1989) showed infarctions with MRI in the region supplied by the superior cerebellar artery in four patients, three of whom had had negative CT scans. The rarity of infarction was shown, however, by Broderick and Swanson (1987) who were able to find only 20 examples of stroke occurring with an attack among almost 5000 patients at the Mayo Clinic. Good recovery was usual, only two being left with moderate disability and 14 with mild or minimal disability.

Bogousslavski et al. (1988) made a careful comparison between 22 patients who suffered a stroke during an attack, and matched migraine patients who had had strokes remote from attacks. A second control group consisted of non-migraineurs with stroke. Only 9% of the study group had cardiovascular abnormalities as potential sources of emboli, compared with 86% of controls. Involvement of the posterior cerebral circulation was more frequent at 41% and 9%, respectively. The mean number of migraine attacks was similar to that in the controls with migraine, but the duration of attacks had been significantly longer. All such features suggested that the strokes occurring in the course of attacks were intimately related to the pathophysiology of the migraine process, namely that they were probably attributable to prolonged oligaemia in the territory responsible for the auras.

Findings of possible relevance have come from brain imaging. Earlier CT studies reported mild generalised and focal atrophy in a considerable proportion of patients, but these lacked comparison with controls (Mathew et al. 1977; Sargent et al. 1979; du Boulay et al. 1983). Moreover no association was observed with the severity or duration of migraine or the presence of complicating factors. Of more significance, Hungerford et al. (1976) found evidence of infarction in six of 53 patients with very severe migraine, three of the infarctions corresponding in site to aspects of the clinical history. Of the 13 patients with permanent neurological sequelae 11 showed some abnormality on the scan.

MRI scanning has also revealed abnormalities, chiefly scattered areas of high T_2 signal intensity in the subcortical white matter, sometimes with larger cortical changes resembling infarcts in patients with complicated migraine (Soges et al. 1988; Ziegler et al. 1991). Igarashi et al. (1991) investigated 91 patients with common or classic migraine, and found that 40% showed small white foci of this nature. They were usually bilateral and without correspondence to the side of headache or aura. The incidence rose with age, positive findings occurring in all patients over 60. Twenty-nine per cent of those under 40 showed the abnormalities, compared with 11% of age-matched controls suffering from tension headache, psychiatric disturbance or epilepsy. Most such lesions were situated in the centrum semiovale and frontal white matter, but they extended to deeper white matter in patients over 40. No relationship could be found to duration, severity or type of migraine, or with consumption of ergotamine.

The significance of such findings is uncertain. In appearance the lesions resemble the 'unidentified bright objects' (UBOs) found with ageing, hypertension and other arteriosclerotic risk factors, but were seen in the absence of such factors in the younger migraine patients. An origin in the repeated attacks of hypoperfusion during auras seemed unlikely, because no relationship could be discerned with the presence or absence of auras or with the duration of the condition. Igarashi *et al.* (1991) suggest, nonetheless, that the MRI findings may reflect early pathological brain changes of a nature yet to be clarified.

The occasional cases of dementia in association with migraine are discussed below (p. 407).

Aetiology and pathology

The precise cause of migraine remains uncertain. An inherited predisposition seems likely in view of the high familial concentrations reported (Dalsgaard-Nielsen 1965), though careful epidemiological surveys suggest that this may have been overstressed (Waters 1971). Allergic factors have often been proposed but rarely upheld. Hormonal influences are suggested by the high remission rate in pregnancy, the exacerbation on taking the contraceptive pill and the small group of cases with attacks clearly related to the menstrual periods. Even in the latter, however, precise correlations with hormonal levels remain elusive (Epstein *et al.* 1975). There is often evidence of sodium and water retention with attacks, patients noticing weight gain and oedema beforehand and polyuria as the headache subsides, yet diuretics have little prophylactic value. The role of hypoglycaemia has been studied in cases provoked by fasting and cases preceded by abnormal sensations of hunger; no clear correlations have emerged with blood glucose levels, but there are indirect indications of an abnormal central response to carbohydrate depletion in certain subjects (Hockaday *et al.* 1971, 1973; Rao & Pearce 1971).

Much of the above therefore appears to be dealing with epiphenomena to attacks rather than revealing the fundamentals of the disturbance. Pearce (1969) suggests that the basic abnormality may lie in a periodic central disturbance, or functionally labile threshold, of hypothalamic activity. This could have effects on the autonomic control of the vasculature, and at the same time provide a mechanism whereby emotional disturbance could influence the pattern and timing of attacks.

The pathophysiological mechanisms responsible for the headache have been explored in a long series of studies summarised by Lance (1993). There is good evidence that headache is associated with dilatation of the cranial arteries, the principal component coming from the extracranial or scalp arteries. An important additional factor appears to be the development, later in the attack, of a sterile inflammatory reaction in and around the affected vessels, with the accumulation of substances which sensitise them to pain. Pain may also be derived in part from meningeal and other intracranial vessels, accounting for

accentuation by coughing, sneezing and head movement (Blau & Davis 1970).

The mechanisms behind the production of neurological prodromata remain incompletely understood. Vascular theories, by way of intracranial vasoconstriction as a prelude to the extracranial vasodilatation, vie with theories which view the disturbance as arising primarily within the brain parenchyma. Cerebral blood flow studies using intracarotid xenon or SPECT have shown oligaemic changes very clearly during the course of classic migraine attacks, but there is considerable dissociation between their time course and that of the development of focal symptoms (Lauritzen 1987). Moreover vasoconstrictors (such as ergotamine) given early in the attack can sometimes cut short the aura as well as preventing the headache. The reduced perfusion typically starts posteriorly in the brain, then spreads anteriorly over the course of 15–45 minutes to involve parietal and temporal regions independently of the territories of supply of the larger cerebral vessels. The rate of progression at 2–3 mm per minute is closely similar to that of Leao's 'spreading depression'. It is therefore possible that the perfusion deficits represent arteriolar constriction which is *secondary* to some other propagating change in cortical function and that this is fundamental to the pathogenesis of the disorder. In the case of prolonged neurological phenomena, as in hemiplegic migraine, local oedema or hypoxia ensuing on the spasm may be responsible for the symptoms.

The site of the changes responsible for auras must differ widely from one form to another. Teichopsia and homonymous field defects almost certainly originate in the occipital lobes, illusions of altered size, shape and position in the optic radiations, and bitemporal hemianopias from disturbance of chiasmatic vessels. The retinal vessels are clearly involved in some cases of monocular scotoma and the occlusion of retinal arteries has been directly observed. The middle cerebral or internal carotids are likely to be involved in hemiplegic migraine, and the vertebrobasilar system in patients with brain stem manifestations. In fact it is probable that in many attacks a large part of the cerebral vasculature is affected diffusely, the focal symptoms merely reflecting ischaemia in the territory most severely involved—hence the vague but definite symptoms of slowed cerebration and somnolence which are common in attacks.

Biochemical alterations have been identified along with the vascular changes and could conceivably play a primary role in the genesis of attacks. In the early stages catabolites of noradrenaline and serotonin are excreted in excess in the urine, and plasma serotonin has been shown to fall abruptly at the onset of the headache phase. Serotonin is known to constrict scalp arteries, so the fall could be responsible for the vasodilatation of the headache. The effectiveness of pharmaceutical agents such as methysergide and sumatriptan reinforces the view that serotonin plays a central role in migraine, but it is unclear whether this lies in a direct effect on cranial blood vessels or in more central effects on the cortex and pain control pathways (Lance 1993). It remains to be explained, moreover, why attacks should commonly be unilateral in distribution, and some constitutional vascular instability or hypersensitivity to humoral agents must still be postulated.

Psychiatric aspects

Virtually all observers, neurologists and psychiatrists alike, stress the influence which psychological factors may have in migraine and the importance attaching to them in treatment. Migraine is indeed often seen as a model for 'psychosomatic' disorders. A considerable literature has accumulated concerning the personality of migraine sufferers and the role of emotions and conflicts in precipitating attacks. Mental phenomena are also recognised as common accompaniments of the disorder, and may sometimes assume bizarre expression leading to diagnostic difficulty. These aspects will be briefly reviewed.

Personality in migraine

Many accounts stress the driving conscientious personality of migraine sufferers, often with marked obsessional traits and above average intelligence. Such a picture originated with the work of Wolff (1937, 1963) and has clearly accorded with the experience of others (Alvarez 1947; Fine 1969).

Wolff's migraineurs were described as overtly obedient but with traits of stubbornness and inflexibility. Most were ambitious and preoccupied with achievement and success, attempted to dominate their environments, and were exacting and meticulous. Many harboured strong resentments which were linked to their intolerance and superabundance of drive. Sexual dissatisfaction was common. Such features, when present, appeared to furnish optimal conditions for the precipitation of attacks.

Psychoanalysts have highlighted certain other constellations in the personality—repressed hostility, unresolved ambivalence, oral fixation and strongly developed anal sadism resulting in compulsive behaviour and rigidity (Fromm-Reichmann 1937; Sperling 1964). Others have emphasised the significance of sexual conflicts and confusions over sexual identification.

It is unlikely, however, that generalisations can be made about the personality make-up of migraine patients. Sacks (1970) illustrated the variety of emotional needs which attacks appeared to fulfil, and found it impossible to fit his material into stereotypes of obsessive personality or chronically repressed hostility. Special selection would appear often to have been at work where earlier reports were concerned. Selby and Lance (1960) made a rough categorisation of their patients, and considered that the personality range differed little from what occurs in the population generally—23% showed obsessional trends, 22% were hyperactive and found it hard to relax, 13% showed overt anxiety symptoms and 42% were considered 'normal'. Dalsgaard-Nielsen (1965) estimated that a third showed pathological personality configurations, a third showed minor peculiarities — being sensitive, perfectionistic and inclined to bottle up feelings —while a third showed no abnormal traits whatever.

Attempts at achieving unbiased samples of migraine sufferers have been unable to uphold many of the personality features traditionally linked to the disorder. Henryk-Gutt and Rees (1973) surveyed a large population of government employees and matched the migraine sufferers with carefully chosen controls, thus overcoming the selective processes involved in medical referral. Semi-structured interviews and personality inventories were used to explore psychological aspects of the disorder. They obtained no evidence of increased ambitiousness, striving or obsessionality among the migraine subjects, though a history of suppressive parental discipline was significantly commoner than among the controls. Hostility and guilt scores on the inventories showed no clear relationship to migraine. However, 'neuroticism', as measured by the Eysenck Personality Inventory, was significantly higher than among controls, likewise indices of emotionality as manifest in current nervous symptoms, current emotional difficulties, liability to mood swings and tendencies to bottle up anger and resentments. They concluded that while migraine subjects were no more ambitious or obsessional than non-migraine subjects, they were constitutionally predisposed towards increased emotional reactivity and thus to experience a greater than average reaction to a given quantity of stress. This increased reactivity of the autonomic nervous system could conceivably provide the predisposing factor for the development of attacks.

Waters' (1971) survey of a community-based sample was also informative. No evidence was found to support the contention that migraine is especially common among persons of higher intelligence, though it was noted that a higher proportion of the more intelligent sufferers had consulted doctors about their headaches. Similarly, there was no indication that migraine was especially frequent among persons in social classes I and II, but again there was a tendency for a higher proportion of migraineurs in these social classes to have consulted their doctors.

A failure to corroborate specific personality features among migraine sufferers as a group does not, of course, diminish the importance which may attach to such features when they are apparent in the individual. Clearly the type of personality structure outlined by Wolff and others will, when present, readily lead to conflicts and contradictions with the environment. And as described below, psychological precipitants can be closely relevant to the pattern and timing of attacks.

A special association with affective and anxiety disorders has been reported by Merikangas *et al.* (1990), in a prospective study of a cohort of 27- and 28-year-olds in Zurich. Sixty-one of the 457 subjects were deemed to suffer from migraine, and these showed a significant excess of major depression, bipolar spectrum disorder (i.e. cyclothymia and hypomania), generalised anxiety and social phobia. The association with anxiety disorders was particularly strong. Retrospective data suggested a characteristic time course, with anxiety often manifested in childhood, followed by the development of migraine some years later, and then by discrete episodes of depression in early adult life. Depressive personality disorder and dysthymia were not, however, increased among migraine sufferers.

Psychological precipitants

Many observers place psychological factors high on the list of features that may provoke episodes of migraine. It is common to find that periods of stress, or the anticipation of stress, are associated with attacks. Sustained emotional tension seems to be more important than acute emotional disturbance, the crucial factor being the degree to which feelings are sustained, bottled up and inadequately expressed (Rees 1971). Frustrations and resentments may operate powerfully in this way. Another well-documented finding is the tendency for some patients to develop attacks during the 'let down period' after intense activity and striving. Consequently some have attacks quite regularly when a harassing day is over, at weekends or on the first day of a holiday. Many patients, however, insist that the majority of their attacks are entirely without discernible precipitants. Emotional disturbance therefore appears to be a common, but by no means a universal, factor.

Some two-thirds of clinic-based samples report that emotional precipitants are important, though rarely as the sole invariant factor (Selby & Lance 1960; Dalsgaard-Nielsen 1965). Henryk-Gutt and Rees (1973), in their community survey, found about 60% in whom problems at work or problems with interpersonal relationships

were regarded as direct precipitants. Relief from strain was noted as a factor in about a third. In controls with non-migrainous headaches such features were less commonly blamed. In almost half of the migraine subjects the disorder had had its onset during a period of emotional stress. The subjects were then asked to keep records of their attacks for a 2-month period, noting any special events or emotions coinciding in time with the attacks. Over half of the episodes recorded proved to be related to emotionally stressful events. Other precipitants such as alcohol, food or hunger were by comparison very rare. In approximately one-third of attacks no cause whatever could be discerned.

Psychiatric features associated with attacks

Feelings of irritability and anxiety may last for several hours as a prelude to attacks. More rarely patients may experience unusual health and vigour, sometimes amounting to elation. A rebound of energy is also described in the wake of attacks, with feelings of buoyancy and increased drive. Others by contrast remain listless and fatigued for several days. Such features may sometimes occur with sufficient regularity to suggest that they are part and parcel of the pathophysiology of the disorder.

Mental changes are almost universal during the attack itself. Anxiety and irritability are common early on, with drowsiness and lethargy as the headache continues. Depression can be severe. Cerebration is typically slowed, with poor concentration and poor ability to think coherently. Klee (1968) made a detailed analysis of patients with migraine severe enough to warrant hospitalisation, and found that attacks were accompanied by marked impairment of memory in 10%, clouding of consciousness or delirium in 8%, pronounced anxiety in 8%, complex visual and auditory hallucinations in 6%, changes of body image in 6% and severe depression in 4%. Altogether 22% of patients experienced at least one mental symptom severely enough to affect them greatly in the course of their attacks.

Alterations of consciousness range from blunting of alertness, through states of marked lethargy and drowsiness to frank loss of consciousness. The latter is the so-called 'migrainous syncope', sometimes occurring during the aura and sometimes later in the attack. Typically the patient lapses into unconsciousness over a period of several minutes, appears as though sleeping deeply, then emerges from the episode in the same gradual fashion. Such attacks have been described as characteristic of basilar artery migraine (Bickerstaff 1961b) but can also be seen with hemiplegic migraine and other varieties

(Hockaday & Whitty 1969). On rare occasions there may be short-lived periods of coma with incontinence or even epileptic fits at the height of attacks.

Mental 'confusion' can be marked. Sometimes it represents a focal disturbance of cerebral function with dysphasic, apraxic or agnosic manifestations. Disturbance of memory can be the main component as described below. Or there may be elaborate 'dreamy states', probably reflecting temporal lobe dysfunction, with feelings of *déjà vu*, timelessness, depersonalisation or forced reminiscence.

A 44-year-old man suffered very occasional attacks of migraine from adolescence, ushered in by scintillation scotomata. In one attack a profound dream-like state followed the visual phenomena thus — 'First I couldn't think where I was, and then I suddenly realised that I was back in California. . . . It was a hot summer day. I saw my wife moving about on the verandah, and I called her to bring me a coke. She turned to me with an odd look on her face, and said 'Are you sick or something?' I suddenly seemed to wake up, and realised that it was a winter's day in New York, and there was no verandah and that it wasn't my wife but my secretary who was standing in the office looking strangely at me.' (Sacks 1970)

Other examples clearly represent acute organic reactions due to generalised cerebral dysfunction, with disorientation and clouding of consciousness. Medicaments administered for treatment of the attack may sometimes be partly responsible. Such states may be coloured by anxiety, restlessness and complex visual and auditory hallucinations. A paranoid element may be marked. The condition may amount to a frank delirium, lasting throughout the headache for several hours or days. Very occasionally the headache fails to materialise and the mental disturbance then appears as a psychotic episode in itself ('mental migraine equivalent'). The range and diversity of the pictures seen is illustrated in the examples below:

A 50-year-old woman had suffered migraine from the age of 16, increasing in severity from the age of 43. For the past 5 years pronounced mental changes had accompanied attacks, in that her memory became faulty and she felt extremely depressed and hopeless. In particularly severe examples consciousness was clouded, with disorientation and restlessness. During several of her severe attacks she had had the experience of seeing her deceased adoptive mother, and in one attack imagined that she saw and talked to her deceased biological mother, lying in a hospital bed as she had done when last she saw her. During the course of these hallucinations she was very anxious, definite about the experiences but unable to remember all the details afterwards. Since the onset of the mental components she had noticed that some reduction in memory tended to persist between attacks. (Klee 1968)

A boy of 16 had been prone to migraine attacks since childhood, taking many different forms. Commonly they started with paraesthesiae in the left leg and right hand. As these died away he developed distortions of hearing, then bilateral scintillation scotomata in both lower half-fields of vision. Other attacks started with tingling in the epigastrium associated with an intense sense of foreboding. Those occurring at night often had a nightmarish quality with feelings of compulsion and restlessness leading on to a profound hallucinatory state — hallucinations of being trapped in a speeding car and of figures made of metal advancing upon him. As he emerged from these he became conscious of paraesthesiae then intense headache. This patient also suffered 'syncopal' attacks during severe auras, with simultaneous fading away of sight and vision, a sense of faintness and then unconsciousness. (Sacks 1970)

A 37-year-old housewife had suffered attacks of migraine from 19, increasing in severity since the age of 32. Attacks began with headache, later proceeding to paraesthesiae in the right hand and leg with weakness of the limbs and a variety of visual phenomena. They often lasted for 3 or 4 days. During a particularly severe attack which lasted for a week she had to be admitted to a mental hospital. On the preceding day she had become increasingly restless with clouding of consciousness, had heard neighbours making unpleasant comments about her and believed she had been stuck with knives. For the first few days in hospital she was disorientated, restless and appeared hallucinated both visually and aurally. She heard children's voices and the voice of her general practitioner, and believed her legs had been amputated. This psychotic episode disappeared within a few days and she was amnesic for it afterwards. Her last clear memory was of lying down to sleep at home, and the next of waking in hospital. (Klee 1968)

The hallucinatory elements may sometimes dominate the picture, as in one of Klee's patients who saw greyish-coloured Red Indians, 20 cm high, crowding round in the room in which he lay. On another occasion he picked up hallucinatory musical instruments from the floor. Another patient saw 'white living creatures', stationary and rather indistinct, apparently unaccompanied by clouding of consciousness or disorientation.

Florid examples of confusion are probably rare, at least in adults. But in children it seems not uncommon for migraine to present in this fashion. Gascon and Barlow (1970) observed four children who showed acute organic reactions lasting from 6 to 24 hours. Although headache developed in every case it was usually not detected until the mental disturbance had receded. Ehyai and Fenichel (1978) found five similar examples among 100 consecutive cases of childhood migraine, with episodes of agitated confusion lasting from several minutes to hours, and succeeded by diffuse EEG changes indicative of cerebral ischaemia. Such attacks tended to recur on follow-up but were eventually replaced by typical migraine.

Paranoid psychosis is very rare as a fully developed manifestation, and is usually seen as an elaboration of an acute organic reaction. However, Bhatia (1990) has described a patient with Capgras' syndrome, setting in during the headache despite normal orientation and memory, and persisting for several weeks. In the patient reported by Fuller *et al.* (1993) psychotic features were in the forefront of the picture, four episodes occurring over a 17-year period and each setting in within 24 hours of migraine attacks:

A 69-year-old man woke on the day following a severe episode of migraine, complaining that his wife and brother-in-law were changing before his eyes, that their arms were lengthening and that they each had only one eye. Familiar things looked strange, and he thought the house had been replaced by a cleverly produced copy. The next day he saw threatening words on the walls, and refused to enter certain rooms because of evil in them.

On admission to hospital he was agitated and suspicious, but orientated in time and place. There was mild impairment of recent memory, and his speech was disjointed with paraphasia and neologisms. He saw red piranha fish on the floor which disappeared when he stamped on them, and the doctors' arms appeared to be elongated. On one occasion he saw his hospital bed being swallowed up into the floor. He had ideas of reference, and bizarre delusions that his wife had been killed and that the staff were systematically butchering other patients on the ward. He believed that the ward had been 'towed across country' to another location (reduplicative paramnesia). A CT brain scan was normal, but EEGs showed bisynchronous frontal delta activity at 2–3 Hz. His mental state gradually became normal over the next 10 days, and he was able to recall the content of the hallucinations with full insight into their unreal nature.

He had suffered from migraine since the age of 16, attacks beginning with tingling in the lips and left arm, dysarthria and flashing lights. At 53 an attack was followed by an episode of paranoid psychosis lasting for 3 weeks, and similar episodes occurred at the ages of 64 and 65. In one of them he was initially disorientated in time. His mother suffered from migraine, and she too had had attacks followed by paranoid hallucinatory episodes later in life.

Amnesia may feature prominently in some episodes, either along with the visual aura or as a variant of classic attacks. When occurring as a relatively isolated phenomenon it may reflect changes in the hypothalamic or hippocampal regions. Nielsen (1930, 1958) described examples lasting from 20 minutes to several hours, sometimes associated with typical headache but sometimes occurring as migraine equivalents. During attacks it was common to find that isolated thoughts and ideas came to the mind unbidden while wanted material could not be recalled. Islands of thought failed to associate one with another, leading to patchiness of memory:

A 37-year-old doctor complained of episodes of mental disturbance lasting 3–6 hours at a time, and occurring once or twice per year from the age of 18. They began with a feeling of mild depression, then strangeness, then mental confusion. Through-

out the attack he remained perfectly orientated, yet was unable to organise his thinking and had large defects in his memory. Facts and events seemed isolated and devoid of normal associations. He was unable to remember things for more than half a minute and found it difficult to converse as a result, repeating questions and appearing absent-minded to onlookers. Close questioning revealed migraine attacks with scotomata and fortification spectra occurring in between such episodes. The more typical attacks were also associated with very mild confusion.

(Nielsen 1930)

A woman of 24 had attacks beginning with fortification spectra in the right half-field, leading after a few minutes to severe anterograde amnesia and inability to direct her thoughts. Independent ideas came to her mind spontaneously, but she was unable to follow them through or gain associations before they disappeared again. Everything looked strange, and topographical orientation was considerably disturbed. This would last for 20 minutes then merge with headache, nausea and vomiting if the attack was to be complete. More commonly, however, the attacks consisted of the mental disturbance alone, following the visual spectra but without further progression thereafter.

(Nielsen 1958)

Caplan *et al.* (1981) have reported an association between the syndrome of transient global amnesia (p. 413) and migraine, describing 12 migraineurs who experienced a typical amnesic episode. Six were cases of common migraine and six of classic migraine. Of the latter, three experienced their classic aura accompanying the attack and headache followed it; two more had pounding headache during the attack. Altogether nine of the 12 experienced headache in the course of the amnesic episode. The evidence which increasingly points to pathophysiological mechanisms similar to those of migraine in a substantial proportion of patients with transient global amnesia is discussed on p. 417.

Body image disturbances may occur just before, during or after attacks of headache. Parts of the body are felt to be magnified, diminished, distorted, reduplicated or absent. Some examples were described in Chapter 2 (pp. 72 and 73). Lippman (1952) reported several examples, all in classic migraine, including patients in whom the abnormal sensations could constitute the entire attack without headache developing. One patient felt as though the neck or hip were extending out on one side, another that the left ear was ballooning out for 15 cm or more, another that the head had grown to tremendous proportions and had become light, floating up to the ceiling. One patient felt alternating enlargements and diminutions in the size of the right half of the body, coming and going throughout the headache period. Patients who feel exceedingly tall or extremely minute during attacks are suggestive of *Alice in Wonderland* and Lewis Carroll was known to have suffered from migraine.

Lippman (1953) also described experiences of physical duality (autoscopy, p. 73) in association with migraine. During attacks such patients felt a conviction of having two bodies, usually for several seconds at a time, before, during or after the headache. Qualities such as observation, judgement and perception were typically transferred to the 'other' body which for the moment seemed the more real of the two, but throughout the experience the patient remained aware of the actual body and its position in space. Feelings of fear, mild wonder or amazement were common accompaniments. This striking phenomenon is best illustrated by some of Lippman's examples:

A woman of 37 wrote: 'Until . . . 5 years ago, I felt the queer sensation of being two persons. This sensation came just before a violent headache attack and at no other time. Very often it came as I was serving breakfast. There would be my husband and children, just as usual, and in a flash they didn't seem to be quite the same. They were my husband and children all right — but they certainly weren't the same.... There was something queer about it all. I felt as if I were standing on an inclined plane, looking down on them from a height of a few feet watching myself serve breakfast. It was as if I were in another dimension, looking at myself and them. I was not afraid, just amazed. I always knew that I was really with them. Yet there was "I" and there was "me" — and in a moment I was one again!'

Another patient might develop attacks when walking. She would feel as if from the hips downwards the walking continued but with no volition or direction — the 'control' was in the upper self, way up above, totally indifferent to the legs' destination. During such experiences she would try to move over to a doorway or building until she could focus on 'myself' and become one again. Such episodes always occurred during episodes of headache or just after recovery.

Another patient while performing some habitual activity had the distinct impression of being two people — one going through the actions of eating or reading, the other suspended above and to one side, perceiving or contemplating herself in a detached way. This experience would come and go in a flash.

(Lippman 1953)

Affective disturbance may sometimes greatly exceed the usual irritability and depression of attacks. Klee (1968) noted examples of profound anxiety and depression. Sacks (1970) referred to sudden eruptions of 'forced mood' occurring in the course of an aura — feelings of foreboding or states of awe, rapture or sudden hilarity. They were marked by the suddenness of onset, their senselessness and their overwhelming quality. Most were brief, lasting for only a minute at a time.

Periodic mood changes have also been described interictally in patients who experience affective disturbance as part of their attacks. Episodes of depression or elation may occur, lasting for hours or days at a time, and differing from manic–depressive mood swings chiefly by their brevity (Moersch 1924; Sacks 1970). These have been interpreted as representing the affective component of attacks devoid of headache or other aural manifestations. Clearly the distinction from primary emotional disorders will often be difficult in such cases.

Other psychiatric abnormalities have been described, usually as rarities or striking instances. The literature is reviewed by Moersch (1924) and Bruyn (1968a). Conversion hysteria may be seen at the height of attacks, or states of dissociation with multiple personality. Automatisms have been described, apparently similar to those occurring with epilepsy except for a more gradual onset and the accompanying headache and malaise (Nielsen 1958). Disinhibition, obsessions, phobias and compulsions may occur in association with attacks. Kleptomania has sometimes been claimed as an integral part of the disturbance, either occurring in association with headache or as a migraine equivalent.

Progressive mental impairment has occasionally been noted in sufferers from severe migraine, though a causal connection has not been clearly established. The association would certainly appear to be rare. Gowers (1888) stated that some permanent failure of mental power could occasionally be observed after many attacks attended by intellectual difficulties, and Flatau (1912) reported several patients with restricted powers of concentration and memory continuing between attacks. Symonds (1951) considered it probable that in some cases there might be slight but cumulative brain damage as a result of successive small infarctions. An example is reported by Bradshaw and Parsons (1965):

A 39-year-old nursing sister had had migraine from the age of 7, increasing after a period of worry some years before. After injecting herself with ergotamine tartrate during one attack she developed a right hemiplegic episode with dysphasia. This improved slowly over 5 weeks but left a slight residual deficit. Angiography and other investigations showed no abnormalities. Follow-up showed unequivocal evidence of progressive impairment of mental faculties, leading to memory impairment, falling standards of work, lack of insight and emotional instability. Further migraine attacks had continued, some with right-sided paraesthesiae. Her mother had had right hemiplegic migraine, and from the age of 52 had shown mental changes which progressed to gross dementia over the course of several years.

More recently, Pedersen (1980) has described three patients with cortical atrophy and marked signs of reduced intellect. No other causes could be found to account for this, and two of the patients had shown a marked increase in frequency of attacks prior to the onset of the dementia.

With regard to psychometry, Klee and Willanger (1966) found evidence of slight impairment in six of eight patients, and Zeitlin and Oddy (1984) have reported impairments in comparison to a carefully matched control group. In the latter study 19 patients with histories of migraine extending over 10 years were matched to controls in terms of age, sex, social class, verbal IQ and education. All were under 50 with a mean age of 36 years. Significant impairments were revealed on choice reaction time tests, the Trail Making Test and Paced Auditory Serial Addition Test (PASAT), and on recognition memory for words. No associations emerged, however, with measures of the severity of migraine or the use of ergotamine.

'Chronic migrainous disability'

Occasional sufferers from migraine may enter a phase in which very frequent, severe and unremitting headaches develop. Typically this is coupled with malaise, anorexia, sleeplessness and loss of weight. Depression of considerable severity is usually an integral part of the picture. Overmedication may prove to be partly responsible, but in many cases psychological influences are clearly at work in initiating or perpetuating the disorder.

The deterioration may be decisively linked to the development of a depressive illness, the migraine and the affective disorder thereafter reinforcing each other. In other patients it may be difficult to discern which components have been primary in initiating the vicious circle once the condition has become entrenched. Some will prove to have been 'caught in a malignant emotional bind of one sort or another' and to be reacting to chronically difficult life situations (Sacks 1970). The attacks may then be observed to bring about a range of reactions—regression, withdrawal or exploitation—which in turn initiate autonomic and other pathological mechanisms which exacerbate and perpetuate the condition.

The interdependence of emotional disturbance and migraine is highlighted in such examples, and a conjoint approach by psychological and physical measures is usually essential for resolution of the situation.

Differential diagnosis

Migraine headaches must first be differentiated from other causes of pain in the head and face—chronic sinus disease, glaucoma, hypertension and raised intracranial pressure. In the majority of cases the history will be sufficient to allow such a distinction, aided by physical examination or simple investigations. More difficulty may be encountered in making a firm distinction between migraine and tension headaches, both of which are common, chronic and frequently incapacitating. This issue is considered separately below.

Problems with neurological diagnosis are likely to arise in cases of 'complicated migraine' where marked neurological deficits accompany or follow attacks. Here a neurological opinion is essential, even though a basis in structural cerebral pathology will emerge in only a minute proportion of cases. An angioma must be considered when the deficits well outlast the headache, and especially when attacks of hemiplegic migraine involve one side of the body exclusively. Ophthalmoplegic attacks limited to one side will raise the possibility of an aneurysm of the internal carotid or posterior communicating arteries. In basilar migraine the prominence of brain stem deficits may suggest the possibility of some brain stem lesion. And even classic migraine attacks may warrant investigation if they first declare themselves in adult life, particularly if the auras tend to occur alone without much by way of headache.

On occasion difficulty can arise in distinguishing migraine from epilepsy (p. 291), and indeed the two may occur together. When loss of consciousness occurs with migraine it is usually gradual in onset and a good deal less profound than in epilepsy. Even when sudden, it is usually succeeded by headache far exceeding that which follows an epileptic attack. Doubt can also arise over the complex auras of migraine, especially when these occur as isolated events. However, visual phenomena are far commoner in migraine than in epilepsy and often assume their highly specific form. Paraesthesiae are rarely bilateral in epilepsy, and proceed with much greater rapidity than in migraine. The most ambiguous situation is represented by the rare dream-like states of migraine, especially when accompanied by depersonalisation, terror, rapture or other alterations suggestive of complex partial seizures (Sacks 1970).

Patients presenting with episodes of confusion may be suspected of delirium due to toxic or metabolic factors. Long-lasting acute organic reactions may be diagnosed as transient paranoid reactions. Episodes coloured by marked mood disturbance may resemble the swings of manic–depressive disorder, especially when preceded or followed by a rebound of elation and hyperactivity. Episodes of syncope in migraine may be regarded as hysterical dissociation, particularly when the impairment of consciousness is not profound and is preceded by a dramatic train of symptoms. In all such variants the true situation is usually revealed by the development of headache later in the attack or by a history of more typical migraine attacks in the past.

Migraine versus tension headache

Tension (or 'muscle contraction') headache is probably almost as frequent as migraine. Moreover the two may coexist in a substantial proportion of patients. The difficulties sometimes encountered in making a clear distinction are widely recognised, yet the differentiation must be attempted if specific anti-migrainous therapy is to be employed. Diagnostic difficulty is most likely to arise with common migraine where characteristic prodromata to attacks are lacking.

While emotional factors are important in the genesis of both forms of headache, the mechanism of their operation is different. Tension headache seems to depend essentially on sustained contraction in the muscles of the scalp, forehead and neck. The intracranial and extracranial vasculature is not primarily involved, though vascular reactivity within the muscles, or the accumulation of pain-provoking substances, may make a contribution.

Comprehensive accounts are provided by Friedman et al. (1954), Martin (1966) and Lance (1993). Tension headache usually arises and coexists with emotional conflicts or states of anxiety and depression. The patient may be aware of such a derivation, though in long-lasting examples the emotional disorder may come to be regarded as secondary to the headaches themselves. Frequent concomitants are fatigue, insomnia, lack of interest and difficulty with concentration. Close questioning will often reveal evidence of tension or depression persisting between the headaches, whereas attacks of migraine usually occur against a background of relative well-being. In migraine, moreover, there is often a long history of intermittent attacks dating well back to childhood or adolescence.

Tension headaches, like migraine, vary widely in intensity, frequency and duration but certain characteristics help in the distinction. There are usually no prodromata and the onset and offset tend to be gradual. Tension headaches are commonly of daily occurrence, which is very rare in migraine, and they are often day-long in duration. Undulations in severity may occur throughout the day, diurnal variation sometimes being the key to an origin in depressive disorder. They are usually bilateral in distribution, generalised over the head or with an accent on the frontal, occipital or posterior cervical regions. Examination may reveal tenderness over the scalp or on palpation of the trapezius and posterior cervical muscles.

The quality is typically dull and steady, described as a sensation of tightness, pressure or constriction around the head. Again many variations may be seen in the classic picture. Sudden jabs of pain can be superimposed upon a steady ache, or throbbing may occur at times. Anorexia is common, and nausea may be felt when the headache is severe though actual vomiting is rare. Some degree of photophobia may be present. Pronounced relief may be obtained with alcohol, whereas migraine headaches are almost invariably worsened by this.

The points of value in distinguishing between migraine and tension headaches were indicated in Friedman et al.'s (1954) analysis of 1000 cases of each. A family history of headache was present in 65% of migraine sufferers and 40% of patients with tension headaches. Onset had been over the age of 20 in 45% of the former and 70% of the latter. The frequency was daily in only 3% of migraine yet 50% of tension headaches, and less than once per week in 60% and 15%, respectively. Prodromata occurred in 60% of migraine patients but only 10% of patients with tension headaches. The character was throbbing in 80% and 30%, respectively, and the distribution bilateral in 20% and 90%, respectively. Vomiting occurred in 50% of migraine patients and 10% of tension headache patients. No differences could be found with regard to precipitants, mood changes or the gradualness of onset or ending. In all cases of tension headache emotional causes could be identified, usually environmental demands which exceeded the patient's capacity to cope. As with migraine the conflicts were variable in nature but often seemed to centre around the control of hostile impulses.

Treatment

Medical details of treatment are dealt with in neurological text books but may be briefly outlined here. Many attacks are adequately controlled by rest and simple analgesics such as aspirin, paracetamol or ibuprofen, provided these are taken at an early stage. Metoclopramide (Maxolon) may usefully be taken as an antiemetic.

Ergotamine tartrate usually gives pronounced relief in more severe attacks, again when taken very early in the course. Oral preparations may contain certain adjuvants in addition to ergotamine, such as caffeine (in Cafergot) or caffeine and cyclizine (in Migril). Patients commonly appear to find some preparation which suits them better than others. Preparations are available for use sublingually, by inhaler and by suppository. Prochlorperazine (Stemetil) suppositories may be used when vomiting is severe.

Ergotamine preparations must be strictly avoided in patients with peripheral vascular disease, coronary disease, hypertension or in pregnancy. They should be restricted to those under 40 and when attacks occur less than monthly (Davies & Rose 1987), and the dose must be carefully controlled to a maximum of 1–2 mg per dose or 6 mg per week. In addition to the well-known toxic effects of overdosage there is risk of habituation and tolerance from excessive self medication. A paradoxical effect may indeed emerge, in which the drug relieves the headache for which it is given, but at the same time leads to increasing frequency of headaches so that consumption steadily rises. Lucas and Falkowski (1973) drew attention to the special dangers of such a course in emotionally disturbed patients, and showed the benefit that could result from withdrawal of medication.

Sumatriptan (Imigran), a recently introduced 5-HT$_1$-like receptor agonist which mediates selective vasoconstriction in the cranial arterial bed, has proved to be remarkably effective in treatment of the acute attack, with the advantage that it can work even if given several hours after the onset of headache (Drug & Therapeutics Bulletin 1992b). In addition to relieving headache it has beneficial effects on nausea and photophobia. It may be taken orally or in prefilled syringes for subcutaneous injection. The principal disadvantage is the high cost of treatment, also a tendency for headache to recur within 48 hours. It is contraindicated in patients with ischaemic heart disease, uncontrolled hypertension and in pregnancy. The subcutaneous injection must not be given to patients with hemiplegic migraine.

Prophylactic drug therapy may be indicated when two or more attacks are regularly experienced per month. Tranquillisers such as diazepam may be tried initially, and amitriptyline has been shown to be successful even when clinical evidence of depression is absent (Gomersall & Stuart 1973). However, propranolol (Inderal) is widely regarded as the drug of first choice, and has been shown to be effective in a high proportion of patients. Other beta blockers such as metoprolol or atenolol are also used. Pizotifen (Sanomigran), a serotonin antagonist, is a useful alternative, though weight gain and drowsiness are troublesome side effects. Sodium valproate has recently been shown to be effective (Jensen *et al.* 1994).

Methysergide (Deseril), another serotonin antagonist, enjoyed a vogue as a potent prophylactic, but is probably no more effective than propranolol. It must only be taken under close supervision, with a month's suspension of treatment every 4–6 months, on account of its danger of leading to retroperitoneal or pleuropulmonary fibrosis. It can also produce peripheral vasoconstriction, sometimes affecting a single large vessel alone.

Older traditional prophylactics such as belladonna combined with a small dose of phenobarbitone and ergotamine (Bellergal tablets) have an unproven place in treatment.

Pharmacological aspects are, however, merely a part of the total management required in patients with migraine of disabling severity. Attention may need to be directed towards a host of factors specific to the individual—regularisation of sleep and meal times, judicious avoidance of stress where this is possible, and perhaps attention to provocative substances in the diet. In addition social and psychological factors will usually warrant close consideration when attacks have become frequent and incapacitating.

Psychotherapy in the formal sense would appear to be indicated in only a small proportion of patients. What is more commonly required is a sound doctor–patient relationship, through which an understanding can be gained of the emotional problems and life situations which provide the settings for attacks. The ability of the patient to handle emotional tension, and to learn how to avoid situations which lead to it, will often prove to be a major factor in preventing attacks or in breaking a vicious circle. It will usually be unrealistic to seek to persuade a driving and overcommitted person to change his life style, but he may respond to advice to moderate his work, delegate duties or to arrange for regular periods of rest and relaxation.

It is important to detect and treat depressive or anxiety states which are aggravating the situation. One must similarly be alert to sources of emotional turmoil which have arisen, especially conflicts at work or in interpersonal relationships. When the patient's personality and life situation are well understood, the attacks may be seen as providing oblique expression for various feelings and moods which are denied expression in other ways — imposing a halt after prolonged activity, allowing temporary respite for the working through of stresses and conflicts, providing an outlet for repressed anger, or fulfilling a self-punitive role in chronically depressed individuals (Sacks 1970). The principal motivational determinants are often apparent without recourse to intensive psychotherapy, but in some instances there may be indications for embarking on this. Examples of striking success from analytically orientated therapy have been reported in selected groups of patients by Fromm-Reichmann (1937) and Sperling (1964).

Mitchell (1971) has indicated the value which may be obtained from behaviourally orientated techniques in reducing the frequency and severity of attacks. Training in relaxation has been shown to produce enduring improvement, likewise hypnosis aimed at reducing tension or apprehension (Lance 1993). Biofeedback has been reported to show striking success with certain patients (Fischer-Williams *et al.* 1981; Kogeorgos & Scott 1981), though the coincident use of relaxation makes the specificity of such treatment uncertain. Electromyographic feedback, of value with tension headaches, often fails with migraine; electrothermal feedback, in which for example the patient is trained to raise the distal finger temperature, appears to be the most promising technique with headaches of vascular origin.

Subdural haematoma

The majority of subdural haematomas follow head injury, though spontaneous cases occasionally arise in patients with blood dyscrasias or on anticoagulants. Blood accumulates in the subdural space from rupture of veins running between the cortex and the dural venous sinuses. It becomes encysted between the dura and arachnoid and may swell by osmosis to reach a very large size. Localising signs often remain minimal, however, since the brain is compressed from without. The collections usually lie over the frontal or parietal lobes and are bilateral in a third to a half of cases.

Those which declare themselves acutely after head injury present either with failure to regain consciousness or with fluctuating confusion and torpor often lapsing into coma. Hemiparesis and ocular changes are usually evident, but neurological deficits can be surprisingly slight and overshadowed by the mental disturbance. Quite often the haematoma is suspected only because the patient's recovery from the injury is slower than expected.

It is the chronic subdural haematoma, however, which is notorious for leading to mistakes in diagnosis, particularly among the elderly. The antecedent head injury may be trivial and go unrecognised, and there may be few clear pointers to the presence of a space-occupying lesion within the skull. Sometimes there is a latent interval of days, weeks or months after injury before the declaration of symptoms. Very occasionally a year or more may elapse.

In classic examples there is vague headache which sets in gradually and may or may not be localised. It may be present only intermittently or occasionally be entirely absent. Dullness, sluggishness and difficulty with concentration slowly increase in severity. Lapses of memory and episodes of mental aberration occur. The level of consciousness fluctuates widely, with periods of apparent normality alternating with periods of drowsiness, changing from day to day or even from hour to hour. The variability in the mental state is often the most important indicator of the condition. Physical signs may be few, with inequality of the pupils, transient ocular paralyses or upgoing plantar responses. Pyramidal tract involvement may progress to hemiparesis, and a grasp reflex may be present. Papilloedema remains absent in a large proportion of cases. Epileptic fits may occur but are rare. Ultimately the patient lapses into intermittent mutism or semicoma, but even at this stage evidence of neurological involvement can be surprisingly slight.

Wide variation may be seen from the typical picture. Occasional patients present with severe headache but no physical signs, others with episodes of confusion and restlessness. In long-standing cases there may be insidious failure of intellect progressing to generalised dementia. In a retrospective survey, Black (1984) analysed the mental changes recorded in 79 patients discharged from hospital with subdural haematomas. In 20% mental symptoms had been the initial manifestation, and 58% had developed them by the time of admission. Delirium occurred in 24 patients, with lethargy and fluctuating clouding of consciousness. Dementia was present in seven, coma in six and three patients showed depression with minimal changes in consciousness or intellect.

Problems with diagnosis are particularly severe among the elderly where the classic picture has been found to be the exception rather than the rule, occurring in only five of 52 examples reported by Bedford (1958). The typical story was of an aged person, already somewhat enfeebled, recently becoming mentally confused. Drowsiness was not always present, and concomitant disease such as pneumonia, uraemia or cardiac failure provided further diagnostic distractions. Stuteville and Welch (1958) found that a history of trauma could not be elicited in almost a quarter of patients, or when present it was often trivial and considered a symptom rather than the cause. Falls are commonplace in old age, likewise minor neurological signs such as a positive Babinski response or pupillary abnormalities. The diagnosis may therefore be overlooked until the patient declines and becomes somnolent or comatose. Despite the utmost vigilance only 40% of Bedford's cases were diagnosed during life.

In a psychiatric hospital autopsy study, Cole (1978) found subdural haematomas to be the commonest form of space-occupying lesion. Six acute and eight chronic haematomas were discovered among 200 routine autopsies, yet the diagnosis had been made before death only once. In the chronic cases, particularly, signs were often minimal and fluctuation of consciousness had rarely been conspicuous. A terminal seizure or sudden death had sometimes been the first indication of a change in the patient's condition. In the elderly a cerebrovascular accident had often been held responsible when neurological deficits were present.

Apart from dementia, differentiation must be made from cerebral infarction, cerebral tumour and alcoholism. Important features distinguishing subdural haematomas from strokes are the slow steady increase in neurological deficit, the presence of some lack of responsiveness, and lack of improvement mentally despite comparatively slight physical disability (Carter 1972). Sometimes the two occur together when cerebral infarction has led to a fall with striking of the head. Cerebral tumour may be closely simulated when there is evidence of raised intracranial pressure. The fluctuating course of the drowsiness and mental confusion can then be an important differentiating feature. Chronic alcoholism may lead to similar drowsiness and intermittent mental aberration, and alcoholics are liable to head injuries which are then forgotten. Thus seven of the 14 examples of subdural haematoma discovered by Selecki (1965) among patients admitted to a psychiatric hospital were in deteriorated chronic alcoholics.

Further examples of diagnostic difficulty are provided by Chambers (1955):

A man in his forties entered hospital twice on account of severe intractable headache. Because of certain problems in his environment he was at first diagnosed as suffering from tension headaches. The cerebrospinal fluid was normal in content and under normal pressure. The only neurological sign was drift of the left arm. When closely questioned his family admitted that he had behaved oddly, on one occasion for example walking naked through the house in front of the children. Air encephalography showed lack of subarachnoid air on the right, and on the evidence of these few findings burr holes were made. A subdural haematoma 5 cm thick was removed from the right frontal area and he made a complete recovery.

A 70-year-old mother became excited on hearing that for the first time her family were not coming to visit at Christmas. She fell backwards from a rocking chair, striking her head, but was not rendered unconscious. Over the next few weeks she became depressed, sullen, somnolent and lacking in appetite. For 3 months she was treated as a case of depression superimposed on senility until she finally had a convulsion. A large subdural haematoma was then disclosed.

Investigations are usually crucial for the diagnosis. Skull X-ray may reveal shift of the midline structures. The EEG is abnormal in 90% of patients, with diminution or suppression of alpha rhythms over the affected hemisphere or unilateral slow activity (Kiloh *et al.* 1981). It is a guide to laterality in 75% of cases, but there can be abnormal rhythms bilaterally or even localisation to the wrong side of the head.

The CT scan will usually provide definitive evidence, showing displacement of midline structures, obliteration of the ventricle on the ipsilateral side and a low density area underlying the skull. Care must be taken, however, particularly with bilateral haematomas which can sometimes be missed by CT (Davenport *et al.* 1994). The clotted blood is initially more dense than brain, becoming hypodense as it liquefies; it therefore passes through an isodense phase during the transitional period. Clues may lie in the generalised absence of sulci and a small ventricular system, but such signs are often equivocal. The issue is sometimes resolved with contrast enhancement, or better still with MRI. The latter has been shown to be greatly superior to CT, particularly in the demonstration of small

subdural collections (Kelly *et al.* 1988). When CT or MRI are not available, and the index of suspicion is high, alternative investigations may be required. A radioisotope scan may show crescentic uptake over the hemisphere, or angiography the characteristic displacement of vessels. Exploratory burr holes will sometimes be needed to resolve the issue decisively.

Lumbar puncture must be avoided when a subdural haematoma is suspected. The cerebrospinal fluid is often under increased pressure but may be otherwise normal. The protein may be raised and xanthochromia may be present. Red blood corpuscles are found if a leak has occurred into the subarachnoid space.

Evacuation of the haematoma can lead to excellent results, particularly in early cases. Much depends, however, on the presence of complicating pathologies, and the prognosis often proves to be poor in the elderly. Forty-three per cent of Stuteville and Welch's (1958) cases died postoperatively. Among 30 survivors Wortis *et al.* (1943) found that half recovered virtually completely, though some of these were left with emotional dullness. The remainder showed impairments of memory and intellect, dysphasia, or persistent euphoria with severely impaired behaviour. Mehta (1965) similarly stressed the high morbidity among survivors, particularly by way of organic mental impairments.

Giant cerebral aneurysms

The great majority of aneurysms giving rise to subarachnoid haemorrhage are small, rarely exceeding 1 or 2 cm in diameter. Massive aneurysms are distinctly uncommon, but when present can give rise to much diagnostic confusion and are often not even considered in differential diagnosis.

Best known is the aneurysm of the intracavernous portion of the internal carotid artery, which may compress surrounding nerves leading to ophthalmoplegias and sensory loss of trigeminal distribution. It occasionally ruptures to give rise to a pulsating exophthalmos.

Those situated on the circle of Willis at the base of the brain rarely rupture, but can produce local pressure effects simulating basal space-occupying lesions. Bull (1969) reported 22 such cases collected over a similar number of years. Common complaints were of visual disturbance or headache. In six patients, however, mental changes predominated; dementia was the presenting feature, usually but not invariably accompanied by neurological signs such as cranial nerve deficits or hemiparesis.

Morley (1967) reviewed the literature concerning unruptured vertebrobasilar aneurysms, which can lead to a variety of pictures simulating multiple sclerosis, posterior fossa tumours or vertebrobasilar ischaemia. Three of his own five cases had at first been diagnosed as psychiatrically unwell — vague symptoms of headache, nondescript dizziness, slowed speech and a muted facial expression had led to an impression of depressive illness. Mental impairment was also sometimes evident.

Transient global amnesia

The syndrome of transient global amnesia consists of episodes, abrupt in onset, in which the patient displays profound memory difficulties despite remaining alert and responsive to the environment. Attacks usually last for several hours after which memory functions gradually return to normal. Several large-scale studies have shown that the prognosis is essentially benign. The pathogenesis remains obscure and it seems likely that there are several causes; a basis in cerebral thromboembolism is now considered uncommon, and a proportion of cases show evidence of a link to migraine.

Attention was first drawn to the condition by Bender (1956, 1960) and Poser and Ziegler (1960). It was independently described by Fisher and Adams (1958, 1964) who gave it its name. The condition appears to be not uncommon and derives much of its importance to neurologists and psychiatrists from the mistakes in diagnosis that are liable to be made.

Clinical features

Most patients are affected in late middle or old age, and males appear to outnumber females. Abruptly and entirely without warning the memory apparatus ceases to function, with the result that current experiences fail to be recorded in memory. The patient may sense that something is wrong, or may merely betray the abnormality to onlookers by remarks or behaviour. As the attack continues it becomes evident that the patient cannot memorise the events of his immediate situation, also that he has a patchy retrograde amnesia for the days, weeks or even years preceding the onset of the attack. Thus he has difficulty in locating himself in time or place, and in ascertaining his relationship to what is happening around. Furthermore, whatever information is given cannot be held in the mind for long. A state of anxious bewilderment typically results, with repeated stereotyped questioning of onlookers and sometimes expressions of considerable fear and concern. Some patients, however, appear to lack insight and sit quietly, though puzzled, through most of the attack.

In contrast to the difficulty with recent memory and the inability to store new information, recall appears to be normal for events from the distant past. A temporal gradient may be discerned, with better recall of long-distant items than those occurring within the preceding months or years. Knowledge of personal identity remains unimpaired, and relatives and acquaintances of long standing are recognised normally. The memory deficit is 'global' in the sense of affecting all modalities — visual impressions, verbal material, thoughts, events, etc. Confabulation is rarely observed.

The detailed descriptions of Fisher and Adams (1964) and the recent extensive study by Hodges (1991) indicate that most functions other than memory remain substantially intact throughout the attack. There is no drowsiness, inattentiveness or other evidence of impairment of consciousness. The attention span is normal as judged by the digit repetition test. The patient may be able to continue working for some minutes on an assigned task. Thinking appears to be coherent within the limits allowed by the memory disorder. Understanding and production of language are normal, and perceptual competence well preserved. Habitual acts such as dressing, eating and even driving are performed without difficulty. Most patients have found their way normally about familiar environments, and several have driven home while attacks were continuing.

Gordon and Marin (1979) were able to make detailed observations on a patient during an attack. He showed normal immediate recall, as tested by the digit span, but an almost total inability to store new information. Cueing was of no help with this anterograde amnesia. There was an extensive though patchy retrograde gap, with no knowledge of the President of the USA or his predecessor, and vague awareness of a 'catastrophe' affecting President Kennedy (13 years before) but no knowledge of its nature. Other cognitive functions were carried out normally. The failure to recall or recognise information from the distant past, which was perfectly available to the patient when the attack was over, implied an impairment of retrieval as well as of consolidation.

More recently Hodges and Ward (1989) have reported detailed neuropsychological examinations on five patients studied during attacks. They were able to confirm normal immediate memory functioning as tested by the digit span, intact language and visuospatial functioning, and the lack of any clouding of consciousness or blunting of attention. The profound anterograde memory impairments involved both verbal and nonverbal material. Retrograde memory tests showed variable results, but in general confirmed an extensive and temporally graded deficit affecting both personal and public events, often but not always extending over several decades. Kazui *et al.* (1995) have shown that procedural learning and priming effects remain intact during attacks.

The episodes commonly last from one to several hours or rarely for several days. In seeking to establish agreed diagnostic criteria for the syndrome Hodges (1991) suggests that 24 hours should be accepted as the upper limit of duration, in conformity with that used for transient ischaemic attacks (p. 380). In his own material of 114 cases the great majority of attacks lasted for 1–8 hours.

As the attack begins to subside the retrograde gap shrinks, distant events returning before those most closely related to the onset, and the patient gradually shows evidence that current experiences are beginning to register. A further hour or more may elapse before memory appears to be fully restored to normal. After recovery a dense amnesic gap remains for the period of the episode, together in most cases with a permanent retrograde amnesia of several minutes to several hours. Other than this there are no overt sequelae in the typical case.

Thus the attacks are in essence a highly circumscribed failure of the memory apparatus, lasting usually for several hours and proving to be reversible. Other accompaniments, by way of neurological signs or systemic disturbances, have in most cases been conspicuous by their absence. Occasionally, however, when opportunities have arisen for detailed observation, there has been evidence of dizziness, tinnitus, headache, mild paraesthesia, diplopia or ataxia. By the strict diagnostic criteria proposed by Hodges (1991), patients with accompanying focal symptoms or signs are excluded. Non-focal symptoms are permitted, however, and in Hodges' large series 20% suffered from headache, nausea or vomiting during or immediately after their attacks.

Hodges and Ward (1989) were able to show that resolution of the memory disturbance was often slower than was clinically apparent. Though the patients and their families felt that complete recovery had occurred, testing in five patients showed persisting verbal and non-verbal memory deficits at 24 hours, with continuing improvement over the following week. Slight further improvements were demonstrated at 6 months, by which time all but one patient performed within the normal range. The issue of more enduring impairments of a subtle nature is discussed on p. 415.

Typical examples are as follows:

A man of 67 developed his attack immediately after a prolonged interview with two journalists who had noticed nothing amiss. He turned to his family after bidding the visitors goodbye, looking puzzled and asking 'Who are they? What are they doing here?' He then asked how it happened that certain members of his family were present (they had come for a visit the previous day). He was obviously worried and appreciated that he could not remember or collect his thoughts. For the next hour and a half he repeatedly asked similar questions — 'What are they doing here? What are you doing here? Do you see anything wrong with me?' There was no dysarthria or dysphasia. He tested his arms and legs periodically to assure himself that they functioned normally. He did not remember that the journalists had made their appointment a few weeks previously, nor did he recall special events of the day before or of the morning hours preceding the interview.

As recovery occurred he first recalled the events of the day before, then of the evening before, and finally he recalled fetching wood for the fire 1 hour prior to the interview. After 1.5 hours he lay down and slept for an hour, following which he appeared to have recovered fully. A retrograde amnesia remained permanently for the period of the interview (1.5 hours), and the hour prior to this. He also proved subsequently to remember very little of the day following the attack, although he appeared to his family to have recovered in 3 hours.

(Fisher & Adams 1964)

A 76-year-old housewife was in good health when, without premonitory symptoms, she suddenly appeared confused and disorientated, asking questions such as 'Where am I?', 'What happened?', etc. There was no disturbance of sight, speech or motor power. When admitted to hospital 3 hours after the onset she was fully alert, and answered routine questions about her family and past history correctly, but was restless and anxious, frequently interrupting the conversation with stereotyped questions such as the above. She did not know where she was and forgot immediately after being told. She was muddled as to the time, date and year. After the initial examination the doctor left the room for a few minutes and when he returned she did not recognise him. A retrograde amnesia was present, covering the preceding week, whereas memory for remote events was intact. The patient seemed to be aware of the memory defect and did not confabulate. No abnormal signs were found on neurological examination. Ten hours after admission the patient's memory functions began to return, and during the following 2 days the retrograde amnesia cleared.   (Bolwig 1968)

Precipitating factors, though not universal, have been mentioned in several series—physical exertion, exposure to cold as in sea bathing or to heat as when taking a bath. Occasional examples have set in during or after sexual intercourse, or after painful procedures such as dental extractions. Emotional stress, for example receiving bad news or being involved in a violent argument, had occurred during the preceding 24 hours in 14% of Hodges' (1991) series. Altogether Miller et al. (1987) observed notable antecedents in a third of their 277 patients.

Single attacks appear to be the rule, though recurrence occurs in a significant number of patients. The proportion has been widely variable in different series, no doubt due to differing inclusion criteria. The two largest series to date are those reported by Miller et al. (1987) and Hodges (1991); 14% of Miller et al.'s patients had recurrences during the next 6.5 years, and 15% of Hodges' during almost 3 years' follow-up. This latter proportion fell to 8% after excluding cases in whom recurrence was due to epilepsy (p. 417). A much higher rate of subsequent attacks was reported by Heathfield *et al.* (1973), eight of whose 19 patients had further episodes at intervals varying from several days to several years. Lou (1968) reported one patient with nine attacks and another with three attacks over periods of several months. As described below it has emerged that patients with multiple attacks are at increased risk of developing epilepsy, suggesting that in this subgroup the aetiology may often be different from the remainder.

The question of residual impairment after attacks has also been variously reported. Clearly the great majority of patients recover completely, as judged by the patients themselves and their relatives and friends. In some patients with multiple attacks, however, persisting memory difficulties have been described (Steinmetz & Vroom 1972; Mathew & Meyer 1974). This runs counter to general experience, and it is possible that some of these patients were suffering from amnesic strokes. CT scanning was not available at that time to exclude thalamic or posterior cerebral infarctions. Mazzucchi *et al.* (1980) found minor impairments on psychometric testing in a group of 16 patients who had suffered single episodes when examined on average 8 months later; in comparison to controls they performed less well on verbal memory tests despite feeling that they had recovered completely, and their verbal intelligence scores were significantly lower than performance intelligence scores.

The situation has been clarified by Hodges and Oxbury (1990), who tested 41 patients along with carefully selected controls at 6 months post-attack. All of the patients had conformed to strict diagnostic criteria—witnessed attacks, no clouding of consciousness or loss of personal identity, absence of epileptic features or accompanying focal symptoms or signs, no recent head injury and resolution of the attack within 24 hours. Neuropsychological evaluation at 6 months showed no evidence of intellectual decline, but verbal memory tests showed mild but consistent deficits compared to controls. This could not be attributed to a subgroup alone, but reflected a general shift in the distribution of scores. Tests of remote memory, both autobiographical and impersonal, also showed slight impairments. Non-verbal memory, by contrast, appeared to be fully intact. It would seem therefore that though the patients and their families are unaware of it, subtle deficits are prone to persist at least for many months.

CT scanning in patients with 'pure' transient global amnesia is usually normal. Hodges (1991) found that 12% of 95 cases showed small white matter lacunes or periventricular lucencies, but in no case did these involve memory-related structures. The only instance of infarc-

tion was in a patient already known to have had a stroke. The EEG is also typically normal, though minor and non-specific abnormalities have been reported in a varying proportion of patients.

Differential diagnosis

Though varying as to detail, the main features of the attacks are remarkably similar from one example to another. Unless one is conversant with the syndrome, however, a range of diagnoses will usually be considered.

A short-lived episode may raise the possibility of temporal lobe epilepsy. Complex partial seizures begin abruptly in a similar fashion, involve a suspension of memory recording and leave an enduring amnesic gap. Patients with repeated episodes will be particularly suspected of epilepsy, and this may indeed prove to be the diagnosis in some of them as discussed on p. 417. Several patients, moreover, have shown electroencephalographic abnormalities in the region of the temporal lobes (Steinmetz & Vroom 1972; Heathfield *et al.* 1973). However, most complex partial seizures are brief, lasting minutes rather than hours, and may be ushered in by aural manifestations which are totally lacking in transient global amnesia. During a complex partial seizure there is usually evidence of clouding of consciousness, poor appreciation of the environment and purposeless or 'automatic' behaviour. By contrast, patients with transient global amnesia remain fully in touch with their surroundings, are alert and show evidence of awareness of what they are doing and experiencing. They respond to questions appropriately and behave normally apart from the obvious memory defects. Recovery of normal mental function is gradual after an attack of transient global amnesia whereas it is usually abrupt after a complex partial seizure.

Hypoglycaemic attacks may likewise set in abruptly, lead to a period of confused behaviour, and leave an amnesic gap for what has transpired. However, behaviour is usually inappropriate or even disorderly during the attack, and motor coordination is likely to be impaired with ataxia, clumsiness or dysarthria. Nevertheless, when a patient is seen in the course of an attack, hypoglycaemia should be excluded, and when there is room for doubt glucose should be administered.

Many patients will be suspected of suffering from minor strokes. Cerebral ischaemia on a vascular basis may indeed be the mechanism behind occasional episodes, as discussed below. It should be noted, however, that attacks of transient global amnesia only rarely show ancillary evidence of cerebral ischaemia by way of associated neurological deficits, and that strokes rarely lead to extensive temporary amnesia unless other manifestations are marked.

A brief episode of delirium or some acute intoxication may at first be considered a possibility. Alcoholism will sometimes be suspected. However, the suddenness of onset in persons who were normal a moment before, the restriction of the abnormalities to memory defects, and the lack of clouding of consciousness or perceptual disturbance should allow a differentiation. When the history of the onset is not available a period of post-traumatic confusion may be suspected. Very occasionally, episodes of amnesia may be the presenting feature of an encephalitic illness.

A psychological origin for the amnesias is probably quite often entertained, especially when follow-up fails to reveal the development of organic disease. However, the setting and the manifestations of the attacks are quite unlike amnesic episodes due to psychological causes. A stereotyped setting will, of course, raise the strong possibility of psychogenesis as in the following example:

A 28-year-old man experienced five amnesic episodes over the course of a year, lasting from 30 minutes to 14 hours at a time. None were witnessed, and all had occurred from the moment of locking his office door after a stressful day at work. After three of the attacks he regained awareness while sitting on a railway station awaiting a train to Aylesbury. After another he regained a vague recollection of being in Aylesbury and visiting his old home there. He could not be encouraged to divulge reasons for the recurrent preoccupation with Aylesbury, but readily accepted that it indicated a psychogenic basis for the attacks. He had lived there until moving to Kent 2.5 years previously. Current stresses included serious illness in his father, his wife's second pregnancy and a threat of foreclosure on the mortgage involving his new home.

Psychogenic amnesia is uncommon in the age group principally affected by transient global amnesia, obvious psychological precipitants rarely come to light, and most patients are said to be of normal personality and good premorbid stability. The duration of attacks of transient global amnesia is typically several hours, whereas psychogenic episodes often last for days or weeks. The structure of the memory defect itself, with demonstrably faulty new learning and a time-related retrograde gap, is entirely consistent with an organic origin. The retention of knowledge of personal identity throughout the attack is also at variance with what is often found during psychogenic amnesias. The memory difficulties are not restricted to matters of personal concern or specific themes, there are no inconsistencies in performance, and no evidence of gain. The patients are not suggestible during attacks, but behave appropriately and typically seek to remedy the amnesic gaps by anxious questioning.

Croft *et al.* (1973) indicated the relative frequency of transient global amnesia among 39 patients referred by general practitioners to a neurological clinic. All had experienced a transient amnesic episode. Twenty-four (62%) proved to be examples of transient global amnesia, seven were epileptic, two had occurred in the context of migraine and two were the prelude to encephalitic illnesses. Only four were considered psychogenic in origin, but this may have reflected the special selection inherent in neurological referral.

Nature of the disorder

One of the fascinations of the disorder is that in the majority of instances the cause remains unknown. Despite numerous observations, often on large and carefully selected series, no unifying aetiological factor has come to light. Fisher and Adams considered that both an unusual type of local cerebral seizure and a transient ischaemia of the hippocampal–hypothalamic system were tenable hypotheses, though there were difficulties in the way of either interpretation. If epileptic in origin the attacks were distinctly unusual in form, as already outlined. Many, indeed the majority, seemed not to recur; and epilepsy beginning so late in life would be expected to have a lesional origin yet such is not revealed.

A basis in cerebral thromboembolism was suggested by the fact that the majority of patients are elderly, that recurrence is relatively uncommon, and that attacks are occasionally followed by permanent memory impairments. However, the transience of the memory disorder in most cases and the generally excellent long-term prognosis are hard to reconcile with ischaemic stroke. In some series, but not in others, a high prevalence of hypertension or other risk factors for infarction have been reported (e.g. Mathew & Meyer 1974). In the remarkable family reported by Corston and Godwin-Austen (1982), where four brothers had suffered attacks, it seemed likely that the reason was a summation in the family of risk factors for vascular disease — hypertension, diabetes and heart disease.

Although the evidence remains conflicting, recent studies have served to discount a basis in cerebral thromboembolism, at least when patients with accompanying neurological signs are excluded. Hinge *et al.* (1986) followed 74 such patients for a mean of 5.5 years, and found that the rates of death and of cerebrovascular morbidity were no different from those expected in the Danish population of equivalent sex and age. In the large series of 277 patients from the Mayo Clinic, Miller *et al.* (1987) found no increased risk for stroke during an average follow-up of 6.5 years. Most decisively, Hodges (1991) matched 114 cases, carefully selected as described on p. 414, with patients who had suffered transient ischaemic attacks and with healthy community-based controls. In comparison with the latter the amnesic patients showed no increased prevalence of risk factors such as hypertension, ischaemic heart disease, cardiac dysrhythmias, diabetes, peripheral vascular disease, alcohol consumption or smoking. On follow-up only two deaths occurred, both due to non-vascular causes, compared with 33 deaths among the transient ischaemic attack controls of which 21 were due to vascular factors. The standardised mortality was seven times greater among the transient ischaemic attack controls. Strokes occurred in only two patients compared to 32 of the transient ischaemic attack controls, this again representing a sevenfold increase in incidence among the latter when standardised for length of follow-up. On such data a basis in cerebrovascular pathology must be regarded as very unlikely, at least for the great majority of cases. However, it still remains a possible explanation for occasional examples, namely those atypical cases (excluded by Hodges) in whom neurological deficits accompany attacks or where noteworthy deficits persist.

Two features relevant to aetiology emerged from Hodges' study. First, eight of the 114 patients (7%) became epileptic during the follow-up period, usually within a year, even though none of these had a history of epilepsy prior to their first attack of amnesia. Most developed complex partial seizures, usually with episodes of altered consciousness consisting of blankness or automatism followed by periods of amnesia. This subgroup was characterised by multiple attacks of transient global amnesia at presentation, and by attacks of unusually brief duration, mostly lasting for less than an hour. Presumably in this small group the presenting attacks also represented seizures and the epileptic features had gone unnoticed at the time. CT scans and EEGs carried out at presentation had, however, been unremarkable.

The second important finding was the high prevalence of migraine, occurring in almost a third of the patients with transient global amnesia. This was the only factor that occurred significantly more often than in the normal controls and the patients with transient ischaemic attacks. An association with migraine was noted in 14% of Miller et al.'s (1987) patients, and headache and nausea were reported in 17% of episodes. Crowell et al. (1984) noted that five of their 12 patients were migraineurs, and regional cerebral blood flow studies showed impaired vasomotor responses of migrainous type in five of the seven patients tested. It seems possible, therefore, that in a substantial proportion of cases the underlying pathophysiological mechanism may share features in common

with migraine; 'spreading depression' (p. 402) is a likely contender (Olesen & Jorgensen 1986). Again, however, it is unlikely that this accounts for the majority of examples of the syndrome.

In very occasional cases still other mechanisms appear to be responsible. Typical attacks have been reported after head injury, subdural haematoma, hydrocephalus, polycythaemia and diazepam overdosage (Hodges 1991). Several cases have occurred in patients with cerebral tumours, usually with atypical features, and several have followed cerebral (especially vertebral) angiography.

It seems, therefore, that a number of aetiological factors are likely to be operative in transient global amnesia. A small subgroup appears to represent epilepsy, albeit of late onset and without a lesional basis, and a larger group to be allied in some fashion with migraine. Less 'pure' cases, with concomitant neurological defects, may represent thromboembolic phenomena, and occasional examples may have a basis in other cerebral pathology. In the remainder, which represent the majority, the cause is still unknown.

Despite these varying aetiologies, the uniformities in the clinical picture, with circumscribed and transient memory failure, suggest that the pathophysiological basis of attacks may ultimately share much in common or indeed may be identical from one case to another. On the basis of present anatomical knowledge of the memory apparatus one must postulate some reversible affection of the diencephalic–hypothalamic system or the inferomedial parts of the temporal lobes. SPECT scanning carried out during the course of attacks by Kazui et al. (1995) showed hypoperfusion restricted to the latter situation in all three cases studied.

Systemic lupus erythematosus

Systemic lupus erythematosus (SLE) is a member of the so-called 'collagen diseases' or 'connective tissue disorders', along with rheumatoid arthritis, rheumatic fever, scleroderma and dermatomyositis. To some extent there may be overlap between variants of SLE and these other conditions, though in the main it is established as a specific disease entity.

The change in our conception of the disease, from a fulminant and rapidly fatal disorder to one that can run a chronic course with relapses and remissions, owes much to the establishment of the LE test as a diagnostic measure by Hargreaves et al. in 1948. It is now recognised as a not uncommon disease with markedly pleomorphic manifestations. Cerebral involvement has been reported increasingly, and mental symptoms are known to be prominent in a high proportion of cases. It is evident, moreover, that very occasionally neuropsychiatric complications can set in early, before the involvement of other systems is clinically obvious. Hence it has become important to include appropriate screening tests in the detailed evaluation of certain neurological and psychiatric patients as described below.

The aetiology remains incompletely understood. An inherited predisposition may be partly at work, and a great deal of evidence supports an immunological basis for the development of tissue lesions. Whether the hypersensitivity reactions are to external toxins or the result of an autologous autoimmune process is not entirely clear, though the latter is favoured. Many of the pathological features of the disease appear to be due to deposition of antibody–antigen complexes with resultant complement fixation and inflammation of the tissues.

General clinical features

The disease is markedly more common in females with a female : male ratio of 9 : 1. It mainly occurs in young adult life, with a mean age of onset of 30 years, but the range is wide.

The clinical manifestations are described by Dubois (1966) and Byron and Hughes (1983). The onset is usually insidious with the development of fatigue, malaise and low-grade intermittent fever. A migratory arthritis or arthralgia ultimately develops in the majority of cases, closely resembling that of rheumatoid arthritis or rheumatic fever. Diffuse muscle aching is a common accompaniment. Skin changes are frequent, though the classic butterfly eruption over the nose and cheeks is by no means always seen. SLE and discoid lupus erythematosus are now regarded as poles of a spectrum, sometimes occurring separately and sometimes with an admixture or transitional forms in the same patient. Other skin manifestations include purpura, Raynaud's phenomenon and alopecia. Photosensitivity of the skin may be pronounced.

Lymphadenopathy, oedema and anaemia are often disclosed. Of the viscera the kidneys are probably most frequently involved, also the pleura, lungs, heart and pericardium. Liver involvement is exceptional and gross splenomegaly rare. Anorexia, nausea, abdominal pain and vomiting are common. Hypertension is often considerable in degree and retinopathy may develop.

Thus SLE is a multisystem disease, the majority of its manifestations being attributable to vascular lesions or more directly to disturbances of connective tissue. Its manifestations are polymorphous, sometimes involving one organ or system predominantly and often changing

considerably over time. Nervous system involvement, as described below, is no exception in this regard.

The *course of the disease* may be acute, subacute or chronic. Chronic progression with repeated exacerbations and remissions appears to be a frequent pattern, and treatment with steroids is usually successful in tiding the patient over crises and perhaps in delaying fresh progressions. It can be a recurrent mild illness with prolonged asymptomatic intervals. Five-year survival rates have improved from 50% reported in the 1950s to greater than 90% in the 1990s, with 15-year survivals in excess of 80% in some series (Gladman 1992). This is probably attributable to earlier diagnosis, better treatment and the more frequent recognition of mild forms of the disease. Nevertheless central nervous system involvement still ranks with renal failure among the commoner causes of death.

Laboratory investigations

Anaemia is often accompanied by leucopenia, especially lymphopenia, and occasionally by thrombocytopenia. The erythrocyte sedimentation rate (ESR) is raised in about 90% of cases, showing an approximate correlation with the current stage of activity of the disease. Sometimes, however, it can remain high when the disorder is in full remission, and very occasionally a normal ESR is found in the presence of active SLE. Plasma protein abnormalities are common, with lowered serum albumin and raised serum globulins. Serum complement concentrations are reduced, especially in the presence of renal disease. Serological tests for syphilis such as the WR, TPHA and VDRL (pp. 342–3) are liable to give false positive results in 10% of cases though the TPI and FTA will be negative. Examination of the urine will often reveal proteinuria or abnormal sediments.

The LE cell test, which consisted of looking for characteristic changes in polymorphs after incubation with the patient's blood, has been superseded by more sensitive and specific serological markers. The detection of antinuclear antibodies by indirect immunofluorescence is the most sensitive screening test, identifying over 95% of cases (Venables 1993). Antibodies to double-stranded DNA are more specific to the disorder, being virtually restricted to SLE. Antibodies to ribosomal-P proteins are also highly specific, occurring with higher frequency when the disease is active than when quiescent (Sato *et al.* 1991). Earlier suggestions that they might be a marker for cerebral involvement (Bonfa *et al.* 1987) have not, however, been confirmed. Biopsy of skin lesions, or occasionally renal biopsy, may give valuable confirmation of the diagnosis.

Electroencephalographic changes are common whether or not neuropsychiatric changes are present. They are usually diffuse and non-specific though focal changes may occur (Dubois 1966). The cerebrospinal fluid shows an elevated protein and occasional lymphocytes in approximately half of the patients with neuropsychiatric manifestations (Johnson & Richardson 1968).

A high incidence of cerebral atrophy has been shown by CT scanning, but this is not universal even in the presence of neurological complications (McCune & Golbus 1988). Sometimes, moreover, the CT appearances of atrophy are attributable to steroid medication in the absence of cerebral disease (p. 141). MRI detects lesions in a greater number of patients as described on p. 421.

Nervous system involvement

Neuropsychiatric manifestations are now being reported in up to 60% of patients with SLE, when comprehensively studied and followed for reasonably long periods of time. Indeed Hughes (1974) suggests that central nervous system involvement may be overtaking renal disease as the major clinical problem in the disorder, in that it carries a high mortality and the response to treatment is uncertain.

Valuable reviews of the psychiatric and neurological features are provided by Dubois (1966), O'Connor and Musher (1966), Johnson and Richardson (1968), Estes and Christian (1971), Bennett *et al.* (1972) and McCune and Golbus (1988). Mental disorders are repeatedly stressed as the commonest of neuropsychiatric manifestations, with acute and chronic organic reactions, schizophrenic and affective psychoses, changes of personality and a variety of neurotic reactions. The majority of mental disturbances appear to be transient, usually clearing within 6 weeks and rarely outlasting 6 months, though episodes are often recurrent (Gurland *et al.* 1972). Seizures are also common. Neurological findings may include cranial nerve palsies, peripheral neuropathy, movement disorders, intracranial ischaemic events, or more rarely spinal cord involvement leading to paraparesis.

The relative frequency of such changes was shown by Estes and Christian's (1971) survey of 150 patients followed closely over several years. Forty-two per cent showed disorders of mental function, with organic mental syndromes in 21%, functional psychoses in 16% and neurotic reactions in 5%. Seizures occurred in 26%, cranial nerve abnormalities in 5%, peripheral neuropathy in 7%, tremor in 5% and hemiparesis in 5%.

It is clear that the neurological and psychiatric features

of SLE lack any characteristic form or pattern but are as varied as other manifestations of the disease. The most that can be said is that they show a tendency to appear in the later stages, and to develop during relapses of the disorder when other systemic features are in evidence. This is not invariable, however, and central nervous system involvement can sometimes be the primary manifestation, antedating other clear-cut evidence of the disease by months or years (Siekert & Clark 1955). Psychiatric disturbance can also be the presenting feature. Lim *et al.* (1988) reported a patient who presented with acute behavioural change, paranoid ideas and a degree of impairment of consciousness, and who was soon afterwards found to have SLE with renal involvement. Three further psychotic episodes coincided with recrudescences of physical symptoms. Hopkinson *et al.* (1992) discovered three cases of SLE on routine screening of 296 admissions to acute psychiatric units.

Multiple neuropsychiatric manifestations often occur together. The bizarre nature of the syndromes produced can readily lead to mistakes in diagnosis unless the possibility of the disease is borne in mind and appropriate investigations performed. Patients presenting with neurological symptoms may be suspected of multiple sclerosis, sometimes for several years before multisystem involvement is noted (Dubois 1966). Psychotic developments may similarly be misinterpreted in the early stages, or lead to diagnostic difficulty when they appear in a patient who is apparently in full remission. Fessel and Solomon (1960) suggested that all psychotic patients who have a raised ESR and positive serology for syphilis, with no apparent reason, should be fully explored immediately for SLE.

Organic mental syndromes are the most frequent of the mental abnormalities, occurring at some time or another in approximately 30% of patients (Heine 1969). Acute organic reactions ('lupus psychosis') account for the great majority. These are usually brief, lasting for hours or days, then subsiding completely. They are often recurrent, appearing with fresh relapses of the disease and clearing as it goes into remission. The picture may be of quiet confusion and clouding of consciousness, or more florid delirium with visual and auditory hallucinations and excessive motor activity (Johnson & Richardson 1968). Paranoid delusions, mood disturbances and hallucinations may be in the foreground, leading to a diagnosis of schizophrenia if the organic mental features are overlooked (Guze 1967). The degree of disorientation and memory impairment may fluctuate markedly from time to time.

Overt evidence of chronic cerebral dysfunction is a good deal less common, but deterioration of intellect and memory can occasionally progress to a picture of dementia (Johnson & Richardson 1968; Burton *et al.* 1971). Clark and Bailey (1956) found memory deficits in many patients, often associated with changes of personality, anxiety and emotional lability. More subtle deficits may emerge on neuropsychological investigation, and may be indicative of subclinical central nervous system involvement. Carbotte *et al.* (1986) found evidence of impairment on a battery of tests in two-thirds of 62 patients seen consecutively, compared with 17% of patients with rheumatoid arthritis and 14% of healthy controls. Those with a history of clear neurological, schizophrenic or major affective syndromes were twice as liable to show impairment as those without, independently of whether such manifestations were currently active or quiescent.

Affective disorder and schizophrenia are substantially less common than organic psychiatric disturbances. The pictures are often hard to classify with precision since an admixture of organic and non-organic features may occur together. Clearly, however, classic depressive, hypomanic and schizophrenic illnesses can occur. Major depression appears to be much the most common. Guze (1967) found 10 episodes of affective illness and five of schizophrenia-like disorder in 101 patients. Others who have reported a high incidence of schizophrenia may have overlooked the presence of minor memory deficits or clouding of consciousness in patients with paranoid delusions.

Neurotic reactions are probably a good deal commoner than their reported incidence. Anxiety, depression, withdrawal and episodes of depersonalisation have all been stressed. O'Connor and Musher (1966) observed severe anxiety and depression in 19 of 150 patients, and a further two had episodes of 'hysteria'. Such acute neurotic reactions were usually short lived. The anxiety may fluctuate markedly from day to day, without associated change in the physical condition and without clear relation to the current life situation (Clark & Yoss 1956; O'Connor 1959). Similarly, patients may complain of overwhelming feelings of impending disaster which are quite unwarranted by the state of their disease (Clark & Bailey 1956).

Depressive reactions tend to be more gradual in onset, lasting for several weeks or months then resolving slowly (Heine 1969). Ganz *et al.* (1972) compared patients with SLE and with rheumatoid arthritis, and showed that depression was chiefly responsible for the increased incidence of psychiatric disorder in the former disease. Depressive symptoms were twice as common as organic mental symptoms, occurring in 51% and 22% of SLE patients, respectively.

Seizures have been reported in up to 50% of cases, usually grand mal but also focal epilepsy and temporal lobe seizures. Status epilepticus can lead directly to death. Seizures are most common in the terminal stages but sometimes appear early in the disease. Occasionally they accompany an acute exacerbation and then do not recur (Dubois 1966). A rare source of diagnostic uncertainty is the occasional epileptic patient on treatment with hydantoins or primidone who develops an SLE-like syndrome which regresses on withdrawal of the drug.

Cerebrovascular accidents occur in some 5–10% of patients, resulting in a variety of focal neurological deficits (McCune & Golbus 1988). Arteritis of medium-sized vessels may be responsible, or thrombotic occlusions or emboli.

Cranial nerve disorders are among the commoner neurological signs. Usually they set in suddenly without prodromata and most are transient. Disorders of external ocular movement, pupillary abnormalities and vertigo are the most frequent, more rarely disorders of the fifth, seventh and bulbar nerves. Visual field defects are often partly due to retinal changes. Papilloedema may result from a local retinal lesion and optic atrophy may follow.

Peripheral neuropathy is usually symmetrical and distal, with both sensory and motor deficits. A Guillain–Barré form may occur, or occasionally a mononeuropathy.

Movement disorders include tremors, parkinsonian rigidity, ataxia due to brain stem lesions and choreoathetosis. All are relatively rare. Choreiform movements in association with SLE may at first be diagnosed as Sydenham's chorea.

Hemiparesis is rare. Most examples arise in the course of the disease but it can be the initial manifestation (Bennett *et al.* 1972). Dysphasia is occasionally seen. Paraparesis due to transverse myelitis of the cord is also infrequent.

Headache is perhaps the most common of all neurological problems encountered in the disease, often with features typical of migraine (McCune & Golbus 1988). Common or classic migraine had developed since the onset of the illness in seven of 40 patients in Lim *et al.*'s (1988) series, and within the first 5 years in five.

Aetiology of neuropsychiatric manifestations

Pathological changes in the brain have been abundantly described in SLE, chiefly in the form of disease of the small blood vessels leading to scattered infarctions and haemorrhages. The smaller arterioles and capillaries are principally affected with evidence of inflammatory, destructive and proliferative changes. A true 'vasculitis' is rare, the usual finding being fibrinoid degeneration in the vessel walls or hyalinisation with necrosis (Johnson & Richardson 1968). This may be associated with microglial proliferation around the capillaries or with microhaemorrhages due to extravasation of erythrocytes and fibrin. The vascular changes are especially prevalent in the cortex and brain stem. Infarcted areas are usually small and multiple, though extensive areas of softening and large intracerebral haemorrhages occasionally occur.

Many of the neuropsychiatric manifestations clearly depend directly on the cerebral pathology. Johnson and Richardson (1968) observed a correlation between seizures and microinfarcts of the cortex, and between cranial nerve lesions and infarcts in the brain stem. The small size of the typical lesions accorded with the transient nature of the clinical symptoms. Johnson and Richardson further hypothesised a relationship between acute confusional states and widespread cortical pathology. A higher incidence of cerebral atrophy has been shown on the CT scan in the presence of neuropsychiatric features (Ostrov et al. 1982), similarly more severe abnormalities of cerebral blood flow and regional cerebral metabolism (Bresnihan et al. 1979). In the presence of diffuse cerebral disorder, MRI may show symmetrically distributed areas of increased signal intensity in the subcortical white matter (Bell et al. 1991). These may reverse with treatment. Patients with focal signs by contrast are liable to show focal MRI change and atrophy in regions corresponding to the major cerebral vessels, and these are unaltered by steroid treatment.

Clinicopathological correlations at autopsy are, however, far from exact. O'Connor and Musher (1966) found that gross impairment of central nervous system function could exist with no demonstrable lesions at autopsy, and conversely patients without neuropsychiatric manifestations could show widespread cerebral pathology. Other factors such as uraemia, electrolyte disturbance and hypertension may therefore make their own contributions to mental disturbance.

An additional mechanism may depend on immunological reactions which implicate brain tissue. Gamma globulin deposits have been identified in the choroid plexus of patients with mental disturbance but not in controls (Atkins et al. 1972). These appeared to be immune complexes derived from the blood, similar to those deposited in the glomerulus in lupus nephritis. Lymphocytotoxic antibodies may also have special affinity for neural tissue, and levels have proved to be higher in patients with cerebral manifestations than in those without (Bluestein & Zvaifler 1976; Bresnihan et al. 1979). Antineuronal antibodies have also been found in the serum. Episodes of cerebral vasculitis may thus allow brain-reactive antibodies to gain access to the cerebral parenchyma, accounting at least in part for the neuropsychiatric manifestations.

Considerable attention has been given to the possible role of steroids in precipitating confusional episodes, with a consensus of opinion that they can only rarely be held responsible (Dubois 1966; O'Connor & Musher 1966; Guze 1967). Thus similar episodes were often reported before steroids were introduced, they continue to be reported in patients not having such treatment, lowering of the dose has an inconsistent effect, and episodes do not necessarily recur when steroids are given again during later relapses. Nevertheless, the possibility must be borne in mind that steroids may occasionally have an aggravating or precipitating effect.

The genesis of schizophrenia-like episodes remains uncertain. In some examples the presence of disorientation or drowsiness points to possible organic determinants, and some may be provoked by steroid administration. Even in cases without such features, Lim et al. (1988) concluded that pathological changes in the brain were likely to play some part. Thus the patients in their series who showed psychotic episodes invariably had evidence of previous or current neurological disorder. Moreover, psychotic episodes were not observed in a control group of patients with rheumatoid arthritis or inflammatory bowel disease, who had been chosen because of their similarly variable chronic disability and treatment with steroids, yet absence of cerebral involvement.

Affective disorders and neurotic developments are almost certainly tied to the stresses of a debilitating and chronic illness. In Lim et al.'s (1988) study, mentioned above, episodes of depression and anxiety were commoner in SLE patients than controls, but the SLE patients were experiencing more social stress in terms of employment and family relationships. High psychiatric symptomatology scores, mainly due to anxiety and depression, correlated significantly with measures of social stress, but not with the presence of neurological disease or abnormalities on MRI.

Others, however, have noted that the incidence of affective disorders and neurotic reactions seems to be higher than with other medical conditions (Baker 1973). The reversibility of such disturbances, and their reappearance later in the illness, have similarly suggested that they may be intrinsically related to the disease process itself. Gurland et al. (1972) emphasise the difficulty in speculating about mechanisms when there is so much uncertainty about the frequency and form of psychiatric symptomatology in SLE, and when sampling problems are clearly implicit in most of the studies reported.

Treatment

The treatment of SLE is best undertaken by experts if an

optimal outcome is to be achieved. Current practice is outlined by Venables (1993) and Snaith and Isenberg (1996). In addition to specific treatment, patients should be warned to avoid undue exposure to the sun, and intercurrent infections should be treated promptly since they can lead to exacerbations. Preparations containing oestrogen, such as the contraceptive pill, are best avoided.

Steroids are the mainstay of treatment for the systemic effects of the disease and are also important in managing certain neuropsychiatric developments. Prednisolone is used most commonly. A high dosage may be required during exacerbations of the disorder, but this can be reduced to maintenance levels or discontinued entirely during phases of quiescence. Immunosuppressive drugs such as cyclophosphamide or azathioprine may also be used with caution during serious exacerbations, including acute organic reactions (Brook & Evans 1969). Cyclosporin can be effective in patients unresponsive to conventional immunosuppression, though renal toxicity is high.

The management of neuropsychiatric manifestations can prove difficult, though fortunately most episodes are transient and self limiting. Special attention must be paid to clouding of consciousness or mild intellectual impairment in what appear at first sight to be non-organic disturbances. The EEG and examination of the cerebrospinal fluid can be helpful in deciding on the likelihood of an organic cerebral cause, but are not an accurate guide in every case (Bennett *et al.* 1972). Other causes must be carefully considered — uraemia, electrolyte disturbance, hypertension, infection or steroid administration. In a prospective survey of 36 episodes of cerebral disturbance, Wong *et al.* (1991) considered that active SLE was responsible in less than a quarter, infection, steroids or hypertensive encephalopathy accounting for the remainder.

When confusion or delirium appear with fresh relapses of the disorder, steroids may help considerably in their resolution. On other occasions, however, they may stand to aggravate rather than help the clinical picture, some psychotic episodes responding to a reduction of current dosage. Particular difficulty can arise when a patient in good remission on maintenance therapy develops a marked personality change or psychosis. Dubois (1966) then recommends an initial attempt at gradual steroid withdrawal, but with readiness to give large doses immediately if the mental picture worsens along with systemic recrudescence. McCune and Golbus (1988), by contrast, suggest the opposite approach, namely doubling the steroid dosage for 3 days in case active cerebral vasculitis is responsible, then tapering off if there is no improvement and little other evidence of active disease. The monitoring of DNA and other specific antibodies can also be useful in helping to decide between a steroid-induced psychosis and a psychosis attributable to the disease process itself.

Phenothiazines will often be given, with or without steroids, for acute psychotic disturbances. Antidepressants may be required and electroconvulsive therapy is not contraindicated.

Polyarteritis nodosa (periarteritis nodosa, panarteritis nodosa)

Polyarteritis nodosa is characterised, like SLE, by involvement of many systems of the body and not infrequently implicating the nervous system. The cause is unknown but a hypersensitivity or autoimmune reaction is suspected. There may be a preceding history of streptococcal infection, and on rare occasions it may follow the administration of phenytoin, sulphonamides or other drugs.

The underlying pathology is a focal arteritis of small and medium-sized vessels. The larger arteries may also suffer due to involvement of their nutrient vessels. Highly characteristic focal dilatations are seen along affected vessels and whitish-grey nodules may be apparent macroscopically. A cellular reaction occurs at the site of the changes in and around the vessel walls. Necrosis of the artery wall leads to rupture, and intimal proliferation causes thrombosis.

The onset is usually in middle age but the range is wide. Males predominate over females. The disorder may declare itself abruptly or insidiously, and tends to run a subacute or chronic course with relapses and remissions.

Early symptoms consist of headache, malaise, weakness and a low-grade intermittent fever. Rhinorrhoea, coughing and wheezing are frequent. Weight loss may be profound and multisystem involvement is usually soon apparent. Renal insufficiency leads to severe hypertension in a high proportion of cases, and crises of abdominal pain result from infarctions in the mesenteric vessels and their tributaries. Arthritis and myositis are common. Pleuritic pain and pneumonitis may develop, and cardiac involvement leads to myocardial infarction, congestive cardiac failure and pericarditis.

Skin lesions include purpura, ecchymoses, subcutaneous nodules, necrotic ulcers and superficial gangrene. In addition to hypertensive retinopathy the eyes may show evidence of scleritis, keratitis, choroiditis, retinal artery occlusion or optic atrophy.

Laboratory investigations usually disclose anaemia, a raised ESR, and reversal of the albumin/globulin ratio. There are, however, no specific laboratory tests for the disorder. Leucocytosis is common, sometimes with eosinophilia. Most cases show uraemia, albuminuria and abnormal sediment in the urine. The chest X-ray may show pulmonary infiltration or a pleural reaction. The cerebrospinal fluid is sometimes under increased pressure, with elevation of protein, pleocytosis or xanthochromia. Arteriography via the aorta may reveal a diagnostic picture by way of multiple small aneurysms, focal dilatations, or infarcted areas in the kidneys or other abdominal organs. Biopsies from skin, liver, kidney or small nerves serve to confirm the diagnosis.

The disease formerly carried an extremely poor prognosis, death usually being attributable to renal failure or to coronary, mesenteric or cerebral infarction. Treatment with steroids and immunosuppressive drugs, usually in combination with one another, now offers hope of delaying or even halting progression. Hypertension warrants vigorous management and anticoagulants may be indicated.

Nervous system involvement

Peripheral neuropathy is the most frequent neurological finding and is more often seen with periarteritis nodosa than with any other collagen disease (Aita 1972). It is quite commonly a presenting feature. The nerves suffer via their nutrient arteries, leading to multiple infarctions along their course. The result is usually a mononeuropathy or multiple mononeuropathy, with paraesthesiae, weakness and wasting. Symmetrical polyneuropathy occurs more rarely.

Cerebral manifestations appear in up to half of cases eventually, but usually in the later part of the illness. Cranial nerve lesions are common, especially blurring of vision, vertigo, tinnitus and disorders of external ocular movement. Focal cerebral or cerebellar infarctions may lead to hemianopia, hemiparesis or ataxia. A local mass of brain necrosis may simulate a tumour, and spontaneous subarachnoid haemorrhage may occur. Headache is common, sometimes attributable to hypertension and sometimes to arachnoiditis at the base of the brain. Epileptic seizures may result from uraemia, hypertension or focal lesions in the brain.

Mental changes can figure prominently and occurred in 26 of 114 cases from the Mayo Clinic (Ford & Siekert 1965). The usual picture was of confusion and disorientation, sometimes with visual hallucinations and delusions. Delirium, 'mania' and paranoia were seen occasionally. Forgetfulness was noted in many patients, and seven showed marked intellectual deterioration. Eight showed a fluctuating impairment of consciousness varying from somnolence to coma.

Occasional cases are reported in which polyarteritis nodosa appears to be largely confined to the nervous system. MacKay et al. (1950) described a patient who for 2 years showed intermittent diplopia, hemiparesis and cranial nerve disorders accompanied by a low pyrexia, then developed depression and progressive dementia leading to death over several months. At autopsy the typical changes of polyarteritis nodosa were largely confined to the brain and cord.

Giant cell arteritis (temporal arteritis, cranial arteritis)

Giant cell arteritis is a disease of later years, appearing rarely before 60 and with a mean age of onset at 70. The temporal arteries are the site of a subacute inflammatory reaction with necrosis, granulation and giant cell formation. Intimal proliferation leads to thrombosis. The ciliary arteries, which supply the optic nerve and disc, are involved in about 30% of cases. The occipital vessels and the aorta and its main branches may also be affected. The disease is related to polymyalgia rheumatica and the two may occur together.

Clinically there is often a prodromal phase of vague malaise with muscle and joint pains lasting for several weeks or months. A low pyrexia may develop and weight loss and depression may be marked. Characteristic headache then appears, sometimes abruptly, situated principally over the affected vessels in the temporal region. The temporal arteries may be palpable and exquisitely tender. Suffering is usually intense, with throbbing or lancinating pain and severe insomnia.

The acute stage lasts for a week or two but tenderness may persist rather longer. At any time in the early days or weeks the serious complication of ciliary artery obstruction may follow, leading to impairment or loss of vision in one or both eyes. Hence the importance of prompt diagnosis and treatment. Ophthalmoplegias may also occur. The systemic disturbance continues throughout the stage of headache and visual complications, and may last for many months more. Peripheral neuropathy and muscle pain and wasting may occur. Infarctions can follow from involvement of the carotid or vertebral vessels. McCormick and Neuberger (1958) describe the brain lesions which may be observed at autopsy, including involvement of small intracerebral vessels by giant cell arteritis.

Mental disturbances sometimes feature prominently during the illness, with confusion, delirium, memory impairment and drowsiness proceeding to coma (Cloake 1951). Vereker (1952) described examples in the literature with restlessness, disorientation, severe memory difficulties and episodes of delirium, often with abrupt resolution after several weeks. Coma is a serious development, but patients can recover after several days. Vereker also stressed the frequency of severe depression in the disease, and considered that in many examples it was attributable to cerebral arterial disease rather than being secondary to the headache. Russell (1959) found that seven of 35 patients were depressed and four were confused during the stage of headache.

The ESR is greatly raised and there may be a leucocytosis. However, in about 10% of cases the ESR may be normal in the early stages (Russell & Graham 1988). Biopsy of an inflamed artery serves to confirm the diagnosis. Steroids meet with dramatic success in treatment and must not be delayed. They are given in high dosage initially then reduced after 1–2 weeks to maintenance levels which are continued for 6–12 months or sometimes indefinitely. Mason and Walport (1992) discuss the regimens involved. Anticoagulants may also be indicated in the acute stages.

Granulomatous angiitis of the nervous system

Granulomatous angiitis of the nervous system (GANS) represents another form of giant cell arteritis. The cause is unknown. Though rare it is important to neurology and psychiatry in that it can affect the nervous system alone without evidence of vasculitis elsewhere. Moreover, clues to its presence are not regularly forthcoming from laboratory investigations, and angiography followed by biopsy are usually essential for the diagnosis.

Sigal (1987) reviewed the 61 cases in the literature to that date. Men are affected slightly more often than women, with a mean age of onset of 46 years. The range is wide, however, with cases reported in childhood and old age.

Presentation is often remarkably non-specific, with the acute or subacute onset of headache, confusion and memory disturbance. Alterations of personality and other psychiatric symptoms can be to the fore. Nausea occurred in a third of Sigal's patients and severe muscle weakness in half. Hypertension and fever were present in a quarter. Focal neurological signs may develop with limb pareses, incoordination or aphasia, but these are not seen in every case. Cranial nerve lesions affect the facial or abducens nerves predominantly, and papilloedema may be present. Seizures and losses of consciousness may occur. The picture may initially suggest encephalitis, cerebral tumour, meningovascular syphilis or sarcoid of the nervous system.

The ESR is usually but not always raised, and the cerebrospinal fluid typically shows increased protein and a lymphocytic pleocytosis. Occasionally, however, this too can be normal. The EEG shows diffuse or focal slowing in some 80% of patients. CT or MRI may indicate infarcts or foci of oedema.

Clearly, however, such investigations are insufficient for diagnosis or for excluding the condition, and when suspected angiography will always be required. This shows diffuse or localised changes in large and small arteries, with irregularities, beading and aneurysmal formation. Biopsy is essential for the definitive diagnosis, revealing an inflammatory process in the arteries and arterioles of the brain parenchyma and leptomeninges. Intimal thickening and fibrosis are accompanied by multinucleated giant cells. Significant vasculitis is rarely seen other than within the cranium, although spinal cord and temporal arteries may be affected.

The prognosis was extremely poor before the advent of steroid medication. This, with cytotoxic agents such as cyclophosphamide and azathioprine, now brings hopeful prospects of treatment.

A related disorder, also discussed by Sigal (1987), is the cranial arteritis which can develop some weeks or months after herpes zoster infection of the eye ('delayed contralateral hemiplegia'). This is typically restricted to the distribution of the middle cerebral artery on the affected side. In addition to hemiplegia, cranial nerve involvement and muscle weakness are common, though confusion and other psychiatric symptomatology are less often in evidence.

Other forms of vasculitis which may remain confined to the nervous system include Cogan syndrome and Eales' disease, both occurring in young adults. Cogan syndrome consists of episodes of interstitial keratitis and vestibular and auditory symptoms. Focal neurological abnormalities and organic mental syndromes may develop. Eales' disease is restricted to the peripheral retinal vessels, often leading to visual loss.

Thromboangiitis obliterans (Buerger's disease)

Thromboangiitis obliterans is virtually confined to males, presenting usually between 25 and 40 years of age. The cause is unknown, but tobacco smoking shows a strong association with the development of the disorder and markedly aggravates the symptoms.

The pathology consists of a panarteritis affecting all layers of the vessels and implicating both arteries and veins. The medium-sized vessels of the legs are predominantly affected. An acute inflammatory response is followed by fibrosis and scarring. Intimal proliferation leads to thrombosis, often with recanalisation later. A relapsing–remitting course is characteristic, affecting short segments of the vessels at a time so that lesions in all stages of activity are found at different sites.

The common presentation is with intermittent claudication, leading eventually to gangrene of the toes. Superficial venous thromboses frequently occur. The affected limb is pulseless, cyanosed and cold. Nocturnal pain is typically relieved by hanging the leg downwards out of bed.

Many cases remain confined to the peripheral circulation but cardiac, visceral and cerebral involvement can occur. A chronic intermittent course is usual, extending over many years with remissions and fresh progressions, though ultimately with considerable residual disability. The blood pressure remains normal throughout.

Cerebral involvement is rare but well attested. The literature is reviewed by Perk (1947), Davis and Perret (1947) and Cloake (1951). In some reported cases the nature of the responsible pathology in the cerebral vessels must be open to doubt, but in others clear confirmation has been obtained at autopsy of typical changes in the arteries of the brain.

Cerebral manifestations usually appear only when the peripheral disease is well established, though in occasional cases they have been the presenting feature. The possibility of the disease should therefore be borne in mind when young adult males develop cerebrovascular symptoms, especially in the absence of hypertension. It further seems possible that in occasional cases a cerebral form of the disease may exist alone.

The vessels principally affected are the internal carotids and the anterior and middle cerebral arteries (Cloake 1951). Infarctions follow in the corresponding territories. In the early stages the deficits may be slight and transient, suggesting that they are due to episodes of spasm or emboli. Transient pareses and paraesthesiae may be accompanied by confusion and memory impairment. Episodes of giddiness, diplopia, visual flickering or speech disturbance may last for minutes or days and recur in different forms. Epileptic fits are common and headache of migrainous type may occur. Later there are major and more lasting syndromes of cerebral infarction, and a trend towards increasing emotional and intellectual deterioration. Dementia can ultimately be profound with an end-state similar to that of multi-infarct dementia.

Very occasionally florid mental disorders occur in the course of the disease, with acute organic psychoses, paranoia or psychotic depression. Perk's (1947) case showed a predominantly manic picture, lasting for many months along with transient diplopia, fits and episodes of unconsciousness.

The course is variable once cerebral symptoms have been declared. Survival may sometimes be seen for up to 15 years, though few patients seem to survive for more than 5 years.

Other forms of vasculitis

The spectrum of vasculitis is wide, as reviewed by Fauci *et al.* (1978). Several varieties can be recognised and categorised as distinct entities, but in others there is overlap between one disease and another. All share in common inflammation and necrosis of blood vessels; in some this is the predominant manifestation, whereas in others it occurs in association with other pathologies. Most are associated directly or indirectly with immunopathological mechanisms. The American College of Rheumatology has put forward criteria for classification which depend on both clinical and laboratory manifestations (Hunder *et al.* 1990).

The forms of vasculitis which may involve the nervous system are reviewed by Sigal (1987). *Wegener's granulomatosis* shows cerebral involvement in 25–50% of cases, usually in a setting of active sinusitis, otitis or lung disease. Headache and cranial nerve palsies are common, and subarachnoid haemorrhage or hypertensive encephalopathy may occur. The antineutrophil cytoplasmic antibody (ANCA) test is positive in the serum in most cases when the disease is active (Ramirez *et al.* 1990). *Lymphomatoid granulomatosis* may present with neuropsychiatric features which antedate other manifestations by several years—confusion, cranial neuropathies and cerebrovascular syndromes. *Takayasu's arteritis* predominantly affects the aortic arch and its branches, and may present with strokes, seizures or syncope. *Systemic rheumatoid vasculitis* very occasionally involves the nervous system, leading to focal neurological deficits, cranial nerve palsies, seizures or dementia. In all reported cases joint disease has already been well established when cerebral symptoms appear. *Vasculitis due to drug abuse* is considered on pp. 619–20.

Finally, the patients reported by Chynoweth and Foley (1969) are worth considering in some detail, in that suspicion of a collagen vascular disorder led to a trial of treatment with steroids with gratifying results in all three cases. The patients had presented with dementia, together with a raised ESR and altered serum proteins. Other features indicative of collagen vascular disorder included fluctuating confusion, headaches, muscle cramps, transient disturbances of vision and variable neurological signs. In view of the importance of detecting treatable causes of dementia an example from their series is given below, illustrating the rather minor clues which led to a trial of steroid therapy:

A woman of 58 complained of headaches and epistaxes which were attributed to sinus infection. The following year she developed cramp-like pains in the limbs and back, double vision and occasional difficulty with speech. Transient episodes of disorientation occurred during which she failed to recognise her friends or her own bedroom. Examination showed mild nominal dysphasia with impairment of memory and difficulty in performing simple calculations. Deterioration occurred, with bouts of trembling and falling and increasing depression.

In hospital, 2 years from onset, the ESR was raised at 30 mm per hour and an air encephalogram showed cortical atrophy. Her mental state fluctuated considerably, with a return to normal over several weeks but relapsing soon thereafter. She became distractible, disorientated and had marked memory difficulties. The ESR remained elevated and the cerebrospinal fluid showed 2 lymphocytes/ml, a protein of 75 mg/100 ml and a positive Pandy test. The EEG showed diffuse abnormalities with paroxysmal slow waves. Serum proteins were normal and no LE cells were found.

Over the next few months she became progressively confused with confabulation and paranoid delusional ideas. Fluctuation continued but with overall deterioration. Ultimately she was doubly incontinent, abusive, aggressive and with profound loss of orientation and memory. A diagnosis of presenile dementia secondary to cerebrovascular disease was made.

After 2 months in her local psychiatric hospital the ESR remained elevated at 19 mm per hour, there was a slight polymorph leucocytosis, and electrophoresis of serum proteins now showed an increase in alpha-2 globulin and mucoprotein. A trial of steroids was considered worthwhile. Hydrocortisone was commenced intramuscularly for 1 week then followed by prednisone orally. Within 24 hours of starting treatment her mind became clearer and she recognised her surroundings. Within 1 week she was up and about and appeared to have recovered completely. The EEG showed progressive improvement, and psychological testing confirmed normal memory functioning though with slight residual impairment of visuospatial memory. She was discharged and remained well 1 year later, still taking prednisone 5 mg daily.   (Chynoweth & Foley 1969)

Thrombotic thrombocytopenic purpura

Autoimmune or 'idiopathic' thrombocytopenic purpura may follow viral infections in children as a short self-limiting illness, or pursue a chronic relapsing course in adults (Machin 1996). Thrombotic thrombocytopenic purpura is a more serious condition, usually developing between the ages of 20 and 50 years and showing a female preponderance (Gordon-Smith & Contreras 1996). This typically runs a fulminant course with renal involvement, fever, haemolytic anaemia and widespread small vessel occlusions in many organs. Neuropsychiatric features are often conspicuous, with headache, confusion, convulsions and coma, also pareses and visual symptoms result-

ing from blockage of small cerebral vessels by platelet aggregates and fibrin thrombi (Davies-Jones 1989; Walton 1993b). These can be the presenting signs in up to 60% of cases. Symmetrical cranial nerve involvement is said to be characteristic, and delirium and stupor may simulate encephalitis (Miller 1966b). Hypertension is common. Bleeding into the brain may be preceded by neck stiffness and headache.

The finding of purpura on examination, along with thrombocytopenia and renal manifestations, is likely to be diagnostic. High dosage of steroids combined with splenectomy may be helpful, also immunosuppressive therapy and plasma exchange, but in severe examples the prognosis is poor.

Polycythaemia rubra vera

Polycythaemia is a member of the myeloproliferative disorders, showing an increase in red cell mass and usually with an excess of white blood corpuscles and platelets as well. It presents mainly in middle or later life, and with a slight male preponderance. Sometimes it declares itself insidiously, or it may present with acute complications such as a cerebrovascular accident or major thrombotic episode (Weatherall 1996). Patients may experience angina or claudication, or suffer recurrent emboli or venous thromboses. Complaints of pruritus are common. The facies is typically plethoric with injected conjunctivae, and splenomegaly and hepatomegaly are often present.

Neuropsychiatric features can be prominent and have been reported in half to three-quarters of cases (Silverstein et al. 1962). Impairment of the cerebral circulation leads to headache, impaired concentration, dizziness, vertigo and visual blurring. Episodes of confusion may progress to dementia. The increased blood viscosity predisposes to transient ischaemic attacks and cerebral infarctions. Murray and Hodgson (1991) reported a patient who developed a severe depressive illness with psychotic features after a series of transient ischaemic attacks, ultimately with good resolution after electroconvulsive treatment. Other cerebral symptoms occasionally include chorea, narcolepsy and seizures.

Willison et al. (1980) showed that patients with high-normal or above-normal haematocrit values (range 0.46–0.77) were impaired on tests of alertness when compared with controls matched for age and occupation — tests of digit copying, counting backwards, letter cancellation and coding. After venesection the haematocrit values fell from a mean of 0.54 to 0.45 and the test scores improved. The extent of improvement correlated significantly with increases in cerebral blood flow as measured by ^{133}Xe inhalation.

The prognosis can be good in the absence of major complications. Treatment is by repeated venesection to gently lower the packed cell volume, sometimes along with myelosuppressive agents such as busulphan, hydroxyurea or ^{32}P. In some cases transformation takes place to leukaemia or myelosclerosis.

Chapter 10: Senile Dementias, Presenile Dementias and Pseudodementias

The clinical syndrome of dementia has many causes, both cerebral and extracerebral, as outlined in Table 4 (p. 153). Prominent among them are certain intrinsic degenerative diseases of the brain occurring in middle or late life which have attained the title of dementia as signifying specific disease entities. These, the so-called 'primary dementias', will be the subject of the present chapter. Later in the chapter the 'pseudodementias' will also be discussed—an important group of conditions in which an apparent dementia occurs in the absence of physical pathology and in the context of non-organic psychiatric disorder.

By far the commonest of the primary dementias is Alzheimer's disease, chiefly by virtue of its sharply rising incidence with age. Among presenile dementias, namely those with onset before the age of 65, it is also probable that Alzheimer's disease is more frequent than other varieties. Next in frequency is 'multi-infarct' or 'arteriosclerotic' dementia, both in the senile and presenile age ranges. This is traditionally discussed along with the primary dementias, even though strictly speaking it represents a secondary rather than a primary degenerative brain process. Lewy body dementia, a more recently described variety, may also prove to be common, as discussed on p. 450. Pick's disease, other frontal dementias, Huntington's disease and Creutzfeldt–Jakob disease constitute the best known of the remaining primary dementias and are all much less common. When the distinctive pathologies of the above conditions fail to be revealed at autopsy in a patient with a primary dementing illness it is usual to speak of a 'simple' or 'non-specific' primary dementia.

The general clinical picture is similar in all—a progressive disintegration of intellect, memory and personality, with symptoms of the chronic organic reaction as described in Chapter 1. The different conditions are distinguished to some extent by the rapidity of their course or by associated symptoms and signs, as will be described when the individual disorders are considered in turn. Quite often, however, the precise diagnostic category is revealed only by careful postmortem examination of the brain, and even then a measure of uncertainty can remain in some cases. There is considerable dispute over the nosological distinctions which can be made among several of the rarer subvarieties. Future work may be expected to clarify these issues, but unfortunately clinical information is all too often sparse by the time the brain comes to histological or biochemical examination.

All of these diseases share a uniformly hopeless prognosis and the chief aim in diagnostic practice must be to distinguish them from the 'secondary dementias', i.e. to search for the other causes of chronic organic reactions which may have some therapeutic issue.

It is perhaps because of this emphasis in clinical enquiry that the primary dementias were formerly neglected in neurological and psychiatric research. No doubt enthusiastic enquiry into their aetiology was also impeded by the evidence of genetic predisposition where several are concerned, and by the similarities in pathology with the normal processes of senescence. Thus Gowers' concept of 'abiotrophy' was often applied, with the implication that they represent merely a precocious ageing of the central nervous system, sometimes on a familial basis, and due to limited viability of the cells concerned. There is a risk, however, of falling into error here since diseases may represent an intensification of the ageing process without owing much, or anything, directly to it. There has now been a start with more intensive research, particularly in relation to Alzheimer's disease, and some lines of enquiry are afoot which may ultimately prove to be fruitful. These are outlined in some detail on pp. 441–9.

In the first place experience with other disorders has shown that genetic causation is not incompatible with possibilities for therapeutic intervention. Where a single dominant gene is responsible, as in Huntington's disease, a specific biochemical abnormality may be discovered and prove to be remediable. Where polygenic inheritance is likely the genetic factor will probably to be quantitatively graded in severity, and some additional exogenous cause may be required before the disease becomes manifest. With regard to the parallels drawn with senescence, recent studies have served to sharpen the distinctions between normal ageing and the dementing diseases on both clinical and pathological grounds, even in Alzheimer's disease where the parallels in pathology were always most readily drawn. Most hopefully of all, the traditionally static techniques of neuropathological examination are being supplemented by neurochemistry, immunocytochemistry and detailed quantitative approaches which seek to explore the genesis of the salient changes in the nervous system. Altogether it has now become clear that causation could lie at least in part in biochemical aberration, toxic influences or subtle deprivations which may one day prove to be remediable. Possibilities even of infection have been raised in view of the transmissibility of prion diseases such as Creutzfeldt–Jakob disease. All of these and related matters will be considered in further detail below.

Senile dementias

Dementia setting in after the age of 65 has usually been considered separately from that occurring in younger patients. The organisation of clinical services for the elderly, and the development of the specialities of geriatrics and psychogeriatrics, have served to reinforce the practice. Unfortunately, in consequence, 'senile dementia' has tended to acquire nosological status as a separate and distinct entity in clinical and even in some research writing. In fact the dementias of the elderly can have several causes, as at any other age, and with advancing age multiple causes will sometimes be operative together.

The most common pathology displayed at autopsy in elderly demented patients is closely similar to, if not identical with, that of Alzheimer's disease in younger persons. Formerly this was labelled as 'parenchymatous senile dementia', but more recent practice is to speak of 'senile dementia of the Alzheimer type' (SDAT). The change in terminology reflects the increasing body of evidence that the conditions are likely to be identical whether setting in before or after the age of 65 years. A second large group consists of the arteriosclerotic or multi-infarct dementias, whereas a third is determined by an admixture of these two common forms of pathology. The relatively small remainder of cases is likely to show a range of other causative pathologies, or the brain may be normal apart from the changes expected with age. Lewy body dementia is reported to be common in some series of patients (p. 450) and will, perhaps, come to rank as another major cause of dementia in the elderly.

The difficulty in applying precise nosological labels during life has impeded clarification of the clinical, genetic and other allegiances of the dementias of the elderly. Opportunities have been rare for the long-term follow-up of patients to allow clinicopathological correlations on any extensive scale. Special difficulties arise, moreover, from the fact that plaques and tangles accumulate in the brain as age advances, even in the healthy aged population. This has led to uncertain lines of demarcation, even at the pathological level, between what should be regarded as relevant or irrelevant to the development of dementia as older age groups are considered.

In the present chapter the sections on Alzheimer's disease and multi-infarct dementia will describe the clinical picture and underlying pathology of these conditions in some detail. First, however, it will be useful to consider certain aspects of the dementias of the elderly separately, bearing in mind that the major proportion of such cases is likely to represent SDAT.

Prevalence and forms

Epidemiological studies show that the prevalence of dementia rises markedly with age, from about 2% in persons aged 65–70 years to approximately 20% in those over 80 (Royal College of Physicians 1981). In addition to such cases of 'moderate to severe' dementia there are perhaps two to three times as many patients at any one time with mild forms of the disorder. As a consequence of increasing longevity in the population the prevalence of dementia has therefore risen and continues to rise alarmingly. Terry and Katzman (1983) estimated that there were approximately 1.3 million persons with severe dementia in the USA, that is with a degree of impairment that precluded independent living, and a further 2.8 million who were still able to live semi-independently. Altogether dementia now probably ranks as the fourth or fifth most common cause of death in the USA (Katzman 1976).

The implications of a problem on such a scale for the cost and provision of care are clearly enormous. Kay et al. were able to show in 1970 that admission rates to hospital for the elderly demented exceeded the rates for all other psychoses combined, likewise that their demands on hospital and residential facilities outstripped those due to all other forms of disability in old age. Yet statistics from institutions underestimate the size of the problem. The Newcastle-upon-Tyne survey of a random sample of people living at home, coupled with a census of institutions in the same area, disclosed that fewer than one-fifth even of the more severe cases were in hospitals or homes for the elderly (Kay et al. 1964). Of demented patients in the community, moreover, only a small proportion are known to their general practitioners (Williamson et al. 1964).

Accurate data on the relative prevalence of different forms of dementia in the elderly are obviously hard to obtain. Autopsy information, based largely on hospitalised patients, has consistently shown that an Alzheimer pathology is the most common variety encountered and occurs in some half to two-thirds of patients. A vascular basis is present in perhaps a quarter; this will sometimes coexist with Alzheimer changes, each contributing to the dementia. Thus Tomlinson *et al.* (1970) found the following distribution in their autopsy material on 50 patients: definite Alzheimer pathology in 50%; definite arteriosclerosis in 12% and probable arteriosclerosis in 6% more; and a mixture of Alzheimer and arteriosclerotic pathology in 18%. The remaining 14% could not be classified into any of the above three categories, some representing probable Alzheimer's disease (6%), some showing no evident pathology (4%) and the others a probable traumatic or Wernicke basis (4%).

It is difficult, however, to judge how far these findings may be extrapolated to the elderly demented generally. Different forms of institution tend to cater for different types of patient; those dying in geriatric and psychiatric facilities, for example, may not be strictly comparable with each other, and those who remain in the community may present a different spectrum again. The nosological status of patients with less severe and less rapidly progressive forms of dementia has not been clarified directly. Nevertheless the clinical impression remains that SDAT and multi-infarct dementia account between them for the great majority of cases, other varieties being distinctly uncommon after the age of 65. Those patients in whom no clear pathological basis for their dementia can be demonstrated at autopsy—4% in Tomlinson *et al.*'s (1970) series and 12% among those reported by Blessed (1980)— remain puzzling and a challenge to further research. The quite recent description of Lewy body dementia (p. 450 *et seq.*) is an indication that not uncommon varieties may still remain to be discovered.

Aetiology of SDAT

Despite the close neuropathological similarities between SDAT and the brain changes seen with normal ageing, it can now scarcely be doubted that a disease process is involved. Thus epidemiological surveys show that even in extreme old age the great majority of persons remain free from clinical evidence of dementia; it seems probable that there are genetic determinants for its development; and most persuasively of all there are ever-increasing indications that SDAT is similar in virtually all essentials to Alzheimer's disease occurring in younger persons. Key factors in the aetiology of the one are therefore likely to

apply to the other, hence the current emphasis of research in many centres into the origins of such pathology.

The rival theories concerning the pathogenesis of Alzheimer's disease are outlined on p. 441 *et seq.* Here it is only necessary to note that where opportunities have arisen to compare research findings in presenile and senile cases the results have been very similar. Detailed observations concerning the structure of plaques and tangles yield equivalent results whatever the age of the patient, and cholinergic deficits are pre-eminent among the brain biochemical changes. Certain exceptions in the biochemical data are discussed on p. 445 but do not yet amount to a serious challenge to the unitary nature of the disorder. Whatever may ultimately emerge as decisive for the pathogenesis of presenile Alzheimer's disease may therefore be expected to apply with equal force to SDAT as well.

Genetic studies have had to contend with a measure of diagnostic uncertainty, especially when based on living probands. Nevertheless, evidence of genetic predisposition for SDAT was soon forthcoming. Kallmann's (1956) investigation of 108 twin pairs showed that 43% of monozygotic twins were concordant for 'parenchymatous senile dementia', compared with 8% of dizygotic twins and 7% of siblings. Larsson *et al.* (1963) studied the incidence of the disorder in the first-degree relatives of 377 cases, with the striking finding that their morbidity risk was about four times that of corresponding age groups in the general population. They concluded that a dominant autosomal gene was probably responsible, with partial penetrance. Polygenic inheritance seemed unlikely since forms intermediate between dementia and normal ageing were not found among the relatives.

Other significant findings from Larsson *et al.*'s survey were that there was no increased risk for other psychoses among the relatives, and that the incidence of multi-infarct dementia was actually lowered. A puzzling feature was the lack of presenile Alzheimer's disease in over 2000 first-degree relatives in Larsson *et al.*'s study; others, however, have found such cases (Constantinidis *et al.* 1962), also cases of SDAT among the relatives of patients with presenile Alzheimer's disease (Lauter & Meyer 1968).

Heston *et al.*'s (1981) careful genetic survey took origin from 125 probands, all with autopsy proof of Alzheimer-type pathology. The onset had been below the age of 65 in approximately 40% of cases and at 65 or over in the remainder. The risk for parents and siblings proved again to be elevated some fourfold over general population estimates. Here, however, age of onset appeared to be an important consideration, in that a relatively early onset (below 70 years) together with the presence of an affected parent greatly increased the risk to sibs; conversely when the illness began only after the age of 70 the risk to sibs appeared to be little if at all elevated. This important study is discussed further on p. 437. Preliminary evidence that certain clinical features of the dementia may indicate special genetic risk await confirmation; Breitner and Folstein (1984) suggest that familial aggregations of dementia may be largely confined to patients who show language disorder and apraxia as part of the clinical picture.

An important conceptual change has been to ask whether SDAT, even in cases which are not obviously familial, may nonetheless be very strongly determined by genetic factors. It is likely that genetic expression of the disorder increases in late old age, but many persons at risk will have died of other causes before such expression is declared, thus obscuring the evidence. Using data from pooled studies and life tables to estimate the age-specific incidences in relatives, the cumulative risk among first-degree relatives has been shown to approach 50% by the age of 90 (Mohs et al. 1987; Breitner 1994). This would be consistent with transmission as an autosomal dominant trait. Such considerations lend added importance to attempts to define the gene or genes responsible, as described on pp. 447–8.

Attention has also been directed at the possibility of loss of chromosomal material in elderly demented patients by searching for hypodiploid cells in peripheral lymphocytes. Hypodiploidy has been found to increase with age in females, and less certainly in males (Martin 1982). Several studies have reported a further increase in females suffering from dementia (Nielsen 1968, 1970a; Jarvik et al. 1974a, 1974b), though this has not been uniformly confirmed (Martin et al. 1981).

Interesting findings also emerged from the neurophysiological work of Levy et al. (1970, 1971), which raised the possibility that the dementia may represent only one facet of a more general degenerative process affecting the nervous system at several levels. Patients with SDAT, when compared with patients of the same age without mental impairment, were found to have slowing of motor conduction along the ulnar nerve distally in the arm. There was a high correlation between the severity of the dementia and the degree of peripheral slowing, and re-testing 1 year later showed that increase in dementia was associated significantly with further slowing. The latencies and morphological characteristics of somatosensory evoked responses were also found to be altered in SDAT, though here the site of slowing was probably within the brain itself rather than in peripheral pathways.

The frequent finding of folate deficiency among elderly persons is discussed in Chapter 12, but it is unlikely that this contributes on any widespread scale to the development of dementia in old age. A role for cerebral anoxia has sometimes been championed, especially in view of the frequency of cardiac disease and dysrhythmias in the elderly (Lancet 1977), but evidence for an aetiological connection between cardiac disorder and SDAT has not been forthcoming (Emerson et al. 1981). Socioeconomic factors are certainly important in dictating admission to hospital and residential care (Sainsbury et al. 1965) but do not seem to influence the incidence of the disease.

Clinical features of SDAT

The onset is usually in the seventies or eighties and females preponderate over males to a considerable extent. In Larsson et al.'s (1963) large Swedish material the mean age of onset was 73 years for males and 75 for females. The early stages are rarely seen in hospitals or clinics and many patients already have advanced dementia by the time they come to attention.

The general clinical picture follows that described for Alzheimer's disease on p. 438 et seq., except that the onset may be particularly hard to discern and parietal lobe symptomatology is less regularly conspicuous. Among older patients it is probable that the disorder can sometimes follow a relatively protracted course as a result of more 'benign' development of the pathological changes.

The early stages are commonly overlooked by relatives and even by medical attendants. Failing memory and lack of initiative and interest tend to be regarded as no more than an accentuation of the normal processes of ageing. An exaggeration of such traits as obstinacy, egocentricity and rigid adherence to old habits may be viewed likewise. Thus the family will often adapt insensibly to the patient's gradual decline in a manner that scarcely impinges on their attention. Old people, moreover, may already have adopted a circumscribed routine within which cognitive failure is slow to be exposed.

The diagnosis of dementia in such early stages can present considerable problems. Follow-up of a large community cohort of elderly persons 2–4 years later showed that only six of 20 'borderline demented' subjects had indeed progressed to unequivocal dementia (Bergmann 1977). The misdiagnoses had mostly occurred in persons of low social class and low intelligence, and in those who were relatively incoherent at interview. The distinction from depression will often be far from clear-cut, likewise the discernment of what may be expected by way of memory failure with age.

In this last respect Kral (1962) has attempted to distinguish a 'benign' form of memory failure ('benign senescent forgetfulness') from that due to dementia. The former is said to be patchy and variable, with difficulty over the recall of names and places but with relative ease of recall of experiences. In dementia, by contrast, the memory disturbances are soon more severe. At first they may selectively affect recent rather than remote events but this distinction rapidly becomes obscured. Whole segments of experience are blotted out and the patient becomes increasingly disoriented in time and place. He may imagine he is living in the remote past or in some other location, forget the names of his children or spouse or the death of close relatives and friends. Islands of memory may stand out for a time, but are frequently displaced in time and distorted in context.

In a follow-up over 4 years of 40 normal elderly persons, 20 patients with benign forgetfulness and 34 patients with dementia, Kral (1978) indicated that valid distinctions could be drawn. Those with benign forgetfulness showed similar mortality rates and longevity to the normal group, with mean survival times of 24 and 25 months, respectively, whereas the demented patients fared significantly worse with an average survival of 15 months.

O'Brien et al. (1992) have in the main confirmed the benign nature of the disorder. Sixty-four patients with benign senescent forgetfulness from the Maudsley Hospital memory clinic were followed up for an average of 3 years. Six had developed clinically recognisable dementia, which was little more than expected from the age structure of the population under scrutiny. The remainder showed a small but significant decline in Mini-Mental State scores, which was in keeping with normal ageing.

The more recent concept of *Age Associated Memory Impairment* appears to be not so very different. Crook et al. (1986) have proposed the term for persons over 50 who complain of gradual-onset memory dysfunction in everyday activities (e.g. remembering names following introductions, misplacing objects, remembering multiple items to be purchased or recalling information quickly or following distraction), whose subjective difficulties are substantiated on well-standardised memory tests, and who show an absence of dementia, psychiatric disorder, drug or alcohol abuse, or medical or neurological disorders affecting cognition.

Interesting results have come from attempts to study the very early stages of dementia in elderly persons. In an important Swedish study a group of 374 non-demented 70-year-olds was followed up 5 and 9 years later, and comparisons made on a number of tests and ratings performed at the initial examination (Persson et al. 1991; Persson & Skoog 1992). Those who progressed to dementia had shown significantly reduced memory for recent events, difficulties in word finding and a lowered number of remembered dreams per week. They had also been slower to complete certain cognitive tests, and had scored lower on a trait reflecting mental energy. It was thus confirmed that cognitive changes of an insidious nature mark the earliest phases of the disorder. Moreover comparisons between subjects who had become demented early and late during the follow-up period indicated that there may often be a long subclinical period before the dementia becomes clinically obvious.

While the onset of dementia is insidious it not infrequently comes to attention as a result of some acute disturbance. An intercurrent illness may have taxed the reserves of the failing brain beyond their limit or resulted in an acute episode of delirium. Or a sudden change of environment or the loss of a partner may have abruptly revealed the inroads made by the disorder. Other cases come to notice as a result of the social disorganisation produced by the dementing process — the patient may wander away and get lost, become suddenly abusive on account of paranoid delusions or harm himself due to some clumsiness or accident.

Once firmly established, the disintegration of intellect and personality proceeds relentlessly. Confusion becomes more prominent at night and the patient sleeps badly. Repetitive futile behaviour is characteristic and restlessness may become extreme. Psychotic features are common, usually of a paranoid nature and sometimes with grotesque hypochondriacal delusions. Emotions become blunted, though outbursts of anger may occur if routines are disturbed. Habits deteriorate with loss of sphincter control, so that the patient is sometimes found to have been living in appalling conditions by the time of admission to hospital. The appearance becomes decrepit and shrunken, and the gait slow, shuffling and tottery. The general physical enfeeblement is said to be in contrast to presenile Alzheimer's disease, in which physical deterioration is often delayed until the dementia has reached a very advanced degree.

The frequency with which various psychiatric and behavioural symptoms are encountered in SDAT has been charted by Burns and Levy (1992) in a survey of a representative sample of patients from a defined geographical area. The average age of the patients was 80 years and the mean duration of illness 5 years. One hundred and seventy-eight patients were examined, all meeting NINCDS–ADRADA criteria (pp. 439–40).

Seventeen per cent had experienced hallucinations at some time, visual hallucinations being slightly more common than auditory. Thirty per cent had shown misidentification syndromes, 12% failing to recognise others, 6% believing events on television to be real, 4% failing to recognise themselves in a mirror and 17% believing that there were others in the house. Sixteen per cent had been deluded at some point, usually with simple delusions of suspicion or theft, and an additional 20% showed paranoid ideation. Almost two-thirds had at least one symptom of depression, and a quarter appeared to be depressed to the observer. Those who complained of depression were less cognitively impaired than those who did not. Mania by contrast was exceedingly rare, and only 4% appeared to have elevated mood.

As found by Teri et al. (1988), behavioural disturbance occurred more commonly as the severity of dementia increased, especially wandering (19%), incontinence (48%) and aspects of the Klüver Bucy syndrome. Seventy-two per cent of patients showed at least one symptom of the latter — misrecognition (44%), apathy (41%), rages (36%), hypermetamorphosis (31%), binge eating (10%), sexual disinhibition (7%) or hyperorality (6%). Patients with symptoms of the Klüver Bucy syndrome were especially likely to have temporal lobe atrophy on computerised tomography (CT) scans, likewise the 20% who showed aggression.

Neurological abnormalities were uncommon, with the exception of a snout reflex in 41% of cases. A grasp reflex was seen in 7% and extensor plantars in 4%. Extrapyramidal signs were present in 15%, tremor in 6% and myoclonus in 5%. Three per cent had a history of epileptic fits since the onset of the illness.

It was formerly considered that focal symptomatology was rare in senile dementia but this has now been reconsidered. Lauter and Meyer (1968) reported a high incidence of dysphasia, apraxia, agnosia and disturbance of spatial orientation when patients were examined systematically. Blessed's (1980) series was followed to autopsy, and almost a third of those with typical Alzheimer pathology had shown evidence of parietal lobe symptomatology during life. It is clear therefore that these features are common, though not universal, in SDAT. Seltzer and Sherwin (1983) attempted a direct comparison between patients with onset of Alzheimer's disease before or after the age of 65, confirming a higher prevalence of language disorder among the younger patients. However, much may depend on the severity with which the disease process is developed, the more severe afflictions tending to compromise the parietal lobe to an extent that has issue in clinical symptoms. McDonald (1969) was able to show that parietal lobe symptoms were commoner among the rather younger patients who developed the disease and conferred a poorer overall prognosis. Hare (1978) similarly found a poorer outcome in their presence, and Kaszniak et al. (1978) found increased mortality in the presence of expressive language difficulty. Naguib and Levy (1982a) have shown that survival may be shorter when there is decreased absorption density in the parietal region on CT scans.

Such observations deserve attention because they are relevant to the question of the distinction between the presenile and senile forms of Alzheimer's disease as discussed on p. 449. Those who see no reason for the distinction are not surprised at the occurrence of focal parietal lobe symptomatology in SDAT. Those who have wished to uphold the distinction, such as Sourander and Sjögren (1970), separate off those patients who display marked focal signs as 'late-onset Alzheimer's disease' and place the remainder in a distinct nosological category. The latter may be designated as 'parenchymatous' or 'simple' senile dementia.

The relationship between SDAT and functional psychiatric illness in late life was discussed by Post (1968). His studies discounted the idea that neurotic or depressive symptomatology is a frequent prodromal manifestation of SDAT. Nor does he regard SDAT as an important cause of sexual transgression against juveniles in old men. The late appearance of paraphrenic symptoms is perhaps more commonly associated with SDAT, but this may be partly due to the difficulty sometimes encountered in distinguishing clinically between the early stages of the two disorders.

Rather more suggestive findings emerge in relation to premorbid personality adjustment. When the dementia is accompanied by florid paranoid or affective symptoms the subject will more commonly have shown evidence of an abnormal personality earlier in life; those whose dementia pursues a simple downward course are found to have been more stable (Post 1944). Thus the clinical features of the illness appear to be influenced pathoplastically by factors in the previous personality. Both Post (1968) and Oakley (1965) have also stressed the frequency with which obsessional traits emerge in the earlier history, such as rigidity of outlook, obstinacy and overconscientiousness. The validity of such associations must, however, wait upon proper random comparisons of unselected series of patients, since special features in the personality may obviously dictate referral to hospitals and other institutions.

The EEG usually shows little more than an accentuation of the normal changes with ageing. With increasing age alpha activity is reduced in frequency and abundance, theta activity tends to appear in the temporal regions, and even random delta activity may emerge (Kugler 1964; Kiloh et al. 1981). In SDAT such changes may be marked, sometimes with total abolition of alpha and prominent theta and delta activity. However, the changes lack specificity, and occasionally advanced dementia can exist alongside a normal EEG. Localised theta activity in the temporal regions of elderly subjects must be interpreted conservatively, and will usually warrant no definite conclusion about the presence of cerebral pathology.

Brain imaging in SDAT

Cerebral atrophy detected on CT or magnetic resonance imaging (MRI) scans will be obvious in many patients, though as described on p. 139 overlap with age-matched controls prevents this from being used as a firm diagnostic criterion. The significance of white matter lucencies on CT, and areas of high signal intensity on MRI, is discussed on p. 460.

Attempts have recently been made to refine the value of structural scans by concentrating on the medial temporal lobe regions, since these are known to be affected early in the disease. Le May *et al.* (1986) performed discriminant function analyses of ratings of temporal lobe regions, and Jobst *et al.* (1992) derived a direct linear measure of the width of the medial temporal lobe by scanning patients at an angle of 20 degrees caudad to the standard head alignment. The latter procedure appears to hold special promise, yielding little overlap between patients and controls when scanned late in the disease, and with indications of good discrimination at earlier stages.

MRI carried out in the coronal plane allows direct measurement of hippocampal volumes. Seab *et al.* (1988) found these to be reduced by 40% in SDAT patients without overlap with controls, whereas considerable overlap occurred on global measures of brain atrophy. The latter, but not the former, correlated with severity of dementia, suggesting that hippocampal atrophy may be an early and sensitive sign of the disorder whereas cortical atrophy becomes important in determining symptoms later. In Kesslak *et al.*'s (1991) small sample hippocampal and parahippocampal atrophy did prove to correlate with severity of dementia, and also, interestingly, with the degree of impairment of sense of smell.

Changes in cerebral blood flow and metabolism have been clearly demonstrated by functional imaging techniques. Early studies by Ingvar (1970) and Simard (1971) showed reductions in blood flow in proportion to cognitive failure, and this has been confirmed by more recent positron emission tomography (PET) and single photon emission computerised tomography (SPECT) techniques. Frackowiak *et al.* (1981), using PET, demonstrated substantial decreases in both cerebral blood flow and oxygen utilisation in SDAT, affecting both grey and white matter and implicating the parietal and temporal regions most severely. Sequential studies showed further decline with clinical deterioration, frontal hypometabolism appearing when deterioration was advanced. By contrast the visual cortex and the primary sensorimotor cortex were relatively spared. Such findings have been confirmed in PET investigations of glucose metabolism (Benson *et al.* 1982; Duara *et al.* 1986) and in studies of regional cerebral blood flow using SPECT (Gemmell *et al.* 1989; Montaldi *et al.* 1990). Frackowiak's study showed, moreover, that blood flow and oxygen utilisation remained closely coupled in all brain areas studied, thus disproving the idea that chronic brain ischaemia might underlie the dementia.

The reductions of blood flow in SDAT outstrip what is seen in age-matched controls, despite the significant relationships observed between decline in flow with age in cognitively intact subjects (Zemcov *et al.* 1984; McGeer 1986; Martin *et al.* 1991). Martin *et al.* performed PET scans on healthy volunteers aged 30–95, and pixel by pixel linear regression analysis showed declines in cingulate, parahippocampal, superior temporal, medial frontal and posterior parietal cortices bilaterally. They suggest that this loss of cerebral function with age in limbic and association cortex may represent the cerebral substrate of the cognitive changes that occur during normal ageing.

To some considerable extent it has been possible to relate areas of maximal hypometabolism in SDAT to particular patterns of neuropsychological failure. Using FDG-PET, Chase *et al.* (1984) observed relationships between hypometabolism in the left peri-Sylvian region and language impairment, right posterior parietal region and visuospatial impairment, left angular gyrus and dyscalculia, and frontal hypometabolism in relation to personality change and attentional deficits. Haxby *et al.* (1988) found that frontal hypometabolism correlated with poor verbal fluency and attentional skills, whereas parietal hypometabolism was associated with impairment in verbal comprehension, arithmetical ability and visuospatial functioning. In a follow-up of mildly affected patients over several years, Haxby *et al.* (1990) showed that asymmetries in hypometabolism between the left and right hemispheres remained directionally stable over time, and predicted the relative degree of impairments of language and visuospatial functions that eventually appeared. Burns *et al.* (1989) used SPECT to show that SDAT patients with aphasia and apraxia had lower cerebral blood flow than those without in the lateral temporal and posterior parietal lobes; and that in the group as a whole praxis correlated with posterior parietal activity, memory with left temporal lobe activity, and language with activity throughout the left hemisphere. McKeith *et al.* (1993) found that the association between memory impairment and reduced temporal uptake applied equally on the left and on the right.

Finally it is of interest that Geaney *et al.* (1990) have demonstrated improvements in cerebral blood flow in the posterior parietotemporal regions of elderly demented patients in response to infusions of physostigmine. Two HMPAO-SPECT studies were performed in eight patients and controls, with or without cholinergic stimulation from physostigmine. Significant focal increases in flow were observed in these regions in the demented patients, but not in controls, adding to the evidence that the cholinergic deficits in dementia may be at least partially reversible.

Course and outcome of SDAT

The overall course is usually steadily and smoothly progressive, in contrast to the step-like progression often seen in multi-infarct dementia. Death tends to follow within 5–7 years of the appearance of the disease, but precise estimates are difficult to obtain because many cases are not seen in hospitals. Certainly among those admitted to psychiatric hospitals life expectancy is poor, though there appears to have been a steady decline in mortality over the past 40 years as documented by Christie (1994). Roth (1955) found that almost 60% of patients were dead within 6 months and 80% within 2 years. Shah *et al.* (1969) reported rather better survival, at least where female patients were concerned, and Blessed and Wilson (1982) showed further gains. Christie and Wood (1990), in a sample gathered from the Crichton Royal Hospital between 1984 and 1986 found a mortality of only 9% at 6 months and 35% at 2 years. The reasons for this seeming gradual improvement in survival are unclear, but it is probably largely attributable to modern standards of care and in particular to antibiotics.

Heston *et al.*'s (1981) elderly patients with SDAT usually survived for less than 7 years, but occasional patients could live for more than 20 years after the first appearance of the disease. In the Burns and Levy (1992) study described on p. 432, mortality was 3.5 times that expected for the general population, with the following features predictive of decreased survival: male sex, advanced age, longer duration of illness, presence of physical illness, poorer cognitive function and depression. Apraxia appeared to predict earlier death, in keeping with other evidence that parietal lobe symptomatology confers a poor prognosis (p. 433). Misidentification syndromes, strangely, were significantly associated with longer survival.

Death is often due to intercurrent infection, or may follow upon a gradual period of 'vegetative extinction' which cannot be attributed to any exact cause. In consequence death certifications may fail to document the existence of dementia, reporting only pneumonia, cardiac failure or some other physical disorder occurring prior to death. At autopsy the body and viscera are said commonly to be atrophied in addition to the changes within the brain. Several studies have stressed the marked and progressive reduction in body mass index in patients with SDAT, as reviewed by Wolf-Klein and Silverstone (1994) and confirmed in a recent longitudinal population-based investigation (Cronin-Stubbs *et al.* 1997). The weight loss has emerged as substantially greater than in patients with heart disease or cancer. The responsible mechanisms remain unclear, but inadequate food intake seems unlikely to be the explanation. Whether it depends on metabolic or endocrine factors, or possibly on hypothalamic pathology, remains to be explored.

Pathology of SDAT

The pathological changes within the brain appear to be identical in form and distribution to those occurring in presenile Alzheimer's disease as described on p. 440. Here it may be noted, however, that they are said to be generally less severely developed in elderly demented persons. Sourander and Sjögren (1970) made detailed comparisons between the pathological findings in patients with presenile Alzheimer's disease, patients with parenchymatous senile dementia and elderly patients dying from other causes. A striking finding was that the reduction in brain weight was much more severe in presenile Alzheimer's disease than in the elderly dements; and a quantitative assessment of the frequency of neurofibrillary tangles showed them to be considerably more frequent in all brain regions studied in the presenile patients.

Vascular changes may coexist with the Alzheimer pathology as in old age generally—arteriosclerosis of large vessels and hyaline degeneration of small vessels, though these are by no means characteristic of the brain in SDAT. Amyloid changes may also be observed in small cortical arterioles in which the entire vessel wall has the appearance of a thick almost homogeneous tube (Corsellis 1969b). Occasional small infarcts are probably not uncommon as a result. In some cases, perhaps 10–20% of elderly dements generally, a clear admixture of Alzheimer change and arteriosclerotic pathology will be found to have contributed to the picture as described on p. 430.

Distinction between SDAT and normal ageing

All components of the cerebral pathology of SDAT may also be found in aged persons who have appeared to be mentally intact up to the time of death. Thus it has been argued that cerebral atrophy and its attendant histological changes are so common in later life that the structural state of the brain, as at present revealed, is of doubtful significance in relation to the disease process (Rothschild 1956). Some other qualitative differences might be waiting to be discovered, or alternatively it might be the mode of the patient's reaction to the ageing processes within the brain which holds the key to dementia. The relevance of the brain changes to dementia has now been clarified, first from the comprehensive studies of Corsellis (1962) and from the series of reports from Newcastle upon Tyne (Roth *et al.* 1967; Blessed *et al.* 1968; Tomlinson *et al.* 1968, 1970; summarised by Roth 1971).

Corsellis (1962) examined the brains of a large group of aged patients who had died in a psychiatric hospital, and found a high level of agreement between the clinical diagnosis during life and the severity of the neuropathological changes. Both parenchymatous and vascular changes tended to become more common with advancing age, but the great majority of those diagnosed as suffering from dementia showed cerebral pathology of at least moderate severity compared to only a quarter of those who had suffered from 'functional' mental disorders. It was possible to conclude that the occurrence of a progressive dementia was more often than not reflected in the ultimate appearance of the brain when fully and comprehensively examined.

The Newcastle workers undertook prospective studies, beginning with clinical and psychometric observations during life, and comparing these with quantitative measures of neuropathological changes after death. The subjects included elderly dementing patients, patients with 'functional' psychiatric illness, and mentally well-preserved persons who had died from accidents or other acute illnesses. The non-dementing elderly subjects frequently showed senile plaques in the cortex, and neurofibrillary changes in the hippocampi. Outfall of cells and granulovacuolar degeneration were also seen in some degree in the absence of dementia. But quantitative estimates of the number of plaques, or of the severity of neurofibrillary changes, proved to correlate very highly indeed with scores of intellectual and personality impairment. In fact the relationship between impairment and mean plaque count was broadly linear. Moreover, plaques were present in all layers of the cortex in demented subjects, but often restricted to the superficial layers in those who had shown no intellectual decline. Very large conglomerate plaques were far commoner in demented than in normal subjects.

Wilcock and Esiri (1982) confirmed the Newcastle findings and focused particular attention on the significance of neurofibrillary change. Ball (1976) had already demonstrated an enormous increase in the number of tangle-bearing neurones in the hippocampi when SDAT patients were compared with age-matched controls, and Wilcock and Esiri sought to relate this to the severity of the dementia. Counts of both plaques and tangles were made in the cortex and hippocampi in patients with SDAT and in controls of equivalent age. Tangle formation proved to be highly correlated with the severity of dementia prior to death in the majority of areas sampled, in addition to distinguishing reliably between demented and non-demented subjects. Plaque counts showed significant associations of a similar nature but less impressively so. Tangle counts, moreover, correlated with the severity of choline acetyltransferase reductions in the brain (Wilcock et al. 1982). It would appear, therefore, that the extensive development of neurofibrillary tangles

may be of particular significance as a histological marker of SDAT. Tomlinson (1982) concludes from his considerable experience that while tangles can be found in the hippocampal pyramidal layer and occasionally in the hippocampal gyrus in healthy aged subjects, it is extremely rare to find them in the neocortex at any age in the absence of dementia.

Thus it appears that SDAT arises clinically when the pathological changes of senescence develop beyond a certain degree of severity. Thresholds in terms of mean plaque counts or neurofibrillary change could be established with reasonable clarity in the Newcastle studies, below which destructive changes appeared to be accommodated within the reserve capacity of the brain and above which dementia became manifest. The finding of such quantitative relationships is impressive evidence for upholding the significance to be attached to the neuropathological changes, and the demonstration of regional effects goes some way to supporting a distinction between SDAT and normal ageing.

It remains possible, of course, that additional differences remain to be discovered and that these will highlight even more clearly the distinctions that can be drawn. As discussed on p. 443 there is increasingly clear evidence of profound cell loss from the cortex when SDAT patients are compared with age-matched controls (Terry et al. 1981; Terry & Katzman 1983). Changes in the morphology of dendrites (Scheibel 1978) and reductions in their fields of arborisation (Buell & Coleman 1979, 1981) may prove to be of especial significance for dementia (p. 443). The biochemical changes found in SDAT are described on p. 444 et seq. Here again it is noteworthy that while cholinergic function declines with age, the scale of the deficits found in dementia outstrips in large degree what might be expected from ageing processes alone.

Other evidence which may be presented for regarding SDAT as distinct from normal ageing includes the genetic information outlined on pp. 430–1, as well as the more dubious distinctions that can be drawn between the detailed nature of the psychological disabilities seen in the two conditions. Dorken (1958) has contrasted the orderly relationship in the decline of various abilities in normal old age with the more chaotic state of affairs in senile dementia, and Botwinick and Birren (1951) point out that the intellectual skills most vulnerable in normal senescence are not necessarily those which differentiate between normal and demented subjects. The issues involved are comprehensively discussed by Miller (1974, 1977) who concludes that it is unlikely that the psychological changes in dementia are merely analogous to accelerated ageing. The most clear-cut experimental evidence for this has come from studies of the rate of forgetting on a picture recognition test (Huppert & Kopelman 1989). Normal ageing was found to be associated with a mild acquisition deficit, as well as a significant increase in forgetting rate when tested 24 hours and 1 week later. By contrast, demented patients given the same test showed a severe acquisition defect but normal forgetting rates once initial learning had been accomplished (Kopelman 1985a).

The problems which surround the distinction between SDAT and multi-infarct dementia are discussed on pp. 455–8.

Alzheimer's disease

Alzheimer's disease was first described early in this century (Alzheimer 1907, 1911) and is now believed to be the commonest of the primary dementing illnesses. Alzheimer's 1911 paper has been usefully translated in full by Förstl and Levy (1991). Characteristics of the disorder when it appears in the elderly have been described just above. In what follows, presenile Alzheimer's disease will be given special consideration.

Aetiology

The great majority of cases appear to arise sporadically, though a slight but definite familial tendency has emerged when large series have been investigated. Sjögren et al.'s (1952) evidence suggested a multifactorial mode of inheritance. Much more rarely it seems to be transmitted as a regularly manifest dominant trait in occasional families (Pratt 1967). Here the usual female preponderance is said not to occur, and there are sometimes features peculiar to the family concerned — muscular twitching, spastic paraplegia or marked amyloidosis of cerebral vessels. An example has been described in a mother and identical twin sons who died in early adulthood after rapidly progressive dementia (Sharman et al. 1979).

Heston et al.'s (1981) genetic study, taking origin from autopsy-proven cases of Alzheimer's disease, revealed secondary cases among first-degree relatives in 51 of 125 families. Sixty per cent of the probands were thus isolated cases despite large family memberships in certain instances. The increased risk to relatives was largely confined to patients whose dementia had begun below the age of 70, but was then increased fourfold; indeed the risk to siblings when onset had been before 70 years of age and when a parent had already shown the disease approached 50%, resembling autosomal dominant inheritance in these unusual families. Interesting further associations emerged: among the relatives of younger

probands there appeared to be an increased risk of Down's syndrome, of myeloproliferative disorders such as lymphosarcoma, reticulum cell sarcoma and Hodgkin's disease, and of immune system disorders. Heyman et al. (1983, 1984) have confirmed a significant increase in Down's syndrome in the families of probands, and point also to a possibly increased incidence of thyroid disorder in the past histories of affected females. It would seem therefore that presenile Alzheimer's disease may be associated with a genetic factor leading occasionally to substantial familial aggregations of dementia, and conferring vulnerability to other disorders as well. The important molecular genetic work which has sought to identify the genes for familial Alzheimer's disease (FAD) is described on pp. 447–8.

The association with Down's syndrome is particularly striking in that patients with mongolism are unusually prone to developing the neuropathological features of Alzheimer's disease, including the typical paired helical filaments in neurofibrillary tangles (Jervis 1948; Malamud 1964, 1972; Olson & Shaw 1969; Burger & Vogel 1973; Ball & Nuttall 1980). It has been claimed, indeed, that it is rare for Down's syndrome patients to survive beyond middle age without such features developing in the brain. Wisniewski et al. (1978) have obtained some evidence of deterioration in institutionalised Down's syndrome patients over the age of 35 which may reflect this developing pathology, and Yates et al. (1980a) have shown cholinergic deficits in the brain similar to those occurring in Alzheimer's disease (p. 444).

The interesting suggestion has been made that an underlying defect in microtubule organisation, reflecting a disturbance of tubulin protein, may explain this association. Erratic functioning of the spindle mechanism could lead to the initial disturbance of chromosome division producing mongolism, and equally have issue in the development of neurofibrillary tangles. The increased incidence of chromosomal aneuploidy in Alzheimer's disease could be further evidence of the basic defect (Cook et al. 1979; Nordenson et al. 1980).

McMenemey (1963a) suggests that the genetic tendency may operate by allowing other extrinsic influences to bring the disease process into being. It is such additional influences which may ultimately be identified, and which are now being vigorously pursued along a number of research pathways. These important and mostly relatively recent developments are described in some detail on p. 441 et seq.

The question of precipitation is not uncommonly raised by relatives who may note an apparent onset after head injury, operations or admission to hospital for other causes. A detailed history will then usually show that the illness had already been in existence, and the so-called precipitant has merely revealed the true state of affairs. The possibility must be recognised, however, that minimal brain damage from head injury, infection or anaesthesia may sometimes have served to worsen the situation, and may have been decisive in pushing the patient below a threshold at which he was previously coping.

A more definite link between head injury and the development of Alzheimer's disease has been suggested from several case control studies, involving patients both in the senium and the presenium (Heyman *et al.* 1984; Amaducci *et al.* 1985; Mortimer *et al.* 1985; Graves *et al.* 1990). The interval between the injury and the development of dementia had often been several decades, and recoveries in the interim had usually been complete. The mechanisms whereby trauma could predispose to dementia later in life are far from clear, though it has been suggested that a decreased neuronal reserve consequent upon injury may serve to unmask brain ageing prematurely. The work by Corkin *et al.* (1989), discussed on p. 186, would support such a hypothesis. Alternatively, disruption of neuronal membranes may have led to increased beta amyloid production. In a recent report Roberts *et al.* (1991) examined 16 patients who survived for only 6–18 days after head injury, and were able to show extensive deposits of beta amyloid in the cortex of six, mostly in their forties and fifties. They suggest that induction of amyloid precursor protein mRNA may be a normal response to neuronal stress, but that it may lead to disease in susceptible individuals.

The validity of the link remains at present uncertain, and it is hard to discount the effects of selective reporting by the families of Alzheimer patients. A methodologically sound study of 274 case control pairs by Chandra *et al.* (1989) found no evidence of head injury as a risk factor for Alzheimer's disease. On the other hand a recent meta-analysis of 11 case control studies involving over 1000 cases has upheld the association in male patients (Mortimer *et al.* 1991; Mortimer 1994).

A report by Hollander and Strich (1970) is also of interest in this regard. Six patients were described in whom dementia of acute onset became manifest within hours or days of some catastrophic illness such as subarachnoid haemorrhage, head injury or major cardiac surgery. The brains showed the pathological features of Alzheimer's disease along with widespread amyloid angiopathy. It seemed that the acute illnesses had probably played some part in the sudden mental deterioration which occurred, and the amyloid changes, at least, appeared to have been of very rapid evolution. Hollander and Strich suggest that generalised metabolic precipitants, or disturbance of the cerebral circulation, should more often be taken into account in assessing the aetiology of Alzheimer's disease.

Clinical features

The onset of presenile Alzheimer's disease is usually after the age of 40, though rare cases have been reported at younger ages. Females preponderate over males in a ratio of 2 or 3 : 1.

The beginning is usually insidious and can be dated only imprecisely. The slow development of the intellectual deterioration often allows the patient to preserve considerable social competence until the disease is well advanced. Fortunately it is usual for the patient to lose insight into the changes within himself from an early stage.

Three main phases to the disease are commonly distinguished. The first, often lasting for 2 or 3 years, is characterised by failing memory, muddled inefficiency over the tasks of everyday life and spatial disorientation. Disturbances of mood may be prominent but psychotic features are rare. The mood disorder may take the form of perplexity, agitation and restless hyperactivity. Others by contrast have stressed aspontaneity and apathy from the early stages (Sjögren *et al.* 1952).

The second stage brings more rapid progress of intellectual and personality deterioration and focal symptoms appear. An accent on the parietal lobes is common with dysphasia, apraxia, agnosia and acalculia. Extrapyramidal disorders are also characteristic with disturbance of posture and gait, increase of muscle tone and other typical features of parkinsonism. Such parkinsonian signs were present in almost two-thirds of Pearce and Miller's (1973) patients. Extensor plantar responses may be seen and facial weakness is not uncommon. Florid psychotic symptoms of a delusional or hallucinatory nature may occur, but usually only when the dementia is far advanced.

The third or terminal stage consists of profound apathetic dementia in which the patient becomes bedridden and doubly incontinent. Gross neurological disability may sometimes develop, such as spastic hemiparesis or severe striatal rigidity and tremor. Forced grasping and groping may be seen, along with sucking reflexes. Grand mal fits are not uncommon. In the terminal phase of the disease bodily wasting may be rapid despite adequate preservation of appetite. Before this, however, somatic manifestations of senility usually remain in abeyance despite the steadily progressive dementia.

The clinical features which have been stressed as distinguishing Alzheimer's disease from other forms of presenile dementia include the following:

Memory difficulties are reported as the earliest feature more regularly than in any other presenile dementing process, and are said to precede changes in mood and behaviour in virtually every case. This was confirmed in the important study by Sim *et al.* (1966) who used cerebral biopsy to establish the pathological diagnosis in a large series of patients. Emotional changes such as anxious hyperexcitability or aspontaneity have also been regarded as characteristic, likewise dysphasic, apraxic and agnosic difficulties. Lauter and Meyer (1968) found the latter in virtually every patient below 59 years of age, though progressively less often in older age groups. Disturbances of gait and other extrapyramidal manifestations are regarded as equally typical of Alzheimer's disease.

Other features regarded as characteristic include early spatial disorientation, a progressive reduction in spontaneity of speech and increased muscular tension. Gustafson and Nilsson (1982) have partially validated a weighted scale, using these and other features, for distinguishing Alzheimer's disease from other forms of presenile dementia.

The frequency of epilepsy has sometimes been quoted as a distinctive feature and has been reported in up to 75% of cases. Minor seizures may occur early in the disease, though grand mal fits appear to be mainly a late development. Sim *et al.* (1966) found that early fits were actually more frequent in presenile dementias other than Alzheimer's disease.

Sourander and Sjögren (1970) drew attention to the frequency of behavioural abnormalities suggestive of temporal lobe dysfunction in presenile Alzheimer's disease, particularly phenomena reminiscent of the Klüver Bucy syndrome in animals after bilateral temporal lobe excision (p. 23). Visual agnosic difficulties were often the first focal deficits to be noted, especially inability to recognise the faces of relatives or the self in a mirror. Late phenomena included strong tendencies to examine and touch objects with the mouth (hyperorality), and tendencies to be stimulus-bound to contact and touch every object in sight (hypermetamorphosis). Hyperphagia was often a terminal phenomenon, with indiscriminate eating of any material available. The emotional changes of apathy and dullness were similarly reminiscent of the pathological tameness of monkeys with the Klüver Bucy syndrome. Such manifestations were observed in over three-quarters of patients with Alzheimer's disease, and in some of them the full gamut of phenomena was displayed. The human counterpart of the Klüver Bucy syndrome has been occasionally observed with other cerebral disorders such as arteriosclerosis, Pick's disease and cerebral tumours, but Sourander and Sjögren considered that in most cases it formed an essential part of the symptomatology of Alzheimer's disease. They also stressed that the seizures which occur are often temporal lobe in origin with characteristic chewing, smacking and lip-licking movements.

The EEG shows abnormalities more frequently in Alzheimer's disease than in any other form of dementia. Several investigations have demonstrated abnormal records in every case (Letemendia & Pampiglione 1958; Liddell 1958; Swain 1959), and Gordon and Sim (1967) confirmed that changes are likely to be seen even in very early examples with minimal dementia. The early stage consists of reduction of alpha activity which may sometimes disappear entirely. This is particularly characteristic of Alzheimer's disease and is perhaps of some value in distinguishing it from other varieties. Later diffuse slow waves appear, typically irregular theta activity with superimposed runs of delta. Focal or paroxysmal features are rare, even in patients with epileptic fits. The degree of abnormality appears to be more marked in patients in whom the disease is rapidly progressive (Swain 1959), and to worsen with the increase in dementia (Gordon & Sim 1967; Gordon 1968). CT and MRI scans show diffuse cerebral atrophy in a large majority of cases, with pictures analogous to those seen in late-onset Alzheimer's disease (pp. 433–4).

The overall findings of Sim *et al.* (1966) may be quoted as providing the best available comparison of the early and late manifestations of Alzheimer's disease in relation to other forms of presenile dementia. Biopsy during life allowed 35 patients with Alzheimer's disease to be compared with 21 patients suffering from other dementing processes. The non-Alzheimer patients were considered to represent a mixture of Pick's disease and several other forms. Features occurring early in Alzheimer's disease but often late in the other group included impairment of memory, apraxia and generalised disturbances in the EEG. Features occurring late in Alzheimer's disease but early in other cases included fits, incontinence, confabulation, personality change, delusions and hallucinations, and gross focal neurological disturbances such as spasticity, hemiparesis, striatal rigidity and tremor.

Finally, in seeking operational criteria for the clinical diagnosis of Alzheimer's disease for use in research, the following rules have been put forward by a working group established by the National Institute of Neurological and Communicative Disorders and Stroke and the Alzheimer's Disease and Related Disorders Association (NINCDS-ADRDA criteria) (McKhann *et al.* 1984):

I *For the diagnosis of **probable** Alzheimer's disease:*
Dementia established by clinical examination and documented by the Mini-Mental Test, Blessed Dementia Scale or similar examination and confirmed by neuropsychological tests.
Deficits in two or more areas of cognition.
Progressive worsening of memory and other cognitive functions.
No disturbance of consciousness.
Onset between 40 and 90 years.
Absence of systemic disorders or other brain diseases to account for the progressive deficits in memory and cognition.

II *Such diagnosis is supported by:*
Progressive deterioration of specific cognitive functions such as language, motor skills and perception.
Impaired activities of daily living and altered patterns of behaviour.
Family history of similar disorder, particularly if confirmed neuropathologically.
Laboratory results of normal lumbar puncture, normal EEG pattern or non-specific EEG changes, evidence of atrophy on CT with progression on serial observations.

III *Other features consistent with such diagnosis*, after excluding other causes of dementia:

Plateaus in the course of progression.

Associated symptoms of depression, insomnia, incontinence, delusions, illusions, hallucinations, catastrophic outbursts, sexual disorders, weight loss, and other neurological abnormalities (especially with more advanced disease) including increased muscle tone, myoclonus and gait disorder.

Seizures in advanced disease.

CT normal for age.

IV *Features that make such diagnosis unlikely:*

Sudden apoplectic onset.

Focal neurological signs such as hemiparesis, sensory loss, visual field deficits and incoordination early in the course.

Seizures or gait disturbances at the onset or very early in the course.

V *Diagnosis of **possible** Alzheimer's disease:*

May be made on the basis of the dementia syndrome, in the absence of other neurological, psychiatric or systemic disorders sufficient to cause dementia, and in the presence of variations in the onset, presentation or clinical course.

May be made in the presence of a second systemic or brain disorder sufficient to produce dementia, which is not considered to be *the* cause of the dementia.

Should be used in research studies when a single, gradually progressive severe cognitive deficit is identified in the absence of other identifiable cause.

VI *For the diagnosis of **definite** Alzheimer's disease:*

The clinical criteria for probable Alzheimer's disease and histopathological evidence obtained from biopsy or autopsy.

VII *Classification of Alzheimer's disease for research purposes* should specify features that may differentiate subtypes of the disorder, such as familial occurrence, onset before 65 years, presence of trisomy 21 and coexistence of other relevant conditions such as Parkinson's disease.

In a prospective study of 50 elderly patients followed to autopsy, Burns *et al.* (1990) have shown the value of the NINCDS-ADRADA criteria. Of 32 patients diagnosed as 'probable' Alzheimer's disease this was correct in 28, and of 18 'possible' cases the diagnosis was confirmed in 14 (i.e. sensitivities of 88% and 78%, respectively). Mistakes mainly involved Lewy body dementia in the former and vascular dementia in the latter.

Course and outcome

The disease runs a progressive course with death following some 2–8 years after onset. In Heston *et al.*'s (1981) material a trend could be seen for survival to increase a little from a mean of 7 years in those under 49, to 8.5 years for those aged 55–74. In more elderly groups the survival was on average shorter, presumably due to deaths from competing causes, but even so the span could sometimes exceed 20 years. Seltzer and Sherwin (1983)

made direct comparisons of 'relative survival time' between patients with onset before and after the age of 65 (by comparing observed length of survival for each individual with his expected survival from actuarial tables), and found significantly shorter survival for those in the presenile category.

Rare cases are described in which the disorder becomes arrested for a time, but these must be regarded as exceptional. Neither remissions nor fluctuations characterise the disease.

Pathology

The typical picture is of a grossly atrophied brain, without immediately obvious variation from one cortical region to another. Histologically there is extensive degeneration and loss of nerve cells accompanied by secondary glial proliferation. The striking features of senile plaques and neurofibrillary tangles are much in evidence. The vascular system is usually normal or displays only minimal changes, though sometimes amyloid angiopathy may be seen as described below.

The cortical atrophy, though generalised, tends to affect the frontal and temporal lobes more severely than the parieto-occipital regions. Variants on the typical picture are very occasionally seen, for example restricted lobar atrophy similar to that in Pick's disease or a lack of any gross shrinkage despite extensive microscopic degeneration. Neuronal degeneration affects the outer three cortical layers particularly. An accent is often found on the limbic areas and especially on the hippocampi and amygdaloid nuclei. Affected neurones may show an accumulation of lipofuscin pigment, or granulovacuolar degeneration in which minute vacuoles surround a central granule in the cytoplasm. The white matter shows axonal degeneration, hyperplasia of astrocytes and fibrous gliosis.

Senile plaques (neuritic plaques) are almost universally seen in Alzheimer's disease (Plate 10). They are usually found densely throughout the cortex and can readily be identified by silver staining. The hippocampi and amygdaloid nuclei are again particularly affected, the latter perhaps more severely than any other part of the brain (Corsellis 1970). The subcortical grey matter is much less severely affected and plaques are not seen in the white matter itself. They appear as irregular masses ranging from 50 to 100 μm in diameter. A central argyrophilic core is usually surrounded by a clear halo, and then an outer ring of filamentous material consisting of dystrophic neuronal processes containing paired helical filaments. Amyloid material is present in the core. Microglial cells can often be identified within the disintegrating tissue of the plaque, and astrocytes tend to collect around its margin. Within the substance of the plaque unmyelinated neuronal processes, including synaptic boutons, can be identified by electron microscopy (Terry & Wisniewski 1970).

Neurofibrillary tangles are also present and are usually considered essential for the diagnosis. They are again shown by silver impregnation and occur diffusely in the grey matter and particularly in the hippocampi. They lie within the nerve cells themselves, often displacing the nucleus or filling the cell body entirely (Plate 10). A major component of the tangle is tau protein, derived from the microtubules of the cell and existing in an abnormally phosphorylated form (p. 442).

Another focus of interest has been the occurrence of amyloid-like material in the brains of patients with Alzheimer's disease. This is most readily shown after treatment with Congo red when the material becomes birefringent. Divry (1927) first demonstrated the material in the centre of the senile plaque, and it has since been found in the neurofibrillary tangles and in the walls of intracortical arterioles. Heavy involvement of the vasculature (amyloid angiopathy, congophilic angiopathy) has formed a special feature of certain familially occurring variants (Corsellis & Brierley 1954). On electron microscopy even the smallest plaques are found to contain wisps of the material, whereas larger (and presumably older) plaques may simply consist of amyloid alone (Terry & Wisniewski 1970).

Despite this abundance of distinctive features the neuropathological diagnosis of Alzheimer's disease is not always straightforward. There can be a good deal of heterogeneity in the severity and distribution of lesions, and in older subjects it may be hard to decide whether the histological changes exceed what is to be expected with ageing generally. An admixture with vascular and other pathologies may also be encountered. Lantos and Cairns (1994) review the attempts that have been made to seek agreement on firm criteria for the pathological diagnosis.

Pearson et al. (1985) have made a careful study of the regional distribution of pathology in Alzheimer's disease, charting the frequency of plaques and tangles in different areas. This has confirmed a marked accent of pathological change in the association areas of the temporal, parietal and frontal lobes, whereas the motor, somatosensory and primary visual cortex are virtually unaffected. Changes also invariably involve the olfactory areas of the brain, in striking contrast to other primary sensory areas, along with the uncus, medial amygdala and hippocampal formation.

Pearson et al. suggest that the severe and constant involvement of the olfactory regions may indicate that they are the primary seat of the disease process, with spread thereafter along well-defined anatomical connections to the association areas of the cortex and to the hippocampus. It is therefore interesting that a deficit in the sense of smell has been established as a marked and early feature of Alzheimer's disease (Corwin et al. 1985; Serby et al. 1985; Knupfer & Spiegel 1986).

Following this lead, Talamo et al. (1989) have examined the olfactory mucosa of Alzheimer patients at autopsy, revealing the presence of abnormal neuritic processes with increased reactivity to neurofilament antibodies. Tabaton et al. (1991) have demonstrated tau-reactive filaments in biopsies of the olfactory mucosa in patients diagnosed during life, thus possibly indicating a means for antemortem confirmation of the disease.

Other than this, extracerebral pathology has been remarkably little studied in the disorder. The reason for the striking terminal loss of weight, often unrelated to inadequate intake of food, is unknown (p. 435).

Research findings

The past two decades have witnessed an accelerating investment of research into Alzheimer's disease, spurred on by the emergence of a number of promising leads. The Medical Research Council in the UK nominated research into the dementias as a priority area in 1977 (Medical Research Council 1977) and the Royal College of Physicians commissioned a review of the current state of knowledge in 1981 (Royal College of Physicians 1981). Since then the volume of research publications on dementia has increased enormously (Lishman 1994). There is now no dearth of avenues for study—the difficulty is rather to choose from among a number of quite different pointers towards the pathogenesis of the disorder. In addition to genetic effects, toxic, biochemical and immunological theories can find support, but none at the moment can claim primacy over the others. Research proceeds in parallel into presenile and senile Alzheimer's disease, though with the latter providing the more abundant clinical material.

Histology

Histological studies continue with the aim of determining what are the significant tissue elements involved in the disorder, and which of them may reflect primary steps in its evolution. The intensity of development of senile plaques and neurofibrillary tangles correlates closely with the severity of dementia (Tomlinson et al. 1970; Wilcock & Esiri 1982), but their precise significance remains uncertain and is subject to continuing exploration. Questions of nerve cell and synaptic loss can now be approached directly by quantitative techniques which bring important additional information. Close attention is also concentrated on the beta amyloid which accumulates within the senile plaques and around blood vessels, and which could prove to play a fundamental role in the disorder.

Both tangles and plaques have been studied in detail in the hope of throwing light upon their genesis. Electron microscopy shows that the tangles of Alzheimer's disease consist of twisted bundles of paired helical filaments (Kidd 1963), chemically and immunologically closely related to the normal microtubules and neurofilaments which make up the cytoskeleton of the cell (Iqbal *et al.* 1978; Grundke-Iqbal *et al.* 1979). They are found not only in diseased cell bodies, but also in the abnormal dendritic and axonal processes which accumulate around senile plaques. An important discovery is that a major constituent of the tangle consists of tau protein in an insoluble and abnormal form (Wischik *et al.* 1988a, 1988b). Tau protein is closely associated with the microtubules of the cell and appears to be essential for their assembly and stability. Thus, when it is sequestered in the form of paired helical filaments, transport processes along axons are likely to fail disastrously.

Careful studies have shown that abnormal processing of tau appears to be specific to Alzheimer's disease, and that phosphorylated tau and paired helical filament tau are increased more than 20-fold in comparison with healthy age-matched controls (Harrington *et al.* 1994). This compares with a more modest twofold increase in the accumulation of beta amyloid (see below). Altogether over 80% of tau protein in the Alzheimer brain is in the truncated insoluble form compared with less than 5% in control brains, and most of the insoluble fraction appears to be integral to the paired helical filaments (Mukaetova-Ladinska *et al.* 1993). It remains uncertain, however, whether the abnormal processing of tau is a primary step in the development of Alzheimer's disease, or whether it takes place only after the paired helical filaments have accumulated (Harrington & Wischik 1994).

Tangles consisting of paired helical filaments are not unique to Alzheimer's disease—they are found in dementia pugilistica, postencephalitic parkinsonism, subacute sclerosing panencephalitis and Down's syndrome, indicating that a variety of pathological processes can lead to their development. Those seen in other conditions, for example progressive supranuclear palsy, are now known to be distinct, consisting of straight filaments alone. The significance to be attached to the tangles of Alzheimer's disease therefore remains uncertain — they could reflect some fundamental derangement unique to the disease or merely represent a secondary and non-specific reaction within the cell.

The origin of senile plaques is likewise open to debate. They could result from metabolic derangements in the neuropil, and histochemical studies have shown increased enzyme activity around their margins (Friede 1965). Their frequent proximity to blood vessels and their amyloid content have suggested that immunological processes could be important to their development. It is possible that amyloid deposition may be the initial step, this leading in some manner to the aggregation of abnormal neurites around their margins. Others, however, have favoured the view that the nidus of formation is the damaged neurite itself (Terry & Wisniewski 1970, 1972). Ultrastructural studies of material from cortical biopsies have suggested that the first stage of plaque formation may be the appearance of small groups of degenerating terminal dendrites containing large numbers of mitochondria. Amyloid material then appears in the form of wisps between the neurites and condenses to form the central core. In this view it may well be that the paired helical filaments of the neurofibrillary tangles are the primary structural abnormality, embarrassing cell function centrally and, by interfering with axoplasmic flow, causing the neuritic processes to degenerate and contribute to plaque formation.

The amyloid depositions have become the focus of intense research interest themselves. Amyloid has long been recognised as an integral part of the picture in Alzheimer's disease, in the core of plaques, in neurofibrillary tangles and in the walls of blood vessels. It has proved to be distinct from the amyloid that accumulates in the systemic amyloidoses, but in common with that shows a beta-pleated secondary protein structure. In consequence it is often referred to as beta amyloid protein (but also as Aß amyloid, A4 amyloid or ßA4 in view of its relative molecular mass of 4 kDa). The protein was isolated from plaque cores by Masters *et al.* (1985) and from cerebral blood vessels of Alzheimer patients by Glenner and Wong (1984). It was then characterised in detail, and its amino acids sequenced as a chain which is variably 39–42 amino acids in length. Kang *et al.* (1987) were able to show that it is derived from a much larger molecule (the amyloid precursor protein or APP) which is a normal constituent of nerve cell membranes and also occurs in other tissues of the body. This precursor is encoded by a single gene on chromosome 21.

A number of reasons have arisen to underline the potential importance of beta amyloid in Alzheimer's disease. Recent antibody-labelling studies have shown that it is deposited much more widely in the brain than was previously recognised (Lantos & Cairns 1994). Such deposits take a variety of forms, including subpial, punctate, granular and laminar deposits throughout the neocortex, hippocampus, central nuclear masses, cerebellum, brain stem and cord. In effect Alzheimer's disease can be regarded as a beta protein amyloidosis of the central nervous system. Another pointer to its importance has come from the discovery, albeit in very rare families, that mutations in the APP gene appear to be causal for the development of familial Alzheimer's disease (p. 448). In these cases, at least, it seems indisputable that APP protein plays a crucial role in the pathogenesis of the disorder. Meanwhile, it has been shown that beta amyloid can exert neurotoxic effects on neurones in tissue culture (Yankner *et al.* 1990), further indicating that it may be an important cause of neuronal damage when accumulating in the brain.

Cell counting within the brain has been important in determining whether neuronal loss in the disease exceeds that to be expected as a result of ageing alone. If it does not there could be reason to doubt whether Alzheimer's disease represents a primary neuronal disorder; whereas if cell loss is indubitable the development of tangles, plaques and other features could perhaps be of secondary importance.

The relation of neuronal loss to age has itself turned out to be complex, with certain brain regions showing different stability from others. Brody (1955) claimed substantial decrements in the cortex from childhood to the eighth decade, some areas such as the superior temporal gyrus showing losses of up to 50% while others such as the postcentral gyrus were relatively stable. Henderson *et al.* (1980), using an automated technique, found losses of up to 60% for large neurones in all cortical areas sampled over an equivalent age range, and without this regional variability. The Purkinje cells of the cerebellum clearly decline with age (Hall *et al.* 1975), but in the brain stem the situation is variable— losses occur in the locus caeruleus, whereas counts in many cranial nerve nuclei appear to change very little (Brody 1978; Tomlinson 1979).

In presenile Alzheimer's disease substantial cell losses were reported by Colon (1973) and Brun and Englund (1981), but among elderly patients the situation was initially unclear. Shefer (1973) found substantial decrements in SDAT, but Terry and co-workers were at first unable to confirm this (Terry *et al.* 1977; Terry 1979). More recent studies, however, are unequivocal — major neuronal losses are found in frontal, parietal and temporal areas in SDAT, affecting mainly the larger neurones and amounting to a reduction of some 40% relative to age-matched controls (Terry *et al.* 1981; Terry & Katzman 1983).

Mountjoy *et al.* (1983) have reported similar findings, though with the interesting observation that cell loss was less marked in the most elderly dements in their series, no longer being significant in those over 80 years of age. Others have confirmed that the percentage cell loss in relation to age-matched controls becomes progressively less in older Alzheimer patients, this applying to cell counts in many areas — the temporal cortex, hippocampus, locus caeruleus, nucleus basalis and the raphe nuclei (Mann 1985; Mann *et al.* 1985).

Nevertheless it has been shown that cortical cell loss is fundamental to cognitive failure. In a study of biopsy material from Alzheimer patients, Neary *et al.* (1986b) found that the degree of cognitive impairment correlated more strongly and consistently with measures of pyramidal cell loss in the cortex than with plaque or tangle counts. Significant correlations were also observed with indicators of activity in the cells that remained, namely measures of nuclear and nucleolar volume and of cytoplasmic RNA. With regard to non-cognitive features of the disease, Förstl *et al.* (1992) have observed that depressed patients with SDAT show lowered neuronal counts in the locus caeruleus. This may indicate that a noradrenergic deficit represents the organic substratum for depression in the disorder.

Dendritic changes have been reported with age and in dementia and could be of special significance. The dendritic tree represents 70–90% of the total membrane area of the neurone, and any curtailment will stand markedly to diminish synaptic connectivity. Scheibel (1978) has described loss of spines, degeneration of basal branches and later of terminal arches, as a widespread affection of pyramidal cells in the frontal and temporal cortex of elderly deteriorated patients. Furthermore, in cases of presenile Alzheimer's disease, clusters of new dendritic growth have been observed, perhaps in an attempt at compensation, but organised in a haphazard and 'lawless' fashion (Scheibel & Tomiyasu 1978).

Computer-assisted methods have been employed for tracing the extent and complexity of the dendritic trees deriving from individual nerve cells, with particularly interesting results. Buell and Coleman (1979, 1981) have obtained strong indications that in healthy elderly persons the dendritic domains become *more* extensive, with increased branching and larger terminal segments than in persons of middle age. This would seem to imply a continuing growth of the dendritic trees attaching to neurones which remain healthy, extending well into old age and perhaps compensating for the decline in total neuronal numbers. In elderly dements, however, the size of the dendritic trees was significantly reduced compared to those found in elderly controls (Buell & Coleman 1981; Flood & Coleman 1986). SDAT may therefore represent a failure of normal dendritic growth, or perhaps even a net regression of existing dendritic domains. The factors which govern dendritic extension and division may thus be fundamentally at fault.

Most recently attention has been focused on the density of synapses in the Alzheimer brain, with rather striking results. Hamos *et al.* (1989) used immunohistochemical markers of two major protein constituents of synaptic terminals (synapsin and synaptophysin), and showed a marked decrease in density in the molecular layer of the hippocampus. Direct visualisation of synapses on electron microscopy has confirmed such findings in lamina III of the frontal cortex (DeKosky & Scheff 1990; Scheff *et al.* 1990). Moreover, in these latter studies it was possible to show that synaptic counts in biopsy specimens correlated significantly with scores on the Mini-Mental State examination, suggesting that the loss is directly related to the decline in cognitive function in Alzheimer's disease. There were also indications of a compensatory process at work, in that as the number of synapses decreased the mean size of those remaining increased, with the net result that in the biopsy samples the total synaptic contact area was broadly maintained. In autopsy material, however, synaptic loss was more severe and had outstripped such capacities for compensation.

Biochemistry

Biochemical studies of brain tissue obtained at autopsy, chiefly from patients with SDAT, have revealed key changes that occur in brain proteins, enzymes and other constituents. Bowen *et al.* (1973) showed lack of a specific brain protein (neuronin S6) in the cortex, also biochemical indices reflecting neuronal loss and glial reactivity (Bowen *et al.* 1979). The most promising approach, however, has been the study of substances involved in synaptic transmission, culminating in the focus of attention on the cholinergic system.

Investigations from several centres combined to highlight a widespread deficiency in cholinergic transmission, both in presenile and senile Alzheimer's disease (Davies 1977; Perry *et al.* 1977; Spillane *et al.* 1977; White *et al.* 1977). The enzymes responsible for the synthesis of acetylcholine (choline acetyl transferase, ChAT) and for its degradation (acetylcholinesterase, AChE) emerged as remarkably deficient, with reductions amounting to 30% of normal levels in many areas. The balance of evidence suggests, moreover, that the density of the principal receptor-binding sites remains relatively normal. Nicotinic receptors are reduced (Perry *et al.* 1989), also presynaptic M_2 muscarinic receptors (Mash *et al.* 1985), but the important postsynaptic M_1 muscarinic receptors remain largely intact (Bowen *et al.* 1979). This latter observation has opened up prospects for treatment with cholinergic substances, as described on p. 502 *et seq.*

ChAT levels decline with age, at least in the hippocampus, but not to an extent that could account for the decrements seen in SDAT (Perry *et al.* 1977). In multi-infarct dementia analogous deficits do not occur (Perry *et al.* 1978; Wilcock *et al.* 1982). The reduction in ChAT has been demonstrated in biopsy as well as autopsy samples (Spillane *et al.* 1977; Bowen *et al.* 1979); and in fresh tissue samples a parallel reduction in acetylcholine synthesis has been confirmed (Sims *et al.* 1980; Francis *et al.* 1985). ChAT is reduced in proportion to the severity of the dementia prior to death, and in relation to the concentration of senile plaques and neurofibrillary tangles displayed on histological examination (Perry *et al.* 1978; Wilcock *et al.* 1982). The evidence combines to suggest therefore that cholinergic deficits are an integral and meaningful part of the Alzheimer disease process, not merely related to non-specific agonal factors.

Further research has shown that there are deficits in other neurotransmitters too, which is not surprising in view of the pleomorphic symptoms of the disease. The other systems are not, however, involved with the same consistency or severity, and show less clear-cut correlations with key pathological features. Noradrenaline and its metabolites are depleted in many brain regions, the levels in some areas being significantly related to the severity of dementia prior to death (Adolfsson *et al.* 1979; Mann *et al.* 1980; Arai *et al.* 1984; Francis *et al.* 1985). Dopamine-β-hydroxylase, the marker enzyme for noradrenaline, is also reduced, though not consistently in all patient samples studied (Cross *et al.* 1981). Cortical dopamine levels appear to be normal, but the serotonergic system is clearly affected. Reduced concentrations of 5-hydroxytryptamine (5-HT) (and 5-hydroxyindoleacetic acid) have been shown in the cortex, also a markedly reduced density of 5-HT_2 receptor-binding sites (Cross *et al.* 1983, 1984; Arai *et al.* 1984; Reynolds *et al.* 1984). The serotonergic deficits lack association with the degree of cognitive impairment, but they may be related to behavioural changes such as aggression and perhaps to depression (Palmer *et al.* 1988).

It is clear that these transmitter deficiencies reflect cell loss, not only in the cortex, but also in the subcortical nuclei which give rise to ascending cortical projections. In the cholinergic system, for example, the reductions in ChAT greatly exceed estimates of cell loss in the cortex, indicating that cholinergic *terminals* must also be involved. These are derived from projections from the basal forebrain nuclei—the medial septal nucleus, the diagonal band of Broca and the nucleus basalis of Meynert in the substantia innominata. The nucleus basalis of Meynert, which gives rise to the main cholinergic projection, has proved to be profoundly depleted of cells in Alzheimer's disease (Whitehouse *et al.* 1982; McGeer *et al.* 1984).

Equivalent evidence has emerged in relation to the noradrenergic deficits. Significant cell depletion has been shown in the locus caeruleus, which provides the main noradrenergic input to the cortex (Tomlinson *et al.* 1981; Mann *et al.* 1984). Surviving cells in the nucleus, moreover, show reduced nucleolar volume and reduced cytoplasmic RNA indicative of diminished activity (Mann *et al.* 1980). Cell loss and neurofibrillar tangles are found in the dorsal raphe nucleus of the midbrain, which may similarly account for the cortical losses in serotonin (Curcio & Kemper 1984; Yamamoto & Hirano 1985).

It was accordingly tempting to postulate that the primary seat of disturbance in Alzheimer's disease might be subcortical in location. Neuronal degeneration in the cortex could be largely secondary, as a result of transynaptic degeneration due to loss of ascending inputs. What had long been seen as an essentially cortical disease process might thus have its roots elsewhere. Rossor (1981) postulated such a model, whereby Alzheimer's dementia could be viewed as a disease of the 'isodendritic core', i.e. of subcortical neuronal systems which project to the cortex along biochemically defined pathways. An analogy was drawn with Parkinson's disease which involves the dopaminergic projections from the substantia nigra to the corpus striatum; and with progression of either disease extension might occur to the other neural projections, accounting for the later appearance of dementia in some Parkinson's patients (p. 653) and of extrapyramidal dysfunction in Alzheimer's disease (p. 438).

Further information has, however, undermined such ideas. Neuronal loss in the cortex outstrips what could be accounted for by losses entirely connected with the ascending projections; and strict relationships have not been upheld between the severity of cortical ChAT depletion and cell counts in the nucleus basalis of Meynert. Moreover, the additional neurotransmitter deficits discussed below point increasingly to the implication of intrinsic cortical neurones in the disease process. Cortical pathology is therefore reinstated as having a primary role in Alzheimer's disease, and much of the degeneration in the subcortical nuclei is now regarded as secondary to this.

A bewildering variety of changes have been reported in other neurotransmitters, with some conflicts of evidence from one laboratory to another. In many cases this is due to technical difficulties in making reliable observations on autopsy-derived material. Reviews are provided by Rossor (1987) and Dewar and McCulloch (1994).

Gamma aminobutyric acid (GABA) is widely distributed in the cortex as an inhibitory neurotransmitter, chiefly in local interneurones, and therefore stands to give information about intrinsic cortical pathology. It appears to be reduced in the temporal cortex in younger cases (Rossor et al. 1982, 1984), but other than this few consistent changes have emerged. Glutamic acid decarboxylase (GAD), the marker enzyme for GABA, is reduced in autopsy but not in biopsy samples, and may therefore reflect non-specific agonal changes.

Of the peptides, somatostatin is markedly reduced (Davies et al. 1980; Ferrier et al. 1983). Such a change may occur late in the disease since biopsy samples have given normal results (Francis et al. 1987). Somatostatin receptors have also been found to be depleted (Beal et al. 1985). The two other main cortical peptides, cholecystokinin (CCK) and vasoactive intestinal polypeptide (VIP), have in general been found to be normal. Substance P, however, is depleted (Quigley & Kowall 1991).

Glutamate transmission has attracted special interest in view of the possible role of glutamate-mediated excitotoxicity, especially in cells which are already compromised in some degree. Moreover glutamate is the principal transmitter associated with pyramidal cells in the cortex and hippocampus. The estimation of glutamate levels at autopsy is, however, unreliable and results have been conflicting. Some evidence has been obtained of a reduction in free glutamate in cortical and subcortical areas (Ellison et al. 1986), and of loss of presynaptic glutamatergic terminals (Cowburn et al. 1988a, 1988b). Dewar and McCulloch (1994) review autoradiographic studies which have shown reduced glutamate binding in superficial cortex and discrete areas of the hippocampus. The rather indirect evidence for a role of glutamate-induced excitotoxicity in Alzheimer's disease is outlined by Zorumski and Olney (1992). Thus excitotoxins have been shown to cause degeneration of cholinergic neurones in the basal forebrain and to selectively kill somatostatin neurones in cortical cell cultures; furthermore cultured spinal neurones develop paired helical filaments when exposed to glutamate.

As more detailed biochemical evidence has emerged it has seemed probable that the deficits encountered are more severe in younger than older Alzheimer patients. Thus Rossor et al. (1981, 1982, 1984) have shown that patients dying in their eighties or nineties have a relatively pure cholinergic defect, principally involving the temporal lobe and hippocampus, whereas those dying in their sixties and seventies have more severe and widespread deficits extending to the frontal cortex as well. The younger group also showed depletions in noradrenaline, GABA and somatostatin, which were rarely reduced in the very old. Tagliavini and Pilleri (1983) found that neuronal losses from the nucleus basalis of Meynert were more profound in presenile than senile Alzheimer's disease (while present in both), and no losses whatever could be detected in a small group of very elderly patients with 'simple' senile dementia. Bondareff et al. (1981b, 1982), investigating neurone counts in the locus caeruleus, have found a bimodal distribution—those with low counts being significantly younger at death than those in whom counts were normal. It is difficult to decide, on present evidence, how far these age-related differences merely reflect the more 'malignant' course of the disease process when it occurs at a younger age, or whether in time they will point to subdivisions within a 'syndrome' of Alzheimer's disease. Particular interest will attach to the clinical–biochemical correlations which emerge from further studies, and to the impact the findings may have on the current unitary theory of presenile and senile Alzheimer's disease.

Aluminium toxicity

Toxicity from aluminium has been suspected since 1965 when Klatzo *et al.* showed that intracerebral injections of aluminium salts could induce neuronal tangles in cats and rabbits. Such tangles consist of straight filaments and lack the classic paired helical structure, but nevertheless this seemed at one time to offer a potential animal model for Alzheimer's disease. Crapper *et al.* (1978) found that similar tangles were induced when aluminium was added to cultured human foetal neurones. And elevated aluminium levels were demonstrated in the brain in Alzheimer patients, the levels being highest in regions markedly affected by neurofibrillary degeneration (Crapper *et al.* 1976).

Perl and Brody (1980), using a spectrometric method, were able to detect foci of aluminium actually within the nuclei of hippocampal neurones affected by neurofibrillary degeneration, adjacent tangle-free neurones being unaffected. More recently aluminium and silicon have been identified in high concentration in the cores of senile plaques (Candy *et al.* 1986; Edwardson & Candy 1990). The association of aluminium with both major neuropathological features of Alzheimer's disease is certainly a striking finding. Further evidence came from reports of progressive dementia in patients exposed to high aluminium levels, and from the realisation that aluminium is responsible for the deterioration seen in patients suffering from dialysis encephalopathy as discussed on p. 558.

Nevertheless, the aluminium hypothesis remains controversial, as discussed in Rifat and Eastwood (1994). Some have failed to replicate the finding of raised aluminium levels in Alzheimer brains; and it is possible that aluminium may accumulate in plaques and tangles as a secondary effect, rather than playing a primary role in the disorder. In patients dying from dialysis encephalopathy the brain does not show neurofibrillary tangles, nor any deficit in cholinergic activity. A clinical study which appeared to show benefit from a chelating agent in Alzheimer's disease (Crapper McLachlan *et al.* 1991) has also been criticised on methodological grounds.

In spite of these caveats the leads already available have prompted further extensive work into the possible pathogenic effects of aluminium in drinking water:

Flaten (1986) found that rates of death attributed to dementia in Norway were significantly correlated with aluminium concentrations in different geographical regions. Martyn *et al.* (1989) then used CT scan information for the labelling of Alzheimer's disease in 88 county districts in England and Wales; the risk appeared to be 1.5 times higher in districts where concentrations exceed 0.11 mg/l compared to districts where concentrations were below 0.01 mg/l. Michel *et al.* (1990) screened elderly community residents in the Gironde region of France, and found that local aluminium concentrations correlated with the percentage of patients meeting NINCDS-ADRADA criteria for Alzheimer's disease. Finally, Neri and Hewitt (1991) have reported a case-control study in which over 2000 patients discharged from hospitals in Ontario with Alzheimer's disease were matched with patients of the same age and sex who had non-psychiatric diagnoses. The relative risk of developing Alzheimer's disease increased across the four levels of aluminium concentration in the drinking water in the patients' areas of residence.

All such studies are open to criticism on a number of grounds, but nonetheless offer sufficient evidence to keep the question of possible aluminium neurotoxicity open. It would seem reasonable to suppose that aluminium may rank among several other environmental factors which can contribute to the development of Alzheimer's disease, probably against a background of genetic susceptibility.

Infection

An infective aetiology for Alzheimer's disease has been considered in view of the known transmissibility of Creutzfeldt–Jakob disease (p. 473). The evidence so far is, however, slender and the leads obtained to date must be viewed with caution. In Gajdusek's laboratory three out of 35 cases of Alzheimer's disease proved to be transmissible to chimpanzees, two being examples of familial Alzheimer's disease and all having shown atypical features in one way or another (Traub *et al.* 1977). All, moreover, produced on transmission the picture of spongiform encephalopathy, typical of Creutzfeldt–Jakob disease, not the histological features of Alzheimer's disease itself. Three other aberrant transmissions were obtained from cases of progressive supranuclear palsy, Leigh's disease and dementia of an unknown type (Goudsmit *et al.* 1980). The possibility therefore arises that the inocula may have been contaminated, and certainly numerous other attempts to transmit the disease have been uniformly unsuccessful. The conclusion at present must be that transmissibility in Alzheimer's disease has not been demonstrated with any reasonable degree of certainty.

Other lines of evidence are, however, intriguing. Wisniewski *et al.* (1975) showed that plaques similar to those of Alzheimer's disease could be induced in mice by inoculation with the 'scrapie' agent. Moreover, the brains so infected show a reduction in ChAT activity similar to that occurring in Alzheimer's disease (McDermott *et al.* 1978a). The remote possibility therefore remains that species-specific factors may have prevented the demonstration of Alzheimer pathology in the chimpanzee in the experiments described just above.

Interest also attaches to the demonstration of neurofibrillary tangles in tissue cultures of human foetal cortex after adding extracts of brain tissue or cerebrospinal fluid from patients with Alzheimer's disease (De Boni & Crapper 1978; Crapper McLachlan & De Boni 1980). The latent interval observed has seemed consistent with the presence of some infectious agent, though spontaneous degenerative processes in the cultures cannot be excluded.

Immunology

Immunological factors have been suspected from several lines of evidence. Ageing is associated with a decline in both cell-mediated and humoral-mediated immune mechanisms, and Alzheimer's disease might conceivably represent a profound accentuation of such a process (Nandy 1978).

There is a good deal of evidence that amyloid is deposited in tissues under conditions of altered immunity, and immunoglobulins have been identified in the amyloid of the plaques (Ishii & Haga 1976). Moreover the close relationship of plaques to blood vessels, especially when these are heavily affected, suggests that the deposition may originate from the blood stream (Behan & Behan 1979). Abnormalities in certain serum protein fractions have been identified in patients with Alzheimer's disease, similar to those that occur in primary and secondary amyloidosis (Behan & Feldman 1970). In generalised amyloidosis the brain is very rarely affected, but in Alzheimer's disease there may be some concurrent disruption of the blood–brain barrier, and evidence exists for this (Wisniewski & Kozlowski 1982).

Abnormalities of serum immunoglobulins have been reported in patients with SDAT when compared with age-matched controls, and some significant correlations have emerged between immunoglobulin levels and tests of cognitive function (Eisdorfer et al. 1978; Cohen & Eisdorfer 1980; Eisdorfer & Cohen 1980). There are also indications of an age-related increase in antineural antibodies in the serum, with higher titres in dements than in age-matched controls (Nandy 1981). It is difficult, however, to decide whether such observations are secondary to the cerebral pathology rather than reflecting primary aetiological mechanisms. The more recent and often conflicting research findings in these areas are reviewed by Sweet and Zubenko (1994).

Aisen and Davis (1994) discuss further evidence that inflammatory and immune mechanisms may be involved in tissue destruction in Alzheimer's disease, suggesting indeed that they could play a part from the earliest stages of the disorder. Modern serological studies provide evidence of inflammatory activity by way of an 'acute phase response', with elevation of C-reactive protein and α_1-antichymotrypsin in the serum. The latter has also been identified in the amyloid of senile plaques. Cytokines, which mediate the acute phase response, appear to be involved in the pathophysiological process. Thus the serum of Alzheimer patients contains elevated levels of tumour necrosis factor, and brain tissue shows an increase in microglial cells which react immunologically for interleukin-1. Activated microglial cells accumulate around senile plaques, and the plaques themselves show immunoreactivity for interleukin-6.

Such findings may be indicative of an acute phase response taking place within the brain. And a fundamental role for inflammatory–immune mechanisms is suggested by the presence of complement proteins and α_1-antichymotrypsin from the earliest stages of plaque formation. Disruption of the blood–brain barrier could be part of the initiating sequence, serving to expose previously protected brain antigens to the immune system.

The study of human leucocyte antigen (HLA) typing in Alzheimer's disease has sometimes pointed to certain unusual distributions of HLA subtypes (Behan & Behan 1979; Harris 1982). It is possible, therefore, that some immunological deficit predisposing to the disorder may be conferred by the patient's genetic constitution. The demonstration of an increased incidence of immune system disorders among the relatives of patients with Alzheimer's disease (Heston et al. 1981), and of an increased incidence of thyroiditis, hypothyroidism and Grave's disease in the histories of female probands (Heyman et al. 1983, 1984), lends some support to the hypothesis that autoimmune factors may be important in the disorder. Recent evidence that the onset of SDAT in elderly twin pairs is inversely associated with prior use of corticosteroids or non-steroidal anti-inflammatory drugs is a further intriguing pointer in this direction (Breitner et al. 1994).

Molecular genetics

Molecular genetic research has yielded important and continuing advances. The field was opened up when St George-Hyslop et al. (1987) found linkage to DNA markers on chromosome 21 in four kindreds with early-onset familial Alzheimer's disease (FAD). Chromosome 21 was selected for study because of the known associations between Alzheimer's disease and Down's syndrome, but the linked probes did not map to the region implicated in the latter disorder. Soon afterwards the gene coding for APP was identified, and this proved to be very close to the FAD markers (Goldgaber et al. 1987; Kang et al. 1987). Initial speculation that the FAD gene and the APP gene might be identical was rendered unlikely when recombinations between the two were demonstrated in certain families (Tanzi *et al.* 1987). Moreover families were discovered in whom no linkage whatever could be shown to chromosome 21, indicating that genetic heterogeneity must exist (St George-Hyslop *et al.* 1990).

Further work has revealed linkages to other chromosomes in certain families — to chromosome 19 in late-onset familial disease (Pericak-Vance *et al.* 1991) and to chromosome 14 in early-onset cases (Mullan *et al.* 1992; Schellenberg *et al.* 1992). The linkage to a particular marker on chromosome 14 was found to be especially close and to apply in many of the families who also showed linkage to chromosome 21.

Meanwhile attention was refocused on chromosome 21 by Goate *et al.* (1991), who demonstrated a point mutation in the APP gene in two families, consisting of a substitution of isoleucine for valine at codon 717. This was the first mutation to be established in Alzheimer's disease. It was confirmed that this segregated with the disease in a number of additional families, supporting its pathogenic role. A different mutation at the same point was discovered by Chartier-Harlin *et al.* (1991), and several others have followed since, all in close proximity to the region coding for the beta amyloid sequence (Mullan 1992; Clark & Goate 1993). These discoveries, though applicable in only a small proportion of families, are of great importance, strongly suggesting that in these cases, at least, beta amyloid deposition may be the central event in the pathogenesis of the disorder.

Further work on chromosome 19 has centred on the gene coding for apolipoprotein E (ApoE). This is of special interest in that it applies to late-onset disorder, and to sporadic as well as familial forms of the disease. The ApoE gene occurs in three common forms, E_2, E_3 and E_4, which occur in various combinations. A highly significant association has emerged between possession of the E_4 allele and both familial and sporadic forms of late-onset Alzheimer's disease (Poirer *et al.* 1993; Strittmatter *et al.* 1993). It would seem that some 80% of familial and 60% of sporadic late-onset cases have at least one $ApoE_4$ allele, compared to 30% of control subjects. Moreover, an increased risk has been demonstrated in relation to increased 'dosage' of E_4 alleles, suggesting that they act in a partly additive fashion (Corder *et al.* 1993). Thus among 42 late-onset families the proportion of affected individuals increased significantly with the number of E_4 alleles present, from 20% of subjects with genotype 2/3 or 3/3, to 47% with 2/4 or 3/4, and to 91% of those with genotype 4/4. The mean age of onset decreased in similar fashion, from 84 years in subjects with no E_4 allele, to 75 in the presence of one and 68 when two E_4 alleles were present.

The ApoE alleles have important additional associations. E_4 is possibly related to an increased risk of ischaemic heart disease, and E_2 has been found to be especially frequent in those who survive to be centenarians (Schächter *et al.* 1994; van Bockxmeer 1994). Indeed there is evidence that the E_2 allele may be protective against the development of late-onset Alzheimer's disease (Corder *et al.* 1994). Other interesting associations include a significant increase of the E_4 allele in Lewy body dementia (Harrington *et al.* 1994) and in patients with motor neurone disease of bulbar onset (Al-Chalabi *et al.* 1996). No such increase has been found in Parkinson's disease, with or without dementia, or in Huntington's disease (Harrington *et al.* 1994; Marder *et al.* 1994).

With regard to Alzheimer's disease, ApoE has been immunochemically localised to senile plaques, vascular amyloid and neurofibrillary tangles, and $ApoE_4$ binds particularly tightly to beta amyloid and tau proteins. There may, therefore, be prospects for developing therapeutic strategies by finding substances which interfere with such interactions (Scott 1993). Nevertheless some 40% of people with Alzheimer's disease do not possess an E_4 allele, so other aetiological factors and probably other genes must also be at work (Owen *et al.* 1994). Whether future advances will bring possibilities of predictive testing in families strongly affected remains to be seen.

Finally, a mutation on chromosome 1 has been identified in Volga German kindreds with early-onset familial Alzheimer's disease (Levy-Lahad *et al.* 1995a, 1995b). Of particular interest is the finding that the gene is closely similar in chemical sequence to that on chromosome 14 in other early-onset families, suggesting that the proteins they encode may have analogous functions.

Ageing research

Research into ageing proceeds along with that into dementia. The number of parallels that can be drawn between neural ageing and dementia is impressive (Lishman 1991, 1994). With increasing age there is a decline in neuronal numbers, an increase in plaques and a decrease in many neurotransmitters and their synthesising enzymes. Moreover the older the Alzheimer patient is at death, the smaller is the divergence from age-matched healthy controls on most of these parameters. In the very elderly there may be little in the brain to distinguish Alzheimer patients from non-dements of equivalent age.

With regard to clinical features there are slower rates of progression in older patients, less evidence of focal brain failure and, from Heston *et al.*'s (1981) data, less evidence over the age of 70 of the operation of genetic influences. Moreover, when representative samples of the elderly population are examined, decline in cognitive function appears to lie on a continuous distribution rather than with the bimodality that would be expected if dementia and ageing were dichotomous (Brayne 1994).

In this manner arguments can be marshalled in favour of a neural ageing hypothesis as the basis for Alzheimer's dementia, accelerated ageing accounting for most of the observed changes on clinical, neuropathological or biochemical examination. Such a conception will, of course, be challenged if some clear-cut marker should be established which distinguishes incontrovertibly between Alzheimer patients and non-demented elderly persons. Current discoveries in molecular genetics, outlined above, perhaps hold promise of providing such evidence. The work of Jobst et al. (1994), on sequential CT scanning of Alzheimer patients and healthy ageing controls, also points in this direction. Preliminary data indicate a remarkable acceleration of medial temporal lobe atrophy in Alzheimer's disease, so rapid that it appears to reflect some catastrophic event or cascade process superimposed upon normal age-related changes.

In the last analysis the distinction between 'ageing process' and 'disease' may yet be found to be an artificial dichotomy drawn from older concepts. The nature of ageing processes within the brain, and the genetic and environmental factors which accelerate or retard them, may prove to be amenable themselves to neurobiological research.

Finally, the intriguing suggestion has recently come forward that education may be *protective against dementia*. Orrell and Sahakian (1995) review the several studies supporting such an association and the possible neural mechanisms that may underlie it.

The most persuasive evidence comes from a prospective population-based study in Rotterdam in which 7528 participants over the age of 55 were carefully screened for dementia (Ott et al. 1995). The prevalence of dementia rose sharply with age as expected, but additionally showed highly significant associations with the level of education attained. This applied to all dementias combined, also to Alzheimer's disease and vascular dementias considered separately. As an example, persons with the lowest grade of education (primary education only) had a fourfold relative risk of developing Alzheimer's disease compared with those with the highest grade (medium level vocational training to university level). Indicators of cardiovascular disease were examined as possible confounding factors but did not substantially decrease the association, either in the dementias as a whole or in diagnostic subgroups.

Possible contributions to the association must include lowered socioeconomic status among persons with poorer education, leading to poorer physical health, also a degree of diagnostic bias in that early dementia may more easily be missed in highly educated persons. In Ott et al.'s study it is further possible that despite the fairly high participation rate (73%) the non-response may have been in some degree selective. Nevertheless the detailed results are impressive.

Orrell and Sahakian (1995) discuss two explanations which are not mutually exclusive. Education may be 'neuroprotective' in that keeping neurones active may stimulate beneficial mechanisms such as DNA repair. Secondly it may increase brain reserves by augmenting the density of neocortical synapses, thus allowing greater compensation to occur in the presence of brain pathology and delaying the onset of mental symptoms.

Distinction between Alzheimer's disease and SDAT

Most authorities hold the view that Alzheimer's disease and parenchymatous senile dementia are identical in all respects other than age of onset (Lauter & Meyer 1968; Corsellis 1969b; Terry & Katzman 1983). In the neuropathological picture no distinguishing features, taken individually, have come to light, and certainly few neuropathologists would claim to be able to distinguish between the two on examination of the brain. Hence the present practice of referring to 'presenile Alzheimer's disease' and 'senile dementia of the Alzheimer type' as explained on p. 429.

Nonetheless Sourander and Sjögren (1970) believed that distinctions could be drawn. Their comparisons between the pathological findings among older and younger patients are discussed on p. 435, with indications of less severe cerebral atrophy and less intense pathological change among the elderly. They were led to conclude that Alzheimer's disease represents something other than merely an early occurrence of parenchymatous senile dementia, at least in so far as the intensity of neuropathological features is concerned.

Recent neurochemical findings have also pointed to differences between younger and older patients, the former tending to show more severe and widespread cholinergic deficits and more definite depletions in other neurotransmitters (p. 445). There are indications also from PET scan studies that the derangement of brain metabolism may be more focal in presenile cases and more global in the elderly, but such findings are as yet insubstantial (Small et al. 1989; Mielka et al. 1991). Differences are also suspected in certain key subcortical nuclei which play an important role in relation to brain biochemistry (p. 445). As with the neurohistological features, however, it is hard to exclude the possibility that all such findings merely reflect a greater overall severity of the dementing disease process in the young compared to the old. How far further biochemical and ultrastructural studies will challenge the basic similarities between presenile and senile Alzheimer's disease remains to be seen, though present indications still tend to favour a unitary disorder.

Other strands of evidence which may indicate a difference are equally debatable, but may be summarised as follows. Certain genetic evidence has implied a distinction as discussed on pp. 430–1. Physical senescence is said to be absent in Alzheimer's disease until the terminal stage of rapid emaciation, whereas in SDAT physical deterioration often parallels the mental disintegration throughout. This, however, may be no more than a reflection of the greater impact on physical health of any disease process in persons of advanced age. It was formerly taught that disturbances such as dysphasia and apraxia were characteristic only of presenile Alzheimer's disease, though this view has recently come under review (p. 433). Seltzer and Sherwin (1983) have nevertheless found that language disorder is significantly more common, and length of survival reduced, in patients with presenile as compared to senile Alzheimer's disease.

Lewy body dementia (diffuse Lewy body disease, cortical Lewy body dementia, senile dementia of the Lewy body type, SDLT)

Lewy bodies, which are the hallmark of the brain stem pathology of Parkinson's disease, have been found sometimes to occur diffusely in the cerebral cortex and to be accompanied by dementia. After an initial report from New York (Okazaki et al. 1961) patients were described from Japan, and more recently the condition has attracted attention in the UK and the USA. The nosological status of the disorder, and particularly its relationship to Alzheimer's disease, remains uncertain, likewise the confidence with which it can be diagnosed during life. Some regard it as part of the spectrum of Parkinson's disease (Gibb et al. 1987) and others as a variant of Alzheimer's disease (Hansen et al. 1990). In both clinical and pathological terms it appears to bridge the two conditions.

The current interest in the disorder derives from the frequency with which such pathological findings have emerged, especially when immunocytochemical techniques are employed for detection of Lewy bodies in the cortex. In two recent series, from Nottingham and Newcastle upon Tyne, the condition has emerged as possibly second only to Alzheimer's disease as a cause of dementia in the elderly, occurring in some 20% of cases coming to autopsy (Byrne et al. 1989; Perry et al. 1990d). However, virtually all examples to date have been reported from neuropathological laboratories in special centres, so sampling procedures may have played a part in determining estimates of its frequency.

This relatively new conception as a basis for dementia is clearly of great importance. It may help to explain why a considerable proportion of Alzheimer patients develop extrapyramidal symptoms, and cortical Lewy bodies may

make a significant contribution to dementia in patients with Parkinson's disease. Conceivably in some cases the condition may constitute a distinct neurodegenerative disorder, though arguments can be marshalled against this (Gibb 1990).

Clinical features

Males have outnumbered females in some though not all series, with onset typically in the sixties or seventies. The clinical features, and particularly the mode of presentation, have varied in different reports, depending no doubt on the source from which the patients were referred for pathological examination. In some the commonest presentation has been with extrapyramidal features, in others with dementia, and in some with confusional states or psychotic symptomatology. With progression of the disorder both dementia and extrapyramidal features are usually in evidence, though dementia can be the sole manifestation throughout.

Byrne et al. (1989) reported 15 cases from 57 autopsies carried out on patients who had shown dementia or extrapyramidal disorder or both. Six had presented with classic parkinsonian features then progressed to cognitive impairment 1–14 years later; three presented with both parkinsonian features and cognitive impairment together; and six presented with dementia alone, all of whom developed extrapyramidal features later. Gibb et al.'s (1989a) patients presented with dementia more often than with parkinsonism, Perry et al.'s (1990d) mostly with confusional states complicating the dementia, and many of Birkett et al.'s (1992) had first been diagnosed as having paranoid illnesses. Six of the 21 patients reviewed by McKeith et al. (1992) did not develop extrapyramidal features at any stage.

The dementia is typically cortical in type, with progressive memory impairment and the development of dysphasia, dyscalculia and dyspraxia. It has been suggested that the detailed pattern of neuropsychological deficits may be useful in aiding the distinction from 'pure' Alzheimer's disease—impairment is said to be more severe on tests of visuospatial and frontal lobe function when patients with Lewy body dementia are compared with Alzheimer patients at a similar stage of dementia (McKeith et al. 1995). Periodic acute organic reactions are commonly superimposed, even from the early stages. Distinct day-to-day fluctuations in mental competence have been emphasised, also prominent behavioural disturbance with psychotic features. Both auditory and visual hallucinations occur in many patients, particularly the latter, also paranoid delusions and severe depressive symptoms. In some cases such psychiatric symptoms may precede other manifestations of the disorder by many months.

The reasons for the marked fluctuations in the clinical picture remain obscure. The exacerbations appear to be partly related to decreased attention, but are not invariably associated with drowsiness or delirium, nor with specific changes on the EEG (Lennox 1992). They cannot be clearly attributed to toxic, metabolic or iatrogenic processes, and as the dementia worsens they tend to disappear.

The motor manifestations show the typical features of Parkinson's disease, with bradykinesia, rigidity, tremor, mask-like facies and stooped posture. Involuntary movements are sometimes reported, also myoclonus, quadriparesis, dysarthria and dysphagia (Burkhardt et al. 1988). Orthostatic hypotension may occur, and falls and unexplained losses of consciousness are often seen (McKeith et al. 1992).

McKeith et al. (1992) have described the spectrum of clinical features in detail, making a retrospective case note comparison between 21 cases of Lewy body dementia and 37 cases of Alzheimer's disease proven histologically. The Lewy body patients tended to show milder cognitive impairment at presentation, and more often showed marked fluctuations at any stage. Episodes of clouding of consciousness occurred in 80% of patients. Visual hallucinations were commoner than in the Alzheimer patients, and were often complex, vivid and rapidly moving. One patient saw an express train going through his room, another gypsies climbing through the window. Auditory hallucinations and persecutory delusions were also frequent. The fluctuating nature of such symptoms and their tendency to worsen at night suggested an acute confusional state superimposed on the dementia. Fluctuation was also observed in memory, language and visuospatial abilities; lucid periods with near normal memory capacity were sometimes recorded until late in the disease. Almost half of the Lewy body patients had falls or transient and unexplained losses of consciousness which were rare in the Alzheimer patients. Depression was significantly more common in the Lewy body patients and was sometimes the reason for the initial referral.

Extrapyramidal features in this series were no commoner at presentation than in the Alzheimer group, but developed more frequently and more severely later on. An important observation was that they almost always appeared to be directly related to the prescription of neuroleptic medication. Moreover, the Lewy body patients appeared to be unusually susceptible to severe reactions to neuroleptics such as chlorpromazine or haloperidol, developing first sedation then the acute onset of rigidity accompanied by postural instability and falls. Rapid deterioration led to death in many cases. There were no such acute reactions in the Alzheimer patients.

Hansen et al. (1990) and Förstl et al. (1993) have also made comparisons between Lewy body dementia and Alzheimer patients, but in both reports the Lewy bodies were an unexpected finding in patients who had conformed to strict criteria for the diagnosis of Alzheimer's disease during life. They are therefore likely to represent patients on a different part of the spectrum of Lewy body dementia. Hansen et al. found poorer performance among the Lewy body patients on tests of attention, verbal fluency and visuospatial function, and they more often showed mask-like facies and other extrapyramidal features. Förstl et al. found no differences between the groups in terms of duration, severity of cognitive impairment, hallucinations or fluctuating course, but extrapyramidal features were commoner and frontal cerebral atrophy on CT scans more marked.

Operational criteria for the diagnosis of the syndrome have been put forward by Byrne et al. (1991) and by McKeith et al. (1992), differing somewhat in the emphasis placed on extrapyramidal disturbance, but likely ultimately to help in refining conceptions of the disorder.

Many cases will be suspected during life as suffering from acute or subacute organic reactions on account of the marked fluctuation in cognitive status, and careful screening will be required to exclude an infective, metabolic or toxic reaction superimposed upon the dementia. Multi-infarct disease may be suspected, especially in the presence of hypertension. When extrapyramidal disturbance is pronounced from the early stages the patient may be diagnosed as having Parkinson's disease with superadded dementia.

Investigations are usually uninformative. The cerebrospinal fluid is usually normal except for occasionally elevated protein. Electroencephalography often shows abnormal but non-specific tracings with diffuse slowing. Neuroimaging reveals diffuse cerebral atrophy in most cases, but this may not be severe.

Course and outcome

On present evidence it would seem that the clinical course, though widely variable, is shorter than with Alzheimer's disease. In McKeith et al.'s (1992) series the time from onset of symptoms to death was a mean of 1.8 years in the Lewy body group and 4.8 years in the Alzheimer patients. Those who suffered adverse reactions to neuroleptic treatment fared particularly badly, surviving a mean of less than 1 year. Burkhardt et al.'s (1988) review, by contrast, suggested a rather longer course, ranging from 1 year to even 15–20 years in occasional cases. Lennox (1992) suggests that the average survival time from the onset of dementia is approximately 6 years.

Pathology

At autopsy the brain usually shows mild cortical atrophy and ventricular enlargement. Pallor is detected in the substantia nigra and locus caeruleus.

The distinctive pathological finding is the occurrence of numerous Lewy bodies in the cortex. They are also found in the substantia nigra, other brain stem nuclei and basal forebrain regions, though often less in number than in Parkinson's disease. In Parkinson's disease occasional Lewy bodies can sometimes be detected in the cortex, but not in anything approaching the numbers seen in Lewy body dementia.

Lewy bodies consist of rounded eosinophilic inclusions within neurones. They are easily detected in the brain stem, where they stain deeply with haematoxylin and eosin stains, and where the pale halo around the filamentous core is highlighted by the surrounding neuromelanin (Plate 11). In the cortex, however, they are less eosinophilic and less clearly circumscribed, making their detection less straightforward. The use of anti-ubiquitin antibodies has been an important advance (Plate 12), permitting reliable estimates of Lewy body frequency and proving to be twice as sensitive as conventional stains in revealing them in cortical areas (Lennox et al. 1989b).

In the cortex they are found in greatest numbers in limbic areas including the medial temporal cortex, insula and anterior cingulate gyrus, though the hippocampus is largely spared (Lennox 1992). Rather lower densities are found in neocortical parts of the frontal, temporal and parietal lobes, where they mainly occur in the small and medium-sized neurones of the deeper layers. The relative distribution has tended to vary in different reports, perhaps accounting for differences in clinical presentation. Psychotic features may owe much to limbic involvement. Lennox et al. (1989a) reported a strong correlation between the density of cortical Lewy bodies and the severity of dementia in their cases, but this was not found by Perry et al. (1990d).

In rare cases Lewy bodies have been found without any accompanying Alzheimer-type pathology (Birkett et al. 1992) but this is exceptional ('pure Lewy body dementia'). There is usually mild to moderate senile plaque formation, though neurofibrillary tangles are typically few or even absent. The severity of Alzheimer pathology is usually described as well below what would be expected in Alzheimer's disease and insufficient to make such a diagnosis on its own. Moreover, the relative distribution

of Lewy bodies and Alzheimer pathology do not mirror one another closely. Again the severity of Alzheimer changes appears to reflect the form of clinical presentation, neurofibrillary tangles being more conspicuous in those patients whose illness has closely resembled Alzheimer's disease during life (Hansen et al. 1990).

Varying degrees of cell loss are reported in the cortex, though less severely than in Alzheimer's disease. Cell loss is also seen in the substantia nigra and other subcortical nuclei, though less than in Parkinson's disease. Severe reductions in choline acetyltransferase activity have been found in the temporal neocortex, exceeding even that found in Alzheimer's disease (Perry et al. 1990e). This may be attributable to the combined effects of Alzheimer and Lewy body pathology in the nucleus basalis of Meynert. Caudate dopamine levels are also depleted, paralleling the neuronal loss in the substantia nigra (Perry et al. 1990c).

Interesting results have come from comparisons between patients who have experienced hallucinations and those who have not. ChAT activity is significantly lower in the parietal and temporal cortex in the presence of hallucinations (Perry et al. 1990a), but conversely monoaminergic markers (dopamine and serotonin metabolites and serotonin S_2 binding) are significantly decreased in patients who have not hallucinated (Perry et al. 1990b). This has suggested that an imbalance between monoaminergic and cholinergic transmitters in the temporal lobes may be responsible for hallucinations in the disorder.

In a considerable number of cases spongiform vacuolation has been found in the medial temporal lobe regions, indistinguishable from that seen in the spongiform encephalopathies (Burkhardt et al. 1988; Hansen et al. 1990). The significance of this finding remains unclear.

Distinction between Lewy body dementia and Alzheimer's disease

The clinical picture can obviously sometimes resemble Alzheimer's dementia very closely, as shown by those cases detected at autopsy in patients who have conformed to strict clinical criteria for Alzheimer's disease during life. Förstl et al. (1993) suggest that the diagnosis of Lewy body dementia should be considered even in patients satisfying NINCDS-ADRDA criteria when they show marked parkinsonian features and a frontal accentuation of atrophy on CT scans.

In other patients the diagnosis will be suspected when there are marked fluctuations in performance from day to day, or when dementia is accompanied by acute or subacute organic reactions for which no other cause can be found. A preponderance of psychotic features by way of hallucinations and paranoid ideation may also raise suspicion, though these are not so uncommon as previously thought with Alzheimer's disease alone (p. 432). The prominent development of extrapyramidal features, either early or late in the course must also bring the condition to mind, likewise severely adverse reactions to the administration of neuroleptics.

Multi-infarct dementia (arteriosclerotic dementia, vascular dementia, arteriopathic dementia)

The dementias which rest on a vascular basis are considered here rather than in the chapter on cerebrovascular disorders since they enter into the differential diagnosis of other dementing illnesses. Both in the senile and presenile age ranges they appear to be second only to Alzheimer's disease as a cause of progressive intellectual impairment. It is probable, however, that there is a considerable tendency to overdiagnose this category during life. Corsellis (1969b) pointed out that in the middle-aged adult the clinical diagnosis is encountered much more often than is justified by the eventual pathological findings. In the aged patient with SDAT the diagnosis may also be made erroneously, since the relatively common minor infarctions of later life will readily produce clinical evidence of focal disorder when the reserves of the brain are reduced.

The presence of arteriosclerosis in the peripheral or retinal vessels cannot be taken as a firm guide towards the diagnosis. Peripheral changes are common with advancing age and will frequently be found when the dementia has some other basis; conversely, after middle age, cerebral arterial pathology cannot be excluded even when there is no evidence of arteriosclerosis elsewhere. Hypertension is perhaps a more reliable guide but can similarly be misleading. Nevertheless in St Clair and Whalley's (1983) survey of autopsy-proven cases the blood pressure had been significantly higher in those with multi-infarct dementia (mean 173/98) than in those with Alzheimer's disease (mean 137/85).

A major difficulty in clarifying the pictures to be expected lies in the pleomorphic forms that the vascular dementias may take. One large and prominent group rests on major infarctions of cerebral tissue, sometimes few in number but strategically situated to disrupt key cortical systems. 'Single infarct dementia', for example, can result from angular gyrus lesions (p. 493) or lesions in the intralaminar nuclei of the thalamus (p. 384). Posterior cerebral and parietal lobe infarctions can also give rise to pictures resembling dementia. Alternatively, there may be numerous scattered softenings, individually small in effect but combining together to produce an additive

result. In the latter category the accent of pathology may be cortical, subcortical or both. When the subcortical 'lacunar state' affects the basal ganglia and pons the dementia may show distinctive associated features (p. 384). Rarer subvarieties include dementias which owe much to diffuse white matter demyelination ('subcortical arteriosclerotic encephalopathy') as discussed on p. 458.

Aetiology

The ultimate cause will usually lie with the causes of atheromatous disease and hypertension generally, for which textbooks of medicine should be consulted. Hachinski et al. (1974) stressed that the evolution of the dementia depends not on progressive chronic ischaemia, i.e. a relentless strangulation of the brain's blood supply, but essentially on the accumulation of deficits from infarcts large and small. Hence they preferred the term 'multi-infarct dementia' to 'arteriosclerotic dementia', in order to underline such a pathogenic mechanism. They concluded, moreover, that the majority of infarcts were due to thromboembolism from the extracranial arteries and the heart, and that only in a small minority of cases could atherosclerosis of the cerebral arteries be primarily blamed for the cerebral softenings. In Tomlinson et al.'s (1970) autopsy-proven cases ischaemic cortical lesions involving the territories of the middle and posterior cerebral arteries appeared to be particularly significant.

Others, however, have laid emphasis on the role of hypertensive small vessel disease in leading to dementia. Hypertension is associated with fibrinoid necrosis and microaneurysm formation along the walls of small arteries and arterioles, leading on to local occlusions and perianeurysmal haemorrhages. It affects particularly the long perforating arteries to the deep white matter and subcortical nuclear masses, resulting in numerous 'lacunar' infarcts in the central brain substance. The relative frequency of these two main forms of pathogenesis remains debatable, as discussed by Liston and La Rue (1983). Not uncommonly both forms of pathology will be found together, since hypertension itself predisposes to widespread atherosclerosis.

Other associated disease processes may contribute to the arterial pathology in certain cases, diabetes mellitis being prominent among them. Collagen vascular disorders, leukaemia or polycythaemia may occasionally play a part. Cardiac conditions predisposing to embolisation include rheumatic valvular disease and atrial fibrillation; carotid stenosis or occlusion is another important source.

Finally, any full consideration of dementia with a vascular basis should take account of dementias due to ischaemic–hypoxic lesions such as those following cardiac arrest or profound hypotension (p. 548), and those which follow haemorrhagic lesions such as subarachnoid haemorrhage or chronic subdural haematoma. For this reason the term 'vascular dementia' is nowadays sometimes preferred to 'multi-infarct dementia' as a more all-embracing term (Román *et al.* 1993; O'Brien 1994a).

Clinical features

Multi-infarct dementia is found with almost equal frequency in males and females, with perhaps a slight excess in males. It usually begins during the late sixties and seventies, though well-confirmed examples are occasionally seen in patients in their forties.

Arteriosclerosis will often be obvious in the peripheral and retinal vessels and hypertension will usually be severe, but these alone do not provide firm guidelines to the diagnosis. Attempts have been made to define the characteristics of the dementing process itself which will enable it to be distinguished from other forms of senile and presenile dementia, but in fact the clinical distinctions remain far from well established.

The onset is frequently more acute than in Alzheimer's disease, and a substantial number of cases only come to medical attention after a frank cerebrovascular accident has occurred. When the onset is gradual, emotional or personality changes may antedate definite evidence of memory and intellectual impairment. Other common early features include somatic symptoms such as headache, dizziness, tinnitus and syncope which may be the main complaints for some considerable time.

Once established the cognitive impairments characteristically fluctuate in severity, varying from day to day and sometimes even from hour to hour. In large measure this may be due to episodes of clouding of consciousness which are a feature from the early stages. Clouding is common towards nightfall and may lead to florid nocturnal delirium. Birkett (1972) confirmed that fluctuations tended to distinguish multi-infarct dementia from SDAT, but even so two of his patients who showed striking fluctuations proved ultimately to have the latter disease.

Apoplectiform features punctuate the progress of the disorder and are due to episodes of cerebral infarction. Commonly they consist of abrupt episodes of hemiparesis, sensory change, dysphasia or visual disturbances. At first they are transient and followed by gradual restitution of function, but later each leaves more permanent neurological deficits in its wake. Each episode is usually followed by an abrupt increase in the severity of the dementia. Lacunar infarcts may lead to a variety of neurological defects including ataxia, dysarthria and motor and sensory disturbances, culminating in the picture of

pseudobulbar palsy (dysarthria, dysphagia and emotional incontinence) together with bradykinesia and *marche à petit pas*. Very occasionally, however, lacunes may be associated with gradual mental deterioration without conspicuous focal signs (p. 384).

Other features which suggest multi-infarct dementia include the patchy nature of the psychological deficits that result. Thus the basic personality may be well preserved until late in the disease, whereas in other dementing illnesses this is undermined from an early stage. Capacity for judgement may persist for a surprisingly long time, and a remarkable degree of insight is sometimes retained. As a result the patient often reacts to awareness of his decline by severe anxiety and depression.

Other emotional changes include lability, no doubt due to lesions in the basal parts of the brain, and a tendency towards explosive emotional outbursts. Episodes of noisy weeping or laughing may occur on minor provocation, often without accompanying subjective distress or elation.

Birkett (1972) found that neurological abnormalities predicted arteriosclerosis more accurately than any mental feature. Even in the absence of gross defects, such as dysphasia or hemiparesis, there will often be minor focal signs. The tendon reflexes are often unequal, the plantars extensor or the pupil reactions impaired. Parkinsonian features may be conspicuous, likewise evidence of pseudobulbar palsy as described above. Epileptic seizures are found in about 20% of cases, and attacks of syncope are common.

The EEG shows a picture similar to that of Alzheimer's disease (p. 439), but the changes tend to be more severe. Advanced examples can, however, sometimes show normal records. A distinctive feature may be the appearance of focal abnormalities in the region of local cerebral thromboses—a low amplitude delta focus may emerge if the infarction is sufficiently extensive, and some asymmetry may persist for several weeks thereafter. Frontal delta activity may appear when there are episodes of delirium. Harrison *et al.* (1979) found that the EEG more often showed focal or lateralising abnormalities in patients diagnosed as having multi-infarct dementia than in equivalently impaired patients with Alzheimer's disease. The occurrence of paroxysmal activity or of a normal EEG is also commoner in the former than the latter (Erkinjuntti & Sulkava 1991).

The CT or MRI scan will usually show evidence of cerebral atrophy, sometimes marked in degree. Areas of low attenuation, consistent with old and recent infarctions, may be revealed. Multiple small lacunar infarcts will often escape direct detection on CT, but loss of central brain substance shows as ventricular dilatation. Radue *et al.*

(1978) found that in general the CT scan was unreliable in differentiating multi-infarct dementia from Alzheimer's disease, though patients with the former were more likely to show low attenuation areas, unequal Sylvian fissures and focal enlargements of the ventricles. Altogether the scan findings were equivocal in 80% of patients, though useful in predicting the type of dementia in the remainder. MRI imaging can give firmer information by virtue of its superior ability to reveal small infarcts, particularly lacunar infarcts in the deep white matter. The issue of white matter low attenuation (leukoaraiosis) in multi-infarct dementia is discussed on p. 460.

The cerebrospinal fluid shows an elevated protein in perhaps a quarter of cases, especially when there has been a recent episode of cerebral infarction or in the presence of uraemia or congestive cardiac failure.

Course and outcome

Perhaps the most reliable distinguishing characteristic of multi-infarct dementia is the course which it pursues. This is rarely smoothly progressive as in Alzheimer's disease, but punctuated by abrupt step-like progressions. Acute exacerbations are sometimes followed by improvement for a time, and in the early stages, at least, periods of remission may last for months at a time. These features depend on the pathogenesis of the disorder in terms of repeated cerebral infarctions.

The time to death varies widely. Sometimes the course is brief and stormy, but in general progress is slower than in Alzheimer's disease. The average duration after diagnosis is perhaps some 5–7 years, though many cases survive much longer. Among patients admitted to psychiatric hospitals Roth (1955) was able to demonstrate an improved survival compared to those with SDAT after 6 months, though by 2 years the differences were diminished and 70% of the multi-infarct patients were dead. Shah *et al.* (1969) confirmed improved survival among patients with multi-infarct dementias where females were concerned, with 65% of hospitalised females surviving at 2 years (compared to 32% of females with SDAT). Death is attributable to ischaemic heart disease in approximately 50% of patients, others dying of cerebral thrombosis or renal complications.

Pathology

The brain may show localised or generalised atrophy, with thickened adherent meninges and sometimes with evidence of subdural haemorrhage. The ventricles are dilated and cyst formation may be evident to the naked eye. Scattered infarctions are seen with areas of softening and scarring. Sometimes occlusion of a major vessel will have affected a large part of a hemisphere.

The detailed picture is summarised by Corsellis (1969b). Vessels of all sizes are usually implicated in the arteriosclerotic process. The main arteries at the base of the brain are thickened, tortuous and rigid, often with yellowish patches and nodular expansions of the wall. Their lumina are greatly reduced or even obliterated by intimal thickening and subintimal plaques of atheromatous material. Small vessels within the substance of the brain show greatly thickened walls with a fibrosed or 'onion skin' appearance. Frequently the walls are necrotic and disintegrated. Perivascular rarefaction may produce a sieve-like appearance, particularly in the striatum and thalamus.

Microscopy shows the effects of both ischaemia and infarction. Loss and chromatolysis of nerve cells is extensive, sometimes occurring in streaks or patches within the cortex. Irregular patches of demyelination may be seen in the white matter. Small scattered infarcts are revealed, with cyst formation and reactive gliosis. Small cystic softenings are particularly common in the pons, and micro-infarcts in the hippocampi. In the 'lacunar state' multiple cavities with irregular contours are found in the central brain regions, particularly in the basal ganglia, internal capsules and thalamus. Larger areas of infarcted brain tissue show necrotic degeneration with masses of granular phagocytes, or at a later stage sclerosis with dense glial and fibrocytic infiltration and distortion of brain substance.

Arteriosclerotic changes are likely to be seen elsewhere in the body, especially in the heart and kidneys, and the heart is commonly enlarged at autopsy. Quite often one or more of the main arteries supplying the brain is found to be stenosed and atherosclerotic, either the carotids in the neck or the vertebrals within the bony channels of the skull.

Distinction between multi-infarct dementia and Alzheimer's disease

The distinction between multi-infarct dementia and Alzheimer's disease can be unclear during life, particularly in the elderly, and has also been debated in terms of neuropathology. It has been suggested that vascular and parenchymatous changes occur so commonly together with advancing age that a valid distinction is hard to maintain. The situation has again been clarified by the investigations of Corsellis and Tomlinson as described on pp. 435–6.

Corsellis (1962) concluded that in the majority of elderly patients the parenchymatous and vascular forms of dementia could be broadly distinguished from each other in terms of the neuropathological findings. When the severity of each type of pathological process was examined in his material, overlap was found in only 20% of the brains examined. The Newcastle studies reported by Tomlinson *et al.* (1970) and Roth (1971) support this conclusion. First of all, within the group of subjects diagnosed on clinical grounds as having vascular dementia, it was possible to show a quantitative relationship between the dementia score during life and the extent of cerebral softening measured at autopsy. A marked threshold effect was seen, 50 ml of softening differentiating to a high degree between arteriosclerotic dements and non-dements. This measure allowed an assessment to be made of the contribution which vascular changes might make to the cerebral disorder in SDAT. In fact a high level of discrimination was found — 94% of patients diagnosed as having parenchymatous dementia had less than a total of 50 ml of softening, whereas 73% of patients diagnosed as having arteriosclerotic dementia had more than 50 ml of softening. There was, of course, some degree of overlap, as might be expected from two such relatively common degenerative processes of old age. Thus cases diagnosed clinically as having vascular dementia, but proving at autopsy to have less than 50 ml of softening, frequently also showed plaque formation to a substantial degree. There was also evidence that the two types of pathological change, when appearing together, could augment each other to a significant extent in the production of dementia. In Tomlinson *et al.*'s (1970) material the principal softenings in patients with vascular dementia were cortical in location; lacunar infarcts could often be present as well but these were also frequent in elderly patients without dementia.

The other evidence supporting a distinction between multi-infarct dementia and Alzheimer's disease may be summarised as follows:

There is evidence of a genetic contribution to SDAT, yet no excess of multi-infarct dementia has been found among the relatives of probands studied (Larsson *et al.* 1963); females are affected in excess of males in SDAT but not in multi-infarct dementia, though this may represent no more than the greater tendency to longevity in females; the length of survival after hospitalisation is rather longer in multi-infarct dementia than SDAT, and whereas the cause of death in the former is frequently ischaemic heart disease or definable arteriosclerosis in other organs, the precise cause is often uncertain in SDAT.

Distinguishing clinical features may be summarised thus: a relatively sudden onset favours multi-infarct dementia; the step-like course is characteristic, and is seen

from an early stage in conjunction with episodes of cerebral infarction which leave transient or permanent neurological deficits. In Alzheimer's disease, by contrast, the course is smoother and more gradual. Acute episodes of clouding of consciousness or delirium are much commoner in multi-infarct dementia. Psychological deficits tend to be patchy with, for example, good preservation of insight and personality, whereas the disintegration in Alzheimer's disease is global. There is greater mood lability with multi-infarct dementia, and a greater tendency towards conspicuous depression and anxiety. Hypertension and fits are much commoner in multi-infarct dementia than Alzheimer's disease, and somatic complaints such as headache and dizziness feature more often in the history. On neurological examination both gross and subtle evidence of focal cerebral disorder is common, likewise evidence of arteriosclerosis elsewhere in the body.

Most difficulty in clinical differentiation is likely to occur in those patients who lack a history of stroke, or in whom the onset is insidious and the course evenly progressive. Such problems may be encountered in some 20% of patients with multi-infarct dementia (del Ser *et al.* 1990; Erkinjuntti & Sulkava 1991). In the absence of a history of stroke there will usually have been indicators of other acute cerebrovascular episodes antedating the dementia, such as short-lived periods of impaired consciousness, confusion or memory disturbance.

The 'ischaemic index' drawn up by Hachinski *et al.* (1975) has been widely employed as a guide to distinguishing between multi-infarct dementia and Alzheimer's disease. Features in the clinical history and on examination are given a weighted score as follows: abrupt onset (2), step-wise deterioration (1), fluctuating course (2), nocturnal confusion (1), relative preservation of personality (1), depression (1), somatic complaints (1), emotional incontinence (1), history of hypertension (1), history of strokes (2), evidence of associated atherosclerosis (1), focal neurological symptoms (2) and focal neurological signs (2). Patients scoring 7 or above are classified as having multi-infarct dementia and those scoring 4 or below as having parenchymatous dementia. The separation of patients on such a basis can be valuable in refining groups for research purposes, and when used with caution can give some guidance to diagnosis in the individual case. The index was drawn up, however, on relatively young and mildly affected patients; a very considerable degree of overlap may be expected in the elderly and when the dementia is more advanced.

Radue *et al.* (1978) and Harrison *et al.* (1979) showed certain broad differences in EEG and CT scan findings when patients were separated on the basis of the Hachinski index (pp. 454–5), though cerebral blood flow studies have given conflicting results. Hachinski *et al.*'s (1975) own study, using the intracarotid xenon method, showed significant reductions in overall blood flow among patients scoring in the multi-infarct dementia range, and this was confirmed by Harrison *et al.* (1979). Frackowiak *et al.* (1981), however, found no difference in cerebral blood flow or oxygen utilisation using PET when patients were separated in this manner.

The attempts that have been made to validate the index on autopsy-proven material have shown reasonable predictive accuracy, with sensitivities and specificities exceeding 70% for identifying groups with Alzheimer's disease alone or vascular dementia alone (Rosen *et al.* 1980; Mölsä *et al.* 1985; Wade *et al.* 1987). However, the capacity of intermediate scores of 5 or 6 to indicate patients in whom both forms of pathology are present ('mixed dementia') has proved to be very limited. Such studies have also revealed considerable room for further improvement in the items to be included. Rosen *et al.* (1980), for example, found no value attaching to depression, fluctuating course, nocturnal confusion or the presence of atherosclerosis elsewhere, and prediction was improved when such items were excluded. Mölsä *et al.* (1985) showed the potential for improving discrimination by assigning new weights to the items. In general the index has emerged as more useful for excluding patients with vascular pathology from the Alzheimer group than for making a firm diagnosis of multi-infarct dementia (Fischer *et al.* 1991).

The use of brain imaging techniques, particularly MRI and SPECT, can help to make the distinction during life, though prospective studies with autopsy confirmation are needed to explore their credentials further. MRI may be helpful in pointing to small infarcts in the deep white matter which are missed on CT scans, or in confirming marked leukoaraiosis (p. 460). O'Brien (1994a) suggests that an entirely normal MRI scan virtually excludes a vascular basis for dementia. In some comparisons, however, MRI has proved to be disappointing in separating cases diagnosed according to Hachinski's criteria. Ebmeier *et al.* (1987) found MRI to be poor and SPECT to be superior in this regard—bilateral posterior parietal areas of hypoperfusion were evident in 19 of 21 patients diagnosed as suffering from Alzheimer's disease but only in four of 18 with supposed multi-infarct dementia.

Geaney and Abou-Saleh (1990) suggest that when dementia is relatively advanced and a SPECT scan is normal it is unlikely that the patient is suffering from Alzheimer's disease, while multi-infarct dementia remains a possibility. And though the parietotemporal deficits of Alzheimer's disease may be asymmetrical in degree, asymmetry affecting other areas favours multi-infarct dementia, this being especially likely when the areas of hypoperfusion coincide with infarcts seen on CT or MRI.

PET scanning has yielded similar pointers, typically showing more focal and asymmetrical areas of hypometabolism in multi-infarct dementia than in Alzheimer's disease (Benson *et al.* 1982; Kuhl *et al.* 1985b). Herholz *et al.* (1990) have attempted to derive ratios of affected to unaffected regions of the brain in working towards such a distinction.

Finally, an important step has been the publishing of research diagnostic criteria for vascular dementia which include a synthesis of both clinical and neuroimaging information. These are analogous to the NINCDS-ADRADA criteria for Alzheimer's disease described on pp. 439–40, and though awaiting validation from autopsy studies they seem likely to advance understanding considerably. Two such sets of criteria are available—from the State of California Alzheimer Disease Diagnostic and Treatment Centres (ADDTC criteria) (Chui *et al.* 1992), and from the neuroepidemiology branch of the National Institute of Neurological Disorders and Stroke in association with the Association Internationale pour la Recherche et l'Enseignement en Neurosciences (NINDS-AIREN criteria) (Román *et al.* 1993), respectively. The latter will be outlined as the more comprehensive of the two.

I *The NINDS-AIREN clinical criteria for **probable** vascular dementia require:*

1 Dementia diagnosed according to defined operational criteria and documented by neuropsychological testing. Among the exclusion criteria are aphasia or major sensorimotor impairments which preclude such testing. Dementia in this context implies cognitive decline from a previously higher level of functioning, whether it has a stable, ameliorating or progressive course. The decline must be manifest in impairment of memory and in two or more other cognitive domains. The resulting deficits must be severe enough to interfere with activities of daily living which are *not* due to the physical effects of stroke alone.

2 The presence of cerebrovascular disease, as detected by focal deficits on neurological examination consistent with stroke (whether or not there is a history of stroke), together with evidence of relevant cerebrovascular disease on brain imaging (CT or MRI). The latter includes multiple large vessel infarcts, a single strategically placed infarct, multiple basal ganglia or white matter lacunes, or extensive periventricular white matter lesions. Severity standards are set for excluding trivial infarcts, occasional lacunes or minor periventricular lucencies.

3 A relationship between 1 and 2 must be manifest, either by onset of the dementia within 3 months of a recognised stroke,

or by abrupt deterioration or stepwise progression in cognitive function in the absence of a history of stroke.

II *Clinical features consistent with probable vascular dementia include:*
The early presence of gait disturbance (*marche à petit pas*, magnetic, apraxic-ataxic or parkinsonian gait).
A history of unsteadiness and frequent unprovoked falls.
Early frequency or urinary incontinence.
Pseudobulbar palsy.
Personality and mood changes.
Psychomotor retardation, perseveration and difficulty in shifting and maintaining sets.

III *Features that make a diagnosis of vascular dementia uncertain include:*
Early onset of memory deficit and progressive worsening of memory and other cognitive functions in the absence of corresponding focal lesions on brain imaging.
Absence of focal neurological signs other than cognitive disturbance.
Absence of cerebrovascular lesions on CT or MRI.

IV *Clinical criteria for **possible** vascular dementia include:*
1 Dementia with focal neurological signs, but absence of confirmation of cerebrovascular disease on brain imaging.
2 Absence of clear temporal relationship between dementia and stroke.
3 Patients with subtle onset and variable course (plateau or improvement) of cognitive deficits and evidence of relevant cerebrovascular disease.

V *Criteria for **definite** vascular dementia require:*
1 Clinical criteria for probable vascular dementia.
2 Histopathological evidence of cerebrovascular disease obtained from biopsy or autopsy.
3 Absence of neurofibrillary tangles and neuritic plaques exceeding those expected for age.
4 Absence of other disorder capable of producing dementia.

The NINDS-AIREN criteria sidestep any attempt to define 'mixed' cases of Alzheimer's disease and vascular dementia. Instead the term 'Alzheimer's disease with cerebrovascular disease' is applied to patients who fulfil the NINCDS-ADRADA criteria for possible Alzheimer's disease and who also present clinical or brain imaging evidence of relevant cerebrovascular disease.

Subcortical arteriosclerotic encephalopathy
(chronic subcortical leucoencephalopathy, Binswanger's disease)

This rare form of vascular dementia was first described by Binswanger (1894) under the title 'encephalitis subcorticalis chronica progressiva'. The cognitive failure in such patients appears to be attributable to pronounced changes in the white matter and the cerebral cortex is often little if at all affected.

Olszewski (1962) suggested the name subcortical arteriosclerotic encephalopathy in his review of the earlier lit-

erature. The condition derives from pathological changes affecting the long perforating vessels to the deep white matter and subcortical nuclear masses, resulting in multiple small areas of infarction (lacunes) together with the cardinal feature of diffuse demyelination of the white matter. The arcuate fibres beneath the sulci are by contrast spared, and the cortex itself is substantially intact. The white matter changes are usually extensive, demyelination being associated with pronounced fibrillary gliosis. Possible pathogenic mechanisms include diffuse ischaemia consequent on subacute hypertensive encephalopathy (Caplan & Schoene 1978), or chronic hypoperfusion in the watershed area between the territories of the cortical medullary arteries and the long perforating branches to the white matter (Loizou *et al.* 1981).

Clinical features stressed from the outset were of a slowly evolving dementia associated with focal neurological deficits, usually in hypertensive patients in their fifties or sixties. Caplan and Schoene (1978) clarified the picture from a description of autopsy-proven cases. They noted persistent hypertension, a history of acute strokes, a lengthy course, and dementia accompanied by prominent motor signs and usually by pseudobulbar palsy. The distinctive clinical manifestation, however, was the *subacute* progression of focal neurological deficits. Such deficits commonly developed in a gradual fashion over some weeks or months, the picture then stabilising with long plateau periods lasting for months or occasionally years. This feature appeared to separate the Binswanger patients from those whose dementia rested on large vessel occlusions or on a lacunar state without accompanying white matter demyelination. The dementia varied considerably in its manifestations — some patients showed a phase of ebullience and lack of inhibition, others progressive loss of spontaneity. Memory disorder was not invariably prominent as in senile dementia of the Alzheimer type.

The interest has been to relate this apparently rare condition to the observation of diffuse white matter lucency on the CT scan in certain dementing patients (leukoaraiosis) as described immediately below. Previously the diagnosis had necessarily been based on autopsy findings alone. Loizou *et al.* (1981) attempted to identify patients with the syndrome using a combination of Caplan and Schoene's (1978) clinical features and the typical CT scan appearances. Fifteen patients were found, showing the following characteristics:

The onset was between 50 and 70 years, with a slight male preponderance and durations varying from 1 to 12 years. Twelve of the 15 patients were hypertensive. Eight had presented with neurological features (acute or resolving strokes, ataxia or apraxia) and were found to be demented, and seven had presented with dementia (all with neurological deficits). The dementia commonly showed an insidious loss of memory, slowly evolving to global intellectual impairment with prominent affective changes. It was often less incapacitating than motor symptoms such as gait disturbance, dysarthria or the full picture of pseudobulbar palsy. The neurological deficits could arise in an acute or subacute fashion, and stepwise deterioration in motor and mental functions was often observed.

White matter low attenuation was present on all CT scans and could sometimes be observed to progress over 6–18 months despite treatment of hypertension. In addition, nine patients showed subcortical lacunar infarcts in the internal capsule and basal ganglia, and three showed infarcts in the cortex. Ventricular dilatation was common, but the cortical sulci were normal in six and only mildly to moderately enlarged in the remainder.

Bennett et al. (1990) have put forward criteria for the diagnosis of Binswanger's disease for use in research. The patient must be demented and show bilateral subcortical radiological abnormalities (of a specified nature and extent) on CT or MRI. Large or multiple cortical lesions contributing to the dementia must, however, be absent. Additionally, at least two of the following three features must be present: (i) a vascular risk factor or evidence of systemic vascular disease (e.g. hypertension, diabetes, history of myocardial infarction); (ii) evidence of focal cerebrovascular disease (e.g. history of stroke, presence of focal pyramidal or sensory signs); or (iii) evidence of subcortical cerebral dysfunction (e.g. parkinsonian or 'senile' gait, parkinsonian or gegenhalten rigidity, spastic bladder). The validity of such criteria was tested on both autopsy-proven and prospectively followed patients and found to be reasonably satisfactory.

In discussing differential diagnosis Loizou et al. (1981) point out that the clinical picture is very similar to that of pseudobulbar palsy resulting from the subcortical lacunar state (p. 384). The CT scan appearances appear to differ, but it remains possible that the two conditions may merely represent different stages in the natural history of subcortical arteriosclerosis. Patients with multi-infarct dementia due to extracranial thromboembolism may also present with a not dissimilar picture; five of Loizou et al.'s patients had initially been diagnosed as such, then reclassified in view of the subacute evolution of the neurological deficits and the CT scan appearances. The slow and insidious development of the dementia may cause confusion for a time with Alzheimer's disease.

Leukoaraiosis

The term leukoaraiosis was introduced by Hachinski et al. (1987) to denote diminution of white matter density in the periventricular regions as revealed on brain imaging. When first detected on CT scans it was thought to be rare, occurring in some 2% of routine scans on patients with cerebral atrophy (Valentine et al. 1980). Most of those affected were hypertensive and two-thirds showed evidence of dementia. The white matter low attenuation was bilateral and usually symmetrical, always affecting the regions around the frontal horns of the ventricles and usually spreading backwards to involve parietal and central regions as well. Zeumer et al. (1980) found similar changes in 15 patients, all with progressive dementia and histories of transient, usually recurrent, neurological deficits. All but one were hypertensive and two showed pseudobulbar palsy. Microinfarcts were visible in the basal ganglia in a third of cases. One of the patients came to autopsy and showed the histological features of Binswanger's disease. It therefore seemed likely at the time that this might be a neuroradiological marker of the condition.

With increased awareness and improved scan techniques, however, the incidence was found to rise considerably. Goto et al. (1981) reported CT lucency in 8% of hospital patients, with a steady rise in incidence after the age of 50. Only half of Goto et al.'s patients were demented. George et al. (1986) found white matter lucency in 30% of elderly demented patients, even after excluding those with a history of stroke or hypertension severe enough to require medication. Sixteen per cent of healthy elderly subjects showed analogous CT findings, and in both groups the incidence and severity rose markedly with age.

Workers from Ontario (Inzitari et al. 1987; Steingart et al. 1987a, 1987b) examined the associations of leukoaraiosis in large groups of demented and non-demented aged subjects. The demented patients were classified as presumed SDAT, mixed SDAT and vascular dementia, or multi-infarct dementia, on the basis of clinical findings and scores from the Hachinski index. Leukoaraiosis was observed in 33% of the SDAT patients, 38% of mixed dementia patients, all five of the patients with multi-infarct dementia and 11% of the non-demented elderly (mean age 71 years).

Both the demented and the non-demented subjects who showed leukoaraiosis were significantly older by some 5 years than those who did not. Weakness of the limbs and abnormal plantar responses were also significantly commoner. An association with certain vascular risk factors was present in both groups, namely a history of stroke, higher systolic blood pressure and, in the demented group, the presence of infarcts on the scan. Among the SDAT patients a relationship could be discerned with the severity of cognitive impairment in those who were mildly to moderately demented, but in advanced cases any contribution from the white matter changes appeared to have become eclipsed.

In the non-demented elderly there was again a relationship to poorer cognitive performance, especially on tests of verbal memory and orientation for time. Gait impairment and the presence of certain primitive reflexes were also commoner when leukoaraiosis was present.

Subsequent investigations have shown that the leukoaraiosis is commonly more extensive in multi-infarct dementia than in Alzheimer patients, sometimes extending to over half of the total white matter area. In the non-demented elderly it tends to be restricted, especially to small regions around the frontal and occipital horns of the ventricles (Erkinjuntti & Sulkava 1991).

Thus white matter lucency appears to represent a pathological process with relevance to cognitive dysfunction in the elderly, and to be associated with vascular risk factors. It is commoner and more severe in vascular dementia than in Alzheimer's disease, though the overlap is too great to allow its use as a diagnostic marker. It also seems to be much too common to be regarded as indicative of Binswanger's disease, narrowly defined, since this is known from autopsy studies to be relatively rare. Its occurrence in a substantial proportion of patients with otherwise typical SDAT is of considerable interest.

This last observation serves to blur the distinction between vascular and parenchymatous dementia to some degree, and is a further reminder that both vascular pathology and Alzheimer changes may commonly reinforce one another. Amyloid deposition in blood vessels may be the responsible factor in SDAT patients, rendering them susceptible to the harmful effects of elevated blood pressure and atherosclerosis. The white matter will bear the brunt of such changes since it lacks a collateral blood supply. Hypotension may also be aetiologically relevant, leading to hypoperfusion in the long medullary arteries. This may be the consequence of congestive cardiac failure, cardiac dysrhythmias, over-treatment of hypertension or impairment of autoregulation with age (Román 1987).

Already in 1981 Janota had described white matter demyelination in seven demented patients at autopsy, two of whom had seemed to follow the insidious course of Alzheimer's disease during life. Brun and Englund (1986) have strongly reinforced this observation. Among 20 presenile and 28 senile cases of Alzheimer's dementia they detected white matter changes at autopsy in addition to the typical Alzheimer changes in the cortex. White matter demyelination was found in a half to two-thirds of patients, extending symmetrically from the periventricular regions towards the periphery. Areas of pallor were obvious macroscopically on whole brain slices stained for myelin. Under the microscope these resembled 'incomplete infarctions', with patchy myelin loss, mild reactive gliosis and stenosis of arterioles and smaller vessels. The stenosis was due to hyaline changes in the vessel walls rather than hypertensive vessel disease; the picture therefore differed from the classic pathology of Binswanger's disease in this respect as well as in the absence of complete infarctions. Hypoperfusion within the white matter was thought to be aetiologically relevant since many of the patients had cardiovascular disease, usually with hypotension or episodes of dysrhythmia. The small vessel disease would then stand to compromise blood flow locally. Janota et al. (1989) have found indications that extensive white matter pallor in Alzheimer's disease may betoken a particularly severe process and earlier death.

It is interesting, therefore, that the story of white matter lucency in dementia has altered very considerably, from a suspected marker of Binswanger's disease, through an attribute of most cases of multi-infarct dementia, to an indicator of vascular contributions to Alzheimer's disease. The significance of such changes in non-demented elderly subjects remains to be clarified. Its association in such subjects with vascular risk factors and some degree of cognitive impairment suggest that it may be a marker of early vascular dementia, or it may prove to be heterogeneous in aetiology. Kirkpatrick and Hayman (1987) explored the autopsy findings in 15 clinically healthy subjects who showed white matter changes on MRI. In eight there were areas of perivascular demyelination, perhaps attributable to chronic low-grade vascular insufficiency, while four showed small vascular malformations and three had diverticulae of the ventricles extending into the white matter.

MRI complements the findings obtained with CT, but by virtue of its greater sensitivity the MRI changes tend to lack specificity. T_2-weighted MRI shows the CT lucent areas as bright white images which in severe cases may surround the entire ventricular margins (Kinkel et al. 1985). Such 'periventricular hyperintensities' are detected in a high proportion of elderly subjects, both with and without dementia, and small 'caps' to the tips of the ventricles may occur at all ages as a variant of normal. The considerable literature dealing with the significance of such changes is discussed by Mirsen and Merskey (1994).

Differential diagnosis must include leukoencephalopathies such as metachromatic leucodystrophy (p. 758), as well as hydrocephalus when the ventricles are enlarged (p. 746). The periventricular lucency seen in the latter condition can lead to considerable diagnostic difficulty. Multiple sclerosis must also be considered when the changes are asymmetrical or patchy in distribution.

Pick's disease

Pick's disease is a great deal less common than

Alzheimer's disease, though it was first described earlier in 1892. It is now established as a separate disease entity, sometimes familial and with a distinct neuropathological picture. Its relationship to the larger group of 'frontal lobe dementias' (p. 463) remains, however, to be clarified. The relative incidence of Pick's and Alzheimer's diseases has varied considerably in different reports, from one in three in Minnesota, to one in five in Sweden, one in seven in Scotland and one in 50 in New York (Glen & Christie 1979). Interesting geographical differences between the two disorders have been described in Sweden, with most cases of Pick's disease coming from the region of Stockholm and most cases of Alzheimer's from near Gothenburg (Sjögren *et al.* 1952).

There have been few clues towards causation apart from the evidence of strong genetic allegiances in certain families. Sjögren *et al.* (1952) suggested determination by a single autosomal dominant gene, possibly along with other genes which modify its manifestations. Most cases, however, appear to arise sporadically. In a family study of 11 autopsy-proven cases Heston (1978) found evidence of dominant inheritance in one family but not in any other. Groen and Endtz (1982) have been able to report 25 patients, 14 with proof at autopsy, in a single large family followed over six generations. Brown (1992) estimates from the literature that perhaps some 20–50% of cases are familial.

With regard to the pathophysiology of the disorder Constantinidis *et al.* (1977) found increased concentrations of zinc in the brain and red blood corpuscles in several cases, together with increased excretion of zinc in the urine. Biochemical studies have failed to show the cholinergic brain deficits typical of Alzheimer's disease, though muscarinic cholinergic binding sites may be reduced (Yates *et al.* 1980b). Kosaka *et al.* (1982) found some autopsy evidence that head injury might occasionally evoke or intensify Pick's disease, especially when involving the frontal or temporal lobes.

Clinical features

Women have been affected more often than men in some, though not all, reports. The onset tends to be rather later than in presenile Alzheimer's disease, with a peak between 50 and 60 years, though cases have been reported at all ages from the twenties onwards. The course of the illness is also said to be somewhat slower, though accurate data on a large number of cases are not available.

The most distinctive clinical feature is a tendency to begin with changes indicative of frontal lobe damage. Thus the early abnormalities often concern changes of character and social behaviour rather than impairment of memory and intellect. Drive becomes diminished and episodes of tactless or grossly insensitive behaviour may occur. Lack of restraint may lead to stealing, alcoholism, sexual misadventures or other ill-judged social conduct. From an early stage the expression becomes fatuous and vacant, manners deteriorate and indolence may become extreme. A tendency to indulge in foolish jokes and pranks has often been noted. Insight is impaired early and to a severe degree.

With progress of the disease, impairment of intellect and memory become obvious and slowly increase in severity. The predominant mood often remains as a fatuous euphoria, or apathy may be interspersed with brief periods of restless overactivity. Delusions or hallucinations are relatively rare and epileptic fits uncommon.

Speech becomes markedly perseverative, and a prominent reduction in vocabulary with stereotyped repetition of brief words or phrases is said to be characteristic. Dysphasic disturbances may progress to jargon and periods of mutism may occur. Apraxia and agnosia sometimes appear, but less commonly than in presenile Alzheimer's disease. Gait and muscle tone are also less frequently affected, but occasional cases show marked parkinsonian features in association with an accent of the pathological changes on the basal ganglia. Robertson *et al.* (1958) have reported transient attacks of hyperalgesia similar to that of the 'thalamic syndrome', but how far this is characteristic of Pick's disease is uncertain. Cummings and Duchen (1981) stressed the early appearance of features of the Klüver Bucy syndrome—oral tendencies, overeating with weight gain and tendencies to touch and seize objects within the field of vision—contrasting this with its late appearance in Alzheimer's disease (p. 439). In the late stages the general disintegration of intellect and personality is indistinguishable from that of other advanced dementing processes.

The EEG shows a considerably lower incidence of abnormalities than in Alzheimer's disease (Swain 1959; Gordon & Sim 1967; Johannesson *et al.* 1979). The record may be entirely normal, or when abnormalities are found they are often mild in degree. The general picture is similar in form to that of Alzheimer's disease (p. 439) but the reported changes do not conform to any consistent pattern. Contrary to expectation there is usually little discernible accent on the frontal or temporal regions.

The CT or MRI scan appearances may sometimes be sufficiently characteristic to suggest the diagnosis (Plate 13). In typical cases marked atrophy affects the anterior portions of the frontal and temporal lobes, with considerable enlargement of the frontal horns; by contrast, the bodies of the lateral ventricles and the sulci over the parietal and occipital lobes are much less affected. The scan may, however, resemble that seen in Huntington's chorea, especially when caudate atrophy is marked. Groen and Endtz (1982) have made the interesting observation of frontal atrophy in four out of 12 offspring in a large family affected by hereditary Pick's disease, one of the four developing clinical evidence of the disorder a year later. MRI scanning will show the distribution of atrophy more clearly than CT, in particular on coronal cuts which allow the temporal lobe atrophy to be visualised directly. PET investigations have revealed sharply circumscribed metabolic deficits in the frontal lobes and basal ganglia (Kamo *et al.* 1987; Salmon & Franck 1989). These may be sufficiently distinctive to suggest a differentiation between Pick's and Alzheimer's diseases during life.

Pathology

In classic cases the gross appearance of the brain is characteristic. Some degree of generalised atrophy is combined with striking circumscribed shrinkage of certain lobes, most commonly the frontal and temporal lobes. In the frontal lobes the convexity or the orbital surface may be affected alone, and in the temporal lobes the posterior half of the superior temporal gyrus may stand out as relatively spared. The distribution of atrophy varies considerably from case to case, but major involvement of the parietal lobes is unusual and occipital atrophy extremely rare. The gyri are roughened and brownish, often with a characteristic 'knife-blade' appearance.

The ventricles are dilated, often with great enlargement of the horn of the lateral ventricle beneath the site of maximal cortical atrophy. The basal ganglia and thalamus also show atrophy, sometimes pronounced in the caudate nucleus, but the cerebellum is usually spared.

Microscopy shows neuronal loss, accompanied by dense astrocytic proliferation and fibrous gliosis in the cortex and underlying white matter, hence the older term of 'lobar sclerosis'. The neuronal loss is chiefly in the outer layers of the cortex in affected areas, and a striking feature may be the presence of normal neurones quite near to severely degenerated cells. Characteristic 'Pick cells' ('balloon cells') may be seen but are not a constant feature — the affected neurones are swollen and oval in shape, with a loss of Nissl's substance and displacement of the nucleus towards the periphery. 'Pick bodies' consist of irregular filamentous inclusions within neurones, which are argentophilic and immunoreactive to both tau and ubiquitin antibodies (Lantos 1992a). Eosinophilic inclusions ('Hirano bodies') may also be seen, also granulovacuolar changes.

In the majority of cases senile plaques and neurofibrillary tangles are conspicuous by their absence. Vascular changes are not characteristic. The middle cortical layers may have a spongy appearance similar to that in Creutzfeldt–Jakob disease. Loss of myelin in the white matter of affected lobes is usually considerable.

A variant of the typical picture has been described as Pick's disease type II or progressive subcortical gliosis (Neumann & Cohn 1967). Histological examination shows pronounced and severe gliosis in the subcortical white matter, while that within the cortex itself is less marked than in the classic disease. Glial proliferation is also marked in the subcortical nuclear masses, the brain stem and the ventral columns of the cord. Loss of cortical neurones is not a prominent feature, and those which are affected are shrunken rather than swollen.

Constantinidis *et al.* (1974) have suggested a division based on the presence or absence of argyrophilic inclusions and neuronal swellings. Patients with both features had predominant atrophy of the temporal lobes, those with swellings but no inclusions had atrophy mainly affecting the frontal lobes, whereas those with neither feature could have atrophy in either location. The last group corresponded to the type II cases of Neumann and Cohn.

The usefulness of noting these variants lies in the clues they may provide to aetiology. In type II Pick's disease the primary change would appear to be the overwhelming proliferation of astrocytes in the subcortex and elsewhere, with only secondary embarrassment of neuronal function.

Differential diagnosis at autopsy must include corticobasal degeneration (p. 668), which presents a not dissimilar pathological picture with cortical cell loss, gliosis and Pick cells. However, the cortical atrophy is frontoparietal rather than frontotemporal, and the clinical picture is distinctive. Pick bodies are occasionally found in primary progressive aphasia (p. 752), and sometimes frontotemporal degeneration is seen in conjunction with motor neurone disease (p. 708). During life the distinction from 'dementia of frontal lobe type', discussed just below, will usually be impossible; the validity of the distinction between the two is indeed uncertain, since it is accepted that a substantial proportion of patients with Pick's disease lack both Pick cells and Pick bodies.

Distinction between Pick's disease and Alzheimer's disease

In addition to the distinctions which can be drawn on pathological grounds, certain differences in the clinical picture have traditionally been emphasised. In most cases, however, the true diagnosis is revealed only at autopsy.

In Pick's disease changes of character and disposition are often noted from the onset, whereas memory disturbance is almost invariably the presenting feature in Alzheimer's disease. Incontinence occurring early in the course of the dementia has also been regarded as indicative of Pick's disease, and may similarly be due to the accent of pathology on the frontal lobes.

Parietal lobe symptomatology in the form of dysphasia, apraxia and agnosia is said to be much less common in Pick's disease than in Alzheimer's disease, likewise disturbances of gait and other extrapyramidal features. Aspects of the Klüver Bucy syndrome may be detected early in Pick's disease but are in general a late development in Alzheimer patients (Cummings & Duchen 1981).

The facile hilarity and aspontaneity of Pick's disease has been contrasted with the depressed anxious mood and overactivity of Alzheimer's disease (Stengel 1943b), though Sjögren et al. (1952) have emphasised aspontaneity in the latter condition also.

The preservation of a normal EEG, even in the presence of moderately advanced dementia, will suggest Pick's disease, likewise atrophy restricted to the anterior half of the brain as revealed by CT or MRI scanning. Intermediate pictures will, however, quite often be encountered. PET scanning holds the promise of more reliable differential diagnosis (p. 462).

It appears, therefore, to be chiefly in the mode of onset of the disorder and in the neurological concomitants that a clinical differentiation is to be sought. The differentiation is more easily made in the earlier than the later stages, since ultimately any differences become submerged.

Frontal lobe dementia (fronto-temporal dementia, dementia of frontal lobe type (DFT), frontal lobe degeneration of non-Alzheimer type (FLD))

While Pick's disease has been accepted as something of a rarity, recent evidence suggests that dementia presenting with frontal features may not be so very uncommon. The term 'frontal' or 'fronto-temporal' dementia is used to signify those dementias which depend principally on degeneration within the anterior parts of the brain, as detected by mode of presentation, neuroimaging procedures or autopsy examination. They are of special importance to psychiatry because of their tendency to present with behavioural disorder and change of personality.

Surveys have suggested that these may constitute up to 10–20% of the dementias setting in during the presenile period of life, and autopsy examination has shown that only a small proportion have the classic histological features of Pick's disease. The nosological status of the remainder is at present uncertain. They may represent a distinct clinicopathological entity, or they may yet be related to Pick's disease in view of the known variability in its neuropathological picture.

Attention was drawn to such cases by Brun (1987) and Gustafson (1987) in Sweden, and independently by Neary et al. (1988) in the UK. The Swedish material was derived from postmortem examination of a large series of demented patients. Among 349 cases with full neuropathological examination, Gustafson et al. (1992) found 33 patients with frontal dementia, five (1.4%) showing the pathological changes of Pick's disease and 28 (8%) lacking both Pick bodies and Pick cells. Neary et al.'s patients were recruited from clinical practice, and though lacking postmortem confirmation showed anterior cerebral dysfunction on SPECT scans. Twenty-six such patients were seen in a neurological clinic over a 5-year period, compared with 112 patients with Alzheimer's disease. The similarity of the clinical features in both series suggests that essentially similar patients are being reported. Both, moreover, showed a familial incidence in approximately 50% of cases. Other than this, few clues have emerged with regard to aetiology.

Clinical features

The onset is usually in the presenile period with a range from 45 to 70 years (Gustafson et al. 1992). There was a small preponderance of males in Neary et al.'s (1988) series.

As with Pick's disease the onset is insidious, usually with deterioration of personality and behaviour. Cognitive changes may not be obvious for some considerable time, though deficits in memory and concentration are usually found on testing. The typical presentation is with blunting of emotions, apathy and a change towards egocentricity. Disinhibited behaviour and lapses of judgement may be early signs. Lack of insight is usually conspicuous from the beginning. Traffic accidents due to inattention and carelessness, and a tendency to drink excessively, are not uncommon.

Some patients show inertia and aspontaneity, others restless overactivity and marked distractibility. Gustafson et al. (1992) emphasise impulses to explore the environment, to touch things and to try to use objects on sight—features similar to the 'utilization behaviour' of Lhermitte (p. 106) and to the Klüver Bucy syndrome (p. 23). In keeping with the latter, gluttony may sometimes be marked.

Dissolution of language is often striking and progressive

even in the absence of other obvious cognitive deficits. Verbal aspontaneity, echolalia and stereotyped comments and phrases progress ultimately to mutism. Expressive defects of this nature appear to exceed receptive language dysfunction until late in the disease. Orientation in place and time are by contrast well preserved, likewise visuospatial abilities. Performance on memory tests is often poor, in contrast to the evidence of reasonably well-preserved memory in day-to-day situations. Neary *et al.* (1988) suggest that this reflects a strategic failure to utilize memory effectively, rather than an inability to acquire and retain new information. Tests of frontal lobe function, such as verbal fluency and card sorting, show pronounced deficits from early in the disorder.

Neglect of personal appearance and hygiene are often conspicuous, and incontinence of urine is common. Hallucinations and delusions were observed in 20% of Gustafson *et al.*'s patients.

Other aspects which have been especially noted include marked hypochondriasis, often bizarre in nature and sometimes based on sensory distortions such as hyperaesthesia. Compulsive behaviour and rituals have also been stressed, and can be of unusual intensity:

A woman of 42 gradually lost her interests and became inefficient at work. She complained of stomach pains for which no cause could be found. Some months later she began repetitive checking behaviour and counting rituals and became progressively untidy and withdrawn. The following year it was apparent that her memory was impaired and her verbal fluency was poor, though she still remained fully orientated. Two years later she was withdrawn, incontinent and mostly mute. She sat swaying and rocking, often singing in a fatuous manner. Marked frontal atrophy and ventricular enlargement were apparent on the CT scan. The EEG remained normal.

An accountant of 40 showed a 2-year decline in efficiency at work and self care, and developed severe compulsive behaviour. He would check that the front door was closed up to 10 times per hour. A diagnosis of obsessional neurosis was made, though it was noted that insight was lacking. His mood tended to be jovial. During the following year he developed child-like behaviour with yelps and shouts, and became gluttonous, often stealing from other people's plates. When seen 4 years from onset new learning was poor but he gave the dates of past events correctly. He was orientated for place and year but was wrong for the month. He performed very poorly on proverb interpretation. The EEG was normal, but the CT scan showed severe frontal atrophy.

Neurological examination typically shows no abnormalities, other than the emergence of primitive reflexes such as grasping, pouting or sucking (Neary *et al.* 1994). The plantar reflexes may be extensor. Fascicular twitchings are sometimes observed, and some patients develop dysarthria and dysphagia. Late in the disease the patient may become immobile through akinesia and rigidity.

The EEG is usually normal, even late into the disease. Brain imaging may show atrophy largely confined to the frontotemporal regions, usually with ventricular enlargement. Functional brain imaging can have special importance in revealing diminished blood flow or metabolism selectively affecting the anterior brain regions, even when structural scans show little abnormality:

A professional man of 44 had been suspended from work because of poor performance and certain errors of judgement over the preceding year. A neurologist suspected early dementia, but other consultant neurologists and psychiatrists considered him to be normal. It was thought that the problem might lie with over-critical colleagues rather than with himself.

His wife, however, described a gradual change of personality, with rigidity of habits and a tendency towards irritability and agitation. On occasion he had been embarrassing in social situations, making insensitive comments of a personal nature to casual acquaintances. She described marked lacunae in his distant memory, for example for a holiday they had taken some years ago. He admitted to memory problems but in other respects considered that he was well.

Examination showed normal mood and he made good rapport. He was fully orientated and well informed about recent events, but seemed totally amnesic for significant episodes from his past life. He made occasional paraphasic errors and his verbal fluency was poor. Physical examination showed no abnormalities.

The EEG was normal, and a CT scan showed only marginal abnormalities over the left Sylvian fissure and possible dilatation of the left anterior horn. These were considered to be of doubtful significance. SPECT scanning, however, showed clear evidence of hypoperfusion over both frontal lobes.

Follow-up over the next 2 years showed very gradual deterioration, with increasing lack of initiative, disinhibition and obsessionality. Psychometric testing revealed increasing naming difficulties and problems with card sorting. His mother had suffered from a slowly progressive dementing illness of a similar nature.

Course and outcome

Gustafson *et al.*'s (1992) series is the largest to date with pathological confirmation of the disease. The total duration of the illness showed wide variation from 3 to 17 years. The mean of 8.1 years was somewhat shorter than in the cases of classic Pick's disease in their series (10.5 years).

Differential diagnosis

The subtle nature of the behavioural change in the early stages, and the lack of conspicuous cognitive defects, often lead to long delays before the correct diagnosis is made. A personality disorder may be suspected, especially when some life event appears to have provoked the change in demeanour. Other patients are suspected of alcoholism, or of hypomania when there is elevated mood and disinhibition. Agitation and hypochondria may give the impression of an anxiety or depressive state, and compulsive features may lead to the diagnosis of obsessive–compulsive neurosis. It is not uncommon for the patient to have received treatment for such disorders before the organic nature of the illness becomes evident through progressive lack of self care and the advent of clear cognitive deficits.

Pick's disease will often be considered until autopsy fails to show its characteristic histological features. As already discussed it remains uncertain how far the two conditions represent distinct clinicopathological entities. Huntington's disease may be suspected when personality change and psychotic features are prominent, and especially when other family members are affected. Differentiation from Alzheimer's disease will rarely be difficult, though occasional Alzheimer patients present with behavioural change and with anterior rather than posterior hypoperfusion on SPECT scans (Neary et al. 1987).

Difficulty may be encountered with patients who develop the progressive language disorder of primary progressive aphasia (p. 752). The presence of muscle wasting and weakness will raise the likelihood of frontal dementia in association with motor neurone disease (p. 708).

The Swedish and Manchester groups have recently published agreed clinical criteria upon which the diagnosis should be based (Brun et al. 1994).

Pathology

Gustafson et al. (1992) emphasise that the cerebral atrophy is milder and less circumscribed than in classic Pick's disease and is not of the 'knife-blade' variety. Changes in the basal ganglia and thalamus were not evident macroscopically in their cases.

Microscopy showed loss of neurones with slight gliosis and fine spongiform change in the frontal and temporal lobes, most severely developed over the frontal convexity. The insula and anterior cingulate regions were also involved. In occasional cases the corpus striatum and posterior parts of the brain were also affected, but to a relatively slight extent. Pick cells and Pick bodies did not occur. Alzheimer changes were absent except occasionally in older patients. The white matter in the anterior regions showed mild loss of myelin and gliosis.

Mann et al.'s (1993) material, by contrast appeared to be heterogeneous in histopathology, suggesting the presence of distinct subgroups. All showed loss of large cortical neurones in the frontotemporal regions, but one group showed mild gliosis along with spongiform change in the superficial laminae, while another showed severe gliosis and absence of spongiosis. A third group showed severe striatal atrophy with variable cortical involvement. Brun et al. (1994) have published a consensus statement jointly from the Swedish and Manchester groups outlining the neuropathological criteria which should be met before the condition is diagnosed at autopsy.

Huntington's disease

Huntington's disease has attracted a great deal of interest and attention. Choreiform movements are combined with the dementia, serving as a clinical marker which has allowed its genetic background to be studied with care. Since Huntington's original account in 1872, cases have been reported from all over the world and no race appears to be immune. The responsible mutation has clearly arisen repeatedly.

Prevalence varies markedly from one investigation to another. Very high figures have been reported from Tasmania, while in parts of Japan the disease appears to be extremely rare. Myrianthopoulos (1966) considers that 4–7 cases per 100 000 of the population is a reasonable overall estimate. In the UK, surveys have indicated 5.2 cases per 100 000 for the West of Scotland (Bolt 1970) and 6.3 per 100 000 in Northamptonshire where detailed pedigrees have been kept for many years (Oliver 1970). An astonishingly dense focus is known to have existed for a long time in the Moray Firth area of Scotland, with the equivalent of 560 cases per 100 000 in a small fishing community on the east coast of Ross-shire (Lyon 1962).

Aetiology

The disease is associated with a single autosomal dominant gene with a virtually 100% rate of manifestation. Approximately half of the offspring of an affected person can therefore be expected to develop the disorder, with equal incidence in males and females. It is only very rarely known to have skipped a generation. Cases in Massachusetts and Connecticut have been traced back to emigrants from England, principally to three men and their wives who left from Bures in Suffolk in 1630 and thereafter produced 11 generations of choreics (Vessie 1932). Subsequent work has, however, cast doubt upon some of the genealogies in Vessie's study (Harper & Morris 1991).

A family history is not always forthcoming, even

among classic examples. In Heathfield's (1967) North London survey a family history was lacking in one-fifth of cases. This may be the result of several factors—the early death of a parent, illegitimacy, lack of an adequate history, or concealed and circumscribed knowledge within the immediate family circle. The spontaneous appearance of new mutations from time to time is also very probable.

Genetic counselling is the only method at present available for curtailing the disease and is indicated on humanitarian and economic grounds. In Barette and Marsden's (1979) survey most relatives stated that they preferred to know the painful facts as soon as possible, and the majority were then prepared to restrict their families or have no children whatever. Only 7% said that they would have preferred to remain in ignorance. Unfortunately, however, the major part of reproductive life is often over when the disease comes to medical attention, and there are some indications that fertility may be increased among affected as compared to unaffected sibs. As the patient deteriorates he is less likely to use contraception and hypersexuality is said sometimes to occur. This, added to the social disorganisation often encountered in Huntington families, can make effective prevention a most difficult task. In Bolt's (1970) survey, for example, 15 children were found to have been produced by three of the patients since the onset of their disease. Despite such difficulties a fall in the number of births at risk has been documented in a South Wales population followed prospectively, and this may have owed a good deal to regular support and counselling (Harper et al. 1981). Prenatal testing is now available by molecular genetic techniques to detect whether or not a foetus is at risk, and therapeutic abortion will generally be undertaken when the result is positive. This difficult and sensitive area is discussed by Craufurd (1989).

Carrier identification

The search for a reliable means of detecting carriers in the presymptomatic stages of the disease has been pursued energetically for many years and in a multitude of directions. Spectacular success has at last been achieved through the medium of molecular genetics, culminating in the pin-pointing of the pathogenic mutation itself (Huntington's Disease Collaborative Research Group 1993). It is already clear, however, that the availability of a genetic marker for the disease raises ethical problems of considerable magnitude, and can prove to be a source of increased suffering for many family members. Thus while a negative result brings relief to the person tested, a positive result can mean many years of anxious anticipation for a disorder still several years away from making its

appearance. Adverse effects in terms of job and marital prospects, and with respect to insurance, are added sources of concern.

The gene mutation for Huntington's disease lies on the short arm of chromosome 4. Its identification represented the culmination of remarkable and sustained collaboration between several teams in the UK and USA. Already some 10 years earlier Gusella et al. (1983) had discovered a restriction fragment length polymorphism (RFLP) on chromosome 4 which was closely linked to the disease. Other similar markers proved to be even closer to the abnormal gene itself (Gilliam et al. 1987; Wasmuth et al. 1988). These were all sufficiently close to allow their use in prediction with 96–99% accuracy, but even this small area of doubt raised special problems for genetic counselling. It was also necessary to test the parents and at least one grandparent in order to determine whether the DNA marker travelled with healthy or diseased family members, and only a minority of subjects at risk had the appropriate family members living (Harper 1986).

With the discovery of the abnormal gene itself these particular problems have been largely overcome. The pathogenic mutation consists of an unstable region near one end of the gene, consisting of multiple repeats of a cytosine/adenine/guanine (CAG) trinucleotide sequence. When normal the gene ends with 11–34 such repeats, but when pathogenic for Huntington's disease the repeats are much longer. Cases have now been reported with repeats ranging from 37 to 120 in number.

The distinctive finding of an expanded repeat sequence for pathogenic effect mirrors what is found in the genes for myotonic dystrophy (p. 717), fragile-X syndrome and spinal–bulbar muscular atrophy. Moreover, an inverse correlation is shown between the length of the repeat and the age of onset of the disorder, the correlation being especially strong in juvenile cases (Harper 1993). Longer repeats in genes inherited through the paternal line provide a likely explanation for the high incidence of paternal inheritance in juvenile-onset cases (p. 471), and the possibility of expansion of the repeat during paternal transmission supports the observed trend for 'anticipation' of the disease in male family members. So far this mutation has been found in almost all Huntington patients tested, including apparently isolated cases (Harper 1993). The few patients not showing the abnormality have mostly proved to have erroneous diagnoses, or at least to be atypical in some respects. The predicted protein product derived from the gene mutation has been named 'huntingtin', and intensive work now centres on the possible mechanisms of its pathogenic effects.

Valuable experience was gained when the earlier more approximate markers were offered for use in genetic counselling (Brandt et al. 1989; Tyler et al. 1992a, 1992b). The ethical issues raised included the capacity of the patient to cope when identified as positive, the strain thrown on marriage, and the potential misuse of the information gained in terms of employment and insurance prospects (Craufurd & Harris 1986; Craufurd 1989). On this account guidelines were set up both internationally and in the UK concerning precautions and standards to be adopted (World Federation of Neurology: Research Group on Huntington's Chorea 1989, 1990; Craufurd & Tyler 1992). In addition to careful inclusion and exclusion criteria, full pre- and post-test counselling was regarded as mandatory, covering such matters as explanation of the limitations and implications of the test, the subject's motivation for seeking it, the evaluation of coping strategies and the identification of social supports.

Similar social and ethical problems will continue to surround the use of mutation analysis for detecting the pathogenic gene itself, and additional new issues have arisen. As Simpson and Harding (1993) point out, a natural barrier to hasty decisions has been removed now that there is no need to test other family members. Moreover, persons who have not wished to be tested may discover that they are at risk by virtue of a son or daughter undertaking the test. Further difficulties may surround the reversal of an earlier test result which was inaccurate because of recombination between the gene and the linkage marker used. Scourfield et al. (1997) review a range of other problems which are prone to arise with testing in psychiatric patients. Careful counselling, and the involvement of other family members, will therefore continue to be strongly indicated. It furthermore remains desirable to test an affected relative whenever a positive result is obtained, to confirm beyond doubt that this mutation is the cause of the disease in the family concerned.

Prior to this recent development many other approaches had been employed in attempts at carrier identification but without conspicuous success. Psychometric testing showed some, though limited, predictive value (Lyle & Quast 1976; Lyle & Gottesman 1977), and electroencephalographic abnormalities were found in a high proportion of relatives at risk (Patterson et al. 1948). A levodopa challenge test was used by Klawans et al. (1973, 1980), whereby those harbouring the abnormal gene were liable to develop facial chorea and/or limb dyskinesia after several weeks on the drug, but follow-up soon showed it to be unreliable as a predictor (Myers et al. 1982).

Biochemical studies

The clear genetic determination of the disorder has suggested that an inborn error of metabolism might be responsible, and accordingly extensive biochemical enquiries have been undertaken. These sometimes uncovered isolated abnormalities, but until relatively recently most biochemical studies were disappointing.

Earlier findings are reviewed by Myrianthopoulos (1966) and Slater and Cowie (1971). Calcium, magnesium and trace elements such as copper have been investigated, the latter by analogy with Wilson's disease, but the total evidence remains contradictory. Phospholipids, glycolipids, neutral lipids and acid mucopolysaccharides have been found to be normal in the blood, whereas alterations in brain lipids are almost certainly secondary to the neuropathological changes. Urinary amino acids have shown no consistent abnormalities. Perry et al. (1969) found low levels of certain amino acids in the serum, including tyrosine, and Ottosson and Rapp (1971) showed significant lowering of phenylalanine and tyrosine in patients with the established disease, but such changes may prove to be secondary rather than causative. Immunological studies have shown elevation of various globulin fractions, but so many different fractions are implicated that the changes are likely to be non-specific.

More recent studies on brain material obtained at autopsy have produced more interesting findings. Perry et al. (1973) found reduced levels of GABA in the basal ganglia and substantia nigra of brains from patients with Huntington's disease when compared with brains from neurologically normal persons. GABA is an inhibitory synaptic transmitter, so its lack could be significant in relation to the movement disorder. Bird et al. (1973) and Bird and Iverson (1974) confirmed the deficiency in further patients when compared with controls, and showed a marked reduction of the enzyme responsible for the synthesis of GABA (glutamic acid decarboxylase, GAD) in the putamen and globus pallidus. Levels were normal in the frontal cortex, thus indicating a selective loss of GABA-containing neurones from the basal ganglia. It is now known that GABA receptors are depleted in the striatum from early in the disease, and before there is extensive cell loss and atrophy (Walker et al. 1984).

Cholinergic neurones are also severely deficient in the striatum, as reflected in low levels of choline acetyltransferase and of cholinergic receptors. The dopaminergic system is, by contrast, spared (Spokes 1980). Indeed dopamine (and noradrenaline) have proved to be elevated in the striatum and substantia nigra, perhaps as a consequence of the low GABA levels since GABA inhibits the release of dopamine in the nigrostriatal system.

A model is therefore proposed whereby the intact nigrostriatal pathway in Huntington's disease releases approximately normal quantities of dopamine onto a considerably reduced population of striatal neurones, leading to net dopamine overstimulation of those that remain (Spokes 1980; Marsden 1982). Dopamine overactivity in the striatum is known to provoke chorea (p. 651). This could therefore be the key neuropharmacological feature of Huntington's disease, at least where the movement disorder is concerned; and a similar excess of dopamine in the mesolimbic system may underlie the behavioural manifestations and psychoses seen with the disease. Further biochemical changes could, however, prove to be involved, and the levels of peptides such as substance P and angiotensin-converting enzyme are also low in the basal ganglia.

Clinical features

The onset is usually in the fourth and fifth decades, with an average in the mid forties. Variation is wide, however, and onset may occur in childhood and in extreme old age. In general the age of onset among sibs tends to be closer than among members of different families, but the correlation is not sufficiently close to be of value in genetic counselling. There is evidence that the disease follows a more severe course when onset is early rather than late, also that emotional disturbance is more prominent as a premonitory feature. There is some suggestion of other changes in manifestation with age of onset—striate rigidity predominating in the early twenties, choreic symptoms in middle age and intention tremor after the age of 60. Special features of the disease in childhood will be considered below.

Considerable variation may be seen in the relationship between the neurological and psychiatric features. In the typical case involuntary movements precede dementia, though the reverse can also be seen. Occasionally several years may separate the appearance of the two components, or the two may begin and proceed throughout together. Certainly once both are well established each tends to worsen in conformity with the other.

Very occasionally chorea may be the sole manifestation. Dementia without chorea has similarly been recorded, even when chorea was prominent in previous generations of the family. Other variations include the form the neurological abnormalities take, progressive rigidity with parkinsonism replacing the typical choreic movements in up to 10% of cases. All such variations usually appear sporadically; despite some indications in the literature it is not well established that in different families the form of the disease tends to breed true.

Presenting symptoms

The presenting symptoms were almost equally divided between neurological and psychiatric features in Heathfield's (1967) survey. Neurological presentations were usually with choreiform movements, or less often with unsteadiness of gait, a tendency to fall or general clumsiness. Psychiatric presentations could be with symptoms of incipient dementia, but even more commonly with change of disposition, emotional disturbance and paranoia.

Most observers agree that psychiatric changes are often present for some considerable time before chorea or intellectual impairment develops. A change in personality may be marked, the patient becoming morose and quarrelsome, or slowed, apathetic and neglectful. These are well recognised as premonitory symptoms by those who have practical dealings with communities in which the disease is rife (Lyon 1962). Paranoid developments may be the earliest change, with marked sensitivity and ideas of reference. Sometimes a florid schizophrenic illness may be present for several years before the true diagnosis becomes apparent. Depression and anxiety may be marked from the outset.

Neurological features

The neurological features often go unrecognised at their first appearance. The typical early choreic movements consist of randomly distributed and irregularly timed muscle jerks, brief in duration and unpredictable in their appearance. At first the patient is merely thought to be clumsy or fidgety. Early movements may be no more than the twitching of a finger, or fleeting facial grimaces which pass for mannerisms. The movements usually start in the muscles of the face, hands or shoulders, or are first manifest in subtle changes of gait. Speech is often affected early with slight dysarthria. For some time the patient may conceal the involuntary nature of the movements by exploiting them to perform some habitual activity such as smoothing the hair or the clothes.

With worsening of the disease the pathological nature of the motor disturbance becomes abundantly obvious. The movements are abrupt, jerky, rapid and repetitive but variable from one muscle group to another. They may be aggravated by voluntary movement but may also occur spontaneously. The face shows fleeting changes of expression and constant writhing contortions which give a grotesque appearance. The fingers twitch, the arms develop athetoid twisting movements and the proximal musculature is affected with shrugging of the shoulders. It is characteristic, however, that even late into the disease the movements largely cease during sleep.

The gait is sometimes affected by a curious dance-like ataxia which results from the variable choreic influences on the lower limbs—the weight tends to be carried on the heels while the toes are dorsiflexed, and often a foot will remain suspended off the ground for longer than usual. Eventually the patient walks with a wide base, exaggerated lumbar lordosis, wide arm abduction and zigzag progression due to lurching of the trunk. Progress is interrupted by pauses and even backward steps, and accompanied by a great increase in choreiform movements of the upper limbs.

Hemichorea, massively affecting one half of the body, may be seen. Involvement of the diaphragm and bulbar muscles may lead to jerky breathing, explosive or staccato speech, dysphagia and difficulty in protruding the tongue.

In addition to such involuntary movements Folstein et al. (1986) emphasise a characteristic disorder of voluntary activity which can be an important aid to diagnosis. The rhythm and speed of fine motor movements is disturbed, with conspicuous slowness in the performance of tasks. Disturbances of eye movement have also been reported, often from early in the disease and with gradual worsening over time. Patients have difficulty in initiating fast saccades when asked to glance quickly at objects in the periphery, also impairments of smooth pursuit and gaze fixation (Quarrell & Harper 1991).

In some patients extrapyramidal rigidity may be present, or spasticity with pyramidal signs. As mentioned above some cases develop striate rigidity rather than chorea, perhaps especially when the onset is at an early age ('Westphal variant'). This is commonly associated with akinesia, tremor and cogwheel rigidity, and occasionally progresses to torsion dystonia. Fits are more frequent in this variety than in the generality of cases (16% compared to 3%) (Myrianthopoulos 1966).

Dementia

The cognitive impairment is commonly insidious in development. Brandt and Butters (1986) and Folstein (1989) summarise the studies which have sought to characterise the dementia in detail. General inefficiency at work and in the management of daily affairs is usually the presenting feature, rather than obvious memory impairment. A prevailing apathy, setting in early and impeding cognitive functioning has been stressed as characteristic (McHugh & Folstein 1975). In consequence the patient's performance on everyday tasks is usually more slipshod than psychological testing would predict during the early stages of the disorder.

Slowing of cognitive responses is usually marked from an early stage. Rigidity is observed in thinking and behaviour, with difficulty in changing easily from one activity to another. Memory impairment can usually be demonstrated when carefully sought out, even in patients examined within a year of onset of the chorea (Butters et al. 1978). But it is rarely conspicuous as in Alzheimer's disease, and it gradually becomes submerged in general

difficulties with attention, concentration and organisation of thought. The relative sparing of memory as the disease progresses is consonant with the pathological finding that the limbic areas of the brain are often less affected than in other dementing processes. Disorientation in time and place tends similarly to be a late development.

Detailed investigation into the nature of the memory deficits shows certain distinctive features as outlined by Brandt and Rich (1995). Thus the predominant difficulty appears to lie with deficient retrieval strategies rather than acquisition deficits, in that free recall can be markedly impaired in the presence of near-normal multiple-choice recognition. The retrograde amnesia is usually severe and generalised, being equally impaired across the decades and not showing the temporal gradient of Korsakoff's syndrome. This again reflects impaired retrieval processes.

With regard to implicit (procedural) memory there is an interesting difference from the deficits seen with Alzheimer's dementia; lexical priming is well preserved (e.g. on word-stem completion tasks) while the acquisition of motor and perceptual skills is impaired. This pattern is the reverse of that seen in Alzheimer's disease (p. 32), probably reflecting the accent of neuronal loss in the basal ganglia.

Focal psychological features are also rare in comparison with other primary dementias (Bruyn 1968b; McHugh & Folstein 1975). Word-finding difficulties can occur, and verbal fluency is severely affected from the early stages, but dysphasia, dyslexia, apraxia and agnosia are seldom detected. Tests of visuospatial functioning are, however, typically poorly performed. Judgement is often severely impaired as part of the widespread intellectual decline, but insight is commonly retained for a considerable length of time. The patient may thus be aware of his mental changes, complaining that he feels dulled, slow and forgetful and that his thinking is muddled.

These clinical impressions were confirmed by Aminoff et al. (1975), who examined 11 patients with the disease an average of 6 years after onset, and when all were sufficiently impaired to have warranted premature retirement from work. The intellectual deterioration was found to be global, with a pattern of results on psychometric testing which approximated to that of the decline normally occurring in old age. Memory was not selectively impaired, and no patient showed focal symptoms such as dysphasia or dyspraxia. Seven of the 11 were fully orientated for time, place and person, and nine retained full insight into their condition.

Distractibility is a marked and characteristic feature, and can be seen as the counterpart of the disturbed motor patterns. Depression may be severe, especially while insight is retained, and suicide is a considerable risk in the early stages. The eventual mood, however, is of apathy or fatuous euphoria, and inertia and self neglect become pronounced. Episodes of restlessness and irritability or outbursts of excitement may occur from time to time, and some patients become difficult to manage on account of spiteful, quarrelsome or violent behaviour. A picture resembling akinetic mutism may mark the terminal stages.

The special features of the dementia in Huntington's disease—poor cognitive ability generally but a lack of language disorder or other focal cortical deficits—has suggested that it owes much to subcortical rather than cortical pathology. The pronounced apathy which accompanies and develops along with it is also typical of subcortical dementia as outlined on p. 667.

Affective and psychotic disturbance

Affective and psychotic features become obtrusive in many cases, often early in the course or even preceding the onset of chorea or dementia. Most common is major depressive illness, sometimes recurrent and usually responsive to drugs or electroconvulsive therapy. A schizophrenic or paraphrenic picture may also be seen. Delusions of persecution can be pronounced, with religiosity and sometimes grandiosity. Ideas of reference are perhaps accentuated by the attention attracted by the involuntary movements and bizarre facial expressions.

Folstein *et al.* (1983) surveyed the incidence of affective disorder among 88 patients (from 63 kindreds) drawn from a defined geographical area in Maryland. Forty-one per cent showed major affective disorder, 32% being depressive and 9% bipolar. This development had antedated the Huntington's disease by 2–20 years in almost two-thirds of cases. It appeared, moreover, to be confined to certain families, suggesting that the association may represent genetic heterogeneity within Huntington's disease. Five probands with affective disorder and five without were subjected to detailed family studies; affective disorder accompanied the Huntington's disease significantly more often in the families of the former than the latter, and was also somewhat commoner among unaffected family members. Suicide had already been stressed by Huntington (1910), and has been found to account for 7% of deaths among non-hospitalised patients (Reed & Chandler 1958).

The schizophrenia-like pictures can also be an early development. McHugh and Folstein (1975) prefer the term 'delusional–hallucinatory states', noting the emergence of psychotic symptoms from a pervasive delusional mood. They describe the typical progression as follows: the patient is overwhelmed by a vague impression of an uncanny change in reality which becomes laden with meaning of an uncertain nature. Delusions and hallucinations distil from this, often welling up suddenly and usually lasting for several months. Treatment with neuroleptics can lead to considerable improvement. McHugh and Folstein suggest that the admixture of dementia with such a picture may account for many of the reports of severe personality change and paranoid features among patients with Huntington's disease.

Behavioural change

Change of behaviour and/or personality was noted in 42% of 65 patients identified in the Oxfordshire region (Watt & Seller 1993). Aggression and violence, usually against the spouse, was the most common change, followed by suspiciousness and outbursts of temper. Aggression was particularly common among men and quarrelsomeness among women.

Investigations

The EEG characteristically shows poorly developed or complete loss of alpha rhythms. There may be generalised low voltage fast activity or random slow activity, but this too may disappear as the disease progresses. In consequence the record may become entirely flat. Occasionally, however, a normal record may be obtained even in the presence of advanced dementia.

CT and MRI scans show dilated ventricles, often particularly affecting the frontal regions. Atrophy of the heads of the caudate nuclei may be clearly apparent, with loss of the normal convex bulging into the lateral walls of the frontal horns (Plate 14). Various linear measures have been proposed for establishing this feature as an aid to diagnosis, but they are not sufficiently specific to be of value in the individual case (Shoulson & Plassche 1980). In addition MRI studies have shown significant reductions in the thalamus and the medial temporal lobe structures (Jernigan *et al.* 1991b).

Functional imaging techniques can be of particular value by revealing marked hypometabolism in the caudate and putamen. Kuhl *et al.* (1982, 1985a), using PET, showed that this developed early in the disease and before tissue loss was evident on CT scans. By contrast, metabolic values were often normal in other brain regions despite severe disability and CT evidence of atrophy. Caudate hypometabolism was also observed in occasional subjects at risk of Huntington's disease, even while they were asymptomatic. Mazziotta *et al.* (1987) confirmed this in a large group of at-risk persons; 31% showed bilateral reductions in caudate glucose metabolism, which was close to the 34% estimate for the likelihood of developing the disease when age and other factors were taken into account. Smith *et al.* (1988) and Gemmell *et al.* (1989) showed that reductions of cerebral blood flow may be detected with SPECT in the caudate nuclei in a large proportion of patients. This, being more widely available, is likely to find clinical application in uncertain cases.

The value of PET scanning in remedying a false diagnosis of Huntington's disease was illustrated in a woman of 55. For the past 10 years she had shown a slowly progressive dementia, along with increasing motor disorder by way of a stiff, unsteady gait, writhing of the hands and choreiform movements of the face. The antecedent family history was at that time uncertain, but her sister in New Zealand was known to suffer from an entirely similar illness. The motor disorder in both cases had been judged to be typical of Huntington's disease. The EEG showed moderate diffuse theta and occasional delta waves.

CT scanning, however, showed well-preserved caudate nuclei, despite very pronounced cortical atrophy and ventricular dilatation. Her sister's scan was remarkably similar. Doubts about the diagnosis were further reinforced when vigorous efforts to trace the family history revealed longevity in the parents and their many siblings, with no evidence of dementia or movement disorder in any of them. The parents proved to be first cousins.

It was therefore concluded likely that the illness represented a recessively inherited dementing disorder, with adventitious movements attributable to the neuroleptics which had been administered for many years. In confirmation that Huntington's disease was unlikely, PET scans showed excellently preserved metabolism in the caudate nuclei, but with poor metabolism in both frontal lobes and both thalami.

Course and outcome

The course after the first definitive manifestations is generally much longer than with other primary dementing illnesses. The average duration is reported as 15–20 years, but with wide variation, some cases showing very slow progression over several decades.

Special features in childhood

Huntington's disease may occasionally set in during childhood or adolescence, though the true diagnosis will sometimes only be made post mortem. In several respects the disease tends to differ from the adult form, yet the pathological changes at autopsy are the same (Hayden 1981; O'Shea & Falvey 1991). Muscular rigidity and tremor are commoner than choreiform movements, the mental deterioration tends to be rapid, and epileptic fits occur in more than half of the cases. The time to death is in general much shorter than with adult cases.

After developing normally the child begins to fail at school and shows difficulties with concentration. Change of personality and anxiety are common. He may become

clumsy, ataxic and dysarthric. The absence of chorea readily leads to other diagnoses even in families known to harbour the disease. Friedreich's ataxia may be suspected, or Wilson's disease or postencephalitic parkinsonism. When a change of personality is the predominant manifestation this may all too easily be ascribed to external factors, especially when the onset is at the approach of adolescence:

A 25-year-old man was admitted to a hospital for the mentally handicapped. He was judged to have low intellect and to suffer from a personality disorder. He showed ataxia, tremor, dysarthria and muscular rigidity, but these were thought to be due to the neuroleptics he had been given. He was illegitimate and the fate of his father was unknown.

His mother insisted that he had been a bright and inquisitive child, and that until the age of 11 he had progressed well at school. From then on he had shown unwillingness to work and increasingly aggressive behaviour. On leaving school he obtained simple labouring jobs, and was repeatedly arrested for thefts and other misdemeanours. From 18 he became increasingly withdrawn and developed dysarthria. During several hospital admissions thereafter he had been variously regarded as psychopathic or mentally subnormal, and was treated with a variety of neuroleptics. At 22 he was arrested for indecent exposure and other sexual offences.

Psychometric assessment was difficult, but he obtained an IQ equivalent of 67 on the coloured progressive matrices, compared with a verbal reasoning score of 103 recorded when he was 11. Detailed review 2 years later showed a parkinsonian gait, dysarthria and markedly increased tone in the limbs. There were jerking tremors around the mouth and in the fingers of the left hand. He spoke only monosyllabically, but proved to be fully orientated in time and place.

An EEG revealed the absence of alpha rhythm and a very low amplitude tracing. The CT scan showed flattening of the heads of the caudate nuclei (Plate 14). Over the next few weeks he declined abruptly, and postmortem brain examination showed the typical pathology of Huntington's disease (Plate 15).

(Brooks *et al.* 1987a)

It has been known for some time that 'juvenile-onset' cases, i.e. those setting in before the age of 20, are more likely to demonstrate paternal than maternal transmission. Osborne *et al.* (1982), for example, found that children with onset before the age of 10 had an affected father approximately four times as frequently as an affected mother. This puzzling feature now finds an explanation from recent discoveries in molecular genetics, as described on p. 466.

The death rate of children in the first decade is known to be high in Huntington families, and has often been vaguely ascribed to 'mental deficiency' or 'spinal paralysis' (Oliver & Dewhurst 1969). The infant mortality is also high, and Oliver and Dewhurst suggest that this may be partially due to undiagnosed cases occurring even in infancy. Such deaths are often attributed to birth injury, spasticity or quadriplegia. Social factors, however, are also likely to be important in contributing to the infant mortality, since Huntington families are often disadvantaged and sometimes severely disorganised (see below).

Other psychiatric associations

The frequent occurrence of change of personality and emotional disturbance as premonitory symptoms of the disease has already been mentioned, also the marked psychotic features which may accompany the dementia. The association with severe depressive illness may have special genetic determinants (p. 470). In addition certain other psychiatric associations deserve emphasis.

A large number of psychiatric abnormalities, sometimes severe in degree, are reported when detailed studies of Huntington families are undertaken. Some families are severely disorganised on account of a multitude of pathologies, involving both the patients themselves and their relatives. Epilepsy, schizophrenia, mental defect and a variety of other degenerative brain diseases have been reported. How far these may represent common genetic determinants remains to be established. It is possible that to some extent assortative mating between patients from Huntington families and those with other physical and psychiatric handicaps may contribute to the frequency of such disabilities.

Minski and Guttmann (1938) noted a variety of psychopathological features in the relatives of cases, particularly a personality characterised by explosive irritability and readiness to take offence. Suicide has been reported to be frequent even among members unaffected directly by the disease (Bickford & Ellison 1953). It is unclear how far this may be due to endogenous mental illness or the result of knowledge of the consequences of the condition. Watt and Seller (1993) found that a third of first-degree relatives of patients gave a history of depression, mainly reactive to stresses within the family or to the onset of definitive illness in a family member. No support was obtained for a direct pathogenic effect of the Huntington gene in leading to depression or to personality disturbance in as yet unaffected persons.

Dewhurst et al.'s (1970) study of 102 patients illustrates vividly the psychosocial consequences of the disorder. Ten attempted suicide and 13 self mutilation; 19 were alcoholics and 18 had had convictions for serious criminal offences. Of those who had married 38% subsequently divorced or separated, usually because of social or intellectual deterioration in the patient. Sexual disturbances were common — excessive demands, sexual assault, sexual deviation, impotence and frigidity. Notably there was often a history of promiscuity with the production of

illegitimate offspring. The children were sometimes found to be at risk from their parents with examples of serious neglect.

Oliver (1970) showed that unaffected siblings from Huntington families could also become victims of their disturbed environment. Ninety-three out of 150 either died young, became psychotic or suffered such disturbance as psychopathy, chronic alcoholism, criminality or divorce.

Mistakes in diagnosis

Huntington's disease may be mistaken for many other psychiatric and neurological illnesses, certainly in the early stages. Surveys have shown that over a third of cases may be wrongly diagnosed initially (Bolt 1970; Dewhurst et al. 1970).

In a systematic study of patients in Maryland, Folstein et al. (1986) found that 11% had been given some other diagnosis, mainly because the existence of a diagnosed family member was not known to their doctor. Systematic interviewing of relatives revealed 47 cases additional to the 212 already known, and in half of these there had been some other false diagnosis. Moreover 15% of the 212 cases reported by community physicians proved on review not to have Huntington's disease, but to be suffering from other neurological and psychiatric conditions. Sometimes tardive dyskinesia consequent upon medication had led to the mistake. An example of a false diagnosis of Huntington's disease as a result of neuroleptic-induced dyskinesia is described on p. 471.

Psychiatric misdiagnoses are the most common, especially a label of schizophrenia or paranoid psychosis. When schizophrenic features are obtrusive the chorea may readily be ascribed to 'schizophrenic mannerisms' or to the medications given. Affective psychosis, anxiety state and personality disorder may be the initial diagnosis. Other forms of dementia will often be suspected when a family history is not forthcoming, and the motor abnormalities which develop may then be ascribed to dyskinesia induced by phenothiazines.

Bolt (1970) found that diagnoses of neurosis or affective psychosis were almost invariably revised before the patient's death, but sometimes a diagnosis of schizophrenia or paranoid psychosis was not. A diagnosis of some other form of dementia or of neurological disease was much less likely to be corrected.

Neurological mistakes include multiple sclerosis, Wilson's disease, Parkinson's disease, neurosyphilis, cerebellar disorders and ataxia due to drug abuse. Arteriosclerotic or senile chorea may be misleading in the elderly — distinguishing features include the absence of a family history, and mental changes which are less conspicuous or progressive; moreover these are often vascular in origin and can therefore be abrupt in onset and with a tendency towards resolution. The rare syndrome of 'hereditary chorea without dementia' (benign familial chorea) may also be misleading (Quarrell & Harper 1991). This autosomal dominant disorder usually presents in childhood and mainly affects the head, face and upper limbs. In most families there is little progression beyond childhood, though worsening has occasionally been seen throughout adult life (Schady & Meara 1988). Intellect remains unimpaired.

The childhood form is liable to be mistaken for mental subnormality, Friedreich's ataxia, Wilson's disease, epilepsy, spasticity or birth injury. Sydenham's chorea may be simulated, but is usually sudden in onset and associated with other rheumatic manifestations.

Whenever the picture of Huntington's disease is atypical, and particularly when seizures, areflexia or muscle wasting are present, neuroacanthocytosis should be suspected (p. 757). The examination of fresh blood films may then immediately clarify the diagnosis.

Pathology

The brain is usually small and atrophic though this varies greatly in degree. It is in general hard to correlate the intensity of pathological changes with the severity of mental symptoms. The frontal lobes are often the site of maximal cortical change. Marked dilatation of the ventricular system is characteristic, especially of the frontal horns, along with striking atrophy of the caudate nuclei. Instead of bulging into the lateral ventricles these may be represented by a mere rim of tissue along the ventrolateral edge of the dilated anterior horns (Plate 15). The putamen is also atrophic, though the globus pallidus usually escapes in large degree.

Microscopic examination shows cell loss accompanied by gliosis. This can usually be detected in the cortex even when atrophy is not severe. It is particularly marked in the frontal lobes. Severe cell loss is invariably present in the caudate and putamen together with much astrocytic proliferation. The loss of small nerve cells is particularly striking. Similar changes of less degree are sometimes found in the globus pallidus, substantia nigra or cerebellar nuclei.

The white matter shows diffuse loss of nerve fibres, often with consequent narrowing of the corpus callosum. Vascular changes are not marked and cannot be incriminated in the pathogenesis of the disorder.

Creutzfeldt–Jakob disease

This rare disease is the best known of the human spongiform encephalopathies ('prion diseases'). It was first described by Creutzfeldt in 1920 and by Jakob in 1921. It has a worldwide incidence varying from 0.3 to 5 cases per million of the population, with some 30 new cases per year occurring in the UK (Will 1993). Siedler and Malamud's (1963) important contribution reviewed the cases reported to that date. Recent accounts are presented by Lantos (1992b) and Anderson (1993). The disorder consists essentially of a dementing illness which runs a very rapid course, usually accompanied by a number of prominent neurological symptoms and signs. Florid psychiatric symptoms, by way of delusions or hallucinations, are also often seen. The neuropathological changes typically include an accent on structures additional to the cerebral cortex itself — the subcortical nuclear masses, cerebellum, brain stem and cord, though a good deal of variability is seen from one example to another.

So many different pictures have been reported that the nosological status of the disease has sometimes been in doubt. To some extent the term has run the risk of being applied to any atypical presenile dementia which runs an unusually rapid course. More recently, however, the identification of abnormal forms of 'prion' protein in the disorder, and the discovery of distinctive changes in the prion gene are revolutionising our conceptions, and under the focus of present interest greater clarity is being achieved.

Aetiology

The disease usually arises sporadically, though review of a large number of cases worldwide showed that a positive family history is obtained in some 15% of cases (Masters *et al.* 1979). This appears to rest on autosomal dominant transmission in certain families, though the possibility of lateral transmission of an infective agent in genetically susceptible hosts has not been disproved.

A chief stimulus to interest in the condition came from the demonstration that it was transmissible to animals (Gibbs *et al.* 1968). Certain similarities between kuru and Creutzfeldt–Jakob disease had suggested that since the former was transmissible to chimpanzees by brain inoculation the latter should be investigated similarly. A homogenate of brain tissue obtained at biopsy from a patient was accordingly inoculated into a chimpanzee, and the animal developed a fatal neurological disease 13 months later. The clinical and neuropathological pictures were remarkably similar in man and animal and appeared to represent essentially the same disease (Beck *et al.* 1969a, 1969b). These observations were amply confirmed with biopsy material from further human cases, with transmissions to chimpanzees, monkeys, cats, guineapigs, mice and hamsters (Gajdusek 1977). Serial passage from animal to animal proved successful, including transmission through purely peripheral routes—intravenously, intramuscularly, subcutaneously and intraperitoneally. Experimental evidence of oral transmission has also been forthcoming (Kimberlin 1986).

Creutzfeldt–Jakob disease is thus part of the group of 'transmissible spongiform encephalopathies' which includes kuru (p. 751) and Gerstmann–Sträussler syndrome (p. 751) in humans and a considerable range of conditions in animals—scrapie in sheep and goats, chronic wasting disease in elk and deer, transmissible mink encephalopathy, bovine spongiform encephalopathy (BSE) and analogous conditions recently reported in domestic cats. All show transmissibility to experimental animals, long incubation periods, a considerable degree of species specificity, and lead to closely similar pathological changes in the brain. It seems likely, moreover, that in all of these diseases similar or even identical transmissible agents may be involved.

The transmissible agent

The precise nature of the agent has, however, remained elusive and is still subject to debate. It passes a 100 nm filter and is remarkably resistant to heat, formalin, ultraviolet light and X-rays, does not evoke an immune response and does not have a cytopathic effect in tissue cultures. In these respects it differs markedly from conventional viruses and even from 'viroids'—naked pieces of RNA without protein which are responsible for certain plant diseases. An additional puzzle is that any complete explanation must account both for transmissibility under experimental conditions and the genetic liability which is seen in both Creutzfeldt–Jakob disease and the Gerstmann–Sträussler syndrome.

Current interest has come to centre firmly on 'prion' protein as playing a central role in these disorders. The prion ('proteinaceous infective particle') was so-labelled by Prusiner (1982), when enrichment of brain fractions from scrapie-infected sheep revealed the presence of a distinctive glycoprotein. It then emerged that this protein (PrPsc) was an isoform of a naturally occurring protein (PrPc), differing only in its solubility and resistance to digestion by proteases, and furthermore that it was encoded by a single gene on chromosome 20. The exciting series of steps which ultimately clarified the situation are described by Prusiner (1987), Weissmann (1991a) and Brown et al. (1991). In consequence it is now common to use the term 'prion diseases' in place of the former label of spongiform encephalopathies.

In essence it appears that PrPc is a membrane protein highly conserved in evolution, occurring in many organs of the body and perhaps subserving important receptor and 'housekeeping' roles. In the transmissible spongiform encephalopathies it accumulates in the brain in abnormal form, constituting the amyloid plaques often visible in such disorders. After some initial confusion it became clear that such amyloid, though similar in appearance, was quite distinct from the A_4 amyloid which occurs in Alzheimer's disease.

The challenge has been to explain the 'infectivity' of prion protein and to understand the relationship between pathogenic forms and those which occur naturally in the brain. A consensus now suggests that the introduction of small quantities of PrPsc to the brain initiates a cascade reaction whereby healthy PrPc becomes gradually converted to the pathogenic form, with resultant disruption of cerebral function. The matter is not, however, decisively settled. Some still maintain that the accumulation of abnormal prion protein may be the product of infection with as yet unidentified nucleic acid-bearing agents (Somerville 1985). Weissmann (1991b) has presented a model which attempts to encompass both points of view.

A main difficulty for the 'prion-only hypothesis' has been to account for the many 'strains' of transmissible agent known to exist even within the domain of scrapie, and the species barriers which are found when prion protein from one species is introduced to another. It is here that striking evidence has come from molecular genetic experiments. Normal mice initially show much longer incubation times when infected with hamster scrapie than when infected with mouse scrapie, though this effect becomes attenuated after multiple passages. But the situation is altered when transgenic mice are artificially created by the introduction of the hamster prion gene (Prusiner et al. 1990; Prusiner 1991). Incubation times for hamster scrapie are then dramatically reduced. In elegant experiments the converse has also been shown to obtain. In other words the relative species barrier can be broken by genetic manipulation of the host prior to infection. Genetic mechanisms in the host may thus be fundamental in determining relative susceptibility, and in contributing to the spurious appearance of a 'mutating' infective agent. Moreover these experiments illustrate that the development of spongiform encephalopathy involves a direct interaction between the normal PrPc of the host and exogenously administered PrPsc.

The prion gene

Further molecular genetic studies have concentrated on the prion gene itself. This has emerged as abnormal in many patients suffering from Creutzfeldt–Jakob disease or the Gerstmann–Sträussler syndrome. In a family with Creutzfeldt–Jakob disease Owen et al. (1989) found a mutation consisting of a 144 base pair insertion in the prion gene, and Hsiao et al. (1989) found a point mutation at codon 102 in two families with the Gerstmann–Sträussler syndrome. Another mutation at codon 200 was shown to be consistently present among Libyan Jews with Creutzfeldt–Jakob disease, apparently accounting for the great excess of the disorder in this particular population (Hsiao *et al.* 1991). Clusters of the disease in Slovakia also show the same mutation (Goldfarb *et al.* 1990). Other point mutations have been found in other familial cases as described by Collinge and Palmer (1994). The potential pathogenicity of such mutations was clearly demonstrated by Hsiao *et al.* (1990); transgenic mice created to carry the codon 102 mutation spontaneously developed spongiform degeneration some 5–6 months later, similar in all respects to the picture seen in mouse scrapie.

The suggestion is that such prion gene abnormalities predispose to the production, at some point, of PrPsc in the individual at risk. Once this has occurred further conversion of PrPc to PrPsc will occur by a chain reaction, rendering the disease overt. Among sporadic cases of Creutzfeldt–Jakob disease, homozygosity for a polymorphism at codon 129 has been identified at frequencies greater than chance, again probably indicative of special vulnerability (Palmer *et al.* 1991). Homozygous polymorphisms at this site have been found in patients succumbing to Creutzfeldt–Jakob disease after the administration of pituitary-derived growth hormone, also in the recent cases thought to derive from eating BSE-infected beef (see below).

A scenario therefore exists which could explain both the familial nature of Creutzfeldt–Jakob disease in some 15% of cases, and a selective vulnerability in some persons to its more common sporadic appearance. However, other than in the tragic iatrogenic examples described below, the source of the initiating event in sporadic cases remains unknown. In some there may have been aberrant post-translational processing of PrPc leading to the production of molecules of PrPsc, or these may have arisen through some metabolic or toxic derangement. Unidentified somatic mutations may occasionally be responsible. The disturbing possibility nonetheless remains that Creutzfeldt–Jakob disease may sometimes be transmitted by an 'infective' process in man. The evidence remains indirect, but certain interesting and important observations have been made.

'Infectivity' in humans

Thus small but apparently definite geographical clusters of cases have been reported in persons unrelated genetically to one another. Matthews' (1975) survey of 46 cases in England and Wales showed a markedly uneven geographical distribution, with several clusters which bore no relation to urban density. A small rural community in the Midlands produced three patients who had probably had contact with one another, and an area in eastern England yielded five. Galvez *et al.* (1980) reported a remarkable example of a woman who developed the disease after marrying into a family with several affected members. Such evidence is little more than anecdotal, but striking in view of the rarity of the disease.

The possibility of contracting Creutzfeldt–Jakob disease through eating animal products was raised early on by analogy with scrapie in sheep (Gibbs *et al.* 1980; Roos 1981). Special concern arose at Kahana *et al.*'s (1974) discovery of a very high incidence of Creutzfeldt–Jakob disease among Libyan Jewish immigrants to Israel, thought possibly to be related to the eating of sheep's eyeballs, but significant family clusterings and distinctive changes in the prion protein gene have been shown to be responsible (Alter *et al.* 1978; Neugut *et al.* 1979; Hsiao *et al.* 1991).

BSE and Creutzfeldt–Jakob disease

Most recently public concern has been strongly aroused in connection with the outbreak of BSE in British cattle in 1986, and the possibility that this might provide a vehicle for the development of spongiform encephalopathies in humans. The reporting of occasional cases in domestic cats and dogs, and the experimental transmission of BSE to pigs, has fuelled such concerns. BSE appears to have arisen through the feeding of scrapie-infected carcasses to cows, and this apparent breech of the species barrier is disturbing. However, carefully argued reviews of the potential risk to human beings initially suggested that the risk, though potentially present, was infinitesimal in degree (Lancet 1990b; Harrison & Roberts 1991, 1992).

Since then Creutzfeldt–Jakob disease has occasionally been reported in dairy farmers who have had contact with BSE-infected herds (Smith *et al.* 1995), although there have been conflicting opinions about whether this exceeds chance expectation (Delasnerie-Laupretre *et al.* 1995; Gore 1995). Cousens *et al.* (1997) report recent epidemiological evidence of a significant excess among occupationally exposed persons, though none showed the 'new-variant' form of CJD (see below). More worrying has been the recent appearance of the disease in a group of unusually young patients in the UK which has had an explosive impact in increasing public alarm (Collinge & Rossor 1996; Will *et al.* 1996). During 1994 and 1995, 10 patients between the ages of 16 and 39 developed what appears to be a new variant of the disorder, eight of whom have died at a median age of 29 years. Previously the identification of the disease in patients less than 30 years of age has been exceptional. Other unusual features of the so-called *new-variant CJD* include a rather protracted course (median 12 months to death), presentation often with anxiety, depression and behavioural changes leading to psychiatric referral, and the development of ataxia early and myoclonus later in the course than commonly seen. The EEG, though abnormal, lacks the features characteristic of the condition. The neuropathological picture is also unique in several respects and consistent across all cases; the presence of spongiform change and PrP plaques confirms the diagnosis, but the plaques are large and strikingly abundant, stain strongly on immunocytochemistry for PrP, and show distinctive morphological features reminiscent of the 'florid' plaques of scrapie and those seen in kuru. All cases studied to date are homozygous (for methionine) at the polymorphic residue at codon 129 (Collinge et al. 1996). By August 1997 the total of definite and probable cases of new-variant CJD had risen to 21, of whom 20 have died (Warden 1997).

Improved ascertainment seems unlikely as an explanation for this remarkable group of cases. Direct proof of a link with BSE has not been forthcoming, but the observation of a potentially new form of Creutzfeldt–Jakob disease must be regarded as consistent with such a link (Will et al. 1996). Exposure of the human population to the BSE agent is likely to have been maximal in the 1980s, and especially towards the end of the decade before the ban on the use of specified bovine offal was introduced. This would be consistent with an incubation period of 5–10 years for the newly reported cases.

Clearly continued vigilance and on-going surveillance is essential, also strenuous efforts to determine experimentally whether the specific prion strain responsible for BSE has unusual potential for cross-species transmission. It may prove possible through strain-typing to determine directly whether this prion strain has indeed infected humans. A pointer in this direction has already been obtained with the demonstration of a characteristic pattern of PrP conformation and glycosylation in experimentally transmitted BSE and these recent human cases (Collinge et al. 1996). Meanwhile the impact on the beef industry in the UK has been disastrous, with marked repercussions in Europe and continuing political upheavals (Warden 1996a).

Iatrogenic transmission

Iatrogenic transmission, by contrast, is fully proven. Creutzfeldt–Jakob disease has several times been accidentally transmitted from patient to patient by ophthalmic or neurosurgical procedures, and more recently by the administration of pituitary-derived growth hormone and gonadotrophins. Duffy et al. (1974) reported transmission by corneal transplantation, and Bernoulli et al. (1977) by the inadvertent use of contaminated depth electrodes. Foncin et al. (1980) reported a patient who developed the disease 2 years after an intracranial operation carried out in the same operating theatre that had been used 3 days

earlier on a patient with the disease. Retrospective evidence has incriminated similar neurosurgical transmission in three of the eight patients included in Nevin et al.'s (1960) series (Masters et al. 1979; Will & Matthews 1982). The implantation of cadaver-derived dura mater grafts has been followed by the development of Creutzfeldt–Jakob dementia, and the deaths of a neurosurgeon, a neuropathologist and two histopathology technicians raise the question of accidental workplace infection (Brown et al. 1992). However, a recent consensus report concludes that there is as yet no established evidence that health care workers as a group bear a higher risk than other members of the population, and, specifically, no proven case in which a transmissible encephalopathy has developed in relation to contact with patients (Budka et al. 1995a).

A serious threat has arisen from the development of the disease in patients who, many years earlier, had received courses of injection of growth hormone prepared from pooled pituitary glands obtained at autopsy. Such cases were reported from the UK and USA (Gibbs et al. 1985; Koch et al. 1985; Powell-Jackson et al. 1985), leading to the abrupt withdrawal of the treatment in 1985. Other cases have continued to accumulate, however, some 28 now being reported from around the world. More recently cases in Australia have apparently originated from the administration of pituitary-derived gonadotrophins (Healy & Evans 1993). The incubation periods from such peripheral routes of infection have varied widely from 4 to 30 years, with a mean of 15 years, this being very considerably longer than the 1–2-year interval in the neurosurgical cases. The clinical patterns also tend to differ, with an accent on cerebellar disturbance and the late development of dementia in the peripheral cases, while presentations with dementia predominate after neurosurgical transmission (Brown et al. 1992). In a molecular genetic analysis of the six UK patients whose disease followed growth hormone administration, Collinge et al. (1991) have shown the common occurrence of homozygosity for a polymorphism at codon 129 on the prion gene, suggesting that genetic susceptibility is likely to play some part in such a development. Recent fears of contracting the disease via blood transfusions appear to be unfounded (Esmonde et al. 1993; Klein & Dumble 1993).

Short of transmission by the above means, the risk of acquiring the disease by day-to-day infection appears to be remote. Masters et al. (1979) concluded from their vast experience that the potential for transmission by noninvasive bodily contact must be judged as very low. Certain reasonable precautions are recommended, nonetheless, in those who come into contact with patients with the disease (Corsellis 1979; Advisory Group on the Management of Patients with Spongiform Encephalopathy (Creutzfeldt–Jakob Disease) 1981; Budka *et al.* 1995a):

The isolation or barrier nursing of patients is not considered to be necessary. However, wounds and sores must be dressed with strict sterile precautions, similar care being observed when taking blood or cerebrospinal fluid. Equipment must not be re-used thereafter and should be incinerated. Attendants should wash thoroughly if exposed to saliva, nasopharyngeal secretions, urine or faeces, and skin puncture in attendants must be very carefully avoided.

At operation or autopsy, tissues must be handled with special care, likewise blood, cerebrospinal fluid or biopsy material obtained from patients. Even formalin-fixed specimens should be regarded as potentially infective. Tissues and body fluids have been divided into four classes of decreasing infectivity on the basis of experimental transmissions (Budka *et al.* 1995a): high infectivity for brain, spinal cord and eye; medium infectivity for spleen, lymphoid tissue, organs with a lymphatic component (e.g. ileum and proximal colon), placenta, pituitary, dura mater and cerebrospinal fluid; low infectivity for peripheral nerves, bone marrow, liver, lung, pancreas and thymus; and no detectable infectivity for muscle, kidney, fat, bone, blood, milk and bile.

Disposable drapes, dressings and where possible disposable instruments, should be used for any operation. Otherwise steam autoclaving at specially prescribed temperatures and pressures is recommended for sterilising glassware or instruments; for chemical decontamination of non-autoclavable materials and surfaces 2N NaOH solution should be used for 1 hour, or alternatively 5% NaOCl for 2 hours (Budka *et al.* 1995a). Personnel involved in autopsies must wear safety gloves, disposable aprons and eye and mouth protection; tissue blocks must be handled with special care and soaked in concentrated formic acid for 1 hour followed by fresh formaldehyde for at least 48 hours.

Even remotely suspected patients must not be used as blood, tissue or organ donors, or as sources for the preparation of biological products to be used in human beings. Corneal grafts are not to be taken from any demented patient, from those dying in psychiatric hospitals or from patients who die from obscure undiagnosed neurological diseases.

Clinical features

Both sexes appear to be equally affected though a female preponderance has sometimes been reported. The onset is usually in the fifth or sixth decades but cases are reported with onset at any adult age.

The clinical features are very diverse from case to case. A prodromal stage is usually described, lasting weeks or months and characterised by neurasthenic symptoms. The patient complains of fatigue, insomnia, anxiety and depression, and shows a gradual change towards mental slowness and unpredictability of behaviour. Occasionally the mood is mildly elevated with loquacity and inappropriate laughter. Already at this stage there may be evidence of impaired memory and concentration, the limbs may appear to be weak and the gait unsteady. Frequently, however, objective findings are lacking and a 'functional' psychiatric disorder is suspected. This is especially likely in patients in whom the early symptoms remit for several weeks at a time.

An instructive example was reported by Keshavan *et al.* (1987). A 38-year-old man became forgetful and disorientated from Christmas 1983, but this was attributed to heavy alcohol consumption and depression. His marital situation and business affairs had become chaotic. When admitted to a psychiatric hospital 6 months later his mental state showed marked fluctuations, with disorientation and bizarre memory disturbances alternating with periods of lucidity. He was emotionally labile and gave approximate answers to questions, and the presumptive diagnosis was of hysterical pseudodementia. In August 1984 the EEG showed mixed theta and delta activity, attributed to possible alcoholic encephalopathy, but a CT scan was normal. No abnormal neurological signs could be detected apart from a pout reflex and a shuffling gait.

During the following month he deteriorated markedly and became regressed in his behaviour. In October he was referred for a further opinion, at which stage it was impossible to test cognitive functions because of extreme distractibility. He was perplexed, gazed vacantly and spoke in a slurred incoherent babble. At this stage neurological examination revealed gross apraxia, generalised myoclonic jerks and choreoathetoid movements. He was incontinent of urine and faeces. The CT scan now showed some evidence of atrophy, and the EEG showed prominent slow waves maximal over the left frontotemporal region. He then followed a downhill course until his death in March 1985, when autopsy confirmed the diagnosis of Creutzfeldt–Jakob disease.

Intellectual deterioration or neurological defects soon become prominent. The latter are extremely variable but are liable to involve motor functions, speech or vision. Myoclonic jerks are almost invariably seen. There may be ataxia of cerebellar type, spasticity of limbs with progressive paralysis, extrapyramidal rigidity, tremor or choreoathetoid movements, depending on the brain regions principally involved. Involvement of the anterior horn cells of the cord may lead to muscular fibrillation and atrophy, especially of the small hand muscles, resembling amyotrophic lateral sclerosis. Speech disturbances are common with dysphasia and dysarthria, likewise parietal lobe symptoms such as right–left disorientation, dyscalculia and finger agnosia. Vision may be severely affected with rapidly progressive cortical blindness. Apart from this, sensory changes are usually absent. Brain stem involvement may lead to nystagmus, dysphagia or bouts of uncontrollable laughing and crying. Epileptic fits may occur.

Attempts have been made to classify this bewildering variety of phenomena though with little success. A given case may show a succession of different neurological features as the disease progresses. A broad classification into those which begin with cerebellar symptoms and those with parietal lobe symptoms has been suggested, similarly into cases with and without spinal cord or visual cortex involvement.

Intellectual deterioration follows or appears along with the neurological defects and evolves with great rapidity. An acute organic picture may be present initially with clouding of consciousness or frank delirium. Auditory hallucinations and delusions may be marked, and confabulation is often seen. Ultimately a state of profound dementia is reached, accompanied by gross rigidity or spastic paralysis and often a decorticate or decerebrate posture. Repetitive myoclonic jerking of muscle groups is often still evident late in the disease. Emaciation is usually profound by the time death occurs.

The cerebrospinal fluid is usually normal throughout, though the protein is very occasionally elevated. A recently described immunoassay for a particular protein (protein 14-3-3) in the cerebrospinal fluid appears to have high specificity for the disorder in patients with clinical evidence of dementia (Hsich *et al.* 1996). The CT scan may show cortical atrophy and ventricular enlargement but this is rarely gross in degree. Indeed the CT scan can be essentially normal when the dementia is well advanced, a feature which may be of some importance in differential diagnosis (Galvez & Cartier 1984). The EEG is almost always markedly abnormal. A variety of changes have been reported and different findings may emerge at different stages of the illness. Initially there is some diffuse or focal slowing. Later paroxysmal sharp waves or slow spike and wave discharges appear; these are bilaterally synchronous and may accompany the myoclonic jerks. Ultimately a characteristic pattern emerges of synchronous triphasic sharp wave complexes at 1–2 Hz, superimposed on progressive suppression of cortical background activity (May 1968; Elliott *et al.* 1974). The triphasic discharges are at first intermittent, but evolve to a periodic picture at rates of one to two per second. The latter changes may be helpful in diagnosis, though usually only late in the course of the disease.

Course and outcome

The course is much more rapid than with most other primary dementing illnesses, the great majority of patients dying within 2 years. Among 185 cases of sporadic Creutzfeldt–Jakob disease identified since 1990 in the UK the median duration to death was 4 months (Will

et al. 1996). Death is usually preceded by a period of deepening coma which lasts for several weeks.

Pathology

The brain may appear to be somewhat atrophied but often there is little abnormal to detect macroscopically. Histological examination shows great variability from case to case, but the essential features consist of neuronal degeneration, great proliferation of astrocytes and a characteristic spongy appearance of the grey matter. In some varieties the latter may be so pronounced that it is visible to the naked eye. The degenerated neurones often show an accumulation of lipid material. Neuropathological diagnostic criteria for the disease have recently been presented (Budka *et al.* 1995b).

The accent of the pathology may fall on different regions, accounting for the various clinical pictures that are seen. The cortex is nearly always involved, though often with relative sparing of the parietal and occipital lobes. The hippocampi may also escape. In different cases there may be a marked emphasis on the corpus striatum, thalamus, cerebellum, substantia nigra, brain stem and spinal cord. The corticospinal tracts and also the extrapyramidal pathways are often severely degenerated.

The 'status spongiosus' of the cortex is highly characteristic, showing as a finely meshed vacuolation under the microscope. The vacuoles then enlarge and coalesce to form microcysts (Lantos 1992b). Severely affected areas have the appearance of being riddled with tiny cavities (Plate 16). In some varieties this is widely disseminated. Electron microscopy shows the presence of vacuoles within the cytoplasm of neurones and astrocytes, particularly within dendrites, and the accumulation of abnormal cytoskeletal protein. Status spongiosus is not entirely pathognomonic for Creutzfeldt–Jakob disease, having occasionally been reported in senile dementia of the Alzheimer type, Pick's disease, Wilson's disease and other degenerative conditions.

There are usually no senile plaques or neurofibrillary tangles as in Alzheimer's disease, no massive circumscribed atrophy as in Pick's disease, and no evidence of an inflammatory reaction. However, some cases show extracellular amyloid plaques especially in the cerebellum. The cerebral vessels appear healthy, or if cerebrovascular disease is present this appears to be incidental. Immunocytochemistry using antibodies to prion protein gives a positive reaction which can be useful diagnostically in uncertain cases.

Subvarieties of the disease

Several subvarieties have been described, depending

partly on the detailed neuropathological picture and partly on clinical features. Present views on classification are far from unanimous, however, and some varieties may yet prove to be distinct clinical entities.

One in particular has been labelled *subacute spongiform encephalopathy* (Jones & Nevin 1954; Nevin 1967). The age of onset is some 10 years later than that of the classic disease, and the beginning tends to be abrupt without the usual prodromata. The course is extremely rapid with a fatal ending after 3–6 months. Visual failure due to degeneration of the striate cortex has been a prominent feature in over a third of reported cases. Extrapyramidal changes are well developed with progressive hypertonus, likewise irregular shock-like myoclonic jerks which come to involve the entire body musculature. The EEG is always markedly abnormal as described above.

At autopsy the brain shows more severe and widespread cortical atrophy than in other forms of Creutzfeldt–Jakob disease, and an emphasis is seen on the occipital lobes which is otherwise exceptional. The brain stem and cord are spared. Status spongiosus is widely disseminated in the grey matter and usually extremely well developed.

Another very rapid form has been named the *ataxic form of subacute presenile polioencephalopathy* (Brownell & Oppenheimer 1965). This is regarded as a nosological entity within the Creutzfeldt–Jakob group. It presents initially with rapidly progressive cerebellar ataxia. This is followed by dementia and abnormal motor movements in the form of rhythmic myoclonic jerking, leading ultimately to generalised muscular rigidity. The principal findings at autopsy are selective degeneration of cells in the granular layer of the cerebellum, variable status spongiosus, and cell loss and astrocytosis in the cortex, thalamus and striatum. It would appear to be this variety of the disease which first proved to be transmissible on intracerebral inoculation, as described on p. 473.

The *amyotrophic form*, which presents with muscle wasting, can sometimes run a relatively chronic course. This variety was at first thought to be non-transmissible to animals, though more recent evidence has changed this view (Connolly *et al.* 1988).

The possibilities of overlap with Alzheimer's disease in rare examples have also been stressed from time to time (Matthews 1981, 1982). Cases diagnosed as Creutzfeldt–Jakob disease during life with dementia, myoclonus and the typical electroencephalographic changes, can occasionally show Alzheimer pathology and nothing more at autopsy. Conversely, Creutzfeldt–Jakob pathology may on rare occasions be detected in patients who have died after unremarkable dementing illnesses, with little to raise suspicion of the disease during life.

The full range of expression of inherited prion disease has yet to be established, and there are already indications that such disorders may be considerably more common than hitherto recognised. Patients formerly diagnosed as suffering from familial Alzheimer's disease, for example, have been found to harbour characteristic prion gene mutations, likewise a family whose members had attracted diagnoses of Alzheimer's, Huntington's and Pick's dementia in addition to Creutzfeldt–Jakob disease (Collinge *et al.* 1989, 1992). A noteworthy feature in this family was the occurrence of long-standing antisocial personality disorder preceding the onset of dementia in some affected individuals.

In another case with characteristic prion gene abnormalities, full autopsy examination failed to reveal the histological hallmarks of spongiform encephalopathy, suggesting that even the neuropathological picture may be extremely variable (Collinge *et al.* 1990). It thus seems that patients dying from a variety of dementing illnesses may have an inherited prion disease when this has not been suspected clinically or even at autopsy. The true incidence of such disorders, and their range of phenotypic expression, is likely only to be determined by greater knowledge of prion gene variants and the systematic use of molecular genetic screening in patients.

Pseudodementias

In a number of conditions a clinical picture resembling organic dementia presents for attention yet physical disease proves to be little if at all responsible. These disorders are conveniently grouped together as the 'pseudodementias'. The main varieties include the Ganser syndrome, hysterical pseudodementia, simulated dementia, depressive pseudodementia and other rarer forms as discussed below. The distinction from organic dementia can sometimes be difficult, at least for a time. It must also be remembered that in the early stages of organic brain disease a patient may occasionally react in such a way that his dementia is suspected of being more apparent than real—in other words a pseudodementia may turn out in fact to be a 'pseudo-pseudodementia'.

While it is helpful to consider the several varieties separately it must be stressed that the dividing lines between them are often far from clear. Several mechanisms may contribute to the genesis of the clinical picture, sometimes in relatively pure culture but sometimes in combination with one another. Thus mechanisms of hysterical dissociation may operate to some degree in depressive pseudodementia; covert affective disorder may make a contribution to hysterical pseudodementia; and conscious simulation will only rarely be entirely divorced from the operation of hysterical and other neurotic defensive mechanisms. In dealing with an individual case of pseudodementia, therefore, it will be necessary to keep several possible factors in mind. It will often not suffice to seek out simple pointers such as obvious motivation or coincident depressive illness as the total explanation. This has been illustrated particularly well by the chequered career of the Ganser syndrome, which is considered in some detail immediately below.

The Ganser syndrome

In 1898 Ganser described three prisoners who showed an unusual clinical picture, including the feature which now bears his name—the Ganser response ('answering past the point', 'approximate answers', 'vorbeireden'). The condition has been the focus of interest, controversy and misunderstanding ever since, as reviewed by Whitlock (1967b) and Enoch *et al.* (1967). Uncertainty surrounds its nosological status and the mechanisms behind its appearance.

Clinical features

The phenomenon which from the outset attracted most attention was that of answering past the point. A clear example occurs in one of Ganser's original cases:

'In what city are we? In Berlin, in Russia. What are you doing here? We wanted to go hunting, and we unhitched our horses. How many noses do you have? I don't know. Have you any nose at all? I do not know if I have a nose. Have you eyes? I have no eyes. How many fingers do you have? Eleven. How many ears? (He first touches his ears, and then he says: Two). How many legs does a horse have? Three. An elephant? Five. After being shown a coin and asked, What is that? the answer is: A map which a person hangs on his watch chain. Glancing at the eagle stamped on a coin: I don't know that person. Is it Kaiser Wilhelm? He was shown a dollar and was asked: Do you know a dollar? He said, I don't know a dollar. That is a toy which one gives to children. What is your name? My name is Fürst (incorrect)'.

(Ganser 1898)

Another example is provided by Kiloh (1961):

A man of 25 became fully accessible some hours after a head injury but for a period replied as follows to questions: What is the colour of your pyjamas?—Red (in fact they were blue). What is the colour of the chair in the corner?—What corner? I don't know what a corner is. I don't see a chair. Look again!—Red (yellow). What year is it?—1938 (1958). What year were you born?—1933. How old are you?—That makes me five. What is the date?—The second day of the 12th month (12 February). Which is the 12th month?—January.

The patient's responses to questions are markedly inaccurate and often absurdly so. But they seem to betray a knowledge of the purpose of the question, and by their close approximation to the correct answer imply that this too was at some level available to the patient. Approximate answers may be seen in response to simple addition, counting, the naming of colours or simple questions about everyday matters. Sometimes the patient may answer in a way quite contrary to the evidence before him, for example stating that it is midnight when the sun is shining clearly through the window. The absurd responses are usually given with full deliberation and apparently serious intent, and false responses may be quite inconsistently interspersed with accurate answers.

A difficulty with the concept of 'approximate answers' is that they require an element of subjective interpretation on the part of the examiner. In some rare examples, when asked to count fingers or add an ascending series of digits, the patient may consistently give one in excess or one less than the correct answer throughout the series, but such clear instances are rare. Short of this it can be difficult to decide how approximate an answer must be to deserve the appellation. Anderson and Mallinson (1941) foresaw a tendency for the term to be applied to any random answer and proposed the definition: 'that false response of a patient to the examiner's question where the answer, although wrong, is never far wrong and bears a definite and obvious relation to the question, indicating clearly that the question has been grasped by the patient'. Moeli's (1888) early description was that 'the answer is wrong it is true, but it bears nevertheless some relationship to the sense of the question and shows that the sphere of appropriate concepts has been touched upon'.

Whitlock (1967b) has suggested that it is often not the approximateness but the absurdness of the answers which is so striking. The playful childish character of the responses may have something in common with the 'buffoonery syndrome' of schizophrenia. On other occasions the replies may be akin to other forms of schizophrenic thought disorder, or may resemble the confused responses seen in clouding of consciousness or early dementia. They may sometimes resemble confabulations, though usually the randomness and absurdity of the replies differs sharply from the factual and circumstantial detail of the confabulation response.

The apparent dementia which accompanies the approximate answers is usually incomplete, inconstant and often self contradictory. Disorientation is invariably present, but the apparently gross disturbance of intellect fails to be reflected in the patient's overall behaviour. Thus he usually proves capable of adapting to the demands of daily life in a way that the severe organic dement would not. Motor behaviour may range from dazed stupor to histrionic outbursts of excitement, and the mood may vary from apathetic indifference to anxious bewilderment.

Other features shown by Ganser's original patients are often overlooked. All had prominent hallucinatory experiences, hysterical stigmata of various types, and showed evidence of fluctuating disturbance of consciousness. Resolution of the disorder was abrupt, the abnormal mental state clearing suddenly along with the hysterical conversion symptoms. All were left with a complete amnesia for the period of the illness.

Nosological status

Cases closely similar in all these respects have been reported from time to time, for example those described by May *et al.* (1960), but the complete syndrome is undoubtedly very rare. Much more commonly patients are reported who show approximate answers along with other mental abnormalities, or exhibit aspects of the syndrome superimposed upon other psychiatric disorders. A partial or complete Ganser state may be seen in the course of depressive and schizophrenic psychoses, after head injury, in the course of early dementia, in general paresis or in a wide variety of toxic states including alcoholism. It seems, however, that it can also occasionally appear in subjects without other definable psychiatric disorder and in response to purely emotional traumas.

Hence the difficulty with the nosological status of the syndrome. It has been suggested that it should rank as a distinct nosological entity along with other excessively rare and exotic psychiatric disorders, or alternatively that it should be viewed as a preformed mode of reaction which is determined by the individual's defensive structure and which may be called forth by a variety of different stresses and disease processes. Either way the problem remains how much must be present to justify applying the label. There is much to commend Scott's (1965) distinction between the *Ganser symptom* (approximate answers) and the *Ganser syndrome*, the first being common and the second extremely rare, while both may be found in a wide variety of psychiatric illnesses. Whitlock (1967b) suggests that the diagnosis of the syndrome should imply, in addition to approximate answers, at least some evidence of impairment of consciousness, a sudden termination and subsequent amnesia for the episode.

Mechanisms

With regard to the mechanisms underlying the development of Ganser symptoms, these have been variously regarded as akin to hysterical conversion reactions, malingering, organic confusion and psychotic thought disorder.

Ganser entitled his original contribution 'an unusual hysterical confusional state', and stressed the presence of a variety of other hysterical phenomena. He insisted, however, on the pleomorphism and severity of the acute illness episodes which he had witnessed, and did not commit himself to an hysterical aetiology for the total picture. Since then, the reporting of other examples in response to purely psychological stresses, and the appearance of approximate answers in patients with obvious hysterical pseudodementia, have led many authorities to view hysterical mechanisms as fundamental to the development of the condition. The hallucinations in most reported examples have seemed to be analogous to the pseudohallucinations of hysterical states, the content usually being immediately related to current conflicts in the patient's mind. It must be conceded that hysterical mechanisms are likely to contribute in large measure, but in many cases these may have been released by brain damage or other psychiatric illness. It is unfortunate therefore that the 'Ganser syndrome' has often come to be regarded as synonymous with 'hysterical pseudodementia'.

The older and more restricted views of 'hysteria', with the implication of overt gain as a motivating force, will not of course always be found to apply. Gain may be obvious in prisoners awaiting trial, or in the considerable number of cases where compensation is at stake, but in many others more complex dynamic factors may be at work. Anderson and Mallinson (1941) claimed that the precipitating situation could be internal to the patient, sometimes no more than a 'wrathful conscience', and with no external threat or disgrace which could be identified. Other suggested motivations include the wish to be insane, the protection of self esteem or an essay at absolution (Scott 1965). May *et al.* (1960) described Ganser patients who paradoxically had in common the prospect of release from freedom-restricting situations. Here, what looked like imminent gain had apparently been perceived as threat. Obviously these expanded possibilities are to a large extent inferential, and must run the risk of sometimes being applied when other factors are primarily at work.

Many patients with the Ganser syndrome have been suspected of malingering, that is of deliberately feigning their approximate answers and other symptoms. The phenomenon of approximate answers has struck some observers as so bizarre that conscious simulation has seemed the only reasonable explanation. In fact Ganser was himself at pains to point out that he rejected any suspicion of deliberate simulation, and that the patients made an exceedingly convincing impression of being genuinely ill. He noted that they made no spontaneous absurd remarks, but only in response to questions. They seemed convinced that what they said was correct, and seemed unwilling to have anyone think their answers false or themselves foolish or simple minded.

Other observers have felt less able to absolve their patients from all trace of simulation, and motivation 'near the level of consciousness' has often been inferred even when the syndrome accompanies other frank psychiatric illness. The fact that Ganser's original three patients were prisoners has perhaps caused selective reporting of cases from the prison population, and this in turn may have given spurious emphasis to the possibilities of deliberate simulation. The Ganser syndrome has, indeed, sometimes been labelled 'prison psychosis'. Scott (1965) reported that it still occurred in UK prisons but extremely rarely, typically in prisoners awaiting trial but also in sentenced prisoners who later developed schizophrenia. Most cases nowadays are in fact probably to be found in patients in mental hospitals, and include a fair proportion of law-abiding citizens.

The striking frequency with which the condition is found in conjunction with some form of trouble — domestic, sexual, financial, or legal—should not of course argue more in favour of simulation than of hysteria, nor should the two be regarded as mutually exclusive.

McGrath and McKenna (1961), in their interesting attempt at a psychological formulation of the mechanisms behind approximate answers, saw them as the result of defence mechanisms of an unusual character, operating in patients who fail to carry through an initial wish to feign non-comprehension. 'The typical (approximate) answer is a compromise, simultaneously carrying on the original attempt to simulate and attempting to regain the lost reality by convincing both the patient himself and others that apprehension of the environment is still operating. The result of the message is a contradictory one, conveying "I am insane, yet sane". Hence the confusion in the diagnostic constructions put upon this relatively rare state.'

A contribution from cerebral dysfunction is attested by the large number of cases reported after head injury, or occurring in the course of other acute and chronic organic reactions. Of Ganser's original three cases, two had suffered head injury and the third was recovering from typhus fever. Among the more typical cases in the literature evidence of fluctuating impairment of consciousness is found almost without exception, and a dense amnesia for the episode remains after it has resolved. In general it can be said that the organic character of much of the disturbance, as well as the organic antecedents, have impressed many observers. It is likely that in many cases an admixture of organic and psychogenic factors are operating together, the organic process serving to actualise whatever more complex mechanisms underlie the Ganser state. In this connection it is noteworthy that even in the presence of obvious cerebral dysfunction there is frequently a psychogenic setting to the development of the disorder.

The conjunction of typical Ganser states with schizophrenia and depression was increasingly reported after Ganser's original observations. Sometimes catatonic phenomena and other typical schizophrenic features have been found to accompany Ganser manifestations, and sometimes the Ganser state has appeared merely as a prelude to a developing schizophrenia. Hence the idea has gained ground that mechanisms akin to psychotic thought disorder might underlie the process. Schizophrenic thought disorder may occasionally come close to 'approximate answers'. Sometimes these seem to be due to a childish playful attitude on the part of the patient, as in the 'buffoonery syndrome'. In others they may represent catatonic phenomena of the nature of forced responsiveness, in that the patient is obliged to respond to the question immediately and says the first thing that comes into his head (Fish 1962). Anderson and Mallinson (1941) reported three examples of Ganser's syndrome, two in the course of endogenous depression and one with schizophrenia, and suggested that here depersonalisation was the common factor which led to the development of Ganser symptoms. These ideas have not, however, stood the test of time, and hysterical or allied mechanisms continue to be given precedence, even in cases with obvious concomitant psychosis. The latter is seen merely to release the more specific Ganser tendency, and to colour it accordingly. Certainly Ganser episodes are mostly transitory when they occur in the course of other psychoses, and, as with organic brain disease, a psychogenic precipitant can frequently be discerned.

In summary, therefore, it may be said that the Ganser syndrome represents a definite but exceedingly rare disorder, characterised by approximate answers, some disturbance of consciousness and subsequent dense amnesia for the episode. While the syndrome itself is rare the symptom of approximate answers is not. Both the Ganser syndrome and Ganser symptoms are more commonly found in association with other psychiatric disorders than in isolation, occurring in the course of both organic and non-organic psychiatric illness. Evidence of psychogenesis is frequently to be found, even in cases complicated in such fashion. The disorder would appear to rest principally on a complex psychogenic basis, in which hysterical mechanisms or mechanisms closely allied to them are largely responsible, though contributions due to brain dysfunction and psychotic thought disorder cannot be excluded in certain cases. It seems probable, however, that when these features are seen in association with the Ganser manifestations they have served principally as releasers rather than as prime determinants of the condition.

Hysterical pseudodementia

Of all the forms of pseudodementia there is probably least difficulty in distinguishing the typical case of hysterical pseudodementia from true organic dementia. On occasion, however, there can be protracted difficulty in making this differentiation. There may also be an added psychogenic component in the early stages of organic cerebral dysfunction, and it is then that most difficulty is likely to arise.

Hysterical pseudodementia is mostly seen in persons of limited intellectual endowment. Sometimes the patient is mute or monosyllabic in his replies. Short of this his account is grossly incoherent, he appears disorientated and fails on simple tests of cognitive function. The symptom of 'approximate answers' may be seen, but perseveration does not occur and clear examples of concrete thinking will rarely be detected.

Careful observation will usually soon reveal much that is inconsistent or self contradictory in behaviour. Responses to commands may be grossly inaccurate, the patient producing an unconvincing and theatrical display of non-comprehension and inability to perform. The wrong reply or action may be followed later by the correct one, or patchy performance may fail to correspond to any hierarchy of increasing difficulty. The patient is usually found to be highly suggestible, so that the level of performance is readily influenced by the way in which he is handled. Unlike organic dementias, memory may appear to be markedly deficient for the most elementary aspects of knowledge and experience, and even simple skills may apparently be lost. Most impressively of all, such patients may settle into ward routines and find their way about in a manner quite inconsistent with the degree of disability displayed at interview. Personal care, habits of eating and standards generally may be observed to be little impaired, with normal competence in the everyday things of life.

Sometimes, though by no means invariably, other hysterical conversion symptoms will be present, such as sensory loss, paralysis or other stigmata of classic type. In the great majority of cases the patient's attitude is bland and unconcerned, with an incurious detachment to his predicament ('belle indifference'). He may show a fatuous cheerfulness or a state of sullen apathy. In general his emotional responses are superficial and in large degree unconvincing.

In more severe degrees of 'hysterical puerilism' or 'hysterical infantilism' the patient may enact a desire to regress to the helpless state of infancy, losing the ability to walk and talk, eating with his fingers, making inarticulate noises and wetting the bed. Such florid states are relatively rare, and the abundant evidence of superficial motives and of previously unstable personality will usually serve to dispel real diagnostic difficulty.

Hysterical amnesia forms part and parcel of the picture in most cases of hysterical pseudodementia, though it may also occur in relative isolation. The cardinal features of psychogenic amnesia have already been described in Chapter 2 (p. 33) along with the points which serve to differentiate it from organic amnesic states. Kennedy and Neville's (1957) series of 74 patients presenting with abrupt failure of memory, with or without loss of personal identity, remains one of the most comprehensive surveys to date:

The patients had either presented themselves at hospital or at police stations and were examined in the acute phase of the disorder. In 43% psychogenic mechanisms appeared to operate alone, in 41% psychogenic and organic factors together, and in 16% organic factors alone. Sometimes brain disease was present along with an obvious psychological precipitant, and neither aetiology precluded the other. Altogether more than a third had some evidence of brain damage on complete examination; many had epilepsy but others were suffering from the effects of head injury, chronic encephalitis lethargica, early presenile dementia, multiple sclerosis, neurosyphilis or raised intracranial pressure.

Kennedy and Neville suggested that brain damage appeared to predispose to the development of primitive mental mechanisms of escape, or lower the threshold at which stress would bring them out. The flight was typically from simple situations to do with difficulties in marriage, bigamy or debt, but could also be from mental pain as in examples suffering from endogenous depression. The great majority of their cases of psychogenic amnesia, when seen and managed in the acute stage, recovered within a few hours or several days.

In cases of hysterical pseudodementia there is frequently an antecedent history of severe personality instability, if not of previous hysterical conversion reactions. The problem, of course, is that such retrospective evidence is often not available when the patient first presents for attention. Typically the condition arises in response to emotionally traumatic events or personally threatening situations, though sometimes the psychogenic derivation may be complex and not immediately obvious. In routine civilian practice domestic disharmony, financial troubles or complications of sexual encounters rank high on the list of causes, while in the army disciplinary measures will often be found to be pending. The patient may have wandered away in a fugue-like state, sometimes for several days on end, after which he presents for attention with loss of personal identity and other evidence of intellectual malfunction. At other times the condition may be witnessed to set in abruptly, as after head injury or when the patient is apprehended for some misdemeanour. Some of the most entrenched examples occur in head-injured patients when litigation is in progress over claims for compensation.

The points of difference between hysterical pseudodementia and the Ganser syndrome are implicit in the account of the latter given above. The presence of clouding of consciousness and abundant evidence of approximate answers will lead most observers to apply the term Ganser syndrome, and particularly so when the episode occurs in conjunction with organic or psychiatric disorder. Approximate answers alone should not, however, be used as the basis for the distinction. It is generally agreed that the whole reaction appears more superficial with hysterical pseudodementia than in the Ganser syndrome, and that some element of conscious malingering is more often to be detected along with it. Ganser episodes are typically brief, with sudden spontaneous termination even in patients who progress ultimately to schizophrenia or other mental illness, while hysterical pseudodementia not infrequently runs a prolonged and relapsing course, particularly when the underlying conflicts cannot be revealed or resolved.

The distinction between hysterical and depressive pseudodementia rests principally on the absence of melancholic changes or typical psychomotor retardation, and in the general superficiality of the emotional display. In depressive pseudodementia the cognitive disabilities are likely to appear more genuine, and can often be traced to the patient's difficulty with attention and concentration.

The features which may point to conscious simulation rather than hysterical pseudodementia are discussed in the section that follows.

Simulated dementia

Most authorities agree that entirely conscious simulation of dementia, or indeed of amnesia, is very rare indeed, though self-confessed cases have been recorded from time to time. Motivation is gross and obvious when adequate information is to hand, though of course this is likely to be carefully concealed from the examiner.

As with hysterical pseudodementia, careful observation usually soon reveals much that is out of keeping with genuine cognitive impairment. The simulant, after all, is presenting his own notion of the condition he seeks to portray, and through ignorance will usually fail to show the complete picture (Bluglass 1976). An isolated symptom, such as loss of memory or loss of speech, will be more commonly encountered than a complex syndrome.

Formal examination may be impossible on account of mutism or total lack of cooperation, and it will then be necessary to judge the patient's behaviour when he feels under less careful scrutiny. He may be observed to cope with the necessities of daily life in a manner quite inconsistent with the impression made at interview. In more productive examples the patient will often overdo his part, mixing up incoherent and absurd answers with a theatrical demonstration of insanity and talking no sense at all.

Interesting attempts have been made to assess the responses of healthy subjects who have been asked to feign mental illness. The broad conclusion from such experiments is that convincing simulation of dementia for more than a very brief period is virtually impossible, even among reasonably sophisticated subjects. Anderson et al. (1959), for example, asked 18 psychology students to simulate mental disorder, and compared the results with the clinical picture shown by 25 patients with organic dementia and 10 patients with hysterical pseudodementia. No normal subject was able to feign dementia in a convincing manner. The length and thoroughness of the examination was an important factor in revealing the spuriousness of the simulations; fatigue was observed to 'increase the pull of reality', and responses became more and more normal as the examination progressed. A special focus of interest was the occurrence of approximate answers and confabulations; simple 'near miss' answers were given on occasion by all three groups but most often by the patients with hysterical pseudodementia, while gross confabulations occurred with almost equal frequency in the simulants, the dements and the pseudodements. Perseveration was a more useful distinguishing feature, being prominent in the organic cases but very rarely observed in simulation or pseudodementia.

Benton and Spreen (1961) discuss differences in performance on a visual memory test between subjects simulating brain damage and patients with true brain damage. Significant differences between the groups were observed where certain qualitative aspects of performance were concerned; the simulators made more errors of distortion than the patients in reproducing visual designs, and fewer errors of omission, perseveration and size. Hunt (1973) summarises work on certain scales incorporated in the Minnesota Multiphasic Personality Inventory which prove sensitive to experimentally induced malingering, and which could, at least in theory, have practical value in pointing towards deliberate attempts at feigning mental illness.

Gudjonsson and Shackleton (1986) have examined differences in the pattern of scores between 'fakers' and 'non-fakers' on Raven's Progressive Matrices. The 60 items of the test consist of five series which become progressively more difficult. Fakers were shown to have a significantly smaller decrement across the five series of sets, as a result of faking errors on disproportionately more of the easy items at the start.

A useful approach which may be employed when simulated amnesia is suspected is described by Brandt (1988). A list of 20 words is read to the subject, who is then asked to recognise each of them in a forced-choice recognition test. Each of the 20 words is presented anew along with a distractor word, and the subject must say which was in the list he has already heard. Genuinely amnesic patients, though performing badly, will not fall below the chance level of 50% obtained by simply guessing; any performance significantly below this will indicate a deliberate withholding of knowledge. One may also examine the 'serial position effect' on free recall of a list of items. In normal subjects items at the beginning or the end of a list are better recalled than those in the middle ('primacy' and 'recency' effects). Organic amnesics typically show normal recency but much attenuated primacy effects. The simulant will be most unlikely to mirror the organic pattern closely or consistently; his overall scores may be low, but the serial position curve may be expected to be normal in shape. Lezak (1995) and Pankratz (1988) describe other neuropsychological measures which may be useful in various circumstances in the detection of simulation.

The distinction between simulation and hysteria usually provides most difficulty, and the decision reached will often depend to a considerable extent on the orientation of the examiner. The patient who is simulating will be likely to have a markedly abnormal personality, and hysterical mechanisms may be mobilised in his performance. Thus even the simulant may be partly deceiving himself, with the result that the boundaries between fully conscious feigning of dementia and hysterical pseudodementia are probably far from definite, and the two will be inextricably mixed in many cases.

In attempting to apportion the roles of simulation and hysteria, Kräupl-Taylor (1966) makes the important clinical point that the malingerer is likely to be anxiously on guard to avoid inconsistencies in his behaviour, and will get angry or upset and attempt to explain away his slips when these are pointed out to him. With the self deception of the hysterical pseudodement, on the other hand, there is often a carelessness about the inconsistencies shown, and his reaction may be bland, uncaring or even puzzled when these are brought to his attention. The inconsistencies themselves are likely to be more crude and obvious, and will often be closely tied to the conflict-inducing situation — the hysterical patient, for example,

may recognise a neighbour while disclaiming recognition of his wife in a way that would not occur with conscious simulation.

Suggestibility is another feature which may help towards the differentiation. Kennedy and Neville (1957) found that their patients with psychogenic amnesia were markedly suggestible during interview, but the small group who later confessed to malingering had hardly been suggestible at all. Finally, the simulant is also much more likely than the hysterical patient to use his resources to defeat full inquiry, and to fail to cooperate in any close investigation.

As already stressed, however, the distinction will often be blurred, and the situation may fail to be resolved in a considerable proportion of cases. Kräupl-Taylor (1966) points out that even retrospectively the evidence can be equivocal — the dependence of the syndrome on a critical situation, and the fact that the patient has stood to gain from his behaviour, is likely to be found equally in hysterical pseudodementia and in malingering. Even a confession from the patient himself will not always be final proof, since some will confess under pressure when there is strong evidence of organic or psychological causation (Kennedy & Neville 1957). It will often be helpful to keep the criteria of Farrell and Kaufman (1943) in mind before deciding firmly on a diagnosis of simulation — namely the absence of obvious disease, *a firm impression that the individual is consciously aware both of what he is doing and of his motive for so doing, and that he is fixed in carrying out a purpose to a preconceived result.*

Depressive pseudodementia

Pseudodementia due to affective disorder is the form that most commonly leads to mistakes in diagnosis. The depression may activate hysterical mechanisms in the predisposed patient, so that signs of hysterical pseudodementia accompany the other manifestations of the illness. Sometimes successive attacks of depression may regularly produce a similar clinical picture.

More commonly, however, and particularly in the elderly, it is the psychomotor retardation coupled with withdrawal of interest from the environment which leads to a misleading impression of dementia. The patient becomes slow to grasp essentials, thinking is laboured, and behaviour becomes generally slipshod and inefficient. Events fail to register, either through lack of ability to attend and concentrate or on account of the patient's inner preoccupations. In consequence he may show faulty orientation, impairment of recent memory and a markedly defective knowledge of current events. The impression of dementia is sometimes strengthened by the patient's decrepit appearance due to self neglect and loss of weight (Kiloh 1961), or when the elderly depressive becomes tremulous and assumes a shuffling gait (Post 1965). Some patients tend to emphasise the physical components of the disorder in their complaints and fail to report the change of mood; or when depression and agitation are detected these may be regarded as secondary to the supposed dementing process.

An alternative formulation, which has gained ground in recent years, is to view the above picture as reflecting true cognitive failure rather than merely a misleading impression of such. Folstein and McHugh (1978) suggest that the term *'dementia syndrome of depression'* more accurately reflects the verifiable cognitive deficits encountered in certain elderly depressives, and attribute the disorder to the interaction between ageing processes within the brain and the neurochemical changes induced by depression. Resolution of the latter could nonetheless allow a return of cognition to normal. In this view the label *pseudodementia* becomes a misnomer since the temporary impairment is real. Evidence in favour of a cerebral basis to the condition in elderly subjects is discussed below.

Whatever the correct nosological status may be, patients are certainly not infrequently encountered in whom an initial impression of dementia proves to have been due to depression. Kendell (1974) analysed the stability of psychiatric diagnoses in England and Wales over a 5-year period as reflected in statistical returns to the Department of Health and Social Security, and found that 8% of the diagnoses of dementia were later changed to depression. Follow-up studies of patients discharged from hospital have shown even more pointedly how commonly mistakes may be made (Nott & Fleminger 1975; Ron *et al.* 1979). Thus in Ron *et al.*'s survey, described on p. 492, five of 51 patients discharged with a firm diagnosis of presenile dementia were found later to have been suffering from affective disorder alone, and in several more depression had combined with other factors to give the misleading impression.

Rabins *et al.* (1984) showed clearly how treatment of depression could improve cognitive function in patients who appeared to be both depressed and demented. Eighteen such patients, who fulfilled DSM-III criteria for both major depression and dementia, were matched with demented controls and patients with major depression alone. All were being hospitalised during the same 1-year period.

The great majority were traced 2 years later. Treatment of depression had led to pronounced improvement in the 'depressed/demented' group, all but two of them showing a rise to normal scores on the Mini-Mental State examination. The demented controls had deteriorated as expected, and the non-demented depressives had maintained their normal scores.

There are obvious risks in this clinical situation, since the depression can easily be viewed as a reaction to cognitive impairment rather than vice versa. The problem of differentiation is likely to be particularly difficult with cases of mild impairment, since in early dementia there is often a lack of collateral support from electroencephalographic or neuroimaging procedures. Moreover it is in mild and early cases of dementia that depression is most likely to occur (Reifler *et al.* 1982).

Post (1965) reported a typical example of severe cognitive impairment in the course of a depressive illness:

A retired schoolmaster had had a first depressive illness at 63, recovering with electroconvulsive therapy. At 69 he was readmitted with a 6-week history of increasing agitation. He was very restless and apprehensive, looked perplexed and miserable, and believed that a cancer was closing up his throat. He also thought that the police were about to arrest him for some trivial sexual misdemeanour in his youth. There were no physical abnormalities, but the patient appeared to be confused: he did not know the name of the hospital, thought it was situated in Edenbridge instead of Eden Park, and that he had been previously admitted 1 year ago. He gave the year (1950) variously as 1918, and 1952. He failed to learn his psychiatrist's name. In addition he telescoped the dates of various events in his life, placed the First World War correctly, but was unable to give the dates of the 1939 war, and thought MacDonald had preceded Churchill as prime minister. These failures were not due to lack of cooperation, as he was consistently able to repeat correctly eight digits forwards and six backwards, and he also gave excellent immediate renderings of a brief story. He recovered after four electroconvulsive treatments, and a week or two later his performance on tests of memory function was in keeping with his educational background and almost faultless. He continued to enjoy his retirement, but at the age of 73 had to be admitted once again on account of agitation and a fear that he had a growth in his neck. Cognitive impairment was again noted, clearing together with the agitated depression after five electroconvulsive treatments.

(Post 1965)

Bourgeois *et al.* (1970) present further examples of apparent dementia in a setting of severe depression, all responding to electroconvulsive treatment even where antidepressant medication had failed.

Mechanisms

Precisely what factors govern the liability of some patients to manifest such prominent cognitive disturbance in association with depressive illness is not known. Those who do so may have some personal predisposition, since not infrequently the situation recurs in subsequent attacks. The problem may rest on matters of cerebral metabolism, levels of arousal or other variants in the biological background of the depressive illness process. Impairment of cortical arousal, as measured by barbiturate sedation thresholds, has been studied in elderly depressives by Hemsi *et al.* (1968) and Cawley *et al.* (1973), and appears to provide a partial explanation for those who show cognitive difficulties.

The tendency is certainly particularly common in later life. Elderly depressives may sometimes score like patients with brain damage on tests of learning new material, even when not showing striking clinical signs of confusion. In consequence too great a reliance on the assessment of intellectual functions alone can be misleading in the depressed elderly patient, as described in Chapter 3 (p. 115). It is probable, moreover, that the biological processes of ageing within the brain are related to the development of cognitive failure with depression, just as they appear sometimes to facilitate the emergence of depression itself. It has been shown, for example, that elderly depressives may have larger ventricles than controls (Jacoby & Levy 1980b), and decreased brain absorption density as measured on CT scans (Jacoby *et al.* 1983). Such features appear to characterise those patients whose first depression has only appeared in old age. Hendrickson *et al.* (1979) have shown delays in the latencies of auditory evoked responses in elderly depressed patients, similar in direction though less in degree to those seen in dementia. There is reason to suppose therefore that ageing processes affecting the brain, such as cerebral neuronal loss, may combine with the neurochemical concomitants of depression to lead to the cognitive failure.

A further pointer towards organic pathology in old age depression has been provided by Abas *et al.* (1990). Twenty elderly depressives were examined on an extensive battery of psychological tests, including computerised tests which permitted measures of speed of response. Seventy per cent showed impairment, particularly on memory and measures of latency. Significantly, on recovery from depression a third continued to show impairment when compared with matched healthy controls, even though the majority of tests had shown improvement. The impairments that persisted were on measures of slowing and on a number of tests of memory and learning. Increased size of the cerebral ventricles on CT scanning correlated with poor ability on the tests which recovered incompletely, but not with those which showed a return to normal.

It is important nonetheless to consider the possibility that in some elderly patients the cognitive failure seen with depression may be the harbinger of a dementia that is to follow later. Earlier follow-up studies had indicated that elderly depressives were no more at risk of dementia than the general population (Post 1962), but more recent observations have cast some doubt on this. Reding *et al.* (1985) followed 28 depressed non-demented elderly patients over a 3-year period, and found that more than half went on to develop frank dementia, usually in the context of Alzheimer's, Parkinson's or multi-infarct disease. More particularly Kral (1983) followed up 22 depressive pseudodements, of mean age 77, for 4–18 years. Twenty had become demented, compared to the four or five who would have been expected to do so. Thus a proportion of elderly patients who show cognitive failure with depression may be in the very early stages of progressive cerebral disease which becomes manifest in diagnosable form only some years later.

Clinical differentiation

The following clinical points may be helpful in making the important differentiation between depressive illness and degenerative brain disease in patients where the situation is uncertain (Post 1965; Roth & Myers 1969; Wells 1979, 1982):

The onset of affective disorder is typically acute and recent, whereas that of dementia is insidious. A careful history in depressive pseudodementia may strongly suggest that up to the time of appearance of depressive symptoms there had been no decline whatever in abilities or memory. Arie (1983) stresses the importance of seeking evidence of depression from relatives or nurses who see the patient around the clock; they may witness transient emergence from incoherence or inaccessibility and the utterance of depressive statements. In the history it can be important to search for a potentially relevant life event. The depressed patient will often communicate a sense of distress, whereas in dementia the emotions tend to be shallow. In particular, patients with depression will often complain of their cognitive difficulties with vigour and feeling in a manner distinctly unusual for dementia. In the standard interview it may be noted that questions about the presenting complaints are handled well and that large amounts of historical information are organised without difficulty, whereas replies to direct and specific questions meet with a strangely inadequate response. A tendency to counter questions by 'Don't know' responses is frequently observed, in contrast to the attempts to confabulate or make facile excuses for failure in the patient who is organically confused. Performance on tests of cognitive function may be inconsistent in depressive pseudodementia, with surprising preservation of certain areas and topics. Inattention will usually emerge as the principal defect, along with slowed mental processing and paucity of verbal elaboration (Caine 1981). Defects of higher cortical function such as dysphasia or dyspraxia will be conspicuous by their absence. Finally, in cases which most resemble dementia the family pattern of illness is often also atypical.

Mention must be made of the special problem that exists when depressive illness complicates the picture in patients with brain damage. The situation in patients recovering from head injury is discussed in Chapter 5 (p. 185), but difficulty may also arise with other forms of cerebral insult as in the following case:

A 43-year-old woman of good previous intelligence and stable personality was referred to hospital with a 6-month history of insomnia, difficulty in thinking clearly, forgetfulness when shopping and difficulty in managing her home. Three weeks before admission she had developed an acute episode of agitation with incoherent and muddled speech, and from that time she had become progressively out of touch with those around her. On examination she was perplexed and anxious but showed no noteworthy evidence of depression. Her talk was incoherent, she was disoriented for time, and psychometric examination revealed a full scale IQ of 60 (verbal scale 68, performance scale 59). The EEG showed some reduction of activity over the right central area and slow waves in the posterior temporal regions. The air encephalogram showed dilatation of the right lateral ventricle with some cortical atrophy over the surface. A diagnosis of presenile dementia was made, and after an unsuccessful trial at home she was transferred to a mental hospital in another part of the country. There she could be visited by her sisters while her husband continued to rear the children alone.

Some 6 years later she was re-referred for assessment at the request of her relatives. They had noted great variability in her condition, and although most of the time she had continued to be incoherent and perplexed she had not deteriorated further as expected. On weekend leaves from hospital in recent months she had even shown short-lived spells of near normal behaviour.

Examination now showed her to be slow, incoherent and perplexed as before, often losing the thread in simple sentences and with obvious difficulty in assembling her thoughts. Now, however, she was correctly oriented and showed definite evidence of mild depression. Her level of performance fluctuated remarkably from day to day, and sometimes she proved capable of answering questions and holding brief conversations on simple matters. The air encephalogram showed persistent cortical atrophy on the right and the ventricles were slightly larger than before, but repeat psychometric testing showed considerably better scores (a full scale IQ of 91, verbal scale 97, performance scale 84). However, tests of new learning ability remained firmly in the organic range.

She was started on imipramine and this was followed by slow improvement. Later six electroconvulsive treatments were given with further improvement still. Lucid intervals became increasingly prolonged and she began for the first time to take some interest in her affairs and predicament. Unfortunately it emerged that in the intervening years her husband had established a liaison with his housekeeper and he now refused to have her home, but despite the distress of this discovery she achieved a job

as a typist and eventually left hospital to live in a hostel nearby. She remained well during the next 12 months, apart from occasional brief relapses to her former incoherent state after particularly distressing episodes in relation to her family situation. She then died suddenly of a subarachnoid haemorrhage and autopsy was not obtained.

It would seem that in this patient some episode, possibly of a vascular nature, had led initially to the brain damage which came to light and which had suggested the diagnosis of presenile dementia. Over the ensuing years her level of function had been still further impaired by affective disorder, which nonetheless responded gratifyingly to appropriate treatment and with substantial and sustained improvement in cognitive function.

In the following patient brain damage had again led to undervaluing of the role of depression in the clinical picture, and undue emphasis had been placed on the results from the CT scan. The patient also illustrates the value that can attach to observation after a period of sleep deprivation as discussed below:

A woman of 62 was admitted to hospital with a clear depressive illness, the third such episode over the past 20 years. She failed to respond to treatment and made two serious suicide attempts. In one she put a plastic bag over her head and took an overdose of phenelzine, in the other an overdose of sodium amytal. After the first she had a transient right hemiparesis resolving over 2 days, and after the second the plantar reflexes were up-going for 2 days. After both she was deeply unconscious for a while.

For the next year she was markedly withdrawn, apathetic and self neglectful. She seemed capable of everyday tasks but totally lacking in motivation. Psychometric testing showed reasonable results, but a CT scan revealed extensive right frontal lobe infarction, presumably dating from one of the suicide attempts. Her behaviour was now interpreted as reflecting brain damage, her inertia and self neglect being seen as frontal in origin.

At this point she was referred for a second opinion. The diagnostic dilemma was dramatically resolved after two nights of sleep deprivation, carried out as a diagnostic test. She became perfectly well as the depression lifted transiently. More vigorous antidepressant medication was resumed, and over the next few months she was successfully rehabilitated.

Abreaction and sleep deprivation

Some patients can obviously present severe and protracted difficulties over the question of diagnosis, particularly those who are mute or bordering on stupor. When the situation remains uncertain after careful in-patient observation, the response to light abreaction with intravenous sodium amytal or diazepam can be informative (Patrick & Howells 1990). Abundant evidence of depressive thought content may be revealed or memory difficulties may clear substantially, whereas in organic dementia the confusion would be exacerbated. Perry and Jacobs

(1982) review the value of the procedure and give guidance over matters of technique.

Attempts at sleep deprivation have also been recommended in this situation (Letemendia *et al.* 1981). A period of 40 hours of maintained wakefulness can result in a temporary reversal of mood in depressive pseudodementia and a dramatic return to normal intellectual function. Though only briefly maintained this can provide the decisive information on which to base future treatment strategies. Electroconvulsive therapy, as indicated above, can at times be effective when antidepressant medication has failed, and will frequently warrant a trial when results from these procedures are encouraging.

Electrophysiological measures can also assist in the differentiation between depressive pseudodementia and dementia with depressive features, and can be combined with the sleep-deprivation strategy just described:

Reynolds *et al.* (1988) analysed electroencephalographic sleep data in elderly subjects, showing first that depressed and demented subjects could be distinguished with reasonable reliability by discriminant function analysis of four features — rapid eye movement (REM) sleep latency, per cent REM sleep, loss of spindles and K complexes during non-REM sleep, and early morning wakening. The same predictor variables were then applied to patients with depressive pseudodementia or dementia with depressive features, and permitted correct classification in almost two-thirds of cases.

The same group (Buysse *et al.* 1988) examined the effect of one night's sleep deprivation, along with monitoring of mood and EEG, on eight patients with depressive pseudodementia and 18 with dementia and depressive features. Both groups had similar pretreatment depression scores. The pseudodements showed a significant drop in Hamilton depression scores after sleep deprivation, with a median 4-point change. All decreased by at least 2 points, whereas only four of 14 dements showed an improvement of this order. None of the pseudodements showed a worsening of depression, while six of the dements did. The differences between the groups were significant. The value of mood monitoring along with sleep deprivation was demonstrated, in that a 2-point change in the Hamilton ratings was barely obvious clinically.

After sleep deprivation the pseudodements showed a marked REM sleep rebound, most obvious at the beginning of the second night's sleep, whereas this did not develop in the dements. The duration of the first REM period on night two permitted discrimination between the two groups with 90% accuracy.

Other forms of pseudodementia

Hypomania rather than depression may very occasionally produce a picture which is mistaken for dementia. Distractibility may be so severe that the patient cannot follow a coherent train of thought, and answers may be so random that he appears to be grossly disorientated with failing memory. Playfulness may also lead to false replies to questions. When at the same time the affective component of the picture is incompletely developed, considerable difficulty with diagnosis may be encountered. Such cases are rare, but an example has been reported by Kiloh (1961):

A man of 58 had been behaving strangely for 4 weeks, claiming that he had won £100 000 on the football pools and extracting paste stones from cheap jewellery and attempting to sell them as valuable diamonds. He was restless and overactive and broke several windows on being removed from his lodgings.

On admission to hospital he appeared grossly confused. He gave hopelessly inaccurate answers to calculations, to the date, and gave long rambling stories about his earlier activities, each totally different from the others. He was thought to be confabulating and the diagnosis of a Korsakoff syndrome with an underlying dementia was made. On psychiatric examination it became apparent that he was elated and many of his ideas were distinctly grandiose in quality. Although he was dirty and neglected, behaviour was in most respects out of accord with his apparently gross memory defect. Furthermore he gave an accurate account of the facts leading up to his admission, even though he insisted that this had occurred 9 years ago. He was clearly well in touch with his surroundings and his replies merely reflected a playfulness dependent on a somewhat simple sense of humour. He was, in fact, suffering from a manic illness and there was no real evidence of any intellectual impairment.   (Kiloh 1961)

Episodes of mania in the elderly are particularly liable to produce a picture which at first sight suggests dementia (Carney 1983). The overactivity is mistaken for agitation, and incoherence and physical deterioration can combine to suggest an organic cerebral process.

Schizophrenia may likewise lead to difficulty, for example when a patient with advanced schizophrenic deterioration presents for attention at a hospital where he is unknown. The poverty of ideas, blunting of emotion and unkempt appearance may strongly suggest dementia, especially when habits are deteriorated and hoarding rituals have become established. Elderly patients with late paraphrenia can present a particularly misleading picture (Roth 1981). Years of self-induced isolation coupled with entrenched paranoid ideas may have led to a situation of chaos and disorganisation in their homes. Moreover their delusions and hallucinations can be so bizarre and insightless that dementia immediately springs to mind. Naguib and Levy (1987) have demonstrated mild cognitive disorder and ventricular enlargement in patients with late paraphrenia, these seeming to be indicative of ageing processes in the brain which have helped to precipitate the condition. As with depressive pseudodementia, therefore, undue reliance on psychometric testing can sometimes prove to be misleading, and all aspects of the clinical picture must be taken into consideration when making the diagnosis.

In schizophrenia both concrete thinking and perseveration may be much in evidence, and proper assessment of cognitive functions may be very difficult. The so-called 'buffoonery syndrome' perhaps comes closest to simulating dementia (Bleuler 1924). As the name implies such patients show a tendency to clowning and fatuous jocularity, give bizarre, inaccurate replies to questions and fail hopelessly on tests of cognitive function. The distinction from hysterical pseudodementia may be difficult, and hysterical as well as schizophrenic mechanisms are probably operative in many examples.

In uncertain cases the clinical distinction between schizophrenia and dementia usually rests on identifying first-rank symptoms of schizophrenic illness, or cardinal aspects of schizophrenic thought disorder. Schizophrenic thinking, although grossly disordered, is usually adequate for the day-to-day tasks of living, and the 'hard core' of basic cognitive functions which deteriorate early in organic dementia can usually be shown to be intact. In very occasional cases, however, the distinction can be extraordinarily difficult. Recent research has underlined the severity of cognitive disturbance in some schizophrenic patients, and neuroimaging may indicate substantial cerebral atrophy (see Chapter 2). Follow-up will often clarify the situation, in that the cognitive deficits of schizophrenia will rarely be progressive.

Forms of neurotic reaction other than hysterical dissociation may also lead to pictures resembling dementia. Severe obsessional ruminative states occasionally entrap the patient to an extent that leads to self neglect, and may block his ability to demonstrate that intellectual functions are intact. In severe anxiety neurosis the patient may come to focus on minor defects of memory, difficulty with concentration and a host of physical symptoms, and be rendered incapable of cooperating fully on tests of cognitive ability. Reactive depression, in addition to liberating hysterical features, may also lead to states of pathological regression and dependence which fortify the impression of failing cognitive function; such an example was described in Chapter 5 (p. 193).

Assessment and differential diagnosis

Every patient suspected of a primary senile or presenile dementia requires comprehensive evaluation. This will in all cases require certain investigatory procedures in addition to the routines of history taking and clinical examination. The label of a primary dementing illness carries a hopeless prognosis, and unless every care is taken in applying it serious mistakes may later be revealed.

The principal aim must be to exclude a remediable cause for the patient's symptoms. Altogether the yield of treatable conditions is likely to be low, but those that are discovered are vitally important. Moreover, even if a primary dementing process is confirmed, other concomitant disorders may still be aggravating the situation and will sometimes have caused the patient to present at this particular time.

Conditions amenable to treatment include pathologies within the skull such as cerebral tumour, subdural haematoma, normal-pressure hydrocephalus and general paresis, also certain systemic disorders which may be impairing cerebral function indirectly. The latter include the several causes of cerebral anoxia, myxoedema, hypoglycaemia, metabolic derangements due to renal or hepatic disease, vitamin deficiencies, alcoholism and intoxication due to various drugs and chemicals. The tendency, especially in the elderly, for a depressive illness to masquerade as dementia or to aggravate its manifestations must also be remembered.

This range, even of the commoner differential diagnoses, is very large, and cannot be adequately appraised in the out-patient clinic. In-patient evaluation should be regarded as mandatory for every patient suspected of presenile dementia; many patients with dementia in old age will require admission, though in the very elderly it will not always be justified to pursue investigations to the limit as discussed on p. 496. In the hospital setting a more comprehensive history can be obtained, the patient's behaviour can be closely observed and investigations can be planned and carried out more efficiently than on an out-patient basis.

The value of comprehensive in-patient evaluation has been shown by several surveys, as indicated in Table 17. These represent consecutive series of patients admitted to hospital with a presumptive diagnosis of dementia from the UK (Marsden & Harrison 1972), the USA (Freemon 1976), Scotland (Victoratos *et al.* 1977) and Australia (Smith & Kiloh 1981). Remarkably similar findings emerge with regard to the relative incidence of different forms of pathology. The series were from neurological units and represent a broad spectrum of patient ages, some 80% or more being below the age of 65; they should be interpreted, therefore, as indicating what might be expected in presenile rather than senile dementias.

The first point to note is that some 15% of the patients were judged not to be demented after full evaluation, but to be suffering from some other organic psychosyndrome or from nonorganic psychiatric disorder. Almost half of the total were presumed to have Alzheimer's disease, establishing this as the single most important cause of dementia. Multi-infarct dementia follows next, with an equal number where alcoholism is thought to have played a part. Huntington's disease and Creutzfeldt–Jakob disease make a relatively small contribution to the total numbers. Lewy body dementia had not attracted attention at this time, nor had AIDS dementia appeared on the scene.

Tumours and normal-pressure hydrocephalus are not infre-

Table 17 Final diagnosis in patients presumed to be demented after evaluation in hospital (see text).

	Study 1 (Marsden & Harrison 1972)	Study 2 (Freemon 1976)	Study 3 (Victoratos et al. 1977)	Study 4 (Smith & Kiloh 1981)	Total	% of total
Total cases admitted	106	60	52	200	418	
Dementia confirmed						
Cause unknown (presumed Alzheimer's disease)	48	26	31	84	189	45%
Multi-infarct dementia	8	5	5	22	40	10%
Alcohol contributing	6	4	1	30	41	10%
Huntington's disease	3	4	—	5	12	3%
Creutzfeldt–Jakob	3	—	1	—	4	<1%
Tumour or subdural haematoma	8	3	5	3	19	5%
Normal-pressure hydrocephalus	5	7	1	8	21	5'%
Post head injury	1	1	1	5	8	<2%
Myxoedema/neurosyphilis/ post encephalitis	1	3	1	3	8	<2%
Other	1	—	4	4	9*	2%
Total	**84**	**53**	**50**	**164**	**351**	**84%**
Dementia uncertain	6	—	—	—	6	1%
Diagnosis uncertain	2	—	2	—	4	1%
Other organic psychosyndrome						
Korsakoff's syndrome	—	—	—	11	11	3%
Drug toxicity	2	5	—	1	8	<2%
Delirium	—	—	—	2	2	<1%
Dysphasia/epilepsy/hepatic failure	1	1	—	2	4	<1%
Total	**3**	**6**	—	**16**	**25**	**6%**
Non-organic psychiatric disorder						
Depression	9	1	—	11	21	5%
Hypomania/mania	1	—	—	2	3	<1%
Schizophrenia	—	—	—	7	7	<2%
Hysteria	1	—	—	—	1	<1%
Total	**11**	**1**	—	**20**	**32**	**8%**

*Includes: 2 epilepsy, 2 cerebral anoxia, 1 post-subarachnoid haemorrhage, 1 giant aneurysm, 1 Parkinson's disease, 1 cerebellar degeneration, 1 Kufs' disease.

quent. Among the eight tumours in Marsden and Harrison's series three were benign, three had no abnormal neurological signs and seven showed global impairment of intellect without focal psychological deficits. The rarity of examples of myxoedema, B_{12} deficiency and other well-recognised causes of dementia may have been the result of out-patient screening for more obvious medical illnesses.

Non-organic psychiatric disorder masquerading as dementia proves to be remarkably common in the UK and Australian series, and amounts to 8% of cases overall. Depression is most often responsible.

In discussing such results Wells (1978) concludes that potentially correctable disorders (depression, drug toxicity, hydrocephalus, benign intracranial masses) may be expected in some 15% of patients, with an additional 20–25% in whom some

useful intervention will be possible — control of hypertension, withdrawal of alcohol or genetic counselling. Thus prospects for helping are by no means rare when the precise diagnosis is pursued energetically. In elderly demented patients the results will of course be less impressive; Smith and Kiloh (1981) estimated that 21% of their patients below the age of 65 had potentially treatable conditions, compared with only 5% of those aged over 65 years. The situation in the very elderly will be even less rewarding (Walstra et al. 1997a, 1997b). Though excess disability due to remediable physical and psychiatric disorders was often discovered in Walstra et al.'s patients, treatment rarely had much impact on the dementia itself. Altogether, of 170 patients with a mean age 79, reversible dementia was of the order of 1% when outcome after treatment was fully assessed.

Analogous surveys of patients admitted to psychiatric hospitals are not available but might be expected to show a higher incidence of non-organic psychiatric disorders. Two follow-up reports of patients *discharged* from psychiatric units with a firm diagnosis of presenile dementia have yielded striking results. Nott and Fleminger (1975) enquired into the long-term outcome of 50 patients discharged with such a diagnosis; of the 35 traced 5–25 years later, 15 had deteriorated as expected and many of these had died, but two remained unchanged and no less than 18 had actually improved. Thus the diagnosis had been erroneous in more than half of the patients. The presence of memory disorder on initial evaluation had been a central source of error, but abnormal results on psychometry and indications of atrophy on air encephalography had also contributed. The patients wrongly diagnosed as demented consisted mainly of people with marked personality difficulties and severe neurotic or affective disorders, most of whom continued thereafter to show chronic psychiatric disability of a non-organic type.

Ron *et al.* (1979) carried out a similar 5–15-year follow-up, obtaining information on 51 patients discharged from the Bethlem Royal and Maudsley Hospitals with a diagnosis of presenile dementia. Eighteen were alive, and the diagnosis was rejected in 16 (31%). Seven of the 16 proved in retrospect to have been suffering from a non-organic psychiatric disorder alone, mostly affective illness. The other nine showed non-progressive brain damage or Parkinson's disease, or had had transient acute organic reactions; many had had a complicating affective illness as well. The results of psychometry and air encephalography had again often lent spurious support to the clinical impression of a progressive dementing process. Both studies therefore illustrate the surprisingly large margin of error liable to occur in the diagnosis of dementia in psychiatric units, and the need to take special care over the evaluation of the total psychiatric setting in which the presumed dementia occurs. Ron *et al.* were able to show that certain key psychiatric features discriminated strongly between patients who had demented and those who had not — the presence of depressed mood during admission, a history of previous affective disorder and evidence of an abnormal premorbid personality.

A broad attitude to the question of differential diagnosis must be maintained throughout all stages of the clinical enquiry. The history provides important clues, similarly the physical and mental state examinations. Psychometric assessment can be very helpful, especially in borderline cases, and in confirming or refuting the global nature of the patient's intellectual difficulties. Certain ancillary investigations will always be needed, as set out below. In the majority of cases the definitive diagnosis will soon become apparent, but occasionally the picture will be perplexing and the search may need to be far ranging. The problem may then conveniently be considered in relation to the broad diagnostic categories outlined in Chapter 4—organic versus non-organic mental illness, acute versus chronic organic reactions and diffuse versus focal lesions —before embarking on a systematic consideration of specific disease entities. With observation in hospital those non-organic psychiatric disorders which masquerade as

dementia will usually be detected before investigations have proceeded very far, but this is not invariably so.

Occasionally complete investigation will leave one with probabilities rather than certainties, and it will then be necessary to see what course the disorder takes with time. In early cases of primary dementia all investigations can be negative. Lack of clear confirmation of the diagnosis will mean that it is essential to keep the patient under regular review, with readiness to investigate anew if later developments are in any way unusual.

History

The *family history* can be of prime importance in Huntington's disease, particularly in very early cases and when the presentation is atypical. A family history may occasionally be forthcoming with other forms of primary dementia, but not sufficiently often to help materially with diagnosis. A marked family history of affective disorder may occasionally help towards the identification of depressive pseudodementia.

The *antecedent history* may contain clues of great significance. Even slight head injury can lead to a subdural haematoma, especially in elderly, arteriosclerotic or alcoholic subjects. This may declare itself only after a considerable latent interval. Normal-pressure hydrocephalus may likewise be traceable to prior head injury, subarachnoid haemorrhage or meningitis.

Recent fits, faints or episodes of collapse will indicate the possibility of a cerebral tumour, a cerebral infarction, episodic hypoglycaemia or an undiagnosed myocardial infarction which has led to cerebral anoxia. Previous episodes of transient neurological disturbance will raise the question of multi-infarct dementia or multiple sclerosis.

Special care must be taken whenever there is a previous history of anaemia, heart disease or chronic pulmonary disorder which may now be leading to cerebral anoxia. The recent administration of an anaesthetic may be significant, or any episode of carbon monoxide poisoning or prolonged coma due to drug overdosage.

Recent illnesses must be viewed in relation to their effects on cerebral function, in particular hepatic or renal disease which may have led to metabolic disturbance, or infective processes which may have resulted in a cerebral abscess.

Dietary neglect may have produced vitamin B or folic acid deficiency, either as a primary aetiological factor or as a complication of the dementing process. A history of gastrectomy may be especially significant in relation to vitamin B_{12} deficiency.

Alcoholism deserves careful and sometimes pressing

enquiry. The progressive inefficiency and deterioration of habits in alcoholic subjects can present as a possible dementing process, and Korsakoff's syndrome can at first sight be mistaken for global intellectual impairment. The possibility that a true alcoholic dementia may exist is discussed on p. 603. Drug abuse should be suspected when the picture fluctuates from time to time or when there is a history of similar episodes in the past. A history of intravenous drug abuse, or any indications of male homosexuality, will bring the possibility of HIV infection to mind. Medication recently prescribed should also always be determined. In obscure cases the patient's occupation warrants consideration, with enquiry about the possibility of chronic poisoning from lead, manganese or other chemicals.

Finally, attention should be paid to any history of markedly unstable traits in the previous personality, of previous episodes of mental illness, or of conflict situations antedating the onset of the illness. These may be the essential clues to certain cases of pseudodementia.

Certain symptoms are of importance. Headache, visual disturbance or vomiting will raise the possibility of a space-occupying lesion. Epileptic fits, especially with a focal onset, must similarly be noted with care. Other complaints which may indicate focal rather than diffuse cerebral disease include special difficulty with language, trouble in recognising people or objects, or inability to carry out habitual acts and manipulations.

Benson and Cummings (1982) have drawn attention to the 'angular gyrus syndrome' which may easily be confused with Alzheimer's disease on account of the number of features they have in common. Such patients present with posterior aphasia, alexia with agraphia, Gerstmann's syndrome and constructional deficits, usually in consequence of a cerebral infarction. The abrupt onset, if known, will give the clue, likewise the preservation of memory and topographical orientation.

Malaise, loss of energy and anorexia will suggest anaemia, uraemia or occult malignant disease. A cough of recent onset and severe loss of weight will suggest carcinoma of the lung, which can sometimes present with dementia in the absence of secondary cerebral deposits. Sensitivity to cold will immediately raise the possibility of myxoedema, and excessive thirst or bone pain may suggest parathyroid disorder.

The *mode of evolution of the illness* is of great diagnostic importance. Separate note must be taken of the nature of the principal early difficulties, the duration up to the time of presentation, the definiteness or indefiniteness of onset, and the steadiness or otherwise of progression.

An onset with memory disturbance is characteristic of most primary dementias, especially Alzheimer's disease which is the commonest form. In the elderly this may for a time be hard to distinguish from the 'normal' memory difficulties of old age; the dysmnesia of senescence typically progresses very slowly, and occurs in a setting of relative preservation of other cognitive processes, whereas in dementia other aspects of intellect usually soon come to be implicated. Any onset with symptoms other than memory disturbance should always raise suspicion. Marked affective disturbance or change of personality may be seen with Pick's disease, other frontal dementias or Huntington's disease, but may equally be indicative of a frontal lobe tumour or general paresis.

A short duration immediately raises the possibility of a secondary dementia — due to cerebral tumour, covert cerebral infarction, AIDS or some extracranial cause. In most primary dementing illnesses the symptoms are of long duration, usually of many months by the time the patient presents for attention.

A definite date for the onset is also rarely obtained in the primary dementias, which tend to begin so insidiously that neither the patient nor his family can give a precise timing to the earliest manifestations. With cerebral tumours, by contrast, there is usually some episode or symptom which can later be recalled as the first indication of the illness. This information can be important in tumours which are unaccompanied by headache or other evidence of raised intracranial pressure, or, for example, in frontal meningiomas which can present with global dementia and lack all focal signs.

An abrupt onset coupled with neurological defects which later resolve will strongly suggest a cerebrovascular accident. Alvarez (1966) has stressed the importance of 'little strokes' which may lead to intellectual impoverishment yet produce no identifiable focal signs whatever; here the clue is provided by the fact that the disturbance can be traced to a precise point in time. Caution is needed, however, before ascribing the patient's dementia entirely to such causes, and when rapid dementia follows a minute infarct some additional pathological process such as the parenchymal changes of SDAT may be expected to be present as well. Lewy body dementia will be suspected when marked extrapyramidal features precede or follow the dementia, when there are pronounced fluctuations with lucid intervals, or when the patient develops seriously adverse reactions to neuroleptic drugs.

Steady progression without remission is typical of all the primary dementias with the exception of multi-infarct dementia. Marked fluctuations from time to time must therefore immediately suggest that one may be dealing not with a chronic but an acute organic reaction, or at least with an acute component superimposed upon the basic dementing process. Considerable difficulty can sometimes be encountered in differentiating between a subacute organic reaction and dementia, especially multi-infarct dementia. The elderly are unusually vulnerable to the effects of anoxia or metabolic derangements, and the responsible somatic disease may not be very obvious. A markedly intermittent course, with periods of possible clouding or delirium, should therefore be noted with care, and will indicate the need for a survey of the cardiac, pulmonary, renal, hepatic and endocrine systems. Fluctuations and periods of remission will also raise the possibility of a subdural haematoma or drug abuse. An intermittent course with discrete episodes of abnormal behaviour may suggest hypoglycaemia, and when severe this can leave enduring dementia in its wake.

Examination

The *physical examination* is usually much more important than the mental state evaluation in pointing to remediable causes of dementia, or in revealing systemic disorders which may be aggravating the situation. The general appearance may suggest myxoedema or malnutrition. Inspection of the skin and tongue may indicate dehydration, vitamin depletion or anaemia. A patient who looks unwell will be suspected of metabolic disorder, malignant disease or some infective process. Common foci of infection in the elderly include low-grade pneumonia or bronchitis, and in women cystitis. Among younger patients who look unwell AIDS should be suspected. A low-grade intermittent pyrexia may raise the possibility of subacute encephalitis, cerebral abscess, collagen vascular disorder or, on rare occasions, multiple embolisation in association with subacute bacterial endocarditis (Roth 1981). The cardiovascular state always requires appraisal with regard to hypertension, arteriosclerosis, congestive cardiac failure and the patency of the carotid arteries in the neck. In elderly males the possibility of prostatic enlargement should be explored.

The *neurological examination* will rarely reveal marked localising signs in the primary dementias, with the exception of multi-infarct dementia and the rare cases of Creutzfeldt–Jakob disease. Evidence of focal paresis or sensory loss in association with a slowly progressive dementia therefore immediately raises the possibility of a space-occupying lesion. Considerable care must sometimes be taken to exclude visual field defects or unilateral anosmia, which can be difficult in patients who are less than fully cooperative.

Examination of the optic fundi may reveal evidence of raised intracranial pressure. The pupil reactions may betray general paresis, and nystagmus will suggest barbiturate intoxication. A Kayser–Fleischer ring at the corneal margins will indicate Wilson's disease. Pronounced ataxia in association with memory disturbance will suggest the residue of Wernicke's encephalopathy, and peripheral neuropathy will raise the possibility of alcoholism or heavy metal poisoning.

Evidence of dysarthria, minor dysphagia or a brisk jaw jerk may indicate early pseudobulbar palsy, and should be carefully assessed when cerebral arteriosclerosis is suspected.

Early incontinence and unsteadiness of gait are important pointers towards normal-pressure hydrocephalus. Close observation may sometimes be required for the detection of the early choreiform movements of Huntington's disease, and myoclonic jerking in association with dementia will raise the possibility of Creutzfeldt–Jakob disease. Evidence of Parkinson's disease or multiple sclerosis must not be overlooked. The prominent development of parkinsonian features, either early or late in the course, will suggest Lewy body disease. Rigidity, tremor or dystonia in the younger patient will raise suspicion of Wilson's disease.

The *mental state evaluation* is principally directed at establishing the global nature of the intellectual disorder. Care must be taken to avoid mistaking dysphasia, circumscribed amnesic difficulties or parietal lobe symptomatology for global dementia. Somnolence, in the absence of uraemia or other metabolic disorder, will suggest hypothalamic damage. A marked degree of emotional lability with pathological laughing and crying will suggest a vascular process with an accent on the basal regions of the brain. Any suspicion of clouding of consciousness will immediately raise the possibility that one is dealing with an acute organic reaction rather than dementia, or that there is some complicating toxic, infective or metabolic disorder present.

The mental state evaluation is equally important for the detection of pseudodementia. Inconsistencies in the patient's performance may raise the question of a Ganser state, hysterical pseudodementia or even on rare occasions simulation. The patient's attitude to his symptoms and the degree to which his purported disabilities interfere with daily life can be observations of crucial importance. Affective changes sometimes need to be sought out with care. A marked depressive component may indicate depressive pseudodementia, or concurrent depression may be aggravating the situation in a patient with organic cerebral disease. The help that may sometimes be obtained by abreaction in reaching the correct diagnosis is discussed on p. 488. Careful interviewing may reveal schizophrenic symptomatology in the patient who is markedly withdrawn or bizarre in conduct.

Psychometric testing will often be of value (p. 108). It may help in the distinction between organic and non-organic psychiatric illness and with the question of diffuse versus focal cerebral disorder. In very early cases psychometry provides a measured baseline against which future progress can be assessed.

Diogenes' syndrome. Patients are occasionally found to be living in a state of extreme squalor and gross physical neglect, yet prove to be free from any psychiatric disorder sufficient to account for it. In particular their cognitive functions may emerge as relatively or completely intact. This has been designated 'Diogenes' syndrome' or 'senile self neglect', though the nosological status of the condition remains uncertain (Clark *et al.* 1975; Cybulska & Rucinski 1986; Bergmann 1991). Some may be in the early stages of a dementing illness while others appear to be suffering essentially from personality disorder. Quite often such patients prove to be solitary and reclusive individuals who are reacting to stress, bereavement or loneliness. Hoarding rituals may have become entrenched, and serious medical illness or disability is not uncommon.

Orrell *et al.* (1989) have reported marked frontal lobe dysfunction on neuropsychological examination in some instances, raising the possibility that frontal lobe dementia (p. 463) may occasionally be responsible. Reports of such patients underline the need for careful assessment of elderly patients even when first appearances are strongly suggestive of advanced Alzheimer's disease.

Investigations

In the primary dementias there are no specific abnormalities in the blood, urine, cerebrospinal fluid or on skull X-ray. The only exception is Creutzfeldt–Jakob disease where specific changes in the protein of the cerebrospinal fluid have recently been reported (p. 478). Investigations are therefore principally directed at detecting remediable conditions or uncovering systemic disorders which may be worsening the clinical picture.

Every patient with dementia requires the following investigations as a minimum: estimation of haemoglobin, full blood count, erythrocyte sedimentation rate, serological tests for syphilis, blood urea, serum electrolytes, serum proteins and liver function tests. Routine urine examination should be supplemented by microscopy and where necessary culture. Chest X-ray should always be performed for the evaluation of cardiac and pulmonary status and as a screen for primary or secondary carcinoma. Skull X-ray is required for the detection of possible pineal shift or raised intracranial pressure. The EEG should be performed routinely; evidence may emerge to raise suspicion of a focal cerebral disorder, or the pictures seen with the primary dementias may be obtained and give some support to the diagnosis. The latter, however,

lack specificity as discussed in Chapter 3 (p. 131), and must never be relied upon alone. An entirely normal EEG will lead one at least to reconsider the possibility of a pseudodementia.

Where CT scanning is available this should also be carried out routinely, though pressures on services for the elderly may sometimes make this impractical. MRI will give even greater information. Special indications for scanning will include any remote suspicion of a cerebral tumour or subdural haematoma, the presence of focal neurological signs, a history suggestive of cerebral infarction or head injury, or clinical pointers towards normal-pressure hydrocephalus. In the primary dementias cerebral atrophy will be revealed in a high proportion of cases, with ventricular dilatation and prominence of cortical sulci but without distortion or displacement of the ventricular system. The distribution of atrophy may point towards a diagnosis of Pick's disease or other frontal dementia (pp. 461 and 463), or marked shrinkage of the heads of the caudate nuclei may indicate Huntington's disease (p. 470). Evidence of old and recent cerebral infarctions may suggest a vascular basis for the dementia. Sometimes, however, the CT or MRI scan may be entirely normal, especially in early cases, and conversely some degree of atrophy may be found in persons not suffering from dementia. The results can be interpreted only in conjunction with the total clinical findings, and the latter must be given precedence when discordant results emerge. The question of the significance of cerebral atrophy as revealed by brain imaging is discussed further in Chapter 3 (p. 138 *et seq.*).

Bradshaw *et al.* (1983) investigated the yield from CT scanning in 500 consecutive patients referred with suspected dementia over an 18-month period. Most had evidence of atrophy or infarction, but 82 (16%) had entirely normal scans. Forty-two patients (8%) had tumours, six hydrocephalus and four subdural haematomas. Thus 10% had potentially treatable conditions, and this represented 5% of those without symptoms such as headache and without focal neurological signs. The yield of treatable conditions was as high in those over 65 as in younger age groups.

Sometimes it will be advantageous to supplement CT or MRI with the functional imaging techniques of SPECT or even PET. In patients suspected of very early dementia, or when the differential diagnosis from depressive pseudodementia is uncertain, the demonstration of characteristic patterns of regional brain hypometabolism can add important information. Posterior parietotemporal deficits in regional blood flow or metabolism, though not pathognomonic, may add to a suspicion of Alzheimer's dementia (p. 434), while sharply circumscribed frontal deficits may indicate Pick's disease (p. 462). The value of SPECT in delineating 'dementia of the frontal lobe type' is described on p. 464, and the use of SPECT and PET in relation to

Huntington's disease on pp. 470–1. Functional imaging techniques will rarely be used clinically to differentiate Alzheimer's disease from multi-infarct dementia, though there are indications that they could be superior to MRI for such a purpose (Ebmeier *et al.* 1987).

Further tests will very often be required and many clinicians will wish to include several of the following as routine when facilities are available: estimation of serum B_{12}, folate, sugar, T_3 and T_4, cholesterol, lipids, calcium, phosphorus and barbiturate levels. Serum protein electrophoresis may be indicated, also immunoglobulin assay and the estimation of antinuclear antibodies. The electrocardiogram may show evidence of dysrhythmia, heart block or recent myocardial infarction. When a vascular dementia is suspected further tests may include coagulation studies, Doppler ultrasonography of the carotids and echocardiography. Guidance to the choice of these more extended investigations will have been obtained from the history and clinical examination.

Lumbar puncture should be undertaken if the cause for the dementia remains uncertain and when there is no reason to suspect a cerebral tumour or raised intracranial pressure. Examination of the cerebrospinal fluid can be decisive in the diagnosis of general paresis in cases when the blood serology has been negative. Dementia can also occur with syphilitic arteritis which has produced scattered cerebral infarcts. The first indication of a subdural haematoma may come from an elevated cerebrospinal fluid pressure, increased protein or xanthochromia. Subacute and chronic forms of encephalitis may likewise be detected only after examination of the fluid.

In most cases of primary dementia the cerebrospinal fluid is entirely normal. It has been uniformly normal in autopsy-proven cases of Alzheimer's disease, though occasionally the protein may be elevated in Creutzfeldt–Jakob disease and sometimes in cases of multi-infarct dementia when there has been a recent cerebral infarction, uraemia or congestive cardiac failure. A positive immunoassay for protein 14-3-3 appears to be highly specific for Creutzfeldt–Jakob disease in the presence of dementia (p. 478).

Most of the above procedures cause relatively little discomfort or inconvenience and are readily carried out. The chief difficulty usually arises when CT scanning is not available and a decision must be made about further radiological procedures which are upsetting to the patient. Echoencephalography may be undertaken as a screening test for focal brain lesions, or alternatively a radioisotope scan. But arteriography or air encephalography may then be needed, the latter remaining definitive for excluding a cerebral tumour or normal-pressure hydrocephalus.

Air encephalography will be required for the complete investigation of younger demented patients in the absence of facilities for a CT scan; in the elderly, however, it must be performed more circumspectly, especially when the physical condition is poor. When all other evidence is consonant with a primary dementing process, and there is no focal component to the clinical picture, it will usually be judged unwarranted to subject a frail and elderly person to the distress of the investigation.

The further investigations required when normal-pressure hydrocephalus is strongly suspected — for example intracranial pressure monitoring — are discussed on p. 746.

Very occasionally it will be deemed advisable to exclude other rare conditions which can give rise to dementia. Wilson's disease is detected by the estimation of serum caeruloplasmin and confirmed by liver biopsy (p. 663). Neuroacanthocytosis requires the examination of fresh blood films (p. 757) and metachromatic leucodystrophy the estimation of arylsulphatase-A in the blood or urine, or biopsies of the peripheral nerve or rectal wall (p. 759). Kufs' disease is detectable by skeletal muscle or rectal biopsy (p. 760), Whipple's disease by lymph node or jejunal biopsy (p. 760), and mitochondrial myopathies by a search for 'ragged red fibres' in skeletal muscle biopsy. A search for sarcoid may involve X-ray of the phalanges, biopsy of the lymph nodes or skin lesions, and the Kveim intradermal test (p. 763). When Creutzfeldt–Jakob disease or the Gerstmann–Sträussler syndrome are suspected it can be valuable to screen the patient for characteristic prion gene mutations (pp. 474–5). Tonsillar biopsy, examined by immunohistochemistry and Western blot analysis, has recently been proposed as a means of identifying the abnormal prion protein in Creutzfeldt–Jakob disease, and may prove to be of value in allowing early clinical or possibly preclinical diagnosis of the condition (Hill *et al.* 1997). For the diagnosis of granulomatous angiitis of the nervous system (p. 424) angiography will usually be essential, followed by cerebral biopsy.

Other than this, cerebral biopsy is rarely used as an aid to diagnosis. Changes typical of Alzheimer's disease may be revealed, or on rare occasions Creutzfeldt–Jakob disease or subacute encephalitis may be discovered. Short of cerebral biopsy there are very few investigatory procedures which can give information of much value in differentiating one form of primary dementing illness from another, but in the present state of knowledge such distinctions are of little practical value to the patient.

Neary *et al.* (1986a) report experience in carrying out biopsies in 24 patients with presenile dementia, 20 from the right temporal lobe and four from the right frontal lobe. One patient showed transient weakness of the left arm, resolving over 7 days, and eight showed postoperative confusion resolving over 1–7 days in all but one case. The latter patient, aged 69 and the oldest of the series, continued to have fluctuating confusion over the ensuing months. Neuropsychological ratings showed that all except this patient had regained their previous levels of functioning prior to discharge from hospital.

On return home the relatives of four out of 20 patients reported deterioration early on, two with subsequent improvement. This was matched by two similar reports by relatives of 20 patients who had not been biopsied. Five patients had infrequent epileptic seizures, occurring 2 months, 1 year and 3 years postoperatively, and not requiring long-term anticonvulsants. Follow-up at 6-monthly intervals in a subsample gave no suggestion of acceleration of cognitive decline.

The procedure was considered safe when patients were carefully selected as being physically well, when a minimal time was spent under anaesthesia and when minimal samples were taken. It should be noted, however, that Neary *et al.*'s patients were relatively young, with ages ranging from 43 to 69 years.

If future research should bring promising leads in the treatment of individual conditions, biopsy may ultimately become better justified and more widely practised.

Management of the senile and presenile dementias

The first step in management is always full medical evaluation along the lines already discussed. This is necessary for the firm establishment of the diagnosis, the exclusion of remediable conditions which have masqueraded as primary dementia, and to check on any concurrent disease which may be aggravating the symptoms. In cases where the first evaluation has given equivocal results this must be borne in mind during follow-up, with readiness to reopen investigations if the course is in any way unusual.

Early problems in management

After establishing the diagnosis, both the disease and the person suffering from it must be kept in mind. In early cases, particularly of presenile dementia, difficult decisions will often have to be made over such questions as continuation with work and how fully to explain about prognosis. On both issues much will depend on factors specific to the individual and his family.

Continuation with employment may occasionally be possible for a surprising length of time when the work makes little demand on the intellect and social competence is preserved. Simple assembly work, for example, may continue to be feasible even though memory lapses are occurring in unfamiliar situations. Unfortunately, however, it is often in the field of work that the earliest evidence of the disease has emerged. Certainly work involving responsibility or the need for informed decisions should be terminated as soon as the diagnosis is unequivocally established.

A housewife may continue to cope for some considerable time with the help of simple props and tactful aid from other members of the family. Advice at a very simple level, such as the provision of shopping lists or the setting aside of more time for routine tasks, may delay the point when independence must be relinquished. Regular visits from a friendly neighbour during the day can similarly be invaluable.

On the question of prognosis there is usually little to be gained by attempting to explain this in detail to the patient. Often he will not raise the subject at all; quite commonly the difficulty is in trying to persuade him that something is amiss and that an alteration is needed in his way of life. Some simple formula is usually most appropriate and kindest to the patient, telling him for example that 'there appears to be some trouble which has caused your memory to be faulty, and we are going to try to remedy it'. More detailed explanations are likely to be forgotten. If, however, the affective tone of the consultation is gloomy this may well persist and colour the patient's attitude to his disability.

With the relatives it will usually be necessary to be entirely frank, particularly if long-term family decisions are to be made. Here again, much will depend on a sensitive appreciation of the nature of the person who will have to bear responsibility for the patient. Some will genuinely want to know the outlook, others will find it easier to learn about it gradually from the course of events. Since one cannot hope to be accurate it is wise and humane to err in the direction of too favourable rather than too pessimistic a forecast; the latter may needlessly destroy morale just when it is most needed in the earlier phases of the disorder. Thus it is reasonable to emphasise the variability in the rate of progress of such disorders from one patient to another, and to stress that one must wait to observe what course is followed in each particular example.

It is important, if the point is pressed, to emphasise how commonly the patient's own appreciation of his decline becomes blunted with the progress of the disease.

Finally, an issue that should be addressed as early as possible concerns the establishment of Power of Attorney, whereby the patient's financial affairs are placed in the hands of another. The timing of such a step and its explanation to the patient can require much tact and care. The common form of Power of Attorney loses its force when the person who created it becomes incapable mentally, but provisions are now available to draw up an Enduring Power of Attorney (EPA) which outlasts such complications. MacFarlane (1988) and Jacoby (1996) discuss the issues involved. In the absence of an EPA drawn up at a time when the patient is still capable of understanding its nature and effect, it will eventually be necessary to apply to the Court of Protection (in England and Wales) to appoint a receiver when the patient becomes incapable of managing his affairs; this is a more cumbersome and costly procedure. The important question of testamentary capacity in relation to the drawing up of a Will is discussed by Jacoby and Bergmann (1996).

Social work care

The management of the dementing patient and his family is an area in which the social worker can give a great deal of help. At a practical level maintenance in employment may be secured for a while. An understanding employer may be persuaded to make allowances, or to readjust the nature of the demands made upon the patient. When gainful occupation is no longer feasible attendance at a day centre may be arranged, improving at the same time the morale of the patient and the family.

Among the elderly, in particular, it will often be necessary to exploit community resources to the full, with provision of home helps, 'meals on wheels' or domiciliary laundry services. The assistance of community nurses or health visitors may be required. Voluntary organisations can provide invaluable help, such as the local branches of the Alzheimer's Disease Society, Age Concern or the National Association for Mental Health (MIND). Informal church and community groups are often well placed to give support. These will more readily offer help when a social worker is at hand to advise and coordinate activities. Much will depend on knowledge of what is available in the vicinity.

In addition, and very importantly, the family can be helped in their own understanding and management of the patient. It is important to explain in some detail the nature of the patient's disabilities and the areas in which he is liable to fail. The need to avoid sudden changes of surroundings and routines should always be stressed, and the family's natural inclination to take the patient for a holiday or complete change of scene must sometimes be discouraged. A proper appreciation of the causes of failure and of aberrant behaviour will do much to relieve the onlooker's distress. Unhelpful attitudes of irritability or hostility towards the patient may be prevented, likewise attitudes of excessive compassion and concern. Again valuable support and advice can be obtained by relatives from the Alzheimer's Disease Society in the UK (or the Alzheimer's Disease and Related Disorders Association in the USA). Many families and carers will benefit from the

detailed practical advice on the management of day-to-day problems contained in the guides now increasingly available, for example those by Mace and Rabins (1981), Gilleard (1984), Jacques (1988) and Lay and Woods (1989). The effectiveness of a simple practical guide in reducing levels of stress among carers was shown by Toner (1987).

Macmillan (1960) has discussed the common progression seen in the families of elderly demented patients, whereby responsibility is at first willingly accepted but later this becomes increasingly irksome. A similar pattern may be discerned with presenile dementia. A state of partial rejection ultimately develops, and this may suddenly become intensified by some stressful incident such as wandering away, soiling or an outburst of paranoid hostility. The situation can be greatly ameliorated by ongoing social work support, and the need for institutionalisation may then be considerably delayed. It is important, however, that the family should know that when it is finally necessary, admission to some form of long-term care will be arranged. Temporary respite admissions may also help the family to cope, or better still attendance at a day centre from an early stage.

The burden experienced by families caring for a demented relative has come under detailed scrutiny in several important reports (Argyle *et al.* 1985; Eagles *et al.* 1987; Gilleard 1987; Levin 1991; Levin *et al.* 1994). Among the behavioural problems which tax carers most severely are restlessness by day, sleeplessness, aggression, wandering, incontinence and impairment of communication. Such strains have been shown to be decisively reduced when there is adequate access to domiciliary services, day care and periodic respite admissions.

When the patient can no longer be managed at home optimal placement must be arranged. Much will depend on local facilities and the extent to which social, psychiatric and geriatric services have become organised. Preparation should ideally be made well in advance of the time when this is likely to be required, though this is not always possible. Alternatives to hospitalisation will often suffice, since after full evaluation and attention to remediable abnormalities most patients need little by way of direct medical attention. The more expensive models of hospital care are not always optimal and may sometimes be counterproductive; small homely units may do more to maintain self-help skills and delay total dependence. A residential home for the elderly or a nursing home is often ideal. Sheltered accommodation for married couples is sometimes a possibility. The needs of different patients are widely variable, and should ideally be matched by a similarly broad range of resources.

Huntington's disease presents particular problems and

challenges for social work care, not least on account of the dread of the disorder among as yet unaffected relatives. Martindale and Bottomley (1980) illustrate some of the issues involved in the long-term counselling of patients and their families. Self-help groups — the Huntington's Disease Association in the UK and the Committee to Combat Huntington's Disease in the USA—provide valuable support and information about services available in addition to funding research.

Psychological aspects of management

In the early stages supportive care can do much to help the patient. A positive relationship with a physician or general practitioner has an important part to play in alleviating distress, and while insight is retained the patient should not be made to feel abandoned. Skilled help may be required to enable him to reach a new adjustment and to persuade him to relinquish tasks which are no longer possible. The aim must be to achieve such things without a catastrophic lowering of self esteem.

Kennedy (1959a) describes how dementing patients commonly develop a sense of ill-formulated inferiority, and react thereto in a variety of ways. Intimate knowledge of the patient and of his style of coping can often help to avert, or at least defer, the more florid forms of reaction.

Some patients tend to react by what Kennedy describes as 'dependent decline', with greater than necessary dependence on those around and premature abdication of responsibility. Others react by 'defensive limitation' with restriction of activities, hoarding of material assets, suspicious attitudes and self isolation. Others 'overcompensate', becoming interfering and dogmatic, and tend to dwell on the past with insistent repetition of anecdotes. Some 'retreat from reality', with refusal to retire from work. 'Projective decline' involves the blaming of others for mistakes and transgressions, and in more florid form extends to the development of frank paranoid delusions. Other forms of maladaptation involve egocentric demanding behaviour, exaggeration of deafness or immobility, reactive depression, hypochondriasis or paranoia.

Of central importance is the handling the patient receives from those in daily contact with him, whether members of his family, nurses or occupational therapists. Wells (1971b) usefully distinguishes three aims in management—the restitution of lost functions, the reduction of the patient's need for functions irretrievably impaired, and the optimal utilisation of those which remain.

The first, the *restitution of lost functions*, is unfortunately rarely possible. It is largely a matter of medical treatment (as discussed below) with measures to promote optimal physical health and some rather dubious benefits which may accrue from certain drugs. But with the others—the reduction of need for functions lost and the optimal use of those which remain—considerable headway can be made by skilled and tactful interaction with the patient.

Reduction of need for functions lost. An accurate assessment of functions irretrievably lost is essential, so that the patient may be steered away from attempts to perform impossible tasks. Immediate stress is often the cause of anxiety, outbursts of aggression or paranoid reactions. An anonymous author writing in the *Lancet* (Lancet 1950) describes with great sensitivity her interactions with her dementing father, and how the origin of illusions, delusions and episodes of grossly disturbed behaviour could be helped by the correct approach:

'He was still potentially rational. His delusions were not determined by a warped mental outlook, but were a reasonable attempt to make sense out of what was subjectively a hopelessly confusing situation. In days gone by I had learned to follow his train of thought intuitively, and could still keep close to him in spite of his difficulty with speech. I found that if I got him away from other people and steered his mind to topics which he had handled with ease in the past he became rational quite quickly. I sometimes led him into interesting discussions on subjects which he knew and cared about, and when he got the sense of being on familiar ground, where he could still tread firmly, the black cloud of depression lifted and he became his old self. As soon as he returned to the strain of new and unfamiliar situations he relapsed.'

Thus whenever possible conversation should be restricted to subjects within the patient's capability, and his own leads should be followed rather than venturing upon new topics. New and disturbing experiences should be kept to a minimum, and the daily routine structured as simply as possible. Extra time must be set aside for necessary tasks, preferably with someone at hand to remind the patient what to do and how to do it.

The environment should be manipulated as far as possible to maintain calm and non-taxing surroundings, and matters arranged so that the patient is rarely confronted by his inadequacies. Things frequently required can be placed prominently and near at hand. The disposition of furniture in the room should not be changed, and a clock and a calendar should be hung conspicuously on the wall. It may be helpful to label the lavatory with a printed notice. Goldfarb (1972) discusses the ordered use of such props and supports; the more protective the setting the less will be the occasions on which the patient's autonomy and self esteem are challenged.

Williams (1956) showed experimentally that in dealing with demented patients the provision of extra cues can help to maintain behaviour at an improved level. Such cues may be the repetition of orders or the supplementing of instructions by visual example. What the patient lacks is often not so much the ability to behave in a fitting manner, as the ability to select or abstract what is relevant from all the information available. Thus in Williams' experiments the performance of patients could often improve on tests of perception, or even of intellectual activity, when they were supplied with additional cues or helped to focus attention upon those cues normally available.

Clearly these requirements will at some point be better met in a hospital or nursing home than in the patient's own home. The strain imposed on the family should not be allowed to continue too long on the false assumption that he will be happier there. Skilled supervision ultimately becomes essential, and in the correct milieu these principles of management can be carried out much more effectively and extensively. The nurse or attendant must be prepared to repeat instructions, explain the surroundings with a minimum of words, repeatedly say who he or she is and become the focal point around whom the patient can orientate his thoughts (Kennedy 1959a). Again the environment should be stabilised as far as possible, with the minimum of changes of staff. Strong multi-colour decorations may help to improve orientation. Similarly, the patient should be allowed to have familiar possessions around him.

The *optimal use of residual functions* is a separate aim. The patient should be encouraged to continue with social activities and to take regular exercise. Adequate periods of rest must be interspersed with gentle urging towards activity. His surroundings should be stimulating within his restricted range of abilities and despite the need for constancy. Without this the patient's own diminished self motivation can easily lead to underutilisation of faculties which remain.

Occupational therapy requires a careful selection of tasks in order to avert frustration and help in the readaptation of the failing brain. The skill lies in helping towards disengagement from work beyond the patient's capabilities, and guidance towards substitute activities which are still within his range. It is thus the reverse of the common aims of occupational therapy in patients who are being rehabilitated for work. Simple domestic tasks are often most fitting, or repetitive craft work which can give a sense of achievement without making demands on intellect or memory.

Attempts must be made to combat social isolation. Continuing ties with the family should be encouraged, even when admission to long-term care has become necessary. Socialisation may be fostered and communication improved by conjoint tasks and group activities. Simple games, quizzes and assembly work in groups can be of considerable benefit.

Cosin *et al.* (1958) were able to demonstrate the effectiveness of simple occupational and social activities in improving, at least in the short term, the general level of behaviour of elderly patients with dementia. Domestic activities, particularly when involving cooperation with others, produced the most noticeable stimulation and satisfaction. Bower (1967) similarly reported the effects of an enriched environment in slowing, or even reversing, outward evidence of the dementing process for a time.

'*Reality orientation*' and related programmes of management have been introduced in many centres where the long-term care of demented patients is undertaken. Such enterprises hinge largely on the principles outlined above, but seek to involve the staff in regularly prescribed periods of intensive interaction with the patients. These in turn have the aim of stimulating the patient into reusing neglected patterns of functioning, of reorienting him to his environment and of restoring a sense of purpose and identity.

Informal reality orientation involves only the day-to-day interactions between staff and patients; repeated opportunities are taken to remind the patient who and where he is, of the time and day, and of what is happening around him. The repeated communications with the patient must be slow, clear and direct. In effect he relearns then continually rehearses essential items of information. More formal treatment takes place in groups, occupying perhaps half an hour per day and usually in a specially set-aside room. Here stimulating materials are kept to hand, with large colourful illustrations of everyday objects and the day, month and year clearly displayed to view. During reality orientation sessions the patients are encouraged to greet one another, rehearse names and dates, identify objects, and where possible discuss outstanding items of news. A daily diary of basic information may be kept, followed by spelling and counting games and simple group activities. The precise techniques adopted must be geared to the levels of ability of the patients concerned.

Brook *et al.* (1975) have described the effectiveness of sessions such as these in improving socialisation in the ward and sometimes even in diminishing incontinence. The active engagement of the therapists with the patients was shown to be important for success. Woods (1979) compared reality orientation sessions with unstructured discussion groups in which equivalent staff attention was given, and found that the former led to greater improvement on tests of information, orientation and memory. In general, however, the gains from treatment tend to be small and evanescent, and improvements in cognitive function usually prove to be closely tied to the content of the training sessions. Generalisation to other aspects of behaviour and to other situations has often been disappointing in the long-term view. Powell-Proctor and Miller (1982) provide a comprehensive review of the techniques and the benefits which may be expected.

Other procedures include '*reminiscence group therapy*', in which patients are specifically encouraged to engage in familiar over-learned activities, listen to familiar music and re-enact well-practised social situations. Bewilderment may be lessened and group cohesion improved. Reminiscence therapy with the individual patient usefully concentrates on rehearsing details of past life events, or working with family photograph albums and personal memorabilia.

Miller (1977) and Woods and Britton (1977) review further specialised treatment approaches, including attempts at behavioural modification by token economy regimes. All share common factors, including the active participation of both staff and patients, the need for a consistent approach, and the desirability of near-continuous operation if maximal gains are to be achieved. The importance of these newer treatment approaches lies in the demonstration that dementing patients are capable of responding to properly structured interactions with those who care for them, and hopefully thereby of attaining improvement in the quality of their day-to-day existence.

Medical aspects of management

Medical aspects of care can assume importance in a high proportion of patients. Optimal physical health must be maintained if the patient's deterioration is to be slowed and the best use made of residual functions at any given stage. Attention to adequate nutrition, hydration and vitamin replacement can sometimes meet with gratifying improvement. The elimination of infection is a matter for repeated checks, particularly chronic infection within the lungs or urinary tract. Any tendency towards congestive cardiac failure, cardiac dysrhythmia or anaemia must be treated energetically. Hypertension, when severe, will warrant appropriate management. Special care must be taken to guard against iatrogenic disorders, particularly electrolyte imbalance due to diuretics and toxicity from other drugs.

In multi-infarct dementia there will often be a special case for strict control of hypertension, and sometimes for treatment with anticoagulants or aspirin to guard against embolisation. Other vascular risk factors such as hypercholesterolaemia or diabetes will need special attention. Vasculitis may require treatment with corticosteroids.

Adequate physical exercise must be encouraged, sometimes with the aid of physiotherapy. Orthopaedic complications may need attention in the elderly. Adequate daily activity will induce normal fatigue and lessen the incidence of disturbed and restless nights. It will also help defer the time when nursing in bed, and hence the terminal stages, are reached.

Psychotropic medication will often be needed to allay agitation and depression. In general, however, one will wish to avoid using drugs with strong anticholinergic effects for prolonged periods of time, in view of the known cholinergic deficits in Alzheimer's disease. Phenothiazines may transform the problems of management in a disturbed

and restless patient, and paranoid symptoms may lose distressing force and intensity. Unlike barbiturates, phenothiazines are relatively safe among elderly and brain-damaged subjects and less likely to aggravate confusion. A very small dose of haloperidol can be useful for short periods of time. Antidepressant and anxiolytic drugs can also be effective, especially in multi-infarct dementia where emotional instability and depression are particularly common.

For sedation at night chloral hydrate, chloral betaine (Welldorm), promethazine (Phenergan) or temazepam are greatly preferable to barbiturates or nitrazepam. Chlormethiazole (Heminevrin) can also be employed. Pearce and Miller (1973) make the further important point that restlessness and insomnia are often prompted by pain, and simple analgesics are more effective than hypnotics if a painful hip, knee or back is keeping the patient awake. Similarly, faecal impaction or a distended bladder may require attention and should be borne in mind when agitation appears without obvious cause.

Alzheimer's disease

Specific drug treatment, aimed at delaying the degenerative process or improving cognitive performance, has so far proved to be disappointing. Numerous claims have been made, but to date no substance has proved its worth in routine clinical practice. Where gains have been reported these appear to have been evanescent and usually small in degree. The more enthusiastic reports have often been from uncontrolled or poorly controlled investigations, and of course even severely demented subjects will demonstrate placebo effects when exposed to increased attention, encouragement and stimulation. Nevertheless, there is a place for trying the effects of some of the less expensive preparations, certainly in the early stages and even if for little more than the benefit of their placebo effects. The development of cholinergic enhancement therapies, described on p. 503 *et seq.*, currently appears to hold promise of modest success in certain patients, and this approach warrants continuing exploration and refinement. The other lines of treatment which have had their vogue are reviewed by Kopelman and Lishman (1986), Drug and Therapeutics Bulletin (1990) and Whalley and Bailey (1994).

High potency vitamin preparations have been advocated enthusiastically from time to time. Krawiecki *et al.* (1957) reported memory improvement after intramuscular Parentrovite in a double-blind study on elderly patients with dementia, as well as some increase in activity, spontaneity and interest.

Ribonucleic acid has been given in attempts to encourage cell regeneration and revival. Improvements have been claimed in patients with dementia, especially vascular dementia (Cameron & Solyom 1961; Cameron 1963; Cameron *et al.* 1963). Memory, self care and emotional stability were said to improve. However, a carefully controlled attempt to reproduce these findings was not successful (Nodine *et al.* 1967). Magnesium pemoline is another interesting substance thought to act as a catalyst to RNA and said to assist learning in small animals. This too has been reported to lead to improvement in dementia (Cameron 1967), but the situation is again far from clearly established.

Anticoagulants have sometimes been advocated (Walsh 1969a, 1969b) but their value is unproven. Moreover they are associated with risk of haemorrhage, particularly in the elderly.

Hyperoxygenation has attracted interest as a result of the work of Jacobs *et al.* (1969). Thirteen elderly demented patients were exposed to oxygen under 2.5 atmospheres of pressure, for 90 minutes twice a day for 15 days. A double-blind crossover trial showed significant improvements in psychological test scores and ward behaviour, persisting well beyond the increase of Po_2 in the blood or tissues. Similar findings were reported in less severely affected out-patients by Edwards and Hart (1974). Thompson *et al.* (1976), however, found entirely negative results.

Central nervous system stimulants have been tried in small groups of patients. Pentylenetetrazol (Metrazol) was shown to increase visual discrimination learning in mice, bringing renewed interest to its use in geriatric patients. Prien (1973) listed the many studies in humans, some finding beneficial effects and others not. Leckman *et al.* (1971) reported the only controlled trial with a trend towards positive results where intellectual functions are concerned. Rather more positive findings have emerged with pipradol (Meretran), though this has been less extensively evaluated. Turek *et al.* (1969) showed in a controlled trial that it produced significant improvement in ward behaviour among hospitalised elderly patients with dementia.

Attention was turned to *vasopressin* when De Wied showed its role in relation to memory in the rat (De Wied & van Ree 1982; De Wied 1984). The administration of vasopressin analogues to patients with dementia has, however, proved disappointing, with any beneficial effects attributable to enhanced mood and attention rather than to improved cognition *per se* (Kaye *et al.* 1982; Peabody *et al.* 1986). Other neuropeptides such as analogues of somatostatin and adrenocorticotrophic hormone have also proved disappointing (Whalley & Bailey 1994).

Other treatments discussed by Villa and Ciompi (1968) include procaine and novocaine injections, pyrithoxin (Encephabol), the nucleosides cytidine and uridine, and *meclofenoxate* (centrophenoxine, clofenoxine, ANP$_{235}$, Lucidril). The last has been shown to bring about the disappearance of the lipofuscin granules which accompany age changes in the neurones of the guinea-pig (Nandy & Bourne 1966; Nandy 1968), and there are reports that in senile patients it may reduce confusion, apathy and memory disturbance. Gedye *et al.* (1972) showed a small but significant improvement with meclofenoxate on an automated learning task in a small group of patients with mild to moderate dementia. Other drugs with similar actions on lipofuscin deposition include kavain and magnesium orotate (Lancet 1970). So far the value of all these agents remains unproven.

More recently, low dosage of L-*deprenyl* (selegiline) at a level which selectively inhibits monoamine oxidase B, has been reported to help in terms of mood, activity and social interaction, this being accompanied by improved performance on a cognitive task reflecting sustained effort (Tariot *et al.* 1987). The non-steroidal anti-inflammatory drug, *indomethacin*, has been reported to slow decline in cognitive function in a small preliminary study (Rogers *et al.* 1993), likewise *nimodipine*, a calcium channel blocker (Van Rooijen *et al.* 1995).

A large number of *vasodilator substances* have been tried, both in vascular and other forms of dementia. Two in particular, cyclandelate and Hydergine, have been subjected to careful studies. *Cyclandelate* (Cyclospasmol) was used in a double-blind crossover trial by Fine *et al.* (1970) on 40 elderly patients with dementia considered to be due to cerebral arteriosclerosis. Significant improvements were observed in orientation, communication and socialisation. Young *et al.* (1974), in a similar trial on patients with vascular dementia, found slight improvements in memory, apraxia and certain subtests of the Wechsler Adult Intelligence Scale (WAIS), and concluded that a modest but real gain in ability to cope with everyday life was achieved. Davies *et al.* (1977), however, were unable to confirm such benefits. It appears that the drug increases cortical perfusion rates, and there are claims that it brings about a redistribution of blood flow to especially ischaemic areas.

Hydergine is the proprietary name for a combination of several hydrogenated ergot alkaloids. Several double-blind trials on patients with vascular dementia and SDAT have indicated significant improvements in mood and attitude, self care and the relief of physical symptoms such as anorexia, dizziness and incoordination (Gerin 1969; Triboletti & Ferri 1969; Banen 1972). Improvement in cognitive functioning has been less consistently reported, but there have been claims of improved alertness, memory and orientation (Ditch *et al.* 1971; Jennings 1972; Rao & Norris 1972). Roubicek *et al.* (1972) noted concurrent improvement in EEG patterns. However, in a study by Thompson *et al.* (1990) the possibility of adverse effects on cognition and behaviour was raised. Yesavage *et al.* (1979) and Wittenborn (1981) provide further reviews. Hydergine is thought to improve neuronal metabolism through its influence on enzyme systems, thereby increasing cerebral blood flow as a secondary effect.

Naftidrofuryl (Praxilene) is another vasodilator which has attracted some favourable reports (Drug & Therapeutics Bulletin 1972). Judge and Urquhart (1972) carried out a double-blind trial on geriatric patients with severe intellectual impairment, and found improved scores on certain tests of cognitive function but no benefit on activities of daily living or recent memory. Gerin (1974) found improved social behaviour and memory in a small group of patients with cerebral arteriosclerosis. A review of subsequent studies in demented patients has failed to find clear evidence of benefit (Drug & Therapeutics Bulletin 1988a).

In Europe *piracetam* (1-acetamide-2-pyrrolidine, Nootropil), a cyclical derivative of GABA, has been widely promoted for use in dementia, largely on the basis of observed effects in animals. It has been shown to improve animal learning, to protect from anoxia and to increase the amplitude of transcallosal evoked potentials, thus possibly enhancing associative cognitive functioning. Controlled trials in patients with dementia have produced equivocal results, some indicating improvement and some showing no benefit whatever (Gustafson *et al.* 1978). It is possible that it may have some stimulant effect on attention and memory in mildly affected patients (Reisberg *et al.* 1981), and recent studies (see below) suggest that it may enhance the effects of choline when the two are given together.

Cholinergic treatment has attracted a good deal of attention following the demonstration that cholinergic transmission is profoundly affected in Alzheimer's disease (p. 444). Measures designed to augment brain acetylcholine levels have been pursued with vigour, especially since it seems that the cholinergic receptors are largely intact. There is evidence, moreover, that the cholinergic system is important in relation to memory functions even in healthy persons, giving added weight to its relevance in dementia:

Drachman and Leavitt (1974) found that central cholinergic blockade with scopolamine impaired learning and retention in normal subjects, producing deficits similar to those seen in aged drug-free controls. Sitaram *et al.* (1978) confirmed this, and also showed that the learning of word lists was slightly but significantly enhanced after orally administered choline or injected arecholine. Mohs *et al.* (1979) demonstrated similar improvement in the memory of healthy volunteers during the slow intravenous infusion of physostigmine, an anticholinesterase which crosses the blood–brain barrier and impedes the breakdown of brain acetylcholine. All such effects are slight and transient, but illustrate how manipulation of the central cholinergic system can influence memory processes.

Unfortunately, however, attempts at remedying the cholinergic deficits in patients with Alzheimer's disease have so far met with only limited success. The various strategies employed are summarised by Levy (1994). Substrate loading has been tried with choline, lecithin (phosphatidyl choline) and acetylcarnitine; trials of cholinergic agonists have involved deanol, arecoline and RS86; other means for enhancing acetylcholine production include nerve growth factor, the beta carbolines, and the 5-HT$_3$ inhibitor odansetron. Acetylcholinesterase inhibitors have included physostigmine, tetrahydroaminoacridine, and more recently donepezil and velnacrine. These last approaches appear to hold most promise of success.

The numerous trials reported in Corkin *et al.* (1982) showed that little benefit could be expected from feeding choline or lecithin. Sporadic improvements were sometimes observed but were generally minor in degree. Greater effectiveness was sometimes achieved when choline and piracetam were given together (Friedman *et al.* 1981; Ferris *et al.* 1982). In Little *et al.*'s (1985) lecithin trial favourable results were obtained only in older subjects whose biochemical deficits are known to be largely restricted to the cholinergic system. Livingston *et al.*'s (1991) trial of acetyl-l-carnitine showed possible slight gains in those taking the active preparation.

Among choline agonists, dimethylaminoethanol (Deanol) has given essentially negative results (Worral & Dewhurst 1979). RS86 has proved to be toxic, and arecoline has shown limited benefit even when introduced directly into the ventricles (Harbaugh *et al.* 1984). Trials of nerve growth factor face similar problems of administration (see below). The beta carbolines and odansetron are currently under investigation in full-scale clinical trials.

Physostigmine infusions were shown at an early stage to yield short-term benefit on memory (Smith & Swash 1980; Davis & Mohs 1982), but not in a manner that could be useful therapeutically. Nevertheless such results served to focus attention on the use of acetylcholinesterase inhibitors. Frequent 2-hourly dosage of physostigmine by mouth was shown to give some benefit (Thal *et al.* 1983; Beller *et al.* 1985), and longer-lasting oral acetylcholinesterase inhibitors were accordingly sought out.

A trial of such a substance (*tetrahydroaminoacridine, THA, tacrine*) on 17 patients attracted widespread interest when marked therapeutic benefit was claimed (Summers *et al.* 1986). In addition to improvements on global assessment and tests of orientation and name-learning, worthwhile changes were reported in activities of daily living. Dramatic improvements were reported among 12 patients on long-term treatment, one patient resuming most of her home-making tasks, another golf and another part-time employment. No serious side effects were encountered.

However, the trial was severely criticised on several grounds—unclear methodological details, the inclusion of non-blinded results, the use of concurrent medication and the validity of the assessment procedures employed (Herrmann *et al.* 1987; Kopelman 1987c; Pirozzolo *et al.* 1987; Small *et al.* 1987; Tariot & Caine 1987). Further careful trials have followed, with less dramatic though sometimes modestly favourable results. The problems to be surmounted in achieving adequate evaluations have proved to be considerable, and paradoxically some of the negative results may also be traced to troubles with trial design (e.g. Chatellier & Lacomblez 1990; Gauthier *et al.* 1990).

The Maudsley Hospital study (Eagger *et al.* 1991a, 1991b, 1992; Eagger & Levy 1992) found significant symptomatic improvement with tacrine in patients with mild to moderate Alzheimer's disease:

Sixty-five patients completed a 3-month crossover design with a 1-month washout period, the dosage of tacrine being gradually increased up to 150 mg per day along with lecithin at 10.8 g per day. Significant improvements were obtained in Mini-Mental State and Abbreviated Mental Test scores, improvements in the former reflecting significant changes in orientation, attention/calculation and recall subscores. Results from the Cambridge Neuropsychological Test Automated Battery (CANTAB) were more heterogeneous, and indicative of effects on perceptual, attentional and executive functions rather than on memory itself. Case note analysis based on carers comments also clearly favoured the patients taking the drug. Improvement was correlated with the plasma tacrine levels obtained, but there was little evidence of a rise in plasma choline concentrations.

On detailed analysis it was clear that the overall results were largely due to substantial improvement in a subgroup of rather less than half of the sample, while the others showed no change or actually deteriorated. The level of improvement attained on key outcome measures was roughly equivalent to the deterioration that might have been expected over a 6–12-month period. In general, cognitive improvement occurred during the first 2 weeks of treatment, reaching its maximum at 1 month. When continued long term as an open study, the improvements were maintained for 1–2 years and were then followed by inevitable deterioration.

Adverse peripheral cholinergic effects included nausea, vomiting, other gastrointestinal symptoms, transient dysphoria, headache and irritability — most occurring at doses of over 100 mg per day and being severe in some 10% of cases. A dose-dependent elevation of liver enzymes occurred in rather less than half of the patients, in all cases reversing on lowering the dose or stopping the drug. The monitoring of liver function tests at 2–4-week intervals was recommended for all patients taking tacrine.

Other trials continue, with both positive and negative results (Davis *et al.* 1992; Farlow *et al.* 1992; Wilcock *et al.* 1993). A recent Australian study (Maltby *et al.* 1994) found little demonstrable benefit after 9 months of treatment, and only 17 of the 32 patients could tolerate the maximum dose of 100 mg per day. The large USA multicentre trial on 663 patients, by contrast, successfully used doses of up to 160 mg per day, and recorded significant improvements on several outcome measures including objective cognitive tests and quality of life assessments (Knapp *et al.* 1994). At week 30 of the trial, 42% of patients on 160 mg per day were found to be improved, compared with only 18% of those on placebo. Significant dose–response trends were observed, and it was recommended that individual patients be titrated to their maximum tolerated dose.

The usefulness of tacrine in clinical practice is thus still *sub judice*. High dosage would appear to be essential for therapeutic effect, and reports are conflicting about how easily this can be achieved. Clearer indications of possible benefit, optimal dosage and the potential for identifying likely responders, may be expected to emerge as the results of other current studies become available.

Donepezil hydrochloride (Aricept, E 2020), though introduced more recently than tacrine, is the first long-acting acetylcholinesterase inhibitor to be licensed for the treatment of Alzheimer's disease in the UK and USA. It has been available on prescription since early 1997. Donepezil is a piperidine-based acetylcholinesterase inhibitor, with a highly specific effect on acetylcholinesterase within the brain and little by way of peripheral activity, consequently having less troublesome side effects. In particular liver toxicity has not been observed. The dose is 5 mg orally each evening, increasing after 4 weeks to 10 mg per day. Side effects may include diarrhoea, muscle cramps, fatigue, nausea, vomiting, insomnia and dizziness, all being usually mild in degree and subsiding during the early weeks of treatment.

Rogers *et al.* (1996) examined the efficacy of donepezil in a double-blind parallel-group design in 141 patients with mild to moderate Alzheimer's disease. Dose-related improvements were shown on the cognitive subscale of the Alzheimer's Disease Assessment Scale and the Mini-Mental State Examination, improvements on the former being statistically significantly greater with donepezil 5 mg per day than with placebo. There was a 50% reduction in the proportion of patients showing clinical decline on the drug relative to placebo during the 12-week trial period (11% and 20%, respectively). Significant correlations were observed between plasma drug concentrations and the above test scores and on patient-rated quality of life scores. Significant correlations were also noted between measures of red blood cell acetylcholinesterase inhibition and cognitive improvement.

Other acetylcholinesterase inhibitors under active investigation include *velnacrine*, *galanthamine* and *huperazine*.

Cholinergic deficits, though predominating, are of course only one of several neurotransmitter deficiencies in Alzheimer's disease. Too much should therefore not be expected of attempts directed at this aspect of cerebral failure alone. Even within the realm of memory, for example, it is clear that the deficits in Alzheimer patients go well beyond what could be expected from a pure cholinergic deficit. In elegant experiments Kopelman and Corn (1988) have shown that cholinergic blockade in normal subjects is without effect on aspects of primary memory which are severely implicated in Alzheimer's disease, nor does it affect the recall of temporal context or of long-established semantic knowledge. Replacement of more than one neurotransmitter may accordingly be required for optimal improvement in memory and other cognitive functions, and even then expectations will need to be realistic in view of the severely depleted neuronal population which occurs in the disease. In fact it is far from clear that the effects of tacrine rest on its anticholinesterase actions alone. In addition it interacts with muscarinic and nicotinic receptors, inhibits monoamine oxidase and blocks potassium channels with possible subsequent effects on other neurotransmitters.

Other potential approaches to treatment in Alzheimer's disease remain at present largely theoretical. Neurotrophic factors such as nerve growth factor could offer benefit in view of their role in promoting growth and survival of nerve cells. Furthermore nerve growth factor has been shown to be trophic to cholinergic neurones in the basal forebrain, and to produce a specific increase in choline acetyl transferase activity in the cortex of experimental animals. However, it does not cross the blood–brain barrier and alternative modes of delivery raise serious problems. Olson *et al.* (1992) tried the effect of slow intraventricular infusion in a single patient over a 3-month period, with seeming transient improvement in verbal memory. Related chemical compounds may yet become available which offer more realistic hopes of therapeutic application, and as other trophic factors are discovered they may prove to have therapeutic potential.

Methods to arrest the accumulation of beta amyloid or tau protein accumulation could ultimately come to light through current molecular biological research. Cytokines such as interleukin-1 appear to be involved in the pathway leading to amyloid production, and interleukin antagonists could perhaps prove of value.

Also theoretical is the promise inherent in transplantation of foetal cholinergic cells from the basal forebrain region into the hippocampus. Experiments have shown the feasibility of such an approach in the experimental animal, and have demonstrated improvement in learning which is proportional to the degree of outgrowth of acetylcholinesterase-containing cells (Björklund & Stenevi 1977; Dunnett *et al.* 1982, 1988; Gage *et al.* 1984). Promising as these experiments may seem, application in the clinical field on any widespread scale is clearly beset with immense practical and ethical problems.

Lewy body dementia

The management of Lewy body dementia is outlined by Lennox (1992). When patients present with parkinsonism and then develop dementia, antiparkinsonian therapy should be reduced where possible to avoid unwanted effects on cognitive function. Anticholinergic drugs are especially liable to exacerbate confusion and hallucinations, since cholinergic enzyme levels are particularly low in the disorder. Simplification of the regimen to

a single drug such as levodopa, used cautiously, is generally to be recommended, though this too can provoke hallucinations and behavioural disturbance. A trade-off may need to be achieved between decreased mobility and increased lucidity.

Where dementia is the presenting feature management poses equal problems once parkinsonism has developed. The relief of extrapyramidal rigidity may then be at the cost of the patient wandering or falling, and levodopa should probably be restricted to patients with mild cognitive impairment. Cholinergic enhancement strategies may be of value, and may perhaps be expected to meet with more success on cognitive function than in Alzheimer's disease in view of the severe and relatively selective cholinergic deficits in Lewy body dementia. Levy *et al.* (1994) have already presented preliminary data which suggest this may be so.

In the management of psychotic features it is necessary to proceed with great caution before administering neuroleptics in view of the deleterious reactions described on p. 451. They are not, however, absolutely contraindicated. Small doses of thioridazine or sulpiride are best used initially. Chlormethiazole and lorazepam have also been found to be valuable, the latter for short-term use only (McKeith *et al.* 1995). Depression, by contrast, usually responds well to antidepressant therapy, and the improvement in mood may be paralleled by enhanced cognitive performance. Electroconvulsive therapy is not contraindicated.

Huntington's disease

Further specific treatment may help in Huntington's disease for the control of choreic movements. Phenothiazines are widely employed for this purpose and have been shown to be effective. Perphenazine, trifluoperazine, thiopropazate and sulpiride have been especially commended. Barr *et al.* (1988) demonstrated the value of low doses of haloperidol at 1.5–10 mg per day. Tetrabenazine can help considerably but causes sedation and severe depression. It is uncertain whether such agents act merely by calming emotional tension, and perhaps by creating an element of muscular rigidity which opposes the choreic movements, or whether they exert more direct beneficial effects on central neurotransmitter systems. The phenothiazines and butyrophenones may act by dopamine receptor blockade, whereas tetrabenazine depletes neuronal stores of dopamine and other amines as well.

Benzodiazepines have been recommended, both for control of chorea and emotional lability. Diazepam and clonazepam have proved to be effective. Here there is little to support any direct central action on the basal ganglia. When muscular rigidity is the predominant abnormality, as in patients with juvenile onset, this may respond to antiparkinsonian drugs such as levodopa, amantadine or bromocriptine.

Morris and Tyler (1991) review other treatments which have shown little consistent effect—chelating agents, procaine amide, lithium, GABA-ergic drugs such as baclofen, and a variety of cholinergic therapies. Pallidectomy and thalamotomy have sometimes led to improved control of abnormal motor movements but have fallen into disfavour. Heathfield (1967) considered that such operations had a place in younger patients with minimal mental changes and severe chorea, but unfortunately they appear to carry a risk of aggravating the dementia.

Creutzfeldt–Jakob disease

In Creutzfeldt–Jakob disease there have been occasional reports of benefit from treatment with amantadine, one patient appearing to have been cured completely. Unfortunately, however, negative results are also frequently observed, and it is hard to be certain about the diagnosis in patients who have responded. A trial of treatment with the drug is nevertheless worth consideration since the outlook is otherwise hopeless.

Braham (1971) first reported a patient who showed temporary improvement on the drug. The clinical course and the electroencephalographic findings had been typical of the disorder, and the patient was stuporose by the time treatment with amantadine was commenced. Marked improvement began 2 days later, relapse accompanied a few days' interruption of treatment, and improvement occurred again on restarting it. The rapidity of the effect suggested a biochemical rather than an antiviral action in producing these results.

Sanders and Dunn (1973) reported two further patients treated with some success. In one who showed temporary improvement the disease was confirmed later at autopsy; the other in whom the disease was never proven appears to have been cured:

A man of 69 showed rapid onset of confusion and loss of memory, and within 6 weeks had become stuporose and incontinent, with extrapyramidal rigidity in the limbs and widespread muscular fasciculation. The cerebrospinal fluid was normal and the EEG showed diffuse slow activity. Amantadine, 200 mg per day, produced a markedly beneficial response within several days. The extrapyramidal rigidity lessened and he began talking rationally. The improvement was sustained for 2 months. Thereafter he deteriorated and pursued a downhill course over the next 2 months despite increasing doses of amantadine. At autopsy, histological examination of the brain showed changes consistent with early Creutzfeldt–Jakob disease.

A woman of 55 had a more protracted illness with listlessness, depression and obvious intellectual impairment. She developed diplopia and later became ataxic with frequent falls. A year after onset there were pyramidal signs in the legs, the cerebrospinal fluid was normal and the EEG showed runs of theta and frontal delta waves. Marked tremor appeared in the limbs and tongue. She was agitated, emotionally labile and showed confusion and disorientation which fluctuated from day to day. Eighteen months after onset she was severely demented and doubly incontinent, with extrapyramidal rigidity in the legs. Her speech was rapid and indistinct and she was unable to stand, walk, dress or feed herself. Four days after starting amantadine she was more alert, and after 10 days she was beginning to walk. After 2 weeks she was well orientated and able to carry on a rational conversation. Progressive improvement led to the disappearance of all abnormal signs within 2 months. Follow-up showed maintained improvement, normal results from psychological testing and a normal EEG. After 18 months the amantadine was stopped and she remained well 1 year later. Further follow-up (Sanders 1979) showed that she still remained well.

Sanders and Dunn, like Braham, felt that a metabolic rather than an antiviral action of the drug was involved in these patients, especially since in the first example the response appeared to be dose related. Terzano *et al.* (1983) tried amantadine in four patients, three with autopsy confirmation of the disease. Five patients who received supportive treatment only served as controls. Three of the treated patients showed appreciable though transient improvements in level of wakefulness, motor impairment and mental performance after receiving the drug, in contrast to the uniformly progressive course in the other five. Beneficial effects on the EEG were observed in two, with reduced background slow activity and a reduction of periodic discharges. However, the time to death after the initiation of therapy was not significantly different between the two groups. Others who have tried amantadine have found no benefit (Ratcliffe *et al.* 1975; Kovanen *et al.* 1980). Interferon has also been given without success. Further experience may clarify whether positive responders are truly examples of Creutzfeldt–Jakob disease or represent some other disorder.

Patients suspected of *subacute sclerosing panencephalitis* will warrant a trial of treatment on steroids (p. 363), similarly patients whose dementia is thought to be based in some collagen vascular disorder. Examples of the latter reported by Chynoweth and Foley (1969) are described on pp. 425–6.

Chapter 11: Endocrine Diseases and Metabolic Disorders

The relationship between endocrinology and psychiatry has attracted a good deal of attention for obvious reasons. Endocrine disorder can be accompanied by prominent mental abnormalities, as for example in myxoedema and hyperthyroidism, and epochs of life marked by endocrine change such as pregnancy and the menopause appear to be associated with special liability to mental disturbance. In the reverse direction it is now clear that primary emotional disturbance is accompanied by changes in neuroendocrine regulatory functions of a complex nature.

Historically it is interesting to note that treatment by means of hormones has often been viewed as a possibility in psychiatry. Kraepelin (1896) at one time proposed that dementia praecox was basically an endocrine disorder. Others have speculated on the role of hormones in regulating the 'biological background of psychic life', noting their influence on such matters as impulsivity, attention, arousal and their role in numerous drives in animals as well as humans (Bleuler 1967). Patients on substitution therapy are said to 'lose something in their personal profile' due to lack of the complex interplay between emotions and hormonal levels. On this general question, however, there is as yet no clear evidence.

More recent interest centres on the way hormonal influences during intrauterine life and immediately after birth can come to alter fundamental aspects of behaviour and brain development. Experimental work in animals has clarified the morphological basis by which thyroxine lack during early development impairs the maturation of behaviour (Eayrs 1968). And it is now apparent that prenatal steroid hormones have a decisive influence in animals on sexual differentiation and a wide range of sexual and social behaviours (McCarthy 1994; Signoret & Balthazart 1994). In human beings, Money and Ehrhardt (1968) reported that girls affected by androgens *in utero*, either due to spontaneous hyperadrenocortical activity or as a result of progesterone given to pregnant mothers, showed an increased tendency towards tomboyish behaviour later in their development. Such findings, if well confirmed, may open a further chapter in the relationship between endocrinology and psychological functions in human beings.

During the past two decades there has been an explosion of interest in peptide hormones, their regulation and their possible relevance to psychiatry. Thyrotropin-releasing hormone (TRH), corticotrophin (adrenocorticotrophic hormone, ACTH) and other hypothalamic peptides have proved to be under delicate control from neural as well as endocrine feedback processes. The activity of the hypothalamic–pituitary axis has come under detailed scrutiny in mental disorder, with evidence of, for example, impaired cortisol production in response to dexamethasone (Carroll 1976a; Carroll *et al.* 1981) and impaired growth hormone response to clonidine and other drugs in endogenous depressive illness (Checkley 1992). Such disturbances appear to reflect central, presumably hypothalamic, alterations accompanying the emotional disorder. Pituitary neuropeptides related to ACTH and vasopressin are now known to affect learned behaviour in animals (De Wied *et al.* 1976). Through them it can be expected that the pituitary plays an important role in motivational, learning and memory processes. The opiate peptides (the endorphins and enkephalins) are obviously an immensely important discovery with potential relevance to addictive behaviour and the control of chronic pain (Rees 1981).

The purpose in what follows is not to explore these many aspects in detail, but rather to concentrate on the clinical psychiatric manifestations of primary endocrine disorder. It may be said that in all of the conditions considered below, occasional individuals will react in such a way that psychiatric manifestations gain prior attention and the endocrine disturbance goes unnoticed. With some conditions, for example myxoedema and Addison's disease, the psychiatric abnormalities are regularly intrusive to such a degree that there is a constant risk of mistaken diagnoses.

The other metabolic disorders to be discussed — hypoglycaemia, anoxia, uraemia, electrolyte disturbance and hepatic disorder — similarly illustrate the importance of the correct biochemical milieu for the proper functioning of the central nervous system. They are quite often encountered by psychiatrists working in general hospitals and their psychological manifestations have accordingly received increasing attention in recent years. Porphyria is included as a rare but striking example of an inborn error of metabolism with important psychiatric features.

Hyperthyroidism

Hyperthyroidism affects females much more commonly than males in a ratio of approximately 6 : 1. It is commonest in the second and third decades of life but the range is wide. The cause may lie in a hyperplastic nodule or secreting adenoma of the thyroid gland, but more commonly the gland is diffusely overactive (Graves' disease). Goitrous enlargement may or may not be present.

Attention has been directed to the role of stress and emotional disturbance in precipitating hyperthyroidism, also to the psychological constitution of those who develop the disorder. The onset is often abrupt and may be seen to follow directly upon some stressful event or emotional crisis. It is hard, however, to exclude the possibility that such emotional traumas may themselves have been the by-products of early and unsuspected thyroid overactivity. Jadresic (1990) reviews the evidence from several studies, including Gray and Hoffenberg's (1985) failure to find an association between stressful life events and the onset of thyrotoxicosis. More recently, Wisna et al. (1991) have reported a significant excess of negative life events compared with controls in the 12 months preceding the diagnosis of Graves' disease, but this study has been criticised on a number of methodological grounds (Harris et al. 1992). The issue would therefore appear to remain sub judice.

With regard to predisposition, opinions have varied widely. Mandelbrote and Wittkower (1955) emphasised instability of the premorbid personality in persons subject to hyperthyroidism. Robbins and Vinson (1960), however, considered that the role of personality factors had been overstressed. Gurney et al. (1967) found that hyperthyroid patients as a group fell somewhere between neurotics and normals in terms of previous stability, with a similar family and personal history of psychiatric disorder to the neurotics but with greater previous stability on a number of other indices. It is clearly difficult to make accurate assessments of personality from the patient's own account since this will be biased by the changes of mood that occur in the course of the illness (Jadresic 1990).

Common psychological accompaniments

Psychological disturbance of some degree is universal with thyroid overactivity. The patient becomes restless, overactive and irritable, sometimes with hyperacuity of perception and over-reaction to noise. Heightened tension leads to impatience and intolerance of frustration, and emotional lability may develop with unreasonable or histrionic behaviour. Depression can be prominent, though unaccompanied by retardation. Kathol et al. (1986) found that almost a third of 29 consecutive patients seen in an endocrine clinic met DSM-III criteria for major depression. Eighty per cent had generalised anxiety. The picture of 'apathetic hyperthyroidism' with anergia and mental slowing occurs mainly in elderly patients and is discussed on p. 511.

The over-arousal leads to distractibility so that concentration is impaired and effort cannot be sustained. In addition, careful examination may reveal definite cognitive impairments of which the patient is unaware, in the form of difficulty with simple arithmetic or difficulty with recent memory (Whybrow et al. 1969).

The emotional disturbance can reach a degree which leads to difficulty in clinical management, though modern antithyroid drugs have proved invaluable in circumventing the problems which arose when urgent thyroidectomy was the treatment of choice. States of extreme anxiety or irritability may emerge as a direct extension of the heightened emotional tension, or paranoid features may appear as an aspect of the disturbed mental state. Whybrow et al. (1969) found that seven out of 10 consecutive hyperthyroid patients in a general hospital showed psychiatric abnormalities severe enough to constitute a 'psychiatric illness', even though none had been referred or considered as 'psychiatric problems'. Nevertheless hyperthyroidism does not appear to be exceptionally frequent among hospitalised psychiatric patients. McLarty et al. (1978) found eight patients with thyrotoxicosis after surveying the entire population of two psychiatric hospitals, a total of over 1200 persons in all. In six the hyperthyroidism had been unsuspected prior to the survey, and in five it seemed to be contributing to the mental illness.

Psychoses

Other developments include the organic, affective and schizophrenic psychoses which sometimes accompany hyperthyroidism. Occasionally these are the presenting feature and lead directly to psychiatric referral.

Acute organic reactions accompany 'thyroid crises' and show the typical picture of delirium, usually accompanied by fever. They were formerly one of the commonest forms of major mental illness encountered in the disease, but are now relatively rare owing to modern methods of treatment. They constitute a grave emergency and warrant urgent intervention. Diagnostic confusion is unlikely to arise on account of the abundant evidence of hyperthyroidism accompanying their development. The rare 'apathetic hyperthyroidism' (p. 511), however, can sometimes progress to stupor or coma, and here diagnostic difficulties may be encountered.

Affective and schizophrenic psychoses are sometimes indistinguishable from their naturally occurring counterparts. Mania is said to be more frequent than depression, and often the progression to mania can be seen as a direct outgrowth from the characteristic mental changes of the endocrine disorder. Schizophrenic illnesses of all types have been reported — hebephrenic, catatonic and paranoid — and have sometimes been found to outnumber affective psychoses.

It is no longer believed that a specific 'thyroid psychosis' exists, but it is generally agreed that a distinctive colouring may be lent by the hyperthyroidism. Thus a manic component may accompany otherwise typical schizophrenic symptomatology, and agitation is often profound in the presence of depression. Most observers are also agreed that paranoid features are especially common whatever form the psychosis may take.

The diagnostic distinctions between the affective and schizophrenic reactions are often blurred, and an admixture of organic psychiatric features is relatively common. A seemingly schizophrenic psychosis may sometimes represent covert organic disorder, the essential evidence for which may be overlooked as in the patient reported by Greer and Parsons (1968):

A man of 28 developed a short-lived schizophrenia-like illness with a paranoid delusional system, ideas of reference and influence, and auditory and visual hallucinations. Orientation and memory were apparently intact, but a contribution due to organic cerebral disorder was suggested by the presence of *déjà vu* and panoramic memory at the height of the illness.

Psychotic developments have been reported in up to 20% of cases, though this may reflect special selection and the inclusion of acute organic reactions in earlier series. Johnson (1928) found only 24 examples of psychosis among over 2000 patients referred for thyroidectomy when patients with obvious confusion or delirium were excluded. Most were depressive states with hallucinations and delusions. The majority had a personal or family history of mental disorder, and the psychosis had usually been in evidence long before symptoms of hyperthyroidism appeared. This prevalence, at little more than

1%, would suggest a chance association in most instances, with the hyperthyroidism merely aggravating an established mental disorder. In a careful survey of a number of patients with manic–depressive psychosis who had also had thyrotoxicosis, Checkley (1978) was unable to detect clear time relationships suggestive of a link between the two. He argued that if the hyperthyroidism had so little effect on the course of the affective disorder in patients long subject to manic–depressive episodes, it would seem unlikely to serve as a precipitant in patients without such liability.

Dunlap and Moersch (1935) reported 143 patients with mental disturbance accompanying hyperthyroidism; over 70% were organic psychosyndromes, but 26 patients showed manic–depressive psychoses (mostly depressions), two had dementia praecox and two were paranoid. Bursten (1961) found 10 examples of psychosis among 54 hyperthyroid patients seen in a general hospital during a 4-year period. Five were schizophrenic, three were organic reactions, one was a depressive illness and one a psychosis of undetermined type. From the same source of referral six examples of psychosis were observed among an equivalent number of patients with diabetes matched for age and sex, and only two among an equivalent number of patients with cholecystitis.

Neurological accompaniments

The commonly associated tremor at 8–12 Hz is best seen in the outstretched hands; it persists during movement and is absent at rest. The well-known signs of lid-lag and upper lid retraction may be accompanied by exophthalmos due to swelling of the retro-orbital tissues. There may then be impairment of convergence (Moebius' sign). The tendon reflexes are usually brisk, some patients showing clonus and positive Babinski responses.

Epileptic fits are occasionally precipitated, thyrotoxicosis being a contributory factor in about 1% of new-onset fits in adults (Kaminski & Ruff 1989). Abend and Tyler (1989) review the electroencephalographic changes seen in up to 50% of patients, these usually being reversible when the euthyroid state is attained. A proximal myopathy may develop with weakness, wasting and myalgia, and a significant association exists between thyrotoxicosis and myasthenia gravis. Occasional thyrotoxic patients suffer from recurrent attacks of 'periodic paralysis' (p. 721).

Investigations

Laboratory investigations are essential for confirming the diagnosis of hyperthyroidism. In the majority of cases they give unequivocal results: raised serum thyroxine

(T_4) and triiodothyronine (T_3) as measured by radio-immunoassay, coupled with a raised 'free-thyroxine index'. The latter is calculated when the free T_4 cannot be measured directly, since total T_4 is much influenced by the levels of thyroxine-binding proteins in the serum.

In a small number of cases, however, the results may be borderline or even self contradictory. The clinical features then require careful appraisal, and referral for specialist investigation is usually indicated. Such borderline cases will often prove to be suffering from primary emotional disorder rather than hyperthyroidism, but further tests are nonetheless essential.

The estimation of serum thyroid-stimulating hormone (thyrotropin, TSH) is invaluable for confirmation of the diagnosis. With recent sensitive methods using mono-clonal immunoassay, levels below 0.01 mU/l are almost invariably found with symptomatic hyperthyroidism (McGregor 1996). On rare occasions it may be necessary to test for an impairment of the TSH response to an injection of thyrotropin-releasing hormone (TRH), though this is seldom now required.

Special difficulty may be encountered with psychiatric patients in that thyroid function tests can be transiently abnormal after admission to hospital. Among 480 newly admitted psychiatric patients, Cohen and Swigar (1979) found abnormalities in total thyroxin, thyroxine-binding capacity and free T_4 in 9% of the patients, usually returning to normal within a few weeks. They labelled this 'acute stress hyperthyroidism'. Low T_4 levels were found in a similar proportion, also often resolving spontaneously.

In the syndrome of 'T_3 toxicosis' there is an isolated excess of triiodothyronine which can produce clinical signs of thyrotoxicosis despite normal levels of total and free serum T_4.

Differential diagnosis

The differential diagnosis between hyperthyroidism and anxiety neurosis is a classic and often difficult exercise. Physicians and psychiatrists need to be aware of the pitfalls. The presenting mental symptoms can be virtually identical in both conditions; both show tachycardia, fine finger tremor, palpitations and loss of weight, and both may appear to have been precipitated by stressful events. The presence of previous neurotic symptomatology in thyrotoxic patients and their families can lead to further blurring of the diagnostic criteria between the two conditions.

Careful analysis of the features shown by large numbers of patients with hyperthyroidism has clarified the physical symptoms and signs which are of most

importance in indicating this disorder (Wayne 1960) and it is useful to refer to such data in doubtful cases. The symptoms, in descending order of discriminating value, were sensitivity to heat and preference for cold, increased appetite, loss of weight, sweating, palpitations, tiredness, 'nervousness' and dyspnoea on effort. The signs, in order of importance, were cardiac dysrhythmias (chiefly auricular fibrillation), hyperkinetic movements, tachycardia exceeding 90 beats per minute, a palpable thyroid gland, a bruit audible over the thyroid, exophthalmos, lid retraction, hot hands, lid-lag and fine finger tremor. These lists show how closely anxiety neurosis may be simulated.

Gurney *et al.* (1967) focused more closely on the problem by reviewing the features found in euthyroid patients with psychiatric disorder but who were initially referred with suspected thyrotoxicosis. Such patients, when compared with thyrotoxics, had an increased frequency of psychological precipitants for the illness, a lower age of onset, more frequent hysterical symptoms and panic attacks, and more neurotic features in the personality.

Thus hyperthyroidism will usually be readily suspected when the patient gives a clear history of sensitivity to heat and a preference for cold, and this deserves careful specific enquiry. Similarly the classic signs of exophthalmos, lid retraction and lid-lag will clarify the situation when such are present. Precipitation by stress will be found more commonly and more impressively in anxiety neurosis. But perhaps the most decisive feature in differentiating the two conditions is the preservation or otherwise of appetite in face of steady loss of weight; in hyperthyroidism appetite is characteristically increased whereas in anxiety states it is reduced.

In the presence of frank psychosis, diagnostic difficulties are liable to be increased and the hyperthyroidism may sometimes go unrecognised for a considerable time. It is necessary to beware of the occasional case of hyperthyroidism in which fluctuations occur with periods of spontaneous resolution. Repeated episodes of affective disorder may be particularly misleading:

A man of 40 was admitted to hospital with a typical attack of hypomania which responded satisfactorily to chlorpromazine during the next 3 weeks. Ten days later he was re-admitted with a relapse after discontinuing the medication, but once again he responded rapidly to chlorpromazine. Three months later he developed marked weakness and depression, and for the first time appeared to be physically unwell. It was noted that he had a persistent tachycardia, a warm moist skin and possibly an enlarged thyroid gland. Investigations confirmed hyperthyroidism, and retrospective enquiry revealed steady loss of weight and increased appetite since shortly before the first episode of hypomania. The admission notes on the two previous occasions had shown a tachycardia which had been overlooked at the time.

Special diagnostic difficulty is likely to be encountered when thyrotoxicosis is accompanied by depression. 'Apathetic hyperthyroidism', though rare, may easily be overlooked. The typical picture is of a middle-aged or elderly patient with considerable weight loss and apathy or depression (Lahey 1931; Thomas *et al.* 1970). Cardiovascular symptoms may overshadow other evidence of thyrotoxicosis, and eye signs in particular tend to be absent. The physical appearance may resemble senility. In younger patients, too, depression can be the presenting feature. Folks and Petrie (1982) describe a woman of 23 presenting with depression, insomnia and early morning waking, who after an overdose of amitriptyline was found to be thyrotoxic. The affective disorder resolved as the hyperthyroidism came under control. Taylor (1975) reported a patient who was found to be thyrotoxic during a second attack of psychotic depression, the first having responded to electroconvulsive therapy; here the depression likewise abated when the thyroid disorder was treated.

Alcoholism may be wrongly blamed for the tremulousness and emotional lability of hyperthyroid patients. Davis *et al.* (1971) reported three men with previously stable records who were found to have been indicted for larceny shortly after the onset of thyrotoxicosis. In two of them alcoholism had been suspected by the employers on account of tremulousness, weakness and inattention at work, and loss or threatened loss of employment had precipitated their crimes.

Aetiology of mental disturbances

The common psychological accompaniments of hyperthyroidism are probably the direct result of increased T_4 levels and subsequent metabolic derangements within the central nervous system. This is supported by the uniformity of the common mental changes from case to case, their fluctuations with exacerbations of the disorder, and the rapid subsidence of symptoms with antithyroid treatment. In Kathol *et al.*'s (1986) investigation generalised anxiety disorder, but not depression, showed a strong relationship with measures of the free-thyroxine index. Cerebral catecholamines may be intimately involved, particularly increased sensitivity of beta adrenergic receptors. Thus beta adrenergic blocking agents can be shown to improve psychiatric symptoms in hyperthyroidism despite unaltered levels of thyroid hormones (Trzepacz *et al.* 1988). The acute organic reactions are likely similarly to have an origin in brain metabolic disturbance and usually appear only at peaks of thyrotoxicosis.

The precise aetiology of psychotic developments is incompletely understood. Constitutional predisposition is usually invoked to explain severe affective or schizophrenic disorders, but even so the situation may be complex. The psychosis may be precipitated by the metabolic derangement or by the resulting emotional turmoil; alternatively, an ingravescent psychosis may have served to precipitate the thyrotoxicosis. Simple coincidence may account for the two developments, but the parallel course which they sometimes pursue suggests that a causal relationship of some sort is likely to exist quite commonly. At all events, once the processes are under way they doubtless augment one another.

During treatment with antithyroid drugs, such as carbimazole, an acute organic psychosis may make its first appearance, presumably in response to the toxic effects of the drug or a period of drug-induced hypothyroidism (Brewer 1969; Herridge & Abey-Wickrama 1969). Other cases are reported in which schizophrenia-like psychoses make an appearance at such a time. Bewsher *et al.*'s (1971) case illustrates the difficulties that can be encountered in deciding on the precise aetiological factors at work:

During the fifth week of treatment with carbimazole a woman became acutely psychotic with paranoid delusions, auditory hallucinations and marked overactivity, producing bursts of song and whoops of excitement. Initially she was febrile (38°C, 100°F) and showed a tachycardia, but there was no evidence of recurrence of thyrotoxicosis. Memory and orientation were normal throughout and the level of consciousness was unimpaired. The paranoid delusions slowly resolved over several months during which chlorpromazine was given and carbimazole continued. The patient was euthyroid at the time the psychosis developed and remained so throughout its resolution. Follow-up over the next 2 years showed no recurrence. It was suggested that the psychosis had been precipitated by the fairly rapid alteration in the level of circulating T_4 from severe excess to normality over the preceding 4 weeks, and perhaps by virtue of the effects of this transition on cerebral catecholamines.

Outcome of mental disturbances

The result of treatment is in general satisfactory, with resolution of emotional disorder as the patient is rendered euthyroid. Sometimes, however, emotional instability persists, and in most cases is probably attributable to premorbid tendencies in this direction. Kathol *et al.* (1986) found that depression and anxiety resolved in the great majority of cases with antithyroid treatment alone. Occasionally, however, additional psychotropic medication will prove to be necessary. The acute organic psychoses usually also respond rapidly as the thyrotoxicosis comes under control. Schizophrenic psychoses may run a more variable course, but as with other psychoses in which a precipitating cause is apparent the prognosis will usually be better than for schizophrenias which arise spontaneously.

Hypothyroidism (myxoedema)

Myxoedema is of great importance in psychiatric practice and notorious for leading to mistakes in diagnosis. It is liable to be overlooked on account of its insidious development, and the minor and diffuse nature of the early complaints. Mental symptoms are almost universally present by the time the patient seeks advice, and many examples come before the psychiatrist. It is only by keeping the disorder in mind that early cases, or sometimes even advanced examples, will be detected.

As with hyperthyroidism, myxoedema is very much commoner in females than males, in a ratio of approximately 8 : 1. It presents most frequently in middle age though the range is wide. The physical accompaniments deserve first consideration since these will usually prove to be the features which raise suspicion.

Physical features

The appearance in classic examples is characteristic, with a pale puffy complexion and baggy eyelids. The skin is dry and rough, with a non-pitting oedematous appearance over the face and limbs and in the supraclavicular fossae. The patient may have noticed increased loss of hair, which has become lank and dry in texture. Speech is slow, and the voice often coarse, thick and toneless. The whole disposition of the patient tends to be sluggish and inert. It must be appreciated, however, that all such features may not be apparent in early stages of the disorder.

The pulse is usually slowed and angina is not infrequent. Appetite is diminished, the patient is often constipated, and hearing, taste and smell may be impaired due to deposits of mucoid material. Intolerance of cold is often a prominent early complaint. Menorrhagia is common in females, and impotence in males. Vague generalised aches and pains of a rheumatic nature may occur. Very occasionally muscular weakness may be the initial manifestation. On examination the ankle reflexes may be slowed with marked delay in the relaxation phase.

Common psychological accompaniments

The typical picture is of mental lethargy, general dulling of the personality and slowing of all cognitive functions. In the earlier stages the patient is subjectively aware of such changes, and complains of a thickness in the head or of 'feeling in a fog'. Ready fatigue may be a conspicuous feature, and relatives may have noted increasing psychomotor retardation with the patient taking progressively longer to perform routine tasks. Memory is often affected from an early stage, with failure to register events and forgetfulness for day-to-day happenings.

With further progression there is marked inability to sustain mental exertion and increasing slowness of uptake and grasp. The profound loss of interest and initiative carries the risk of delaying medical attention, since the patient may cease to complain and come to spend her time in a state of sluggish indifference.

The typical mood change is towards apathy rather than depression, though the distinction is not clear-cut. Irritability is a frequent feature, and some patients become markedly agitated and aggressive.

Psychoses and dementia with myxoedema

It is against the background of these changes that the more severe psychiatric disturbances of myxoedema occur. An organic psychosis may develop acutely or run a subacute course over several weeks or months. More commonly, memory impairment develops insidiously and may progress over several years to advanced dementia. A severe depressive psychosis may emerge, or a typical schizophrenia may be precipitated. It is generally agreed that there is no form of psychosis specific to myxoedema, but rather a variety of 'reaction types' which may be called forth differently in different individuals. The only unifying feature, upheld by many observers, is the frequency of a paranoid colouring whatever form the psychosis may take.

In Asher's (1949) classic paper on 'myxoedematous madness' five patients showed an organic reaction with hallucinations and persecutory ideas, five showed the picture of schizophrenia with a marked paranoid colouring, two presented as advanced dementia and two with depressive features.

Organic psychoses usually show the features of delirium, with florid delusions and hallucinations, mental confusion and impairment of consciousness. Delusions of persecution may be gross and bizarre. Auditory hallucinations appear to be particularly common. The condition may run a fluctuating course, but even when clouding of consciousness cannot be established there is usually evidence of impairment of cognitive function, particularly of recent memory.

Dementia develops as an extension of the mental impairment characteristic of the condition generally. It progresses insidiously in a manner indistinguishable from a primary presenile dementia, and may have reached an advanced degree by the time the diagnosis is made. Oli-varus and Röder (1970) considered myxoedema to be the most important, and the most frequently overlooked, of the metabolic causes of reversible organic intellectual impairment.

A 53-year-old woman developed dizziness and a constant diffuse headache after a mild head injury. Four months later she was admitted to hospital for repair of a rectal prolapse, but the opera-tion was deferred because she was found to be confused and deluded. The EEG revealed diffuse slow activity with occasional sharp waves in the frontotemporal regions.

Full examination of the mental state showed her to be men-tally sluggish, slightly depressed and with marked intellectual impairment. This was confirmed on psychological testing. There was slight left facial weakness and incoordination of the left arm. Her husband explained that in recent years she had had increas-ing difficulties with her job as a teacher, mainly because the pupils made fun of her lapses of memory. In the last 4 months she had become slowed and sluggish, with increasing inability to concentrate or remember.

Angiography failed to reveal a cerebral tumour and a diagnosis of presenile dementia was seriously considered. Air encephalo-graphy, however, showed little evidence of cortical atrophy. Signs of myxoedema were then noted and the diagnosis was confirmed.

Within 3 weeks of starting replacement therapy she reported improvement, with decreased fatigue and improved memory. She was able to do crossword puzzles which she had given up several years before. Two months later psychometric testing con-firmed marked intellectual improvement and showed only slight residual impairment of memory. She resumed her work without difficulty and remained well on follow-up.

(Olivarus & Röder 1970)

Depressive and schizophrenic psychoses may or may not be accompanied by organic mental features, though these are usually found when sought out with care. Paranoid symptoms again figure prominently. The depressive psychoses are often severe, with agitation or bizarre hypochondriasis, and may prove to be particularly resis-tant to treatment until the myxoedema is discovered. Schizophrenic psychoses will in general be coloured by mental slowing, and often include features indicative of organic cerebral impairment.

Neurological accompaniments

The slowing of the tendon reflexes has already been men-tioned. This may serve as a useful confirmatory sign, and with careful measurement has been used to monitor the progress of treatment.

Jellinek (1962) drew attention to the occurrence of fits, faints and cerebrovascular accidents in myxoedematous patients. Four patients were reported with grand mal

attacks which responded to thyroid replacement, others with attacks of syncope, and others with unusual confusional episodes which suggested temporal lobe dysfunction. Millichap (1974) has reported further examples.

A man of 57 had sudden attacks which lasted a few minutes and consisted of varying sensations of familiarity and unfamiliarity: 'You know where you are but things face the wrong way'. On one occasion, when quite near home, he crossed the road away from his intended route and walked straight into a flow of moving traffic. He came to, in a state of panic, in the centre of the road. The attacks stopped when thyroxine was commenced.

Another patient had 'blackouts' in which she would become briefly confused and talk nonsense. On one occasion she was accused of being drunk by a taxi driver when she refused to pay her fare. These attacks also ceased when she started thyroid treatment.
(Jellinek 1962)

Cerebrovascular accidents were found to have occurred in several of Jellinek's patients, and evidence of attacks of transient cerebral ischaemia in several more.

Jellinek and Kelly (1960) described other cases of myx-oedema presenting with cerebellar disturbance in the form of ataxia, tremor, dysarthria and nystagmus, and remitting promptly with replacement therapy. Wise *et al.* (1995) have confirmed such pictures and reported patients with other unusual presentations. One presented with shock-like pains in the feet and an altered sleep pattern, another with myalgia and weakness in the calf muscles. The myopathy of myxoedema typically affects the proximal musculature with weakness, cramps and sometimes wasting. Sleep apnoea may occur as a result of obesity or upper airway obstruction.

Myxoedema coma is a grave condition which carries a high mortality. It typically develops in association with superimposed infection, surgery or trauma (Kaminski & Ruff 1989). It should be suspected in any patient with severe impairment of consciousness and hypothermia. The skin feels icy cold, and a low-reading rectal ther-mometer is required to confirm the hypothermia. Respi-ration may be sluggish, and cardiac failure or dysrhythmia are features of serious significance.

Investigations

As with hyperthyroidism it is essential to confirm the diagnosis by laboratory tests before starting treatment. The total and free T_4 levels are low, though the serum T_3 may be normal. Elevated plasma TSH will indicate primary thyroid failure, whereas normal basal levels will suggest a pituitary origin. The latter is confirmed by an absent, subnormal or delayed response to TRH (McGregor 1996). The estimation of circulating autoantibodies to thyroglobulin and thyroid peroxidase may help to establish the cause, for example Hashimoto's thyroiditis.

The serum cholesterol is elevated, the heart is usually enlarged and the electrocardiogram shows a low-voltage tracing with flattened or inverted T waves. The EEG shows lowered voltage and slowing of the dominant frequencies; occasionally it is normal despite severe myxoedema but this is rare. The protein in the cerebrospinal fluid may be moderately raised.

Differential diagnosis

Not uncommonly the myxoedema is first recognised only after a considerable lapse of time. Early dementia or intractable depression are probably the diagnoses most frequently entertained, or the patient may have been labelled as neurotic, hypochondriacal or personality disordered. Occasionally such patients are found to have spent some time in a vain quest for medical help before the correct diagnosis is made.

The suspicion of myxoedema is usually derived from the characteristic facial appearance or other physical symptoms and signs, but unless the disorder is specifically considered these may easily be overlooked. In the 14 cases reported by Asher (1949), all with florid mental illnesses, the myxoedema had been missed by the referring doctor in every case. In the more severe psychotic illnesses organic features are usually evident in the mental state but not invariably so.

Even without overt evidence of myxoedema, psychiatric patients may warrant investigation if they have a history of thyroidectomy or of having required thyroid medication in the past. These were the factors that prompted investigation in five of 18 myxoedematous patients surveyed by Tonks (1964) in a psychiatric hospital. Patients on long-term lithium therapy are also at increased risk of developing hypothyroidism and require periodic checks of serum thyroxine levels.

Aetiology of mental disturbances

The mental symptomatology in myxoedema can be largely ascribed to changes in cerebral metabolism. Such changes are reflected in the electroencephalographic findings described above, and these can be observed to improve with substitution therapy. Cerebral blood flow has been shown to be considerably reduced as a result of diminished cardiac output, while the cerebral metabolic demands for oxygen and glucose are unaltered (Scheinberg *et al.* 1950; Sensenbach *et al.* 1954; O'Brien & Harris 1968). The relative cerebral hypoxia that results is worsened by the anaemia which frequently coexists. The cerebral changes therefore appear to be largely secondary to the effects of thyroxine deprivation on other organs such as the heart, rather than the direct result of thyroxine lack on the brain itself.

Such abnormalities probably go much of the way towards explaining the mental slowing and dulling which form an integral part of the disorder. The acute organic psychoses are likely to be due to some additional aspect of the intracerebral metabolic disturbance. Distinctive colouring by way of mood disorder or paranoia will perhaps be derived from premorbid personality factors.

Cases of major affective disorder and schizophrenia are likely to owe a good deal both to organic factors and to matters of constitutional vulnerability. In the rare examples where organic features are entirely absent from the mental state the cerebral metabolic defect has probably served merely as a precipitant. But the situation is not entirely straightforward, since patients with purely depressive symptomatology have been found to respond to thyroxine after other forms of treatment have failed entirely (Michael & Gibbons 1963).

'Non-myxoedematous hypometabolism'

Kurland *et al.* (1955) reported a syndrome of 'metabolic insufficiency', in which the basal metabolic rate was low in spite of a normal serum protein-bound iodine and radioactive iodine uptake. Such patients frequently complained of fatigue, lethargy, sensitivity to cold, musculoskeletal pain and diminished sexual potency. Treatment with thyroxine was ineffective, but triiodothyronine was said to raise the basal metabolic rate and lead to striking clinical improvement. The condition gained popularity and came to be rather commonly diagnosed.

Levin (1960), however, performed a careful double-blind trial of thyroxine, triiodothyronine and placebo in patients fulfilling the diagnostic criteria, and neither treatment could be shown to have definite effects on symptoms or on the basal metabolic rates. The patients' complaints were more typical of neurotic disorder than of myxoedema, and Minesota Multiphasic Personality Inventory (MMPI) scores showed a high degree of psychological maladjustment in the individuals concerned. It would seem therefore that the syndrome is unlikely to be a clinical reality, and that triiodothyronine is not effective treatment. Some neurotic patients clearly have low basal metabolic rates, but so also do some members of the general population.

Outcome of mental disturbances

The treatment of myxoedema is usually highly rewarding. The patient gradually regains vitality, physical symptoms diminish and mental processes return to their usual speed and efficiency.

The great majority of patients with serious psychiatric developments can also be expected to respond, even those with overt dementia, provided too long an interval has not elapsed. Jellinek (1962), however, stressed that several of his cases were left with measurable defects of intellect and memory after being rendered euthyroid, mostly those who had remained undiagnosed for very long periods of time or where treatment had been inadequate.

Where response to thyroxine is concerned, the frankly organic psychoses can in general be expected to do better than psychoses with predominantly 'functional' symptomatology. This was confirmed by Tonks (1964), who surveyed 18 hypothyroid patients in a psychiatric hospital during a period of treatment with thyroid preparations alone; the proportion who made complete and lasting recoveries was much higher among patients who showed evidence of disturbance of consciousness, by way of disorientation or confusion, than among those who did not. The duration of the illnesses was also important, in that no patient with a mental illness exceeding 2 years had a satisfactory response to the trial of thyroid replacement therapy alone. The only clearly organic condition which failed to respond was a patient with chronic progressive dementia and aphasia of 7 years' duration.

Additional measures in the form of phenothiazines, antidepressant medication or electroconvulsive therapy may be necessary in severe psychotic disorders, and particularly so when organic features are absent from the mental state. It must be borne in mind, however, that phenothiazines carry some risk of precipitating hypothermic coma in hypothyroid patients, as in the case reported by Mitchell *et al.* (1959).

It is necessary to introduce thyroxine with caution at the beginning of treatment, especially in the elderly, because of the possibility of myocardial damage. The starting dose of l-thyroxine sodium should not exceed 50 µg per day. If there is no evidence of cardiac failure or angina this may be increased by 25–50 µg per day every 2–3 weeks until the maintenance dose of 100–150 µg per day is reached.

Very occasionally the initiation of treatment is accompanied by the emergence of psychotic disorder, which interestingly usually takes the form of mania. Josephson and Mackenzie (1980) refer to 18 examples in the literature, 12 being manic illnesses and the others mixed affective or depressive disorders. The symptoms usually began within 4–7 days of starting thyroxine treatment, resolving over 1–2 weeks irrespective of further therapeutic intervention. All recovered completely. Such patients often had a personal or family history of psychiatric disorder and had frequently been depressed or delusional prior to starting treatment.

Cushing's syndrome

Cushing's syndrome is commoner in women than in men, usually starting in young middle age though the range of onset is wide. A tendency has been noted for the disorder to start during pregnancy, at the menopause or at puberty, or while the subject is undergoing a prolonged period of psychological stress.

In the majority of cases, perhaps some 80%, it is due to pituitary overproduction of ACTH, resulting in secondary bilateral hyperplasia of the adrenal cortices. How commonly this in turn is due to a primary abnormality of the pituitary, or a primary hypothalamic disturbance affecting the mechanisms of corticotrophin release, is still not clear, though small pituitary microadenomas are demonstrable in a high proportion of cases (Burke 1983). Occasionally there may be a radiologically demonstrable pituitary basophil adenoma, though this is rarely large enough to cause chiasmatic compression or raised intracranial pressure. Rarer causes include adrenal tumours—benign adenomas or malignant carcinomas — or ectopic ACTH production from malignant tumours elsewhere. Apart from differing levels of circulating ACTH, the endocrine abnormalities are the same whether due to adrenal or pituitary disease — a sustained excessive production of cortisol, obliterating the normal diurnal rhythm, and usually excessive production of adrenal androgens as well. Chronic alcoholics may occasionally develop a typical Cushing's syndrome which resolves within days or weeks when the alcohol intake stops (Smals *et al.* 1976; Morgan 1982); it can therefore be wise to rule out alcoholism as a cause.

The great majority of cases present for medical attention on account of the physical disorder which develops, but psychiatric features are strikingly frequent and can be severe. Moreover occasional cases have been reported to present with psychiatric illnesses from the outset as discussed below, and the endocrine disorder may then be recognised only after a considerable delay.

Physical features

The physical changes include the well-known moon face, buffalo hump and purple striae on the abdomen and thighs. Truncal obesity is almost always present, and insidious weight gain is often the earliest sign. The complexion is plethoric and hirsutism may be marked. Excessive bruising is common. Skin pigmentation may develop from the direct action of excessive ACTH on melanocytes. Hypertension is often severe and mild glycosuria may appear. Amenorrhoea is usual in the female, and impotence, testicular atrophy or gynaecomastia in the male. Other noteworthy features include liability to intercurrent infections, osteoporosis leading to backache or vertebral collapse, and muscular weakness particularly involving the legs which can sometimes be extreme.

Psychiatric features

Among patients reported from general hospitals, psychiatric disturbance has often been found in more than 50% of cases (Michael & Gibbons 1963). Trethowan and Cobb's (1952) series of 25 consecutive patients seen in a general hospital is typical — four were severely disturbed and psychotic, six moderately disturbed and eight mildly disturbed; three had relatively insignificant psychiatric symptoms but only four could be declared mentally normal. Jeffcoate et al. (1979) surveyed 40 patients of whom 22 were depressed, five severely, and four who showed other psychiatric disorders (mania, chronic anxiety and an acute organic reaction). Only a third were judged to be free from mental disorder. Whybrow and Hurwitz (1976), in a review of the literature up to that time, suggested that some 35% of patients develop depression, 16% disturbed cognition and 9% psychotic illness. Less than 4% appeared to show euphoria, in contrast to the situation when exogenous steroids are administered for therapeutic purposes (p. 628). Starkman et al. (1981) reported a particularly high frequency of psychiatric symptoms in 35 patients examined prospectively before the start of treatment. All 35 were fatigued, 30 showed irritability, 29 impairment of memory, 26 depression, 24 decreased libido, 24 insomnia, 23 anxiety and 23 impairment of concentration. Irritability was the earliest symptom in most cases, often antedating the physical manifestations. Depression could be of sudden onset and was usually intermittent rather than sustained, rarely lasting for longer than 3 days at a time. Social withdrawal was common, seemingly often due to feelings of shame at the physical appearance.

Depression is widely reported as the most frequent psychiatric symptom, and paranoid features are also very common. A range of other mental abnormalities is seen— emotional lability with gross overreaction to emotional stimuli, uncooperative behaviour or sudden outbursts of restless hyperactivity. These may be noted from very early in the development of the illness. Acute anxiety may also figure prominently, or states of apathy verging on stupor.

Fatigue and asthenia derived from the physical disorder often colour the psychiatric picture.

Cohen's (1980) study was important in that a consecutive and unselected series of 29 patients with Cushing's syndrome were examined closely from the psychiatric point of view. Twenty-five of them (86%) showed a significant degree of depression, this being mild in seven, moderate in 13 and severe in five. Almost half of the series had a family history of depression or suicide, or a past history of early bereavement or separation; six had had a major emotional disturbance shortly preceding the onset of the endocrine disorder, and in five this had consisted of a loss (bereavement, separation or broken engagement). These are all factors of known importance in the genesis of depression, raising at least the possibility of an aetiological link between Cushing's syndrome and depressive illness. Moreover, depression was particularly common among the 21 patients with a pituitary origin for their Cushing's syndrome; and all six patients with a disturbing life event preceding it fell into this group. It was, by contrast, uncommon to find severe psychiatric disturbance in the eight patients with adrenal adenomas or carcinomas.

The severe psychoses accompanying Cushing's syndrome are again mostly depressive in nature. Typically they are florid illnesses with delusions and auditory hallucinations and often with paranoid symptoms. Retardation tends to be severe, sometimes bordering on stupor. Anxious agitation may replace the retardation in other cases, or there may be acute brief episodes of grossly disturbed behaviour. Marked fluctuations in the severity of the condition appear to be characteristic.

Acute organic reactions are rare, but an element of disorientation or transient impairment of consciousness may be detected in severe examples of the disease. Classic schizophrenic psychoses are also rather uncommon though a schizophrenic colouring may be lent to the total picture. Johnson (1975) reviewed the occasional cases of schizophrenia in the literature and presented an unusual example of his own:

A woman of 50 had had a chronic schizophrenic illness with first-rank symptoms for 25 years. This had been extensively treated with insulin comas and electroconvulsive therapy. Signs perhaps suggestive of Cushing's syndrome — excessive bruising and pigmentation — had been noted some 19 years before the florid endocrine illness was declared. Despite the length of the psychiatric history, bilateral adrenalectomy led to a dramatic and sustained improvement in her mental state. It was concluded that in all likelihood she had had a primary schizophrenic illness, partly in remission as a result of earlier treatment, then exacerbated by the developing Cushing's syndrome.   (Johnson 1975)

The chief diagnostic hazard lies with those patients who develop psychotic features early in the illness. These may dominate the picture to such an extent that the endocrine disorder goes unnoticed. Two of Spillane's (1951) patients were apparently psychotic from the outset and long before the physical changes were sufficiently marked to suggest Cushing's syndrome.

One of Spillane's patients, a man of 26, had developed a paranoid psychosis which was treated with electroconvulsive therapy and continuous narcosis. It was not until 2 years after the first hospitalisation that Cushing's syndrome was diagnosed. It was on his return home after being invalided from the army that his mother noted a pronounced change in his appearance, with obesity, a bullneck and a plethoric complexion.

Trethowan and Cobb (1952) similarly reported a woman of 31 who had developed obesity, marked muscular weakness and amenorrhoea for a year before becoming excited, overactive and disorientated. Two further acute psychotic episodes occurred before Cushing's syndrome was diagnosed. Another of their patients was diagnosed as schizophrenic for several months, and another as hysterical for a year before the physical changes led to investigation of Cushing's syndrome.

Cognitive impairments have rarely been investigated systematically in Cushing's syndrome. A report by Whelan et al. (1980), involving neuropsychological testing of 35 unselected patients before treatment, indicated some degree of diffuse cerebral dysfunction in almost two-thirds of the sample. Thirteen patients showed essentially normal results on an extensive battery of tests, 10 showed mild impairments, eight moderate and four severe and frequent deficits. No aspect of cognitive functioning was spared, though impairments tended to be more marked on non-verbal tests (visual–ideational, spatial–constructional and visual memory tasks) than in the field of language and verbal reasoning. Patients may therefore be more impaired in cerebral functioning than is evident in conversation or on purely verbal assessments. The deficits sometimes extended beyond purely cognitive functions, with poor performance on tests of manual dexterity and somatosensory discrimination.

Mauri et al. (1993) carried out a carefully controlled investigation of 25 patients, and emphasised a selective disturbance of memory functions. Patients with depression or other psychiatric disorders had been excluded, also patients with a past history of head injury or drug abuse. Significant impairments were revealed on a number of memory tests, particularly in older subjects, and approximately half reported mild impairment of memory and attention in everyday-life tasks. Other cognitive functions were, by contrast, spared, apart from impairment on the Digit Symbol Substitution Test (DSST)

reflecting problems with attention and/or visuomotor functions. In a small subgroup who were retested 6 months after removal of their pituitary adenomas significant improvement was noted in both memory and DSST performance.

Radiological evidence of cerebral atrophy has also been found in a considerable proportion of patients (Momose et al. 1971), occurring as commonly in those below 40 as in older groups. Cerebellar atrophy was often conspicuous despite a lack of clinical signs. Computerised tomography (CT) scanning has shown atrophy, reversible with treatment and perhaps attributable to electrolyte and fluid changes or protein loss (Heinz et al. 1977). Ventricular enlargement and cortical atrophy have also been reported at autopsy (Soffer et al. 1961).

Aetiology of mental disturbances

The depression so characteristic of Cushing's syndrome is doubtless partly reactive to the physical disfigurements and discomforts produced by the disease. But a more direct connection is suggested in those cases where affective disorder is an early or even presenting feature, and by the frequency with which the depression reaches 'psychotic' intensity.

Cohen's (1980) observations (p. 516) are particularly interesting in this regard. The common finding of factors predisposing to depression in the histories of his patients may merely illustrate their vulnerability to depression in the face of physical illness; or it may indicate something more — a close pathophysiological link between the genesis of depression and the genesis of some forms of Cushing's syndrome. Thus it is noteworthy in his series that depression was significantly more common in primary pituitary than primary adrenal forms of the syndrome, a difference that had already been discerned by Carroll (1976b) from cases in the literature. Disturbing life events, antecedent to the development of the endocrine disorder, were confined to this form of the disease. More discriminating controlled studies will be necessary, however, before concluding that Cushing's syndrome may sometimes be stress induced.

The depression of Cushing's syndrome has often been contrasted with the elevation of mood characteristically seen when steroids or ACTH are administered for therapeutic purposes. Whether the difference is due to differing plasma levels of biologically active steroids, or to the long-continued chronic elevation of steroids in Cushing's syndrome is not known. Neither Cohen (1980) nor Kelly et al. (1983) could relate the severity of depression to the levels of circulating cortisol in their patients; yet its alleviation after surgical removal of the hyperplastic adrenals suggests that it must owe a good deal to some substance they produce. Hypothalamic factors may also be presumed to play a part in view of the complex neuroendocrine relationships now apparent in the control and regulation of the hypothalamic–pituitary axis (p. 507). In cases of pituitary origin additional factors could be the increased levels of beta endorphin and methionine enkephalin which are secreted along with ACTH (Fava *et al.* 1987).

The mechanism whereby hypercortisolaemia leads to cognitive impairment is largely unknown, but could conceivably depend on hippocampal damage. Thus Starkman *et al.* (1992) found indications on magnetic resonance imaging (MRI) of reduced hippocampal volume in three of 11 patients with Cushing's disease, the reduction in volume of the hippocampal formation correlating significantly with measures of verbal memory impairment and negatively with the levels of plasma cortisol. The hippocampal formation contains the highest proportion of corticosteroid-binding sites in the brain, which may make it particularly vulnerable in Cushing's disease.

Outcome

A successful psychiatric outcome can be expected when the endocrine disorder is effectively treated. The physical and mental symptoms usually improve in parallel until the patient regains her former stability. Depression is regularly observed to recede after adrenalectomy, pituitary operation or treatment with metyrapone, often starting to abate within days or weeks though sometimes taking as long as a year to clear completely (Jeffcoate *et al.* 1979; Cohen 1980; Kelly *et al.* 1983). Needless to say, when psychiatric disturbance has long antedated the Cushing's syndrome there may be little or no change when the latter is remedied.

With florid psychotic illnesses the results can be dramatic, as in the following examples:

A woman presented initially with physical symptoms of Cushing's syndrome, but on admission to hospital developed an acute psychotic picture with auditory and visual hallucinations and delusions about changing her sex. This was thought to have been precipitated partly by the mounting anxiety surrounding her admission to hospital. She became markedly paranoid and agitated, developed confusional episodes and showed bizarre catatonic motor phenomena. The entire condition responded well to bilateral extirpation of the hyperplastic adrenal glands and her mental state returned to normal within a few days of the operation. Follow-up 3 years later showed that she remained entirely well. (Hickman *et al.* 1961)

A soldier of 23 with a good service record became abruptly confused and hallucinated, and showed severely disturbed behaviour with grandiose and religious delusions. He was diagnosed as schizophrenic and treated extensively with electroconvulsive therapy. It was not until 1 year from the start that Cushing's syndrome was diagnosed. He continued to be severely disturbed, but pituitary irradiation 18 months and 2 years after onset led to transitory amelioration of the psychotic symptoms. Two and a half years after onset bilateral adrenalectomy was performed, and thereafter there was steady and gradual improvement until full premorbid stability was regained. (Hertz *et al.* 1955)

Details of management of the endocrine disorder, and of the distinction between pituitary and adrenal causes, will not be dealt with here. There are rival claims and special indications for bilateral adrenalectomy, pituitary operation and pituitary irradiation. Metyrapone can be useful in suppressing cortisol production.

Addison's disease

Addison's disease usually presents in early adult or middle life. It results from autoimmune destruction of the adrenal cortices or from diseases such as tuberculosis which involve the glands bilaterally. The output of all adrenal steroids is low — glucocorticoids, mineralocorticoids and androgens. Loss of sodium is accompanied by retention of potassium and extracellular dehydration. The blood sugar is usually low.

Physical features

The onset of symptoms is gradual, and the usual presentation is with general weakness, loss of appetite and loss of weight. Tiredness is an almost universal complaint. Pigmentation develops mainly on exposed skin surfaces. The voice is often soft and whining. Loss of libido is common, with impotence in the male and amenorrhoea in the female. Resistance to stress is lowered and sensitivity to infections increased. There is often pronounced intolerance of cold and the body temperature is usually subnormal. Hypotension is almost always present, syncope is common and symptoms of hypoglycaemia may appear at higher levels of blood sugar than is usual. There is an increased liability to convulsions, and the EEG is often abnormal with diffuse high amplitude slow activity. Potassium retention may lead to hyperkalaemic periodic paralysis (p. 721).

These several features deserve emphasis because the correct diagnosis is often delayed, sometimes until a severe 'Addisonian crisis' has occurred with considerable threat to life. The Addisonian crisis consists of a sudden exacerbation of symptoms with pyrexia, vomiting, epigastric pain, dehydration and profound hypotension. It may occur spontaneously or in response to infection, chilling or drugs such as morphine or anaesthetic agents.

Psychiatric features

Psychiatric abnormalities are present almost without exception in patients with Addison's disease. The commonest changes are those which might be expected in persons suffering from chronic physical exhaustion — depression, emotional withdrawal, apathy and loss of drive and initiative. There are sometimes sudden fluctuations of mood, or episodes of marked anxiety and irritability. Based on his own experience and on cases from the literature, Cleghorn (1965) described the mental symptoms as apathy and negativism in 80% of cases, depressive withdrawal and irritability in 50%, suspiciousness in 15%, agitated behaviour in 10% and paranoia with delusions in 5%.

Difficulties with memory are a major feature in up to three-quarters of cases (Michael & Gibbons 1963). Mild dementia may be simulated on account of the mental anergia, poverty of thought and general air of indifference. Considerable perceptual impairment may be seen as well, with increased thresholds to tactile, auditory and olfactory stimuli (Leigh & Kramer 1984). Drowsiness can be conspicuous though some patients show restlessness and insomnia. The severity of the changes may fluctuate from time to time, varying directly with the severity of the endocrine disorder.

Addisonian crises are sometimes preceded by increasing irritability and apprehension. Nightmares and episodes of panic lead on to acute organic reactions with clouding of consciousness, delirium, stupor and epileptic fits. In Addisonian stupor the patient is obviously unwell, lies curled up in bed resenting interference, and is collapsed and cold with dehydration, falling blood pressure and peripheral circulatory failure.

Psychotic pictures of a depressive or schizophrenic nature are rare, in contrast to the situation in Cushing's disease. Cleghorn (1951), however, reported examples of acute and chronic paranoia, hallucinatory states and schizophreniform psychoses. Such disturbances may be evanescent. They are sometimes intimately related to impending crises. McFarland (1963) reviewed reports of 10 patients with schizophrenia, six with affective psychosis and one with organic psychosis, concluding that the form of psychotic development is unpredictable. One of his patients presented with hypomania; this masked the adrenal disorder until the patient lapsed into coma after electroconvulsive treatment, when severe hyponatraemia was discovered.

Differential diagnosis

Addison's disease must be differentiated from hypopituitarism and from other chronic debilitating diseases. Weight loss, hypotension and pigmentation may all be seen, for example, in carcinoma, tuberculosis, malabsorption or malnutrition. It is therefore essential to investigate adrenal function adequately before making the diagnosis.

Hyponatraemia is present in about 90% of cases of primary adrenal insufficiency, and hyperkalaemia in 65% (Edwards 1996). Normal blood levels of sodium and potassium therefore do not preclude the diagnosis entirely. Similarly, basal plasma cortisol levels and urinary free cortisol levels cannot be relied upon to exclude the diagnosis since these often lie within the low normal range (Edwards 1996). The definitive tests for primary adrenal failure are either the simultaneous measurement of plasma cortisol and plasma ACTH, showing that the latter is disproportionately elevated in comparison to the former, or measurement of the plasma cortisol response to the 'synacthen test'. This involves the intramuscular injection of tetracosactrin, an ACTH analogue, then examining the rise in plasma cortisol that follows. In primary hypoadrenalism there is little or no response; in hypoadrenalism secondary to pituitary failure the response is delayed with much higher values at 24 hours than at 4 hours. The estimation of plasma renin activity can also be of value, levels being raised in primary adrenal failure in consequence of mineralocorticoid deficiency.

From the psychiatric point of view an erroneous diagnosis of neurosis or early dementia may easily be made. The depression and generalised weakness is often attributed to neurasthenia, especially when pigmentation is slight and the serum electrolytes are normal. The impression of neurosis is strengthened by the anorexia, irritability and diminished libido, and by the fluctuations which occur from time to time. Dementia, or a chronic amnesic syndrome, is suggested when memory difficulties are in the forefront of the picture.

Outcome

Adequate replacement therapy is usually highly successful in alleviating both physical and mental disturbances. The patient's sense of well being is quickly restored, and appetite and energy gradually return to normal. It has been observed that Addisonian patients are unusually sensitive to the mood-elevating effect of steroids (Cleghorn 1965). Glucocorticoids appear to be more important than mineralocorticoids for reversing the mental symptoms and abolishing the electroencephalographic abnormalities, indicating that these do not rest entirely on disturbances of electrolyte and water balance (Reichlin 1968). Cleghorn (1951) found that apathy, depression and irritability often persisted on treatment with desoxycorticosterone acetate and salt alone, but could resolve when cortisone was added later. Further treatment with androgens appeared to give no additional benefit.

Phaeochromocytoma

Phaeochromocytomas are tumours of the chromaffin cells of the adrenal medulla. Occasionally they are found ectopically in relation to the sympathetic ganglia lying along the aorta or in the cervical and thoracic chains. Most are benign and some occur familially. Some association with neurofibromatosis has been noted; also with hyperparathyroidism and medullary carcinoma of the thyroid (multiple endocrine adenomatosis, MEA type 2) (p. 528). In Hutchison et al.'s (1958) series the age of presentation varied from 9 to 51 years.

Clinical features

The tumours secrete an excess of adrenaline and noradrenaline, the relative proportions differing in different cases. The output may be paroxysmal or continuous. Accordingly the clinical features are subject to great variation.

Hypertension is always present during attacks and commonly persists in between (Ross 1972a, 1972b). The paroxysms that occur are usually the presenting feature. They last anything from 5 minutes to several hours at a time, and consist usually of severe palpitations, flushing or blanching, sweating, dizziness and tremulousness. A violent tachycardia is common, sometimes with substernal pain and acute dyspnoea. Nausea and vomiting may occur. The acute rise of blood pressure can be accompanied by agonising headache and may precipitate a cerebrovascular accident, epileptic fit or myocardial infarction. Death may result from ventricular fibrillation. After a severe attack the patient is left exhausted for hours or sometimes days.

Marked mental symptoms regularly accompany attacks. Intense fear is often present at the start and the patient may be overwhelmed with a feeling of impending death. Anxiety usually remains severe throughout the attack, and a period of excitability and confusion can follow. Attacks are precipitated by physical exertion, change of posture or raised intra-abdominal pressure, but also sometimes by emotional factors. Quite commonly they are triggered by a recognisable stimulus such as excitement, shock or panic. Sometimes, however, there are no discernible precipitants.

While the above is the classic picture, with well-marked

episodes, cases may also present surreptitiously. Attacks are sometimes minor in nature, or mentioned only in passing as feelings of faintness, palpitations or episodes of sudden anxiety. Hence the great importance of carrying out appropriate investigations whenever the disorder is remotely suspected.

Examination reveals marked hypertension during attacks and usually also in between. Papilloedema may very occasionally be present, with haemorrhages and exudates in the retina. Transient glycosuria may accompany the attacks, and a considerable proportion of patients show diabetes mellitus (Hutchison et al. 1958).

Investigations

The essential investigation is the demonstration of greatly increased levels of catecholamines in the plasma or urine, or of their metabolites in 24-hour samples of urine (metadrenaline, metnoradrenaline and vanilmandelic acid). When the index of suspicion is high, repeat estimations may have to be undertaken. Bravo and Gifford (1984) discuss the relative merits of urinary and plasma estimations. Twenty-four-hour urinary specimens can occasionally be misleading, since the amount of free catecholamines and their metabolites varies according to the levels of synthesising and metabolising enzymes within the tumour. On the other hand, a single plasma estimation may miss the occasional patient with truly episodic secretion. Plasma must be withdrawn with the patient fasting and resting supine for at least 30 minutes, also with the cannula in place well beforehand. In borderline cases a suppression test is useful: pentolinium or clonidine cause an immediate fall in plasma catecholamines and blood pressure when a phaeochromocytoma is present. Provocation tests formerly used various procedures to demonstrate an abrupt rise of blood pressure; these have now been largely abandoned since they can give misleading results and are potentially dangerous.

Differential diagnosis

Many patients referred as possibly having phaeochromocytomas prove to be suffering from some other condition. In Evans et al.'s (1951) series, 10 out of 20 suspected cases were suffering from anxiety or hysteria, often with episodes of hyperventilation. Other cases prove to be suffering from vascular headache, epilepsy, agitated depression or alcoholism (Hutchison et al. 1958).

More serious mistakes may occur in the reverse direction in that the phaeochromocytoma is missed. Essential or renal hypertension are probably the commonest misdiagnoses. Hyperthyroidism is often suggested by the patient's hypermetabolic state and associated heat intolerance. Any patient with hypertension in whom hyperthyroidism is suspected should immediately be screened for phaeochromocytoma. Other misdiagnoses include temporal lobe epilepsy, hypoglycaemic attacks and paroxysmal cardiac dysrhythmias (Ross 1972b).

From the psychiatric point of view an anxiety state may be very closely simulated, especially when emotional factors are known to trigger attacks. In two patients reported by Doust (1958), anxiety states of considerable duration had been attributed to psychological factors alone. One showed no obvious acute episodes and was normotensive. In a patient described by Gillmer (1972) a diagnosis of endogenous depression was made initially and the true condition was revealed in an unusual manner:

A woman of 61 with a strong family history of affective disorder complained of depression and anxiety for 18 months which had recently intensified greatly. She had severe insomnia and marked psychomotor retardation alternating with periods of acute anxiety and agitation. Blood pressure was 180/100 and there were minor hypertensive retinal changes. Treatment with antidepressants, chlordiazepoxide and electroconvulsive therapy was commenced. After the first electroconvulsive treatment she complained of severe headache associated with sweating and tachycardia, and the blood pressure was found to be 120/60. In view of the drop in blood pressure 6-hourly recordings were instituted before further electroconvulsive therapy was given. During the period of observation it was found that bouts of severe headache, dizziness and sweating were associated with peaks of greatly elevated blood pressure, for example to 300/170. A phaeochromocytoma was confirmed and removed successfully.

A patient seen personally illustrates another unusual mode of presentation, and underlines the importance of screening tests:

A 57-year-old man presented with a 1-year history of decline in work performance, loss of confidence and a change towards becoming quiet and subdued. This appeared to follow an accident at work when, as a senior ship's pilot, he had grounded a large vessel. After a second similar accident he was referred for investigation.

There was a 13-year history of diabetes mellitus, currently being treated with 44 units of insulin per day. Two years previously he had been treated briefly for hypertension with propanolol. Searching questions revealed two possible episodes of transient neurological dysfunction; for a few days after the first grounding he had appeared disorientated and had shown problems with direction when driving, and a year before that there had been tingling in the left arm and dragging of the left foot for a few hours.

On examination he was found to be depressed, apathetic and poorly informed about recent items of news. He was fully orientated but performed poorly on tests of memory and showed word finding difficulties. The blood pressure varied from 140/95 to 180/130. There were no neurological abnormalities.

The CT scan showed some diffuse cerebral atrophy, generalised white matter low attenuation, and two small cerebral infarctions—in the head of the right caudate nucleus and in the right cerebellar hemisphere. It was considered that the likely diagnosis was an early multi-infarct dementia in the setting of hypertension and diabetes mellitus. However, as part of a thorough screening procedure 24-hour urine collections were obtained and showed greatly elevated levels of vanilmandelic acid, metadrenaline and metnoradrenaline. A body scan showed bilateral suprarenal masses.

At operation bilateral phaeochromocytomas were removed. Evidence of diabetic retinopathy rapidly receded thereafter and he was soon able to dispense with hypoglycaemic agents. The blood pressure remained within normal limits or only mildly elevated without antihypertensive treatment. Repeat psychometric testing showed steady gains in general intellectual competence, the full-scale IQ rising from 99 to 114 during the first postoperative year. Word finding difficulties resolved completely, though difficulties with new learning persisted. He regained a good deal of his former vitality though remaining quieter than formerly. Repetition of the CT scan showed persistence of the white matter low attenuation, and some dilatation of the anterior horn of the right lateral ventricle adjacent to the infarct in the caudate nucleus.

In this patient the phaeochromocytomas had clearly been responsible for diabetes of many years standing, and for the hypertension that had more recently been discovered. The diagnosis was only made, however, after episodes of silent cerebral infarction had led to difficulties in a demanding work situation. There had at no point been indications of episodic changes in blood pressure or anything remotely resembling anxiety attacks.

Acromegaly

Overproduction of the pituitary growth hormone results from an adenoma, or rarely simple hyperplasia, of the eosinophil cells of the anterior pituitary gland. Skeletal overgrowth develops insidiously, affecting mainly the hands, feet, skull and lower jaw. Headache is often marked and incapacitating, kyphosis is common and joint pain may be severe. Hypertension, hypogonadism and diabetes mellitus usually occur. Loss of libido is a frequent early sign. Chiasmatic compression is relatively rare.

With regard to psychological accompaniments Bleuler (1951b) set the stage by a study of 22 patients from the Burghoelzli clinic in Zurich. He described alterations of personality by way of lack of initiative and spontaneity, sometimes interrupted by brief periods of impulsive behaviour, also changes of mood towards cheerfulness and self satisfaction. Brief swings of mood were regarded as characteristic, sometimes with spells of anxiety.

Bradyphrenia was observed in advanced cases and somnolence was common. Egocentricity and lack of consideration of others could be a problem for members of the family.

These impressions have rarely been checked in systematic studies. Anecdotal reports have emphasised depression and anxiety, coupled with loss of self confidence and concern over body size (Avery 1973). Margo (1981) reported a patient with a chronic depressive illness beginning 12 years before the acromegaly was diagnosed and with prominent psychomotor retardation from the outset. Sivakumar and Williams (1991) described a patient who showed pronounced depression and marked behavioural changes by way of pathological gambling out of keeping with his previous personality. This appeared to represent a loss of impulse control.

Psychotic disorders appear to be rare. Pye and Abbott (1983) described a patient who developed ideas of reference, visual hallucinations, delusions that her food was poisoned and voices urging her to harm her children, shortly before her acromegaly was diagnosed. Spence (1995) reported a patient with persecutory delusions and visual and auditory hallucinations in the context of depression. This was accompanied by an episode of impulsive stealing.

It is hard in such examples to know how far simple coincidence may be responsible. Abed et al.'s (1987) survey of 51 acromegalic patients used standardised assessments, and failed to find any general increase in psychiatric morbidity, nor a specific increase in depression when compared with the rates in other population studies. Indeed the scores were significantly lower than in certain other samples, and the interviewer was impressed with the optimism and even elation shown by many of the subjects. No overall relationship could be found between growth hormone levels and psychiatric morbidity; however, females showed significantly higher morbidity rates than males, and 10 of the 11 subjects who scored above the cut-off points for psychiatric illness were women.

The instruments used in Abed et al.'s study were unsuited to the measurement of personality change so this aspect remains to be elucidated. Patients are described as sometimes reserved, touchy and irritable, with emotional lability and traits of obstinacy. How far such features may be understandable as reactions to disfigurement, headache and limb pain, or whether they depend on metabolic changes or basal brain compression has not been clarified.

Neurological complications include mild proximal myopathy, and occasionally carpal tunnel syndrome due to hyperplasia of tendons and ligaments coupled with synovial oedema (Pickett et al. 1975). Hypersomnia may be a consequence of sleep apnoea occasioned by airway obstruction due to macroglossia and hypertrophy of the pharyngeal soft tissues (Perks et al. 1980; Seggev et al. 1986). In some cases, however, the daytime somnolence remits rapidly on treatment of the acromegaly, suggesting that it is not solely due to airway obstruction.

The mainstay of treatment is the removal of the responsible pituitary adenoma, usually by the transsphenoidal route (Wass 1993). With large tumours there is a risk of loss of pituitary function and other complications, and radiotherapy may then be employed. Bromocriptine improves symptoms in many patients, but carries a small but definite risk of precipitating a schizophrenic or hypomanic psychosis (Le Feuvre et al. 1982; Turner et al. 1984). Octreotide, a long-acting analogue of somatostatin, has proved to be even more effective in suppressing growth hormone secretion.

Hyperprolactinaemia

The commonest secreting tumour of the pituitary is a prolactin-secreting adenoma, leading to amenorrhoea and more rarely galactorrhoea in women, and to impotence and infertility in men. There is often a very considerable delay in recognising the tumour as the cause (Franks et al. 1977). In women it is usually a microadenoma, less than 1 cm in diameter, whereas in males it is commonly larger and may present with headache or visual field disturbance (Abrams & Schipper 1989). Even microadenomas can now be identified in a high proportion of cases by magnetic resonance imaging (Naheedy et al. 1987). Short of direct visualisation the tumour may be revealed by displacement of the infundibulum, focal bulging of the pituitary gland or focal erosion of the floor of the sella turcica.

Prolactin secretion is normally under tonic inhibition from the hypothalamus, the major inhibitory factor being dopamine secreted by neurones in the tuberoinfundibular region. Loss of such inhibition can be an important indicator of hypothalamic disease. Other important causes of hyperprolactinaemia include drugs which block dopamine receptors, notably neuroleptics. It may also accompany Cushing's disease, perhaps through stimulation of prolactin secretion by beta endorphin.

Fava et al. (1987) review studies showing high levels of anxiety and depression in women with the disorder, this being greater than in controls suffering from amenorrhoea but with normal prolactin levels. Up to a third of patients have been found to satisfy DSM-III criteria for major depression. In males the evidence for a relationship with affective disorder is less clear, suggesting that the effects of prolactin may in part depend on its interaction with gonadal hormones.

In general the depression responds poorly to antidepressants, but is ameliorated by the fall of prolactin induced by bromocriptine. Tumour size is also decreased by the drug. Transsphenoidal adenomectomy can be effective when a tumour is identified, likewise radiotherapy. Treatment with bromocriptine may very occasionally result in the development of a psychosis as in the treatment of acromegaly (Turner *et al.* 1984). Such reactions may occur in the absence of a personal or family history of psychiatric disorder, and usually remit on stopping the drug or reducing the dosage:

A 38-year-old woman with hyperprolactinaemia due to prolactinoma was treated with 7.5 mg bromocriptine daily for 7 months. During this time she became increasingly depressed, anxious and tearful and became convinced that she was being followed. She described people talking about her in the street and attempting to try keys in the lock of her door. She stopped taking bromocriptine because of her mood state and lost her schizophreniform symptoms within a month.

(Turner *et al.* 1984)

Hypopituitarism (Simmond's disease)

The commonest cause of hypopituitarism was formerly ischaemic necrosis of the anterior pituitary gland as a result of postpartum haemorrhage (Sheehan's syndrome). The cause is now usually a pituitary tumour, in particular a prolactin-secreting tumour in adults or a craniopharyngioma in children. A rare cause is head injury with fracture of the base of the skull.

Physical features

The condition is commonly of long duration, sometimes extending over many years when first presenting for attention. Leading symptoms include weakness, ready fatigue and marked sensitivity to cold. There is loss of libido, with amenorrhoea in females and impotence in males. Loss of weight is common, but despite the earlier name of 'pituitary cachexia' it is not universal. Nor is it extreme until the terminal stages of the disorder (Sheehan & Summers 1949). In cases with pituitary neoplasms, weight may actually be gained if hypothalamic function is disturbed. Anorexia is common but in some cases appetite is well preserved.

Cardinal signs on examination are a thin dry skin, which fails to tan normally and may become wrinkled as in premature ageing; a dull expressionless face and loss of pubic and axillary hair. The body temperature is often subnormal, the pulse slow and the blood pressure low.

Psychiatric features

The mental picture can be equally striking. The frequency of psychiatric disorder was shown by Kind's (1958) survey of cases from the literature and from his own experience. Ninety per cent showed psychiatric symptoms and in half these were severe.

Depression may be marked, sometimes with outbursts of irritability. Drive and initiative are impaired, and the patient comes to spend progressively longer in bed. Virtually all patients show apathy, inertia and somnolence in some degree. Ultimately most are dull and drowsy, prone to self neglect and indifferent about their state. The degree of psychological change commonly seen is greater than in other chronic debilitating diseases, and the patient's poor physical condition is therefore unlikely to be the complete explanation.

Impairment of memory may occasionally figure prominently and give rise to an impression of a dementing process. Other severe psychiatric complications include episodes of delirium in relation to impending metabolic crises, or more rarely chronic paranoid hallucinatory psychoses.

Metabolic crises may lead on from delirium to hypopituitary stupor or coma which is always a grave complication. Such severe developments usually set in only several years after the physical disorder has made its first appearance. The following case reported by Blau and Hinton (1960) illustrates the problems that may arise:

A woman of 46 was admitted with drowsiness, neck stiffness and a moderate pyrexia of 2 days' duration. She opened her eyes to her name but would not obey commands and resisted examination. Meningitis was diagnosed at first, but scanty pubic and axillary hair soon led to the diagnosis of Simmond's disease.

Falling blood pressure required intravenous noradrenaline in addition to intravenous glucose and hydrocortisone. She emerged from the semicomatose state but remained incontinent and uncooperative and proved to be deluded about her attendants. Violent behaviour necessitated transfer to a psychiatric hospital 2 weeks later, and over the next month she fluctuated from apathy to outbursts of restlessness with aggressive shouting. Memory and orientation were faulty and she was unable to concentrate for long. During the next few weeks she settled into a calm rather foolish euphoria and was correctly orientated for most of the time.

She was followed up with regular treatment with cortisone. Three months after recovery from the coma her mental state and intellectual functions were back to normal. She had recovered her libido, which had deteriorated along with her general health since the birth of her child 10 years previously.

In this case the episode of coma appeared to result from a combination of intercurrent infection, hypoglycaemia, hypotension and hypocorticoidism. The transient organic psychosis which followed it was probably due to reversible cortical damage resulting from some of the latter factors.

A more typical example was reported by Khanna *et al.* (1988):

A 28-year-old woman presented with a history of abnormal behaviour and irrelevant talk during the preceding 5 days. This had been sudden in onset and progressive. She suspected others of taking away her belongings and heard bizarre threatening sounds and voices 'from inside her abdomen'. She was neglectful of personal care and incontinent of urine. On examination she was dehydrated, markedly pale, mildly hypotensive and showed loss of axillary and pubic hair. She was disorientated in time, place and person and showed disturbance of immediate and recent memory. The provisional diagnosis was of delirium.

Her last child had been born 18 months previously along with excessive blood loss requiring transfusion. Failure of lactation and persistent amenorrhoea had followed the delivery. Thereafter she became slowed in household work, complained of weakness and fatigue, intolerance of cold, poor appetite and almost complete loss of libido. For 2 weeks prior to hospitalisation she had had frequent vomiting.

She was treated with rapid intravenous infusions to correct her dehydration and hyponatraemia. Within 48 hours she improved markedly and became fully orientated. Memory and intellectual function improved gradually on prednisolone and thyroxine and she regained her physical strength. She remained well on follow-up 3 years later.

Thus, as with adrenal cortex hypofunction, hypopituitarism rarely leads to functional psychoses, but commonly to acute organic reactions in association with crises of metabolic disturbance. In both endocrine conditions alterations of mood form an integral part of the clinical picture and take the form of apathy, anergia and indifference. In all these respects the psychiatric accompaniments and complications are in contrast to those of Cushing's disease, where functional psychoses are common and where the usual mood change is towards depression and emotional lability.

Differential diagnosis

Hypopituitarism must be differentiated from myxoedema, in which the facial appearance of the patient is very different, and from Addison's disease in which pigmentation is a prominent feature. In questionable cases full endocrine assessment is essential before embarking on the appropriate replacement therapy.

From the psychiatric point of view, neurosis and dementia may sometimes be closely simulated, but the principal differential diagnosis is from anorexia nervosa. Many of the early reported cases of hypopituitarism seem in retrospect to have been anorexia nervosa and vice versa (Sheehan & Summers 1949). Now that the situation has been clarified, however, there is rarely clinical doubt, even though both share the cardinal feature of amenorrhoea. Severe weight loss is rare except terminally in hypopituitarism, whereas it is usually a presenting feature in anorexia nervosa. Similarly appetite may sometimes be well preserved in hypopituitarism. Loss of pubic and axillary hair is unusual in anorexia nervosa, and the fine downy facial hair of anorexia nervosa is rare in hypopituitarism. The psychological features of the two conditions are also very different: in hypopituitarism the patient is dull, apathetic and somnolent, whereas in anorexia nervosa the patient is typically restless and surprisingly active; distinctive attitudes to food and to the body image are lacking in hypopituitarism, whereas they form an important constellation of symptoms in anorexia nervosa. When serious doubt exists full endocrine assessment will clarify the differential diagnosis.

Outcome

Response to replacement therapy is usually good. Within a few days the patient experiences return of interest and energy, and most lose their symptoms entirely. In cases of very long duration, however, apathy and lack of drive may persist in some degree. Cortisol or prednisolone alone may suffice, though thyroxine is sometimes given in addition. Gonadal steroids may be required to restore libido and potency in the male. Textbooks of medicine should be consulted for further details.

Diabetes insipidus

The syndrome of diabetes insipidus consists of polyuria with secondary polydipsia, resulting either from a deficiency of circulating antidiuretic hormone (ADH, vasopressin) or a lack of action of the hormone on the kidney. ADH is synthesised in the supraoptic and paraventricular nuclei of the hypothalamus, whence it is transported to the posterior lobe of the pituitary and then gains access to the circulation. It acts to increase the reabsorption of water by the distal convoluted tubules of the kidney, resulting in the production of a more concentrated urine.

In cranial (neurogenic) diabetes insipidus ADH is produced in insufficient quantity. In the nephrogenic form the kidney fails to respond normally to that available. Both result in the production of large volumes of dilute urine, normally accompanied by thirst. The urine osmolality is low, but the plasma osmolality is usually only slightly raised provided the thirst mechanisms are intact and the patient drinks adequately. If thirst does not occur, or if fluid intake is prevented, a dangerous degree of hypernatraemia and dehydration may develop.

Cranial diabetes insipidus can set in at any age without apparent cause, usually as an isolated abnormality but occasionally with other indications of hypothalamic disorder. The onset is typically abrupt. In very rare examples the condition is familial, being inherited as a Mendelian dominant. Other cases result from head injury with damage to the pituitary stalk, then often being transient, or follow pituitary surgery or yttrium implantations. Primary or secondary tumours involving the hypothalamus may be responsible.

Nephrogenic diabetes insipidus can occur as a rare sex-linked recessive disorder affecting males, and usually presenting soon after birth. Causes in adults include hypercalcaemia, potassium depletion and the prolonged intake of excessive amounts of water, all of which can impair the action of ADH on the nephron. A variety of drugs, including lithium, may also be responsible. Polyuria from lithium treatment can develop when plasma levels are within the therapeutic range; some 40% of patients on lithium experience thirst, with perhaps 12% developing polyuria (Ledingham 1983). In most cases this resolves within several weeks of withdrawing the drug.

The differential diagnosis of diabetes insipidus must include primary renal disease, diabetes mellitus, and the polydipsias induced by drugs such as chlorpromazine or thioridazine which may stimulate drinking by a direct action on the hypothalamus. The major diagnostic problem, however, is to distinguish diabetes insipidus from compulsive water drinking as described below.

The treatment of neurogenic diabetes insipidus consists of administering vasopressin. For transient states, as after head injury, aqueous vasopressin may be given subcutaneously. In the chronic condition the synthetic analogue desmopressin (desamino-D'-arginine vasopressin, DDAVP) is preferable on account of its longer duration of action and diminished pressor activity. This can be administered as a nasal spray. Nephrogenic diabetes insipidus is treated by thiazide or amiloride diuretics combined with indomethacin (Baylis 1996).

Compulsive water drinking
(psychogenic polydipsia)

Compulsive water drinking may be associated with a wide range of psychopathology—neurosis, personality disorder or psychosis. In psychotic patients it is frequently delusionally motivated. Among the nine examples described by Barlow and De Wardener (1959), long-standing personality disorder was common, often with hypochondriasis and depression. Six of the patients had had hysterical conversion episodes and some had histories of compulsive eating. Denial and evasion were sometimes a prominent part of the picture. Illowsky and Kirch (1988) estimate that polydipsia and polyuria without identifiable medical cause occur in 6–17% of psychiatric patients, especially those with chronic schizophrenia.

The clinical syndrome that results can simulate diabetes insipidus closely. In both conditions the fluid intake and output are raised and the urine osmolality is low. With compulsive water drinking, however, the plasma osmolality is also likely to be low. Hyponatraemia may develop when the water intake is so excessive that it exceeds the kidneys' ability to excrete it. There may be other evidence of psychiatric disorder to give the clue, or the onset may be clearly related to a depressive phase or period of emotional stress. The onset will often be gradual rather than abrupt, and consumption may tend to fluctuate from hour to hour or day to day in contrast to the steadily increased intake of diabetes insipidus. Nocturnal polyuria will often prove to be absent.

Not infrequently, however, the distinction can be difficult, and such difficulty can persist during fluid-deprivation studies. In normal subjects fluid deprivation over an 8-hour period leaves the plasma osmolality unchanged, while the urine osmolality rises to twice that of the plasma (Hall 1983). In diabetes insipidus the plasma osmolality rises, but that of the urine remains relatively low. The test may indeed have to be discontinued if the patient loses more than 3% of body weight. In compulsive water drinking the initial plasma and urine osmolality are low, and the plasma osmolality rises to normal at the end of the test. However, the urine osmolality may fail to rise to twice that of the plasma, since the prolonged excessive water intake may have led to a secondary nephrogenic diabetes insipidus. Prolonged water deprivation (carefully monitored) for 2–4 days may be necessary to allow the return of normal renal function, or this may be even longer delayed. Hypertonic saline infusion with measurement of the plasma ADH response may ultimately help towards clarifying the diagnosis, likewise a carefully supervised therapeutic trial of desmopressin (Baylis 1996).

When compulsive water drinking is mistaken for diabetes insipidus and treated with ADH, hyponatraemia and symptoms of water intoxication (p. 559) can develop. Water intoxication also seems to be a special hazard in compulsive water drinking associated with psychosis; numerous examples of such a complication have been described in schizophrenic patients, sometimes presenting acutely with vomiting, impairment of consciousness or fits (Jose et al. 1979; Khamnei 1984; Singh et al. 1985; Grainger 1992). Fatalities have been reported from time to time (Vieweg et al. 1985).

Both Jose *et al.* (1979) and Khamnei (1984) noted that a high proportion of patients with water intoxication secondary to polydipsia were psychotic, sometimes with evidence of inappropriate ADH secretion. In other cases there have been indications of enhanced renal sensitivity to vasopressin (Goldman *et al.* 1988; Emsley *et al.* 1989). How far such features may reflect hypothalamic or other disorders intrinsic to the psychosis is, however, uncertain. Multiple factors may often be at work, including the effects of medical illnesses or drugs (Fowler *et al.* 1977; Illowsky & Kirch 1988).

Special attention has been drawn to the role of psychotropic medications in leading to the syndrome of inappropriate ADH secretion (SIADH) (p. 559), including tricyclic antidepressants, tranylcypromine, fluoxetine, paroxetine, phenothiazines, haloperidol, thiothixine and carbamazepine (Sandifer 1983; Grainger 1992; Committee on Safety of Medicines 1994). In half of the cases reviewed by Sandifer, hyponatraemia had developed within a week of starting medication, usually but not always in association with SIADH. When hyponatraemia is found in a patient taking psychotropic medication it is important to test the response to a water load while on and off the drug, after ensuring that the serum sodium has been restored to normal. The drug may then be exonerated as the cause.

It is clearly important to enquire for a history of polydipsia in any psychotic patient who presents with seizures or lowering of consciousness. Similarly the discovery of polyuria with a low urinary specific gravity should always lead to careful observation of the patient's water intake. This may on occasion be skilfully concealed. Treatment must aim at restricting fluid intake, along with attempts to obtain maximal control of the patient's psychiatric disorder. Where long-term fluid restriction proves to be impractical, or when an offending medication must be continued, demeclocycline has proved to be beneficial in controlling both the hyponatraemia and the polydipsia, even in the absence of classic SIADH (Illowsky & Kirch 1988).

Klinefelter's syndrome

Klinefelter's syndrome results from the presence of at least one additional X chromosome in the nucleus in the male. It may present with infertility or delayed sexual maturation, or the hypogonadism may be discovered on routine examination. The usual karyotype is 47 XXY, revealed on buccal smear examination. Other variants occur, however, and in mosaicism the abnormal cell line may be restricted to testicular or other tissue.

Examination shows small testes and a variable degree of androgen deficiency, manifest as gynaecomastia or scanty beard growth. Azoospermia or oligospermia are always present and irreversible. The urinary gonadotrophin levels are raised.

Psychiatric features

A high prevalence of psychiatric disorder has emerged in this condition. Intelligence is often low, personality and behaviour are frequently abnormal, and there is a probable excess of psychotic illness. Some psychiatric features appear to be attributable to the endocrine disorder, others to be more directly related to the chromosomal abnormality.

Early reports of an excess of Klinefelter's syndrome among patients in mental subnormality hospitals led to the view that severe impairment of intellect was characteristic. It is now appreciated, however, that even superior intelligence may occasionally be encountered (Swanson & Stipes 1969). The usual picture is of mild impairment only, though perhaps a quarter of patients presenting at infertility clinics fall within the subnormal range. The greater the number of additional X chromosomes in the karyotype the more severe the mental retardation (Forssman 1970).

It seems clear that genetic rather than hormonal factors are operative in reducing the level of intelligence. No relationship has emerged between the degree of hypogonadism and the IQ levels obtained; and patients with hypogonadism due to other causes tend to show intelligence within the normal range. Thus Pasqualini *et al.* (1957) and Wakeling (1972) found a mean IQ of approximately 80 among their Klinefelter patients, compared with a mean of 100 among hypogonadal patients, despite a tendency towards more severe endocrine disorder in the latter.

Interesting findings have emerged from more detailed psychometric studies, which show impaired verbal abilities in comparison with non-verbal abilities. Thus Netley and Rovet (1982a) found mean verbal and performance WISC IQs of 85 and 101, respectively, in their sample of 33 children with XXY karyotypes. The verbal IQs were significantly lower than in unaffected sibling controls, and a 'sentence verification test' confirmed the presence of specific language impairments. Similar results were reported by Graham *et al.* (1988), who also found expressive language disorder with problems in word finding and the production of syntax. Achievement on a variety of reading and spelling tasks was impaired. In many respects this pattern is the reverse of what is found in subjects with Turner's syndrome (p. 528).

The altered intellectual functioning may be due at least

in part to impaired cerebral maturation or other brain abnormality consequent upon the genetic defect. A high prevalence of EEG abnormalities has been reported in the condition, chiefly slowed alpha frequencies but also slow wave dysrhythmias and paroxysmal features (Hambert & Frey 1964). Epilepsy is also commoner than chance expectation. Netley and Rovet (1982b) found that almost a quarter of 33 children with the condition were left-handed.

The personality in Klinefelter patients is sometimes abnormal. A variety of pictures has been described, ranging from markedly antisocial conduct to passivity and social withdrawal. Common descriptions are of patients lacking in drive and initiative, with severe restriction of interests and generally indolent, insecure and dependent. At the same time tolerance of frustration tends to be impaired, with explosive irritability and outbursts of aggression. Poor school and work records, marital instability and impoverished social relationships are said to be common.

Nielsen's (1969) review showed histories of alcoholism in 6% and of criminal behaviour in 12% of patients. A small excess of XXY patients has emerged in surveys of institutions caring for severely disturbed criminals, along with the more usual excess of XYY or XXYY karyotypes (Swanson & Stipes 1969). Schiavi et al. (1984), however, failed to support any excess of violent or aggressive behaviour among Klinefelter (or XYY) subjects in their comprehensive survey from Copenhagen. The prevalence of criminal convictions was slightly higher than for XY men, but this difference disappeared on controlling for intelligence and parental socioeconomic status. Moreover the great majority of the offences committed did not involve personal violence.

The endocrine disorder may play a part in hindering personality maturation and contributing to some aspects of personality difficulties. Thus patients with hypogonadism due to other causes are typically shy, timid and markedly lacking in drive. They tend, however, to show more stable histories and temperaments than Klinefelter patients, and lack any excess of criminal behaviours. Wakeling (1972) compared 11 Klinefelter patients and nine other hypogonadal patients seen in a psychiatric hospital; both groups showed insecurity and low tolerance of frustration, but passivity was more marked in the hypogonadal patients and impulsive erratic behaviour in the Klinefelter patients. The latter, moreover, frequently had histories of prepubertal maladjustment, with a higher incidence of unsettled schooling, neurosis and behaviour disorder in childhood. It appears, therefore, that in Klinefelter's syndrome delayed cerebral maturation may make a contribution, over and above the androgen deficiency,

in leading to poor social adjustment and disturbed personality functioning.

Sexual problems, as might be expected, are not uncommon. Potency tends to be low and to show an early decline, especially when features of hypogonadism are marked (Pasqualini et al. 1957). Androgen treatment can be successful in restoring libido and potency (Beumont et al. 1972). Occasional reports have described homosexuality, transvestism, exhibitionism and paedophilia in Klinefelter patients, but there is little to suggest that deviation is characteristic of the syndrome (Orwin et al. 1974). Sexual pathology, when it occurs, probably again reflects the restricted personality development and incapacity for deep interpersonal relationships. The more extreme examples of deviant sexual practice have usually occurred in severely antisocial or psychotic individuals.

Mental hospital surveys, reviewed by Forssman (1970), have indicated a threefold increase in Klinefelter patients compared with the general population. This appears mainly to be due to psychotic illnesses of a schizophrenic nature. Nielsen (1969) found that 6% of patients recorded in the psychiatric literature had been given a diagnosis of schizophrenia, and another 7% had psychoses of an uncertain type but almost all with paranoid delusions. Well-documented examples of schizophrenia in association with Klinefelter's syndrome are provided by Pomeroy (1980) and Roy (1981). The increased risk of mental illness may represent another facet of the increased vulnerability to stress of the Klinefelter patient, or may have more direct genetic determinants.

There is little to suggest an increased incidence of organic psychiatric illness. Jablensky et al. (1970) have described a patient who demented rapidly in his early forties, showing diffuse white matter degeneration and adrenal cortical atrophy at autopsy; this, however, may well have represented a chance association with Klinefelter's syndrome.

Turner's syndrome

The XO karyotype is associated with oestrogen deficiency and hence failure of sexual maturation. Primary amenorrhoea is accompanied by short stature and a variety of skeletal abnormalities including cubitus valgus and arching of the palate. The facial appearance is often characteristic with a small jaw, fish-like mouth and low set ears. The neck is short and may be webbed. Congenital renal abnormalities and coarctation of the aorta are common. The classic case shows a 45 XO karyotype, though other X chromosome abnormalities occur. The concentration of follicle-stimulating hormone (FSH) in the urine is raised.

Psychiatric interest in the condition has largely centred on the cognitive functioning of such patients. Mental retardation, chiefly mild in degree, was once regarded as common, but it now seems probable that verbal intelligence, at least, is normally distributed. Superior intelligence can certainly be encountered.

Money (1963, 1964) drew attention to the common finding of lower performance than verbal intelligence in patients with the syndrome, the means in his sample being 88 and 105 respectively (on the WISC or WAIS). This was paralleled by inferior scores on tests of perceptual organisation when compared with scores on verbal comprehension — discrepancies which became more marked at the higher intelligence levels. Visuospatial ability appeared to be particularly poor.

In some respects this disparity can be seen as an accentuation of the usual female as opposed to male pattern of differential cognitive abilities, which brings interest to Money's suggestion that it might be a specific cognitive consequence of the abnormal chromosomal condition. Garron and Vander Stoep (1969) review further evidence that Turner's patients have poor ability at drawing geometrical designs from memory, at drawing human figures and in certain aspects of left–right orientation.

The more recent study of 18 patients by Murphy *et al.* (1993) has confirmed significantly greater verbal–performance discrepancies than in controls, with lower scores on most aspects of the WAIS except for verbal comprehension. The greatest difference was in visuospatial ability. Among a subset of patients with XO mosaicism, visuospatial ability was negatively correlated with the percentage of lymphocytes containing the XO karyotype.

It remains uncertain how far such deficits reflect impairment of cerebral maturation due to genetic or endocrine factors, but quantitative MRI analysis of specific brain regions has shown interesting differences from controls (Murphy *et al.* 1993). Even after allowing for differences in head size the Turner's syndrome patients showed significantly smaller cerebral hemisphere volumes, parieto-occipital brain matter volumes, and smaller hippocampi, lenticular nuclei and thalamic nuclei bilaterally. On many of these measures the mosaic patients occupied an intermediate position. Among the group as a whole there was a significant right–left asymmetry in parieto-occipital brain matter volumes, that on the right being reduced. Occasional reports have suggested the presence of neuropathological abnormalities at autopsy, including atrophy, white matter heterotopias or small focal infarcts, chiefly affecting the right side of the brain (Reske-Nielsen *et al.* 1982).

With regard to personality, feminine sexual identification and interests are usually normal, and gross psychopathology appears to be rare (Garron & Vander Stoep 1969). Libido tends to be low, however, and many descriptions stress childish, meek and overcompliant behaviour. Traits of passivity and immaturity in the personality are congruent with failure of sexual maturation (Kihlbom 1969; Nielsen 1970b). Such features may also be partly determined by the infantilising response called forth by the patients' short stature and child-like appearance.

Neurotic traits may emerge, but severe emotional disorder appears to be rare despite the handicaps imposed by the physical defects and sterility. In contrast to the situation in Klinefelter's syndrome, there is no suggestion of an increased prevalence of antisocial behaviour or of psychotic illness. It would seem, therefore, that the lack of an X chromosome has substantially less effect than the possession of an additional X chromosome where mental health is concerned (Forssman 1970).

Hyperparathyroidism

Hyperparathyroidism has gained recognition as a rather rare but important cause of psychiatric morbidity. It is important because the diagnosis may be missed, resulting in many years of chronic mental ill health, yet treatment of the endocrine disorder can bring prompt relief. The cause is usually a benign adenoma of one of the parathyroid glands. Sometimes multiple tumours are present, and occasionally the condition may occur familially. More rarely there may be diffuse hyperplasia of all parathyroid tissue. In 'multiple endocrine adenomatosis' ('pluriglandular syndrome'), parathyroid adenomas are accompanied by endocrine tumours of the pancreas and pituitary (MEA type 1) or by phaeochromocytomas and medullary carcinoma of the thyroid (MEA type 2). Secondary hyperparathyroidism can result from renal failure due to elevated parathormone levels and impaired activation of vitamin D.

Women are affected more often than men. Cases usually present in middle age though the range of onset is wide. Calcium and phosphorus are mobilised from the bones and excreted in excess in the urine.

Physical features

Renal calcification is present in about two-thirds of cases in the form of renal calculi or diffuse nephrocalcinosis. The typical X-ray changes of osteitis fibrosa are present in many of the remainder.

In the great majority physical complaints are the predominant feature, with pain, fracture or deformity of bones, renal colic or profound muscular weakness. The myopathic syndrome consists of proximal muscular weakness and wasting, hypotonia and discomfort on movement. Other common symptoms which may suggest the condition are increased thirst, polyuria, dull diffuse headache, anorexia and nausea. On examination corneal calcification may be seen close to the corneoscleral junction as linear aggregations of granular material.

Psychiatric features

Mental symptoms are also common and were found in two-thirds of Petersen's (1968) series, even after excluding patients who had been referred specifically because of psychiatric disturbance. In a third the mental abnormalities were severe. Watson (1968) found that a very small but important group presented with mental symptoms alone, and showed neither renal stones nor bone disease. In Karpati and Frame's (1964) series four out of 33 patients had psychiatric complaints which dominated the picture to the extent that they had been referred initially for psychiatric or neurological consultation:

A woman of 40 presented with depression which had proved resistant to drugs and psychotherapy for several years before hyperparathyroidism was diagnosed. A woman of 64 had a 2-year history of agitated depression with tremulousness, disorientation, confusion and severe headache. A man of 43 presented with increasing nervousness and obsessive–compulsive features which subsided after operation. The fourth patient presented with a confusional state accompanied by severe headache.

Gatewood et al. (1975) reported five further examples, all presenting with problems that seemed to be mainly psychiatric, and four of them showing no evidence of bone or renal pathology:

A 63-year-old man developed persistent confusion following a cholecystectomy, which subsided within 2 weeks of discovering and removing a parathyroid adenoma. A 65-year-old man presented with a 14-month history of progressive depression, fatigue, lethargy and periods of confusion, and was similarly cured. A 56-year-old woman had been treated for 4 months for catatonic schizophrenia and improved gradually without medication after operation. A 74-year-old woman with endogenous depression similarly recovered without antidepressants. And a 75-year-old diabetic with a recent history of syncope, confusion and drowsiness made a remarkable recovery from what had initially been thought to be a cerebrovascular accident.

The commonest mental change is depression with anergia. The patient gradually becomes tired, listless and dull, with marked lack of initiative and spontaneity. In Petersen's (1968) series 36% of patients showed such changes, and almost all of these had been unable to work on account of lack of energy during the months preceding operation. Tension and irritability sometimes accompanied the depression, and explosive outbursts were occasionally seen.

Even among patients who do not complain of such symptoms at the time, they can often be recognised retrospectively when operation has restored the metabolic state to normal. Anderson (1968) found that three-quarters of patients reported that they felt better postoperatively, with higher spirits and greater energy than for many years before. It seemed that the chronicity of the disorder, which had often been present for 10 or more years when diagnosed, had made it difficult for the patient to appreciate the mental changes subjectively at the time.

Organic mental symptoms were present in 12% of Petersen's cases, chiefly impairment of memory or general mental slowing. This may be an insidious and chronic development, or may herald an acute organic reaction as part of a 'parathyroid crisis'. Such acute organic psychoses occurred in 5% of cases, with spells of mental confusion, or acute delirious episodes with hallucinations, paranoia and aggressive behaviour. Stuporose states may also occur, or recurrent convulsions leading to coma. Hockaday et al. (1966) described a patient who presented with stupor, and Cooper and Schapira (1973) reported a patient in whom stupor supervened during the course of a depressive illness. Both of these showed flexibilitas cerea at some point in their course.

Numann et al. (1984) have shown that even in patients without specific neuropsychiatric complaints operation can be followed by significant improvement on tests of verbal memory and cognition. Very occasionally the degree of intellectual impairment can give rise to a mistaken diagnosis of presenile dementia.

Non-organic psychoses appear to be rare in hyperparathyroidism, and when present are probably coincidental. However, a clear example of paranoid psychosis was reported by Alarcón and Franceschini (1984); the florid psychosis was unaccompanied by organic features in the mental state and subsided rapidly after removal of a parathyroid adenoma. Kleinfeld et al. (1984) refer to a case with mania as the sole clinical manifestation.

Investigations

Confirmation of the disease is usually obtained by finding a raised serum calcium. Repeat estimations may sometimes be required. The serum phosphate may be low but is sometimes normal. Blood must be taken while the patient is fasting and without venestasis, and account must be taken of the serum albumin level. Radioimmunoassay for parathyroid hormone levels can provide further confirmatory evidence, though a normal result does not exclude the condition. A hydrocortisone suppression test can also be useful—in hyperparathyroidism the administration of steroids usually fails to lower the plasma calcium, whereas this occurs in hypercalcaemias of other origin.

The serum alkaline phosphatase is raised when the bones are involved. Renal stones or calcification may be detected on X-ray, and typical changes may be seen in the bones. The hand X-ray can be particularly informative. Radiography of the skull may occasionally show calcification in the caudate nuclei and frontal lobes, though this is very much less common than in hypoparathyroidism since the calcium deposits are usually finely distributed. The EEG shows widespread slow activity, sometimes with paroxysms of frontal delta waves at high levels of serum calcium.

Differential diagnosis

The disorder should be borne in mind in patients who show chronic affective disorder, neurotic disability or minor intellectual impairment in association with suspicious physical symptoms. Neurotic ill health together with polydipsia and polyuria is a not uncommon mode of presentation. Petersen (1968) suggested that hyperparathyroidism should always be considered 'when lack of initiative, depression and thirst appear during a prolonged, insidiously developing and diagnostically unclear change of personality'.

Patients with fluctuating confusion or delirium may cause special diagnostic difficulties. When the acute organic reaction is recognised the main hazard is concentrating on a fruitless search for some intracranial cause (Henson 1966). In the presence of stupor, the electroencephalographic finding of widespread slow waves may provide the important clue to the metabolic derangement (Moure 1967; Cooper & Schapira 1973).

Neurological disorders are more frequently simulated. Headache, vomiting, fits and drowsiness can lead to a suspicion of cerebral tumour, or profound muscular weakness may suggest a primary muscular disorder. Cerebral arteriosclerosis, subdural haematoma, uraemia and phaeochromocytoma are other misdiagnoses that have been reported. Patten and Pages (1984) describe two patients who presented with severe muscle weakness, atrophy and fasciculation, one being first diagnosed as having amyotrophic lateral sclerosis. They suggest that all

patients with this condition should be checked for hyperparathyroidism.

Aetiology of mental disturbances

The cause of the psychiatric disturbance appears to lie chiefly or even exclusively with the elevation of serum calcium. Unlike the other endocrinopathies a relatively straightforward quantitative relationship is found between the severity of the psychological disturbance and this simple measure of serum chemistry. In Petersen's (1968) careful review, affective disorder and disturbances of drive corresponded to a serum calcium of 12–16 mg/100 ml, acute organic reactions with florid delirium appeared at 16–19 mg/100 ml, and somnolence and coma were found with levels exceeding 19 mg/100 ml. Such a sequence of changes could sometimes be traced in the single patient. Bleuler (1967) pointed out that the psychiatric disorders of hyperparathyroidism are more constant from person to person, and less dependent on the dynamics of the personality, than are the psychiatric pictures seen with most other endocrine disorders. This is no doubt because they depend upon a widespread ionic intermediary, and not upon the direct cerebral effects of a hormone which can influence brain functions in a more complex manner.

The level of circulating parathormone does not appear to be directly responsible, since mental symptoms can improve rapidly when the serum calcium is lowered by peritoneal dialysis (Petersen 1968). Nor can a relationship be discerned with the level of serum phosphorus or serum alkaline phosphatase, or with the duration of the disorder. The possible role of hypomagnesaemia remains unclear. Other factors may make a contribution, such as hypertension or renal failure due to nephrocalcinosis, but in the majority of cases these are clearly of subsidiary importance (Karpati & Frame 1964).

Outcome

Removal of the parathyroid adenoma usually brings relief to disorders of affect and drive, also to acute organic psychoses. The mental disorder is commonly found to be wholly reversible, with rapid resumption of former mental health. Headache is abolished and muscular strength increased. The time to recovery has been found to be independent of the duration of the disease and of the severity of the mental changes, and to parallel closely the fall in serum calcium. The rare psychotic states of long duration, with thought disorder and paranoia, may respond less satisfactorily, but probably owe a good deal to premorbid vulnerability. With severe depressive illness antidepressant medication may be required to obtain complete resolution, as in a patient described by Noble (1974):

A woman of 50 developed a severe depressive illness for the first time in her life. This responded well to electroconvulsive therapy. Eighteen months later she became apathetic and retarded, failed to respond to antidepressants, and during a course of electroconvulsive therapy became dehydrated and incontinent. A parathyroid adenoma was discovered while this was being investigated. Its removal, however, left her profoundly apathetic and unwell, despite the return of the plasma calcium to normal. After 4 weeks she was started again on tricyclic antidepressants which now led to progressive and full recovery.

Postoperatively, care is needed to guard against hypocalcaemia and plasma calcium should be monitored daily for the first few days. Preoperative preparation is required in patients who have significant bone disease, with the administration of vitamin D and calcium supplements (Kanis 1996). Acute anxiety may herald tetany, usually between the 10th and 14th postoperative days. Sometimes short-lived psychiatric disturbance sets in within a few days of the operation even though hypocalcaemia cannot be demonstrated, presumably occasioned by the abrupt drop in extracellular calcium which has occurred. Karpati and Frame (1964) reported such examples showing catatonia, acute agitation or mental confusion. Mikkelson and Reider (1979) described patients with fluctuating paranoid psychoses, hallucinations and stupor, with onset 4–12 days after operation and subsiding within a few days or weeks.

Hypoparathyroidism

Hypoparathyroidism, like hyperparathyroidism, has come to be recognised as a cause of remediable psychiatric disorder, especially since the comprehensive survey of the literature by Denko and Kaelbling (1962). This is replete with examples of failure to diagnose the condition, sometimes over very many years, yet treatment offers an excellent chance of reversing both the physical and psychiatric changes.

The commonest cause is removal of the parathyroid glands at thyroidectomy, or interference with their blood supply in the course of other operations on the neck. In other cases the aetiology is obscure; the parathyroids are found to be absent or degenerated, sometimes in more than one member of a family and occasionally in association with Addison's disease (idiopathic hypoparathyroidism). An autoimmune basis is suspected. The deficiency of parathormone leads to a low serum calcium and a raised serum phosphate. Calcium deposits may occur in the skin and the brain.

Two allied conditions occur more rarely:

In *pseudohypoparathyroidism* the parathyroid glands function normally but the tissues are resistant to the effects of parathormone. The same abnormalities are found in the serum chemistry despite elevated plasma hormone levels, and calcium deposits are found similarly in the soft tissues including the brain. It is due to loss of the actions of parathormone on calcium and phosphate, and the reduced formation of 1,25-dihydroxyvitamin D with consequent defects in mobilisation of calcium from bone and reduced calcium absorption from the gut (Spiegel 1989). Various subtypes are recognised according to the associated physical features and the location of the putative defect leading to hormonal resistance. Type Ia (Albright's osteodystrophy) is usually inherited as an autosomal dominant, showing additional traits of short stature, shortening of some of the metacarpals and a characteristic rounded facies. This normally presents early in life and may show resistance to multiple hormones. Type Ib usually shows a normal physical appearance, and resistance is limited to parathormone. It can be both sporadic and familial. Type II is rarely if ever familial and shows a different form of resistance. Parathyroid hormone infusion produces a normal rise in urinary cyclic adenosine monophosphate (cAMP) but a blunted phosphaturic response.

Pseudo-pseudohypoparathyroidism is identical to Albright's osteodystrophy in the associated traits, but hormonal resistance is lacking so the serum calcium and phosphate are normal. Spiegel (1989) discusses the confusion that has surrounded the term. It is best restricted to the relatives of patients with type Ia pseudohypoparathyroidism who show the associated physical features of Albright's osteodystrophy but produce a normal rise in urinary cAMP excretion in response to parathyroid hormone infusion. Diagnosis on the basis of serum calcium alone can be misleading since patients with hormonal resistance are sometimes normocalcaemic. Moreover the severity of hormonal resistance can vary widely within a family and may represent a polygenic trait.

Physical features

Hypoparathyroidism should be suspected in patients with symptoms of chronic tetany, or when ocular cataracts develop at an unusually young age. A history of operation on the neck should bring the possibility of the condition to mind. Symptoms can sometimes be present for many years before it is diagnosed, as in the remarkable example reported by Bellamy and Kendall-Taylor (1995). Thyroidectomy in childhood had been followed by epilepsy from the age of 27 and episodes of nocturnal stridor 10 years later, yet the patient's hypocalcaemia was detected only at the age of 47 after some years of progressive weakness accompanied by paraesthesiae and spasms in the hands and feet.

Tetany occurs in the form of numbness and tingling in the hands and feet or around the mouth. With more severe degrees the patient experiences muscular cramps and stiffness in the limbs, carpopedal spasms or laryngeal stridor. In carpopedal spasms the metacarpophalangeal joints are flexed and the interphalangeal joints of the thumb and fingers are extended to produce a characteristic posture of the hand ('main d'accoucheur'). Epilepsy can be the first and sometimes the only manifestation. In addition to cataracts the patients may have a dry coarse skin, scanty hair, trophic changes in the nails and poor dental development. Calcium deposits may be detected in the skin, or appear on skull X-ray as calcification in the region of the basal ganglia. Clinically useful signs include twitching of the facial muscles on tapping the facial nerve below the zygoma (Chvostek's sign), and the production of carpopedal spasm by temporarily occluding the circulation to the arm (Trousseau's sign). Very occasionally papilloedema may be observed.

Psychiatric features

A wide variety and a high incidence of psychiatric disturbances have emerged in hypoparathyroidism. Denko and Kaelbling (1962) estimate that at least half of the cases attributable to surgery have psychiatric symptoms, and that the frequency is probably higher still in idiopathic hypoparathyroidism.

The most frequent disturbances are organic psychiatric syndromes. Acute organic reactions with features typical of delirium are prone to develop in surgical cases, where the biochemical changes are likely to be abrupt. More chronic and insidious developments are not uncommon in idiopathic hypoparathyroidism, where the biochemical changes have developed gradually and have been much longer in operation. Such patients may show sustained difficulty with concentration, emotional lability and impairment of intellectual functions. Robinson *et al.* (1954) reported a patient with idiopathic hypoparathyroidism who presented first with status epilepticus and seeming presenile dementia, which illustrates the clinical problems involved:

For 7 years a woman of 61 had suffered from depression, commencing shortly after the death of her husband, and had gradually lost interest in her appearance and surroundings. Sometime after the onset bilateral cataracts had been removed. For several years she had experienced occasional numbness and tingling in the legs, and some 3 years previously skull X-ray had shown calcification in the basal ganglia. However, she had not reattended hospital for follow-up at this time. For 2 years there had been episodes of urinary incontinence, and for 6 months 'fainting spells' in some of which twitching of the limbs had been observed. For 5 weeks there had been considerable mental deterioration with confusion and loss of memory.

She was admitted to hospital with status epilepticus which subsided with treatment, and she was then found to be disorien-

tated, apathetic and doubly incontinent. Evidence of self neglect was extreme. She showed dysarthria, fine lateral nystagmus, diminished tendon reflexes and feeble extensor plantar responses. On the 10th day there were attacks of tetany and carpopedal spasm and Chvostek's sign was positive. The electrocardiogram showed prolonged Q–T intervals and low T waves. She was treated with intravenous calcium gluconate, oral dihydrotachysterol (A.T.10) and calcium lactate. Within a few days she had improved, becoming continent, orientated and taking an intelligent interest in her surroundings.

She remained well and her mental state did not deteriorate, but 3 months after treatment she developed choreiform jerks of the limbs and twitching in the face, presumably as a result of lesions in the calcified basal ganglia.

An important point stressed by the authors was that the patient showed no evidence of tetany on clinical examination until 10 days after her acute presentation.

Another remarkable example was reported by Eraut (1974):

An 80-year-old man was admitted to hospital on account of numerous falls at home. He could give no account of himself, but his wife reported that he had been deteriorating for many months and had been confused and forgetful for a long time. Cataracts had been extracted 14 and 20 months previously. While in hospital the previous year mild dementia had been noted. He was disorientated in time and place, could answer simple questions but could not respond to commands. There were no neurological abnormalities. A chest infection responded to antibiotics, but he remained demented. Three weeks after admission he had a grand mal fit, and when started on phenytoin became tremulous and totally unresponsive. This was followed by tetanic spasm of the left hand and laryngeal stridor, whereupon tests confirmed the presence of idiopathic hypoparathyroidism.

Treatment with dihydrotachysterol led to considerable improvement within a few days. He was discharged well recovered mentally, capable of lucid conversation and showing reasonable memory for recent and past events.

'Pseudoneurosis' is described as the next most common change, both in surgical and idiopathic hypoparathyroidism, and occurs in all age groups. Children show temper tantrums and night terrors, and adults become depressed, nervous and irritable with frequent crying spells and marked social withdrawal. The emotional disturbances may fluctuate in degree or show periods of spontaneous resolution.

In this connection the concept of 'partial parathyroid insufficiency' is interesting. Fourman *et al.* (1963) showed that in a quarter of patients who had undergone thyroidectomy the plasma calcium was merely at the lower limit of normal, but could be provoked to fall to definitely subnormal values by calcium deprivation or intravenous administration of edetic acid. About half such patients had mental symptoms in the form of tension and anxiety, panic attacks, depression and lassitude. Often there were no other pointers to parathyroid insufficiency and the symptoms were therefore indistinguishable from those commonly found in middle-aged neurotic women. Fourman *et al.* (1967) later assessed the relevance of such symptoms by a double-blind trial of calcium citrate tablets and placebo, and confirmed that calcium was significantly effective in reducing psychiatric symptom scores. The most consistent changes were with regard to depression and diminution of appetite.

More rarely, psychotic illnesses of manic–depressive or schizophrenic type may be seen, particularly in cases due to surgery. Again spontaneous remissions or response to other forms of treatment may delay diagnosis of the underlying condition.

In pseudohypoparathyroidism and pseudo-pseudohypoparathyroidism intellectual impairment is by far the most frequent psychiatric abnormality, occurring in approximately half of reported cases. Several such patients have been discovered in hospitals for the feeble minded, and Denko and Kaelbling (1962) suggest that the serum calcium should be investigated in every patient with mental retardation. Pollard *et al.* (1994) have recently reported a 13-year-old girl of normal intelligence with type II pseudohypoparathyroidism who presented with an episode of apparent hysterical paralysis and rapid cycling bipolar mood disorder.

Investigations

The serum calcium is low, the serum phosphate raised, and the urinary excretion of calcium and phosphate diminished. The serum alkaline phosphatase is normal. Skull X-ray frequently shows calcification in the region of the basal ganglia as symmetrical bilateral punctate opacities. Electroencephalographic abnormalities may be present even in the absence of epilepsy, usually generalised but sometimes surprisingly focal (Watson 1972).

In pseudohypoparathyroidism the same abnormalities of serum chemistry are found, but a distinction can be made by examining the effect of an infusion of parathyroid hormone on the excretion of phosphate and cAMP in the urine.

Differential diagnosis

The diagnoses which may be mistakenly entertained include mental retardation, presenile dementia, neurosis, hysteria, idiopathic epilepsy and cerebral tumour.

A diagnosis of neurosis or hysteria is suggested by the peculiar and intermittent nature of the symptoms, including bizarre paraesthesiae and muscular spasms. Moreover the patient may give a vague and perplexing account with

obvious difficulty in observing and describing the symptoms. Attacks may be triggered by emotional influences, since hyperventilation will lead unusually readily to tetanic symptoms. Hypochondriasis is readily suggested by the generally heightened level of anxiety, the vagueness of the complaints and the occurrence of periods of spontaneous remission. As a result patients with hypoparathyroidism are sometimes found to have carried a label of psychogenic disorder for several years before the true diagnosis is made. In other cases well-defined mood swings have led to an initial diagnosis of manic–depressive disorder (Denko & Kaelbling 1962).

Epileptic attacks may be thought to be idiopathic in origin, and the serum calcium should be determined in every epileptic patient when the precise cause of the attacks remains uncertain. Occasionally increased intracranial pressure and papilloedema are encountered in patients with hypoparathyroidism, this reversing with correction of the serum calcium; cerebral tumour may be closely simulated, especially when fits are present and alteration of personality has occurred.

Outcome

The response to correction of the serum biochemistry is usually gratifying. Neurotic symptoms are reported to clear in the majority of cases even though some weeks may elapse before the patient feels entirely well.

Acute organic reactions may be expected to improve promptly. Chronic cognitive impairments may also be completely reversed. Denko and Kaelbling (1962) noted that when adequate details were given, about half the cases of idiopathic hypoparathyroidism with intellectual impairment were reported to improve whereas very few cases were unchanged or worse. Patients with pseudohypoparathyroidism may also improve cognitively when the serum chemistry is corrected, but rarely to a spectacular extent. This is perhaps because such patients have been damaged intellectually while still immature, or perhaps because there is an associated genetic cause for their cognitive impairment.

Details of long-term management will not be dealt with here. This usually requires vitamin D or equivalent preparations such as dihydrotachysterol in addition to oral calcium.

Diabetes mellitus

Diabetes mellitus results from an absolute or relative deficiency of insulin production by the pancreas, causing disturbed carbohydrate metabolism with hyperglycaemia and glycosuria. Secondary changes are prone to occur in the metabolism of protein and fat, the latter leading to ketosis and acidosis. It is a syndrome rather than a disease entity. The requirements of insulin may be found to be in excess of normal pancreatic production, owing to cellular resistance to the action of insulin or excessive gluconeogenesis. Hence it is probable that factors other than decreased insulin production contribute to the severity of diabetes in many patients, with the anterior pituitary and adrenal glands also playing a part.

The onset can be at any age from infancy to old age, with approximately half of cases appearing before 50 and another quarter between 50 and 60 years. The disorder tends to be rapid in onset in the young, but usually insidious in development and milder in older persons. A division is made into type I (insulin dependent) and type II (non-insulin dependent) diabetes. Type I typically occurs in young thin patients, shows absolute insulin deficiency and is ketosis prone; type II is usually found in older obese patients, shows relative insulin lack and tissue resistance to insulin effects, and is not ketosis prone (Windebank & McEvoy 1989).

It is well established that genetic mechanisms are operative in both forms of the disease, and interesting progress has recently been made in relation to type I diabetes (Bennett et al. 1995; Kennedy et al. 1995; Bell & Hockaday 1996). Multiple loci are clearly involved, including loci on chromosome 6 in the human leucocyte antigen (HLA) region, and on chromosome 11 in close relation to the insulin gene itself. The insulin gene is flanked upstream by multiple repeats of a 14 base pair sequence, variations in length of the sequence correlating with disease susceptibility, perhaps through a direct effect on transcription of the insulin gene. Genetic influences in type II diabetes are especially apparent in patients who are not overweight, including, it seems, changes in mitochondrial DNA.

Textbooks of medicine should be consulted for the general clinical associations of the disorder and the principles of management by diet, insulin and oral hypoglycaemic agents.

Psychiatric attention to diabetes has been sporadic, and few systematic surveys have been made of the emotional and other mental complications. However, valuable reviews were produced by Wilkinson (1981) and Tattersall (1981). In clinical practice it is clear that the diabetic who is poorly endowed or emotionally unstable can pose a considerable therapeutic problem, since cooperation in treatment is essential if adequate control is to be achieved. Moreover, there are indications that psychological stresses can be important in aggravating the disorder or precipitating episodes of loss of control, and there are even suggestions that emotional factors may sometimes bring the disorder into being.

These issues will be discussed below, along with the question of brain damage in diabetic patients. When evidence of brain damage emerges this may be attributable to episodes of hypoglycaemia or diabetic coma, or alternatively to the high incidence of atherosclerosis which exists in diabetics. The picture of diabetic coma, and certain common neurological complications, will also be briefly described.

Emotional influences on the course of diabetes

A considerable body of evidence shows that emotionally stressful experiences can produce fluctuations in levels of blood glucose and ketone bodies, both in diabetic and non-diabetic persons. Early experimental observations in this area are summarised by Hinkle and Wolf (1952a, 1952b). The magnitude of such changes is much greater in diabetics, and if of long enough duration they appear capable of leading to ketosis and hyperglycaemia in some cases and to hypoglycaemia in others. It has proved difficult, however, to define the extent to which such factors may be operative in the actual disease.

Stress, either physical or emotional, has often been blamed as the initial cause. Examples of the sudden manifestation of diabetes in relation to dramatic stresses are scattered throughout the literature, also attempts at constructing a characteristic personality profile which has rendered the diabetic unusually susceptible to stress. Treuting (1962) reviews the theories that have been elaborated, suggesting for example that diabetes is a disorder of adaptation and that persons showing it have reacted to various life crises with a physiological response that is appropriate to starvation. However, no increased incidence of the disorder emerged in battle casualties from the First and Second World Wars, and it now seems most unlikely that stress can bring the disorder into being in people who would otherwise never have developed it. It remains possible, nonetheless, that stress may sometimes change a latent case of diabetes into an active one, i.e. that physical or emotional stresses may play a part in determining the time at which the disorder is declared.

A rather less controversial area is the effect of emotional influences on the course of the established disease. Diabetic patients may sometimes show a close relationship between disturbing life experiences and episodes of loss of control, even to the extent of developing ketotic coma. Hinkle and Wolf (1952a, 1952b) observed 64 diabetics, giving special attention to their prevailing attitudes and the relationships important to their emotional security. In long-term studies extending over several years, periods of exacerbation and remission were correlated with events in the life situation. Events which were consciously or unconsciously interpreted by the patients as threatening to their security appeared to be particularly liable to lead to loss of control. Case histories were presented to illustrate how admissions to hospital for coma could regularly follow stressful situations, as in the following example:

An adolescent girl from a disturbed home background had 12 admissions for diabetic acidosis and coma during 5 years, all following acutely stressful life situations. 'To each of these stresses—fights between her parents, arguments with her mother, change to a new school, the departure of her sister ("the only one who loved me")—she reacted as if it were a threatened deprivation of love and security. They aroused in her resentment, which she felt afraid to express, and were accompanied by the rapid development of thirst, polyuria, ketosis and coma. On several occasions . . . she expressed her hopelessness and rebellion by stopping her insulin when the ketosis developed. On other occasions she expressed her resentment and hopelessness by failing to sterilise her equipment, and the subsequent infections led to hospital admissions. In half of these instances, however, diabetic coma followed swiftly upon the onset of a stressful life situation, despite the fact that no infection was present and the insulin dose was not altered. It may be remarked in passing that this patient was typical of the group in that the exacerbations of the diabetic state were in all instances closely related to situational and interpersonal conflicts . . .'. Close supervision and help with her emotional problems led in this case to better control of the diabetes. (Hinkle & Wolf 1952b)

The uncertainty in such examples concerns the extent to which the direct metabolic consequences of the emotional upheavals are responsible, rather than secondary effects due to abandoning dietary regimes or insulin requirements. Thus some patients may overeat or resort to alcohol when under stress, and others may omit insulin or neglect sterile precautions. In occasional cases comas may be deliberately induced to secure attention or as a means of escape into the shelter of hospital. Indeed, Tattersall (1981) has termed insulin-dependent diabetes 'the manipulator's delight'.

Hinkle and Wolf, however, argued strongly for a more direct influence of life experiences upon the metabolic disorder and hence on the course of the disease. When it appeared that a certain personal conflict was connected with variations in the diabetic state, they tested this in short-term experimental settings. Baseline observations were made, then the suspected topic of conflict was vigorously introduced into discussion. Control studies were made in which neutral topics were discussed. In this way psychological stress was shown to lead to ketonaemia and increased water, glucose and chloride excretion, in addition to alterations in fasting blood sugar levels.

Baker and Barcai (1970) felt able to demarcate a small number of 'super-labile' juvenile diabetics in whom emotional arousal led directly to ketoacidosis, mediated by an increased ketone response to endogenous catecholamines. Beta adrenergic blockade was apparently successful in inhibiting the metabolic decompensation in such patients, producing marked therapeutic benefit. Tattersall (1981), however, doubts whether organic *a priori* causes are common. In the usual 'brittle diabetic', whose life is constantly disrupted by episodes of hyper- and hypoglycaemia, physiological, psychological and social problems come in time to be inextricably intertwined. Depression and reactions of frustration and futility breed carelessness in self management and distrust of prescribed routines. An emotional origin often appears to be paramount in leading to this vicious circle.

Whatever the mechanisms, many agree that life experiences and emotional factors can have an important bearing on the course of diabetes, and that this is particularly important in juveniles and adolescents (Treuting 1962). Attempts at demonstrating the influence of life events have indeed been partially successful despite difficulties in methodology. Grant *et al.* (1974) studied 37 adults over 8–18 months, and found a trend towards an association between important life events, particularly those of an unpleasant nature, and fluctuations in diabetic control. Bradley (1979) reviewed 114 patients retrospectively, and found a significant association between the number of life events experienced over a 12-month period and the incidence of glycosuria, changes in prescription and number of clinic attendances. Insulin-treated patients appeared to be more vulnerable in this regard than those receiving oral hypoglycaemic agents. Accordingly it may sometimes be necessary to pay careful attention to psychological and psychosocial aspects of the patient's situation if optimal control of the diabetes is to be achieved.

Psychological problems

In several ways the situation imposed by diabetes is unusual in comparison with other chronic diseases. The patient must often face interminable dietary restrictions and daily self-administered injections, yet is usually symptom-free so gets no perceptible reward. He has responsibility, which is rare in other illnesses, for judging unusual situations and adjusting the dose of insulin required. Repeated hospitalisations can stigmatise him from an early age. Such factors can contribute to neurotic developments or disturbed family relationships, and hypochondriacal attitudes may come to be established.

Certain types of behaviour are said to be common in diabetics, but many are of a nature which would be unremarkable but for the fact that they complicate therapy.

Thus some show an unusual need to eat and find great difficulty in adhering to dietary regimes. This may be intensified during periods of loneliness, depression or tension. Explosive rebellion may be seen in adolescents, with wilful neglect of treatment.

In children the disorder lends itself to incorporation in disturbed parent–child relationships. The anxiety of the parents may be transferred to the young child, or a perfectionistic mother may gain control over the illness at the cost of behaviour difficulties. The child on his part may utilise the diabetes to manipulate the home environment, using food as a weapon or form of retaliation. Surveys of diabetic children have been undertaken to explore possible psychological effects in detail, though with varying results (Sterky 1963; Swift *et al.* 1967; Gath *et al.* 1980). In general adjustment has seemed remarkably good, though the sample investigated by Swift *et al.* showed minor abnormalities on measures of dependence/independence, self perception, manifest and latent anxiety and sexual identification.

In adult life employment or marriage prospects may stand to be affected. Pruritis and decreased sexual interest may contribute to emotional complications, and impotence and amenorrhoea can be early complaints even in undiagnosed diabetics. Surridge *et al.* (1984) found indications of delayed psychosexual development when diabetes sets in at an early age. Earlier reports of the frequency of impotence in men and anorgasmia in women (Kolodny 1971; Kolodny *et al.* 1974) may have been an overestimate, but there can be little doubt that such problems often occur. Disturbances of ejaculation are also probably common (Fairburn *et al.* 1982). The physical handicaps later imposed by ocular and other complications bring further problems of their own.

A major fear among many insulin takers is the occurrence of a hypoglycaemic attack. They particularly dread attacks which lack the adrenergic warning, and in which loss of self control or bizarre behaviour may occur. It now seems clear, moreover, that 'subclinical' hypoglycaemia is commoner than previously suspected in diabetics, as a result of overtreatment, and that this may account for considerable chronic disability.

Thus Gale and Tattersall (1979) found, from overnight metabolic studies, that nocturnal hypoglycaemia occurred in 22 of 39 poorly controlled insulin-treated patients. This was often sustained for periods of several hours. Overt hypoglycaemic symptoms by day had been very mild or absent. The features occurring in such a situation included lassitude and depression in 15 patients, undue difficulty in waking in 11, early morning headache in seven and nocturnal fits in two. By day the worst affected appeared pale, apathetic, torpid and demoralised.

Others complained of lethargy, depression and difficulty in concentration. Reduction of insulin dosage relieved or abolished all such problems without loss of overall diabetic control. Schwandt *et al.* (1979) have described similar examples. Nine out of 45 unstable diabetics turned out to have been chronically overtreated with insulin; their symptoms included excessive appetite, polydipsia, vertigo, mood swings, irritability and chronic fatigue.

Descriptive studies have shown that all forms of mental illness may occur in association with diabetes but there is little evidence about prevalence and forms. Apart from disturbances associated with overt or covert hypoglycaemia there is probably little that is specific. Increased fatigue and diminished energy were the most prominent mental symptoms in Surridge *et al.*'s (1984) survey, also depression and irritability. However, carefully controlled observations do not appear to have been carried out. Surveys of psychiatric hospital populations have sometimes indicated a higher prevalence than expected of diabetes mellitus (Waitzkin 1966a, 1966b; Clayer & Dumbrill 1967), but chiefly of the late-onset non-insulin-dependent form. This may merely reflect the age and tendency to obesity among long-stay patients; chlorpromazine, moreover, may lead to hyperglycaemic responses on the glucose tolerance test.

Finally, in the management of manic–depressive illness in diabetics it may sometimes be necessary to consider the possibility that insulin requirements increase during markedly depressive phases:

Crammer and Gillies (1981) reported a woman with long-standing manic–depressive disorder which for some years had been cyclical, occurring approximately every 20 weeks. For several years she had also had late-onset diabetes, well controlled with oral hypoglycaemic drugs. During a particularly severe depressive episode the diabetes became out of control, requiring soluble insulin injections. Electroconvulsive therapy relieved the depression, but coincidentally the insulin requirement declined dramatically. With recurrence of the depression the same changes were seen, again resolving on recovery. During her manic phases, by contrast, no changes in diabetic treatment were required.

Kronfol *et al.* (1981) reported a similar example of a patient who required increased insulin during recurrent phases of a depressive illness.

Brain damage in diabetes

When a diabetic patient develops organic psychiatric disorder the question arises how far this may be attributable to some aspect of the diabetic process. Episodes of hypoglycaemia or diabetic coma may have contributed to brain damage, or associated atherosclerosis may be responsible.

In very young children Ack *et al.* (1961) produced some evidence that intelligence may be impaired, possibly as a result of damage to the immature brain by episodes of hypoglycaemia or acidosis. Thirty-eight diabetic children were compared with their siblings on the Stanford Binet test, and those with onset below the age of 5 years were found to score an average of 10 points lower than the controls. By contrast those with onset over the age of 5 were unaffected. The result may have reflected some degree of brain damage, or merely the psychological impact of a chronic disease at such a young age.

Ives (1963) surveyed 380 adult diabetics in a general hospital and found that 45 were mentally abnormal. Eighteen showed 'organic brain syndromes', 14 were mentally deteriorated, nine had personality disorders and four were psychotic. Hypertension was commoner in the mentally impaired patients than in the group as a whole, suggesting that cerebral atherosclerosis was probably the responsible factor. In others the mental abnormalities may have been coincidental, but episodes of diabetic coma and hypoglycaemia had been more frequent in the total group of 45 than in the remainder.

Bale (1973) compared 100 patients from a diabetic clinic with age- and sex-matched controls drawn from visitors to the hospital. All patients were under 65 years of age and had had diabetes for 15 years or more. On the Walton Black New Word Learning Test 17 diabetics, but no controls, scored in the brain-damaged range. A significant relationship was observed between low scores on the test and the apparent severity of past hypoglycaemic episodes. The frequency of cerebrovascular accidents was higher in the diabetic group than the controls, but only one patient with a cerebrovascular accident scored within the brain-damaged range. It thus appeared that mild cognitive difficulty was not uncommon in long-standing diabetics, and that hypoglycaemic episodes rather than cerebrovascular disorder might be the principal factor responsible.

Two more recent studies have addressed the issue. Wredling *et al.* (1990) selected 17 insulin-dependent diabetics with histories of recurrent severe hypoglycaemic episodes and compared them to 17 diabetics without such histories. The two groups were comparable in terms of sex, age, duration of diabetes, injection frequency, dose of insulin and socioeconomic parameters. On neuropsychological evaluation the group who had had hypoglycaemic episodes performed significantly less well on tests of finger tapping, digit span, Necker cube reversals and maze learning.

Langan *et al.* (1991) tested 100 insulin-dependent patients on an extensive psychometric battery, after excluding those who had evidence of other causes of brain damage including cerebrovascular disease. A questionnaire was used to assess the number, frequency and severity of hypoglycaemic episodes experienced. Significant correlations were found between the frequency of severe hypoglycaemias and an index of intellectual decline (discrepancy between NART and WAIS IQ), all of the WAIS performance subtests and a choice reaction time test. Speed of information processing as measured by the PASAT (p. 198) correlated with the estimated number of hypoglycaemic episodes sustained during the patient's lifetime. No such relationships could be discerned for measures of verbal memory or verbal IQ. Contrasting groups were then identified with and without a history of severe hypoglycaemias: though balanced in terms of premorbid IQ and duration of diabetes the former were significantly slower on choice reaction time tests and showed a greater IQ decrement.

All such findings, while strongly suggestive of a pathogenic role for hypoglycaemia, are not of course conclusive. It is possible that the association between impaired cognitive capacity and hypoglycaemic episodes reflects the poorer management of diabetes by patients who are less well-endowed intellectually. Deary and Frier (1996) review these and other studies and conclude that the verdict remains at present 'unproven'. Prospective studies over a considerable period of time will be needed to clarify the situation decisively.

A patient reported by Mace (1987) raised the possibility of memory impairment secondary to self-induced hypoglycaemias. A 29-year-old computer manager had abused many drugs and drunk excessively from his teens, and diabetes was diagnosed at 25. He developed severe hypoglycaemic episodes, some with convulsions and automatisms and prolonged bouts of disinhibited behaviour. In hospital it was noted that such episodes were frequent when he was left to measure and administer his own insulin, but stopped when it was given under nursing supervision. He denied deliberate abuse of insulin, but phials and syringes were found concealed among his possessions along with other drugs. His memory was clearly faulty for events of the previous year, and testing confirmed the presence of severe verbal memory deficits. It was difficult to know how far the insulin hypoglycaemias had contributed to this rather than the abuse of alcohol and other drugs.

The role of arterial disease is clear in patients who develop cerebrovascular accidents and will often be incriminated in those who develop dementia. Diabetes is recognised as a key risk factor for atherosclerotic brain infarction, along with hypertension and heart disease (Dyken *et al.* 1984). Its impact was clearly demonstrated in the Framingham prospective study of middle-aged and elderly persons, in relation to stroke, cardiovascular disease and claudication (Kannel & McGee 1979).

Careful autopsy studies have also confirmed the association with cerebral atherosclerosis. Alex *et al.* (1962) showed that cerebral infarctions were one and a half times as common in diabetics as controls, with a greatly increased frequency of proliferative lesions in the small cerebral vessels. Grunnet (1963) graded the severity of atheroma in the circle of Willis in 107 cases, and showed an increased frequency and severity in all age groups when compared to controls. Between the ages of 30 and 70 years the incidence was almost doubled. The duration of diabetes and the presence or absence of hypertension were not closely correlated with the severity of such changes, but they seemed to be related to high blood cholesterol levels and frequent acetonuria.

Cerebral blood flow studies have indicated another mechanism whereby the risk of cerebrovascular damage may be increased in diabetics (Dandona *et al.* 1978). Even when resting levels are normal, the reactivity of the vessels to carbon dioxide inhalation is unusual in a high percentage of patients. The expected increase in cerebral blood flow may fail to occur, or paradoxically there may be a substantial fall. This failure to compensate appropriately in response to increased cerebral metabolic demands may in the long term make its own contribution to brain damage.

Reske-Nielsen and Lundbaek (1963) found both diffuse and focal changes in the brains of long-standing diabetics, partly attributable to vascular disease and hypertension but possibly also deriving in part from the effects of metabolic disturbances on the neurones. Diffuse degeneration was observed in neurones and nerve fibres of the cerebrum, cerebellum and brain stem, and gliosis was often considerable. Such changes may account for Perlmuter *et al.*'s (1984) finding that older non-insulin-dependent diabetics performed worse than controls in terms of memory and learning, even after excluding those with overt dementia or cerebrovascular disease.

Diabetic coma

The development of *ketotic coma* is a serious medical emergency, still responsible for some 10% of deaths due to diabetes each year (Windebank & McEvoy 1989). Very occasionally patients may present in this way without being known diabetics, but usually the ketosis develops in a patient with the established disorder which has got out of control. Insulin may have been omitted, or there may have been precipitants by way of infection, physical trauma, gastrointestinal disturbance or alcohol excess. The role that has been claimed for emotional precipitants has already been discussed.

Prodromal symptoms consist of weakness, thirst, dull headache, abdominal pain, nausea, vomiting and drowsiness. The onset may be abrupt or insidious. It is sometimes very gradual over several hours, so that a patient with a dangerous level of ketosis may still be fully ambulant. Air hunger and heavy laboured breathing develop. The patient becomes increasingly listless and in about 10% of cases sinks into coma, sometimes after a period of restlessness, irritability and confusion.

The pulse is rapid and feeble and the blood pressure low. Dehydration is marked, the face flushed, and acetone may be smelled on the breath. Investigations reveal large amounts of sugar and acetone in the urine, and elevated sugar and ketone bodies in the blood. Acidosis is marked and the blood urea is raised. Cerebral oedema and disseminated intravascular coagulation are grave developments. Management is discussed by Hammond and Wallis (1992).

On initial examination the picture may be hard to distinguish from hypoglycaemic coma or from advanced renal failure. Overdosage with salicylates can also give a closely similar picture. In older subjects the differential diagnosis must sometimes include a cerebrovascular accident, since glycosuria may also occur in such a situation.

Hyperosmolar (non-ketotic) coma is principally encountered in older type II diabetics. There is no associated ketoacidosis, but extremely high levels of serum osmolality and glucose are seen, sometimes developing over several days or weeks. It often arises as a complication of infection or other medical problems and mortality is again high. The presenting picture may be of gradually increasing lethargy and impairment of consciousness, but unlike ketotic coma seizures and focal neurological signs are common. The patient may at first be thought to be suffering from an acute stroke, presenting with hemiparesis, aphasia or simple or complex hallucinations (Guisado & Arieff 1975). The condition is usually reversible with correction of the metabolic abnormalities. Autonomic changes can include hyperpnoea and hypertension.

Neurological complications

Peripheral neuropathy can be a severe and distressing complication. In the middle aged and elderly sensory changes usually predominate, with paraesthesiae, pain and cramps in the calves, absent knee and ankle reflexes and diminished vibration sense. Loss of postural sense may lead to ataxia. In younger patients the affection may be more severe, with both motor and sensory disturbances involving all four limbs. Both forms tend to improve when the diabetes is properly controlled. Microvascular changes in the vasa nervorum may be responsible, or some as yet incompletely understood metabolic complication.

Isolated 3rd or 6th cranial nerve palsies are not uncommon, and are probably attributable to focal infarctions in the cranial nerve trunks. These usually clear spontaneously after a few weeks or months. In elderly diabetics pupillary changes may include miosis, irregularity and a sluggish reaction to light, sometimes amounting to the classic Argyll Robertson pupil (pseudotabes). Lesions in the midbrain are presumably the cause.

Other complications include a variety of forms of radiculopathy, amyotrophy, myelopathy and autonomic disturbances.

Insulinomas and other forms of hypoglycaemia

Though rare, insulin-secreting tumours of the pancreas are an important cause of hypoglycaemia, especially to the psychiatrist. The disorders which they produce are extremely varied and usually intermittent with normal health between attacks. Problems of differential diagnosis are therefore considerable and will be dealt with in some detail. The discovery of the condition is often long delayed, resulting in prolonged ill health and very occasionally in irreversible brain damage.

Pathology and pathophysiology of insulinomas

Insulin-secreting tumours gained recognition in the late 1920s. By far the most common are benign adenomas of the islet cells. Those found during life are usually 0.5–5 cm in diameter, whereas those seen at autopsy are often microscopic in size. A tumour too small to be palpated at operation may therefore be responsible for symptoms. Two-thirds are found in the body and tail of the pancreas rather than the head, and multiple tumours are common. Rarely ectopic insulinomas occur in the vicinity of the duodenum or porta hepatis.

The great majority are benign, but approximately 10% are malignant and can metastasise to other parts of the body. Microadenomatosis throughout the pancreatic tissue is another rare possibility, or diffuse insular hyperplasia without tumour formation. These latter conditions sometimes occur familially along with adenomas of the parathyroid, pituitary or other endocrine glands as part of the 'pluriglandular syndrome' (MEA type 1) (p. 528).

The type of tumour which produces insulin is composed of beta cells. Other forms of islet-cell tumour may be non-functioning or 'ulcerogenic', the latter being associated with gastric hypersecretion and peptic ulceration (Zollinger–Ellison syndrome).

The primary defect in insulin-secreting tumours appears to be inability to control the storage and release of insulin, rather than simply excessive production. The result is a constant slow excessive release coupled, for unknown reasons, with sudden excessive discharges. In consequence the plasma insulin level shows large and abrupt fluctuations.

Syndromes of hypoglycaemia

Marks (1981a), from whom much of the present account is taken, demarcates four categories of disturbance all of which may be seen with insulinomas. He prefers the term 'neuroglycopaenia' when referring to clinical syndromes, and reserves the term 'hypoglycaemia' to describe the level of sugar in the blood. Correlations between the two are not exact, and occasionally profound lowering of blood sugar may be found without apparent effect on brain function.

Acute neuroglycopaenia

This is the common syndrome that follows overdosage with insulin or oral hypoglycaemic agents, though similar attacks may occur with insulinomas. The patient experiences vague malaise with anxiety and panic, or an unnatural detached feeling akin to depersonalisation. This is accompanied by feelings of hunger, palpitations and restlessness, and is shown objectively by tachycardia, tremor, flushing, sweating and ataxic gait. Angina may be precipitated if coronary artery disease exists. Brief episodes of unconsciousness may occur and epileptic attacks can be provoked. Occasionally focal neurological disturbances such as diplopia, hemiparesis or dysphasia may be seen without obvious diffuse cerebral disturbance. In severe examples progression occurs to coma.

Subacute neuroglycopaenia

This also occurs episodically and is more characteristic of insulinomas. Subjective symptoms are slight, and all of the above features may be only minimally developed. Instead there is clumsy performance at habitual tasks, and behaviour that is out of character for the person affected. He may behave in a disinhibited, foolhardy or aggressive manner which closely resembles alcoholic intoxication. Others become apathetic and withdrawn, with slurred speech and somnolence. Disorientation and mental confusion are usually in evidence but consciousness is retained until late.

The degree of functional impairment is out of proportion to subjective discomfort, and the person typically lacks realisation of the changes within himself. Moreover negativism is a common feature, so that he may fail to seek help or take appropriate action even if partially aware of the disturbance. Often it is only after recovery that the person realises he has been unwell at all.

Chronic neuroglycopaenia

This, though rare, is virtually confined to patients with insulinomas. There are no dramatic symptoms or signs but a change of personality tends to develop insidiously. Defective memory and intellectual deterioration ultimately lead to severe dementia. Emotional changes may be prominent, with irritability, apathy or emotional lability, and psychotic features with paranoid delusions may develop. The course may be punctuated with episodes of acute or subacute neuroglycopaenia, or may be uniformly smooth so that the possibility of hypoglycaemia goes unsuspected. The symptoms and signs are unaltered by food, and little further deterioration is observed with fasting unless this is very prolonged.

Hyperinsulin neuronopathy

Peripheral neuropathy may develop, with paraesthesiae in the hands and feet and wasting of muscles. The wasting is usually in the distal musculature but can sometimes be proximal. The cause of the hypoglycaemia is almost always an insulinoma. It may occasionally be the presenting feature of the illness, but is more commonly overshadowed by preceding coma or other acute disturbances.

Clinical manifestations of insulinomas

Insulinomas occur equally in males and females. They present usually between the ages of 20 and 50, though cases are reported at all ages including childhood. Familial examples are described, perhaps as part of the pluriglandular syndrome. Episodes of odd behaviour and disturbances of consciousness are the main reasons for referral. Symptoms have commonly been present for months or years by the time the diagnosis is made, sometimes for as long as 30 years. Very occasionally long remissions may be detected in the histories.

Almost any psychiatric syndrome may be simulated, depending partly no doubt on the make-up of the individual. The detailed content of attacks may differ from one occasion to another and diagnostic confusion is common. The essential clue usually lies in the episodic and recurrent nature of the attacks. An added difficulty is that organic features are not always in evidence, the change of consciousness sometimes being so slight that it passes unnoticed except to those familiar with the patient.

Typically attacks of subacute, or less often acute, neuroglycopaenia occur as described above. These gradually increase in frequency, initially occurring at intervals of several weeks or months but often occurring several times per week by the time of presentation. Attacks may commence abruptly, or with a slow build-up of weakness, ataxia and increasing confusion. During witnessed attacks one may see sweating, nystagmus, incoordination or focal neurological signs such as hemiparesis or positive Babinski responses. Actual coma is rare except in the most severe episodes.

At first attacks are commonest at noon or late afternoon, and only later do they occur more characteristically before breakfast and during the night. Only a quarter of patients give a clear history of a relationship to fasting and only 10% to exercise, while relief by eating is even more rarely noticed by the patient (Marks 1981b).

Typically the patient has complete amnesia for the content of the attacks, and occasionally for additional periods during which behaviour was seemingly normal. Between attacks he usually feels quite well.

In a small proportion there is progressive mental or physical disability with little or no history of episodic disturbance. This has already been described under the heading of chronic neuroglycopaenia.

The diagnostic problems are well illustrated by cases in the literature:

A man of 44 suffered from attacks of confusion with bizarre behaviour over a 5-year period, each lasting from a few minutes to several hours, and increasing in frequency until they were occurring four or five times a week. He had a partial or complete amnesia for most of what happened during attacks. Initially they were interpreted as hysterical fugue states.

On one occasion, when motoring home from a funeral, he abruptly began to drive at breakneck speed and seemed quite unaware of his passenger. On another he wandered in a semi-confused condition about the corridors at work for 2 hours, carrying on coherent conversations with certain people he met but ultimately removing his shirt and staring foolishly at people who tried to talk to him. Once when chopping wood he suddenly clutched his axe in a menacing manner and wandered about the neighbourhood with a dazed and glassy-eyed expression; after this he was taken to hospital where his speech was confused and mumbling and he showed constant grotesque and purposeless movements. He then abruptly recovered with amnesia for the entire episode.

In the attack which led to the correct diagnosis he had frightened a fellow employee by brandishing a knife. This informant was able to give a clear description of many episodes, describing marked pallor, sweating, limpness, unsteady drunken behaviour and double vision, and emphasising their liability to occur after excessive exertion or towards the end of the morning.

Before removal of the insulinoma, detailed studies were made of the interrelationships between the patient's behaviour and blood sugar levels. During prolonged starvation experiments it was possible to demonstrate intermittent disturbances of awareness which became progressively more marked even though the blood sugar values were essentially unchanged. Periods of acute motor excitement with confusion and aggressive behaviour could similarly begin and end without significant changes in the blood sugar.

(Romano & Coon 1942)

A 27-year-old man was referred as a psychiatric emergency on account of bouts of aggressive and destructive behaviour. He showed disorientation and inappropriate behaviour during attacks, with sweating and violent tremor, and had no subsequent recollection of what occurred. He had always been backward and had had a head injury at 18. His father had shown similar bouts of violent behaviour.

The initial differential diagnosis had included aggressive psychopathy, mental subnormality with behaviour disturbance, and post-traumatic epilepsy. Prolonged fasting provoked a typical attack at 16 hours, associated with hypoglycaemia and relieved by glucose. At laparotomy multiple islet-cell tumours were found. A diagnosis of multiple endocrine adenomatosis (pluriglandular syndrome) was made since hyperparathyroidism was also present. His father had died with 'islet-cell-secreting tumour of the pancreas and calcification of the kidneys'.

(Carney *et al.* 1971)

A physicist of 32 had attacks consisting of inappropriate aggressive behaviour, sometimes involving attacks on people or destruction of his own belongings. Attacks might last for 30 minutes to 1 hour and were succeeded by dense amnesia for what had occurred. If they did not end in an epileptic fit or simple unconsciousness, they would lead on to a period of emotional disturbance and confusion for which memory would subsequently be incomplete and fragmentary. The EEG showed some inconstant theta activity arising mainly in the temporal leads. A 12-hour fasting blood sugar was normal at 84 mg/100 ml.

He was regarded as suffering from temporal lobe epilepsy but anticonvulsant treatment was ineffective. Subsequent and more thorough blood sugar studies indicated an islet-cell tumour and this was confirmed at operation.

(Whitty, Stores & Lishman 1977)

Investigation of insulinomas

The finding of a low blood glucose is essential to the diagnosis. The exact level at which symptoms of cerebral dysfunction may be expected is somewhat variable, but they usually do not appear until the level is below 2.2 mmol/l (Marks 1981c). The range is wide, however, depending on the rate of fall and other concurrent metabolic factors.

If an actual attack is witnessed blood should be taken immediately for glucose estimation, also where possible for the measurement of plasma insulin and C-peptide levels (see below). The ability of intravenous glucose to bring prompt relief should then be assessed. If spontaneous attacks do not occur while the patient is under observation, an attempt may be made to provoke an attack by fasting, coupled if necessary with exercise. Routine overnight fasts may need to be repeated on a number of occasions, but will fail to reveal significant changes in perhaps 10% of cases; the fast may then need to be prolonged for up to 72 hours. Close supervision is of course necessary, and with any attack that occurs the efficacy of intravenous glucose to terminate it should be tried immediately blood has been withdrawn. The hypoglycaemia seen with insulinomas is characterised by inappropriately high levels of plasma insulin. At a fasting glucose level below 2.5 mmol/l, a plasma insulin concentration greater than 5 mU/l is diagnostic of insulinoma (Turner 1996). C-peptide levels are also inappropriately raised; C-peptide is secreted molecule for molecule along with insulin by the pancreas, providing a very useful measure of pancreatic beta cell function.

In equivocal cases a 'suppression test' may circumvent the need for prolonged fasting and brings important evidence of its own. Patients with insulinomas show increased sensitivity to a slow infusion of insulin, and more importantly fail to suppress the production of C-peptide in the normal manner.

The availability of refined plasma insulin measurements and C-peptide assays has rendered most other tests superfluous, for example tolbutamide or glucagon stimulation tests. These also carry a certain hazard. It should only rarely be necessary nowadays to do an exploratory laparotomy to search for an undisclosed tumour.

Electroencephalography

The earliest change to be detected is the appearance of delta rhythms on overbreathing. Then spontaneous theta and delta waves occur, and later asynchronous irregular waves and a flattened tracing. The abnormalities are often most marked over the temporal lobes. In hypoglycaemic coma the EEG consists of high voltage delta waves as in other comas of metabolic origin. After severe hypoglycaemic episodes, abnormalities may persist in the EEG for several days and then revert to normal.

These sequential changes were studied in the course of therapeutic insulin comas, formerly used for the treatment of schizophrenia. The electroencephalographic response to hypoglycaemia appears to vary considerably in different subjects, though the same individual may show closely similar responses in each episode of a series. In general, the correlation between the symptoms provoked and the electroencephalographic changes is closer than that between symptoms and blood sugar levels.

The value of the EEG in helping towards a diagnosis of

insulinoma is controversial. Rose (1981) considers it useful to take serial records during fasting, and if symptoms occur with a low blood sugar and an abnormal tracing intravenous glucose can then be shown to restore the record to normal within minutes.

After removal of the insulinoma the EEG soon returns to normal, including the response to overbreathing.

Differential diagnosis of insulinomas

The following psychiatric and neurological conditions may often be suspected before the true diagnosis is revealed:

Neurotic disorder is suggested by the occurrence of transient symptoms which are described vaguely and diffusely, often variable from time to time, and unbacked by physical signs when the patient is examined between attacks. Episodes of anxiety, panic and depersonalisation may suggest anxiety neurosis; transient disturbances of consciousness with periods of amnesia may suggest hysteria. The latter may also be diagnosed when transient neurological features such as dysphasia or hemiparesis follow attacks. The differentiation between neurosis and essential reactive hypoglycaemia is discussed on p. 543.

Personality disorder may be suggested by a history of episodes of aggressive or antisocial conduct, for which the patient claims amnesia or only a hazy recollection. Aggressive psychopathy may be diagnosed in more extreme examples.

Manic–depressive or schizophrenic psychoses may very occasionally be diagnosed. Rare cases of insulinoma have been reported to present with acute depressive psychoses, no doubt as a result of individual predisposition. In other cases the bizarre nature of the behaviour during attacks may suggest an ingravescent schizophrenia, and in chronic neuroglycopaenia thought disorder and paranoid delusions may be prominent.

Presenile or senile dementia may be closely simulated in cases with chronic deterioration of intellect and personality. Superimposed episodes of acute and transient disturbance may resemble the step-like course of multi-infarct dementia. These are serious diagnostic mistakes since the brain damage that occurs may ultimately become irreversible.

A space-occupying lesion may be suspected when attacks provoke epilepsy, or when headache and focal neurological symptoms accompany clouding of consciousness. Subdural haematoma may be considered in view of the negative or equivocal neurological findings between attacks.

Carotid artery stenosis may be suggested by attacks of dysphasia or hemiplegia, or vertebrobasilar insufficiency when vertigo and diplopia are prominent features.

Epilepsy is a relatively rare form of presentation of hypoglycaemia except in childhood. But any episodic and recurrent neurological disorder is likely to raise the question of epilepsy, and the content of attacks may closely resemble the automatisms of complex partial seizures.

Intoxication with alcohol is often suspected when attacks are witnessed by on-lookers and the picture may be very similar indeed. When the patient is known to be alcoholic, episodes of amnesia may be ascribed to 'alcoholic blackouts'. Intoxication with other drugs may similarly be suspected.

Other metabolic disorders such as uraemia or liver failure may be closely simulated, or endocrine disorders such as thyrotoxicosis, hypoparathyroidism or phaeochromocytoma.

Peripheral neuropathy has already been mentioned as a rare form of presentation. Narcolepsy may sometimes be considered, or attacks of somnolence may suggest the Kleine–Levin syndrome

Among disorders of the cardiovascular system, angina, vasovagal attacks, orthostatic hypotension and Stokes–Adams attacks may all come under suspicion.

The differential diagnosis from other forms of hypoglycaemia is considered below. Of particular importance in psychiatric practice are *essential reactive, alcohol-induced* and *factitious hypoglycaemia.*

Other forms of hypoglycaemia

An important step when hypoglycaemia is confirmed is to differentiate between the various conditions with which it may be associated. The old classification into organic and functional hypoglycaemia has outgrown its usefulness, since the former rests entirely on finding some identifiable cause. When an insulinoma was missed at operation the case would have been erroneously labelled as functional; and the cause remains elusive in some of the organic forms which are important in general medicine.

The most useful classification in practice is into hypoglycaemias which are provoked by fasting and those which are not. The latter are labelled the 'stimulative hypoglycaemias' since they develop only in response to some identifiable stimulus. The distinction is helpful since attempted provocation by fasting always forms the first step in investigation.

Fasting hypoglycaemias

The fasting hypoglycaemias include those due to insulinomas and those associated with liver disease and endocrine disorder. Fasting hypoglycaemia may occur with all varieties of liver disease, both trivial and serious, and shows little correlation with the severity of the hepatic disorder. Among endocrine disorders Addison's disease and hypopituitarism are the commonest causes.

Other causes, unlikely to come before the psychiatrist, include glycogen storage disease, neonatal hypoglycaemia and the so-called idiopathic hypoglycaemia of childhood. The differentiation of these conditions from insulinoma requires careful medical investigation; the absence of raised plasma insulin levels during fasting and the presence of normal C-peptide suppression after insulin administration ultimately provide the distinction.

Stimulative hypoglycaemias

Essential reactive hypoglycaemia

This is the commonest form of stimulative hypoglycaemia and must be carefully distinguished from insulinoma. The most important clinical difference is that symptoms resembling acute neuroglycopaenia occur after ingesting food but are not provoked by fasting. They do not occur before breakfast, whereas this is common with insulinoma. In effect the disorder represents an exaggeration of the normal physiological response to the ingestion of carbohydrate.

Females are affected more frequently than males, and most cases occur between the ages of 30 and 40 years. It appears to occur particularly in asthenic and emotionally labile persons, and may be associated with minor psychiatric instability in a manner which initiates a vicious circle.

Common symptoms are episodes of weakness, faintness, palpitation and irritability, often in association with feelings of hunger, nausea, headache and vertigo. The patient may complain of 'blackouts', but objective evidence of impairment of consciousness is rare. An interesting medicolegal example, in which a patient committed a serious offence but had no knowledge of it afterwards, is described by Bovill (1973). The symptoms are commonest in mid morning, usually 2–5 hours following food, though the patient rarely comments spontaneously on such an association. Exercise may provoke or aggravate the symptoms, but food or glucose do not bring decisive relief. Between attacks the patient often reports that he feels run down and is functioning below his optimum. The episodes may occur intermittently over several years, but do not show the progression in frequency and severity characteristic of insulinomas.

Fasting blood glucose levels are normal, but a 6-hour glucose tolerance test will show an excessive fall 1.5–4 hours after glucose ingestion. The diagnosis should be made only when both hypoglycaemia and symptoms of neuroglycopaenia are reproduced during the procedure.

A pronounced rise of plasma cortisol in response to the rebound hypoglycaemia will add confidence to the diagnosis.

It is often uncertain whether the degree of reactive hypoglycaemia demonstrated in such patients should be considered abnormal. Many authorities suggest that only a minority have a true defect of glucose homeostasis as a cause of symptoms. A number of examples probably represent neurotic disorder, and since reactive hypoglycaemia in some degree is just as likely to occur in neurotic as non-neurotic individuals one must be cautious in attributing the symptoms to the blood sugar changes which are demonstrated.

Ford et al. (1976), for example, found that among 30 patients referred as possible examples of the syndrome, only 18 showed reactive hypoglycaemia on testing. Moreover, half of the sample were markedly psychiatrically unwell, mostly with depression or anxiety neurosis. Many showed hysterical or obsessional personality patterns. While the patients attributed their emotional distress to hypoglycaemia the overall findings ran counter to this. Thus the number and severity of symptoms experienced—emotional lability, depression, headache, tremor, tachycardia, weakness, dizziness—were unrelated to the degree of hypoglycaemia shown on glucose tolerance tests. Moreover, whether or not they had demonstrated reactive hypoglycaemia their scores for emotional disturbance on the MMPI were similar. Careful histories often showed a close association between the onset of the complaints and some precipitating stress.

Ford et al. concluded that while essential reactive hypoglycaemia remained a definite clinical entity, causing genuine somatic discomfort, it was nevertheless considerably overdiagnosed in the face of multiple non-specific complaints. Patients with unstable or obsessional personalities may come forward with symptoms that would be tolerated with less anxiety by other persons; when a glucose tolerance test is then performed the symptoms may all too easily come to be attributed to any hypoglycaemia revealed, incidental though this may be.

Rennie and Howard (1942), moreover, described a group of patients suffering from tension states and depression in whom the reactive hypoglycaemia appeared, in fact, to be secondary to the psychiatric disorder. After appropriate psychiatric treatment the patients were found to have lost their presenting symptoms, but in addition repetition of glucose tolerance tests often showed that these too had returned to normal.

Clearly therefore the interrelationships between psychiatric disorder, physical symptoms and low blood sugar levels are complex. It is nevertheless worth trying the effect of a high-protein low-carbohydrate diet in the more marked examples of the disorder, and especially when there is no overt neurosis towards which treatment can be directed.

Alcohol-induced hypoglycaemia

Hypoglycaemia may occur in response to various drugs

and poisons of which alcohol is the most important. Inhibition of gluconeogenesis by alcohol appears to be the predominant factor, though impaired response of the pituitary–adrenal axis, and enhanced insulin secretion following an oral glucose load, can also play a part.

The true importance of alcohol-induced hypoglycaemia has been recognised relatively recently. It occurs mostly in chronic alcoholics, usually 6–36 hours after a large intake, and quite often presents with hypoglycaemic coma. It may sometimes develop sooner, then running a considerable risk of being overlooked in the face of obvious intoxication. Recovery is usually prompt after the administration of glucose though hydrocortisone may be required as well. It is possible that the condition accounts for a considerable number of deaths in alcoholic subjects.

Recurrent attacks are rare but have been reported (Fredericks & Lazor 1963; de Moura *et al.* 1967). It is uncertain whether some special sensitivity to alcohol has been acquired in such cases, since the alcoholic history is often of long duration before the complication makes its appearance.

An especially severe form of alcohol-induced hypoglycaemia is liable to occur in insulin-dependent diabetics. Arky *et al.* (1968) first drew attention to this, reporting patients who were repeatedly admitted to hospital in hypoglycaemic states after an alcoholic debauch. Their five patients illustrated the severity of the neurological damage that could result from hypoglycaemia of such combined origin—two died without recovery from coma and three were left with permanent memory impairments or dementia.

Factitious hypoglycaemia

The clandestine use of insulin or sulphonylureas to induce hypoglycaemic symptoms can pose a difficult diagnostic problem. It is seen predominantly among nurses and other paramedical personnel, or in close relatives of diabetics who have access to the agents. It has also been noted among teenage female diabetics who misuse their insulin (Lancet 1978). Some patients addicted to heroin have described obtaining insulin from the same sources of supply.

The hypoglycaemias may be induced for the benefit of the symptoms experienced or as part of attention-seeking behaviour. Sometimes the practice appears to be allied to Munchausen's syndrome, the patients submitting to laparotomy and even subtotal pancreatectomy.

The presentation is with symptoms suggestive of insulinoma. Many patients are admitted in coma. Scarlett *et al.* (1977) found that symptoms had been present for 2 months to 6 years among their seven insulin abusers, two of whom had had subtotal pancreatectomies before the true cause was discovered. One had been diagnosed as diabetic for 17 years and this had probably always been erroneous. Another described the exquisite pleasure of going to sleep after injecting insulin, not knowing whether she would regain consciousness. A sinister facet of Scarlett *et al.*'s series was that two patients had also given insulin to their children, one with a fatal result.

Jordan *et al.* (1977) described patients abusing sulphonylurea and presenting in a similar manner. One of their patients began taking her husband's chlorpropamide while severely depressed, another was an alcoholic whose hypoglycaemia was at first ascribed to alcohol. Jordan *et al.* estimated that the problem had become as common as genuine insulinoma, requiring therefore the utmost care to screen for factitious hypoglycaemia before such a diagnosis was made.

The risk of error is increased by the finding of inappropriately raised plasma insulin during the hypoglycaemic episodes, both with insulin and sulphonylurea abuse. However, C-peptide levels (p. 541) will be low when exogenous insulin has been taken, and this will immediately raise suspicion of the practice. After oral hypoglycaemic agents the picture can be virtually indistinguishable from insulinoma since C-peptide levels are likely to be raised as a result of beta-cell stimulation; the diagnosis must then be made by demonstrating the drugs in the blood or urine.

Under the heading of *pseudoneuroglycopaenia* Marks (1981a) describes a quite separate group of patients with disturbed personalities, also paramedical workers or relatives of diabetics, who present with attacks simulating acute neuroglycopaenia, sometimes gradually proceeding to coma. Here the blood glucose and EEG remain normal throughout the episodes. Recovery occurs spontaneously or may be provoked by saline injection. The situation is considered to represent an hysterical conversion reaction.

Other stimulative hypoglycaemias

After gastrectomy the 'dumping syndrome' occurs during or immediately after a meal; other similar forms of disturbance may be some hours delayed. The symptoms resemble those of essential reactive hypoglycaemia. Glucose tolerance tests again often produce conflicting results, and the true relationship of symptoms to reactive lowering of blood sugar remains uncertain.

A number of drugs other than alcohol may provoke hypoglycaemia. The effect of salicylates can be profound, especially in children, leading occasionally to fatal results. They potentiate the effect of oral hypoglycaemic agents. Propanolol and other non-selective beta blockers can have a similar effect. Among poisons those present in certain toadstools are markedly hypoglycaemic.

Finally under the heading of stimulative hypoglycaemia, the reactions liable to occur in insulin-treated diabetics must be remembered. Some diabetics are particularly prone to insulin-induced hypoglycaemias and others are incautious of diet.

In the stimulative hypoglycaemias fasting fails to produce abnormal blood sugar levels and the other confirmatory tests for insulinoma will be negative, the sole exception being sulphonylurea abuse as described above.

Treatment of hypoglycaemia

Sugar or glucose tablets should be carried by patients awaiting investigation when hypoglycaemic attacks are known to occur, and relatives should be instructed about the urgent need to give glucose in the earliest stages of an attack. In severe reactions, or if the patient is comatose, glucose should be given intravenously, 10–20 g as a 33.3% or 50% solution.

Treatment of hypoglycaemic coma is always a grave emergency. Whenever its presence is considered a possibility intravenous glucose should be given immediately after withdrawing blood for laboratory investigations. The response is usually rapid, though it may sometimes be slow if the coma has been of long duration or the patient is markedly hypothermic. The possibility of coincident hypoadrenalism or hypopituitarism must then be borne in mind, and parenteral hydrocortisone should be tried. The response may be dramatic if irreversible brain damage has not occurred.

The essential treatment for insulinoma is surgical removal at the earliest opportunity after the diagnosis is established. Sometimes more than one adenoma is present and re-operation may occasionally be necessary. When the diagnosis of hyperinsulinism has been fully confirmed by tests, yet no tumour is palpable, subtotal pancreatectomy is indicated. If operation is refused, or if the tumour proves to be malignant, palliative treatment may help for a while in the form of large doses of steroids or diazoxide, together with constant food intake at 3-hourly intervals during the day.

Patients with essential reactive hypoglycaemia should not be given repeated doses of glucose, but must be encouraged to take frequent meals which are high in protein and fat.

Outcome of hypoglycaemia

The immediate outcome for most attacks is excellent. The symptoms usually resolve spontaneously even without specific treatment. Sometimes, however, neurological and psychiatric manifestations may outlast the actual period of hypoglycaemia. Dysphasia, hemiparesis and stupor have been reported to persist for hours or even weeks after restoring the blood sugar to normal, also negativism, restlessness, apathy and prolonged behaviour disorder (Markowitz et al. 1961). Such disturbances are thought to rest on a vascular basis which ultimately resolves. Recovery from hypoglycaemic coma may similarly be delayed for hours or even weeks in occasional cases. After prolonged coma recovery may be incomplete, with evidence of permanent brain damage and dementia (Arky et al. 1968).

The outcome after surgery for insulinoma is excellent in the great majority of cases. The typical patient who has presented with intermittent episodes of neuroglycopaenia ceases to have such attacks, whatever form they have taken, and normal health is restored.

While this is the experience of most observers, occasional reports have indicated a less favourable picture on prolonged follow-up. Markowitz et al. (1961) followed six early cases after a lapse of 25 years, and found that five had shown either persisting or newly acquired mental disturbances in the interim. These were sometimes severe, including manic–depressive psychosis, irrational or erratic behaviour and other aberrations of personality, and were thought possibly to represent the aftermath of brain damage sustained during the hypoglycaemic episodes. A surprisingly high incidence of peptic ulceration and haemorrhage had also developed, even though ulcerogenic pancreatic tumours had not appeared to be present.

The rarer presentations in the form of chronic psychosis or intellectual deterioration may be expected to improve to some degree after operation, but here recovery is seldom complete. In these cases, as after prolonged episodes of hypoglycaemic coma, irreversible brain damage often proves to have occurred. Thus among 100 patients with psychosis or 'long-term insanity' in the detailed review by Laurent et al. (1971), 37 showed little or no improvement after removal of the hypoglycaemic tumour. The longer the duration of symptoms before the diagnosis, the greater was the risk of permanent mental disability.

Cerebral pathology of hypoglycaemia

The pathological changes in the brain after acute episodes of hypoglycaemia have mostly been studied in cases of insulin shock. The brain may show oedema and vascular congestion. Survival after profound hypoglycaemic coma may be associated with ventricular dilatation, cortical atrophy and shrinkage of the hippocampi.

Microscopically the neurones show ischaemic cell changes and associated gliosis. The cell damage may occur in scattered foci, but is more typically laminar with emphasis on the third and fifth layers (Brierley 1981). Relative sparing of the visual cortex is usual, but the corpus striatum and hippocampus appear to be especially vulnerable, much as in anoxia (p. 548). However, with hypoglycaemia the Purkinje cells of the cerebellum are said to be less prone to be affected (Richardson *et al.* 1959).

The pathology that may result from more minor degrees of intermittent hypoglycaemia has not been documented, nor the changes that result from long-continued chronic neuroglycopaenia. The pathological basis for the rare examples of persistent neuropsychiatric disability short of gross dementia is therefore incompletely understood.

Cerebral anoxia

Barcroft (1920) distinguished four main varieties of anoxia — anoxic, anaemic, stagnant and metabolic — which serve as a framework for reviewing the clinical conditions in which cerebral anoxia can occur. These are shown in Table 18 along with a fifth category of 'overutilisation anoxia'.

Anoxic anaemia

Anoxic anoxia is due to deficient oxygenation of the arterial blood. It may result from respiratory insufficiency in pulmonary diseases such as chronic bronchitis, emphysema or pneumonia, from the administration of general anaesthetics, from asphyxia or drowning, or from lack of oxygen in the inspired air at high altitudes.

A respiratory cause, and particularly a respiratory infection, must be constantly borne in mind when unexplained mental confusion appears in the elderly, or when a fluctuating acute organic reaction is superimposed upon a known dementing process. The anoxia which results from respiratory disease is often further complicated by the accumulation of carbon dioxide (hypercapnia) as described on p. 562.

General anaesthesia inevitably carries a hazard of anoxia. In particular, minor degrees which would be tolerated by a fit person may prove disastrous when the blood volume is low (Dinnick 1964). Thus anaesthesia contributes to some of the acute delirious episodes which appear postoperatively, especially those which emerge immediately upon recovery. A mild degree of persistent dementia may very occasionally make its first appearance after the administration of an anaesthetic for some relatively minor surgical procedure. This is particularly likely in the elderly or arteriosclerotic in whom the reserves of cerebral function have already been precarious.

Bedford (1955) reviewed a population of over 1000 geriatric subjects who had had operations in the preceding 15 years, and found that in more than a third the relatives claimed that the patients had 'never been the same again'. The statement proved to be unjustified in the majority, but in approximately one case in 10 there was reason to think that the anaesthetic may have contributed to memory difficulties or intellectual impairment. In 18 cases seen personally, Bedford found a severe dementia which appeared to have followed anaesthesia directly. Other more minor forms of intellectual disability were found, as in the case of a surgeon who had been obliged to cease work on account of memory difficulties.

In contrast to Bedford's findings, Simpson *et al.* (1961) were able to identify only one out of 681 elderly patients who suffered permanent intellectual impairment following anaesthesia. This was a careful prospective investigation involving assessments both before and after operation, and comparisons between those who had had local and general anaesthetics. Simpson *et al.* concluded that when patients deteriorate after operation the great majority do so by virtue of reasons unrelated to brain damage or anaesthetic agents. Progression of the original disease or the development of new disease can usually be identified as the responsible factor.

Anaemic anoxia

Anaemic anoxia results from deficient oxygen-carrying power of the blood as in carbon monoxide poisoning.

Table 18 Causes of cerebral anoxia.

Anoxic anoxia	Chronic bronchitis, emphysema, pneumonia, pulmonary embolism, general anaesthesia, asphyxia, drowning, high altitudes
Anaemic anoxia	Carbon monoxide poisoning, gastrointestinal bleeding, severe anaemia
Stagnant anoxia	Cerebral arteriosclerosis, peripheral circulatory failure (shock), cardiac surgery, congestive cardiac failure, cardiac arrest, paroxysmal dysrhythmias, myocardial infarction
Metabolic (toxic) anoxia	Hypoglycaemia, cyanide poisoning, carbon disulphide poisoning
Overutilisation anoxia	Epileptic seizures

Abrupt blood loss may be the cause as in haematemesis or unsuspected gastrointestinal haemorrhage. Severe anaemia is an important cause which runs an especial risk of being overlooked:

A man of 70 was admitted to hospital with a 12-month history of jerking movements of the head and arms, and loss of weight and appetite for 2 years. He was noisy and restless by day and night, and emotionally labile with frequent laughing and crying. At night he was agitated and confused and moaned continually. There were incessant coarse movements of the limbs and head but no definite parkinsonian features. The EEG was markedly abnormal with a diffuse excess of theta and paroxysmal delta activity. He was thought to be suffering from presenile dementia secondary to cerebral arteriosclerosis.

His haemoglobin was found to be only 6.1 g/100 ml, probably as a result of chronically bleeding haemorrhoids. Three pints of blood were transfused and he improved remarkably, with resolution of the involuntary movements and of the mental abnormalities.

Four months later the appearances of dementia and the motor abnormalities returned in the course of a transient depressive illness, but on this occasion responded well to antidepressant medication. The EEG now showed only mild abnormalities in the form of generalised theta activity on overbreathing. He remained well when followed up during the next 2 years.

Carbon monoxide produces much of its effect by inactivating the oxygen-carrying power of the haemoglobin molecule. Since carboxyhaemoglobin is relatively stable the effects of exposure to carbon monoxide may be longer-lasting and more profound than a transient reduction in oxygen supply *per se*. But carbon monoxide also acts directly on tissue cells by inhibiting the oxydo-reduction enzyme system, contributing an element of metabolic anoxia as well.

Stagnant anoxia

Stagnant anoxia is due to arrest or reduction of blood flow. It occurs in cerebral arteriosclerosis, or more acutely in peripheral circulatory failure due to shock. Important cardiac causes are heart surgery, congestive cardiac failure, temporary cardiac arrest, episodes of severe dysrhythmia as in paroxysmal ventricular tachycardia, and myocardial infarction. A silent coronary infarction can be particularly misleading. Abrupt loss of consciousness at the onset may be misdiagnosed as a cerebrovascular accident, especially if epileptiform jerking has occurred. An episode of severe collapse followed by confusion, but leaving behind no residual neurological signs, should therefore be viewed with suspicion (Slater & Roth 1969). The myocardial infarction is especially prone to be overlooked in hypertensive patients whose blood pressure may drop to normal levels after the episode.

With stagnant anoxias there are additional complicating factors. In addition to oxygen lack there is a deficiency of glucose supply to the brain, and accumulation of waste products leading to acidosis and other local metabolic derangements.

Metabolic or 'toxic' anoxia

Metabolic or 'toxic' anoxia occurs when there are factors which interfere with the utilisation of oxygen by the tissues even though there is no lack of oxygen supply. This is seen with hypoglycaemia and with poisoning by substances such as cyanide or carbon disulphide. As mentioned above carbon monoxide has a histotoxic effect in addition to reducing the oxygen-carrying capacity of the blood.

Overutilisation anoxia

Overutilisation anoxia exists when there is an increased demand in relation to supply. This occurs locally in the brain during epileptic seizures.

Clinical features

The clinical picture varies with the individual situation, depending on the rate at which anoxia develops, its duration and the degree of concomitant physical exertion. Individual tolerance also varies widely, with more severe effects and a greater likelihood of sequelae in persons who are already existing near the threshold of neuronal reserve. Coexisting hypotension is often an important, and sometimes a crucial, factor in determining the severity of brain damage, as after temporary cardiac arrest (Brierley 1970).

Most forms of cerebral anoxia are transient events, presenting with impairment of consciousness of varying severity, confusion, disorientation or delirium. There may be muscular twitching or tremor, and epileptic fits may occur. In sustained hypoxia, as at high altitudes, mental obfuscation may develop more gradually and personality change may be the obtrusive feature as described below. In either event the diffuse nature of the cerebral affection is apparent.

Unless the anoxia is sufficiently prolonged or severe to cause death there are rarely enduring sequelae. A dense amnesic gap for the acute condition is usually all that remains. In a minority, however, permanent memory difficulties may result, or more global impairment of intellect extending even to severe dementia. Neurological sequelae may consist of extrapyramidal disturbances with parkinsonism or athetosis. Hemiplegia, blindness or pseudobulbar palsy may very occasionally remain. After the anoxia which follows abrupt systemic hypotension there may be a monoplegia and sensory loss affecting the arm predominantly, due to the selective involvement of neurones at the borderland territories of supply of the anterior and middle cerebral arteries (see below). Parietal lobe deficits may also be severe.

The psychological changes produced at high altitudes and the clinical complications of carbon monoxide poisoning are considered in more detail below. The sequelae of cardiac surgery are also briefly reviewed.

Cerebral pathology

The pathological changes in the central nervous system in fatal cases have been described by Hoff *et al.* (1945) and Richardson *et al.* (1959). They are usually remarkably similar regardless of the cause, and resemble those seen after hypoglycaemia (p. 545). Brierley (1976) presents a comprehensive review.

If death occurs within a few minutes there is little to be detected other than scattered petechial haemorrhages. Cerebral oedema occurs early, and changes in cerebral blood flow raise the intracranial pressure further in a manner which aggravates the situation (Brock 1971). If the patient survives long enough there may be widespread degeneration and necrosis of nerve cells with corresponding glial proliferation. The cells of the third, fourth and fifth cortical layers are particularly susceptible (laminar cortical necrosis), also the Purkinje cells of the cerebellum and the cells of the corpus striatum. Bilateral necrosis of the globus pallidus is often a marked feature. The hippocampus and the parastriate cortex are also characteristically affected severely. Areas of subcortical demyelination eventually become apparent if the patient survives for more than a few weeks. The subcortical U fibres are, however, characteristically spared.

The biochemical changes set in train by hypoxic brain damage, and the particular role of glutamate excitotoxicity in leading to cell damage and death, are gradually being clarified by experimental studies. Some of the principal findings to date are described on pp. 164–5. Closely similar biochemical changes appear to ensue whether the brain damage is hypoxic or hypoglycaemic in origin, or the result of direct brain trauma.

A different pathological picture results when blood flow to the brain has been abruptly curtailed despite a sustained normal arterial oxygen tension. Thus the sudden systemic hypotension occasioned by temporary cardiac arrest, or severe myocardial infarction, may lead to ischaemic neuronal destruction in restricted areas of the brain. Brief periods of ischaemia cause selective cell

necrosis in the hippocampus and cerebellum, the CA_1 zone of the hippocampus being particularly affected. Longer and more severe episodes of hypotension produce infarcts largely confined to the boundary zones between major arterial territories in the cerebrum and cerebellum. Brierley (1970, 1976) reviews the experimental and clinical evidence on the matter. Changes can be minimal or absent in the hippocampi and diffuse laminar cortical necrosis does not occur. Boundary zone necrosis is often most severe in the parieto-occipital regions where the territories of the anterior, middle and posterior cerebral arteries meet. Involvement of the subcortical white matter is roughly proportional to the severity of the cortical lesion, sometimes extending inwards as far as the wall of the lateral ventricle. Accompanying lesions in the basal ganglia are variable but often circumscribed and severe. In the cerebellum the lesion is at the junction of the superior and posterior inferior cerebellar arteries, forming a wedge with its base at the cortical surface and its apex in the central white matter.

Such classic boundary zone lesions may sometimes be combined with diffuse ischaemic changes, depending on the speed of development and severity of the hypotension. If the fall in cerebral perfusion pressure is abrupt and considerable, ischaemic necrosis will tend to be confined to the boundary zones; if it is slow and relatively moderate the changes will often be more generalised, since the accompanying vasodilatation will allow a more uniform distribution of the available but inadequate blood flow. Coincident respiratory failure will often also have occurred in examples encountered clinically, and a combination of the two factors — primary hypoxia and systemic hypotension — will often have been operative together.

The electroencephalographic changes in anoxia are identical with those of hypoglycaemia as described on p. 541.

Anoxia at high altitudes

The psychological changes produced at high altitudes have received a good deal of attention, with renewed interest in view of the current vogue for climbing without supplementary oxygen. Important early observations were made on expeditions such as the International High Altitude Expedition to Chile (McFarland 1932, 1937) and in experiments conducted in low pressure chambers where high altitudes could be simulated (Haldane *et al.* 1919; Barcroft 1925). Aviation experiences, particularly during the First World War, underlined the importance of this area of study. The earlier literature is comprehensively reviewed by Van Liere and Stickney (1963).

The slow ascent in mountaineers allows a process of adaptation. Individual variability is marked, some subjects being affected at 2500 m and some only at 4500 m. Hypoxia due to the decline in partial pressure of oxygen in the inspired air is accepted as the principal cause, though fatigue, extreme cold, mountain glare and isolation will also contribute to the picture.

Ryn (1988), reporting on a group of Polish alpinists, has described the typical progression from states of dysphoria or sometimes elation at 3000–4000 m, to features of an acute organic reaction at over 7000 m. The early dysphoria shows as apathy, depression, mental exhaustion and slowing of thinking processes. Some subjects, by contrast, show elevation of mood coupled with irritability, argumentativeness and impulsivity. At rather higher levels there may be cyclic alternations between the two pictures. The symptoms of the acute organic reaction at 7000 m include a marked decrease in motor and mental activity, clumsy behaviour and a blunted awareness of dangers. Periods of dense amnesia lasting from minutes to days may occur, also excessive somnolence. Brief lapses of consciousness are followed by confusion, purposeless activity and ataxia. Occasional subjects become severely disorientated, especially towards night-time, with fearfulness and visual and auditory hallucinations. West (1986) quotes examples of bizarre subjective experiences, such as seeing pulsating cloud-like objects in the sky, or strong feelings that a second person is present. Disturbances of judgement and faulty reasoning can impose serious risks to the climber and others. Headache, nausea, anorexia and tachycardia are common additional features.

A prolonged stay at high altitudes may be accompanied by an entire change of personality. Along with episodes of mental confusion there is progressive indifference and apathy, mild depression and persistent inability to concentrate. Refreshing sleep is hard to obtain, and insomnia worsens the emotional and intellectual abnormalities. Dreams are frequently of an unpleasant and frightening nature, though at still higher altitudes dreaming apparently ceases to occur.

On return to normal altitudes there are rarely enduring deficits of a conspicuous nature. An early report by Pugh and Ward (1956), however, described residual memory difficulties in a mountaineer who had climbed to 8500 m without additional oxygen. Townes et al. (1984) made careful observations on members of the 1981 American Medical Research Expedition to Everest, testing them before and after the ascent, and found evidence of mild transient deficits in memory, learning and verbal expression. These had disappeared at the 1-year follow-up. However, impairments in finger tapping speed persisted at 1 year suggesting that motor deficits might be longer-lasting.

Townes et al.'s subjects had used supplementary oxygen, unlike those reported by Regard et al. (1989). Eight world-class climbers who had reached summits of over 8500 m were tested an average of 7 months later. In comparison to controls several were still mildly impaired on tests of concentration, verbal and figural memory and cognitive flexibility (Stroop test and concept matching tasks). By contrast perceptual ability, reaction times, language and visuospatial abilities were within normal limits. They regarded their results as indicative of long-lasting frontotemporal dysfunction; this was supported by EEG abnormalities in the temporal regions in the two most severely affected subjects.

Among aviators flying without oxygen the onset of symptoms is more dramatic, appearing often at 3000 m though depending again on the rate of ascent and individual susceptibility. Difficulties are universal above 6000 m without additional oxygen, and complete loss of consciousness is likely to occur at 7500 m. The first manifestations are variable — fatigue and mental slowing, euphoria, or surly and pugnacious behaviour. Headache, nausea and vomiting are again usually in evidence. Motor control soon becomes impaired and reaction times are slowed.

The subject is typically unaware of the change in himself and becomes oblivious of danger. He may feel his mind to be unusually keen and develop a dangerous fixity of purpose from which he cannot be dissuaded. Thus foolhardy and reckless behaviour is common. Birley (1920) reports some interesting examples of altered judgement in pilots during the 1914–18 war. One returned from a high photographic reconnaissance flight well pleased with his effort until it was found that he had taken 18 exposures on the same plate; others had attacked enemy formations without any plan of campaign, making tactical errors of which they would not ordinarily be guilty. One officer had been known to wave his hand in friendly greeting to the enemy.

Experimental observations in the decompression chamber, or with re-breathing apparatus, have amply confirmed these changes and shown their essential dependence on cerebral hypoxia. Severe exposures can lead to loss of consciousness without warning. Less severe degrees produce a picture closely resembling alcoholic intoxication, with headache, drowsiness, confusion, muscular weakness and incoordination. An initial stage of euphoria is again often seen with feelings of self satisfaction and unusual power. The lifting of inhibitions sometimes leads to hilarious silly behaviour, anger or outbursts of uncontrolled laughter. Both the quantity and quality of mental work are affected; reasoning is slow, calculations faulty and writing shows perseverative errors. Distractibility becomes marked and attention to detail is lost. Choice reaction times are affected earlier than simple reaction times, but these too are slowed as neuromuscular control deteriorates. Visual and kinaesthetic perception are impaired, and later auditory perception also. Memory and learning ability can be shown to decline from an early stage. The lack of subjective awareness of the changes and the dangerous loss of initiative which accompanies them have also been fully confirmed.

Carbon monoxide poisoning

In addition to attempted suicide with domestic gas supplies, carbon monoxide poisoning may occur accidentally in connection with slow combustion stoves, bathroom geysers and car exhaust fumes in enclosed spaces. Domestic risks have been greatly diminished in the UK since the introduction of North Sea gas which is not in itself poisonous, but carbon monoxide is still produced if faulty equipment leads to incomplete combustion. In industry poisoning is seen in connection with blast furnaces and when explosions occur in mines.

The clinical picture was fully documented by Bour *et al.* (1967). Lowered efficiency and self control lead imperceptibly to loss of consciousness without any intervening delirium. Complete unconsciousness is usually rapidly attained, resulting in coma of variable duration. Diffuse hypertonicity is common, with trismus and up-going plantar responses. Paroxysms of decerebrate rigidity may occur. Hypotonic forms are rare and carry a graver prognosis. Sphincter and swallowing difficulties are often present, and the corneal and pupillary reflexes may be abolished. The complexion is plethoric, and hyperpnoea is often extreme with a forceful expiratory phase. The classic 'cherry red' colour is in fact rare. The cerebrospinal fluid is normal.

In Shillito *et al.*'s (1936) series of 21 000 cases two-thirds were successfully resuscitated. If death is to follow this is usually within a few days, but sometimes survival extends for several weeks or months. Very occasionally the patient recovers for 10–15 days before a fatal relapse. Long persistence of coma after removal from the contaminated atmosphere carries an unfavourable prognosis, likewise prolonged circulatory collapse, fluctuating pyrexia, hyperglycaemia, uraemia or acidosis.

After-effects

As coma regresses the patient shows a period of disorientation and confusion. Sometimes there is a brief phase of irritability and restlessness, but usually the predominant features are apathy and general inertia. Approximately one-fifth of patients show prolonged delirium, ranging from several hours to several weeks (Smith & Brandon 1970). Hallucinations and delusions are conspicuous by their absence (Shillito *et al.* 1936). Speech is slowed and difficult for a time, and thought processes reduced. Amnesic difficulties are usually much in evidence and often the last to clear:

A woman of 70 was admitted in coma and only several weeks later had recovered sufficiently to respond to simple commands and reply to questions. For the next 2 weeks she was grossly disorientated in time, giving the year variously as 1888 or 1918, and being equally wide of the mark for her age. Another week passed before she realised she was in hospital, yet insisted it was in Armagh, the place of her childhood, though in fact she was in Belfast. At this stage she was able to repeat the months of the year correctly, and could repeat four digits, but could retain nothing of a name and address after a 3-minute interval. She could remember the names of her brothers and sisters and recall some episodes from her childhood. Two weeks later she had improved remarkably. She was then consistently orientated in time and place, had good general insight and was able to recall the circumstances leading right up to her accidental coal gas poisoning.
(Allison 1961)

Sometimes a classic Korsakoff syndrome emerges, or alternatively the patient's profound inertia, indifference and slowing of cerebration may cause the memory to appear to be more defective than is really the case ('une sorte d'indifference amnestique' – Ajuriaguerra and Rouault de la Vigne 1946). Agnosia, constructional apraxia or dysphasia may also be seen later in recovery.

Extrapyramidal signs which are absent during the stage of coma may emerge on recovery, with cogwheel rigidity of the musculature, athetosis or immobility of facial expression. Transient hemiplegia is not uncommon, and 8th nerve affections may produce deafness and vertigo. In most cases the neurological abnormalities gradually clear along with the psychological disturbances, though sometimes this may take several weeks or months. The degree of recovery from early severe disability can sometimes be remarkable:

A 24-year-old woman was admitted to hospital in deep coma. There were repeated tonic seizures, breathing was laboured and she required a tracheostomy. After several days in coma she passed into a muttering resistive state for some weeks, then became mute and unresponsive for 3 weeks more. At this stage she showed a quadriparesis and bilateral extensor plantar responses. Six weeks later she began to show some recovery of consciousness and ability to move, but remained confused and severely aphasic. Four months after the initial exposure, however, there had been a good deal of recovery; she was then talking well and was discharged from hospital. She continued to improve in a remarkable fashion, and by 8 months there was only a moderate hemiparesis and slight mental impairment.

(Richardson *et al.* 1959)

Latent interval

A strange feature, repeatedly noted in large series of cases, is the occurrence of a latent period between recovery from coma and the onset of profound neurological or mental disorder (Bour *et al.* 1967; Choi 1983; Lee & Marsden 1994). This may also follow other forms of cerebral anoxia, as after anaesthesia or cardiac arrest (Plum *et al.* 1962). Apparently normal health is regained, but 2–10 days later, or even after several weeks, there is an abrupt relapse with the appearance of extrapyramidal disturbance and personality and cognitive changes. Delirium or coma may recur. Sometimes the patients have been discharged or even returned to their jobs in the interim. Complete recovery is again often attained:

A man of 37 was accidentally gassed while intoxicated. He was unconscious for 2 days but for the rest of the week seemed entirely recovered. On the seventh day he began to act peculiarly, became unresponsive to questions and the right plantar response was found to be up-going. Several weeks later he was still dull, apathetic and disorientated, but thereafter improved and was ultimately discharged fully recovered.

A woman of 51 was unconscious for 2 days, but was discharged at the end of a week fully recovered apart from a general feeling of weakness. After 2 weeks, however, her gait became unsteady, and she became confused and bewildered. Her face was blank and expressionless and she developed a coarse tre-mor of the hands. She gradually improved over the next few months, with disappearance of the mental and neurological abnormalities.

(Shillito *et al.* 1936)

A latent interval of this nature has been reported in 3% of patients and in 12% of those who are hospitalised (Choi 1983). The apathy, mutism and indifference which develop may then be falsely interpreted as reflecting psychiatric disorder, especially if the patient has attempted suicide (Zagami *et al.* 1993). Delayed sequelae tend to be commoner when the initial period of unconsciousness has been prolonged, but Choi observed several examples in patients who had remained mentally clear during the acute episode. The ultimate outcome is often reasonably good, 75% of the patients reviewed by Choi recovering within a year, while the remainder showed no improvement or died. Parkinsonism or mild memory impairment persisted in a fifth of those who recovered.

The underlying pathology appears to be demyelination within the cerebral hemispheres though the mechanism responsible is unclear. In 15 patients reported by Chang *et al.* (1992) MRI invariably showed confluent regions of high signal intensity in the centrum semiovale and periventricular white matter. Ten also showed alterations in the thalamus and putamen suggestive of iron deposition, and nine showed bilateral ischaemia or necrosis of the globus pallidus. Repeat imaging in three patients whose clinical symptoms improved showed decreases in the extent and intensity of the white matter changes. In Hayashi *et al.*'s (1993) patient an area of demyelination apparent on CT in the centrum semiovale was observed to enlarge during the latent period, suggesting that the white matter damage was progressive throughout.

Enduring sequelae

The majority of patients are left only with an amnesic gap for the period of coma, together with a variable amount of retrograde amnesia and patchy memory for part of the period of recovery. The commonest neurological sequelae are extrapyramidal disturbances, usually parkinsonian in nature or sometimes athetotic. In the most severe examples the patient is left in an akinetic mute state. This carries a grave prognosis and a high mortality. Global impairment of intellect is uncommon but permanent defects of memorising may be seen. Neurological disabilities are almost invariably evident when gross mental impairments remain, though occasional patients are described with purely cognitive and behavioural deficits (Gordon & Mercandetti 1989; Mendez & Doss 1995).

It was formerly claimed that persistent sequelae were rare. Thus over a 10-year period Shillito *et al.* (1936) found that 21 000 cases of carbon monoxide poisoning had occurred in New York City with 14 500 recoveries, but only 39 patients (0.27% of survivors) could be identified who had been hospitalised with enduring defects. It seemed therefore that the great majority of patients either succumbed or recovered completely. Lee and Marsden (1994) point out, however, that carboxyhaemoglobin levels were not measured in Shillito's survey, so that patients with intoxication by drugs or alcohol and minimal carbon monoxide exposure may have been included. Most of those with permanent sequelae had been deeply comatose for hours or days, and had often required long periods of assisted respiration when first discovered. Van Amberg (1942) found that recovery within an hour of removal from the contaminated atmosphere carried a uniformly good prognosis.

The investigations of Smith and Brandon (1970, 1973), however, revealed a more serious picture. Two hundred and six cases of carbon monoxide poisoning were traced from a defined geographical area (Newcastle-upon-Tyne), 42% being accidental and 58% due to suicide attempts. Of the 135 survivors, three patients (2.2%) were severely affected at the time of discharge, all showing dementia and one with parkinsonism in addition. Two others had spastic hemiplegia, though it was possible that this had developed immediately before exposure.

Follow-up was then undertaken among those who had been domiciled within the city at the time of poisoning. Seventy-four patients were traced at an average of 3 years after the event. Eleven had died (15%), three from suicide and eight from other causes. Eight (11%) had evidence of gross neuropsychiatric damage which was directly attributable to the poisoning, in the form of cognitive disability, personality change or severe neurological abnormalities. In some cases deficits such as parkinsonism, dementia or personality change had become evident only after discharge from hospital, emphasising the importance of following every case for sufficient time to allow for the emergence of delayed sequelae. Five of the eight showed a severe global deterioration of intellect.

Of the 63 alive at follow-up, 27 patients (43%) complained of impaired memory and this correlated highly with objective deficits on the Wechsler Memory Scale. Twenty-one (33%) showed a deterioration of personality subsequent to the poisoning, with a marked association between personality and memory deficits. The commonest personality change was towards increased irritability, verbal aggressiveness, violence, impulsiveness and moodiness, a constellation described by the authors as 'affective incontinence'. Thus, over and above the 11% with gross sequelae, a large number appeared to have suffered milder brain damage, resulting in personality and affective change with associated mild cognitive impairment. This was a great deal more common than in a matched control group of patients who had survived barbiturate overdosage. The level of consciousness on admission to hospital correlated significantly with the development of gross neuropsychiatric sequelae and with complaints of memory impairment.

An example from Smith and Brandon's (1973) series with severe personality change was as follows:

A 33-year-old miner of good premorbid stability was accidentally exposed to carbon monoxide in a coal mine explosion. He was comatose when found some minutes later, and subsequently was delirious, irritable and aggressive for 4 hours. Oxygen was given and he was discharged from hospital the same day. Subsequently he was forgetful, had difficulty in coping with his previous level of work, was increasingly irritable, restless and argumentative, and on occasion was violent towards his wife. He was more impulsive and outspoken, more anxious and more prone to paranoid misinterpretations. His physical energy was markedly diminished. In the month before interview he had been charged with indecent assault on five young girls. His wife verified his previous mental stability and the deterioration of memory and personality subsequent to exposure. An independent witness, unaware of the patient's fate after the accident, attested to his previously stable personality. Financial compensation had never been considered.

Lee and Marsden (1994) attempted to determine features that might predict the level of disability 1 year later among 31 patients who developed neurological sequelae. Eight had shown a progressive course to a persistent vegetative state, whereas 23 had relapsed after a latent interval. The former were significantly younger than the latter, and the mean duration of coma had been significantly longer (10 days and 2 days, respectively). Levels of carboxyhaemoglobin, however, did not differ between the groups. None of the eight vegetative patients improved.

Among the 23 with delayed sequelae two patterns could be seen — relapse to a parkinsonian state with behavioural and cognitive impairment (nine cases) or relapse to a bed-bound state with mutism, apathy and severe rigidity (14 cases). Such relapses occurred rapidly over the course of several days. The majority of the former, but less than half of the latter, improved over subsequent months. Occasional patients in either group showed a second phase of deterioration. A third of the CT scans were normal at the start, and contrary to previous reports the presence of features such as white matter low density or globus pallidus lesions were not good predictors of outcome. Follow-up scans could show new lesions or progressive changes even in patients who improved. Bruno *et al.* (1993) similarly found that MRI changes did not correlate well with clinical outcome.

Cerebral pathology

Lapresle and Fardeau (1967) describe the characteristic changes in the brain in cases of carbon monoxide poisoning coming to autopsy. The most frequent lesion is necrosis of the globus pallidus, sometimes limited to a small and circumscribed portion bilaterally. Similar lesions are common in Ammon's horn, again variable in extent and sometimes affecting Sommer's sector only. The cerebral cortex shows necrotic foci with intense capillary proliferation and degeneration or disappearance of nerve cells, but the typical laminar cortical damage seen with other forms of anoxia is rare. The cerebellum also shows necrosis but the Purkinje cells are relatively spared, again in contrast to their special vulnerability in other forms of anoxia.

Lesions are common in the white matter of the centrum ovale. Here foci of necrosis can be extensive and coalescent with areas of demyelination. The latter appears to be particularly characteristic of cases which have shown a latent interval during their clinical course. Axis cylinders then tend to be relatively preserved even when demyelination is extensive in the deep white matter and periventricular areas.

Vascular lesions are widespread, with endothelial swelling leading to thrombosis and miliary diapedetic haemorrhages. Sometimes there is marked general vasodilatation. Cerebral oedema occurs regularly in the early stages and may contribute to the ischaemic changes. The lesions of the globus pallidus and Ammon's horn are thought to rest on a common vascular basis.

Brucher (1967) discusses the aetiology of the lesions. The cerebral pathology differs from that of anoxia due to other causes in certain important respects—laminar cortical damage is rare, the Purkinje cells are relatively preserved and lesions are prominent in the white matter. This suggests that carbon monoxide may have a specific histotoxic action in addition to its effect in reducing the oxygen-carrying capacity of the blood. Alternatively both the white matter changes and the lesions in the globus pallidus could depend critically on circulatory failure, i.e. hypoxia compounded by systemic hypotension and acidosis (Ginsberg 1985). Hence the importance in treatment of prompt attention to hypotension and the acid–base balance in addition to the administration of oxygen. A haemorrhagic origin for the pallidal lesions is supported by MRI findings indicative of the presence of methaemoglobin within them (Silverman et al. 1993).

Chronic carbon monoxide poisoning

From time to time it has been claimed that intermittent exposures to low concentrations of carbon monoxide can have a cumulative effect, resulting in chronic disability. In Scandinavian countries during the 1939–45 war this became a focus of concern among persons handling 'producer gas' or driving vehicles in which this was the source of power (Grut 1949). Other industrial occupations at possible risk are foundrymen, gas workers and blast-furnace workers.

Proponents of the disorder point out that breathing as little as 0.05% of carbon monoxide in the inspired air leads to symptoms after several hours, and that experiments with animals show pathological changes in the central nervous system after prolonged sublethal exposures (Beck 1936). Beck reported 97 patients who had suffered many weeks or months of exposure to domestic gas, vehicle exhaust or blast furnace fumes, and concluded that a definite clinical syndrome was produced. The chief complaints were of dull frontal headache, vertigo, nervousness, generalised weakness, neuromuscular pains, anorexia, digestive disturbances, dyspnoea, palpitations, tremulousness, weakness of the legs with ataxia, and paraesthesiae of the extremities. Almost all showed prominent mental manifestations and many were 'confirmed neurotics'. Psychological symptoms included depression, restlessness, anxiety, mental retardation, memory deficits and periods of confusion. Drowsiness and insomnia were common. Some showed speech defects, tinnitus, visual disturbances or impairment of the sense of smell. Four patients showed parkinsonian features.

The syndrome, however, has come heavily under suspicion (Lindgren 1961), and evidence for an objective physical basis has not been forthcoming (Slater & Roth 1969). Hunter (1978) pointed out that carbon monoxide is not a cumulative poison and that small amounts are readily ventilated out of the blood; he therefore concluded that there was no such clinical condition as chronic carbon monoxide poisoning. However, the subject remains under review in view of risks to health from urban atmospheric contamination (e.g. Goldsmith & Landaw 1968). It is also important to beware of minor exposures resulting from chronically malfunctioning domestic equipment. The occurrence of fatigue, headache, diarrhoea and flu-like symptoms amongst several members of a household, or recurring at a particular time and place, should raise suspicion of possible minor intermittent exposure (Drug & Therapeutics Bulletin 1988c). Evidence incriminating intermittent exposure to carbon monoxide as the cause of increased liability to atherosclerosis in smokers is also relevant in this regard (Astrup 1972).

Sequelae of cardiac surgery

During the early era of open heart surgery complications by way of anoxic brain damage and stroke were frequent, occurring in over 20% of patients (Hotson 1989). Improvements in surgery and in the techniques for extracorporeal circulation have substantially reduced the incidence of disabling sequelae, but more sensitive measures show that after-effects of a subtle nature are still not uncommon. Moreover, as confidence in coronary artery bypass surgery has grown the operation is offered to patients at greater risk by virtue of age, advanced ischaemic heart disease or arteriosclerosis elsewhere.

The principal risks are from cerebral hypoperfusion during operation, and embolism caused by material dislodged from the aorta and cardiac chambers. Major embolism leading to stroke is commoner when the heart needs to be opened as for valve replacement, but may also occur after coronary bypass surgery. Multiple microembolism is a great deal commoner, resulting from the passage of air, platelet aggregates, fibrin or fat into the cerebral arterial tree.

It can often be difficult to apportion the blame between microembolism and hypoperfusion in leading to some of the common diffuse cerebral sequelae described below. Early neuropathological studies showed evidence of both, with scattered embolic infarcts and anoxic changes most prominent in the hippocampus. Major advances in reducing such complications have come from the incorporation of microfilters in the extracorporeal circulation, from adequate heparinisation and haemodilution, and from maintenance of the mean arterial blood pressure during operation above 50 mmHg.

Clinically obvious sequelae

The more obvious sequelae include stroke, ophthalmic abnormalities and postoperative confusion or delirium. Shaw *et al.* (1985) examined 312 patients immediately after coronary bypass surgery and found neurological changes in 61%. Serious morbidity was, however, rare. Definite stroke occurred in 5% though this was rarely severely disabling. Ophthalmic abnormalities were found in 25% by way of retinal infarcts, visual field abnormalities, or reductions in visual acuity for which no definite cause was discovered. Three per cent showed prolonged depression of consciousness not attributable to sedative drugs, and 1% a delirious state with hallucinations and paranoia. One patient sustained fatal cerebral hypoxic damage. Primitive reflexes were detected in 39%, chiefly palmomental and pout reflexes, and 12% had sustained brachial plexus injuries from torsion or compression during surgery.

Postoperative delirium is usually transient, resolving within a few days. Sometimes it follows a lucid interval of 2 or 3 days and the cause may then be uncertain. It has been reported in over a quarter of subjects in some series (Mayou 1986). Sleep disturbance, medication and the relative sensory deprivation induced by the stay in an intensive care unit are probably often contributory factors.

'Soft' neurological signs and neuropsychological deficits

The high prevalence of primitive reflexes noted by Shaw *et al.* may reflect hypoxic–ischaemic damage. Other minor neurological signs may be detected immediately postoperatively, such as transient nystagmus, impairment of coordination or depressed reflexes. These almost invariably recover within a few days. Neuropsychological assessment has likewise shown that early deficits are common, with falls from preoperative levels in 80% of patients (Shaw *et al.* 1986). Such deficits chiefly involve

problems with attention and concentration, psychomotor speed and verbal learning. Almost half of those who had deteriorated in Shaw *et al.*'s sample made no complaints of impairment, and only 10% were overtly disabled in everyday ward activities. However, dysfunction on testing correlated significantly with the presence of new palmomental reflexes, suggesting that it was likely to be due to diffuse brain damage of a subtle nature.

Sotaniemi *et al.*'s (1986) long-term follow-up study raised the strong possibility that such deficits were not always evanescent. Forty-four patients who had had valve replacements were examined 10 days postoperatively for minor neurological signs and at 8 weeks for neuropsychological change. Almost three-quarters showed *improvement* on neuropsychological testing, while a quarter were impaired in relation to preoperative performance. At follow-up 5 years later the group with early neurological signs or psychometric impairment were more liable to report some degree of memory difficulty, and showed significantly poorer performance on testing than the remainder. When divided into those who had had short or long perfusion times during operation, the latter performed significantly less well at 5 years, irrespective of the presence or absence of early neurological signs.

The immediate postoperative outcome thus appears to have implications for long-term psychological performance, with predictive value attaching even to asymptomatic early deficits. A good deal of effort has accordingly been devoted to exploring their possible origins.

Studies from the cardiothoracic unit at the Middlesex Hospital, London, have compared patients undergoing coronary bypass surgery with controls having major vascular or other thoracic surgery (Smith *et al.* 1986; Newman *et al.* 1987; Treasure *et al.* 1989). Transient neurological dysfunction as reflected in 'soft' neurological signs was found in some 60% of bypass patients at 24 hours compared with 20% of controls. This, however, may have been largely related to the dosage of analgesics and sedatives employed. Deterioration on a battery of neuropsychological tests was detectable in almost three-quarters of bypass patients at 8 days, and was significantly more likely to occur with older age, longer time on extracorporeal circulation and lower perfusion pressures. By 8 weeks significant recovery had taken place but deficits persisted in over a third. Similar neuropsychological changes were observed in half of the controls but these patients were somewhat older. Cerebral blood flow measurements using intravenous ^{133}Xe showed significant reductions in the coronary bypass group at 8 days, returning to preoperative levels at 8 weeks. This mirrors Henriksen's (1984) finding with single photon emission tomography. There were no significant changes in blood flow in the comparison group.

Follow-up of a substantial proportion of these bypass patients showed that the deficits present at 8 weeks tended to remain relatively stable, being still detectable 12 months later (Newman *et al.* 1990). Patients with enduring deficits were again significantly older than those without, and had had significantly longer periods on extracorporeal circulation. So far these results could reflect either microembolism or haemodynamic factors related to perfusion, since the influence of both will stand to increase with the duration of extracorporeal perfusion.

Investigating possible influences further, the same group has examined the effects of different forms of oxygenation during extracorporeal bypass, and the effects of introducing arterial line filters. A sheet membrane oxygenator, in comparison with a bubble oxygenator, produced a marked decrease in retinal microembolism as assessed by retinal fluorescein angiograms, also a trend towards reduction in neuropsychological deficits on the eighth postoperative day (Blauth *et al.* 1989). Comparisons between patients randomised to the presence or absence of a 40 μm micropore filter in the extracorporeal circulation showed that it significantly reduced the incidence of neuropsychological deficits at 8 days (Pugsley *et al.* 1994). Doppler ultrasound, used to monitor the presence of microemboli in the middle cerebral artery, confirmed that they were reduced when the filter was used, and the number detected correlated with the likelihood of the patient having neuropsychological deficits later. Clearly, therefore, microemboli, whether gaseous or particulate, make a contribution to the subtle deficits detected postoperatively. The extent to which other aspects of the perfusion process may contribute through hypoxic brain damage remains uncertain.

In a small preliminary study Toner *et al.* (1994) have performed MRI imaging before and after bypass surgery. One week postoperatively four of 15 patients showed additional MRI changes by way of punctate hyperintense areas which could have been due either to microembolism or perfusion-related ischaemia. Åberg *et al.* (1982, 1984) have produced biochemical data which point towards the influence of hypoxia–ischaemia; adenylate kinase, a marker of cell membrane disruption, was shown to be elevated in the cerebrospinal fluid in patients who had had extracorporeal bypass 24 hours earlier, and to correlate with the extent of the ensuing neuropsychological deficits.

Cardiac transplantation carries all of the above risks, with additional problems due to postoperative immunosuppression and the attendant risk of infections. Hallucina-tions, delusions and disorganised behaviour can occur during the first 2 weeks, and multiple factors will often contribute to such pictures including the administration of steroids and sedatives. When developing later than this, psychotic disturbances will often be indicative of intracranial infection (Hotson & Pedley 1976).

Uraemia

Uraemia may result from primary disease of the kidneys or from extrarenal causes. Any process which results in a prolonged and severe reduction of blood flow through the kidneys can produce potentially reversible renal failure due to tubular damage, for example shock or dehydration following operations, burns or crush injuries. The uraemia is then often aggravated by the increased protein catabolism that ensues.

Disordered mental functioning forms a prominent part of the syndrome of uraemia, both in chronic renal failure and in these more acute disturbances. In Stenbäck and Haapanen's (1967) large consecutive series of patients seen in a renal unit, mental manifestations occurred in 60%, rising to 75% when the blood urea exceeded 250 mg/100 ml. Mental changes were as common in the acute as in the chronic uraemic patients.

Presentation with psychiatric features

Uraemic patients are usually obviously unwell, but occasionally the mental changes can be the most prominent manifestation and lead directly to psychiatric consultation. This is more likely when the uraemia has developed slowly. The picture may simulate neurasthenia with symptoms of lethargy, anorexia and depression. Or early dementia may be suspected in view of sluggish comprehension and difficulty with memory. Elderly demented patients may suffer additional mental impairment from unsuspected uraemia, sometimes as a result of prostatic hypertrophy and an associated hydronephrosis. More rarely an acute organic reaction may be the first indication, and uraemia must be constantly borne in mind in the differential diagnosis of delirium of uncertain aetiology.

Common psychological accompaniments

By far the commonest mental disturbance is progressive torpor and drowsiness with the insidious development of intellectual impairment. Stenbäck and Haapanen (1967) describe the following sequence of changes:

The first complaint is usually of feeling generally

unwell, with fatigue and incapacity for physical or mental effort. The difficulty with concentration is characteristically episodic, so that the patient performs well for short periods of time but cannot sustain mental activity. There may be no other definite features on examination at this stage, though headache and anorexia are usually prominent complaints.

With further progression memory becomes obviously impaired, and episodes of disorientation and confusion appear. Listlessness and apathy prevail but an anxious restlessness may sometimes be seen. Depression and emotional withdrawal are usually marked. There may be petulant demanding behaviour, with negative attitudes towards treatment and hostility towards attendants, which later clears with clinical improvement. Both the impairment of consciousness and the changes of mood typically fluctuate markedly, with lucid periods during which behaviour returns to normal. Neurological accompaniments include fascicular twitching, tremor, multifocal myoclonus and muscle cramps. Flapping tremor of the outstretched hands may be observed, similar to that of hepatic encephalopathy (p. 564). On recovery there is patchy or complete amnesia for the periods of disorientation and confusion.

Episodes of acute delirium appear in a third of cases, with apprehension, bewilderment and fleeting hallucinations which may be terrifying in content. As with delirium due to other causes the picture changes rapidly from time to time and paranoid developments are common. Eventually more profound impairment of consciousness develops with increasingly sluggish comprehension and reaction, slurring of speech, incontinence and ultimately coma.

Epileptic fits develop in about a third of cases, more frequently in acute than chronic uraemia. They are usually a late feature unless hypertension is present at an early stage. The combination of clinical signs of cerebral depression together with excitability, as manifest in seizures, is rare in other metabolic encephalopathies (Raskin 1989). When the blood pressure is very high there may be episodes of hypertensive encephalopathy, with severe headache and transient attacks of blindness, dysphasia or monoplegia.

Peripheral neuropathy is common in chronic renal failure. Sensation is impaired distally and symmetrically, reflexes are diminished and intense painful paraesthesiae sometimes occur (Mawdsley 1972). Even in the absence of clinically overt neuropathy impairment of peripheral nerve conduction can often be shown. The 'restless legs syndrome' (p. 640) develops in a considerable proportion of patients, with or without overt neuropathy, presenting with unpleasant sensations in the lower limbs, worse

in the evenings and relieved by movements (Raskin 1989).

Psychoses with uraemia

Occasionally, and presumably depending on the premorbid constitution, the picture may closely simulate a schizophrenic or affective psychosis. Baker and Knutson (1946) reported a patient initially diagnosed as suffering from catatonic schizophrenia, but with rapid fluctuations between psychotic and normal periods. Menninger's (1924) patient presented with mounting paranoia over many months, culminating in a florid psychotic illness with clear organic features. Psychotic depression may likewise occur, and occasional manic reactions have been observed. In all of these, close examination will usually betray organic mental symptoms. The obvious impairment of physical health, with weakness, weight loss and anorexia, should alert one to the true situation.

Depression may usually be treated safely with tricyclic antidepressants, though patients receiving dialysis will warrant careful monitoring of blood levels (Rosser 1976). Phenothiazines should where possible be avoided on account of their enhanced liability to induce dystonia and other movement disorders in the presence of uraemia.

'Acute azotaemic psychotic encephalitis'

At one time it was believed that certain conditions existed in which an acute psychotic illness was accompanied by uraemia but was not directly caused by it. A primary cerebral pathology was thought to lead on the one hand to the psychosis and on the other to the uraemia. In the French literature an 'acute azotaemic psychotic encephalitis' was described, presenting with acute delirium and fever and progressing to coma and usually death, with evidence of degenerative and inflammatory lesions in the central nervous system. The case was vigorously argued that the uraemia was secondary to lesions in vegetative centres of the nervous system rather than their cause, just as uraemia might occasionally complicate epidemic encephalitis or delirium tremens (Marchand 1953). The 'fatal catatonia' of German workers was viewed similarly (Stauder 1934; Arnold 1949).

More recent knowledge allows most of these cases to be seen as examples of acute renal failure secondary to extrarenal causes, with the psychotic manifestations being attributable to the uraemia in the usual way. Alternatively, acute renal failure may have complicated a psychosis already brought about by other factors. It is noteworthy that the illnesses often followed operations, deliveries or acute infections. Links have been drawn with the 'neuroleptic malignant syndrome' of present-day practice (p. 626).

Investigations

The blood urea is raised and electrolyte disturbances are common. Sodium depletion can be marked, the serum phosphate elevated, and bicarbonate and calcium reduced. In the later stages the serum potassium may rise. Anaemia can be considerable in patients with chronic uraemia.

Electroencephalographic changes develop roughly in proportion to the severity of the clinical condition, and are rarely absent when the blood urea exceeds 60 mg/100 ml (Tyler 1968). They resemble the changes seen in hepatic decompensation, namely lowering of voltage with loss of well-developed alpha activity, then progressive slowing and disorganisation with runs of waves occurring at 5–7 per second which ultimately replace all other activity. Secondary hyperparathyroidism may play a part in contributing to the slowing (Raskin 1989). Epileptiform changes frequently appear.

The pressure of the cerebrospinal fluid is usually slightly raised, sometimes with moderate elevation of protein but without increase of cells.

Aetiology of mental disturbances

Mental and neurological changes become commoner with increasing elevation of the blood urea, but there is by no means a simple linear relationship. Nor can urea be regarded as responsible for all or even the majority of the symptoms that result; considerable improvement can follow dialysis when urea is present in the dialysis fluid, and experimentally urea has not been found to have a strong neurotoxic effect. Other abnormalities must therefore play a direct aetiological role, with the level of blood urea serving mainly as an indicator of the severity of overall metabolic disturbance. Nevertheless estimation of the blood urea remains an important clinical indicator for monitoring the progress of the patient's condition.

Other derivatives of protein such as uric acid may play a part, as may other toxins so far unidentified. Electrolyte disturbances are certainly important in many cases. Changes in sodium, potassium, calcium, chloride, phosphate, acid–base balance and osmolality can all be blamed in individual instances. The rapidity of the shifts appears to be the essential factor, whether this is in the direction of normality or abnormality (Tyler 1968).

Drugs have been strongly incriminated as a cause of mental disturbance in patients with chronic renal failure, accounting for over a third of the episodes in some series

(Richet & Vachon 1966; Richet et al. 1970). Sedatives and antibiotics appear to be mainly responsible, either by virtue of accumulation when the drug is excreted by the kidneys, or as a result of increased susceptibility of the central nervous system in the uraemic patient.

Arterial hypertension brings its own contribution by way of transient neurological disturbances, fits and headache. In many cases a part is played by raised intracranial pressure, changes in cerebral blood flow and cerebral oxygen utilisation, and altered permeability of small blood vessels.

Neary (1976) has drawn attention to other causes of neuropsychiatric disturbance in patients with chronic renal failure. The risk of intracranial infection is increased in uraemia, especially when immunosuppressive drugs are used after renal transplantation; encephalitis due to herpes simplex or cytomegalovirus may be hard to diagnose in the prodromal stages, leading to behavioural disturbance and change of personality. Low-grade meningitis can lack the typical physical signs and present as depression with chronic headache. The use of anticoagulants in maintenance haemodialysis may result in a subdural haematoma.

The psychological stresses associated with haemodialysis or transplantation bring a range of problems of their own. Salmons (1980) has reviewed the problems inherent in such management of chronic renal failure, with disruptions in work, daily life and family relationships. Not surprisingly there is a high incidence of depression, anxiety and disturbed sexual functioning among such patients. Short-lived psychotic episodes may be observed, usually in clear consciousness but often marked by 'organic' features such as visual hallucinations or loosely held delusions. Steroids administered after transplantation may make an important contribution to such developments (p. 628). The risk of brain lymphoma is very considerably increased after transplantation, largely but not entirely attributable to immunosuppressant treatment (Raskin 1989).

Disturbances occasioned by dialysis

Gradual improvement usually follows dialysis, with return of mental clarity a short while after chemical normality has been achieved. Occasionally, however, the time lag may be several days in duration.

If the patient is lucid beforehand he usually remains so, provided time is taken over the procedure. However, too rapid dialysis carries a hazard of worsening the clinical situation (dialysis disequilibrium syndrome). Headache, muscle twitching, fits and confusion may develop, sometimes progressing to coma with signs of brain stem compression (Peterson & Swanson 1964; Mawdsley 1972). This is commoner when the initial level of blood urea has been very high, and usually occurs towards the end of the dialysis.

The exact cause is unknown, but is probably related to rapid changes in blood biochemistry and the acid–base balance. In some cases the cause appears to lie in the more rapid clearance of urea and other osmotically active substances from the blood than from the central nervous system, resulting in an osmotic gradient which draws water into the brain and cerebrospinal fluid sufficiently to raise the intracranial pressure. Electroencephalography carried out during dialysis shows changes consistent with such an hypothesis and reversible with hypertonic fructose (Kennedy *et al.* 1963). Similar disturbance may result from quite another mechanism, when glucose enters the blood from the dialysing solution and provokes reactive hypoglycaemia (Rigg & Bercu 1967).

Another serious complication of dialysis has been traced to the aluminium content of the water used in preparing the dialysate. This, known as *'dialysis encephalopathy'* or *'dialysis dementia'*, was formerly one of the commonest causes of death in certain units (Burks *et al.* 1976). The earliest signs were difficulty with speech or episodes of confusion appearing during the dialysis procedure. Over time the mental difficulties became permanent, with dysarthria, dysphasia, apraxia and slowly progressive generalised dementia. Paranoia, bizarre behaviour and episodes of delirium were sometimes prominent. Neurological accompaniments were flapping tremor, facial grimacing and myoclonus. Focal seizures and various pareses often occurred.

Slow worsening of the disorder usually led to death. Treatment was ineffective and progression could continue despite restoration of normal renal function by transplantation. At autopsy the changes in the brain were slight and non-specific.

Most patients developing the disorder had been on haemodialysis for several years. It was found that the aluminium content of the brain, and especially the grey matter, was increased fourfold in such patients compared with uraemics dying from other causes (Alfrey *et al.* 1976; McDermott *et al.* 1978b). This was at first ascribed to the aluminium in the phosphate-binding gels employed, but it eventually emerged that the regional incidence of encephalopathy in various centres correlated with the aluminium content of the water used as dialysate (Parkinson *et al.* 1979). Since taking steps to circumvent the problem the disease has now virtually disappeared.

In areas where the incidence was high an association could be shown between duration of time on dialysis and certain measures of cognitive impairment, even before the severe disorder was declared (English *et al.* 1978). The EEG was similarly often markedly abnormal for many months before signs appeared.

Cerebral pathology

Gross lesions in the central nervous system are rare in the absence of marked hypertension. The most constant change is scattered neuronal degeneration, with chromatolysis and vacuolisation of nerve cells. In chronic cases this progresses to pyknosis and areas of cell loss. Olsen (1961) systematically examined the brains of 104 patients dying of uraemia, and found such changes most frequently in the brain stem nuclei, reticular formation and cortex, though variable in location from case to case. He was unable to confirm other features which have traditionally been emphasised, such as focal glial proliferation, areas of demyelination and cerebral oedema.

Changes in the cerebral vessels with thrombosis and infarction are common, but correspond to hypertension and arteriosclerosis rather than to uraemia itself. A general haemorrhagic tendency may be seen when other factors are present to explain it.

In general, therefore, the cerebral pathology shows little that is specific for uraemia, and the picture is dominated to a high degree by the disease processes responsible for the uraemia and the secondary complications that develop.

Electrolyte disturbances

A delicate balance must be maintained in the chemical environment, both intracellularly and extracellularly, to maintain the proper functioning of the central nervous system. In this certain relatively simple components have been identified: the correct acid–base balance must be preserved, the proper gradient of sodium and potassium across the cell membrane, and the correct concentration of calcium and perhaps magnesium ions. These factors may be disturbed separately or together in many disease processes and mental symptoms may follow.

The metabolic dynamics involved in the production of mental symptoms are often complex, since disturbance of one aspect of electrolyte balance can have repercussions upon others. Alterations in cerebral blood flow may follow and complicate the situation further. Nevertheless the correct appreciation of the primary disturbance is of the utmost importance if appropriate treatment is to follow.

Electrolyte disturbance plays a prominent part in certain endocrine disorders and in uraemia as already described. It complicates respiratory disorders, and can assume great importance postoperatively when the patient is maintained on intravenous fluids for long periods of time. A variety of other causes will be mentioned below where appropriate.

Water depletion

Water depletion can arise from simple unavailability as in shipwreck, or may be seen clinically in the presence of severe weakness from any physical illness, in severe dysphagia and in coma. Intense thirst and dryness of the mouth is coupled with a greyish ill appearance and loss of weight. Signs of dehydration are less obvious than in sodium depletion since the greatest loss is from the intracellular compartment. The plasma sodium, chloride and urea tend to rise. Increasing mental confusion gives way to delirium and coma. The administration of water relieves the situation, but if intravenous fluids are required a 5% glucose solution should be given. Seizures may occur with high sodium levels, or due to brain oedema during too rapid rehydration.

The elderly are especially at risk in view of their narrow limits of physiological balance, diminished capacity for renal tubular absorption, and liability to chronic debilitating disease. Jana and Romano-Jana (1973) have described four cases of 'hypernatraemic psychosis' in which elderly patients were admitted to a psychiatric hospital in a confused and disorientated state. Discovery of a raised serum sodium led to the intravenous administration of hypotonic fluids with rapid restoration of normal mental function. All four had been ambulatory on admission and did not complain of excessive thirst. The cause of the dehydration remained uncertain, but diminished fluid intake may have been occasioned by primary emotional disturbance and cognitive changes.

Water intoxication

Overhydration may result from excessive infusion of 5% glucose solution postoperatively, from the administration of excessive quantities of vasopressin, or if too much water is drunk in the presence of renal failure. An important cause in psychiatric patients can be compulsive water drinking, as described on p. 525. The serum osmolality and sodium are low.

Anorexia, nausea and vomiting are early signs, with marked lassitude and changes of mood. Headache and blurring of vision may occur. Later there is impairment of consciousness, delirium and coma. Muscle cramps and twitches are sometimes seen, and epileptic fits are common.

Sodium depletion

Sodium depletion occurs in tropical climates when common salt is omitted during the process of acclimatisation. Clinically it is seen after severe vomiting and diarrhoea from any cause, in Addison's disease, in salt-losing nephritis and pyelonephritis, and postoperatively when patients are maintained on intravenous glucose alone. Severe hyponatraemia may follow extensive burns. The syndrome of 'inappropriate antidiuretic hormone secretion' (SIADH) has many causes, chief among which are carcinoma of the lung, duodenum or pancreas, the sequelae of encephalitis, stroke, brain tumour or trauma, and a number of drugs including hypoglycaemic agents, thiazide diuretics and psychotropic agents as described on p. 526 (Illowsky & Kirch 1988). Hyponatraemia and hypotonicity of the plasma are accompanied by continuing excretion of sodium in the urine.

The classic symptoms and signs of heat exhaustion include weakness, dizziness, pallor, profuse sweating, diminution of urine, rapid pulse and respiration, low blood pressure and cramping pains in the abdomen and limbs. The onset is usually sudden, and the response to sodium chloride by mouth is dramatic. However, the picture can be misleading when it sets in very gradually. Saphir (1945) described 10 cases which were missed until the serum chloride was estimated. The resemblance to neurosis was striking, and in some patients malingering had been suspected. Prominent mental complaints included irritability, depression without cause and intense anxiety.

When associated with medical diseases the presenting features are usually of lassitude, apathy and weakness. Giddiness and hypotensive faints are common, with muscle cramps and weakness. Anorexia develops with nausea and vomiting. The patient appears dehydrated but thirst is rarely a prominent complaint. Mental confusion ultimately appears with disorientation, delusions and hallucinations. If untreated the condition progresses to coma. The occurrence of fits is an ominous sign with a mortality of over 50% (Riggs 1989).

Treatment consists of giving salt by mouth, or when necessary intravenous saline. The administration of water alone or glucose in water can be dangerous, as the hypotonicity is aggravated further. The danger of over-rapid correction of severe hyponatraemia in causing central pontine myelinosis is described on p. 586.

Potassium depletion

The normal renal mechanisms for the conservation of potassium are relatively inefficient, and accordingly potassium deficiency is liable to develop in any disease associated with chronic starvation or anorexia. The commonest cause is again inadequate intake when patients are maintained postoperatively on intravenous fluids. Gastrointestinal causes include hyperemesis gravidarum, chronic diarrhoea due to ulcerative colitis, malabsorption syndromes such as steatorrhoea, or the long-continued use of purgatives. Other causes include Cushing's disease, the massive diuresis which may arise in diabetes mellitus, the diuretic phase of acute renal insufficiency, or the rarer potassium-losing nephritis and renal tubular acidosis. It may also result from the administration of diuretics, ACTH or adrenal steroids. Excessive transfer of potassium into the cells may occur after myocardial infarction, in familial periodic paralysis, and when diabetic ketosis is treated vigorously with glucose and insulin.

Judge (1968) has reported that potassium deficiency may arise in elderly persons simply because their diet contains inadequate amounts. Depression, apathy, weakness, paranoid ideation and disturbance of sleep rhythm follow. The serum potassium level may sometimes be normal, yet improvement in mood, alertness and activity follows supplementation. Others may have just sufficient potassium in the diet, but a secondary deficiency is produced by an attack of diarrhoea and vomiting, an acute infection or a small cerebrovascular accident. In addition such persons may take a purgative or be given a diuretic which aggravates the deficiency.

The usual presentation in all cases is with lethargy, apathy and depression which can be profound in degree. Anorexia, constipation and abdominal distension are common accompaniments and paralytic ileus may develop. Severe muscle weakness may extend to flaccid paralysis with rhabdomyolysis and myoglobinuria.

Hysteria may be diagnosed, especially since the tendon reflexes are sometimes preserved until very low potassium levels are reached. Moreover, in familial periodic paralysis (p. 721) emotional stress may precipitate an attack. Mitchell and Feldman (1968) report an example of a patient with renal tubular acidosis who was first thought to show conversion hysteria:

A woman of 30 complained of marked weakness of the arms and legs after a fall some hours earlier, and was unable to walk. There was a long previous history of anorexia, occasional vomiting, constipation and muscle spasms, and there had been several similar falls in preceding months. Marital difficulties were prominent and a hysterical conversion reaction was diagnosed. She slowly regained strength and was discharged after 4 days.

One month later she was readmitted with extreme weakness of several hours' duration, and complained of sleeping excessively and frequent headaches. The serum potassium was low at 2.4 mEq/l but again spontaneous recovery occurred. Two days later there were similar complaints, the serum potassium was

1.8 mEq/l and the electrocardiogram showed typical changes. There had been no evidence of impairment of consciousness at any stage.

Apprehension and irritability are sometimes marked and an anxiety state may be simulated. Emotionally induced hyperventilation may be thought to be responsible for paraesthesiae, vague muscle discomfort and transient visual disturbances. Very occasionally a typical acute organic reaction is seen with disorientation, confusion, impairment of memory and delirium.

The electrocardiogram shows characteristic changes which may alert one to the situation—a small T wave, prolongation of the Q–T interval and depression of the ST segment. A low serum potassium confirms the diagnosis but is not always found in the early stages.

Potassium chloride or bicarbonate should be given orally. Nasogastric or intravenous infusion of potassium chloride may be needed if oral intake is impossible, but this must be undertaken with great care.

Potassium excess

Hyperkalaemia occurs with acute renal failure, in severe crises of Addison's disease and in diabetic coma. It can be induced by potassium-sparing diuretics and angiotensin-converting enzyme (ACE) inhibitors (Drug & Therapeutics Bulletin 1991b). Cardiac toxicity precludes the appearance of nervous system manifestations in most cases, with bradycardia due to heart block, ventricular dysrhythmia or fibrillation and ultimately ventricular asystole (Riggs 1989). The most frequent neurological manifestation is flaccid muscle weakness akin to that seen with potassium depletion. The dullness and lethargy of patients with Addison's disease is probably mainly related to sodium depletion.

Hypercalcaemia

The clinical manifestations of hypercalcaemia have already been described in the section on hyperparathyroidism (p. 529). Malignancy is another important cause — carcinoma with secondary bone deposits, multiple myeloma and Hodgkin's disease. The hypercalcaemia is then often due to a combination of increased bone destruction caused by metastases, and bone resorption occasioned by a variety of humoral factors secreted or induced by the tumour. Of these, parathyroid hormone-related peptide is particularly important and has been demonstrated with squamous cell carcinoma of the lung and carcinomas of the breast and kidney (Meader & Vella 1992). Other causes include sarcoidosis, hyperthyroidism, the excessive administration of vitamin D, and the prolonged ingestion of calcium especially when taken as milk with an antacid ('milk-alkali syndrome'). Long-term treatment with lithium may very occasionally produce hypercalcaemia by elevating the level of parathyroid hormone (Christiansen et al. 1976).

Petersen (1968) reported six examples, mostly due to vitamin D intoxication, with clinical pictures similar to those seen with hyperparathyroidism. Thirst, asthenia, depression and tension states were the main manifestations, and three patients showed acute organic psychoses. Weizman et al. (1979) found that seven of 12 patients with hypercalcaemia due to malignant disease had prominent psychiatric symptoms. Three showed depression or anxiety, sometimes severe, three developed acute organic reactions and one an acute paranoid psychosis. In all cases the mental symptoms disappeared within 2–6 days of the serum calcium being restored to normal. There is obvious risk of viewing the emotional disorder as a reaction to the basic disease, or of ascribing organic mental symptoms to intracerebral complications.

Hypocalcaemia

Hypocalcaemia may result from a deficiency of calcium or vitamin D in the diet, producing rickets in children and osteomalacia in adults. Hypoparathyroidism, chronic steatorrhoea and chronic nephritis are other possible causes. Anticonvulsant therapy leads to hypocalcaemia in a substantial proportion of epileptic patients. Acute severe forms are usually the sequelae of thyroid or parathyroid surgery, or arise as a complication of acute pancreatitis (Riggs 1989).

In children there is a characteristic triad of convulsions, laryngeal stridor and carpopedal spasm (p. 532). In adults the usual complaint is merely of painful cramps or tingling paraesthesiae in the limbs. The characteristic signs of latent tetany and the common mental manifestations are described in the section on hypoparathyroidism (pp. 531–3).

Tetany due to alkalosis is described below.

Hypomagnesaemia

The clinical pictures attributable to magnesium depletion are ill defined and controversial, largely because magnesium deficiency is usually associated with other concurrent metabolic derangements. It may arise after prolonged parenteral feeding, in chronic alcoholism, in delirium tremens, and in cases of severe malnutrition or malabsorption associated with diarrhoea and vomiting. Renal loss of magnesium occurs in diabetic acidosis and renal tubular necrosis, also with cisplatin use in children (Hayes et al. 1979).

Vallee et al. (1960) found that a picture identical with hypocalcaemic tetany could result, with convulsions, carpopedal spasm, Chvostek's and Trousseau's signs, and athetoid movements of the limbs. They described such cases in which the serum calcium was normal and parenteral magnesium sulphate promptly abolished the symptoms. Hanna et al. (1960) presented three cases of pure magnesium deficiency with a rather different picture. Convulsions were present, but tetany in the sense of spontaneous muscle cramps was absent. The most marked manifestations were depression, irritability, vertigo, ataxia and muscle weakness. Fishman (1965) described myoclonic jerks and bizarre multifocal seizures. Other reports have included tremors, fasciculation, choreiform movements, mild confusion and disorientation, delirium of sudden onset and stupor, all of which may be reversed by intramuscular magnesium sulphate (Flink 1956; Hammarsten & Smith 1957; Randall et al. 1959; Hall 1973). Shils (1969) kept volunteers on magnesium-deficient diets for periods of many months, resulting in lethargy, tremors, fasciculations and spontaneous carpopedal spasms, all responding to the administration of magnesium. However, all symptomatic subjects had developed secondary calcium depletion despite adequate intake and absorption, as well hypokalaemia. The contribution of magnesium deficiency alone could therefore not be determined. More recent evidence on the subject is reviewed by Tucci (1981) and Riggs (1989).

Hypermagnesaemia is rare, occurring when there is excessive intake in a setting of impaired renal function. Depression of the nervous system results in lethargy, confusion and loss of the tendon reflexes, proceeding in severe cases to flaccid paralysis due to blockade of neuromuscular transmission.

A number of workers have investigated serum magnesium levels in patients with schizophrenia. Elevated magnesium has often been reported, but also lowered levels or no difference from controls. Alexander and Jackson (1981) review the inconsistent findings in the literature.

Low serum zinc

Zinc deficiency is rare, but occurs in certain malnourished populations and in countries where bread with a high phytate content is consumed. It can be found with regional enteritis and with malabsorption syndromes. The excretion of zinc is increased in liver disease, diabetes, some renal diseases and with certain drugs (Lancet 1973; Drug & Therapeutics Bulletin 1988b).

The syndrome most closely tied to low serum zinc is diminished acuity of taste and smell (hyposmia, hypogeusia), first described by Henkin *et al.* (1971) and shown to be responsive to the administration of oral zinc sulphate. Many such patients had developed the hypogeusia soon after a respiratory illness, while in others it appeared spontaneously. The strong perversions of taste and smell that were sometimes present could precipitate emotional disturbance including profound depression.

Henkin *et al.* (1975) monitored the low serum zinc produced by histidine in the treatment of six patients with progressive systemic sclerosis. They were able to follow the sequential appearance of anorexia, dysfunction of taste and smell, and ultimately the development of neurological and psychiatric features. The patients became dizzy and unsteady, with cerebellar symptoms in the form of ataxic gait and intention tremor. Several were irritable and easily upset, with depression and periods of weeping. Others showed memory impairments, lethargy, auditory and visual hallucinations and pronounced emotional lability. The disturbances correlated with the degree of lowering of serum zinc and with indicators of total body zinc loss. All were quickly reversed following the administration of zinc sulphate.

Staton *et al.* (1976) described a young male patient presenting with a picture resembling catatonic schizophrenia who responded rapidly to zinc administration after failing to respond to other treatments:

He had presented with auditory and visual hallucinations, loose associations, blunted affect and disorientation in time and place. Drooling, negativism and catatonic postures became established. Phenothiazines were ineffective and led to severe extrapyramidal disturbance. After some months electroconvulsive therapy was tried and produced only transient improvement. A low serum zinc and high serum copper were discovered and oral zinc sulphate and pyridoxine were commenced. Thenceforward he made excellent progress and remained well 1 year later.

Alkalosis

Metabolic alkalosis results from repeated vomiting as in pyloric stenosis, or the ingestion of large quantities of sodium bicarbonate given, for example, in the treatment of peptic ulcer. An important cause from the psychiatric point of view is the respiratory alkalosis which results from overbreathing. Attacks of hyperventilation are common in states of anxiety and in histrionic patients under stress. Hyperventilation also follows the ingestion of large quantities of salicylates.

In the cases associated with vomiting there is often apathy, delirium and stupor, but concomitant potassium and water depletion may often play a part. Tetany is liable to occur, because the proportion of ionised calcium is reduced even though the total serum calcium is normal.

The sequence of changes seen with hyperventilation are reviewed by Wyke (1963). Experimental studies show that hyperventilation increases suggestibility and facilitates the induction of hypnosis. At an early stage perception is increased, but later dulled. As consciousness becomes impaired and awareness of the environment diminishes the EEG begins to slow, and high voltage delta waves ultimately appear. Impairment of memory and calculation develop when the dominant frequency reaches 5 Hz. Psychological studies show impaired performance on tests of reaction time, manual coordination and word association, and there is often subsequent amnesia for events of the period.

When hyperventilation accompanies anxiety the emotional instability is increased, creating a vicious circle. Vertigo and paraesthesiae further reinforce the patient's concern. Mental confusion may become marked, and myoclonic jerks or epileptic phenomena may be precipitated. In severe cases the condition may progress to loss of consciousness.

It is uncertain whether these clinical phenomena depend directly on the lowering of carbon dioxide tension in the blood, or on the rising pH and other metabolic changes in the environment of the neurones. Hypoxia resulting from vasoconstriction of the cerebral arterioles may make a further contribution. The decrease in the ionised calcium of the blood is almost certainly responsible for the tetanic phenomena.

Acidosis

Metabolic acidosis may result from renal failure or from diabetes mellitus with ketosis. In chronic diarrhoea there may be loss of sodium bicarbonate in the stools. Respiratory disorders such as emphysema or status asthmaticus which lead to underventilation similarly cause acidosis due to carbon dioxide retention.

In metabolic acidosis the most prominent result is stimulation of the respiratory centre with deep and rapid respiration. Consciousness is progressively impaired and mental confusion or delirium are seen in varying degree. The precise clinical picture in the individual case is largely determined by the underlying condition and other associated metabolic derangements.

Respiratory acidosis (*hypercapnia*) provides a more distinctive clinical picture. Inhalation of 6–7% carbon dioxide can be shown to impair psychological functioning and lead to perseverative responses. In chronic respiratory disease mental dulling and drowsiness are common, and it has long been known that if oxygen is given alone this can sometimes impair consciousness further and precipitate mental confusion and irrational behaviour. This was at first ascribed to overoxygenation, but is now recognised to result from the increased carbon dioxide retention which occurs as dyspnoea is relieved.

Westlake *et al.* (1955) reviewed the clinical findings in carbon dioxide retention due to emphysema. Mental disturbances were usually present when the blood pH was below 7.2 or the arterial tension of carbon dioxide above 100 mmHg, ranging from mild impairment of consciousness with irritability, disorientation and confusion, to delirium with auditory and visual hallucinations. Headache, muscle twitching and sweating were common accompaniments. When the pH fell below 7.1 or the tension of carbon dioxide rose above 120 mmHg, there was increasing lethargy and drowsiness leading ultimately to coma. The intracranial pressure was often raised, and papilloedema was sometimes seen. The disturbances were usually transient, because the pH is ultimately restored by renal activity, but in a minority of cases the outcome could be fatal.

The mental changes are thought to be due to the direct action of acidaemia or hypercapnia on the metabolism of cortical neurones. The rise of intracranial pressure is ascribed to the accompanying cerebral vasodilatation. The EEG shows delta waves, sometimes paroxysmal or episodic, at high arterial levels of carbon dioxide.

Hepatic disorder

Striking neurological and psychiatric changes may be seen in patients with liver disease. The range and extent of these features were clearly defined in the classic paper by Summerskill *et al.* in 1956. An important point was the demonstration that neuropsychiatric disorder could sometimes dominate the picture, even when unequivocal evidence of liver disease was not immediately obvious. The correct diagnosis might therefore easily be overlooked.

Seventeen patients were reported, mostly with portal cirrhosis. Neuropsychiatric symptoms were the presenting feature in eight patients in whom liver disease had not previously been suspected. Four had been admitted to psychiatric hospitals initially, and in three others a psychiatric opinion had been sought. Only three were jaundiced and only seven had large livers. Five showed little biochemical evidence of liver dysfunction. The signs of most value in supporting the diagnosis were palmar erythema, spider naevi, finger clubbing and loss of body hair. Foetor hepaticus was prominent in every patient and the spleen was constantly enlarged.

Since then the topic appears to have received less attention than it deserves, but new interest attaches to it in view of improved methods of treatment of liver disease which allow much longer survival. Collis and Lloyd (1992) provide a valuable recent review.

Psychiatric features of hepatic encephalopathy

The manifestations are extremely variable, making it hard to demarcate a single entity of 'hepatic encephalopathy'. Essentially the picture is of a chronic organic reaction, characterised by acute exacerbations and remissions and accompanied by neurological abnormalities which also wax and wane. Neurotic or psychotic features may be prominent, depending on the premorbid personality, and change of personality may feature in large degree. The disturbances may persist for many years, sometimes with complete remissions for long periods of time, or the condition may become chronic and constant ('acquired chronic hepatocerebral degeneration') (Victor *et al.* 1965). The picture then resembles dementia, often with persistent motor abnormalities by way of pyramidal and extrapyramidal disturbance.

Impairment of consciousness is always present during exacerbations of the disorder. Warning signs are a fixed staring appearance and reduction of spontaneous movements. Hypersomnia is an early feature, sometimes with overpowering attacks of sleepiness by day and inversion of sleep rhythm. Later this progresses to periods of marked confusion, semicoma or coma, though deterioration can be arrested at any level. Coma at first resembles normal sleep, but later progresses to total unresponsiveness.

Rapid changes in the level of consciousness are accompanied by delirium with hallucinations, mainly in the visual modality. Episodic 'twilight' states with sudden onset and ending may also occur. One patient reported by Summerskill *et al.* (1956) experienced panoramic scenes in bright colours of frightening bears and wolves, and synaesthesia so that a dripping tap in the right peripheral field of vision was experienced as a cold drip on the right cheek. Recent memory is impaired in proportion to the impairment of consciousness, and confabulation is sometimes much in evidence. Dense amnesias with retrograde loss follow periods of coma.

The mood often shows abrupt swings, sometimes with depression, sometimes euphoria. Personality changes may be marked and are sometimes the presenting feature. During exacerbations uninhibited behaviour may be released, or previous traits of irritability or joviality are exaggerated. Between exacerbations an enduring disturbance of personality is characteristically seen, reminiscent of frontal lobe disorder with blunted affect, loss of drive and initiative, incongruous jocularity, tactlessness, defective insight and loss of finer aspects of social judgement. Murphy *et al.* (1948) noted similar changes and found that 'the jaundiced, pot-bellied cirrhotic patients are usually the jovial clowns of the ward'. Such patients would often insist on going home or claim perfect health despite all evidence to the contrary.

Other features include short-lived depressive episodes, hypomanic reactions, anxiety attacks or obsessive–compulsive behaviour. Occasionally paranoid reactions which have set in during episodes of confusion persist on recovery.

Episodes typical of acute schizophrenia or hypomania have also been reported, sometimes in the absence of impairment of consciousness, but usually accompanied by other signs of hepatic encephalopathy (Read *et al.* 1967). These may develop as little as weeks or months after portal–systemic anastomotic operations. They are rare, however, and their causal relationship to liver dysfunction remains in doubt.

Neurological features

The neurological abnormalities are more specific, and tend to worsen or remit in parallel with the psychiatric symptoms.

Motor disorders are the outstanding feature. There may be little to detect in remission other than mild exaggeration of tendon reflexes, unobtrusive tremor and a characteristic blank or grimacing facial expression. But at some stage almost every patient shows the characteristic *flapping tremor* (asterixis) which is brought into evidence when the arms are held outstretched. This consists of rapid bursts of flexion–extension movements at the metacarpophalangeal and wrist joints, superimposed upon a fine 6–9-per-second tremor. It is aggravated by fatigue, anxiety and excitement but is absent at rest. The disorder is characteristic but not entirely specific for hepatic encephalopathy, and is occasionally seen in uraemia, respiratory failure or severe heart failure (Sherlock & Dooley 1993).

Deterioration is accompanied by a combination of extrapyramidal and pyramidal features — dysarthria, ataxia, gross tremor, muscular rigidity, hyperreflexia and clonus. The plantar reflexes usually remain flexor until the stage of coma is reached, so that the unusual combination of rigidity, clonus and down-going plantar responses is frequently seen. In deep coma the muscles become flaccid and reflexes may be abolished.

These gross neurological disorders can remit abruptly and dramatically from one day to the next along with the psychiatric features. Serial tests of handwriting may serve as an indicator of progress. Other neurological abnormal-

ities include dysphasia with perseverative speech disturbances, blurring of vision, diplopia and nystagmus. Constructional apraxia has been stressed as an early and sometimes persistent feature.

Read *et al.* (1967) have described some less common syndromes of neurological defect. One small group of patients developed progressive paraplegia, and another cerebellar dysfunction along with parkinsonian features. Occasional patients developed myoclonus or epilepsy, or were at first suspected of cerebral tumours on account of dementia coupled with focal neurological signs.

Investigations

Biochemical evidence of liver dysfunction will usually be found but may sometimes be relatively slight.

The EEG can be of help in diagnosis and prognosis and shows a close correlation with the grades of neuropsychiatric disturbance (Parsons-Smith *et al.* 1957; Kennedy *et al.* 1973). Changes occur early in the progression towards coma, and even before psychological abnormalities have appeared. The earliest change is slowing of the alpha rhythm and the appearance of 5–7-per-second theta waves, most marked in the frontal and temporal regions. Theta comes to replace the alpha activity increasingly as consciousness is progressively impaired. Later, characteristic triphasic waves are seen, the appearance of which suggests a poor prognosis. Further deterioration is shown by decrease in amplitude, blunting of the triphasic waves and periods of flattening.

These changes are not specific for hepatic failure, and occur with many other metabolic derangements — uraemia, hypokalaemia, anoxia, carbon dioxide retention, hypoglycaemia, B_{12} deficiency and in the early phases of raised intracranial pressure — but in the conscious patient with liver disease they are virtually diagnostic of impending coma.

Lumbar puncture reveals cerebrospinal fluid under normal pressure. The protein is sometimes raised during coma but there is no pleocytosis (Sherlock & Dooley 1993). Glutamic acid and also glutamine may be increased.

Brain imaging may show minor degrees of cerebral atrophy, chiefly sulcal widening over anterior brain regions. This is more evident in patients with chronic persisting encephalopathy than in those with relapsing–remitting episodes (Zeneroli *et al.* 1987), but it is sometimes seen even in seemingly well-compensated patients (Tarter *et al.* 1986a; Moore *et al.* 1989). Such findings have been observed in non-alcoholic cirrhotics, confirming that they are unlikely to be due to alcoholism alone (Tarter *et al.* 1986a; Bernthal *et al.* 1987). In some investigations the degree of atrophy has shown significant relationships to biochemical indices of liver dysfunction and to certain measures of psychological deficit, but such correlations have not been striking.

Psychometric studies have confirmed the presence of deficits in encephalopathic patients with an accent on attentional processes (Elsass *et al.* 1978). Among cirrhotic patients generally, cognitive performance has been shown to be poor, especially on measures of memory and visuospatial ability (Tarter *et al.* 1986b, 1988). By contrast verbal abilities are generally well preserved. Again such impairments are found in both alcoholic and non-alcoholic patients, and sometimes with significant relationships to biochemical measures of liver dysfunction. Arria *et al.* (1990) have shown that psychometric impairments are more prominent in cirrhotic patients with low vitamin E levels, suggesting that impaired absorption of vitamin E and perhaps of other nutrients may make its own contribution to cognitive deficits.

Subclinical hepatic encephalopathy

Efforts have been made to detect patients with 'subclinical' or 'latent' hepatic encephalopathy so that appropriate measures may be undertaken to avert its full development. Thus even among patients without EEG abnormalities, and with normal psychiatric or neurological examinations, it has been observed that certain changes may herald the development of encephalopathy later. The sensitivity of visual evoked potentials in this regard was shown by Zeneroli *et al.* (1984), and the value of the WAIS Block Design Test and the Trail Making Test by Gitlin *et al.* (1986) and Sood *et al.* (1989). Davies *et al.* (1991) recommend the use of a simple screening battery including the drawing of a five-pointed star, and a 'number connection test' which is a modified version of the Trail Making Test. Weissenborn *et al.* (1990) compared the relative sensitivities of EEG patterns, visual evoked responses, P_{300} latency and the number connection test. The last two appeared to be optimal in the detection of impending encephalopathy.

Differential diagnosis

Summerskill *et al.*'s (1956) original patients had received various diagnostic labels including neurotic anxiety, hysterical ataxia, depression, frontal lobe tumour, cerebral arteriosclerosis, narcolepsy, psychomotor epilepsy, multiple sclerosis, Wilson's disease and parkinsonism.

The fluctuations in severity differentiate the condition from dementia, but may closely simulate drug intoxication. The distinction from Wilson's disease (p. 661) can be important; the neurological disturbance is then non-fluctuating, the motor abnormalities usually consist of choreoathetoid movements rather than a flapping tremor, and a Kayser–Fleischer corneal ring is virtually always present.

Delirious episodes may at first suggest delirium tremens, though hallucinations are less vivid and the patient is rarely fearful. The differentiation from alcoholic intoxication can be difficult because the two may coexist.

Depression may be misdiagnosed in view of the fixed facial expression, psychomotor retardation and depressive swings of mood. Catatonia may be suggested by episodes of mutism and stupor. Moreover psychoses of an affective, schizophrenic or paranoid type may be precipitated at an early stage.

Finally, in the presence of known liver disorder which is under treatment, the disturbances must be distinguished from those due to hyponatraemia caused by a low sodium diet and the administration of diuretics.

Aetiology of mental disturbances

It is now established that the neuropsychiatric disturbances are similar whatever the underlying liver pathology. Hepatocellular failure, portal hypertension or surgically induced portal–systemic anastomosis all lead to essentially similar pictures. The feature they share is a circulatory pathway by which portal blood may enter systemic veins and reach the brain without being metabolised by the liver (Sherlock & Dooley 1993). In primary hepatocellular failure the shunt is through the liver itself, because the cells cannot metabolise the contents of the portal blood completely. In cirrhosis the shunt is via the collateral vessels which become established. The mental disturbance is therefore essentially due to cerebral intoxication by intestinal contents which have failed to be metabolised by the liver.

The precise toxin responsible is uncertain, but it is clearly nitrogenous in nature. Thus the picture can be decisively influenced by the level of protein in the diet. A large intake of protein produces exacerbations and may even precipitate coma, while rigid protein restriction ameliorates the condition. The ammonium ion itself was at one time thought to be directly responsible, but this now appears unlikely.

Other metabolic disturbances may aggravate the situation by making the brain more susceptible to toxic influences. Acid–base imbalance, electrolyte disturbance, hypotension and anoxia may all contribute in this way. Not uncommonly acute episodes are found to have been precipitated by haemorrhage into the gastrointestinal tract, infection, injudicious sedation or the administration of a potent diuretic.

Treatment

Treatment is a matter for specialist medical supervision and is described by Sherlock and Dooley (1993). The fundamental requirement is rigid restriction of dietary protein, often coupled with oral antibiotics to decrease bacterial ammonia formation in the gut. Enemas and purgation may help. Lactulose and lactitol have proved to be beneficial, likewise the benzodiazepine antagonist flumazenil (Ferenci *et al.* 1989). Branched-chain amino acid supplements are possibly useful in patients who cannot tolerate sufficient protein in the diet to prevent a negative nitrogen balance (Horst *et al.* 1984). Bromocriptine is employed in patients with long-lasting encephalopathy who prove resistant to other measures.

Liver transplantation now offers hope to patients with end-stage liver disease. Powell *et al.* (1990) demonstrated its effectiveness in improving cognitive and neurological function in a patient with chronic progressive encephalopathy after many years of portal–systemic shunting:

A 44-year-old woman had developed splenomegaly at 19 years of age and severe bleeding from oesophageal varices 2 years later. Liver biopsy showed 'post-necrotic scarring' and portacaval anastomosis was performed. During her thirties she developed intermittent confusion and abnormal behaviour, and had several admissions with ascites, oedema and recurrent chest infections.

When seen at 44 she was unable to perform simple household duties or shop or manage her finances. Her speech, memory and gait had deteriorated progressively over the preceding 2 years. Though orientated, memory and arithmetic were poor, likewise abstracting and visuospatial ability. She was unable to write her name and address without making spelling errors. Neurological examination showed dysarthria, coarse tremor and clasp-knife rigidity in the legs. Her gait was ataxic.

After liver transplantation her cognitive and neurological status was considerably improved at 3 months, with further gains after a year. By then she was fully independent in all aspects of daily living and managed her household and finances normally. Detailed testing showed some residual deficits and dysarthria persisted, but the tremor had resolved and her gait was normal.

Nevertheless transplantation may be attended by psychosocial problems as discussed by Heyink *et al.* (1990). Of 29 patients seen at an average of 3.5 years after operation, 10 had had serious problems by way of depression and three had made suicide attempts. There had often been difficulties in coming to terms with altered status and function within the family after many years of invalidism, in adjusting to altered appearance occasioned by steroids, and in coping with worries about rejection of the organ. Six patients had difficulties in adjusting to the presence of the new liver within their bodies, feeling it to be strange or having fantasies about the donor. Such problems were generally found to be more intrusive than the physical consequences, though they mostly ameliorated with time.

Outcome

In the early stages, at least, the mental and neurological features are usually found to be reversible, including quite severe degrees of cognitive impairment. Frequently the therapeutic result is excellent. The prognosis depends principally on the extent of liver cell failure. Acute hepatitis has the worst prognosis, whereas a favourable outcome can be expected in chronic disorders with relatively good liver cell function but extensive collateral circulation. The prognosis is always better if a precipitant such as infection or haemorrhage can be identified and treated.

Cerebral pathology

In cases coming to autopsy the brain is usually normal macroscopically though it may be oedematous. The most striking histological change is diffuse proliferation and enlargement of astrocytes in the cerebrum, cerebellum, putamen and globus pallidus. The neurones themselves show relatively minor alterations.

Such a picture appears to be virtually specific for liver disease. It can develop within a few days of the onset of encephalopathy and bears an approximate relationship to the duration and severity of neuropsychiatric symptoms. In chronic cases there may be cerebral softening with cortical thinning, and neuronal degeneration is most marked in the deeper layers of the cortex (Victor *et al.* 1965).

Other psychiatric disorders with liver disease

Surveys have shown that in addition to hepatic encephalopathy, patients with liver disease are vulnerable to a range of other psychiatric disorders. Ewusi-Mensah *et al.* (1983) examined 71 patients with alcoholic liver disease and 71 with non-alcoholic liver disease, using the life-time version of the Schedule for Affective Disorders and Schizophrenia. Two-thirds of the former and one-third of the latter had, or had a history of, psychiatric illness. Depression, anxiety disorder and antisocial personality were all commoner in the alcoholics. Sarin *et al.* (1988) in a similar comparison reported psychiatric morbidity in three-quarters of alcoholics with liver disease and a quarter of non-alcoholic cirrhotics. The commonest diagnoses according to Research Diagnostic Criteria were anxiety neurosis (34%) and depression (27%). Patients with a past or present history of hepatic encephalopathy were excluded from the latter survey. Among the alcoholics no differences could be found in relation to the severity of the liver disorder, those with hepatitis scoring as highly as those with cirrhosis. No schizophrenic psychoses were seen in either series.

Trzepacz *et al.* (1989) made a prospective study of 247 consecutive candidates for liver transplantation, all with end-stage liver disease. By DSM-III criteria 17% had delirium, 20% an adjustment disorder (mainly depression), 5% major depression and 1% dementia. Nine per cent showed alcohol abuse or dependence and 2% other drug misuse. All subjects and their families scored highly in terms of stress, this centring largely on uncertainties regarding the impending transplant. Such figures underline the important role for psychiatric services in units which care for patients with liver disorder, and the need for counselling when transplantation is being considered.

Acute porphyria

The classification of the several varieties of porphyria is discussed by Kappas *et al.* (1989) and McColl *et al.* (1996). The commonest form in the UK is the Swedish or 'acute intermittent' type. This is inherited through an autosomal dominant gene on chromosome 11, resulting in a 50% reduction of porphobilinogen deaminase activity. The other major form is the South African type, 'porphyria variegata', with a similar though genetically distinct basis. The deficiency is in protoporphyrinogen oxidase activity. This can declare itself either by light-sensitive skin lesions of a bullous or erythematous nature, or in a manner similar to the acute intermittent type (see below). When in the latter form this too is occasionally seen in European countries. The third acute form is 'hereditary coproporphyria' with not dissimilar modes of presentation, due to deficiency in coproporphyrinogen oxidase activity. Other rare varieties of little relevance to psychiatry include the 'symptomatic porphyria' secondary to severe liver disease, and 'congenital erythropoietic porphyria' which is associated with skin lesions and haemolytic anaemia. All represent inherited or acquired disorders of the many different enzymes involved in haem biosynthesis.

The historical researches of Macalpine and Hunter (1966, 1969) and Macalpine *et al.* (1968) have brought special interest to the disorder. Evidence has been presented which suggests that George III's prolonged and puzzling mental illness may have been associated with porphyria, and the disease has been traced in the Royal Houses of Stuart, Hanover and Prussia back to Mary Queen of Scots. Doubt has, however, been cast on these conclusions (Levy 1970). Porphyria has also been proposed as the basis for van Gogh's illnesses (Loftus & Arnold 1991).

Clinical features of acute intermittent porphyria

The clinical features of the acute intermittent type declare themselves at any age from puberty onwards, but mostly in the third decade. Since the disease often exists in latent form a family history may not be forthcoming. Indeed with the advent of porphobilinogen deaminase determinations it is now apparent that some 90% of persons who inherit the biochemical defect remain clinically unaffected throughout their lives (Kappas *et al.* 1989). Symptoms are more common in females than males.

Attacks may take many forms which renders diagnosis difficult. Valuable reviews of the clinical features are provided by Stein and Tschudy (1970), Kappas *et al.* (1989) and McColl *et al.* (1996). Typical symptoms consist of acute abdominal pain, or pain in the chest, limbs or back, often associated with nausea, vomiting, headache and severe constipation. Epileptic fits occur in some 20% of cases, and status epilepticus may develop. Hypertension is a common accompaniment and may persist between attacks. A rapidly developing and predominantly motor peripheral neuropathy may ensue or can be the presenting feature, with weakness, diminution or loss of tendon reflexes, numbness, paraesthesiae or pain in the limbs. This can progress to severe paralysis with embarrassment of respiration. After an attack weakness or wasting may occasionally persist as an enduring disability.

Mental disorder accompanies attacks in 25–75% of cases, and psychiatric symptoms can dominate the picture. The patient becomes emotionally disturbed, sometimes acutely depressed or anxious and sometimes restless and violent. Marked emotional lability is common with histrionic, demonstrative behaviour. Clouding of consciousness and confusion may progress to delirium, with hallucinations, delusions and noisy disturbed behaviour. Coma sometimes develops abruptly. Psychotic developments may resemble schizophrenia and paranoid reactions are not uncommon.

Precipitation of attacks

The majority of attacks are precipitated by identifiable factors though some appear to arise spontaneously. The main precipitants include inadequate nutrition, endocrine factors, alcohol excess, intercurrent illnesses and infections, and a wide range of drugs.

The importance of nutrition is shown by attacks which

occur while on reducing diets, especially when these lead to precipitous loss of weight. Some unusually sensitive persons may experience attacks after missing several meals (Kappas *et al.* 1989). Endocrine influences are shown in the increased frequency of attacks at the time of the menses and their decline after the menopause. Synthetic oestrogens and progesterone are known to induce attacks. Among drugs barbiturates are notorious for the grave risk of aggravating the disorder if given in an attack to sedate the patient. Thiopentone given in the course of laparotomy may endanger life by precipitating paralysis and respiratory failure. Other drugs which may precipitate or worsen attacks include anticonvulsants (carbamazepine, phenytoin, primidone, sodium valproate and succinimides), nortriptyline, tranylcypromine, diazepam, nitrazepam, meprobamate, sulphonamides, erythromycin, ergot preparations, phenylbutazone, metoclopramide, tolbutamide, clonidine, methyldopa, chloroquine and the contraceptive pill. Those judged safe include aspirin, narcotic analgesics, penicillin, streptomycin, tetracycline, propranolol, chlorpromazine, paraldehyde, and probably chlormethiazole (Moore & Disler 1988; Kappas *et al.* 1989; McColl *et al.* 1996).

There has been much discussion of the role played by emotional disturbance in precipitating attacks. This was reviewed by Ackner *et al.* (1962) who found the evidence to be inconclusive. In their group of 12 patients, only three of the many episodes occurred at times of acute or chronic emotional stress. The patients and their relatives did not consider stress to be causally related, and detailed enquiry revealed many stresses in the past which had failed to provoke attacks.

Premorbid stability

Similar controversy surrounds the background of emotional instability which has been said to characterise porphyric patients. It has been claimed, for instance, that porphyria occurs specifically if not exclusively in patients with severe neurosis or personality disorder, and that a family history of psychiatric disorder is very common (Roth 1945).

Ackner *et al.* (1962) failed to confirm these features. The previous mental health and stability of their patients was unremarkable between attacks, and only one had a family history of mental illness. There was no strong evidence of abnormal personalities among the relatives. Ackner *et al.* suggest that the evidence for personality disorder is often confused with evidence of episodic disturbed behaviour during attacks, and that the latter is liable to add to a general impression of emotional instability. In fact it was surprising how little effect the disabling and capricious disease had had upon most of the patients in their series, despite frequent hospitalisations with mistaken labels of hysteria and personality disorder.

Investigations

The diagnosis is confirmed by the detection of excess porphobilinogen and *d*-aminolaevulinic acid in the urine and possibly also in the serum, and the demonstration of reduced porphobilinogen deaminase activity in erythrocytes. Quantitative tests are preferable to qualitative screening tests on urine samples, which should be collected without acid and refrigerated to protect them from light. Porphobilinogen is itself colourless, but may change to a red uroporphyrin after standing, acidification or heating. Freshly voided urine may therefore be colourless, or pale pink varying to deep mahogany depending on conditions at the time.

The absence of raised porphobilinogen and *d*-aminolaevulinic acid in the urine does not exclude the diagnosis, since some patients fail to hyperexcrete; conversely low porphobilinogen deaminase activity does not entirely confirm that the attack was a manifestation of the disease because many gene carriers are asymptomatic. The correct diagnosis thus depends on both sets of estimations coupled with knowledge of the clinical history. Caution is also required on account of the false positive results that can occur in the urine with certain febrile illnesses, in lead poisoning and in patients receiving phenothiazine drugs (Reio & Wetterberg 1969).

In the South African variety and in coproporphyria, examination of the stools is more reliable than the urine, excess porphyrins producing a brilliant pink fluorescence in extracts under ultraviolet light.

In the acute intermittent variety there is a tendency for the porphyrin metabolites to reach a peak during exacerbations of the disorder and to decrease to low or negligible levels between attacks. This, however, is by no means invariable and persistently elevated levels may occur. Ackner *et al.* (1961, 1962) failed to find a clear relationship between the levels of porphobilinogen and *d*-aminolaevulinic acid in the urine and the presence or absence of symptoms. The excretion of the two compounds fluctuated considerably over time, sometimes with quite high levels in symptomless cases and sometimes with no marked increase in output during mild attacks.

The widespread belief that there is a necessary association between increased excretion and acute attacks therefore appears to be erroneous. It may have arisen because the chance production of coloured urine is quite often the first pointer to the diagnosis in patients who have suffered from unexplained symptoms for a considerable time. In any case a coloured urine should not necessarily be expected in acute attacks, since the colour depends on physical characteristics of the urine and does not reflect the levels of excretion.

The EEG often shows abnormalities during attacks, with slowing of dominant frequencies and an excess of intermediate slow activity. Sometimes, however, it remains entirely normal. Isolated records are therefore of little help in the diagnosis, but serial recordings can occasionally be useful in confirming the organic origin of symptoms in attacks of uncertain nature.

Differential diagnosis

Porphyria is notorious for leading to mistakes in diagnosis, and patients are sometimes admitted repeatedly to psychiatric units before the condition is discovered.

An impression of psychiatric illness is reinforced by the patient's emotional instability during attacks, and the long history of intermittent physical complaints for which no cause has previously emerged. Diagnoses of personality disorder or severe neurosis are commonly made. Hysteria may be suspected when the patient complains of weakness of the limbs and varied aches and pains unbacked by physical signs. Psychotic developments may likewise obscure other aspects of the disorder and lead to a primary diagnosis of depressive illness or acute schizophrenia.

Other patients are admitted to general medical wards with suspected appendicitis on account of abdominal pain and vomiting. Intestinal obstruction may be diagnosed when there is severe constipation. Laparotomy therefore features in the history of many porphyric patients. Other cases may be mistaken for the acute ascending polyneuropathy of Guillain–Barré, or the combination of fits and hypertension may suggest hypertensive encephalopathy.

Treatment and outcome

The chief aim must be prevention of attacks by educating the patient about adequate nutritional intake and the drugs which must be avoided. Abstention from alcohol should be advised. Any infection which arises must be treated immediately. On occasion the onset of an attack can be aborted by increasing carbohydrate intake.

The symptomatic treatment of the acute attack is described by Kappas *et al.* (1989) and McColl *et al.* (1996). Vomiting may be controlled with phenothiazines, and pain with dihydrocodeine or if necessary pethidine or morphine. The drugs of choice for emotional disturbance are chlorpromazine, promazine or trifluoperazine. Epileptic seizures are perhaps best treated with chlormethiazole, though most will settle spontaneously as the attack resolves. Barbiturates must be avoided under all circumstances.

Intravenous haematin is now used increasingly and appears to be effective in curtailing attacks. Adequate intake of carbohydrate should always be ensured, if necessary by giving dextrose intravenously. Electrolyte imbalance may need attention, especially lowering of the serum sodium in the face of persistent vomiting. It is known that inappropriate secretion of antidiuretic hormone is liable to accompany attacks. A careful watch must also be kept for threatened respiratory embarrassment. Tracheotomy and assisted respiration may occasionally be needed in the more severe attacks.

The duration of attacks varies widely from a few days to several months. The majority subside completely without enduring defects. Some patients, however, are left severely crippled with weakness or muscular wasting, and some remain psychotic for long periods of time. Ultimately there is usually full physical and mental recovery.

Chapter 12: Vitamin Deficiencies

Severe chronic malnutrition is accompanied by well-known psychological changes—apathy, emotional lability, retardation, impairment of memory and sometimes acute psychotic illness. Such manifestations have been described in prisoners of war by Helweg-Larsen *et al.* (1952). During periods of famine interest becomes focused on food alone and cultural and social inhibitions are prone to disappear.

In adults all such effects usually prove to be reversible when the deprivation is relieved, though in long-term follow-ups of prisoners of war persistent states of fatigue, depression and lability of affect have been well described (Thygesen *et al.* 1970). A small proportion also appear to be vulnerable to the later development of spinal cord lesions and parkinsonism (Gibberd & Simmonds 1980). Persistent impairments of memory and concentration have sometimes been ascribed to brain damage occasioned by the severe starvation, with impressions that cerebral atrophy and premature dementia may occasionally supervene (Thygesen *et al.* 1970).

In infants and young children, by contrast, there is firmer evidence that starvation is liable to damage the brain. Winick (1976, 1979) reviews the evidence that early malnutrition can retard brain growth substantially with curtailment of cell division, myelination and the arborization of dendrites. All brain regions appear to be vulnerable. Enduring effects on intellectual development are therefore probable, especially when the malnutrition has dated from the early months of life. Definitive evidence is obviously hard to obtain in human subjects, but studies of children suffering from severe protein malnutrition (kwashiorkor) have suggested that they fail to reach their intellectual potential. Champakam *et al.* (1968) and Gopalan (1970) reported a 7–8-year follow-up of 19 such children, first seen and treated when 18 months to 3 years old; on psychometric testing they found marked impairments, especially with regard to perceptual and abstracting abilities in comparison to carefully matched controls. In a similar follow-up of 32 such children Mehta *et al.* (1975) showed that their IQs were impaired in proportion to the severity of the malnutrition when hospitalised; there was no correlation between the children's IQ and that of their mothers, suggesting that the previous malnutrition had been responsible rather than genetic influences.

Under normal circumstances malnutrition of this degree is rarely encountered in Western societies. But even in populations where the general standard of nutrition is high there are persons prone to inadequate or imbalanced intake of food who may present with vitamin depletion. The mentally retarded and the chronically mentally sick often live precariously in the community and vitamin deficiencies may add to their symptomatology. The aged population is similarly at risk, especially when depression or early dementia impair standards of self care. Alcoholics face the multiple hazards of inadequate intake, poor absorption and special demands made on vitamin reserves for the metabolism of alcohol. These are all groups of persons who are particularly liable to come before psychiatric attention. Patients with chronic gastrointestinal disease and malabsorption are another group at risk, while any physical illness may deplete reserves. Profound deficiencies may be revealed postoperatively, especially in patients maintained for a considerable time on intravenous fluids.

Of all the vitamins it is the members of the B complex, and particularly thiamine and nicotinic acid, which have proved to be of most importance in psychiatric practice. Other deficiencies will often coexist in chronic malnutrition, but specific roles for vitamins A, C and D have not been clearly identified in relation to mental disorder. Vitamin B_{12} and folic acid have been increasingly studied in relation to psychiatric illness and this evidence will also be reviewed.

Vitamin B deficiency

Laboratory studies provide a firm basis for expecting functional and pathological changes in the central nervous system as a result of vitamin B deprivation. Many components of the B complex are known to play an essential role in metabolic processes within the brain: thiamine pyrophosphate (TPP) is a coenzyme involved in carbohydrate metabolism, particularly the oxidation of pyruvate, and may also be necessary for the proper transmission of nerve impulses; nicotinic acid and its amide act as constituent parts of coenzymes which are necessary for glucose metabolism; riboflavine acts similarly; pantothenic acid is concerned with the formation of acetylcholine; and pyridoxine becomes converted into pyridoxal phosphate which is a coenzyme fundamental to several enzyme systems concerned in brain metabolic processes.

It was not until the 1930s that the full significance of vitamin B deficiency in relation to psychiatric disorder began to be appreciated, although mental disorder had been recognised as an integral part of the syndrome of pellagra from its earliest descriptions. In the 1930s, however, the various constituents of the B complex were identified, and careful observation soon extended awareness of their functions. Experimental studies showed that deprivation could lead to psychological symptoms well before definitive manifestations were declared in other systems of the body. Acute and severe depletion of vitamin reserves also proved to be responsible for fulminating neuropsychiatric disorders which had not previously been thought to be nutritional in origin.

The wide natural dispersion of the B vitamins has made it difficult to work out precise relationships in naturally occurring disorders, and multiple deficiencies will often operate together. Sometimes, however, the evidence linking specific deficiencies to specific clinical pictures has been clarified by noting the therapeutic response to vitamins given singly. Thiamine and nicotinic acid have emerged as the vitamins of greatest importance in neuropsychiatric disorders, with others such as pyridoxine, pantothenic acid and riboflavine contributing mainly to ancillary symptoms. Moreover with both thiamine and nicotinic acid it is clear that different syndromes of deficiency can follow, depending on the severity of depletion and the time over which it has operated.

Thiamine (B₁) deficiency classically leads to beriberi, with neuropathy, cardiac failure or peripheral oedema. This is the picture that results from chronic depletion of fairly severe degree. Over shorter time spans a neurasthenic picture may result, with fatigue, weakness and emotional disturbance, well before these physical features have been declared. Acute and fulminating depletion can lead instead to the picture of Wernicke's encephalopathy (p. 575), usually when overwhelming demands have been made on reserves which are already low. The changes in Wernicke's encephalopathy may be confined to the central nervous system, and other evidence of vitamin lack may be entirely absent.

Nicotinic acid (niacin) deficiency shows a similar range of disorders. Subacute deficiency produces the syndrome of pellagra (p. 573) with gastrointestinal symptoms, skin lesions and psychiatric disturbance. In the early stages, however, a neurasthenic picture may be seen in relative isolation. Acute and sudden depletion may again lead to a picture of 'encephalopathy' (p. 574), sometimes with little or nothing in other systems to provide the clue to vitamin deficiency.

Pyridoxine (B₆) deficiency can lead to convulsions in infants, either in those on deficient diets or in those with unusually high requirements. Pronounced abnormalities appear in the EEG and mental deterioration may ensue. Both the symptoms and the electroencephalographic changes may resolve within minutes of injection of the vitamin. Lack of pyridoxine may also contribute to the neuropathy seen with severe malnutrition. Experimental deficiency in adults, or the feeding of pyridoxine antagonists, has been found to lead to irritability, confusion and lethargy (Fabrykant 1960). More recently, with the availability of sensitive and reliable assays, pyridoxine deficiency has been suspected of playing a part in contributing to depressive illness (Carney *et al.* 1979, 1982). Among patients admitted to a psychiatric unit deficiencies of pyridoxine, and perhaps of riboflavine, have emerged in a higher proportion of those with affective disorder than with other psychiatric conditions. Pyridoxine deficiency has also been incriminated as the mechanism leading to depression in patients taking oral contraceptives; in such a context pyridoxine replacement was shown to be effective in relieving the depression in a double-blind cross-over trial (Adams *et al.* 1973).

Riboflavine (B₂) deficiency produces glossitis, angular stomatitis, lachrymation and photophobia. It may also cause a normochromic, normocytic anaemia. In an experimental study of severe and specific riboflavine restriction in healthy volunteers, Sterner and Price (1973) found weakened hand grip on dynamometer tests after several weeks, and 'personality changes' as reflected in scores on the Minnesota Multiphasic Personality Inventory (MMPI). Changes in the hypochondriasis, depression and hysteria scores appeared to reflect increasing lethargy, hypersensitivity and a multitude of minor somatic complaints.

Pantothenic acid deficiency has been incriminated in leading to sensory neuropathy and the 'burning feet syndrome'. However, as in the case of riboflavine, a role in naturally occurring neurological or psychiatric disorder has not yet been clearly established.

It is important to note that various aspects of vitamin B

deficiency may prove to be commoner than expected among a wide range of psychiatric patients (Carney *et al.* 1979, 1982). Among 172 successive admissions to a psychiatric unit, 30% were considered to be deficient in thiamine, 27% in riboflavine and 9% in pyridoxine as assessed by red cell enzyme functions (see below). More than half were deficient in at least one of the three, despite being drawn from a reasonably affluent community. Thiamine deficiency was mainly encountered in patients who could be expected to have neglected their diets — alcoholics, drug addicts, schizophrenics and depressives. Those with pyridoxine deficiency, by contrast, often showed little evidence of malnutrition, and as mentioned above there was a significant association with depressive illness. Controlled studies will be required to determine whether such vitamin deficiencies may sometimes play an aetiological role in the genesis of depressive disorder, or indeed in contributing more widely to psychiatric morbidity.

In clinical practice, thiamine deficiency can be investigated by means of the pyruvate tolerance test. The fasting pyruvate level may be raised or normal, but after glucose administration it rises excessively. However, the test is of limited value since pyruvate metabolism may be blocked in a number of other conditions—thyrotoxicosis, pyrexia, congestive cardiac failure, anoxia and various intoxications (Thompson 1967). Whole blood thiamine estimations can be performed by microbiological methods, but the measurement of red cell transketolase is a simpler and perhaps more reliable procedure (Williams 1976). Moreover, the red cell enzyme activity can be measured with and without the presence of added thiamine *in vitro*, providing an indication of the extent to which bodily stores have been chronically depleted. Equivalent assessments of other vitamin-dependent red cell enzymes can reveal riboflavine deficiency (glutathione reductase) or pyridoxine deficiency (aspartate aminotransferase).

Experimental studies of vitamin B deficiency

Volunteer subjects have been kept on diets deficient in B vitamins, with the object of determining the earliest clinical features of deprivation. The findings are in broad agreement from one study to another, particularly in emphasising the prominence of mental symptoms. Jolliffe *et al.* (1939) observed anorexia, lassitude, precordial pain, palpitations, dyspnoea and muscle cramps, but were unable to induce the neuritic symptoms of beriberi. Elsom *et al.* (1940) observed a marked psychological disturbance in one subject who became depressed and irritable, wept frequently without cause and withdrew from social contacts. Defective memory and difficulty with concentration

were prominent complaints. This was considered to represent more than a simple reaction to physical malaise, and to reflect a true change in cerebral functioning. Riboflavine was without effect on the symptoms, thiamine caused partial improvement, but full relief was only obtained on giving yeast containing all components of the B complex. O'Shea *et al.* (1942) in a similar experiment found measurable cognitive impairment on Porteus Maze scores which was relieved by thiamine and by yeast.

Williams *et al.* (1940, 1943) carried out a series of experiments with a diet severely deficient in thiamine but considered to contain adequate amounts of other vitamins. After several weeks all subjects developed neurasthenic symptoms — generalised weakness, depression, anorexia and insomnia. A few developed apathy, forgetfulness and difficulty with thinking, while others reported giddiness, paraesthesiae and soreness of muscles. Physical activity was greatly decreased and capacity for work fell progressively. Less severe but more prolonged deficiency led to emotional instability with moodiness, quarrelsomeness, depression and numerous somatic complaints. The patients were made to serve as their own controls during periods with and without thiamine replacement, and a valid relationship between mental symptoms and thiamine deficiency appeared to be upheld.

Brozek and Caster (1957) confirmed such psychological effects by more precise dietary techniques for producing severe thiamine depletion. General weakness and extreme anorexia were associated with marked irritability and depression, and scores on the hysteria, hypochondriasis and depression scales on the MMPI deteriorated considerably. Continuation of the diet led ultimately to peripheral neuropathy. Tests of manual speed, coordination and reaction time were impaired, but general intelligence was unaffected. The reintroduction of thiamine restored appetite promptly and produced a dramatic change in the attitude of the subjects, but the peripheral neuropathy was slower to improve.

Kreisler *et al.*'s (1948) study appears to be unique in attempting to evaluate the effects of induced vitamin B deficiency in patients already mentally ill. This was a prolonged experiment with chronically hospitalised schizophrenic and demented patients. The observations were largely impressionistic, but indicated both aggravation of pre-existing psychotic disorder and the development of new mental changes. Moderate restriction over 1–2 years was associated with gradual diminution of activity, dulling of affect and loss of interests. Severe restriction sometimes led to the explosive onset of serious emotional disturbances with loss of inhibitory control, exaggeration of pre-existing hypomanic or depressive features, and the emergence of paranoid trends. Recovery on giving yeast extract containing the full range of B vitamins was said to be often dramatic and sudden. Clearly these interesting findings would require confirmation by properly controlled investigation, though the ethical problems raised would probably be insurmountable.

Mental changes in pellagra

Multiple vitamin deficiencies are probably operative in pellagra, but lack of nicotinic acid is by far the most important and its administration can rapidly relieve the symptoms. The characteristic triad includes gastrointestinal disorder, skin lesions and psychiatric disturbance. Gastrointestinal disturbances include anorexia and diarrhoea. Skin changes include roughening and reddening of the dorsum of the hands and pigmentation over bony prominences. Stomatitis and glossitis are also often seen.

The prodromal features are similar to those encountered in experimental thiamine deficiency. General deterioration of mental and physical health may antedate more definite manifestations by weeks or months, and indeed pellagra was sometimes thought to be a neurotic disorder before its relationship to vitamin deficiency was discovered. Most prominent is a subjective feeling of incapacity for mental and physical effort, coupled with a multiplicity of other vague complaints—anorexia, insomnia, nervousness, apprehension, dizziness, headache, palpitations and paraesthesiae. Characteristically these fluctuate markedly from one day to the next. Irritability and emotional instability may dominate the picture. Depression can be severe with considerable risk of suicide. At a later stage the mental processes are obviously retarded, memory is faulty and confabulation may appear.

Such changes are well known in areas where pellagra is endemic, and the patients themselves often recognise them as prodromata of the more florid manifestations of the disease. They are likely to be misconstrued, however, when sporadic cases arise. Spies et al. (1938) made careful observations on patients attending a pellagra clinic who had recurrences each spring over a number of years, and were able to confirm the prompt response of such 'neurotic' symptoms to nicotinic acid. Discontinuation of treatment without the patients' knowledge caused recurrence of the complaints. Thiamine by contrast helped peripheral neuritis when this was present, but not the subjective complaints and emotional disturbances.

Longer-continued and more severe nicotinic acid deficiency leads to the florid psychiatric manifestations of pellagra. These sometimes develop without the above prodromata. They are often associated with gastrointestinal and skin changes but may nonetheless dominate the picture. The commonest is an acute organic reaction with disorientation, confusion and impairment of memory. Wild excitement and outbursts of violent behaviour may occur, depression is often conspicuous, or paranoia may develop with hallucinations and delusions of persecution. Occasionally chronic untreated pellagra may progress with a picture akin to Korsakoff's syndrome, or as a slowly increasing generalised dementia.

The acute psychotic pictures again respond to nicotinic acid, often in a dramatic fashion. Calm and rational behaviour may be restored within hours of vitamin replacement, or more commonly over the course of several days. It is very rare indeed for treatment to fail in acute cases, though with chronic mental disablement less success can be expected (Spies et al. 1938; McLester 1943). Neurological disturbances are usually a late development, showing as tremor, ataxia and sometimes dysarthria and dysphagia. A sensorimotor peripheral neuropathy is common with paraethesiae, pain and tenderness, chiefly in the distal leg muscles.

The early symptoms of pellagra presumably depend on reversible biochemical changes within the neurones, but these can ultimately lead to structural changes. In established pellagra the pathognomonic finding is central chromatolysis ('retrograde cell degeneration') in the Betz cells of the motor cortex, usually also involving cells of the pontine, dorsal vagal, gracile and cuneate nuclei (Leigh 1952). The nuclei of the affected neurones are displaced to the periphery and the Nissl bodies disappear from the centres. Other brain stem neurones may be involved, likewise the anterior horn cells of the cord. The Purkinje cells of the cerebellum are by contrast spared. Degeneration of the posterior and lateral columns of the spinal cord is sometimes a prominent feature (Spillane 1947).

Hartnup disease

This rare inborn error of metabolism results in nicotinic acid deficiency despite a normal dietary intake, due to reduced availability of its precursor, tryptophan. Pellagra-like features occur as episodic attacks during childhood, then tend to subside during adult life. Increased renal clearance of neutral amino acids, including tryptophan, is accompanied by defective absorption of tryptophan from the gut. The abnormal amino aciduria is the most constant diagnostic feature; indoles also appear in the stools and urine, derived from the action of the intestinal flora on unabsorbed tryptophan (Brenton 1996).

Some cases are asymptomatic and discovered only on routine screening. Other patients present with a photosensitive skin rash, often accompanied by psychiatric disturbance, cerebellar ataxia or other neurological abnormalities. Oral nicotinamide helps substantially during attacks, though these tend to subside spontaneously.

Psychiatric features range from emotional lability in the milder cases to apathy, irritability, depression, confusion and delirium in the more marked examples (Hersov & Rodnight 1960). The coexistent photosensitive skin rash is an important clue to the underlying biochemical abnormality.

Acute nicotinic acid deficiency encephalopathy

This syndrome gained recognition as a result of a series of reports of patients who presented with various forms of acute organic reaction, and proved to show an excellent response to large doses of nicotinic acid (Cleckley et al. 1939; Jolliffe et al. 1940; Sydenstricker 1943; Gottlieb 1944). Since that time it seems largely to have disappeared from the British and American literature, though there is evidence, discussed below, that examples are still quite frequent in countries where nicotinic acid is not given routinely as part of parenteral multivitamin therapy.

Nicotinic acid was initially tried empirically because some of the patients had shown glossitis, but other evidence of vitamin depletion was not invariably present. A great number were chronic alcoholics, and others were the elderly infirm who had been living alone on inadequate diets. A third important group were patients without a clear history of dietary deficiency, who developed the disorder in the course of acute physical illness or after surgical operations or delivery.

The picture was of stupor or delirium, often catastrophic in development and carrying a high mortality. Weakness and lethargy were common but anxiety and agitation could be marked. A noteworthy feature was the development of extrapyramidal disturbance, with cogwheel rigidity and often grasping and sucking reflexes. Glossitis or stomatitis were frequently but not always present. In some patients the neuropsychiatric picture was the sole manifestation.

Cleckley et al.'s (1939) patients all had a history of malnutrition. The majority were elderly and suffering from other organic diseases which might easily have been considered an adequate cause for the mental symptoms. More than half had advanced arteriosclerosis. Nicotinic acid was found to produce a striking and dramatic improvement, and was felt to be life saving in many cases:

A man of 78 was admitted to hospital after several weeks of increasing weakness and lethargy. For 8 days he had been bedfast and stuporose. He was found to be mildly delirious with a slight pyrexia, and showed marked hypertension, advanced arteriosclerosis and right-sided heart failure. The tongue was dry, bright red and atrophic. A liquid high-vitamin diet with intravenous dextrose and digitalis had no effect on his mental state. Sodium nicotinate was commenced, 100 mg intravenously, and on the second day he became alert and attentive. By the fourth day the mental state had returned to normal and all signs of glossitis had disappeared. He remained well until he died of a cerebral haemorrhage 3 months later.

Jolliffe et al. (1940) were able to report 150 cases from Bellevue Hospital, New York. All were alcoholics who had been admitted with severe impairment of consciousness or delirium. Half showed stomatitis or other evidence of a partial pellagrinous state. Some had evidence of scurvy, polyneuritis or oculomotor disturbance as in Wernicke's encephalopathy but this was by no means invariable. Cogwheel rigidity of the limbs was a marked part of the picture in many cases. Thiamine was without effect, but nicotinic acid in large dosage produced recovery usually in 3–5 days. Mortality was drastically reduced by such treatment, from 90% to 14%. Those who survived were often left with memory deficits. The syndrome was ascribed to a marked depletion of nicotinic acid, developing acutely in patients already partially depleted but before classic pellagrinous manifestations had become established.

Sydenstricker (1943) referred to analogous cases seen in general hospitals, often postoperatively or after delivery, or when fever and infection had suddenly imposed increased metabolic demands. Some had been suffering from gastrointestinal diseases and some had been maintained for several days on intravenous fluids. After a short period of confusion the patients developed acute delirium with excitement and hallucinations. The tongue was often dry and red, but there were sometimes no physical signs whatever of vitamin deficiency. The response to nicotinic acid or nicotinamide was again rapid. These cases were considered to represent the most severe and acute examples of nicotinic acid deficiency, when sudden metabolic demands had exhausted scanty reserves.

Gottlieb (1944) confirmed these findings and added further cases seen in alcoholics, in the elderly malnourished and postoperatively:

A woman of 56 was admitted in alcoholic coma and resuscitated. Three days later she became confused, restless and irrational, and deteriorated over the next 3 days with noisy behaviour and gross disorientation. Apart from nystagmus there was no physical abnormality. Nicotinic acid produced dramatic improvement within 24 hours and she remained well thereafter.

A woman of 62 was admitted with confusion, disorientation and incontinence of urine. Her memory had been failing for 2 weeks. Her tongue had been sore for 10 days and the angles of her mouth had been cracked for some 3 months. There was no history of alcoholism but she had been neglecting her food since the death of her son 1 year earlier. She was given oral thiamine and nicotinic acid for 10 days without improvement, but then responded rapidly to nicotinic acid given intramuscularly.

A patient reported by Slater (1942) is important because evidence of organic brain dysfunction was minimal:

A man of 52 was admitted with complaints of numbness in the legs but there was no evidence of peripheral neuritis on examination. In hospital he became acutely psychotic, believing he was to be punished for his sins and that there was a spirit under the counterpane. He showed flexibilitas cerea and echopraxia, and the picture resembled schizophrenia closely. He remained fully orientated and without intellectual impairment, but a clue to the organic nature of the psychosis was provided by marked perseveration and some dysarthria. He deteriorated physically, with abdominal distension, diarrhoea and the development of a raw red tongue. Dramatic improvement followed the administration of nicotinic acid and ascorbic acid, with resolution of the psychotic illness. Prior to the illness he had had a period of prolonged malnourishment on account of a gastroenterostomy and subsequent gastrectomy.

It is interesting that reports of the syndrome are now so rare. Its apparent demise in the UK and North America is possibly because nowadays high potency vitamin therapy almost invariably consists of multiple vitamin replacement (Lishman 1981). This became established as a routine from the 1950s onwards. Parentrovite injections in the UK (more recently Pabrinex), and Solu-B or Bejectal in the USA, contain ample nicotinamide in addition to thiamine. In the treatment of alcoholics and other depleted patients the syndrome may therefore be concealed.

It appears, nonetheless, to be still evident in other countries. M.S. Kayatekin (personal communication, 1981) observed three patients in Turkey with severe and prolonged confusion in the wake of delirium tremens which cleared promptly on giving nicotinic acid. Treatment with parenteral thiamine, riboflavine and pyridoxine had been without effect. Ishii and Nishihara (1981) have produced clear evidence that the syndrome persists in Japan. They discovered the classic brain changes of pellagra in 20 of 74 necropsies on alcoholics. The condition had gone unsuspected during life, presumably because most of the patients lacked skin lesions indicative of pellagra:

These patients had presented in a surprisingly uniform fashion. They had been hospitalised with a diagnosis of delirium tremens, then went on to develop extrapyramidal rigidity, hyperreflexia, gait disturbance and double incontinence. Gastrointestinal symptoms appeared in the form of diarrhoea, constipation or vomiting. Progressive deterioration led to death within a few weeks or months. The mental accompaniments were variable, including confusion, hallucinations, delirium, anxiety, depression, excitement and neurasthenia. Several patients had

polyneuropathy but only one had shown signs of Wernicke's encephalopathy. Glossitis was a fairly common feature. Treatment with thiamine, pyridoxine and vitamin B_{12} had been ineffective. Nicotinic acid or nicotinamide had not been given.

Ishii and Nishihara suggest that when an alcoholic patient develops neurological signs, particularly extrapyramidal rigidity, in addition to mental and gastrointestinal symptoms, nicotinic acid deficiency must be strongly suspected even in the absence of skin lesions. Gait disturbance, incontinence and hyperreflexia are further important features differentiating the syndrome from uncomplicated delirium tremens. In many cases it may be expected that thiamine deficiency will be operative in addition; however, only two of Ishii and Nishihara's 20 patients showed the pathology of Wernicke's encephalopathy in addition to that of pellagra.

More recently 22 cases have been reported among alcoholics from France (Hauw *et al.* 1988; Serdaru *et al.* 1988). Neurological features included marked oppositional hypertonus ('gegenhalten') and myoclonus along with confusion and clouding of consciousness. At autopsy chromatolysis was observed in neurones of the brain stem and cerebellar dentate nuclei, typical in all respects of nicotinic acid deficiency. During the same period 111 cases of Wernicke's encephalopathy had been identified at autopsy. Thiamine and pyridoxine had been given without niacin and sometimes appeared to aggravate the neurological state. Typical cases were as follows:

A 52-year-old man was admitted because of weakness and weight loss. He was given thiamine and pyridoxine because of his drinking habits, and thereafter developed confusion and hypertonus. Three weeks later he showed marked oppositional hypertonus and startle myoclonus of the limbs and face. The tendon reflexes were brisk and the right plantar reflex extensor. The EEG showed diffuse slow activity. His level of consciousness deteriorated and he died from aspiration pneumonia a few days later.

A 52-year-old man was admitted because of rapidly evolving ataxia of gait. Two days later he developed delirium tremens. Rehydration and the administration of thiamine and pyridoxine produced some improvement, but 5 weeks later he deteriorated despite continued parenteral vitamin therapy. The mental state fluctuated, along with marked oppositional hypertonus and irregular asynchronous myoclonus. There were bilateral grasp reflexes. He deteriorated over the ensuing weeks with swallowing disturbances, dysarthria, weight loss and ultimately coma, dying from aspiration pneumonia.

Wernicke's encephalopathy

Wernicke's encephalopathy represents the acute neuropsychiatric reaction to severe thiamine deficiency. It may be defined as a disorder of acute onset characterised by nystagmus, abducens and conjugate gaze palsies, ataxia of gait, and a global confusional state, occurring together or in various combinations (Victor *et al.* 1971). Wernicke first described the condition in 1881 under the title of 'polioencephalitis haemorrhagica superior', reporting two cases in chronic alcoholics and one in a patient with persistent vomiting after sulphuric acid poisoning. Initially it was ascribed to an inflammatory process in the central nervous system, but abundant evidence has since accumulated to show the role of thiamine deficiency. Alexander (1940) was able to demonstrate lesions in the brains of thiamine-deficient pigeons which were similar in distribution and type to those of Wernicke's encephalopathy, and Jolliffe *et al.* (1941) clearly established the efficacy of thiamine in relieving the ophthalmoplegias and in improving clouding of consciousness in human subjects. Nicotinic acid, by contrast, failed to do so. The precise relationship of Wernicke's encephalopathy to alcoholism, to beriberi and to Korsakoff's psychosis remained, however, to be clarified.

Wernicke's encephalopathy and alcoholism

Alcoholism is an important but not an exclusive cause of the disorder. It leads to thiamine deficiency by several routes — the replacement of vitamin-containing foods by alcohol, impaired absorption of thiamine from the gut, impairment of storage by the liver, decreased phosphorylation to thiamine pyrophosphate (TPP), and excessive requirements for the metabolism of alcohol. Among alcoholics partial gastrectomy appears to be a significant additional risk factor (Price & Kerr 1985). However, Wernicke's encephalopathy is known to occur in a number of other conditions all closely connected with thiamine deficiency. Campbell and Russell (1941) could find a definite history of alcoholism in only five of 21 cases, and Spillane (1947) listed the following additional causes in his review of the literature — carcinoma of the stomach, pregnancy, toxaemia, pernicious anaemia, vomiting, diarrhoea and dietary deficiency. Very occasionally the condition has developed in association with anorexia nervosa (Ebels 1978; Handler & Perkin 1982), and it has been reported after a self-imposed 'hunger strike' in a paranoid patient (Pentland & Mawdsley 1982). Other causes have included prolonged intravenous feeding, renal dialysis, hyperemesis gravidarum (Bergin & Harvey 1992) and severe malnutrition in a chronic schizophrenic patient (Spittle & Parker 1993). In a patient reported by Schmidtke (1993) alcoholism was compounded by cerebral anoxia following attempted suicide by hanging.

Rimalovski and Aronson (1966) reported a large autopsy series and found that unequivocal evidence of alcoholism had been recorded in only 50% of patients. In most of the remainder the cause appeared to be carcinoma, especially of the oesophagus, or widespread tuberculosis. Lindboe and Løberg (1989) found that almost a quarter of their autopsy cases were non-alcoholics, this rising to 40% in active acute cases. Most of the non-alcoholic patients had suffered from severe cachexia due to a variety of underlying diseases. Nevertheless in the largest series reported from the USA, Victor *et al.* (1971) found that all but two of their 245 cases were suffering from established alcoholism. They therefore still regarded Wernicke's encephalopathy as essentially a disease of alcoholics, at least in American urban society.

It seems, however, that not all alcoholics are equally at risk, for reasons that remain to be fully explored. Many neglect their diets severely without developing an overt encephalopathy, whereas others may do so quite early in their alcoholic careers. A young alcoholic was reported by Turner *et al.* (1989) who presented with Wernicke's encephalopathy at the age of 18. Even from place to place the prevalence of the Wernicke–Korsakoff syndrome appears to be remarkably uneven. First admissions to hospital with the condition have ranged from 65 per million population in Queensland, Australia, to 8 per million in New York. And at autopsy it has emerged in 2.8% of persons in Western Australia, 2.2% in Cleveland, Ohio, 1.7% in New York, 0.8% in Oslo and 0.4% in France (Harper *et al.* 1989, 1995). No obvious correlations can be discerned with the per capita consumptions of alcohol in these different countries. Numerous factors are likely to be involved — the beverage consumed, its thiamine content, patterns of drinking and patterns of dietary neglect.

There may, however, be an important additional factor by way of personal susceptibility. Thiamine is important in relation to several key enzyme systems of the body and brain. It is first phosphorylated to TPP which acts as a coenzyme, i.e. combines with proteins to form the effective enzyme system. This applies to enzymes such as transketolase which is essential for the maintenance and synthesis of myelin, and to the pyruvate dehydrogenase complex and the alpha ketoglutarate dehydrogenase complex, both of which play key roles in brain glucose metabolism and energy production (Langlais 1995).

The question therefore arises whether persons vulnerable to thiamine deficiency could have an *inborn abnormality* by way of reduced affinity between TPP and the enzymes with which it must combine. Kaczmarek and Nixon (1983) and Pratt *et al.* (1985) have shown that transketolase is heterogeneous, existing as a number of 'isoenzyme variants', some differing in their affinity for TPP (Greenwood *et al.* 1984). Certain variants have seemed to be specific to Korsakoff patients (Blass & Gibson 1977; Nixon 1984). It has been difficult, however, to exclude the possibility that such variants are the product of damage to the enzyme system rather than genetically transmitted defects. Nevertheless Mukherjee *et al.* (1987) have presented some preliminary evidence which favours genetic transmission of reduced binding between TPP and transketolase in certain families.

Other enzymes which depend on TPP for their proper functioning appear to have been little explored in relation to the syndrome. Pyruvate dehydrogenase and alpha ketoglutarate dehydrogenase are just as essential as transketolase to brain cell survival, and all three have been shown to be greatly reduced in samples from the cerebellar vermis in Wernicke–Korsakoff patients (Butterworth *et al.* 1993). Reductions in alpha ketoglutarate dehydrogenase were particularly severe, and Butterworth *et al.* suggest that this could be the trigger for a series of metabolic events which culminate in neuronal death.

Wernicke's encephalopathy and beriberi

The relationship with beriberi proved more of an embarrassment, since the classic neuritic and cardiac forms of the disease seemed rarely to be associated with encephalopathy despite their dependence on thiamine deficiency. During the Second World War, however, experience in prisoner of war camps gave ample opportunity for observing relatively acute deficiency syndromes in large numbers of subjects. In epidemics of beriberi psychological changes were often found to be prominent, with irritability, depression and disturbance of memory (Cruickshank 1961). More particularly, De Wardener and Lennox (1947) were able to report 52 typical cases of Wernicke's encephalopathy from a prisoner of war camp in Singapore, most of whom at the same time showed neuritic, cardiac or oedematous signs of beriberi. Their classic paper was based on records which spent 2 years of the war buried in a Siamese cemetery; it was entitled 'Cerebral beriberi (Wernicke's encephalopathy)', and effectively bridged the gap between the two conditions.

Response to thiamine was in general excellent in this series. Gross examination of the brains in fatal cases confirmed pathological changes in the distribution typical of Wernicke's encephalopathy. The authors proposed that the encephalopathy appeared when particularly acute and severe thiamine depletion was superimposed upon partial deficiency, whereas other forms of beriberi generally resulted from less severe and more prolonged lack of the vitamin. In almost all of their cases the encephalopathy had set in when some other factor, such as epidemic diarrhoea, had intensified the vitamin deficiency. The situation was thus analogous to that seen with nicotinic acid, where severe acute depletion produces profound evidence of cerebral dysfunction and more chronic deficiency leads to the orthodox syndrome of pellagra.

Wernicke's encephalopathy and Korsakoff's syndrome

The relationship between Wernicke's encephalopathy and Korsakoff's syndrome has also gradually been clarified. Korsakoff gave the first comprehensive account of the amnesic syndrome that bears his name in 1887, shortly after Wernicke's description of his syndrome, but the close relationship between the two was not appreciated at the time.

All of Korsakoff's cases had polyneuritis which led him to propose the name 'psychosis polyneuritica'. The great majority of cases were reported in alcoholics and the cause was thought to be some toxic effect of alcohol. Shortly thereafter cases were reported without alcoholism or neuropathy in patients suffering from puerperal sepsis, typhoid or intestinal obstruction. By the 1930s other known causes included gastric carcinoma, intractable vomiting and severe dietary deficiency. Thiamine deficiency therefore came under suspicion as the common metabolic link. Bowman *et al.* (1939) tried the effect of parenteral thiamine and reported encouraging results; disorientation and confabulation responded in many cases, but the memory deficits were largely unaltered.

Meanwhile evidence accumulated to suggest a clinical link between Wernicke's encephalopathy and Korsakoff's syndrome. Features of the two disorders were sometimes seen together, and the former was noted often to lead on to the latter. De Wardener and Lennox's (1947) cases were again important here, showing clear evidence of memory deficits in association with ataxia and ophthalmoplegias. The acuteness of their cases also allowed the memory deficits to respond unequivocally to thiamine in many cases. The link between the two conditions was finally consolidated when the site of the cerebral lesions in Korsakoff's syndrome was clarified. Malamud and Skillicorn (1956) eventually provided clear evidence that in patients dying with Korsakoff's syndrome the location of cerebral pathology appeared to be identical with that seen in Wernicke's encephalopathy, the two merely differing in the acuteness or chronicity of the pathological process.

The amnesic syndrome can, of course, result from a variety of brain lesions which have nothing to do with thiamine deficiency, as outlined on p. 25. But where the nutritionally depleted subject is concerned, Wernicke's encephalopathy and Korsakoff's syndrome now appeared to be merely different facets of the same pathological process. In effect, Wernicke's encephalopathy emerged as the acute organic reaction of which Korsakoff's syndrome represented the residual and sometimes permanent defect. Confirmation came from the comprehensive clinicopathological study of Victor *et al.* (1971) which they published under the composite title of 'The Wernicke–Korsakoff syndrome'. Of 186 alcoholic patients who survived the acute illness and were observed for long enough to assess the development of amnesia, 84% developed a typical Korsakoff syndrome. Other cerebral pathology may make additional contributions to the fully developed picture, as discussed on p. 582, but lesions in the Wernicke location appear to be fundamental to the amnesic deficits displayed. The possibility that a direct toxic action of alcohol on the nervous system may also contribute to Korsakoff's syndrome is considered on p. 583.

Clinical features

Victor *et al.*'s (1971) observations on 245 patients form the basis for much of the description that follows. These clinical and pathological data are also found in the second edition of their monograph (Victor *et al.* 1989).

Wernicke's encephalopathy typically declares itself abruptly, though sometimes it may be several days before the full picture is manifest. The commonest presenting features are mental confusion or staggering gait. The patient may also be aware of ocular abnormalities with complaints of wavering vision or diplopia on looking to the side. This well-known triad of confusion, ataxia and ophthalmoplegia confers a highly characteristic stamp to the syndrome when it appears in full, but all parts are not always seen together. In an admittedly retrospective analysis of 97 autopsy-proven cases, Harper *et al.* (1986) found that the classic triad had been present in only 16%; 28% had shown two of the signs and 37% only one, but in 19% no feature of the triad was documented. A high index of suspicion is therefore necessary if the condition is not to be missed.

Other common features include prodromal anorexia, nausea and vomiting. A marked disorder of memory is frequently in evidence and has been insufficiently emphasised in most descriptions. Special attention has also been called to lethargy and hypotension which, in the presence of an acute organic mental syndrome, may indicate Wernicke's encephalopathy despite the absence of other definitive signs (Cravioto *et al.* 1961). Rare presentations may be with hypothermia, stupor or coma (Kearsley & Musso 1980).

The age range is evenly distributed throughout adult life, with males affected approximately twice as often as females. This ratio is considerably lower than for alcoholism generally and may be partly a reflection of differences in patterns of drinking. The pattern which leads to Wernicke's encephalopathy appears to be steady drinking extending over months or years and coupled with inadequate intake of food. In Victor *et al.*'s (1971) series delirium tremens or other withdrawal syndromes had occurred at some time in the past in 40% of cases, withdrawal fits in 10% and liver disease in 10%, indicating the general severity of alcohol abuse.

On examination Victor *et al.* observed the following signs:

Ocular abnormalities were present in 96% of patients on initial examination. The commonest findings were nystagmus, sixth nerve palsies producing lateral rectus weakness, or some form of conjugate gaze paralysis. The pupils usually showed little more than sluggishness of reactions. Ocular signs can be remarkably evanescent, resolving speedily with treatment or even on feeding thiamine-containing foods. This no doubt accounts for the much lower prevalence of ocular abnormalities reported in cases viewed retrospectively.

Ataxia was observed in 87% of patients who were testable, varying from inability to stand without support to minor difficulties with heel–toe walking. By contrast intention tremor in the legs or arms was relatively rare.

Peripheral neuropathy was present in 82% of cases and usually confined to the legs. In addition to objective signs there were often subjective complaints of weakness, paraesthesiae and pain.

Serious malnutrition was evident in 84%. Common signs were redness or papillary atrophy of the tongue, cheilosis, angular stomatitis, telangiectases, and dryness and discoloration of the skin. Two-thirds of the patients showed evidence of liver disorder and a quarter were bedridden when first seen. Overt signs of beriberi were rare but resting tachycardia and dyspnoea on effort were common.

An *abstinence syndrome* was found at inception in 13%, with epileptic fits, hallucinoses or delirium tremens.

Mental abnormalities were observed in 90% of patients, the rest presenting with ataxia and ophthalmoplegia but remaining lucid throughout. The commonest mental disturbance was a state of *quiet global confusion* with disorientation, apathy and derangement of memory. Many were drowsy, sometimes falling asleep in mid-sentence, and others showed marked indifference and inattention to their surroundings. Against the prevailing view, however, almost all were readily rousable and impairment of consciousness was rarely profound or persistent.

In the typical case spontaneous activity and speech were minimal, and remarks irrational and inconsistent. Grasp, awareness and responsiveness were markedly impaired. Misidentifications were extremely common and made without hesitation. Physical and mental fatiguability was pronounced, and concentration was difficult for the simplest task. By contrast a small proportion were alert, responsive and voluble, despite obvious confusion and defects of memory.

Evidence of *delirium* was sometimes seen, with perceptual distortions, vivid hallucinations, insomnia, agitation and autonomic overactivity. In a small number this amounted to frank delirium tremens, but was always evanescent and usually not severe. Hallucinations were rare in the remainder. Loosely knit delusions appeared occasionally and sometimes persisted for weeks after the confusion had cleared.

Assessment of memory was often difficult, but *in testable cases a defect of memorising was discovered or else became evident as soon as the major confusion subsided*. It was often hard to determine the point at which confusion of thought receded and the memory defect became the most prominent abnormality, since the two usually blended imperceptibly in the course of the illness. The memory disorder could easily be overlooked; while confused the patients were often markedly evasive, and later covered their defects by spontaneous facile chatter. In a small number (14%) a typical Korsakoff memory defect was clearly evident from the outset, being the most prominent mental abnormality at the time of initial examination.

Confabulation was common early in the disorder but was not found in every case. In those who showed it, moreover, it could not be elicited on every occasion. The origin could often be traced to confusion of thought or perceptual disorder, and it was sometimes hard to separate confabulations from misidentifications and misinterpretations. As the global confusion receded, and the memory defects became clearly established, the confabulation could often be traced to translocations in time of genuine past experiences.

Features more particularly stressed by De Wardener and Lennox (1947) included *emotional abnormalities* which appeared in two-thirds of their prisoner of war patients. Typically these set in soon after the ocular abnormalities had become well established. Apprehension was the common early change, with anxious insomnia and fear of the dark. Later this gave way to apathy, and later still to depression with emotional lability. Occasional patients showed marked excitability. De Wardener and Lennox's cases also more frequently experienced hallucinations, and more frequently progressed to coma.

Investigations

Diffuse slowing was found on electroencephalography in half of the patients tested by Victor *et al.* (1971). Sometimes, however, the tracings were entirely normal in marked and classic examples of the syndrome.

The cerebrospinal fluid may be abnormal with a mild elevation of protein. The blood pyruvate level may be expected to be raised in the acute phase of the disease. Transketolase studies can be informative, as described on p. 572.

In occasional examples, computerised tomography (CT) scanning has shown symmetrical areas of decreased attenuation in the region of the thalamus (Escobar *et al.* 1983; McDowell & Le Blanc 1984). In the latter study the lesions were observed to improve after several weeks of treatment with thiamine. Magnetic resonance imaging (MRI) can show such lesions more clearly (Plate 17), and may also identify atrophy of the mamillary bodies (Charness & DeLaPaz 1987; Bigler *et al.* 1989) or hyperintensities surrounding the third ventricle and aqueduct (Gallucci *et al.* 1990). Meyer *et al.* (1985) have demonstrated reductions in both grey and white matter cerebral blood flow, which improves with treatment. The most prominent reductions in Hata *et al.*'s (1987) patients were in the region of the hypothalamus and basal forebrain nuclei, but the thalamus, basal ganglia and limbic system also showed hypoperfusion.

Course and response to treatment

The unique value of Victor *et al.*'s (1971, 1989) series is that a substantial proportion of the patients who survived the acute stage remained under close medical observation for many months or years thereafter. Altogether 17% died during the acute stage, a quarter were followed for at least 2 months, and more than half were followed for periods of 2–13 years. The long-term outcome with thiamine replacement was accordingly greatly clarified.

Sixth nerve palsies always recovered, often starting to resolve within hours though sometimes taking several days or weeks to disappear completely. Other ocular abnormalities responded similarly, with the exception of horizontal nystagmus which was a permanent residuum in two-thirds of the patients. Ataxia usually began to improve within the first week, but often took a month or two for maximum resolution. In a quarter of patients the ataxia showed no improvement whatever, and altogether more than half were left with permanent unsteadiness of some degree. Thus residual ataxia and nystagmus can sometimes be useful signs in pointing to the origin of an obscure chronic amnesic syndrome. Polyneuropathy improved only very slowly over several months, and diminution or absence of tendon reflexes was another common permanent sequel.

The global confusion always recovered in survivors, beginning usually within 2–3 weeks and clearing completely within 1–2 months. As the confusion receded the amnesic defects stood out more prominently. Of 186 patients followed for long enough to assess the presence or absence of the Korsakoff state, 84% developed the typical amnesic syndrome. The few who escaped had all shown relatively brief acute illnesses and had lost their confusion within a week. In addition the authors drew attention to the small but important group who presented with the Korsakoff amnesic defect from first contact along with ocular and ataxic signs (some 10% of the total), and their further very small group of nine cases (4%) who had apparently developed the amnesic syndrome without ophthalmoplegia or ataxia at any time.

Follow-up of the Korsakoff patients showed complete recovery in a quarter, partial recovery in half, and no improvement whatever in the remainder. Complete recovery was observed even in some very severe examples. The onset of recovery was commonly delayed for several weeks or months, and once started it sometimes continued for as long as 2 years.

In the chronic amnesic stage anterograde and retrograde amnesia were the dominant features, but continuing minor impairments of perceptual and cognitive function could usually be discerned by careful examination. The retrograde amnesia was often of several years' duration, though with islands of preservation and without a sharply demarcated beginning. Confabulation was rarely encountered in the chronic stage. The patients were typically inert, apathetic and lacking in insight, though fully alert and responsive to their surroundings. They were mostly neglectful of appearance, and tended to spend their days in complete idleness. A very few were gregarious or overtalkative. Most were placid, bland and detached in attitude, and emotional reactions were hard to arouse. Sustained anxiety or depression were rare, though brief periods of anger or irritability might be seen from time to time.

Pathology

The pathological changes are remarkable for their predilection for certain circumscribed parts of the brain. Symmetrical lesions are found predominantly in the neighbourhood of the walls of the third ventricle, the periaqueductal region, the floor of the fourth ventricle, certain thalamic nuclei (including especially the paraven-

tricular parts of the medial dorsal nuclei, the anteromedial nuclei and the pulvinar), the mamillary bodies, the terminal portions of the fornices, the brain stem, and the anterior lobe and superior vermis of the cerebellum. By contrast, obvious lesions are rarely seen in the cerebral cortex, corpus striatum, subthalamic and septal regions, cingulate gyri or hippocampal areas. Victor et al. (1971), however, found that convolutional atrophy was conspicuous enough to be remarked upon in 27% of their cases who came to autopsy.

Microscopically the lesions tend to involve all neural elements—neurones, axis cylinders, blood vessels and glia—but with variability from case to case and from one location to another. In general, myelinated fibres tend to be affected more severely than the neurones themselves. Astrocytic and histiocytic proliferation is found in the areas of parenchymal loss. Proliferation of blood vessels and petechial haemorrhages may occur, but the latter may often represent terminal events.

The distribution of lesions is virtually identical in patients dying in the acute stages of Wernicke's encephalopathy and in patients who have shown a chronic Korsakoff syndrome, differing only in the chronicity of the glial and vascular reactions.

In seeking a correlation between symptoms and lesions, Victor et al. (1971) suggested that the ophthalmoplegias result from lesions in the third and sixth cranial nerve nuclei and adjacent tegmentum, nystagmus from lesions of the vestibular nuclei, and ataxia from lesions of the vestibular nuclei and the anterior lobes and vermis of the cerebellum. Amnesia in their material appeared to be particularly closely associated with lesions in the medial dorsal nuclei and pulvinar of the thalamus; mamillary lesions which have traditionally been regarded as crucial for the development of amnesia were less constant (Victor 1964; Victor et al. 1971, 1989). The question of the precise anatomical basis for the amnesic deficits in Korsakoff's syndrome is discussed in more detail in Chapter 2 (p. 25).

Subclinical Wernicke's encephalopathy

The foregoing description applies to patients who have come dramatically to medical attention on account of an acute, often fulminating, disorder. It seems probable, however, that milder variants may exist, or indeed that damage may sometimes develop surreptitiously in the Wernicke location without clear clinical indicators of the process (Lishman 1981). The evidence is somewhat indirect but the pointers towards it deserve careful consideration.

Cravioto et al. (1961) and Grunnet (1969) found patients with the classic lesion at autopsy who had died without exhibiting Wernicke's classic signs. Comparison of patients dying in the 1930s and 1960s suggested that the clinical presentations had become less severe, perhaps as a result of the wider availability and prescription of vitamins. The lesions at autopsy tended to be more circumscribed in the recent cases, and more often subacute or chronic in nature. Most significant of all, the condition could remain undiagnosed prior to death.

This last point has been strongly reinforced by Harper (1979, 1983). Over the course of 9 years in Perth, Australia, 131 cases of Wernicke's encephalopathy were diagnosed at autopsy, representing almost 3% of all brains examined in the hospital or referred by the city coroner. Only 26 of these 131 cases had been suspected during life, despite the fact that most had been examined in teaching hospitals. The great majority of affected persons were known to be alcoholics, and several had died suddenly and unexpectedly. A considerable range was encountered in the acuteness or chronicity of the lesions, with the not uncommon conjunction of acute histological changes superimposed on chronic pathology within the same brain regions. Two-thirds showed chronic pathological changes alone.

Some alcoholics may therefore harbour covert, undiagnosed pathology of the Wernicke type over a considerable period of time. Whether this evolves insidiously or in stepwise fashion is unknown. It may sometimes represent the cumulative effects of repeated minor episodes of Wernicke's encephalopathy which have largely gone unnoticed at the time.

In favour of the idea is the noted resistance to treatment of many alcoholic Korsakoff states, even when thiamine is administered from the earliest stages. This contrasts with the gratifying responses observed, for example, in De Wardener and Lennox's (1947) nutritionally depleted prisoners of war. The alcoholics appear often to have acquired an entrenched structural pathology which may well have been evolving for some time. Those cases in which the Korsakoff syndrome develops insidiously, without an obvious Wernicke episode (p. 583), could equally be explained on such a basis. Finally, one might argue that a lesion dependent on biochemical changes secondary to vitamin deficiency is rather unlikely to obey an 'all or none' law, especially when the vitamin depletion has been operative for many years; that the lesion should either declare itself fully or fail to develop entirely would seem to be unlikely.

It could conceivably be the case that covert pathology of this nature makes a contribution to the memory deficits encountered in alcoholics generally. Some support for this idea has been obtained from CT scan studies. Chronic changes in such a location might be expected to lead to widening of the third ventricle; Acker et al. (1987) found that performance on a battery of memory tests was significantly related to the width of the third ventricle in a group of detoxified non-Korsakoff alcoholics. Not dissimilarly, Jacobson (1987) divided a sample of non-Korsakoff alcoholics into those with good and poor memory, according to performance on the Logical Memory Test, and compared their scans with those of Korsakoff patients and normal controls. Both the lateral and the third ventricles tended to be larger in alcoholics with poor rather than good memory, the values in the former approaching the values found in Korsakoff patients and the latter the values found in normal controls. The difference in third ventricular size was statistically significant. Although these are indirect approaches to the problem, it would seem that impaired memory in the alcoholic subject is related to changes of some sort in the deeper structures of the brain.

The issue is of potential therapeutic importance. If a substantial number of alcoholics develop a thiamine-dependent pathology well before it is clinically apparent, high potency vitamin therapy should find wider prophylactic application. The feasibility and desirability of routinely supplementing alcoholic beverages with thiamine has indeed received consideration (Centerwall & Criqui 1978; Weinstein 1978; Bishai & Bozzetti 1986; Finlay-Jones 1986; Rouse & Armstrong 1988). Price et al. (1987) conclude that fortification of flour alone, as practised in the UK and the USA, is insufficient for prophylaxis in problem drinkers. Reuler et al. (1985) estimate that the supplementation of alcoholic beverages in the USA would merely cost the consumer an additional 0.1 cent per litre of wine. The identification of persons at special genetic risk (pp. 576–7) could also prove to be important. These, however, are matters to be clarified by future research.

Treatment

Wernicke's encephalopathy represents an acute medical emergency and warrants energetic treatment from the moment the diagnosis is made. Doses of thiamine as small as 2–3 mg can modify the ophthalmoplegias, but much larger doses are indicated to minimise the chance of disabling sequelae, particularly since associated hepatic disorder may interfere with utilisation of the vitamin. A dose of 50–100 mg of thiamine hydrochloride should be given intravenously (after taking blood for pyruvate or transketolase estimation if the diagnosis is in doubt), and this should be accompanied by at least an equal amount intramuscularly. Intramuscular injections should be continued daily until a normal diet is resumed. In view of the possibility of other concurrent vitamin deficiencies, Pabrinex (which in recent years has replaced Parentovite) is usually employed intravenously or intramuscularly in place of thiamine alone. Intravenous injection should always be carried out slowly over 10 minutes on account of the risk of anaphylactic reactions. Each injection of Pabrinex contains thiamine hydrochloride 250 mg, nicotinamide 160 mg, riboflavine 4 mg, pyridoxine hydrochloride 50 mg and ascorbic acid 500 mg. In the occasional patient who seems refractory to thiamine replacement, determination of the serum magnesium level may be indicated. Traviesa (1974) showed that hypomagnesaemia impaired both the biochemical and clinical response to treatment. The syndrome of nicotinic acid deficiency encephalopathy (p. 574) must also be kept in mind when response has been lacking or incomplete to the replacement of thiamine alone.

Other aspects of management must include attention to infection, dehydration or electrolyte imbalance as a result of vomiting. Strict bed rest is mandatory in the acute stages, since sudden collapse and death can occur due to abrupt cardiac decompensation. Signs of congestive cardiac failure call for rapid digitalisation. Disturbed behaviour, and particularly that due to coincident delirium tremens, will require appropriate sedation (p. 603).

Oral vitamin supplements are usually continued for several weeks after the acute illness has resolved, though the value of this is uncertain. In patients with enduring ataxia, polyneuritis or memory disturbance, high potency vitamin injections should be pursued energetically as long as improvement is occurring.

Korsakoff's syndrome

The emergence of Korsakoff's syndrome as an often permanent aftermath of Wernicke's encephalopathy has been outlined above. The clinical picture and the neuropathological basis for the amnesic defects are described in Chapter 2 (pp. 29–32 and 25). Here, certain more recent considerations with regard to the pathogenesis and the nosology of the condition remain to be discussed.

First, it has become evident that the classic lesion at the base of the brain is often associated with more widespread cerebral pathology, including cortical shrinkage and ventricular dilatation. The contribution which this may make to certain aspects of the clinical picture warrants careful appraisal. Second, the rarity of a fully fledged Korsakoff syndrome as a residue of thiamine deficiency in non-alcoholics raises the possibility that a direct neurotoxic action of alcohol may play some part in the evolution of the condition. Finally, there is evidence that Korsakoff's syndrome may be misdiagnosed to a considerable extent in clinical practice, and that an overlap with alcoholic dementia may be more widespread than is often appreciated.

Cortical pathology

Cortical pathology was widely described in the earlier literature before the diencephalic basal brain lesion came to be fully appreciated (Lishman 1981). Thereafter interest in cortical aspects showed a pronounced decline. Neuroimaging studies have, however, re-emphasised that supratentorial changes are common. Jacobson and Lishman (1990) compared 25 Korsakoff patients, gathered from hospitals around London, with non-Korsakoff alcoholics of similar age. On CT scans the Korsakoff patients had wider third ventricles, as might have been expected from their diencephalic lesions, but also significantly larger lateral ventricles, Sylvian fissures and interhemispheric fissures. The widening of the interhemispheric fissures, measured between the frontal lobes, was particularly marked and showed significant correlations with certain tests of frontal lobe function (Jacobson 1989). Shimamura et al. (1988) found atrophy in frontal sulcal and peri-Sylvian areas on CT in comparison with normal controls, the frontal atrophy correlating with impairment on memory and other tests. Jernigan et al. (1991c), using MRI, showed greater grey matter losses in the medial temporal and orbitofrontal cortex when Korsakoff patients were compared with non-amnesic alcoholics.

Further evidence of cortical involvement has come from functional brain-imaging studies. Hunter et al. (1989) examined 10 Korsakoff patients with HMPAO-SPECT, revealing impaired blood flow in the frontal regions which correlated significantly with deficits on tests of memory and orientation. Glucose metabolism as measured by FDG-PET was reduced overall by 20% in Kessler et al.'s (1984) patients, with hypoperfusion in numerous cortical areas in addition to the thalamus and basal ganglia. Joyce et al.'s (1994) results are particularly intriguing in that care was taken to control for atrophy on CT scans; FDG-PET showed robust hypometabolism in only three regions—the anterior cingulate, posterior cingulate and precuneate areas — in comparison to normal controls. These represent components of the 'Papez circuit' known to be involved in memory functions. It is interesting that cingulectomy, carried out for the relief of obsessional and other psychiatric disorders in the 1950s, was reported to lead to a transient Korsakoff-like amnesic–confabulatory syndrome during the early postoperative period (Whitty & Lewin 1960).

At autopsy Victor et al. (1971) noted convolutional atrophy in a quarter of cases; Harper (1983) found ventricular dilatation and cortical atrophy in 34%, the latter most commonly involving the frontal lobes.

A substantial cortical component to the pathology could be relevant to the considerable range of cognitive deficits detected in Korsakoff patients on detailed psychological testing, sometimes exceeding those in matched non-Korsakoff alcoholics (Jacobson *et al.* 1990). It could also explain some of the striking clinical aspects of the syndrome, in particular the apathy, lack of initiative and profound lack of insight which the majority of patients display. As discussed on pp. 31–2, these are not inevitable concomitants of severe memory disorder, and can be entirely absent in amnesic syndromes of other aetiologies. Many such features would appear to reflect frontal lobe damage. Using sophisticated neuropsychological tests Joyce and Robbins (1991) have demonstrated deficits in frontal lobe function in Korsakoff patients which are independent of their memory impairments. Oscar-Berman *et al.* (1992) have shown consistent impairments on delayed-response tasks, of a type known to be sensitive to prefrontal cortical damage in primates, when alcoholic Korsakoff patients are compared with non-Korsakoff alcoholics and control subjects. It is possible, moreover, that certain aspects of the memory disorder itself are influenced by the presence of cortical pathology: Butters (1984) reviews the evidence that frontal lobe damage may confer such matters as impairment of temporal recency judgements and failure to release from proactive interference on memory testing.

Neurotoxic action of alcohol

A role for the direct toxic action of alcohol in leading to Korsakoff's syndrome has been raised from time to time. It could be relevant to the aspects discussed just above, since a good deal of evidence points to alcohol neurotoxicity where cortical changes are concerned (p. 607). A more difficult question is how far thiamine deficiency alone can account for the chronic amnesic deficits which constitute the core feature of the syndrome. Certainly thiamine replacement is not regularly effective in reversing the memory difficulties; and as Freund (1973) pointed out there is a remarkable lack of evidence that permanent memory disorder can follow thiamine deficiency unaccompanied by alcohol abuse. There have been occasional recent reports of a persistent Korsakoff syndrome following severe vomiting, malabsorption or prolonged intravenous feeding, but in a close examination of these Kopelman (1995) concludes that the evidence for a non-alcoholic nutritional cause must still be regarded as equivocal.

The inevitability of the link between an overt episode of Wernicke's encephalopathy and Korsakoff's syndrome may also be challenged on the basis of clinical experience. In many Korsakoff patients there is evidence of a pre-existing Wernicke encephalopathy, as reported by Victor *et al.* (1971), but in others no such history is forthcoming. Some patients appear to develop their amnesic difficulties insidiously, in the context of chronic continuing inebriation. Such patients would be under-represented in Victor *et al.*'s sample, since most of their patients were incepted as cases of Wernicke's encephalopathy then followed through to the korsakovian development.

Thus while the relationship between thiamine deficiency and Wernicke's encephalopathy cannot be doubted, there is less clear-cut evidence to incriminate thiamine exclusively in the chronic Korsakoff state. Alcohol neurotoxicity can vie with avitaminosis as a possible cause; or a conjunction of the two together may be necessary for the development of the fully-fledged syndrome. This may be why the condition remains elusive except in alcoholic patients. The possibility that an unusual susceptibility to both thiamine lack and alcohol neurotoxicity may be necessary for the development of the chronic Korsakoff state is discussed in some detail by Lishman (1990). An alternative explanation is to view the amnesic difficulties as firmly linked to thiamine deficiency, but accepting that in alcoholics this may often have been operative over a considerable period of time. In other words alcoholism may tend to be associated with a 'subclinical' Wernicke pathology which, by the time it becomes overt, has led to fixed and irreversible structural changes (pp. 580–1).

Continuity hypothesis

It is interesting in this connection that certain continuities are now being discerned between the memory deficits seen in Korsakoff's syndrome and those found in chronic alcoholics generally. Ryback (1971) was the first to point out that such were likely to exist. Butters and co-workers have reported detailed comparisons between alcoholic Korsakoff patients and groups of abstinent non-Korsakoff alcoholics on a wide range of memory tests (Butters & Cermak 1980; Ryan & Butters 1980). The non-Korsakoff alcoholics were divided into those with and without complaints of memory impairment. On standard memory tests (such as the Wechsler Memory Scale or the Benton Visual Retention Test) only those alcoholics who reported memory difficulties were impaired, overlapping in scores with the Korsakoff patients; the remainder performed well and were indistinguishable from controls. But on more demanding experimental memory tests (paired associate learning tests and the Brown–Peterson test), even the alcoholics who had no memory complaints were also significantly impaired.

Subtle but definite 'subclinical' memory deficits thus appear to be widespread in the alcoholic population, and these become more pronounced in alcoholics who complain of memory difficulties. In the latter the severity of the deficits can overlap in some degree with those seen in Korsakoff's syndrome. Continuities are also apparent in measures of third ventricular width as detected on CT scans (p. 581). Either alcohol neurotoxicity or 'subclinical' thiamine deficiency could be the common link. Bowden (1990) has argued strongly for the latter, suggesting that in neuropsychological research a rigid distinction between Korsakoff and non-Korsakoff alcoholics should no longer be regarded as valid.

Nevertheless, there remain certain clear-cut differences between the Korsakoff and non-Korsakoff patients in broader clinical terms — the latter are aware of their memory deficits, make efforts to compensate for them, are not disorientated, and show little by way of a retrograde memory gap.

Diagnosis

The diagnosis of Korsakoff's syndrome requires clear evidence of a marked memory disorder along with good preservation of other cognitive functions. Subtle deficits will often be revealed by special testing as outlined on p. 31, particularly with regard to visuoperceptive functions and abstracting ability, but performance on standard intelligence tests should be substantially intact. This was well illustrated by Butters and Cermak's (1980) comparison of intelligence test scores (Wechsler Adult Intelligence Scale, WAIS) in a group of Korsakoff patients and a group of intact normal controls. The latter were carefully matched for age, socioeconomic class and educational background. With the sole exception of the digit–symbol subtest, no significant differences could be discerned in any aspect of test performance. In measures such as the Wechsler Memory Scale, by contrast, Butters and Cermak state that Korsakoff patients can generally be expected to score some 20–30 points below the expectation derived from their IQs.

In clinical practice, however, such careful distinctions are not always observed. In a retrospective survey of 63 alcoholic patients admitted to the Maudsley Hospital, Cutting (1978b) found that 50 had been labelled as having Korsakoff's syndrome and 13 as having alcoholic dementia. The Korsakoff patients proved, however, to be heterogeneous. Those with a relatively acute onset mirrored the classic syndrome, with an isolated memory deficit and a poor prognosis as judged by capacity to resume independent existence. Seventeen of the 50, however, shared several characteristics with the alcoholic dements. Their symptoms had been several months in evolution, they tended to be older, females predominated over males, and some two-thirds were capable of improvement on follow-up. Psychological test profiles, where available, showed that the gradual-onset group, like the alcoholic dements, were impaired across a wide range of cognitive functions in addition to their memory problems. This suggested that several patients with more global dementia had been falsely labelled as suffering from Korsakoff's syndrome.

Jacobson and Lishman (1987) have provided additional evidence of heterogeneity within the syndrome. They obtained separate indices of the severity of memory impairment and of 'generalised intellectual decline' in their sample of 38 chronic Korsakoff patients. The former was derived from the discrepancy between the WAIS IQ and the Wechsler Memory Quotient, the latter from the discrepancy between the WAIS IQ and the National Adult Reading Test which yields an approximate estimate of premorbid IQ (p. 111). When the two indices were plotted against each other a marked scatter was apparent; some two-thirds of patients showed clear memory impairment with little fall from premorbid IQ (i.e. the classic Korsakoff pattern), others showed both mild memory and mild intellectual decline, whereas 10% showed little memory impairment but marked intellectual decline. Thus it appeared that there was an admixture of patients in the sample, with at one extreme a group who might more properly have been labelled as demented. The transition across the sample as a whole was gradual, not abrupt. Females featured disproportionately among those with generalised impairment as was the case in Cutting's survey. Certain relationships could be discerned with CT scan parameters — widening of the third ventricle tended to be associated with more severe memory deficits, and widened interhemispheric fissures with greater fall from premorbid intellectual functioning.

It would seem therefore that Korsakoff's syndrome is not so sharply circumscribed from generalised impairment as is generally thought. It appears to shade, through various transitional forms, into something that might more properly be termed 'alcoholic dementia' (p. 603). Certainly the label of Korsakoff's syndrome would appear to be more commonly applied in clinical practice than is strictly warranted.

Treatment

In the established chronic Korsakoff state treatment will often prove to be disappointing. Cutting (1978b) reviews the differing reports in the literature, some finding no patients whatsoever with a significant response to thiamine and others obtaining improvement in up to 70%. The results in Victor *et al.*'s (1971) large series are described on p. 580. The possibility of occasional substantial improvement means, nevertheless, that high dosage thiamine replacement must always be attempted, by the parenteral route, and must be pursued over many months if benefit continues to be observed.

Benefit has been reported in a double-blind trial of clonidine, a specific alpha noradrenergic agonist (McEntee & Mair 1980; Mair & McEntee 1986). A small but statistically significant improvement was obtained on measures of memory functioning in a group of chronic Korsakoff patients. This accords with the demonstration that the primary metabolite of noradrenaline (3-methoxy 4-hydroxy phenylglycol, MHPG) is substantially reduced in the cerebrospinal fluid of Korsakoff patients, in proportion to the severity of memory impairment (McEntee & Mair 1978; McEntee et al. 1984). The distribution of the lesions in the diencephalon and brain stem stands to disrupt the pathways of monoamine-containing neurones, so these biochemical findings could reflect an important component in the genesis of the memory failure.

Others, however, have failed to confirm any lowering of MHPG in the cerebrospinal fluid (Martin et al. 1984), and O'Carroll et al. (1993) were unable to replicate McEntee and Mair's finding of improvement in memory with clonidine in a rather older and more chronic sample of patients. Intravenous infusion of clonidine, however, was shown in these patients to increase verbal fluency and to be accompanied by increased blood flow to the anterior cingulate region (Moffoot et al. 1994).

Martin et al. (1989) found significant improvements on the Wechsler Memory Scale with fluvoxamine in a small group of Korsakoff patients, this correlating with the reductions that occurred in 5-hydroxyindoleacetic acid in the cerebrospinal fluid. Again, however, O'Carroll et al. (1994) have been unable to confirm this finding in a larger sample.

The occasional report that inhalation of vasopressin helps the Korsakoff memory impairment (Le Boeuf et al. 1978) also stands in need of further investigation. This may well be a non-specific effect, since vasopressin has also been found to improve attention, concentration and memory in non-brain-damaged healthy volunteers (Legros et al. 1978). Gash and Thomas (1983) suggest, indeed, that vasopressin may primarily affect arousal and motivation rather than memory processes per se.

Other nutritional disorders associated with alcoholism

The syndrome of Wernicke's encephalopathy can be confidently ascribed to thiamine deficiency. Other disorders in alcoholics are suspected of being nutritional in origin though the evidence is less complete. Of those considered below peripheral neuropathy is almost certainly due in part to vitamin deficiency, but here and in the others a direct toxic effect of alcohol may also be responsible. The question of 'alcoholic dementia' raises special issues, so far unresolved, and is considered on p. 603 et seq. in Chapter 13.

Peripheral neuropathy

Alcoholic peripheral neuropathy may sometimes be symptomless and manifest only by loss of the ankle reflexes, but in most cases there are prominent complaints of sensory disturbance. It begins usually in the feet with numbness, pins and needles, burning sensations and pain. Sensory ataxia may be prominent. Weakness may progress ultimately to foot drop with wasting of the leg muscles. Cutaneous sensory loss is most marked peripherally in the hands and feet, and intense hyperaesthesia may be elicited on stroking the skin. The calf muscles are often very tender. Oedema of dependent parts may develop along with dystrophic changes of the skin and nails.

The condition often accompanies Wernicke's encephalopathy or Korsakoff's syndrome, and some 50% of patients with neuropathy show residua of these disorders. It may also present as an isolated abnormality, or in association with delirium tremens. The main cause appears to be deficiency of thiamine, though other deficiencies may be important as well. Pyridoxine and pantothenic acid deficiency can produce neuropathy and are likely to be involved in some alcoholics. A toxic role for alcohol itself, or other toxic substances in alcoholic beverages, has been proposed, but slow recovery is usual with vitamin therapy even though drinking continues.

Cerebellar degeneration

Victor et al. (1959) have described a remarkably uniform cerebellar syndrome in alcoholics, with ataxia of stance and gait as the principal abnormalities. The arms are little affected, and nystagmus and dysarthria may be absent. The typical course is gradual evolution over several weeks or months after which the disorder remains static for many years. More rarely, slow progression occurs over a number of years. The resemblance to cerebellar degeneration seen with bronchial carcinoma can sometimes be close (p. 740), and a chest X-ray is obviously important in every case. CT or MRI may reveal cerebellar cortical atrophy. Gillman et al. (1990) have shown hypometabolism in the superior cerebellar vermis with FDG-PET.

Pathological changes are largely restricted to the anterior and superior aspects of the vermis and cerebellar hemispheres. The cell loss affects the Purkinje cells especially. Victor *et al.* (1989) suggest that the ataxia of Wernicke's encephalopathy, at least in its chronic form, is based on a similar type of lesion. They therefore favour a nutritional cause, rather than a direct toxic effect of alcohol. There is little evidence to favour the latter, Estrin (1987) finding that estimates of annual and life-time consumption were *lower* in alcoholics with cerebellar degeneration than in those without. Karhunen *et al.* (1994) have shown a small inverse correlation between Purkinje cell counts and size of daily intake in moderate drinkers, but the variation was wide suggesting important differences in individual susceptibility.

A similar cerebellar syndrome was reported by Skillicorn (1955) in alcoholics, with gross cerebellar atrophy demonstrable on air encephalography. Skillicorn's cases sometimes showed evidence of intellectual deterioration, and diffuse cerebral atrophy was found in addition to the cerebellar lesion.

Amblyopia

In rare cases retrobulbar neuritis may develop in alcoholics, progressing over 1 or 2 weeks but rarely extending to complete blindness. Dimness of central vision, especially for red and green, is the more common result. An associated peripheral neuropathy is usual. The smoking of strong pipe tobacco is often incriminated in addition to the alcoholism, and deficiencies of both thiamine and vitamin B_{12} appear to be responsible. Acute blindness is more commonly seen as a result of methyl alcohol consumption, and is then attributed to the direct toxic effects of the poison.

Marchiafava–Bignami disease

This rare disorder was formerly thought to be restricted to Italian males but this is now known to be erroneous, likewise the belief that it was especially related to the drinking of wine. It presents with ataxia, dysarthria, epilepsy and severe impairment of consciousness, or in more slowly progressive forms with dementia and spastic paralysis of the limbs. Delmas-Marsalet *et al.* (1967) reviewed the literature and presented cases with full neuropathological examination. Extensive demyelination affects the corpus callosum and adjacent subcortical white matter, the optic tracts and the cerebellar peduncles. The mortality is high, but patients sometimes survive for several years. Recovery is rare. Characteristic findings have been reported in the corpus callosum on CT or MRI (Kawamura *et al.* 1985). A nutritional origin is suggested by the symmetry and constancy of location of the lesions

within the central nervous system, and the frequent history of dietary deprivation. The fact that virtually all cases have occurred in alcoholics suggests that alcohol may also play a part in causation (Victor *et al.* 1989). The precise factors involved remain uncertain.

Central pontine myelinosis

This is an acute and often fatal complication of alcoholism, presenting with obtundation, bulbar palsy, quadriplegia and loss of pain sensation in the limbs and trunk. Vomiting, confusion, disordered eye movements and coma are common. Some patients show the 'locked in' syndrome with mutism and paralysis but relatively intact sensation and comprehension (Adams & Victor 1993). The lesion lies in the centre of the basis pontis, varying in extent and sometimes involving other neighbouring structures. It consists essentially of a focus of demyelination, usually demonstrable with MRI.

A nutritional origin has again been strongly suspected (Cole *et al.* 1964). Many cases are seen in association with Wernicke's encephalopathy and polyneuropathy. However, it may also occur with liver disease not due to alcohol, with Wilson's disease, and after liver transplantation or haemodialysis (Compston 1993). Other causes include severe burns, hyperemesis gravidarum and diuretic therapy which have led to hyponatraemia. It has emerged that over-rapid correction of low serum sodium is a common cause in such situations, the pons being unusually vulnerable to rapid changes in electrolyte balance due to its close admixture of white matter bundles and richly vascular grey matter (Leslie *et al.* 1980). This has led to the relabelling of the condition as the 'osmotic demyelination syndrome' (Sterns *et al.* 1986).

Subacute necrotising encephalomyelopathy (Leigh's disease)

This rare disorder appears to be heterogeneous, some examples being inherited as autosomal recessives and others representing variants of mitochondrial encephalomyopathy (p. 761). A disorder of thiamine metabolism is suspected in many cases. Deficiencies of pyruvate dehydrogenase and other respiratory chain enzymes have been demonstrated, also a factor in the blood and urine which inhibits the synthesis of thiamine triphosphate. Treatment with very large doses of thiamine and thiamine propyldisulphide have been thought to induce remissions, though without altering the overall course (Pincus *et al.* 1971). At autopsy necrotic lesions in the brain stem and basal ganglia resemble those of Wernicke's encephalopathy in form and location, except that the mamillary bodies are spared.

Leigh (1951) first described the condition in a 7-month-old infant who died after a rapidly progressive neurological disorder. Many cases have since been reported, as reviewed by Monpetit et al. (1971) and Pincus (1972). Most have occurred in the first 2 years of life, though later childhood onset is occasionally seen. The picture is of progressive psychomotor retardation with feeding difficulties, respiratory disorder, hypotonia and weakness, leading to death usually within 4 years and often within 1 year. Neurological features are usually marked with oculomotor deficits, loss of vision, ataxia, corticospinal tract signs, seizures and movement disorders. The extreme variability of the picture makes diagnosis during life difficult unless the pathology has already been demonstrated in a sibling.

More recently, several autopsy-proven cases have been reported in adults, as reviewed by Plaitakis et al. (1980). Their own patient showed the insidious development of strabismus, visual loss, a broad-based gait and impairment of intellect from early schooldays onwards, but remained active until he was 20. Thereafter he pursued a rapidly downhill course with death after a period of stupor.

A review of the large pedigree associated with this patient showed that several family members were affected and to a markedly variable degree. Mental retardation was commoner than specific neurological manifestations; some patients showed severe neurological affliction, others only subtle deficits. The onset could be abrupt or insidious, and in some cases the course was chronic and remittant. Plaitakis et al. suggest that the genetic defect has variable degrees of expression, resulting in a wide spectrum of disorder. Mild examples would stand to be missed at autopsy.

Vitamin B_{12} deficiency

Pernicious anaemia may be accompanied not only by the neurological complication of subacute combined degeneration of the cord, but also by mental abnormalities. Depression or anergia may be the earliest manifestation of the anaemia, and apathy and somnolence may be marked when anaemia is severe. In addition a number of other psychiatric disturbances have from time to time been attributed directly to the B_{12} deficiency—affective disorder, schizophrenia, paranoid states, episodes of disorientation and delirium, and progressive dementia. Interest was renewed in these phenomena by Holmes (1956) and Smith (1960) who reported several patients in whom mental symptoms apparently responded dramatically to B_{12} replacement. Moreover the mental manifestations

had sometimes antedated the first signs of anaemia or cord disease by many months or years.

This is clearly an important subject for careful evaluation. If covert B_{12} deficiency can truly be responsible for mental disturbance, it will be important to identify and treat it at the earliest opportunity before irreversible structural changes occur in the brain. Unfortunately it has proved difficult to establish firmly whether causal relationships exist and how widely they may apply, and the field remains controversial.

Surveys of psychiatric populations have often shown a large number of patients with low serum B_{12} levels. Edwin et al. (1965) found that 15% of a large group of patients had values below 150 pg/ml and 6% below 100 pg/ml. Both organic and non-organic types of mental illness featured among the patients with low values, and few had pernicious anaemia on examination of the blood. Carney and Sheffield (1970) found a similar incidence of low values among new psychiatric admissions. Shulman (1967a) found that 12% of new admissions to a psychogeriatric unit had values below 150 pg/ml, compared to 5% of elderly non-psychiatric patients assessed by the same laboratory. By contrast, however, Henderson et al. (1966) screened 1000 unselected psychiatric patients and found low B_{12} levels in only nine individuals, which is probably no higher than in the general population.

An additional difficulty is that the low levels of B_{12} which are discovered may sometimes be the consequence rather than the cause of the abnormal mental state, since B_{12} deficiency can result from inadequate nutrition. The daily requirements of B_{12} are small, and it would normally take many years before simple dietary lack became manifest in this way. However, a low serum iron or folic acid can contribute to lowering of the serum B_{12}, hence the latter may sometimes result from a mixed nutritional deficiency in depressed or demented patients who have neglected their diet.

In an attempt to resolve the problem, Zucker et al. (1981) reviewed numerous case reports in the literature, using strictly defined criteria before accepting a causal link between B_{12} deficiency and psychiatric disturbance. As a result they found 15 patients where the relationship seemed well established. Among their requirements were the absence of other organic causes for the mental symptoms, a non-relapsing course, poor response to other treatments, and a positive and well-maintained response to B_{12} administration. Criteria for the diagnosis of B_{12} deficiency were also specified with care. The psychiatric pictures in the patients so identified were heterogeneous, though with a preponderance of organic mental symptoms, depression, paranoia, irritability and episodes of assaultive behaviour. Marked psychiatric disorder could sometimes occur in the absence of neurological abnormalities or anaemia. Zucker *et al.* concluded in particular that the combination of severe depression with organic mental symptoms should lead to screening tests for B_{12} deficiency.

Non-organic psychiatric disorders

Where affective disorders and schizophrenia are concerned there is a lack of critical evidence, other than that just cited, to support a causal relationship with B_{12} deficiency. Little has been done by way of controlled investigations. Minor mood disorder in association with pernicious anaemia may represent no more than a reaction to the non-specific effects of the physical disease. In cases of schizophrenia, severe affective disorder or paranoia, there may sometimes be no more than precipitation in the predisposed individual, or mere coincidence, or a secondary nutritional origin as outlined above. In many cases vitamin B_{12} has been administered along with other treatments so that its effectiveness in therapy is hard to determine.

Shulman (1967b) found four cases of affective disorder with low levels of B_{12} among his geriatric admissions, but all had shown considerable improvement with other forms of treatment before the results of the B_{12} estimations were known. In a separate study (Shulman 1967c) a group of patients with pernicious anaemia was compared with a group suffering from other forms of anaemia after matching for age, sex and haemoglobin level. The overall frequency of psychiatric symptoms was similar in each, and several patients from both groups had had an initial psychiatric referral on account of symptoms which were regarded as neurotic in origin. Depression was sometimes marked, but showed no clear relationship to B_{12} lack; it often resolved before the first injection had been given, i.e. as soon as the patient was told the diagnosis and reassured about prognosis. In a retrospective survey such improvements might well have been attributed to replacement therapy. Nevertheless it was interesting that almost half of the patients with pernicious anaemia reported an increased sense of well being when re-examined after treatment, whereas this was rare in patients with other forms of anaemia.

Organic psychiatric disorders

There is more convincing evidence that B_{12} lack is related to organic psychiatric symptoms. In Shulman's (1967c) prospective study, approximately three-quarters of the patients with penicious anaemia showed objective impairment of memory on a simple learning test. On re-testing after treatment the majority had returned to normal, sometimes within 20 hours of the first injection.

Edwin *et al.'s* (1965) review indicated that low serum B_{12} was more commonly found in elderly demented patients than in controls of similar age. Occasional patients with presenile dementia and low serum B_{12} have been reported to improve with replacement therapy (Henderson *et al.* 1966; Hunter *et al.* 1967a), though many failures are also recorded (Edwin *et al.* 1965; Shulman 1967b). Too much would not, of course, be expected of treatment when the dementia was of very long standing, even if B_{12} deficiency had been the initial responsible cause. B_{12} lack as a cause of dementia appears, however, to be far from common. In a consecutive series of 170 elderly demented patients low B_{12} levels were identified in 26 cases, but B_{12} supplementation led to improvement in only one patient and this may in fact have reflected recovery from a respiratory tract infection (Teunisse *et al.* 1996).

More short-lived disturbances might prove reversible, however, and an interesting example was reported by Strachan and Henderson (1965):

A housewife of 60 was admitted with a provisional diagnosis of presenile dementia or stuporose depression. For 4 months she had complained of generalised weakness and vague epigastric discomfort, and had shown purposeless chewing and spitting movements. In recent weeks she had become distant and confused. On examination she lay silent in bed, was disorientated in all spheres, incontinent of urine and faeces, and able to obey only simple commands. There were no abnormal signs in the central nervous system, but the EEG was abnormal with diffuse theta and right centroparietal delta waves. The blood and cerebrospinal fluid were normal. On this occasion she improved spontaneously over the course of 3 weeks and returned to normal.

Five years later she was readmitted with a similar picture of 1 week's duration, and the EEG was even more abnormal with replacement of the alpha rhythm by high voltage theta and delta waves. This time a low serum B_{12} of 64 pg/ml was discovered, along with a histamine-fast achlorhydria but a normal blood and bone marrow. She again improved spontaneously and was discharged before the B_{12} result was known. On recall to the hospital she was now orientated, but her relatives noted that her memory remained poor and that she was lacking in interest in her home and pastimes. The EEG remained abnormal. Vitamin B_{12} produced gradual improvement with return of her normal energy, memory and interests, and this was paralleled by steady improvement in the EEG picture.

Vitamin B_{12} deficiency was likewise incriminated in a patient with an acute organic reaction reported by Smith and Oliver (1967); here, moreover, the possible role of folate administration in leading to the fall in B_{12} levels was illustrated:

A woman of 53 was started on iron and folic acid when anaemia was discovered 11 months earlier. She was admitted to hospital with depression, glossitis and minor symptoms of peripheral neuropathy. Four days later she abruptly became psychotic with confusion, auditory hallucinations and delusions that others were talking about her and that she was about to undergo a serious brain operation. The B_{12} level was 62 pg/ml. After an injection of 1000 µg her mental state began to improve within 24 hours and became normal within a few days. The symptoms of peripheral neuropathy improved over the next few weeks.

There is abundant evidence of cerebral disorder in B_{12} deficiency to serve as a basis for organic psychiatric disturbance. A cerebral pathology is known to occur in pernicious anaemia, similar to that which affects the cord in subacute combined degeneration (Adams & Kubik 1944; Davies-Jones 1989). This consists essentially of diffuse and focal areas of degeneration in the white matter, with relatively little gliosis or change in the neurones, and should therefore be reversible at least in the early stages. The EEG in pernicious anaemia is abnormal in a high proportion of cases (Walton et al. 1954; Kunze & Leitenmaier 1976). Mild abnormalities show as excessive slow activity, and severe abnormalities as delta activity which is sometimes paroxysmal or focal. Such abnormalities bear no simple relationship to the severity of the anaemia but appear to reflect a specific defect of cerebral metabolism. The majority of abnormal records are reversible with treatment, improvement sometimes starting within 7–10 days of the first B_{12} injection. Metabolic studies have also revealed impaired uptake of oxygen and glucose by the brain, especially in the presence of mental symptoms such as forgetfulness, confusion and disorientation, and again responding to replacement therapy (Scheinberg 1951). These too were unrelated to the severity of anaemia and appeared to be a specific result of B_{12} deficiency. Similar disturbances of metabolism may accordingly be expected in patients with low serum B_{12} even in the absence of pernicious anaemia.

Such observations make it important to consider B_{12} deficiency in the differential diagnosis of all patients with unexplained acute organic reactions or dementing syndromes, and to pursue treatment vigorously at the earliest opportunity.

Routine screening

It has been suggested that routine screening of psychiatric populations might bring to light remediable cases of B_{12} deficiency which would otherwise be missed. But the definitive investigation, namely estimation of the serum B_{12} level, clearly cannot be provided for every psychiatric patient.

Various preliminary screening procedures have been proposed. Shulman (1967a) recommended the routine estimation of haemoglobin and examination of blood films before selecting patients for further investigation. This, however, would miss cases presenting with mental symptoms in the pre-anaemic phase. Strachan and Henderson (1965) suggested confining attention to patients with a histamine-fast achlorhydria, but this examination can be difficult to perform on psychiatric patients. Henderson et al. (1966) recommended a test of antigastric antibodies, which is essentially a serum test for the Addisonian state and only an indirect indicator of B_{12} deficiency. It therefore applies only to patients with incipient pernicious anaemia, and not to those with other causes of B_{12} deficiency such as inadequate nutrition. Moreover many false positives are obtained.

In practice the routine screening of psychiatric populations remains of doubtful value. It would seem preferable to confine attention to those at greatest risk, namely any patient with an organic psychiatric illness of uncertain cause, and those who complain of unexplained fatigue or are found to be anaemic. In addition Hunter et al. (1967b) have stressed the importance of assessing B_{12} levels in any psychiatric patient with a history of gastric surgery. Among 20 psychiatric patients with a history of gastrectomy they found five to have low levels of B_{12}, and in four the psychiatric illness was considered to be primarily due to this. Patients with regional ileitis or malabsorption syndromes such as steatorrhoea will also warrant screening. The estimation would further be indicated in any patient who is known to have subsisted for a considerable time on an inadequate diet. Low B_{12} levels are particularly common in vegans.

Finally, symptoms indicative of subacute combined degeneration of the cord must, of course, arouse suspicion in any psychiatric patient:

Early symptoms consist of distal paraesthesiae in the feet and hands, sometimes bizarrely described as feelings of coldness, tightness, constriction or swelling. Constrictive feelings may be experienced around the chest or abdomen. Motor weakness and sensory ataxia may first be described as fatiguability and unsteadiness when walking. Findings on examination include impairment of superficial sensation, often of 'glove and stocking' distribution, loss of vibration and joint position sense, and a positive Romberg's sign. The ankle reflexes are usually absent because of concomitant peripheral neuropathy, but the knee jerks eventually become exaggerated and the plantars up-going.

Treatment

Hydroxocobalamin (Neo-Cytamen) has largely replaced cyanocobalamin (Cytamen) in the treatment of B_{12} deficiency, since it is better retained in the body and maintenance injections are required less frequently. In the treatment of uncomplicated pernicious anaemia six intramuscular injections of 1 mg are usually given at 3-day intervals, before proceeding to maintenance therapy at 1 mg 3-monthly. With subacute combined degeneration of the cord it is customary to give at least twice the loading dose in the early weeks of treatment, and this is equally advisable in patients with suspected cerebral involvement.

Folic acid deficiency

Folic acid deficiency has also become the focus of considerable psychiatric interest. Like B_{12} deficiency it may result in megaloblastic anaemia, though the metabolic interrelationships between the two vitamins are complex and incompletely understood. It has become clear that megaloblastic anaemia due to folate deficiency is commoner in the UK than was previously thought, occurring particularly in pregnancy, in old people who are incapacitated, and in those suffering from psychiatric disorder (British Medical Journal 1968). Accordingly surveys have been made of the prevalence of folate deficiency in psychiatric populations with interesting results. A level of 5 ng/ml is usually accepted as the lower level of normal for serum folic acid, with 2.5 ng/ml representing definite abnormality, though to some extent each laboratory must set its own cut-off point. Read et al. (1965) found that 80% of entrants to an old people's home showed values below 6 ng/ml, and Shulman (1967a) showed a similar proportion among elderly patients admitted to a psychiatric hospital. Hurdle and Picton-Williams (1966) found values below 5 ng/ml in 30% of elderly patients admitted to a geriatric unit with a variety of physical and mental disorders. Even allowing for a possible fall of serum folate with age these proportions are remarkably high. The most common disorders associated with the deficiency appeared to be the organic psychosyndromes of old age.

In younger psychiatric patients low serum folates also appear to be common. Hunter et al. (1967a) found that half of a group of psychiatric hospital admissions of all ages had values below 3 ng/ml. Carney (1967) surveyed 423 consecutive psychiatric admissions of all ages and found that 25% had values below 2 ng/ml. In the latter study a normal control group was selected from the hospital staff, and differences were significant not only for the patients with organic psychoses and epilepsy but also among those with endogenous depression.

Firmer evidence has come from studies of red cell folate levels, which are a better guide to long-term folate stores and less vulnerable to the effects of drugs. Carney et al. (1990) surveyed 285 consecutive patients seen in a psychiatric unit and found borderline (<200 ng/ml) and definite (<150 ng/ml) red cell folate deficiency in 31% and 12% of patients, respectively. The levels in patients with depression were significantly lower than in other groups, but alcoholics were also severely affected.

In all such surveys it is hard to assess the causal significance of the low folates that are found. In the majority of cases deficient nutrition may have been responsible and, as with B_{12} deficiency, this may often be secondary to the mental disorder itself. Or if a causal relationship does exist, the psychiatric disturbance must, at least, often establish a secondary vicious circle by impairing food intake further. Where serum as opposed to red cell folates are concerned, low levels may be the consequence of taking alcohol, barbiturates and possibly other drugs.

Nevertheless in a retrospective survey of a large number of patients, Carney and Sheffield (1970) found evidence to suggest that greater improvement had occurred when the folate deficiency was treated than when it was ignored. The results were most clear with organic psychosyndromes, but appeared also to apply to the quality and speed of recovery of patients with depression and schizophrenia. In the same population the remedying of B_{12} deficiency, when this was discovered, appeared not to be of benefit. More recently Godfrey et al. (1990) have reported a double-blind placebo-controlled trial of adding methylfolate to standard psychotropic medication in 41 patients with low red cell folates and acute psychiatric disorders. Methylfolate was used because this is the form in which folate is actively transported across the blood–brain barrier. Twenty-four of the patients were suffering from depression and 17 from schizophrenia. Over the course of the trial methylfolate supplementation was associated with significant improvement in clinical outcome in both patient groups, which was more evident at 6 months than at 3 months.

It seems possible therefore that even if not directly causal, the folate deficiency may often add its own contribution and worsen the clinical picture in a number of psychiatric conditions.

In addition to these general surveys, particular attention has been focused on folate deficiency in three conditions—depression, dementia and epilepsy.

Depressive illness

The finding of especially low folate levels in depressed patients when compared with other psychiatric groups is of especial interest. Shorvon et al. (1980) paid special attention to the mental status of patients presenting in a general hospital with megaloblastic anaemia due to either B_{12} or folate deficiency. The commonest disturbance in the low folate group was depression, occurring in 50% of patients compared with only 20% of those with B_{12} deficiency.

There are also indications that folate-deficient depressives may have more severe affective disorders and respond less well to conventional treatment. Thus among 100 patients with severe depressive illness Reynolds *et al.* (1970) found evidence that those with low serum folates improved less well with antidepressant drugs or electroconvulsive therapy than the others, as judged by scores on depression inventories at the time of discharge. The differences, though small in size, were statistically significant. A study of out-patient depressives attending a lithium clinic lent some support to these findings; patients with low serum folates showed a higher affective morbidity at the time of the folate assay and also over the preceding 2 years (Coppen & Abou-Saleh 1982).

A causal relationship between folate deficiency and depression is also consistent with biogenic theories of affective disorder. Methylfolate is required for the synthesis of *S*-adenosyl methionine (SAM), which is involved in numerous methylation reactions in the nervous system, including the synthesis of monoamines and neurotransmitters. Moreover SAM has been shown to have antidepressant properties of its own (Reynolds *et al.* 1984; Reynolds 1991).

Dementia

The folate level in the cerebrospinal fluid is known to be several times higher than that in the serum, suggesting that folic acid is likely to be important in cerebral metabolism. It is therefore interesting that occasional case reports have pointed to a close relationship between folic acid deficiency and organic psychiatric illness. Anand (1964) described a patient with megaloblastic anaemia, myelopathy, impairment of memory and moderate dementia of 'frontal lobe type', who showed no response to B_{12} but improved in all respects after starting folic acid. Read *et al.* (1965) similarly described an 82-year-old patient with megaloblastic anaemia due to nutritional deficiency in whom mental confusion and double incontinence improved with folic acid. Two further striking examples were provided by Strachan and Henderson (1967), both with advanced dementia. In each case the folate deficiency followed chronic malnutrition, and the dementia responded gradually to treatment with folic acid; there was a coincident megaloblastic anaemia in both cases but the blood picture returned to normal several months before the mental symptoms resolved:

A 70-year-old widow was seen in domiciliary consultation because of mental deterioration of several months' duration. She was grossly disorientated for time and place and showed a severe defect of recent memory. She had been subsisting on tea and biscuits. In hospital she tended to lose herself in the ward and found it impossible to retain the names of members of staff. There were no neurological abnormalities, the haemoglobin was 69% with a few macrocytes, and the sternal marrow showed megaloblasts. The serum B_{12} was normal, but the folic acid was 2.7 ng/ml. The EEG was moderately abnormal with slowed dominant activity at 7 Hz and fluctuating slower waves.

She was started on folic acid 20 mg daily by mouth together with ferrous sulphate. One month later she was discharged to an old people's home virtually unchanged. When re-examined 2 months later, however, there was considerable improvement — she was clean and tidy, orientated for time and place, recognised the nurses and showed excellent awareness of current events. Learning ability was now within normal limits for her age. The EEG had improved. Nine months later she had maintained her improvement and detailed psychological testing showed further gains in cognitive function.

A 69-year-old widow was admitted with confusion of 3 months' duration, and shortness of breath. She had been living for over a year on tea, toast and biscuits. She lay inert in bed, surveying the scene around in perplexed fashion, gave the year as 1891 and did not know her address. She could not cooperate on tests of memory and tended to confabulate. She was incontinent of urine and faeces.

The haemoglobin was 30% with many macrocytes, and the bone marrow was megaloblastic. The serum B_{12} was normal, and the folate 0.6 ng/ml. The EEG showed widespread theta and random irregular slow waves at 2 Hz. The blood urea, electrolytes and cerebrospinal fluid were normal.

Folic acid was given, 260 µg daily intramuscularly, and packed cells were transfused. After 1 month the haemoglobin had risen to 72% but there had been no definite improvement in the mental state. A month later she knew her age and date of birth, was orientated for time and place, and serial EEGs showed progressively more normal records in parallel with her clinical improvement. Six months later she was readmitted for assessment. She was neatly dressed, fully orientated, gave a good account of her life and previous medical history, and showed an excellent knowledge of current affairs. Psychological testing showed no evidence of intellectual impairment. Her improvement was maintained when seen 2 years later.

(Strachan & Henderson 1967)

Melamed (1979) reviews further examples of patients with organic psychiatric syndromes, often in association with spinal cord damage or peripheral neuropathy, who responded to folate replacement. Nevertheless the rarity of such patients is surprising in view of the frequency of nutritional folate deficiency. Melamed suggests that long-standing folate deficiency, or individual susceptibility, may be necessary before such effects are declared.

While severe mental impairment is rare, it seems possible that some degree of cerebral dysfunction may be commoner than generally suspected. Among patients presenting in a general hospital with very low folate levels, Reynolds *et al.* (1973) found that cognitive abnormalities were significantly commoner than in controls.

Shorvon *et al.* (1980) found that approximately a quarter of patients with megaloblastic anaemia showed organic mental changes, the proportion being similar when low folate and low B_{12} were responsible. Botez *et al.* (1977) found some evidence pointing to minor changes on CT scans in their low folate patients, and were able to demonstrate significant improvements on psychometric tests after folic acid replacement.

With regard to the general problem of dementia in the elderly, Sneath *et al.* (1973) studied 113 consecutive admissions to a geriatric unit, of whom 14 were diagnosed as suffering from dementia. These patients had significantly lower red cell folates than the remainder. Moreover, where red cell folates were low in the patients as a whole, there was a small correlation between scores of mental impairment and the red cell folate level. The likely explanation seemed to be that dementia had led to the folate deficiency, by virtue of poor dietary intake, but the possibility could not be excluded that folate deficiency might of itself have led to impaired mental function.

Epilepsy

In epilepsy there is universal agreement that a low serum folate, with or without megaloblastic anaemia, can result from the administration of anticonvulsant drugs. Phenobarbitone, phenytoin and primidone all appear to be responsible, and it has been suggested that there may be a causal relationship between their antifolate and anticonvulsant properties. In one series of treated epileptics attending an out-patient clinic over three-quarters showed subnormal serum folate levels, and over one-third had megaloblastic haemopoiesis. The serum B_{12} levels were within the normal range but tended to be low when the folic acid was low (Reynolds *et al.* 1966a; Reynolds *et al.* 1966b).

Moreover, folate levels appear to be lower in mentally abnormal epileptics than in those who are free from psychiatric symptoms, whether measured in the serum, red blood corpuscles or cerebrospinal fluid (Reynolds *et al.* 1969; Reynolds *et al.* 1971a; Edeh & Toone 1985). The differences have sometimes been found to be particularly large where dementia is concerned, but also to apply to depression and schizophrenia-like illnesses. Snaith *et al.* (1970) found levels to be low in small groups suffering from schizophrenia, depression, neurosis and personality disorder when compared to mentally healthy epileptics, but could find no clear relationship to any particular form of psychiatric disturbance.

The usual difficulties are encountered in assessing the significance of these findings, and in deciding how far the folate levels may be causally related to the psychiatric

abnormalities. Reynolds (1967a) treated a group of folate-deficient epileptics with folic acid in an uncontrolled investigation, and found that the mental state improved over the ensuing months in the great majority. Improvement was seen in energy, drive, alertness and sociability, mood swings were lessened and aggressive behaviour reduced. But half of the patients showed a coincident increase in fit frequency or severity which sometimes necessitated termination of treatment. Reynolds (1967b) also drew attention to a possible relationship between schizophrenia-like episodes in patients with temporal lobe epilepsy and disturbances of folate or B_{12} metabolism induced by treatment with anticonvulsant drugs.

Subsequent controlled trials have, however, so far failed to confirm these findings. Grant and Stores (1970) carried out a double-blind trial on in-patient epileptics with low serum folates, and found that folic acid was without significant effect on tests of speed of thought and action, personality, behaviour or fit frequency. Norris and Pratt (1971) confirmed these negative findings where fit frequency was concerned, and suggested that the occasional examples — even of status epilepticus on starting folic acid — were probably due to chance. Smith and Obbens (1979) reviewed the continuing uncertainty surrounding folate supplementation and seizures, concluding that while most patients were unaffected, individual epileptics could undoubtedly suffer adverse consequences.

Thus while an association between lowered folate and mental disturbance in epileptics appears to be firmly established, a causal relationship remains to be definitely proved. The results of giving the vitamin are also uncertain. Blood–brain barrier effects appear to be important in determining the effects of administered folic acid, and differing durations of treatment may go some way towards explaining discrepant findings to date (Reynolds 1973, 1991).

Routine screening

Again the problem arises whether psychiatric patients should be screened routinely for folic acid deficiency. Estimation of folate levels would seem to be indicated in any patient with an acute or chronic organic mental illness of uncertain aetiology, and a case can be made for including it as a routine investigation for every patient diagnosed as suffering from senile or presenile dementia. The same applies to epileptic patients on anticonvulsant drugs who show marked psychomotor retardation or psychiatric disturbance. The large number of patients with depressive illnesses makes routine screening impractical in most settings. Nevertheless estimations of folic acid should be performed whenever there is a history of subsistence on an inadequate diet, of malabsorption syndromes such as steatorrhoea, or in the presence of megaloblastic anaemia. Patients who show a surprisingly poor response to treatment will also warrant investigation.

Treatment

A trial of treatment with folic acid, 5 mg three times per day, is well worth while when deficient levels are found. It should, however, always be preceded by careful screening for B_{12} deficiency. The serum B_{12} tends to fall when folic acid is started (Reynolds *et al.* 1971b), suggesting that the two vitamins are intimately involved in the metabolic disturbances and that some patients may need treatment with both. Moreover there is danger of precipitating or aggravating neurological disturbances by giving folic acid in patients with undiagnosed pernicious anaemia.

Chapter 13: Toxic Disorders

Alcohol, drugs and certain metals and chemicals are the exogenous toxins that will be considered in this chapter. The effects of toxins derived from invading microorganisms have been briefly considered on pp. 368–9, and the toxic products of disordered metabolism in uraemia and hepatic dysfunction in Chapter 11.

Alcohol is the toxin most commonly encountered in psychiatric practice, though the effects of drug abuse must now be frequently considered in the differential diagnosis of acute psychiatric disturbance. Poisoning due to metals and other chemical compounds is largely the province of industrial medicine, but must also be borne in mind in occasional patients who present with psychiatric illness of uncertain aetiology.

Effects of alcohol on the nervous system

Alcohol is remarkable for the range of nervous system disorders that it can produce and for the diversity of mechanisms by which they come about. First there is the direct toxic effect of alcohol present within the body, which acts as a depressant of central nervous functioning; a further series of disorders including fits, hallucinoses and delirium tremens are largely due to alcohol withdrawal; associated nutritional defects lead to Wernicke's encephalopathy, Korsakoff's psychosis, peripheral neuropathy and perhaps cerebellar degeneration; and liver disorder or hypoglycaemia may ensue with their own neuropsychiatric complications. In addition there is evidence that alcohol and/or its metabolites may exert lasting neurotoxic effects. The distinction between these mechanisms cannot be considered absolute for all of the syndromes concerned, but in general reaches broad agreement. The nutritional disorders associated with alcoholism have been considered in Chapter 12, and the direct toxic effects and withdrawal effects will be considered below.

Alcohol intoxication

Alcohol acts as a central nervous system depressant in a manner analogous to that of anaesthetic agents, though acting very much more slowly and with a greatly reduced margin between the level producing surgical anaesthesia and the level which depresses the respiratory centres to a dangerous extent. Its initial action is probably on the reticular formation, leading to increased excitability of the cortex. Later there are depressant effects on the cortical neurones as well.

The early effects are to produce inebriation, usually with subjective exhilaration, excitement and loquacity. Personality factors and environmental factors are important at this stage, lively company leading usually to boisterous cheerfulness, whereas alcohol taken alone may intensify feelings of loneliness and depression. Cultural influences are also clearly important in helping to shape the outward evidence of intoxication (Edwards 1974).

Soon there is reduction of psychological efficiency and motor control, which is often at variance with subjective feelings of superiority and skill. Thinking becomes slowed and superficial, with poverty of associations and impaired judgement and reasoning. Learning and retention become faulty, and remote memory unreliable. Acuity of perception is reduced, attention impaired and distractibility increased. Muscular control is impaired at an early stage and reaction times delayed. Later dysarthria, frank incoordination and ataxia appear.

With more severe intoxication there is progressive loss of restraint, self control becomes undermined and irregularities of behaviour appear. Emotions of hilarity, sadness or self pity may gain the upper hand, or there may be marked irritability and hostility. With very high blood levels there is increasing drowsiness, leading finally to coma. In alcoholic coma the breathing is slow and stertorous and the temperature subnormal. The pupils may be contracted or widely dilated and the tendon reflexes weak or absent.

A fairly close relationship exists between the intensity of the effects and the level of alcohol in the blood. A level of 150–250 mg/100 ml is usually associated with very obvious signs of intoxication, and the legal maximum for drivers in the UK is set at 80 mg/100 ml (17.4 mmol/l). Arguments can be marshalled, however, for setting it considerably lower (Guppy 1994). The situation is complex, however, depending on the rate of rise to a given level and also the length of time that alcohol has been in the body. Thus a quick rise will produce effects at a lower level of blood alcohol than a gradual rise, and for a given rate of rise the effects will be less marked if alcohol has been present at a constant level for some time before. Isbell *et al.* (1955) found slowing of rhythms on the EEG when signs of clinical intoxication appeared, but later this effect diminished even though the blood level rose higher still. Tolerance within the central nervous system may be obvious in habitués, who absorb more quickly from the gastrointestinal tract yet at the same time become resistant to the early effects. Prolonged ingestion can also lead to metabolic adaptation; there is evidence to suggest that during periods of long-continued chronic intoxication the subject metabolises alcohol at an increased rate (Isbell *et al.* 1955).

'Pathological intoxication'

On occasion irrational combative behaviour may develop abruptly during the course of intoxication. In marked examples it presents as an outburst of uncontrollable rage and excitement leading to destructive actions against other persons and property. This is the 'pathological reaction to alcohol', 'pathological intoxication', 'acute alcoholic paranoid state' or 'manie à potu', much discussed in the earlier literature. As typically described the behaviour is out of character for the individual concerned, the duration is short and there is subsequently amnesia for the entire episode. Banay (1944) and May and Ebaugh (1953) review the condition.

It was sometimes maintained that such responses could follow the ingestion of relatively small amounts of alcohol, and that the normal associated phenomena of intoxication could be minimal or absent. The condition accordingly attained considerable medicolegal importance. It was regarded as an acute organic reaction or a short-lived paranoid psychosis released by alcohol in especially susceptible persons. Special attributes of personality were held to be responsible, or periods of strain or great exhaustion. Tendencies to epilepsy or hypoglycaemia were sometimes invoked.

There have, however, been few critical studies relating to the condition or its antecedents. Coid (1979), in a thorough review, found virtually nothing to support the notion that small amounts of alcohol could trigger such outbursts, and little to suggest that they could develop in persons of stable disposition. The nosological status of the condition seemed very doubtful. He considered that the label should be dropped, and that the conception could be of little use in courts of law in cases of alcohol-related violence.

There is perhaps some evidence to suggest that brain-damaged persons may be particularly liable to display reactions of this nature. Morozov *et al.* (1973) examined 105 persons who had committed infringements of the law in a condition of 'pathological intoxication' and 100 in 'simple intoxication'. Ninety-one per cent of the former showed evidence of organic changes in the central nervous system, mainly traumatic in origin, compared to 50% of the latter. This may, of course, reflect no more than the well-known increased susceptibility to severe intoxication in the presence of brain damage.

Attempts to study pathological intoxication directly have led to conflicting results. Bach-y-Rita *et al.* (1970) gave intravenous infusions of alcohol to 10 men with a history of violent outbursts when intoxicated, but in no case was the abnormal behaviour reproduced. In a similar experiment, however, Maletzky (1976) obtained the expected reactions in 15 of 22 cases. Nine became violent with inappropriate rage, four became psychotic with hallucinations and delusions, and two showed a mixture of both. The remainder developed normal intoxication only.

Maletzky's experiment is important in demonstrating that large amounts of alcohol were necessary before the disturbed behaviour occurred, the mean blood alcohol level at the time being 195 mg/100 ml. Many subjects showed changes in the EEG during the course of the infusion, but these did not correlate with the abnormal behavioural responses. In general the disturbed behaviour was superimposed on the normal phenomena of intoxication, but occasionally signs of the latter were slight. In some cases a witness to the disturbance could well have been blind to the causative agent. Maletzky's further impression that the behavioural responses were out of keeping with the personality of the subjects when sober is hard to evaluate. Further controlled studies would obviously be necessary to clarify the point.

Alcoholic 'blackouts'

Special interest attaches to the abnormalities of memory which may follow a period of severe intoxication. An amnesic gap will of course follow any bout of drinking which is carried to the point of severe impairment of consciousness, but the alcoholic 'blackout' is a phenomenon of a more specific kind. It consists of a dense amnesia for significant events which have occurred during a drinking episode, when at the time outward behaviour perhaps seemed little disordered. Usually the gap extends for a period of several hours, but very occasionally it may cover several days. The subject may have carried on a conversation and gone through quite elaborate activities, for all of which there is no trace of memory next day. On rare occasions grossly abnormal or even criminal conduct may have occurred during the episode, and the amnesic gap can then become a matter of medicolegal importance (Sweeney 1990). The onset, as judged by subjective recall, is usually abrupt, and the end of the amnesic gap may be equally sharp if sleep does not follow directly.

Goodwin *et al.* (1969a, 1969b) presented a detailed description of the nature of blackouts in 64 alcoholic subjects. They confirmed that behaviour during the episode was usually similar to behaviour during any heavy drinking bout, except that some subjects tended to travel long distances as in fugue states. Thus a quarter of their patients had found themselves in strange places with no recollection of how they got there. The wives of two patients claimed that they could tell when a blackout was in progress on account of a glassy stare, belligerent behaviour or the repetition of questions which showed that experiences were failing to register. *En bloc* blackouts, as just described, were distinguished from 'fragmentary' losses in which the subject was unaware that events had been forgotten until he was told about them later. Sometimes in this milder variety the memories might return with the passage of time, and sometimes recall was facilitated by further drinking. Thus many subjects had had the experience of hiding money or alcohol when drinking, forgetting it when sober, and later having the memory return in a subsequent drinking bout.

Such episodes can represent profoundly disturbing experiences for an alcoholic. They are commoner, apparently, after the ingestion of spirits than after wine or beer (World Health Organization Report 1955). The sharpness of the rise and fall of the blood alcohol level has been thought to be more important than the height attained, and sometimes the episodes have been reported to follow the drinking of medium or even quite small amounts. Jellinek (1952) drew attention to their frequency in the histories of established alcoholics, usually dating from a time before the drinking had got out of control. He suggested that repeated experience of the phenomenon might be a prodromal sign of alcohol addiction, and that its occurrence after only medium alcohol intake represented heightened susceptibility or sensitivity to the effects of alcohol in the prospective addict. Goodwin *et al.* (1969a, 1969b) were unable to confirm these features in their careful study. The occurrence of blackouts was directly associated with the severity and duration of alcoholism. They appeared only late in the course of the

illness, and well after physical dependence and loss of control had become established. Blackouts were very rarely seen unless large amounts of alcohol were being consumed, chiefly in the form of spirits. Goodwin *et al.* also noticed a fairly strong association with a prior history of head injury.

Tarter and Schneider (1976) investigated the possibility that alcoholics subject to blackouts might have some enduring impairment of memory when sober, but with negative results. Those with frequent blackouts performed as well as those in whom blackouts were rare on a wide battery of memory measures. The quantity of intake on a given occasion again seemed to be the discriminating factor—the group with many blackouts had a significantly greater tendency to drink to intoxication or until falling asleep, and showed a significantly higher frequency of craving, tolerance and loss of control.

The pathogenesis of these episodes remains uncertain. They have been attributed to psychogenic mechanisms of repression, especially in view of the emotional setting in which some of the attacks are known to occur. Malingering has been suspected in the occasional cases where they have been used as a defence against charges of criminal behaviour. The majority, however, must be accepted as organically determined. An interesting suggestion is that they may represent the effects of 'state-dependent learning'. It has been shown that animals trained in a drugged state may 'remember' their training better when retested in a comparable drugged state, indicating that learning depends for its optimum expression on restoration of the original conditions in which the learning was acquired. Goodwin *et al.* (1969c) have demonstrated an analogous situation in volunteers trained and tested under the effects of alcohol. For some tasks learning transfer proved to be better when the subject was intoxicated in both the first and the second test sessions, than when he was intoxicated in the first but sober in the second. This accords with the observation cited above that events during an alcoholic blackout may sometimes be recalled under subsequent alcoholic intoxication.

Another study has added further information by investigating short-term memory and 24-hour recall during a 2-week period of sustained intoxication (Tamerin *et al.* 1971):

Thirteen alcoholic patients, all with a long history of 'blackouts', were tested each day for registration (5 seconds recall) and short-term memory (1 and 5 minutes recall) of simple test material, and were also asked a set of standard questions about the activities of the day before. During periods of moderate intoxication registration was substantially normal, but short-term memory was considerably impaired. More severe intoxication showed a significant fall in registration and a more profound decrement in short-term memory. Ability to recall the events of the preceding day was significantly reduced on days following moderate intoxication and more so on days following severe intoxication. The decrement was also related to the duration of intoxication, in that it tended to become worse as the days of the experiment went by. Deficits in 24-hour recall were also more frequent and severe the worse the short-term memory had been when tested on the preceding day. Conversely, 24-hour recall was always normal in subjects who had shown intact short-term memory the day before.

Marked individual susceptibility was revealed, however, with the same blood alcohol level affecting different subjects to a different extent. Only six of the 13 subjects showed 'blackouts' — defined as ability to answer less than 30% of the questions concerning the previous day's activities. Three of the subjects were particularly vulnerable in this regard. No relationship was discovered to factors commonly thought to be important such as age, intelligence, history of head injury, presence of EEG abnormalities, duration of drinking history or history of delirium tremens.

This investigation therefore clearly reinstates the importance of an organic basis for the blackout. State-dependent effects were excluded in this particular setting because 24-hour recall was tested while the subjects were still intoxicated. The correlates of individual vulnerability remain an important question for further investigation.

Treatment of intoxication

An acute episode of intoxication rarely calls for specific medical treatment, but severely intoxicated persons should be kept under close observation in case alcoholic coma should supervene. Gastric lavage is usually unnecessary since alcohol is rapidly absorbed from the stomach. If there is a possibility that drugs have been taken as well, however, lavage will be indicated. Episodes of paranoid or combative behaviour may, on occasion, require sedation with major tranquillisers, but there are obvious hazards involved in adding one cerebral depressant to another. In actual management the most important factor is usually the handling that the patient receives from those around, who must attempt to react in as good-natured and unprovocative a way as possible. Kelly *et al.* (1971) have shown that intravenous injections of high potency vitamins B and C can reduce the subjective effects of intoxication and improve performance on reaction time tests, apparently by virtue of a direct effect on the central nervous system, but this will rarely need to be exploited in practice.

Alcoholic coma represents a medical emergency and should be managed in hospital. Care is needed to exclude coincident head injury and its complications, gastrointestinal bleeding, hepatic failure, pneumonia or meningitis. Blood should be taken to confirm the presence of significant amounts of alcohol and to exclude barbiturate intoxication or alcoholic hypoglycaemia (pp. 543–4). A clear airway must be maintained, analeptic drugs may be indicated, and peripheral circulatory failure may require intravenous fluids, vasopressor drugs and steroids. If glucose-containing fluids are transfused thiamine must always be given in case Wernicke's encephalopathy should be precipitated. Intravenous fructose or even peritoneal dialysis may occasionally be indicated to accelerate the rate of fall in blood alcohol levels (O'Neill *et al.* 1984).

Abstinence or withdrawal syndromes

An important group of manifestations occur against a background of severe alcohol abuse but make their appearance usually after a period of complete or relative abstention. It seems, therefore, that they depend not on the direct toxic effects of alcohol present at the time, but rather on a fall in the level circulating within the body (Victor & Adams 1953; Isbell *et al.* 1955). They include tremulousness, hallucinosis, fits and most important of all delirium tremens.

The precise mechanisms underlying these disorders are far from clear. Where hallucinosis and delirium tremens are concerned several complex factors are probably at work. But all share in common the tendency to occur shortly after drinking has stopped or been abruptly curtailed. The clearest evidence comes from the experiments of Isbell *et al.* (1955), who kept 10 subjects continuously intoxicated for periods of 6–12 weeks while a high calorie diet was given along with full vitamin supplements. No fits or delirium occurred while consumption continued, but on withdrawal all developed an abstinence syndrome characterised by tremors, weakness, nausea, vomiting, hyperreflexia and fever. Two had seizures, two experienced transient auditory and visual hallucinations, and three developed frank delirium tremens. The intensity of the withdrawal symptoms was related to the amount of alcohol that had been taken and the duration of consumption. Only one of the subjects who had persisted with continuous drinking beyond 7 weeks escaped without fits or hallucinations. Serial EEG records had shown slowing during the period of acute intoxication, but on withdrawal became normal for a while; 16–33 hours later the alpha rhythm diminished and random spikes and bursts of slow waves appeared coincidentally with the more severe withdrawal effects. This was therefore an unusually clear demonstration that withdrawal is a factor of prime importance in producing these phenomena, and also that nutritional deficiency is unlikely to be causally related.

The discovery of the different stages of sleep brought new evidence concerning alcohol withdrawal (Greenberg & Pearlman 1967; Gross & Goodenough 1968). Increasing levels of alcohol suppress the rapid eye movement (REM) phase of sleep (p. 725) and the dreaming associated with it. With continuation of drinking some readjustment occurs, but on withdrawal an abrupt rebound is seen with a great excess of REM sleep. Immediately prior to an attack of delirium tremens REM sleep may occupy the whole of the sleeping time. It has been suggested that the vivid hallucinations of delirium tremens may represent a 'spilling over' of this active dream material into waking life. The essential mechanisms remain to be clarified, but certainly there appears to be an important relationship between the nature of the sleep disturbances associated with alcohol withdrawal and the clinical manifestations that occur.

A further interesting hypothesis has been put forward by Ballenger and Post (1978) who draw analogies with the phenomenon of 'kindling' in rats and other animals:

It has been shown that brief bursts of electrical brain stimulation, carried out at daily intervals and at constant intensity, can result in enduring changes in brain excitability (Goddard *et al.* 1969). Much theoretical interest attaches to the process. Stimulation which is initially subthreshold in its effect gradually acquires increased potency with daily repetition. After-discharges appear, increase, and spread widely to subcortical brain structures, eventually manifesting epileptiform spikes and then sustained epileptic discharges. Behavioural concomitants likewise develop, first in the form of motor automatisms then progressing to seizures in response to the stimulation. Stimulation within the limbic areas of the brain elicits kindling most reliably, and repeat stimulation at intervals of 24 hours appears to be the optimal rate for its development.

Ballenger and Post point out that similar kindling effects can result from the administration of metrazol and other drugs, and suggest that repeated heavy alcohol intake may have analogous effects. Intoxication and withdrawal are accompanied by minor dysrhythmias as described just above. Limbic system hyperirritability accompanying each episode of withdrawal may thus conceivably increase by the kindling process and spread widely in subcortical structures. Long-term changes in neuronal excitability may accordingly underlie the progressive escalation of withdrawal symptoms from tremors, to seizures, and ultimately to delirium tremens. Direct electrophysiological evidence for the hypothesis is necessarily lacking in humans, since depth electrode studies would be required. But Ballenger and Post have presented other data consistent with the hypothesis. In a survey of the incidence and forms of withdrawal phenomena in a large group of alcoholics, they demonstrated a stepwise escalation in the severity of the symptomatology as the years of alcohol abuse increased. Similar stepwise behavioural changes in response to stimulation are observed during kindling in animals.

Hemmingsen and Kramp (1988) review experimental work indicative of changes in membrane phospholipids and synaptic structure following repeated alcohol withdrawal. They suggest that withdrawal reactions consist essentially of two components — physical signs such as tremor which are determined by the degree of physical dependence developed during the most recent drinking bout, and seizures, hallucinations and delirium which reflect long-term central nervous system dysfunction accruing over many years of repeated intoxication and withdrawal. A combination of both factors may be operative in some of the withdrawal phenomena encountered.

From clinical evidence it would appear that tremulousness, nausea and transient hallucinations in clear consciousness are among the earliest withdrawal phenomena, occurring often within 3–12 hours of cessation of drinking. Fits occur somewhat later after an interval of 12–48 hours, and the full syndrome of delirium tremens usually only after 3–4 days (Victor & Adams 1953). It is well established that a prolonged period of indulgence is necessary for the more severe effects to occur. With all withdrawal phenomena temporary alleviation follows the taking of alcohol again. All are essentially benign conditions with the exception of delirium tremens.

Alcoholic tremor

This, the commonest withdrawal effect, is usually associated with general weakness, nausea and irritability. In mild form it can occur after a single night's abstinence and after a period of drinking of only several days. In severe form it usually occurs 12–24 hours after stopping, and only after several weeks of continuous drinking. The patient is alert, startles easily, suffers insomnia and craves the relief which further alcohol will bring. Usually the disorder subsides over several hours or days, but after severe attacks it may be 1 or 2 weeks before the patient is composed and can sleep without sedation.

Hallucinosis

Approximately a quarter of tremulous patients have disordered sense perception, ranging from transitory misperceptions of familiar objects to illusions and hallucinations (Victor & Adams 1953). Hallucinations usually occur in both the visual and auditory modalities, are generally fleeting and emerge in clear consciousness. The absence of disorientation, confusion and psychomotor overactivity is important in distinguishing the condition from delirium tremens. It is usually a benign condition, lasting often less than 24 hours and rarely for more than a few days.

Sabot *et al.* (1968) found that the hallucinations are often accompanied by simple auditory and visual sensory disturbances which seem to facilitate their appearance. Tinnitus is common with auditory hallucinations, antedating their appearance and persisting after they have cleared. Visual disturbances in the form of blurring, flashes and spots are usually reported by patients with formed visual hallucinations. The visual hallucinations are mostly of small animals such as rodents and insects, characteristically moving rapidly on the walls, floor or ceiling. Larger animals or human beings may also be seen, or fleeting half-formed images of faces.

As with tremulousness, withdrawal of alcohol appears to be the chief factor leading to transient hallucinations. Occasional patients, however, develop hallucinations while continuing to drink, and in these it has been suggested that thiamine deficiency may be a contributory cause (Morgan 1968). Blackstock *et al.* (1972) followed this possibility further, but were unable to demonstrate a significant difference in indicators of thiamine levels between alcoholics with or without a recent episode of hallucinatory disturbance.

The term *alcoholic hallucinosis* is sometimes used in a more restricted sense to refer to the relatively rare condition in which verbal auditory hallucinations occur alone, again in a setting of clear consciousness. Most examples clear within a few days, but the disorder may sometimes be prolonged. As such the picture may strongly resemble schizophrenia, and a good deal of discussion has centred on its nosological status.

The auditory hallucinations often commence as simple sounds such as buzzing, roaring or the ringing of bells. Gradually they take on vocal form, usually the voices of friends or enemies who malign, threaten or reproach the patient. The hallucinations may consist of a single derogatory remark repeated with relentless persistence, or the patient may be assailed by a combination of accusations and admonitions. He may be discovered arguing angrily with his voices, or he may complain to the police about them. Sometimes the voices command the patient to do things against his will, and their compelling quality may be such that he is driven to a suicide attempt or some episode of bizarre behaviour. Usually the voices address the patient directly, but sometimes they converse with one another about him, referring to him in the third person as in schizophrenia. Secondary delusional interpretations follow upon the hallucinatory experiences,

and the patient comes to believe firmly that he is watched, hounded or in danger.

The result is an illness which at first sight resembles acute paranoid schizophrenia. The delusions will be found, however, to follow only upon the hallucinatory experiences and not to arise autochthonously. Schizophrenic thought disorder is not seen, nor incongruity of affect, and insight is regained immediately the voices begin to wane. The syndrome must, of course, be viewed separately from the picture seen in established schizophrenic patients who also drink. Such patients may similarly develop abrupt auditory hallucinations when drinking and during withdrawal, since drinking bouts may aggravate the schizophrenic process. The distinction is made on the basis of the preceding history and the features in the mental state as just outlined.

Victor and Hope (1958) review the divergent views about the implications of the illness, ranging from the belief that it represents a form of schizophrenia released by alcohol, to the view that it represents an independent psychosis induced by drinking for many years. Of their 76 examples 90% showed hallucinations which were benign and transient, the great majority clearing within a week. Hallucinations became chronic in only eight patients, persisting then for months or years. In four of the latter the disorder ultimately resolved without the development of more serious psychiatric illness; only in the remaining four was there progression to a true schizophrenia-like illness with ideas of influence, emotional withdrawal and persistent paranoid delusions. Family histories gave no indication of special allegiance with schizophrenia, and the previous personality tended to be cyclothymic rather than schizoid. This applied even in those rare cases which did prove ultimately to develop a schizophrenia-like illness.

In these important respects the findings were in broad agreement with Benedetti's (1952) large series. Eighty per cent of 113 cases cleared within a few weeks or months, usually leaving no psychiatric defect whatever. The great majority of these cleared within a few hours or days. The remaining 23 became chronic, some developing typical schizophrenia and the others a chronic amnesic syndrome or dementia. Six months appeared to be the cut-off point beyond which remissions could not be expected. In the group as a whole a family history of schizophrenia was a great deal lower than among the relatives of schizophrenics, though possibly somewhat higher than in the general population.

There is therefore little to suggest that auditory hallucinosis is merely latent schizophrenia made manifest by alcohol. The mechanisms involved remain uncertain, beyond the fact that prolonged indulgence in alcohol is a necessary precursor and that abstinence is frequently observed prior to its onset. Of the 76 cases reported by Victor and Hope (1958), only 15 began while the patient was still drinking, and three of these were reducing their intake substantially at the time. In the remainder the hallucinations began after drinking had stopped entirely, usually setting in 12–48 hours later. The factors which determine the occasional prolongation of the hallucinosis or transition to a schizophrenia-like illness remain unknown, but there is some indication that repeated attacks may make the patient ultimately more vulnerable to the type of attack which leads on to schizophrenic deterioration.

Phenothiazine drugs are usually effective in treatment. Electroconvulsive therapy may terminate the attack abruptly in those cases which persist beyond a few weeks.

Alcoholic convulsions ('rum fits')

The consumption of alcohol can precipitate fits in a person suffering from epilepsy, and sometimes this happens after a 'normal' evening's drinking. Commonly the fit then occurs next morning during sobering up. Quite distinct from this are the withdrawal fits which may occur in persons without special epileptic predisposition. These occur only after heavy consumption, and usually within 12–48 hours of the termination of a long-continued bout. They are usually seen only after several years of established alcohol addiction. Very occasionally they occur while consumption continues, presumably as a result of transient falls in the blood alcohol level.

Mostly the fits occur in bouts of two to six at a time, and very occasionally status epilepticus may be precipitated. The fits are usually grand mal in type. If a focal component exists this is likely to be the result of trauma in addition to alcoholism. In almost 30% of cases the fits are followed by delirium tremens. Conversely 30% of cases of delirium tremens and 10% of cases of auditory hallucinosis are preceded by fits (Victor & Adams 1953).

The EEG is abnormal at the time of the fits, but reverts to normal thereafter. It remains normal in the intervals between, thus discrediting the wide belief that they represent a latent epileptic process which has been brought to light (Victor 1966).

In addition to withdrawal seizures, and seizures precipitated by alcohol in persons suffering from epilepsy, it has been proposed that alcohol may sometimes provoke fits directly ('alcoholic epilepsy'). Thus patients may be observed in whom seizures are closely associated with alcohol intake, sometimes repeatedly, and in the absence of other predisposing factors. The uncertain nosological status of this group, which is certainly very small, is discussed by Brennan and Lyttle (1987).

Delirium tremens

Delirium tremens represents by far the most serious of the alcohol withdrawal phenomena with a mortality of up to 5%. Some large series of cases have been reported to show a lower mortality, but have probably included many partial and incomplete forms.

Definition

The fully developed syndrome consists of vivid hallucinations, delusions, profound confusion, tremor, agitation, sleeplessness and autonomic overactivity. Defined in this way delirium tremens is relatively uncommon, and was found to represent only 5% of a consecutive series of 266 patients admitted to Boston City Hospital with an obvious complication of alcoholism (Victor & Adams 1953). By contrast in the same series acute tremulousness occurred in 34%, transient hallucinosis with tremor in 11%, auditory hallucinosis in 2%, fits in 12% and the Wernicke–Korsakoff syndrome in 3%.

Before diagnosing delirium tremens McNichol (1970) requires the presence of hallucinations along with at least two of the following: confusion and disorientation, tremulousness, increased psychomotor activity, fearfulness and signs of autonomic disturbance. He recognises three grades in the development of the complete syndrome: first, mental sluggishness with tremor and evidence of residual intoxication; later, emotional lability, agitation, fearfulness, increased psychomotor activity, autonomic disturbance, nightmares and disorientation; and finally the onset of definitive delirium tremens with the appearance of hallucinations. The presence of autonomic hyperactivity (tachycardia, sweating, fever) can be of considerable diagnostic importance in pointing towards the condition when the cause of a delirious state is not immediately obvious.

Clinical features

Delirium tremens frequently presents in a dramatic manner and appears to have had an explosive onset. But when opportunities arise for observing during the evolution of the illness a prodromal phase is commonly seen. The onset is usually at night, with restlessness, insomnia and fear. The patient startles at the least sound, has vivid nightmares and wakes repeatedly in panic. Transient illusions and hallucinations may occur even at this stage, and typically arouse intense anxiety even though insight may still be largely retained.

As the illness becomes more fully declared the face is anxious or terror stricken. The patient is tremulous, and if out of bed is usually seen to be ataxic. There is evidence of dehydration with dry lips, a coated tongue and scanty urine. Restlessness is extreme, with agitated activity by day and night, preventing sleep and leading ultimately to dangerous physical exhaustion. Autonomic disturbance shows in perspiration, flushing or pallor, dilated pupils, a weak rapid pulse and mild pyrexia. Epileptic seizures occur in up to a third of cases, virtually always preceding the delirium (Victor & Adams 1953).

Illusions and hallucinations occur in great profusion, principally in the visual modality but also auditory and haptic. Spots on the counterpane may be mistaken for insects, and cracks on the ceiling for snakes. Visual hallucinations typically consist of fleeting, recurrent and changeable images which compulsively hold the patient's attention. Rats, snakes and other small animals are said to be typical, and can appear in colourful and vivid forms. They are frequently Lilliputian in size, and invested with rapid ceaseless activity. The author has observed a patient who followed intently, and with excited comments, a game of football performed for half an hour on end by two teams of normal-coloured miniature elephants in a corner of his room. Other hallucinations may be normal in size, such as threatening faces or fantastic scenes depicting terrifying situations. Sometimes the hallucinations are amusing or playful in nature, and recapture some of the bonhomie of the patient and his companions during drinking spells. The patient's occupation and experience may colour the perceptual disorders, the station master seeing trains rapidly approaching him, or the factory worker seeing his bench before him and going through the motions of his work activities.

Auditory hallucinations are commonly of a threatening or persecutory nature. Vestibular disturbances are frequent, and felt by the patient as rotation of the room or movement of the floor. Insects may be felt to be crawling over the skin, perhaps as an elaboration of paraesthesiae.

A marked feature is the intense reality with which the hallucinatory experiences are imbued, and the strong emotional reactions they produce. Apprehension and fear are typical, but amusement and even jocularity may be seen. Sometimes apprehension and amusement are mixed together in a characteristic and paradoxical manner. As with the hallucinations themselves the affective state is often changeable from one moment to another, though fear or even terror is usually uppermost.

The degree of impairment of consciousness varies widely from case to case and in the same patient from one moment to another. It is rarely profound except in the terminal stages, though the true level may be very hard to judge. Diminished awareness of the environment is coupled with overarousal in a characteristic fashion. The patient appears to be alert and over-responsive, but his responsiveness usually proves to be closely tied to his own internal stimuli; he may startle easily but is otherwise largely unaware and indifferent to what proceeds in the real world around him. Disorientation and confusion are very obvious, but the degree of inattention and distractibility may give the impression that consciousness is more severely impaired than is actually the case. When attention can be held fleetingly it is sometimes possible to show that memory and other intellectual functions are intact to a surprising degree.

Speech is usually slurred and with paraphasic errors. In severe examples it may be incoherent and fragmented. Delusions are secondarily elaborated on the faulty perceptual experiences, but are usually fragmented, transitory and as changeable as the hallucinations. Suggestibility is marked and adds to the frequency with which illusions occur; pressing on the eyeballs may cause the patient to see whatever one tells him he sees, and when presented with a blank piece of paper he may proceed to 'read' it on instruction.

The EEG typically shows fast activity in delirium tremens as described on p. 131. In this it is in marked contrast to the picture seen in most other forms of delirium where slowing of the dominant rhythms is the characteristic pattern.

Outcome

The disorder is usually short lived, lasting less than 3 days in the majority of cases. Very rarely recurrent phases may be seen over a longer period of time. Typically it terminates in a prolonged sleep after which the patient feels fully recovered apart from residual weakness and exhaustion. In rare cases a prolonged attack of delirium tremens may clear to reveal an amnesic syndrome, when Wernicke's encephalopathy had been present and unnoticed during the acute stage.

Death when it occurs is usually due to cardiovascular collapse, infection, hyperthermia, or self injury during the phase of intense restlessness. Any infective process, and particularly pneumonia, markedly increases the mortality.

Aetiology

The precise pathophysiology is unknown. Cerebral oedema was formerly thought to be responsible but has not been adequately confirmed. A primary disorder of the reticular formation is strongly suggested by the clinical components of profound inattention coupled with alertness, overactivity and insomnia. The remarkable association with disturbance of REM sleep has already been described (p. 598).

Cerebral blood flow studies have indicated a state of increased central nervous system excitability during the course of delirium, in keeping with the characteristic fast frequencies seen on electroencephalography. Hemmingsen *et al.* (1988) performed xenon-SPECT studies in patients with actual or impending delirium tremens, with repeat examination on recovery. Increased hemispheric blood flow correlated significantly with the presence of visual hallucinations and psychomotor agitation, and decreased when the acute phase subsided.

A low serum magnesium has been found in delirium tremens (Flink *et al.* 1954) but is not accepted as causal. Adrenal insufficiency has also been blamed, but steroids are not markedly effective in treatment. Low levels of thiamine and nicotinic acid have been found in proportion to the severity of the symptoms (Kershaw 1967), though this probably reflects the severity of the underlying alcoholism rather than a directly causal relationship. Thus the condition is known to be capable of recovering on water alone, and in the experimental studies of Isbell *et al.* (1955) high vitamin supplements given intramuscularly did not prevent its appearance.

Withdrawal of alcohol is the factor most clearly incriminated in the aetiology of the condition, and in the majority of cases can be detected in the antecedent history. Premonitory symptoms often set in within a day or two of cessation of drinking, but the full-blown syndrome usually appears only after 3 or 4 days of abstinence. Refeeding with alcohol has been shown to ameliorate the condition. Nevertheless some cases undoubtedly begin during a bout of heavy consumption, and reduction of intake below some critical value must then be postulated.

However, all authorities do not agree about the essential role of alcohol withdrawal. Lundquist (1961) could find evidence of abstinence antedating the onset in only a quarter of cases, and in half of these there was some other complicating factor such as trauma or infection. Those who question the role of withdrawal suggest that the patient has commonly stopped drinking because of nausea or distaste for alcohol, these symptoms being the first sign of a developing illness. Certainly it can be shown that trauma or infection are present from the outset in up to half of cases, many others having liver failure, gastrointestinal bleeding or hypoglycaemia. Lundquist (1961) found biochemical evidence of acute liver damage in up to 90% of patients with delirium tremens, and much more commonly than in non-delirious alcoholics.

A multifactorial aetiology will probably prove to be the complete explanation. Alcohol withdrawal may well be the principal factor in the majority of cases, but this would

appear to act by way of complex metabolic and neurophysiological pathways. Hence in some patients equivalent disturbances may sometimes come about by other means.

Treatment

Treatment of minor withdrawal symptoms can often be undertaken on an out-patient basis with the help of sedation from chlordiazepoxide or chlormethiazole. However, patients with a history of withdrawal seizures, and those with any indication of impending delirium tremens, should be admitted to hospital immediately. Management will in essence consist of close nursing observation at regular intervals, so that the dosage of sedative drugs can be titrated against the symptoms displayed. Edwards (1982) recommends chlordiazepoxide up to 40 mg three or four times per day, starting if necessary with an intramuscular dose of 50–100 mg. Treatment with chlormethiazole is an alternative. The drugs are then gradually tailed off over several days at a rate which prevents significant recrudescence of withdrawal symptoms.

With *established delirium tremens* treatment must always be in hospital, preferably in a setting where the medical and nursing staff are experienced with the procedures involved. The necessary steps are described by Rix (1978) and Edwards (1982). Fluid replacement and adequate sedation are the first essentials, with careful examination to detect complicating pathologies which aggravate the delirium and greatly worsen prognosis.

Head injury and infection must always be borne in mind. Skull and chest X-ray will be required. Coincident intoxication with barbiturates or other sedative drugs may lead to particularly severe withdrawal manifestations. Hypoglycaemia, hepatic failure, uraemia and electrolyte imbalance will need to be excluded. Wernicke's encephalopathy must be detected early and treated vigorously. Cardiac failure, gastroduodenal bleeding or bleeding from oesophageal varices may be present. A close watch must be kept at all stages for seizures or circulatory collapse.

The intensity of treatment required will obviously depend on the severity of delirium which has become established. When the syndrome is well developed half-hourly recordings of temperature, pulse and blood pressure should be made, along with a record of fluid intake and output. At least 6 litres of fluid per day will be required, of which 1.5 litres should be given as normal saline. If adequate oral intake cannot be ensured intravenous administration must be started with 5% glucose solution or glucose in saline. Hypokalaemia is a special risk. Hypomagnesaemia may occur.

Adequate sedation is essential, and the dosage should be monitored closely against the patient's clinical state and level of consciousness. Chlordiazepoxide or chlormethiazole are now regarded as the drugs of choice in this situation. Chlordiazepoxide may be required in dosage of up to 400 mg daily or even more in divided doses. Initially it may be given by intramuscular injection—100 mg every 6 hours over the first 24 hours. Dosage reduction should then proceed smoothly over the next 5 days if possible. In patients who are very disturbed, a slow intravenous injection of diazepam may be employed in a dosage of 10–15 mg given at not more than 5 mg per minute. Chlormethiazole is preferred in several centres, with a starting dose of up to 2 g orally four times per day. Slow infusion of a 0.8% solution can be given by intravenous drip (Glatt *et al.* 1966; Glatt & Frisch 1969). Other sedatives such as phenothiazines, butyrophenones or paraldehyde should where possible be avoided.

Other treatment must always include high potency vitamin preparations as a prophylactic against Wernicke's encephalopathy or nicotinic acid-deficiency encephalopathy. Phenytoin or carbamazepine should be given routinely when there is a past history of withdrawal seizures. Cardiovascular collapse, vomiting or hyperthermia will require appropriate management.

'Alcoholic dementia' and cerebral atrophy in alcoholics

The conception of alcoholic dementia has had a chequered history, figuring prominently in early textbooks of psychiatry but later yielding pride of place to Korsakoff's syndrome (Lishman 1981). Nowadays the idea of a genuine dementia caused by alcohol is quite commonly viewed with caution. Many patients labelled as alcoholic dements are indeed suffering from Korsakoff's syndrome (though it seems possible that the reverse also obtains as described on p. 584). Others are merely displaying profound social disorganisation in the context of chronic continuing inebriation. When opportunities arise to assess the latter after a period of total abstinence, intellectual functions may turn out to be substantially intact. Other alcoholics who dement are suffering essentially from a coincident vascular dementia or a dementia of the Alzheimer type.

Nevertheless clinical experience suggests that the long-continued abuse of alcohol may sometimes lead directly to an end-state of dementia. The data in Table 17 (p. 491) show that alcohol is suspected of being at least a contributory cause in a substantial number of demented patients seen in hospital; it features approximately as often as multi-infarct dementia in many of the series shown. One

must appreciate, moreover, that for every patient who has reached the stage of being investigated for a frank dementing picture, many others may be suffering from milder, and perhaps protracted, earlier stages of such disorder.

Adequate epidemiological studies are not available to clarify the problem directly. Only a proportion of alcoholics come before treatment services, and a comprehensive follow-up of those who do can present formidable problems. It is possible, moreover, that those who suffer marked cognitive impairment are particularly liable to be lost to view as time goes by. There have been few surveys of 'skid row' alcoholics who may be expected to represent the more deteriorated subjects.

Edwards (1982) estimates that among alcoholics attending any ordinary type of treatment facility upwards of 50% of patients aged over 45, and with a lengthy drinking history, will be found on careful assessment to show some degree of cognitive impairment. At one end of the spectrum there will be no more than minor impairments of memory, concentration and judgement, and at the other the fully developed picture of dementia. Among patients coming forward for treatment in Australia, some 8–9% have been considered to warrant the label of dementia on the basis of progressive failure of memory, loss of intellect and deterioration of personality (Wilkinson *et al.* 1971; Horvath 1975).

Psychological evidence

Clinical psychologists have presented a now substantial body of evidence which shows that severe alcoholics, even after thorough 'drying out', remain compromised on a broad range of psychological functions. These extend well beyond memory deficits alone — problems with visuospatial competence, abstracting ability and complex reasoning. Such deficits can be demonstrated even when verbal ability is well preserved, which of course can produce a misleading impression at interview. Again it is noteworthy that they have emerged in subjects presenting themselves for treatment; the cognitive status of those out of contact with medical services has for obvious reasons not been determined.

In an early study Fitzhugh *et al.* (1960, 1965) compared a group of abstinent alcoholics with brain-damaged and non-brain-damaged controls after matching for age and education. The alcoholics scored on the Wechsler Adult Intelligence Scale (WAIS) like the non-brain-damaged group, but on certain tests more specifically related to brain damage (the Trail Making Test and tests from the Halstead Battery) they were comparable to the brain-damaged sample. Similar psychometric evidence, suggesting varying degrees of brain damage in alcoholics despite preserved IQ, has been reported by Goldstein and Chotlos (1965),

Jones and Parsons (1971) and Long and McLachlan (1974). It has emerged in alcoholics from middle and upper socioeconomic classes with higher than average IQ (Smith *et al.* 1973). Thus formal intelligence tests such as the WAIS may sometimes give a misleading impression of the capabilities of the alcoholic patient.

The more recent and often complex psychological literature is reviewed by Goldman (1983), Tarter and Edwards (1985), Parsons (1987), Grant (1987) and Evert and Oscar-Berman (1995). Numerous variables among the populations under survey must be taken into account, not least the duration of abstinence prior to testing. Psychological assessments during the first few weeks of abstinence show substantial recovery of intellectual and memory functions, so assessment of the stable cognitive state must be deferred for some considerable time. Continuing restitution of function may indeed proceed for a period of several months. Nevertheless it seems that even after a year of abstinence psychological deficits persist on tests of psychomotor speed, perceptual–motor functioning and visuospatial competence, also measures of abstracting ability and reasoning. Careful tests of memory function can likewise remain impaired, to the extent that a continuum of memory impairment has been postulated, ranging from normality at one extreme to the fully-fledged picture of the Korsakoff amnesic defect at the other (Ryback 1971; Ryan & Butters 1980) (p. 583). New learning capacity has been found to remain impaired after a minimum of 5 years' abstinence, likewise capacity for complex figure–ground analysis (Brandt *et al.* 1983).

Deficits on tests related to frontal lobe function, such as the category subtest of the Halstead–Reitan Battery or the Wisconsin Card Sorting Test, are particularly noteworthy. Frontal dysfunction could be relevant to aspects of the personality change encountered in alcoholics — the circumstantiality, plausibility and weakness of volition—which may contribute significantly to relapse. Thus Gregson and Taylor (1977) found that an alcoholic's cognitive status on admission to hospital was the best single predictor of his response to treatment. Goldman (1990, 1995) reviews other evidence pointing in this direction. A vicious circle may often be established, with worsening cognitive status contributing to the potentiation of the addiction.

The psychological impairments established in the majority of surveys have usually been no more than mild or moderate in degree. This, along with their tendency to ameliorate with abstinence, has probably led to the concept of alcoholic dementia becoming unfashionable. It is no longer unusual, however, to accept a dementia that is capable of improvement. The alternative term, *reversible alcoholic cognitive deterioration*, has perhaps something to commend it, though with the proviso that the reversibility may not always be complete. Moreover, with a high prevalence of such deterioration among the alcoholic population it is not unlikely that this will sometimes come to be severely developed, perhaps on the basis of special vulnerability in certain individuals. The stage will certainly be set, as the alcoholic gets older, for the brain damage occasioned by alcoholism to couple with other pathologies — those of ageing, trauma, vascular changes

and hepatic dysfunction — leading to more serious and irreversible change.

Neuropathology

Direct appraisal of cerebral pathology in alcoholics, over and above that concerned with the classic Wernicke lesion, has met with conflicting findings. Cerebral atrophy, mild or moderate in degree, was reported in a high proportion of Courville's (1955) chronic alcoholics at autopsy, as well as in half of Neuberger's (1957) and all of Lynch's (1960). Other reports, however, do not find it or do not comment upon it. On microscopy Courville found arachnoidal thickening and cell degeneration and loss, affecting mainly the smaller pyramidal cells of the superficial and intermediate laminae. Disintegration of nerve fibres was also observed. Lynch (1960) described a similar histological picture in 11 chronic alcoholics with adequate nutritional status, when compared with a group of non-alcoholic subjects of the same age and sex. Commenting on the negative reports in the literature, he attributed this to a waning of neuropathological interest in the cortex of alcoholics, with the accent of pathological enquiry centring increasingly on the Wernicke lesion at the base of the brain and on changes in the cerebellum. He also stressed how difficult it is to chart changes, degenerations and loss in such a complex and crowded area as the cortex.

More recent quantitative studies on brains obtained at autopsy have confirmed that atrophy or 'shrinkage' is indeed often detectable. Thus in comparison with controls brain weight is slightly but significantly reduced in the alcoholic (Harper & Blumbergs 1982; Torvik *et al.* 1982), and the pericerebral space over the cortex is enlarged (Harper & Kril 1985). This emerges whether or not there is evidence of nutritional brain damage, perhaps pointing to the role of alcohol neurotoxicity. The amount of white matter in the cerebral hemispheres is reduced, and the ventricles enlarged by over a third, a figure not dissimilar from that found in computerised tomography (CT) studies as discussed below (Harper *et al.* 1985; de la Monte 1988). The thickness of the corpus callosum is also significantly reduced by approximately 20% (Harper & Kril 1988).

Detailed cell counts have indicated a 22% reduction in the number of neurones in the superior frontal cortex, along with reduction in the size of neurones in the motor and cingulate cortices (Harper *et al.* 1987; Kril & Harper 1989). Other cortical areas seem not to have been extensively examined. A quantitative study of the extent of dendritic arborisations in layer III pyramidal neurones from the frontal and motor cortex has shown significant reductions in mean dendritic length, number of branches and mean width of basal dendritic fields (Harper & Corbett 1990).

These painstaking studies have thus revealed a morphological basis, albeit subtle in nature, which may be responsible for the cognitive impairments so common in alcoholics.

Neuroimaging

Several earlier reports suggested that cerebral 'atrophy' might be commoner than expected on air encephalography. These have been summarised by Ron (1977). Lereboullet *et al.* (1956), for example, were able to assemble 77 alcoholics with 'indubitable atrophy' on air encephalography after rigorously excluding those with head injuries or other causes which could have accounted for it. Twelve went on to autopsy and a close correspondence was observed between the radiological and postmortem findings.

Air encephalography was, of course, difficult to justify except on specially selected subjects, and adequate control comparisons were hard to achieve. The significance and the generality of the findings thus remained in doubt. Certain studies were nevertheless impressive, such as those of Haug (1968) and Brewer and Perrett (1971), with between half and three-quarters of subjects showing cortical changes or ventricular enlargement. Haug found that the changes were most marked when personality deterioration was severe and intellect was impaired.

CT scanning has allowed a more thorough-going appraisal of the situation, and several surveys have been conducted on large populations of alcoholics (Bergman *et al.* 1980a, 1980b; Cala *et al.* 1980; Ron *et al.* 1980, 1982; Carlen *et al.* 1981; Lishman *et al.* 1987). The non-invasive nature of the procedure has allowed representative samples of alcoholics to be investigated and compared with normal controls, and dilatation of the sulci, fissures and ventricles has been found to be common.

The conclusions to be drawn from these more recent studies are as follows. Some 50–70% of severe chronic alcoholics show indubitable evidence of cortical shrinkage or ventricular dilatation or both. Involvement of the frontal lobes of the brain has sometimes been particularly evident. The changes can be found in quite young alcoholics, appearing well within the first decade of alcohol abuse, though they become more marked in the older age groups studied. Planimetric measures of lateral ventricular size show on average some 50% enlargement compared to age-matched controls. This has emerged even in identical twins discordant for a history of alcoholism (Gurling *et al.* 1984). Atrophy of the cerebellar vermis can also be seen in a high proportion of subjects. However, personal susceptibility to such developments appears to vary widely, in that approximately a third of subjects continue to show normal scans despite long-continued and severe drinking histories. There are indications that the female brain may be more vulnerable than the male to the development of such CT changes (Jacobson 1986).

Magnetic resonance imaging (MRI) has confirmed the ventricular enlargement and the increase in cerebrospinal fluid over the cortical surface which is apparent on CT scans. In Jernigan *et al.*'s (1991a) MRI study the cortical changes were particularly impressive, and were associated with significant reductions in grey matter in medial temporal, superior frontal and parietal regions. Subcortical grey matter was also reduced, particularly in the caudate nucleus and diencephalon.

These cerebral changes clearly antedate clinical evidence of mental impairment, being demonstrable after excluding patients with clinically obvious cognitive deficits. They often appear to set in early during the alcoholic career, and after developing to a certain degree it is possible that they fail to progress further. In seeking clinical associations of the CT scan findings few have emerged other than age and duration of abstinence. The duration and severity of alcohol abuse appear to bear little relation to the severity of the cerebral changes once age has been taken into account, though there is some indirect evidence that episodic drinking may be less harmful in this respect than steady continuous drinking.

The most decisive influence, where the drinking history is concerned, has proved to lie with the duration of abstinence. It has been shown that with increasing length of abstinence prior to scanning the CT changes become less pronounced; and follow-up over an interval of 1–3 years has confirmed that abstinence in the interim is the factor most closely associated with whether or not the scans will show improvement (Ron *et al.* 1982; Ron 1983). Even after several years of abstinence, however, as in samples recruited from Alcoholics Anonymous, some degree of persistent ventricular enlargement appears to remain (Jacobson 1986; Lishman *et al.* 1987).

Studies using MRI, which allows more accurate measurement of cerebrospinal fluid volumes, have confirmed significant decreases in both ventricular size and subarachnoid spaces during the early weeks of abstinence (Schroth *et al.* 1988). Coincident measurement of T_2 values for white matter have served to discount dehydration and rehydration of the brain as the sole explanation; other effects such as increased protein synthesis or increased dendritic growth after withdrawal from alcohol may be more important factors.

This partial reversibility with abstinence is, of course, strong evidence against the possibility that the cerebral changes revealed on the scan may have antedated, and predisposed to, the onset of the alcoholism.

Psychometric testing carried out in conjunction with scanning has indicated, as expected, that a considerable proportion of the alcoholics score poorly on many tests. The concordance between measures of functional and structural change has, however, usually proved to be low. Bergman *et al.* (1980a, 1980b) found some evidence that impairment of memory and general intelligence was associated with the degree of ventricular enlargement, and that the Halstead Impairment Index was associated with cortical status. All such correlations were, however, low. Acker *et al.* (1984) found remarkably few associations on an extensive battery of tests once care had been taken to control for age and estimates of premorbid intellectual competence.

Investigation of regional brain CT absorption densities, as opposed to obvious structural change, has produced more promising results—verbal fluency, for example, showing a small but significant relationship to density measurements in the frontal white matter, and verbal memory to density in medial thalamic regions (Lishman *et al.* 1987). Gebhardt *et al.* (1984) reported a similar finding in the thalamus. Chick *et al.* (1989), using MRI, have shown significant relationships between impairment on the Bexley Maudsley Category Sorting Test (p. 121) and T_1 relaxation times, these being most robust in frontal white matter.

It would seem, therefore, that the major structural changes revealed by neuroimaging are largely independent of functional deficits, and that sophisticated methods of scan analysis are required to reveal significant correlations with psychometric performance. This would suggest that cerebral shrinkage *per se* is a poor indicator of functional competence, and that this is more closely tied to parameters reflecting the tissue characteristics of the brain. The practical implication is that reliance cannot be placed on scan appearances of ventricular or sulcal enlargement in evaluating the competence of the individual alcoholic patient.

Other evidence

Further evidence of cerebral disorder in alcoholism has come from studies of evoked brain potentials, cerebral blood flow and functional imaging techniques. Brain stem evoked potentials and event-related potentials have proved to be abnormal in alcoholics, independently of the presence of overt signs of brain damage (Porjesz & Begleiter 1987). While the former recover with abstinence the latter appear not to do so. Begleiter *et al.* (1980) found that the P_{300} component of the event-related potential was smaller in alcoholics with demonstrable cerebral atrophy than in those without.

Risberg and Berglund (1987) review regional cerebral blood flow studies which reveal progressively decreased cortical perfusion in older alcoholics, particularly in frontal regions. Ishikawa *et al.* (1986) have reported diffuse reductions in grey matter flow, improving with abstinence. Hata *et al.* (1987) used xenon-enhanced CT to show that hypoperfusion also involves deep cerebral structures, including the thalamus and hypothalamus, even in the absence of Wernicke–Korsakoff features. Such changes were also reversible in some degree with abstinence.

Positron emission tomography scanning has revealed a 20–30% decrease in cerebral glucose utilization involving frontal, temporal and parietal areas, the latter most severely (Wik *et al.* 1988). Subcortical cerebral structures were also affected. Melgaard *et al.* (1990) found that alcoholics had a greater number of low flow areas on SPECT scanning than controls, whether or not the CT scan was abnormal. Relationships could be discerned with the severity of the alcoholism and with the presence of intellectual impairment or cerebral atrophy.

Neurochemical investigations appear to have been less thoroughly pursued in the alcoholic brain than would have been expected. Nevertheless impaired cholinergic function has been shown in brain samples obtained at autopsy (Antuono *et al.* 1980; Nordberg *et al.* 1980), of a nature similar to those encountered in Alzheimer's disease (p. 444). Deficits have likewise been shown where several brain biogenic amines are concerned (Carlsson *et al.* 1980).

Morphometric evidence indicative of both macroscopic and microscopic brain changes at autopsy have already been described on p. 604.

Possible causes

These various findings are all pointers to the vulnerability of the alcoholic brain; a vulnerability that is clearly more of a risk in some individuals than others. The determinants which allow occasional alcoholics to escape brain changes and functional deficits despite severe dependence, while others develop them from an early stage, remain at present unknown. Genetic factors may play a considerable role. In susceptible individuals, however, the brain malfunction may contribute not only to decreased tolerance but also to loss of control; and if some alcoholics have impaired control on an organic basis from early in their drinking careers this could be an important factor in perpetuating the addiction. When susceptibility to the cerebral disorder is marked, this can be seen as paving the way to a later alcoholic dementia.

Several factors may be operative in contributing to such functional and structural deficits — dietary neglect, repeated episodes of head trauma, liver disorder, alcoholic comas with anoxia or hypoglycaemia, and/or the direct toxic action of alcohol on the central nervous system. Their relative contributions have been hard to determine. In the principal neuroimaging studies outlined above care has usually been taken to exclude patients with known cerebral trauma, episodes of drug overdosage or other possible reasons for the development of cerebral atrophy. Even so, accumulating minor insults may have made a contribution. A role for dietary neglect in contributing to psychological impairments has sometimes been highlighted (Guthrie & Elliott 1980) but would seem unlikely as the whole explanation. The brain weights in Harper and Blumbergs' (1982) study were as low in those without histological evidence of nutritional brain damage as in those with changes indicative of a Wernicke's encephalopathy; by contrast Harper and Kril (1985) found that the 'pericerebral space' was more greatly increased in the presence of Wernicke's encephalopathy or liver disease (p. 604). Severity of liver damage, as assessed by biopsy, has shown some association with the degree of cortical shrinkage on the CT scan (Acker *et al.* 1982), but the relationship was weak and has not emerged in other investigations (Lee *et al.* 1979; Carlen *et al.* 1981).

Laboratory evidence lends support to the possibility that a direct toxic action of alcohol on the brain may play a considerable role. Leonard (1986) and Charness *et al.* (1989) review its effects on neuronal membranes, cell transport systems and neurotransmitter functions. Studies in mice and rats have shown that brain changes can be induced after a period of several months on a diet supplemented with alcohol (Riley & Walker 1978; Walker *et al.* 1980a, 1980b). Marked alterations in dendritic morphology were found in the hippocampal pyramidal neurones, dentate granular layers and cerebellar vermis, proceeding to cell degeneration and loss. These effects were produced despite the maintenance of good nutrition in all other respects. West *et al.* (1982) showed, moreover, that alcohol inhibits the reactive sprouting of dendrites in the rat hippocampus which constitutes the normal response to injury. McMullen *et al.* (1984) found that ingestion of alcohol by well-nourished rats leads to reduction of branching in dendritic domains, and a reduction of thickness in corresponding dendritic strata. Abstinence then allows regrowth of dendritic branching and a return to normal thickness of the strata. King *et al.* (1988) have shown similar reversible alterations in the density of dendritic spines in the rat hippocampus.

Such observations could be relevant to the pervasive CT scan changes encountered in alcoholics, and might help to explain the slow reversal of cortical shrinkage that has been observed with abstinence. As discussed on p. 443, the plasticity inherent in the adult brain with regard to dendritic growth and sprouting has come to be appreciated (Buell & Coleman 1979, 1981; Flood & Coleman 1986), continuing growth of the dendritic domains appearing to compensate for an age-related decline in neuronal numbers. Dendritic growth may stand to be compromised in the alcoholic subject, with a return to normal levels when prolonged abstinence has been assured. Other factors may also be involved, such as changes in protein or lipid synthesis (Harper 1989; Harper & Kril 1990).

Victor and Adams (1985) and Victor *et al.* (1989) dispute the existence of a primary alcoholic dementia, and suggest that most patients carrying such a diagnosis merely show the lesions of the Wernicke–Korsakoff syndrome at autopsy. Torvik *et al.* (1982) found such lesions in 12% of alcoholics dying in institutions in the Oslo area, mostly with chronic inactive pathology. Among the 20 in whom there was adequate documentation of psychiatric status prior to death, 15 had a 'more or less pronounced global dementia in addition to a severe memory defect'. Eight of these patients had been labelled during life as having a presenile or senile dementia, but in fact only two showed Alzheimer changes and one the changes of multi-infarct dementia at autopsy.

It therefore seems possible that the Wernicke–Korsakoff lesion may sometimes itself be responsible for pictures of dementia. Lishman (1986, 1990) has suggested that it may do so by encroaching on key neurochemical nuclei at the base of the brain, with consequent disruption of monoaminergic and cholinergic inputs to the cortex. The locus caeruleus is often implicated in the Wernicke–Korsakoff lesion, and Halliday *et al.* (1993) have shown substantial depletions of serotonergic neurones in the brain stem in alcoholics. Depletion of neurones has been demonstrated in the nucleus basalis of Meynert in Korsakoff patients (Arendt *et al.* 1983) and in patients diagnosed as suffering from alcoholic dementia (Akai & Akai 1989).

Pursuing this hypothesis further it is possible to amass evidence that the basal regions of the brain are vulnerable not only to thiamine lack but also to the direct toxic action of alcohol (Lishman 1990). Alcoholics are likely to vary considerably in their vulnerability to each form of insult, perhaps by virtue of genetically controlled biochemical factors. There may often be a complex relationship between such basal brain changes and the cortical changes revealed on neuroimaging, each contributing in some degree to cognitive deficits, and combining to account for their reversibility or permanence in individual patients.

A dual system of this nature could also explain the spectrum of cognitive changes encountered in patients labelled as suffering from Korsakoff's syndrome, ranging from circumscribed memory deficits to more global impairment in a proportion of cases (p. 584). Those with special vulnerability to both thiamine lack and alcohol neurotoxicity will be at very special risk of damaging the basal brain regions severely and irreversibly; this may be why a chronic Korsakoff syndrome is relatively rare even among severe alcoholics, likewise pictures of advanced and irreversible dementia.

Barbiturates

Acute barbiturate intoxication may be the result of a suicide attempt or of self medication to gain relief from severe tension and anxiety. Chronic intoxication is mostly seen in barbiturate addicts. Both oral and intravenous addiction reached a peak in the 1970s but are now uncommon as a result of more stringent prescribing practices. Addiction is associated with increasing tolerance so that ultimately enormous quantities can be consumed, often along with addiction to alcohol and other drugs.

Acute intoxication

A short period of confusion and drowsiness gives way to deepening coma. The pulse and respiration are slowed, the blood pressure lowered, and the body temperature often subnormal. The tendon reflexes are diminished, or absent in deep coma. The plantar responses may be upgoing. Nystagmus is a prominent feature in the earlier stages together with tremors of the tongue and lips. Death may result from respiratory failure or peripheral circulatory collapse.

During recovery signs of cerebellar disturbance are marked, with nystagmus, ataxia, asynergia, dysarthria and hypotonia. A muddled euphoria is often seen while consciousness is returning, and a period of hypomania may persist after all neurological features have cleared.

Estimation of the blood barbiturate level serves to confirm the cause of the acute intoxication or coma. The EEG may also be useful in showing generalised fast beta activity during the first 24 hours after overdose, unlike most other severe intoxications which produce slowing of rhythms in parallel with reduction of the level of consciousness.

Chronic barbiturate intoxication

Chronic barbiturate intoxication produces drowsiness, fluctuating confusion, dysarthria and ataxia which may closely resemble drunkenness due to alcohol. Withdrawal effects are also similar with epileptic fits and delirium. It is important to consider addiction in patients who present with intermittent confusion of obscure origin, or who develop fits or delirium of uncertain aetiology on admission to hospital. An important clue may lie in the patient's unwillingness for investigations and his strenuous objection to hospitalisation.

The clinical picture was described by Curran (1938, 1944) and clarified by the experiments of Isbell and associates on volunteer subjects serving narcotic sentences (Isbell *et al.* 1950; Fraser *et al.* 1958). While intoxicated the patient is somnolent and muddled, with difficulty in concentration and periods of disorientation. The usual mood change is towards euphoria with restlessness and periods of excitement and irritability. Neurological features include nystagmus, dysarthria, tremulousness, and ataxia of gait and stance. The abdominal reflexes are typically depressed or absent.

A prominent feature is the variability from day to day and even from hour to hour. This was observed by Isbell *et al.* (1950) among volunteers even though the daily intake was constant. The degree of somnolence was variable and periods of severe confusion could alternate with periods of lucidity. Behaviour could be facetious, petulant or hostile, changing from one moment to the next. Different subjects also varied in their response; some showed swings between elation and depression, some became seclusive and withdrawn, and others were combative, abusive or paranoid.

The withdrawal syndrome was also clarified by Isbell *et al.* Prior to their studies there had been reports of withdrawal fits and delirium in barbiturate addicts, but in these cases there had often been coincident addiction to other drugs and alcohol. Isbell *et al.* (1950) and Fraser *et al.* (1958) were able to observe the effect of abrupt withdrawal after keeping subjects intoxicated with barbiturates alone for long periods of time.

On withdrawal there was first seeming improvement during the initial 8–12 hours. Minor withdrawal manifestations then appeared in the form of anxiety, tremor and distortions of visual perception, usually accompanied by dizziness, nausea and profound insomnia. The pulse and respiration rates were raised and there was often mild pyrexia. More severe manifestations appeared on the second or third day with one or more grand mal convulsions, sometimes followed by acute delirium. This closely resembled delirium tremens, usually terminating after several days but sometimes proving to be protracted and dangerously exhausting. Complete recovery was usually attained within 1 or 2 weeks. The degree of physical dependence and severity of the withdrawal syndrome were closely dependent on the dosage employed during the period of intoxication.

Little is known regarding *possible long-term effects* of barbiturate abuse on the central nervous system. It appears that the question has rarely been addressed directly, no doubt because of difficulties in the systematic follow-up of subjects. Moreover polydrug abuse has been a common pattern in barbiturate addicts, with a large number of sedative, narcotic and stimulant drugs often featuring in the histories of patients.

Grant and co-workers (Grant & Judd 1976; Grant *et al.* 1976) attempted to investigate the problem in subjects abusing multiple drugs, predominantly those of the sedative–hypnotic class. As judged by neuropsychological testing and electroencephalography, almost half showed evidence of mild to moderate generalised cerebral impairment during the early weeks of treatment. Abstracting ability and perceptuomotor control were principally affected, with relative preservation of general intelligence, memory and verbal abilities. The psychological deficits were often evident after many weeks of abstinence, sometimes appearing to persist even beyond 5 months. It was difficult, however, to exonerate the effects of further drug abuse during the follow-up period. Possibilities of cerebral vascular disease among injecting drug addicts could also be relevant, as discussed on pp. 619–20.

Electroencephalographic changes

The EEG during chronic intoxication shows augmented amplitude and an increased percentage of fast frequencies. After withdrawal dramatic changes occur, with high voltage paroxysmal discharges or bursts of high amplitude waves at 4–6 Hz during the first 12–48 hours (Isbell *et al.* 1950). Records during and after fits are similar to records obtained with the grand mal fits of idiopathic epilepsy. Within 30 days of withdrawal the pattern has usually returned to normal.

The electroencephalographic changes seen with more modest doses of barbiturates were investigated by Oswald and Priest (1965). Amylobarbitone 400 mg nightly produced an initial fall in the proportion of REM sleep, which had returned to normal after a week. Increasing the dose to 600 mg again led to a transient reduction. Withdrawal after a total of 18 nights was then followed by a rebound increase in REM activity accompanied by insomnia and nightmares. The increased REM persisted for several weeks after the last dose had been given.

Differential diagnosis

When barbiturate abuse was common considerable diagnostic problems were prone to arise. The nystagmus, incoordination and ataxia could suggest cerebellar disease or multiple sclerosis. Forgetfulness and a markedly unkempt appearance sometimes led to an impression of presenile dementia. It was usually the fluctuations in behaviour and the patient's surreptitious attitude which raised the possibility of drug abuse. Alternatively, the patient could be diagnosed as suffering from severe neurosis or personality disorder when the principal abnormalities were persistent insomnia and irritability. Other intoxications or metabolic disorders were often suspected until the blood was examined for barbiturate content.

Withdrawal fits could also be misleading, likewise the delirium that was prone to develop 2 or 3 days after the patient was admitted to hospital.

Treatment

The treatment of an acute overdose of barbiturates requires immediate admission to hospital, with facilities at hand for mechanical respiration and dialysis if required. Induced vomiting or gastric lavage must be carried out urgently, and measures may be needed to control peripheral circulatory failure. Deepening or prolonged coma may necessitate artificial respiration and the use of dialysis.

The detoxification of chronic addicts must be carried out gradually and with care because of the risk of inducing status epilepticus. It should be undertaken in hospital. Throughout the withdrawal period the patient is observed for evidence of tremor, agitation, tachycardia and postural hypotension, and these are controlled by judicious dosage of pentobarbitone or phenobarbitone (Ghodse 1995). After a stabilisation phase incremental reductions are made over a period of 2–3 weeks. Phenothiazines and other drugs with epileptogenic properties should be avoided during withdrawal. If convulsions should occur these are best treated with intramuscular sodium amylobarbitone, and the rate of withdrawal will require readjustment.

Benzodiazepines

The benzodiazepines are effective agents for the short-term relief of anxiety, for night-time sedation and for reducing muscle spasticity. They have powerful anticonvulsant properties though the rapid development of tolerance limits their use in epilepsy. Unfortunately widespread use has led to considerable problems by way of dependence, especially among psychiatric patients, and discontinuation can lead to severe withdrawal effects. These have proved often to mimic the symptoms for which the drugs were initially prescribed, with an exacerbation of anxiety and insomnia which can lead to further prescribing and escalation of dosage. Moreover, patients who continue to take therapeutic doses over long periods of time may show an admixture of beneficial and withdrawal effects, perhaps owing to the uneven development of tolerance to different benzodiazepine actions (Ashton 1986). Accordingly the drugs are now prescribed more cautiously, and preferably for no more than 2–4 weeks at a time.

Some persons become addicted as a result of faulty prescribing, while others abuse the drugs for their sedative effects. They are then usually taken intermittently, often in high dosage and along with alcohol and other drugs. Strang *et al.* (1994) have charted the use of benzodiazepines by addicts in the UK, more than half of whom had injected them intravenously. Temazepam has apparently replaced flurazepam and diazepam as the most frequently injected variety. The use of gel-filled temazepam capsules by injection is associated with particularly severe morbidity.

All forms of benzodiazepine act by binding to benzodiazepine receptors in the central nervous system, these being closely associated with gamma aminobutyric acid (GABA) receptors. Their sedative effects appear to be mediated by promoting the inhibitory actions of GABA on serotonergic and other neurones. The duration of action varies widely, diazepam and alprazolam (Xanax) having relatively long half-lives, and oxazepam (Serax) and lorazepam (Ativan) being shorter acting. Among night sedatives nitrazepam and flurazepam (Dalmane) have longer effects than temazepam, lormetazepam and triazolam (Halcion). The risk of physical dependence is greater with shorter-acting benzodiazepines, and particularly with lorazepam on account of its potency.

The psychiatric complications attending their use are best considered first in terms of their sedative actions, and then the withdrawal phenomena, though as described above an admixture of the two may sometimes coexist.

Sedative effects

A chief virtue of the benzodiazepines has been their capacity to relieve anxiety without undue sedation. Tolerance develops rapidly with regular repeat administration, both to their sleep-inducing properties and their sedative effects. However, the anxiolytic action is also prone to diminish, hence the tendency to seek increased dosage as time goes by.

Despite such tolerance sedation can occur, especially with escalating dosage, leading to slowed cerebration, increased reaction time and decreased vigilance. This can be hazardous in persons using machinery or when driving. When used for night sedation 'hang-over' effects may be troublesome, particularly in older persons, and especially with long-lasting preparations such as nitrazepam. Severe sedation, from cumulative dosage or excessive intake, can result in a picture of intoxication with slurred speech, ataxia, emotional lability and poor memory and concentration. Impairment of judgement may be compounded by a paradoxical increase in hostility and aggression, ranging from excitement to outbursts of anger and antisocial behaviour. Very large doses lead to

coma with respiratory depression, though fatalities from overdosage have proved to be rare.

A good deal of interest attaches to the amnesic effects that may be produced, especially with intravenous administration. This has been utilised prior to surgery or uncomfortable investigatory procedures. Wolkowitz *et al.* (1987) gave incremental doses of diazepam intravenously to volunteers, revealing marked effects on attention and word list recognition. At higher dosage the effects could be so profound that the subject could not remember that a word list had been given. By contrast access to information acquired prior to the injections was totally spared. Lister (1985) and Hartman (1988) review other studies which have shown impaired recall of new material, apparently due to deficient acquisition into long-term memory. The severity and duration of the memory effects varies according to the particular drug used, the dose and the route of administration, but beyond this the pattern appears to be qualitatively the same — impairment of acquisition without effects on retention or retrieval. In some circumstances the drugs may even facilitate retrieval. How far these effects depend on sedation, reflecting attentional processes rather than memory *per se*, remains uncertain.

It is also unclear whether long-continued use can lead to neuropsychological impairment. Observations suggesting that this is so have usually been on patients taking other medications in addition. Lucki *et al.* (1986) studied patients who had taken benzodiazepines continuously for a mean of 5 years, mostly in normal therapeutic dosage. In comparison with matched controls seeking treatment for anxiety-related disorders there were few demonstrable effects. The free recall of word lists was unaffected, also performance at digit–symbol substitution and letter cancellation tasks. Impairment was found only on the critical flicker–fusion threshold. Such results would appear to reflect tolerance to the amnesic and other psychological effects of the drugs with long-term use.

Withdrawal effects

It is now clear that physical as well as psychological dependence occurs with benzodiazepines, unpleasant symptomatology often following reduction of dosage or discontinuation. Such dependence can set in remarkably quickly and with normal therapeutic dosage. Withdrawal of regular night sedation can precipitate nightmares, vivid dreams and 'rebound insomnia', accompanied by increased REM sleep for several weeks. Discontinuation of daytime treatment has been shown to lead to agitation, dysphoria and perceptual changes in a third to a half of patients (Tyrer *et al.* 1981, 1983). Such reactions may occasionally occur after as little as 6 weeks on the drugs (Murphy *et al.* 1984). Adverse reactions are commoner with abrupt than gradual withdrawal, after high dosage and prolonged use, and with shorter-acting forms of benzodiazepine. Much individual variability clearly exists in that half or more of subjects are unaffected.

The pictures encountered are reviewed by Owen and Tyrer (1983) and Edwards *et al.* (1990). Somatic symptoms of anxiety tend to be accompanied by restlessness, emotional lability, impaired concentration and depersonalisation. Insomnia is often severe. Panic attacks and paranoid feelings may occur. Weakness, dizziness, tremor, muscle twitching, palpitations, headaches and sweating are common, likewise gastrointestinal symptoms including nausea, anorexia, abdominal discomfort and diarrhoea. More specific symptoms include perceptual disturbances in many modalities — sensations of movement or tilting in the visual field leading to feelings of unsteadiness ('perceptual ataxia'), also tinnitus and unusual tactile sensations. Blurring of vision, facial burning and hot and cold feelings may be accompanied by muscle pain and aching. Increased sensitivity may be experienced to light, sounds, smells and taste.

The symptomatology is highly variable from one patient to another but is often deeply distressing. The usual time course is for symptoms to develop within 3–10 days of stopping treatment, though with compounds of short half-life they can appear much more quickly. Lorazepam has been associated with particularly early and severe withdrawal effects. The more florid manifestations last on average 5–20 days, but anxiety and its attendant features can persist for 6–12 months.

More severe and dangerous manifestations can follow abrupt withdrawal from large dosage. Confusion and hallucinations may progress to delirious states closely similar to delirium tremens. Grand mal fits are a serious risk, sometimes with status epilepticus.

Management of withdrawal

After careful assessment of the reasons for commencing the medication, and of the possible need for continuing alternative treatment, the dosage of benzodiazepines should be very gradually tapered. Edwards *et al.* (1990) recommend that this should extend over 6–8 weeks at least, and in some cases for considerably longer. When the patient is on a short-acting compound substitution with diazepam may facilitate withdrawal. Propanolol may help to ameliorate some of the somatic symptoms, and clonidine has been claimed to be useful. Sedative antidepressants may be indicated when depression is severe. Anxiety management techniques have been shown to be valuable, and self-support groups have come to be widely established.

Opiates

The major and most valuable property of opiate drugs is pain relief but they are widely abused on account of their euphoriant effects. Administration is followed by a state of mental detachment and feelings of extreme well-being. They also have sedative effects, leading to difficulty with concentration, drowsiness and sleep (Ghodse 1995). After large doses depression of the respiratory centres can cause respiratory arrest and death. The characteristic sign of 'pinpoint' pupils may betray covert addiction.

Opium is obtained from the opium poppy (*Paver somniferum*) and processed in various forms. Morphine is a major constituent, little favoured by addicts because of its liability to cause nausea and vomiting. Heroin (diamorphine) is prepared from morphine by acetylation and has a particularly marked euphoriant effect. Other semisynthetic and synthetic opioids include methadone (Physeptone), widely used in the maintenance treatment of addicts, also pethidine, dipipanone (Diconal), dihydromorphine (Dilaudid) and dextromoramide (Palfium). All have addictive potential. Codeine and dihydrocodeine may be used by addicts to supplement their supplies or to avert abstinence symptoms. Several drugs have mixed opioid agonist and antagonist properties and are sometimes abused, for example pentazocine (Fortral) and buprenorphine (Temgesic).

The central actions of opioid drugs have been clarified by the identification of opiate receptors in the brain. These exist as several subclasses and are found widely throughout the animal kingdom. It is now known that 'endogenous opioids' are present in the nervous system—encephalins, endorphins and dynorphin — these having important modulating effects on pain perception. There is evidence that repeated administration of exogenous opioid drugs leads to suppression of endogenous opioid activity, also to resetting of opioid 'mu' receptors and their adenylate cyclase second messenger systems (Kosten 1990).

With repeated use tolerance develops rapidly so that dangerously large doses come to be taken. Severe psychological dependence may then disrupt the addict's life by constant drug-seeking behaviour. Physical dependence becomes apparent when administration is disrupted or curtailed. The early opiate abstinence syndrome consists of craving, anxiety, sweating, restless sleep and running eyes and nose. More severe degrees show as gooseflesh ('cold turkey'), shivering, muscle twitching, dilated pupils and aching in the bones and muscles. Abdominal cramps develop later with vomiting, diarrhoea, increased pulse and blood pressure, severe insomnia and low-grade fever. Consciousness is unimpaired throughout. The withdrawal syndrome tends to reach a peak during the third and fourth days, usually subsiding within a week. Though extremely unpleasant it is rarely life threatening. Morphine and heroin cause the most severe dependence.

Psychiatric disorder

Apart from the general risks attaching to intravenous injection, and the ever-present danger of overdosage, the use of opiates appears to be relatively free from adverse effects on the central nervous system. Pethidine is unusual in that high doses can result in excitation, tremors, dilated pupils and convulsions (Madden 1990). Other opiates are associated with a high incidence of depression, often leading to the concomitant use of alcohol (Roszell et al. 1986), but little evidence has been obtained of neuropsychological impairment. Fields and Fullerton (1975), for example, failed to identify impairments on the Halstead–Reitan Battery among young heroin-addicted veterans when compared with non-drug users. Hill et al. (1979) compared 70 heroin addicts with 23 alcoholics and 14 non-addicted subjects on Raven's Matrices and on the Category Sorting and Tactual Performance tests from the Halstead–Reitan Battery, finding that they tended to fall between the two groups on certain items. Longer opiate careers were associated with greater impairment, but this appeared to be largely reversible in subjects who abstained. There were few indications of abnormality on CT scans.

Carlin (1986) reviews these and other studies, concluding that there is little clear evidence that opiate abuse is associated with cerebral impairment. Considerable difficulties are encountered, however, in discerning the possible contributions of individual substances when polydrug abuse is so common a pattern. Thus it is hard to make definitive statements on the issue, in contrast to the obvious cerebral toxicity of several other abused substances. This may in itself be a significant observation.

Cannabis (Indian hemp, hashish, marihuana)

The relationship between cannabis and psychiatric disorder is controversial and has tended to become an emotive topic. There is still uncertainty about the prevalence of seriously adverse psychological reactions to the drug, and case reporting has perhaps highlighted the rare and exceptional. It is certain, however, that some individuals can present with marked mental disturbance occasioned by cannabis, and this must nowadays be increasingly considered in psychiatric differential diagnosis. Both acute and chronic forms of adverse reaction have been described. The main point of contention is how far these reflect special vulnerability in the patient rather than the direct toxic properties of cannabis on the nervous system.

Evidence has, however, been forthcoming of a toxic effect of tetrahydrocannabinols on certain brain structures in experimental animals, notably the hippocampus (Landfield et al. 1988). Decreased hippocampal neuronal density and increased glial reactivity are seen, and could perhaps account for the memory disorder suspected in long-term cannabis users (p. 616). Interestingly, tetrahydrocannabinol receptors have now been identified in the rat brain — in the hippocampal formation, dentate gyrus and cerebral cortex — which act to inhibit adenylate cyclase activity in a dose-dependent manner (Matsuda et al. 1990).

Cannabis intoxication

The effects of mild intoxication after smoking marihuana are reasonably distinctive and were described in detail by Bromberg (1934) and Allentuck and Bowman (1942). The principal features include a euphoric dream-like state, mild impairment of consciousness and distortion of time sense. More severe intoxication is accompanied by fragmentation of thought processes and often hallucinations.

Almost immediately after inhalation the subject feels light-headed and dizzy, with ringing in the ears and a sensation of floating on air. Sometimes there is transitory anxiety or panic, but this characteristically gives way to feelings of ease and mild elation. The conjunctivae redden and photophobia and lachrymation may develop. Some subjects show tremors, twitching and ataxia. The pulse and blood pressure are usually increased.

Further developments no doubt depend on features in the individual and the circumstances in which the drug is taken. Exhilaration is common, with a vivid sense of happiness, buoyancy and lightness of the limbs. An aphrodisiac effect has been claimed but is not well substantiated. A phase of psychomotor overactivity often ensues with rapid speech which the subject considers to be brilliant and witty. Answers to questions seem to him to be ready formed and surprising in their clarity, but to the observer the performance is usually dull, banal and often confused. By contrast some subjects react to cannabis by becoming markedly apprehensive, querulous or suspicious. Others become lethargic and slip directly into a state of 'delicious and confused lassitude' which sometimes borders on stupor.

Cognitive functions are affected in many subtle ways. The stream of talk tends to be circumstantial and fragmented. There may be difficulty in linking parts to the whole, or sudden interruptions in the stream of thought resembling the blocking of schizophrenia. Time sense is characteristically distorted, often with remarkable subjective lengthening of time spans. Sometimes there is unawareness of the passage of time, or a curious disturbance in which the present does not seem to arise out of the past. Attention, concentration and comprehension are only slightly impaired in the milder stages of intoxication, but memory functions can usually be shown to be faulty (Tinklenberg *et al.* 1970).

With more severe intoxication there are more dramatic symptoms. Waves of ecstasy, perplexity or terror may be experienced, along with feelings of depersonalisation or derealisation. Body image disturbances are often alarming. The subjective evaluation of sensations in all modalities may be changed. Visual disturbances are the most intrusive, with distortion of shapes and intensification of colours. Hallucinatory experiences consist of flashes of light, amorphous forms of vivid colour, geometrical figures, human faces or pictures of great complexity.

As the acute intoxication subsides the subject usually drifts into a dreamless sleep. After-effects are uncommon, though following excessive doses the subject may wake with fatigue or generalised aches and pains. A clear memory is commonly retained of the principal phenomena experienced during the acute intoxication.

Keeler *et al.* (1968) described spontaneous recurrences of marihuana effects after discontinuation of the drug, and considered this to be relatively frequent. In some of their examples the recurrences served to precipitate severe anxiety and necessitated emergency psychiatric treatment. Whether or not such features are due to persistent biochemical effects of the drug is unknown. They appear to be analogous to the 'flashbacks' of LSD experience discussed on pp. 622–3, and to be commoner in persons who have previously used LSD.

One patient was confused under the drug, with disorientation, panic, inability to talk, and hallucinations of coloured spots and designs. For 3 weeks thereafter he experienced intermittent confusion, disorientation and similar hallucinations most often when attempting to sleep.

Another patient found that under marihuana the limbs of trees would appear to undulate and objects would seem to be covered with sparkling points of light. This would return during the day after drug use and the patient looked forward to such spontaneous recurrences.   (Keeler *et al.* 1968)

It seems that tetrahydrocannabinols are responsible for most of the psychological effects of cannabis. Different preparations vary in their potency and probably in their content of other toxic constituents, accounting for the somewhat different pictures reported from one investigation to another. Isbell *et al.* (1967) were able to reproduce the essential manifestations of hashish or marihuana intoxication by giving chemically pure Δ-9-tetrahydrocannabinol to human volunteers, either orally or by smoking.

The question of tolerance has been controversial. This appears not to develop in mild and occasional users, but in countries where regular and heavy consumption is common extremely large doses are tolerated. Abstinence phenomena may then be encountered on abrupt withdrawal in the form of irritability, weakness, insomnia and decreased appetite. Psychological dependence appears to be relatively rare in terms of craving or drug-seeking behaviour.

Acute psychiatric disorder

When taken in moderation it is unusual for individuals to experience more than the relatively benign effects of intoxication described above. Occasionally, however, episodes of acute psychiatric disturbance occur and may bring the patient to medical attention. The pictures that have been described include acute organic reactions and neurotic and psychotic disturbances of variable duration.

It is generally agreed that there is no specific 'cannabis psychosis', but rather that the mental picture is determined by individual predisposition coupled with contributions from the circumstances in which the drug is taken. Many of the more florid disturbances occur in unstable individuals with a past history of psychiatric disorder. Sometimes, indeed, severe abuse may be secondary to the development of an affective or schizophrenic illness, and with the longer-lasting psychotic manifestations it can often be hard to decide how far the drug is responsible. The clearest evidence incriminating the drug directly is with the acute organic reactions described below, which appear to be a great deal commoner in patients using high potency cannabis preparations.

Reactive emotional states were among the short-lived disturbances described by Bromberg (1934) and are probably the commonest form of adverse reaction. These emerge in response to features of the acute intoxication. Acute anxiety culminates in episodes of panic, or hysterical dissociation may lead to fugue-like wandering with subsequent amnesia. A period of mania may grow out of the emotional excitement occasioned by the drug, or suicidal ideas may emerge while the patient is confused.

Such reactions are self limiting, lasting from several minutes to several hours, and are said to occur most frequently in novice users, ambivalent users and users in a strange or threatening situation (Halikas 1974). The frequency of their occurrence, as with all other adverse reactions, is unknown.

Acute paranoid and schizophrenic reactions without clouding of consciousness probably occur mainly in subjects who are especially predisposed. Delusions and hallucinations take on a markedly paranoid colouring, or schizophreniform features may emerge with negativism, posturing and flexibilitas cerea. Such disturbances gradually subside as the drug is cleared from the body, though a few may progress to longer-lasting psychotic illnesses.

Ghodse (1986) reviews studies which suggest that such reactions may differ in subtle ways from ordinary paranoid schizophrenia, though this is far from well proven. Patients with cannabis-induced paranoid psychoses tend to show more by way of hypomanic features, with rapidity of thought and flight of ideas, and an absence of characteristic schizophrenic thought disorder. Violent and panicky behaviour is common, and insight better preserved. However, in a detailed comparison of cannabis-positive and cannabis-negative acute psychotic patients, McGuire *et al.* (1994b) could detect no differences in terms of psychopathology, mode of onset or Present State Examination syndrome profiles. Response to antipsychotic medication is usually swift with an excellent short-term outcome, though relapse may occur on using cannabis again.

In the rare example that persists for weeks or months, the illness may already have been present before the drug was taken, or the cannabis may have served to precipitate an illness which then follows its own independent course. Spencer (1970) reported several examples with certain features in common, and without a family or previous history of psychotic illness, and concluded that these at least were directly due to the repeated use of cannabis:

The illnesses began abruptly and coincidentally with acute intoxication. The patients developed severe psychomotor over-activity, pressure of thought and flight of ideas. Many were markedly aggressive. Elation was coupled with incongruity and lability of mood. Bizarre grandiose delusions were common, also passivity phenomena and ideas of reference and influence, but hallucinations were conspicuous by their absence. Consciousness was clouded in the first few days but then cleared rapidly so that the major part of the illness occurred in clear consciousness. All patients showed dense amnesia extending from prior to the onset of the illness until admission to hospital or apprehension by the police, and this amnesic gap remained as a permanent sequel. The acute phase required hospitalisation for 1–2 months, gradually giving way to flattening of affect and residual thought fragmentation which sometimes appeared to persist indefinitely. Insight was gained into the florid delusional beliefs, but many of the patients remained odd and some suspicious in demeanour after all other features had cleared.

Acute organic reactions or 'toxic psychoses' bear a more convincing relationship to cannabis use. They are rarely reported from the UK where usage tends to be mild and casual, but appear to be not uncommon in countries where high potency preparations are taken in large dosage.

Talbott and Teague (1969) reported 12 examples among soldiers in Vietnam. Ten occurred in soldiers of previously stable personality and in all of them the disturbance followed the first admitted exposure to the drug. All showed disorientation, impairment of memory, confusion, reduced attention span and tangential or disjointed thinking. Affect was labile with marked anxiety and fearfulness. Delusions, hallucinations and paranoid symptoms figured prominently, though the latter may have been partly determined by the environmental stress to which the men were exposed. The disorders were self limiting and all subjects returned to duty within a week.

A 26-year-old soldier became aware of a burning choking sensation in his throat immediately after smoking marihuana. Shortly thereafter he felt apprehensive and suspicious. This rapidly increased in intensity and he became fearful that 'Nationals' were out to harm him. He fled in terror to his quarters where a doctor was called to see him. On examination he was anxious, disorientated for time, and showed wave-like fluctuations in the intensity of his paranoid fears. At its worst his fear of the 'Nationals' reached delusional intensity. Affect was appropriate but labile. Thinking was rapid and disjointed, as if he were experiencing a multitude of changing thoughts of dissimilar nature but with a common apprehensive quality. There were no hallucinations. Coordination was impaired on the finger–nose and heel–knee test and Romberg's sign was positive. Tendon reflexes were symmetrical and hyperactive. The conjunctivae were reddened. He improved rapidly and was returned to duty within 48 hours. There was no recurrence during the next 3 months.

(Talbott & Teague 1969)

Chopra and Smith (1974) reported similar pictures from Calcutta, observing that a dose–response effect appeared to exist. Thus the reactions were commoner in patients using high potency preparations, and the higher the potency the shorter the period of use before the reaction occurred. Most patients recovered within hours or days, with recurrence among those who reverted to cannabis use though not among those who abstained. Chaudry *et al.*'s (1991) patients showed pictures dominated by 'mania-like' symptoms—grandiosity, excitement and hostility — along with disorientation and paranoia. These again resolved completely, usually within several days of starting neuroleptics.

Chronic psychiatric disorder

It has been claimed that excessive use of cannabis over long periods of time can result in a chronic psychotic illness akin to schizophrenia, and to an insidious personality change ('amotivational syndrome') with social and sometimes intellectual deterioration. Decisive evidence has been hard to obtain, and most reports of such associations are usually viewed with caution. When chronic psychoses have developed there may have been important predisposing factors or even pre-existing illness; and where social decompensation is concerned much may be due to social or subcultural influences. A study by Halikas *et al.* (1972) showed clearly how it could be erroneous to attribute causal significance to the drug. One hundred regular cannabis users were interviewed along with 50 non-user friends of the group. A high prevalence of psychopathology was found in both samples, approximately half of each fulfilling criteria for some psychiatric diagnosis. Moreover almost every diagnosed psychiatric illness among the users had begun before the first exposure to cannabis.

Nevertheless there is a theoretical possibility that cannabis could have cumulative effects. Tetrahydrocannabinols and their metabolites are fat soluble, and remain for long periods in body tissues from which they are slowly released back into the blood stream. Repeated exposure at intervals of less than 8–10 days may, therefore, result in the accumulation of substances with adverse psychological effects. The reports that cannabis may make its own contribution to lasting mental disorder therefore warrant close consideration.

There have been examples of *prolonged depersonalisation* lasting for months after cannabis use, sometimes after relatively brief exposures (Edwards 1963; Szymanski 1981; Keshavan & Lishman 1986). The patients often considered their chronic symptoms to be identical with those experienced during acute intoxication, adding to the suspicion that neurobiological factors could be responsible.

With regard to *chronic psychoses*, Thacore (1973) presented detailed clinical histories of four Indian patients in whom long-term ingestion of 'bhang', a mild cannabis preparation, seemed to be responsible for long-lasting schizophrenia-like illnesses. The patients were characterised by disturbance of thinking, fearfulness, hostile perception of the environment, delusions of persecution and auditory and visual hallucinations, but these occurred in clear consciousness and with little or no disturbance of memory. The data strongly suggested a causal relationship between excessive consumption of bhang and the development of the psychoses; the latter continued and fluctuated with continuing and fluctuating cannabis ingestion, but remitted whenever cannabis was stopped or greatly curtailed.

This may illustrate a common mechanism, in that such patients may effectively maintain themselves in a chronic psychotic state by the repeated evocation of short-lived psychotic reactions of the type already discussed. In others the use of cannabis may exacerbate the symptoms of an already present schizophrenia. There is little to suggest, by contrast, that cannabis can cause a chronic psychosis that persists after the drug is discontinued (Ghodse 1986, 1995).

The strongest evidence favouring a link with schizophrenia comes from a prospective study of Swedish conscripts, followed up through national hospital registers 15 years later (Andréasson *et al.* 1987, 1989). Those who had been users of cannabis at conscription showed a markedly increased risk of developing schizophrenia later when compared with non-users. Moreover the risk increased in proportion to the level of cannabis exposure. It appeared to be unrelated to other drug use or to prior evidence of mental disorder, though the numbers in which such factors could be explored was small. Thus the authors' conclusion that cannabis may be an independent risk factor for schizophrenia has generally been viewed with reserve.

The concept of an *amotivational syndrome* derives from the observations of Kolansky and Moore (1971, 1972). They proposed that chronic alterations of personality might result from biochemical or structural changes in the central nervous system induced by persistent marihuana use. Cognitive changes were also involved. Their initial report concerned 38 adolescents and young adults:

Several who had smoked marihuana four or five times per week over many months showed neurological impairment — slurred speech, staggering gait, hand tremor and disturbances of perception. Most of the others showed cognitive and emotional changes. Attention and concentration appeared impaired. A frequent complaint was of difficulty in converting thoughts into words, with the result that speech tended to be discursive. In the emotional sphere most subjects showed anxiety, depression, apathy and general indifference. Some showed hyperactivity and agitated behaviour. Paranoid developments and social withdrawal were common.

Social and ethical standards had often fallen so that promiscuity and venereal disease were frequent and the incidence of unwanted pregnancies was high. Personal cleanliness had deteriorated along with work and study habits. Eight patients showed frank psychotic developments with paranoid ideation, delusional systems, hallucinations, inappropriate affect and outbursts of aggression. The more florid features slowly disappeared on cessation of smoking, but some individuals were left with mild intellectual blunting or residual memory defects which seemed destined to be permanent. Unfortunately there was no attempt at objective psychometric assessment of such persisting cognitive impairments.

Kolansky and Moore stressed that none of the patients had shown evidence of psychiatric disturbance or personality deviation prior to starting use of the drug. Those who showed no more than aggravation of previous neurotic difficulties were excluded from the report, similarly those in whom a predisposition to psychotic illness could be discerned. Such judgements, however, are notoriously hard to make with confidence, and the report was criticised on this and other grounds (Benson 1971).

Subsequently, Kolansky and Moore (1972) described a further series of adults who had smoked cannabis for periods of 16 months to 6 years. Here the organic impairments were stressed again:

A distinctive clustering of symptoms was described, including chronic headache, reversal of sleep rhythm and 'mental and physical sluggishness'. Confusion appeared to be attributable to difficulty with recent memory, coupled with slowed time sense and incapacity for sustained thought processes. Apathy was associated with poor reality testing, loss of interest in life goals and disturbed self awareness. The intensity of the symptoms and the presence of delusions seemed to be directly related to the frequency and length of time of cannabis use. Flattening of affect was often marked; this was interpreted by the patient as representing a new philosophical calm, but in fact was liable to give way readily to anger under duress.

Again the symptoms were said to have begun only after starting cannabis, and to tend to fade out 3–24 months after discontinuation. The stereotyped nature of the symptoms was cited as evidence that they were caused by the effects of the drug on the central nervous system. In addition to reversible toxicity on a biochemical basis, Kolansky and Moore suggested that structural cerebral changes might occur in some instances.

The lack of controls, and of objective measures of impairment, have led Kolansky and Moore's conclusions to be viewed with considerable reserve. Studies soon afterwards found no evidence of impairment on neuropsychological testing among students taking marihuana when compared with their fellows (Grant *et al.* 1973; Culver & King 1974). These reports may, however, have given an overoptimistic view in that it is likely that dosages were relatively mild.

There is now evidence that *cognitive impairment*, at least for some time after exposure, may not be uncommon where heavy usage or high potency preparations are concerned. Mendhiratta *et al.* (1978) found impairments on a wide range of functions among 'charas' smokers and 'bhang' drinkers, tested a minimum of 12 hours after the last exposure to the drug; in comparison to controls they were impaired on tests of reaction speed, concentration,

time estimation and perceptuomotor ability. Those using charas, the stronger preparation, were the more severely impaired. Block *et al.* (1990) compared heavy users and non-users in Iowa, after equating earlier performance at school, and showed impairments in verbal expression and mathematical ability. Solowij *et al.* (1991) studied selective attention using event-related potentials and found evidence of impaired information processing.

Memory impairment has become the focus of special attention as reviewed by Reed and Grant (1990) and Deahl (1991). In a well-controlled investigation of a small group of adolescents, for example, Schwartz *et al.* (1989) found significant deficits on tests of both auditory–verbal and visual–spatial memory. Some improvement was observed after 6 weeks of supervised abstinence, but selective memory deficits appeared to persist to this time. Schwartz *et al.* point out that the potency of cannabis preparations available in the USA has steadily increased since the time of the earlier negative studies.

The possibility of structural brain changes appeared at first to find some support from neuroradiological evidence, again controversial, presented by Campbell *et al.* (1971). Ten young patients with histories of regular cannabis smoking were reported to show cerebral atrophy on air encephalography. Linear measurements of ventricular size were significantly increased in comparison to a control group, and three patients showed dilated sulci over the convexity of the hemispheres. Presenting complaints included generalised headache, impairment of recent memory, episodes of amnesia, poor concentration and loss of efficiency at work. Some showed poor memory, difficulty with thinking and obvious lack of insight. Other causes of cerebral atrophy in so young a group of patients could not be discerned.

However these findings came under criticism on several grounds—the nature of the controls, the adequacy of the radiological evidence and the lack of objective assessments to substantiate the impression of organic mental deficits (Bull 1971; Lancet 1971; Brewer 1972). Subsequent CT scan and cerebral blood flow studies have been essentially negative (Co *et al.* 1976; Kuehnle *et al.* 1977; Ashton 1987).

Amphetamines

The amphetamines comprise a group of drugs with analogous effects to adrenaline on the body. Hence they are often referred to as 'sympathomimetic amines'. They stimulate the central nervous system and also activate the sympathetic nervous system. Medical usage is now largely restricted to the treatment of narcolepsy (dextroamphetamine sulphate, racemic amphetamine sulphate, methylphenidate, p. 726), though the latter drug is also used in children with attention deficit hyperactivity disorder. Ephedrine, the earliest member of the group, is mainly employed as a nasal decongestant, and its derivatives are ingredients of over-the-counter cold cure remedies—pseudoephedrine (Sudafed), phenylpropanolamine (Triogesic) and phenylephrine. Other related compounds have been used for the treatment of obesity though this is now discouraged (phenmetrazine (Preludin), diethylpropion (Apisate), phentermine (Duromine), etc.).

Many patients have become dependent as a result of careless prescribing, and all drugs in the group may be abused for their stimulant and euphoriant effects. The use of methylamphetamine (Methedrine) by intravenous injection presented particular problems during the 1960s. Stricter prescribing controls are nowadays offset by illegal manufacture.

Physical and psychological effects

The principal effects are to produce elevated mood and increased energy, alertness and self confidence. Feelings of hunger and fatigue are reduced, the pupils are dilated, and the heart rate and blood pressure increased. Palpitations and dry mouth are common. With larger doses the subject becomes restless, talkative and often irritable. Rapid speech and overactivity are accompanied by ataxia and marked insomnia. Violent behaviour may be released. Severe toxicity is associated with dizziness, cardiac dysrhythmias, chest pain and sometimes convulsions. Hyperthermia is a serious risk and hypertension may lead to cerebral or subarachnoid haemorrhage.

Tolerance develops rapidly both to the euphoriant and the cardiovascular effects with repeat administration. Hence the dose must be increased to obtain mood elevation and large amounts come to be tolerated. Continued administration in narcoleptics does not, however, appear to diminish the awakening effects of the drugs.

Psychological dependence occurs rapidly when the drugs are abused, leading to intense craving and drug-seeking behaviour. Physical dependence is manifest in a rebound effect on REM sleep upon withdrawal (Oswald & Thacore 1963; Lewis et al. 1971). Lassitude and depression may then persist for several days, but this may be mainly the consequence of overactivity and lack of sleep while taking the drug.

Psychiatric disorder

Repetitive stereotyped behaviour of the type seen with cocaine abuse (p. 619) may emerge with chronic amphetamine ingestion, and tactile hallucinations may similarly lead to scratching and picking at the skin. Delusions concerning the presence of insects under the skin may again emerge.

However, the most dramatic complication is the development of an acute psychiatric disturbance which at first sight has none of the hallmarks of an organic toxic reaction. This is particularly common after injection of methylamphetamine. The classic picture is of an acute paranoid illness virtually indistinguishable from paranoid schizophrenia (Connell 1958). Disorientation and other organic mental symptoms may occur fleetingly after very large doses, but in the addict are usually conspicuous by their absence. Certainly in the fully-developed paranoid reaction it is very rare indeed to find evidence of cerebral impairment. The rapidity of onset, the dream-like quality of the experiences, and the brisk emotional reaction with an emphasis on fear are aspects of the condition which tend to differentiate it from endogenous schizophrenia. Stereotyped repetitive behaviour may give the clue, and outbursts of aggression may be prominent. Bell (1965) stressed that visual hallucinations predominate over auditory hallucinations to an extent that is unusual for schizophrenia, and formal thought disorder is rarely seen. However, none of these features allow a truly confident differential diagnosis. It is therefore essential to search for amphetamines in the urine when the condition is suspected.

Amphetamine-induced hallucinations usually subside over 1 or 2 days but delusions may persist for a week or longer. Persistence of the acute illness for more than a week after urinary tests have confirmed complete clearance of the drug from the body therefore makes the causal connection unlikely.

Similar psychotic reactions have been reported with the appetite suppressant phenmetrazine, though disorientation, inattention and difficulty with concentration are more usually in evidence (Bartholomew & Marley 1959). Classic examples in all respects have been described with ephedrine (Whitehouse & Duncan 1987).

Finally, when used by injection there is a risk of producing cerebral vasculitis as described on pp. 619–20. In several reports amphetamines have been especially incriminated in leading to this potentially serious complication.

Cocaine

Cocaine addiction has escalated dangerously, both in the USA and more recently in the UK. The appearance on the illegal market of cheap and particularly addictive forms of the drug ('crack') has come to pose especially severe problems.

The use of cocaine has a long history and it was formerly regarded as relatively safe for recreational purposes. This scenario has, however, changed dramatically, with increasing numbers of persons suffering profound social and physical consequences of addiction. The alkaloid is obtained from the leaves of the coca bush (*Erythroxylum coca*) which is grown extensively in Columbia, Bolivia and Peru. Coca paste, a crude derivative of the leaves, may be smoked, but most of the crop is converted into cocaine hydrochloride and sold as a powder, often mixed with various adjuvants. This can be inhaled into the nose (sniffing or snorting) or injected intravenously.

Freebase forms are derived from the hydrochloride as preparations suitable for smoking, a simple process yielding the form known as 'crack'. Tiny pellets of crack, representing pure crystalline cocaine, are sold remarkably cheaply and rapidly lead to the most severe form of addiction. Animal experiments have shown that cocaine is a powerful primary reinforcer, largely mediated through the dopaminergic system, leading the animal to work for drug reward to the exclusion of food and often until death. The use of freebase forms in humans can have a similar compelling quality.

Acute effects

In whatever form it is taken cocaine is a powerful stimulant and euphoriant, leading to increased energy and wakefulness for a time and feelings of great well-being. Intravenous use produces an intense 'rush' or 'high' almost instantaneously, gradually receding over 20–30 minutes. The smoking of crack has a similarly rapid effect, peaking after 5 minutes or so then abating quickly leaving the addict craving another dose. Nasal inhalation leads to a more gradual onset of euphoria, since vasoconstriction occurs within the nasal mucosa. The effects then typically wear off over an hour or so. While under the influence of the drug the subject shows enhanced alertness and mental acuity and feels increased confidence in social interchange. Cocaine is often regarded as an aphrodisiac because of the elation and disinhibition experienced, but higher doses lead to impotence and decreased sexual desire.

The stimulant effect upon the sympathetic nervous system leads to tachycardia, raised blood pressure, increased temperature and dilated pupils. Important effects are also exerted on the dopaminergic system, especially in mesolimbic and mesocortical areas. Large doses can result in a dangerous degree of hypertension, cardiac dysrhythmias or grand mal convulsions. Adulterants by way of procaine or lignocaine increase the risk of cardiovascular complications or status epilepticus. Other toxic

effects include muscle twitching, nausea and vomiting, irregular respiration and hyperpyrexia.

Sudden fatalities can occur from myocardial infarction, ventricular fibrillation or cerebral haemorrhage. Other deaths result from central nervous system depression with circulatory and respiratory failure, loss of reflexes and delirium. Unexplained deaths are thought to be due to toxic effects upon the myocardium. Persons with a congenital deficiency of pseudocholinesterase are at special hazard from even small doses since cocaine is broken down in the body by this enzyme.

Severe malnutrition is common in regular abusers who often present with multiple vitamin deficiencies. The powerful local anaesthetic effect of cocaine serves to obscure pain, so that dental neglect can reach extreme degree. Many addicts therefore present in a severely deteriorated state.

Ghodse (1995) discusses the issues of tolerance and dependence. It was formerly thought that tolerance did not occur, based on experience of occasional recreational users of the drug. It is now clear, however, that users of freebase forms can come to tolerate immense and frequently repeated doses, with adaptation to the convulsant and cardiovascular effects. It is less clear whether tolerance develops to the euphoriant properties though this is likely.

Psychological dependence develops rapidly and soon becomes a major problem. Even the casual weekend user is prone to find that little is enjoyable without the drug, and progresses to more frequent and dangerous forms of administration. As the dosage increases dysphoric effects emerge in the wake of elation, with depression, irritability, anxiety and profound insomnia. Severe craving and intense drug-seeking behaviour can then become entrenched. Withdrawal results in a state of depression, apathy and increased appetite, with lethargy and disinterest often persisting for many weeks. Suicidal feelings are not uncommon. Physical aspects of withdrawal include disturbed sleep patterns, tremors and muscle pain, but the major physiological disruptions seen with opiate and sedative withdrawal do not occur.

Psychiatric disorder

Estroff and Gold (1986) divide the psychiatric effects of cocaine into four successive stages—euphoria, dysphoria, hallucinosis and psychosis. The euphoria, already described, shows symptoms analogous to mania with heightened pleasure, hyperactivity and increased speed of intellectual functioning. Disinhibition and impulsive behaviour are common, including a proneness to violence. The second stage, dysphoria, resembles major depression with anxiety, misery, apathy and irritability, occurring when cocaine levels are falling or when the addict is craving another dose. Restlessness and hostility can be prominent. Alcohol or other drugs may be used to combat such phases.

Cocaine hallucinosis usually begins with visual and auditory misperceptions. Harmless objects and noises appear to be threatening and the person is hypervigilant and increasingly concerned. Halo effects may appear around lights, or sensations of movement at the periphery of the visual field. Hallucinations then emerge in several modalities — lights sparkling at the periphery of vision ('snow lights'), voices calling the user's name, and the classic tactile hallucinations of insects felt crawling under the skin. The last usually develop only after several days of intensified use (Siegel 1978). At this stage partial insight is retained into the unreal nature of the hallucinations and delusions.

Cocaine psychosis represents further progression to extreme paranoia. It is usually preceded by a transitional period of increasing suspiciousness, ideas of reference, dysphoria and compulsive behaviour (Weiss *et al.* 1994). The patient is restless and talkative, and everyday events are misinterpreted in delusional fashion — he believes others are plotting against him or about to attack him, or that he is being followed by the police or drug dealers. He may act on such beliefs with unusual aggressiveness, damaging property or becoming homicidal or suicidal. Insight is lost into the unreal nature of the hallucinatory experiences; he may pick and scratch at his skin in the search for insects or even claim to see them. A further characteristic feature is repetitive stereotyped behaviour, such as dismantling and reassembling a watch or radio over and again, or compulsively arranging and rearranging a set of objects (Ghodse 1995). Consciousness is fully preserved throughout and there is no disorientation.

Such pictures are strikingly similar to the paranoid psychoses seen with amphetamine intoxication (p. 617), but come to medical attention less often because they are usually of briefer duration. The major manifestations usually subside within 24 hours, though Manschreck *et al.* (1987) have reported examples lasting for days or weeks among freebase smokers. Severe examples usually arise in the context of chronic addiction but can follow a single large dose. The manifestations are probably closely related to elevated dopamine activity in the brain.

In addition to these classic pictures, other forms of psychiatric disturbance are not uncommon. There is a high prevalence of depression among users of cocaine, particularly during attempts at discontinuation. It remains unclear how far this reflects the cerebral effects of the drug or the social disturbances induced by addiction. Transient episodes of paranoia have emerged as frequent in surveys of addicts, with up to two-thirds reporting them at some time (Weiss *et al.* 1994). Persons already suffering from psychiatric disorder are more vulnerable to becoming addicted, and this may shape the effects of the drug. Mania may be precipitated in cyclothymic persons, or schizophrenia exacerbated after quite low doses. Those with a predisposition towards panic disorder may experience their first or worst panic attack (Weiss *et al.* 1994).

The cognitive sequelae of cocaine addiction have received little attention, and it is possible that any impairments detected are mainly related to loss of sleep and depression. Herning *et al.* (1990) review occasional reports of transient deficits in information processing during withdrawal, also impaired blood flow to the prefrontal cortex. Herning *et al.*'s own study followed a small group of patients during the first few weeks of abstinence, showing increased P_{300} latencies on the first day and slowed reaction times on a short-term memory test during the next 3–4 weeks. O'Malley and Gawin (1990) have reported mild deficits in concentration, memory and abstracting ability in recently abstinent patients, and persistent impairment of motor skills.

Neurological complications

The risk of convulsions and cerebrovascular accidents following acute administration has already been mentioned above. Among 996 emergency room visits by cocaine abusers in San Francisco, Lowenstein *et al.* (1987) reported seizures in 29, focal neurological syndromes in 12, headache in 10, transient losses of consciousness in six and stupor or coma in three. The time from administration to the development of seizures varied from minutes to several hours, two patients presenting with status epilepticus. The focal motor and sensory syndromes were often transient, resolving within hours or days, though they sometimes reflected the occurrence of subarachnoid or intracerebral haemorrhage. Transient loss of consciousness appeared to be due to syncope, sometimes consequent upon cardiac dysrhythmia. All such events could occur in new or occasional users as well as in chronic addicts. Mody *et al.* (1988) have reported occasional patients presenting with anterior spinal artery thrombosis, medullary infarction or transient ischaemic attacks, again sometimes after first exposure to the drug.

Cerebral vasculitis represents another hazard. This was first suspected in intravenous drug users from angiographic findings — irregular segmental constrictions in intermediate-sized arteries and complete obstruction in smaller vessels (Lignelli & Buchheit 1971; Rumbaugh *et al.* 1971). Citron *et al.* (1970) found autopsy evidence of multiorgan involvement resembling polyarteritis nodosa. Polydrug abuse was the common pattern in such cases, and impurities in the injected material, or sepsis, could have been chiefly responsible. As such reports accumulated it seemed that methylamphetamine injection might be the common denominator, but there is now autopsy and biopsy evidence to incriminate cocaine as well. The patient reported by Fredericks *et al.* (1991) developed an acute encephalopathy shortly after intravenous cocaine administration, and brain biopsy revealed an extensive vasculitis primarily involving the small arteries. The patient had no history of amphetamine or heroin abuse.

Treatment

Treatment of acute toxic reactions may require barbiturates or diazepam to control severe agitation, overstimulation or seizures (Estroff & Gold 1986). Propanolol helps with tachycardia and hypertension, and further drugs may be needed to deal with cardiac dysrhythmias. Impending circulatory and respiratory failure will warrant urgent supportive measures. Respiratory depression may indicate that opiates have been taken as well, requiring the administration of naloxone. Chlorpromazine or haloperidol may be needed for the control of psychotic reactions.

Approaches to treatment of the addiction are outlined by Ghodse (1995). Gradual stepwise reduction of dosage is not appropriate, as used in opiate and sedative detoxification, because of the brevity of effect of each dose of cocaine. The drug is therefore discontinued abruptly and the ensuing symptoms treated appropriately. Diazepam or propanolol are used for dysphoria and agitation, and antidepressant drugs for depression. Depression, though transient, can be severe and the risk of suicide is sometimes considerable.

Attempts are under way to determine which drugs might best assist the patient to abstain by blocking the major effects of cocaine. Desipramine and bromocriptine both appear to reduce craving, the latter perhaps by restoring depleted dopamine reserves. 'Cue-precipitated craving' can be especially strong with cocaine abuse, persisting long after use of the drug has been abandoned (Strang *et al.* 1993).

Lysergic acid diethylamide (LSD-25, lysergide)

LSD is an indole derivative of ergot and can be manufactured synthetically. It is the most powerful hallucinogen known, doses as small as 25 µg usually having a demonstrable effect on humans. In other species its range of effects is extraordinary — it makes cats afraid of mice, reduces spiders' ability to build webs, causes fish to maintain a vertical nose-up position and swim backwards, and induces catatonia in pigeons (Louria 1968). Chromosomal changes have also been reported, with increased chromosomal breaks and rearrangements of chromosome material, though studies of patients receiving LSD for therapeutic purposes have failed to confirm such findings (Robinson *et al.* 1974). The mode of action on the brain is thought to lie with inhibition of the serotonergic system, by the stimulation of presynaptic 5-hydroxytryptamine (5-HT$_2$) receptors and consequent feedback effects on serotonergic neurones (Kosten 1990).

Soon after its discovery it enjoyed a vogue in experimental psychiatry for the study of 'model psychoses' which could be induced in normal subjects. Thereafter it was employed as an adjunct in psychotherapy, for abreaction and to assist in the recall of long-forgotten experiences. As a result the acute effects of its administration were closely studied and formed the basis of a good deal of theoretical speculation. Nowadays administration under medical supervision is rare, but the drug continues to be widely taken on an illicit basis. The benefits claimed by users include augmented aesthetic sensitivity, enhanced creativity, the occurrence of transcendental experiences, the acquisition of new insights, and aphrodisiac effects. None of these has been properly substantiated. It is widely abused by unstable individuals in search of dramatic experiences, and often by those who abuse other drugs as well. As a drug of abuse LSD carries the special hazard that it can easily be administered surreptitiously without the subject's knowledge, resulting in profoundly disturbing effects which may sometimes lead to psychiatric referral.

When taken at intervals of more than a week the reaction is just as intense with the same repeated dose; however, when taken daily tolerance develops rapidly, but is lost just as quickly when discontinued for a few days (Isbell *et al.* 1956). There is no evidence that LSD is a drug of addiction in the sense of creating physical dependence, and there are no withdrawal effects on discontinuation. The danger lies rather in psychological dependence on the effects that are produced.

Acute effects of ingestion

The acute effects are well described by Isbell *et al.* (1956) and by Freedman (1968). There is some variation in individual susceptibility, but striking psychological changes usually follow doses in the range of 20–120 µg. The predominant effects with small doses are autonomic changes and alterations of mood, while larger doses produce perceptual distortions, vivid hallucinations and striking subjective changes in the body image. These remarkably intense phenomena are usually not accompanied by clouding of consciousness or demonstrable impairment of intellectual processes; indeed a heightened state of awareness is maintained, and thought processes characteristically remain clear. The subject becomes preoccupied with the phenomena which he is witnessing and experiencing, but usually retains insight into the fact that they are due to the drug. In these respects the 'toxic' state resulting from LSD and related hallucinogens is very different from the acute organic reactions induced by most other agents.

The autonomic effects are the first to appear. They include dilatation of the pupils, piloerection and some rise in body temperature. The tendon reflexes are often increased, and muscular tremors and twitching develop in severe reactions. Weakness, somnolence and giddiness may be marked. The earliest mood changes are of euphoria or anxiety. Euphoria is usually the predominant change and may extend to feelings of ecstasy, but this can be followed later by sudden swings to depression, panic or a profound sense of desolation. Some subjects become active and excited, while others are quiet, passive and withdrawn. Some are overwhelmed with a sense of mystical experience. Others become paranoid and hostile to their surroundings. Much probably depends on the premorbid personality of the subject, his expectations and the setting in which the drug is taken.

Perceptual distortions, illusions and hallucinations are mainly in the visual sphere but can affect all modalities. Vision may be blurred or astonishingly enhanced and vivid. The perception of depth and distance is changed, size and shape distorted, and colour greatly intensified. Hearing may be dulled or hyperacute, clothing may feel like sandpaper, or the body may feel extremely light or heavy. Synaesthesia often occurs and is fascinating to the subject—sensory data are transformed from one modality to another so that sounds or tactile stimuli appear as bursts of light or scintillating moving spectra. Hallucinations are again mainly visual and occur in both unformed and formed varieties—kaleidoscopic patterns of light in intense and changeable colour, or complex visions of animals and people. Tactile paraesthesiae, metallic tastes and strange smells are not uncommon, but auditory hallucinations are rare.

Distortions of the body image can figure prominently and take bizarre forms. Customary boundaries become fluid, so that the patient feels he is one with the chair upon which he is sitting or merged with the body of another. His own hands and feet may appear to be transformed into claws or the extremities of a dead person.

Sometimes intense somatic discomfort is experienced with feelings of being twisted, crushed or stretched. Depersonalisation and feelings of unreality may extend to the impression of being outside of one's own body, difficulty in recognising the self in a mirror, or difficulty in deciding whether a thought refers to a real event or is merely a spontaneous thought.

Despite these experiences the subject is able to respond to questions, and conceptual and abstract thinking can usually be shown to be substantially intact. Except in the most severe reactions a large measure of critical self judgement is preserved. However, as the effects of the drug increase, external reality becomes progressively less intrusive and self control may be lessened, occasionally with dangerous results as described below. Frank delusions may occasionally be expressed but an organised delusional system rarely develops.

Formal intelligence tests may show some decrease, mainly where verbal subtests are concerned (Isbell *et al.* 1956). The Minnesota Multiphasic Personality Inventory shows a large increase in scores on the psychasthenia, schizophrenia and paranoia scales. Anxiety questionnaires similarly show a marked rise in scores. The effect of LSD on the EEG is not to slow it, as with agents which produce impairment of consciousness, but to change it towards a pattern associated with increased arousal and vigilance, namely diminution or abolition of alpha activity and an increase in low voltage fast frequencies.

The effects of the drug are usually apparent within 30 minutes of ingestion, rising to a maximum 1–4 hours thereafter. The reaction subsides gradually over the next 8–16 hours and there is usually no residuum on waking next morning. After the vivid effects of the drug experience, however, the real world often appears to be drab and dull, and natural events lack the urgent and compelling quality of what has gone before. Some degree of depression and disillusionment may thus be an understandable aftermath.

Acute adverse reactions

Among habitual users the great majority of LSD experiences are apparently without adverse effect. Occasionally, however, profoundly disturbing results accompany the acute effects of the drug, and lead to emergency medical referral or trouble with the police. Adverse effects appear to be commoner in unstable subjects. Certainly a large proportion of those coming before psychiatrists have a history of previous psychiatric care (Ungerleider *et al.* 1966). It has been estimated that less than 0.1% of normal subjects experience seriously adverse reactions when LSD is taken under medical supervision; among patients undergoing psychotherapy the incidence rises to 0.2–1.0%, and among psychotic subjects to 1–3% (Louria 1968). The frequency among illicit users is unknown but is probably higher still. Much may also depend on the circumstances in which the drug is taken, on impurities in the preparations used and on injudicious doses.

The pictures that result have been described by Frosch *et al.* (1965), Ungerleider *et al.* (1966), Bewley (1967) and Freedman (1968). They may be divided into acute emotional disturbances, the acting out of impulses, and acute psychotic reactions.

Acute emotional disturbances are the most common, especially an acute panic reaction in which the subject feels overwhelmed by experiences beyond his control. He may feel that he is going insane or react in terror to homicidal impulses. He may present himself at hospital seeking relief, or be brought by friends who fear he will come to harm. There is no impairment of consciousness though recollection of the details of the LSD experience may be hazy. Rapid recovery occurs as the drug effects wear off, usually within 8–12 hours, though sometimes 1 or 2 days are required to regain normality.

Other acute emotional disturbances include depression, paranoia and outbursts of explosive anger. Profound depression very occasionally leads to attempted or successful suicide. Acute paranoia may cause the subject to flee about the streets in terror or lead to episodes of explosive anger.

The acting out of impulses is facilitated as self control becomes diminished. The subject may become unmanageable, run amok, attempt to disrobe or make overt homosexual advances. Sociopathic individuals are more prone to commit acts of violence and attempted homicide has been reported. Feelings of invulnerability may lead the patient to take unwarranted risks with danger of bodily harm. Patients who have fallen from windows or roofs have sometimes apparently acted on the belief that they would float down unharmed.

Acute psychotic reactions are commonly longer lasting, and the majority of Ungerleider *et al.*'s (1966) patients remained in hospital for more than a month. Most are schizophrenia-like illnesses with hallucinations, delusions and overactive behaviour. Less commonly they take the form of acute organic reactions with confusion, disorientation and marked emotional lability. The latter, however, may often be the product of multiple drug abuse. Muller (1971) has described the dramatic response which may occur to electroconvulsive therapy when such psychotic reactions are prolonged.

Hatrick and Dewhurst (1970) reported two interesting examples in which psychotic illnesses followed a latent interval, well after the effects of acute intoxication had

subsided. The illnesses were nevertheless coloured by phenomena reminiscent of the acute phase of intoxication. Both patients were said to have been previously stable and well adjusted, and the illnesses followed a single exposure to LSD:

A student of 19 had a pleasant 'trip' lasting 8–9 hours and was her usual self next day. Two weeks later she developed a severe depressive illness requiring admission to hospital. This was accompanied by confusion about the time sequence of recent events. As the depression cleared schizophrenic features were revealed, with tangential thought disorder, depersonalisation, feelings of unreality and disturbed ego boundaries. She experienced uncertainty about objects in her perceptual field, and had difficulty in realising she had a body. Heightened visual perception was associated with these disturbances and everything was described as wonderful and beautiful. She improved rapidly after electroconvulsive treatment and had no recurrence during 2.5 years of follow-up.

A secretary of 21 had been given LSD surreptitiously in her drink, producing various perceptual disturbances and a vivid dream. She remained well for 2 weeks thereafter but then began to have nightmares in which she saw stabbing scenes in gory detail. These represented a sequence from a film she had attended while still under the effects of LSD. She also experienced hypnagogic hallucinations of a horrifying nature. Thereafter she developed a severe agitated depression with persecutory auditory hallucinations. Electroconvulsive treatment produced rapid benefit and she remained well when seen 4 months later.

Features which may be of diagnostic significance in LSD-induced psychoses are discussed by Dewhurst and Hatrick (1972). A particularly striking aspect may be the wide variety of schizophreniform, affective and neurotic symptoms present in the same patient. Suggestive symptoms include regression to childhood, loss of time sense, grandiose delusions of a pseudophilosophical nature, and a wealth of visual hallucinations and perceptual disturbances. Visual hallucinations are said to be more intense than in other acute organic reactions and may be specific, transient and recurring. Auditory hallucinations tend to have a more startling, personal and realistic quality than in schizophrenia. The emotional response is usually constantly shifting with apprehension, panic, elation or depression in rapidly changing sequence. When an LSD-induced psychosis presents as hypomania, euphoria may alternate with panic which is an unusual combination in primary affective illness. Many patients with suicidal ruminations have irrational compulsive urges to self destruction, arising suddenly and sometimes unbacked by other depressive symptoms.

Recurrences of the LSD effect (flashbacks)

Occasionally there may be a simple prolongation of the

LSD state lasting several days, with undulating anxiety and persisting visual aberrations, but Frosch *et al.* (1965) have described more remarkable phenomena in which the LSD experiences recur for many weeks or months after discontinuation of the drug. Sometimes it is merely bewilderment or fear which recur in milder form, but quite commonly sensory phenomena are involved as well. Two of Frosch *et al.*'s patients experienced depersonalisation and perceptual distortions 2 months later. Another had many transient episodes of catatonia and visual hallucinations over the course of a year, similar to those that had been induced by LSD.

Horowitz (1969) suggests that perhaps as many as 5% of users experience mild recurrences from time to time, and others have put the estimate much higher. Sensory recurrences have been reported in all modalities, but the visual system is most often involved. Horowitz described three main varieties. The commonest consists of the repeated intrusion into awareness of some image derived from the LSD experience. This arrives unbidden and is outside voluntary control. It may be accompanied by distortion of time sense or reality sense. It is usually the same image that recurs, often of a frightening nature, and considerable psychiatric disturbance can occasionally be provoked. The second variety consists of the spontaneous return of perceptual distortions — halo effects, blurring, shimmering, reduplication, distortion of planes, changes of colour, micropsia or macropsia. Thirdly, there may be an increased sensitivity to spontaneous imagery for some time after taking LSD. Such imagery is more vivid than usual, less readily suppressed, and occupies a greater proportion of the subject's thought and time than formerly.

Abraham (1983) added additional phenomena, notably geometric pseudohallucinations, false perceptions of movement in the peripheral field, flashes of colour, intensified colours, and 'trailing phenomena' in which afterimages remain immediately behind an object as it traverses the visual field. Symptoms were sometimes reported as long as 8 years after the last exposure to LSD. Common precipitants in Abraham's series were emergence into a dark environment, staring at a blank wall or the subsequent use of marihuana. Benzodiazepines were found to be useful in treatment.

Several explanations have been put forward to account for recurrences but none has been substantiated. Brain damage has been blamed, or the release of some stored metabolite, or neurophysiological changes in the mechanisms underlying imagery formation and suppression. Abraham (1982) has obtained evidence that LSD users are impaired on tests of colour discrimination when examined an average of 2 years after their last exposure, and that those experiencing flashbacks are particularly

affected. Further visual studies have shown depressed critical flicker frequencies and reduced sensitivity to light during dark adaptation in past users of LSD (Abraham & Wolf 1988). The tendency for recurrences to accompany periods of stress and anxiety has suggested that they may represent a form of conditioned response or learned reaction to anxiety. Psychodynamic theorists have viewed the recurrent imagery as representing screen images to conceal emotional conflict, or as symbolising the breakthrough of repressed ideas.

Late adverse reactions

The use of LSD as an adjunct to psychotherapy was known to lead, very occasionally, to long-lasting psychiatric complications. States of anxiety and bewilderment could last for several weeks or months, or prolonged depression could follow when feelings of guilt or shame had been mobilised. More serious psychotic developments were attributed to the release of overwhelming conflict-laden material. Cohen and Ditman (1962, 1963) documented similar prolonged adverse reactions after illicit use of the drug, lasting often for several months and sometimes for up to 2 years.

The psychoses that follow are usually of schizophrenic type. Catatonic and paranoid forms have been reported, often with elements similar to those seen during acute LSD intoxication. Visual hallucinations may be prominent, highly coloured and mobile, and euphoria and grandiosity are often much in evidence. Such reactions can follow a single dose of the drug. Many of the reported examples have been in long-standing schizophrenic subjects, and in them the drug has presumably served merely to precipitate a recurrence. The majority of the remainder have been in persons with unstable personalities. The important question of whether prolonged psychoses can be provoked in persons without special predisposition remains unanswered.

Rosenthal (1964) drew attention to a further rare type of prolonged reaction, consisting of visual hallucinosis in clear consciousness. Rosenthal considered this to be specifically related to multiple exposures to LSD over a considerable period of time. The condition is often heralded by a change in the experience produced by the drug, typically a change to unpleasant reactions which may have led to its discontinuation. Spontaneous visual hallucinations then commence and continue for many months. The hallucinations are similar in form and content to those experienced under the drug—droplets of colour, shimmering panels and brightly coloured shape distortions. Cats, crabs, insects and corpses may also be seen. Pleasant hallucinations were often under semivoluntary control, in that the patient could make them more or less intense by efforts of concentration, but the unpleasant phenomena were intrusive and liable to provoke severe anxiety. The patients continued to recognise the unreality of the hallucinations, and there was no evidence of thought disorder or other schizophrenic phenomena. Occasionally, however, a secondary delusional system was elaborated to explain the hallucinations.

Other hallucinogens

Other drugs with similar hallucinogenic properties to LSD will not be discussed in detail. Many are derived from plants and enjoy a vogue in certain parts of the world. *Mescalin* comes from a cactus grown in Mexico and nearby parts of the USA, and *psylocybin* and *psilocin* from mushrooms ('magic mushrooms') found in a variety of regions. Mace, nutmeg and the morning glory plant contain other hallucinogenic substances.

A range of synthetic compounds with hallucinogenic and amphetamine-like activity have also been widely abused—dimethyltryptamine (*DMT*), dimethoxyamphetamine (*DMA*) and dimethoxymethylamphetamine (*DOM*). *Phenyclidine* (PCP, 'angel dust') is related to pethidine and has been widely abused in North America. Its use is particularly hazardous on account of a tendency to precipitate convulsions and coma, and its unpredictable psychological effects including outbursts of violent bizarre behaviour and prolonged psychoses.

Ecstasy

Ecstasy (3,4-methylene-dioxymethamphetamine, MDMA) is one of the new class of 'designer drugs', manufactured in attempts to side-step legal controls, though it has now been banned in the UK and the USA. It is a synthetic derivative of amphetamine and was once marketed as an appetite suppressant. In the UK it is mainly used in the context of 'raves' — parties organised for energetic dancing — as a euphoriant and to promote feelings of closeness to others. Along with mild stimulation it has some hallucinogenic potential. From time to time it attracts widespread publicity from the sudden tragic deaths that occur, occasionally on first contact with the drug.

Tolerance occurs gradually with repeated use, some habitués taking as many as 10–20 tablets during the course of a weekend (Winstock 1991). It does not, however, appear to cause physical dependence.

Toxic effects include appetite suppression, nausea, muscle aches, trismus and bruxism. Insomnia may occur, likewise tachycardia and hypertension, all resolving

within 48 hours. The more serious complications include hyperpyrexia, often compounded by vigorous dancing, and states of collapse possibly due to dehydration and hyponatraemia. Convulsions, rhabdomyolysis, disseminated intravascular coagulation and acute renal failure have all been reported (Fahal *et al.* 1992; Henry 1992). Recurrent hepatitis has also been described with repeated use (Shearman *et al.* 1992). Acute adverse reactions can require urgent medical intervention with active cooling measures, control of seizures, rehydration and sometimes forced diuresis with mannitol (Screaton *et al.* 1991).

Two cases of mutism and stupor lasting for 48 hours were reported by Maxwell *et al.* (1993), both patients showing hyponatraemia. One had evidence of inappropriate antidiuretic hormone secretion and had drunk large quantities of water. This may be the mechanism underlying occasional reports of prolonged coma, sometimes with a fatal outcome, and apparently due to water intoxication with cerebral oedema.

Psychiatric disorder

Psychiatric adverse reactions include short-lived episodes of panic (Whitaker-Azmitia & Aronson 1989), dysphoric reactions lasting 2–3 days and occasionally severe depression (Benazzi & Mazzoli 1991). Feelings of paranoia accompany the euphoriant effect in up to 40% of cases (Winstock 1991). Longer-term reactions have included flashbacks of pleasurable feelings and of perceptual distortions, the latter accompanied by intense anxiety, often recurring over several weeks or months (Creighton *et al.* 1991). McGuire and Fahy (1991) have reported examples of chronic paranoid psychoses and morbid jealousy after heavy misuse.

In a recent report McGuire *et al.* (1994a) describe a consecutive series of 13 patients referred for psychiatric treatment, eight being psychotic, two experiencing hallucinations and other complex visual phenomena, and one each with severe depression, recurrent panic attacks and chronic depersonalisation. All of the psychotic patients had been regular users of the drug for a mean duration of 1 year. Half presented within a week of discontinuation, the others after several weeks or months. The phenomenology was closely similar to that of other psychotic patients, with persecutory delusions as the most prominent feature but also delusions of reference and bodily change. Auditory hallucinations were less common and usually fleeting. Some patients experienced visual illusions and flashbacks. Two of the eight responded to neuroleptics within 2–4 weeks, whereas treatment was only partially effective in the remainder.

The patients with predominantly visual phenomena

showed a mixture of illusions, hallucinations and palinopsia, persisting for over a year. One had set in during regular use, the other 2 weeks after a single dose. The first patient was seen by the present author:

This was an 18-year-old girl who had taken 1–2 tablets of ecstasy at weekends over several months. After some weeks each ingestion would be followed for 2 hours or so by visual disturbances— shimmering in the air, shadowy images and eventually complex illusions in which writing would appear from the patterns of the carpet. At times she also saw disembodied faces, miniature people and running spiders.

These phenomena lasted longer after each dose of ecstasy, and became continuous after 6 months at which point she stopped the drug. They were still present when seen a year later. She saw masses of brightly coloured 'cartoon-like' spiders running here and there, especially when looking at shadowy corners of the room. Patterns and objects appeared to move when she looked at them, and she saw brightly coloured patterns when her eyes were closed. She frequently experienced palinopsia — when moving the hand across her field of vision she saw numerous after-images which then moved to join up with her hand. Sometimes when staring at an object she could make it move 'in her mind'.

These disturbances were perhaps becoming gradually milder and she was learning to ignore them in some degree. She had full insight into the unreal nature of the hallucinations. She had not used other drugs or alcohol and had no psychiatric or medical history. Formal neurological and ophthalmological examination showed no abnormalities and brain MRI was uninformative. Chlorpromazine and Prothiaden had no effect on the symptoms.

The great majority of McGuire et al.'s patients had used other drugs in the past, but the present disturbances had clearly developed in the context of ecstasy abuse. Half had a family history of psychiatric morbidity and some had had adverse reactions to other drugs, suggesting that ecstasy may merely have precipitated the present problems. However, the occurrence of visual phenomena and flashbacks in several patients suggested a more direct toxic role for the drug.

Ecstasy is known to be a selective serotonergic neurotoxin, producing a rapid decrease in brain 5-hydroxytrptamine and 5-hydroxyindoleacetic acid in experimental animals (McKenna & Peroutka 1990). Low levels can persist for as long as 12 months after repeat administration, especially in the frontal cortex, hippocampus and striatum. Structural damage has also been shown in non-human primates, affecting serotonergic fibres in the cortex and cell bodies in the dorsal raphe nucleus (Ricaurte et al. 1988). The degree of damage has proved to be cumulative and dose related. The serious possibility therefore arises that ecstasy may cause irreversible damage to the serotonergic system in certain individuals, perhaps conferring long-term vulnerability to psychiatric disorder (Green & Goodwin 1996).

Toxic effects of other drugs

Many other drugs can produce toxic effects on the central nervous system and lead to psychiatric disturbance. The number involved is legion, and the variety of their effects too great to be discussed in detail here. Comprehensive reviews of drug toxicity are presented by Dukes (1992), and aspects of particular relevance to psychiatric practice are dealt with by Tornatore et al. (1987), Ciraulo et al. (1989) and Lipowski (1990). These cover the adverse reactions seen with steroids, insulin, narcotics, analgesics, hypnotics, anticonvulsants, tranquillisers, anticholinergic agents, antiparkinsonian drugs, rauwolfia alkaloids, antihypertensive drugs, digoxin, diuretics, antituberculous drugs, other antibacterial agents, androgens, oestrogens and oral contraceptives. Only some of these will be considered below.

Sometimes the toxic reaction is an idiosyncratic response to the drug given in normal therapeutic dosage, or to several drugs being prescribed in combination. For this reason it is essential to review the patient's current medication when dealing with psychiatric illnesses of obscure origin, and particularly when these take the form of acute organic reactions. Sometimes the cause is excessive self medication, either in error or when the patient is addicted. The range of drugs which are surreptitiously abused tends to increase steadily.

The commonest form of disturbance is an acute organic reaction of variable duration, usually with features typical of delirium and often with prominent hallucinations. Neurological and other systemic signs specific for the drug in question may be in evidence. Some drugs, however, are associated primarily with mood changes or psychotic reactions in clear consciousness as described below.

The elderly are especially at risk of adverse drug reactions. Concomitant physical illness or incipient dementia will reduce the margins by which delirium is provoked. Common offending drugs are digoxin, minor and major tranquillisers, antihypertensives and diuretics. Hypnotics such as nitrazepam readily accumulate, leading to daytime confusion. Anticholinergic agents — antispasmodics, tricyclic antidepressants, phenothiazines and antiparkinsonian drugs—are particularly liable to induce confusion or memory impairment in the elderly (Potamianos & Kellett 1982). Anticholinergics have also been clearly incriminated as a major factor leading to postoperative delirium (Tune et al. 1981).

Antidepressants

Among psychotrophic drugs, severe reactions may occasionally be seen with antidepressant medication or combinations of antidepressant drugs. These are reviewed by Connell (1968) and McClelland (1986). Minor degrees of disturbance are probably quite frequent; Davies *et al.* (1971) reported episodes of impaired memory and orientation in 13% of patients taking tricyclic antidepressant drugs, rising to 35% in those over 40 years of age. Withdrawal reactions may occasionally be seen when monoamine oxidase inhibitors, or more rarely tricyclic antidepressants, are stopped abruptly, with nausea, gastrointestinal upset, headache, anxiety and panic (Drug & Therapeutics Bulletin 1986a).

Lithium

Lithium can have serious effects on central nervous system functioning. A fine tremor, representing an exaggeration of normal physiological tremor, must often be accepted, likewise some minor forgetfulness and lethargy. When such symptoms develop in patients on long-term lithium treatment the possibility of an induced hypothyroidism must be borne in mind (p. 514). More marked symptoms — muscle fasciculation, coarse tremor, ataxia, incoordination or extrapyramidal signs — call for abrupt cessation of treatment. The development of confusion or impairment of consciousness constitutes a medical emergency; the severe encephalopathic reactions which can then ensue sometimes prove to be irreversible or to result in permanent brain damage. Increasing confusion is accompanied by seizures, cerebellar signs, marked generalised tremor or decerebrate rigidity. States of stupor or coma may be prolonged. For reasons that are unclear such reactions may sometimes set in despite normal serum concentrations of lithium (Spiers & Hirsch 1978; Newman & Saunders 1979). Upon recovery there may be long-lasting cerebellar and extrapyramidal deficits (Sellers *et al.* 1982; Schou 1984). Smith and Kocen (1988) have described two patients in whom the clinical picture closely resembled Creutzfeldt–Jakob disease, with rapid onset of dementia, rigidity and in one case myoclonic jerks. The EEG picture closely supported such a diagnosis. In both cases discontinuation of lithium led to resolution of the symptoms and the EEG abnormalities over the course of 2–3 weeks.

The *combination of lithium and haloperidol* was specially incriminated by Cohen and Cohen (1974) in leading to severe reactions. Two of their patients were left with permanent parkinsonian–cerebellar deficits and dementia, and two with persistent dyskinesias. Loudon and Waring (1976) reported similar though milder reactions of this nature, and Spring (1979) described severe neurotoxic developments from the combination of lithium with thioridazine. Sometimes the same combination of drugs

has been given previously without ill effect as in the following example:

A patient reported by Thomas (1979) had been maintained on lithium within the normal therapeutic range for many years. Haloperidol was then added on account of a hypomanic swing, in a dosage of 1.5 mg three times per day. Two days later she developed gross extrapyramidal signs with marked rigidity and orofacial dyskinesia. She became severely confused and disorientated, and the EEG showed diffuse slow waves. Both drugs were stopped, with gradual resolution of the extrapyramidal disturbance over the course of the next 3 months. She was left, however, with persistent evidence of brain damage by way of disorientation and memory impairment. This patient had experienced the combination of lithium and haloperidol 3 years previously without adverse effect.

Such reports must be viewed in the context of the many patients treated safely on the same combinations of drugs. Nevertheless close monitoring of the clinical situation and of serum lithium levels would seem essential whenever lithium is coupled with other neuroleptic agents. Episodes of sleep-walking have also been reported after adding neuroleptics to patients established on lithium; Charney *et al.* (1979) reported 10 examples, involving haloperidol, thioridazine, chlorpromazine and other neuroleptics, usually occurring within a few days of starting the second drug. Neurotoxicity has also been reported when lithium is given with carbamazepine, phenytoin or methyldopa (Beeley 1986).

Neuroleptic malignant syndrome

The extrapyramidal disorders associated with the phenothiazines and butyrophenones are described in Chapter 14 (p. 639 *et seq.*). The neuroleptic malignant syndrome is a more recently recognised complication of such drugs, seemingly rare but of great importance in that it is not infrequently fatal. Reviews of the condition are provided by Caroff (1980), Cope and Gregg (1983), Addonizio *et al.* (1987) and Kellam (1987). It has been described sporadically since the 1960s but the syndrome still lacks clear definition. Buckley and Hutchinson (1995) review its uncertain nosological status. An excess of cases has sometimes been described in patients below the age of 40 but the age range is wide. Males appear to be affected more commonly than females.

The patient develops severe extrapyramidal rigidity and akinesia, usually setting in abruptly or over the course of several days. Pyrexia is a characteristic accompaniment, along with autonomic disturbances by way of sweating, sialorrhoea, tachycardia, hyperventilation and labile blood pressure. Muscular rigidity is the cardinal feature, but may be accompanied by tremor, oro-bucco-lingual dyskinesias and sometimes dysphagia and dysarthria. Fluctuating impairment of consciousness can lead to confusion, stupor or coma. Agitation is common and may be severe. Dehydration and prostration can become extreme. Common laboratory findings include a leucocytosis, raised creatinine phosphokinase activity and abnormal liver function tests, but these are not invariable. The EEG sometimes shows diffuse slowing but is usually normal. The CT scan is uninformative. The picture may be mistaken for encephalitis or meningitis, but cerebrospinal fluid examination is negative. Catatonia may be diagnosed on account of the stupor, posturing or waxy flexibility. Anticholinergic intoxication should be considered in the differential diagnosis (Howells 1994). Death is estimated to occur in up to 20% of cases, usually from cardiorespiratory failure, pneumonia or renal failure secondary to rhabdomyolysis and myoglobinuria.

The syndrome has been reported in association with butyrophenones, phenothiazines and thioxanthines, though perhaps most commonly with haloperidol and depot fluphenazines. It sets in usually within the first two weeks of treatment. It may begin shortly after the first dose, though a puzzling feature is its occasional development after many months on the drugs. Earlier courses of the identical drugs may have been given without adverse effect. In a small but important subgroup an identical syndrome has developed in parkinsonian patients when antiparkinsonian medications such as levodopa or amantadine are withdrawn (Kellam 1987). Rare examples have been reported following lithium, metoclopramide, carbamazepine, desipramine, dothiepin, tetrabenazine and other non-neuroleptics (Buckley & Hutchinson 1995).

Medically ill psychiatric patients appear to be at increased risk, many examples developing in patients with dehydration, malnutrition or concomitant neurological disease (Sternberg 1986). Indeed Levinson and Simpson (1986) have questioned the unitary nature of the syndrome, suggesting that a number of examples merely represent extrapyramidal reactions complicated by fever due to remediable medical conditions. Dehydration with electrolyte imbalance and infections such as pneumonia appeared to be the factors most often responsible.

Treatment consists of the withdrawal of all neuroleptic medication immediately the condition is suspected, along with intensive supportive measures to maintain respiratory, renal and cardiovascular function. Dehydration or electrolyte imbalance must be remedied, and a thorough search made for infections and other medical conditions which may be complicating the picture. Active cooling measures may be required. Benefit has been reported from treatment with dantrolene sodium, a peripheral

muscle relaxant, and from the dopamine agonist bromocriptine (Granato et al. 1983; Miyasaki & Lang 1995). Electroconvulsive treatment has sometimes been found to be rapidly beneficial, though obviously this must be undertaken with care (Davis et al. 1991). From Davis et al.'s review such treatment appears to be safe, with the proviso that neuroleptics are discontinued beforehand.

The disorder usually lasts for 5–10 days after stopping the drugs, or rather longer with depot preparations. Resolution is typically complete in those who recover, though occasional patients are left with neurological residua (Miyasaki & Lang 1995). When treatment of the original psychiatric disorder continues to be necessary, alternative drugs such as carbamazepine or lithium should be tried. If it is essential to reintroduce phenothiazines those with low potency should be given initially. Careful monitoring of the blood pressure and temperature will then be necessary, with vigilance if extrapyramidal rigidity should develop. There are indications that 'rechallenges' with neuroleptics are, in fact, often safely accomplished provided a gap of at least 2 weeks is left after resolution of the syndrome (Rosebush et al. 1989). Clozapine should be considered when conventional neuroleptics cannot be tolerated (Weller & Kornhuber 1992).

Dopamine receptor blockade in the basal ganglia or hypothalamus has been postulated as the cause, though with little direct supportive evidence. Significantly decreased levels of homovanillic acid, the major metabolite of dopamine, have however been found in the cerebrospinal fluid, both during active phases and after recovery from the syndrome (Nisijima & Ishiguro 1990). Some evidence also points to serotonergic involvement (Buckley & Hutchinson 1995). At autopsy no specific abnormalities have yet been discovered.

Attention has been drawn to certain similarities between the condition and the 'fatal catatonia' (p. 556) of the pre-neuroleptic era (Caroff 1980; Kellam 1987). Some examples of adverse reactions to the combination of lithium and haloperidol (p. 626) may also represent variants of the syndrome, particularly the cases reported by Cohen and Cohen (1974) where extrapyramidal dysfunction was accompanied by fever, leucocytosis and elevated serum enzymes. On present evidence the condition would seem to represent an idiosyncratic reaction to the neuroleptic medication, though it remains possible that this may merely have served as a trigger to some largely independent pathogenic process.

Withdrawal effects

Withdrawal effects must be considered where drugs with a depressant action on the central nervous system are concerned. Drugs other than alcohol or barbiturates can lead to severe withdrawal phenomena including epileptic fits, hallucinations and periods of delirium. Such pictures have been reported for glutethimide (Doriden) and ethchlorvynol (Placidyl) in patients admitted to hospital for investigation of long-standing intermittent confusion (Lloyd & Clark 1959; Hudson & Walker 1961). Similar results may follow withdrawal from paraldehyde, meprobamate, methaqualone (Mandrax) and carbromal (Granville-Grossman 1971). The withdrawal effects that can be seen with benzodiazepines are described on pp. 610–11.

Analgesics

Chronic analgesic abuse may readily cause diagnostic confusion. Bizarre behaviour and hyperventilation may lead to a mistaken diagnosis of hysteria. When consciousness is severely impaired diabetic coma may be suspected. Greer *et al.* (1965) reported examples of chronic salicylate intoxication producing pictures of confusion, amnesia, agitation, stupor and coma. Some patients were hallucinated, paranoid and combative. Hyperventilation and tinnitus were important signs, also coarse irregular tremors of the hands and ataxia of gait.

Murray *et al.* (1971) drew attention to another possible hazard of chronic analgesic abuse. Of eight patients who had consumed very large doses of compound analgesics containing phenacetin, four showed definite evidence and two possible evidence of dementia. Neuropathological studies of the brains of nine other analgesic abusers showed a surprisingly high frequency of histological changes typical of Alzheimer's disease even though cerebral atrophy was absent. These interesting findings merit further investigation.

Steroid therapy

Mood changes accompanying steroid therapy more often consist of mild elation than depression, and are much commoner than confusion or delirium (Granville-Grossman 1971). The elation and social activation seen while on steroids may be replaced by depression when the drugs are withdrawn (Carpenter & Bunney 1971). More florid reactions have been reported in up to 10% of patients given steroids in large dosage — excited elated behaviour, intense anxiety with panic attacks, severe depression, or transient psychoses with perceptual abnormalities, hallucinations, derealisation and paranoia. Such reactions are often deeply alarming to the patient, but generally subside within a few weeks when the drugs can be withdrawn.

Their determinants will often be complex when the steroids are given for conditions which implicate the central nervous system. Hall *et al.* (1979), however, restricted attention to the psychoses seen in patients in whom there was no reason to suspect a cerebral lesion. They found that the clinical pictures defied formal classification, often representing a complex admixture of affective, schizophreniform and organic features. Moreover a single episode in a given patient could show a great variety of symptoms from one moment to another, and little was characteristic except this changeability. A common constellation of symptoms was emotional lability, anxiety, distractibility, pressured speech, insomnia, perplexity, agitation, hypomania, auditory and visual hallucinations, delusions, intermittent memory impairment, mutism and body image disturbance. The onset was usually within 3 weeks of the start of treatment, mostly within 5 days, and response to phenothiazines was excellent. Electroencephalographic changes of a non-specific type commonly accompanied the disturbances, reverting to normal on recovery. There was no evidence that a history of previous psychiatric illness was a predisposing factor.

Other drug reactions

An important group of drugs are those which produce mood changes or psychotic reactions without evidence of confusion or impairment of consciousness. With reactions of this type it is less likely that the essentially 'toxic' nature of the disturbance will be appreciated. Rauwolfia alkaloids were an early example, leading to severe depressive mood changes unaccompanied by organic mental symptoms. The rauwolfia reaction may develop only after several weeks or months on the drug, and has been attributed to a fall in cerebral monoamines. The acute psychotic reactions that can occur with amphetamines or cocaine, in the absence of impairment of consciousness, are discussed on pp. 617 and 619.

Solvent abuse

The abuse of commercially available solvents by inhalation has caused increasing concern during recent decades. In the UK it is mainly confined to adolescent males, usually in the form of 'glue sniffing' which is carried out sporadically as a small-group activity. At this level serious complications are rare, but the solitary abuser who indulges regularly and over long periods can develop adverse consequences.

A variety of agents may be employed from one subculture to another, differing in their toxicity. Glues contain toluene as the main volatile constituent, also acetone, xylene and *n*-hexane. Polystyrene cements are similar. Paints, varnishes and lacquers contain trichloroethylene and methyl chloride in addition to toluene. Cleaning fluids may contain carbon tetrachloride, trichloroethylene and trichloroethane. Butane may be inhaled from lighter refills, or acetone and amyl acetate from nail polish remover. Aerosols contain fluorinated hydrocarbons ('freons'). Petrol contains hydrocarbons and tetraethyl lead.

Acute effects

Glue is commonly inhaled from a plastic bag, the 'sniffing' being adjusted for maximal euphoriant effect. Cleaning fluids or petrol may be sniffed from a rag or directly from the tin. Aerosols may be sprayed directly into the mouth, a particularly hazardous procedure.

The result is a period of euphoria and exhilaration, setting in rapidly and accompanied by giddiness and disorientation. This phase may be prolonged for several hours by judicious adjustment of sniffing. Hallucinations may occur, chiefly in the visual modality and often frightening in nature. Spatial distortions, macropsia, micropsia and body image disturbances are commonly experienced. At a deeper level of intoxication there is blurring of vision, ataxia, marked confusion and drowsiness progressing to coma. Disinhibition and feelings of omnipotence during the phase of intoxication may lead to risk-taking, accidents and aggressive antisocial behaviour. Amnesia for the events of the episode is common upon recovery.

The habitual abuser may be detected by nasal and lachrymal secretions and a perioral rash, glue stains on clothing, or a change to listlessness, moodiness and sullen withdrawn behaviour. Anorexia is sometimes marked. Blood toluene estimations can be useful in confirming suspicion of the practice, remaining positive for several days after the last exposure (King et al. 1981).

Adverse consequences

The great majority of glue sniffers do not come before medical attention, and at the level of mild sporadic use appear usually to escape long-term physical damage. However, a considerable number of deaths have been reported, often due to inhalation of vomit or suffocation from the plastic bag. Inhalation of trichloroethane or aerosol propellants may lead to sudden death from ventricular fibrillation. Tolerance can develop if regular abuse persists over many months so that very large quantities come to be employed. Physical dependence by contrast appears to be uncommon, though Watson (1979a, 1979b) has described a withdrawal syndrome after some months of intensive sniffing.

The danger lies chiefly in those vulnerable individuals for whom inhalation becomes a regular and entrenched habit. The motivation to continue can then be extremely

strong. A number of complications, some serious, have now been reported, both with glue sniffing itself and with abuse of other solvents. Much may depend on individual susceptibility to the chemicals involved.

Toluene encephalopathy has been described from several centres. It may present acutely with ataxia, hallucinations, convulsions and coma, or as a chronically evolving cerebellar disorder with evidence of diffuse brain damage. The latter appears to be largely restricted to adult abusers. An early example was reported by Grabski (1961) and followed up by Knox and Nelson (1966):

After some years of regular toluene inhalation a 21-year-old man presented with confusion, inappropriate laughter and long periods of staring into space. He showed the classic titubating gait and intention tremors of cerebellar dysfunction. Over the years he became increasingly slowed and forgetful. On occasions when he stopped inhaling for several days the ataxia would remit considerably. Eight years later he was still abusing toluene and was ataxic, tremulous and emotionally labile. Air encephalography showed diffuse cerebral atrophy.

A similar example was described by Lewis *et al.* (1981):

A man of 28 had abused toluene for 14 years. After 6 years his hands began shaking, followed gradually by difficulty in walking, blurred vision and considerable loss of weight. He showed scanning speech, nystagmus, labile affect and tangential thinking. Psychotic features were absent but there had been an episode of paranoia some years before. There were coarse tremors of the extremities, head and neck, poor finger–nose coordination and a wide-based gait. Psychometric testing showed an IQ of 62 with slowness, perseveration, and poverty of reasoning, judgement and logic. Immediate memory was severely impaired along with evidence of expressive and receptive dysphasia. The EEG showed slow wave abnormalities in the temporal areas. The CT scan showed symmetrically enlarged ventricles, prominent cortical sulci and enlargement of the cisterns around the brain stem and cerebellum.

King *et al.* (1981) have drawn attention to acute encephalopathy in children occasioned by glue sniffing. Of 19 examples four presented with coma, three with convulsions, three with ataxia, seven with euphoria and hallucinations, and two with behaviour disturbance and diplopia. Thirteen recovered completely, five still showed personality changes and psychological impairment on discharge, and one showed persisting evidence of cerebellar damage:

A child of 11 presented with a 1-week history of headache, vomiting, abnormal behaviour, slurred speech and unsteadiness of gait. He was thin, apyrexial, and with superficial ulceration of the lips and nostrils. Examination showed euphoria, dysarthria, coarse rotatory nystagmus, moderate intention tremor and severe ataxia of gait. He denied glue sniffing but blood toluene assay was positive, and it was later confirmed that he had been sniffing for several months. CT scan and lumbar puncture showed no abnormalities. The EEG showed diffuse slow waves. His condition remained unchanged over 72 hours then improved slightly over the course of 3 weeks. The EEG became normal. On follow-up 1 year later cerebellar signs persisted despite confirmatory evidence that he had abstained from further sniffing (King *et al.* 1981).

Fornazzari *et al.* (1983) attempted a comprehensive survey of 24 adolescent and adult toluene abusers admitted to hospital. Eleven showed intention tremor, 11 ataxia, and five had obvious memory impairment. Psychological testing revealed deficits in those patients with neurological dysfunction but not in the remainder. CT scans during the second week showed abnormalities in seven of the 14 examined — widened cortical sulci, enlarged ventricles and marked prominence of the cerebellar sulci. Half of the patients remained in hospital for a 2-week period, but with little amelioration of their neurological abnormalities or psychological deficits. Many of the more mildly affected patients discharged themselves prematurely, however, and these may have subsequently improved. Interestingly none of the patients showed withdrawal symptoms or distress while in hospital, despite a clear history of daily toluene abuse for many years.

Among adult paint sniffers in the USA, Streicher *et al.* (1981) found muscle weakness and peripheral neuropathy in addition to mental changes. Memory difficulties, alteration of personality, depression, irritability, lethargy and paranoia have also been described (Wyse 1973). Korman *et al.* (1980) compared a large group of solvent abusers seen in emergency room practice with polydrug (non-solvent) abusers, and found them to be significantly worse with regard to memory, abstracting ability and capacity for insight and judgement. Ron (1986) reviews the available evidence concerning short- and long-term neuropsychological deficits in solvent abusers and concludes that definitive studies remain to be undertaken. The better controlled investigations suggest that if impairment is lasting it is usually mild and limited. Ron also reviews isolated reports of optic neuropathy or sensorineural hearing loss in toluene abusers. While peripheral neuropathy is rare with toluene, a predominantly motor neuropathy may follow abuse of *n*-hexane.

Escobar and Aruffo (1980) reported a patient who came to autopsy after 12 years of inhaling glue and paint thinner. Diffuse cerebral and cerebellar atrophy were obvious, with thinning of the corpus callosum and shrinkage of the basal ganglia. Cell loss and reactive gliosis were accompanied by diffuse demyelination in the subcortical white matter. The cerebellum showed severe Purkinje cell loss.

Anaemia may complicate solvent abuse, likewise gas-

trointestinal disturbances including haematemesis. Impairment of renal and hepatic function may be found (Will & McLaren 1981). The chlorinated hydrocarbons—trichloroethylene, trichloroethane and carbon tetrachloride—are particularly hazardous in this regard.

Petrol sniffing carries additional hazards as reviewed by Poklis and Burkett (1977) and Kaelen *et al.* (1986). Intoxication is liable to continue for some hours after exposure, and prolonged or rapid inhalation may lead to a phase of violent excitement followed by coma. Chronic inhalation leads ultimately to loss of appetite and weight, neurasthenic symptoms, and muscular weakness and cramps. EEG abnormalities and other evidence of brain damage have been described, perhaps largely caused by minor constituents such as benzene and xylene rather than by the hydrocarbons themselves.

A special complication is encephalopathy due to the tetraethyl lead added to petrol (p. 633). Law and Nelson (1968) described an example in a woman of 41, presenting with a chronic paranoid psychosis along with memory impairment. Robinson (1978) reported a girl of 15 who presented with hypomania and combative behaviour after some months of deterioration in school work. Both patients responded to treatment with chelating agents. Kaelen *et al.*'s (1986) patient died following acute encephalopathy; autopsy showed severe cerebellar atrophy with loss of Purkinje cells, neuronal loss in the hippocampus, and chromatolysis of cells in the cerebral cortex and reticular formation.

Heavy metals and other chemicals

Lead

It has been suggested that lead poisoning may have contributed to the decline of the Roman Empire after the introduction of lead pipes for the supply of drinking water (Gillfillan 1965). There was a high prevalence of mental retardation, sterility and infant mortality among influential Romans, and the bones of wealthy Romans have been found to have a high lead content.

Domestic water supplies remain at risk in areas where the water is soft, and some outbreaks have been traced to beer or cider which has stayed overnight in lead pipes. In children lead poisoning may result from chewing lead-containing paint on toys or furniture. Industrial causes have been greatly reduced as a result of stringent precautions, but a risk exists in the following occupations — painting, plumbing, ship building, lead smelting and refining, brass founding, pottery glazing, vitreous enamelling, the manufacture of storage batteries, white lead, red lead, rubber, glass and pigments, and among compositors who handle type metal. The list is important because a history of exposure is often the crucial factor in arousing suspicion of the disorder.

Overt lead poisoning is now a great deal rarer than earlier in the century. However, a new focus of interest has come to centre on possibilities of 'subclinical' lead poisoning, more specifically on the relationship between quite low lead levels in the body and effects on intelligence in children. This is discussed on pp. 632–3.

Clinical manifestations

The principal manifestations include abdominal colic, 'lead neuropathy' and 'lead encephalopathy'. Children are more seriously affected than adults, particularly where cerebral effects are concerned. Useful reviews are provided by Rodgers *et al.* (1934), Byers (1959) and Lee (1981).

Lassitude is almost invariably the earliest symptom. Aching in joints and limbs is also common. Gastrointestinal disturbances then appear, with anorexia, constipation and attacks of severe intestinal colic. The child is pale and often irritable. Acute phases of disturbance tend to be precipitated by intercurrent infection or other sources of acidosis which mobilise lead from the bones.

'Peripheral neuropathy' was formerly common in adults but has always been rare in children. It is now very rare in both. It is unique in being a purely motor disturbance, perhaps with the primary effect on the muscles themselves though ultimately the nerves are involved as well. The muscles chiefly affected are those most used, resulting in the classic picture of wrist drop and paralysis of the long extensors of the fingers. Less commonly there is weakness and wasting of the shoulder girdle muscles or of the dorsiflexors of the foot.

Lead encephalopathy is the most serious manifestation. In adults it may present with episodes of delirium, often in association with fits. During crises the blood pressure is elevated. In chronic encephalopathy the patient is dull, with poor memory, impaired concentration, headache, trembling, deafness or transitory episodes of aphasia and hemianopia (Hunter 1959). Hartman (1988) reviews evidence that 'subclinical' exposure in adults can lead to complaints of fatigue, sleepiness, depression and apathy, with cognitive dysfunction appearing at slightly higher blood lead levels. Memory and visuomotor functions appear to be affected early, also psychomotor speed and dexterity. Mapou and Kaplan (1991) suggest that the fundamental impairment is in attentional and motor functioning, and document such deficits in a stained glass artist suffering from chronic lead exposure.

Korolenko *et al.* (1969) described a picture of acute delirium developing against a background of chronic headache, depression, lowered capacity for work, physical weakness, vertigo and hyperaesthesia for visual and auditory stimuli. During the delirious phase hypnagogic visual hallucinations appeared in profusion in Korolenko *et al.*'s patients, also isolated visual and auditory hallucinations while awake. Disorientation persisted for several days after the hallucinations had ceased, then cleared to leave a worsened form of the chronic asthenic syndrome.

The most pronounced manifestations, however, are seen in children, and cerebral involvement is reported in about half of those affected. The encephalopathy may sometimes set in very rapidly. The intracranial pressure rises abruptly with headache, projectile vomiting, visual disturbances and severe impairment of consciousness. Convulsions and muscular twitching are common, and acute delirium may lead on to coma. Ocular and limb pareses may develop. Papilloedema is often seen, and meningeal irritation may cause neck stiffness and head retraction. The cerebrospinal fluid is under increased pressure, the protein is raised and a moderate pleocytosis may be found. Death can result from medullary compression.

Diagnosis

In the diagnosis of lead poisoning there is no one sign which is pathognomonic. A lead line on the gums may be produced by subepithelial deposits of lead sulphide, especially when the teeth are carious. This is rare, however, in children. Anaemia is always present and usually accompanied by basophilic stippling of the erythrocytes. In young children, X-ray of the long bones shows a dense band in the lines of provisional calcification. Repeated examinations of the blood and urine may reveal a raised lead content, but single readings can be misleading with falsely high or low results. Coproporphyrins are increased in the urine.

Lead encephalopathy should be considered in children who develop fits of obscure origin, and when headache and papilloedema are discovered without obvious cause. Anaemia in association with colic or peripheral neuropathy should similarly raise suspicion. Diseases which may be simulated include encephalitis, cerebral tumour, tuberculous meningitis, uraemia and hypertensive encephalopathy.

Treatment

Most of the lead is held in storage in the bones, and as a temporary measure storage can be promoted by giving calcium lactate and extra milk in the diet. Chelating agents can be used to promote the urinary excretion of lead and have proved to be a considerable advance in treatment (Byers 1959). Disodium calcium ethylene-diamine-tetra-acetate (calcium versenate, EDTA) is given parenterally. Lead replaces the calcium in the compound and the circulating unionized chelate is excreted by the kidneys. Symptoms are rapidly relieved since the chelate is much less toxic than the ionized metal in the body fluids. In consequence chelating agents have been regarded as life saving in the management of acute lead encephalopathy. More recently meso-2,3-dimercaptosuc-cinic acid ('succimer'), an analogue of dimercaprol, has been employed as an oral chelating agent with low toxic-ity, and is being evaluated in children who are found to have elevated blood lead levels (Norman & Bordley 1995).

Outcome

The risk of permanent intellectual disablement is consid-erable among the survivors of lead encephalopathy. Chil-dren may be left with mental retardation, cerebral palsy, fits, or blindness due to optic atrophy. Of 40 children seen by McKann (1932), encephalopathy developed in 24, with death in nine and permanent cerebral damage in five of the survivors. Of 20 cases of mild lead poisoning in infancy, Byers and Lord (1943) found that only one child progressed satisfactorily at school thereafter. Byers' (1959) follow-up of 45 children treated with chelating agents showed that four had died, eight were feeble minded and seven showed other persistent psychiatric abnormalities. Perlstein and Attala (1966) reviewed a large group of 425 children who had suffered lead poison-ing, finding permanent sequelae in 39%. This rose to 82% among those who had presented with encephalopathy. The adult reported by Mapou and Kaplan (1991) showed measurable gains in attentional and motor functioning after chelation, though a degree of impairment persisted.

Cerebral pathology

The cerebral manifestations have been attributed to a combination of intense cerebral oedema and vascular changes. There is proliferation of the endothelium of small blood vessels, sometimes with occlusion of the lumen, and the development of perivascular nodules of hypertrophied glial cells. Cerebral ischaemia may result from the acute rise of intracranial pressure and lead on to cerebral atrophy. In chronic cases the meninges become fibrosed and hyperplastic, and arachnoiditis obstructs the flow of cerebrospinal fluid (Akelatis 1941). Internal

hydrocephalus is often marked in patients who show residual cerebral impairment.

Subclinical lead poisoning

The conventional estimate of what may constitute a 'safe' blood lead level in children has gradually been lowered downwards during recent decades. Once set at 50 or 60 μg/100 ml, some now urge that it should be 25 μg/100 ml. And even below this level there is concern that intellectual development may still be hampered. The debate has been hard to resolve, not least because the cor-relation is known to be poor between blood lead levels as measured and the presence or absence of overt toxic symptoms. Furthermore, blood lead levels cannot be taken as a reliable index of past absorption.

Nevertheless public concern has been raised by the finding from screening programmes of higher than expected blood lead levels in many children, principally those from inner city areas. High levels of lead have been found in dust, dirt and soil, which perhaps constitute the principal sources. Moreover, the majority of air-borne lead appears to derive from additives to petrol; hence the campaigns in the UK and the USA to promote the use of lead-free petrol.

The evidence that body lead levels may be causally related to impaired intelligence or behaviour in children is highly suggestive, and the case has gradually become better proven. Methodological difficulties in resolving the issue have, however, proved to be considerable. Rutter (1980), Needleman (1982) and Taylor (1991) provide comprehensive reviews.

Lansdown et al. (1974) were able to show that blood lead levels in a large population of children were related to the proximity of their homes to a lead works, but no relationship could be demonstrated to measures of mental functioning. Estimates of intelligence and of behavioural disorder were much more closely related to social factors in the homes of the children concerned.

More reliable evidence came from Needleman et al.'s (1979) survey in the USA. Acknowledging the vagaries of blood lead estimations, lead levels were measured in the dentine of shed teeth. Over 2000 children were examined in all. When those in the top tenth percentile for dentine lead were compared with those in the lowest tenth percentile, small but significant differ-ences emerged in intelligence, particularly verbal intelligence, on measures of auditory and speech processing, in reaction times, and on most items of teachers' ratings of classroom behav-iour. The latter, measuring distractibility, impulsivity and capac-ity for concentration and organisation, varied in a dose-related manner with the dentine lead levels across the whole sample of children. Thus lead exposure, at doses below those which would produce symptoms, appeared to be associated with minor psy-chological deficits and impaired classroom performance. After controlling for the influence of various social factors these associations remained significant.

Yule *et al.* (1981) provided further evidence from a preliminary UK study. One hundred and sixty-six children living near a lead works in outer London had previously been shown to have blood lead levels ranging from 7 to 33 μg/100 ml. On tests of intelligence, reading and spelling carried out during the following year, significant associations emerged with the blood lead levels. These largely persisted after controlling for social class. Children with lead levels of 13 μg/100 ml and above, when compared with those of 12 and below, showed an average difference of 7 points on the WISC full-scale IQ. Taylor (1991) reviews more recent studies from Edinburgh, North Carolina, Italy, New Zealand and elsewhere, with variable but often significant results in terms of impairment of cognition or behaviour.

These findings, while important, must be viewed with some caution. A large number of studies have shown a close correlation between blood lead levels and social factors, since poverty increases exposure. It is therefore hard to prove a causal relationship between lead levels and intelligence in children, as opposed to a common association of each with a host of intervening social and genetic factors. Rutter (1980) concluded that it is likely that psychological impairment occurs in some asymptomatic children who show repeated blood lead levels of 40–80 μg/100 ml, and possible, though less certain, that impairment sometimes occurs with levels below 40 μg/100 ml.

Recent follow-up studies have perhaps provided the firmest evidence of all. Needleman *et al.* (1990) found that adolescents whose dentine lead had been elevated 10 years earlier had a higher risk of reading disability and of terminating their schooling prematurely, also lower vocabulary scores and poorer eye–hand coordination than those who had had low levels. Bellinger *et al.*'s (1992) prospective study indicated that higher blood lead levels at the age of 24 months were significantly predictive of lower global scores on the WISC-R and measures of educational attainment at the age of 10. Even over the range of 0–25 μg/100 ml, a 10 μg increase in blood lead at 24 months was associated with a 5.8 point reduction in WISC IQ at 10. Tong *et al.*'s (1996) follow-up of children from a lead smelting town in Australia has recently lent strong support to this finding.

Tetraethyl lead

Tetraethyl lead is added to petrol as an antidetonant and may be absorbed through the skin and respiratory tract. Symptoms of poisoning have been reported among those involved in its manufacture or in the cleaning of large petrol storage tanks.

The clinical picture has been described by Machle (1935) and Boyd *et al.* (1957) and differs from other forms of lead poisoning. After severe exposures acute symptoms may begin within hours, but in less severe cases there is often a delay of several days. Prodromata consist of anorexia, nausea, marked weight loss and a metallic taste in the mouth. Other prominent complaints include headache, vertigo, muscular pains and generalised weakness. The patient is anxious and excitable, and has marked insomnia with terrifying dreams. At this stage the condition may easily be mistaken for an anxiety state.

In the fully developed reaction the mental manifestations increase and come to dominate the picture. Severe delirium is accompanied by acute terror, misidentifications and hallucinations. Episodes of mania may be seen with flight of ideas. Coarse jerky tremors involve the limbs, lips and tongue, and brief epileptic fits may occur. The precise pattern of the acute psychosis is remarkably variable from one person to another. In the most severe examples coma and death may supervene. Otherwise, the condition subsides after several weeks with complete recovery, though convalescence is sometimes protracted and an anxiety state may persist for a considerable time. The neuropathological picture is described on p. 630.

Mercury

Chronic mercury poisoning can occur in many settings. It is a hazard among workers involved in recovering the metal from the ore, in chemical workers, thermometer makers and photo engravers. Groups of cases were reported among fingerprint experts employing a mercury and chalk mixture (Agate & Buckell 1949) and among repairers of direct current electric meters (Bidstrup *et al.* 1951). Mercury was also extensively employed in the felt hat industry, where the toxic effects no doubt contributed to the epithet 'mad as a hatter' and to Lewis Carroll's choice of the hatter in *Alice in Wonderland*. Warkany and Hubbard (1951) made a signal contribution by discovering that the mercury contained in teething powders was the common cause of acrodynia (pink disease) in infants and young children. Kew *et al.* (1993a) have recently reported a case of mercury intoxication in an adult caused by pills prescribed for eczema by an Indian ethnic practitioner.

Clinical manifestations

Physical symptoms include stomatitis, spongy bleeding gums and excessive salivation. A coarse tremor may develop in the hands, face and tongue, characteristically interrupted by coarse jerking movements (hatters' shakes). A sensorimotor peripheral neuropathy is common, sometimes with prominent sensory ataxia, also varying degrees of visual field constriction.

Psychological symptoms are often an early manifestation. In particular a constellation of symptoms known as 'erythism' has been repeatedly noted. In this the sufferer is nervous, timid and shy, blushes readily and becomes embarrassed in social situations. He objects to being watched and seeks to avoid people. He becomes irritable and quarrelsome, sometimes to the extent that he is obliged to give up work. Such symptoms are usually accompanied by lassitude, tremulousness, ataxia and some degree of impairment of intellectual capacity. Of 32 men involved with finger printing in the Lancashire Constabulary, Agate and Buckell (1949) found seven with tremor and four who showed evidence of past or present erythism:

A detective sergeant of 45 was trained in fingerprint work and sent to a division where he investigated up to 300 crimes per year. During this time he became a 'nervous wreck', could not hold a cup without spilling it, and found court appearances acutely distressing because he could not stand still or answer questions without embarrassment. During the early war years the crime rate declined and his symptoms improved, but they worsened again immediately the crime rate rose in the postwar period. On examination he showed a marked tremor and several teeth were loose.

Bidstrup et al. (1951) found definite evidence of erythism in 10 and probable evidence in eight of 161 men engaged in mending direct current electric meters:

One employee had noticed tremor of his hands for a year and had become irritable, short tempered and easily embarrassed. He had developed a stammer for the first time in his life. A few months later he became unsteady on his feet and his whole body developed a tremor. His writing became almost illegible. He was ultimately diagnosed as suffering from multiple sclerosis. At this point he read in the daily paper about the above findings in the Lancashire Constabulary and told his general practitioner that he too handled mercury. Six months after transfer to another job he had recovered completely.

Kark et al. (1971) report another example with prominent neurological symptoms:

A man who had worked for 2 years extracting mercury from batteries showed a gradual decline in memory and loss of interest, becoming less talkative and active. He developed gingivitis, decreased visual acuity and insomnia. Tremor ultimately made eating and drinking impossible, and he was virtually unable to stand on account of titubation and truncal ataxia. On examination he showed dysarthria, constricted visual fields and diminished acuity of both hearing and vision. There were constant choreiform movements of the face and fingers. The EEG showed diffuse theta activity and the air encephalogram revealed cere-bral atrophy. He recovered slowly on treatment with chelating agents.

Neuropsychological testing has shown identifiable deficits in persons chronically exposed to mercury, often persisting for many years. Ngim et al. (1992), for example, found that dentists with a history of contact with mercury vapour were significantly poorer than controls on tests of motor speed, visual scanning, visuomotor coordination and memory. Performance correlated inversely with the cumulative dose of exposure. None showed overt toxic signs but their blood mercury levels were raised. Hartman (1988) and O'Carroll et al. (1995a) review studies on mercury miners and plant workers which have shown impairment of motor coordination, reaction time and short-term memory. O'Carroll et al.'s own patient suffered exposure while cleaning a tank containing phenylmercury ammonium acetate which releases inorganic mercury in the body, and was chronically disabled thereafter by muscle spasms, shakiness, anxiety and depression. Psychological testing 3–4 years later showed marked and specific deficits in attention and concentration, with performance well below expectation on verbal fluency, Trail Making and Stroop tests and on the Paced Auditory Serial Addition Test (PASAT). MRI showed no abnormality, but SPECT scanning revealed focal hypermetabolism in the posterior cingulate cortex.

Acrodynia is a serious disease of infants and young children. The hands and feet are reddened with desquamation of the skin, itching, burning and evanescent rashes. In severe cases the hair and even the nails may be lost. The child is restless and miserable, showing periods of apathy alternating with extreme irritability. Anorexia, insomnia and photophobia are prominent. On examination there is hypotonia with diminished tendon reflexes and peripheral sensory loss. There is a tachycardia and the blood pressure is raised. The cause was unknown, though a toxic agent had long been suspected. Warkany and Hubbard in 1951 found mercury in the urine in a large number of cases, and proposed that exposure to mercury in hypersensitive infants was the responsible factor. This has since been well established (Dathan 1954), the source being mainly from teething powders, worming pills, ointments or nappy powders. Fortunately the condition is now very rare indeed.

Organic mercury compounds

Organic mercury compounds are associated with marked neurological and psychiatric disturbances, especially the ethyl and methyl derivatives which are used in the manufacture of fungicides. From time to time certain accidents have resulted in large outbreaks of poisoning with a heavy mortality. In the Minamata Bay epidemic in Japan, 83 persons were affected, most patients dying or suffering permanent severe disability (Kurland *et al.* 1960). Inorganic mercury derived from industrial processes had been discharged into rivers, methylated by aquatic microorganisms, and eaten by fish which then became poisonous. More recently Amazonian riverside communities have been affected in Brazil as a result of mercury used in the course of gold mining (British Medical Journal 1992). In Iraq several outbreaks resulted from the distribution of grain treated with fungicides, intended for planting but made into bread by mistake. In the 1972 epidemic 6500 persons were admitted to hospital and there were 459 deaths (Bakir *et al.* 1973).

Sensory disturbances are in the foreground with numbness of the hands, deafness, blurred vision and narrowing of the visual fields progressing to blindness (Hunter 1978). Ataxia and dysarthria may be severe, often in association with sore gums and salivation. Involuntary movements and convulsions are common. Mental dullness is accompanied by restlessness, progressing over the course of weeks or months to coma. Many cases are fatal. At autopsy selective cortical damage is seen in numerous areas, with neurone loss, porosity of the underlying white matter and swelling of oligodendrocytes (Hay *et al.* 1963). Extensive spongiosis of the cortex may occur in childhood cases (Takeuchi *et al.* 1979). Severe destruction may also be seen in the cerebellum, basal ganglia and calcarine region (Feldman 1982).

Manganese

Manganese poisoning is predominantly an occupational disease. It occurs in manganese ore workers and in those involved in steel manufacture, dry battery manufacture, bleaching and electro-welding. Despite the large number of people at risk manganese poisoning is relatively rare, and it is probable that a large quantity must be absorbed over a long period of time before harmful effects are produced. Individual sensitivity also appears to be important in that some subjects exposed for an equally long period show no ill effects. The chief route of entry is by inhalation of the dust, fumes or vapour. Possibilities of adverse effects from environmental contamination have been raised from time to time, especially from the manganese contained in anti-knock agents added to lead-free petrol.

The foetal and neonatal nervous system may be unusually susceptible. Learning difficulties have been tentatively linked to the use of infant feeding formulas with a high manganese content (Cawte 1985).

Clinical manifestations

The early manifestations usually develop insidiously with headache, asthenia, torpor and hypersomnia. Impotence is common. Psychological abnormalities then become pronounced and may first draw attention to the disorder. There have been reports of marked emotional disturbances in up to 70% of cases, especially episodes of persistent and uncontrollable laughter and crying (Fairhall & Neal 1943). There may be strong impulsions to run, dance, sing or talk which the patient finds difficult to resist. Impulsive acts and stupid crimes are a special risk in the early phases (Penalver 1955). Other abnormalities include forgetfulness, mental dullness, marked irritability and outbursts of aggression. Neuropsychological assessment in refinery workers has shown constructional apraxia, correlating significantly with levels of exposure to manganese dust (Brown *et al.* 1991). Very occasionally an acute psychotic picture is seen with severe excitement, agitation, hallucinations and delusions (Abd El Naby & Hassanein 1965).

Parkinsonism develops later with typical mask-like facies, slow monotonous speech and slowing of voluntary movements. Nocturnal leg cramps are a prominent feature. Fine tremor or gross rhythmical movements develop in the hands, limbs and trunk. The gait becomes typically parkinsonian with retropulsion and propulsion. A characteristic 'cock-step' gait has been described — a peculiar broad-based slapping walk, with the legs held stiffly on tip-toe and wide apart. On examination muscular rigidity is found, with increased reflexes and ankle clonus. Cerebellar deficits may also be present. Sensory disturbances are rare. Chronic headache and severe insomnia may accompany the neurological developments.

Severe examples have been misdiagnosed as paralysis agitans, Wilson's disease, postencephalitic parkinsonism or multiple sclerosis. Wilson's disease may be closely simulated since liver damage may also be present.

Removal from exposure at an early stage usually allows considerable recovery to occur. The psychological symptoms resolve quickly but disturbance of speech and gait may persist. In well-established cases the neurological disabilities may prove to be irreversible and the patients are left permanently disabled. A considerable number have been observed to worsen neurologically even after removal from exposure (Abd El Naby & Hassanein 1965). Treatment with levodopa may sometimes improve the motor abnormalities (Huang *et al.* 1989).

At autopsy the basal ganglia are found to be mainly affected, with cell loss, gliosis and shrinkage. This is most marked in the globus pallidus. The thalamus may also be involved. Diffuse changes are found elsewhere including the cerebral cortex and brain stem, and slight generalised cortical atrophy may be seen (Canavan *et al.* 1934). In advanced cases the peripheral nerves and muscles may show degenerative changes (Penalver 1955).

Arsenic

Arsenic poisoning is encountered in the ore-refining industry, the fur industry, and in the manufacture of glass, insecticides and weed killers. Medicinal poisoning was formerly seen when Fowler's solution was prescribed over long periods of time. Acute poisoning may follow the accidental ingestion of insecticides, disinfectants and rat poisons. A case of sensorimotor peripheral neuropathy resulting from powders prescribed for eczema by an Indian ethnic practitioner has recently been reported (Kew *et al.* 1993a).

Acute poisoning results in vomiting, diarrhoea and violent abdominal cramps. Headache, delirium and fits develop, and coma and death may follow within 2 or 3 days.

In chronic arsenic poisoning the picture is different. Early signs include dermatitis, conjunctivitis, lachrymation and coryza. Keratosis and skin pigmentation may be extensive, with characteristic white lines across the nails (Mee's lines). Anorexia and weight loss are common, but the abdominal cramps and diarrhoea of acute poisoning are often absent. Headache and vertigo are accompanied by apathy, drowsiness and impairment of mental acuity. At this stage the mental changes can be the leading clinical manifestations, sometimes closely simulating neurotic disorder (Ecker & Kernohan 1941). Later restlessness, excitability and confusion become marked. Severe memory disturbance can occasionally produce the picture of Korsakoff's syndrome. Peripheral neuritis is common, with paraesthesiae, burning pain in the limbs and conspicuous sensory signs. Distal leg weakness may develop with loss of the ankle reflexes.

Thallium

Thallium has been widely used as a rodent poison and pesticide. Ginsburg and Nixon (1932) described an outbreak of poisoning in the USA caused by eating barley bread made from contaminated grain. Reed *et al.* (1963) reported 72 cases in children in Texas who had ingested pesticides.

Tingling in the hands and feet develops within 24 hours of ingestion, followed by severe paroxysmal abdominal pain and vomiting. Headache, tachycardia, stomatitis, salivation and offensive breath are other early features.

Involvement of the nervous system follows within a few days. After small doses ataxia and paraesthesiae develop and may progress to frank peripheral neuropathy. Retrobulbar neuritis is often seen. Tremor, chorea, athetosis and myoclonic jerking are also common. Mental abnormalities may be pronounced, with impairment of consciousness, paranoia and depression (Grinker & Sahs 1966). After large doses cerebral involvement is severe, with cranial nerve palsies, delirium, hallucinations, fits and coma. Death often follows from respiratory paralysis.

Alopecia develops some 10 days after ingestion and dystrophic changes appear in the nails. Toxic damage occurs in the kidneys and hypertension is common.

Follow up by Reed *et al.* (1963) showed that sequelae were limited to the nervous system, both peripherally and centrally, and occurred in half of the survivors. The enduring deficits consisted of features derived from the acute stage—ataxia, tremor, abnormal motor movements, fits and visual disturbance. Thompson *et al.* (1988) have reported a patient with cognitive impairment persisting at 7 months, though with some improvement 6 months later. Memory was particularly affected, along with performance subtests of the WAIS.

Bismuth

An encephalopathy induced by bismuth salts has been described. Most reports have come from Australia, Belgium and particularly France, but it may be expected that cases will arise elsewhere. Weller (1988) has reported a mild example from the UK. The cause is excessive ingestion of bismuth preparations taken for gastrointestinal and skin disorders. Most patients have been between the ages of 40 and 70, with more women affected than men.

Collignon *et al.* (1979) analysed reports of 99 cases in the literature and describe seven patients of their own. Neurological abnormalities are prominent during the prodromal phase—disturbances of gait and balance, tremors, myoclonic jerks and other disorders of movement. Headache, insomnia and apathy may be accompanied by difficulties with thinking and memory. Some patients show marked oscillations between depression and euphoria. Buge *et al.* (1981) report occasional patients with visual hallucinations and persecutory delusions. Such prodromata can last for several weeks or months.

The acute encephalopathy then presents with confusion and clouding of consciousness, often accompanied by considerable excitement and agitation. Disturbances of memory and praxis sometimes dominate the picture and myoclonic jerks are almost universal. Up to a third of patients suffer generalised seizures. Motor neurological abnormalities are marked while the blood bismuth levels are high. Von Bose and Zaudig (1991) report a recent example in which rapidly progressive dementia, intermittent delirium, ataxia and myoclonus led to an initial diagnosis of Creutzfeldt–Jacob disease.

As the acute organic reaction subsides the patient may recover completely, or be left with short-term memory difficulties or more global defects of intellectual function. These can persist for more than a year in certain cases. Collignon *et al.* (1979) stress apraxic and agnosic deficits which may remain along with the memory disorder. The picture may mimic the presenile or senile dementias or chronic subdural haematoma, or may suggest the presence of a frontal lobe lesion.

Buge *et al.* (1981) have described characteristic CT scan appearances during the acute phase, with hyperdensities in the cerebral cortex, cerebellum and basal ganglia due to the presence of bismuth there. These disappear slowly over 2–3 months on recovery, though enlargement of the cortical sulci may sometimes persist.

Organophosphorus compounds

Complex esters of phosphoric acid and its derivatives are widely used in industry, horticulture and agriculture. Prominent among them are pesticides such as parathion and malathion, also diazinon and chlorfenvinphos used in sheep dip. Chemical warfare agents include sarin, tabun and soman. Contamination of whisky with tri-orthocresyl phosphate occurred during prohibition in the USA, and contaminated cooking oil occasioned an outbreak of peripheral neuropathy in Morocco (Smith & Spalding 1959). Organophosphate poisoning from pesticides is currently under consideration as a contributory factor in some cases of 'Gulf war syndrome' (Jamal *et al.* 1996; Warden 1996b; David *et al.* 1997; Landrigan 1997).

Such compounds are potent inhibitors of acetylcholinesterase, first binding to phosphorylation sites then altering membrane function in a manner which can lead to delayed neurotoxicity. They also interact with adrenergic, dopaminergic and serotonergic mechanisms (Bradwell 1994).

Acute toxic effects consist of cholinergic crises with miosis, bronchoconstriction, diarrhoea, bradycardia and cardiac dysrhythmias. Many patients show weakness due to depolarisation block of neurotransmission, with areflexia and fasciculations (Donaghy 1993). Tremors, ataxia, confusion and agitation may develop, sometimes with bulbar signs and convulsions. Respiratory failure is the usual mode of death. In less severe cases a progressive sensorimotor polyneuropathy follows the acute symptoms after a delay of 1 or 2 weeks. Severe quadriparesis

may result. Cognitive deficits have been identified in several epidemiological studies, often persisting for several years after acute exposure (Steenland 1996).

Less intense and intermittent exposure may lead to chronic complaints of nausea, headache, cramps and dizziness, sometimes with muscle fasciculations and difficulty in focusing the eyes. Tiredness and hypersomnia are prominent, almost half of Metcalf and Holmes' (1969) patients complaining of fatiguability and drowsiness. Hartman (1988) and Steenland (1996) review neuropsychological studies which have shown impairments of sustained attention and information processing. Levin *et al.* (1976) found heightened levels of anxiety on the Taylor Manifest Anxiety Scale among commercial insecticide sprayers, despite the absence of overt toxic symptoms.

Florid psychiatric pictures resulting from chronic exposure were described by Gershon and Shaw (1961) in 16 patients. Most were farmers or greenhouse workers who had used pesticide sprays without adequate protection. After some years of exposure seven developed depressive illnesses, five schizophrenic reactions and four presented with cognitive difficulties. Most had had episodes of acute poisoning in the past with classic symptoms and signs. Bradwell (1994) has reported a farm worker chronically exposed to weed killers and pesticides who suffered repeated episodes of acute organic psychosis, also periods of depression and mania over several years, all against a background of chronic anergia and hypersomnia.

Methyl bromide

Methyl bromide is a colourless, odourless gas which is sold as a liquid in pressurised containers. It is used as a fire extinguisher, refrigerant, fumigant and insecticide, and occasional cases of poisoning have been described. Severe exposures are fatal with acute pulmonary oedema, renal failure and convulsions (De Jong 1944). Brief exposures are followed by headache, nausea and vertigo, then a characteristic interval occurs of hours or even days during which the patient is symptom-free. This may be followed by the explosive onset of headache, muscular twitching, convulsions, delirium, visual disturbances and somnolence progressing to coma (Baker & Tichy 1953). Chronic mild exposure may be followed by peripheral neuropathy.

Carbon disulphide

Carbon disulphide is used in industry, mainly as a rubber solvent and in the manufacture of rayon. Many cases of poisoning were reported in France after its introduction in the 19th century. Braceland (1942) reported examples from the USA and found that a high proportion of rayon workers were affected by the fumes.

The commonest toxic effect is peripheral neuritis affecting both motor and sensory nerves and producing aching cramp-like pains in the limbs (Hunter 1978). Visual changes also occur, with central scotomata and concentric narrowing of the visual fields. Auditory symptoms include tinnitus and deafness, and dizziness may occur. Mental changes may be profound and can be the presenting feature. Braceland (1942) described both insidious changes of personality and acute toxic psychoses.

Personality changes consist of mood swings, irritability and outbursts of inexplicable rage. The worker may be exhilarated when breathing the fumes in the factory but depressed when at home. Constant fatigue may progress to a state of profound apathy. Headache, anorexia and insomnia are usually marked, and loss of libido is common. Later there may be difficulties with memory, and auditory and visual hallucinations may occur.

In Braceland's survey one worker was found to be confused and disorientated with obvious memory difficulties. He had been nervous and irritable for several months and complained of feeling in a fog. He was subject to rapid mood changes and had overwhelming impulses to anger from time to time. He could sleep for only 2 hours at a time and had recurrent dreams of a violent and anxious nature. There was complete loss of libido. Another worker was similarly affected and had experienced auditory and visual hallucinations. Another was extremely agitated and was subject to intermittent visual hallucinations.

The more acute psychoses were usually sudden in onset and sometimes closely resembled episodes of mania. These appear to be uncommon today, now that levels of exposure in the workplace have been regulated. Severe confusion was accompanied by noisy aggressive behaviour, delusions and hallucinations. Most cleared rapidly on admission to hospital, but some could last for many weeks or months. Residual memory defects occasionally persisted. Examples of acute schizophrenia-like psychoses were also reported, probably in those who were specially predisposed.

Hartman (1988) reviews the cognitive effects of chronic exposure. Motor speed, reaction time, vigilance and visuoconstructive abilities have proved to be affected, sometimes showing significant correlations with duration of exposure. In part this could be the consequence of cerebral arterial disease, since carbon disulphide is markedly associated with increased atherosclerosis.

Chapter 14: Movement Disorders

The movement disorders form a substantial part of neurological practice and have gradually attracted increasing psychiatric interest. This is partly on account of their psychiatric concomitants, for example a high incidence of depression in Parkinson's disease and of behavioural disturbance in the opening stages of hepatolenticular degeneration. More than this, however, biochemical research, particularly in relation to dopamine metabolism, has revealed analogies between the changes thought to underlie certain movement disorders and those postulated to occur in major psychiatric illnesses. Basic research on such issues has been stimulated very considerably. We are, in effect, learning to value the lessons for psychiatry that can be gained from the study of extrapyramidal disease, and to appreciate the importance of subcortical activity in contributing to many aspects of mental life.

An additional spur to interest is the need to be conversant, in day-to-day clinical practice, with the wide range of movement disorders induced by neuroleptic medication. The management of the syndromes that result, and the unravelling of underlying mechanisms, have led neurologists and psychiatrists to areas of common endeavour.

Other movement disorders, such as spasmodic torticollis, writer's cramp, blepharospasm and Gilles de la Tourette's syndrome, reflect the striking influence that mental factors may bring to bear on motor dysfunction. So close is this interaction that psychogenic factors may appear to be solely responsible for causing such conditions, yet other evidence suggests that cerebral malfunction may be primarily to blame. Marked psychosensitivity need carry no implications for psychogenesis *per se*, yet attempts to discern the true situation can prove to be difficult. In the discussion of such disorders below the arguments advanced in both directions will be presented.

Drug-induced disorders

Soon after the introduction of phenothiazines to psychiatric practice it became apparent that extrapyramidal movement disorders ranked high among the unwanted effects of treatment. Until the introduction of clozapine, the successive development of new neuroleptics failed to solve the problem, in that all major tranquillisers appeared to share these side effects in some degree. Their propensity to disturb extrapyramidal function proved, indeed, to be roughly proportional to their antipsychotic effect, though earlier ideas that the two were necessarily linked to one another have not been upheld.

Among the phenothiazines, those with a piperazine side chain (e.g. trifluoperazine) show more marked extrapyramidal effects than those with aliphatic or piperidine side chains (e.g. chlorpromazine, thioridazine). The butyrophenones (haloperidol, benperidol, droperidol) are particularly potent in this regard. The thioxanthenes (e.g. flupenthixol) may induce the whole range of disorders considered below, whereas reserpine's effects are usually limited to parkinsonism. Disturbance of dopaminergic mechanisms within the brain has been clearly incriminated as the major factor in leading to these effects, and clarification of the detailed mechanisms involved has had important consequences for the management of some of the more serious disorders.

Clinical pictures

Four main syndromes have been delineated, namely parkinsonism, akathisia, acute dystonic reactions and the group of disorders at present subsumed under the term 'tardive dyskinesia'. Tardive dystonia and tardive akathisia have been recognised more recently. Precise estimates of the incidence of all such conditions have been hard to obtain, on account of variations in prescribing practice and differences in the populations surveyed. It is now firmly established, however, that the drugs are to be blamed rather than inherent aspects of the psychiatric disorders themselves. Exactly analogous movement disorders are induced whether the neuroleptics are given for schizophrenia, affective disorder, neurotic disability or for the control of chronic pain. It must be granted, however, that the stereotypies and mannerisms of chronic schizophrenia can at times lead to diagnostic difficulty and even obscure for a while the development of the extrapyramidal symptoms.

The clinical pictures encountered are fully described in comprehensive reviews by Marsden *et al.* (1975) and Miyasaki and Lang (1995), and may be summarised as follows.

Parkinsonism

Parkinsonian features usually develop insidiously, often within a week and almost always within the first month of treatment. The development of parkinsonism is broadly dose dependent, increasing as higher levels of neuroleptics are achieved. It emerges, however, in only some 20–40% of persons, individual susceptibility being important. The incidence increases with age, as with idiopathic Parkinson's disease.

All of the features of idiopathic Parkinson's disease (p. 646) may be induced. Bradykinesia is the earliest and commonest sign, with muscular rigidity and disturbance of posture and gait developing later. Tremor is a good deal less common than with the idiopathic disease, the exception being the occasional appearance late in the course of treatment of fine perioral tremor ('rabbit syndrome'). The latter generally sets in after months or years of therapy as with tardive dyskinesia.

With continuation of the drugs the parkinsonian features may gradually subside as tolerance develops. Short of this they will usually resolve over the course of several weeks when the drugs are stopped. Marsden and Jenner (1980) stress, however, that occasional patients continue to show parkinsonism for as long as 18 months after cessation of therapy. In the rare examples that fail to recover thereafter one may usually presume that idiopathic Parkinson's disease had already been present.

With the more severe extrapyramidal reactions provoked by potent neuroleptics, the clinical picture may occasionally come to resemble 'catatonia'. Gelenberg and Mandel (1977) described a group of patients showing negativism, withdrawal, posturing and waxy flexibility, of gradual onset usually in the first few weeks of treatment. Incontinence of urine was sometimes observed. Behrman (1972) has described mutism, sometimes progressing to the full syndrome of akinetic mutism. Such developments may easily be confused with worsening of schizophrenic symptomatology, leading to increase in dosage of the offending medication. Stopping the drugs, by contrast, can lead to slow resolution.

Akathisia

Akathisia consists of motor restlessness accompanied by subjective feelings of inner tension and discomfort referable chiefly to the limbs. It often coexists with parkinsonian features but is possibly even more common. The symptoms can be considerably distressing and are a frequent cause of poor drug compliance. The patient complains of being driven to move, of pulling sensations in the legs and an inability to keep them still. The disorder usually appears within the first few days of treatment but may only develop as higher dosage is achieved. Barnes (1989) has produced a rating scale for assessment of both the observable and subjective components of the syndrome. Sometimes the latter are lacking (pseudo-akathisia), chiefly in patients with negative psychotic symptoms (Barnes & Braude 1985).

Braude *et al.* (1983) investigated motor restlessness in detail by ratings of subjective sensations and objective manifestations in a large group of patients on antipsychotic medication. A principal components analysis served to delineate the akathisia syndrome more precisely. Mild examples presented mainly subjectively; inner restlessness was a common and non-specific symptom, but complaints clearly referable to the legs characterised the akathisia group. Moderate akathisia showed in addition a tendency to rock from foot to foot or to walk on the spot, along with coarse tremor or myoclonic jerks in the feet. The severe akathisia group showed difficulty in maintaining their position, for example shuffling or tramping the feet when sitting, rising repeatedly when seated, or walking or pacing when attempting to stand still. In the most severe forms patients may be unable to tolerate any position, whether sitting, lying or standing, for more than a few minutes.

Continuation of the drugs may allow the symptoms to subside, but this is not invariable. An extrapyramidal origin is postulated, but the evidence for this is mainly inferential.

Akathisia must be distinguished from the *restless legs syndrome* (Ekbom's syndrome) which may resemble it closely. This is seen in the absence of neuroleptic medication, usually in patients who are otherwise in normal health. However, associations have been noted with iron-deficiency anaemia, uraemia and pregnancy, and it is unusually common among patients with fibromyalgia or rheumatoid arthritis (Yunus & Aldag 1996). Physical examination typically shows no neurological abnormality, though a small proportion of patients have peripheral neuropathy. The condition is sometimes familial.

An important difference from akathisia lies in the presence of marked leg discomfort, with creeping sensations, dysaesthesiae or sensations of cold or weakness, usually most pronounced in the calves (Parkes 1986a). The desire to move arises directly from such discomforts which are temporarily relieved by getting up and walking about, whereas in akathisia the motor restlessness appears to derive directly from psychological impulses (Clough 1987). The discomfort usually occurs while at rest in the evening or while trying to sleep, often leading to pronounced insomnia. Nocturnal myoclonus may be present. Among many treatments used clonazepam, carbamazepine, chlorpromazine and levodopa are perhaps the most effective.

Acute dystonia

Acute dystonic reactions are considerably rarer than the above reactions, affecting perhaps some 2% of patients. They develop abruptly and early in the course of treatment, within a few days of oral treatment or within hours of intramuscular injection. The more potent piperazine phenothiazines and the butyrophenones are chiefly responsible. Young adults and children appear to be particularly susceptible, and males have outnumbered females in most surveys.

The patient is seized with strong sustained or intermittent muscular spasms which are frequently painful and deeply alarming. Deviation of the eyes, blepharospasm, trismus and grimacing are common. Severe examples show tongue protrusion, dysphagia and respiratory stridor. Extension to the neck and trunk can lead to torticollis, retrocollis, writhing and opisthotonos. Continuous slow writhing may affect the limbs, with dystonic postures of hyperpronation and adduction.

Marked examples may be mistaken for status epilepticus or tetanus by the inexperienced observer. Hysteria may be diagnosed when muscular spasms are remittent. The disorder is self limiting and usually of no more than several hours duration, though therapeutic intervention will often be indicated for the relief of acute distress.

Tardive dyskinesia

As experience was gained of long-term neuroleptic medication it became apparent that a range of movement disorders make their first appearance only late in the course of treatment. These have attracted considerable attention, on account of their sometimes seriously disabling nature and because in a proportion of patients they can prove to be irreversible. The term 'tardive dyskinesia' is used to refer to such late developments rather than to any phenomenologically distinct dyskinetic picture.

The commonest site of the abnormal movements is around the mouth and tongue, which become involved in a more or less continuous flow of choreiform activity (orofacial dyskinesia, bucco-linguo-masticatory dyskinesia). The tongue protrudes, twists and curls, along with incessant chewing, pouting and sucking movements of the lips, jaw and cheeks. In severe examples talking and eating can be hampered. The upper face tends typically to be spared, but may show tic-like blinking or blepharospasm. The neck may be affected with twisting dystonic movements.

Involvement of the trunk, arms, hands and legs may also be observed (Kidger *et al.* 1980). The distal extremities show choreiform and athetotic movements, with finger twisting and spreading, tapping of the feet and dorsiflexion of the toes. Abnormalities of gait and posture show as lordosis, rocking and shoulder shrugging. Grunting and disturbance of the respiratory rhythm may be in evidence. Factor analysis applied to ratings of involvement of different body regions has suggested that there may be relatively independent subvarieties, affecting, respectively, the jaws and tongue, the face and lips, and the extremities and trunk (Glazer *et al.* 1988). These may possibly have differing aetiological and prognostic connotations.

Altogether the picture may come to involve a complex admixture of tics, chorea, athetosis, dystonia and myoclonic jerks. Rhythmic tremor is not, however, seen. It may worsen dramatically with emotional stress and it decreases with drowsiness. Choreiform movements appear to be commoner in the elderly, and dystonic pictures in the young. Age also influences the topography, orolingual movements being especially common in the elderly.

A similar disorder is known to occur spontaneously in the elderly, as the relatively rare 'senile chorea'. In patients on long-term neuroleptics, however, tardive dyskinesia is far from uncommon. Variable estimates have resulted from different surveys, depending among other factors on readiness to include very minor degrees of movement disorder. The working party appointed by the American Psychiatric Association (Task Force on Late Neurological Effects of Antipsychotic Drugs 1980) concluded that between 10 and 20% of people given antipsychotic drugs for a year or more could be expected to develop a clinically appreciable tardive dyskinesia, the rate probably being higher in the elderly. Disabling degrees are, however, rare. In the great majority of cases the patient will have been on neuroleptics for at least 2 years when the disorder makes its first appearance and often for considerably longer. A minimum period of exposure appears to be 3–6 months. In addition to neuroleptics, the condition may follow the prescription of antiemetics such as metoclopramide which also acts through dopamine receptor blockade.

Among the predisposing factors highlighted in certain surveys are age, sex and evidence of brain damage. There is a marked increase in incidence after the age of 40, and a female preponderance has repeatedly emerged among the elderly. The influence of pre-existing brain damage has been less uniformly upheld, but a history of exposure to electroconvulsive therapy or leucotomy has been found to increase the risk, likewise evidence of cognitive dysfunction or negative symptoms in schizophrenia (Waddington & Youssef 1986; Barnes 1987). In McClelland *et al.*'s (1991) long-term follow-up of hospitalised patients the development of facial dyskinesia was significantly associated with ventricular enlargement on computerised tomography (CT) scans. Patients with organic psychiatric disorders have shown an especially high prevalence (Yassa *et al.* 1984).

The evidence that patients with affective disorders may be more at risk than patients with schizophrenia is reviewed by Barnes (1987), likewise indications that depressive symptomatology in the course of schizophrenia may confer additional risk. There is some evidence that prolonged exposure or exposure to high dosage of neuroleptics may increase the chance of developing the condition, but this is disputed. The Yale study, in which a large cohort of patients was followed prospectively for evidence of developing the condition, has been exceptional in finding a clear positive relationship to neuroleptic dose (Morganstern & Glazer 1993). It is clear, however, that most patients will have received large total quantities before tardive dyskinesia supervenes. The concomitant administration of anticholinergics appears to increase the severity of the disorder but probably does not alter the risk of its development. A noteworthy feature is that the first signs very often make their appearance when the drugs are discontinued or the dosage is lowered.

A disturbing aspect of the condition is its liability to persist despite stopping the medication. A majority of patients will improve substantially, usually within months but sometimes taking 1 or 2 years for complete resolution. Between a quarter and a half of patients may be expected to improve markedly within a year (Task Force 1980). In children complete recovery can be predicted, but in some 30% of adults the condition seems destined to be permanent, especially in the elderly. It may, however, pursue a fluctuating course, and some patients experience spontaneous remission (Barnes 1987).

Important aspects of differential diagnosis include schizophrenic stereotypies and mannerisms, senile chorea, Huntington's disease, Wilson's disease and rheumatic chorea.

Tardive dystonia

Burke *et al.* (1982) have described a syndrome of 'tardive dystonia' which appears to be attributable to antipsychotic medication. As with tardive dyskinesia it typically follows several years of treatment with the drugs, and once established it tends to be persistent. The nature of the movement disorder is, however, quite different. The dystonia consists of sustained slow twisting movements affecting the limbs, trunk, neck or face. Among younger patients generalised dystonia is the usual picture, whereas in older patients the movements are often confined to the face, neck or arms. Unlike tardive dyskinesia it typically causes severe distress to the patient and can result in significant neurological disability.

Among Burke *et al.*'s 42 examples the age of onset varied from 13 to 60 years, after an average duration of exposure to drugs of 3–7 years. The onset was usually insidious, progressing over some months or years then becoming persistent and static. One patient was sufficiently disabled to be chronically confined to bed. All classes of antipsychotic medication could be incriminated—phenothiazines, butyrophenones and thioxanthenes.

The picture in generalised cases was indistinguishable from idiopathic torsion dystonia (p. 670), though all lacked a family history of such a condition. The possibility that they simply represented a chance association of this disorder appearing while on antipsychotic medication was considered to be remote, especially since a proportion showed the oral choreic movements of tardive dyskinesia along with their dystonia. Focal cases could present pictures identical to torticollis, blepharospasm or oromandibular dystonia. Pharmacological differences from tardive dyskinesia were shown in that anticholinergic agents, rather than causing exacerbation, could sometimes be observed to improve the dystonic movements. Treatment was, however, mostly disappointing. An increase in the offending medication could lead in some cases to temporary amelioration but this was short-lived.

Further experience has been reported by Kang *et al.* (1986) and Burke and Kang (1988). Among 67 patients the median duration prior to onset was 5 years. However, 20% had developed relatively early within 1 year of starting neuroleptic drugs, the shortest exposure being 3 weeks. Two-thirds began with a focal onset in the face and neck, 15% remaining confined there and the others extending elsewhere. Only one patient showed generalised dystonia from the start. Most progressed to a plateau after several months, and by the time of maximal severity 15% were focal, 72% segmental and 13% generalised in distribution. Sustained postures could sometimes be seen in addition to the slow twisting movements, sometimes relieved by small tactile manoeuvres as in dystonia generally (pp. 670 and 673). Strange paradoxes could be seen, with some activities alleviating the condition while other movements aggravated it. The movements generally abated during sleep. Classic oro-bucco-lingual dyskinesia was present in 20% of patients and had featured at some point in the histories of rather more than half.

Follow-up for a mean of 2.5 years showed that half of the 67 patients had improved on various therapies, but the degree of disability remaining was often considerable. Five of the 42 withdrawn from neuroleptics had remitted completely, but only after substantial periods off the drugs (11 months to 5 years). Another eight could be considered as having successful results from therapy.

Davis et al. (1988) have extended the spectrum of disorders encountered, reporting three patients with laryngospasm as part of the clinical picture, sometimes developing abruptly and requiring tracheostomy, and two patients with spasmodic dysphonia.

In all cases differentiation must be made from Wilson's disease by appropriate diagnostic studies, also from other symptomatic dystonias when there are abnormal neurological signs. A primary blepharospasm, oromandibular dystonia or torticollis must be considered when there are no dyskinetic movements. The distinction from classic tardive dyskinesia can at times be difficult and both may occur together; the distinction is chiefly important because of the different options presented for treatment (p. 645). Finally, it is important to beware of mistaking the picture for a psychogenic disorder, particularly when the movements are bizarre or influenced transiently by emotion, suggestion or an amytal interview.

Tardive akathisia

A syndrome of 'tardive' or 'chronic' akathisia has been distinguished from the acute form, usually developing after some years on neuroleptics. It may coexist with features of tardive dyskinesia, including orofacial dyskinesia and choreoathetoid movements of the limbs; and like tardive dyskinesia it may worsen on dose reduction whereas acute akathisia tends to be aggravated by increase in dosage.

Burke *et al.* (1989) have presented the features seen in 52 cases. The condition had developed after a mean of 4.5 years on dopamine antagonists, but in a third had developed within a year. Complex stereotyped movements consisted of marching on the spot, frequent crossing and uncrossing of the legs, trunk rocking, grunting, moaning and face rubbing or scratching. Half of the patients managed to stop neuroleptics, and the symptoms then persisted for a mean of 2.5 years. The younger patients did better than the old. Attempts at therapy were frequently disappointing (p. 645). The condition can be profoundly disabling, leading to inner torment, irritability and inability to concentrate.

Pathophysiology

The pathophysiology of the neuroleptic-induced movement disorders appears to lie with various aspects of the dopamine–acetylcholine balance within the brain, more particularly within the corpus striatum. Earlier views have, however, become progressively more complex, with the discovery of both inhibitory and excitatory dopamine receptors in the striatum, and the demonstration of feedback striatonigral pathways which may be mediated in part by cholinergic or GABA-ergic mechanisms. The maintenance of correct dopamine and acetylcholine levels in the striatum is clearly under highly complex control and stands to be disturbed in a multitude of ways. Hence, no doubt, the variety of movement disorders encountered when this balance is altered by drugs. Discussions of the theories put forward in attempts at explanation are provided by Marsden and Jenner (1980), Baldessarini and Tarsy (1980) and Miyasaki and Lang (1995).

Among their many pharmacological actions, all neuroleptics have powerful effects on cerebral dopamine mechanisms. These correlate highly with their antipsychotic potency. It is clear, however, that the induction of extrapyramidal motor disorder is not a necessary prerequisite for benefit to psychosis, the latter conceivably hinging on effects within the mesolimbic dopamine projections (arising in the tegmentum of the midbrain and terminating in limbic forebrain structures) rather than on actions within the nigrostriatal system. The phenothiazines, butyrophenones and thioxanthenes act specifically to block cerebral dopamine D_2 receptors. Reserpine and tetrabenazine operate differently, interfering with the intraneuronal granular uptake and storage of dopamine. Clozapine differs from the typical antipsychotics, in that it has weak effects on striatal dopamine D_2 receptors, a high affinity for D_4 and D_1 receptors, and a relatively strong blocking effect on serotonin S_2 receptors (Hirsch & Puri 1993).

Drug-induced parkinsonism appears to be chemically closely analogous to naturally occurring Parkinson's disease. The blockade of dopamine receptors within the striatum amounts to 'chemical denervation', resulting in relative dopamine deficiency. Anticholinergic drugs can accordingly be of benefit by helping to restore the correct dopamine–acetylcholine balance.

The genesis of akathisia is little understood, but may rest on dopamine receptor blockade in brain areas other than the striatum. It is interesting that this is the only form of movement disorder which may develop within a few hours of starting treatment, i.e. within the time frame of dopamine receptor blockade with neuroleptics. It is clear, however, from pharmacological responses that other neurotransmitters must also be involved, including central adrenergic systems (p. 644).

The mechanisms underlying acute dystonic reactions also remain obscure. Their peak incidence at 24–48 hours from the initiation of therapy is well after the peak onset of dopamine receptor blockade. They may reflect interference with *pre*synaptic dopamine mechanisms; or there may be a mismatch between excess release of dopamine and coincident hypersensitivity of dopamine receptors. Neuroleptics principally occupy D_2 receptors, and the increased dopamine turnover may be expressed through overactivation of unblocked D_1 receptors. Again, however, it is likely that other neurotransmitter systems are also implicated.

There is probably not a unitary pathophysiology for tardive dyskinesia; various patterns of movement emerge after varying lengths of treatment and differ in their persistence. It has been especially difficult to explain why drugs which block striatal dopamine receptors should eventually produce forms of dyskinesia known to be associated with dopamine overactivity in the striatum. Thus the choreiform movements of tardive dyskinesia resemble those seen as a complication of levodopa therapy in Parkinson's disease, and the administration of levodopa or of anticholinergic drugs exacerbates the condition. The prolonged blockade may have led to this end result by virtue of increased dopamine turnover coupled with up-regulation of receptor numbers, possibly with an imbalance between the D_1 and D_2 receptors. Alternatively, hypersensitivity of D_2 receptors may cause them to respond abnormally to the dopamine reaching them. Hypersensitivity of this nature probably accounts for the worsening of the condition on withdrawal of neuroleptics and the success of their reintroduction in ameliorating the condition. However, attempts to demonstrate dopamine receptor supersensitivity by positron emission tomography (PET) or at autopsy have been relatively unsuccessful.

Animal studies have indicated that over the course of prolonged neuroleptic administration, dopamine receptor blockade may actually slowly disappear, giving way to supersensitivity in its place. The latter, moreover, can be shown to persist for many months after withdrawal, providing an analogy to the possible situation in tardive dyskinesia in humans (Clow et al. 1979a, 1979b). It remains difficult, nevertheless, to reconcile the very late appearance of tardive dyskinesia with the supersensitivity known to develop soon after starting neuroleptics, and it is likely that complex interactions with other neurotransmitters are also in part responsible. A role for GABA neurones in the striatum has been suggested (Gerlach & Casey 1988).

No convincing pathology has been described in the brain to account for those tardive dyskinesias which become irreversible. Structural or neurotoxic changes in the neurones, affecting their membranes or the cell respiratory mechanisms, must nevertheless be postulated in such cases.

Management

Parkinsonism

Anticholinergic drugs are of value in controlling drug-induced parkinsonism. It often transpires, however, that once parkinsonian features have come under control, the antiparkinsonian medication can then be withdrawn without recrudescence of the motor disorder. It should therefore be tapered off after 3 months for a trial period. Certainly if the risk of producing a severe tardive dyskinesia is to be minimised it would seem important to give anticholinergic medication as sparingly as possible, and only when the parkinsonism causes definite disability. Long-continued anticholinergic administration as a routine adjunct to neuroleptic treatment is now considered to be contraindicated. Levodopa should theoretically help drug-induced parkinsonism, but has been little used to date, perhaps because of adverse effects on the psychosis.

Akathisia

When akathisia is a persisting and disabling complaint the most decisive remedy is reduction of drug dosage (Braude et al. 1983). Benzodiazepines may help in some degree, also anticholinergic agents when drug-induced parkinsonism is present as well. The most encouraging results, however, appear to be obtained with beta blockers such as propanolol, which can reduce both subjective and objective manifestations of the syndrome (Adler et al. 1986). If the above procedures are without effect and the symptoms are very disabling it may be necessary to change the neuroleptic to clozapine.

Acute dystonia

For acute dystonic reactions anticholinergic drugs are best given parenterally. Benztropine (Cogentin), diphenhydramine (Benadryl) and procyclidine (Kemadrin) can be administered intravenously and are often dramatically effective. Intravenous diazepam can also help. For milder reactions it is important to remember the efficacy of non-specific calming of the patient, or simple sedation with diazepam. The previous occurrence of dystonic reactions constitutes one of the few indications for the prophylactic prescription of anticholinergic drugs from the start of a course of neuroleptic medication.

Tardive dyskinesia

The management of tardive dyskinesia must take into account every effort at prevention. There is no firm evidence that any particular phenothiazine, butyrophenone or thiothanxene is less hazardous than others in this regard, though some think the risk is less with thioridazine, oxypertine or sulpiride. Dosage and duration of neuroleptics should be kept to a minimum, and long-term maintenance therapy strictly reserved for patients in whom definite benefit can be expected. In practice this usually means patients with chronic schizophrenia of a type liable to manifest on-going positive symptoms in the absence of medication. The task force of the American Psychiatric Association recommended that all patients on long-term treatment should be reviewed at 6- or 12-month intervals (Task Force on Late Neurological Effects of Antipsychotic Drugs 1980). Whenever considered safe and feasible at these reviews the drugs should be gradually reduced until stopped completely for a 2-week period. Such 'drug holidays' have not been shown to be helpful in themselves in preventing tardive dyskinesia, and there have even been suggestions that they may increase the risk (Goldman & Luchins 1984). Nevertheless they allow assessment of continuing responsiveness to the drug and facilitate detection of the earlier stages of the disorder. Mild and early examples are perhaps most likely to subside, but even if they do not the patient will be left with less severe disability. Anticholinergic drugs as an adjunct to treatment should be avoided whenever possible.

Once tardive dyskinesia is detected anticholinergic drugs should be discontinued immediately. The next step is to reduce the dosage of neuroleptics gradually and if possible stop them altogether. This may lead to an initial worsening of the condition, but in favourable cases it will be a temporary exacerbation. Some 30–50% of patients will improve as a result, but this may occur only gradually over a number of months or years. If the mental state does not permit total withdrawal it may be possible to settle for a lower dose, or a change to a less potent neuroleptic such as thioridazine or sulpiride. In severely psychotic patients a change to clozapine may be indicated.

When the movements persist other treatments may be tried, but the number advocated indicates that none is universally successful. Drugs which deplete striatal dopamine such as reserpine or tetrabenazine are probably the treatments of first choice (Teoh 1988), but should be avoided in patients with pre-existing depression. Cholinergic agents such as physostigmine and lecithin, or GABA-enhancing drugs such as baclofen and sodium valproate may sometimes help. Benzodiazepines may be useful by virtue of their sedating effect. Propanolol, clonidine and the calcium channel blocker diltiazem have occasionally produced success (Ross et al. 1987). More recent treatments evaluated by double-blind comparisons include clonazepam (Thaker et al. 1990) and vitamin E used as a free radical scavenging agent (Elkashef et al. 1990).

Quite often, however, it will be found that no available therapy ameliorates the condition and one must merely hope for spontaneous resolution. The temptation to control the dyskinesia by reintroducing neuroleptics at increased dosage is strictly to be avoided, except in those rare cases where life is threatened by the severity of the involuntary movements. While it may be highly efficacious in producing short-term relief, this merely postpones the problem by reinstating the original pathogenesis and can be expected to worsen the ultimate disability. Clozapine in high dosage is perhaps an exception in this regard, preliminary studies showing that when given long term it can be effective in suppressing the condition (Casey 1989).

Tardive dystonia

Tardive dystonia presents equally severe management problems and the results of treatment are often disappointing. The first step should be to taper or discontinue the causative drugs or change to alternative therapy. Anticholinergic drugs such as benzhexol can help, though at the expense of worsening any coincident tardive dyskinesia. Reserpine or tetrabenazine are probably the most effective treatment, producing improvement in two-thirds of Kang et al.'s (1986) patients. Diazepam, lorazepam or baclofen may also be successful on occasion, different patients responding to different drugs.

Rarely it may be necessary to continue with the offending neuroleptic drug, for example when severe dystonia is causing pain or muscle damage as indicated by raised levels of serum creatine phosphokinase; or it may be necessary to reintroduce it when a drug-free period of 4–5 years has not achieved remission and all other treatments have failed (Burke & Kang 1988). Clozapine holds special promise and has been reported to help after fruitless attempts with other drugs, leading to slow improvement over several months (Lamberti & Bellnier 1993). It would certainly appear to be the drug of choice in patients whose psychosis requires the continuation of neuroleptics (Friedman 1994). The combination of clozapine and clonazepam has sometimes proved to be particularly effective (Shapleske et al. 1996).

Tardive akathisia

Treatment of tardive akathisia can be particularly difficult, not least because discontinuation of neuroleptics may lead to transient worsening. This should nevertheless be attempted, even though few cases will benefit substantially. Burke et al. (1989) found that reserpine and tetrabenazine were the most successful drugs to try, though only a third of their patients achieved complete resolution of symptoms. Anticholinergics and beta blockers were without effect, though lorazepam improved occasional patients markedly. Sometimes the reintroduction of neuroleptics at higher dosage may need, ultimately, to be tried.

Parkinson's disease and the parkinsonian syndrome

The cardinal neurological deficits which make up the syndrome of parkinsonism are tremor, muscular rigidity, bradykinesia and postural abnormality. A large number of other associated features are also characteristic as described below.

By far the commonest form is idiopathic parkinsonism or paralysis agitans, as described by James Parkinson in 1817. This owes its origin to a specific degeneration of pigmented cells in the brain stem, particularly those of the substantia nigra. An hereditary tendency towards the disease has recently been newly reconsidered (Golbe 1990; Hawkes 1996); in certain very rare families it has followed the pattern of autosomal dominant inheritance (Golbe *et al.* 1990). Environmental 'toxins' are also possibly operative (p. 648). Idiopathic parkinsonism is usually diagnosed when no evidence can be found from the history or examination for the presence of other diseases which could be aetiologically relevant.

The same clinical picture may be induced by certain medications such as reserpine, phenothiazines, butyrophenones and methyldopa ('drug-induced parkinsonism'). This tends to remit slowly over several weeks or months when the offending drug is withdrawn. A similar syndrome, 'postencephalitic parkinsonism', was a common aftermath of the pandemics of encephalitis lethargica which occurred almost 80 years ago (p. 352). Cases could appear up to 20 years after the original infection which was sometimes very mild. An early age of onset suggested the postencephalitic variety, also oculogyric crises, abnormal pupil reactions or continuing marked sleep disturbance.

Many other conditions that affect the basal ganglia may cause akinetic rigid syndromes along with other features resulting from diffuse brain damage, for example repeated head injuries in boxing, cerebral syphilis, anoxia due to cardiac arrest, or poisoning with carbon monoxide or manganese. Such a syndrome may appear as part of other degenerative disorders such as progressive supranuclear palsy, multiple system atrophy, Alzheimer's disease, Lewy body dementia, Wilson's disease or cerebral arteriosclerosis. The latter, however, is no longer recognised as a cause of Parkinson's disease *per se*, and the category of 'arteriosclerotic parkinsonism' has fallen into disrepute (Eadie & Sutherland 1964; Pallis 1971). Certainly the clinical features that were used to delineate this form of the syndrome were variable from one observer to another. An arteriosclerotic origin tended to be blamed when the onset had been acute or progression had occurred in a step-like manner, when progressive dementia coincided with or preceded the parkinsonism, or when pseudobulbar palsy or pyramidal deficits were present. *Marche à petit pas* seemed also to be characteristic of the variety. It is hard, however, to establish a causal relationship to cerebral arterial disease when this exists, and the two disorders probably simply occur together by coincidence. In Eadie and Sutherland's (1964) study no more clinical evidence of arterial disease could be found in a large group of parkinsonian patients than among equivalent age-matched controls.

Hoehn and Yahr (1967) reviewed 802 patients from a neurological clinic and considered 84% to be idiopathic, 15% secondary (mostly postencephalitic but also 'arteriosclerotic', toxic and metabolic in origin) and 1% to show uncertain evidence of being either primary or secondary.

Clinical features

The idiopathic disease is slightly commoner among men than women. The mean age of onset is 55 years with two-thirds of cases beginning between 50 and 59 (Hoehn & Yahr 1967). Excellent accounts of the clinical features and natural history are given by Selby (1990) and Pearce (1992).

Tremor is the presenting feature in about three-quarters of the idiopathic cases, consisting of four to six per second alternating contractions of opposing muscle groups. It is present at rest but ceases during sleep, and may become less marked when the limb is engaged in voluntary movement. It is worsened by excitement, anxiety and fatigue. Most typically it appears in the hands as flexion–extension movements affecting the metacarpophalangeal joints of the fingers and thumb. It is common also in the jaw and tongue and may come to affect the head or the lower limbs. In some cases it is predominantly or entirely unilateral.

Rigidity affects the large and small muscles of the limbs, trunk and neck, involving agonists and antagonists equally and through the whole range of passive movement. In these respects it is quite unlike the spasticity that results from corticospinal tract damage, and feels to the examining hand to have a 'lead pipe' or 'plastic' quality. When tremor is also present, the rigidity is broken up ('cogwheel rigidity'). Rigidity, like tremor, can be predominantly unilateral. It persists during sleep and is unaffected by emotional factors.

Bradykinesia consists of poverty and slowness of movement. This is not due solely to rigidity since stereotactic surgery can relieve rigidity without improving bradykinesia. Bradykinesia is not always sufficiently emphasised in descriptions of the disorder yet can be the most disabling aspect to the patient. Sometimes it dominates the entire picture. It shows in slowness in the initiation and execution of motor acts, and poverty of automatic and associated movements such as the normal swinging of the arms when walking. Fleminger (1992b) has shown that it can be distinguished by certain dual task performance tests from the motor retardation of depression. Bradykinesia probably accounts for many of the classic features of parkinsonism — the mask-like face, infrequent blinking, clumsiness of fine finger movement, crabbed writing and monotonous speech. The striking disorder of prosody evident in the speech of Parkinson patients has been shown to be related to motor control, not loss of linguistic knowledge or associated depression (Darkins *et al.* 1988). The gait is affected in many characteristic ways with slowness, shuffling, difficulty in starting and turning and impaired equilibrium. It may show an episodic quality, causing periodic freezing of action or episodes of complete immobility.

More than any other feature bradykinesia can be profoundly affected by the patient's mental state. There are numerous reports of severely disabled patients achieving surprising feats of motor behaviour in response to fear, excitement or other environmental stimulation.

Postural changes show as a characteristic flexion of the trunk and neck bringing the chin to the chest, with arms adducted at the shoulders and flexed at elbows, wrists and knuckles. The typical 'festinant' gait appears to be a product of the abnormal posture along with difficulty in controlling the centre of gravity. Postural instability leads to frequent falls.

Other features include oculomotor abnormalities, excessive salivation, seborrhoea, constipation, urinary disturbance, subjective sensory discomfort and marked fatigue. Infrequent blinking is common in all forms of parkinsonism, and paresis of convergence may occur. The latter is particularly common in postencephalitic parkinsonism which may also show oculogyric crises (pp. 352–3). Sialorrhoea is mainly the result of difficulties in coping with normal quantities of saliva on account of dysphagia. Constipation is a major symptom of the disease and a cause of much distress. Urinary frequency and incontinence are frequent complaints. Sensory discomforts include feelings of tightness, pain and cramp in the limbs and back. The fatigue associated with the disorder is often particularly distressing and disabling. It has been found to correlate better with coexistent depression than with the severity of motor symptoms but is often independent of both (Friedman & Friedman 1993).

In the detection of early cases the following observations can be useful. The patient shows difficulty when asked to maintain a steady rhythmic movement, as in tapping or making polishing movements. The handwriting often reveals changes at an early stage, as do attempts to draw parallel lines or spirals. The glabellar tap reflex is elicited by tapping over the root of the nose between the eyebrows; parkinsonian patients are said to blink in response to each tap no matter how often or at what frequency, and fail to habituate as normal subjects do. Observation of the gait can also be revealing in early cases when attention is directed at the lack of arm swinging, difficulty in turning sharply or the exacerbation of tremor in the hands.

Course and outcome

Idiopathic parkinsonism is usually a progressive disease. Hoehn and Yahr (1967) found that a quarter of patients were severely disabled or dead within 5 years of onset and two-thirds within 10 years. A small number, however, show very slow progression and remain without severe disablement after 20 years or more. The mortality is estimated to be three times that of the general population of the same age and sex. Older treatments did not influence prognosis but it is possible that levodopa therapy has prolonged life expectancy. Common causes of death are cardiac and cerebral vascular disease, bronchopneumonia and neoplasia. The prognosis in terms of rate of progression and mortality is better for postencephalitic cases and worse for those labelled as arteriosclerotic.

Pathology and pathophysiology

Parkinson's disease is associated with lesions in component parts of the extrapyramidal nervous system. The most striking finding is degeneration and loss of neurones in the pars compacta of the substantia nigra, seen macroscopically as nigral pallor. The surviving neurones characteristically show Lewy bodies within their cytoplasm which are the pathological hallmark of the condition. These are inclusion bodies with characteristic eosinophilic staining surrounded by a clear halo (Plate 11). Gibb and Lees (1989) were able to demonstrate Lewy bodies in the remaining pigmented nuclei of the substantia nigra in every case that conformed to strict clinicopathological criteria for idiopathic Parkinson's disease.

Neuronal loss and Lewy body formation are also found in other brain stem nuclei, especially the locus caeruleus, raphe nuclei and dorsal vagal nucleus, as well as in the hypothalamus and nucleus basalis of Meynert. In up to a third of cases they are also apparent in the parahippocampus and temporal neocortex (Gibb & Lees 1987). Glial scarring is seen in the brain stem in the islands from which neurones have disappeared. Cellular degeneration is often apparent in the globus pallidus, putamen and caudate, possibly by virtue of trans-synaptic degeneration. Diffuse cortical atrophy has been reported to be common, and possibly greater than would be expected for healthy individuals of equivalent age (p. 655).

In postencephalitic parkinsonism the pigmented cells of the substantia nigra and locus caeruleus are similarly lost, but neurofibrillary changes rather than Lewy bodies are seen in those that remain.

The cardinal biochemical feature of parkinsonism is striatal dopamine deficiency, resulting from loss of dopaminergic fibres in the nigrostriatal tract which passes from the pars compacta of the substantia nigra to the caudate and putamen. In consequence dopamine concentrations in these regions may be reduced to 10–20% of normal levels. The net result is increased inhibitory striatal input to the globus pallidus, and thence changes in many parts of the extrapyramidal system which conspire to the development of the parkinsonian picture (Stacy & Jankovic 1992).

The connections of the basal ganglia, and the neurotransmitters involved in these, are complex and probably as yet incompletely understood (Stacy & Jankovic 1992; Harding 1993a). Multiple parallel loops are present in the extrapyramidal system, two of which predominate. The striatum (i.e. the caudate nucleus and putamen) receives glutamatergic projections from all parts of the cortex which pass to their small spiny neurones. These neurones use GABA and a variety of peptides as their neurotransmitters. They project to the lateral globus pallidus and from there to the subthalamic nucleus. This in turn sends glutamatergic projections to the internal segment of the globus pallidus, which projects to the ventrolateral nucleus of the thalamus and back to the cortex.

The second major loop involves GABA-ergic projections from the striatum to the pars reticulata of the substantia nigra, and dopaminergic projections back from the pars compacta of the substantia nigra in the dense nigrostriatal pathway. The striatum also contains large cholinergic interneurones; dopamine and acetylcholine appear to be antagonistic in their effects in the striatum, any condition which alters the balance in the direction of marked cholinergic dominance leading to parkinsonism. It is clear, however, that dopamine deficiency will also alter the balance of excitatory and inhibitory activity in many parts of the extrapyramidal system, and that the evolution of parkinsonian symptoms will depend on changes in several of its components.

The losses of dopamine in the striatum can be detected by brain imaging with PET. The presynaptic uptake of ^{18}F dopa is reduced in the caudate and putamen in comparison with age-matched controls, the degree of decline correlating with severity of locomotor disability (Brooks et al. 1990). The posterior part of the putamen is most severely affected with reductions averaging 45% of normal, the anterior putamen and caudate being less markedly involved (62% and 84% of normal levels, respectively). This pattern differs from that seen with progressive supranuclear palsy (p. 666) which shows equally severe reductions in all parts of the putamen and caudate. There is also evidence from studies with ^{11}C raclopride that the density of D_2-binding sites is slightly up-regulated in the putamen in untreated Parkinson's disease, but without change in the caudate (Sawle et al. 1990).

In addition to the nigrostriatal pathway, other dopaminergic neurones in the ventral tegmental area of the brain stem project to the cortex and limbic structures. There is evidence that these 'mesolimbic' and 'mesocortical' pathways are also impaired in Parkinson's disease, which may be relevant to some of the psychiatric complications discussed below.

Interesting evidence has recently been obtained concerning the possible origin of the selective degeneration of dopaminergic neurones in the substantia nigra in the disease. The discovery that MPTP (1-methyl-4-phenyl 1,2,3,6 tetrahydropyridine) taken by drug addicts could result in parkinsonism (Langston et al. 1983) has led to the hypothesis that environmental toxins could conceivably play a part. MPTP induces neuronal death via its metabolite MPP+, which has been shown to inhibit NADH-CoQ$_1$ reductase (complex I), the first enzyme of the mitochondrial respiratory chain (Nicklas et al. 1985). Complex I was then shown to be selectively deficient in the substantia nigra of patients with Parkinson's disease, with normal activities of this and other respiratory chain enzymes in other brain areas (Schapira et al. 1989, 1990a, 1990b). No such abnormality was present in patients with multiple system atrophy which also leads to parkinsonism, suggesting that it may be causally related to Parkinson's disease rather than a consequence of the neuronal degeneration. Possible mechanisms by which MPP+ causes neuronal damage are discussed by Marsden (1990). It is taken up and concentrated in mitochondria, leading to depletion of adenosine triphosphate (ATP) and alterations in cellular calcium content. It may also induce the formation of free radical species, resulting in oxidative stress and consequent lipid membrane peroxidation.

Additional evidence comes from the finding of abnormalities in sulphur metabolism and N-methylation in the disease (Steventon et al. 1989; Green et al. 1991). Both reflect deficiencies in the metabolic pathways for removing toxins from the body, suggesting that patients with Parkinson's disease may have been unusually susceptible to environmental toxins with MPP+-like activity. Support for such an idea comes from the observation that several environmental toxins can cause parkinsonism, for example carbon monoxide and manganese. Genetic susceptibility to these or other widespread toxic agents could conceivably play a role in the genesis of the disorder.

Differential diagnosis

The diagnosis is usually apparent once the disease is reasonably well advanced but mistakes can occur in the early stages, particularly if tremor is absent. In elderly patients the signs may be overlooked and complaints of back or limb pain may lead to a diagnosis of arthritis or osteoporosis. Alternatively, the presentation may be with unexpected falls which are attributed to vertebrobasilar insufficiency. Strictly unilateral rigidity in the absence of tremor can raise suspicion of a cerebral tumour. Marked bradykinesia may at first raise the question of myxoedema or depressive illness. In patients with evidence of intellectual deterioration the parkinsonian features may be overlooked in favour of a diagnosis of presenile or senile dementia. Marked parkinsonian features are indeed not uncommon in Alzheimer's disease (pp. 433 and 438).

Rapid fluctuations in the early stages can suggest a psychiatric disorder by way of neurosis, hysteria or even malingering. Such suspicion will be increased if the family report that the patient can function entirely normally in the face of a stressful situation. In the presence of known psychiatric disorder under treatment with neuroleptic drugs, considerable difficulty may be encountered in distinguishing side effects of therapy from the ingravescent development of idiopathic Parkinson's disease. Here it can be important to remember that the parkinsonian side effects of neuroleptic drugs usually make their appearance early in the course of therapy, then often tend to subside (p. 640). In cases of doubt withdrawal may be necessary for very long periods, sometimes for a year or more, before the true situation is clarified.

Benign essential tremor (juvenile, adult or senile — Minor's disease) may lead to difficulties with diagnosis. This can begin at any age, a positive family history is often forthcoming and improvement with alcohol is characteristic. The hands are principally affected, the tremor disappears when the limbs are inactive, and titubation of the head is commoner than in Parkinson's disease. There is no bradykinesia or rigidity and the condition is static or perhaps very slowly progressive over several decades.

Other neurological diseases which must sometimes be considered include Huntington's disease and Wilson's disease. The rigid and akinetic forms of Huntington's disease may at first resemble Parkinson's disease. Wilson's disease must be carefully excluded when parkinsonian symptoms begin in adolescence or early adult life. The rigidity of Wilson's disease is similar to that of parkinsonism, but the involuntary movements are more varied including choreic jerking, athetoid and dystonic move-

ments, or flapping tremor of the outstretched hands. Other degenerative conditions which must be borne in mind include progressive supranuclear palsy (p. 666), corticobasal degeneration (p. 668) and multiple system atrophy (p. 668). Diffuse Lewy body disease (p. 450) may sometimes present with parkinsonian features alone. Quite surprisingly it has recently been found that almost a quarter of patients diagnosed as suffering from Parkinson's disease are wrongly so labelled: out of 100 cases coming to autopsy 24 had been misdiagnosed, showing the pathological features of progressive supranuclear palsy, multiple system atrophy, Alzheimer's disease or basal ganglia vascular disease (Hughes et al. 1992).

Treatment

The treatment of Parkinson's disease has undergone dramatic changes. Anticholinergic drugs are still in use but a vogue for stereotactic operations has now largely given way to treatment with levodopa. Useful reviews of current management are provided by Bakheit (1990) and Quinn (1995). Treatment will be considered only briefly here, but certain aspects of drug treatment and stereotactic operation will be dealt with in more detail in the following sections on psychiatric aspects of the disease.

There is no clear evidence that modern therapy alters the underlying pathology of the disease as opposed to suppressing the clinical manifestations. Nevertheless a large proportion of patients can obtain a gratifying degree of relief from their more disabling symptoms, certainly during the earlier stages of the disorder. Some severely crippled patients are enabled to lead relatively independent lives. Specific therapies must be accompanied by general measures to keep the patient active for as long as possible, with physiotherapy or the use of simple mechanical aids. Psychosocial aspects often need attention, especially since the degree of physical disability may be considerably worsened by stress or concurrent depression.

Anticholinergic drugs are still used alone in mild cases and are usually continued thereafter when further measures need to be instituted. The best known are benzhexol (Artane, Pipanol), benztropine (Cogentin), orphenadrine (Disipal), procyclidine (Kemadrin) and biperiden (Akineton). Their effect is variable. Mobility is usually improved, with some decrease in rigidity and tremor. Bradykinesia is usually little affected. Atropine-like side effects limit the dose that can be employed.

Oculogyric crises in postencephalitic parkinsonism are sometimes reported to diminish with anticholinergic drugs. *Amphetamine* and *chlordiazepoxide* have also been found to help in this regard. Prolonged crises can often be terminated by intramuscular *ethopropazine* (Lysivane).

Amantadine hydrochloride (Symmetrel) stimulates dopamine release in the central nervous system, and is indicated if anticholinergic drugs fail and the patient is only mildly disabled. Among the severely disabled it finds application in patients who cannot tolerate levodopa. Amantadine helps with bradykinesia and postural instability in addition to improving rigidity. Mobility may thereby be considerably improved.

Selegiline (Eldepryl, Deprenyl) inhibits monoamine oxidase B, one of the enzymes responsible for the breakdown of dopamine in the brain. It has limited antiparkinsonian action, but when used with levodopa can potentiate and prolong its action, sometimes helping with mild dose-related fluctuations of response. It may also allow the dose of levodopa to be reduced. However, it can sometimes worsen dyskinesias and aggravate psychiatric adverse reactions.

Selegiline became widely regarded as the treatment of first choice for newly diagnosed patients because it proved to be 'neuroprotective' in animals, preventing damage to the nigrostriatal system when they were exposed to the toxin MPTP (Heikkla *et al.* 1984). Evidence was obtained, moreover, that Parkinson's disease progressed more slowly in patients who started on treatment with selegiline, in that the need for levodopa was delayed for almost a year in relation to controls (Parkinson Study Group 1989; Tetrud & Langston 1989), though it remained unclear whether this reflected neuroprotection or merely mild symptomatic benefit. These results have, however, come under critical re-evaluation, and more recent evidence has even pointed to increased mortality among patients treated with the combination of levodopa and selegiline, casting doubts on the advisability of its long-term use in the disease (Calne 1995; Lees 1995).

Levodopa (L-dopa) is now well established as a highly effective drug with a wide range of activity on different parkinsonian symptoms. It is a logical form of treatment, L-dopa being the immediate precursor of dopamine which is known to be deficient in the brain. Approximately one-third of patients can be expected to obtain marked relief, one-third moderate benefit, and the remainder show a modest or disappointing response. Perhaps some 15% do not respond at all; in such cases the possibility of some alternative diagnosis such as progressive supranuclear palsy or multiple system atrophy should be considered.

Levodopa is therefore widely regarded as the treatment of choice in patients who can tolerate it. A synergistic action is seen when given in conjunction with anticholinergic drugs and perhaps with amantadine as well. It may take several months before maximal benefit is obtained,

and it cannot be said to have failed until it has been tried for 6 months or preferably a year. The variability of response seen from one individual to another cannot yet be accurately predicted.

Levodopa is now always given in combination with a peripheral dopa-decarboxylase inhibitor such as carbidopa (in Sinemet) or benserazide (in Madopar). This prevents its metabolism in the gastrointestinal tract, reducing nausea and vomiting, and allows higher blood levels to be achieved with smaller doses. Moreover the combined preparations increase the turnover of dopamine in the nigrostriatal system more selectively than does levodopa alone, and maximal benefit is obtained earlier.

Rigidity is helped and tremor also improves but less consistently. Propanolol or some other beta blocker may further help the latter. Outstanding benefit is seen where bradykinesia and postural instability are concerned, both of which are rarely responsive to anticholinergic drugs. Thus facial mobility is improved, salivation lessened and the voice strengthened. Gait, handwriting and ability to do fine manipulative tasks all improve. The overall result can be dramatic with the patient able to do such things as shaving, knitting or getting out of bed unaided when these have not been possible for some considerable time.

Unfortunately as time goes by the efficacy of levodopa may diminish. In general, over a 5-year period a third of those who responded initially retain their benefit, a third lose some and a third lose all their gains becoming worse than they were before (Marsden & Parkes 1977). This is most probably due to progression of the underlying disease. Variations in benefit may emerge for hours or days at a time, or the effects of each dose may become shorter-lasting. The first sign of fluctuation may be early morning bradykinesia when the effects of the previous day's dose have worn off. 'End dose deterioration' then appears, with bradykinesia or tremor returning as each dose is due. In time this shows as the 'on–off' effect, with swings from complete relief to total immobility, often occurring with startling rapidity and sometimes many times a day (Marsden & Parkes 1976). By this time peak dose dyskinetic movements have also usually developed. In extreme form the patient may be precipitated within minutes, or even seconds, from a state of dyskinetic mobility to one of profound rebound parkinsonism (Quinn 1995).

Tests carried out serially during on and off phases have shown some mild impairment of cognition and adverse swings of affect during the latter phases (Brown *et al.* 1984). In a detailed study of nine patients experiencing severe on–off phenomena, Nissenbaum *et al.* (1987) found that four had clear-cut depression and anxiety when 'off', one also showing features of elation and disinhibition when 'on'. In a questionnaire survey two-thirds of 31 such patients reported some degree of parallel mood change, usually towards depression when akinetic but also with feelings of irritability, aggressiveness and frustration. In rare cases hallucinations and delusions may accompany the transient depressions:

A 69-year-old woman on treatment with Sinemet progressed after 7 years to severe and abrupt changes characteristic of the on–off phenomenon. One year later she began to experience parallel fluctuations in mood. In the 'off' condition she showed depressed mood, agitation, hypochondriacal and nihilistic delusions, and an unshakable belief that something dreadful was about to happen. She had ideas of guilt, and auditory and visual hallucinations. Although agitated she remained fully orientated and could retain information provided her attention could be sustained. In this condition she was chair-bound. When mobile and 'on' she had a mildly depressed mood, but was not agitated, deluded or hallucinated, and had partial insight into the psychotic phenomena experienced when immobile.

(Nissenbaum *et al.* 1987)

A 35-year-old man who had taken Sinemet for 4 years developed manic features during 'on' phases alternating with depression when 'off'. During 'on' phases he showed choreoathetoid movements and became overactive and talkative. He was extremely elated and expressed grandiose ideas that he would marry several women and live for 100 years. On reverting to severe immobility he showed profound depression and nihilistic thought content and expressed the wish to be dead. Between the fluctuations in mood and movement he improved, exhibiting neither mood abnormalities nor dyskinesias. There was no past or family history of affective disorder. His condition was ameliorated by giving smaller doses of medication more frequently.

(Keshavan *et al.* 1986)

Considerable improvement may be obtained by giving the drug in small divided doses, even 2- or 3-hourly through the day, or by the use of sustained release preparations. Other approaches are to add selegiline, or to partially substitute an agonist drug such as bromocriptine or pergolide. Apomorphine can find a special place in the treatment of refractory on–off oscillations as described below.

Adverse effects commonly include anorexia, nausea, vomiting and hypotension. These can usually be overcome by starting with low dosage and increasing very gradually. The gastrointestinal effects can be largely avoided by the use of combined preparations of levodopa with a selective extracerebral decarboxylase inhibitor (Sinemet or Madopar). Tremors, tachypnoea, flushing and cardiac dysrhythmias may also be troublesome, but the commonest dose-limiting factor is the appearance of dyskinetic movements. Such dyskinesias can take any form, including orofacial dyskinesia, chorea, dystonia or athetosis of the limbs, analogous in form, and probably in pathophysiology, to the movements seen in tardive dyskinesia (p. 641). Three main varieties are recognised: 'peak dose dyskinesia' with choreic or dystonic movements, 'diphasic dyskinesia' occurring at the beginning and end of the dose and often being ballistic in character, and 'off period dystonia' with fixed, often painful, spasms mainly involving the feet. A compromise quite often has to be sought between the severity of such adventitious movements and the degree of relief of parkinsonian disability. The psychiatric effects of levodopa are considered on p. 658 *et seq.*

Bromocriptine (Parlodel) acts as a direct stimulant of dopamine receptors. Only about a third of patients obtain a response to bromocriptine alone, but when given along with levodopa it allows a smaller dose of the latter to be employed. Some prefer to use it initially on its own in order to defer the introduction of levodopa with its attendant long-term risks of fluctuation in response and dyskinesias. Early combination therapy with levodopa and bromocriptine has some advocates. It finds a special place in the management of patients who experience fluctuations in response to levodopa as described above.

Bromocriptine must be used with caution in the presence of peripheral vascular disease since it is derived from ergot, and it is contraindicated in the presence of ischaemic heart disease. Postural hypotension can be a problem when starting treatment, also nausea and vomiting which are helped by domperidone. Psychiatric side effects are similar to those seen with levodopa (p. 658 *et seq.*).

Other dopamine agonists include lisuride (Revanil) and pergolide (Celanace), the latter with a longer duration of action and effects on D_1 as well as D_2 dopamine receptors. Both are again ergot derived, and similar contraindications apply. Indications for their use parallel those for bromocriptine, some patients appearing to derive more benefit from one drug than another. A high incidence of psychiatric complications, particularly hallucinations, has again been reported.

Apomorphine has a special place in the treatment of late-stage fluctuations in response to levodopa when other approaches have failed, and can on occasion be life-saving (Stibe *et al.* 1988; Hughes *et al.* 1993). It is also a D_1- and D_2-receptor agonist but must be given by subcutaneous injection. Oral domperidone is given concurrently to prevent vomiting. Patients and their relatives can be instructed to inject the drug when 'off' periods occur, relief occurring within 15 minutes and lasting for up to an hour. Continuous daytime infusion can be achieved through a portable pump.

The injections work with high reliability and tolerance does not develop, but drowsiness and local reactions at the injection sites can be troublesome. Adverse psychiatric complications have been rare, in contrast to those encountered with continuous lisuride infusions.

Catechol O-methyl transferase inhibitors are currently under trial. This is one of the enzymes that metabolise levodopa and dopamine. Entacapone acts peripherally and tolcapone both peripherally and centrally. Both appear to have a dose-sparing effect and to prolong the effects of levodopa.

Psychotropic drugs often have an important part to play in management. The relief of depression and anxiety can itself lead to a considerable improvement in physical disability, but over and above this the tricyclic antidepressants may have a more direct effect on parkinsonian symptomatology. Imipramine or amitriptyline are usually employed along with anticholinergic drugs or levodopa, but in mild cases may prove to be effective on their own. The antidepressant nomifensine was regarded as particularly appropriate by virtue of its dopaminergic activity, but has now been withdrawn on account of toxic effects. Diazepam is used when anxiety is the predominant manifestation. Monoamine oxidase inhibitor antidepressants must not be given in association with levodopa.

Stereotactic surgery declined abruptly in popularity after the introduction of levodopa, but still finds an occasional place in patients with tremor or rigidity which are predominantly unilateral and when bradykinesia is minimal. The optimal site for stereotactic destruction has been extensively debated. Common targets have included the globus pallidus, the ventrolateral nucleus of the thalamus and the pallidofugal fibres in the ansa and fasciculus lenticularis.

The relief of tremor and rigidity can be impressive but the gains in terms of functional ability are often disappointing. This is probably because the bradykinesia of the disorder is unaffected. Thus the festinant gait, postural imbalance and mask-like face persist unaltered. Side effects of the operations further limit their usefulness — occasional patients suffer speech disturbance, impairment of balance or some degree of paresis or mental deterioration.

Neural transplantation has been shown to be successful in restoring function in primates with lesions of the dopamine pathways, and limited experience has been obtained in patients with Parkinson's disease (Hitchcock 1992; Lindvall 1994; Hauser *et al.* 1995). Despite occasional reports of striking success with autologous transplantation of tissue from the adrenal medulla this approach has proved disappointing, and the use of foetal dopaminergic cells appears to hold more promise. This, however, raises considerable ethical problems.

Adrenal medullary transplantation seems commonly to be followed by behavioural complications in the immediate postoperative period, including sleep disturbance, hallucinations, delusions, confusion and mood changes (Stebbins & Tanner 1992). Techniques of this nature may yet find a place in the management of younger patients whose disease is difficult to control by other means, but continuing improvements in drug therapy may overtake their further development.

Psychiatric aspects of parkinsonism

Interest in the psychiatric aspects of parkinsonism has increased as a result of advances in knowledge of the disease. The advent of stereotactic surgery focused renewed attention on the problem of intellectual impairment in the disorder, and the demonstration of disturbance of amine metabolism has brought new interest to its association with depression.

There is a good deal of disagreement in different reports regarding the frequency of mental symptoms, depending no doubt upon the particular population under scrutiny. Thus behavioural disturbance is likely to be more common when a substantial number of postencephalitic cases are examined, and intellectual impairment will be more frequent when patients with 'arteriosclerotic parkinsonism' are included in the sample. The difficulties of achieving anything like a reliable estimate are increased by the problems inherent in distinguishing these different varieties one from another.

Mjönes (1949) reviewed the earlier work in detail. Three main groups of mental disturbance gradually came to be recognised and were sometimes regarded as an integral part of the pathological picture—a change of personality towards suspicion, irritability and egocentricity, an impairment of memory and intellect, and psychotic developments with depression, paranoia and sometimes visual hallucinations. Some felt that there was a typical paralysis agitans psychopathy, others a characteristic psychosis. Some found a great excess of dementia, others of depression. Mjönes' own investigation of 262 cases of paralysis agitans revealed mental symptoms in approximately 40% of cases. 'Organic' changes predominated over 'reactive' changes, the former consisting of impaired memory and intellect, the latter of depression with irritability, egocentricity and hypochondriasis. Transitional forms were also encountered in which the relative contributions of organic or reactive elements were uncertain.

More recent studies have served to underline the associations with depression and cognitive impairment, the latter chiefly in later-onset Parkinson's disease. It now seems indubitable that the risk of dementia is increased above expectation and several theories have been advanced to account for this. A typical personality change, or a characteristic form of psychotic reaction, are no longer recognised. Those psychoses which do emerge are largely seen in the context of treatment with levodopa and other drugs. These matters are dealt with in detail in the sections that follow.

Cognitive impairment and dementia

The question of cognitive impairment in Parkinson's disease has attracted a great deal of interest, particularly since the advent of treatments which may be effective in prolonging life. There is no doubt that some patients show impairment of cognitive function, sometimes severe and pervasive enough to amount to an easily recognised progressive dementia. Others by contrast remain intellectually intact despite gross physical disablement. The issue which has been hard to resolve is whether, as a group, patients with idiopathic Parkinson's disease are more prone to develop such difficulties than would be expected by virtue of their age alone. The present consensus is that the risk of dementia is definitely increased, perhaps some two- or threefold. Possible reasons for this have turned out to be complex, and are gradually being disentangled as discussed below.

Brown and Marsden (1984) review the differing estimates of the prevalence of dementia in Parkinson's disease, ranging from 10% to over 80%, and the possible reasons for such wide discrepancies:

Sampling errors are compounded by difficulties in excluding other causes of akinetic–rigid syndromes during life, in particular in separately idiopathic Parkinson's disease from 'arteriosclerotic parkinsonism' (p. 646). If some examples of parkinsonism merely reflect an accent of diffuse cerebral vascular disease on the basal ganglia, then the cognitive impairments encountered could be due to the widespread cerebral changes in this group. When, on the other hand, cognitive impairment is used as a criterion for separating arteriosclerotic from idiopathic parkinsonism, the idiopathic cases will tend to be reported as intact.

Problems with the definition and assessment of dementia are also considerable, and the criteria employed have varied from one study to another. Some have sought to identify the clinical syndrome of dementia, using behavioural criteria and brief mental state tests, whereas others have used batteries of psychological tests to look for specific cognitive deficits. With both approaches the assessment of parkinsonian patients can raise special difficulties. Behavioural criteria must allow for the curtailment of activities occasioned by the disease; psychological testing must take into consideration slowness of response which may be largely attributable to motor handicap. Care must be taken to allow for what is to be expected in any ageing group of persons, and to differentiate cognitive failure from the depression which is common with Parkinson's disease. Drugs taken for treatment of the condition may further complicate assessments.

Earlier studies served mainly to focus attention on the problem. Riklan et al. (1959) examined 220 consecutive patients referred for stereotactic surgery, using a battery of measures for assessing cognitive and personality functioning. Duration of illness was unrelated to scores on any test, but muscular rigidity and autonomic dysfunction were associated with decreased intellectual productivity and perceptual difficulties. But the most striking relationships were between the degree of voluntary movement impairment and a wide range of psychological deficits—loss of drive and energy, impairment of intellectual and perceptual functions, and pervasive personality and emotional disorders. This was thought to reflect not only central factors but also the psychosocial consequences of the disease.

Pollock and Hornabrook (1966) estimated that 20% of a large unselected series of patients showed significant mental deterioration, the majority being in the group labelled as arteriosclerotic but some being examples of idiopathic Parkinson's disease. They stressed that intellectual impairment could exist alongside mild parkinsonism, many patients being a burden to their families on account of dementia rather than their motor disabilities. Mindham (1970) found that one-third of parkinsonian patients admitted to a psychiatric hospital showed cognitive impairments, this being equally frequent among idiopathic and arteriosclerotic cases. Celesia and Wanamaker (1972) claimed that 40% of 153 patients with idiopathic Parkinson's disease showed some evidence of cognitive impairment, this correlating in frequency and severity with the duration of the disease.

An impressive early survey was carried out by Marttila and Rinne (1976) involving all traceable patients with Parkinson's disease in a defined area of Finland. Of 144 patients, 29% were thought to be demented, 50% of these being mildly, 30% moderately and 20% severely affected. Patients with evidence of arteriosclerosis were more often demented than those without (56% and 18% of cases, respectively). There was a clear rise with age, from 20% among the under seventies to 65% among the over eighties. The severely physically disabled showed dementia more often than the mildly affected, increasing severity of rigidity and bradykinesia showing a positive correlation with the degree of intellectual decline. This association pointed to a role of subcortical structures in the pathophysiology of the dementia.

Lieberman et al. (1979) found moderate to marked dementia in one-third of 520 patients, this being 10 times the prevalence in spouses used as controls. The demented patients, in addition to a later onset, had become more physically disabled in a shorter time and had responded less well to levodopa. Two distinct forms of Parkinson's disease, with and without dementia, thus seemed a possibility. Lees and Smith (1983) restricted attention to mildly disabled patients, all under the age of 65 and with normal CT scans. Comparisons with age-matched controls showed no impairment on tests of intelligence or memory, but revealed significant deficits on the Wisconsin Card Sorting Test and a verbal fluency test. Frontal cognitive deficits were therefore highlighted.

More recent surveys have attempted to allow for the various sources of artefact outlined above, in particular adopting stringent criteria for the diagnosis of dementia. The great majority have confirmed an increased prevalence of dementia in the disease. Rajput *et al.* (1984) reviewed the Mayo Clinic records of all Parkinson patients seen over a 13-year period, charting dementia only when this had been diagnosed on at least two separate occasions. For every patient two sex- and age-matched controls were selected from residents in the area. Of the 138 new Parkinson patients seen, 13 (9.4%) were demented, compared with 2.9% of controls. When none of the three matched individuals showed dementia at the time the parkinsonism was first recognised these were followed further, and dementia emerged more frequently among the patients than the controls.

Mayeux *et al.* (1988a) performed a similar review of records from a medical centre in New York. Among 339 patients with idiopathic Parkinson's disease 10.9% were demented according to DSM-III criteria. The demented patients were significantly older than the remainder, had a later age of onset and a more rapid progression of physical disability. When the parkinsonism had begun after the age of 70 dementia was noted almost three times as often as when the onset had been earlier. Among patients over 60 years old the prevalence was judged to be almost four times that expected for a population of equivalent age.

Equivalent results were obtained from a register-based survey of patients in the Netherlands, incepted with a hospital discharge diagnosis of Parkinson's disease and followed an average of 8 years later (Breteler *et al.* 1995). In comparison with a reference group of patients with non-cerebral diseases the risk of developing dementia during this period was increased threefold.

The most clear-cut evidence, however, has come from Mindham's group, who have reported the first truly prospective study of dementia in idiopathic Parkinson's disease (Biggins *et al.* 1992):

Serial assessments were made of cognition, mood and level of disability in a group of 87 patients and 50 healthy matched controls over a 4.5-year period, each subject being examined at 9-month intervals. The mean age of the patients was 64 years. Patients were excluded if they had a history of stroke, hypertension or transient ischaemic attacks, or when there were indica-

tions of other neurological disorder. An extensive battery of psychometric tests was administered at each examination, along with rating scales for depression, anxiety and physical disability. The accumulated data sheets were reviewed at the end of the study, blind to whether the subject was a Parkinson patient or control, and diagnoses of dementia were made according to DSM-III criteria. Judgements were made as to the assessment at which these criteria were first satisfied.

Five of the 87 patients (6%) were considered to have been demented from the outset of the study, and 10 more became demented during the follow-up period. No control subject did so. After allowing for patients who dropped out during the course of the survey the cumulative incidence of dementia over this period was 19%. Comparisons between those who demented and those who did not showed that the former were older, older at onset of Parkinson's disease, had a longer duration of illness, and lower initial performance on certain cognitive tests. This last might indicate that their dementia had already been present in milder form while not yet meeting DSM-III criteria.

It therefore seems clear that dementia, identifiable clinically, is increased above expectation in Parkinson's disease, even when care has been taken to exclude vascular and other pathologies which might have contributed towards it. Cognitive impairments, insufficient in themselves to lead to such a diagnosis, seem also to be common, though there is insufficient information to judge how often these may be a prelude to dementia.

Psychometric studies show a wide spectrum of deficits among cognitively impaired parkinsonian subjects, as reviewed by Ross *et al.* (1992). In some the picture resembles 'subcortical dementia' (p. 667), particularly with respect to memory functioning, and executive function deficits are often prominent suggesting disruption of frontal–subcortical connections. In others, however, there are language and other impairments which point to cortical dysfunction. Sometimes, indeed, the clinical picture appears to overlap with that of Alzheimer's disease. Ross *et al.* conclude that the heterogeneity of the pictures seen suggests that there are multiple dementia syndromes in Parkinson's disease, associated with varying structural and biochemical pathology.

The causation of these deficits remains uncertain and a number of possibilities must be considered. First, they may be due in part to the classic pathology of Parkinson's disease and the dopamine deficiency that ensues. The subcortical nature of the dementia in many examples would fit with such a pathogenesis, especially since mesolimbic and mesocortical projections are known to be involved along with disruption of the nigrostriatal system. Such projections arise from the medial substantia nigra and the ventral tegmental area, and these have been found to be particularly severely affected in Parkinson patients with dementia (Rinne *et al.* 1989). Neuronal counts and noradrenaline levels have also proved to be reduced in the locus caeruleus in the presence of dementia, suggesting that diminished noradrenergic inputs to the cortex may make an additional contribution (Gaspar & Gray 1984; Chui *et al.* 1986; Cash *et al.* 1987). Together these observations support a subcortical origin for the dementia.

To a notable degree, however, dementia is rare in younger patients with Parkinson's disease, even though in all other respects the course and pathology of the disorder appears to be similar whatever the age of onset (Gibb 1989). Dementia has emerged as exceptional with onsets below the age of 50, even with disease of long duration, and it becomes commoner with later onsets, especially after 70 years. Indeed the factor of age of onset has emerged as one of the firmest risk factors for the development of dementia.

With age there is increasing likelihood of finding Alzheimer-type pathology in the cortex, and certain studies have suggested that this may play a major role in producing the dementia. Alvord *et al.* (1974) and Hakim and Mathieson (1978, 1979) found Alzheimer changes to be commoner in patients with Parkinson's disease than in age-matched controls, and Boller *et al.* (1980) found the prevalence of plaques and tangles in the cortex to rise as the severity of dementia increased. A cortical pathology of Alzheimer type might thus be accelerated in the presence of Parkinson's disease and account for the cognitive deficits seen. However, further detailed studies have given conflicting results and this hypothesis is now regarded as uncertain (Jellinger & Riederer 1984; Gibb 1989).

A third possible explanation involves the nucleus basalis of Meynert. Perry *et al.* (1985) demonstrated marked cholinergic deficits in the cerebral cortex of Parkinson patients, which in the temporal neocortex correlated with the severity of mental impairment assessed prior to death. The cholinergic deficits were of a similar order to those seen in Alzheimer's disease, despite the dementia being milder, but lacked correlation with the degree of tangle and plaque formation. Rather they correlated with the extent of neuronal loss in the nucleus basalis of Meynert. This was always pronounced with losses of up to 70% in the presence of parkinsonian dementia. Thus the cortical cholinergic deficits seemed not to be explicable in terms of cortical pathology, but more probably resulted from degeneration of cholinergic axons associated with the loss of cells in the Meynert nucleus. Such loss might itself be due to a pathological process analogous to that inducing changes in the substantia nigra.

This striking set of observations has been both con-

firmed and refuted in other studies, as reviewed by Ross *et al.* (1992) and Chui and Perlmutter (1992). And it has become apparent that, at least in some cases, dementia can occur in Parkinson's disease in the absence of either Alzheimer-type pathology in the cortex or cell loss in the nucleus basalis of Meynert.

These various possible contributions to dementia are discussed in detail by Dubois and Pillon (1992). It seems probable that many of the cognitive changes are largely due to subcortical pathology, with dopamine deficiency being compounded by loss of inputs from noradrenergic and cholinergic nuclei. In the older patient with Parkinson's disease and severe dementia, concomitant changes of Alzheimer type in the cortex are likely to make an additional contribution.

Structural brain imaging has not contributed substantially to this cortical/subcortical debate. Air encephalography (Selby 1968) and CT scanning (Sroka *et al.* 1981) have shown a high prevalence of cerebral atrophy in patients with Parkinson's disease, and in several studies ventricular enlargement has correlated with the presence of cognitive impairment (Huber & Glatt 1992). Third ventricular width and the intercaudate distance have also shown such associations, whereas the contribution of cortical atrophy usually disappears on controlling for age. To this extent structural imaging supports the relevance of subcortical pathology. Magnetic resonance imaging has not clarified the situation further (Huber *et al.* 1989).

PET and SPECT scans have by contrast tended to underline the importance of cortical pathology, showing deficits in metabolism in the frontal and parietal regions which are marked in the presence of dementia. Metter *et al.* (1990), using FDG-PET, found essentially the same pattern of hypometabolism in parkinsonian dementia and Alzheimer's disease, with global reductions in brain metabolism and an accent on the parietal regions. These could be observed to progress with worsening of the cognitive impairment. Peppard *et al.* (1992) showed widespread cortical and subcortical reductions in glucose metabolism in non-demented Parkinson patients, though with significant further reductions in the cortical regions in the presence of dementia. The temporoparietal regions were again particularly affected. It remains unclear, however, whether such patterns reflect intrinsic cortical pathology, or the cortical effects of deafferentation from subcortical structures.

Finally a fourth element has been added now that it is appreciated that Lewy bodies are often found in the cerebral cortex as well as in the brain stem nuclei. How far diffuse Lewy body disease (p. 450 *et seq.*) may make its own contribution to cognitive failure in patients with Parkinson's disease remains to be determined, but no doubt this may operate as a substantial additional factor.

Affective disorder

An association between parkinsonism and depression is

well established. The depression is sometimes clearly reactive in nature, setting in immediately the patient is informed of the nature of the disease, or developing later as an understandable response to the limitations and discomforts imposed by the disablement. Mindham (1974), for example, was able to show a significant correlation between the severity of the leading signs of parkinsonism and the severity of depression in a group of patients attending a neurological clinic. This relationship persisted during treatment with levodopa, those improving physically showing a fall in the severity of affective symptoms.

However, there are also indications that depression may sometimes bear a more integral relationship to the disease process itself, reflecting in some way the causative brain pathology. The high prevalence of depression has impressed many observers and it has seemed to be commoner than in equivalently disabling illnesses. In several investigations it has failed to show a proportionate relationship to the degree of disability, and quite often it has been found to respond to antidepressive treatment (including electroconvulsive therapy) while the physical disability persists unchanged. Rather strikingly, Fleminger (1991) showed that depression and anxiety were both commoner when unilateral Parkinson's disease affected the left rather than the right side of the body, which is the reverse of what might have been expected if the symptoms were purely a response to functional disability. Schiffer et al. (1988) found that the depression was often atypical in form, frequently coexisting with panic disorder or generalised anxiety.

Warburton (1967) examined 140 parkinsonian patients referred for thalamotomy and compared them with matched controls suffering from a variety of surgical and medical conditions. Depression was significantly commoner among the parkinsonian patients, particularly among the females. Fifty-six per cent of the males and 71% of the females showed some degree of depression. No relationship could be observed to age, duration of illness or degree of physical handicap.

Mindham (1970), in a retrospective survey of 89 parkinsonian patients admitted to a psychiatric hospital, found that in almost two-thirds the psychiatric diagnosis had been of an affective disorder. Several patients improved in mood with appropriate psychiatric treatment even though their physical condition remained unaltered.

Celesia and Wanamaker (1972) found some degree of depression in one-third of 153 patients with idiopathic Parkinson's disease, the severity again being independent of the degree of motor disability or duration of disease. Horn (1974) confirmed a significant relationship between parkinsonism and depression using an objective rating scale for mood disorder. This relationship was indepen-

dent of age, duration or measures of severity of handicap, suggesting an integral association with the disease process itself.

Robins (1976), in a carefully controlled study, supported such an interpretation. Forty-five patients with Parkinson's disease were matched for age and sex with chronically disabled people drawn from the same institutions (patients with hemiplegia, paraplegia and arthritis). The groups resembled each other with regard to the frequency of a pre-illness history of depression or of neurotic symptoms. The duration of disablement was similar in both but the degree of handicap greater in the non-parkinsonian group. Nevertheless the patients with Parkinson's disease were significantly more depressed than the controls as measured by the Hamilton rating scale. In neither group did the severity of disability affect the presence or absence of depression, suggesting that the latter was not solely reactive in nature. Mayeux et al. (1981) examined 55 patients using their spouses as controls. Forty-seven per cent of the patients were deemed depressed, compared with 13% of controls, the depression being mild in two-thirds and moderate to severe in the remainder.

In a large postal survey Gotham et al. (1986) were able to show that depression was related to the degree of impairment in activities of daily living, but even so much of the variability was left unaccounted for. Individual differences in coping style and the availability of social support were probably also influential. The symptom profiles observed included pessimism, hopelessness, decreased motivation and increased concern over health; by contrast guilt, self blame and worthlessness were usually absent.

With regard to treatment antidepressant medication can be highly effective in relieving both physical and mental symptoms (p. 652). Electroconvulsive treatment is not contraindicated, and may result in pronounced motor benefit while alleviating the affective disorder (Lebensohn & Jenkins 1975). Sometimes, indeed, improvement in parkinsonian features has been observed to antedate the improvement in depression during a course of electroconvulsive therapy (Asnis 1977). Rasmussen and Abrams (1992) and Faber (1995) review the evidence that such treatment can improve the motor symptoms of Parkinson's disease, at least temporarily, even in the absence of depression.

In the great majority of cases depression follows the onset of the disease, but patients are occasionally encountered where it is the presenting feature. Kearney (1964) reported two examples in whom the first symptom was depression combined with anxiety and agitation. In the first the depressive illness responded well to electroconvulsive therapy, then returned 1 year later when it was apparent that parkinsonism was developing. The second patient became increasingly depressed over several months with complaints about his legs which he could not describe accurately; he thought he had Parkinson's disease and sought many consultations with negative result until 6 months later when the definitive signs appeared.

To the extent that depression appears to be closely tied to the parkinsonian disease process it is tempting to suppose that common biochemical factors may be operative. In depressive illness, as well as in Parkinson's disease, deficiencies of noradrenaline, dopamine and 5-hydroxytryptamine (5-HT) have been postulated to play a part. Fleminger's (1991) finding that left-sided Parkinson's disease is associated with greater depression than right-sided disease suggests that dopamine deficiency in the right cerebral hemisphere may be especially liable to provoke depression. Mayeux *et al.* (1984, 1988b) suggest, however, that a reduction in brain 5-HT may be the important factor, showing that the cerebrospinal fluid content of its major metabolite (5-hydroxyindoleacetic acid) is significantly lower in depressed than non-depressed Parkinson patients. Oral administration of 5-hydroxytryptophan, a serotonin precursor, was found to alleviate the depression in the absence of changes in motor symptoms or activities of daily living. It is possible therefore that serotonergic antidepressants such as fluoxetine may be particularly helpful in the disorder.

Finally, increased tearfulness has been found to be common in patients with Parkinson's disease, sometimes with 'emotionalism' as indicated by sudden weeping with loss of normal social control (Madeley *et al.* 1992). Almost half of a group of patients with idiopathic Parkinson's disease reported being more tearful since the onset, and 10% showed emotionalism of the type following cerebrovascular accidents (pp. 386–7). Such disturbances were sometimes evident in the absence of lowered mood or cognitive impairment.

Personality changes

Increasing disability may understandably lead to irritability, as in any disease which results in restriction of activities and dependence upon others. Egocentricity, querulousness and an exacting attitude towards those around have often been stressed, likewise a change towards suspiciousness or even frank paranoia. However, the prevalence of such changes is hard to assess. Obsessional traits in the premorbid personality may become exaggerated, and hypochondriasis can be marked. Euphoria by contrast appears to be distinctly rare, and

when present is probably closely tied to intellectual deterioration.

There does not appear to be any form of personality change specific for parkinsonism. The majority of the features outlined above are generally held to be accountable in terms of individual vulnerability and the psychological and social stresses which operate upon the disabled person.

Psychoses

The commonest psychotic disorder in parkinsonism is affective in nature. This is almost always depressive, Mindham (1970) finding no examples of mania in a retrospective survey of 89 patients admitted to a psychiatric hospital. Only two had schizophrenic illnesses, one with postencephalitic and one with arteriosclerotic parkinsonism. Davison and Bagley (1969) note that reports of schizophrenia-like psychoses in association with idiopathic Parkinson's disease are rare and review the occasional examples in the literature. Crow *et al.* (1976) report four further cases, two with postencephalitic and two with idiopathic parkinsonism.

Mjönes (1949) could find no support for the idea of a special paralysis agitans psychosis. Many of the earlier examples, with florid delusions and auditory and visual hallucinations, were no doubt the product of overmedication with hyoscine, atropine or other solanaceous drugs. Even nowadays acute organic reactions in parkinsonian patients are most often due to medication as discussed below. Celesia and Wanamaker (1972) observed acute psychotic episodes in 12% of 153 patients, the majority being attributable to drugs and most occurring in patients who showed impairment of cognitive function. Bell *et al.* (1991) found a similar prevalence of psychosis—13% in 393 patients—with less than a third being unrelated to medication. On follow-up the non-drug-related psychoses proved usually to be transient and were frequently associated with the development of dementia. The psychoses which may develop in response to treatment with levodopa and dopamine agonists are discussed below.

Psychiatric complications of anticholinergic drugs

Anticholinergic drugs may produce an acute organic reaction which sometimes leads to diagnostic difficulty. Porteous and Ross (1956) reported mental disturbance in 20% of patients treated with benzhexol (Artane), sometimes in response to small doses. Symptoms included confusion, excitement, agitation, paranoid delusions, hallucinations and suicidal intentions, all rapidly disappearing when the drug was withdrawn. The disorder was usually evident soon after starting the drug, but could sometimes be gradual in evolution with risk that the relationship to treatment would be overlooked. Stephens (1967) and Crawshaw and Mullen (1984) have reported misuse of benzhexol in high dosage for its hallucinogenic properties, sometimes with outbursts of severe pathological excitement. Adverse reactions in parkinsonian patients are mostly seen in the elderly. They are also especially common when anticholinergics are added to levodopa, even in low dosage (De Smet *et al.* 1982).

Duvoisin and Katz (1968) recommend treating such reactions with physostigmine, a parenteral anticholinesterase which gains access to the central nervous system. Symptoms such as confusion, agitation, hallucinations, ataxia and dysarthria were promptly reversed by the drug in patients who had developed toxic reactions to scopolamine, atropine and antiparkinsonian medications.

Amantadine in high dosage may likewise provoke acute organic reactions and sometimes epileptic fits.

Psychiatric aspects of treatment with levodopa and dopamine agonists

A great deal of psychiatric interest has centred on the psychiatric consequences of treatment with levodopa. Closely similar disorders have emerged with dopamine agonists such as bromocriptine, lisuride and pergolide. Adverse reactions range from acute organic reactions and affective disorders to psychotic developments. The latter may occur in conjunction with delirium or in clear consciousness. Beneficial effects include a feeling of increased well being and temporary improvements on tests of cognitive function.

Goodwin (1971) reviewed reports to that date of adverse psychiatric reactions to levodopa, varying in incidence from 10% to 50% of patients treated. Mental complications were next only to gastrointestinal disturbances and movement disorders as side effects. Confusion and delirium had developed in 4% of patients treated, a similar proportion showing depression, restlessness and agitation, or delusions and paranoia. Hypomania had occurred more rarely, and hypersexuality had developed in occasional patients. Other reactions included lethargy, anxiety, impulsivity, insomnia and vivid dreaming.

Brief episodes of tension and restlessness may accompany the ingestion of each dose from the early phases of treatment, but the more severe reactions tend to set in only after many months on the drug. Jenkins and Groh (1970) emphasised the abrupt appearance, often with little warning, of the mental complications, and the rapid

worsening that could occur. As experience of long-term treatment has accrued it has become apparent that the prevalence of abnormal mental reactions increases as time goes by. Barbeau (1971) noted changes of intellect and behaviour in a fifth of patients maintained on the drug for over 2 years, and Sweet *et al.* (1976) found that agitation, hallucinations and delusions increased from 10% of patients initially to 60% after 6 years of treatment. Some of the more dramatic changes in mood accompany the swings of motility which develop as part of the 'on–off' effect as described on pp. 650–1.

The psychoses that arise with levodopa are not uncommonly the reason for limitation of dosage. Klawans (1988) suggests that they are prone to occur in two situations — either during the early weeks of treatment in patients with a previous history of psychiatric illness, or after several years in patients who lack such a history. The commonest manifestation consists of visual hallucinations typically of relatives, neighbours or animals, recurring frequently and especially at night. These are usually preceded or accompanied by vivid dreams and sleep disturbances. Insight into their unreal nature may be preserved for a time. Auditory and tactile hallucinations also occur but are much less common. Such disturbances may be accompanied by confusion and agitation, amounting sometimes to frank delirium, but typically they occur in a setting of fully preserved consciousness.

Delusions are prone to develop only later, being rare before 2 years of treatment with levodopa have elapsed (Cummings 1992b). They are typically persecutory in nature, often taking the form of a paranoid–delusional system. Again these usually emerge with a clear sensorium but are occasionally part of a confusional state. They are more frequently encountered in the elderly or in the presence of cognitive impairment.

Both hallucinations and delusions usually resolve with reduction of dosage, but if not low dosage of neuroleptics should be tried with caution. Clozapine has been especially commended for its effectiveness and lack of liability to aggravate extrapyramidal disturbance (Friedman & Lannon 1989; Duncan & Taylor 1996). It is especially valuable when antiparkinsonian medications cannot be adjusted downwards without compromising the patient's functional status, and may even lead to improvement of parkinsonian symptoms. Risperidone can be a useful alternative. Electroconvulsive therapy has also been shown to be effective with non-confusional psychoses, leading to sustained remissions despite the continuation of dopaminergic drugs (Hurwitz *et al.* 1988).

Dopamine agonists are equally liable to provoke psychotic reactions, and may do so when they are added to levodopa on account of fluctuations in effect (Lang *et al.* 1982; Critchley *et al.* 1986). Lisuride infusions appear to be accompanied by a particularly high incidence of visual hallucinations and paranoid delusions. Bromocriptine has been observed to induce paranoid psychoses when given to non-parkinsonian patients for the regulation of the menstrual cycle (Taneli *et al.* 1986), also schizophreniform and hypomanic psychoses when given to patients with acromegaly or prolactinomas (Turner *et al.* 1984). Again the psychotic symptoms usually resolve within a few days of partial or complete withdrawal.

Acute confusional states are mostly encountered in the context of intellectual impairment and treatment with multiple drugs. Severe delirious reactions may be accompanied by aggressive and even violent behaviour. Such reactions should be managed first by the withdrawal of any concurrent anticholinergic medication, then discontinuation of selegiline, amantadine and dopamine agonists (Quinn 1995). The dosage of levodopa should then be gradually tapered.

It is unclear whether long-term treatment with levodopa conspires towards cognitive decline, or merely enables patients to survive long enough for this to be revealed. Sometimes resolution of the parkinsonism may unmask a dementia not previously apparent. Sweet *et al.* (1976) followed a large group of patients for several years; the prevalence of dementia, judged clinically, fell after starting levodopa, but with continuation over the years new cases appeared and established cases could be observed to worsen.

Patients with already-established dementia seem usually to show little change on instituting treatment (Yahr *et al.* 1969; Markham *et al.* 1974). Some, however, deteriorate abruptly, with changes that may be transient or permanent. Sacks *et al.* (1970, 1972) describe the alarming adverse reactions which may occasionally emerge in such a situation, with the abrupt appearance of agitated hallucinatory delirium accompanied by chorea, akathisia and motor unrest. Some patients proceeded to stupor or coma, with or without the preceding phase of excitement. The disturbances could persist for a week or more after withdrawal of levodopa. Those who had had severe confusional episodes showed worsened intellectual deficits for many months afterwards.

By contrast, patients who have been dulled from previous medication may show abrupt improvement on starting levodopa. Others, irrespective of previous medication, may appear to think more quickly and clearly. The effect has been construed as part of an overall alerting and activating effect of the drug, but usually proves to be evanescent. Nevertheless improvements on psychometric tests have been documented after starting on optimal regimens of treatment, independently of physical or affective changes, and persisting some years later (Loranger *et al.* 1972a, 1972b; Fisher & Findley 1981).

Affective responses have proved to be variable, a proportion of patients experiencing improvement in mood but others developing severe depression, apprehension and anxiety. Many patients experience increased well being on levodopa, with renewal of interest in family life and the environment, replacing earlier feelings of depression and apathy. The mood elevation can sometimes extend to mania, with elation, overactivity and increased libido. Those who develop depression have sometimes failed to obtain motor benefit but have sometimes responded well. A depressive state prior to starting levodopa has emerged as the most important predisposing factor. Pre-existing anxiety may also be exacerbated, leading to feelings of impending disaster. Responses of this nature are also observed after starting treatment with dopamine agonists.

Sexual interest and activity may improve with levodopa or dopamine agonists, usually in the context of dramatic improvement in mobility. Among 19 patients Bowers *et al.* (1971) found activation of sexual behaviour in six; in the majority this seemed to be part of a general motor improvement, though occasionally there appeared to be a specific stimulation of the sexual drive. In one patient the increased sexual behaviour resulted from disinhibition associated with an acute toxic reaction to the drug. Hypersexuality has been reported in a minority of patients, sometimes in the presence of hypomania. Deviant sexual behaviour has very occasionally been unmasked, including episodes of sadomasochistic behaviour and exhibitionism (Quinn *et al.* 1983).

These various psychiatric effects are clearly variable from one individual to another and no uniform set of mental changes has emerged. The factors responsible are likely to include genetic vulnerability, the pretreatment psychiatric state, the extent of neurological and central dopaminergic involvement, and perhaps the presence of diffuse brain damage. Older age, high dosage and the concurrent administration of anticholinergic and dopaminergic medication are clear risk factors. A previous history of psychiatric illness appears to constitute a special hazard where affective and some psychotic reactions are concerned. Some have proposed that levodopa is contraindicated in patients with prior severe mental illness, but in practice a cautious trial of this and other drugs will frequently be undertaken in patients with such a history.

Finally, mention must be made of the astonishing effects of levodopa observed among long-term survivors of encephalitis lethargica (Sacks 1973). Institutionalised patients who had spent 20 years or more in states of 'trance' or immobility due to advanced parkinsonism were often dramatically liberated, experiencing virtually a total return to physical and mental health for a time. Sooner or later, however, the majority encountered a variety of difficulties, with the reactivation of symptoms and behaviour patterns from an earlier stage of the disease. Profound motor blocking set in, or a great excess of tics and urges. States of mounting excitement and ecstasy gave way eventually to exhaustion, depression and a recrudescence of the parkinsonism. Sacks' vivid case studies illustrate the profound and far-reaching effects which levodopa had on the mental life of his patients, in addition to its remarkable effects on the motor system.

Psychiatric consequences of stereotactic surgery

The vogue for stereotactic surgery in Parkinson's disease provided an unusual opportunity for examining large numbers of patients before and after circumscribed lesions of the basal ganglia. Extensive psychological studies were pursued, usually with a view to exploring the functions of such regions in relation to intellect, mood or personality. The results were unfortunately often conflicting, though some interesting general findings emerged as reviewed by Crown (1971).

Transient deficits in certain cognitive functions were a common sequel, usually with a return to preoperative status in the months that followed. The side of the lesion was sometimes found to affect the nature of the immediate postoperative deficits. Riklan and Levita (1970), for example, found verbal impairments after left-sided ventrolateral thalamic lesions, and spatial–perceptual impairments after right-sided lesions. Asso et al. (1969) showed transient impairments in auditory–verbal learning but found no convincing relationship to the laterality of the lesion. Samara et al. (1969) were able to examine the exact site of the lesion at autopsy in the brains of 27 patients and correlated the results with the language deficits which had resulted. They demonstrated convincingly that a lesion strictly confined to the ventrolateral thalamic nucleus could be followed by language deficits. When these occurred the lesion had almost always been in the left dominant hemisphere. Dysarthria could result from a lesion on either side but was usually associated with bilateral operations.

Riklan et al. (1962) showed changes in figure drawing, compared to preoperative performance, in a group of patients having operations on the globus pallidus and thalamus. For several months postoperatively there was a significant decrease in the 'humanisation' apparent in the drawings, involving such factors as facial expression, shape and body details. This was interpreted as reflecting the level of self or ego development, in turn related to conceptions of the body image. It seemed possible that the basal ganglia might play a role in the integration of the body image, perhaps through their interactions with the parietal lobes.

Discrepant findings emerged where emotional reactions were concerned. Hays et al. (1966) found that depression commonly improved after operations on the ventrolateral thalamic nucleus, with an elevation of mood that was largely maintained during the following year. This could not be attributed solely to improvement of motor function and appeared to be a specific consequence of the operation. By contrast Asso et al. (1969) found a high incidence of anxiety and depression in the first 9 months after operation and elevation of mood was rare. These differing results doubtless owed much to the preoperative or premorbid psychiatric status of the patients concerned, and perhaps also to the exact sites of the lesions involved.

Premorbid personality and psychological precipitation of Parkinson's disease

As with certain other neurological diseases there have been occasional suggestions that the premorbid personality of patients with Parkinson's disease has characteristic features. Closely associated is the proposition that psychological influences may be important in the development of the disorder. None of the observations in this area can be regarded as well founded, but neither can it be said that they have been decisively disproved.

Certain striking qualities in patients with Parkinson's disease have been stressed — their industriousness, rigid moralistic attitudes and habitual suppression of aggression prior to the appearance of the disease. Sands (1942) and Booth (1948) championed the view that persons of a particular psychological make-up were at special risk of developing the disorder. Sands (1942) described what he called the 'masked personality', finding a marked discrepancy between the outward appearance of coping and the turmoil within. Premorbid histories showed the patients to have been exemplary citizens, successful in their undertakings and externally calm, undemonstrative and stable. Close acquaintance, however, revealed a subjective state of tension which was suppressed and concealed from outsiders. With the development of parkinsonism a decompensation could often be observed, exposing the inner turmoil in the form of complaints, demands and self-centred behaviour. Sands suggested that the habitual suppression of emotion, doubtless involving intense physiological activity in many parts of the brain, may have led in some way to the degenerative changes responsible for the disease.

Booth (1948) developed such concepts further in a clinical study of 66 patients supplemented with Rorschach protocols. Some were postencephalitic and some 'senile degenerative' in origin. He concluded that the personality structure had been more decisive for the development of parkinsonism than the immediately obvious pathogenic mechanism; the latter had merely served to precipitate or actualise the disorder. Features stressed by Booth included a habitual impulse to action and a striving for success, independence and authority. Tension was prone to arise between this and the equally strong drive towards social conformity. But such tensions, like other emotions and impulses, were firmly suppressed. Regarding their success in life, he found this to be usually the result neither of great intelligence nor of unusual vitality, but attributable to aggressive perseverance and instinctive social conformity. An externally virtuous and docile disposition concealed hostile and sadistic impulses of unusual strength.

Such a character structure would be vulnerable to frustration in a number of ways. In many examples the first clinical symptoms of parkinsonism were preceded by a situation which had imposed a serious handicap to the execution of self-willed strivings and activities — arthritis, exhaustion, economic losses or professional disappointments. In other patients psychological conflicts could be identified as precipitants. Booth saw the major symptoms of parkinsonism as reflecting the original personality and its conflicts—rigidity, for example, being the product of a balance between overcoming obstacles and submission to restrictive influences, and the parkinsonian posture being related to unconscious hostility. Psychotherapy, in conjunction with antiparkinsonian medication was claimed to meet with success in alleviating the symptoms.

There has been little support for these ideas from more recent studies. Diller and Riklan (1956) attempted an objective assessment of personality and background in a large number of patients referred for stereotactic surgery, but found nothing that could be regarded as characteristic for Parkinson's disease. Smythies (1967) compared 40 consecutive patients referred for surgery with control groups on a questionnaire relating to childhood disturbance, premorbid neurotic symptoms and life adjustment. No excess of premorbid emotional disability could be discerned, and no unusual difficulties in life adjustment antedating the illness. Pollock and Hornabrook (1966), however, were impressed with the high proportion of teetotallers among their large unselected series of parkinson-

ian patients, and found that many lacked hobbies and showed narrow intellectual horizons. Poewe et al. (1990) compared groups of patients with Parkinson's disease and benign essential tremor with healthy controls, using Cattell's personality inventory and a structured interview. Both patient groups were significantly more likely to be introverted, rigid, pedantic and self reproachful than the controls, confirming previous impressions of personality. However, the similarity between the parkinsonian and tremor patients suggested that such traits were merely the product of chronic disability.

More interesting findings have come from comparisons between pairs of monozygotic twins, one of whom had Parkinson's disease and the other did not (Duvoisin et al. 1981; Ward et al. 1984). The affected members tended to describe themselves as more nervous, quiet, serious and introspective, whereas their co-twins were more outgoing and light-hearted. Moreover a group of traits showed significant differences before the onset of the Parkinson's disease—the affected twin was less commonly the leader, less aggressive, more self controlled and less confident. These differences in personality sometimes dated well back into adolescence and early adult life. It seemed possible therefore that neurochemical differences between the twins might have existed from early in their lives, or that there had been some error of foetal development in the member destined for the disease.

Twin studies have also been employed to detect risk factors for the illness. The only possible association that has emerged is that affected twins have smoked less often and less heavily than their co-twins (Ward et al. 1984; Bharucha et al. 1986), which is interesting in that animal studies have indicated a dopaminergic effect of smoking on the brain. Baron (1986) reviews the epidemiological evidence from many case-control studies which also suggest that smoking may be protective, though with occasional negative reports (Golbe et al. 1986). It is possible, however, that differences in smoking habits reflect no more than differences in personality.

Hepatolenticular degeneration
(Wilson's disease)

Hepatolenticular degeneration is a rare inherited disorder affecting both the liver and the central nervous system. Since its description by Wilson in 1912 understanding of the condition has advanced very considerably, and it is known to be linked to abnormalities of copper metabolism. This has led to treatment with penicillamine which meets with considerable success in the amelioration of symptoms. Familial concentrations of the disorder have always been recognised. A high consanguinity rate is found among the parents, who are themselves unaffected, and it is now clear that the fundamental biochemical abnormality leading to the illness is inherited as an autosomal recessive. The responsible gene has been mapped to the long arm of chromosome 13 (Bowcock *et al.* 1987).

Clinical features

The onset is usually in childhood or adolescence, but may be delayed as late as the fifth decade of life. Approximately half of patients are symptomatic by the age of 15. The presentation may be with hepatic disorder, neurological disorder or both together. In addition, as discussed below, a considerable proportion present initially with psychiatric disturbance. Bearn (1957) estimated that some 40% of cases first show hepatic dysfunction, 40% neurological symptoms, and perhaps 20% psychiatric illness or behavioural disorder. There is a marked tendency for the liver disorder to be the first to appear when the onset is in childhood.

Hepatic involvement is almost invariable but may sometimes be found only on liver biopsy or at autopsy. Jaundice or hepatosplenomegaly can be the presenting features, or later there may be ascites, ankle swelling or haematemesis from rupture of oesophageal varices.

The neurological disorder is confined to the motor system and takes the form of extrapyramidal disturbance with a characteristic accent on the facial and bulbar muscles (Harding 1993a). There may be rigidity, tremor, athetoid writhing movements and abnormal dystonic postures of the limbs. In the early stages the disabilities may be transient and sensitive to emotional influences, leading to an erroneous impression of conversion hysteria. A flapping tremor may be seen at the wrists, or characteristic 'wing beating' at the shoulders when the arms are abducted and the elbows flexed. The facial expression is stiff and motionless, often with open mouth and a rigid silent smile. Bulbar symptoms take the form of spastic dysarthria and dysphagia.

Occasional patients develop epileptic seizures, usually of Jacksonian type. Dening *et al.* (1988) found that seizures were 10 times as frequent as in the general population. Hemiplegia is not uncommon. Periods of coma or semicoma may develop, persisting for several weeks but not necessarily heralding a fatal outcome.

Variations in the clinical picture depend to some extent on the age at presentation (Bearn 1957). In young subjects dystonia or spastic rigidity tend to dominate the picture and tremor may be slight. The course is then liable to be acute and rapidly progressive. In adults tremor pre-

dominates and rigidity may be unobtrusive, with a milder course and slower progression. A good deal of overlap occurs, however, and mixed pictures are common. In the earlier literature the term 'lenticular degeneration' was used for cases showing spasticity, rigidity and dystonia, and 'pseudosclerosis' for cases with marked tremor and dysarthria.

The Kayser–Fleischer ring is a diagnostic sign of great importance. It is situated at the margin of the cornea, brown or greyish-green in colour, and often evident to the naked eye. It is readily detected on slit-lamp examination. Absence of a Kayser–Fleischer ring makes the diagnosis of Wilson's disease improbable in the presence of neuropsychiatric symptoms, but it may be absent in purely hepatic forms of the disease.

The CT and MRI scans have been found to show a characteristic picture (Williams & Walshe 1981; Aisen *et al.* 1985). Ventricular dilatation, cortical atrophy and enlargement of the cisterns around the brain stem are common, and may be accompanied by typical hypodense areas in the basal ganglia on CT. This combination is considered to be specific for Wilson's disease. The hypodense areas are most frequent in patients with neurological disability, but can also be seen in those presenting with hepatic disorder or even in presymptomatic cases. MRI characteristically shows symmetrical focal areas of increased signal, especially in the lenticular nuclei (i.e. putamen and globus pallidus) but also in the thalamus, caudate nuclei, dentate nuclei and brain stem (Aisen *et al.* 1985). Focal white matter lesions may sometimes be observed. Rescanning after treatment with chelating agents (p. 664) may show resolution of the changes. PET scanning has shown diffusely reduced brain metabolism with a particular accent on the lenticular nuclei (Hawkins *et al.* 1987).

Other features include abnormalities of renal function, with aminoaciduria in a high proportion of cases. The urine may also contain sugar or protein, or unusual quantities of uric acid, calcium or phosphate. Degenerative changes around joints are commonly seen on X-ray examination, even in young persons, and fractures and fragmentations of the bones of the hands and wrists may be detected. Episodes of haemolytic anaemia may occur, presumably due to sudden release of copper from the tissues.

Course and outcome

Remissions may be seen in the earlier stages, and even thereafter marked fluctuations in severity can occur. Ultimately, however, severe crippling results from spasticity and dystonic contractions. Dysphagia is often profound, and intellectual deterioration is common in the later stages. The prognosis is worse the younger the age of onset. Formerly children rarely survived for more than 4 years, whereas adults might survive without severe disablement for 12 years or more. Death usually occurs from liver failure, rupture of oesophageal varices, inhalation or intercurrent infection.

With treatment this gloomy outlook has been altered as described below.

Pathology

Smith (1976) describes the pathological findings as follows. The brain is usually normal externally, but on section the corpus striatum is found to be shrunken and brownish or brick red in colour. The putamen often shows cavitation. Microscopically neuronal loss is seen in the caudate and putamen, and the latter contains large numbers of astrocytic nuclei, many having a characteristic enlarged and vesicular appearance ('Alzheimer nuclei'). By contrast the globus pallidus often shows relatively little change. Pericapillary concretions which stain for copper may also be detected. Other abnormal elements include large phagocytic 'Opalski' cells, possibly derived from histiocytes.

The thalamus, the subthalamic nuclei and the brain stem nuclei may also show Alzheimer nuclei and Opalski cells. Phagocytes containing iron pigment are commonly found in the substantia nigra. Degeneration of the dentate nuclei and superior cerebellar peduncles has occasionally been observed.

Foci of degeneration are not uncommon in the cerebral cortex, especially in the frontal lobes. Diffuse loss of neurones and fibres may occur, or status spongiosus involving both the cortex and the white centres of the convolutions. Astrocytic and oligodendrocytic proliferation may be seen.

The liver may be enlarged in the early stages but is usually smaller than normal at autopsy. It is coarsely cirrhotic, varying in colour from yellow to brown or brick red depending on the relative amounts of copper storage, fatty degeneration and bile staining. Microscopically the picture is of multilobular cirrhosis. The spleen is usually enlarged.

Biochemical abnormalities

Abnormalities of copper metabolism appear to be fundamental to the development both of the hepatic and cerebral lesions, though the underlying defect of copper homeostasis is still unclear (Starosta-Rubinstein 1995). The liver and brain contain a marked excess of copper in the disease, the basal ganglia being particularly heavily affected. The Kayser–Fleischer ring in the cornea is due to deposition of copper there, and levels may be raised in the kidneys and other tissues. The total serum copper is usually low and the excretion of copper in the urine is high, though measurement of these is of little value for diagnosis.

Scheinberg and Gitlin (1952) showed that the caeruloplasmin content of the serum was low or even absent in the disease, and this has emerged as a finding of great importance. Caeruloplasmin is a globulin which is synthesised in the liver. Ninety per cent of the serum copper is normally bound to caeruloplasmin, the remainder being loosely attached to serum albumin. This free copper is the toxic pool, probably representing the part in transition to other body regions, and it is raised in the disease. While important as a screening test, low values of caeruloplasmin are not invariable, some 5% of patients having normal levels and 10–20% of heterozygotes showing a deficiency (Starosta-Rubinstein 1995). Levels may also be reduced in protein-deficiency states and in the presence of liver disease. When the index of suspicion is high, and caeruloplasmin is normal, a radioactive ^{64}Cu incorporation test can be valuable, revealing a lack of uptake of orally administered copper into newly synthesised caeruloplasmin. Definitive diagnosis can depend on liver biopsy which reveals elevated copper levels and the histological changes of nodular cirrhosis.

With the advent of effective treatment special attention must be directed towards the detection of asymptomatic but vulnerable individuals in the families of patients so that prophylactic treatment can be commenced. Once the disease has been diagnosed all siblings of the patient should be examined: 25% will be at risk and 50% will be heterozygote carriers. Discovery of a low caeruloplasmin should then lead to liver biopsy, which in the heterozygote may show a mild increase in liver copper, though not in the range of Wilson's disease, and the liver histology is normal (Harding 1993a).

The exact pathogenesis of the disorder remains uncertain. The low caeruloplasmin is no longer thought to play a primary role, and there is not a close correspondence between the severity of the disease and the extent to which caeruloplasmin is lowered. There seems rather to be a defect in hepatobiliary copper excretion, allowing excessive accumulation of copper in the liver until free copper enters the blood stream and is deposited in other organs (Starosta-Rubinstein 1995). There may additionally be an abnormal affinity of certain tissues for copper. The primacy of the liver abnormality in the disorder is supported by the success that may follow liver transplantation as described below. Whatever the precise pathogenic mechanism, the net consequence is a positive body copper balance which must be reversed if treatment is to be effective.

Treatment

The aim of treatment is to eliminate excessive copper from the body and prevent its reaccumulation. It must begin as soon as the diagnosis is made and continue for life. Dimercaprol (BAL) was the first chelating agent to be tried (Denny-Brown & Porter 1951). Results were encouraging but the injections were painful and liable to lead to toxic reactions.

D-penicillamine is now the treatment of choice, though sensitivity reactions can limit its use—fever, rashes, lymphadenopathy and bone marrow suppression. Prednisone cover may allow a restart to be made if bone marrow suppression has not occurred (Starosta-Rubinstein 1995). During the early weeks of treatment the neurological state may worsen as copper is mobilised from the tissues. This may occasionally extend over several worrying months (Walshe 1986). Late side effects can include skin changes, renal damage, systemic lupus erythematosus, myasthenia gravis, optic neuritis, bone marrow suppression and loss of the sense of taste. The treatment should ideally be combined with a low copper diet, avoiding such items as liver, shellfish, nuts, chocolate, mushrooms, dried fruits and whisky.

When problems arise with D-penicillamine a change may be made to the alternative chelating agent trientine (triethylene tetramine dihydrochloride), or to zinc acetate or sulphate which decrease copper absorption from the gut. Acutely ill patients may be unable to wait the 2–6 months necessary for chelating agents to work, and plasma exchange may then be indicated or peritoneal dialysis with albumin added to the dialysate.

Clinical improvement may not be obvious for 6 months or even a year in some patients, but with maintenance of treatment progressive gains can continue for several years (Walshe 1968; Goldstein et al. 1971). Most patients make an excellent recovery from both hepatic and neurological disorder; a small proportion, however, fail to respond to penicillamine or any other drug and follow a steady downhill course to death over several weeks or months (Walshe 1986).

Neurological improvement is often more rewarding than hepatic improvement, but all aspects of the picture can respond. Tremor, rigidity, dystonia, dysarthria and dysphagia may all gradually resolve and some patients become entirely symptom-free. In general improvement

is more complete the earlier treatment has been commenced. Dramatic results have been reported from states of hopeless incapacity to relative independence, though such cannot always be achieved.

Psychiatric symptoms have been found to improve as well, some more impressively than others. This is discussed below.

Occasional patients will warrant liver transplantation, which effectively treats the Wilson's disease as well as the liver failure, restoring copper excretion to normal. Polson et al. (1987) have reported its success in reversing severe neurological manifestations, this occurring with unusual rapidity in one of their patients:

A man of 30 had a 14-month history of hepatic and neurological impairment. Despite treatment with penicillamine he developed increasing dysarthria, dysphagia, akinesia and rigidity of the limbs, requiring continuous nursing care. After transplantation liver function became virtually normal from 4 weeks onwards, and neurological recovery began 2–3 months later. By 8 months postoperatively no neurological signs were detectable.

Psychiatric manifestations of Wilson's disease

Psychiatric symptoms can form a prominent part of the clinical picture along with the neurological defects. On this account it is not uncommon for patients to present to psychiatrists before their disease is diagnosed, with a risk that treatment will be dangerously delayed. Dening and Berrios (1989a) recommend that serum caeruloplasmin should be measured in all psychiatric patients who show personality change, especially towards disinhibited, bizarre or reckless behaviour, in those who show neurological signs not accounted for by medication, and in patients with unexplained hepatic disease. Dysarthria and other bulbar symptoms will be a strong indication for investigation in patients below middle age, likewise deterioration in school or work performance in children or young adults. The following case illustrates the diagnostic difficulties that can arise:

A 17-year-old girl developed emotional lability, nervousness, difficulty with handwriting and deterioration in school performance. She was at first thought to be suffering from adolescent adjustment problems. Chlorpromazine was prescribed, leading to increasing tremor, and she became withdrawn. Abnormal liver function tests were noted, likewise mild extrapyramidal dysfunction, but both were ascribed to the drug. She was later hospitalised with a diagnosis of schizoaffective disorder. Finally she was noted to show excessive drooling, a mask-like face, dysphagia, choreoathetoid movements, dystonia, spasticity, splenomegaly and Kayser–Fleischer rings. A diagnosis of Wilson's disease was confirmed 22 months after the first manifestations. Two years of treatment with penicillamine left her still dysphonic and with severe motor disability.   (Cartwright 1978)

Wilson (1912) stressed the prominence of psychiatric symptoms in his initial description and believed them to be a fundamental part of the clinical picture. He noted psychotic and hysterical manifestations, later adding affective change and disordered behaviour (Wilson 1940). Impairment of mental function seemed often to be more apparent than real, being to a large extent suggested by the patient's appearance and dysarthria.

These various aspects have been reiterated in subsequent descriptions, though until recently it has been difficult to obtain a comprehensive picture. Most examples have been reported anecdotally by psychiatrists or in small series examined by neurologists. Scheinberg *et al.* (1968) found that more than a quarter of 49 patients had significant psychiatric disorder as the first indication of their illness, and almost two-thirds at some point in the course, mostly personality and emotional disturbance. Loss of impulse control could be marked, also depression, anxiety, irritability and excitability. Many patients showed evidence of cognitive impairment, but in general emotional and behavioural disorders predominated. Inose (1968) drew attention to fluctuating disturbances of consciousness with episodes of delirium, especially in the later stages. Knehr and Bearn (1956) demonstrated intellectual impairment on psychological testing in all seven patients examined, with good preservation of language but substantial difficulties with conceptual thinking. More recently Medalia *et al.* (1988) have compared groups of patients with and without neurological impairment on a battery of psychological tests. The former were poorer on memory tests than the latter, but the deficits were mostly mild. Performance on tests reflecting motor impairment was also poor, but ability at naming and card sorting was intact. There were no indications of neuropsychological deficits in patients who had never shown neurological symptoms when compared with normal controls.

Particular attention has been given to psychotic phenomena, with reports of depressive, hypomanic and schizophrenic pictures, sometimes as transient episodes and sometimes as enduring accompaniments of the neurological deterioration. Beard (1959) felt that most reports of schizophrenia were probably incorrect, and should more properly be viewed as examples of acute or chronic organic reactions, but reported a convincing example of his own. Davison and Bagley (1969) considered that there was a more than chance association with schizophrenia, and that an organic basis was likely — in most reported cases the psychosis and the neurological abnormalities had appeared at about the same time, a family history of schizophrenia was uncommon, and the psychosis tended to progress towards dementia.

These impressions have been considerably refined by a series of publications on the large number of patients referred to Dr John Walshe at Cambridge, representing the largest series available in the UK (Dening & Berrios 1989a, 1989b, 1990). The careful documentation employed, and the application of operationally defined criteria for the assessment of psychiatric disorder increase the validity of the findings, even though matters of special selection cannot be excluded. The principal conclusions are that personality change and 'incongruous behaviour' are undoubtedly common in Wilson's disease, while psychotic phenomena are rare. Irritability, aggression and depression appear to be frequent, likewise cognitive impairment of mild degree. Many of these psychiatric features appear to have an organic cerebral basis.

Dening and Berrios (1989a) first assessed 195 cases by retrospective case note review. Half were rated as showing some psychiatric disturbance at index admission and 20% had seen a psychiatrist before the disease had been diagnosed. In half of these an organic condition had been suspected and appropriate action taken, but not in the remainder. Reasons for referral included deterioration in school or work performance, outbursts of abnormal behaviour and strange disorders of movement.

Personality change, in terms of alterations in life style, relationships or behaviour, was judged as present or possible in a quarter of patients. A similar proportion showed incongruous behaviour by way of disinhibition, bizarre or reckless behaviour, often leading to forensic problems. Evidence of such behavioural abnormality was significantly associated with high scores on ratings of neurological symptomatology, especially dysarthria. Irritability emerged in 18% and showed similar associations, and aggression was noted in 14%. Cognitive impairment was present or suspected in almost a quarter, being generally mild, and depression in 21%. Depression showed associations with long duration of admission and the presence of family problems but little relationship to neurological symptoms.

By contrast delusions and hallucinations occurred in less than 2% of patients, casting doubt on any significant relationship between psychotic illness and Wilson's disease. Disorientation was relatively rare at 7% and closely associated with liver failure.

A more intensive prospective study was made of 31 consecutive attenders at the clinic (Dening & Berrios 1989b). These ranged in severity from patients who had never been symptomatic to patients who were mute and bedridden. More than half were rated as abnormal on the Personality Assessment Schedule, the main factor on factor analysis reflecting traits such as impulsiveness, irresponsibility and aggression. A third were 'cases' as judged by scores on the General Health Questionnaire. No psychotic symptoms were observed. Only four patients scored below the threshold for cognitive impairment on the Mini-Mental State Examination, and in general such impairment was not severe.

Disorders of personality and behaviour were again significantly related to the presence of neurological symptoms, especially dysarthria, bradykinesia and rigidity, strongly suggesting that they had an organic basis. Depressive symptoms were related to hepatic dysfunction. Cognitive impairment, being mild in this sample, showed less marked correlation with neurological disorder than might have been expected; it was evident, moreover, that some patients who seemed superficially to be impaired performed well on psychometric tests.

Finally an attempt was made to assess the response of neurological and psychiatric symptoms to treatment by retrospective review of 129 patients over a mean period of 10 years (Dening & Berrios 1990). Most gains had occurred during the early years of treatment, with significant improvement in cognition and 'incongruous behaviour'. By contrast depression and irritability seemed not to improve. Aspects of neurological disability also decreased significantly, both early and later during treatment, including tremor, rigidity and overall neurological scores. Dysphagia, however, appeared often to persist and dysarthria to have a poor prognosis.

These largely encouraging results from treatment were mirrored in earlier reports. Scheinberg *et al.* (1968) followed 30 patients with both neurological and psychiatric disorder; 25 showed marked resolution of neurological deficits and 14 showed lessened psychiatric disturbance. Goldstein *et al.* (1968) demonstrated gains on serial psychometric testing, often continuing for several years. All improved to some extent, in a manner that generally paralleled their improvement in neurological status but was less dramatic in degree.

Progressive supranuclear palsy
(Steele–Richardson–Olszewski syndrome)

Steele *et al.* (1964) described a group of patients with an unusual progressive neurological disorder showing as an akinetic–rigid syndrome with ocular and mental features. Outstanding signs include supranuclear paralysis of external ocular movements, particularly in the vertical plane and involving downward gaze, dysarthria, pseudobulbar palsy, dystonic rigidity of the trunk and neck, and cognitive impairment. Signs of pyramidal tract and cerebellar dysfunction may also be seen. A tendency to fall over backwards is characteristic. In the later stages the eyes are fixed centrally, and widespread rigidity reduces the patient to a helpless bedridden state. The onset is usually in the sixth decade, with death some 5–10 years later.

Subsequent reports have confirmed the main features of the syndrome (Steele 1972; Maher & Lees 1986; de Bruin & Lees 1992). Treatment with levodopa may sometimes ameliorate the rigidity and ophthalmoplegia for a time, but treatment response is often disappointing.

The pathology shows cell loss, neurofibrillary tangles, gliosis and demyelination, particularly affecting the basal ganglia, brain stem and cerebellar nuclei. The tangles consist of bundles of straight filaments and do not show the paired helical structure seen in Alzheimer's disease. The distribution of changes is remarkably constant and usually there is a surprising lack of cortical involvement. Steele *et al.* (1964) commented on the resemblance of the histological features to those of postencephalitic parkinsonism or the parkinsonism–dementia complex of Guam, though the distribution of changes is different. The aetiology is unknown. Degenerative or viral processes are suspected, but attempts at transmission to primates have been unsuccessful.

Among the psychiatric manifestations cognitive impairment is very common, affecting over 80% of de Bruin and Lees' (1992) patients in some degree. Five of the 67 patients had presented with symptoms leading to an initial diagnosis of Alzheimer's disease, though early aphasia, apraxia and agnosia were never observed. Personality change, abnormal behaviour, emotional lability, depression and social withdrawal were all common.

The most striking cognitive change is bradyphrenia, with slowing of response and lack of initiative. Judgement is often found to be impaired and abstracting ability may be poor. The question of memory impairment in the disease has been controversial, with differing reports in different series. Here the clearest evidence has come from Litvan *et al.*'s (1989) comparison of 12 patients with matched healthy controls. This revealed significant deficits in learning, consolidation and retrieval, also abnormally rapid rates of forgetting. By contrast 'information scanning', which requires the use of short-term memory processes, remained intact. Verbal fluency tests also showed definite impairment.

The memory disorder may owe much to deafferentation of the subcortical–frontal projections, since the cortical neurones themselves are generally spared. D'Antona *et al.* (1985) have shown marked prefrontal hypometabolism on PET scans in comparison with controls of equivalent age. These observations are relevant to the question of 'subcortical dementia' discussed just below.

Ovsiew and Schneider (1993) have reported a patient with autopsy confirmation of the disease in whom a schizophrenic psychosis was a central feature and present from the earliest stages.

Subcortical dementia

While the disease itself is rare, certain observations made on the mental state of such patients by Albert *et al.* (1974) have provoked considerable interest. The pattern of cognitive impairment seen in progressive supranuclear palsy appears to have distinctive features which may reflect the relative confinement of pathology to subcortical structures. Albert *et al.* termed this picture 'subcortical dementia'. In this they made a valuable contribution, by underlining the fact that cognitive failure does not always imply cortical disease. The cortex depends for its functioning on inputs from the reticular activating systems and other subcortical structures, and when these fail the cortex, though intact, may cease to display its potential.

Albert *et al.* contrasted the behaviour pattern in patients with progressive supranuclear palsy with that seen in patients with cortical disease processes. Among five cases seen personally and 42 adequately described in the literature, several key features were evident in the mental state. Though described as 'forgetful' it could frequently be shown that the patient could produce the correct answer if given encouragement and an abnormal amount of time in which to respond. Memory as such appeared not to be truly impaired, but rather the timing mechanism which enables the memory system to function at normal speed. Slowness of thought was similarly prominent; tasks requiring verbal manipulation or perceptual–motor skills were performed incorrectly under normal pressures, but adequately when time was extended. Thus, when the patient was allowed to proceed at his own pace, or when provided with structured situations to elicit responses that did not occur spontaneously, his intellect could prove to be surprisingly intact. Defects of higher cortical function such as dysphasia, agnosia or apraxia were strikingly absent, though calculation or ability to deal with abstract material were sometimes defective. Personality and mood changes fell into two categories — the larger group was indifferent, apathetic and depressed, while the smaller showed progressive irritability and/or euphoria. Brief outbursts of rage were common, and inappropriate forced laughing and crying were often in evidence.

A woman of 65 with the disease showed extrapyramidal rigidity, slowed speech and marked limitation of upward and downward gaze. Her cognitive state was described as follows:

'She was alert, attentive and socially appropriate. Immediate recall of digits was seven forward and five backwards. Recent memory was deficient in an unusual way: her first answer to almost every question was "I don't know". However, if the examiner encouraged her by saying "Sure you know; just take your time", she would correctly respond to 95% of the ques-

tions. The latency between question and response was often inordinately long — in some cases as long as 4.5 minutes (often taxing the patience of the examiner). Remote memory was intact.

Language functions were as follows. . . . No paraphasias were heard. Naming was excellent on confrontation for high and very low frequency words. Although she complained of having difficulty with words, she had no naming defect. She did, however, have a time-related word-finding defect: in 1 minute she was able to find only three words beginning with the letter B. At 5 minutes she had listed 12; at 10 minutes 23; at 15 minutes 33. Tests of repetition, comprehension of spoken and written language, and reading aloud were normal, except for the slow reading rate.

For simple mental calculations her responses were quick and accurate. With more complex arithmetic problems, she was slow but correct. Her proverb interpretations were concrete and she had difficulty finding similarities in two similar objects.'

A 58-year-old woman had dysarthria, a broad-based ataxic gait and striking impairment of upward and downward gaze. 'Evaluation of mental status revealed an awake, generally placid or apathetic woman who reacted in a seemingly angry manner to the examiner's attempts to question her. Despite her apparent anger, she could nonetheless be coaxed to cooperate. Digit span was six forward. Questions designed to test recent and remote memory led to the following situation: either she refused to answer or she answered incorrectly. However, when the examiner waited, either silently or with attempts to encourage her, for longer than normal waiting periods (even as long as 4–5 minutes for a single question) she then gave the correct answer to 70–80% of the questions. This indicated that her stock of knowledge was not impaired as one might otherwise have concluded. Rather, she was delayed in reaching into the stock for the correct answer. Tests of language and gestures revealed no aphasia or apraxia. No inattention or primary perceptual problems were seen. Proverb interpretations tended to be concrete. Her ability to find the categorical similarities between similar items was impaired. Her calculating ability was poor.'   (Albert *et al.* 1974)

Attention was drawn to rather similar pictures in other diseases with subcortical pathology, and the authors tentatively proposed that the common mechanisms underlying them were those of impaired timing and activation. Impaired functioning of the reticular formation, or a disconnection of the reticular-activating systems from thalamic and subthalamic nuclei, might be the cause of slowing of intellectual processes, even though the cortical systems for perceiving, storing and manipulating knowledge remained intact.

The situation in progressive supranuclear palsy, in which the cortex is known to be largely spared, is likely to exist in some other dementing processes also. Parkinson's disease with intellectual impairment (p. 653) is an obvious example; Huntington's chorea is another (pp. 469–70). Normal-pressure hydrocephalus, Wilson's disease and the dementia associated with deep lacunar infarcts (p. 384) have also been viewed in this way (Benson 1982; Cummings 1982). It could conceivably be the case that some variants of the dementias of old age may have a subcortical rather than a cortical origin to the cognitive difficulties, or at least a prominent subcortical component in the aetiology of the clinical picture. An interesting possibility is that the 'normal' effects of old age upon cognitive functioning may reflect subcortical rather than cortical ageing processes (Albert 1978).

These suggestions have attracted a good deal of interest, since it is possible that pharmacological means might be found to help patients with subcortical dementia perform at an improved level. To the extent that subcortical dementias are due to disturbances of activating, alerting or timing mechanisms, then drugs which have an effect on the anatomical or biochemical systems dealing with these mechanisms could prove to have therapeutic value.

Corticobasal degeneration (cortical–basal ganglionic degeneration)

This rare disorder was first described by Rebeiz et al. in 1968. Further series of patients have been reported by Gibb et al. (1989b) and Riley et al. (1990). The condition is reviewed by Watts et al. (1994). It consists of degeneration in defined regions of the cerebral cortex coupled with marked pathology in the striatonigral system and other subcortical nuclei. The clinical presentation can resemble progressive supranuclear palsy (p. 666), while the pathological changes share features in common with Pick's disease (p. 462). A clinical hallmark is the asymmetry of the motor manifestations, such that one limb may become completely incapacitated before symptoms develop on the other side.

It presents usually in late middle or early old age, with akinesia, rigidity, limb apraxia and a combination of supranuclear gaze palsy, myoclonus, limb dystonia or cortical sensory loss. Postural instability may be marked. The myoclonus is induced by action, and is often markedly stimulus sensitive. Ataxia, chorea, blepharospasm and pyramidal tract signs may also be seen. Not infrequently the patient develops an 'alien limb', whereby the hand and arm feel 'foreign' to the patient and tend to wander involuntarily and uncontrollably. This feature is discussed by Sawle et al. (1991) who ascribe it to damage to the medial frontal cortex and supplementary motor area.

Cognitive disabilities may be notably mild or absent even when severe apraxia hampers the majority of voluntary activity. Other patients, however, develop marked parietal lobe deficits by way of dyscalculia, constructional

apraxia or visuospatial impairment. Severe generalised dementia supervenes in perhaps a third of cases. Progressive incapacity leads to death after 4–10 years. Treatment with levodopa is often ineffective, though baclofen may help the rigidity and clonazepam may dampen the myoclonus (Thompson & Marsden 1992).

Pathological findings consist of cortical atrophy with cell loss and gliosis, mainly affecting the peri-Rolandic frontal and parietal regions in contrast to the frontotemporal atrophy of Pick's disease. Subcortical regions are also markedly affected, especially the globus pallidus, putamen, substantia nigra and lateral thalamus. The subthalamic nucleus, red nucleus and locus caeruleus are also involved. Abnormal neurones show marked resistance to staining methods (achromasia) and a swollen appearance similar to the ballooning of Pick cells. Classic Pick bodies are not, however, present. Basophilic inclusions are seen, especially in the substantia nigra, also globose neurofibrillary tangles similar to those of progressive supranuclear palsy.

CT and MRI show ventricular enlargement and cortical atrophy which may be asymmetrical in distribution. Brain imaging with PET has revealed distinctive features which mirror the pattern of pathological involvement (Eidelberg et al. 1991; Sawle et al. 1991). Cortical hypometabolism is evident in the superior temporal, inferior parietal, posterior frontal and occipital association cortices, with a markedly asymmetrical pattern which may be of value in differential diagnosis. [18]F flurodopa uptake is reduced in the caudate and putamen, again in an asymmetrical manner.

Striatonigral degeneration (multiple system atrophy)

Adams et al. (1964) drew attention to this rare disorder, closely similar to Parkinson's disease in clinical manifestations but with a distinctive pathological basis. Affected patients show rigidity, akinesia, slowed movements and a flexed posture. At autopsy the striking features are extensive neuronal loss in the zona compacta of the substantia nigra, but without Lewy bodies, and marked degenerative changes in the putamen and caudate nuclei.

One of Adams et al.'s four cases also showed olivopontocerebellar degeneration. Many cases have since been reported with this striking combination, prominent cerebellar ataxia then preceding the parkinsonian symptoms. Approximately half, moreover, are handicapped by fainting due to postural hypotension, and other signs of autonomic failure may include impotence and sphincter and deglutition disturbances. Such patients show neuronal loss in the intermediolateral tract of the spinal cord and the dorsal vagal nuclei of the brain stem (Shy–Drager syndrome). Dementia may develop but is uncommon. Gosset *et al.* (1983) reviewed 35 cases with both striatonigral degeneration and olivopontocerebellar degeneration, ranging in age from 30 to 75, half of whom also showed progressive autonomic failure. They termed this combination 'progressive multisystem degeneration'. Several patients also showed pyramidal signs, slight muscle atrophy, intention myoclonus and upward gaze palsy.

Nowadays it is usual to group these various conditions together under the title of *multiple system atrophy*, using the term striatonigral degeneration when parkinsonism predominates, Shy–Drager syndrome when autonomic failure is prominent, and olivopontocerebellar atrophy when cerebellar features are outstanding (Quinn 1995). A cytological hallmark by way of oligodendroglial cytoplasmic inclusions has recently been described, and these are present whatever the clinical predominance (Lantos & Papp 1994).

The condition should be suspected when a parkinsonian syndrome coexists with ataxia, vertical gaze palsy, pyramidal signs and autonomic failure. Quinn (1989) considers that it is less rare than commonly supposed, perhaps accounting for up to 10% of patients with parkinsonism. Treatment with levodopa is usually without benefit, presumably because striatal dopamine receptors are lost, and may sometimes worsen the condition.

The dystonias

The dystonias comprise a group of disorders in which sustained muscle spasms invade muscle groups, causing writhing or twisting movements or distorting the body and limbs into characteristic postures. The abnormal movements differ from tics or choreiform movements in being much slower and sustained, and in their tendency to involve the proximal and axial musculature. Reviews of the classification of these disorders and changing conceptions about them are provided by Owens (1990) and Marsden and Quinn (1990).

Almost any body part may be involved. Typically at the onset the dystonia occurs only during some specific motor act, affecting a restricted group of muscles (focal dystonia). It may remain localised, or spread to involve contiguous body parts (segmental dystonia) or virtually all of the body (generalised dystonia). 'Axial dystonia' is a focal dystonia affecting the trunk. 'Hemidystonia' affects one half of the body alone, and 'multifocal dystonia' affects several discrete regions. The different syndromes that result are often specially labelled—torticollis in the neck, blepharospasm in the muscles around the eyes, and dystonia musculorum deformans when the disorder is generalised. Focal and segmental dystonias greatly outnumber other forms; in the large series of almost 1000 cases reported from the Dystonia Clinical Research Center in New York these accounted for some three-quarters of cases, generalised dystonia occurring in less than a fifth (Fahn *et al.* 1987).

All dystonic movements and postures are worsened by attempts to move. When the spasms are continuous they result in characteristic postures which are maintained except during sleep. When intermittent they cause repetitive, often rhythmic, jerks and spasms, for example in torticollis. The shorter the spasms the more 'myoclonic' is the dystonia. Some patients may show an additional component of tremor.

Some dystonias are symptomatic of structural or metabolic brain disease, following in the wake of perinatal hypoxia or kernicterus (athetoid cerebral palsy) or accompanying Huntington's or Wilson's diseases. The symptomatic dystonias tend to be asymmetrical or unilateral, and to show other evidence of brain damage by way of fits, intellectual impairment or pyramidal tract damage. Other dystonias may be induced by drugs such as neuroleptics or levodopa. The range of possible causes is legion as listed by Marsden and Quinn (1990). In the majority of cases, however, no cause is found and the condition is labelled as a primary or idiopathic dystonia. A pathological cause is identified in some 45% of patients with generalised or multifocal dystonia, but only in 10% of those with focal dystonia. Hemidystonia by contrast is due to a structural cause in over 80% of cases, for example a stroke, head injury or brain tumour. It is essential that Wilson's disease, though rare, is excluded in all patients with onset of dystonia below the age of 50.

Age affects the chances of identifying a cause; in Fahn *et al.*'s (1987) series 40% of cases were symptomatic when onset was in childhood, 30% when onset was in adolescence and 13% when onset was over the age of 20. Age also has a marked though ill-understood effect on the likelihood of progression to generalised dystonia — this occurred in 60% of Fahn *et al.*'s patients with onset in childhood, in 25% with adolescent onset, but in only 3% of adult-onset cases. The legs are usually affected first in children, less commonly in adolescents, and very rarely in adults.

An interesting small group of patients has been reported by Burke *et al.* (1980) in whom persistent dystonia developed after a considerable delay of 1–14 years following static cerebral insults such as anoxia, trauma or infarction. In the trauma and infarction cases the body part affected corresponded to the site of the cerebral damage. Schott (1985) has drawn attention to patients who developed segmental dystonias in the wake of quite mild peripheral injuries such as falls, twisting the back or straining the arm or thumb, the movement disorder developing as the symptoms from the injury subsided. The site of the dystonia corresponded closely to that of the initial injury. Such rare examples contribute to the mystery surrounding the genesis of this group of conditions.

The dystonias are of importance to psychiatrists on many counts. Both acute and chronic forms can emerge as side effects of neuroleptic treatment, the latter providing considerable problems of management (p. 645). They are also of interest in that they are markedly 'psychosensitive', being readily aggravated by intercurrent stresses and tensions. This can be so marked that at least in the earlier stages a psychogenic disorder is suspected, this being reinforced when psychological treatment leads to amelioration. Diagnostic mistakes can also arise from the bizarre nature of the movement disorder and the strange postures induced, leading to an impression of simulation, hysteria or catatonic posturing. Strange paradoxes can add to the confusion, as when the patient can run, dance or mount stairs normally while walking provokes considerable difficulty. Some patients can even walk backwards when walking forwards is a problem. Strange tricks or manoeuvres such as the *geste antagoniste* (p. 673) may be discovered by the patient to control the movement disorder. Difficulties with diagnosis are increased by the absence of abnormalities on formal neurological examination and investigation in the idiopathic dystonias, where diagnosis depends essentially on familiarity with the clinical pictures produced.

Not surprisingly, in view of the above, differing opinions have been held about the causation of dystonia from time to time. Many examples, and particularly the focal forms, were long considered to be psychogenic in origin, for example torticollis and blepharospasm. A measure of doubt still exists in relation to some examples of writer's cramp and other occupational cramps as discussed below. But the accumulation of evidence now increasingly favours the view that both focal and generalised dystonias form part of a spectrum, founded equivalently in some subtle disturbance of brain biochemistry which awaits elucidation.

The resurgence of such a view has depended on a number of factors — the demonstration of relationships between the different forms, observation of transitions from one form to another, the similarities in clinical picture between symptomatic and idiopathic cases, and not least the provocation of classic examples by a range of pharmacological agents. Moreover careful control comparisons have increasingly failed to confirm an excess of personality abnormalities or other psychopathology among the persons affected.

Genetic studies have pointed to an inherited vulnerability to idiopathic dystonia and a common origin for the different subvarieties. Fletcher *et al.* (1990) surveyed 100 British families containing 107 members with generalised, segmental or multifocal dystonia (53 generalised dystonia, 46 segmental, 7 multifocal and 1 hemidystonia). Of the index cases 58 had affected relatives. Altogether 79 secondary cases were discovered, almost half being unaware of their problem (generalised dystonia in 15 cases, segmental in 25, focal in 27, multifocal in 6 and tremor in 6). It was concluded that 85% of the cases were caused by an autosomal dominant gene or genes, with approximately 40% penetrance and highly variable expression. About 14% of singleton cases possibly represented fresh mutations. The estimated risk for siblings or children in familial cases was 21%, and the risk in sporadic cases 8–14%. There was no evidence of increased parental consanguinity.

A genetic contribution to adult-onset focal dystonia is less clearly established but also seems probable. Waddy *et al.* (1991) examined the relatives of 40 patients with torticollis, orofacial dystonias and writer's cramp. Ten of them had relatives with some form of dystonia, segregation analysis again suggesting the presence of an autosomal dominant gene or genes with reduced penetrance.

In a small proportion of cases it is nonetheless still accepted, even by experienced observers, that the dystonia is primarily psychogenic in origin (p. 679). And of course in many patients there will be a strong interaction between organic predisposition and the modulating influence of emotional and environmental factors.

Dystonia musculorum deformans
(generalised torsion dystonia)

Dystonia musculorum deformans is the term commonly used for a generalised torsion dystonia of unknown aetiology which leads to severe and progressive crippling. A genetic basis is apparent in many cases. It must be distinguished from the symptomatic torsion dystonia which may follow severe perinatal anoxia or kernicterus; a similar picture may also be the presenting feature in Wilson's disease and was occasionally encountered after encephalitis lethargica.

The idiopathic generalised disease is rare. It occurs both sporadically and familially and particularly among persons with Jewish ancestry. Eldridge (1970) suggested that both autosomal dominant and recessive forms might exist, the latter being common among Ashkenazi Jews. This is now considered erroneous, and dominant inheritance with varying penetrance is proposed for both Jewish and non-Jewish cases. Recent linkage studies have localised the defective gene to the long arm of chromosome 9 in both Jewish and non-Jewish kindreds, close to the genes for gelsolin, arginosuccinate synthetase and dopamine-β-hydroxylase (Ozelius *et al.* 1989; Kramer *et al.* 1990). The greater penetrance in Jews than non-Jews may be due to different mutations operating at this locus. Moreover it is already clear from studies of certain kindreds that other genetic loci must sometimes be involved.

Within families who inherit the major disease other members may show formes frustes of the disorder — abnormalities of gait, abnormal arm postures, minor speech defects, or static postural abnormalities such as pes equinovarus or kyphoscoliosis.

Apart from these genetic allegiances little is known about aetiology. Pathological studies have occasionally reported abnormal findings in the basal ganglia, substantia nigra and elsewhere, but these are regarded as non-specific or even artefactual. However, the evidence points to involvement of the basal ganglia, both by analogy with examples which are symptomatic of known brain lesions and the response which may be observed to stereotactic surgery. The essential abnormality in idiopathic cases is likely to be a biochemical disturbance, though to date few definite leads have been obtained. The most notable abnormality in two cases examined at autopsy by Hornykiewicz *et al.* (1986) was reduced noradrenaline in the lateral and posterior hypothalamus, mamillary bodies, subthalamic nucleus and locus caeruleus.

Clinical features

The symptoms usually commence in childhood or early adolescence. The first symptom is commonly a disturbance of gait, with plantar flexion, inversion and adduction of the foot when walking. At first the picture is sometimes bizarre with respect to the precise functions affected, as already mentioned above. More rarely the initial disturbance may appear in the upper limbs with abnormal postures or actions. A characteristic dystonic posture consists of extension and hyperpronation of the arms, with flexion of the wrist and extension of the fingers. Occasionally the onset is with involvement of the trunk or with torticollis.

In the early stages the motor abnormalities may become apparent only when activity is attempted and nothing unusual can be found on examination at rest. Remissions lasting for several months at a time may occur, all adding to the erroneous impression that the disorder is psychogenic in origin. Indeed an hysterical disturbance is not infrequently diagnosed initially, particularly when there are coexistent emotional problems or adverse environmental factors. Thus patients are occasionally encountered who have undergone years of psychotherapy for 'hysterical spasms' before progression of the disorder

reveals the true state of affairs. The mistake is easily made in view of the rarity of the disorder and the bizarre nature of the symptoms. Other objective signs of a cerebral lesion are absent, with normal tendon reflexes and unimpaired intelligence. Moreover the dystonic postures which can occur in conversion hysteria are sometimes indistinguishable from the transient early disturbances of dystonia musculorum deformans.

Later the muscle spasms occur even when the body is relaxed, producing irregular spontaneous movements or fixed dystonic postures. The movements cease during sleep but plague the patient continually while awake. Other parts of the body come to be affected, usually with symmetrical involvement of all four limbs, the trunk and the neck The proximal muscles tend to be affected more than the distal, and a rotatory element in the axial musculature is typical. The trunk is forced into marked lordosis or scoliosis, and fixed contractures of the limbs lead eventually to severe crippling and permanent deformity. Speech, swallowing and breathing may ultimately be affected. The tendon reflexes become difficult to obtain or may be exaggerated, but the plantar responses remain down-going. There are no abnormalities of sensation.

Rapid progress and widespread involvement is usual when the onset is in childhood or adolescence. Maximum disability is usually reached within 5–10 years, after which the disease tends to arrest or sometimes may even improve very slightly. In about 5% of patients spontaneous remission occurs, usually lasting for only weeks or months but very occasionally being permanent (Harding 1993a).

An important subgroup which must not be overlooked comprises patients with *dopa-responsive dystonia* or *Segawa's disease* (Nygaard *et al.* 1988, 1991). This accounts for an estimated 5–10% of patients with onset in childhood or adolescence. The onset is typically with a curious abnormality of gait, for example walking on the toes with a wide base, progressing thereafter to the axial muscles producing lordosis and scoliosis. Parkinsonian features are prone to develop with bradykinesia, rigidity and tremor, and spasticity with pyramidal signs may be present. Diurnal fluctuations and improvement after sleep have been emphasised, but probably do not discriminate the group from other dystonias. Worsening after exertion is characteristic. In Nygaard *et al.*'s review of 86 cases, 36 were sporadic and the rest had more than one family member affected.

The dramatic response to levodopa sets the group apart. Small doses give immediate benefit, with a return to normal or near normal after several days or months. Minor gait abnormalities may persist, but full functional capacity is usually regained.

Doses as small as 100 mg have proved effective, though the average is in the range of 500–1000 mg. Dyskinesias have not emerged as a problem with long-continued therapy. Patients have responded after remaining untreated for 25–45 years, and the benefit has been sustained in follow-ups of 10–20 years.

Intelligence

In the symptomatic torsion dystonias the responsible cerebral pathology may lead to intellectual impairment or progressive dementia. In the idiopathic disease, however, this is not so. Eldridge (1970) reported that it was common to find exceptionally good intelligence in the Jewish cases. Precocious mental development may have been noted before the appearance of the symptoms and academic performance could be unusually good thereafter despite the gravity of the physical handicap. Unaffected siblings of patients have also been found to have significantly higher intelligence than carefully matched controls (Eldridge 1970).

Treatment

Treatment of dystonia musculorum deformans is often disappointing in the present state of knowledge, but in favourable cases drugs can bring substantial benefit. It is essential that all children and adolescents should have a 3-month trial of levodopa to see if they have the dopa-responsive form, particularly if the dystonia has started in the legs. If this fails the next drug to try is benzhexol, which helps about half of cases, sometimes very considerably (Burke et al. 1986). A start must be made very gradually, building up to high dosage over several months to avoid side effects. In children doses of up to 120 mg per day may prove to be well tolerated. Other drugs which may help if benzhexol fails include diazepam, clonazepam, baclofen, carbamazepine, tetrabenazine, or neuroleptics such as phenothiazines, haloperidol or pimozide. A combination which can be helpful in very severe dystonia is low dosage tetrabenazine with pimozide and benzhexol (Marsden & Quinn 1990). Unilateral thalamotomy can be helpful when the disease is asymmetrical and extremely disabling, but bilateral operations carry risk of impairing speech and swallowing.

Treatment should also be directed towards helping the patient and his family adjust to the profound emotional problems generated by the distressing and long drawn-out illness. Psychotherapy can sometimes be of considerable assistance, especially in view of the good intelligence of many of the patients. Some bring astonishing powers of adaptation to bear in learning to cope with their severe

disablement. The Dystonia Society gives valuable support and information.

Spasmodic torticollis (cervical dystonia)

Spasmodic torticollis is characterised by involuntary spasms of the musculature which lead to repeated dystonic movements of the head and neck, or sustained abnormal postures, or both. The element of sustained spasm in the picture serves in the differentiation from a tic. It may at times represent either a focal or a segmental dystonia, the latter when it spreads to involve the upper limbs.

Clinical features

Males and females are equally affected with an onset mainly between the ages of 30 and 50. A family history of the disorder is rare but emerges in occasional cases (Patterson & Little 1943; Tibbetts 1971). The onset is usually insidious though in some cases it can be related to an acute shock or an episode of emotional disturbance. Local trauma precedes the onset in up to 10% of cases (Sheehy & Marsden 1980). Sometimes a pulling or drawing sensation is felt in the neck for several weeks before the actual movements appear, or pain may be experienced locally.

The movements are typically irregular, forcible and writhing in character, involving several of the neck muscles along with the upper parts of the trapezii. The sternomastoid is usually prominently involved, drawing the head laterally and rotating the chin in a characteristic manner. Less commonly there may be simple lateral flexion, or the head may be pulled directly forwards (antecollis) or backwards (retrocollis). In time the spasms come to be almost continuous and the affected muscle groups may show considerable hypertrophy. Aching may be prominent, and cervical spondylosis may develop from the continual abnormal postures of the neck. Other abnormal movements are occasionally detected — facial twitches and grimaces, blinking, shrugging of the shoulders, or twisting athetoid movements of the upper limbs.

Once the condition is well developed the patient finds himself powerless to relax the offending muscle groups or to resist the abnormal movements except for short periods of time. The movements are noticeably affected by emotional influences, becoming more powerful and frequent under tension, excitement or distress. Any sudden startle or shock is likely to be followed immediately by a spasm. Self consciousness usually aggravates the condition, likewise walking or engaging in strenuous activity.

The movements subside during sleep, and may temporarily come under a greater measure of control when the patient is engaged in activities such as eating or drinking. An unexplained but striking feature is the ability of some patients to control the spasms by resting a hand or finger lightly against the chin, and not infrequently on the side away from which the turning movements are made (*geste antagoniste*).

The course is usually slow progression over many years but the outcome is extremely variable. Some patients are only mildly affected and can continue with their usual occupations, while others become permanently and severely incapacitated. A few show arrest or resolution of the disorder, others show spontaneous remissions varying from a few days to several years. This uncertain natural history adds greatly to the difficulties of gauging the effects of treatment. The picture may also modify as to detail over time, quick movements changing to slower spasms, or spasms giving way to sustained postures. Different muscle groups may come to be implicated, subsequent relapses even involving turning to the opposite side.

Among 103 cases Patterson and Little (1943) found that 13% pursued a static course, 42% were progressive, 40% were recurrent or intermittent, and two patients had complete remissions without treatment. On follow-up 25% were worse, 12% unchanged, 12% slightly improved, 42% much improved and 7% 'cured'. Ten per cent were unable to work, 49% were partially incapacitated for work and 29% were able to work as well as ever.

Meares (1971a) found that patients tended in general to deteriorate in the first 5 years and then become static. After the first 10 years slight improvement might be seen, those who had had the disability for this length of time often showing considerable adaptation to its effects. Remissions had occurred in a quarter of cases but almost exclusively in the first 5 years. Certain factors could be identified which appeared to be associated with an improved prognosis (Meares 1971b). Patients who remitted tended to be younger at onset, with a mean age of 30 compared to 40 for the remainder. They had significantly higher scores on questionnaires measuring neuroticism and anxiety, and rather more evidence of conflict by way of premorbid marital or sexual disturbance. The type of onset also showed some predictive value: the insidious development of a slow turning movement generally signalled a poor outcome, whereas a tic-like jerking onset or a prodromal period of aching in the neck muscles was characteristic of those who remitted.

Aetiology

Theories about aetiology have been widely divergent,

ranging from psychodynamic to organic, with many suggestions that both sets of factors may be at work. The condition is now firmly classified among the dystonias, but that does not entirely end the argument. In some cases the torticollis is clearly intimately related to other dystonic manifestations, whereas in others it develops as an isolated manifestation in a setting of emotional trauma. In these latter it can sometimes be hard to escape the conclusion that psychological factors are primarily responsible, albeit operating in an individual who is constitutionally predisposed. In working towards a better understanding, attempts have been made to subdivide the syndrome into different varieties and to define the characteristics of each:

Brissaud (1895) differentiated a 'mental torticollis' which developed from a coordinated purposive act, which, by frequent repetition in predisposed persons led ultimately to its involuntary reproduction. Signs of mental instability were common in such cases. By contrast 'torticollis spasm' was uncoordinated, painful and sometimes persisted during sleep. Wilson (1940) proposed a purely psychogenic type, sometimes occupational in origin and similar to writer's cramp; a 'torticollis tic' in the nature of a mannerism; an hysterical variety corresponding to Brissaud's 'mental torticollis'; and organic varieties which could follow encephalitis lethargica or local infections irritating nerves.

Hyslop (1949) suggested a division into torticollis of peripheral and of central origin. Peripheral varieties arose from inflammatory conditions affecting muscles or peripheral nerves, from vestibular disorders, or by way of compensation for paresis of external ocular movement. In such examples there was usually fixed involuntary spasm. Central torticollis could be either organic or psychological in origin, extending on a spectrum between these two extremes.

Tibbetts (1971) divided 72 cases into 'typical' and 'atypical' varieties according to the character of the movements involved. The former showed tonic and clonic movements, or sustained severe spasm if tonic alone; the latter showed much preoccupation over little spasm or else movements which were chaotic and inconsistent. There was strong inferential evidence for regarding the typical cases as organic and the atypical cases as psychogenic in origin. Thus the typical cases more often showed neurological abnormalities, facial dyskinesias or other abnormal movements, and more often had pain as the initial complaint. The atypical cases contained a higher proportion with abnormal mental states at onset and a heavier loading for neurosis. They also showed a much higher incidence of remissions and improvements.

It is possible therefore that different varieties of torticollis may owe their origins to dissimilar mechanisms, unified though they may be in their dystonic manifestations. It may be useful to examine the evidence usually quoted in favour of psychogenesis, and then that supporting an organic causation.

Evidence regarding psychogenesis

Earlier studies which purported to show a high prevalence of neurosis or abnormalities of personality lacked adequate control comparisons (Paterson 1945; Herz & Glaser 1949). More recent studies using surgical or healthy controls have signally failed to uphold such findings (Cockburn 1971; Robertson & Trimble 1988). Jahanshahi and Marsden (1988) found no difference from controls who had cervical spondylosis on a large battery of personality inventories, but this postal survey contained a large number of non-responders.

Precipitation by emotional trauma was striking in certain patients reported by Paterson (1945). One, for example, heard a shout, looked up turning his head sideways and saw a load about to fall on him. The torticollis commenced from that moment. In such examples the condition has appeared to represent conversion hysteria or a manifestation of an anxiety state. Herz and Glaser (1949), however, could identify no psychological precipitants in their cases. Cockburn (1971) found that 13 of 46 torticollis patients had had a major psychological trauma during the year before the symptoms began, but so did 10 of the controls.

Alternatively, torticollis has been regarded as conditioned by movements at work (occupational torticollis) in the manner of an overlearned and conditioned response. In five of Paterson's (1945) patients the onset could be traced to some voluntary purposive act which had become involuntarily repeated — for example in a telephonist who had to turn her head to the side during work, and in two men whose disorder set in during army training.

Finally, psychotherapy has met with success in certain patients (p. 675), extending even to complete resolution of the disorder. This, however, is slender evidence in favour of psychological causation, in view of the known sensitivity of dystonic movement disorders to on-going stresses and conflicts.

Evidence regarding organic causation

In the great majority of cases there is no clear evidence of pathology either peripherally or centrally in the nervous system, but small numbers show associations with other neurological disease. Torticollis has sometimes emerged along with parkinsonian features after encephalitis lethargica, or proved to be the initial feature of a progressive torsion dystonia (Eldridge 1970). Indeed its association with other disorders of movement has attracted increasing attention. Poppen and Martinez-Niochet (1951) reported that half of their cases showed additional abnormalities by way of grimaces, blepharospasm, tremors of the limbs or choreoathetoid movements. Tibbetts (1971) found that 10 of his 49 'typical' cases devel-

oped new patterns of movement disorder on follow-up, including facial dyskinesia and dysarthria. Couch (1976) was able to discern dystonic muscular activity extending to other body parts in 80% of patients with spasmodic torticollis of long duration. This was commonest in the shoulders but could involve the arms, trunk and legs as well.

The nature of the torticollis movements strongly supports the inclusion of the disorder among the focal dystonias. The force, duration and timing of the spasms are very similar to those seen in the generalised disease. The induction of short-lived torticollis as a dystonic side effect of treatment with neuroleptic drugs or levodopa is further evidence favouring this view. Detailed analysis of the movements with physiological recording has shown that sustained dystonic activity usually predominates, along with irregular jerking movements and sometimes rhythmic activity (Herz & Glaser 1949; Herz & Hoefer 1949). In some cases the muscles of the back, shoulder girdles and pectorals were also involved. Altogether the complexity of the movements suggested more than a learned pattern of behaviour, and appeared quite unlike the patterns of an hysterical disorder.

Additional information has come from investigations of vestibular function in the disorder. Bronstein and Rudge (1986) found that more than 70% of patients showed a directional preponderance of vestibular-induced nystagmus, in a direction opposite to that of the head deviation. Smooth pursuit and optokinetic nystagmus were occasionally affected. Thus in addition to extrapyramidal disturbance there may be involvement of the vestibular system too, perhaps reflecting breakdown of central connections which signal and control posture. Bronstein *et al.* (1987) further describe three patients in whom torticollis followed unilateral eighth nerve lesions caused by an acoustic neuroma, surgery or basilar artery ectasia.

Autopsy studies have been relatively few and have shown little clear-cut pathology. A variety of changes have been reported in the basal ganglia and substantia innominata, but the significance of the pictures described is uncertain (Tarlov 1970). A structural basis for the syndrome therefore remains elusive, as with the dystonias generally, but some cerebral biochemical basis might yet be brought to light.

In conclusion it would seem that evidence has steadily accumulated in favour of an organic causation and away from a psychological explanation for the fundamentals of the disorder. The abnormal movements appear to be mediated by some disturbance of brain function, possibly biochemically based, and to which the individual is predisposed. The surveys outlined on p. 670 suggest the likelihood of genetic influences. In these respects, views about spasmodic torticollis are following in the same direction as those concerning the other partial and segmental dystonias. In some cases the hypothetical disturbance will be sufficiently severe to become clinically overt without superadded pathology, either physical or psychological in nature; in others emotional influences, well known to aggravate dystonic disorders, may have served to precipitate the opening manifestations, and these may then resolve with psychological treatment.

Treatment

Physical methods such as massage, traction or immobilisation in collars and braces usually meet with disappointing results. Attempts at immobilisation commonly lead to bruising and chafing, and any benefit is promptly lost on removal of the restraint.

Drug therapy has also proved disappointing. Anticholinergics such as benzhexol are sometimes helpful but less so than in the dystonias which set in during childhood. Adults are more prone to side effects, and often cannot tolerate the high dosage required for therapeutic response. Benztropine, diazepam, and neuroleptics such as phenothiazines or haloperidol, may help a proportion of patients in the early stages, but benefits are often transient.

The treatment that has emerged as most useful is injection of botulinum A toxin (BOTOX, Dysport) into the affected muscle groups (Tsui *et al.* 1986; Stell *et al.* 1988; Blackie & Lees 1990). This should be undertaken only in clinics which have special experience of using the technique. It leads to relief from the neck deviations and associated pain in a high proportion of patients.

Careful choice of injection sites is important, the aim being to weaken the most active muscles from among the sternomastoid, splenius capitis and trapezius. Improvement usually follows within a week. Mild neck weakness may be experienced for some days after the injections, also dysphagia which may persist for a week or two. The beneficial effect typically lasts for 2–4 months, after which repeat injections become necessary. Experience has shown the feasibility of continuing treatments over many years, although antibodies to the toxin may ultimately develop and lead to unresponsiveness. The toxin appears to act by preventing the calcium-mediated release of acetylcholine from nerve terminals, probably by interfering with reuptake into presynaptic vesicles. The affected neuromuscular junctions are permanently inactivated, the waning of effect resulting from the establishment of new junctions by a process of sprouting from presynaptic axons.

Alternative approaches include intensive behaviour therapy employing massed practice, aversion techniques or systematic desensitisation to the anxiety induced by the head movements (Agras & Marshall 1965; Brierley 1967; Meares 1973). Biofeedback may meet with substantial success in certain patients, either as an aid to simple relaxation or more directly by electromyograph feedback from the offending muscle groups (Korein & Brudny 1976; Fischer-Williams *et al.* 1981). Psychotherapy directed at the exploration of conflicts, or analysis of the settings in which the movements first appeared, has been reported to produce improvement and even complete relief in occasional patients (Whiles 1940; Paterson 1945). Surgical approaches have included selective division of cervical nerve roots, peripheral denervation, thalamotomy and even sternomastoid myotomy in very disabled patients, but the advent of treatment with botulinum toxin should reduce the need for such invasive procedures.

Writer's cramp

Writer's cramp is one of the numerous 'occupational cramps' in which there develops a specific impairment of some educated motor skill, usually due to spasm in the muscles employed. All affect a particular manual skill which has achieved dexterity through frequent practice, and tend at least initially to spare other movements whether skilled or unskilled. The type of error occasioned by the spasm is reminiscent in many respects of the distinction between an unpractised movement and one which has been brought to deftness through constant repetitions (Critchley 1954).

The condition affects both sexes, with onset usually in the third or fourth decades. In a small proportion the patient reports some accident or injury to the hand or arm immediately before symptoms begin (Marsden & Sheehy 1990). Some 5% describe a similar condition in other family members. The fingers and hand develop spasm when attempting to write, causing the writing to sprawl in a jerky manner or pushing the point of the pen into the paper. At first the disorder appears only when fatigued or after writing for some time, but later it is evident immediately attempts at writing begin. Both agonists and antagonists can often be seen to be involved, sometimes with the spasm extending well along the upper limb. The finger movements are jerky and incoordinated and tremor may be prominent.

The precise picture varies considerably from one patient to another but the outcome in terms of disability is broadly similar. Certain tricks or strategies are often tried to circumvent the problem, with unusual postures and ways of holding the pen. These may bring new faulty habits and divorce the patient still further from the original skill.

To a remarkable extent other manual functions are typically unaffected, with normal preservation of skills such as sewing or manipulating small objects. Here, however, it has become evident that a distinction must be made between 'simple' and 'dystonic' writer's cramp (Sheehy & Marsden 1982; Marsden & Sheehy 1990). In the latter, which may form a substantial proportion of cases, spasms come to interfere with other actions such as sewing, knitting, shaving or using a knife. The forearm tends to pronate and the fingers extend as attempts at writing continue. Among 91 patients seen in a neurological clinic, Sheehy et al. (1988) found that 14 had been impaired in both writing and other manual acts from the start while the remainder began with difficulty in writing alone; 30 of these 77 later progressed to the dystonic variety after a period of months or years. The spectrum of disorders encountered has been further broadened by the description of patients with tremor and myoclonus induced by writing, this also commonly extending to other manual functions (Ravits et al. 1985).

There is no muscular wasting or weakness, and the reflexes are normal. Sensory functions remain intact, but pain, aching and feelings of stiffness often develop in the muscles on account of the spasm. A minority of patients may show subtle neurological signs, such as reduced arm swing or some increase in tone on the affected side. Tremor may be evident in the outstretched arm, or a dystonic posture in the dystonic variety.

It is necessary to distinguish these pictures from those seen with other diseases which affect fine coordinated movements, such as arthritis, carpal tunnel syndrome, Parkinson's disease or early torsion dystonia. Writer's cramp, sui generis, should only be diagnosed when there is no other physical or neurological abnormality to explain it, and when, at least at the outset, actions other than writing are performed with normal facility.

The course may fluctuate but is chronically progressive in the majority of patients. Spontaneous remissions occur in perhaps one in 20 patients, usually during the first 5 years. In general the prognosis is poor with lifelong disability though arrest of progression can occur at any stage. Sometimes the left hand becomes similarly involved after the patient has laboriously trained himself to write with this.

Aetiology

The aetiology has always been a puzzle, especially with the simple variety. Attempts have been made to explain it in terms of psychodynamic and learning theory models. Thus the disability has been viewed as akin to hysteria, arising out of unresolved conflict, particularly ambivalence towards the occupation. The spasms involve both prime movers and their antagonists in a manner resembling hysterical motor abnormality; and the disability may be influenced by external factors in a very remarkable manner—for example in patients who cannot write when sitting but can do so when standing (Walton 1977). It is only very rarely, however, that patients have seemed to gain or take advantage of the symptoms in any degree. Some re-train themselves successfully to write with the left hand and immediately return to work, while those who are cured by re-training or desensitisation rarely appear to develop other substitute symptoms.

Others have pointed to certain personality configurations in the patients which are thought to be aetiologically relevant. Obsessional features are said to be prominent, with striving conscientious attitudes at work and habitual overcontrol of emotions. Crisp and Moldofsky (1965) found that all seven patients whom they studied were of this type. In addition they had special difficulties in expressing aggression. The emotional conflict associated with the onset of the disability frequently centred around the need to write under frustrating but unavoidable circumstances. Bindman and Tibbetts (1977) supported such findings. It was suggested that an excessive predisposition to react with muscle tension in the arm when experiencing anger and frustration may have contributed in an important fashion to the genesis of the disorder.

Most observers, however, have found their patients to be generally stable and well adjusted (Liversedge 1969), and control comparisons using a variety of personality inventories have failed to detect an excess of psychopathology (Marsden & Sheehy 1990). Where anxiety levels have been high, these have usually resolved immediately after treatment has been successful.

The learning theory model proposes that writer's cramp is the outcome of faulty learning processes; or that whatever its origin its persistence may be explained on the basis of the establishment of maladaptive conditioned responses. Close observation often shows that the cramps tend to arise as soon as the pen or hand touch the paper, and become intensified by further movements of the fingers and thumb as writing proceeds. The good outcome which can sometimes be achieved by conditioning and desensitising techniques lends support to such views.

Increasingly, however, writer's cramp is now viewed as a variant of dystonia, representing along with other occupational cramps a subtle and task-specific manifestation of focal limb dystonia. How far this may apply to both simple and dystonic writer's cramp remains uncertain, but the possibility is raised by examples of transition from the one to the other (Goswami & Channabasavanna 1983; Marsden & Sheehy 1990).

Patients carrying the gene for torsion dystonia have sometimes experienced an episode of writer's cramp for months or years in childhood or adolescence (Zeman & Dyken 1968). The condition can also be seen in association with spasmodic torticollis (Meares 1971c). A few patients, particularly those with younger onset, may go on to develop dystonic spasms of the entire upper limb, a torticollis or a generalised dystonia (Marsden & Sheehy 1990). These scattered observations are as yet rather insubstantial, but combine to suggest that writer's cramp should be added to the list of the focal dystonias. The predisposition so engendered may, nevertheless, sometimes need to combine with factors of a psychological nature before the disability becomes overt.

It is not inconceivable that dystonia should sometimes affect one highly practised and finely focused skill alone, while leaving others employing the same muscle groups intact, especially when this is perhaps the most complex skill motorically for the patient. Admittedly, however, this has often been advanced as a principal argument in favour of a psychogenic rather than an organic causation. The possibility would seem especially plausible in relation to the other occupational cramps discussed below, where motor skills particularly valued by the person are concerned; the playing of a musical instrument, for example, is notoriously disrupted by anxiety, and increased tension is a powerful influence in making dystonic tendencies overt. In a most interesting manner the dystonias repeatedly illustrate the interaction of physiogenic and psychogenic influences.

Treatment

Treatment has traditionally involved a prolonged period of rest away from writing, followed by the teaching of relaxation and graded re-educative exercises. Return to work must then be gradual with strict avoidance of fatigue. Unfortunately such measures are likely to meet with incomplete and temporary results. In particular the gains obtained during treatment sessions often fail to generalise adequately to other situations.

Psychotherapy has rarely led to striking benefit. Nevertheless sources of current conflict warrant careful evaluation, especially conflicts in relation to work, and counselling on such matters may bring a measure of relief. Diazepam is sometimes of considerable value in relieving spasm and abating secondary anxiety. Propanolol may help with tremor. Antiparkinsonian drugs have been tried with occasional partial benefit. Hypnotherapy has sometimes been claimed to produce marked improvement when combined with correction of a faulty writing posture (Besson & Walker 1983).

A promising approach has come from behavioural treatment as described by Liversedge and Sylvester (1955). Deconditioning procedures were employed to treat both the spasm and tremor evoked by attempts at writing. Simple apparatus allowed shocks to be delivered to the left hand whenever the pen was gripped too tightly by the right, or when it deviated from a prescribed course of linedrawn patterns. Of 39 patients so treated satisfactory results were obtained in 29, with 50–100% improvement after 3–6 weeks of treatment (Sylvester & Liversedge 1960). Follow-up showed satisfactory maintenance of response up to 4.5 years later in 24 patients, and the five who relapsed had shown greater psychological disturbance than those who did well. Beech (1960) found that reciprocal inhibition could be helpful, proceeding slowly along a carefully constructed hierarchy of situations which only gradually approached the act of writing, and accompanied by relaxation at every stage. A randomised trial comparing relaxation with 'habit reversal', in which patients were taught to practice tightening the muscles that oppose the spasm, showed no benefit of the one procedure over the other (Wieck et al. 1988). The use of biofeedback techniques to bring the increased tension in the muscles to the patients' attention at an early stage has achieved success in certain cases (Reavley 1975; Cottraux et al. 1983).

Finally, botulinum injections have been tried with the intention of weakening the muscles principally involved in spasm, with modest benefit in a proportion of patients (Rivest et al. 1991).

Other occupational cramps

Other examples of restricted disability which centre on educated skilled manual actions are often referred to as 'occupational cramps' or 'craft palsies'. They show many features in common with writer's cramp, and arguments about their aetiology closely parallel the discussion above.

Telegraphist's cramp was formerly the subject of much attention (Ferguson 1971), apparently affecting some 14% of telegraphists using Morse and keyboard techniques in Australia. Factors identified as contributing to it included previously existing neurosis, workload and perhaps adequacy of equipment, training and supervisory practices. Analogous conditions have been observed among typists, tailors, painters and cigar makers. Sheehy et al. (1988) have reported examples of typist's cramp, several progressing to other manual dystonias. Golfers may develop jerks, tremors or spasms ('the yips') especially during putting (McDaniel et al. 1989).

A particularly interesting variety has been described among musicians, often intimately related to the manual demands made by the instrument played. Newmark and Hochberg (1987) reported 57 examples. The chief complaint was of inadequate control of the upper limb which interfered with playing. Persons with primary complaints of pain or trauma, or who had arthritis, parkinsonism or other central nervous system pathology were excluded.

Among 22 pianists the problem concerned flexion of the fourth and fifth fingers during playing, often after light touch upon the keyboard. Four guitarists and one banjo player showed curling of the third finger into the palm, disrupting tremolo passages. Five clarinetists suffered from extension of the third finger, sometimes with coincident flexion of the fourth and fifth fingers. These patterns were stereotyped in relation to the instrument in question, and highly activity-specific.

The remaining patients exhibited a variety of dysfunctions, ranging from problems with individual finger movements to more gross hand movements or spasms of the pectoralis major. In no case did the movement disorder spread beyond the hand, though in a minority other activities were affected, most commonly writing and typing.

The difficulties were insidious in onset, in general were non-progressive and were unrelieved by cessation of playing for up to several years at a time. They had often been preceded by trauma, tendonitis or significant increases in practice time shortly before the onset of symptoms. The authors favoured trauma as the main aetiological factor, peripheral damage setting in train a dystonic disorder as in the patients reported by Schott (pp. 669–70). Sheehy *et al.* (1988) have described similar problems in pianists, and a form of cramp in violinists in which the fourth and fifth fingers of the left hand lose their skill and press into the finger board.

Blepharospasm and oromandibular dystonia
(cranial dystonia, orofacial dystonia)

Blepharospasm consists of an uncontrollable tendency to spontaneous and forcible eye closure. It may begin unilaterally but both eyes are usually soon affected. Repeated contractions of the orbicularis oculi can progress to almost constant involuntary spasm, sometimes rendering the patient virtually unable to see. Spasms are provoked by bright light, embarrassment, attempts at reading or looking upward. Facial grimacing may be extensive in the efforts to keep the eyes open. Some patients find tricks that help—yawning, humming, touching the eyelids or eyebrows, neck extension or forced jaw opening. All spasms disappear during sleep.

It is most common in middle-aged or elderly women, with onset particularly in the sixth decade. For some con-

siderable time, even years, it may be intermittent, and the aggravation by emotional influences may give a strong impression that psychological factors are operative. A considerable proportion of patients show depression around the time of onset (Marsden 1976b). The affected patients are typically stable, however, and without precipitants that could explain the disorder (Bender 1969).

Oromandibular dystonia has a similar range of onset and also more frequently affects women than men. Prolonged spasms affect the muscles of the mouth, jaw and sometimes the tongue (lingual dystonia). They last for up to a minute and are repetitive but irregular in timing. The lower perioral muscles and the platysma may also be involved. The jaw may be forced open or abruptly closed, the lips purse or retract, and the tongue protrudes or curls within the mouth. Severe grimacing occurs and talking and eating may be rendered difficult. The condition can cause great social embarrassment. Spasmodic dysphonia and dysphagia may also be present.

The picture can at first sight resemble the orofacial dyskinesias seen as a late effect of neuroleptic medication (p. 641) but in essence the movements are different (Marsden 1976a, 1976b). Orofacial dystonia consists of repetitive prolonged spasms rather than the incessant flow of choreiform lip smacking, chewing and tongue rolling movements seen in tardive dyskinesia.

The spasms are typically provoked by embarrassment, fatigue or attempts at speaking, chewing or swallowing. Certain tricks may be learned to abort them, such as grasping the lower jaw firmly or shaking the head. In the early stages the capricious nature of the spasms may produce bizarre results, for example in one of Marsden's (1976b) patients who could not speak without provoking spasms but could sing normally, and in another where the reverse obtained.

While each of these two disorders can be seen in isolation, there is a strong tendency for them to be coupled together. Marsden's (1976b) composite material showed blepharospasm alone in 13 cases, oromandibular dystonia alone in nine, and both together in 17. In a more recent series of 264 patients with blepharospasm, 188 (71%) also showed oromandibular dystonia (Grandas *et al.* 1988). When both are present they usually begin contemporaneously, though sometimes the blepharospasm antedates the oromandibular dystonia by several years. The composite picture has been labelled Meige's syndrome, or 'Brueghel's syndrome' since both aspects are well depicted in the famous painting.

The course is usually chronic and protracted, but can be intermittent over many years. Blepharospasm remains mild in some 20% of cases, whereas other patients become profoundly disabled (Tolosa & Martí 1988).

Grandas *et al.* (1988) found that some 10% patients with blepharospasm had experienced a partial or complete remission, lasting from months to several years, but with ultimate recurrence in the great majority. Half of Marsden's (1976b) patients with both blepharospasm and oromandibular dystonia progressed to dystonia elsewhere —to torticollis, dystonic posturing of the arms, respiratory spasms or flexion spasms of the trunk.

Aetiology

The aetiology of both conditions remains obscure, but they are now firmly included within the dystonia spectrum. Blepharospasm was formerly often considered to be psychological in origin, but its frequent association with oromandibular dystonia has served to dispel this view. An organic basis is supported by its emergence as a side effect of treatment with neuroleptics or levodopa, and its occasional development in Parkinson's disease or as a sequel to encephalitis lethargica. Similar associations apply to oromandibular dystonia which may also accompany Wilson's disease. In both conditions the nature of the spasms—prolonged, repetitive and irregular in timing—is typical in all respects of other dystonias.

Continuous chronic blepharospasm has also been reported after head injury or subarachnoid haemorrhage, or in association with cerebral tumours, degenerative conditions or cerebral arterial disease. Rostral midbrain lesions appear to be particularly closely related to its development (Poewe *et al.* 1989). In all such settings blepharospasm can sometimes resemble a psychogenic disorder but for the history and abnormal findings on neurological examination. In the large group of patients reported by Grandas *et al.* (1988) dystonia was observed in other parts of the body in 78% of cases—oromandibular dystonia in 71%, torticollis 23%, laryngeal dystonia 17%, respiratory dystonia 15%, arm or hand 10%, pharyngeal 7%, trunk 2% and leg or foot 2%. A postural tremor was evident in the arms in 12%. A family history suggestive of blepharospasm or dystonia elsewhere was found in almost 10% of cases, suggesting a genetic predisposition.

Whether or not a purely psychogenic form of chronic blepharospasm should be recognised remains uncertain. As an acute disorder blepharospasm may accompany severe depression or anxiety, and forcible eye closure with resistance to eye opening is well recognised in conversion hysteria. Such cases, however, are usually transient, and accompanied by much overt emotional disturbance or other conversion phenomena. It would seem most unlikely that the chronic continuing syndrome could owe much to a psychogenic aetiology, sensitive though it is to psychological influences once it has become established.

Treatment

Treatment can raise very considerable problems. Some two-thirds of patients with blepharospasm are rendered functionally blind, and responses to drug treatment are often ill-sustained. With both blepharospasm and oromandibular dystonia there may be a good response to anticholinergic medication provided this can be tolerated in adequate dosage. Levodopa and lisuride helped a proportion of Grandas *et al.*'s patients with blepharospasm. Tetrabenazine, lithium, or neuroleptics such as haloperidol and pimozide, are also often tried. Severe cases of blepharospasm may require section of branches of the facial nerve, or muscle-stripping operations to remove selected parts of the orbicularis oculi muscles.

Recently injections of botulinum A toxin have achieved a secure place in the treatment of both conditions. For blepharospasm, injections are made into the orbicularis oculi muscles or subcutaneously, producing benefit after 1–3 days which usually lasts for 2–3 months. Side effects are transient ptosis and diplopia. For oromandibular dystonia, injections are made into the appropriate jaw and tongue muscles with EMG guidance. Unwanted side effects are dysphagia and jaw weakness, again usually transient (Brin *et al.* 1995).

Other dystonias and spasms

Other forms of dystonia rarely present to psychiatrists, though *laryngeal dystonia* may sometimes suggest an hysterical aphonia. In the adductor type the voice is choked and strangled, whereas with the abductor type it is breathy and effortful with whispered segments. Drugs are of little help, but skilled botulinum injections can again give substantial relief. *Pharyngeal dystonia* presents with difficulty in swallowing, and *respiratory dystonia* with difficulty in breathing. For details neurological textbooks should be consulted. *Hemifacial spasm* consists of twitching, tonic spasm and often synkinesis of the muscles innervated by the facial nerve. Though not a dystonic manifestation this too can now be treated effectively with botulinum injections to the facial muscles (Brin *et al.* 1995). Other than this the spasms can be helped in some degree by phenytoin, carbamazepine or clonazepam.

Psychogenic dystonia

Finally, despite all that has been done to exonerate the majority of cases of dystonia from a psychogenic aetiology, it seems probable that some cases are determined exclusively by psychological factors. In Fahn *et al.*'s (1987) series of 932 patients from New York, 24 (2.6%)

were eventually labelled as psychogenic. The authors suggest that the rebound in orientation towards dystonia has led to underdiagnosis of such cases. The label should be applied only when there is clear-cut evidence of a conversion reaction or of malingering. The movements and postures will then often resolve with placebo therapy.

Findings indicative of such a situation include false weakness, false sensory complaints, marked psychiatric disturbance such as self-inflicted injuries, or incongruous and inconsistent movements and postures. These last are, of course, difficult judgements to make in view of the bizarre manifestations which so often accompany organically derived dystonia. A major factor suggesting factitious disorder or malingering is complete resolution of the symptoms when the patient is left alone and supposedly unobserved (Fahn 1994b). Transient relief from hypnotherapy or a barbiturate interview does not suffice to make a diagnosis of psychogenic disorder. It is noteworthy that the severity of psychogenic disturbance can be severe enough in some cases to have led to fixed permanent contractures.

Fahn *et al.* (1983) reported five patients who they believed satisfied the criteria for 'hysterical' dystonia. All showed additional findings which led to a suspicion of conversion disorder, e.g. pain induced by light touch, inappropriate weakness or the presence of factitious injuries. And rather than a history of action dystonia preceding the dystonic postures, these had been present from the outset. Further experience of psychogenic dystonia is reported by Fahn (1994b).

In an extraordinary example reported by Batshaw *et al.* (1985) the diagnosis eventually was of Munchausen's syndrome:

A 35-year-old woman presented with severe dystonia, thought variously to be psychologically and organically based, and finally revealed by the patient herself to have been factitious. She had first presented at the age of 29 with dystonic posturing of the right foot and a left torticollis of 2 months duration. This was thought to be psychogenic in origin and she was given psychotherapy over a 3-year period. However, the dystonic symptoms spread and worsened so that by 32 she could not walk. She referred herself to the National Institutes of Health where a diagnosis of torsion dystonia was made. Fixed contractures were present by then. Suspicious features included the lack of a family history, the rather late age of onset, the unusual symmetry of involvement and the paucity of involuntary movements.

Drugs were without benefit and she underwent left and right ventral thalamotomies. Because of aphonia she did not speak for the next 18 months during which she developed trismus leading to the need for gastrostomy. Episodes of acute opisthotomous and tonic–clonic seizures were unaccompanied by abnormalities on the EEG. Intravenous diazepam led to respiratory arrest necessitating tracheostomy. She reported constant pain from dystonic spasms and was given narcotic analgesics.

A nursing home placement was considered, but just before the decision was made she awoke one morning and began to speak normally. She appeared to be deluded and hallucinated but this was thought to be manipulative in intent. She was transferred to a psychiatric unit and a behaviour modification programme was started. She soon began using her arms, and walked for the first time in 2 years though with an equinus gait. She began eating normally, the gastrostomy tube was removed and the tracheotomy closed, and by the time of discharge all evidence of dystonia had disappeared.

She admitted that she had feigned the whole illness, and others earlier in her career. She had started to turn her right foot inwards while working at a school, in order to avoid the responsibility of taking children for a regular 2-mile walk without assistance. She remained well when followed up 12 months later.

Gilles de la Tourette's syndrome
(Tourette's syndrome)

Gilles de la Tourette's syndrome, though relatively rare, has attracted a good deal of attention, chiefly on account of the striking nature of the clinical picture. Multiple tics are accompanied by forced involuntary vocalisations which can sometimes take the form of obscene words or phrases (coprolalia). One of the chief interests of the condition has centred on this verbal component which has been interpreted as giving a clue to the underlying psychopathological mechanisms. However, it now seems unlikely that psychopathological factors are sufficient in themselves to cause the disorder, even though to some extent they may shape its manifestations. A good deal of evidence suggests that there may be an organic component, or perhaps some form of developmental defect, which is at least partly responsible for the genesis of the condition. Genetic influences seem to be important, and links have increasingly been drawn with obsessive–compulsive disorder.

Clinical features

Valuable reviews of the clinical picture are presented by Shapiro *et al.* (1978), Lees (1985) and Robertson (1989, 1994). The DSM-IV criteria for diagnosis of the syndrome are the presence of both multiple motor and one or more vocal tics at some time during the illness (although not necessarily concurrently); such tics occurring many times a day, nearly every day or intermittently for more than a year and without a tic-free period exceeding 3 consecutive months; an onset before the age of 18 years; marked distress or significant impairment in social or occupational functioning occasioned by the disorder; and the absence of general medical conditions or substances such as stimulants which could account for it. Patients referred for specialist help can certainly be markedly disabled, but it has become increasingly clear that the majority of sufferers are only mildly affected and unknown to health professionals (Robertson & Gourdie 1990). Many of the latter would therefore fail to meet the DSM-IV criteria completely.

The condition is a good deal commoner among boys than girls, in a ratio of approximately 3:1. Onset is rare after 11, the great majority beginning between the ages of 5 and 8. In these respects the syndrome resembles the generality of tics in childhood. Motor tics tend to begin around the age of 7, vocal tics some 4 years later, and coprolalia at the time of puberty. Very occasional examples have been reported with onset in adult life (Marneros 1983), though of course these do not conform to the full DSM-IV criteria above. A family history of simple tics is not uncommon, occurring in 30% of Shapiro et al.'s (1978) patients, but it was formerly considered rare to find other family members with the fully developed syndrome. However, several families have now been reported with multiple members affected (Robertson & Gourdie 1990; Curtis et al. 1992; McMahon et al. 1992; Kurlan et al. 1994).

Simple tics are usually the first manifestation. Tics may be defined as 'sudden, quick, involuntary, and frequently repeated movements of circumscribed groups of muscles, serving no apparent purpose' (Kanner 1957). They are distinct from chorea and other abnormal motor movements in their stereotyped pattern, the same event occurring time and again, and in the ability of the subject to hold the movements in check for a short while at the expense of mounting inner tension. They usually commence around the eyes or in the face, head and neck, spreading later to the limbs and trunk. Before long there are typically multiple tics, often of great force and severity — blinking, grimacing, jerking of the head, shrugging of the shoulders or jerks of the arms and legs. Whole body movements may be involved, leading to bending, jumping, skipping, hopping, stamping or twirling. Compulsions to touch or smell objects, smelling the hands, or to hit and strike objects or the subject's own body are often observed. Complex coordinated movements occasionally appear, such as brief slapping of the face or thighs, or wringing of the hands. The picture may at times be highly bizarre, and the detailed pattern may change over time.

Vocalisations can occur from the outset but are usually added later. Most begin within 5 years of onset. At first they are often inarticulate sounds — sniffs, grunts, barks, throat clearing, snorting or coughing noises which accompany the motor movements. These may then

progress to the enunciation of words, sometimes muttered and barely discernible but sometimes loudly and clearly articulated. The vocal tics commonly occur at the end of sentences or clauses, without impairing the overall speech rhythm.

Common oaths and expletives are frequently involved, or brief obscene phrases of aggressive or sexual content (coprolalia). The obscenities are often uttered loudly, with an unusual cadence or pitch, and sometimes with imprecise pronunciation of phonemes (Lees 1985). The coprolalia occurs without any appropriate stimulus, and in common with other vocal tics it usually breaks through in the pauses between sentences. Some patients repeatedly utter the same swear word over and over again, or use long strings of elaborate obscenities. About a third of patients also utter emotionally charged words of great personal significance, again often spoken oddly with unusual emphasis on particular syllables. One of Lees' patients would occasionally shout the word 'cat', and another 'Elvis'.

The utterance of obscenities commonly sets in at about the time of puberty, but may start as early as 10 or be delayed until well into adult life. It ultimately develops in perhaps a third of patients reported from clinic samples, though with great variation in different reports. Among sufferers generally it is probably quite rare. 'Mental coprolalia' in the form of a compulsion to think obscenities is perhaps commoner than overt coprolalia, and transition from the former to the latter may be observed. Copropraxia consists of the involuntary and inappropriate making of obscene gestures, the commonest in the UK being the palm-backed V sign.

It has been shown that when computer programs generate letters or phonemes in a random manner, second and third order texts appear increasingly more like English language (Nuwer 1982). There is also an unexpected repeated occurrence of physical obscenities, which by the fourth order of processing have largely disappeared. Similar results are obtained with second order German. Thus coprolalia in Gilles de la Tourette's syndrome may conceivably result from a 'short circuiting' in brain function leading to the production of high probability strings of phonemes out of proportion to other words.

Both the tics and the utterances are affected by emotional stress, becoming more severe with anxiety, excitement, anger, boredom or self consciousness. The patient may struggle greatly to conceal the coprolalia, disguising or distorting obscene words so that their true nature is not at first detected. Intense efforts at control may succeed for a while, but at the expense of mounting inner tension and ultimately an explosive recrudescence. The coprolalia tends to cease when the patient is alone but the tics do not. Both are often markedly relieved by alcohol. The tics cease or diminish markedly during sleep and are also said to disappear during sexual arousal (Shapiro *et al.* 1973b). They usually diminish during periods of intense concentration or when the patient is firmly preoccupied with matters which do not arouse anxiety.

Echo-phenomena have often been stressed in the literature but occur in less than one-third of cases. There may be compulsive repetition of words spoken by others (echolalia), or compulsive imitation of actions (echopraxia).

The intelligence of affected persons varies widely but in some series a surprising number have shown superior ability. Most studies have shown the distribution of intelligence to be within normal limits. Robertson (1989) reviews studies which have looked for evidence of specific impairments, noting that language skills appear to be essentially unimpaired whereas visuopractic deficits have emerged with fair consistency. As a result significant discrepancies have often been observed between verbal and performance IQ scores. Attentional deficits have also been highlighted, and may account for Tourette children often falling behind their peers at school despite normal intellectual ability. Channon *et al.* (1992) made comparisons between adult patients with the disorder and matched controls on a variety of attentional tests, demonstrating significant impairments on serial addition, block span sequence, Trail Making and several vigilance tasks. Impairment was found both in sustaining attention and in focusing and shifting sets between salient stimuli. Such deficits were not explicable in terms of depression, anxiety or obsessionality, and showed no relationship to the dosage of drugs taken.

Other features which have often been claimed include a high prevalence of childhood neurotic symptoms and disturbed family backgrounds, but proper controlled comparisons are not available. Similar difficulties surround the reports of antisocial behaviour and conduct disorder in a high proportion of patients, including lying, stealing and aggressive behaviour generally. Inappropriate sexual behaviour, including exhibitionism, has also sometimes been stressed. A high prevalence of self-injurious behaviour has occasionally been reported, including head banging, lip biting and pummelling of the head and chest (Robertson 1992). More serious but rare instances include eye damage and touching hot objects. All such disorders are relatively uncommon in patients seen in the community, so may in part be an artefact of the selective reporting of patients referred expressly because of such problems (Robertson 1989).

More convincing associations have emerged with behavioural disturbances antedating the appearance of the syndrome, including attention deficit hyperactivity disorder (ADHD). These have been reported in up to two-thirds of children, often being the symptoms for which they are referred to a physician. Sleep disturbances including nightmares, somnambulism and night terrors have occurred in up to a third. There is also some evidence that depression and anxiety may be more common in adults with the disorder than in the normal population (Robertson *et al.* 1988, 1993). There is little to suggest any special relationship with psychotic illness, though not surprisingly there have been occasional reports of patients with bipolar affective disorder or schizophrenia.

Increasingly, however, there is evidence of a close association with obsessive–compulsive disorder, to the extent that this is sometimes regarded as an integral part of the condition, perhaps with shared genetic allegiances (p. 686). In addition to ritualistic behaviours and compulsions to touch objects, a high proportion of patients report obsessional thoughts and activities. These sometimes amount to frank obsessive–compulsive illness. Frankel *et al.* (1986) found that half of their patients had significantly elevated scores on a questionnaire for obsessional–compulsive symptoms, many scoring as highly as patients with obsessive–compulsive illness. Robertson *et al.* (1993) similarly showed elevated scores on the Leyton Obsessional Inventory. Obsessional features were observed in two-thirds of the patients reported by Nee *et al.* (1982) and Montgomery *et al.* (1982). The latter study also found a high prevalence of obsessive–compulsive illness among the first-degree relatives of patients.

Caine *et al.* (1988) found that almost half of the children in their epidemiological survey had obsessional ideas, often with associated ritualistic motor behaviour. The commonest included 'evening up', whereby a series of rituals ensured that the body was symmetrical and balanced, also counting games and touching rituals to ward off bad omens. Cummings and Frankel (1985) drew attention to certain similarities between the syndrome and obsessive–compulsive disorder, including age of onset, life-long course with waxing and waning, involuntary intrusive experiences and worsening with depression and anxiety. They advanced the hypothesis that the tics and vocalisations of Gilles de la Tourette's syndrome may be aberrant manifestations of simple motor programmes generated in the basal ganglia, and that obsessions and compulsions represent more complex motor plans initiated by similar anomalous neural activity.

Course and outcome

Over time the severity of the disorder tends to wax and wane, periods of partial remission alternating with exacerbations. The symptomatology may also change as to detail, new tics developing as old ones disappear. Occasionally there may be periods lasting for days or weeks during which the movements remit completely.

Firm information about the longer-term outcome is hard to obtain since there have been few prolonged follow-up studies. Moreover patients will tend to be lost to follow-up as they improve. It seems that the disorder may ameliorate in early adult life, and coprolalia has been said to remit in about one-tenth of subjects without medication (Shapiro *et al.* 1978). The impression, however, is that most patients are destined for life-long disability in some degree.

Bruun and Budman (1992) report a rather more encouraging picture. Of 136 patients who were followed for 5–15 years, 59% had been rated as mild to moderate when first encountered, but at follow-up 91% were now in these categories. More than a quarter had discontinued medication and most others were on lower doses than originally required. Half stated that they had improved spontaneously, most commonly in their late teenage years. A review of several studies suggested that some 30–40% of cases may remit completely by late adolescence, though it cannot be judged whether such remissions are permanent. Anecdotal evidence indicates that elderly Tourette patients rarely exhibit severe symptoms, and it is noteworthy that there have been few reports of elderly patients with the disorder.

The social impact of the illness, at least in the early years, is often disastrous. Some patients withdraw to a considerable extent, while others appear to maintain surprisingly good work records and social relationships despite their disability. Some patients remain only mildly affected all through, clinical impressions of the gravity of the disorder being influenced by those who are referred for specialist help.

Nosology and aetiology

Different views have been put forward about the nosological status of the condition. Some regard it as a rare and distinct disease entity, while others view it as merely the most severe and persistent presentation of the tic syndrome in childhood.

Gilles de la Tourette (1855) himself allied the condition with certain other rare motor and speech disorders reported from various parts of the world—the 'latah' reaction among Malays, the 'myriachit' of Siberia, and the 'jumping Frenchmen of Maine'. It is now realised, however, that this was erroneous. Latah is manifest as echopraxia, echolalia and coprolalia but tic-like phenomena do not occur. Automatic obedience is a prominent feature. It is essentially a severe startle reaction and does not occur without a provoking stimulus. Yap (1952) regards it as a culturally determined fear response found only in primitive cultures where persons have limited powers of control over the environment. Myriachit is similar. The Jumpers of Maine displayed analogous features as part of a religious ritual.

Corbett and co-workers present data which suggest that the fundamentals of Gilles de la Tourette's syndrome differ little from those of childhood tics generally (Corbett *et al.* 1969; Corbett 1971):

Among patients with tics attending child guidance clinics or adolescent departments it was shown that the tics usually began with facial movements, which in severe examples might come to involve progressively more caudal and peripheral parts of the body. The degree of spread could be used in assessing the severity of the tic, those with peripheral involvement tending to be the more persistent. Thus Gilles de la Tourette's syndrome is not unique in its progressive spread.

Almost a quarter of Corbett *et al.*'s patients showed vocal tics along with tics of other parts of the body, thereby satisfying the essential criteria for Gilles de la Tourette's syndrome. These were compared with further patients selected on the basis of coprolalia in conjunction with multiple body tics. The tics associated with vocalisations tended to affect several parts of the body concurrently and were particularly widely distributed and severe when coprolalia was present. In terms of intelligence and frequency of clinical evidence of brain damage, there was little to distinguish Gilles de la Tourette patients from other tiquers, but they showed a higher prevalence of psychiatric symptoms by way of antisocial behaviour and neurotic disturbances. The level of sociopathic factors in the family was several times that in the general patient population attending the hospital, likewise a history of parental mental illness. Both factors were particularly pronounced in those with coprolalia.

On follow-up, patients with vocal tics did less well than those without, and patients with coprolalia did particularly badly in terms of symptom resolution.

Thus on Corbett's data Gilles de la Tourette patients appear simply to represent the more disturbed, severely affected and recalcitrant of childhood tiquers, with coprolalia representing the extreme of the distribution.

The main theories advanced to account for tics are psychogenic formulations, those based on learning theory models, those which view the disorder in terms of developmental defect, and those which postulate some specific brain disorder. Each may accordingly be applied to Gilles de la Tourette's syndrome.

Psychogenic theories

Psychogenic theories regard emotional traumas and conflicts as fundamental to the genesis of tics. Emotional precipitants can sometimes be discerned at the time of onset, and a high prevalence of psychiatric disturbance has been reported in the patients and their families. The tics are seen as the direct or symbolic expression of emotional disturbance, aggression, anxiety or the handling of sexual conflicts.

Psychoanalysts have conceived of tics as the involuntary motor equivalents of emotional activity, allowing repressed impulses, usually of a sexual or sadistic nature, to make their appearance in disguised form (Fenichel 1945). Such impulses have become 'independent of the organised ego', that is to say they lack the normal integration with the totality of the personality. In a similar vein Mahler and Rangell (1943) regarded the symptoms of Gilles de la Tourette's syndrome as expressing the conflict between erotic and aggressive drives on the one hand and internalised censoring controls on the other.

These psychoanalytic conceptions may not seem particularly convincing when applied to tics generally, but it is interesting that in Gilles de la Tourette's syndrome one may meet with vocal and verbal manifestations which lend some support to such views. The noises can often be construed as aggressive or erotic in character, while coprolalia displays such themes in unmistakable form. Morphew and Sim (1969) argued strongly for a psychogenic aetiology for Gilles de la Tourette's syndrome, noting precipitating factors that were largely psychological in nature, and the improvements that could be seen after psychotherapy, leaving home or admission to hospital. Susceptibility to psychological influences need not, however, imply that these are causative. It would seem wiser merely to conclude that Gilles de la Tourette's syndrome may reveal psychodynamic factors at work in an unusually clear fashion, rather than to grant them a primary role in the genesis of the disorder. Some observers with wide experience of the condition have been unable to find evidence of inhibition of hostility or other special personality characteristics, and suggest that any observed psychopathology is most likely to be a product of the illness rather than playing a causative role (Shapiro *et al.* 1972).

Learning theory

The learning theory model views tics as conditioned avoidance responses which have originally been evoked in a traumatic situation, then reinforced by the reduction of anxiety that follows (Yates 1958). Because of stimulus generalisation the anxiety that the tic reduces will eventually be provoked by many more situations so that the tic becomes an increasingly stronger habit. In essence the tic is a simple learned response which has attained maximal habit strength.

Corbett (1971) pointed out that there is a striking similarity between tic movements and the movements seen in the startle response. This applies both to the nature of the movements and their distribution. Thus tics most frequently involve blinking, the face, head and neck, and the limbs, in that order, which parallels the distribution of motor activity during startle. Startle responses, moreover, are sometimes associated with vocalisation, and are easily conditioned to neutral stimuli.

Even if such a model is felt inadequate to explain the origin of the tic, it is easy to see how secondary reinforcing properties may come to attach to it and help to perpetuate the habit. To the extent that problems of aggression and hostility are prominent in patients with Gilles de la Tourette's syndrome the effects of their behaviour on others may sometimes powerfully gratify the habit. Behavioural treatment based on the learning theory model has met with some success (p. 687), though apparently less so with Gilles de la Tourette's syndrome than with simple motor tics.

Developmental theories

A developmental defect has been proposed as the basis of tics and derives support from certain indirect evidence. Such a conception presupposes no necessary special nexus of psychological conflict in the patient, nor some covert form of acquired brain damage, but merely that the normal maturational processes of control over motor movements have not been fully achieved. The patient is accordingly vulnerable to faulty conditioning procedures as set out above, or if he is destined for emotional disturbance his neurosis will be liable to choose the form of a tic on account of his motor lability.

Much of the data presented by Corbett *et al.* (1969) in tiquers fits with a conception of developmental defect. The preponderance in boys accords with their proneness to other developmental disorders. The restricted age of onset between 6 and 8 years suggests a developmental defect, similarly the marked tendency for simple tics to remit at adolescence. Corbett *et al.*'s tiquers showed an excess of other developmental disorders, such as encopresis and speech defects, when compared to the clinic population generally.

It is less clear whether developmental failure could account for the genesis of the more florid manifestations of Gilles de la Tourette's syndrome. The frequency of a family history of simple tics argues in favour of some form of constitutional motor lability, but the tendency for the syndrome to persist through adolescence and indeed well on into adult life would suggest that more than developmental immaturity is involved.

Organic theories

Organic theories presuppose that some specific brain disorder contributes directly to the development of tics. This gained support when tics emerged as a sequel of encephalitis lethargica, sometimes in relative isolation. The question therefore arises whether the generality of childhood tiquers might have suffered some form of subclinical brain damage, even while showing little or nothing abnormal on neurological examination.

Pasamanick and Kawi (1956) explored the possibility of brain damage resulting from prenatal or perinatal factors, by identifying 83 childhood tiquers and tracing the birth records of each. When compared to the next born child, matched for sex, race, maternal age and place of birth, the frequency of complications of pregnancy and parturition was found to have been significantly higher among the children with tics. These results were interpreted in terms of Pasamanick's theory of a 'continuum of reproductive casualty', namely that complications of pregnancy and delivery may lead to brain damage extending in degree from that which is gross and obvious to that which normally evades detection. Depending on the nature and severity of the damage the child may later develop a variety of neuropsychiatric disorders, ranging from epilepsy and mental defect to behaviour disorders or reading retardation. Tics appeared to take their place as part of this spectrum.

Others, however, have argued that the normal or even superior distribution of IQ scores among children with tics, and the absence of other motor abnormalities, make it unlikely that brain damage can play a substantial role.

With regard to Gilles de la Tourette's syndrome the consensus of opinion is that an organic basis awaits to be discovered, though the evidence for this is mainly inferential. The success of treatment with dopamine-blocking agents (p. 687), and the occasional emergence of a not dissimilar syndrome along with tardive dyskinesia after long-term neuroleptic medication (De Veaugh-Geiss 1980; Mueller & Aminoff 1982), point to dopaminergic hypersensitivity as a possible mechanism. To date, however, there has been no direct confirmation of this. Caine (1985) reviews several neurochemical investigations into the disorder, some showing reduced cerebrospinal fluid levels of homovanillic acid, the major metabolite of dopamine, but such findings have been questioned on methodological grounds. More recently Singer has reported increased numbers of presynaptic dopamine carrier sites in the striatum in three Tourette patients studied at autopsy, also reductions of cyclic adenosine monophosphate (AMP) in the cerebral cortex (Singer *et al.* 1991; Singer 1992). A rather striking finding has been reduction in the neuropeptide dynorphin throughout the basal ganglia in a patient with the disorder, with total absence of dynorphin-positive fibres in the dorsal part of the external segment of the globus pallidus (Haber *et al.* 1986). This has since been largely confirmed in further cases (Haber & Wolfer 1992). However, such findings have yet to be incorporated into a coherent neurochemical explanation for the disorder. One report has suggested a histological cerebral abnormality, by way of immature cell structure in the caudate and putamen in a single case (Balthasar 1956). The significance to be attached to this is very doubtful.

Clinical studies by Shapiro, Sweet and co-workers have pointed towards cerebral dysfunction in a high proportion of patients, but their findings were uncontrolled and have not been universally replicated (Shapiro *et al.* 1973a, 1973b, 1978; Sweet *et al.* 1973). Thus they noted histories of clumsiness, perceptual problems or hyperactivity in childhood in many cases, evidence of perseveration or confabulation, and a high prevalence of left-handedness or ambidexterity. Psychometric testing often showed large verbal–performance discrepancies or gave other indications of brain damage. Half of their patients had mild to moderate non-specific abnormalities on electroencephalography, and a similar proportion showed minor asymmetries of motor function on detailed neurological examination. By contrast Lees *et al.* (1984) found abnormalities of this nature in only a small proportion of patients.

Brain imaging has so far not been greatly illuminating, though findings to date support the presence of subtle cerebral defects. CT and MRI scans have proved to be normal in the majority of patients examined, with a few showing mild cortical atrophy, ventricular asymmetry or such unexpected findings as porencephalic or arachnoid cysts (Demeter 1992). Abnormalities in the size of the caudate nucleus and asymmetries in other basal ganglia structures have occasionally been reported (Robertson 1997). PET and SPECT scanning have indicated hypoperfusion in the basal ganglia, thalamus, frontal and temporal cortex, and possibly decreased availability of striatal D_2 receptors (Chase *et al.* 1986; Riddle *et al.* 1992; Robertson 1994; Moriarty *et al.* 1995). Neurophysiological studies have shown that Tourette patients fail to manifest cortical electrical potentials preceding their simple tics, whereas they have a normal premovement negative potential ('Bereitschafts potential') when they voluntarily mimic the same movements (Obeso *et al.* 1981). This suggests that the tics are not generated through the normal cortical motor pathways utilized in willed movement but have a subcortical origin.

In conclusion it seems that none of these approaches to understanding the aetiology of Gilles de la Tourette's syndrome is entirely satisfactory in itself. The study of the disorder illustrates the difficulty inherent in clarifying causes when there is no striking collateral evidence pointing to psychogenic factors or confirming cerebral disorder. Faulty conditioning processes would be most unlikely to result in so bizarre a syndrome when acting on an otherwise normal person; and if developmental immaturity was alone responsible one would expect more impressive evidence in other spheres to confirm it.

Complete explanations are unlikely to be obtained in terms of neurochemical malfunctioning alone, and it seems more probable that both psychological and organic factors interact to produce the final picture. Genetic predisposition has emerged as important as discussed below, and here it could be especially significant that the spectrum of genetic influence appears to embrace both the motor manifestations and aspects of personality functioning, *viz.* the liability to obsessive–compulsive features.

The coexistence in Gilles de la Tourette's patients of multiple motor tics and verbal utterances is at first sight puzzling, but perhaps can be accommodated in what we know of the use of words and body gestures. Both are vehicles of emotional expression and of communication, and must share at some level in their internal representation. Mahler and Rangell (1943) suggest that the cardinal features of Gilles de la Tourette's syndrome can all be regarded as different expressions of dysfunction of the 'system of expressional motility'. Certainly where aggression is concerned the normal processes of development lead from coarse motor expressions of hostile impulses to the more highly differentiated use of language, and the employment of obscenities in connection with aggression is firmly rooted in the culture towards which development proceeds.

Genetics

Though the disorder is often sporadic, recent studies have increasingly supported a genetic contribution, with links between narrowly defined Gilles de la Tourette's syndrome, chronic multiple tics without vocalisations, and obsessive–compulsive disorder. The precise genetic mechanisms remain unclear, but the presence of a single autosomal gene with varying penetrance has been suggested by some investigators. Polygenic inheritance is another possibility, and X-linked modifying genes may account for the increased prevalence among males.

Price *et al.* (1985) investigated 30 monozygotic and 13 dizygotic pairs of same-sex twins where at least one co-twin had Gilles de la Tourette's syndrome. The concordance rates were 53% in the former and 8% in the latter. When the criteria were broadened to include tics of any sort the concordances rose to 77% and 23%, respectively.

The lack of full concordance among monozygotic pairs emphasises the additional role of non-genetic factors, and Leckman *et al.* (1987) were able to show that in non-concordant pairs the unaffected co-twin had always had the higher birth weight. This suggests that prenatal events or exposures may have played a part in actualising the disorder.

Large family studies have shown an increased prevalence of Gilles de la Tourette's syndrome and of chronic multiple tics in the relatives of probands, segregation analysis sometimes suggesting the presence of a major autosomal gene with incomplete penetrance (Robertson 1989). Family studies have also indicated that the same gene may be expressed as obsessive–compulsive disorder. Thus many relatives of Tourette patients describe obsessional–compulsive thoughts and actions in the absence of tics or vocalisations (Robertson 1989); and obsessive–compulsive disorder has been found to be especially common among family members where Gilles de la Tourette's syndrome appears to be an inherited disorder (Cummings & Frankel 1985). Family aggregations have been confirmed in two particularly large pedigrees, one of 122 members from six generations in a British family (Curtis *et al.* 1992), and one of 161 members over four generations in the USA (McMahon *et al.* 1992). Thus while the exact mode of inheritance remains to a large extent uncertain, both family and genetic studies combine to suggest that there is a spectrum of disorder, extending from classic examples of the syndrome to other forms of tic and including also obsessive–compulsive disorder. The search for candidate genes by linkage analysis has not so far yielded definite results.

Treatment

Until the advent of pharmacotherapy the treatment of Gilles de la Tourette's syndrome was mostly disappointing. It was, moreover, difficult to evaluate the effectiveness of interventions on small numbers of cases because of the tendency of the disorder to show spontaneous fluctuations.

Psychotherapy often met with failure but improvements were sometimes reported, very occasionally with seeming total recovery (Mahler & Luke 1946; Eisenberg *et al.* 1959; Kurland 1965). Nevertheless supportive psychotherapy and group counselling procedures find an important place in helping patients to cope with their disability. Abreaction has been attempted with a wide range of drugs, and Michael (1957) reported a patient who underwent a striking remission after a series of carbon dioxide inhalations when intensive psychotherapy had met with no response.

Behavioural therapy can be effective with simple tics, for example 'massed practice' which is based on the theory that voluntary practice of the tics for long periods of time will build up reactive inhibition to their recurrence (Yates 1958). Clark (1966) reported remarkably good results with the technique in two out of three cases of Gilles de la Tourette's syndrome. Coprolalia was eliminated by asking the patient to repeat the most frequently used obscenity as often as possible in a large number of treatment sessions. Others, however, have had less success, finding that practice may aggravate the tics by generating increased anxiety (Sand & Carlson 1973). Techniques in which the patient is taught to practise movements incompatible with the tic, or to substitute a neutral word for an obscenity, have also occasionally helped (Friedman 1980). Cohen and Marks (1977) have reported the value of an operant conditioning programme, involving rewards for tic-free periods of increasing length, which can be implemented in the patient's home. Behavioural techniques also find a special place in the management of severe obsessive–compulsive behaviour when this is part of the condition.

Drugs such as diazepam may help temporarily by reducing anxiety, but dopamine receptor antagonists emerged as the first truly valuable medications. Connell *et al.* (1967) convincingly showed the effectiveness of haloperidol in simple tics in a double-blind comparison with diazepam, and Chapel *et al.* (1964) were among the first to report excellent results in Gilles de la Tourette's syndrome. Haloperidol has since received enthusiastic support and remains among the drugs of first choice. Shapiro and Shapiro (1982) conclude that over 80% of patients gain improvement, though some 13% discontinue it because of side effects. Dysphoria and sleepiness can be troublesome and may outweigh the benefits in terms of tic control. A start is usually made with very small dosage, for example 0.25–0.5 mg daily, thereafter building up very gradually to an end-point of maximal improvement with the minimum of side effects. In many patients 2–3 mg daily is adequate for symptom relief, but sometimes much larger doses are required. Dosage can often later be reduced over several months or years without loss of benefit, sometimes to very low levels.

Pimozide is effective in many patients and is often less sedating, likewise sulpiride which is less prone to provoke extrapyramidal disturbance. Tardive dyskinesia has proved to be more than a theoretical risk in Tourette's syndrome when neuroleptics have been administered over prolonged periods of time (Caine & Polinsky 1981).

Clonidine, a centrally active alpha adrenergic agonist, has also been shown to be effective (Cohen *et al.* 1980), though less regularly so than dopamine antagonists. However, differences in response by individual patients may indicate a trial of several different agents. The anticonvulsant clonazepam and the antidepressant clomipramine have also occasionally shown success, likewise calcium channel blockers such as nifedipine and verapamil. Documented responses have been reported with naloxone, lithium carbonate, tetrabenazine and fluvoxamine (Robertson 1989; Kurlan & Trinidad 1995).

Operative intervention by way of stereotactic surgery to the dentate nucleus of the cerebellum, or the rostral intralaminar and medial thalamic nuclei, has been found to help occasional patients (Hassler & Dieckmann 1970, 1973; Nadvornik *et al.* 1972) but will very rarely be indicated. Even in severely affected patients much can often be achieved by careful adjustment of drug regimens and proper attention to psychosocial aspects of management. Valuable support and information can be provided to patients by the Tourette Syndrome Associations both in the UK and the USA.

Chapter 15: Other Disorders Affecting
the Nervous System

Several affections of the nervous system not falling within the province of the foregoing chapters remain to be considered. Attention will be restricted to those which have attracted some degree of psychiatric interest, either on account of the mental symptoms that accompany them or because they can raise problems of differential diagnosis in the overlapping field between neurology and psychiatry.

Patients with neurological disease sometimes first come before the psychiatrist, usually at an early stage and before there is unequivocal evidence of central nervous system pathology. The incidence of erroneous diagnoses is hard to assess but the findings of Tissenbaum *et al.* (1951) may not be unrepresentative. On reviewing approximately 400 neurological patients attending a Veterans Administration clinic they found that 53 (13%) had been considered to suffer from a psychiatric disorder before the neurological diagnosis was established, the commonest psychiatric diagnoses being conversion hysteria, neurosis or affective disorder. The situation was particularly common among patients with Parkinson's disease or multiple sclerosis. In some instances organic disease had been suspected for some time, though the suspicion of non-organic psychiatric disorder persisted until the underlying disease had progressed much further.

In some neurological disorders psychiatric symptoms are an integral part of the disease process, representing the direct effects of central nervous system involvement on mental functioning. This is most clearly discerned in the numerous disorders which can lead to cognitive impairment, but cerebral pathology may also play a part in determining subtle changes of personality, disorder of affect or even psychotic developments. Where there is evidence on such matters this will be discussed. Other psychiatric disturbances in neurological disease have little to do directly with brain pathology, but reflect the reaction of the patient to his disablement. Neurological disability can pose severe threats to independence and security, or provide obstacles to free communication. Not unnaturally these may tax the individual's capacity for psychological adjustment over time. Emotional symptoms and even frank mental illness may then result, and owe their origin predominantly to the patient's problems and aspects of his social situation. Sometimes, of course, both organic and non-organic factors will be operative together. The correct appreciation of such matters is an essential prelude to planned intervention and help.

Some of the disorders considered below are not uncommon. Others are very rare, but can nonetheless be important in the present context if they are liable to have marked psychiatric sequelae.

Multiple sclerosis

Multiple sclerosis is by far the most frequent of the demyelinating diseases, and indeed is one of the commonest diseases of the nervous system in temperate climates. It is particularly common in the northern hemisphere but rare in tropical and subtropical regions. Although the actual incidence is low the chronicity of the disorder leads it to rank as a major cause of disability.

The aetiology remains unknown despite a large amount of research and a number of tantalising clues. At various times causative theories have involved vascular, infective, dietary and metabolic mechanisms but none can be considered well established. The present consensus is that the disease results from an interplay between genetic and environmental factors, resulting in an immunologically mediated inflammatory response within the central nervous system (Compston 1993). The evidence for genetic susceptibility is convincing, while that for environmental influences is less direct.

Epidemiological data from many parts of the world suggest that racial susceptibility is important in determining the patterns of distribution of the disease. Further evidence of a genetic basis comes from the finding that approximately 15% of patients have an affected relative, and that the lifetime risk for offspring and siblings is significantly increased. When a monozygotic twin is affected the co-twin will develop the disease in 30% of cases. The precise genetic mechanisms have not been clarified but it is likely that multiple genes are involved.

Epidemiological evidence similarly points to the importance of the environment. Compston (1993) reviews data from Australia and New Zealand which indicate that living in the southern hemisphere is relatively protective; and that the protective effect of being black is rapidly eliminated when black persons move to geographical areas of high risk. To date, however, no environmental pathogen has been clearly incriminated.

Clinical features

The onset is chiefly in young adults between 20 and 40 years of age. In the UK females are affected more often than males. The disorder is protean in its neurological manifestations, traditional diagnostic criteria laying emphasis on both the multifocal and relapsing nature of the symptoms and signs. Typically there is evidence, over time if not at a single examination, of disseminated lesions in the central nervous system, which at least in the early stages show a tendency to remission and relapse.

Early manifestations frequently include retrobulbar neuritis, disorders of oculomotor function leading to diplopia or nystagmus, or lesions of the long ascending or descending tracts of the cord producing paraesthesiae or spastic paraparesis. Precipitancy of micturition may be an early symptom, likewise ataxia or intention tremor due to cerebellar involvement. Retrobulbar neuritis is particularly common and can occur as a transient disturbance antedating other manifestations by many years.

The initial symptoms tend to settle within weeks or months, sometimes disappearing completely but sometimes leaving residual disability. Further attacks bring new symptoms or an intensification of those already present. The interval between attacks is extremely variable but in exceptional cases remissions may last for 25 years or more. The majority of cases pursue a relapsing–remitting course of this nature, but some 10% show steady progression of disability from the outset. The latter is the usual mode of progression with onsets after the age of 50 years. Ultimately almost all patients show downward progression with an accumulation of multiple handicaps.

In about a fifth of cases the disease proves to be relatively benign in that there is minimal disability even several years from the onset. However, there can then be sudden deterioration after a period of remaining symptom-free. The outlook is generally better when purely sensory or visual symptoms have been the chief manifestations since the beginning, whereas disorders of motor coordination or balance confer a poorer prognosis.

The most sinister development is the appearance of progressive disease, whether from the outset or after a number of relapses.

On examination typical early pointers to the diagnosis include pallor of the temporal halves of the optic discs, nystagmus, mild intention tremor, exaggerated tendon reflexes, absent abdominal reflexes, extensor plantar responses and impaired vibration and joint position sense. During early remissions of the disease, however, there may be little or nothing to detect by way of abnormal signs. Later there is evidence of multiple lesions particularly affecting the optic nerves, cerebellum, brain stem and long tracts of the cord. Eventually the patient is likely to show some combination of ataxia, intention tremor, dysarthria, visual impairment, dissociation of conjugate lateral eye movements, paraparesis, sensory loss in the limbs and urinary incontinence. The psychological manifestations described below will emerge in a large proportion of cases, some being attributable to lesions in the cerebral hemispheres. Epileptic seizures are a rare manifestation, occurring in about 2% of cases.

Various problems of neurological diagnosis can arise, at least in the early stages, but will not be detailed here. From the psychiatric point of view the principal differentiation that must be made is between hysteria and certain early manifestations of multiple sclerosis as discussed on p. 698.

There are no laboratory findings which are pathognomonic for the disease, but abnormalities occur in the cerebrospinal fluid in a high proportion of cases. About half show a slight increase of mononuclear cells in the acute stages or a moderate elevation of protein. A common finding is an abnormal Lange curve, either paretic or luetic in form. The gamma globulins are typically abnormally high, with the relative proportion of immunogloblin G (IgG) selectively raised in some 90% of cases (Hershey & Trotter 1979). Cerebrospinal fluid electrophoresis commonly shows the striking appearance of oligoclonal bands within the immunoglobulin fraction. False positives may, however, occur with both of these tests.

Halliday et al. (1973) made an important contribution by demonstrating the diagnostic value of studying visual evoked responses in patients suspected of multiple sclerosis. Delayed forms of response from one or both eyes on the presentation of visual patterned stimuli have been shown to correlate highly with the diagnosis, even in patients without a history of optic neuritis and with normal optic discs on ophthalmoscopy. Clearly subclinical lesions of the visual pathways are very common in multiple sclerosis and can readily be detected with such a test. Brain stem auditory evoked responses are also frequently abnormal. Somatosensory evoked responses, recorded over the cervical spine while stimulating the median nerve at the wrist, can similarly detect subclinical abnormalities in the somatosensory pathways.

Brain imaging now makes a major contribution to diagnosis. Computerised tomography (CT) scanning shows ventricular dilatation in a considerable proportion of patients with advanced disease, and may reveal areas of reduced white matter density indicative of plaques (Hershey *et al.* 1979). Magnetic resonance imaging (MRI) is, however, a great deal more sensitive and is the investigation of choice in uncertain cases. In an early comparative study involving 10 patients Young *et al.* (1981) found that five showed a total of 19 plaques on CT; all 10, however, showed lesions with MRI, and a further 112 plaques were revealed.

It is now apparent that 90% of patients with clinically definite multiple sclerosis will show discrete white matter abnormalities on MRI and 98% will have periventricular lesions (Ormerod *et al.* 1987). Lesions can also be shown in the optic nerve, brain stem and spinal cord. Accumulated experience has shown that a normal MRI scan of the brain all but excludes the diagnosis of multiple sclerosis (Armstrong & Keevil 1991). Conversely the presence of multifocal circumscribed areas of altered signal with predilection for the periventricular regions will strongly suggest that the disease is present when clinical features are equivocal (Plate 18). Enhancement with gadolinium-DTPA (p. 142) has an important role in distinguishing active lesions from those that have been present for many years.

Serial studies in individual patients have shown that the earliest change in an evolving plaque is an increase in permeability of the blood–brain barrier, shown by areas of enhancement with gadolinium-DTPA. Such areas precede the onset of more definite changes, and symptoms, by up to 2 weeks (Miller *et al.* 1988; Kermode *et al.* 1990). A mixture of new, evolving and resolving lesions may be seen in the same patient. Moreover MRI lesions are found to occur some 15 times more frequently than new clinical events.

Pathology

The pathological changes within the nervous system consist of scattered sharply circumscribed areas of demyelination, followed later by secondary degeneration of long axonal tracts. Macroscopically the plaques show as greyish translucent areas which may be found in all parts of the neuraxis, chiefly in the white matter but sometimes also in the grey matter of the cortex and spinal cord. Typically the number of lesions greatly exceeds what would

have been expected from the clinical findings. The cerebellum and the periventricular areas of the hemispheres are sites of special predilection.

Microscopically the acute lesions show degeneration of the myelin sheaths while the axis cylinders remain intact. The perivascular spaces contain lymphocytes and macrophages laden with neutral fats. Later the damaged myelin disappears and astrocytes proliferate to form a glial scar. At this stage axonal destruction is observed within the plaque.

Treatment

A good deal can be done to help with symptomatic aspects of the disease (Drug & Therapeutics Bulletin 1986b; Compston 1993). Precipitancy of micturition is helped by propantheline, oxybutynin and tricyclic antidepressants, and painful flexor spasms by baclofen or dantrolene. Intrathecal phenol injections may be indicated when the latter are severe but can impair sphincter control. Physiotherapy helps very considerably with spastic weakness, and re-educative exercises with mild degrees of ataxia. Fatigue is sometimes a serious handicap even in the absence of physical symptoms, and can sometimes be relieved with amantadine (Rosenberg & Appenzeller 1988). Paroxysmal brain stem symptoms such as dysarthria, vertigo or tonic attacks can respond well to carbamazepine.

Recovery from acute exacerbations of the disease is speeded by intramuscular corticotrophin or intravenous infusions of methylprednisolone, which probably act by reducing brain oedema in areas of acute inflammation. Prednisolone may be given orally but its efficacy is less well attested.

Immune suppression can stabilize the course in patients with rapidly progressive disease, and a variety of immunosuppressive agents have been tried in attempts to improve the long-term outlook. Azathioprine and cyclosporin have met with some success in terms of slower deterioration and fewer relapses, but cyclosporin, the more effective drug, leads to adverse effects by way of nephrotoxicity and hypertension. Neither can be recommended for routine treatment. Cyclophosphamide, with or without steroids, has shown inconclusive results. Transfer factor, an immunopotentiating substance, and dietary supplementation with linoleic acid have appeared to slow progress in occasional trials.

More recently there have been encouraging results from long-term trials of treatment with interferon (McDonald 1995). A large-scale trial of interferon beta-1b, given by subcutaneous injection, has shown significantly reduced relapse rates at 2 and 3 years, along with considerably improved MRI appearances in comparison to controls. These were not, however, accompanied by demonstrable effects on measures of disability. A trial of interferon beta-1a, given intramuscularly, has shown significantly delayed deterioration in the treated group; the annual relapse rate was reduced, and the mean number of active lesions seen on gadolinium enhancement was halved at 2 years. Copolymer 1, a synthetic polypeptide with resemblance to myelin basic protein, also appears to reduce relapse rates and perhaps to slow progression of disability.

McDonald concludes that the results of these recent trials give grounds for cautious optimism that we may be near to achieving treatments that delay the progress of the disease. However, it is not yet clear which patients stand to benefit most, nor how decisive the effects will be in terms of long-term disability.

Avoidance of fatigue is usually recommended, and the patient should be counselled that pregnancy may carry special hazards. The psychological management of the patient demands tact and great understanding. As discussed on pp. 699–700 psychotherapy may be indicated in certain patients, not only for support but also in the hope that the resolution of emotional difficulties will help to delay fresh relapses of the disorder.

Psychiatric aspects

It is well recognised that mental changes are common in multiple sclerosis. Some authorities have emphasised intellectual deterioration, others emotional changes. It has sometimes been claimed that the mental picture is characteristic for the disease, euphoria formerly being stressed in this regard. But considerable discrepancies have arisen between one investigation and another and matters of special selection have clearly been operative in many large series.

Attention has also been directed to the possibility that psychological factors may be important in precipitating fresh relapses of the disease. The premorbid personality of sufferers has been said to show certain characteristics, and arguing from slender foundations attempts have been made to suggest a psychogenic aetiology in certain examples. These matters will be considered in detail below (pp. 698–700).

The historical development of psychiatric interest in the disorder is traced by Surridge (1969). Early investigators regarded intellectual deficits as the main disturbance, and towards the end of the 19th century there were numerous reports of acute psychoses occurring in the disease.

Many of these studies, however, were made before multiple sclerosis could be adequately distinguished from cerebrovascular syphilis. Cottrell and Wilson's (1926) study then had an influential effect. In a consecutive series of 100 out-patients they found that emotional changes were strikingly common, usually taking the form of increased cheerfulness and optimism. A sense of physical well-being was frequent among the patients despite their crippled state. In contrast to these affective changes intellectual disorders were minimal or negligible. The triad of change of mood, a feeling of bodily well-being and impairment of emotional control was considered to be of greater diagnostic value than any neurological symptom complex. Brain (1930) added hysterical conversion symptoms as a further characteristic of the disease, suggesting that multiple sclerosis might predispose in some way to the mental dissociation responsible for hysteria. From then onward euphoria and hysteria continued to be emphasised in the English literature as typical of multiple sclerosis.

Meanwhile Ombredane (1929) re-emphasised the occurrence of intellectual deficits, finding abnormalities of intellect and memory in three-quarters of patients on careful investigation. Disturbances of affect were common in the intellectually deteriorated cases, but consisted chiefly of rapid unstable variations in mood rather than constant shifts towards euphoria or depression. Runge (1928) maintained that depression occurred in the early stage but gave way to euphoria as the disease progressed further. Euphoria was seen simply as a concomitant of intellectual deterioration. This view, in sharp contrast to Cottrell and Wilson's findings, became prominent on the European continent thereafter.

More recent investigators have sought to resolve the dilemma by careful surveys of the psychiatric changes in large series of patients. Surridge's (1969) investigation was exceptional for its thoroughness, and in providing a control group suffering from a different progressive disease, namely muscular dystrophy. One hundred and eight patients suffering from multiple sclerosis were visited in their normal places of residence, and separate accounts were obtained from informants to aid in the assessments of mood, intellectual deficits and personality changes. The sample was considered to be representative of patients with multiple sclerosis, except for some possible bias towards more severely disabled cases.

Seventy-five per cent of the multiple sclerosis patients were found to suffer some psychiatric abnormality, compared with less than half of the controls. Intellectual deterioration was present in 61%, varying in degree from mild memory loss to profound global dementia. None of the controls showed intellectual impairment. Abnormalities of mood were found in 53% compared with 13% of controls. Twenty-seven per cent were depressed, 26% euphoric, and 10% showed exaggeration of emotional expression. Euphoria was almost exclusively seen in patients who were intellectually impaired, and a significant correlation emerged between increasing euphoria and increasing intellectual deterioration. Euphoria was also associated with denial of disability which was observed in 11% of the patients. Impaired awareness of disability short of complete denial was found in 31%.

Forty per cent of the multiple sclerosis patients showed personality change compared with 33% of the controls. This was predominantly a change towards irritability, whereas the muscular dystrophy controls often showed increased patience and tolerance. Psychotic disorders were rare.

These findings effectively set the stage for subsequent studies, which have increasingly used neuropsychological assessments and objective rating procedures for charting the changes observed. Control comparisons have amply confirmed the vulnerability of patients to a range of cognitive and emotional complications as will be outlined below. However, considerable difficulties are encountered in reaching firm conclusions about the prevalence of psychiatric disorder in the disease in view of its widely varying manifestations. Dalos et al. (1983) have shown, for example, that much depends on whether patients are studied during remissions or relapses; psychiatric symptoms, mainly anxiety and depression, were present in 39% of patients examined during stable periods and 90% during exacerbations. Certain differences have also emerged between patients with relapsing–remitting and chronic forms of multiple sclerosis, particularly in relation to cognitive deficits (p. 693).

It can be uncertain how far psychiatric manifestations are attributable to brain pathology rather than representing psychological reactions to the threats and limitations imposed by the physical symptoms. Evidence can sometimes be found for a causal role of brain pathology even where seemingly non-organic symptoms such as depression are concerned (p. 695), but other influences are also clearly at work. Ron and Logsdail (1989), for example, found that psychiatric morbidity in their sample was strongly related to the degree of social stress perceived by the patient. This suggests an interactional model whereby the vulnerability created by the presence of brain damage enhances the effects of environmental and personal factors in producing psychiatric disorder (Ron & Feinstein 1992). In seeking to define the organic contribution recent studies have been greatly helped by the availability of sensitive brain-imaging techniques. These have also allowed exploration of the possible contributions of 'covert' brain lesions from early in the disease (p. 693).

Cognitive impairments

Cognitive impairments have been reported with widely varying frequency as reviewed by Rao (1986) and Franklin et al. (1990). Between one-half to two-thirds of patients seem to show deficits in some degree. Much is likely to depend on the stage of the disease at which assessments are made, but even so it is apparent that patients differ markedly in their liability to become impaired. This is perhaps not surprising since the accent of the disease can fall on very different parts of the neuraxis. The severity of impairments also varies widely, from those only detectable on careful testing to pictures of global dementia.

Some studies have found a relationship between cognitive impairment and severity of neurological disability while others have not. Peyser et al. (1980a) showed that cognitive deficits could be present or absent in groups with varying levels of disablement. It is also clear that psychometric evaluation may reveal deficits that have gone unsuspected on more cursory examination. Peyser et al. (1980b) and Heaton et al. (1985) found that half of patients judged to be cognitively intact on routine examination were impaired on psychometric testing. In Heaton et al.'s study 46% of relapsing–remitting and 72% of chronic progressive multiple sclerosis patients were found to show cognitive deficits. The progressive group was more severely impaired and on a wider range of functions.

Verbal skills are often relatively well preserved, which may account for other deficits being overlooked. The functions most markedly affected include memory and learning, and capacities to deal with abstract concepts and problem solving. Attentional processes may be impaired from a very early stage.

Memory impairment has been highlighted as one of the commonest deficits encountered, second only to decline in motor skills. Various studies indicate that 40–60% of multiple sclerosis patients perform below expectation on memory tests when compared to control groups (Grafman et al. 1990b). Again, however, patients vary considerably, some being affected early in the disease while others remain unimpaired. Primary memory as reflected in the digit span appears to remain relatively intact, and rates of forgetting are also largely normal as measured by the Brown–Peterson task. However, secondary memory is often considerably impaired, apparently mainly due to failures of retrieval (Grafman et al. 1990b). Non-verbal memory tends to be as severely affected as verbal memory. The role of attentional deficits in leading to such problems has not been fully explored, but both depression and psychotropic medication have been exonerated as a complete explanation.

Other cognitive processes emerge as defective in a substantial proportion of patients (Rao 1986). Language deficits are rare, except for reductions in verbal fluency. However, marked difficulties may be encountered with psychomotor efficiency and attention and concentration. Problems with abstract thinking, conceptualisation and the shifting of sets may resemble those seen with frontal lobe injuries. Perseveration can sometimes be detected. Mahler and Benson (1990) draw an analogy with the pictures seen in 'subcortical dementia' (p. 667). Such difficulties can emerge in patients who score well on tests of general intelligence, and will then often go unsuspected. In occasional examples the picture amounts to a clinically recognisable dementia.

Thus it is apparent that some patients have not only to adapt to progressive physical disability, but must often do this against a background of diminishing intellect and impaired adaptive capacity. The implications for retraining are obviously important; the presence and severity of impairments such as these may well be crucial in determining the outcome of efforts at rehabilitation.

The course followed by cognitive impairments may be as variable as the neurological symptoms of the disease (Franklin et al. 1990). Some patients experience relapses and remissions, while others show steady progression of their cognitive deficits. Attempts to chart the course of decline in patient groups have therefore yielded conflicting results. An early study by Canter (1951) showed losses on most subtests of the Wechsler Bellevue Battery when 47 patients were retested after an interval of 6 months. Ivnik (1978) similarly found significant deterioration on retesting a small group 3 years later, but this may have been primarily due to sensorimotor dysfunction. In the first truly prospective study, Filley et al. (1990) found remarkably little evidence of progression in a group of 46 patients, only six of 36 test measures showing significant deterioration over 1–2 years. On global clinical ratings, however, seven out of 10 patients with chronic progressive disease showed worsening; of the 36 with relapsing–remitting disease a smaller proportion showed deterioration and this was mainly evident on retesting during a documented relapse. In an interesting single-case study Rozewicz et al. (1996) documented *improvements* over time on arithmetic, naming and comprehension tasks, which paralleled a reduction in cortical lesion size and resolution of a large enhancing lesion in the left parietal lobe.

The high prevalence of mental impairment is hardly surprising in view of the finding that plaque formation is often widespread within the cerebral hemispheres. Brownell and Hughes (1962) were able to demonstrate cerebral plaques in every one of 22 patients coming to autopsy, varying in number from three to 225 with an average of 72 plaques per case. All parts of the white matter tended to be equally involved but large plaques showed a predilection for the periventricular areas. Brain imaging now makes it possible to visualise such lesions during life and relate them to the patients' clinical state. Rao (1990) reviews CT studies which have shown significant relationships between measures of cerebral atrophy and the presence of cognitive impairment, and more discriminating MRI studies which in addition can provide estimates of 'total lesion load'. The latter, which reflects the number of plaques in the cerebral hemispheres, provides the best indicator of performance on tests of recent memory and conceptual reasoning, while atrophy of the corpus callosum tends to correlate with speed of information processing (Rao et al. 1989).

Professor Ron and her colleagues have conducted a series of elegant MRI studies which show that even 'subclinical' brain involvement can lead to detectable cognitive deficits:

Callanan et al. (1989) investigated 48 patients with 'clinically isolated lesions' of the type seen in multiple sclerosis, viz. with clinical evidence of optic neuritis and brain stem and cord lesions, comparing them with controls suffering from rheumatic and neurological conditions not liable to cause brain disease. Subtle cognitive deficits were already apparent in the putative multiple sclerosis group. On MRI 80% of these showed cerebral abnormalities, by way of increased signal in the periventricular rim or discrete lesions in the brain parenchyma, and the extent of such abnormalities correlated with impairment on tests of abstracting ability and auditory attention.

Feinstein et al. (1992c) concentrated on tests of attention and speed of information processing in 42 patients who had recently suffered a first episode of acute optic neuritis, and who in all other respects were neurologically normal. Approximately half of the sample showed abnormalities on brain MRI, and these were more impaired on the tests than patients without cerebral lesions or normal controls. Significant correlations were found between total lesion area and certain measures of attention, particularly the Symbol–Digit Substitution Test. Thus both studies demonstrated that cognitive deficits can be the only manifestation of otherwise silent brain lesions, emerging as more sensitive indicators of cerebral involvement than neurological symptoms and signs.

Finally Feinstein et al. (1992b) followed up 35 of Callanan et al.'s patients 4.5 years later. Approximately half had by then developed clinically definite multiple sclerosis, 13 showing the relapsing–remitting pattern and seven chronic progression. Those who had developed definite signs of the disease showed significant memory deterioration, particularly the group with chronic progression. In the latter cognitive deterioration was also more widespread, and the total lesion scores on MRI were correspondingly greater.

Presentation with dementia is occasionally encountered and can raise important problems of differential diagnosis.

Koenig (1968) described seven patients in whom dementia was the sole or predominant manifestation of the disease, the multiple sclerosis being of a relatively silent variety neurologically. The mental symptoms were indistinguishable from dementia due to other causes, though the onset was usually fairly acute with memory loss, confusion, disorientation, or personality change. Some showed slight fluctuations in the level of mental functioning from day to day. Three showed progressive deterioration and only one had a partial remission. Neurological symptoms of brain stem or cord dysfunction had preceded the dementia or accompanied its onset in four cases, but all showed evidence of disseminated central nervous system disease on careful examination. Koenig suggested that 'silent' or unrecognised multiple sclerosis may be a commoner cause of dementia than is generally recognised. Young *et al.* (1976) reported further examples with intellectual impairment as the presenting symptom or forming a prominent part of the picture from the earliest stages.

Hotopf *et al.* (1994) describe two particularly instructive patients in whom the cognitive changes were at first attributed to psychiatric illness:

A 41-year-old man had a 2-year history of change of personality, becoming quiet, vague and forgetful. He was involved in a series of road traffic accidents and had begun to sleep for long periods. His attitude to his problems was one of bland indifference. There was no family or personal history of psychiatric illness.

On examination he was alert but his affect was strangely inappropriate. He was intermittently disorientated in time and place and there were tendencies to confabulate and perseverate. Concentration, attention and memory were poor, and he had difficulty with verbal fluency and sequential tasks. He made occasional naming errors and paraphasic mistakes when writing. On first contact with the neurological services his mental state had seemed sufficiently bizarre to raise a diagnosis of hysteria, reinforced by his striking lack of concern about his poor performance on tests of cognition.

The only physical signs were an extensor plantar response, which was not present on re-examination, and lack of left arm swinging while walking. Two months later he showed a plantar grasp reflex and a positive glabellar tap. Psychometric testing revealed a verbal IQ of 73 and performance IQ of 63, consistent with moderate to severe decline of intellect. Cerebrospinal fluid examination showed a raised protein with oligoclonal bands and visual evoked responses were abnormal. MRI showed periventricular abnormalities and widespread changes in the hemispheres consistent with multiple sclerosis. Screening tests for other causes of dementia were negative. Over the next 8 years he showed steady deterioration to severe global cognitive deficit, with dysphasia, severe ataxia and incontinence of urine.

The second patient presented at the age of 35 with a 3-year history of difficulties with concentration and memory. He had become increasingly withdrawn but showed no concern over his symptoms. When first seen in a neurological clinic a non-organic psychiatric illness was suspected. He had diabetes, and for 6 months there have been an insidious loss of vision. Neurological findings included bilateral optic atrophy and later some evidence of gait disturbance, but there were no other neurological abnormalities. Cognitive examination subsequently showed disorientation, impaired concentration, poor memory, dyscalculia and reduced verbal fluency. Psychometric testing confirmed these deficits and showed a verbal IQ of 73. Cerebrospinal fluid examination showed oligoclonal bands in the presence of normal total protein, and visual evoked responses were abnormal. MRI revealed changes consistent with multiple sclerosis (Plate 18). Over the next 18 months he continued to show gradual cognitive decline without any marked physical symptoms or signs.

Sometimes the rate of progression of dementia is astonishingly rapid as in the patient described by Bergin (1957):

A woman of 30 developed brief retrobulbar neuritis followed 1 year later by diplopia, ataxia and precipitate micturition. Over 3 months she became severely incapacitated, apathetic, retarded and vague. Examination showed a pale left optic disc, fine lateral nystagmus, slight right facial and arm weakness, incoordination of the legs and up-going plantar responses. The cerebrospinal fluid showed 18 lymphocytes/ml and a paretic Lange curve. One week after admission she became confused, uncooperative and disorientated, doubly incontinent and with gross evidence of intellectual impairment. Two weeks later she could not understand even simple sentences. The EEG showed random irregular slow waves in all areas and the air encephalogram showed moderate ventricular enlargement. Six weeks after admission she was bedfast, making noises but no recognisable words. The only active limb was her left arm which was used to strike out at people and tug at her hair. Within 10 weeks she died and post-mortem examination showed well-defined plaques throughout the brain, cerebellum, brain stem and cord.

Abnormalities of mood

A variety of affective changes are common in multiple sclerosis. Euphoria — a bland elevation of mood out of keeping with the patient's physical condition — was once thought to be the usual picture, but it is now clear that depression is at least as common. Much probably depends on the stage at which the patient is examined and whether some degree of intellectual deterioration has occurred. Depression is often the logical and understandable response to the patient's predicament in the earlier stages, whereas euphoria is more typical as the disease progresses. The transition over time from depression to euphoria can sometimes be observed in the individual patient. Bipolar swings of mood may also occasionally occur, episodes of hypomania sometimes accompanying treatment with steroids (Minden & Schiffer 1990).

Surridge (1969) found depression in 27% and euphoria

in 26% of patients. Kahana *et al.* (1971) in a nationwide survey of cases in Israel found depression in 6% and euphoria in 5%. Cottrell and Wilson's (1926) earlier discordant finding of depression in 10% but euphoria in 63% remains unexplained; this, however, is the view that has tended to persist in clinical teaching. It is possible that an active coping mechanism of denial may quite often be mistaken for euphoria if enquiry is not made into the patient's subjective state.

Depression often appears to be reactive in origin. Thus in Surridge's material the depressed patients showed no special tendency to intellectual deterioration or denial of disability, in sharp contrast to the patients with euphoria. In general therefore the psychological impact of the disability and the patient's awareness of his situation appear to be the main determining factors. Examples of marked depression may be encountered immediately the patient learns the nature of the diagnosis and prognosis (Gallineck & Kalinowsky 1958). Sphincter disturbances constitute an especially severe psychological trauma, increasing dependency and often bringing an end to sexual relationships. Impotence, ataxia and visual disturbances were also among the most distressing of the disabilities experienced by Surridge's patients.

Sometimes, however, the depression may at least in part be physiologically determined. Goodstein and Ferrell (1977) observed three patients in whom episodes of depression predominated from the outset of the disease and before the diagnosis had been established. No precipitants were apparent, and the response to treatment was poor. On this account an organic basis was suspected and multiple sclerosis finally declared itself. Whitlock and Siskind (1980) similarly concluded that depression may sometimes be founded in cerebral pathology. They compared 30 multiple sclerosis patients with equivalently disabled controls suffering from other neurological diseases. The patients with multiple sclerosis were not only more depressed at the time of examination, but had experienced significantly more affective disorder in the year preceding the first signs of the disease. Many had previously been stable people, and the episodes of depression often showed 'endogenous' qualities.

Further evidence against a purely 'reactive' origin for affective disorder comes from the finding that the frequency and severity of depressive episodes can be independent of the severity of the disease as measured by disability scores (Rabins *et al.* 1986). A special relationship is also suggested by epidemiological data. Schiffer and Babigian (1984) found that 62% of multiple sclerosis patients in Munroe County, New York, had had contact with psychiatric services for depression; this was significantly higher than for patients with temporal lobe epilepsy or amyotrophic lateral sclerosis. In the same population the combination of multiple sclerosis and bipolar affective disorder was increased twofold above expectation (Schiffer *et al.* 1986). Joffe *et al.* (1987) confirmed a substantially increased risk for both major depression and bipolar affective disorder in their carefully studied sample. Whether these associations reflect shared genetic determinants or involvement of limbic regions by demyelination remains uncertain. It appears, however, that depression is a good deal commoner in patients with clinical and CT evidence of cerebral involvement than in those with predominantly spinal or cerebellar forms of the disease (Schiffer *et al.* 1983; Rabins *et al.* 1986). Honer *et al.* (1987) in a small group of patients with psychiatric disorder, mainly affective disorder, found that plaques within the temporal lobes were more common than in matched controls without such symptoms.

Irrespective of its derivation the degree of depression in multiple sclerosis can be severe, and suicide has been reported in a considerable number of cases. Kahana *et al.* (1971) estimated that suicide was 14 times commoner among their patients than in the general population of Israel.

Euphoria was defined by Surridge (1969) as a mood of cheerful complacency out of context with the patient's total situation. It differed from the elation of hypomania in not being accompanied by motor restlessness, increased energy or speeding up of thought processes. All but two of the euphoric patients in his series showed intellectual deterioration, and the group as a whole was significantly more disabled than the depressed or normal groups. Braceland and Giffin (1950) had earlier reported that all patients who showed euphoria had evidence of widespread cerebral disorder. In contrast to depression, therefore, euphoria appears to depend essentially on damage to the central nervous system.

This has been fully supported by Rabins *et al.* (1986). In a detailed study of 87 patients those with euphoria were more likely to show clinical evidence of brain as opposed to spinal cord involvement, had more severe disablement, and scored at a lower level on the Mini-Mental State Examination. They were also more likely to have relapsing–progressive or progressive forms of the disease than the relapsing–remitting variety. Among those who had CT scans the ventricles were significantly more often enlarged. Rabins (1990) concluded that euphoria represents a neurologically based inability to appreciate the severity of the deficits present rather than psychologically based denial. He suggested that it may reflect frontal lobe disconnection resulting from involvement of key pathways to and from the frontal regions by periventricular demyelination.

Quite often the initial impression of euphoria proves to be misleading, and the evidence of cheerfulness or complacency subsides as the interview progresses. Indeed Surridge found that eight out of 28 euphoric patients confessed to feeling miserable and depressed despite the strong outward impression that they were unreasonably cheerful. No doubt an element of emotional lability is often associated with euphoria and adds to the difficulty of assessing the patient's true subjective feelings.

Closely related to euphoria is a feeling of increased bodily well-being (eutonia). Cottrell and Wilson (1926) reported this in 84% of patients, Pratt (1951) in only 6%. The phenomenon is possibly related not only to changes of mood but also to denial or impaired awareness of disability.

Disorders of emotional control include true exaggeration of emotional feeling (lability of affect), or an exaggeration of expression which is unbacked by an equivalent degree of feeling (disorder of affective expression). The latter may indeed be incongruous with the underlying mood and is essentially similar to the disorder of emotional expression seen in pseudobulbar palsy. It can be difficult in reports to differentiate clearly between true lability and such disorders of expression. Cottrell and Wilson (1926) found that 95% of their patients showed 'facility and amplification of emotional expression' and 13% rapid changes of mood. Braceland and Giffin (1950) reported emotional lability in 18%. Pratt (1951) found that 6% admitted to laughing and 29% to crying more easily than usual, while 16% were noted to laugh unduly readily but were not aware of this themselves. Surridge (1969) found exaggeration of emotional expression but without concomitant lability in 10% of patients. Intellectual deterioration is the usual accompaniment of all such pictures, which are commonly attributable to lesions in bulbar pathways or the diencephalon. Treatment with tricyclic antidepressants or levodopa can be helpful as described on p. 392.

Personality changes

Many of the personality changes reported in multiple sclerosis consist essentially of the mood changes described above, with or without an element of blunting or indifference attributable to intellectual deterioration. Over and above this there is little firm evidence that multiple sclerosis makes a specific imprint on the personality. Braceland and Giffin (1950) found that it was rather the reverse — in the early stages the patient's reaction was shaped by factors in his own premorbid personality and reflected his habitual modes of response to incapacity or stress. Much could also depend on the particular functions impaired and their significance in personal, marital, economic and environmental terms.

In consequence a great variety of reactions may be seen. Some patients become anxious and depressed from the outset, others irritable and others withdrawn. Some seek to belittle their disability and continue to strive in the face of hardship, while others readily accept a dependent role.

Pratt (1951) could discern no special form of personality change which distinguished multiple sclerosis patients from controls with other organic diseases of the nervous system. Surridge (1969) found that irritability, and to some extent apathy, occurred much more frequently than in muscular dystrophy controls, both tending to coexist with intellectual deterioration. Such changes resulted in great distress to the relatives and were not infrequently the reason why the families could no longer bear the burden of the patient's care.

Harrower (1950, 1954) produced one of the few pieces of evidence which suggest that multiple sclerosis patients may come to manifest certain personality traits with unusual frequency. The results were largely derived from a battery of psychological tests including the Rorschach. A large group of patients was compared with independent control groups—normals, emotionally disturbed patients, parkinsonian patients and patients with poliomyelitis. As a group the multiple sclerosis patients appeared to be unusually willing to adopt the dependent role, to show an absence of anxiety and a minimum of inner conflict. They showed excessive cordiality and a tendency to view the world through rose-coloured spectacles. Though emerging clearly in group comparisons these traits were not universal. On comparing early and advanced cases, Harrower found that the amount of anxiety related to the disease was inversely correlated with the extent of the physical handicap. The foregoing observations therefore probably owe much to the presence of brain damage.

Psychoses

The rarity with which multiple sclerosis patients are admitted to psychiatric hospitals has often been noted (Malone 1937; Pratt 1951). This, however, may be largely because their physical disability prevents the seriously disturbed behaviour which would warrant hospitalisation. Nevertheless psychotic illnesses have been described in the disease, sometimes late in the course but occasionally as a presenting feature.

Malone (1937) reported 10 cases of multiple sclerosis complicated by psychosis—four with dementia associated with outbursts of rage and paranoid beliefs, three with recurrent episodes of psychotic depression, two with hypomania and one with paranoid schizophrenia. Galli-neck and Kalinowsky (1958) reported three patients, one with severe depression, one with catatonia and one with paranoid schizophrenia, all responding successfully to electroconvulsive therapy and appearing to be essentially unrelated to the neurological disorder. They also commented on short-lived organic psychotic reactions developing in the course of the disease. Patients showing alternating mania and depression in association with multiple sclerosis were described by Crémieux et al. (1959) and Whitlock and Siskind (1980).

With regard to schizophrenia Davison and Bagley (1969) identified 39 acceptable cases in the literature, 27 with paranoid–hallucinatory and 12 with hebephrenic–catatonic illnesses. The symptomatology did not differ appreciably from that of other schizophrenic psychoses, except that expansive delusional states seemed to be particularly common, and neurological symptoms such as paraesthesiae were sometimes incorporated into paranoid–delusional systems. The psychoses often developed early in the disease, tending to cluster around the time of the first appearance of neurological abnormalities. This, along with the rarity of a family history of schizophrenia, suggested that the central nervous system disease and the psychosis might not be entirely independent. There was no indication, however, that the overall prevalence of schizophrenia in multiple sclerosis exceeded chance expectation.

Feinstein et al. (1992a) report an attempt to explore the possible contribution of brain pathology to psychotic illness by comparing groups of 10 patients with and without psychosis. These were well matched for age, disability, duration of disease and disease course. The psychoses were equally divided into two broad categories of schizophrenia and affective psychosis. By Present State Examination criteria two had nuclear schizophrenia, two schizoaffective psychosis and one paranoid psychosis; four had mania and one psychotic depression. In all cases the neurological disorder had preceded the onset of psychosis, the mean interval being 8.5 years. On MRI scanning there was a trend for the psychotic group to have a higher total lesion score, particularly in the periventricular regions and in the areas surrounding the temporal horns bilaterally. This reached statistical significance when the left temporal horn and adjacent left trigone areas were combined. Such findings point to a possible aetiological role of brain pathology in contributing to psychotic developments. No differences could be determined in this respect between the schizophrenic and affective psychotic groups.

Presentation with psychosis is rare, but sometimes the neurological abnormalities are so overshadowed by the mental picture that the true diagnosis is missed. Such cases are obviously important. Parker (1956) reported a patient who became apathetic and withdrawn in his early twenties and was diagnosed as suffering from schizophrenia. He showed slight hesitancy of speech and irregular nystagmus but this was ignored at the time. Attempts at treatment and rehabilitation met with no success. A few years later he was fatuous and childish, and by then showed impairment of memory, gross spasticity and pronounced incoordination. He died suddenly and the pathological changes of multiple sclerosis were revealed.

Geocaris (1957) reported four instructive examples of patients admitted with an initial diagnosis of psychosis, three with schizophrenia and one with severe depression, who showed evidence of multiple sclerosis a few weeks or months later. A careful review of the past history in each case showed that symptoms referable to the central nervous system had in fact occurred months or years before the onset of the psychiatric disorder.

Mur et al. (1966) reported three unusual examples in patients over 50 in whom psychotic features dominated the course. One had a paranoid psychosis for 5 years before neurological symptoms appeared in the form of a spastic paresis with dementia; another had a relapsing paranoid syndrome for 11 years accompanied by ataxia of gait and intellectual impairment; and the third had a temporary gait and speech disturbance at the onset of a depressive syndrome which dominated the picture until death. In all three cases the plaques were found to be predominantly in the cerebral hemispheres.

Finally, two patients reported by Matthews (1979) are important in drawing attention to the possibility that acute mental disturbance, remitting completely, may sometimes be the initial manifestation of the disease:

In the first patient, a girl of 19, the presentation was with intermittent confusion and episodes of markedly bizarre behaviour, leading to a diagnosis of probable schizophrenia. No neurological abnormalities were apparent on examination. Epileptic fits developed during a course of electroconvulsive therapy, leading to lumbar puncture which revealed mild pleocytosis in the cerebrospinal fluid. The EEG was diffusely abnormal, and she was treated with phenytoin. Over the course of the next few weeks she recovered completely, the EEG also reverting towards normality. Thereafter she remained well for 3 years. Symptoms typical of multiple sclerosis then made an appearance, the disease following a relapsing and remitting course over the next few years.

The second patient developed depression of acute onset at the age of 24. She became increasingly withdrawn, self neglectful and intermittently incontinent of urine and faeces. The tendon reflexes were noted to be increased in the lower limbs and the plantar responses were extensor. Examination of the cerebrospinal fluid showed abnormalities compatible with multiple sclerosis and the EEG showed a marked excess of slow activity bilaterally. Her mental state varied greatly. At times she was almost normally communicative; at others she gave bizarre replies to questions and had outbursts of shouting and kicking. Treatment with prednisolone led to gradual neurological and mental improvement, the patient becoming entirely normal some 3 months from the onset. Several months after recovery she developed unilateral optic neuritis and bilateral abnormalities of the visual evoked responses, clearly indicative of multiple sclerosis.

The question of possible presentations with psychiatric disorder is clearly of great interest, not least in pointing to the need for neurological examination and a comprehensive review of the past medical history in psychiatric patients. Particular interest would attach to presentations without organic features in the mental state. In a careful review of 91 patients with multiple sclerosis from a defined region of New Zealand, Skegg (1993) found that 19 had been referred to psychiatrists before the disease was diagnosed, often with non-organic symptomatology. Only in two cases, however, did a link between such symptoms and developing multiple sclerosis seem plausible. Skegg's review highlights the difficulty of reaching firm conclusions on the issue.

Hysteria

The relationship between hysteria and multiple sclerosis has absorbed a good deal of attention. In the early stages considerable difficulty can sometimes arise in making a firm diagnostic differentiation. Later in the established disease hysterical conversion reactions have been claimed to be especially common. It has been argued that there may be some fundamental relationship between the two disorders, with common antecedents and perhaps even shared pathophysiological mechanisms. Support for these ideas has not, however, been forthcoming.

Brain (1930) suggested that hysterical conversion symptoms, in the form of paresis and ataxia, seemed to occur more often in multiple sclerosis than with any other organic disease of the nervous system. In two of his cases he noted that hysterical fugues had occurred early in the course of the illness. Pratt (1951), however, could find no evidence that hysteria was a characteristic feature of the disease. In fact conversion hysteria was observed only twice in his series of 100 patients, compared to three examples in controls suffering from other disorders of the nervous system.

Wilson (1940) discounted any special relationship between multiple sclerosis and hysteria and suggested that when conversion symptoms were present this was mere coincidence. But he recognised a 'subjective' or 'predisseminated' type of multiple sclerosis in which the symptoms were solely subjective, and where a diagnosis of hysteria was apt to be made. Typical complaints included paraesthesiae, difficulty in using a limb, giddiness, fatiguability or general shakiness, all unbacked by unequivocal signs of organic nervous disease. Suspicion might nonetheless be aroused by minimal signs such as a defective abdominal reflex, nystagmoid jerking or transient ankle clonus.

Herman and Sandok (1967) reported a patient who illustrates the diagnostic difficulties that can arise, and the impossibility of separating psychogenic from organic symptoms at a certain stage in the disorder. In retrospect conversion symptoms clearly coexisted along with active multiple sclerosis, both aspects relapsing when the patient was subjected to emotional stress:

A 20-year-old enlisted man became homesick and reported to the army doctor with complaints of staggering gait, weakness, numbness and paraesthesiae. On examination he showed astasia abasia, poor coordination easily corrected by reinforcement, decreased sensation in all modalities, 'giving way' on testing muscle strength, and entirely normal reflexes. Examination of the cerebrospinal fluid showed 9 lymphocytes/ml but otherwise laboratory studies showed no abnormalities. The disorder was considered to be non-organic and he was transferred to a psychiatrist who found emotional immaturity and belle indifference. He improved suddenly and dramatically, though many minor complaints persisted.

A few months later he was again admitted with a diagnosis of a conversion reaction, complaining of shocks down his body on neck flexion (Lhermitte's sign). He became asymptomatic when told that he would not be returning to the Far East. Next year after an emotional upset with his father he developed numbness of the left cheek, recurrence of Lhermitte's sign and dragging of the left foot. Examination showed left hypalgesia of non-anatomical distribution, motor weakness of a non-organic type, a bizarre shuffling gait and classic belle indifference. Over the following week, however, severe neurological deterioration occurred with abundant organic signs characteristic of multiple sclerosis. Thereafter he had an episode in which vibration sense was split over the sternum, skull and spine, in association with a hemisensory deficit with transition at the midline.

Premorbid personality

The premorbid personality of multiple sclerosis patients has usually been found to be unremarkable, though certain authors have suggested that there may be a characteristic profile. From a study of 26 patients Grinker et al. (1950) concluded that the majority had shown emotional immaturity throughout their adult lives. An excessive need for affection was coupled with a paramount desire to please and be approved. Frustrations and negative feelings were accordingly repressed, leading to inner tensions. Such a view may, of course, be largely the product of observations on a selected group who have engaged in detailed psychotherapy.

Control studies have produced divergent results. Pratt (1951) compared 100 multiple sclerosis patients with 100 controls, matched for age and sex and suffering from other diseases of the nervous system. He could find no evidence that the premorbid personality was in any way remarkable. Dynamic formulations were not attempted, and comparisons were restricted to certain personality categories and traits. No differences emerged between patients and controls in relation to Sheldon's personality types, the incidence of neurotic traits, or the amount of aggression as measured by the Thematic Apperception Test. No differences were found in the frequency of good or bad childhood environments or of periods of separation from the parents.

Philippopoulos *et al.* (1958), however, produced very different results which are more in line with Grinker *et al.*'s observations. Forty multiple sclerosis patients were compared with 40 controls, matched for age, sex and social background (17 healthy controls and 23 suffering from cervical spondylosis and other cord disease). Striking differences were noted — 70% of multiple sclerosis patients had had unhappy childhood backgrounds compared with 20% of the controls, and only 55% were socially well adjusted premorbidly compared with 85% of controls. Detailed observations suggested that the majority of the multiple sclerosis patients had been emotionally and sexually immature, and deficient in long-term goals. Almost all showed conflicts over aggression and an inordinate need for affection. Forty-five per cent showed hysterical, anxiety or obsessive–compulsive symptoms, 30% showed personality disorders, 10% had been psychotic or borderline psychotic, and only 15% could be regarded as emotionally well adjusted. Thus although no specific personality type emerged, multiple sclerosis appeared to be a disease which occurred predominantly in chronically anxious persons who had shown evidence of emotional immaturity. The implication of these findings, if confirmed, remains uncertain, but the personality constellation described would certainly lead the subjects to be unusually vulnerable to emotionally traumatic experiences, and as described below it is possible that these may influence the course of the disease.

Influence of emotions on the disease

Physical and emotional traumas have often been regarded as precipitants of multiple sclerosis, or as provocative factors which help to determine relapses. Braceland and Giffin (1950) noted that all types of emotional situations tended to be blamed in this way by patients, but judged that most of the psychological precipitants described were unlikely to be significant.

Pratt (1951) attempted to examine the situation in detail. Thirty-eight per cent of multiple sclerosis patients had had some emotional stress in the months antedating the onset, compared with 26% of controls suffering from other nervous system disease. The difference fell just short of statistical significance, but in most cases the stresses had not been unduly severe. With regard to later relapses 25% were preceded by emotional stress, a figure virtually identical with the proportion of controls who had stress antedating their illness. Thus in the group as a whole there was no clear evidence to incriminate emotional factors in causing relapses.

In individual cases, however, a suggestive relationship was sometimes observed. In one patient a relapse occurred within an hour of receiving bad news by letter. In another numbness developed in the legs immediately after a narrow escape from a motor cycle accident, and in another the right arm became useless the morning after breaking off an engagement. Short of major relapses some patients found that emotional disturbances led to transient exacerbation of the symptoms of a pre-existing lesion. This was significantly commoner than among the controls, and the examples were often clear-cut and impressive, usually occurring within minutes of the emotional upheaval. In different patients, for example, worry led invariably to increased unsteadiness, anger to weakness of a leg, fear or quarrelling to weakness of the legs lasting several hours, self consciousness to blurring of vision or exacerbation of diplopia. Pratt suggested that such associations were possibly mediated by vascular mechanisms.

Philippopoulos *et al.* (1958), in the study already outlined, obtained more definite evidence of emotional precipitation, both of the initial manifestations and of subsequent relapses. Eighty-eight per cent of multiple sclerosis patients had had traumatic life experiences preceding the onset, compared with only 17% of the controls with neurological disease. Ten per cent had had an acute emotional trauma, the other 78% prolonged emotional stress, the common feature being the arousal of anxiety. Philippopoulos *et al.* tentatively proposed that exacerbations of multiple sclerosis might be occasioned by emotionally conditioned vasomotor responses or other physical or chemical changes in the central nervous system.

More recent studies have further supported the role of stress. Warren *et al.* (1982) compared 100 multiple sclerosis patients with neurological and rheumatological controls, finding that the former reported more life events during the 2 years prior to onset, and had more often felt themselves to be under unusual stress during that period. Franklin *et al.* (1988) gathered life event data at 4-monthly intervals on 55 consecutive patients with relapsing–remitting disease. Those who reported negative and/or uncontrollable events were almost four times as likely to have a relapse as those who did not.

The most decisive evidence, however, has been produced by Grant *et al.* (1989) who employed the sophisticated Life Events and Difficulties Schedule developed by Brown and co-workers for use in other contexts (Brown & Harris 1978; Brown 1989). This consists of a structured interview which probes systematically for life events and difficulties, sets them in context and focus, and allows ratings in terms of both short- and long-term threat. A cohort of 39 patients was studied, 23 during their first documented episode of the disease and 16 during later relapses. At the time of the interview 16 patients knew of their diagnosis while 23 did not. The interviews concentrated on circumstances during the year preceding the onset of major symptoms. Healthy controls were matched case for case in terms of age, sex, marital status and socioeconomic position.

Over three-quarters of the patients had experienced 'marked life adversity' as rated by the schedule during the 6 months prior to onset, compared with a third of the non-patients. Sixty-two per cent reported 'severely threatening life events' compared with 15% of controls. Both of these differences were highly statistically significant. 'Marked difficulties' had occurred in 49% of patients and 20% of controls. There were no substantial differences between patients experiencing first episodes and those with relapses, nor between those who knew or were unaware of their diagnosis.

When analysed bimonthly, approximately the same proportion of patients and controls had experienced severely threatening events during the preceding 7–12 months; but from 5–6 months onwards there was a marked upswing in the patients, adverse events increasing considerably by 2 months prior to onset. The data were interpreted by the authors as possibly reflecting perturbation of an already unstable immunological system in certain patients, thus accounting for the timing of their symptom exacerbation.

If these findings are accepted, on-going social and psychological support will have an especially important part to play in the management of patients, and may sometimes serve to avert or delay relapses.

Schilder's disease (diffuse cerebral sclerosis, encephalitis periaxialis diffusa)

The generic term 'diffuse cerebral sclerosis' has been applied to a variety of conditions in which widespread demyelination and gliosis occur in the white matter of the hemispheres. Histological examination allows a more precise classification, and it seems that reported cases have included examples of familial leucodystrophy and subacute sclerosing leucoencephalitis in addition to cases pathologically related to multiple sclerosis (Greenfield & Norman 1963). Greenfield and Norman suggest that the latter is the most appropriate restricted use for the term Schilder's disease. Nevertheless some believe that it represents no more than an exceptionally severe variety of multiple sclerosis occurring in early life (Compston 1993). In many previously reported examples in males, the patients were probably suffering from adrenoleucodystrophy (p. 754).

Most cases have been reported in children but adults may also be affected. Both sporadic and familial examples are encountered. The varied neurological manifestations include spastic paraparesis, sensory changes and often progressive cerebral blindness. Central deafness may also occur. Mental functions are affected early and severely, dullness and apathy progressing to dementia and stupor. Acute and widespread demyelination may cause cerebral oedema, raised intracranial pressure and papilloedema (Compston 1993). The disease usually runs a rapid course with death within a few months, though some patients survive for 2 or 3 years. Temporary remissions have been described, and very occasionally recovery (Ellison & Barron 1979). The cerebrospinal fluid shows changes resembling those of multiple sclerosis. Brain imaging usually shows a characteristic picture, with symmetrical, sharply defined, low density lesions in the occipital or frontal regions.

Pathologically the brain shows large areas of brownish or greyish softening in the white matter, usually maximally involving the occipital lobes and spreading forwards through the hemispheres symmetrically (Greenfield & Norman 1963). Affected areas are irregularly rounded and do not encroach on the cortex. Similar focal areas may be found in the brain stem. Microscopically they show complete demyelination, and in the older lesions axonal destruction as well. Astrocytic proliferation is marked. Shrinkage in chronic lesions may lead to local dilatations of the ventricles. In the smaller lesions the picture is indistinguishable from that of multiple sclerosis.

Psychiatric aspects

A point of psychiatric interest has been the occurrence of pictures indistinguishable from schizophrenia in patients who have later shown Schilder's disease at autopsy. Several such reports have now accumulated, mostly in patients who had displayed little or nothing by way of neurological disturbance during life. The cerebral pathological findings were in consequence usually unexpected.

Ferraro (1934, 1943) reported two examples in adolescent boys who had been clinically diagnosed as suffering from hebephrenic schizophrenia. In the first the disorder progressed over 2 or 3 years without neurological abnormalities or features indicative of an organic psychosis at any stage. The second showed fleeting and inconstant neurological abnormalities early in the illness, and obvious intellectual deterioration during the months immediately preceding death 3.5 years later.

Holt and Tedeschi's (1943) patient showed a classic catatonic picture and died within a week. There were no abnormal neurological signs. He had had a previous episode of acute catatonic schizophrenia 18 years previously. Roizin et al.'s (1945) patient similarly showed a picture of catatonic schizophrenia, with auditory hallucinations and periods of stupor alternating with outbursts of impulsive destructive behaviour. There were again no neurological abnormalities and the patient died within a few weeks. Jankowski (1963) described a chronic example in a man of 28 with repeated hospitalisations over 4 years prior to death. Severe affective changes of hebephrenic type developed gradually and without discernible intellectual deterioration. Late in the illness the pupillary reactions to light were lost and he complained of impaired vision, but the cerebrospinal fluid remained normal.

Ramani (1981) has reported yet another example, this time diagnosed by CT scan during life and subsequently confirmed by biopsy:

A man of 34 had suffered from chronic schizophrenia, refractory to treatment, for 5 years. It had started with mood swings, leading on to progressive withdrawal, disorganisation of thinking, and paranoid delusions and hallucinations. He showed bizarre posturing at times and echolalia. There was no family history of schizophrenia. On examination the only neurological abnormalities were bilateral extensor plantar responses and a suggestion of a snout reflex. The CT scan showed large symmetrically situated low density areas in the frontal regions.

In most of these examples the accent of the pathological process was on the frontal lobes of the brain, in contrast to the usual predominant involvement of the occipital lobes. This may have accounted for the atypical presentation and development of the disease.

Tuberous sclerosis (tuberose sclerosis, epiloia)

The classic picture of tuberous sclerosis includes the triad of mental subnormality, epilepsy and adenoma sebaceum. Associated abnormalities may include benign visceral tumours of the heart, kidney or intestine, also retinal tumours (phakomas) which appear on ophthalmoscopy as flat oval or circular patches of a greyish-white colour. These are composed of neuroglia. Other congenital defects may be present such as hare lip or spina bifida. Bodily growth is often considerably retarded. Gomez (1991) discusses the diagnostic significance of the varied clinical manifestations which may present for attention.

The disorder appears to represent a combination of developmental abnormalities of some tissues and overgrowth of others commencing early in foetal life. Ectodermal, endodermal and mesodermal structures can all be involved. It occurs familially with autosomal dominant inheritance, though some two-thirds of cases appear to be due to new mutations (Webb & Osborne 1992). The responsible gene lies on chromosome 9, with weaker evidence for an alternative gene on chromosome 11. However, several pedigrees are negative for both of these loci, confirming that genetic heterogeneity must exist.

Clinical manifestations

The first clinical manifestations are usually in infancy or childhood. Epilepsy or mental defect are the common presenting features. All varieties of epilepsy may be seen—grand mal, petit mal, Jacksonian seizures or temporal lobe seizures. In severe cases the presentation is frequently with infantile spasms (West syndrome, p. 242). However, patients are increasingly reported who first come to attention much later in life, sometimes on account of late-onset epilepsy or sometimes when characteristic skin lesions or X-ray signs have been discovered. Thus it is now recognised that abortive and incomplete cases are perhaps almost as common as the fully developed major disease; epilepsy and adenoma sebaceum may occur without mental defect, or cerebral forms without skin manifestations, or monosymptomatic forms showing adenoma sebaceum alone or visceral tumours alone.

The adenoma sebaceum consists of yellowish-red or brown papules and nodules, chiefly in the nasolabial folds and sometimes extending in a butterfly distribution over the cheeks and bridge of the nose. The name given to the rash is a misnomer since the papules consist largely of hyperplastic connective and vascular tissue (angiofibromas). More critical to the diagnosis are 'hypomelanotic macules', seen typically as leaf-shaped dull white patches, particularly over the trunk and buttocks (Rogers 1979). These may be detected even from infancy by screening with a Wood's lamp which emits light of the appropriate wavelength. Other skin changes may include small pedunculated dermal tags, café-au-lait patches similar to those of von Recklinghausen's disease, and 'shagreen patches' consisting of irregular areas of raised roughened skin several inches in diameter.

In general the earlier the disorder becomes apparent the more rapid is the course. When the disease is declared in childhood it is usually progressive, often with death in the second or third decade. Death is likely to result from status epilepticus, cerebral tumour or renal disease. Exceptions are seen, however, and even the fully developed disease may undergo long periods of apparent arrest. Patients with partial forms may survive with little disability into old age.

The cerebral changes may be detectable radiologically. Skull X-ray may show numerous discrete irregular intracranial calcifications ('brain stones'). Air encephalography could reveal nodular protrusions into the ventricles as a characteristic 'candle guttering' effect. CT scanning is now the investigation of choice for early confirmation of the diagnosis (Houser & McLeod 1979). Calcified subependymal nodules encroaching on the ventricles are the most valuable sign; ventricular dilatation, hamartomatous foci, cortical tubers or astrocytomas may also be seen. More pathological detail is apparent with MRI though the calcifications are less clearly visualised (Houser et al. 1991).

The EEG is usually abnormal in patients with mental subnormality or currently active epilepsy, but can be quite normal in others. No specific pattern is diagnostic. In general it provides a good indication of the severity of cerebral dysfunction. Westmoreland (1979) reported abnormalities in 85% of 138 patients. Epileptiform features were most common but a great variety of other changes occurred. The abnormalities were related to the age of onset of seizures and to the severity of mental subnormality.

Pathology

The striking pathological change in the brain consists of pearly white nodules, 0.5–3 cm in diameter, situated along the ventricular surfaces and sometimes over the cortical surface as well. The nodules are hard, like rubber or potato (hence 'tuberous') and may contain minute calcareous fragments. Histologically they contain dense glial material and curious large cells which are thought to derive from undifferentiated spongioblasts. Frank neoplastic changes may be apparent in the form of glioblastoma multiforme or spongioblastoma. Short of this the nodular protrusions are occasionally sufficiently large to obstruct the flow of cerebrospinal fluid within the ventricles. The intervening brain tissue is often markedly disorganised with abnormal cytoarchitecture, reduction of

neurones and increased gliosis. The cerebellum and cord may be similarly affected.

Psychiatric aspects

In addition to the disabilities which result from epilepsy the principal psychiatric manifestations are intellectual impairment, sometimes progressive, and psychotic disorders.

Mental retardation usually dates from the earliest years of life, but some patients are normal in the early years and then deterioration sets in. The degree of impairment varies from severe subnormality to mild retardation, affecting a high proportion of children in some series (Curatolo et al. 1991). An unusually high incidence of autism has also been reported.

However, examples of the condition are now recognised in which there is no intellectual impairment at all. Kofman and Hyland (1959) reported a man of 62 who showed adenoma sebaceum, a phakoma in the left retina, intracranial calcification and focal epilepsy, but whose intelligence was normal. The adenoma sebaceum had first been noticed at 26 and the fits at 31. There had been no clinical progression over the years that followed. Duvoisin and Vinson (1961) reported three cases, one with an excellent scholastic record and the others with IQs within the average range. Two had presented with unrelated disorders and were diagnosed on account of adenoma sebaceum and intracranial calcification; the third had epilepsy and the air encephalogram showed characteristic intraventricular masses. Other patients dying suddenly with epilepsy have been found to show the characteristic brain changes when these were not at all suspected during life. Among 160 patients reported from the Mayo Clinic approximately one-third proved to be of normal intelligence (Gomez 1979).

Intellectual defect or deterioration may be complicated by marked emotional instability or behaviour disorder. Psychotic pictures are quite commonly seen. Thus Critchley and Earl (1932), reporting institutionalised patients, described the essential psychological feature as a combination of intellectual defect with a 'primitive form of catatonic schizophrenia'. The intensity of the psychosis was independent of the degree of intellectual impairment, though the two were so inextricably intertwined that the relative parts played by each could be difficult to determine. Similarly, Brain et al. (1951) concluded that most epiloic patients finally reached a mental condition comparable to advanced schizophrenia. However, it is now clear that psychotic developments, like the mental defect, are by no means as invariable as these writers believed. Nevertheless the following case reported by Zlotlow and

Kleiner (1965) illustrates the type of schizophrenia-like picture that may be encountered:

The patient had fits from the age of 4 to 7 years but thereafter excelled at school. Pimples developed on the nose and cheeks from 15 onwards. In adolescence he became shy, solitary and withdrawn, and at 20 a severe mental change occurred — he became nervous and easily upset, with frequent tantrums and childish unreasonable behaviour. Seizures became frequent and he appeared slightly dull mentally. Adenoma sebaceum was by this time well developed, the EEG showed abnormalities over the left hemisphere and the air encephalogram showed slight ventricular dilatation.

The mental condition worsened, with fear of leaving the house, feelings that he was losing control of his limbs, and beliefs that people were laughing and talking about him. In hospital at 23 he was retarded, emotionally dull and spoke slowly in whispers. He denied auditory hallucinations but saw 'moving pictures' before his eyes. The IQ was low (70) with evidence of deterioration. He remained seclusive and withdrawn, with frequent mood swings, irritability and overactivity.

At 34 he was regarded as a chronic schizophrenic, often incontinent, speaking incoherently and with long episodes of mutism. Periods of irritable excitement alternated with catatonic stupor. He remained essentially unchanged over the following years. Skull X-ray now showed small calcifications in the pineal region and a number of globular vacuoles in the frontal and temporal bones. The EEG showed much disorganised slow activity. He was untestable psychometrically.

Neurofibromatosis

The neurofibromatoses comprise a number of related conditions characterised by skin pigmentation and tumour formation at a number of sites. Most features arise in tissues of neural crest origin and Schwann cells are the principal components in tumour formation. By far the most common form is von Recklinghausen's disease, now labelled NF_1, with the characteristic development of peripheral neurofibromas. The related disease, NF_2, can lack distinctive skin manifestations and typically presents with bilateral acoustic neuromas (Schwannomas). All other variants are considerably rarer.

Both NF_1 and NF_2 are inherited as autosomal dominants, though in both approximately half of cases represent new mutations. The gene for NF_1 lies on chromosome 17 and has now been identified precisely and cloned (Wallace *et al.* 1990; Marchuk & Collins 1994); that for NF_2 has been localised to chromosome 22 (Rouleau *et al.* 1987; Rouleau 1994).

Clinical manifestations of NF_1

The major defining features of von Recklinghausen's disease consist of café-au-lait spots, peripheral neurofi-

bromas and Lish nodules. However, much of the morbidity and mortality in the condition are dictated by additional complications involving many body systems. Diagnostic criteria have been put forward by the National Institutes of Health and can be of particular importance in genetic counselling (NIH Consensus Development Conference 1988).

The café-au-lait spots are brown macules of varying size which appear during childhood, most affected persons having at least six. Those over 0.5 cm in diameter in children and 1.5 cm diameter in adults are of significance. They may be accompanied by freckling in the axillary or inguinal regions. The peripheral neurofibromas usually develop around the time of puberty and gradually increase in size and number with age. They are largely composed of Schwann cells together with perineural fibroblasts and smaller numbers of other cells. Dermal neurofibromas, derived from terminal nerve branches in the skin, appear mainly on the trunk as soft discrete nodules varying in diameter from a millimetre to several centimetres. Nodular neurofibromas are situated on peripheral nerve trunks and have a firmer consistency. Lish nodules are pigmented hamartomas of the iris, best seen on slit lamp examination.

Other features of less diagnostic significance include macrocephaly in almost half of patients, and short stature in perhaps a third (Huson 1994). Campbell de Morgan spots consist of tiny cherry-red skin angiomas. Slight clumsiness and certain aspects of facial appearance also seem to be characteristic. Riccardi (1981) reported that 30–40% of patients showed speech impediments by way of hypernasality, slowing or imprecise pronunciation. Headaches of various types are common.

Several of the complications that develop involve the nervous system. Plexiform neurofibromas consist of large subcutaneous swellings with ill-defined margins, sometimes causing enlargement of part of the face or a limb and often producing marked cosmetic deformity. Those involving peripheral nerve trunks can be painful. They occasionally undergo malignant change to neurofibrosarcoma. Other complications include spinal root and cranial nerve neurofibromas, malignant change in peripheral nerve neurofibromas, and gliomas particularly of the optic nerve and chiasm. Aqueduct stenosis may lead to hydrocephalus, and there is a small increased risk of epilepsy. Meningiomas are uncommon except in NF_2.

Tumours affecting other parts of the body include rhabdomyosarcoma, phaeochromocytoma and carcinoid tumours of the duodenum. Neurofibromas may be found in the viscera, mediastinum, oral cavity or larynx, sometimes with serious consequences. Skeletal abnormalities include scoliosis, vertebral scalloping, and pseudoarthrosis of the distal long bones. Some 6% of patients develop hypertension.

Neuropathology

In addition to the pathologies described above, the brain may show subtle abnormalities on detailed examination which reflect cortical dysgenesis (Wiestler & Radner 1994). Disturbances of cytoarchitecture are common, with random orientation of neurones and disarray of cortical lamination. Neuronal heterotopias in the subcortical white matter appear to result from disturbed cell migration during embryogenesis. Gyral abnormalities may be seen such as pachygyria or polymicrogyria.

Focal subependymal glial proliferations may project into the ventricular system or contribute to aqueduct stenosis. Areas of fibrillary gliosis have been described in the cerebellum and adjacent leptomeninges, also scattered micronodular vascular proliferations. Neuropathological features of this nature could be relevant to the mental retardation encountered in a proportion of subjects (see below).

Psychiatric aspects

Intellectual impairment has long been recognised in a proportion of subjects with von Recklinghausen's disease though severe degrees of handicap are rare. Ferner (1994) concludes that the majority of persons with NF$_1$ have IQs in the low average range, with about 8–10% scoring below 70. Some, however, can show superior academic ability. Performance IQs tend to be considerably lower than verbal IQs, and specific learning difficulties appear to be common.

Children with NF$_1$ often show underachievement at school. Language development is sometimes delayed and a high proportion have difficulties with reading and writing. In Huson et al.'s (1988) survey in southeast Wales, 10% of 124 patients had attended special schools and a further 17% had required remedial class teaching. Neuropsychological evaluation has shown special problems with language, visuospatial tasks, memory and sustained attention, also difficulties with organisation and planning. Impairments are common with both gross and fine motor coordination in the absence of detectable neurological lesions. Behavioural disorder has also been stressed in childhood, with hyperactivity and impulsive and aggressive tendencies.

In Rosman and Pearce's (1967) autopsy study, abnormalities of cerebral architecture and white matter heterotopias were prominent in all patients with intellectual impairment, with less marked changes in those of normal intelligence. However, MRI studies have shown little relationship between intellectual ability and such features as high intensity lesions on T$_2$ images, suggesting that the cerebral basis of impairment is too subtle to be detected by this means (Ferner 1994).

Other psychiatric disorders have received little attention in neurofibromatosis despite the psychological burden which many subjects must bear. The disfigurement occasioned by the disease can be a grave social handicap, especially when the face is involved. Puzzled or hostile reactions from others are frequently encountered and social ostracism occasionally results.

Despite this the majority of patients seem to be reasonably well adjusted and severe psychiatric disturbance appears to be rare. Samuelsson (1981) reviewed the earlier literature which stressed apathy and depression, also personality disturbance and psychotic states, but these were often in specially selected patients. Samuelsson's own survey involved a thorough psychiatric examination of the 74 cases known to the health services in Gothenburg. Almost a third were considered to suffer from mental illness in some degree, and 13 had had treatment in psychiatric hospitals. The most common diagnoses were of depression, alcoholism and anxiety. One patient showed social phobia. The patients with mental illness were more often mentally retarded than those without, and showed a significantly increased frequency of neurological abnormalities reflecting central nervous system involvement.

Other common complaints were of hostile feelings, sleep difficulties, tiredness and aches and pains. The condition had sometimes had a considerable impact on the patients' lives, including avoidance of sports and other exposures in public, sensitivity about remarks from others, or fear of the nodules becoming malignant. Several patients had decided against procreation.

Samuelsson's study was uncontrolled. Hughes (1994) and Ferner (1994) report an unpublished survey of 103 patients with NF$_1$ which showed that diagnosed psychiatric illness was no more common than in controls matched for age and sex. Moreover there was no significant increase in anxiety and depression as measured by the Spielberger Anxiety Trait Inventory for Children or the Hospital Anxiety and Depression Scale. One-third of the patients had experienced hostile reactions from strangers because of unsightly neurofibromas. The rates of marriage were similar to that of the control group despite such cosmetic problems.

Riccardi (1981) suggests that the psychological burdens experienced in the disease are among the most important elements for patient care. In particular he stresses that frank discussion of the various features and complications serves to decrease adverse concerns, and provides a realistic context for making future decisions.

Friedreich's ataxia

Friedreich's ataxia is the commonest of the spinocerebellar ataxias and one of the commonest of the hereditary diseases of the nervous system. It occurs both sporadically and familially, several siblings sometimes being affected together. Among unaffected family members abortive forms may be found, sometimes showing little more than pes cavus or kyphoscoliosis. The mode of inheritance is recessive, the abnormal gene lying on chromosome 9 (Harding 1993b).

Clinical features

The onset is typically in the first or second decades of life. Unsteadiness of gait may at first be mistaken for the clumsiness of adolescence. With progression the gait becomes broad based and lurching, action tremor appears in the arms and titubation may develop in the head. The trunk may eventually be implicated rendering even sitting difficult.

Nystagmus is present in a fifth of cases, and the speech is dysarthric. Cerebellar dysfunction shows also in generalised hypotonia and asynergia of movement. Weakness and wasting sometimes develop distally in the limbs and the tendon reflexes are eventually lost. The plantar responses are up-going, however, indicating pyramidal tract involvement. Sphincter control is usually unaffected until late in the disease. Posterior column changes are manifest in defective vibration and position sense though other sensory modalities are usually intact. Rombergism is detectable early on.

Characteristic deformities with kyphoscoliosis or pes cavus are found in almost all cases, the latter sometimes long antedating other manifestations. Optic atrophy occurs in about a quarter of cases and sensorineural deafness in 10% (Harding 1993b). Myocardial involvement is common and diabetes is prone to develop.

The disease pursues a slowly progressive course though in occasional cases long stationary periods are encountered. Incomplete and abortive cases also occur in which the condition is static or progresses very slowly indeed. In the typical case severe incapacity with inability to walk is reached within 15 years of onset. Few patients live more than 20 years after the disease is declared, though survival into the sixth or seventh decades is not unknown (Harding 1993b).

Pathology

The brunt of the pathology falls on the long ascending and descending tracts of the cord. Degeneration is most marked in the posterior columns, spinocerebellar tracts and pyramidal tracts. Fibrous gliosis replaces the atrophied fibres. Atrophy may also be seen in the dorsal roots of the cord and the tracts and nuclei of the lower brain stem. The peripheral nerves show loss of large myelinated fibres and segmental demyelination. Purkinje cell loss has been reported in the cerebellum, also atrophy of the dentate nuclei and superior cerebellar peduncles (Oppenheimer 1976, 1979). It can be hard to distinguish primary degenerative changes from those secondary to circulatory disturbances arising from the patient's cardiac disease. The myocardium may show hypertrophy of muscle fibres and fibrosis.

Psychiatric aspects

Psychiatric interest in the disorder has centred chiefly on the intellectual impairment noted in some patients, and on the severe mental disturbances that occasionally arise.

Intellectual impairment has been reported in some series of patients but not in others. The conflicting evidence, reviewed by Davies (1949a), is probably attributable to the differing criteria used for the diagnosis of Friedreich's ataxia and for distinguishing it from other forms of heredocerebellar ataxia.

Friedreich himself noted an absence of mental defect in his cases, but later workers suggested that a considerable proportion showed mental deterioration, possibly associated with an extension of the pathological process to the cerebral cortex. Bell and Carmichael (1939) reviewed 242 families from the literature and noted that mental impairment had been present in almost a quarter. This varied in degree from idiocy to mild dullness, the grade of defect tending to be similar in different retarded members of a given family. Severe retardation appeared mainly to be confined to family members afflicted with the neurological disorder, and had usually been conspicuous from the early stages. Sjögren (1943) concluded that 15% of 84 cases showed oligophrenia and 58% progressive dementia.

Davies (1949a), in a careful study of 20 patients, found no case with mental defect of severe degree. The range of intelligence test scores suggested that mental impairment was no commoner than in the general population, the mean IQ of the group being 101. Some patients, however, showed impairments in recent memory, attention and concentration, with lower scores on the progressive matrices than on a vocabulary test. Similar findings did not emerge in a control group of chronic invalids suffering from rheumatic and cardiac disorders. Davies concluded that Friedreich's ataxia patients are initially no different intellectually from the general population, but that as a group they tend to show mild but significant cognitive decline. This appeared to set in early and then be non-progressive, in that it showed no correlation with age or length of illness.

Personality abnormalities are sometimes marked and an association with juvenile delinquency has occasionally been noted. Some of Davies' patients were extremely irritable with episodes of mute, resentful behaviour, while others showed a surprising contentment and serenity (Davies 1949b, 1949c). A tendency to deny or belittle their disability was sometimes evident. One patient, for example, showed a lofty superiority in the face of severe handicap and affected disdain for a similarly affected sister. Occasionally there was excessive preoccupation with religion or a turning towards mystical modes of expression.

In a disease which appears so early in life it is hard to assign a precise aetiology to personality abnormalities. Davies concluded that the predominant traits were often related to the effect of a disabling disease upon a particular personality, rather than being in any way specific to the illness. Environmental factors appeared to be important, especially in patients confined to home and exposed to the dominance of parents or siblings. Nevertheless the frequent presence of theta rhythms in the EEGs suggested that the disease process may also have interfered with normal cerebral maturation and thus contributed to the personality disturbances shown.

Psychotic developments have also been recognised in patients with Friedreich's ataxia. Many different forms of abnormal mental state are described, but mostly in isolated cases so that the overall incidence is hard to assess.

The form that has attracted most attention is a schizophrenia-like illness characterised by paranoid delusions and outbursts of excitement. Davies (1949b) described a patient who illustrates many of the features stressed in the literature — aggressive impulsive behaviour, paranoid beliefs, nocturnal hallucinations and episodes of clouding of consciousness:

A boy of 15 came from a family in which two members showed pes cavus and two others were subject to attacks of depression. He developed scoliosis, ataxia and titubation of the head at 13. At 15 he became stubborn and irritable, started housebreaking and absconded from home. Four months later he tried to poison his father and bought a rope with which to hang his stepmother. Later that month he was found wandering in a state of confusion.

He had been observed to behave strangely at school where, following a retrosternal 'feeling of excitement', he would bang desks and shout for several minutes, subsequently having no recollection of this behaviour. In bed he had seen visions before falling asleep, often of a diminutive man in ruffles and buckled shoes who would utter the word 'Transformation'.

On admission to hospital he showed advanced features of Friedreich's ataxia, was unhappy and tearful, and claimed that his father and stepmother were plotting against him. Attention, concentration and memory were unimpaired. During 4 months in hospital he remained paranoid and subject to sudden outbursts of rage. The EEG was grossly abnormal with theta waves predominantly in the right temporo-occipital region. Towards the end of his stay he suddenly became euphoric, denied his hatred of his family and was discharged.

He worked well as a laboratory technician for 6 months then again had a fugue-like episode. One month later he attacked his family, threw vitriol over a neighbour, and was committed to a psychiatric hospital.

Such severe psychotic pictures have sometimes been labelled 'Friedreich's psychosis'. It seems unlikely, however, that they are in any way specific for the disease. Some appear to be schizophrenic illnesses, occurring in families already prone to schizophrenia, whereas others may represent the paranoid hallucinatory states of temporal lobe epilepsy. Davies (1949b) and Davison and Bagley (1969) review the evidence available, which is insufficient to decide whether or not any fundamental relationship with organic cerebral disease can be upheld.

Other disturbances which may be encountered include depressive episodes, often reactive in nature and responsive to treatment, and episodes of clouding of consciousness intimately related to epileptic disturbances (Davies 1949b).

Motor neurone disease
(amyotrophic lateral sclerosis)

Motor neurone disease (or amyotrophic lateral sclerosis) is a disorder of unknown aetiology, commoner in males than females and beginning usually between the ages of 50 and 70 years. It consists of a combination of muscular atrophy of lower motor neurone type together with spasticity due to corticospinal tract damage. The precise clinical picture depends on the relative prominence of symptoms of upper and lower motor neurone lesions.

The onset is insidious, usually with atrophy of the small hand muscles. The thenar and hypothenar eminences are often the first to be affected. Slow progression comes to involve the arms and legs symmetrically, atrophy being accompanied by prominent fascicular twitching. Spasticity is usually most marked in the legs, with hyperactive reflexes and up-going plantar responses. The combination of upper and lower motor neurone signs is highly characteristic, exaggerated tendon reflexes being found along with considerable muscular atrophy. There are no sensory changes and the sphincters are rarely affected.

Sometimes atrophy is seen alone without spasticity (progressive muscular atrophy). Sometimes the accent is on the bulbar nuclei from the outset (progressive bulbar palsy), with atrophy and fasciculation of the tongue, paralysis of the vocal cords and difficulty with deglutition and articulation. Lesions of the corticospinal tracts above the medulla frequently produce an added element of 'pseudobulbar palsy' with loss of emotional control, a hyperactive jaw jerk, and spastic dysarthria and dysphagia.

The course is invariably progressive, but the rate varies from case to case. Most patients survive for 2 or 3 years but rarely longer, death resulting from bulbar involvement or weakness of the muscles of respiration. Very occasionally patients are encountered in whom the course is unusually benign. The disappointing results to date of trials of numerous therapies are reviewed by Orrell *et al.* (1994).

The pathological changes consist of degeneration of the anterior horn cells and lateral tracts of the cord with secondary gliosis. The motor nuclei of the brain stem and the pyramids in the medulla also show progressive degeneration. The motor neurones of the cord contain filamentous inclusions and dense bodies which stain with anti-ubiquitin antibodies (Leigh *et al.* 1988; Leigh 1994). Affected muscles show denervation atrophy. In the brain there may be loss of Betz cells and degeneration of the pyramidal layers of the precentral cortex. It would appear that in a considerable proportion of patients abnormal gliosis can be detected in the cortex and subcortical nuclear masses, with atrophy sometimes particularly affecting the frontal lobes (Brownell *et al.* 1970; Hudson 1981).

Information about aetiology is scanty. Toxic, nutritional and metabolic factors have been considered but no firm evidence has been forthcoming. An apparent excess of the disorder in workers in the leather industry has raised the possible role of exposure to solvents (Hawkes *et al.* 1989), and viral infection has been suspected though on indirect grounds (Kelley-Geraghty & Jubelt 1994). Persons with a past history of poliomyelitis may develop new motor neurone deterioration many years later but are not at increased risk of the disease itself (Dalakas 1994). Abnormal glutamate levels have been detected in the brain and spinal cord, also antibodies against gangliosides in a considerable proportion of cases. The significance of all such findings remains, however, uncertain (Harding 1993b).

Some 5–10% of patients have a similarly affected relative, and in occasional families there is a clear pattern of autosomal dominant inheritance. In some such kindreds the gene has been localised to chromosome 21, with mutations sometimes involving the superoxide dismutase gene (Rosen *et al.* 1993). In the majority of cases, however, genetic factors do not appear to be influential. An exception lies in the island of Guam, and neighbour-

ing islands in the Western Pacific, where there is an astonishingly high prevalence of the disease, sometimes with marked familial occurrence. Even so some exogenous factor is thought to be likely in addition to genetic susceptibility. The disorder in Guam bears a close relationship to the 'parkinsonism–dementia complex' as discussed further below (p. 708).

Psychiatric aspects

Precipitation of the disease by physical or emotional trauma has occasionally been suggested but without good evidence (Grinker & Sahs 1966). The majority of patients appear to show little by way of psychiatric disturbance, except perhaps for understandable depression due to their progressive incapacitation, or emotional lability resulting from pseudobulbar palsy. Scattered examples of patients with paranoid or schizophrenic psychoses have been reported, though there is little reason to view such disturbances as an integral part of the disease. Dementia is rare, though increasingly recognised in some degree as discussed below.

Emotional lability and loss of emotional control may be prominent when an element of pseudobulbar palsy is part of the picture. Out of 101 cases Ziegler (1930) reported explosive laughing or crying in 19, all except one of whom had signs of brain stem involvement. Several patients described clearly that their subjective emotional state was at variance with such reactions. One patient, in addition to weeping spasmodically, was prone to violent and uncontrollable outbursts of rage.

Depression in the course of the disease is reported to be common by some observers but surprisingly rare by others. Brown and Mueller (1970), for example, studied 10 patients intensively and found that though all knew about the prognosis none of them spontaneously expressed despair and hopelessness. The lack of depressive affect was sometimes bizarre when patients were discussing their progressive deterioration. Others sought to deny the implications of their disease and went to great lengths to ignore their disability. In premorbid personality and life style Brown and Mueller found indications of an habitual pattern of active mastery over the environment, and a life-long tendency to exclude unpleasant affects from conscious awareness.

Houpt *et al.* (1977), however, were unable to support these impressions in a larger, more representative group. One-third of their patients scored as moderately depressed on the Beck Depression Inventory, and more than a fifth warranted a clinical diagnosis of depression at interview. Hogg *et al.* (1994) have reported the results of a questionnaire survey of 52 patients, finding high scores on the Hospital Anxiety and Depression Scale. Almost half of the sample could be considered depressed, this being significantly related to the severity of physical impairments and dependence on others.

Occasional examples of dementia and psychotic illness in association with amyotrophic lateral sclerosis were reviewed by van Bogaert (1925), Wechsler and Davison (1932) and Davison and Bagley (1969). Dementia is clearly rare, the great majority of patients appearing to retain unimpaired intellect throughout. Careful testing may nonetheless reveal deficits in memory and frontal lobe function, even in patients who are superficially intact (David & Gillham 1986; Ludolph *et al.* 1992). Cortical blood flow and glucose metabolism, especially in frontal areas, have been shown to be reduced on single photon emission tomography and positron emission tomography (Goulding *et al.* 1990; Ludolph *et al.* 1992). Kew *et al.* (1993b, 1993c), using PET, have demonstrated abnormal patterns of activation in prefrontal and other brain areas in response to motor tasks, this being especially marked in patients who perform poorly on frontal lobe tests.

Hudson (1981), Ferrer (1992) and Kew and Leigh (1992) review the literature on patients who develop overt dementia and/or parkinsonism along with the disease. The occurrence of dementia has recently gained increased recognition, being mostly of frontal lobe type (p. 463). Mental features of behavioural, emotional and memory disorder set in insidiously, usually some 6–12 months before wasting begins. However, the two may evolve concurrently, or the wasting may precede the dementia. The clinical picture is typical of other frontal lobe dementias except for its rapid course. The patient is characteristically euphoric and disinhibited, and restlessness and impulsivity are common. Progressive language difficulties lead to stereotyped phrases, echolalia and ultimately mutism, while perceptual and spatial functions usually remain intact. Some patients develop gluttonous behaviour and hypersexuality (Neary *et al.* 1990). In the presence of cognitive impairment the motor manifestations tend to involve the tongue and proximal upper limb muscles predominantly, while the hands and legs are spared, so that the patient remains mobile until late in the disease. A familial incidence has sometimes been noted.

The pathological changes accompanying the dementia are those described on p. 465. Spongiform changes may be apparent in the superficial cortical layers, and it is likely that many cases formerly classified as an amyotrophic variant of Creutzfeldt–Jakob disease (p. 479) were suffering from the present condition. The conjunction between amyotrophic lateral sclerosis and parkinsonism–dementia in the island of Guam (see below)

appears to be different, in particular showing the histopathological hallmark of neurofibrillary tangles.

Paranoid and schizophrenia-like syndromes are likewise rare and probably usually reflect a chance association. Some may represent acute organic reactions to drugs or to coincident metabolic disturbances and infections. Others may have been precipitated in predisposed persons by the non-specific stresses of coping with the disability.

Amyotrophic lateral sclerosis and the parkinsonism–dementia complex of Guam

Amyotrophic lateral sclerosis has been found to occur with extraordinary frequency among the indigenous Chamorro population of the island of Guam in the Western Pacific (Kurland & Mulder 1954). Here the prevalence is 100 times greater than in the USA. Cases tend to occur familially but no clear pattern of inheritance has emerged. In the same population a syndrome characterised by parkinsonism and progressive dementia is also found (Lessell *et al.* 1962), and it is now recognised that the two essentially represent different facets of the same disease process. Both also occur in the neighbouring islands of the Mariana group and in the Kii peninsula of Japan.

The amyotrophic lateral sclerosis is indistinguishable from the classic disease apart from its tendency to be associated with parkinsonism and dementia. The onset also tends to be at a younger age and the course more protracted. The 'parkinsonism–dementia complex' presents with memory deficits and a slowing of mental and motor activity, and progresses to generalised dementia with extrapyramidal rigidity. Some patients develop psychotic disorders in the later stages with delusions, hallucinations and hostile destructive behaviour.

A re-evaluation of 176 patients from Guam confirmed the close interrelationships between the two disorders (Elizan *et al.* 1966). Of the 104 who presented initially with amyotrophic lateral sclerosis, five developed parkinsonism–dementia complex on average 5 years later, five developed parkinsonism alone and two an organic mental syndrome without parkinsonism. Of the 72 who presented with parkinsonism–dementia complex, 27 developed amyotrophic lateral sclerosis on follow-up. In the families concerned, amyotrophic lateral sclerosis and parkinsonism–dementia complex often occurred indiscriminately and in various combinations, giving further evidence of a close relationship between the two syndromes.

The histological pictures similarly show a good deal of overlap. The parkinsonism–dementia complex shows diffuse cerebral atrophy with widespread neurofibrillary changes in the cortex and subcortical nuclei. Atrophy of the globus pallidus is characteristic, also loss of pigment from the substantia nigra (Hirano *et al.* 1961). The cases with amyotrophic lateral sclerosis show similar neurofibrillary changes throughout the brain in addition to the classic cord pathology (Hirano *et al.* 1966). Patients who have shown clinical features of only one syndrome are commonly found to show the pathological changes of both.

The interest in these disorders lies in the clues they might offer to aetiology. An exogenous cause is considered likely in addition to genetic predisposition, and two hypotheses have been explored in detail (Kurland *et al.* 1994). The seed of the cycad plant, used extensively in the Chamorro diet, is known to contain neurotoxins which can induce a not dissimilar picture in animals; and abnormal concentrations of manganese, calcium and aluminium have been detected in the soil and water of regions where the disease is endemic. Neither hypothesis, however, appears to provide a satisfactory explanation on present evidence.

Yase *et al.* (1972) have reported a patient with amyotrophic lateral sclerosis and the pathological changes typical of the combined syndrome who had shown schizophrenia for 5 years before the neurological symptoms were declared. The schizophrenia had fluctuated with periods of stupor and mutism, and was regarded by the authors as symptomatic of the organic cerebral changes.

Myasthenia gravis

Myasthenia gravis is a disorder of the voluntary musculature characterised by abnormal muscle weakness after activity and a marked tendency for recovery of power after a period of rest. It is commoner than chance among patients who have had hyperthyroidism, Hashimoto's thyroiditis or other autoimmune disorders. Thymic abnormalities are usually present in the form of thymus hyperplasia, thymic tumour (thymoma) or more rarely thymus involution. More than two-thirds of cases show characteristic thymic changes with large germinal centres in the medulla, indicative of B-cell activation and proliferation. There is now abundant evidence that the disease is essentially an autoimmune disorder in which circulating antibodies interfere with motor end-plate function (see below).

Clinical features

The disorder can begin at any age but usually appears in the second or third decades. It is more frequent in females than males until late middle age when the sex ratio is reversed. Walton (1993c) reviews the various clinical subtypes, differing in their associations with thymus abnormalities and various human leucocyte antigens (HLAs). The first complaint is usually of ready fatiguability of certain muscle groups, or some symptom of cranial nerve involvement such as diplopia, difficulty with chewing or difficulty with swallowing. The onset is sometimes insidious, sometimes sudden, and precipitation by emotional upset or a febrile illness is not uncommon.

Ocular muscles are usually involved early leading to ptosis or diplopia. Bulbar symptoms are also common, with difficulty in chewing or swallowing which worsens as the meal progresses, or a characteristic fading and slurring of speech after speaking for several minutes. Facial weakness may produce flattening and loss of wrinkles and the smile may have a characteristic 'snarling' quality. The muscles of the neck are often involved, also the shoulder girdles and flexors of the hip. In general proximal muscle groups are more severely affected than distal groups, and the arms more than the legs, but the distribution is variable. The respiratory muscles may fatigue easily on laughing or crying, and in crises of the disorder respiration can be dangerously embarrassed.

The muscular weakness is typically variable from day to day and sometimes from hour to hour. It tends to be worse towards the end of the day, but is sometimes paradoxically most marked on waking in the morning. Ultimately weakness of certain muscle groups may persist even when these have not been exercised for some time. Wasting is occasionally observed. The tendon reflexes almost always remain brisk even when weakness is severe, but may decrease on repeated elicitation. Objective sensory changes are absent but the patient may experience pain in the muscles of the neck and around the eyes, or complain of a feeling of stiffness or paraesthesiae in affected areas.

The course is extremely variable. It is usually slowly progressive but a number of cases prove to be relatively static. Spontaneous remissions and sudden relapses may occur. The 'active' stage is usually limited to the first 4–7 years, and the subsequent course then depends on the extent of disability reached during that period (Simpson 1964). After 10 years the condition appears sometimes to subside.

The diagnosis is usually confirmed by observing the response to anticholinesterase drugs. Edrophonium chloride (Tensilon) may be injected intravenously, with examination for increased muscle strength during the following 30–60 seconds. Electrophysiological tests include the demonstration of an abnormal decrement in compound muscle action potentials on repetitive motor nerve stimulation, or the more sensitive single-fibre electromyography which shows blocking or abnormal 'jitter' (i.e. variations in interpotential intervals). More recently it has become possible to measure the serum level of antibodies to acetylcholine receptors (AChRs) by radioimmunoassay and this provides a valuable indicator of the disorder (Vincent & Newsom-Davis 1985). Such antibodies are found in almost 90% of patients with adult-onset generalised myasthenia, but are lacking in a considerable percentage of cases when the disorder is restricted to the ocular muscles.

It is important to perform tomograms of the anterior mediastinum to detect thymic hyperplasia or the presence of a malignant thymoma, also chest X-ray to exclude bronchial carcinoma leading to the Lambert–Eaton syndrome (see below).

Pathophysiology

Myasthenia gravis has proved to be essentially an autoimmune disorder. The biochemical defect at the neuromuscular junction was at first thought to be due to competitive blocking by circulating antibodies which impaired the effects of acetylcholine at the motor endplate. It is now apparent that there is also damage to acetylcholinergic receptors at the postsynaptic membrane of the neuromuscular junction, brought about by antibodies directed against them (anti-AChRs). In addition structural abnormalities can be demonstrated at the motor end-plate itself; electron microscopy has shown widening of the primary synaptic clefts and simplification of the secondary synaptic clefts and folds (Santa *et al.* 1972; Jennekens *et al.* 1993).

Cultures of thymic lymphocytes from myasthenic patients produce anti-AChR antibodies *in vitro*, particularly those from patients with thymic follicular hyperplasia showing active medullary germinal centres (Ragheb & Lisak 1994). Moreover certain elements within the thymus share strong structural and antigenic similarities with muscle AChRs. It is therefore possible that an early step in pathogenesis consists of sensitisation of anti-AChR antibodies within the thymus itself. In this way evidence can be assembled to suggest that the thymus is involved not only in perpetuating the disease but perhaps in inducing it as well (De Baets & Kuks 1993).

Treatment

Anticholinesterase drugs remain the mainstay of treatment for patients with mild myasthenia or symptoms restricted to a small group of muscles. Neostigmine bromide (Prostigmin) may be given orally three or four times a day, or the longer-acting pyridostigmine bromide (Mestinon) which wanes more gradually. Atropine or propantheline may be needed to counteract muscarinic side effects. Subcutaneous injections of neostigmine methylsulphate may be necessary if absorption is erratic. Edrophonium chloride (Tensilon) has too brief an action for use as maintenance therapy.

More recent developments are summarised by Walton (1993c). There is an increasing tendency to use steroids, usually prednisone, in long-term maintenance therapy, sometimes along with anticholinesterase drugs in low dosage. Prednisone is generally regarded as the treatment of choice in ocular cases. Immunosuppressive agents such as azathioprine or cyclophosphamide are also employed, sometimes meeting with dramatic success. Prednisone and immunosuppressives may be given together in preparation for thymectomy or in patients not suitable for surgery. Plasmapheresis can be remarkably beneficial, but is reserved for patients not responding to other treatments or for use in an emergency. High dose intravenous immunoglobulin G (IgG) has been shown to be temporarily effective in rapidly deteriorating patients with bulbar symptoms and respiratory insufficiency (Durelli 1994).

Thymectomy should be carried out in all patients with radiological evidence of thymic enlargement. This operation was once controversial, but Simpson's (1964) survey showed that it led to a lowered mortality and a greater chance of improvement or remission when compared to medically treated patients. The results were best in patients without thymoma or when the duration had been less than 5 years. Herrmann *et al.* (1963) found that young females benefited particularly. Now, however, it seems that men do just as well as women, and satisfactory outcomes can be observed even in patients of late middle age. The operation is generally thought not to be justified in purely ocular cases. The mechanism by which thymectomy benefits the disease remains uncertain. Improvement is usually accompanied by a fall in anti-AChR antibodies but this is not invariable.

Psychiatric supervision can have an important part to play in patients who develop marked psychological reactions to the disorder. As discussed below the emotional state of the patient may have a considerable influence on clinical progress. Meyer (1966) found evidence that in selected cases psychotherapy might facilitate remission. MacKenzie *et al.* (1969) recommend that in myasthenics who are pursuing a deteriorating course every attempt should be made to investigate and treat possible sources of emotional stress.

Other myasthenic syndromes

Other myasthenic syndromes may be induced by certain drugs, notably phenytoin, streptomycin and penicillamine. The latter in particular may be associated with a rise in anti-AChR antibodies and does not resolve when the penicillamine is withdrawn. *Transient neonatal myasthenia* may occur in children born to myasthenic mothers, usually resolving within weeks or months. *Congenital myasthenia* may be present from birth or become apparent during the first 2 years of life. A variety of anomalies involving acetylcholine and acetylcholinesterase have been demonstrated in such patients, some of the syndromes being familial (Engel 1994). *Juvenile myasthenia* can begin at any age from 12 months to 16 years and in general is similar to the adult disease.

The Lambert–Eaton syndrome is often associated with neoplasia, especially oat-cell carcinoma of the bronchus, sometimes developing several years before the neoplasm is apparent. Perhaps one-third of cases are non-neoplastic. Weakness and wasting, usually insidious, affect the proximal parts of the limbs and trunk, and ptosis and diplopia are not uncommon. Fatiguability is usually less striking than with myasthenia gravis, and autonomic symptoms such as dry mouth are common. Other differences are that the tendon reflexes are diminished or absent but reappear following a sustained muscular contraction, and there may be a 'reversed myasthenic effect' with progressive augmentation of strength during the first few seconds of maximal effort (Erlington & Newsom-Davis 1994). Circulating antibodies to AChRs are absent, but there is evidence of an IgG autoantibody which binds to voltage-regulated calcium channels at neuromuscular junctions. Anticholinesterase drugs lead to little improvement, but guanidine and 3,4-diaminopyridine are of benefit. Prednisone, azathioprine and plasma exchange may be useful in non-neoplastic cases.

Psychiatric aspects

Myasthenia gravis has attracted psychiatric attention on several grounds. Emotional factors have been thought to precipitate the onset in some cases and to play a significant role in aggravating the established disease in others. The psychological make-up of myasthenic patients and their responses to the illness have accordingly been studied in some detail. There is also a possibility that memory may be adversely affected in certain patients. Finally, important problems of differential diagnosis not infrequently arise, and can involve psychiatric as well as neurological disorders.

The psychological responses seen in the illness are discussed by Brolley and Hollender (1955), MacKenzie *et al.* (1969) and Sneddon (1980). The patient is faced with the task of adapting to a disease which produces neither physical deformity nor pain and which has ephemeral manifestations. Interpersonal difficulties may be aggravated by the anxiety and uncertainty which the symp-

toms evoke, and by the tendency for those around to become suspicious of the genuineness of the disorder when there is so little to observe objectively. Patients may be suspected of faking their weakness or of being drunk when the speech is slurred. Meeting strangers can be a source of social embarrassment when facial weakness prevents a smile, likewise eating in public when the jaw must be supported towards the end of a meal.

The individual's reaction to the disease appears to be closely related to his premorbid personality and shows the usual range of responses to physical incapacity. Anxiety can be very marked and the patient's life may come to centre around the schedules of medication. An increase in the dose is regarded as ominous while a decrease leads to fearfulness of symptoms returning. Other patients seek to deny their disability, reducing medication and embarking on too much activity. The dependency induced by the disease often sets in train further psychological reactions. Some patients regress and develop increasing dependence on relatives and doctors. An obsessional attendance on every detail of treatment may result. Others become severely depressed, or hostile and frustrated. The expression of anger is often blunted due to motor weakness so that effective relief from tension may be debarred (Hayman 1941).

Major mental illnesses may occasionally arise. Oosterhuis and Wilde (1964) found that three of 150 myasthenics suffered psychotic episodes of a depressive or schizophrenic nature. Dorrell (1973) reported a patient with recurrent episodes of schizophrenia, apparently in response to the stress of the disease in a person already predisposed to psychosis. Gittleson and Richardson (1973) described a typical paraphrenic illness in a man of 67, but commented on the surprising rarity of reports of schizophrenia in the literature.

The premorbid personality of myasthenics has been described as often unstable but there appear to be no controlled studies on the issue. A high proportion have been observed to come from abnormal backgrounds, or to have had prominent neurotic symptoms before the onset of the illness (Oosterhuis & Wilde 1964; MacKenzie *et al.* 1969). Oosterhuis and Wilde stressed a 'psychasthenic' character structure — overmeticulous, pessimistic in outlook, anxious and phobic — and found scores reflecting a high degree of neurosis on a personality questionnaire.

Precipitation by emotional stress finds wider acceptance by physicians of experience (Simpson 1964, 1968; Chafetz 1966). Specific emotional factors can often be discerned in close relation to the first appearance of symptoms, probably as a result of their aggravating the latent disorder and bringing it to attention. Oosterhuis and Wilde's

(1964) study of 150 cases showed that 8% had had some acute emotional disturbance directly preceding the onset. A further third had had a fairly long-lasting period of emotional stress coexistent with the onset, such as difficulties at work or marital infidelity. Again controlled studies will be necessary before the significance to be attached to these findings is known.

Aggravation by emotional influences has been widely reported once the disease is established. Simpson (1964) noted that double vision could be provoked by embarrassment, or ptosis by emotional disturbance. In Oosterhuis and Wilde's (1964) series 100 patients reported that emotional disturbances worsened their symptoms, 25 denied this and 25 were uncertain. In some cases an increase of ptosis could be observed in immediate response to an emotionally provoking question during the course of taking the history. Several patients had had acute respiratory paralysis in association with severe emotional upsets.

Meyer (1966) reported similar observations, including sudden cataplectic-like intensification of weakness in response to severe rage or fright, or sustained worsening over 1–2 days in patients prone to episodes of anxiety or depression. Some were vulnerable to repeated cycles of aggravation, with weakness provoking anxiety and resentment which in turn further aggravated the disability. MacKenzie *et al.* (1969) added further striking examples from the Mayo Clinic. Half of their 25 patients showed significant exacerbation of weakness following emotional upheavals, anger being the usual provoking factor. The worsening could last from a few minutes to several hours and often required a temporary increase in medication. Three patients showed a major increase in weakness persisting over a prolonged period of emotional tension—one for a week after her son's marriage against her will, another for a week after finalisation of a divorce, and another for 2 weeks after the death of a parent. Conversely improvement could follow when emotional tension was resolved. One patient had had a difficult life with her parents and lost both of them within 2 years; 4 months later the required dose of neostigmine had dropped from 40 to 25 tablets per day despite a full working schedule, and 5 years later, when happily married, she was needing very small doses indeed. Sneddon's (1980) patients had often needed to learn techniques for handling anger-provoking situations in order to remain well. Half, for example, left the room and lay down if they felt themselves becoming angry; others found that crying and swearing relieved the tension and caused less weakness.

The course of the illness can accordingly be seriously affected when emotional disturbance is severe. Collins (1939) reported a man of 24 with known myasthenia who became psychotic with overactivity, elation and paranoid delusions. He died from respiratory crisis 6 days later and the psychosis was regarded as contributing directly to his death.

Meyer (1966) proposed that the emotional reaction of an individual to his disease was an important factor in determining prognosis, and supported this with an impressive analysis of data. Of 99 myasthenics from the Johns Hopkins Clinic, 48 were judged to have had some significant emotional or psychiatric disturbance following the onset of the disease and 51 were without such problems. Follow-up 1–10 years later showed that 46% of the former had died compared to 26% of the latter. Fifty-eight of the survivors were then available for prospective study, 23 with psychiatric problems and 35 without. Over the next 14 years 39% of the former group died compared with 17% of the latter. Anxiety attacks appeared to be of particularly grave significance, increasing the mortality to almost 50%.

The degree of incapacity had been similar in the two groups at the start of the prospective period. Age group analysis showed that the excess mortality among emotionally disturbed patients was evident in each decade and maximal in the twenties and thirties. Further indication of the importance of emotional disturbance in contributing to mortality was obtained from the death certifications of those who had died. Myasthenia gravis had been assigned as the cause of death in five out of nine cases with emotional problems, compared to only one of six cases without.

Cognitive function does not appear to have been comprehensively studied in the disease, though it is possible that memory may be impaired to some degree. Tucker *et al.* (1988) compared 12 myasthenic patients with medical and healthy controls on a number of memory tests, and found significant impairments in both verbal and nonverbal memory. In a second study a myasthenic patient was tested before and after plasmapheresis on two separate occasions, each time showing improvement in memory functioning following the treatment. The authors ascribe such results to deficits in central cholinergic transmission in the disease, for which a certain amount of scattered and indirect evidence can be assembled.

Psychiatric aspects of differential diagnosis

Myasthenia gravis must be distinguished from other neurological disorders including ocular and peripheral neuropathies, brain stem lesions, parkinsonism, motor neurone disease and carcinomatous myopathy. From the psychiatric point of view mistakes may occur in both

OTHER DISORDERS AFFECTING THE NERVOUS SYSTEM 713

directions: patients with weakness and fatigue of neurotic or depressive origin may be suspected of the disease, or conversely patients with myasthenia gravis may initially be diagnosed as suffering from neurosis, conversion hysteria or personality disorder.

Complaints of weakness and excessive fatigue are commonly encountered in routine medical practice and many such patients are mistakenly suspected of myasthenia gravis. Grob (1958) estimated that 20% of patients referred to him as possible myasthenics were in fact suffering from emotional disorders. Schwab and Perlo (1966), in an analysis of 130 patients wrongly diagnosed as having myasthenia gravis, found that by far the greatest proportion (38%) were suffering from a 'chronic fatigue syndrome' attributable to some form of neurosis. Such a mistake is particularly likely to arise when an injection of neostigmine or edrophonium has produced a marked placebo response, and especially if the patient's report of improvement has not been backed by attempts to monitor muscle strength objectively. Sometimes improvement on oral medication alone is accepted as evidence of myasthenia and this can be seriously misleading. Once given the false diagnosis the patient may cling to it and resist attempts at discontinuing medication (Chafetz 1966).

It has been shown that occasional patients not suffering from myasthenia gravis will tolerate enormous quantities of anticholinesterase drugs without ill effect, in a manner previously considered possible in myasthenics only (McQuillen & Johns 1963; Johns & McQuillen 1966). Several such patients were reported, all complaining of weakness and fatigue but without objective signs to confirm it. Complaints of difficulty with chewing, swallowing or phonating were common, but objective evidence of bulbar deficits was uniformly absent. Most in fact had multiple complaints affecting several systems. The psychiatric diagnoses ranged from depression with hysterical features to psychotic illness. Studies of neuromuscular transmission showed no abnormalities, and no withdrawal symptoms followed stopping the drugs.

Examples of the diagnostic difficulties that can arise in this area are as follows:

A 21-year-old girl was diagnosed as suffering from myasthenia gravis. She had a history of fatiguability from the age of 5, and had noted dysphagia and difficulty with chewing since 20. Generalised weakness then forced her to take to bed. On examination ptosis was observed, varying in severity and improving with neostigmine or edrophonium injections. However, photographs showed that the ptosis had been present from the age of 12 months, and placebo injections were found to produce improved strength of grip. Repeat tests with parenteral neostigmine and edrophonium were without effect, and there was no increased

sensitivity to quinine or curare which would be expected in myasthenia gravis. The patient was ultimately diagnosed as suffering from hysteria and schizophrenia.   (Rowland 1955)

A nurse of 31 had been well until 18 months previously. She then suffered a respiratory infection, followed for 3 months by complaints of generalised weakness, diplopia and slurred speech. She returned to work but continued to be readily fatigued. One year before presentation the generalised weakness became progressively worse so that she was obliged to spend most of the day in bed. She improved and again returned to work but complained of difficulty in opening her eyes, diplopia, slurred speech and unsteady gait. An intramuscular injection of neostigmine produced marked improvement lasting 2 hours, but oral neostigmine had little effect. She was then demonstrated to improve markedly with saline taken from a box labelled 'Tensilon'. The issue was squarely faced, but the patient continued to insist that she had myasthenia gravis.   (Schwab & Perlo 1966)

Conversely the diagnosis of myasthenia gravis can easily be missed in the early stages or in mild examples, especially if there is a previous history or current evidence of neurosis. The influence of emotions on the weakness can suggest a psychological disorder, similarly the spontaneous fluctuations that tend to occur. Sometimes the emotional component in patients with true myasthenia gravis is so obtrusive that a clear response is obtained to a placebo. Oosterhuis and Wilde (1964) found that it was common for several months to elapse between the declaration of symptoms and the correct diagnosis, with an interval of more than 2 years in almost a fifth of patients. Mild and atypical cases had sometimes been regarded as hysterical or neurasthenic for 10 or 20 years. Nowadays with the availability of electrophysiological tests and assays for anti-AChR antibodies such mistakes should be a great deal less common.

Neurotic disorder may be suggested by the multiplicity of complaints or by certain characteristics of the early symptoms. An occupational 'cramp' or 'spasm' may be simulated when the initial complaint involves a muscle group which is particularly fatigued in the course of the patient's work (Simpson 1964). Or the first complaint may not be of fatiguability but of other perplexing symptoms. Minimal paresis of ocular muscles may result in 'mistiness' of vision rather than diplopia, slight facial paresis may lead to strange facial sensations, or slight bulbar paresis may produce a feeling of stiffness of the tongue or of something sticking in the throat (Oosterhuis & Wilde 1964). Conversion hysteria may be suspected in patients who develop sudden paralysis of the legs after exertion or sudden episodes of dyspnoea. Moreover patients may occasionally present with a combination of myasthenia gravis and psychiatric disorder as in the following example:

A woman of 36 complained of fatigue, difficulty with deglutition and double vision. She gave the following history. At 18 she had developed a right hemiplegia on waking the day after a violent quarrel with her stepmother. This had resolved over several months. At 20 she had developed difficulty with swallowing after a row with her stepmother, and this recurred thereafter whenever she was nervous. At 24 the right arm became weak after the birth of her child, progressing to total paralysis over 1 week then gradually improving over 3 months. This recurred temporarily after the birth of two subsequent children. At 35 she again noticed weakness of the right arm and leg, this time fluctuating in relation to rest and exertion, and later accompanied by diplopia and difficulty with swallowing.

When examined at the age of 36 she made a theatrical impression. She showed paresis of the left internal rectus, a right hemiparesis with normal reflexes, and a right hemihypalgesia. Neostigmine given by injection in the out-patient clinic caused the diplopia to disappear and enabled her to swallow more easily, but this failed to help when she was studied more closely as an in-patient.

Over the next few years her complaints of weakness, dysphagia and diplopia fluctuated in severity, but increased markedly at 40. She then showed multiple pareses of external ocular movements and a diffuse flaccid paresis of the limbs, right more than left. Placebos did not help but neostigmine produced a good response and thereafter she remained well on medication.

(Oosterhuis & Wilde 1964)

A further instructive example in which a mistaken diagnosis of psychiatric disorder was made was reported by Bail and Lloyd (1971):

A girl of 16 was sent to stay with an aunt because of increasing difficulties in her relationship with her mother. She complained of feeling tired and lacking in energy, and suddenly lost her voice during an emotional religious meeting. This happened several times thereafter. A few months later she developed difficulty in swallowing when her aunt and uncle were about to go on holiday. She required hospitalisation because of aspiration pneumonia and tube feeding became necessary on account of her refusal to eat. Nevertheless otolaryngological and neurological assessments revealed no abnormality and she was referred for psychiatric treatment. A diagnosis of hysteria with severe disturbance of personality and schizoid features was made. Her home background was noted to be disturbed and her mother schizophrenic. She had broken off relations with her boyfriend just before the aphonia began.

She gradually improved but anergia and feelings of weakness persisted. She was hospitalised for a second psychiatric opinion where she complained of seeing double and often treble. There was only a suspicion of general muscle weakness. However, close observation soon showed abnormal fatiguability, and two episodes of unequal ptosis occurred. Myasthenia gravis was eventually diagnosed and the response to neostigmine was excellent. Thymectomy was carried out 5 months later. On follow-up over the next 2 years she proved to be an attractive and outgoing girl with a stable job and a satisfactory relationship with her boyfriend.   (Bail & Lloyd 1971)

Rowland (1955) usefully summarized the clinical approach to be adopted in the diagnosis of equivocal cases. The disease must be considered likely in any syndrome of muscular weakness unaccompanied by alteration of reflexes or sensation and in which strength improves significantly in response to anticholinesterase drugs, except when strong evidence of psychogenesis is forthcoming. The diagnosis of myasthenia becomes more certain if there have been remissions in the past, if weakness is aggravated by fatigue and improved by rest, and if symptoms referable to the cranial nerves are prominent. Placebo injections are valuable prior to all therapeutic tests in equivocal cases, and these will nowadays be supplemented by electrophysiological and antibody tests.

Progressive muscular dystrophies

The progressive muscular dystrophies, or myopathies, comprise a group of genetically determined degenerative diseases primarily affecting the voluntary musculature. Different forms vary in age of onset, distribution of muscles affected and rate of progression. The principal varieties are to a large extent clinically and genetically distinct, though some degree of overlap is recognised. The attempt by Walton and Nattrass (1954) to ascertain all cases in Northumberland and Durham was important as a guide to relative frequency in the UK. Among 105 patients examined personally they found that 48 had pseudohypertrophic dystrophy, 18 limb-girdle dystrophy, 15 facioscapulohumeral, two distal, one ocular, 15 dystrophia myotonica and six myotonia congenita.

However, with present developments in molecular genetics the classification and clinical characterisation of the different forms has improved considerably, and traditional clinicoanatomical divisions are being revised. The common pseudohypertrophic variety, for example, was known to show differing modes of inheritance and to be clinically somewhat heterogeneous, likewise the limb-girdle and distal forms. Walton (1993c), from whom much of this account is taken, now proposes a clinicogenetic classification, the commoner varieties being as follows:

X-linked dystrophies may be divided into the severe (Duchenne) and the benign (Becker), also the rare Emery–Dreifuss type with humeroperoneal atrophy. *Autosomal dominant dystrophies* include facioscapulohumeral and distal varieties, and *autosomal recessives* limb-girdle and distal forms. These will be considered seriatim below. The *myotonic dystrophies* represent a separate group including dystrophia myotonica, myotonia congenita and paramyotonia congenita, and for convenience are described separately on p. 716 *et seq.*

Clinical features and genetics

The Duchenne form was formerly referred to as pseudo-hypertrophic dystrophy and remains the commonest variety. It is due to an X-linked recessive gene, but approximately one-third of affected boys are isolated cases due to presumed genetic mutation. It develops very occasionally in girls when there is a translocation between the short arm of the X-chromosome and some other chromosome; and a variant resembling limb-girdle dystrophy may also be seen in female carriers when one X-chromosome is partially inactivated ('lyonisation').

Duchenne dystrophy becomes apparent towards the end of the third year of life with difficulty in walking and climbing stairs, first affecting the pelvic girdles but soon the shoulder girdles as well. Enlargement of the calf muscles is characteristic, also sometimes affecting the quadriceps and deltoids. Most patients are unable to walk by the age of 10 and become confined to a wheelchair. Progressive skeletal deformity tends to develop as a result of atrophy and contractures. Death usually occurs from respiratory infection or cardiac failure; formerly few patients survived the second decade, but with modern supportive care many now live to their late thirties. Myocardial involvement is invariable but may not be detectable in the early stages. Characteristic changes are seen in the electrocardiogram in a high proportion of cases.

In 1987 the responsible gene on the X-chromosome was identified and cloned, proving to be one of the largest genes known in man (Hoffman *et al.* 1987; Koenig *et al.* 1987). The missing gene product, a protein known as 'dystrophin', is absent or present in only trace amounts in muscle tissue (Hoffman *et al.* 1988). Female carriers of the disease can be detected by DNA studies, complemented where necessary by serum creatine kinase estimations. Prenatal diagnosis of affected male foetuses is also possible (Emery 1993). The attempts that have been made to improve muscle performance by transplantation of normal muscle cells from unaffected relatives have given variable but mostly disappointing results (Dubowitz 1992).

The Becker form of dystrophy affects muscle groups in a similar distribution but is more benign. Onset is usually between the ages of 5 and 25 years and patients may remain ambulant for two or three decades. Though severely disabled some can survive to a normal age. It is about a third as common as the Duchenne form in incidence at birth, and is due to different defects in the same gene. Dystrophin is present but in reduced amounts and often of abnormal molecular size (Emery 1993).

Facioscapulohumeral dystrophy occurs equally in males and females, with onset at any time between childhood and late adult life. The facial and scapulohumeral muscles are the first affected, leading to winging of the scapulae and marked facial weakness which gives a characteristic pouting appearance. Muscular hypertrophy is uncommon. Spread may occur elsewhere, particularly to the anterior tibial muscles producing foot drop. Progression is variable, sometimes leading to severe disability after 20–30 years but sometimes following a benign course with periods of apparent arrest. It is inherited as an autosomal dominant, with the responsible gene now located to chromosome 4 (Wijmenga *et al.* 1990). Scapulohumeral dystrophy is similar but without facial weakness.

Distal muscular dystrophy is rare in the UK and USA but apparently not uncommon in Sweden (Walton 1993c). There it is inherited as an autosomal dominant, with onset usually in middle age. Weakness begins in the small hand muscles and lower legs then gradually spreads proximally. Rates of progression are variable. Autosomal recessive forms have also been described.

Limb-girdle dystrophy affects males and females equally, usually beginning in the second or third decades but sometimes as late as middle age. It is due to an autosomal recessive gene, but sporadic cases are common. Either the shoulder or the pelvic girdles may be affected initially, and enlargement of the calf muscles sometimes occurs. Distinction from the Becker form can be made by muscle biopsy with dystrophin staining. The rate of progression is variable but severe disability is usually present after 20 years.

In all varieties the tendon reflexes are diminished or lost in relation to affected muscle groups. All forms of sensation are intact. Histologically the affected muscles show great variation in the size of individual fibres and a large amount of connective and adipose tissue.

Psychiatric aspects

From the psychiatric point of view the issue which has attracted most attention concerns the level of intelligence of patients with muscular dystrophy, and the possibility that in some varieties intellectual retardation may be an integral part of the picture. There are obvious difficulties in attempting to assess the intellectual potential of children with severe physical handicaps, and in deciding whether educational backwardness should be attributed to innate deficiencies or to the psychosocial consequences of physical disablement. Nevertheless evidence increasingly favours the view that a substantial proportion of patients with the Duchenne form are of low intelligence. There are also indications that this may sometimes reflect cerebral involvement as part of the disease.

Earlier findings were divergent, but the situation has been clarified by psychometric testing. Allen and Rodgin (1960) found that half of their patients had IQs over 95 and half below; but in the latter group intellectual impairment was often severe. No correlation could be found between the degree of intellectual retardation and the severity of physical handicap. Worden and Vignos (1962) found that more than two-thirds of patients with pseudo-hypertrophic dystrophy had IQs below 90, with the total range extending from 134 to 46. The mean for the group was 83 compared to 100 for unaffected siblings. In a group of patients with myotonia congenita, who showed equivalent or even more severe physical handicap, the mean IQ was 118. Again no correlation could be found between level of intelligence and severity of disability, and performance had often been poor from the outset of schooling. Repeat testing on a group of children 2–3 years later showed no significant decrement in intellect as the disease advanced further.

Dubowitz (1965) reported a particularly careful study of 65 patients with pseudohypertrophic dystrophy, aged between 3 and 19 years, involving assessments of reading, writing, arithmetic and general knowledge. On such a basis 46% were estimated to be of average intelligence or above, 22% possibly retarded and 32% definitely retarded. Formal psychometric testing on a group of 27 long-term in-patients showed three with IQs above 100, seven more above 70, 14 between 50 and 70, and three below 50. Thus both scholastic and psychometric indices showed that more than half of the patients had intelligence well below the normal range. Three patients who had been diagnosed very early were followed by repeat testing at frequent intervals; at least one and possibly another showed some evidence of intellectual deterioration over time in that previously acquired skills were later lost.

Two possibilities have been considered to account for the intellectual dullness in such patients—a genetic component determining low intelligence and inherited along with the dystrophic tendency, or some biochemical disturbance that has affected cerebral development. Worden and Vignos (1962) proposed that the brain might be damaged at a vulnerable stage by a by-product of degenerating muscle, and Dubowitz (1965) suggested that there may be some biochemical abnormality which affects both brain and muscle. The latter explanation has received support from the demonstration that an isoform of dystrophin is expressed in the brain which is very similar in structure to muscle dystrophin (Chelly et al. 1990).

Whether or not this could prove to be the responsible factor remains controversial (Emery 1993).

Electroencephalographic evidence of cerebral abnormality has been reported in pseudohypertrophic dystrophy (Perlstein et al. 1960; Niedermeyer et al. 1965), also histological evidence of brain maldevelopment. Rosman and Kakulas (1966) made detailed autopsy studies of seven patients with pseudohypertrophic dystrophy, three of whom had documented evidence of mental retardation during life. One of the latter showed grossly visible malformations of cerebral development, two showed areas of thickened cortex with disordered cortical architecture (pachygyria), and all three showed microscopic 'heterotopias' indicative of arrest of neuronal migration during early development (p. 244). No such changes were apparent in dystrophic patients with normal intelligence.

Other psychiatric disturbances in myopathic patients appear to be surprisingly rare, perhaps because of the gradual process of adaptation which must take place from childhood onwards. Where children are educated together in special schools there is usually said to be little by way of serious behaviour disturbance or neurotic developments. Truitt (1955) found a remarkable absence of depression among 72 boys with pseudohypertrophic dystrophy, but noted a lack of personal identification with their own crippling. Morrow and Cohen (1954), however, found that half of their cases showed emotional immaturity, overdependence and intolerance of frustration, also a tendency to withdraw from people and the environment.

As adulthood approaches the psychosocial consequences of the disorder intrude increasingly, and the patient's psychological adjustment will often be decisively shaped by the milieu in which he lives. The strain thrown on the families of affected individuals may then be very considerable.

There does not appear to be any special association between non-myotonic forms of muscular dystrophy and psychosis, though occasional families have been reported in which schizophrenia and muscular dystrophy appear to coincide. Davison and Bagley (1969) summarize the scattered examples in the literature.

Myotonic dystrophies

In the myotonic dystrophies a variable degree of muscle wasting and weakness is combined with the phenomenon of 'myotonia', namely delayed relaxation of skeletal muscles after voluntary contraction. The commonest is dystrophia myotonica (Steinert's disease), in which the myotonia is accompanied by progressive wasting and weakness of selected muscle groups together with other characteristic features such as cataract, hypogonadism and frontal baldness. Myotonia congenita (Thomsen's disease) is a more generalised muscle affection with myotonia and hypertrophy, setting in very early in life but rarely progressing to serious disablement. Paramyotonia congenita is similar but with the myotonia and weakness appearing only on exposure to cold. Other myotonic disorders include a variant of myotonia congenita with onset later in childhood, and various forms of periodic paralysis which also show myotonic features. The position regarding the classification and interrelationships between these conditions is reviewed by Harper (1989).

Dystrophia myotonica

Dystrophia myotonica is one of the commoner myopathies and certainly the most frequent of the myotonias. It is of particular psychiatric interest because of the high prevalence of mental abnormalities reported in sufferers from the disease. Transmission is by autosomal dominant inheritance. The responsible gene is situated on chromosome 19, and shows an expanded trinucleotide repeat sequence in a similar manner to the gene determining Huntington's disease (p. 466). In the myotonic dystrophy gene the sequence is cytosine/thymine/guanine (CTG). Normal persons have between five and 27 such repeats, but affected persons may have 50–2000.

The discovery of the precise genetic abnormality has been of great importance in clarifying puzzling aspects of the condition. Thus it is widely variable in age of onset, ranging from the time of birth to middle or old age, and the severity of the clinical manifestations is strongly age related. When developing in childhood the muscle weakness is profound and mental retardation is common; presentations in adolescence and early adult life are characterised by myotonia and slowly progressive muscle weakness (the 'classic' form); and onsets in middle or old age may show minimal or even no muscle abnormality and may present with cataract alone. It is now apparent that much of this variability is attributable to the length of the unstable trinucleotide repeat, which has proved to correlate broadly with age of onset and disease severity (Harley et al. 1992b). An explanation is also provided for the phenomenon of 'anticipation', i.e. earlier and more severe appearance in the filial than the parental generation, since the length of the repeat is greater in successive generations. These discoveries stand to be of great value in genetic counselling, also in the differential diagnosis of congenitally abnormal children and of minimally affected persons. It remains unclear, however, why the severe congenital form of the disease shows virtually exclusive maternal transmission. No cases of new mutation have been proven (Harley et al. 1992a).

Clinical features

Males and females are equally affected. The commonest age of onset is between 20 and 25, and 50% of patients will have developed the disorder by this age (Harper 1989). However, the range covers virtually the whole life span as described above. The muscular symptoms in the classic form of the disease consist of a combination of myotonia, weakness, atrophy, and rarely hypertrophy.

The myotonia is usually the first symptom to be declared but is rarely sufficient in itself to lead to medical attention. It chiefly affects the hands, forearms and orbicularis oculi, though the legs may be implicated as well. It is best demonstrated by observing the slowed relaxation of hand grip, or the difficulty in opening the eyes after screwing them up tightly. Delayed relaxation may be noted in the tendon reflexes, or a groove may persist in the tongue after depressing it with a spatula. The smile is sometimes characteristically slow and lingering.

The myotonia is rarely a grave handicap. Involvement of the tongue can cause difficulties with articulation, or sudden falls may result from difficulty in adjusting balance after a trip or stumble. Aggravating factors include exposure to cold or prolonged inactivity. It is characteristically worse on waking and improves as the patient begins to move about. Caughey and Myrianthopoulos (1963) also stress that it is often aggravated by emotional factors such as fright or surprise. One of their patients first noticed the myotonia when his legs seemed to freeze while caught in a burning building, and another when his legs became stiff on the signal to start in a race. Fear, anger or sudden joy may temporarily increase the symptoms so that a wave of stiffness is felt to run through the muscles of the body. Another patient was liable to fall rigidly to the ground whenever she was suddenly excited or surprised. Several had become housebound because of fear of falls in the street.

The atrophy and weakness is selective, symmetrically affecting the facial muscles, masticatory muscles, sternomastoids and distal parts of the arms and legs. Hypertrophy can occur in the early stages but atrophy usually prevails. The facial appearance is characteristic with hollow temples, ptosis, a sad lugubrious expression and a tendency for the mouth to hang partially open. Finger grip is weak and foot drop may occur. The tendon reflexes are normal initially, though diminished or absent as the disease progresses. Sensory changes are rare, but slight sensory disturbances and subjective complaints of pain are occasionally encountered.

The progression of the disability is remarkably variable but usually slow. Rare cases may be completely disabled within a year or two, though most patients remain ambulant for 15–20 years or even longer. In general the muscle weakness and wasting will be much less severe in cases of late onset, and the prognosis can then be remarkably good. In the final stages respiration and swallowing may become embarrassed.

On pathological examination the affected muscles show variation of fibre size, fibrosis and fibre degeneration as in other dystrophic processes. A characteristic finding is multiplication of sarcolemmal nuclei which tend to form long central chains, also sarcolemmal aggregates of mitochondria. Changes have been detected in muscle spindles, with abnormal innervation to the intrafusal fibres and abnormally shaped end-plates (Harper 1989). Nevertheless earlier views that the disease might represent a neuropathy rather than a primary myopathy are no longer held, and such changes are thought to be secondary to splitting of the intrafusal fibres occasioned by the myotonia. Curare-like substances which affect the neuromuscular junction do not alter the myotonia, further suggesting that the basic defect is within the muscles themselves.

The congenital form of the disease differs in important respects from that encountered at later ages. Hypotonia and facial weakness can be present from birth, but myotonia is completely absent. Myotonia dating back to infancy should always suggest myotonia congenita. Talipes equinovarus and mental retardation are common, and in those who survive milestones are usually delayed. Several such infants die from respiratory failure during the first days of life, but once the neonatal period is over the prognosis for life is relatively good (Harper 1989). The hypotonia tends to improve, and the performance of most affected children is more limited by mental incapacity than physical handicap. By late childhood or adolescence, however, the 'adult' features of the disease appear, and death usually follows in early adult life.

Associated defects may involve a number of organs and systems of the body, emphasising that dystrophia myotonica is a generalised disorder with muscle abnormality being but one of its manifestations. Cataract is one of the commonest additional defects — in some series slit lamp examination has revealed lens opacities in almost every case. Other ocular abnormalities may include limitation of eye movements, retinal degeneration or partial constriction of the visual fields. Frontal baldness is common in males and occasionally occurs in females. Endocrine abnormalities include testicular atrophy and hypogonadism in the male, and menstrual abnormalities and infertility in the female. Pituitary–adrenal and thyroid abnormalities have occasionally been reported, also abnormalities of glucose metabolism.

Electrocardiographic abnormalities are found in more than half of patients, including varying degrees of heart block and atrial dysrhythmias. Cardiac failure or sudden death due to cardiac arrest may occur. Smooth muscle dysfunction can involve dilatation of the lower oesophagus, peristaltic incompetence of the small intestine, dilatation of the colon, or a flaccid bladder with urinary retention. Anaesthetics present a special risk, particularly of prolonged respiratory arrest following thiopentone. The serum immunoglobulins are often abnormally low. Skull X-ray may show general thickening of the vault, localised thickening of the frontal bones (hyperostosis frontalis interna), enlarged sinuses or a small sella turcica. Other congenital physical defects include a high narrow palate, hare lip or talipes equinovarus.

The associated abnormalities may sometimes be found as the sole manifestation of the disease among relatives. Such individuals must be regarded as likely to harbour the gene, but whether or not they will develop the disease is unpredictable. Bundey *et al.* (1970) discussed the question of genetic counselling in some detail, and showed that if offspring were still totally symptom-free by the age of 30 the risk of developing the disease was reduced from the usual 50% to 25%. They suggested that any first-degree relative of a patient who asks for genetic counselling should receive a careful neurological examination, supplemented by slit lamp examination for early cataract and electromyography for the detection of myotonic discharges. Electrocardiographic abnormalities and changes on skull X-ray proved less useful for the detection of asymptomatic gene carriers. The availability during recent years of DNA markers very close to the gene has greatly aided genetic counselling and permitted prenatal testing as discussed by Harper (1989). Further marked advances have resulted now that the gene itself has been cloned and sequenced.

Differential diagnosis and treatment

Differentiation from other forms of muscular dystrophy is important on account of the differing prognosis. It can usually be made on the basis of the characteristic distribution of weakness, wasting and myotonia, together with associated abnormalities in other systems as outlined above. The facial appearance may resemble that of facioscapulohumeral dystrophy, though there the limbs are affected proximally rather than distally. Myasthenia gravis may be suspected when ptosis and muscular fatigue are marked. Differentiation from myotonia congenita (see below) can be more difficult when onset is early in life, and indeed the two have sometimes been reported from the same family. Polyneuropathy may be suspected in view of the distal and symmetrical weakness. Peroneal muscular atrophy can usually be distinguished by the associated loss of vibration sense at the ankles.

Nothing can be done to prevent the weakness and atrophy progressing. The myotonia can be helped by several drugs — phenytoin, tocainide and steroids — but this is rarely sufficiently marked and disabling to require treatment. Quinine and procaine amide, which were formerly in vogue, should not be given if electrocardiographic abnormalities are present.

Psychiatric aspects

Psychiatric abnormalities occur in a high proportion of patients and complete the picture of the disease. Klein's (1959) survey from Switzerland showed psychological disorder in over a third of cases, chiefly mental retardation and personality disorder. Others have put the frequency higher and have stressed the social decline which marks families affected by the disease.

Impairment of intellect is common and sometimes severe. It appears to occur predominantly in patients who have developed the disease at a young age. Thomasen (1948) found that one-third of 101 patients with dystrophia myotonica had a 'considerable degree' of mental defect and only one-quarter could be considered of normal intelligence. In adults retardation was more marked when the disease had begun in childhood. In children it was sometimes so severe that they were institutionalised without the true diagnosis being recognised. Calderon (1966) found that almost 80% of children with the disease were mentally impaired in some degree. The deficits were sometimes found to precede the onset of physical disorder, and also appeared in other family members who had no evidence of the disease. Bird *et al.* (1983) tested 29 patients with the Wechsler Adult Intelligence Scale (WAIS) and the Shipley–Hartford Scale and found that one-third had low IQs while three had IQs of over 120. Limited cognitive ability correlated with severity of physical handicap and maternal inheritance of the gene. The most severely affected functions were immediate recall, abstraction and spatial manipulation. An association between intellectual deficit and severity of physical handicap has often been observed but is by no means invariable — severe mental defect may sometimes coexist with mild muscular involvement and vice versa (Zellweger & Ionasescu 1973).

The cause of the intellectual impairment is uncertain. The effects of coexistent hypothyroidism and other endocrine disorders would seem unlikely to play a major role. Genetic influences are probably mainly responsible, occurring as an integral part of the inherited disease process. Assortative mating may contribute further, since patients with dystrophia myotonica often tend to be of lower socioeconomic status and choice of marriage partner may be limited.

There is abundant evidence of cerebral involvement in the disease. Electroencephalographic abnormalities have been reported much more commonly than in other forms of muscular dystrophy. Barwick *et al.* (1965) found abnormal records in 61% of cases compared to 20% of controls, with theta and delta waves and sometimes focal sharp wave discharges. Lundervold *et al.* (1969) reported similar abnormalities in almost 50% of patients. Rosman and Kakulas (1966) found pathological changes in the brain at autopsy in three out of four patients examined, representing all three in whom mental deficiency had been noted during life. Two showed grossly visible malformations of cerebral development, two had areas of disordered cortical architecture, and all three showed microscopic heterotopias indicative of arrest of cortical migration of neurones during early development. The significance of the inclusion bodies detected in the thalamus and elsewhere in the brain by Culebras *et al.* (1973) and Ono *et al.* (1987) remains uncertain. Avrahami *et al.* (1987) carried out CT scanning on 24 patients and found diffuse brain atrophy in three and calcification of the basal ganglia in three. Microcephaly was common, also thickening of the calvarium.

There have been occasional indications, not only of poor initial endowment in the disease but also of deterioration from previous levels of functioning. These, however, have been mainly impressionistic reports. Maas and Paterson (1937) found that 17 of 29 adult patients were of low intelligence, 11 having been retarded from birth and six having deteriorated after normal performance at school. Walton and Nattrass (1954) reported that three of their 15 cases showed 'early evidence of dementia' and another three were themselves aware of slow deterioration of memory and intellect. However, longitudinal follow-up studies were not performed to check the validity of such observations. Bird *et al.* (1983) could not document definite decline in any of their 29 patients, and there was no deterioration on repeat psychometric testing in five cases after intervals of 11–19 years. Malloy *et al.* (1990) carried out a careful study of 20 patients between the ages of 20 and 65, stratified as to age and compared with controls matched for age and education. While the sample as a whole showed cognitive deficits, especially on non-verbal spatial tests, there was no evidence of an abnormal age-related decline. In contrast to the motor deficits, which clearly progressed, the cognitive impairments appeared to be relatively stable.

Serial studies with CT or MRI do not appear to have been carried out to examine the situation further. Using air encephalography Refsum *et al.* (1959, 1967) obtained some evidence of progression of brain atrophy over time in a small number of severely affected patients. The increase in ventricular enlargement appeared to correlate with evidence of clinical deterioration. Such ventricular dilatation could not be ascribed to ageing *per se* since the average age was rather lower in those with progression than those without.

Personality abnormalities and social deterioration are perhaps even commoner than defective intelligence. Thomasen (1948) and Caughey and Myrianthopoulos (1963) laid particular emphasis on reduced initiative and a 'carefree temperament', both of which could contribute directly to social decline. Occasional patients showed concern about their condition and became moody and hostile, but these reactions were exceptional. The great majority showed a surprising equanimity about their physical or social situation. Thomasen found that most were cheerful and rarely got angry despite miserable living conditions. Some were even prone to exaggerated self esteem, and considered they were managing excellently though physically disabled and leading a poor existence.

Reduced initiative was sometimes already obvious in childhood. The affected individual had typically been lazy and uninterested at school, and thereafter failed to complete training and accepted a lowly occupation. This could be noted in retrospect in patients who developed overt signs of the disease only later in life. Women became slovenly and negligent. Men were often content to sit idly at home when only mildly physically incapacitated.

Bird *et al.* (1983), however, have warned against stereotyping sufferers from the disease. They examined 29 patients and found that a third showed prominent personality abnormalities, mainly in the presence of low intellectual ability and advanced physical handicap. However, there was no 'typical' personality type, and the problems that emerged were largely what would be expected in persons with physical and cognitive problems. Unfortunately detailed and objective psychiatric studies appear not to have been carried out on more extensive samples of patients.

Somnolence may be a marked feature in the disease, adding to the impression of apathy and perhaps related to diencephalic dysfunction or alveolar hypoventilation. True fatigue is also prominent in many cases. But some of Thomasen's patients were unable to perform even very light work, and complained of fatigue far exceeding what would be expected from the degree of muscular involvement.

The social decline that can result is usually severe and could be traced in 70% of Thomasen's patients. Caughey and Myrianthopoulos (1963) encountered several families of distinction where the disease, within two or three generations, had led to a marked deterioration in family fortunes and social status. Perron *et al.* (1989) documented the socioeconomic impact of the disease in the Saguenay–Lac-Saint-Jean region of Quebec where it occurs with remarkable frequency. A representative sample of 218 affected persons over the age of 15 was compared with control data from the same population; only 12% were employed compared with 42% of controls, and the mean income for 1982 was reduced by almost two-thirds. The effect on the families was not surprisingly severe—43% were living below the poverty line, which was three times as common as in Canadian families generally.

Psychotic developments have rarely been reported and when they occur are probably coincidental. Maas and Paterson (1937) described one patient with a schizophrenia-like reaction, and one who became paranoid about his wife when impotent. In two others mild grandiosity became exaggerated into a state resembling chronic hypomania. Thomasen (1948) found no examples of psychosis among 101 patients.

Myotonia congenita

Thomsen (1876) gave a clear account of the disease that bears his name in four generations of his own family. Thomasen (1948) subsequently collected all cases in the literature and described three further families, resulting in a total of 157 families with 470 affected persons. It is nevertheless a rare disease. The pattern of inheritance is usually as an autosomal dominant though an autosomal recessive form has also been described. In both the dominant and the recessive forms the gene has been localised to chromosome 7 (Neuromuscular Disorders 1992). Males and females are affected equally.

Onset is usually from shortly after birth and few cases appear after the age of 12. Myotonia is typically the presenting feature and the sole cause of disability for many years. It presents as a painful stiffness or cramp on attempting voluntary movement, most marked after rest and especially troublesome first thing in the morning. The myotonia is widespread throughout the body muscles, unlike its regional distribution in dystrophia myotonica. Involvement of the tongue and jaw may lead to difficulty with speech, chewing and swallowing. Clumsiness on initial movement may lead to frequent falls. Exposure to cold aggravates it, also excitement, tension or emotional disturbance. Most patients find that with repeated movements the stiffness passes off and learn such manoeuvres as limbering up to run.

Generalised muscular hypertrophy is common and atrophy rare. However, the strength is not proportional to the size of the muscles and patients fatigue easily. The tendon reflexes are usually normal. The associated features seen in dystrophia myotonica are rarely encountered, and when present tend to be minimal. Occasional cases have been reported with cataract, minor lens opacities or endocrine disturbance, but it is hard to be sure that these were not cases of early dystrophia myotonica without atrophy.

The course tends to remain static over the years and progression of myotonia or muscular weakness is rarely observed. The disorder is quite compatible with survival to old age. The myotonia is often severe, however, and can require treatment with phenytoin or tocainide.

Psychiatric aspects

Patients with myotonia congenita are usually normal in intelligence and personality. In sharp contrast to dystrophia myotonica social deterioration was not observed in Thomasen's (1948) large material. Mental changes were conspicuous by their absence. Thomsen (1876) himself drew attention to an hereditary psychosis in several members of his own family, describing it as a '. . . kind of imbecility, confusion of ideas combined with a tendency for the mind to wander and vacant brooding; it has most in common with a certain kind of mental weakness which occurs in old age'. Since then, however, most investigators have dismissed any association with psychosis as fortuitous, and in fact there are strong indications that the myotonia and the mental disorder were transmitted independently in different branches of Thomsen's family (Caughey & Myrianthopoulos 1963; Johnson 1967). Johnson (1967) has reported a patient with myotonia congenita who developed two acute psychotic episodes of mixed affective and schizophrenic type. Two of the siblings had myotonia congenita, and the father and several other family members had had acute psychoses; but here again the muscle disorder and the psychotic propensity appeared to be transmitted independently in the family, and no direct relationship could be established between the two disorders.

Paramyotonia congenita

Paramyotonia congenita resembles myotonia congenita except that the myotonia and weakness only appear on exposure to cold. It is transmitted as an autosomal dominant with the responsible gene on chromosome 17 (Neuromuscular Disorders 1992). Typically the disorder develops early in life, worsens at puberty, then tends to improve or vanish in later decades (Caughey & Myrianthopoulos 1963). It often principally affects the muscles of the face, tongue and hands. Involvement of the legs may cause 'cramps' or inability to rise from a sitting position in the cold. Severe weakness is sometimes induced by cold, with or without myotonia, and lasts on rare occasions for several hours at a time. In severe attacks the patient may be bedridden and unable to turn, leading to a suspicion of hysterical paralysis. There is no hypertrophy of muscles, and power and reflexes are normal between attacks.

Psychiatric and social complications appear to be as rare as in myotonia congenita. Associated dystrophic features such as cataracts, testicular atrophy and changes on skull X-ray do not occur.

Familial periodic paralysis

A number of forms of familial periodic paralysis have been described. Some are associated with a low serum potassium and respond to its administration, while others show a normal or high serum potassium and are aggravated by its administration. Among the potassium-provoked varieties there are two myotonic forms; potassium produces weakness in both but cold produces weakness in only one of them. Both are transmitted as autosomal dominants. McArdle (1964) has described the typical clinical pictures and Zellweger and Ionasescu (1973) and Harper (1989) discuss the complex interrelationships between these disorders. Clinical overlap occurs to a considerable extent and may in part be due to the variable expressivity of the respective mutant genes. The important differential diagnoses are from hysterical paralysis or myasthenia gravis, and here knowledge of the family history can be important. Acetazolamide appears to be an effective prophylactic for both the hypokalaemic and hyperkalaemic forms (Riggs et al. 1977).

Narcolepsy

The chief symptom in narcolepsy consists of attacks of daytime somnolence, usually irresistible in intensity and leading to several short episodes of sleep per day ('narcoleptic attacks'). Commonly associated are attacks of cataplexy, in which the patient abruptly loses muscle tone and may fall briefly to the ground, usually in response to some emotionally provoking stimulus. Hypnagogic hallucinations and episodes of sleep paralysis are also characteristic of the syndrome in its most complete expression, and considerable disturbance of nocturnal sleep commonly occurs.

Gelineau gave the first definite description of the disorder in 1880. Thereafter the term came to be applied rather indiscriminately to many varieties of morbid somnolence, some due to structural brain lesions and others associated with psychiatric disorders, resulting in a good deal of nosological confusion and faulty discussion about aetiology. Gradually the condition was separated from these other sleep disorders and established as a distinct disease entity. The great majority if not all cases are without structural brain pathology and probably represent a biochemical disturbance of the sleep mechanisms of the brain. Hereditary associations have been demonstrated. Fresh interest has been brought to the syndrome as a result of present day discoveries concerning the physiological mechanisms involved in sleep as discussed below.

Clinical features

Detailed accounts of the disorder are to be found in Guilleminault *et al.* (1976) and Parkes (1985). The onset is usually between the ages of 10 and 30 years and is rare after 40. The precise time of onset may be hard to determine, relatives often becoming aware of the problem before the patient himself. Males and females are probably equally liable to the disorder. Affected relatives may be found in between a quarter and half of cases.

Approximately three-quarters of cases have at least one of the accessory symptoms in addition to narcoleptic attacks—cataplexy occurs in some 70%, hypnagogic hallucinations in perhaps 30% and sleep paralysis in 25%. The full tetrad occurs in only about 10%. Some authorities have restricted the term to cases with cataplexy in addition to narcoleptic attacks, but this presents difficulties since narcolepsy alone commonly antedates the development of accessory symptoms. In a large series of patients with cataplexy, Yoss and Daly (1960b) found that this had set in at the same time as the narcoleptic attacks in 55%, 1–5 years later in 25% and more than 10 years later in 15%. One may therefore encounter patients in whom daytime sleep attacks constitute the sole manifestation for some considerable time. Cataplexy antedating narcolepsy is distinctly uncommon. Episodes of sleep paralysis as the sole complaint are also rare. Hypnagogic hallucinations, by contrast, are quite frequently encountered in the general population.

Once it has commenced the disorder appears to persist unchanged throughout life, though perhaps with some diminution in severity after middle age. Very occasionally remissions and exacerbations have been described, but in most large series this has not been the case.

Narcoleptic attacks consist of an overwhelming sense of drowsiness, usually leading to a brief period of actual sleep. They are commonly of daily occurrence and with several attacks per day. The period of sleep usually lasts some 10–15 minutes though may be much longer according to circumstances. If the majority of attacks exceed 30 minutes, Roth (1980) classifies the disorder as idiopathic hypersomnia (p. 729). The disorder is said to set in quite often during a period of sleep disruption as in military training, or during a period of emotional upheaval (Zarcone 1973).

The episodes are commoner in situations normally conducive to drowsiness—after meals, in monotonous surroundings and as the day progresses. Usually there is a period of a minute or two during which the patient struggles against actual sleep. But in severe examples attacks can occur in any situation—while talking, eating, working or when engaged in other activities. Attacks while swimming or driving may very occasionally endanger life, though the prodromal drowsiness will almost always serve as a warning. Some patients are extremely irritable when prevented from falling asleep or when suddenly awakened. Typically the patient awakes refreshed, and there is then a refractory period of several hours before the next attack can occur. Some, however, remain drowsy and obtunded on awaking.

The patient may complain either of episodic sleep attacks with reasonable alertness between, or more rarely of fighting a constant battle against drowsiness during the day. Yoss and Daly (1957) divided the syndrome into type I and type II varieties on this basis. The second variety can be a diagnostic problem if there are no accessory symptoms. In fact patients with circumscribed sleep attacks will often be found to have episodes of quite profound drowsiness between, though they may not themselves be fully aware of this. Brief 'microsleeps' lasting 10–20 seconds are also not uncommon, as shown by EEG recordings, yet may not be apparent to the patient or observers.

Cataplectic attacks consist of sudden immobility or decrease of muscle tone, which may be generalised or limited to certain muscle groups. In severe attacks the patient collapses in a flaccid heap and is totally unable to move or speak. Serious falls and injuries may occasionally result. Tendon reflexes are abolished for a while and extensor plantar reflexes have been observed. The patient typically remains fully alert, however, and is aware of what is proceeding around him. Mild episodes may show only as drooping of the jaw, head nodding, or a sense of weakness obliging the patient to sit down or lean against a wall. Objects may be dropped or the knees buckle. Dysarthria, aphonia or ptosis may accompany attacks, and double vision or momentary difficulty with focusing may be the sole manifestation. Pallor and change of pulse rate are sometimes observed. Very occasionally, consciousness may be briefly clouded during attacks but this should be regarded as exceptional (Roth 1980).

The attacks are always of short duration, usually lasting several seconds and rarely more than a minute. They are much less frequent than sleep attacks, rarely occurring more than once per day.

Precipitation by emotional stimuli is usually strikingly evident in the history, in particular precipitation by laughter. But any strong emotion may bring on an attack—surprise, fear, outbursts of anger or feelings of exaltation. Cataplexy may render participation in sports impossible— the excitement inspired by a good tennis shot may bring on an attack, likewise the element of surprise in hunting or fishing (Yoss & Daly 1960b). Many patients learn to avoid provoking situations, and to check any inclination to laugh in order to avoid attacks. Sometimes, however, they can occur without any discernible affective stimulus.

Gelardi and Brown (1967) reported a rare example of a family in which typical laughter-induced cataplexy appeared to be transmitted as an autosomal dominant trait. Eleven members were affected from childhood onwards, with no hint of narcoleptic attacks in eight and questionable narcolepsy in three. Sleep paralysis was an occasional accompaniment.

Hypnagogic hallucinations usually occur in the auditory modality but can be visual or tactile as well. Two or more modalities may be associated in the experience, seeing and hearing quite commonly occurring together. They are experienced during the transition from wakefulness to sleep, or rather less commonly during the phase of recovery from sleep (hypnopompic hallucinations). Not uncommonly they occur simultaneously with episodes of sleep paralysis. They may be experienced in the middle of the night when the patient has roused for a while, and they sometimes accompany daytime narcoleptic attacks. Parkes (1986a) points out that those occurring while falling asleep should more accurately be termed 'pre-sleep dreams', since they are accompanied by rapid eye movement (REM) sleep changes on polysomnography.

Typically the hallucinations are intensely vivid and seem to be real at the time. The patient may react momentarily in accordance with what he is experiencing. Later, however, when fully awake, he almost always recognises their alien character. Lively accompanying affects, especially of terror, are widely reported as characteristic. Roth and Bruhova (1969) stressed the kaleidoscopic nature

and bizarre character of the visions. Zarcone (1973) suggested that the hypnagogic hallucinations of narcoleptics differ from those of normals in their complex dream-like quality and the intensity of the accompanying emotion, whereas in non-narcoleptics the hallucination is usually of a mere word or image with little affective meaning.

Sleep paralysis consists of attacks of transient inability to move which emerge in the stage between wakefulness and sleep. They typically occur while falling asleep, both at night and with daytime sleep attacks. More rarely they occur during awakening. Usually they are infrequent, rarely occurring more than once or twice per week.

The onset is abrupt, with the patient suddenly aware that he can neither speak nor move. The paralysis is flaccid and usually complete, though some patients can open the eyes or even cry out briefly. As with cataplectic attacks the episodes are brief, lasting several seconds and rarely more than a minute. One of Bowling and Richards' (1961) cases, however, had paralysis for more than an hour. The episode is usually dispelled abruptly if the patient's name is called or if he is touched or shaken. Otherwise it resolves spontaneously. Intense alarm is usually provoked. Hallucinatory voices or sounds sometimes accompany the attack and may lead the patient to fear that he is to be harmed or attacked.

Sleep paralysis as the sole symptom is very rare, but 10 such examples were studied by Roth and Bruhova (1969), all occurring in members of two families. The paralysis was accompanied by terrifying dreams, usually preceding the episodes. In one patient the feeling of despair characteristically carried over from the dreams and persisted next morning in the form of severe depression.

Disturbed nocturnal sleep is also characteristic of narcoleptics, occurring in 60–80% of patients. They fall asleep promptly but thereafter are restless, wake again often and may speak, shout or even walk about the room. Sleep myoclonus occurs in up to half of patients. Polygraph recordings confirm frequent periods of wakefulness. Vivid and terrifying dreams are common, occurring in some 60% of patients with narcolepsy and cataplexy and some 20% of patients with narcolepsy alone (Roth & Bruhova 1969). Themes of murder or of being pursued are said to be common. By contrast dreams are rare during daytime sleep attacks.

A variety of *other symptoms* are reported from time to time. Somnambulism is occasionally a pronounced feature. A rapid weight gain at onset may be observed, and libido or potency may become impaired (p. 727). Hypogenitality, a feminine hair distribution, polyuria and polydipsia are very occasionally present. Bouts of amnesia can occur as an occasional complication; the patient suddenly realises he has no knowledge of the past few minutes and has to check what has been done, usually discovering that he has continued to function normally during most of the time. Roth (1980) and Parkes (1986a) also report that automatic behaviour may feature in narcolepsy. The patient tries to overcome his sleepiness and carry on activities but loses awareness of what transpires; he may continue talking without making sense, his handwriting may suddenly change to meaningless scribble, or he may continue walking and wake in fresh surroundings. Such episodes are prone to occur in a third of patients, sometimes closely resembling episodes of transient global amnesia.

Differential diagnosis

The correct diagnosis is of crucial importance if appropriate treatment is to be given. Sometimes the patient's symptoms have long been attributed by relatives or employers to laziness, irresponsibility or emotional instability. There are no abnormalities on physical examination or routine laboratory tests, and the diagnosis rests essentially on a careful history. Polygraph recordings may clarify the situation in uncertain cases, by revealing REM episodes at sleep onset as discussed below.

In mild examples a distinction must be drawn from *normal drowsiness*. The classic accessory symptoms will be present in some three-quarters of narcoleptics, and in most of the remainder the sleepiness will be so excessive that there is little real doubt about the distinction. In borderline examples, however, it can be important to note that attacks of drowsiness are irresistible despite the absence of fatigue, or that attacks occur in inappropriate circumstances.

Fatigue based on anxiety or depression is a common misdiagnosis, especially if the patient presents his complaint as a feeling of tiredness instead of describing periods of excessive sleepiness. Neurosis is liable to be suspected when emotional complications have arisen from disrupted social or economic circumstances. However, narcoleptics rarely complain of muscular and physical exhaustion as do patients with fatigue of emotional origin, and they often awake from naps refreshed whereas the neurotic patient does not. The depressed and anxious patient will rarely complain of drowsiness as such, nor of recurring periods of uncontrollable sleep.

Hysteria may also be suggested. Hysterical dissociation may occasionally take the form of sleep, but this typically follows well-defined precipitants. The hysterical 'sleep' represents an active withdrawal, is usually prolonged, and the patient resists being woken. The question of hysteria or of *schizophrenia* may be raised when hypnagogic

phenomena are particularly vivid or fantastic. Daniels (1934) described such a patient who saw forms appearing at the windows and entering the room, and felt as if snakes, birds and other creatures were moving about in her abdomen and emerging from her mouth. All such symptoms disappeared with ephedrine.

Hypothyroidism may be the initial diagnosis when the patient complains of dullness and fatigue, or *hypoglycaemia* when he describes dizziness or lightheadedness as part of the attacks. *Epilepsy* will be suspected when the episodes are described as 'black-outs', but a careful history will reveal drowsiness before the loss of consciousness and full alertness on recovery. Witnesses will describe an episode of normal sleep from which the patient can be woken and the absence of convulsions. Cataplectic attacks may be mistaken for petit mal akinetic seizures. Precipitation by emotion and the preservation of full alertness are important distinguishing features.

Some patients first seek help on account of diplopia due to latent ocular imbalance brought about by episodes of drowsiness: *multiple sclerosis* or *myasthenia gravis* may then be suspected. Attacks of diplopia or ptosis may also be the principal manifestations of the patient's cataplexy. In older patients cataplexy may be mistaken for drop attacks due to vertebrobasilar insufficiency.

The history will usually readily distinguish narcolepsy from other hypersomnias, such as idiopathic hypersomnia (p. 729), the Kleine–Levin syndrome (p. 732) or the sleep apnoea syndrome (p. 730). The presence of obesity may cause confusion with the latter. Hypersomnia due to structural brain lesions (p. 733) is likely to be long lasting and with other ancillary evidence by way of neurological abnormalities.

Aetiology

The precise cause of narcolepsy remains elusive. It clearly represents a disturbance of the brain stem mechanisms governing sleep, as confirmed by neurophysiological studies, but whether this is primarily biochemical or immunological in origin remains unknown. Animal work shows that the initiation and maintenance of sleep are critically dependent on the balance between catecholamines, serotonin and acetylcholine in pontine areas of the brain stem, and it is possible that other transmitters including peptides are also involved (Parkes 1985). The biochemical abnormality in narcoleptics has not, however, been established. The extremely close association between narcolepsy and DR_2 and DQ HLA antigens (see below) raises the possibility of an immunological basis, especially since DR_2 antigens are widely distributed in the brain, but this too remains to be clarified.

Earlier theories which viewed narcolepsy in psychodynamic or Pavlovian terms have been superseded. The sensitivity of narcolepsy to environmental influences invited psychodynamic explanations in terms of the defensive function of symptoms, attacks serving to protect the patient from unacceptable feelings and impulses and avoiding confrontation with difficulties (Langworthy & Betz 1944; Barker 1948). Such theories were elaborated before clear distinctions had been made between narcolepsy proper and emotionally induced hypersomnias. Pavlovian theories held that the narcoleptic's brain was unusually susceptible to 'cortical inhibition'; in cataplexy inhibition induced by emotion was confined to the motor and postural centres, while in sleep attacks it spread widely to all parts of the cortex (Adie 1926; Levin 1935; Fabing 1946). Sleep paralysis resulted when inhibition failed to irradiate uniformly to all parts of the brain.

More soundly based neurophysiological theories seek to illuminate narcolepsy through what is known of the physiological basis of normal sleep, and in particular through EEG and polygraph observations. It has been established that the routine EEG shows no abnormalities in narcolepsy, beyond the expected changes when the subject is drowsy and the normal sleep changes while asleep. During cataplectic attacks and episodes of sleep paralysis the EEG tracing remains unchanged. But more discriminating assessment of the stages of sleep shows interesting differences from normals.

Polygraph recordings have established that normal sleep consists of two distinct varieties, rapid eye movement (REM) and non-REM sleep. In normal sleep drowsiness first gives way to non-REM sleep of gradually increasing depth. The first REM period occurs after some 50–90 minutes and lasts some 5–10 minutes, then the whole cycle is repeated at approximately 90-minute intervals. Four to six REM periods occur each night, each tending to be longer as the night progresses. Altogether REM sleep occupies some 20–25% of the total night's sleep, becoming more prominent during the final third.

The EEG in non-REM sleep shows four characteristic stages, described by Cooper (1994a) as follows. Stage 1 consists of mixed low voltage frequencies in the fast and theta ranges with a small amount of underlying delta. Towards the end sharp waves may appear at the vertex along with an increase in slow components. This usually occupies 2–5% of total night-time sleep. Stage 2 is characterised by the appearance of K complexes and sleep spindles, together with increasing slow activity in the theta and delta ranges which gradually increases in amplitude. K complexes are discrete wave forms exceeding 0.5 seconds in duration and widely distributed over the scalp, showing a high amplitude negative component followed by a lower positive one. Sleep spindles consist of rhythmic waves at 12–14 Hz which are bilateral, symmetrical and usually bisynchronous. The waxing and waning of amplitude gives the characteristic spindle form. Stage 2 occupies the greatest amount of total sleep time — some

45–55% of the total—and it is from this stage that REM periods often emerge.

Stages 3 and 4 reflect the deepest stages of sleep, showing bisynchronous generalised delta waves at less than 2 Hz which come to occupy over 20% and 50% of the epoch, respectively. Spindles and K complexes can persist into these stages but become increasingly difficult to recognise against the high voltage slow activity. Stages 3 and 4 are often labelled 'slow wave sleep' or 'synchronous sleep', occupying 10–20% of total sleep and being more prominent during the first third of the night.

REM sleep shows an asynchronous mixed frequency EEG accompanied by bursts of rapid conjugate eye movements. Autonomic changes are prominent, with elevation of heart rate, pulse and blood pressure, and penile tumescence. There is a marked decrease in general muscle tone, and extensor plantar responses may occur. Thus REM sleep has been characterised as 'an awake brain in a paralysed body' (Zarcone 1973). It is during this phase that dreaming is liable to occur (Hartmann 1965). When woken from REM sleep the subject typically recalls dreams with narrative visuospatial content, often with the subjective sensation of acting out the dream material; when woken from deep non-REM sleep, by contrast, he may recall isolated images, thoughts or words but these are not connected in dream-like narrative form.

Evidence has accumulated to suggest that non-REM sleep is related to serotonergic mechanisms which bring about inhibition of the brain stem reticular activity. REM sleep appears to be related to catecholaminergic mechanisms, and to be initiated and regulated by areas in the pontine reticular formation, including the locus caeruleus which is responsible for muscle inhibition and areflexia.

Rechtschaffen *et al.* (1963) discovered a distinctive feature in the nocturnal sleep of narcoleptics, namely that a REM period occurred at the onset, or shortly after the onset, instead of after the usual period of 90 minutes or so. Daytime sleep attacks have also been shown to consist of REM-type sleep, almost invariably so when the patient suffers from cataplexy as well as narcolepsy (Dement *et al.* 1964, 1966; Hishikawa & Kaneko 1965; Hishikawa *et al.* 1968). In patients with narcoleptic attacks alone, however, the early REM phase may not be seen, and daytime attacks may be accompanied by non-REM slow wave sleep. Episodes of hallucinations or sleep paralysis have proved to occur exclusively in the sleep-onset REM ('SOREM') periods, and where recordings could be obtained during cataplectic attacks the REM picture was again obtained. Night-time sleep is also generally deranged. In addition to direct or early onset into REM there are often marked phasic REM bursts, poorly regulated sleep cycles, many shifts of phase and frequent awakenings. Altogether SOREM is highly diagnostic of narcolepsy, emerging in over 95% of cases if daytime naps are studied as well as sleep recordings (Parkes 1985).

Thus it seems that the pathogenesis of the narcolepsy syndrome may lie in an abnormality of the triggering mechanism which produces REM sleep in normal individuals. In essence the principal phenomena represent attacks of REM sleep occurring out of proper context. Cataplectic attacks and episodes of sleep paralysis appear to represent a dissociated manifestation of the descending motor inhibitory component of REM aleep, without triggering of the ascending (sleep) component. Hypnagogic hallucinations appear to be a variant of the vivid dreaming normally associated with REM sleep.

However, the pathological mechanisms underlying the REM abnormalities remain unknown. It is unclear whether there is an exceptional reactivity of structures responsible for REM sleep, or a deficiency of the mechanisms producing non-REM sleep, or both. It is likely that the non-REM system is abnormal as well, as witnessed by the frequent periods of drowsiness which occur apart from attacks of sleep, also the frequent failure of nocturnal non-REM sleep to reach the normal depth (Roth & Bruhova 1969).

In very occasional patients narcolepsy has been reported in the presence of structural brain pathology (secondary narcolepsy) but the authenticity of most of these cases is doubtful (Parkes 1985). Indeed the rarity of clear-cut examples would suggest that coincidence has often been responsible. Thus narcolepsy has been described with tumours of the hypothalamus and third ventricle, also with general paresis, cerebral arteriosclerosis and multiple sclerosis. Occasionally it has followed encephalitis or head injury, sometimes after a considerable interval.

Most cases with cerebral pathology are atypical, and are probably more accurately regarded as hypersomnias than narcolepsy, having sleeps of long duration or sustained severe drowsiness. Cataplexy has been extremely rare in such examples. The exception appears to be encephalitis lethargica which has occasionally been followed by cataplexy as well as narcolepsy (Adie 1926; Sours 1963), but again these cases have usually been atypical—in tending to recover and in showing pupillary abnormalities and personality changes. Altogether when narcolepsy and cataplexy are found together it has proved exceptional to find any evidence of structural brain disease.

Genetic factors have emerged as significant in narcolepsy. Among 400 consecutive patients Yoss and Daly (1960a) found a positive family history in approximately a third. Occasional families were found where the disorder appeared to be transmitted as an autosomal dominant. However, Yoss (1970) suggested that the narcoleptic tendency might be polygenically determined and emerge in a graded manner similar to traits such as stature or intelligence. Measurement of pupil size under infrared light allowed the monitoring of ability to remain alert in dark-

ness, and it was found that unaffected relatives of narcoleptics often showed greater drowsiness than normal under such circumstances. The clinically overt disorder may therefore represent one pole of a spectrum, the opposite being represented by persons who remain alert despite unusually little sleep at night.

It has more recently been discovered that there is an almost 100% linkage between narcolepsy and the HLA DR$_2$ antigen in caucasian and oriental subjects, with black narcoleptics showing the strongest association with HLA DQw1 (Cooper 1994b). HLA typing can therefore be of value in confirming the diagnosis, since if the patient is negative for the HLA antigen in question the diagnosis of narcolepsy must be considered very unlikely (Parkes 1986a).

Treatment

The treatment of narcolepsy is outlined by Parkes (1985) and Cooper (1994b). Analeptic drugs are the mainstay of treatment for daytime sleep attacks, though their use is unsatisfactory in a number of ways. High dosage of amphetamines may be required to control attacks, resulting in side effects of insomnia, anorexia, irritability, tremor, hypertension and, on rare occasions, acute paranoid psychoses. Moreover when pushed to high dosage nocturnal insomnia may lead to an increase in daytime drowsiness and sleep attacks. Addiction is an additional risk, though this appears to be rare among narcoleptics.

In practice it is best to try the effect of one of the less potent stimulant drugs such as mazindol or fencamfamin before proceeding to dextroamphetamine sulphate (Dexedrine), racemic amphetamine sulphate (Benzedrine) or methylphenidate (Ritalin). Cross-tolerance does not appear to develop, so alternative preparations can be tried when difficulties arise. Such drugs are known to suppress the REM stage of sleep, and this may possibly be the mechanism of their action in narcolepsy rather than a direct stimulant effect.

These drugs do not improve cataplexy and have little effect on other accessory symptoms. Cataplexy is helped by tricyclic antidepressants such as imipramine and desipramine, and particularly by clomipramine (Anafranil). The latter has been shown to be effective in a dosage considerably lower than is required for antidepressant effect, the cataplexy often lessening within 24 hours of starting treatment. Sleep paralysis and hypnagogic hallucinations are also reduced. Tricyclic antidepressants have no direct effect on narcoleptic sleep attacks, but when employed along with amphetamines they may allow the dosage of these to be reduced. In theory the combination could be dangerous, with risk of hypertensive crises, but Zarcone (1973) employed imipramine with methylphenidate in 45 cases with no apparent harm. Fluoxetine and other 5-hydroxytryptamine re-uptake inhibitors have also been used with success. In the USA gamma hydroxybutyrate has been shown to reduce the frequency of cataplexy, perhaps as a result of improving the quality of nocturnal sleep (Scrima *et al.* 1989, 1990). Diazepam can be useful in controlling disturbed nocturnal sleep, since unlike other sedatives it does not deprive the subject of REM sleep.

Counselling has an important part to play, with advice about acquiring a regular pattern of sleep and daytime activities, and perhaps establishing schedules for daytime naps to ward off spontaneous attacks. Shift work must be avoided, or work where drowsiness or falls could be a hazard. In general untreated subjects should not drive. Psychotherapy will help where social and personal adjustments must be made to the disability.

Psychiatric aspects

In addition to the problems of differential diagnosis, already discussed, the features that have attracted most psychiatric attention are the role of sudden emotions in precipitating cataplexy and the role of emotional conflicts in exacerbating daytime sleep attacks. Interest has also centred on the possibilities that personality change may follow the onset of the disorder, and that schizophrenia-like psychoses may sometimes develop as an extension of the hypnagogic hallucinations.

Susceptibility to psychological factors

Cataplectic attacks usually show such a striking relationship to immediately antecedent emotional stimuli that the causal connection cannot be doubted (p. 723). Laughter is classically regarded as the most common precipitant, but Levin (1953) stressed that aggression is frequently involved, also that laughter may sometimes be based on hostility. Some patients become immediately weak when attempting to discipline their children or when engaging in angry interchanges. Levin suggests that it is the guilt associated with anger, and the conflict between impulses to express or restrain the feeling, which is often the true precipitant. When aggression was justified, and not provocative of guilt, cataplexy seemed less likely to occur.

Smith and Hamilton (1959) suggested that emotional factors played an important part in precipitating other component parts of the syndrome as well. They reviewed the scattered evidence that narcoleptic attacks and even episodes of sleep paralysis could be related to situations of conflict. Among seven cases of their own they found a

close relationship between the intensity of symptoms and current psychological stresses. Situations evoking resentment which could not be expressed seemed particularly likely to bring on both narcoleptic and cataplectic attacks. In four of the seven there appeared to be a definite relationship between sleep attacks and strong feelings of suppressed anger. Less surprisingly the content of sleep hallucinations was sometimes related to underlying conflicts or preceding traumatic events.

Impact on personality

There is little consensus of opinion concerning the personality in narcoleptics. Some have regarded the majority of patients as stable and well adjusted, whereas others have reported a high prevalence of personality abnormalities. Pond (1952b) studied eight cases in detail and found all to be of above average intelligence. An emotional flatness and passivity was noted, however, and few had reached employment positions commensurate with their intelligence. None showed overt neurotic traits or behaviour disorders, but sexual maladjustment was common. All four married men suffered premature ejaculation and the one married woman was frigid.

Smith and Hamilton's (1959) seven patients appeared to have reacted severely to the illness. Withdrawal, loss of confidence and insecurity were often marked. Several were anxious, lonely and depressed. The embarrassing and humiliating nature of the symptoms appeared to account for such developments.

Sours (1963) gave a particularly grave account of the psychopathology in 75 cases. The personality was described as predominantly 'passive–aggressive'. Contrary to other accounts there was a high prevalence of anxiety and depression, and several showed hysterical symptoms. Eight showed schizoid personality disturbances and 10 more developed frank schizophrenic illnesses which required prolonged hospitalisation. Five of the 45 men were impotent.

In a series of 20 patients, 18 from a neurological clinic and two from a psychiatric clinic, Roy (1976) obtained further evidence that psychiatric disability is common. Eight had current evidence of psychiatric disorder and four more a history of such, chiefly in the form of depressive neurosis and personality disorder. Five further patients had had difficulties at work, in marriage and in social life. A striking finding was that nine of the 10 females had been frigid for many years, with failure to achieve orgasm over long periods of time. Of the 10 men one was impotent and another had premature ejaculation.

The impact of the disorder on patients' lives was illustrated in a questionnaire study by Broughton and Ghanem (1976). Many reported recurrent depression, often severe, and almost half described subjective worsening of memory since the onset of the disease. Employment difficulties were common, both on account of sleep attacks and personality difficulties. A surprising number had suffered accidents, either while driving or while engaged in household activities. Recreational pursuits were commonly hampered to a distressing degree.

Roth (1980) reviewed evidence of a special association between narcolepsy and depression, which appeared to be commoner than in the general population. The sleep attacks tended to become more pronounced during phases when the patient was depressed.

Psychoses

Schizophrenia-like psychoses appear to develop in narcoleptic patients more frequently than chance expectation, and often without clear evidence of genetic predisposition. Davison and Bagley (1969) identified 18 acceptable examples in the literature, only one with a family history of schizophrenia. Such psychoses, when short lived, may be attributable to amphetamine medication, but only five of the 18 cases under consideration were on such treatment. Davison and Bagley inclined to the hypothesis that both the narcoleptic syndrome and the psychosis were manifestations of diencephalic dysfunction.

The nosological status of these psychoses, and their relationship to other narcoleptic manifestations, has attracted a good deal of attention. The predominance of visual hallucinations has been noted, often with an emphasis on reptiles and other animals, and sometimes with the patient a spectator of movie-like experiences (Eilenberg & Woods 1962). Though compatible with schizophrenia such features suggest an organically based psychosis. In many examples the psychosis appears to have developed as a direct extension of vivid dreams or hypnagogic experiences. Sleep hallucinosis is, however, by no means an invariable precursor. Davison and Bagley found a history of sleep hallucinations in only 10 of their 18 examples.

Coren and Strain (1965) suggested that two distinct types of psychosis should be recognised. The first is typical of schizophrenia generally, with the classic features of formal thought disorder, inappropriate affect, disturbance of volition and lack of insight into hallucinations and delusional beliefs. These psychoses probably appear in conjunction with narcolepsy by coincidence. The second type is essentially a paranoid–hallucinatory state and is atypical of schizophrenia in many ways. The affect

remains appropriate to thought content, there is no formal thought disorder, and rapport and insight are retained to a marked degree. This is the category in which pre-existing dreams and hypnagogic experiences often become interwoven into the content of the psychosis. Typical examples of this latter group would appear to be as follows:

A girl of 15 had narcoleptic attacks and terrifying nocturnal dreams. The dreams and hallucinatory experiences began to occur by day as well as by night and she came to believe in their reality. After control of the narcolepsy with ephedrine she gained considerable insight though this was not complete.

(Daniels 1934)

A 34-year-old woman suffering from narcolepsy and cataplexy had vivid dreams at night and also during daytime attacks. Hypnagogic hallucinations occurred in auditory, visual and tactile modalities. She ultimately developed recurrent psychotic episodes in the course of which she would believe in the reality of the dreams and hallucinatory experiences. After hallucinating the presence of her husband with another woman she became convinced that he was having affairs for several weeks. She dreamt about having intercourse with partly human, partly animal forms, and developed extensive delusions concerning persecution by hospital staff. She recognised to some extent that she was ill, and would frequently question the reality of her hallucinations. The delusions appeared always to be derived from these. However, with each recurrence of the psychosis the distinction between hallucinations and reality gradually became more difficult until she believed the events depicted had actually occurred. There was no evidence at any stage of loosening of associations, inappropriate affect, or other symptoms fundamental to a diagnosis of schizophrenia.   (Coren & Strain 1965)

Forms that are intermediate between circumscribed nocturnal hallucinations and frank psychosis also appear to occur:

A narcoleptic patient heard doors banging during episodes of sleep paralysis, and people talking who he believed were trying to poison him. He could hear people walking across the room and feel hands trying to force pills into his mouth. Usually these ideas disappeared the moment he managed to open his eyes but on occasion they persisted for an hour or up to a day. He took to sleeping with a pistol and had grilles put on the windows because he was so afraid at night. Even in recounting his story, it seemed that he did not have full insight, and he kept reassuring himself that his wife could not be responsible.   (Thigpen & Moss 1955)

Other sleep disorders

Other syndromes of sleep disturbance have come to be recognised, including 'idiopathic hypersomnia', hypersomnia with 'sleep drunkenness', the sleep apnoea syndromes and the Kleine–Levin syndrome. In addition there are hypersomnias based on identifiable cerebral disease and metabolic dysfunction, and others which appear to be based on psychological factors alone. Brief mention will also be made of the 'parasomnias', including somnambulism and 'night terrors' which very occasionally present for medical attention in adult patients. 'REM sleep behaviour disorder' presents in older adults and must be distinguished from epilepsy.

The relative frequency of these various conditions is indicated by Coleman et al.'s (1982) survey of almost 4000 patients attending sleep disorder clinics in the USA. Half suffered from some form of hypersomnia, a third from insomnia and 15% from a parasomnia. Of the hypersomnias 43% represented sleep apnoea syndromes, 25% narcolepsy, 9% idiopathic hypersomnia, and 5% other hypersomnias including sleep drunkenness and the Kleine–Levin syndrome. Four per cent appeared to be due to psychiatric disorder, mainly depression, 3% to medical or toxic conditions and 2% to drugs or alcohol.

Idiopathic hypersomnia

Under this title Roth (1980) delineated a sizeable group of patients, rarely mentioned in the literature but considered by him to represent an independent nosological entity. Among patients referred to Roth's clinic in Prague this group came second only to narcolepsy in frequency. Others, however, have found it less frequently, and in particular much less commonly than the sleep apnoea syndrome as shown in Coleman et al.'s survey above.

The chief difference from narcolepsy lies in the longer duration of the daytime sleeps which typically last from half an hour to several hours at a time. Cataplexy and the other classic accessory symptoms of narcolepsy are absent. The periods of daytime somnolence lack the irresistible quality of narcolepsy but the patient is nevertheless obliged to fight against sleepiness for a large part of the day. The daytime naps are not refreshing and are typically preceded by long periods of drowsiness (Guilleminault & Faull 1982). 'Microsleep' episodes may be detected by continuous recordings, especially when trying to read or watch television but also at times during conversation. At night the patient falls asleep quickly and sleeps deeply, often with difficulty in waking in the morning. 'Sleep drunkenness' (see below) may be a feature on rising. Prolongation of nocturnal sleep may be present, as well as daytime somnolence. At weekends some patients sleep more or less continuously while undisturbed. Sleep-onset REM is not detected, and daytime sleep is of the non-REM type (Cooper 1994b).

Idiopathic hypersomnia is suspected clinically when the daytime somnolence is the sole symptom, i.e. in the absence of the accessory symptoms of narcolepsy, of snoring at night, or of nocturnal sleep disturbance. Polysomnography confirms the lack of nocturnal apnoeic periods or hypoventilation. A significantly increased amount of stage 2 non-REM sleep may be detected along with a decrease of stages 3 and 4 (Guilleminault & Faull 1982).

The condition sets in usually between the ages of 10 and 20, developing over the course of several months then tending to remain stable as a source of life-long disability. Occasionally the onset may be later, even well into middle age. Males are affected slightly more commonly than females. In some 30% of cases it occurs familially. In all these respects the resemblance to narcolepsy is obvious.

Among Roth's 167 cases, almost half showed psychological difficulties—neurotic problems, personality disturbances and depression. During phases of depression the periods of sleepiness were usually increased. Sixteen per cent had sexual problems, with lack of libido or potency in the men and menstrual disturbances in the women. As with narcolepsy, troubles with education, jobs and recreation were frequent, and often even more severe on account of the long duration of daytime sleeps.

The cause is unknown but presumably rests on biochemical disturbances of the neural mechanisms underlying sleeping and waking. Roth discounted psychogenic factors, likewise any known brain pathology, by his criteria for accumulating the sample. EEG and polygraphic records showed non-REM patterns to be prominent during diurnal sleeps, often proceeding to stages 3 and 4. All night records revealed normal sleep organisation except for its long duration. Treatment consists of the administration of central stimulant drugs, as in narcolepsy, but response to treatment is often poor.

Hypersomnia with 'sleep drunkenness'

Roth et al. (1972) initially reported this as an independent clinical syndrome, representing 30% of the patients in Prague who were referred for investigation of sleep disturbances. Now, however, it is viewed essentially as a variant or complication of idiopathic hypersomnia (Roth 1980).

'Sleep drunkenness' consists of difficulty in achieving complete wakefulness, accompanied by confusion, disorientation, poor motor coordination, slowness and repeated returns to sleep. A large group of patients showed this as a chronic symptom, occurring with almost every awakening and typically persisting as a life-long tendency (Roth et al. 1972). In the great majority daytime hypersomnia was present as well. The patients were rarely capable of waking spontaneously but needed vigorous and persistent stimulation. Even when so awakened they were confused, disorientated and ataxic in a manner resembling drunkenness for between 15 minutes and 1 hour or longer. Many showed impaired efficiency for up to 4 hours.

The majority reported extremely deep and prolonged nocturnal sleep, often failing to wake spontaneously for 16–17 hours. At night they fell asleep rapidly within seconds of retiring. Associated symptoms consisted of headache, recurrent depression, difficulty with concentration or emotional lability. Eight patients had severe personality disorders or showed psychotic features. However, there was no characteristic personality type or psychopathology, and psychiatric symptoms were not invariable accompaniments.

The course appeared to be stationary in the absence of treatment — once declared the disability could last until advanced age. Most patients responded well to analeptic drugs taken by day and immediately before retiring. Alternatively they could be administered immediately after the initial awakening, the patient being allowed thereafter to sleep for half an hour more, after which he would either wake spontaneously or could be easily roused.

In 52 of the 58 examples there was no apparent cause. Six were possibly symptomatic of brain disorder, setting in shortly after severe head injury, encephalitis or a cerebrovascular accident. In the idiopathic cases the pathophysiology remained obscure. Essentially the disorder appeared to represent an extension and intensification of the normal processes of sleep.

Apart from the chronic syndrome described above, sleep drunkenness can also occur as an occasional symptom in healthy persons if, for example, they are suddenly awakened after too little sleep. It is facilitated by fatigue, or the consumption of alcohol or hypnotics before retiring. It has also been described in persons of irritable disposition and in people subject to frequent terrifying dreams. Roth *et al.* (1972) refer to such examples in the older psychiatric and criminological literature, including persons who have become aggressive or even homicidal while in a state of sleep drunkenness.

Sleep apnoea syndromes

The importance of hypersomnias accompanied by alveolar hypoventilation has been increasingly recognised. Best known is the Pickwickian syndrome, so-called by Burwell *et al.* (1956) after the fat boy of *Pickwick Papers*. However, this is merely a special instance of a general class of problems. The topic is comprehensively reviewed by Parkes (1985), Whyte *et al.* (1989) and Douglas (1994).

A division is traditionally made into apnoeas of obstruc-

tive or of central origin, but this is now regarded as being to some extent artificial. The great majority, over 90%, are associated with airway obstruction and it is this that must be detected if treatment is to be successful. The rarer 'central' forms include those associated with lesions of the medulla due to a variety of congenital or acquired pathologies, and the 'Ondine's curse syndrome', seen mainly in infants, in which abnormalities of the respiratory centres are manifest as loss of automaticity of breathing while asleep (Severinghaus & Mitchell 1962). Rare familial forms are probably due to inherited insensitivity of the respiratory centres to hypercapnia. An element of obstructive apnoea usually accompanies these central cases because the pharyngeal and diaphragmatic muscles are responsive to chemical respiratory stimuli.

Obstructive sleep apnoea is usually due to occlusion or narrowing of the upper airway behind the tongue or palate. Fibreoptic endoscopy shows that the lateral walls of the oropharynx oppose during episodes of apnoea, commencing with constriction in the upper oropharynx (Parkes 1985). During inspiration the pressure within the upper airway is always subatmospheric, and the patency of the airway depends on the bracing effect of the surrounding musculature. Since muscle tone drops during sleep there is an enhanced tendency towards narrowing at this time, being greatest when lung volume is minimal at the onset of respiration (Bradley *et al.* 1986). Snoring can result from the turbulent flows engendered, or periods of apnoea when occlusion is complete.

Many of the sufferers from sleep apnoea are obese but this is not invariable. Fat deposition in the submucous tissues around the nasopharynx then contributes to the obstruction. Others may have grossly enlarged tonsils or small mandibular size, the latter often being associated with palatal, tongue or pharyngeal deformity. Rarer causes are myxoedema, acromegaly, failure of the laryngeal abductors as in the Shy–Drager syndrome, or myotonic dystrophy which leads to respiratory muscle stiffness and weakness.

Once apnoea has occurred, normal breathing is only restored following arousal for a few seconds, resulting chiefly from the negative intrapleural pressure as the patient struggles to breath (Douglas 1994). The cycle of recurrent apnoeas and arousals may occur up to 100 times per hour, leading to great disruption of normal sleep patterns.

Most cases of obstructive sleep apnoea present over the age of 40, with a steady increase in prevalence thereafter. Males outnumber females by 10:1. By contrast the rare central forms can affect all age groups and without definite sex distribution. In the USA sleep apnoea has emerged as the commonest diagnosis in patients investigated in sleep clinics for daytime drowsiness, considerably outnumbering cases of narcolepsy (Coleman *et al.* 1982). Equivalent figures do not appear to be available for the UK.

The usual presentation is with excessive daytime sleepiness occasioned by the disrupted nocturnal sleep. A hallmark of the condition is loud snoring or honking at night as reported by sleeping partners, but the absence of snoring does not exclude the condition. Obesity is common, being found in perhaps 50% of subjects, often with a characteristic facial appearance caused by a short thick neck and heavy jowls. The phases of daytime sleepiness are usually profound and often compelling, leading to a significant increase in accidents including road traffic accidents (George *et al.* 1987). Among 80 patients Whyte *et al.* (1989) reported that five had fallen asleep while driving cars, four while driving heavy goods vehicles and one while flying his private plane. The daytime naps are typically of brief duration and are frequent throughout the day. Hypnagogic hallucinations and periods of automatic behaviour may occur.

During sleep, by day and by night, respiratory disturbances give a characteristic stamp to the picture. The breathing becomes periodic, with apnoeic intervals lasting 10–20 seconds during which the level of sleep steadily deepens. Resumption of breathing is accompanied by deep sighing and guttural snoring. While the subject is apnoeic the blood oxygen falls and the blood carbon dioxide rises. Muscular twitching may be marked. Nocturnal sleep is characterised by restlessness, frequent changes of posture, flailing arm movements and repeated awakenings. Nocturia or enuresis may occur. While awake respiratory function studies typically show normal results or there may be persistent alveolar hypoventilation.

Reported complications include pulmonary hypertension resulting from the rises of pulmonary blood pressure during apnoeic periods, and cor pulmonale with right heart failure. Systemic hypertension may develop, likewise cyanosis and polycythaemia. The classic Pickwickian syndrome consists of somnolence with obesity, cor pulmonale and secondary polycythaemia, coupled with daytime hypoxia and carbon dioxide retention. Cardiac dysrhythmias, myocardial infarction and cerebrovascular accidents may contribute further to mortality in marked examples of the syndrome. Not surprisingly a high incidence of unexpected deaths has been reported (MacGregor *et al.* 1970).

These varied adverse effects on health have been widely discussed in the literature, but it can be difficult to apportion the blame between sleep apnoea *per se* and the confounding effects of such variables as obesity and age.

In a systematic review of the evidence Wright *et al.* (1997) conclude that a causal association between sleep apnoea and a range of poor health outcomes has not been firmly established, except with regard to daytime sleepiness and possibly vehicle accidents.

In severe examples mental features can figure prominently. Many patients find morning arousal difficult, with sleep drunkenness, disorientation, headache and motor incoordination (Parkes 1985). Such difficulties may persist during the day with poor memory and concentration. Sackner *et al.* (1975) found a high prevalence of personality disturbance with paranoia, hostility and sometimes agitated depression. Millman *et al.* (1989) reported that almost half of their patients scored highly on the Zung Depression Scale, with sustained improvement once the sleep apnoea had been relieved. Sudden outbursts of violent behaviour and marked anxiety have also been attributed to the condition, likewise sexual problems including impotence.

Greenberg *et al.* (1987) have documented impairments in neuropsychological functioning in sleep apnoea patients, more pervasive and severe than in controls suffering from other causes of daytime somnolence. Tests of attention and motor efficiency were particularly affected. The severity and duration of hypoxaemic episodes correlated significantly with measures of perceptual organisation (Block Design Test) and manual motor speed. Children with sleep apnoea may show a deterioration in school performance and failure to thrive. Guilleminault and Anders (1976) reported that a third of children showed borderline mental retardation when first seen. Such features, and the daytime drowsiness, appear to exceed what might be expected from insomnia and hypoxia alone, and probably owe much to the frequent shifts of sleep phase that occur throughout the night and the loss of deep slow wave non-REM sleep.

In the investigation of suspected examples it can be invaluable to obtain a history from the patient's sleeping partner. The patient himself is often unaware of his snoring and frequent brief arousals. Short of this, direct observation of the patient while asleep can be informative. Useful screening tests include a lateral CT scan of the neck to gauge any generalised airway narrowing, a 24-hour electrocardiogram to detect the bradycardia accompanying apnoeas and the rebound tachycardias that follow, or oximetry to monitor the repeated cycles of desaturation. Rauscher *et al.* (1993) have reported the value of pulse oximetry coupled with indices of weight, height, sex, witnessed episodes of apnoea and reports of falling asleep when reading, in leading to a correct diagnosis of snorers referred to a sleep laboratory.

Polysomnography, however, provides the definitive

diagnosis when facilities are available and permits assessment of the severity of the condition. Overnight recordings allow continuous monitoring of the EEG, the respiratory movements and airflow during sleep. Apnoeas should occur during both REM and non-REM phases to be certain of the diagnosis, but are usually of greater frequency during REM sleep. Hence they are typically more severe during the second half of the night. In practice sleep is sometimes so disrupted that little REM sleep is achieved, and little or no stage 3 or 4 non-REM sleep. Concurrent oximetry allows the severity as well as the frequency of desaturations to be measured.

Treatment should first involve loss of weight when this is indicated, and the strict avoidance of alcohol in the evenings or the use of sedatives or hypnotics. Otolaryngological investigation will often be indicated to explore possibilities of remediable airway obstruction. Contributory factors such as myxoedema, acromegaly or retrognathia should receive attention. No truly effective drug treatment has been achieved, despite earlier hopes from protriptyline, progesterone or acetazolamide.

Patients who fail to respond to simpler measures may, if the condition is severe, be considered for continuous positive airway pressure (CPAP) treatment each night. A pressure of 4–10 cmH$_2$O is applied continuously through a mask fitted over the nose and mouth to prevent the recurrent collapse of the upper airways during sleep. Many patients find that they can adjust to this satisfactorily, with consequent marked improvement in daytime somnolence and both physical and mental symptoms. Surgical procedures have sometimes been employed to tense the lateral pharyngeal walls along with removal of the uvula and parts of the soft palate, but their place in treatment is controversial. Nevertheless, tracheostomy still finds a place in severely compromised patients when CPAP is unsuccessful, or as an emergency when some other operative procedure must be undertaken. Occasional patients with true central apnoeas may require intermittent positive pressure respiration while asleep.

Kleine–Levin syndrome

Levin (1936) drew attention to a rare syndrome of periodic somnolence, often lasting for days or weeks at a time and associated with intense hunger. Mental symptoms by way of irritability, excitement and motor unrest also characterised the somnolent phases. Kleine (1925) had earlier reported several examples. Critchley (1962) carried out a detailed analysis of the 15 cases in the literature at that time and added 11 of his own. In contrast to the other sleep disorders considered above this is a 'long-cycle hypersomnia', the episodes being separated by months or even years of normal health.

The great majority of cases have been in young men and with onset in early adolescence, but up to a quarter of cases are now reported in females (Parkes 1985). A beginning in middle age has very occasionally been described. The onset usually appears to be quite spontaneous, though sometimes a flu-like illness or a period of physical stress has antedated the first attack. Cases following closely upon head trauma have been described (Will *et al.* 1988). The duration of attacks may range from several days to several weeks, most lasting less than a week. Their frequency varies from one to 12 per year with an average of two per year.

Somnolence is the most conspicuous symptom. It may set in abruptly or follow gradually after several days of mounting malaise and tiredness. The patient sleeps excessively by day and night, rousing only to eat or empty bladder and bowels. Incontinence does not occur. He is always rousable, as from natural sleep, but is then liable to be intensely irritable and truculent. When awake he eats voraciously, typically consuming any food in sight. Critchley (1962) preferred the term 'megaphagia' to 'morbid hunger'; compulsive eating in a wolfish and greedy manner is a conspicuous feature, but the patient does not complain of hunger itself and rarely demands food when this is not in sight. Hypersexuality may be observed in a quarter of subjects at this time (Parkes 1986a).

Throughout the attack there are few if any abnormal physical signs. Unexplained fever is sometimes reported, also pupillary changes, nystagmus or an extensor plantar response. Laboratory investigations are usually entirely normal, including examination of the cerebrospinal fluid, though reduced growth hormone secretion has been reported (Chesson *et al.* 1991). The EEG shows the usual changes of drowsiness or sleep, but sleep studies may show an increase in total sleep time to 12–14 hours, reduced sleep latency and REM latency, and a reduction in stages 3 and 4 of non-REM sleep (Pike & Stores 1994). Elian and Bornstein (1969) reported a patient who showed paroxysmal delta and diffuse theta activity during attacks, but this is distinctly unusual. Each episode ends spontaneously, typically in a gradual manner but sometimes abruptly. Partial or total amnesia for the attack is usual.

Mental abnormalities during attacks have attracted much attention. They may be in evidence when the sleeper is roused or wakes spontaneously. Sometimes they also antedate and follow each attack for a short period of time.

Irritability is typically marked, extending at times to

severe aggression when the patient is disturbed. Uninhibited insolent behaviour may emerge, or motor unrest with fidgety behaviour, agitation and tearing at the bed clothes. The bizarreness of behaviour can be an alerting sign; the patient described by Pike and Stores (1994), for example, chased a friend with a carving knife, stole a cucumber, hit a woman in the street with a bag, and repeatedly changed the position of ornaments in the home. Confusion of thought is usually evident too, with disorientation, forgetfulness, depersonalisation and muddled speech. Vivid imagery may be prominent, with waking fantasies which are difficult to disentangle from vivid dreams. Visual and auditory hallucinations may occur. Occasionally the picture has a distinctly schizophrenic colouring: one of Critchley's patients felt responsible for all the events of which he was aware, and believed he could stop a clock with his thoughts and control his own hearing and vision.

Usually the mental abnormalities subside as the period of somnolence ends, but sometimes they persist for days or weeks thereafter. Depression with insomnia is not uncommon for several days. In two of Gallinek's (1954) patients severe depression persisted for several weeks after every attack, with suicidal tendencies, retardation and pathological guilt. A period of elation lasting several weeks has occasionally been reported (Gilbert 1964), also a phase of sexual hyperactivity when the sleep is over (Passouant et al. 1967). Quite often anorexia, headache and malaise follow the attack before the patient feels fully refreshed and regains normal clarity of thought. Thereafter, however, the normal personality is resumed, usually with a partial or total amnesia for what has occurred.

The rarity of the syndrome can lead to diagnostic difficulties. It is probably rarely recognised until several attacks have occurred, especially since the overeating may be overlooked and is often unapparent to the patient himself. Other causes of morbid somnolence are likely to be diagnosed and a primary emotional disturbance may easily be suspected. Disturbed behaviour may dominate the picture, suggesting that the essential problem is a personality disorder or even schizophrenia. When circumstances prevent the patient from taking to bed he may become slovenly, unkempt and very erratic in conduct as in the following case reported by Robinson and McQuillan (1951):

An army officer cadet of 19 came to the notice of the army doctors in an abnormal mental state. He was unkempt, offhand, casual and disinterested, answering vaguely and smiling fatuously. Affect was shallow and inappropriate and he experienced auditory hallucinations. He was clearly confused, cerebration was slow and there was evidence of thought blocking. In hospital he was hostile and insolent. Behaviour was often bizarre and he masturbated openly, grinning broadly. He slept a great deal and his appetite could not be satisfied. After 4 days in hospital the disturbance cleared abruptly, and he again became smart, respectful and well mannered. He was amnesic for the events of the previous days though he realised that he had behaved badly and had been unable to control himself.

A history was then obtained of previous attacks, 2 years and 3 years earlier, each lasting several days and accompanied by somnolence and excessive hunger. In the first he had become strange and distant, avoiding company and seeming unaware of what was said to him. On two successive nights he had micturated into a pair of gumboots. He had sold a bicycle for 25 shillings and spent the money on preserved fruits which he consumed at one sitting. In the second attack he again became drowsy and with an insatiable appetite, and created much disturbance with laughing and shouting. After each attack he had returned abruptly to his normal personality.

Follow-up suggests that the disorder is essentially benign. Attacks appear gradually to lessen in duration, frequency and severity over several years, and ultimately cease. Amphetamines have been claimed to reduce the frequency and severity of the attacks (Gallinek 1962). Lithium proved remarkably effective in preventing attacks in a typical example of the syndrome, with recurrence immediately the drug was withdrawn (Ogura et al. 1976). Similar success with lithium has also been reported in periodic hypersomnia unaccompanied by appetite changes (Abe 1977; Goldberg 1983).

Little can be adduced by way of explanation for the disorder. Physical and mental health are usually normal between attacks, and few patients have shown evidence of significant maladjustment. Discernible precipitants can rarely be discovered for individual attacks. The similarity between one case and another, and the uniform course pursued, have combined to suggest an organic basis. Diencephalic dysfunction is suggested by the combination of sleep and appetite disturbance.

Hypersomnias due to identifiable organic disease

The hypersomnias seen with overt cerebral or metabolic disease differ from the syndromes described above in many respects. They are rarely episodic and lack the transient and overwhelming nature of the narcoleptic attack. Sustained drowsiness is characteristic, or periods of sleep greatly in excess of normal requirements. Sometimes sleep inversion is seen with agitated delirium at night. In contrast to many cases of narcolepsy the sleep of such hypersomnias does not refresh. Depending on the responsible pathology the patient may be roused with ease or difficulty, and to varying levels of alertness. The sleep is usually undisturbed and vivid dreams are rare.

Lesions involving the midbrain tegmentum or posterior hypothalamus are a common cause. The responsible pathology may be a tumour, vascular lesion or degenerative process. Excessive hunger and weight gain may be seen with the somnolence of hypothalamic lesions, likewise polyuria and polydipsia. Prolonged hypersomnia may follow encephalitis lethargica, general paresis or cerebral oedema from any cause. After head injury a variety of sleep disturbances can be seen, including excessive daytime somnolence and sleep apnoea syndromes (Guilleminault *et al.* 1983). These may cause significant disability and raise medicolegal problems. Infective processes such as encephalitis, typhoid, trypanosomiasis or tuberculous meningitis are regularly accompanied by somnolence. Guilleminault and Mondini (1986) have reported patients with prolonged and disabling daytime sleepiness following infectious mononucleosis.

Metabolic disorders such as uraemia occasionally present with somnolence, similarly the encephalopathies associated with anoxia, chronic respiratory insufficiency or hepatic disorder. Endocrine causes include myxoedema, Cushing's and Addison's disease, diabetes mellitus and hyperinsulinism. Rarer causes are industrial toxins and lead encephalopathy. Abed and Bhalla (1991) have reported cases of prolonged hypersomnia following the administration of combined oral and depot neuroleptics, persisting for several months after discontinuation.

Sometimes organic hypersomnias are accompanied by psychiatric symptomatology, chiefly neurasthenic or depressive pictures. A patient described by Roth (1980) showed periodic hypersomnia and manic–depressive psychosis following a head injury, the hypersomnia phases accompanying the depression; while depressed he slept for 20 hours per day, while hypomanic for 3 or 4 hours per day.

The EEG in such conditions generally shows the picture of sleep together with various anomalies in the form of diffuse slow components or bursts of bifrontal or generalised slow waves. The cyclic organisation of REM and non-REM sleep is often modified or disrupted.

Insomnia due to organic disease

Insomnia following cerebral lesions has very occasionally been described. Bricolo (1967) reported a patient who developed total insomnia for 96 hours following bilateral stereotactic thalamotomy for Parkinson's disease. Thereafter he showed inversion of the sleep–wakefulness rhythm which very gradually became more regular.

A remarkable post-traumatic example was described by Webb and Kirker (1981). A 33-year-old woman still showed severe insomnia 2.5 years after a relatively mild head injury. On some nights she claimed she did not sleep at all, while on others she slept for about an hour. In the evenings she felt exhausted but not somnolent. EEG and polygraph recordings on four consecutive nights supported her story, showing brief light sleep for less than an hour and no REM sleep. Hypnotics and sedatives were ineffective in doses that left her alert the following day. Nevertheless, four consecutive nightly doses of L-5-hydroxytryptophan, the precursor of serotonin, were dramatically effective, restoring normal sleep which persisted during several months' follow-up. In the absence of further examples it is hard to interpret such a response, though it remains possible that the drug served to trigger normal sleep mechanisms in the presence of some discrete brain stem lesion.

Fatal familial insomnia is an extremely rare disorder, consisting of progressively worsening insomnia with impairment of autonomic and endocrine functions, and motor signs including dysarthria, ataxia, myoclonus and pyramidal disturbance (Lugaresi *et al.* 1986; Medori *et al.* 1992a). It is inherited as an autosomal dominant with onset in middle age. The sleep disorder is characterised by reduction or loss of both slow wave and REM phases of sleep. Over several months confusion and complex hallucinations ('enacted dreams') give way to progressive memory loss and impairment of consciousness. Death follows a period of coma 6 months to 3 years from the onset. Neuronal degeneration and astrocytosis are most pronounced in the anterior ventral and dorsomedial nuclei of the thalamus, but can extend to other thalamic nuclei, the olives, and the cerebral and cerebellar cortex. Spongiosis is occasionally observed and DNA analysis has shown mutations in the prion protein gene (Medori *et al.* 1992a, 1992b).

Hypersomnias associated with psychiatric disorder

Most studies of patients with hypersomnia reveal cases in which psychological factors are clearly of aetiological importance. The proportion varies, however, according to the orientation of the observer. Roth (1980) points out that during the last century most hypersomnias were thought to be emotional in origin, then organic causes and clear-cut syndromes such as narcolepsy came gradually to be delineated. It still remains uncertain what proportion of cases have a definite psychological causation, as opposed to prominent psychological accompaniments to some other definable cause. Mixed patterns can present especial difficulties, since many of the recognised syndromes described above are strongly influenced by prevailing mood and environmental factors.

The nosology as well as the prevalence of psychogenic hypersomnias remains unclear. In the course of accumulating 88 narcoleptics, Sours (1963) found seven patients with hypersomnia that was symptomatic of organic conditions and 20 with hypersomnia attributable to psychiatric disorder; of the latter nine were regarded as neurotic in origin, two as depressive reactions, two as hysterical and seven as schizophrenic. Smith (1958) suggested that most reported cases of psychogenic hypersomnia would more accurately be labelled as hysterical trances or psychotic stupors.

All agree that hysterical dissociation and depression are the major factors in well-marked examples, with a frequent theme of withdrawal from conflict-laden situations. The somnolence may set in abruptly after traumatic events or emotional upheavals, persisting thereafter for hours or days, or the condition may present recurrently over many months or years.

The following examples almost certainly reflect hysterical mechanisms at work:

One remarkable report concerned a patient who slept for 32 years, but during that time she cried when hearing bad news, would allow only certain persons to attend her and was heard occasionally to speak.   (Fröderström 1912)

A woman of 49 had a history of sleeping attacks for a year, sometimes lasting 36 hours at a time. Hysterical conversion features were present and became intensified during somnolent phases. When confronted with painful topics from her past life, drowsy attacks could be precipitated, but if caught in time and persuaded to expose the conflict-laden material she would return to normal alertness within minutes. She had had an incestuous relationship with her father and had also had a lover throughout her married life. 'Confessional catharsis' led to a great lessening of attacks in the years that followed.   (Spiegel & Oberndorf 1946)

Depressive rather than hysterical mechanisms may have been operative in the following patient:

A 31-year-old teacher had had meningoencephalitis at 3 and was widowed at 22. From the age of 30 she frequently felt ill and suffered from headaches and giddiness when upset. After a 10-year relationship she broke off her engagement saying that her fiancé was not sufficiently well educated. After this she claimed to have slept for a whole week. Since then she had often fallen asleep, sometimes against her will and usually for a whole day. This always occurred after an emotionally upsetting experience. She ultimately improved with psychotherapy and light sedation.
                                                          (Roth 1980)

Hysterical states of somnolence will usually differ in several respects from true sleep. The patient may be unrousable even to painful stimuli, or show gross hysterical stigmata. The prolonged maintenance of certain postures, eyelid tremor, increased muscle tension or contraction of the masseters may be in evidence. EEG recordings made during such states may show wakefulness, perhaps even greater desynchronisation than usual, with a preponderance of fast activity and a good deal of muscle artefact.

Depressive hypersomnias, by contrast, may consist of long periods of genuine sleep; hence the difficulties that may be encountered in reaching a firm diagnosis. It is well recognised that hypersomnia may accompany depression or be the presenting feature (Detre *et al.* 1972; Kupfer *et al.* 1972; O'Regan 1974). In depressive hypersomnias attacks will rarely extend beyond 24 hours at a time, the posture during sleep will be normal and rousing will usually be possible. Many so-called depressive hypersomnias may, however, represent examples of Roth's 'idiopathic hypersomnia' accompanied by depression.

Patients who display negativism, flexibilitas cerea or other catatonic phenomena in the absence of extrapyramidal disease will be suspected of psychotic illness, either affective or schizophrenic in nature.

Unfortunately few modern laboratory studies appear to have been carried out on patients with psychogenic hypersomnia. These would seem essential in working towards adequate differentiation between cases which rest on organic or pathophysiological factors, and those which are primarily due to psychological causes. In the meantime it is necessary to evaluate each patient as fully as possible for neurological and psychiatric disorder. It can be helpful to consider the following aspects individually (Roth 1980): determination from clinical observation of whether or not the attacks represent genuine sleep; evaluation of the course, whether static over years or intermittent, and the effect of external factors upon it; the exclusion of any possible organic cause; assessment of the personality for evidence of pre-existent abnormalities; and the mounting of combined EEG and polygraphic studies, wherever possible during attacks. Where psychiatric factors appear to be causative their alleviation may be decisive in clarifying the diagnosis. Treatment with stimulant drugs carries obvious hazards in any patient whose hypersomnia is due to psychological disturbance.

Somnambulism

Sleep-walking occurs predominantly in males. There is frequently a family history of the disorder and an association with enuresis. The great majority of cases occur in children, and the rare examples coming to attention in adult life are often among servicemen or men under indictment for an offence carried out during an alleged sleep-walking spell. Some 15% of children are alleged to have at least one sleep-walking episode, compared with 2–5% of the adult population (Kales *et al.* 1987).

Behaviour during the somnambulistic episode may sometimes consist of no more than sitting up in bed and making banal repeated movements for a minute or two. More prolonged examples consist of walking aimlessly about, or more rarely running, jumping or searching for something. In the main the behaviour is simple and stereotyped. The subject has a blank expression and movements tend to be repetitive and purposeless, though investigatory eye movements may be apparent and dangerous obstacles are usually avoided. Self injury is rare but serious examples have been reported. Typically the subject behaves as though indifferent to the environment with low levels of awareness and reactivity. However, if spoken to he may answer monosyllabically. Some are suggestible during the episode and carry out simple commands.

There is disagreement about the level of motor performance and dexterity that can be observed. Fenwick (1990b), for example, states that acts can appear to be purposeful, directed and coordinated. The subject may dress or partially undress, open and shut doors and put himself seriously at risk. Cases have been reported in which patients have walked onto fire escapes or allegedly driven cars in a somnambulistic state. The question of violence during sleep-walking is considered further below.

Most attacks last for less that 10 minutes though some may last for half an hour or more. Spontaneous awakening sometimes occurs, but usually the subject returns to bed and continues normal sleep. Attempts at arousal result in gradual return to full awareness, often with marked disorientation and sleep drunkenness. Dream recall is not reported, and there is usually complete amnesia for what has transpired.

In children sleep-walking is usually a benign condition, outgrown in later childhood, suggesting that it rests on delayed cerebral maturation. Kales *et al.* (1980), in a retrospective analysis, showed that when the onset was before the age of 10 years it was usually outgrown by 15. However, the cases which come to attention in adult life appear frequently to be associated with severe psychopathology. Sours *et al.* (1963) studied 14 patients aged between 17 and 27 referred from US Air Force bases. In most the disorder had begun at the time of puberty, and persisted thereafter with attacks every 1–4 months. Traumatic psychological events had seemed to precipitate the onset in many cases—parental death or divorce, a change of school or the birth of a sibling. In some patients each episode was precipitated by interpersonal tensions or other emotional problems. There was strong evidence of disturbed family backgrounds and difficult relationships with the parents. The majority had a past history of acting out behaviour, delinquency and thefts, and many showed evidence of anxiety, depression or depersonalisation. Hysterical conversion symptoms were common. Five of the 14 patients were diagnosed as schizophrenic and four others were markedly schizoid in personality. The remainder were regarded as having character disorders.

Kales *et al.* (1980) similarly found that 29 adults with a present history of sleep-walking showed high levels of psychopathology on the Minnesota Multiphasic Personality Inventory (MMPI), whereas 21 who had outgrown it had essentially normal patterns. In the former the sleep-walking had begun later, was more frequent and had more intense manifestations. It is difficult, however, to know how typical these results may be of adult sleep-walkers generally. Parkes' (1986b) experience is that the majority of adults who sleep-walk have no psychiatric disorder.

The cause of somnambulism remains unclear. An explanation in psychodynamic terms was previously favoured, especially where episodes had an apparent purpose and the content was explicable in terms of current conflicts. The sleep-walking was then viewed as a dissociative state, similar to the hysterical fugue. It is now apparent, however, that sleep-walking rests on an abnormality of the sleep mechanisms of the brain and represents partial arousal out of the deep non-REM stages of sleep. It occurs most often during the first third of the night when stages 3 and 4 predominate — stages during which dreaming is least likely to occur. Kales and Kales (1974) review laboratory studies confirming this in children, and running counter to the popular notion that sleep-walking represents the acting out of a dream. Episodes could sometimes be induced by lifting somnambulists to their feet during non-REM sleep, whereas this did not provoke attacks in children not subject to the disorder.

Conditions that predispose to higher levels of slow wave sleep, such as sleep deprivation, shift work or alcohol consumption can be expected to increase the frequency of sleep-walking (Driver & Shapiro 1993). It may be commoner during periods of stress and anxiety. Attention has also been drawn to the liability of certain drugs, taken at bedtime, to induce somnambulism in susceptible individuals (Huapaya 1979; Nadel 1981). Hypnotics, neuroleptics, antidepressants, tranquillisers, stimulants and antihistamines have been incriminated, often in combinations and sometimes when taken with alcohol. Luchins *et al.* (1978) reported an example, apparently induced by thioridazine and a derivative of chloral hydrate, during which a 44-year-old psychotic woman stabbed her daughter to death. Sleep laboratory studies confirmed the liability of thioridazine to lead to sleep-walking in this patient, which occurred repeatedly out of stage 4 non-REM sleep. The tendency for sleep-walking to be induced by the combination of lithium with other neuroleptics is described on p. 626.

The question of violence towards others during sleep-walking can raise important medicolegal issues and such a defence not uncommonly comes before the courts. Simple aggression usually results from the terror and disorientation of partial arousal from deep slow wave sleep (Parkes 1985). More difficulty is encountered when weapons have been employed or purposeful coordinated behaviour has been implicit in the act. Oswald and Evans (1985) described a 14-year-old boy who stabbed and severely injured his 5-year-old cousin with a knife, and Fenwick (1987b, 1990b) reviews other examples from the literature where violence has occurred. Sleep-walking may also be put forward as a defence against sexual assault.

In appraising such cases, Fenwick (1987b, 1990b) points out that a family history and childhood history of sleep-walking greatly increase the chance that the episode in question is genuine. A first episode occurring in adulthood should be viewed with suspicion. Genuine sleep-walking is most likely to occur within 2 hours of sleep onset; any witnesses are likely to report inappropriate automatic behaviour, usually with an element of confusion; and there will be substantial amnesia for what transpired. Trigger factors such as drugs, alcohol, excessive fatigue and stress will often feature in the episode. Attempts to conceal the crime will be unusual, the natural response on waking being to summon help immediately. It is helpful if the offence can be shown to be motiveless and out of character for the individual. When there is a sexual element in the offence, careful enquiry should be made for sexual arousal with penile tumescence, since its presence would make a sleep automatism highly unlikely.

Sleep-walking has until recently been regarded by the law in England and Wales as a 'sane automatism', leading to acquittal when successfully raised as a defence (p. 298). However, in the recent case of R versus Burgess, 1991, it was agreed that since somnambulism has a genetic cause and arises from internal factors (i.e. a specific stage of sleep) it should be regarded as 'insane automatism' and likely to recur (Fenwick 1993). In consequence the judge may decide on disposal as he thinks fit.

With regard to treatment the most important factor is protection from injury. Doors and windows should be locked and dangerous objects removed. Patients should be advised to avoid situations leading to sleep deprivation, and to avoid taking alcohol before going to bed. Psychiatric treatment is rarely indicated in children, since most outgrow the disorder and in any case are not markedly disturbed. In adults, however, full psychiatric evaluation and treatment may be required. In persistent cases drugs such as diazepam or flurazepam, which suppress stages 3 and 4 of non-REM sleep, may warrant a trial (Kales *et al.* 1987). Their effectiveness has been more convincingly shown with night terrors, discussed immediately below.

Night terrors

Night terrors also arise out of stages 3 and 4 of non-REM sleep, differing sharply in this respect from nightmares which occur during phases of REM sleep (Fisher *et al.* 1973; Kales & Kales 1974). Night terrors and sleep-walking often occur in the same individual and a family history of both is common. Kales *et al.* (1980) suggest that

the two form a continuum, with sleep-walking the mild end and night terrors the more extreme end of a spectrum. The usual time of occurrence is within an hour or so of going to sleep. Episodes are rare after the middle of the night, because stages 3 and 4 of non-REM sleep become shorter later on.

The episode is accompanied by intense anxiety, autonomic discharge, vocalisations by way of screams, moans and gasps, a racing heart and panting respiration. It typically lasts for only a few minutes and the patient is usually amnesic for the event thereafter. If any content is recalled this is usually limited to a single frightening image of being attacked, choked or crushed (Oswald & Evans 1985). Occasionally destructive acts may be carried out such as slashing at objects or hitting other persons (Fenwick 1987b).

Follow-up studies show that most children outgrow the disorder in later childhood. As with somnambulism psychological disturbance is common in affected adults but not in children. Daytime anxiety is also high in adults with the disorder. Diazepam and flurazepam are effective in diminishing night terrors, both in children and in adults. Propanolol can also be markedly beneficial (P. Fenwick, personal communication).

REM sleep behaviour disorder

Schenck *et al.* (1986, 1987) have identified a form of acute behavioural disturbance occurring during sleep which, unlike somnambulism or night terrors, emerges during the REM phases and represents the acting out of altered dreams. This has been confirmed by polysomnographic studies. It seems that in these patients the normal inhibitory outflow from pontine centres to the spinal motor neurones during REM sleep is diminished, allowing motor behaviours to emerge.

Typically the patient develops a progressive sleep disorder, with the abnormal behaviours appearing during the middle or final third of the night and almost always more than 60–90 minutes after sleep onset. The episodes characteristically occur during nightmares of being chased or attacked. Concurrently there has usually been a change in the nature of the dreams experienced, which come to involve motor overactivity and violent confrontations with dream characters. The patient talks, shouts or jumps out of bed during sleep, often injuring himself or grabbing at others in a frenzied or aggressive manner. Such behaviours often clearly represent the attempted enactment of dream material.

A 52-year-old salesman of placid temperament began to talk, yell and sit up during sleep. After 2 years be began to punch, kick and jump out of bed 1–7 nights weekly, often striking and bruising his wife and once punching through a wall. These episodes, which always occurred at least 2 hours after sleep onset, were often the enactment of dreams which had become more vivid, action-filled and violent. 'Usually something is scaring me or is going to hurt my family and I try to protect them. Then I get most violent.'

A 67-year-old man developed a progressive sleep disorder in conjunction with a dementing illness. Limb jerking, moaning and talking appeared every night, with episodes of punching, kicking and running into furniture. On one occasion his wife saw him throw punches while he dreamed he was fighting squirrels in an attic. Both he and his wife had received numerous injuries during sleep.   (Schenck *et al.* 1987)

Schenck and Mahowald (1990) have reported 70 consecutive cases with a marked predominance among older males. The mean age at onset was 53, with a range from 9 to 73 years. Many had initially been suspected of nocturnal epilepsy, obstructive sleep apnoea or various psychiatric conditions. The majority were otherwise healthy, but a third showed evidence of a causal association with central nervous system disorders—dementia, Parkinson's disease, narcolepsy, or occasionally vascular or other brain stem lesions. In some cases there was an apparent association with drug or alcohol withdrawal, or the condition set in after major stressors. In most cases the disorder proved to be gradually or rapidly progressive up to the time of treatment. Three-quarters of the subjects had sustained repeated injuries, mostly bruises or lacerations but extending occasionally to fractures or dislocations.

Schenck and Mahowald (1992) have reported additional cases in narcoleptic patients, these appearing to represent almost 12% of the narcoleptics undergoing polysomnographic studies in their clinic. Treatment with stimulants or tricyclic antidepressants had sometimes induced or exacerbated the condition.

Polysomnographic studies show preservation of the usual distribution and cycling of sleep stages, though sometimes with reduced REM latency, increased REM density and increased stage 3 or 4 sleep. Periodic and aperiodic limb twitching is common during non-REM sleep. The defining characteristic, however, is intermittent loss of the normal electromyographic atonia during REM phases. Seizure activity was never detected in Schenck and Mahowald's cases.

Treatment with clonazepam was rapidly effective in controlling both the disturbing dreams and the problematic sleep behaviours, with only infrequent and minor lapses thereafter. Previous treatments with a variety of sedative–hypnotic drugs had not been helpful. Alternative treatments include desipramine, carbidopa and cloni-dine, and these can be of value in patients with sleep apnoea where clonazepam may be contraindicated.

Neuropsychiatric manifestations of carcinoma

The last few decades have seen the recognition of several neuropsychiatric syndromes which may accompany neoplasia in various parts of the body even when there is no spread of tumour cells to the brain. Thus patients with carcinoma may develop marked nervous system pathology while the tumour remains confined to its original site or at most metastasises to the regional lymph nodes. Mental symptoms figure prominently in such syndromes as well as neurological defects.

The mechanisms underlying such remote effects remain uncertain. Especially puzzling has been the observation that neuropsychiatric manifestations may precede clinical evidence of the primary tumour by a considerable interval of time, sometimes by several years. Moreover the disorders may continue to progress after apparently successful eradication of the neoplasm. Occasionally they make a first appearance some time after removal of the tumour and without evidence of recurrence of the neoplasm itself.

Before considering these remote effects in detail certain aspects of the orthodox involvement of the nervous system by secondary metastatic deposits will be briefly considered.

Metastatic involvement of the central nervous system

Tumours which commonly metastasise to the brain include those of the lung, breast, alimentary tract, prostate and pancreas. Carcinoma of the lung is undoubtedly the most frequent variety today. Melanomas may similarly metastasise to the central nervous system.

Secondary cerebral deposits are usually multiple and fast growing, but occasionally a solitary cerebral metastasis may warrant surgical intervention along with treatment of the primary growth. Not infrequently an intracranial metastasis gives rise to symptoms before the primary lesion, especially when this is in the lung, and sometimes the primary lesion is not discovered until autopsy. The clinical features are those of cerebral tumours generally as discussed in Chapter 6.

An 'encephalitic' form of metastatic carcinoma may very occasionally be encountered, as described by Madow and Alpers (1951). Here there is no tumour formation as such within the brain, but diffuse infiltration of carcinomatous cells throughout the central nervous system — within the brain parenchyma and along the perivascular spaces as well as in the meninges. There is no true inflammatory reaction but the presentation may at first closely simulate an encephalitic process. Of the four cases presented by Madow and Alpers three showed organic mental syndromes, three developed hemiparesis, all had fits and all showed signs of meningeal irritation. The cerebrospinal fluid sometimes contained an excess of cells and protein or could be normal. The lung was usually the site of the primary growth.

Carcinomatosis of the meninges may also produce a misleading picture. Secondary deposits invade the leptomeninges diffusely, particularly at the base of the brain, giving rise to an illness which at first resembles meningitis. Pyrexia and neck stiffness may be prominent features. Headache is usually marked and accompanied by cranial nerve palsies and often visual failure. A period of vague ill health has usually preceded more definite manifestations. Fischer-Williams et al. (1955) stress that severe mental disorder may accompany the neurological defects or even be the presenting feature. Some cases have presented with dementia and others have shown maniacal outbursts or mutism. The cerebrospinal fluid pressure is usually raised, with a moderate pleocytosis and elevation of protein. The detection of carcinomatous cells in the cerebrospinal fluid provides the definitive diagnosis.

Non-metastatic manifestations of neoplasia
(paraneoplastic disorders)

The number of non-metastatic syndromes known to be causally related to cancer is now considerable. The sensory neuropathies were first described (Denny-Brown 1948), then the peripheral neuropathies (Lennox & Pritchard 1950) and shortly afterwards the subacute cerebellar degenerations (Brain et al. 1951). Myelopathies and myopathies have since been recognised. For some time it was thought that pathological changes were restricted to levels caudal to the basal ganglia, but cerebral involvement is now recognised as well. Severe involvement of the limbic areas on the inferomedial surfaces of the temporal lobes is a well-recognised syndrome, producing an illness with prominent memory disturbances and often some degree of dementia.

Obviously the clinical pictures which characterise these non-metastatic complications are many and various. Table 19 represents an attempt at classification modified from Brain and Adams (1965). Strict classification is impossible since the various affections may appear singly or in combination. With the encephalopathies, particu-

Table 19 Neuropsychiatric disorders associated with neoplasms (after Brain & Adams 1965).

1 *Encephalopathies*
 Progressive multifocal leukoencephalopathy (see p. 751)
 Encephalopathy with subacute cerebellar degeneration
 Encephalopathy with brain stem lesions
 Diffuse encephalopathies with mental symptoms
 Encephalopathies presumed due to metabolic disturbance
 Limbic encephalopathy

2 *Myelopathies* (including cases resembling motor neurone disease)

3 *Neuropathies*
 Sensory neuropathy (with degeneration of posterior root ganglia and dorsal columns of cord)
 Peripheral sensorimotor neuropathies
 Subacute optic nerve or retinal degeneration
 Metabolic, endocrine and nutritional neuropathies

4 *Muscle disorders*
 Polymyopathy (mainly proximal, of limb girdles and trunk)
 Myasthenic syndromes including Lambert–Eaton syndrome (p. 711)
 Polymyositis
 Metabolic myopathies

larly, the pathological evidence suggests that a number of syndromes merge into one another as parts of a spectrum. Of the syndromes in the table only those that are likely to be of importance to the psychiatrist will be considered in detail. It should be noted, however, that mental symptoms, including dementia, may feature in all varieties, including cases where neuropathy or myopathy is the predominant part of the clinical picture (Brain & Henson 1958).

From the pathological point of view the accent may be on widely disparate parts of the nervous system. Several of the syndromes show a curious mixture of degenerative and quasi-inflammatory changes within the nervous system, which itself is puzzling from the point of view of aetiology. This is discussed further below.

With regard to prevalence the non-metastatic complications are relatively uncommon and some varieties exceptionally so. Nevertheless they constitute an important part of general hospital neurological practice. Among 1476 cases of carcinoma, Croft and Wilkinson (1965) obtained an overall prevalence of 7% with non-metastatic complications. Carcinoma of the lung produced by far the highest frequency at 16%. Oat-cell carcinomas of the bronchus have repeatedly been shown to be the commonest tumour type involved, with rarer examples from neoplasms of the ovary, stomach, uterus, colon and larynx (Henson & Urich 1982). Hodgkin's disease and lymphoepithelioma of the thymus have also been reported in association with such disorders.

Subacute cerebellar degeneration

This was one of the earlier syndromes to gain recognition (Brain *et al.* 1951). The presenting symptom is usually ataxia of gait, spreading later to all four limbs and often to the trunk. Dysarthria is severe but nystagmus often slight or absent. Muscle weakness, dysphagia, diplopia and sensory symptoms may also occur. The cerebrospinal fluid is often abnormal with a pleocytosis, elevated immunoglobulins and oligoclonal bands. The diagnosis may sometimes be confirmed by the presence in the serum and cerebrospinal fluid of antibodies directed against cerebellar Purkinje cells (Dropcho 1989; Compston 1993).

Mental symptoms figure prominently in the majority of cases. All but one of Brain and Henson's (1958) eight examples eventually showed some degree of dementia, and in two the initial picture was of agitation and depression. Brain and Wilkinson (1965) found mental changes in two-thirds of 17 cases, usually in the form of dementia but also states of agitation and anxiety.

The onset may antedate the appearance of the carcinoma by several months or years, or follow it by a similar interval. In one of Brain and Wilkinson's patients the neurological symptoms first appeared several months after removal of the neoplasm, and recurrence was judged unlikely since the patient survived 6 years without further evidence of the growth. Once started the disorder may progress so rapidly that the patient is bedridden within weeks, while in other cases it may take a year to develop fully. Sometimes arrest may be seen after many months of progression, but remission does not occur. The dementia can continue to progress after the cerebellar affliction has stabilised. Treatment of the neoplasm has no demonstrable effect on the progress of the disorder.

The striking pathological change is the disappearance of the Purkinje cells from the cerebellum. Diffuse degeneration is seen in other cerebellar neurones, and patchy microglial proliferation in the white matter of the cerebral and cerebellar hemispheres. By contrast the dentate nuclei are often little affected. Degeneration may occur in the long tracts of the cord, especially the spinocerebellar tracts and posterior columns, and in the oculomotor and lower cranial nerve nuclei. Meningeal and perivascular lymphocytic infiltration is seen in some cases, and inflammatory changes have been observed in the brain stem and subthalamic region.

Rather similar to the above is *opsoclonus*, consisting of rapid chaotic conjugate eye movements which severely distort ocular fixation and are often accompanied by ataxia (Compston 1993). This can be abrupt in onset, in contrast to subacute cerebellar degeneration, and sometimes progresses to coma and death within several weeks. It may be associated with myoclonus and encephalopathy, but coordination of the individual limbs is preserved. A proportion of cases show a useful clinical response to treatment with corticosteroids, suggesting that the disorder may be due to immune reactions to tumour antigens affecting the brain stem neurones.

Pathological changes involve loss of Purkinje cells and neuronal changes in the inferior olives, along with diffuse mononuclear infiltration of the brain parenchyma and leptomeninges. The disorder is characteristically seen with neuroblastoma in childhood, but also with tumours of the lung, breast and ovary in adults.

Encephalopathy with brain stem involvement

This, the so-called 'mixed form of encephalomyelitis' of Brain and Henson (1958), presents with varied neurological signs including cerebellar disorder, bulbar palsy, disordered external ocular movements, wasting and weakness of the limbs, extensor plantar responses, involuntary movements and posterior column sensory disturbance. Mental changes are again prominent in many examples, including dementia.

The disorder can follow a prolonged course over 2 years or more. In one case the neurological manifestations had been evident for 2 years before serial X-rays revealed carcinoma of the lung.

The pathological changes involve degeneration in the dentate nucleus, the superior cerebellar peduncles, the brain stem nuclei, the motor cells of the cord, and the pyramidal tracts and posterior columns. Inflammatory changes may be conspicuous with perivascular cuffing and cellular infiltrations of the meninges.

Diffuse encephalopathies with mental symptoms

Brain and Adams (1965) gave separate emphasis to a group of patients who present, not with neurological dysfunction, but with psychiatric disorders leading sometimes to psychiatric hospital admission. The mental changes may or may not be associated with evidence of focal cerebral lesions later in their course. A wide range of disturbances can occur. The picture may be of a simple dementia which is usually fairly rapidly progressive, or a disorder of memory with or without confusional episodes. Sometimes mood disorder is the predominant feature with depression, anxiety or agitation and much less evidence of cognitive disturbance.

The cerebrospinal fluid is often normal but the EEG may reveal diffuse changes. A close investigation must always be made into the metabolic, endocrine and nutritional status of the patient since the encephalopathy may be due to disturbance in such factors occasioned by the neoplasm (p. 743). It may also be necessary to search diligently for the primary growth which may so far have escaped detection.

The pathology in this group is described by Brain and Adams as patchy degeneration of the ganglion cells of the grey matter, with gliosis and a variable degree of lymphocytic infiltration. Where memory disorder has been the predominant feature the changes of limbic encephalopathy, described below, may be found. Sometimes, however, remarkably little may be observed in the brain at autopsy.

Encephalopathies presumed due to metabolic disturbance

An important but apparently rare group of cases has been described in which marked mental disorders are associated with carcinoma of the lung yet cerebral changes prove to be minimal or absent on detailed pathological examination (Charatan & Brierley 1956; McGovern et al. 1959). The common feature in such cases was a fluctuating disturbance of consciousness with periods of lucidity, extending over several months prior to death and unaccompanied by neurological abnormalities. Affective disturbances were often prominent in the earlier stages. In all cases the mental disturbance had either preceded or overshadowed the presence of the neoplasm. Here it would seem very likely that metabolic disturbances were fundamental to the development of the mental changes.

The first of Charatan and Brierley's cases was a man of 53 who became depressed and quarrelsome over several months. He later developed paranoid religious delusions and episodes of grossly muddled and odd behaviour. There were no organic features in the mental state and a diagnosis of paranoid schizophrenia was made. After recovering briefly for a week or two he abruptly relapsed, and at this stage carcinoma of the lung was detected. A quick decline led to coma and death.

The second was a man of 43 admitted after wandering from home in a depressed and apathetic state. He had lost his memory but this returned 4 days after admission. The only abnormal sign was some lability of mood. Soon, however, he developed periods of confusion with lucid intervals and deteriorated to death over 4 months. There had been suspicious shadowing of the lung for some months before presentation.

The third was a man of 63 who for 1 year had been slow, lethargic and complaining of feeling tired. Six months before presentation there had been an episode of confused nocturnal rambling, and since then his memory had been failing from time to time. Major epileptic fits had commenced at this time and chest X-ray had shown shadowing of the lung. Gradual decline was accompanied by lucid intervals lasting for a few days at a time. The mental state continued to show marked fluctuation in hospital until he died 2.5 months later.

The EEGs had shown little abnormality in the first two cases, and the cerebrospinal fluid was normal except in the first. In all three the brain was free from metastases and only a marginal gliosis of the white matter could be detected. The livers contained numerous metastases, however, and it was thought possible that liver failure may have contributed to the picture, either with or without other metabolic disturbances occasioned by the neoplasms.

McGovern et al. (1959) added two further examples, both in women:

The first presented with restlessness, apprehension, paranoid ideas and confusion about dates and time of some months' duration. She was profoundly disturbed, averting her face because of shame at things she imagined she had done, and imbuing every sound with fatal significance. She was disorientated, with poor attention and marked difficulties with memory and calculation. The state of severe fear and agitation progressed over 3 weeks to depressive stupor, at which time the chest neoplasm was revealed. She died 2 weeks later after periods of stupor alternating with periods of lucidity.

The second patient had a 6-month history of feeling unwell together with a constant sense of fear, inability to concentrate and occasions when she could not grasp the gist of things properly. There had been two attacks of generalised trembling accompanied by acute terror. In hospital she showed florid depressive thought content and evidence of intellectual impairment. Episodes of delirium gave way to a sustained delirious state for several days, at which point inflammatory changes were discovered in the left lung. Bronchoscopy showed carcinoma of the bronchus. Liver function tests were normal. She improved later to become alert and emotionally composed for several weeks, then episodes of delirium increased until she died some months later.

Again there were no neurological symptoms in either of McGovern et al.'s cases. The brains were entirely normal at autopsy, and metastases were minimal or absent from the livers also. The possible metabolic basis for the mental disturbances remained unclarified.

Limbic encephalopathy

Other patients present with mental disturbance in association with pathological changes largely limited to the limbic grey matter of the brain. The carcinoma is almost always of bronchial origin, often with metastases in the hilar lymph nodes but without direct spread to the brain. In several examples the neoplasm has become evident only at postmortem examination. Strangely the primary growth has not always been discovered even then, the only evidence of cancer sometimes being secondary deposits in the mediastinal lymph nodes. Very occasional examples have been reported with neoplasms of the bladder, mediastinum, thymus and testicle (Bakheit *et al.* 1990).

This form of encephalopathy was comprehensively described by Corsellis *et al.* (1968). The outstanding clinical feature is a marked disturbance of memory for recent events, though some degree of generalised intellectual impairment often develops later. Affective disturbance is frequently prominent early in the evolution of the disorder, usually in the form of severe anxiety or depression. Some patients are hallucinated and some have epileptic attacks, but otherwise impairment of consciousness is not observed. Several patients have shown a coincident carcinomatous neuropathy.

The first report of such a picture in association with carcinoma was included among cases reported by Brierley *et al.* (1960), though the connection was not appreciated at the time. One of their patients with 'subacute encephalitis of later adult life' was a man of 58 who demented over the course of 3 months and died, revealing an intense inflammatory reaction in the brain, most severe in the medial temporal lobe structures. The mediastinal lymph nodes were extensively infiltrated with oat-cell carcinoma though neoplasia had not been suspected during life.

Soon afterwards several similar examples were reported. Yahr *et al.* (1965) described a woman of 61 who developed impairment of memory and difficulty with her secretarial work together with numbness of the limbs. She became depressed, suspicious, confused and severely disorientated. A non-metastatic complication of carcinoma was suspected and at exploratory operation mediastinal lymph nodes were found to contain oat-cell deposits. She deteriorated gradually and died the following year. A small carcinoma of the lung was discovered and the brain showed the typical changes in the medial temporal lobe structures.

Corsellis *et al.* (1968) presented three further examples:

The first, a man of 59, suffered several epileptic fits followed a few weeks later by impairment of recent memory. No cause could be found. He continued to show a gross defect of memorising, but without other intellectual deterioration, until his death 2 years later. At autopsy oat-cell carcinoma was discovered in a mediastinal lymph node, and the medial temporal lobe areas showed degenerative and inflammatory changes.

The second was a man of 50 with known carcinoma of the lung who became mildly demented with some disorientation and impairment of recent memory. The carcinoma was resected but his mental state showed little change. He gradually developed dysarthria and progressive wasting of the small muscles of the hands and feet. At autopsy 2 years later there was no evidence of recurrence of the growth but the brain showed extensive changes in the medial temporal lobe structures, basal ganglia and diencephalon.

The third was a woman of 81 who died after a psychiatric illness of some years' duration, presenting initially as depression and marked in its later stages by dementia and a prominent defect of recent memory. Carcinoma had not been suspected during life but oat-cell carcinoma of the lung was discovered at autopsy. The medial temporal lobe structures were severely damaged along with some involvement of the midbrain and brain stem.

Bakheit *et al.* (1990) review the more recent literature on the condition. Symptoms had predated the diagnosis of malignancy in almost a third of cases, and neurological findings were few unless other brain regions were involved. The CT scan was usually unhelpful in diagnosis, and MRI was normal in two of three cases examined. The EEG can also be normal or show non-specific abnormalities over the temporal lobes, in contrast to the distinctive picture seen with herpes encephalitis (p. 357). The cerebrospinal fluid is usually abnormal with a raised lymphocyte count and raised immunoglobulin level. Oligoclonal bands may be detected. The course in various cases has varied widely from a few weeks to up to 5 years. Treatment of the primary tumour rarely influences the temporal lobe disorder, though rare exceptions have been reported (Burton *et al.* 1988).

The pathological picture shows a combination of degenerative and inflammatory changes which are concentrated on the medial temporal lobe structures — the hippocampus, uncus, amygdaloid nucleus, dentate gyrus, hippocampal gyrus, cingulate gyrus, insular and posterior orbital cortex. The changes can sometimes extend throughout the length of the fornices and involve the mamillary bodies. The rest of the hemisphere and the hindbrain are only slightly affected. The changes consist of extensive neuronal loss, marked astrocytic proliferation and fibrous gliosis, and perivascular infiltration with small round cells and the formation of glial nodules. In no cases have tumour cells been identified within the central nervous system. The severity of the inflammatory component has varied from case to case, but at times has been severe enough to be virtually indistinguishable from viral encephalitis. No inclusion bodies have been seen. Bakheit *et al.* (1990) suggest that immune damage to the limbic neurones is a more plausible explanation than an infective aetiology. Antibody with strong binding to limbic structures has been demonstrated in the serum of a patient.

How commonly mental disturbance in patients with carcinoma may be due to limbic system involvement is hard to assess. As already described some examples are clearly due to more diffuse cerebral pathology or to metabolic disturbances, but where memory failure is a predominant feature the possibility of limbic encephalopathy should be borne in mind.

Mechanisms of non-metastatic complications

The mechanisms underlying the neuropsychiatric complications of carcinoma remain elusive. The rarity of such complications suggests some exceptional factor, either in relation to the tumour or in the subject's reaction to it. The principal theories are that the complications are the consequence of some substance secreted by the tumour; or that they reflect a disturbance in the patient's immunological state which has led to invasion by a virus. More recently it has been proposed that at least some syndromes result from the effects of antibodies, produced in response to tumour antigens and cross-reacting with cytoplasmic components of cells within the nervous system (Dropcho 1989; Compston 1993).

The idea of a specific neurotoxin secreted by the tumour has so far obtained no direct support. Very occasionally removal of the neoplasm has led to improvement in the nervous or muscular symptoms, though this is the exception rather than the rule. Special attention has been concentrated on the hormone-like substances which some tumours, including those of the bronchus, are known to secrete (Lebowitz 1965). Thus hypercalcaemia may be caused by elaboration of an agent with parathormone-like activity and be ameliorated by removal of the primary growth. Cushing's syndrome may result from secretion of an adrenocorticotrophic hormone-like substance, hypoglycaemia from secretion of an insulin-like substance, or hyponatraemia from inappropriate antidiuretic hormone secretion. It is uncertain whether the tumours secrete such hormonally active materials themselves, or produce other substances which serve as releasers for the natural hormones.

In either event this has served as a starting point for exploring the remote effects of tumours on the nervous system. In cases with fluctuating acute organic reactions, as in the encephalopathies described on p. 741, it can be important to investigate the hormonal and metabolic status of the patient as completely as possible. Sethurajan et al. (1967), for example, described a woman with carcinoma of the lung who developed a fluctuating confusional state along with Cushing's syndrome. The mental abnormalities appeared to be directly related to the metabolic derangements produced by adrenal overactivity, and radiotherapy to the lung produced a temporary dramatic improvement in both the mental and endocrine symptoms. There is no evidence to date, however, to link such

hormonal or metabolic abnormalities with the production of fixed pathological changes within the nervous system.

The suggestion that a viral infection may be responsible has arisen from direct observation of the pathological changes in the brain. The idea has also obtained support from the finding of papova virus in the brain in progressive multifocal leukoencephalopathy which is also associated with malignancy (p. 752).

Thus in several of the syndromes discussed above the pathological picture shows inflammatory as well as degenerative changes. The inflammatory component may merely represent a secondary reaction to local products of degeneration, but against such a view is the rarity of such a reaction in other cerebral degenerative processes and the fact that inflammatory changes can be found remote from any area of degeneration. No virus has yet been isolated, however, and the possibility remains hypothetical.

Invasion by a virus or some other opportunistic pathogen would help to explain the lack of any constant relationship between the course of the neuropsychiatric complications and the course of the cancer. Cases in which the complications have first arisen after successful removal of the neoplasm suggest an incubation process of some sort, which once initiated proceeds independently of the tumour. The neoplasm may have disturbed the body's immunological state so as to render it unusually vulnerable to an infective agent, at the same time modifying the pathological reaction to the infection to account for the unusual pictures observed (Adams 1965). Whether the search should be for a latent virus within the brain which has become activated by the tumour, or for some common infective agent which has provoked an abnormal response, remains uncertain. Corsellis et al. (1968) pointed out that the site of cerebral damage in limbic encephalopathy is similar to that caused by herpes simplex infection; disturbed immunological mechanisms may account for the chronic instead of acute progression of such an infection, likewise the unusual features in the pathological picture.

Against any simple infective hypothesis is the striking predominance of one specific type of tumour, viz. the oat-cell carcinoma of the bronchus (Henson & Urich 1982). This has suggested that autoimmune mechanisms may be involved, with antigenic cross-reactivity between tumour cells and nervous system components (Dropcho 1989). The oat-cell tumour may share common antigenic determinants with elements of the nervous system, with the result that immune mechanisms directed against the tumour help to keep it in check while simultaneously damaging neural tissue. Such a mechanism is appealing as an explanation of the limited growth and spread of the tumour in many cases of paraneoplastic disease. The finding of antibodies against Purkinje cells and limbic structures in certain cases has been mentioned on pp. 740 and 742. It remains uncertain, however, whether these are merely 'markers' of the tumour or whether they are truly the cause of the neuronal damage.

The diverse remote effects of cancer on the central nervous system need not of course all share a common mechanism. Some of the encephalopathies may be the result of a virus infection, and others the result of immunological or metabolic derangements.

Depression and carcinoma

Finally, separate attention must be given to reports of affective disorder as a prodromal feature in patients who develop carcinoma. Fras *et al.* (1967) studied 46 consecutive patients with carcinoma of the pancreas, and found that psychiatric symptoms were closely related to the development of the neoplasm in three-quarters. In patients with cancer of the colon, who served as controls, the figure was only 17%. Symptoms of depression, anxiety and premonitions of serious illness were especially common. Nearly half of the 46 patients had developed psychiatric symptoms before any physical complaint, depression being the most frequent and lasting on average 6 months before the neoplasm was declared.

Kerr *et al.* (1969) explored the situation with regard to cancers generally. They traced a group of patients who had been admitted to hospital with affective disorders, and investigated the deaths which occurred during the following 4 years. Of 28 males who had had a depressive illness, seven had died from physical causes and in five the cause was cancer. This was very significantly above the number to be expected on the basis of national statistics. No particular site could be incriminated — deaths had occurred from cancer of the bronchus, prostate, stomach, colon and rectum. By contrast none of the 28 females with a depressive illness had died from cancer.

The five males who died of cancer had not had a previous history of affective disorder, and the depression had evolved without apparent cause. Its course had been unremitting prior to hospitalisation, but electroconvulsive therapy or antidepressants had then produced a complete remission. There had been no evidence of organic mental impairment, and examination had failed to reveal physical disease at the time except for a raised erythrocyte sedimentation rate in two patients. The mean interval between the onset of depression and death was only 2.4 years, strongly suggesting that latent or undiagnosed cancer may have been present during the evolution of the affective illness.

Others have sought by different survey methods to explore the relationship between depression and cancer, but have so far failed to confirm Kerr *et al.*'s findings (Judelsohn 1970; Evans *et al.* 1974). Nevertheless the evidence already at hand underlines the importance of attempting rigorously to exclude physical disease in patients who develop depressive illnesses in middle age, particularly those who do so for the first time and when there is no obvious precipitating factor.

Further evidence of a special association between depressive illness and cancer has come from studies of suicide. Whitlock (1978) reviewed the occasional reports of an unusually high incidence of malignancies in patients committing suicide when compared with community norms. His own survey of 273 suicides in Brisbane revealed 17 malignancies, compared with only two in controls dying from other violent causes (mostly road traffic accidents). The difference was statistically significant. No special site was involved, and intracranial spread had not occurred. In seven of the suicides and one of the controls the disease had not been diagnosed prior to death.

Normal-pressure hydrocephalus
(occult hydrocephalus, communicating hydrocephalus, hydrocephalic dementia)

The term 'hydrocephalus' refers to diffuse enlargement of the ventricular system within the brain. According to conventional terminology it may be divided into obstructive and non-obstructive forms, or communicating and non-communicating forms. In obstructive hydrocephalus there is a block to the free circulation of the cerebrospinal fluid which has led to ventricular enlargement; in non-obstructive forms the enlargement is secondary to atrophy of the brain substance as in Alzheimer's disease (also termed 'hydrocephalus ex-vacuo'). Most forms of obstructive hydrocephalus are non-communicating in the sense that the ventricles do not communicate freely with the cerebral subarachnoid space, whereas in hydrocephalus ex-vacuo such communication is free.

An important variety, however, is at the same time obstructive yet communicating. Here the block is not within the ventricular system but in the subarachnoid space, allowing free egress of the cerebrospinal fluid from the ventricles but preventing its subsequent upward flow over the surface of the hemispheres for absorption at the superior sagittal sinus. The block in such cases is commonly situated in the basal cisterns of the brain. This variety must be very carefully distinguished from hydrocephalus ex-vacuo since it can present with symptoms closely simulating the primary dementing illnesses. It is not infrequently associated with normal pressure within the ventricular system and headache is usually absent.

Such a syndrome has been variously termed normal-pressure hydrocephalus, occult hydrocephalus, communicating hydrocephalus or hydrocephalic dementia.* It owes its delineation to a group of workers who demonstrated cases in whom marked hydrocephalus was associated with a normal or even low intraventricular pressure, sometimes after head injury or subarachnoid haemorrhage but sometimes in patients suspected of a primary dementing illness (Hakim 1964; Adams *et al.* 1965; Hakim & Adams 1965; Adams 1966). Air encephalography showed the absence of any block within the ventricular system, but the air failed to ascend over the surface of the hemispheres betokening obstruction within the basal cisterns or cerebral subarachnoid space. Paradoxically, despite the normal intraventricular pressure, the neurological and mental impairments sometimes proved to be reversible by shunting procedures which reduced the pressure still further.

The discovery of the syndrome is of great clinical importance. It has led to a greater awareness of the caution that must be exercised in diagnosing primary cerebral atrophy, and has delineated a cause of dementia which is amenable to effective treatment.

Clinical features

The clinical features stressed in the early publications have since been amply confirmed. Ojemann (1971) reported clinical experience of 50 such patients. The typical picture is of the development over many weeks or months of memory impairment, physical and mental slowness, unsteadiness of gait and urinary incontinence. However, the precise symptomatology varies rather widely between one patient and another. The syndrome predominantly affects patients in their sixties or seventies though examples have occurred in middle or even young adult life.

The mental changes usually appear first and remain a prominent part of the picture throughout. They range from mild memory disturbance or apathy to severe psychomotor retardation and profound intellectual impairment. Forgetfulness is usually a prominent early feature,

combined with slowing of mental and physical activity, difficulty with thinking and reduced spontaneity—a combination which may lead to a diagnosis of early presenile dementia or depression. Emotional reactions are less vivid and psychic life seems generally impoverished. Insight is limited or absent from an early stage but social comportment is usually well preserved.

With progression of the disorder the patient becomes increasingly disorientated, calculation is impaired, and dysphasia and disturbances of writing and drawing may develop. Memory impairment may ultimately be as severe as that seen in Korsakoff's syndrome, or the global dementia virtually indistinguishable from that of Alzheimer's dementia. Uninhibited or aberrant behaviour is not usually seen, however, and psychotic developments in the form of delusions, hallucinations or paranoia are rare. In very occasional patients, outbursts of aggressive, hostile behaviour may be observed (Crowell *et al.* 1973; Sandyk 1984). Advanced cases sometimes show long periods of mutism, intermittent interruptions of on-going behaviour, or episodes of severe hypokinesia amounting to catatonia-like immobility.

Disturbance of gait may be the presenting feature in itself. In mild examples the patient walks slowly on a broad base with a stiff-legged shuffling gait. There is difficulty with turning and often difficulty with initiating movements similar to that seen in parkinsonism. Falls are frequent. The precise nature of the disturbance is hard to characterise but is often described as an uncertainty, unsteadiness or carelessness in walking. The ill-defined term 'gait apraxia' has been applied. When coupled with the mental symptoms this abnormality of gait is often the feature which leads one to suspect the presence of normal-pressure hydrocephalus. The disturbance may progress eventually to severe difficulty in walking, standing or arising from a seated position, sometimes even to difficulty in turning over in bed. Signs of spastic paraparesis may be evident with hyperactive tendon reflexes and extensor plantar responses. But even when the disability is pronounced it is rare to find frank ataxia of the limbs, dyssynergia or intention tremor of cerebellar type.

Urinary incontinence usually appears only when other symptoms are evident, but may set in surprisingly early in relation to the degree of mental impairment. Again this may have diagnostic importance in bringing the condition to mind. Faecal incontinence is rare and develops only in the most severe examples.

Other features may include slowness of movement in the upper limbs or occasionally some degree of arm tremor or ataxia. Unexplained nystagmus is occasionally present. Late in the course sucking and grasping reflexes may

* None of these terms is entirely satisfactory. The pressure is not always normal, 'occult' hydrocephalus is also used for any hydrocephalus in which the head is not enlarged, 'communicating' hydrocephalus also comprises hydrocephalus ex-vacuo, and dementia is not an inevitable part of the picture.

appear. Headache is rare and when present is usually minimal. Papilloedema does not develop. A history of falling spells with brief impairment of consciousness is common, but frank epileptic seizures have not been reported.

The course without treatment is of slow downward progression with increasing neurological and mental disability. Fluctuations from day to day or from week to week are very characteristic. In some of the more prolonged examples a plateau appears to be reached after many months with a relatively fixed pattern of impairments thereafter. Others progress eventually to coma and death.

Investigations

The findings on investigation are characteristic and necessary to confirm the diagnosis. At lumbar puncture the cerebrospinal fluid is usually under normal pressure and with normal constituents, though this depends on the condition giving rise to the hydrocephalus. The EEG is frequently abnormal, showing non-specific random theta or delta activity.

Before the advent of CT scanning, air encephalography usually provided the decisive evidence by way of symmetrically enlarged ventricles, often reaching huge proportions, but with little or no air in the cerebral subarachnoid space above the basal cisterns. Following the procedure, however, there was a risk of rapid deterioration, sometimes requiring urgent neurosurgical intervention. Isotope cisternography was widely used as an alternative or confirmatory investigation as discussed on p. 136. Angiography could provide the clue in advanced cases by demonstrating the increased circumferential sweep of the anterior cerebral artery occasioned by the distension of the ventricles.

The favoured diagnostic procedure now is CT scanning followed if necessary by a period of continuous intracranial pressure monitoring. The CT scan demonstrates the marked ventricular enlargement, usually with no more than minimal sulcal widening. Periventricular lucency may be seen around the ventricles, particularly over the anterior horns. This last sign can be important in distinguishing the condition from primary cerebral atrophy as in Alzheimer's disease (Jeffreys 1993). The visualisation of widened cortical sulci will also suggest the presence of a primary atrophic process but does not entirely exclude normal-pressure hydrocephalus. MRI scanning finds a special place in the detection of minor obstructive lesions which might otherwise be missed, particularly in the posterior fossa.

When there is doubt about the differentiation from a primary dementia, and in the absence of any obstruction,

it can be useful to perform a tap test by withdrawing 20–30 ml of cerebrospinal fluid by lumbar puncture and observing whether clinical improvement follows (Mendelow 1993). The most reliable method, however, is to monitor the intracranial pressure continuously over a period of at least 24 hours (Jeffreys 1993):

Such monitoring can be done from the surface of the brain but is most accurately performed by inserting a catheter into the lateral ventricle via a frontal burr hole. Continuous recording usually reveals that the pressure is not, in fact, uniformly within normal limits but rises intermittently, particularly during sleep. Alpha waves consist of elevations lasting 30 minutes or more, beta waves lasting for some 2–10 minutes. The identification of such a picture has, moreover, proved to be an important predictor of which patients will show a useful response to shunting. If there are no pressure waves, and the baseline pressure is normal or only marginally raised, a challenge test may be performed, either by abrupt injection of a bolus of normal saline into the ventricles or by continuous slow infusion over several hours. An atrophic brain will cope with these challenges with little alteration of pressure, whereas a patient in need of shunting will show a rise of pressure or beta waves will be induced.

Antecedent causes

In many examples no antecedent cause can be discovered. In others there is a history of subarachnoid haemorrhage, head injury or meningitis which has presumably led to the organisation of adhesions in the basal cisterns of the brain. After subarachnoid haemorrhage organisation of exudate within the arachnoid villi at the superior sagittal sinus may contribute further by obstructing the reabsorption of cerebrospinal fluid (Ellington & Margolis 1969). Very occasionally the typical clinical syndrome may be due to a partially non-communicating hydrocephalus occasioned, for example, by a third ventricular tumour or aqueduct stenosis. A rare cause has been described by Brieg *et al.* (1967) and Ekbom *et al.* (1969): in hypertensive individuals an elongated 'ectatic' basilar artery may indent the floor of the third ventricle and distort the ventricular system upwards and anteriorly, leading to normal-pressure hydrocephalus as described on p. 749.

In Ojemann's (1971) material of 50 cases no cause could be found in 18. These 'idiopathic' cases were all in their sixties or seventies. Of the 32 with known causes, 12 followed subarachnoid haemorrhage, 11 head injury and three meningitis. Five were due to tumours or the after-effects of posterior fossa surgery and one was due to aqueduct stenosis. The age range in this group was wider, from 26 to 69 years.

In the idiopathic cases the symptoms had set in insidiously and no precipitants could be discerned. The essential cause remained obscure, but in three such patients who came to autopsy the basal cisterns were found to be obstructed with fibrous tissue, perhaps due to a forgotten episode of head injury or unrecognised subarachnoid haemorrhage. Those following subarachnoid haemorrhage sometimes evolved from almost immediately after the bleeding or could first present several months later. Similarly after head injury signs of brain dysfunction had sometimes been present from the time of injury but occasionally developed only several months later.

Differential diagnosis

The most important differential diagnosis is from the primary senile and presenile dementias. Thus a substantial proportion of cases have no demonstrable antecedent cause and these tend to occur in patients in their sixties and seventies. McHugh (1966) suggests that the syndrome should be considered in any individual who is declining mentally, particularly if the illness has taken a subacute course over months rather than years or has shown pronounced remissions or exacerbations. It should be strongly suspected if early in the decline there appears a disorder of gait together with inertia, apathy and psychomotor retardation. Urinary incontinence developing before the mental impairments have proceeded very far should also raise suspicion.

A depressive illness may be simulated early in the course, when physical and mental slowness are prominent and intellectual impairment minimal. Several patients reported by Pujol et al. (1989) met DSM-III criteria for major depression. Rice and Gendelman (1973) drew attention to other ways in which the patient may first present to a psychiatrist. In five patients behavioural abnormalities were in the forefront of the picture, sometimes tending to obscure the organic features in the mental state. Examples included personality change with paranoid trends or increasing belligerence, acute agitation and paranoia accompanied by visual hallucinations, and marked anxiety and depression accompanying progressive dementia. In each case the hydrocephalus appeared to have aggravated pre-existing emotional difficulties in the patient in addition to producing intellectual impairment.

When the gait disturbance is the presenting feature differentiation is required from other causes of mild spasticity and ataxia such as cervical spondylosis. Parkinsonism may be suspected initially on account of the pronounced motor slowing. Indeed, the typical parkinsonian syndrome, accompanied by dementia, has sometimes been seen (Sypert et al. 1973). The differential diagnosis must, of course, also include other varieties of obstructive and communicating hydrocephalus and other forms of dementia.

Some of the problems encountered in diagnosis are illustrated in the following cases:

A woman of 66 had had a radical mastectomy for cancer of the breast followed 1 month later by progressive unsteadiness of gait, forgetfulness and intermittent confusion. Within 6 months the memory disorder was pronounced and psychometry showed widespread impairments. There was no evidence of secondary deposits. The cerebrospinal fluid was normal but air encephalography showed gross dilatation of the ventricles with no air over the cortical surface. She worsened precipitately after air encephalography and became drowsy, confused and almost mute. She could no longer walk and nystagmus was present in all directions of gaze. The cerebrospinal fluid now showed what were thought to be neoplastic cells and a diagnosis of carcinomatous meningeal infiltration was made.

Over the next 15 months she did not deteriorate as expected. She gradually became more alert, though she continued to speak little and took little notice of what went on around her. She lay or sat immobile, idle or watching television. On readmission she was grossly disorientated and with marked memory impairments, and showed no initiative whatsoever. She was incontinent of urine and faeces and could not sit or stand unsupported. The ankle reflexes were brisk and the plantars up-going but there were no cerebellar signs. The syndrome of normal-pressure hydrocephalus was recognised and a shunt operation performed. Improvement was evident within 3 days and after 7 weeks her mental state had returned to normal. Control of bowel and bladder was regained, and when seen 9 months later she was walking by herself though still with an uncertain gait.

(Adams et al. 1965)

A man of 49 complained of lethargy, easy fatiguability and vague weakness of the legs. For 6 months his family had noted him to be dull and forgetful. He was found to be slow in motor and verbal responses and with a mild impairment of recent memory. The plantar responses were extensor but there were no other abnormal neurological signs. The cerebrospinal fluid pressure was mildly elevated with a protein of 100 mg/100 ml. Air encephalography showed symmetrical dilatation of the ventricles with a small amount of air over the surface. A tentative diagnosis of Alzheimer's disease was made. In hospital there was considerable improvement in his apathy and inertia but he relapsed after a few weeks at home. Walking became seriously impaired with a stiff-legged gait and several falls. On readmission he was now severely amnesic for recent events and disorientated in time and place. He improved again in hospital but the diagnosis of Alzheimer's disease remained.

Over the next 2 months he gradually declined into severe confusion and was readmitted pending transfer to a long-stay psychiatric hospital. He was now unkempt, apathetic and unconcerned, with great slowness on mental tasks. He walked with a wide-based stiff-legged gait and stumbled on turning. Bilateral grasp reflexes were observed, and a prehensile sucking reflex when the lips were touched. The WAIS IQ was 64, whereas 4 months earlier it had been 101. After lumbar puncture he changed remarkably, becoming alert and quick of mind, fully orientated and able to learn new facts, and the WAIS IQ rose to 105. Gait returned to normal but the plantars remained extensor. A shunt operation was performed with excellent results, and a small mass situated on the floor of the third ventricle encroaching on the entrance to the aqueduct was irradiated. Six months later he was back at his usual clerical job.

(McHugh 1966)

Treatment and response

Treatment involves a shunt operation to lower the cerebrospinal fluid pressure within the ventricles and maintain it at this low level. An indwelling catheter is inserted into a lateral ventricle, incorporating a low-pressure one-way valve, and opening either into the superior vena cava through the jugular venous system (ventriculocaval shunt) or into the peritoneal cavity (ventriculoperitoneal shunt). The latter is now widely preferred. The result, though somewhat unpredictable, is gratifyingly successful in certain cases. Those patients who on intracranial pressure monitoring have shown elevated mean pressures or marked spontaneous pressure waves tend to show the best response (Jeffreys & Wood 1978; Crockard et al. 1980).

Shunt operations, even when dramatically successful initially, are not without their long-term complications (Jeffreys 1993). The catheter may become blocked or infected or shift its position, or the valve may cease to function. The development of a subdural haematoma is not infrequent. Overdrainage can result in headache, lethargy, strabismus, nausea and vomiting, typically relieved by lying down. The 'slit ventricle syndrome', commoner in those who have been shunted since early childhood, presents with a history indicative of intermittent obstruction and is probably also largely a consequence of previous overdrainage (Hendrick 1993).

Among cases with no known cause, Ojemann (1971) found satisfactory improvement after shunting in all patients where a complete block in the subarachnoid space had been demonstrated. The patients with only partial obstruction showed disappointing results, perhaps because some had a primary dementing illness in addition to their normal-pressure hydrocephalus. Pickard (1982) suggests that complete recovery can be expected in about a third of patients, with useful improvement in a further 30%.

The improvement is often manifest immediately on recovery from the anaesthetic, with further gains in the days that follow. Sometimes, however, there is little change during the first postoperative week, gradual improvement then taking place over the next several weeks. The neurological deficits are usually the first to resolve, though gait disturbance sometimes responds only gradually. Incontinence typically clears fairly promptly.

Intellectual deficits tend to improve more slowly, sometimes with maximal gains after several months. In favourable cases intellectual impairments, aspontaneity and apathy can ultimately clear completely. Follow-up with repeat evaluation of cognitive function has shown gains more obvious at 1 year than at 6 months, and well maintained thereafter (Crockard et al. 1980).

In cases following subarachnoid haemorrhage improvement is likely within a few days of shunting, but focal neurological deficits related to the local effects of the haemorrhage will often persist unaltered. The response in cases following head injury is governed by the degree and severity of the underlying brain damage. Salmon (1971) reported nine post-traumatic cases, operated at intervals of 6 months to 8 years after injury. Two were 'much improved' and three 'improved', including two patients who showed some evidence of cortical atrophy as well. The improvements often took place slowly over the course of several weeks.

Shunting has also been tried in presumed cases of Alzheimer's disease with evidence of cortical atrophy in addition to enlargement of the ventricles. Ojemann et al. (1969) found no response in five such patients, but others have reported apparent improvement in patients with Alzheimer's disease, Huntington's disease and other degenerative conditions (Appenzeller & Salmon 1967; Salmon & Armitage 1968; Salmon et al. 1971). However, the results are not sufficiently convincing to commend the procedure and it is no longer undertaken in primary dementing illnesses.

Pathophysiology

The mechanisms behind the development of normal-pressure hydrocephalus are uncertain. It is difficult to explain how the ventricles come to be so greatly enlarged when the pressure within them is normal, or to account for the production of severe neurological and mental deficits which prove to be reversible when the pressure is reduced still further. Several theories exist but none can be considered entirely satisfactory.

With regard to the ventricular enlargement it has been suggested that the pressure may have been elevated at an earlier stage but has subsided by the time the patient is under investigation. This may be so in cases where a definable cause such as subarachnoid haemorrhage has preceded the hydrocephalus, but would seem unlikely in cases without any antecedent history of acute disturbance. In the latter the evolution of symptoms is usually insidious from the outset, and sometimes it has seemed indubitable that symptoms have progressed during the time that the pressure has appeared to be normal. The discovery of periodic rises of pressure in many cases on continuous intracranial pressure monitoring (p. 746) may go much of the way towards resolving such paradoxes.

Some cases may represent arrested hydrocephalus dating back to earlier life. Intellectual failure would then occur more rapidly than in the normal brain in the presence of the minor degenerative processes of later life. This could perhaps apply to patients who show little response to shunting, but would be unlikely to explain those who derive marked and lasting benefit, including a return towards normal in ventricular size.

An alternative suggestion is that the ventricular walls or surrounding supporting tissues may have become altered in some way, allowing progressive enlargement in the face of normal pressure. Geschwind (1968) suggested that pulsatile forces due to intermittent peaks of high pressure may have led to rapid loss of proteins and lipids from the surrounding white matter, altering its ability to withstand the pressure normally exerted upon it. Or changes in the direction of cerebrospinal fluid flow may have had similar consequences. When prevented from rising up to the parasagittal area for reabsorption in the normal way, an excessive amount of cerebrospinal fluid may be absorbed through the ventricular walls, leading to changes in the properties of the surrounding tissues and allowing expansion under normal pressure (Ojemann 1971).

An interesting mechanism appears to be operative in a rare group of cases reported by Brieg et al. (1967) and Ekbom et al. (1969). These patients with hypertension and normal-pressure hydrocephalus were shown to have elongation of the basilar artery, indenting the floor of the third ventricle and producing a characteristic deformity there. A water-hammer effect from the pulsations of the artery may have impaired outflow from the lateral ventricles via the foramina of Monro, thus initiating ventricular distension.

With regard to the production of symptoms and alleviation by shunting, several mechanisms have again been postulated. Hakim and Adams (1965) put forward a theory of 'hydraulic press effect'. They suggested that a normal pressure, when exerted against the greatly increased surface area of the ventricles, would result in a larger than normal total force being expended upon the surrounding cerebral tissues. Symptoms would result from the increased total thrust against important long fibre tracts and nuclei in proximity to the ventricles. The prominence of frontal lobe deficits — apathy, inertia and early incontinence — might thus be due to the especial enlargement of the frontal horns.

Yakovlev's (1947) explanation for the accent of spasticity on the legs in hydrocephalus would also apply — the neurones innervating the legs must sweep round the surface of the ventricles before entering the internal capsule, whereas those destined for the arms and face are laterally placed in the cortex and pursue a more direct route. The hydraulic press hypothesis is supported by the fact that reduction of pressure by as little as 20–33 mm can permit restoration of nervous function and also partially relieve the ventricular distension.

Changes in cerebral blood flow have also been incriminated in the production of symptoms (Greitz 1969). Cerebral blood flow has been shown to be reduced in the disorder to an extent that correlates with the degree of ventricular dilatation, and improvement in cerebral blood flow follows shunting procedures. The decreased blood flow may be the direct result of compression of capillaries and veins, or the consequence of changes in vasomotor centres. Others have suggested that the relative stasis in the enlarged ventricles may lead to an accumulation of metabolites capable of interfering with cerebral function.

These various possibilities await clarification. It is possible that in some cases several factors operate in conjunction with one another.

Other forms of hydrocephalus

The best known form of hydrocephalus is that which declares itself in infancy, resulting from obstruction along the course of the cerebrospinal fluid pathways. This is usually due to developmental defects of the brain, haemorrhage following birth trauma, or an attack of meningitis. When the disturbance is manifest before the cranial sutures have closed there is progressive enlargement of the head. Usual accompaniments are varying degrees of spasticity, mental retardation and sometimes blindness, depending on the severity of the obstruction and the presence or absence of associated developmental brain defects. In some patients the hydrocephalus becomes arrested and intellect may occasionally be surprisingly well preserved. In cases due to developmental defects there are often other congenital abnormalities, particularly spina bifida and meningomyelocoele.

In adults obstructive hydrocephalus is mainly the result of new pathology, such as a tumour strategically situated to impede the cerebrospinal fluid circulation within the brain. It commonly presents with symptoms of raised intracranial pressure but sometimes the initial picture can be misleading. Riddoch (1936) described two patients with tumours of the third ventricle who presented with pictures of dementia without headache or papilloedema. Akinetic mutism may occur (Messert et al. 1966), or there may be a disturbance of gait as the initial manifestation (Messert & Baker 1966).

Occasionally, moreover, adult obstructive hydro-cephalus is attributable to congenital defects or pathology acquired much earlier in life; a partial balance is then achieved between the production and absorption of cere-brospinal fluid. Developmental defects such as aqueduct stenosis or partial obliteration of the foramina of the fourth ventricle can remain latent in this way. McHugh (1964) has drawn attention to examples of such 'occult' hydrocephalus in adults, occasionally remaining un-suspected until autopsy, sometimes decompensating suddenly with an abrupt rise in intracranial pressure, or sometimes progressing insidiously with the development of spastic paraparesis or mental changes. Headache is usual but not inevitable, and a spectrum is likely to exist between the cases considered here and those already described under the heading of normal-pressure hydro-cephalus. A frequent feature is a history of attacks of abrupt loss of consciousness, lasting a few minutes during which the patient lies motionless and flaccid. Such attacks are often preceded or followed by headache and are pre-sumably due to sudden rises of intracranial pressure. The mental changes, which may or may not accompany the neurological developments, can take the form of listless-ness, apathy and inattentiveness, progressing to a picture of dementia and inertia resembling frontal lobe disorder.

Aqueduct stenosis, in particular, may fail to declare itself until adolescence or mid-adulthood. Asymptomatic cases have also been found at autopsy. The stenosis is usually the result of congenital defect, though some can be traced to an episode of meningitis in childhood and others show gliosis of unknown cause. Sometimes a small mass, such as a peri-aqueductal glioma, compresses the aqueduct from without. Nag and Falconer (1966) and Wilkinson *et al.* (1966) discuss the pictures that may present in adult life. Symptoms of raised intracranial pressure may occur, sometimes following an intermittent crescendo pattern succeeded by periods of unconsciousness, but in others such evidence is completely lacking. Some present with unsteadiness of gait or with epilepsy, usually of psy-chomotor type. Others show hypothalamic symptoms such as impotence, amenorrhoea or obesity, due to pres-sure of the distended third ventricle on the pituitary and hypothalamus. Mental symptoms may be the presenting feature, with impairment of memory or generalised dementia. Of the 10 cases reported by Nag and Falconer only five presented with symptoms indicative of raised intracranial pressure, while memory disorder was the initial manifestation in four. Harrison *et al.* (1974) obtained a history of deterioration of memory and con-centration in a third of their cases. This was usually mild, but in two cases was sufficiently marked to be the feature that brought the patient to medical attention.

A man of 52 showed slow progression of gait disturbance and impotence following the death of his mother to whom he was closely attached. Six years later he was hospitalised and the dis-order was ascribed to 'nerves'. Thereafter he developed emo-tional lability, mild memory impairment and occasional urinary incontinence. One year later mental testing was within normal limits except for moderate slowing of responses, but his gait was strikingly abnormal with tiny shuffling steps and difficulty in ini-tiating movement. The cerebrospinal fluid was normal and under normal pressure. Air encephalography showed aqueduct stenosis. Ventriculography showed dilatation of the lateral and third ventricles, and also of the upper 1 cm of the aqueduct. A shunt operation led to excellent resolution of his symptoms. He had had meningitis at the age of 5 and had complained fre-quently of headache throughout adult life.

(Wilkinson *et al.* 1966)

An example reported by Ojemann *et al.* (1969) is also instructive:

A woman of 54 had an 18-month history of progressive change of personality and failure of mental functions. She became disin-terested in people and activities, and showed inattentiveness and difficulty with calculation. Some months later her gait became unsteady and her left hand tremulous, leading to a diagnosis of parkinsonism. Deterioration progressed relentlessly with marked apathy and incontinence of urine. On examination she showed impairment of memory and other intellectual functions, a slight left hemiparesis and spasticity in the legs. On sitting down she took 30 seconds to complete the last 4 inches, and on approaching a step she raised her foot too early and too high. The cerebrospinal fluid pressure was normal, and air encephalogra-phy showed air in the fourth ventricle but none in the aqueduct. Ventriculography displayed large lateral and third ventricles, with gross dilatation of the rostral part of the aqueduct and a nodular mass projecting from the region of the quadrigeminal plate. A shunt operation produced striking improvement and she was entirely normal 1 year after operation.

An interesting association of aqueduct stenosis has been reported by Reveley and Reveley (1983). In the course of examining the CT scans of schizophrenic patients they found three with aqueduct stenosis. Two were known to be hydrocephalic from shortly after birth, while in the third the condition was entirely unsuspected. The signifi-cance of this association remains at present unclear.

The diagnosis rests ultimately on X-ray studies along with CT or MRI. Erosion of the dorsum sellae is shown on plain X-rays in the majority, and the lateral and third ven-tricles are seen to be symmetrically enlarged. The aque-duct is either not displayed or is seen to be very narrow. Intraventricular pressure may be elevated or normal.

Shunt operations can be dramatically successful in relieving the symptoms whether or not the pressure has been raised. A considerable failure rate is seen, however, mainly due to obstruction within the subarachnoid space (McMillan & Williams 1977).

Other disorders producing dementia

Kuru

Kuru is a subacute degenerative disease of the brain leading to dementia. It is restricted to members of the Fore tribe who inhabit the eastern highlands of New Guinea, but has special claims to interest since a transmissible agent is involved. Moreover it holds a certain fascination in that spread has possibly been facilitated by cannibalism. It was the experimental observations on this rare disease that led ultimately to the discovery of transmissibility in Creutzfeldt–Jakob disease discussed on p. 743. The transmissible agent involved is now thought to be abnormal prion protein as with other spongiform encephalopathies.

The disease was first described by Gajdusek and Zigas (1957) and is reviewed by Alpers (1969). Prodromal symptoms of headache, malaise and limb pains lead on to florid symptoms of cerebellar ataxia and tremor. These soon render walking and speech impossible. Strabismus, marked clonus and emotional lability are characteristic features. Progressive intellectual deterioration leads to death usually within 12 months.

The brain shows a variety of neuronal degenerative changes with status spongiosus and marked astrocytosis. These are found diffusely, but the cerebellum is markedly affected and the cerebral cortex may be relatively spared. Amyloid plaques are prominent. There is minimal demyelination and inflammatory changes are absent.

Three factors appear to account for the illness: a genetic predisposition in the Fore people, a transmissible agent, and formerly a possible spread by means of cannibalism. Inoculates of brain tissue from affected persons have been shown to reproduce the disease in chimpanzees, and thence by serial passage from one chimpanzee to another (Gajdusek et al. 1966, 1967).

In the case of kuru, spread may have been greatly helped, until recent years at least, by the practice of cannibalism of dead relatives. With the transmissible agent present in the tissues of affected persons cannibalism would provide an especially hazardous means of increasing the incidence of the disease above that to be expected from genetic sources alone. Until recently kuru claimed the lives of more than 50% of the women of the tribe. It affected women principally, but surprisingly children of both sexes as well. Adult males escaped except in very rare instances. This distribution of cases could be related to the cannibalistic practices of the tribe, in which the women and children ate the viscera and brain but the adult males ate muscle only. Recently the development of new cases of the disease appears to have died out as the practice of cannibalism has ceased (Gajdusek et al. 1977).

It should be emphasised, however, that the cannibalism hypothesis was never firmly proven. Kuru has not been transmitted to chimpanzees by ingestion, only by injection. There may, of course, have been opportunities for 'self inoculation' through cuts and abrasions when infected tissues were handled during the ritual ceremonies of the tribe.

Gerstmann–Sträussler syndrome

This rare disorder was first described by Gerstmann in 1928 and by Gerstmann et al. in 1936. It has attracted attention recently because of its transmissibility to animals, and in view of the molecular genetic abnormalities outlined on pp. 474–5. It represents another example of the transmissible spongiform encephalopathies attributable to prion protein disorder.

The disease usually occurs familially as an autosomal dominant. Onset is mostly in the third or fourth decades though the range is wide. The majority of patients present with cerebellar ataxia, mild dementia appearing some years later during the course of the illness. Gaze abnormalities and dysarthria are frequently present. Other varieties present with dementia from the beginning along with extrapyramidal and pyramidal signs, sometimes closely resembling familial Alzheimer's disease (Hsiao & Prusiner 1990). The boundaries between the condition and Creutzfeldt–Jakob disease are often indistinct, though the duration tends to be longer with a mean of 4–5 years to death.

At autopsy the picture is similar to that of Creutzfeldt–Jakob disease (p. 478), with neuronal degeneration and status spongiosus in the cortex. A distinctive feature is the occurrence of prominent multicentric amyloid plaques in the cerebral and cerebellar hemispheres.

Progressive multifocal leukoencephalopathy

This rare disorder is an occasional complication of chronic diseases affecting the reticuloendothelial system such as lymphoma, Hodgkin's disease, leukaemia or sarcoidosis. It is a not uncommon complication of AIDS (p. 321). Richardson (1961, 1968) describes the typical clinical picture. Most affected patients have been between 30 and 60 years of age. Progressive dementia is accompanied by neurological manifestations indicative of focal involvement of the central nervous system—pareses, ataxia, dysphasia and visual field defects. Rapid mental and neurological deterioration typically leads to death within a few weeks or months, but very occasional cases have shown slow progression over several years. The CT scan shows low density lesions in the central and convolutional white matter, often with a distinctive 'scalloped' appearance to their lateral borders (Carroll *et al.* 1977). Such lesions do not enhance, and are without mass effect. The cerebrospinal fluid is usually normal. Biopsy is important to confirm the diagnosis and to exclude other potentially treatable conditions such as lymphoma (p. 321).

At autopsy scattered crumbling foci of softening are seen as small round greyish areas throughout the brain. They are situated mainly in the white matter, affecting the cerebral hemispheres, cerebellum and brain stem, and showing a special predilection for the junction of cortex and subcortex. Within such areas there is marked demyelination along with relative preservation of the axis cylinders. Perivascular lymphocytic cuffing is usually well developed. A unique stamp is given by the changes observed in the glial cells. Astrocytes are enormously enlarged, with bizarre distorted nuclei which often show abnormal mitoses. The oligodendroglial nuclei often contain inclusion bodies.

Electron microscopy gave the first indication of the presence of virus-like particles in the abnormal glial nuclei (Lancet 1966b; Dayan 1969). Abundant spherical particles could be detected, sometimes in crystalline arrays, together with cylindrical structures resembling those seen in cells infected with papova viruses. It has now been confirmed that the JC papova virus is the responsible agent, gaining access to the brain when immunocompetence is severely undermined.

Treatment is usually without effect, especially in patients with AIDS. Others have very occasionally been reported to respond to cytosine arabinoside (Bauer *et al.* 1973; Marriott *et al.* 1975).

Primary progressive aphasia

A rare form of dementia presents with aphasic symptoms which may continue as the sole manifestation for many years. Global deficits may eventually supervene, but relentlessly progressive impairment of language remains in the forefront of the clinical picture. It now seems likely that the composer, Ravel, suffered from an illness of this nature (Henson 1988).

The condition was first described by Wechsler, though his patient soon developed behavioural disturbance and proved at autopsy to have Pick's disease (Wechsler 1977; Wechsler *et al.* 1982). Other patients were then described with a more purely aphasic course (Mesulam 1982; Kirshner *et al.* 1984, 1987; Green *et al.* 1990; Weintraub *et al.* 1990; Snowden *et al.* 1992). Mesulam and Weintraub (1992) summarise the existing literature. They suggest that the syndrome should be diagnosed only when disso-

lution of language is the sole salient finding for at least 2 years from the outset, other than dyspraxia and dyscalculia, and when other causes (such as stroke or tumour) cannot be identified. Sixty-three patients satisfying these criteria had been reported to that date.

The onset is mostly in the fifties or sixties, with a range from 40 to 75 years. Males outnumber females by 2:1. The language problem usually begins with word-finding difficulties, more apparent to the patient than others. Some patients remain at this stage for prolonged periods, while others progress to a steadily worsening dysphasia. This may be of the fluent or non-fluent variety, with variable comprehension defects, though reading and writing are often relatively spared. Dyspraxic difficulties may accompany the dysphasia, but other cognitive deficits remain absent for a considerable time. Memory, at least in the non-verbal domain, proves to be intact, along with orientation and visuospatial functioning. Daily living activities can be remarkably well preserved, with the patient continuing to drive, keep house and handle his own finances. Social skills also typically remain undisturbed.

Some patients display a relatively isolated progressive aphasia of this nature for 10 years or longer, the mean duration at this stage being 5.2 years in Mesulam and Weintraub's material. Ultimately, however, the patient is likely to become mute and to lose all ability to communicate, at which time it is difficult to assess the intactness of other cognitive functions. Personality and behavioural changes develop in some patients, and memory difficulties with generalised dementia in others. Focal neurological signs occasionally appear, such as right hemiparesis, right body posturing or right arm tremor.

CT or MRI typically show focal atrophy of the left peri-Sylvian region and widening of the left frontal horn, slowly progressive over time. The EEG shows asymmetrical slowing on the left. PET and SPECT scans reveal impaired blood flow and metabolism largely confined to the left frontotemporal regions (Chawluk *et al.* 1986; Tyrrell *et al.* 1990; Snowden *et al.* 1992).

A heating engineer began to experience difficulty in expressing himself at the age of 58, noting hesitancy and lack of fluency when speaking. His writing was slower with spelling and grammatical errors. Four years later he was referred to a neurologist, by which time speech was very slow and hesitant but there was no evidence of cognitive decline. He continued to work at his job and functioned excellently at home. Three years later there was marked deterioration, with no initiation of spontaneous speech, long pauses and frequent paraphasic errors. Memory and judgement remained intact, but there was some evidence of emotional lability.

Nine years after the onset he had recently retired from work. By this stage he could barely repeat single words, while comprehension remained adequate. Some generalised decline was evident in his apathy and inertia, and he had recently made some errors of judgement. He tended to drag his right leg. CT scans showed generalised atrophic features without asymmetry, and a SPECT scan showed markedly reduced frontal flows more marked on the left than the right.

The pathology in such cases has proved to be heterogeneous, some cases showing the picture of Alzheimer's disease and others Pick's disease. In more than half of those examined to date, however, the neuropathological changes have consisted of non-specific neuronal loss with gliosis and some degree of spongiform change, i.e. a picture similar to that seen in frontal lobe dementia (p. 465). The fronto-peri-Sylvian region of the left hemisphere is chiefly affected. Neary *et al.* (1993a) have reported two brothers with the condition, both showing this non-specific pathology. One, who became behaviourally disturbed only towards the end of his illness showed predominantly left frontotemporal atrophy; the other, who developed behavioural change early on, showed bilateral frontotemporal atrophy similar to that of frontal lobe dementia. Neary *et al.* suggest that the clinical manifestations were dictated by the topographical distribution of a common underlying pathology, thus linking the syndrome of progressive aphasia to dementia of frontal lobe type. Neary *et al.* (1993b) regard these diseases as components of a general class of 'lobar brain atrophies' of non-Alzheimer type, which also includes the dementias that can occur with motor neurone disease (p. 708).

It appears, therefore, that primary progressive aphasia reflects brain degeneration with a remarkably selective emphasis on the neural networks subserving language. It is of considerable heuristic interest that Mesulam and Weintraub (1992) report a history of reading and writing difficulties early in the lives of a number of such patients, sometimes with a marked family history of such problems in other family members.

Semantic dementia

A seemingly distinct form of presenile dementia presents as a selective loss of semantic knowledge, i.e. of the meaning of words and objects (Snowden *et al.* 1989, 1994; Hodges *et al.* 1992). The first report of such a condition was in three patients described by Warrington (1975). Though usually presenting as difficulties with language or even 'memory', it becomes apparent that the deficits encompass a profound loss of meaning both in the verbal and non-verbal domains.

Problems with language are usually first in evidence. Speech is effortless, fluent and with normal syntax, though it may be restricted in content through loss of nominal terms. Closer analysis shows profound difficulties with naming and with verbal comprehension. Thus the patient has difficulty in naming objects or pointing to objects or body parts, and in carrying out simple instructions. Tests of verbal fluency show a grossly impaired ability to list examples from a class (e.g. animals or household objects) due to a severely impoverished vocabulary. Paraphasic errors and echolalia may be prominent. By contrast, repetition of heard material is excellently preserved, likewise the recitation of well-known serials. In these respects the form of language breakdown resembles that of transcortical sensory dysphasia (p. 53). In the earlier stages reading and writing to dictation are also preserved, though the patient may not understand what he has read.

The loss of access to meaning is also apparent with non-verbal material. The patient lacks appreciation of the significance of common objects, leading to difficulties in reporting or demonstrating their use. Facial recognition is usually markedly involved (prosopagnosia), with inability to identify people or pictures of celebrities. Errors may be demonstrated when the patient is asked to sort pictures of animals (dogs, cats, birds) into their relevant groups. Despite these defects, elementary perceptual functions remain intact, with ability to copy drawings, match shapes and visual patterns, and even to carry out complex facial matching tasks. Visuospatial and topographical sense remain strikingly intact.

In interesting experiments Snowden *et al.* (1994) have shown that patients perform consistently better in the understanding and identification of personally relevant names of people and places than of those which have little personal relevance, with optimal performance on those which are *currently* relevant. Such distinctions were not evident in a control group of Alzheimer patients. In one patient it was possible to show that object recognition (for example of a kettle or a comb) was better for her own possessions than for alternative examples of the same objects. Such effects may explain the surprising competence which patients may demonstrate in the activities of day-to-day living when formal tests of object recognition are very poor, and the maintenance of a repertoire of personally relevant conversation when language tests show abysmal results.

The patients and their relatives will often attribute the problems to memory failure, and there is a superficial appearance of such. The difficulties prove, however, to be entirely due to loss of semantic knowledge. Orientation in time and place are preserved, and recall of personally relevant day-to-day events (episodic memory) is usually substantially intact. Non-verbal memory may be shown to be entirely normal.

The majority of patients retain adequate social conduct for a considerable time, and show preserved insight with distress at their disabilities. Occasional examples of seemingly confused bizarre behaviour, such as urinating in the bedroom or emptying the dustbin in the garage, may be attributable to failure to appreciate the significance of these locations.

Slow progression over several years leads to diminishing speech and comprehension, and an increasing lack of appreciation of the meaning of objects. Perseverative tendencies become marked. Repetition of language remains little impaired, however, and spatial abilities are typically preserved. Ultimately, lack of initiative and behavioural disturbances similar to those of frontal dementia (p. 463) may make an appearance. Focal neurological signs remain in abeyance.

The EEG is typically normal and brain imaging shows focal atrophy affecting the temporal lobes predominantly. All five cases reported by Hodges *et al.* (1992) showed marked temporal lobe atrophy, and SPECT scans (PET in one case) invariably implicated the dominant temporal lobe.

It is probable that most examples are initially diagnosed as Alzheimer's disease, on account of the seeming memory disturbance and problems with comprehension. The preservation of orientation late into the disease may give the clue, or the intact spatial and topographical abilities. Other patients will be suspected of primary progressive aphasia, but careful examination will show that the problems are not confined to the verbal domain. When behavioural disturbances appear the patient is likely to be suspected of Pick's disease or other dementia of frontal lobe type.

Little is known about the nature of the underlying pathology since the condition is very rare. It is likely that it represents yet another variant of lobar brain atrophy (p. 753), with the clinical features depending on the precise topography of the distribution of pathological change.

Other focal dementias

Very occasionally other focal cognitive deficits are found to remain in the forefront during a cerebral degenerative process. Crystal *et al.* (1982) reported a woman of 57 who developed a right parietal lobe syndrome with numbness of the left hand, pseudoathetosis and impaired position sense in the arm. Astereognosis and agraphaesthesia were marked. Gradual intellectual deterioration followed 2 years later. Biopsy of the right frontal lobe showed numerous plaques and tangles indicative of Alzheimer's disease.

In a 58-year-old patient seen personally (Sahakian *et al.* 1987) the main symptom was of progressive visuospatial impairment over a 7-year period, with comparatively mild deficits in memory and language. She showed left-sided sensory inattention, a left homonymous field defect, severe constructional apraxia and poor topographical orientation. The CT scan revealed widening of the Sylvian fissure and parietal sulci, especially on the right. A trial of physostigmine infusions led to transient improvements in memory and on tests of visuospatial and constructional abilities.

Slowly progressive apraxia was reported by Dick *et al.* (1989) in a man of 55, increasing over a 5-year period and primarily involving finger movements and bimanual activities. Memory, language and visuospatial abilities remained intact. The CT scan showed atrophy affecting both superior parietal lobules, and a SPECT scan showed hypoperfusion in the superior parietal regions especially on the right.

Two patients with progressive upper limb apraxia and gait disturbance are mentioned by Tyrrell and Rossor (1994). In the early stages the gait disturbance was accompanied by a marked fear of falling and intense anxiety, and later both became chair bound; one progressed to generalised dementia after 2 years, while the other showed well-preserved cognitive functioning for 4 years. PET studies revealed hypometabolism in the medial frontal cortex, encompassing the supplementary motor areas.

Other rare syndromes reviewed by Tyrrell and Rossor include patients with progressive orofacial dyspraxia leading to loss of speech and sometimes complete anarthria, also a patient with progressive prosopagnosia extending over a 12-year course. In the former group PET revealed bilateral hypometabolism mainly affecting the inferolateral frontal regions, and in the latter patient hypometabolism was revealed in the superior temporal gyri, especially on the right. Patients whose dementia was heralded by disorders of visual function, such as alexia or visual agnosia, were reported by Benson *et al.* (1988). CT and MRI showed predominant atrophy in the parieto-occipital regions.

The nosological status of such 'focal dementias' remains uncertain. Some may represent variants of well-known cerebral degenerative processes, such as Alzheimer's or Pick's disease, but in others the unusually protracted course suggests some other pathological basis which remains to be clarified. The rarity of such patients, and their sometimes bizarre opening manifestations, can result in considerable delays before the organic nature of the disorder becomes apparent.

Adrenoleucodystrophy

This group of disorders includes neonatal and childhood

adrenoleucodystrophy, Zellweger's cerebrohepatorenal syndrome and adult-onset adrenomyeloneuropathy (Compston 1993). The biochemical abnormality which they share is the accumulation of very-long-chain saturated fatty acids, particularly hexacosanoate, in lipid-containing tissues including the brain. Characteristic lamellar inclusions can be shown in the Schwann cells of the nervous system and the cells of the adrenal cortex. The diagnosis may be made by biochemical assay in body fluids, or ultrastructural examination of nerve terminals biopsied from the skin or conjunctiva. The childhood and adult-onset forms are sex linked, appearing only in males, and may be found in the same family. The neonatal form and Zellweger's syndrome are autosomal recessives.

Adrenomyeloneuropathy presents with spastic paraparesis and sensory loss in the legs due to peripheral nerve involvement, proceeding sometimes to dementia. In rare examples the presentation has been with focal cerebral deficits, the Klüver Bucy syndrome, dementia resembling Alzheimer's disease or spinocerebellar degeneration (Moser *et al.* 1984). Adrenal insufficiency may not be apparent at the time of presentation but Addison's disease develops eventually. Occasionally this precedes the nervous system involvement.

Kraepelin's disease

Kraepelin described the disease which bears his name in 1910, though there is now considerable doubt whether it should be regarded as a clinical or pathological entity. McMenemey (1963b) referred to 17 reported cases in the literature. The onset is usually in the fourth decade but some cases have begun in adolescence. Rapidly progressive mental deterioration is accompanied by restlessness, anxiety, depression and speech defects, and leads to death within 1 or 2 years. Catatonia-like features have accompanied the dementia in many examples and some have begun with an acute catatonic psychosis.

The essential feature at autopsy appears to be destruction of Nissl substance and consequent dissolution of ganglion cells. The changes are patchy in distribution but particularly affect the frontal and central areas and Ammon's horns. Glial proliferation is remarkably slight, and tangles and plaques are not seen.

Schaumberg and Suzuki (1968) reported six members of a family affected by early presenile dementia in whom the pathological changes at autopsy accorded with those described by Kraepelin. Again the picture was of diffuse cortical atrophy and loss of neurones but without more specific features. Nevertheless they agreed that in most reported examples of Kraepelin's disease there have been other plausible explanations for the pathological picture, such as cerebral anoxia or metabolic defects.

Dementia with thalamic degeneration

From time to time patients are reported in whom a progressive dementing illness proves to be associated with unusual and unexpected pathological changes in the brain. One such example is the case described by Stern (1939) where thalamic degeneration was the conspicuous finding at autopsy. Severe generalised dementia proceeded to death within 3 months, during which the patient showed gross memory disturbance, confabulation, perseveration, receptive language difficulties, somnolence and marked inertia. The only neurological signs were loss of the pupillary reflexes to light and accommodation, forced grasping and prominent sucking reflexes.

At autopsy there was no cerebral atrophy. The cortex showed diffuse non-specific degeneration of neurones and some glial overgrowth. But the striking finding was severe degeneration in the thalamus, with complete disappearance of nerve cells in some regions and dense gliosis. The affected areas were bilaterally symmetrical. There were no inflammatory changes and arteriosclerosis was minimal. The symmetry of the process and its circumscribed nature suggested a 'system degeneration' of the thalamus, affecting the phylogenetically most recent parts.

Martin *et al.* (1983) have described a more recent example in a young woman of 21, evolving with severe dementia, amenorrhoea and progressive emaciation. Death followed 3 years later after a short period of coma. She had shown episodes of strange behaviour with blank staring and incoherent mumbling, and she occasionally complained of diplopia. Neurological examination was normal apart from generalised tremulousness and a snout reflex, and the CT scan showed no abnormalities. Neuronal loss and astrocytic gliosis were maximal in the anterior and medial thalamic structures though with some involvement of the pulvinar as well. The rest of the nervous system was intact except for discrete changes in the olivary nuclei.

Martin *et al.* review 12 other cases in the literature of 'pure thalamic atrophy', all showing dementia and/or memory disturbance, sometimes accompanied by ataxia, chorea or athetotic movements. The ages at onset ranged from 18 to 65, with durations to death of 3 months to 20 years. The great majority were male.

It is interesting that a thalamic location has also been reported for tumours and cerebrovascular lesions which lead to dementia (pp. 228 and 384).

Dementia with familial calcification of the basal ganglia (Fahr's syndrome)

Dementia appears to be a common late manifestation in patients suffering from 'idiopathic calcification of the basal ganglia'. This rare syndrome tends to occur familially with a pattern suggestive of autosomal dominant inheritance (Moscowitz *et al.* 1971). The cause remains unknown.

Many affected persons are asymptomatic for long periods of time, though it seems likely that most eventually show some form of extrapyramidal dysfunction. Parkinsonism or choreoathetosis usually develop in late middle age, or more rarely cerebellar ataxia or pyramidal deficits. Progressive impairment of memory and intellect frequently accompany the motor manifestations, with slowing of cognitive processes typical of subcortical dementia (p. 667). Dysphasia and other focal cortical deficits are not observed. In several cases a psychosis indistinguishable from schizophrenia has been reported, often antedating the motor and cognitive manifestations by many years. Francis (1979) and Francis and Freeman (1984) have reported nine patients in four generations of a family in whom a schizophrenia-like psychosis appeared to be the principal accompaniment of the disorder.

Cummings *et al.* (1983) review the literature on the condition, finding indications of two relatively distinct patterns of presentation. Those who present with psychotic episodes tend to do so in their early thirties, those with dementia and motor disorder some 20 years later. Both share the characteristic finding of dense calcification symmetrically involving the basal ganglia and particularly the putamen. The dentate nuclei of the cerebellum and the pulvinar of the thalamus may also be heavily affected.

Other conditions leading to calcification within the basal ganglia must be excluded, the commonest being hypoparathyroidism and pseudohypoparathyroidism. Hyperparathyroidism may occasionally produce a not dissimilar radiological appearance. Investigation of the serum calcium and phosphate serves to make the distinction since these have uniformly proved to be normal. Other causes of calcification such as toxoplasmosis, tuberous sclerosis or the sequelae of encephalitis or anoxia will also need consideration when the familial nature of the condition is not apparent.

In a recent review of the literature, Flint and Goldstein (1992) have cast doubt upon the syndrome as an independent clinical entity. They suggest that it is genetically heterogeneous, and, moreover, that at least some cases are variants of pseudohypoparathyroidism. Some of the associated features of the latter, such as short stature and shortened metacarpals, occurred in their own familial cases and in other reported examples. Flint and Goldstein also conclude that schizophrenia, when carefully delineated, is uncommon and may represent no more than a chance association.

Hallervorden–Spatz syndrome

Dementia is prominent in the majority of patients with this rare extrapyramidal syndrome and can very occasionally be the presenting feature. Late infantile and juvenile forms make up the majority of cases, though a rare adult variant exists. The nosology of the syndrome has become confused as further examples have been reported.

More than one family member tends to be affected though sporadic cases occur. It is considered to be inherited as an autosomal recessive. Dooling *et al.* (1974) describe the typical features as onset at a young age, a motor disorder mainly of extrapyramidal type, the mental changes of dementia, and a relentlessly progressive course leading to death on average 11 years later. Of their 42 examples from the literature, mental changes had been the first manifestations in four. In more than half the onset had been before the age of 10, but one had begun at 30 and two others at 57 and 64 years. The late-onset cases were non-familial and died after 5–6 years. More recently Jankovic *et al.* (1985) have described a familial example with onset at the age of 55.

Motor abnormalities consist mainly of rigidity, dystonia and choreoathetoid movements, though spasticity and pyramidal signs may appear. Dysarthria is almost always present and facial grimacing may occur. Myoclonus and tremor are not uncommon. Abnormalities of posture or movement are the usual presenting symptoms, often interfering with walking. Vision may be impaired due to retinopathy or optic atrophy.

A change of personality sometimes sets in early, with moodiness, depression and outbursts of aggressive behaviour (Sacks *et al.* 1966; Rodzilsky *et al.* 1968). Intellectual deterioration then gradually develops along with the motor manifestations, often progressing to mutism in the terminal stages.

There are no abnormal findings in the blood or cerebrospinal fluid. The EEG shows slowing as the disease advances, sometimes with spikes and sharp waves. The CT scan may resemble that seen in Huntington's chorea, with prominent atrophy of the basal ganglia (Dooling *et al.* 1980). Generalised atrophy of the cortex, brain stem and cerebellum may also be apparent. MRI shows destruction of the central part of the globus pallidus, surrounded by dark signal due to iron deposition ('tiger's eye appearance').

At autopsy the distinctive finding is reddish-brown discoloration of the globus pallidus and pars reticulata of the substantia nigra, due to the accumulation of iron-containing pigment. Microscopy shows loss of neurones in the affected areas with demyelination and gliosis, and numerous oval or rounded structures (spheroids) which are identifiable as axonal swellings. The latter are frequently widely disseminated in the cortex, though this may otherwise show little by way of neuronal loss or gliosis. The Purkinje cells of the cerebellum may be depleted.

Treatment with iron-chelating agents has been tried without success. Levodopa may, however, improve the motor abnormalities for a time.

Neuroacanthocytosis (choreoacanthocytosis)

Neuroacanthocytosis is rare among neurological syndromes in being accompanied by distinctive changes in the peripheral blood. It shows a marked familial tendency, and has attracted interest in view of its pleomorphic features and its resemblance to Huntington's disease. Dementia can occur as a late manifestation.

Acanthocytes are abnormal red blood corpuscles, detected in fresh blood films by their spiny protuberances. They must be carefully distinguished from 'echynocytes' which show a not dissimilar appearance, and from other artefactual changes in red blood cell morphology (Hardie 1989). Acanthocytes are also found in abetalipoproteinaemia (Bassen–Kornzweig syndrome), a condition usually appearing in the first decade of life and accompanied by fat malabsorption, spinocerebellar ataxia and pigmentary retinopathy. These features are attributed to defective absorption of vitamin E. In neuroacanthocytosis, however, lipid metabolism is entirely normal.

The condition usually comes to attention in early middle age though the range of onset is wide. Involuntary movements, chiefly choreic, are accompanied by hyporeflexia or areflexia and sometimes by muscle wasting. Seizures occur in perhaps a half of cases. Steady and slow progression of deficits is the rule over several decades, though there is much variability. Inheritance has appeared to be autosomal recessive or autosomal dominant in different series, and sporadic cases also occur. An association with the McLeod blood group phenotype has suggested a locus on the short arm on the X-chromosome in some cases.

The manifestations were first described by Estes et al.

(1967) and Levine et al. (1968). Scattered examples from several families were then reported, until Hardie et al. (1991) presented 19 cases with a review of the relevant literature. Movement disorder is virtually universal, with choreiform and dystonic movements affecting the orofacial region and sometimes the limbs. In severe examples there may be biting of the tongue and lips, also pseudobulbar features with difficulty with speech and swallowing. Tongue protrusions and severe grimacing may occur. Tics can also be prominent, along with grunting, sniffing and spitting. Vocalisations sometimes develop, usually of monosyllabic words. A peculiar lurching gait may be seen with dipping of the knees and foot flap. A minority of cases progress to an akinetic–rigid state. Muscle wasting and weakness can affect distal or proximal groups, hyporeflexia being common even in its absence.

Among psychiatric features depression, anxiety and obsessive–compulsive disorder are not infrequent. Hardie et al. (1991) also report a characteristic organic personality change, leading to vagueness, distractibility and neglect of appearance and social skills. Wyszynski et al. (1989) review reports of recurrent depression, paranoia, irritability and reclusiveness. Their own patient showed depression with a compulsion to bite her lips and tongue producing considerable self injury. Dementia has been clinically evident in some half of reported cases, but neuropsychological evaluation may show deficits in many more, particularly on tests of attention and planning indicative of frontal lobe disorder.

Investigation in suspected cases must include a careful search for acanthocytes in fresh blood films, repeated if necessary on several occasions since the abnormal cells can be relatively rare in the early stages. The serum creatinine kinase may or may not be elevated. CT scans often show caudate atrophy, or generalised cerebral atrophy in the presence of dementia. MRI may show increased T_2 signals from the basal ganglia.

At autopsy there is extensive neuronal loss and gliosis in the corpus striatum and globus pallidus, also sometimes in the lateral substantia nigra. The caudate nucleus may be virtually depleted of both large and small neurones. The hemisphere white matter shows mild diffuse gliosis, but the cortex itself is spared. In the case examined by Bird et al. (1978) there was no deficiency of choline acetyltransferase or glutamic acid decarboxylase in the cortex or striatum.

Differential diagnosis must obviously include Huntington's disease, especially in patients who show a dominant pattern of inheritance. The presence of seizures, muscle wasting, areflexia or evidence of neuropathy should immediately raise suspicion of neuroacanthocytosis, also good preservation of cognitive function late into the disease. Gilles de la Tourette's syndrome may sometimes be closely simulated, likewise tardive dyskinesia if the patient has been on neuroleptic medication. Estimation of serum lipids will reveal those patients whose acanthocytosis is due to abetalipoproteinaemia.

Metachromatic leucodystrophy

This rare cause of dementia and motor disorder is inherited as an autosomal recessive. It represents an abnormality of neural lipid metabolism, with the accumulation of galactosyl sulphatide in affected tissues. Deposits of the material stain metachromatically. The diagnosis may be confirmed during life by biopsies of peripheral nerve or rectal wall.

Dulaney and Moser (1978) describe infantile, juvenile and adult forms which appear to be genetically distinct. The infantile form represents the classic disease, setting in before the age of 3 and progressing to severe motor and mental retardation, sometimes with blindness. The juvenile form is less common, presenting with motor and mental dysfunction and sometimes resembling a spinocerebellar disorder.

The adult form is rarest of all. Onset in recorded cases has varied from 19 to 46 years, presenting sometimes with dementia and sometimes with psychotic disorder. Motor dysfunction is less prominent and may develop only later in the disease. In adults the course can be extremely protracted over several decades; mistakes in diagnosis are common and unless a sibling has already been affected the condition may go unsuspected during life. Common misdiagnoses are of presenile dementia, schizophrenia or multiple sclerosis. Cummings and Benson (1992) refer to reports of the condition first diagnosed as schizophrenia or presenting with expansive delusions suggestive of mania. When motor abnormalities eventually appear they take the form of pyramidal and extrapyramidal dysfunction with paresis, dystonic movements, dysarthria and parkinsonism. Ataxia, nystagmus and intention tremor are common. Seizures often occur, and peripheral neuropathy is usually present.

Hyde *et al.* (1992) have drawn attention to the special liability of adolescent and early adult cases to present with psychotic disorder, this appearing to be restricted to such an age of onset. Thus of 129 published case reports, 55 patients had had an onset between the ages of 10 and 30 years, and 29 of these (53%) showed psychotic symptoms. This was the most frequent presenting feature in the age group concerned, and seemed considerably more common than with other neurological disorders. No such symptoms were apparent in the 74 cases with juvenile or later adult onset. Typical symptoms included auditory hallucinations, sometimes of voices commenting on the patient's behaviour, complex delusions, fragmentation of thinking, inappropriate affect, bizarre behaviour or catatonic posturing. Many of the psychoses appeared at first to be non-organic, and 15 patients had been diagnosed as suffering from schizophrenia. Two showed mania and three personality change. The false diagnoses sometimes persisted for several years before dysarthria, spasticity and hyperreflexia appeared.

Hyde *et al.* suggest that such psychotic developments may owe much to the disruption of frontal–subcortical connections occasioned by the demyelination. This at first mainly affects the subfrontal and periventricular frontal white matter. As the disease progresses and demyelination spreads more diffusely the psychotic symptoms tend to disappear, being replaced by sensorimotor disturbances and dementia. However, the age of the patient must be an additional determining factor, since a similar distribution of demyelination is seen in the infantile, juvenile and late-onset forms.

A typical diagnostic puzzle was as follows:

A woman of 29 was referred for a second opinion, 2.5 years after admission to a psychiatric hospital with a provisional diagnosis of schizophrenia. Certain organic features in her mental state had then given rise to concern.

Her birth and early development had been normal, and her early schooling had proceeded smoothly. She changed, however, at 11, becoming increasingly disruptive and attention seeking. At 16 she was found to be of average intelligence but thought to have a personality disorder. On leaving school she held jobs for short periods only, and embarked on the life of a vagrant, obtaining money by petty theft and prostitution. Her behaviour became increasingly erratic and bizarre, and she gave birth to two illegitimate children whom she abandoned. All of this was in contrast to her stable family background.

On a number of occasions, while on remand, she was found to be of average intelligence and a label of psychopathic personality was repeatedly applied. At 26 she was found wandering in a dishevelled state which led to her hospitalisation. On examination she was child-like and unable to give an account of herself. She repeated stereotyped phrases such as 'egg but no bacon', smiled fatuously, and would laugh or cry for no reason. She was uncooperative with cognitive testing and the initial diagnosis was of schizophrenia.

Ultimately it was possible to demonstrate grossly impaired short-term memory, poor writing and constructional apraxia. Neurological examination showed primitive reflexes but no other abnormality. However, a CT scan revealed considerable cerebral atrophy and lumbar puncture showed a raised cerebrospinal fluid protein. Her WAIS verbal IQ was 59, and performance IQ was 40.

On transfer to the Bethlem Royal Hospital she showed right–left disorientation, difficulty in following complex instructions and some nominal dysphasia. Such features seemed, however, to be in keeping with her level of global intellectual impairment. Neurological signs remained absent, but by now she was occasionally incontinent.

Extensive investigations revealed grossly deficient arylsulphatase A activity in the white blood cells and cultured skin fibroblasts. Metachromatic granules were present in the urine. The EEG was normal, but the electromyogram showed slowing of sensory conduction in the lower limbs. A repeat CT scan showed more marked changes than before and MRI showed distinctive hyperintensities in the periventricular white matter (Plate 19).

(Fisher *et al.* 1987)

The specific diagnosis depends on showing diminished arylsulphatase A activity in the white blood cells, serum and urine, and demonstration of excessive sulphatide in the urine. However, some individuals with very low levels of arylsulphatase A show atypical pictures or are entirely asymptomatic ('arylsulphatase A pseudodeficiency'). It appears that the locus for the responsible gene is polymorphic, with at least four allelic variants which can be distinguished by careful electrophoresis and immunoblotting (Hohenschutz *et al.* 1989). Certain mutations have also been shown in the gene by nucleotide sequence analysis of cDNA for arylsulphatase A, including a glycine to adenine transition in an adult-onset case (Kondo *et al.* 1991).

Metachromatic deposits within Schwann cells may be detected in biopsy specimens from the sural nerve or rectal wall. Peripheral nerve conduction velocity is reduced. The heterozygote state may also be detected by measurement of arylsulphatase in the white blood cells. Waltz *et al.* (1987) emphasise the importance of brain imaging in bringing the disorder to mind, particularly in patients who present with psychiatric disorder. The CT scan usually shows mild atrophy, with symmetrical decrease in white matter attenuation, especially near the frontal and occipital horns. MRI shows such changes more impressively.

At autopsy severe white matter destruction is seen in the brain, often with cavitation, along with loss of normal myelin sheaths. Accumulations of strikingly metachromatic material appear as spherical granular masses. Similar changes are found in the peripheral nerves and certain visceral organs. The neuronal cell bodies are virtually unaffected, though at the end stage some may show sulphatide accumulations.

Kufs' disease

Kufs' disease, or cerebral ceroid lipofuscinosis, represents a form of cerebral lipidosis in which the abnormal lipopigment deposits consist of a ceroid-like material akin to lipofuscin. The precise nature of the accumulated material

remains uncertain, likewise the pathogenesis of the disorder.

Onset in infancy or childhood has attracted various eponyms (Batten–Bielschowsky or Spielmeyer–Vogt disease) and is usually accompanied by visual symptoms and retinal abnormalities ('cerebromacular degeneration'). These are rare, however, in the adult form which is known as Kufs' disease. Symptoms then begin in adolescence or adulthood, with an insidious dementia accompanied by motor manifestations. Extrapyramidal disturbances and cerebellar disorder appear to be commoner than spasticity in adults. Myoclonic and other forms of seizure are often encountered.

Siakotos (1981) distinguishes autosomal recessive and dominant forms (Kufs type and Parry type, respectively), both with motor symptoms and mental deterioration as the main presenting features. Dementia or behavioural change can be the initial manifestation (Greenfield & Nelson 1978).

In a review of 118 published cases Berkovic *et al.* (1988) accepted only 50 as true examples of the condition. The remainder showed a variety of atypical features or had evidence of other storage diseases (e.g. Niemann–Pick disease or late-onset gangliosidosis). Two main forms of clinical presentation were apparent—type A with seizures and type B with dementia and motor disturbances, though considerable overlap occurred. The seizures typically took the form of progressive myoclonus epilepsy, often with marked photosensitivity, proceeding ultimately to dementia. Neurological signs developed only late in type A patients and consisted of little more than ataxia and dysarthria. Type B patients usually presented with behavioural change, ranging from disinterest to overt psychosis, the organic nature of the condition becoming obvious when dementia or motor disturbances made an appearance. Cerebellar and extrapyramidal features were usually prominent, and tic-like facial dyskinesia particularly so. With both varieties the onset tended to be around 30 years of age though some began in late adolescence. The course of the disease varied considerably, death following a mean of 12 years later. Recessive inheritance predominated, though one family of each type showed autosomal dominance. Of the 50 cases 34 were familial and 16 apparently sporadic. No genetic link appeared to exist between the adult diseases and the younger-onset forms.

The wide variety of motor and mental manifestations makes diagnosis difficult during life when a family history is absent. Berkovic *et al.* (1988) suggest that it should be suspected when an epilepsy of adult onset proves to be intractable, especially if myoclonus is present, or when dementia and behavioural changes are accompanied by dyskinesias involving the face. Rectal biopsy is useful in revealing the abnormal storage material in neurones and smooth muscle from the rectal wall (Brett & Lake 1975). Skin and skeletal muscle biopsies can also yield a reliable diagnosis provided they are examined by electron microscopy (Carpenter *et al.* 1977). Berkovic *et al.* (1988) consider that two ultrastructural features in the material are essential for the diagnosis—'fingerprint profiles' consisting of systems of paired parallel lines, and granular 'osmophilic deposits'. Short of invasive procedures, suspicion of the disorder may be raised by elevated dolichol levels in the urinary sediment.

The characteristic finding at autopsy is a striking distension of nerve cells with autofluorescent lipopigment, along with neuronal degeneration and reactive gliosis. Cells in the basal ganglia, brain stem and cerebellum tend to be more heavily involved than those of the cortex (Dekaban & Herman 1974). A variable degree of generalised brain atrophy may accompany such changes. Visceral involvement is not apparent macroscopically, but histological examination shows deposits in the blood vessels, kidney, liver, heart and other organs.

Whipple's disease

Whipple's disease is a rare multisystem disorder, known to be infective in origin. The responsible organism (*Tropheryma whippelii*) has recently been identified (Relman *et al.* 1992). An immunological defect in the host is likely to play an important part in causation. It is very much more common in men than women, setting in usually in the sixth decade. The classic presentation is with weight loss, lassitude, chronic diarrhoea and malabsorption, often pursuing a chronic course to extreme emaciation. Multiple arthralgias, serous effusions, uveitis, lymphadenopathy and low-grade pyrexia are other common manifestations.

Involvement of the nervous system has come to be recognised increasingly, sometimes after the systemic disorder is well advanced but occasionally as the dominant feature. Neurological involvement has been reported several times when gastrointestinal and other symptoms are minimal (Bayless & Knox 1979). In very rare examples it has represented the sole clinical or pathological manifestation of the disorder (Romanul *et al.* 1977).

The symptoms tend to be non-specific so that diagnosis may be missed or greatly delayed. Pallis and Lewis (1980) describe the common picture as dementia progressing over months or years, external ophthalmoplegias, or myoclonic movements of the head, trunk or limbs. Other patients have presented with focal neurological signs indicative of a space-occupying lesion, or hypothalamic

involvement with somnolence, hyperphagia and polydipsia. Myopathy and peripheral neuropathy have very occasionally been reported (Albers *et al.* 1989).

A slowly progressive dementia has been described in several patients. It may be accompanied by motor disorder, particularly supranuclear gaze palsies or myoclonus though such are not always in evidence (Finelli *et al.* 1977; Feurle *et al.* 1979). Lampert *et al.*'s (1962) patient had a 7-year history of progressive mental deterioration leading to an impression of Alzheimer's disease; there was no history of gastrointestinal disturbance though an attack of arthritis had occurred at the onset.

Evidence of malabsorption or anaemia will often be present. The cerebrospinal fluid may be normal or show pleocytosis and elevation of protein. The CT scan can be negative, though some examples have shown intracranial granulomatous lesions in the form of low density contrast-enhancing areas (Halperin *et al.* 1982). Definitive diagnosis depends on the demonstration of periodic acid Schiff (PAS)-positive material in macrophages which, in the absence of prior treatment, can almost always be revealed by jejunal biopsy. This must be undertaken whenever the disease is suspected. Lymph node biopsy can be informative too, or the characteristic inclusions may be detected in cells from the cerebrospinal fluid. Polymerase chain reaction amplification of the cerebrospinal fluid may nowadays be performed to detect the DNA sequence specific for *T. whippelii* (Grand Rounds, Hammersmith Hospital 1996). Brain biopsy will sometimes be performed, but will stand to be negative in patients with hypothalamic involvement alone.

The findings at autopsy are distinctive. Tissues involved by the disease show PAS-positive granules within macrophages, representing membrane-like structures derived from bacterial walls (sickle particle-containing cells). The bacilli themselves can sometimes be seen by electron microscopy. Central nervous system involvement shows as collections of PAS-positive cells in the brain and cord, often with widespread perivascular nodules and indolent inflammatory changes. In Romanul *et al.*'s (1977) patient the entire cortical ribbon was studded with minute ring-shaped lesions containing PAS-positive material and surrounded by astrocytes. The bacilli could be identified within macrophages in the brain.

Treatment with antibiotics usually meets with a good response where gastrointestinal and other systemic manifestations are concerned. Various regimens have included parenteral chloramphenicol and oral penicillin, tetracycline, streptomycin, ampicillin or co-trimoxazole, with or without steroids. These must often be continued for many months and relapse can tend to occur. In the treatment of neurological complications less success has been reported, though a vigorous attempt should always be pursued. Feurle *et al.*'s (1979) patient showed a good response where confusion, myoclonus and nystagmus were concerned, though paralysis of upward gaze persisted. Albers *et al.* (1989) discuss the various treatment regimens employed, emphasising the importance of using antibiotics which cross the blood–brain barrier if neurological involvement is to be controlled. Ceftriaxone and cefixime have been advocated for the treatment of neurological disorder (Grand Rounds, Hammersmith Hospital 1996).

Mitochondrial myopathy
(mitochondrial encephalomyopathy)

The mitochondrial myopathies are a rather bewildering group of diseases which share in common a primary dysfunction of mitochondrial metabolism. Though first described in relation to skeletal muscle, many other organs may be affected, leading sometimes to dysfunction in the liver, heart, kidney, eye or endocrine system ('multisystem disease'). The central nervous system is frequently involved and neuropsychiatric disorder can be the predominant manifestation ('mitochondrial encephalomyopathy').

The underlying defects in mitochondrial metabolism have been studied in detail, revealing deficiencies in various respiratory chain enzymes, especially complexes I and III. At present, however, the relationship between such defects and the phenotypic manifestations of disease show a good deal of overlap and precise systems of classification have not been achieved. Molecular biological approaches have also revealed certain specific point mutations and deletions in mitochondrial DNA (Di Mauro & Moses 1992), and where maternal patterns of transmission are suspected inheritance may operate via the mitochondrial route (e.g. in MERRF). However, the nuclear genome also encodes extensively for mitochondrial proteins and may often be involved (Shanske 1992). Sporadic mutations are also likely to occur.

A number of clinical syndromes are now well recognised as reviewed by Lombes *et al.* (1989). The Kearns–Sayre syndrome presents with progressive external ophthalmoplegia, pigmentary retinopathy and heart block or cerebellar dysfunction. Onset is in childhood or adolescence. Myoclonus epilepsy with ragged red fibres (MERRF) presents with myoclonus, ataxia and muscle weakness and often progresses to generalised seizures and dementia. Onset is again usually before the age of 20. Mitochondrial encephalomyopathy with lactic acidosis (MELAS) may present in children or adults with stunted growth, seizures and episodic vomiting. Recurrent stroke-

like episodes are characteristic with transient hemiplegias, hemianopias or cortical blindness. Chronic progressive external ophthalmoplegia (CPEO) can be isolated or accompanied by limb muscle weakness. Other varieties are now known to include Leigh's disease (p. 586).

The pleomorphic manifestations of mitochondrial disorders do not, however, fit neatly into distinct subsyndromes. Petty *et al.* (1986) reviewed 66 cases. The onset in the majority was before 20 years of age, but presentations occurred up to the age of 68. Relatives were affected in almost a third of cases. Petty *et al.* made a broad division into three groups. The commonest presentation (55% of cases) was with ptosis, progressive external ophthalmoplegia, and limb weakness induced or increased by exertion. A further 18% presented with limb weakness alone, showing a proximal myopathy with exercise intolerance. These could continue with muscle involvement alone, though a few patients developed neurological manifestations later. The remaining 27% showed predominant involvement of the central nervous system, with features such as ataxia, deafness, involuntary movements and seizures. Retinopathy, external ophthalmoplegia and limb muscle weakness could sometimes be absent. Dementia was common in this last group and was severe in many. Whereas overall prognosis was good in patients without central nervous system involvement the last group fared poorly, half of them becoming dependent on others at a mean of 17 years from onset.

A mitochondrial myopathy will usually be suspected in patients who present with progressive external ophthalmoplegia combined with other symptoms, or when myopathy is accompanied by prominent fatigue. Petty *et al.* suggest that it should also be considered in the absence of such symptoms when there is cerebellar ataxia, deafness or pigmentary retinopathy, and especially when these are combined with involuntary movements or dementia.

Talley and Faber (1989) report a man of 26 suffering from the MELAS syndrome who presented with dementia. Admission to hospital was precipitated by failing memory and social withdrawal 1 month after an episode of status epilepticus. He was short in stature and showed a right visual field defect, diminished hearing and neglect of the right upper extremity. Though initially orientated in time and place he was slowed, and his speech was limited to stereotyped phrases. He was unable to read, perform simple calculations or copy geometric figures. His prevailing mood was of apprehension. The EEG showed diffuse slowing, and a CT scan revealed calcification in the basal ganglia and right thalamus. Lactic acid levels were raised in the blood and cerebrospinal fluid, and muscle biopsy showed diffuse ragged red fibres.

Over the next 3 weeks he became mute, markedly indifferent to what went on around, and with a severe comprehension defect. He developed hemiparesis on the right, and a left visual field defect in addition to the right hemianopia. New findings on CT included lucent areas medially in the left hemisphere. Major seizures developed and he became combative and difficult to manage. Repeated hospitalisations were required on this account over the succeeding 4 years, with periodic stroke-like events, generalised seizures and a fluctuating though declining level of mentation.

The patient's mother was of short stature with bilateral sensorineural hearing loss, easy fatiguability and ragged red fibres on muscle biopsy. His half-sister similarly showed indications of the MELAS syndrome.

The decisive investigation is skeletal muscle biopsy. The appearance of ragged red fibres with the Gomori trichrome stain is almost pathognomonic, representing abnormal accumulations of mitochondria. Histochemical staining techniques and electron microscopy provide confirmatory information; subsarcolemmal mitochondria are abnormal in size and morphology as well as increased in numbers.

Other important investigations include raised resting blood lactate levels, or when normal these are increased on exercise. Electromyography may show myopathic changes, and the cerebrospinal fluid protein may be raised. CT or MRI scans are likely to show cerebral or cerebellar atrophy when there is central nervous system involvement.

Other disorders affecting the central nervous system

Behçet's syndrome

Behçet's syndrome is an uncommon disorder of unknown aetiology predominantly affecting young males. It is rare in childhood and in persons over 50. The classic triple symptom complex consists of oral ulceration, genital ulceration and ocular lesions (uveitis, iridocyclitis, retinal vasculitis), usually occurring in several attacks per year and pursuing a chronic course over many years. Lassitude, malaise and slight pyrexia may accompany attacks but the degree of constitutional disturbance varies. Common additional manifestations include arthritis, thrombophlebitis, erythema nodosum and non-specific skin sensitivity. The overall course is unpredictable, but the illness often abates after one or two decades. Blindness may remain as a permanent sequel.

It is now recognised to be a chronic multisystem disorder with vasculitis as the underlying pathological process (Wechsler & Piette 1992). Diagnostic criteria have been proposed but there is no universally accepted diagnostic test (International Study Group for Behçet's Disease 1990). The 'pathergy test' may be found to be positive,

consisting of the development of a sterile pustule 24–48 hours after needle prick to the skin.

Central nervous system involvement is recognised as a serious additional complication, important not for its frequency but on account of its grave prognosis. No part of the nervous system appears to be immune. A great variety of clinical pictures may result, as described in comprehensive reviews by Wolf et al. (1965) and Alema (1978). The responsible pathological processes are vasculitis and disseminated encephalomyelitis.

The onset is usually abrupt, coinciding with a relapse of orogenital ulceration or uveitis. Failing this there is almost always a well-established history of the syndrome before nervous system involvement sets in. The patient develops headaches, fever, slight neck stiffness and a variety of neurological signs. Brain stem involvement is particularly common with giddiness, ataxia, diplopia, cranial nerve palsies or long tract signs. A typical feature is the episodic nature of such defects, the picture seeming to stabilise after several weeks then relapsing with fresh developments. Recurrent attacks of hemiplegia or paraplegia may lead on to pseudobulbar palsy. Periods of remission may result in temporary improvement, or in rare cases complete recovery. In general, however, serious neurological defects persist. The course has been likened to that of severe forms of multiple sclerosis and differentiation may occasionally present difficulties (Whitty 1958). More recently dural venous sinus thrombosis has been found to be common, often presenting with intracranial hypertension (Wechsler et al. 1992). The cerebrospinal fluid usually shows a slight lymphocytic pleocytosis and increase of protein. When neck stiffness is severe there may be a marked polymorphonuclear response.

Pallis and Fudge (1956) attempted to demarcate three main forms of nervous system involvement—a brain stem form, a meningomyelitic form and a variety with mental symptoms predominating. The last could present either as transient episodes of confusion or in the form of dementia. The patients with dementia usually showed an insidious onset and steady slow progression, sometimes accompanied by features of parkinsonism and sometimes by pseudobulbar palsy. Alema (1978) stressed that both organic and non-organic psychiatric pictures may arise, the former sometimes being accompanied by meningeal signs and cerebrospinal fluid changes. Depression is common among the non-organic disturbances.

Involvement of the central nervous system is usually a serious development. The patient's general condition is often poor, and adverse developments can set in rapidly. The course of each episode is, however, unique and unpredictable. Some patients deteriorate after repeated relapses, some remain quiescent for long periods, and

others decline steadily and die. Wolf *et al.* (1965) estimated the mortality at 40%, more than half of the deaths
occurring within a year of the first neurological signs.
However, the prospective study of 17 patients reported by
Serdaroğlu *et al.* (1989) suggests a much better prognosis,
with only three patients showing worsening after 12
months follow-up. This may be due in part to improved
methods of treatment.

CT scanning may show single or multiple low density
lesions, principally in the subcortical nuclear masses or
brain stem, and often with resolution some weeks later
(Siva *et al.* 1991). Atrophic changes are also common,
with an accent on the posterior fossa cisterns and cerebellar sulci. MRI is more sensitive in revealing focal areas
of altered signal intensity, and is especially valuable in
showing dural sinus thrombosis and allowing assessment
of recanalization (Wechsler *et al.* 1991). Periventricular
lesions similar to those of multiple sclerosis may be seen.
Changes at autopsy include low-grade perivascular
inflammation, scattered areas of demyelination and
necrosis, and patchy cerebral infarction.

The syndrome has been ascribed to infective, vascular
and allergic mechanisms. Steroids have been claimed to
help markedly in some patients, including those with
involvement of the central nervous system, though others
have reported no benefit. Wadia and Williams (1957) recommend that steroids should be given promptly if ocular
or neurological symptoms develop at any point in the
disease, and Alema (1978) concludes that they may have
reduced the mortality from neurological complications.
Immunosuppressive drugs (cyclophosphamide, azathioprine, chlorambucil) may also be of benefit, though side
effects limit their usefulness. Thalidomide has been
shown to be effective for severe recurrent aphthous stomatitis, and cyclosporin for treating ocular manifestations
(Wechsler & Piette 1992).

Sarcoidosis (benign lymphogranulomatosis, Boeck's sarcoid)

Sarcoidosis is characterised by the development of
chronic granulomatous lesions in various parts of the
body. The aetiology is unknown, though an immunologically determined alteration in tissue reactivity appears to
be fundamental to the disease. It may represent some
form of collagen disorder or be caused by some unidentified organism. An atypical response to the tubercle bacillus has been suspected but never confirmed.

The characteristic lesion is the epithelioid cell granuloma or follicle, consisting of a well-demarcated collection
of epithelioid cells with occasional giant cells. The centres
may show necrosis but the caseation seen with tubercular

infection is lacking. The lesions tend to heal spontaneously but provoke surrounding fibrosis. The commonest
site is the respiratory system, presenting with hilar lymphadenopathy or reticular shadowing in the lungs. The
mildness of symptoms often contrasts with the extent of
the lesions, cases sometimes being discovered on routine
chest X-ray. Erythema nodosum is another characteristic
presentation. Ocular manifestations include iridocyclitis
and uveitis. The latter may be accompanied by parotitis
(uveoparotid fever). Other parts of the body commonly
involved are the superficial lymph nodes, spleen, liver
and phalanges of the hands and feet. Overt myopathy is
rare but muscle infiltration is often apparent on biopsy.

The onset is usually between the ages of 20 and 40
years. In general sarcoidosis runs an indolent course with
relapses and remissions, showing a tendency to subside
spontaneously after several years. Individual lesions gradually resolve while others make an appearance, the cycle
sometimes being narrowly confined and sometimes widespread in different organs. Remission can be expected in
some two-thirds of white patients and one-third of black
patients, resolution being less likely in the presence of
extrathoracic disease (Studdy 1996). A minority of
patients are left disabled by pulmonary fibrosis or ocular
complications. Death, when it occurs, may be due to renal
failure or cardiac involvement. Affection of the central
nervous system (see below) can also carry serious
hazards. Treatment with steroids is often effective in
inducing remission and promoting the healing of lesions,
though maintenance therapy must sometimes continue
for many years. Details of the regimens employed in the
various forms of sarcoidosis are summarised by James
(1992).

A low-grade pyrexia is an inconstant accompaniment.
During active phases of the disease there may be a normochromic anaemia, raised erythrocyte sedimentation
rate and eosinophilia. Mild leucopaenia and thrombocytopaenia are sometimes seen. The serum immunoglobulins, especially IgG, are usually elevated and
hypercalcaemia of moderate degree is not infrequent. In
uncertain cases and with unusual presentations chest X-
ray may reveal the characteristic picture, likewise X-ray
of the phalanges. A raised serum alkaline phosphatase
denotes hepatic involvement. Biopsy of skin lesions,
lymph nodes or muscle can give confirmatory evidence.
The Kveim test consists of an intradermal injection of
sarcoid tissue extract; this has fair reliability, yielding a
nodule with the histological features of sarcoidosis.

Involvement of the nervous system is estimated to occur in
5% of patients (Sharma 1975; Stern *et al.* 1985). Neurological dysfunction may be the presenting feature or
indeed the sole clinical manifestation, though cases with

lesions entirely confined to the nervous system are very rare. Among the patients with neurological involvement reported by Delaney (1977) and Pentland *et al.* (1985) this had been the first sign in two-thirds. Other series have been described by Jefferson (1957), Wiederholt and Siekert (1965), Silverstein *et al.* (1965), Matthews (1965) and Stern *et al.* (1985). Heck and Phillips (1989) and Silberberg (1989) provide detailed reviews.

There are no clear demarcations between the various forms of nervous system involvement but certain broad categories can be discerned. The parts most frequently involved are the cranial nerves, meninges, hypothalamus and pituitary.

Lesions of the cranial and peripheral nerves are the commonest neurological feature. The seventh cranial nerve is particularly vulnerable, leading to unilateral or bilateral facial palsies. Involvement of the optic nerves results in blurring of vision, papilloedema, optic atrophy or field defects. The peripheral nerves may be affected singly or in combination. Basal meningitis or brain stem involvement can lead to multiple fluctuating cranial nerve palsies.

Granulomatous meningitis or meningoencephalitis affects mainly the basal brain regions. The meninges become thickened and infiltrated with granulomas and lymphocytes. Lumbar puncture shows an elevated protein and pleocytosis. Chronic headache is accompanied by focal signs as the adjacent chiasm and hypothalamus become infiltrated. An adhesive arachnoiditis can lead to raised intracranial pressure and hydrocephalus. In some cases the meningeal involvement remains entirely subclinical; it was evident in all 14 of Delaney's (1977) autopsied cases, yet had been suspected during life in only nine.

The brain parenchyma may become involved by contiguous spread or by the formation of tumour-like masses of granulomatous material. Involvement of the hypothalamus and third ventricular region leads to somnolence, obesity, hyperthermia and memory difficulties or change of personality. Pituitary dysfunction may show as diabetes insipidus, menstrual irregularities and other endocrine dysfunctions (Winnacker *et al.* 1968). Lesions situated within the cerebral hemispheres may be single or multiple. The cerebellum, brain stem or cord may be similarly affected. Solitary deposits have sometimes been mistaken for neoplasms until biopsy is performed (Jefferson 1957). Focal signs may make an abrupt appearance, and seizures can be hard to control.

Mental disturbance will often be prominent when sarcoidosis affects the central nervous system. Hook (1954) reported patients with a variety of pictures — apathy, lack of judgement and personal neglect progressing over a

year to semicoma; acute agitation and hallucinosis leading to residual dementia; profound memory impairment and irritability. Cordingley *et al.*'s (1981) patient presented with progressive dementia, the only abnormal signs being a wide-based gait and incomplete eye abduction together with nystagmus on lateral gaze. Others have described marked changes of character, fluctuating confusion and a variety of psychotic pictures. In some the disturbance will be occasioned by hydrocephalus consequent upon basal meningitis or obstruction of cerebrospinal fluid flow by granulomatous masses. In others direct brain infiltration will be responsible. Camp and Frierson (1962) reported a patient who presented with headache and progressive failure of memory and intellect who at autopsy showed extensive nodular infiltration throughout the cortex and basal brain regions. In patients with circumscribed failure of memory, as in the following example, localised involvement of the hypothalamus and limbic structures is probably responsible:

A woman developed sarcoidosis at 24, presenting with bilateral hilar lymphadenopathy. Two years later she had a minor seizure and shortly thereafter developed headache, weakness and incoordination. Examination revealed a sensory level at T4 and a myelogram showed obstruction from T4 to T7. The CT scan demonstrated a right frontal granuloma and basal meningeal involvement with mild ventricular dilatation. Dexamethasone produced marked neurological improvement over the following year which was well maintained.

At 28 she became aware of increasing memory impairment over 3–4 weeks, then abruptly became agitated, deluded and doubly incontinent. She was disorientated in time and place and heard hallucinatory voices at night. The acute organic reaction settled over 6–8 weeks on haloperidol and increased dexamethasone, but her memory remained mildly impaired. Psychometric testing at that time showed a WAIS full scale IQ of 78, with scores of 55% on the Wechsler logical memory test and 45% on the Rey–Osterrieth Test.

Some months later her memory deteriorated further and she developed compulsive eating, weight gain and insomnia. At 30 she was obese, mildly ataxic, and with hyperreflexia in the legs and bilateral extensor plantars. There were no psychotic features but she was disorientated in time and showed a severe defect of short-term memory. She could recall nothing of a name and address or of simple geometrical figures. The WAIS IQ was 82, but the logical memory test now gave a score of only 20% and the Rey–Osterrieth Test 30%. The CT scan was unchanged but pulmonary and hepatic involvement were demonstrated. Steroids were increased to high dosage, with improvement 3 weeks later in orientation and on simple tests of recall. She was discharged to a semi-independent life in her own home which she managed to run with the help of memory aids.

(Thompson & Checkley 1981)

A further instructive patient was reported by McLoughlin and McKeon (1991), in whom both memory disorder and bipolar affective disorder appeared to be due to involvement of the limbic system:

A 25-year-old mechanic developed hilar lymphadenopathy, and sarcoidosis was confirmed by mediastinoscopy and lymph node biopsy. This resolved with steroids and he remained well for 6 years until sarcoid meningitis appeared. This too resolved with steroids over a number of months and he remained on prednisolone 15 mg daily thereafter. Three years later, at the age of 34, he developed sensorimotor leg neuropathies and bilateral fifth nerve numbness, but CT scan at this time showed no cerebral abnormalities. Two years later he developed diabetes insipidus and anterior pituitary failure requiring replacement therapy, and the following year was treated with cranial irradiation. Cerebrospinal fluid analysis showed active central nervous system sarcoidosis and MRI revealed minimal cortical atrophy.

The following year he became depressed with anorexia, weight loss and marked guilt feelings about his illness. There was no family history of psychiatric disorder. At the same time he noted that his memory was impaired for recent events. Imipramine relieved the depression, but 12 months later he began to experience marked mood swings alternating between episodes of depression and hypomania lasting for a few days at a time. Three months later lithium was added, by which time the mood swings were alternating every 24–28 hours. Neurological examination was normal apart from bilateral facial sensory impairment. Cerebrospinal fluid analysis showed that the neurosarcoidosis was still active, but repeat MRI showed no change. Psychometric testing confirmed the memory deficit and showed a WAIS-R IQ of 96.

Attempts to stabilise his mood swings with high dosage lithium failed on account of troublesome polyuria, but they nevertheless subsided over several months in hospital. He remained depressed and some months later took an overdose and died.

At autopsy a large granulomatous mass was discovered just anterior to the mamillary bodies at the origin of the pituitary stalk. Histological examination showed that this had infiltrated the dorsomedial nucleus of the thalamus, mamillary bodies, third ventricle, fornices and pituitary stalk. There was patchy basal meningeal fibrosis with isolated meningeal granulomas. The cerebral hemispheres, cerebellum and brain stem were unaffected. Spinal meningeal fibrosis was severe with entrapment of ventral and dorsal roots.

In some cases a combination of structural and metabolic disturbances is likely to shape the psychiatric picture, particularly in the presence of hypercalcaemia or a degree of renal failure. Steroid therapy may make its own contribution to mental disturbances (p. 628).

It can obviously be important, in patients with organic psychosyndromes and neurological defects of obscure origin, to bear the possibility of sarcoidosis in mind. Full investigation along the lines described above will almost certainly produce confirmatory evidence of the disorder, even when nervous system involvement has been the presenting manifestation. The CT or MRI scan may show the intracranial lesions or evidence of basal meningitis, and lumbar puncture may reveal evidence of chronic meningitis. Cordingley *et al.* (1981) suggest that a consistently normal cerebrospinal fluid probably excludes the diagnosis.

The prognosis for patients with neuropsychiatric complications is extremely variable, but in general intracranial involvement should be viewed as a grave development. Some show a remittent picture, others slow and incomplete recovery, while others show progressive disability. A few will die of the neurological manifestations. The outlook, however, is not uniformly poor. Among the 19 patients followed by Pentland *et al.* (1985) half had had an acute monophasic illness which resolved with steroids, and altogether two-thirds showed a surprisingly good outcome 1–16 years later. Those who had shown a relapsing–remitting course had often presented pictures closely simulating multiple sclerosis. Facial nerve palsy is usually transient and shows a good response to steroids. Basal meningitis may slowly ameliorate and subside though the overall response to treatment is poor. In favourable cases intracerebral granulomas can improve or even resolve with steroid therapy, and surgical removal has occasionally been successful.

Electrical accidents and lightning injuries

Contact with powerful sources of electric current may cause sudden death due to ventricular fibrillation or respiratory arrest, sometimes with severe burns where the current enters and leaves the body. The effects of the shock are strongly influenced by the site of contact as well as the strength of the electrical source. Among survivors transient evidence of neurological dysfunction is not uncommon, though persisting sequelae appear to be rare. The mortality in 60 cases reported by Hammond and Ward (1988) was 3%; neurological complications were noted in a quarter and psychiatric sequelae in 18%.

Much of the acute disturbance appears to be due to temporary blockade of neuronal function or vasomotor changes in the brain and cord, though petechial haemorrhages and areas of demyelination and degeneration have been observed. Additional damage may be caused by intense tetanic muscular contractions which sometimes propel the victim for a considerable distance. Acute tetanic spasm of the paraspinus muscles may produce compression fractures of the vertebral bodies. With lightning injuries blast-like lesions may be sustained due to the sudden displacement and return of air in the immediate vicinity of the lightning strike. Reviews of the literature are presented by Langworthy (1936), Alexander (1938) and Silversides (1964). Farrell and Starr (1968) deal with the delayed neurological sequelae and Peters (1983) specifically with lightning injuries.

A period of unconsciousness may last for hours or days, sometimes being delayed for several moments during which the affected person calls for help. The unconsciousness may be accompanied by epileptic seizures or more commonly myoclonic jerking. Cessation of respiration due to bulbar paralysis can require assisted ventilation for many hours. When consciousness is retained the subject may experience intense pain, tinnitus, deafness or visual disturbance, along with tremors, twitching, local paralysis and sensory changes. Confusion and excitement can then be prominent, with retrograde and post-traumatic amnesia much as with head injury. Severe neurological disturbances such as paraplegia, hemiplegia, mutism and aphonia may resolve over hours or days. Transient unilateral parkinsonism has been attributed to damage to the basal ganglia. Fixed dilated pupils during the acute stage are not necessarily an ominous prognostic sign. All patients should have electrocardiographic monitoring for at least 48 hours for the detection of cardiac dysrhythmias, and a watch must be kept for acute renal failure due to myoglobin released from injured muscles (Pruitt & Mason 1996).

More prolonged sequelae include cranial nerve damage with loss of taste, facial paresis and auditory and vestibular disturbances. Very occasionally severe diffuse brain damage may be an enduring aftermath. The most common sequelae, however, are peripheral nerve and spinal cord syndromes which are sometimes days or weeks in developing, perhaps as vascular changes progress. Farrell and Starr (1968) stress that a latent period of months may occasionally intervene. The pictures that have been described include delayed atrophy affecting an arm or leg, quadriparesis, or slowly progressive spasticity with sensory changes ('spinal atrophic paralysis'). The waxing and waning of chronic neurological deficits may sometimes resemble multiple sclerosis. In patients such as these the current may have traversed the spinal cord directly.

Prolonged neuropsychiatric aftermaths include amnesia and impaired cognitive functioning, often compounded by anxiety attaching to the shock and sometimes by compensation issues. Eight of 14 patients reported by Silversides (1964) showed 'psychoneurotic' sequelae by way of headache, fatigue, impotence, anxiety, fear of electricity and apparent personality change. Eleven of 60 patients in Hammond and Ward's (1988) series suffered psychiatric problems similar to post-traumatic stress disorder — insomnia, nightmares, anxiety, headache and difficulty in concentration. The

following patient illustrates the cognitive and personality changes that may occasionally follow:

A 26-year-old man was rendered unconscious for several hours after sustaining a shock from bare wires which made contact with his forehead. On recovery he had throbbing headache, was sluggish in cerebration, and complained of feeling depressed and irritable for several weeks thereafter. A CT scan was normal. Two months later he was still vague and forgetful with delayed responses to questions. Five months after the accident he showed significant impairment of memory, lability of mood and psychomotor retardation. His girlfriend described a marked change of personality with argumentativeness and occasional aggressive behaviour. Cognitive testing showed nominal and expressive dysphasia, impaired right–left discrimination, and difficulty in making simple drawings. He had lost his ability to speak German which he had learned during the previous 3 years. WAIS scores were well below expectation in view of his educational and occupational history.

Two years later his memory remained impaired and he was still mentally sluggish and rather vacuous in appearance. However, there was no longer evidence of dysphasia or drawing difficulties. Simple arithmetic was poor. His mother confirmed a marked change of personality from a bright extroverted person to one who was slow, sullen and withdrawn. Though no longer depressed he was distractible, and had abandoned his reading and former hobbies.   (S Brandon, personal communication)

Brain injury due to diving

Apart from the hazards of anoxia and hypothermia divers are at risk of two main forms of injury to the nervous system, namely toxicity due to gases breathed under high partial pressure and 'decompression illness'. These risks increase in relation to the depth and duration of submersion. They apply equally to caisson workers who may spend several days at a time working at very considerable depths. When explosives are used divers are also exposed to increased risk of blast injury because of the enhanced transmission of pressure waves in water.

There are also concerns that divers, including sports divers, may sometimes sustain a degree of neurological damage even in the absence of obvious events such as decompression illness, though the issue remains controversial. Repeated exposures appear to be a special hazard in persons with a patent foramen ovale or other form of right to left shunt in the circulation. These matters are considered below, much deriving from accounts by Denison (1996) and Wilmshurst (1997).

Gas toxicity

The gases breathed during submersion must be delivered at the same pressure as the surrounding water. Air alone can be safely used to depths of 30–50 m, after which mental aberration becomes increasingly obvious. This is probably due to the narcotic effects of nitrogen dissolved in nerve membranes which impedes neural transmission. The breathing of pure oxygen does not solve the problem, because oxygen is toxic to the lungs when the alveolar pressure exceeds 0.5 atmosphere (5 m of sea water), and to the nervous system when exceeding 2 atmospheres (10 m of sea water). Epileptic convulsions are then liable to occur.

For depths greater than 30 m oxygen–helium mixtures are employed, allowing descents to 500 m or more. Nevertheless at great depths neurological disturbances are prone to arise from the direct effects of gas pressure on nervous tissues (high pressure nervous syndrome). This is manifest as postural instability, somnolence and cognitive dysfunction, often along with tremor, myoclonus and convulsions. Such developments effectively preclude descents below 700 m.

Decompression illness

During submersion inert gases under pressure become dissolved in body tissues; these are nitrogen when breathing air, or helium when breathing oxygen–helium mixtures. In the course of the ascent such gases come out of solution as the ambient pressure falls, tending to form bubbles within the tissues and the blood (gas nucleation). Provided the ascent is sufficiently gradual the extra load of gas diffuses into the blood stream and out of the lungs, but if it is too rapid the bubbles increase in size and number and may come to block blood vessels. This appears to be the principal cause of decompression illness or 'bends', which is a risk with any dives below 10 m unless these are very brief. It is a particular risk after deep 'saturation dives', during which divers are maintained at the pressure of their diving depth for days or weeks on end; chambers are used at the surface for this purpose, to economise in the time which would otherwise be needed for repeated very slow ascents.

Two grades of decompression illness are recognised — 'type 1 bends' consisting of skin irritation and musculoskeletal pain only, and 'type 2 bends' with pulmonary and nervous system manifestations and sometimes circulatory collapse. Pulmonary symptoms consist of sudden chest pain, dyspnoea and cough due to bubble formation within the pulmonary circulation. Neurological symptoms, which occur in about half of cases, consist chiefly of spinal cord syndromes, visual disturbances or vertigo, though central focal deficits may occur. The range of severity is wide, from slight dysaesthesias, ataxia and ophthalmoplegia, to paraparesis, quadriparesis, dysphasia and confusion. Such episodes may be transient or long-lasting and permanent sequelae can result. The episodes are sometimes recurrent, in general resembling thromboembolic cerebrovascular disease except for commonly affecting the cord. The symptoms usually develop some minutes to hours after the dive is over, and must be treated immediately by recompression and the administration of oxygen.

Severe examples of decompression illness may result from a different mechanism, when lung tissue becomes disrupted by the expansion of gases within it (pulmonary barotrauma), allowing gas to enter the pulmonary veins and thus the arterial system. Cerebral gas embolism may then result in severe focal cerebral symptoms. However, the distinction between pulmonary barotrauma and gas nucleation in leading to the various manifestations of decompression illness is far from well established.

Neuropathological effects apparently related to decompression illness have been described by Palmer *et al.* (1987). In an examination of the spinal cords of 11 divers, mostly dying from diving accidents, they found distended empty blood vessels, sometimes with perivascular haemorrhages, and minor chronic changes with foci of gliosis and hyalinisation of blood vessels. In three cases Marchi staining showed tract degeneration, variously affecting the posterior, lateral or anterior columns of the cord. Examination of the brains of 25 divers, again mostly dying from diving accidents, showed distended empty vessels in two-thirds of subjects, presumably caused by gas bubbles (Palmer *et al.* 1992). Perivascular lacunae were present in a third, presumably due to bubble occlusion, along with hyalinisation of blood vessels which may have accrued from periodic rises in luminal pressure. Foci of necrosis were sometimes observed in the cerebral grey matter, and vacuolation in the white matter extending to status spongiosis.

Polkinghorne *et al.* (1988) reinforced the role of vascular factors in decompression illness in a study of ocular fundus lesions using fluorescein angiography. Fundal lesions were found in a high proportion of divers, with changes in pigment epithelium, reduced capillary density at the fovea, lack of capillary perfusion and microaneurysm formation. Such changes were compatible with obstruction to the retinal and choroidal circulation by bubble formation, and could be relevant to the central nervous system effects. The lesions were observed whether or not there was a history of decompression illness, and their severity was significantly related to the length of diving exposure. Hyperbaric conditions may also have made a contribution by virtue of platelet aggregation and increased blood viscosity.

The important recent evidence of multiple hyperintensities on MRI of the brain is discussed below.

Sequelae of diving

A well known long-term effect of diving is the presence of aseptic infarcts in the long bones, evident on X-ray and presumably due to gas embolism. This is commoner with a history of decompression illness but is found in many subjects with no such history. The incidence rises with age and diving intensity. Infarcts near the articular surfaces can be severely disabling, and crippling dysbaric osteonecrosis may occasionally ensue.

The neurological disturbances of decompression illness may fail to resolve completely, and surveys of divers have shown a small but definite prevalence of neurological deficits. Todnem *et al.* (1990) examined 156 commercial divers, aged 21–49, along with 100 controls. Half of the divers had experienced frank episodes of decompression illness. At the time of examination 20% had stopped diving and six had lost their licenses because of neurological problems. Twelve (8%) had had problems with vision, vertigo or reduced skin sensitivity in non-diving situations, and six had been referred to neurological clinics on account of seizures, transient cerebral ischaemia or transient amnesia attacks. No controls had such symptoms. The divers complained significantly more often of symptoms referable to the central nervous system, mainly problems with concentration and memory, and had more peripheral neurological symptoms, chiefly paraesthesia in the hands and feet. On examination significantly more showed hand tremor, or signs indicative of cord damage such as reduced touch and pain sensation in the feet. Seven had a mild peripheral neuropathy. Scores for neurological symptoms and signs correlated significantly with age, amount of diving exposure, and a history of decompression illness.

On investigation 18% of the divers and 5% of controls had abnormal EEGs, with increased temporal slow waves and sharp potentials (Todnem *et al.* 1991). Such abnormalities again correlated significantly with diving exposure and a history of decompression illness, but not with neurological symptom scores. Brain stem evoked potential latencies were also increased in the diving group.

The important question therefore arises whether neuropsychiatric sequelae can be cumulative, either due to repeated episodes of decompression illness or by virtue of repeated exposure to hyperbaric conditions. There appears still to be little consensus on the issue, much of the clinical evidence being anecdotal or poorly controlled (Wilmshurst 1997). The autopsy evidence described above and the neuroimaging studies outlined below certainly raise such a possibility. Moreover the demonstration of brain lesions on MRI in the absence of a history of decompression illness suggests that minor subclinical events, or prolonged exposure to gases under pressure, may sometimes be damaging to the central nervous system.

Palmer *et al.* (1992) review reports of long-term mental changes in caisson workers and divers, including loss of memory, aggressive and antisocial behaviour, retarded reactions, difficulty in concentration and low tolerance to alcohol. Edmonds and Boughton (1985) attempted a survey of intellectual impairment in a group of 30 abalone divers in New South Wales, a population known to be especially at risk of decompression stress and anecdotally reported to contain 'punch drunk divers'. Almost one-third were judged to show impairment on psychometric testing, even though none had neurological deficits. Half reported a history of decompression illness, but impairment was as common in those without. However the psychometric screening battery was extremely brief and no controls were employed.

A recent cause for concern is the demonstration of hyperintensities on MRI in a proportion of divers and caisson workers, presumably due to microinfarcts in the brain (Warren *et al.* 1988; Fueredi *et al.* 1991). Reul *et al.* (1995) studied 52 amateur scuba divers (mean age 38 years), and compared them with 50 controls engaged in other sports; 52% of the divers and 20% of the controls showed hyperintensities, principally in the subcortical white matter and basal ganglia. These were significantly larger and more numerous in the divers. Only three had histories pointing to episodes of decompression illness, suggesting that such lesions may often accrue without clinical indicators of their presence. Others, however, have found no excess of MRI abnormalities in divers compared to controls (Rinck *et al.* 1991; Todnem *et al.* 1991), perhaps due to different selection procedures and imaging protocols.

Knauth *et al.* (1997) report a recent investigation of 87 sports divers, none of whom had a history of decompression illness. Eleven (13%) showed hyperintensities on MRI, but *multiple* hyperintensities occurred exclusively in three subjects with large right to left shunts in the circulation as demonstrated by transcranial Doppler ultrasonography after the venous injection of microbubbles. Ten further subjects with similarly large shunts had normal MRI scans.

Nevertheless the possibility arises that divers with right to left shunts may be at particular risk of accumulating microinfarcts in the brain. The great majority of such shunts are likely to reflect a patent foramen ovale, which may well become functional only under the abnormal pressure conditions of diving. Others could be due to small atrial septal defects or pulmonary arteriovenous shunts.

The significance of interatrial shunts in relation to decompression illness was illustrated by Moon *et al.* (1989), who found that 37% of a group of 30 divers who had experienced such episodes had interatrial shunts on bubble contrast echocardiography, compared with only 5% of healthy volunteer controls. Of the 18 divers who had had serious decompression symptoms 61% had such shunts. Wilmshurst *et al.* (1989) demonstrated an excess of right to left interatrial shunts in divers who had developed neurological decompression symptoms within 30 minutes of surfacing (66% compared with 24% of controls), but not in those whose symptoms developed later.

Further research will clearly be necessary to clarify both the significance of the MRI findings described above and the true extent of diving risk in subjects with right to left shunts. The latter has particular importance in that about a quarter of the normal population is thought to harbour a potentially patent foramen ovale (Denison, 1996).

Hyperostosis frontalis interna (hyperostosis cranii, metabolic craniopathy, endocraniosis, Morgagni's syndrome)

Hyperostosis of the frontal region of the skull was once considered an important clinical sign, indicative of a syndrome with various endocrine and mental manifestations. However, most authorities now consider it to be of no pathological significance, and indeed several major neurological and medical texts make no reference to it. Nevertheless, the condition continues to attract sporadic interest, and there are some indications that it may be commoner than chance expectation in patients with organic psychosyndromes.

The radiological picture is of thickening of the inner tables of the frontal bones, with smooth rounded exostoses projecting into the cranial cavity. Part of the problem in discerning any putative clinical associations lies with the frequency of the condition and with the occurrence of minor variations. It may be found at any age from adolescence upwards, increasing markedly from the third or fourth decades onwards. Females are affected very much more often than males, with a prevalence of perhaps 5–6% overall. Higher estimates at almost 50% for women and 6% for men (Silinkova-Malkova & Malek 1965/66) are probably attributable to the inclusion of subcategories with diffuse thickening of the calvarium, also patients with normal overall skull thickness but reduction and sclerosis of the diploë. It may sometimes appear familially, and has been described in association with dystrophia myotonica (p. 717).

The pathogenesis is unknown. Those who argue for a special association with endocrine dysfunction have claimed an aetiological role via hypothalamic or pituitary dysfunction (e.g. Solomon 1954) though there is no direct evidence of this. Two 'syndromes' have been proposed, Morgagni's syndrome with hyperostosis, obesity and hirsuitism, and the Stewart–Morel syndrome in which neuropsychiatric features predominate. Neither, however, has won wide acceptance.

In most reviews the main features have been headache, obesity, hirsuitism and menstrual disorders. Headache was found in 89% of Silinkova and Malek's series compared with 37% of controls; hirsuitism was present in 37% compared with 14% of controls. Thirst, water retention, sleep disturbances and a variety of rather minor endocrine changes are also described. Among mental features neurotic complaints figure prominently, also disturbances of personality, memory impairment and occasionally dementia. A number of forms of psychosis have been reported. All agree, however, that the condition is very often entirely asymptomatic.

In part the old claims of a special relationship to mental disease may have resulted from the skull being more closely examined in the course of pyschiatric hospital autopsies. Nevertheless, there is some evidence pointing to a higher prevalence of the condition in the mentally ill. Hawkins and Martin (1965) compared skull X-rays from patients seen in a general hospital with those from patients currently resident in a psychiatric hospital. Among the females 5.9% of the former and 10.7% of the latter showed hyperostosis, a statistically significant difference which persisted on controlling for age. Among males there were too few cases for comparison. In neither hospital could the patients with hyperostosis be shown to belong to particular diagnostic categories when matched with unaffected controls.

More recently Walinder (1977) surveyed a large group of women admitted to a psychiatric hospital, finding hyperostosis in 26%. When matched with patients of equivalent age but without the skull changes, dementia emerged as significantly more common in the hyperostosis group. Among the sibs of Walinder's affected patients mental illness also appeared to be significantly more frequent.

Putnam (1974) points to a possibly interesting association, describing a patient with hyperostosis, hirsuitism, diabetes mellitus and borderline hypothyroidism, who was found to have normal-pressure hydrocephalus as a basis for her memory failure and incontinence. A shunt operation improved the mental state. Putnam's review of 11 other cases with normal-pressure hydrocephalus showed hyperostosis in eight.

Agenesis of the corpus callosum

Absence of the corpus callosum, in whole or in part, occurs as a rare developmental abnormality. Other associated defects are usually present—hydrocephalus, microgyria, heterotopias, arachnoid cysts, spina bifida or meningomyelcoele (Merritt 1979). The anterior and hippocampal commissures may be intact even when the corpus callosum is entirely missing.

Most cases have been reported in children, though the condition can come to light at any age. It usually presents by virtue of symptoms attributable to other cerebral malformations — seizures, mental retardation or hydrocephalus. Occasionally, however, it is discovered only at autopsy or in the course of neuroradiological investigations carried out for some other purpose. The discovery of asymptomatic cases is likely to increase now that brain imaging is so frequently performed.

David *et al.* (1993) review the little that is known about causation. Complete agenesis is associated with a wide variety of genetic anomalies, in particular trisomies of chromosomes 8, 13 and 18. It appears sometimes to be the result of intrauterine metabolic disturbances such as hyperglycinaemia, or intrauterine exposure to infections and toxins. Neville (1993) lists a number of metabolic diseases of the nervous system with which it may also occur.

Ettlinger (1977) has summarised the anatomical findings, and detailed reviews are found in Unterhanscheidt *et al.* (1968), Loeser and Alvord (1968) and Probst (1973). All have tended to agree that clinical findings, when present, owe little to the absence of the corpus callosum *per se* and much to the associated anomalies. Epilepsy, spasticity and other motor defects are common, likewise varying grades of mental subnormality. When patients with other malformations are excluded, however, intelligence is not infrequently in the normal range (Lehmann & Lampe 1970).

There has been a renewal of interest in the psychological status of such patients in view of the abnormal functioning known to follow surgical section of the commissures (pp. 41–2). Equivalent evidence of functional disconnection of the cerebral hemispheres has rarely, however, been forthcoming. Some deficits have been demonstrated on tests of bimanual coordination and in crossed-responding to visual stimuli (Jeeves 1965, 1969), in the transfer of maze learning from one hand to the other (Lehmann & Lampe 1970), in cross-location of touch and in the matching of visual patterns between left and right visual fields (Ettlinger *et al.* 1972, 1974). However, all such deficits are variable, and other tests of interhemispheric transfer appear often to be well performed. Compensatory mechanisms must clearly be at work, by way of bilateral speech representation, increased use of ipsilateral inflow pathways, or utilisation of such other commissural pathways as are intact. Kretschmer's (1968) report of two patients who were unable to read in the left half-field of vision, one also being apraxic with the left hand, is exceptional, suggesting that these deficits may have been due to other associated lesions. Milner (1983) provides a valuable review of neuropsychological studies in such patients, concluding that while it is likely that both cognitive and skilled performances can suffer, there are clearly great individual differences from one case to another. In particular, there is no good evidence that acallosal brains are less laterally specialised than normal brains, despite conflicting findings on the issue. Language impairments have been reported in small numbers of patients, the most consistent, interestingly, being in the production and recognition of rhyme (Jeeves & Temple 1987; Temple *et al.* 1989).

David *et al.* (1993) have reviewed the association between developmental defects of the corpus callosum and major psychiatric disturbances. These have included schizophrenia, depression and behavioural disorders of childhood. Of the seven new cases presented four had clear psychotic symptoms, two of these being schizophrenic and one manic–depressive, one had features of Asperger's syndrome, one a personality disorder with depression and conversion symptoms, and one was an adolescent with behavioural problems. No conclusions could be drawn concerning the relevance of the callosal abnormalities to these clinical manifestations, not least because the prevalence of callosal anomalies in the general population is uncertain.

The radiological diagnosis based on the air encephalogram was described by Bull (1967). Marked separation is seen between the lateral ventricles; they show angular dorsal margins, concave medial borders and dilatation of the caudal portions. The third ventricle is widened with a large dorsal extension. Equivalent features can be detected on the CT or MRI scan. Characteristic findings are seen in relation to the pericallosal arteries and other vessels on angiography.

References

The numbers in square brackets after each reference show the page(s) of text on which the item is mentioned.

AARTS, J.H.P., BINNIE, C.D., SMIT, A.M. & WILKINS, A.J. (1984) Selective cognitive impairment during focal and generalised epileptiform EEG activity. *Brain* **107**, 293–308 [262].

ABAS, M.A., SAHAKIAN, B.J. & LEVY, R. (1990) Neuropsychological deficits and CT scan changes in elderly depressives. *Psychological Medicine* **20**, 507–520 [487].

ABD EL NABY, S. & HASSANEIN, M. (1965) Neuropsychiatric manifestations of chronic manganese poisoning. *Journal of Neurology, Neurosurgery and Psychiatry* **28**, 282–288 [635].

ABE, H., WEIS, S. & MEHRAEIN, P. (1993) Degeneration of the cerebellar dentate nucleus and the inferior olivary nucleus in HIV-1 infection: a morphometric study. *Clinical Neuropathology*, **12 (Supplement)**, S7 [323].

ABE, K. (1977) Lithium prophylaxis of periodic hypersomnia. *British Journal of Psychiatry* **130**, 312–313 [733].

ABED, R.T. & BHALLA, D. (1991) Persistent neuroleptic-related hypersomnia: two case reports. *Irish Journal of Psychological Medicine* **8**, 130–132 [734].

ABED, R.T., CLARK, J., ELBADAWY, M.H.F. & CLIFFE, M.J. (1987) Psychiatric morbidity in acromegaly. *Acta Psychiatrica Scandinavica* **75**, 635–639 [522].

ABEND, W.K. & TYLER, H.R. (1989) Thyroid disease and the nervous system. Ch. 16 in *Neurology and General Medicine*, ed. Aminoff, M.J. Churchill Livingstone: New York [509].

ABENSON, M.H. (1970) EEGs in chronic schizophrenia. *British Journal of Psychiatry* **116**, 421–425 [128].

ÅBERG, T., RONQUIST, G., TYDÉN, H., AHLUND, P. & BERGSTRÖM, K. (1982) Release of adenylate kinase into cerebrospinal fluid during open-heart surgery and its relation to post-operative intellectual function. *Lancet* **1**, 1139–1141 [555].

ÅBERG, T., RONQUIST, G., TYDÉN, H., BRUNNKVIST, S., HULTMAN, J., BERGSTRÖM, K. & LILJA, A. (1984) Adverse effects on the brain in cardiac operations as assessed by biochemical, psychometric, and radiologic methods. *Journal of Thoracic and Cardiovascular Surgery* **87**, 99–105 [555].

ABRAHAM, H.D. (1982) A chronic impairment of colour vision in users of LSD. *British Journal of Psychiatry* **140**, 518–520 [623].

ABRAHAM, H.D. (1983) Visual phenomenology of the LSD flashback. *Archives of General Psychiatry* **40**, 884–889 [623].

ABRAHAM, H.D. & WOLF, E. (1988) Visual function in past users of LSD: psychophysical findings. *Journal of Abnormal Psychology* **97**, 443–447 [623].

ABRAMS, G.M. & SCHIPPER, H.M. (1989) Other endocrinopathies of the nervous system. Ch. 18 in *Neurology and General Medicine*. Ed. Aminoff, M.J. Churchill Livingstone: New York [522].

ABRAMS, R. & TAYLOR, M.A. (1976) Catatonia: a prospective clinical study. *Archives of General Psychiatry* **33**, 579–581 [155, 356].

ABRAMS, R. & TAYLOR, M.A. (1979) Differential EEG patterns in affective disorder and schizophrenia. *Archives of General Psychiary* **36**, 1355–1358 [89].

ABRAMS, R. & TAYLOR, M.A. (1980) Psychopathology and the electroencephalogram. *Biological Psychiatry* **15**, 871–878 [89, 128].

ACHTÉ, K.A. & ANTTINEN, E.E. (1963) Suizide bei Hirngeschädigten des Krieges in Finland. *Fortschritte der Neurologie, Pychiatrie* **31**, 645–667 [192].

ACHTÉ, K.A., HILLBOM, E. & AALBERG, V. (1967) *Post-traumatic Psychoses Following War Brain Injuries*. Reports from The Rehabilitation Institute for Brain-injured Veterans in Finland, Vol. 1: Helsinki [190, 191, 192].

ACHTÉ, K.A., HILLBOM, E. & AALBERG, V. (1969) Psychoses following war brain injuries. *Acta Pychiatrica Scandinavica* **45**, 1–18 [190].

ACK, M., MILLER, I. & WEIL, W.B. (1961) Intelligence of children with diabetes mellitus. *Pediatrics* **28**, 764–770 [537].

ACKER, C. (1985) Performance of female alcoholics on neuropsychological testing. *Alcohol and Alcoholism* **20**, 379–386 [121].

ACKER, C. (1986) Neuropsychological deficits in alcoholics: the relative contributions of gender and drinking history. *British Journal of Addiction* **81**, 395–403 [121].

ACKER, C., ACKER, W.L. & SHAW, G.K. (1984) Assessment of cognitive function in alcoholics by computer: a control study. *Alcohol and Alcoholism* **19**, 223–233 [606].

ACKER, C., JACOBSON, R.R. & LISHMAN, W.A. (1987) Memory and ventricular size in alcoholics. *Psychological Medicine* **17**, 343–348 [581].

ACKER, W. & ACKER, C. (1982) *Bexley Maudsley Automated Psychological Screening and Bexley Maudsley Category Sorting Test Manual*. NFER–Nelson: Windsor [121].

ACKER, W., APS, E.J., MAJUMDAR, S.K., SHAW, G.K. & THOMSON, A.D. (1982) The relationship between brain and liver damage in chronic alcoholic patients. *Journal of Neurology, Neurosurgery and Psychiatry* **45**, 984–987 [607].

ACKER, W., RON, M.A., LISHMAN, W.A. & SHAW, G.K. (1984) A multivariate analysis of psychological, clinical and CT scanning measures in detoxified chronic alcoholics. *British Journal of Addiction* **79**, 293–301 [121].

ACKNER, B., COOPER, J.E., GRAY, C.H. & KELLY, M. (1962) Acute porphyria: a neuropsychiatric and biochemical study. *Journal of Psychosomatic Research* **6**, 1–24 [568].

ACKNER, B., COOPER, J.E., GRAY, C.H., KELLY, M. & NICHOLSON, D.C. (1961) Excretion of porphobilinogen and d-aminolaevulinic acid in acute porphyria. *Lancet* **1**, 1256–1260 [568].

ADAMS, C.B.T. (1983) Hemispherectomy—a modification. *Journal of Neurology, Neurosurgery and Psychiatry* **46**, 617–619 [313].

ADAMS, C.W.M. & BRUTON, C.J. (1989) The cerebral vasculature in dementia pugilistica. *Journal of Neurology, Neurosurgery and Psychiatry* **52**, 600–604 [207].

ADAMS, G.F. (1967) Problems in the treatment of hemiplegia. *Gerontologia Clinica* **9**, 285–294 [381, 383, 391].

ADAMS, G.F. & HURWITZ, L.J. (1963) Mental barriers to recovery from strokes. *Lancet* **2**, 533–537 [381, 382].

ADAMS, G.F. & HURWITZ, L.J. (1974) *Cerebrovascular Disability and the Ageing Brain*. Churchill Livingstone: Edinburgh & London [379, 381, 382].

ADAMS, J.H. (1976) Parasitic and fungal infections of the nervous system. Ch. 7 in *Greenfield's Neuropathology*, 3rd edn, eds Blackwood, W. & Corsellis, J.A.N. Edward Arnold: London [361].

ADAMS, J.H. & JENNETT, W.B. (1967) Acute necrotizing encephalitis: a problem in diagnosis. *Journal of Neurology, Neurosurgery and Psychiatry* **30**, 248–260 [357].

ADAMS, J.H., MITCHELL, D.E., GRAHAM, D.I. & DOYLE, D. (1977) Diffuse brain damage of immediate impact type. Its relationship to 'primary brain-stem damage' in head injury. *Brain* **100**, 489–502 [163].

ADAMS, K.M. (1976) Behavioral treatment of reflex or sensory-evoked seizures. *Journal of Behavior Therapy and Experimental Psychiatry* **7**, 123–127 [308].

ADAMS, P.W., WYNN, V., ROSE, D.P., SEED, M., FOLKARD, J. & STRONG, R. (1973) Effect of pyridoxine hydrochloride (vitamin B$_6$) upon depression associated with oral contraception. *Lancet* **1**, 897–904 [571].

ADAMS, R.D. (1965) Discussion of Part IV. Ch. 20 in *The Remote Effects of Cancer on the Nervous System*, eds Brain, W.R. & Norris, F.H., Contemporary Neurology Symposia, Vol. 1. Grune & Stratton: New York [743].

ADAMS, R.D. (1966) Further observations on normal pressure hydrocephalus. *Proceedings of the Royal Society of Medicine* **59**, 1135–1140 [745].

ADAMS, R.D., BOGAERT, L.V. & EECKEN, H.V. (1964) Striato-nigral degeneration. *Journal of Neuropathology and Experimental Neurology* **23**, 584–608 [668].

ADAMS, R.D., FISHER, C.M., HAKIM, S., OJEMANN, R.G. & SWEET, W.H. (1965) Symptomatic occult hydrocephalus with 'normal' cerebrospinal fluid pressure: a treatable syndrome. *New England Journal of Medicine* **273**, 117–126 [745, 747].

ADAMS, R.D. & KUBIK, C.S. (1944) Subacute degeneration of the brain in pernicious anaemia. *New England Journal of Medicine* **231**, 1–9 [589].

ADAMS, R.D. & VICTOR, M. (1993) *Principles of Neurology*, 5th edn. McGraw-Hill Inc: New York [586].

ADDONIZIO, G., SUSMAN, V.L. & ROTH, S.D. (1987) Neuroleptic malignant syndrome: review and analysis of 115 cases. *Biological Psychiatry* **22**, 1004–1020 [626].

ADIE, W.J. (1926) Idiopathic narcolepsy: a disease sui generis; with remarks on the mechanism of sleep. *Brain* **49**, 257–306 [725, 726].

ADLER, A. (1945) Mental symptoms following head injury. *Archives of Neurology and Psychiatry* **53**, 34–43 [173, 174, 175].

ADLER, L., ANGRIST, B., PESELOW, E., CORWIN, J., MASIANSKY, R. & ROTROSEN, J. (1986) A controlled assessment of propanolol in the treatment of neuroleptic-induced akathisia. *British Journal of Psychiatry* **149**, 42–45 [644].

ADLER, M.W. (1987) ABC of AIDS. Development of the epidemic. *British Medical Journal* **294**, 1083–1085 [316].

ADLER, R., MACRITCHIE, K. & ENGEL, G.L. (1971) Psychologic processes and ischaemic stroke (occlusive cerebrovascular disease) 1. Observations on 32 men with 35 strokes. *Psychosomatic Medicine* **33**, 1–29 [396].

ADOLFSSON, R., GOTTFRIES, C.G., ROOS, B.E. & WINBLAD, B. (1979) Changes in the brain catecholamines in patients with dementia of Alzheimer type. *British Journal of Psychiatry* **135**, 216–223 [444].

ADVISORY GROUP ON THE MANAGEMENT OF PATIENTS WITH SPONGIFORM ENCEPHALOPATHY, (CREUTZFELDT–JAKOB DISEASE (CJD)) (1981) *Report to the Chief Medical Officers of the DHSS, the Scottish Home and Health Department and the Welsh Office*. HMSO: London [447].

AGATE, J.N. & BUCKELL, M. (1949) Mercury poisoning from fingerprint photography. *Lancet* **2**, 451–454 [633, 634].

AGRAS, S. & MARSHALL, C. (1965) The application of negative practice to spasmodic torticollis. *American Journal of Psychiatry* **122**, 579–582 [675].

AICARDI, J. (1986) Some epileptic syndromes in infancy and childhood and their relevance to the definition of epilepsy. Ch. 3 in *What is Epilepsy? The Clinical and Scientific Basis of Epilepsy*, eds Trimble, M.R. & Reynolds, E.H. Churchill Livingstone: Edinburgh [242].

AISEN, A.M., MARTEL, W., GABRIELSEN, T.O., GLAZER, G.M., BREWER, G., YOUNG, A.B. & HILL, G. (1985) Wilson disease of the brain: MR imaging. *Radiology* **157**, 137–141 [662].

AISEN, P.S. & DAVIS, K.L. (1994) Inflammatory mechanisms in Alzheimer's disease: implications for therapy. *American Journal of Psychiatry* **157**, 1105–1113 [447].

AITA, J.A. (1948) Follow-up study of men with penetrating injury to the brain. *Archives of Neurology and Psychiatry* **59**, 511–516 [175, 178].

AITA, J.A. (1972) Neurologic manifestations of periarteritis nodosa. *Nebraska Medical Journal* **57**, 362–366 [423].

AJURIAGUERRA, J. DE & HÉCAEN, H. (1960) *Le Cortex Cerebral: Étude Neuro-psycho-pathologique*, 2nd edn. Masson: Paris [181].

AJURIAGUERRA, J. DE & ROUAULT, DE LA VIGNE, A. (1946) Troubles mentaux de l'intoxication oxycarbonée. *Semaine des Hôpitaux de Paris* **22**, 1950–1954 [550].

AJURIAGUERRA, J. DE & TISSOT, R. (1969) The apraxias. Ch. 3 in *Handbook of Clinical Neurology*, Vol. 4, eds Vinken, P.J. & Bruyn, G.W. North-Holland Publishing Co.: Amsterdam [56].

AKAI, J. & AKAI, K. (1989) Neuropathological study of the nucleus basalis of Meynert in alcoholic dementia. *Japanese Journal of Alcohol and Drug Dependence* **24**, 80–88 [607].

AKBARIAN, S., BUNNEY, W.E., POTKIN, S.G., WIGAL, S.B., HAGMAN, J.O., SANDMAN, C.A. & JONES, E.G. (1993a) Altered distribution of nicotinamide-adenine dinucleotide phosphate-diaphorase cells in frontal lobe of schizophrenics implies disturbances of cortical development. *Archives of General Psychiatry* **50**, 169–177 [87].

AKBARIAN, S., VIÑUELA, A., KIM, J.J., POTKIN, S.G., BUNNEY, W.E. & JONES, E.G. (1993b) Distorted distribution of nicotinamide-adenine dinucleotide phosphate-diaphorase neurons in temporal lobe of schizophrenics implies anomalous cortical development. *Archives of General Psychiatry* **50**, 178–187 [87].

AKELATIS, A.J. (1941) Lead encephalopathy in children and adults: a clinico-pathological study. *Journal of Nervous and Mental Disease* **93**, 313–332 [632].

AL-CHALABI, A., ENAYAT, Z.E., BAKKER, M.C., SHAM, P.C., BALL, D.M., SHAW, C.E., LLOYD, C.M., POWELL, J.F. & LEIGH, P.N. (1996) Association of apolipoprotein E$_\varepsilon$4 allele with bulbar-onset motor neuron disease. *Lancet* **347**, 159–160 [448].

ALAJOUANINE, T. & LHERMITTE, F. (1965) Acquired aphasia in children. *Brain* **88**, 653–662 [202].

ALARCÓN, R.D. & FRANCESCHINI, J.A. (1984) Hyperparathyroidism and paranoid psychosis. Case report and review of the literature. *British Journal of Psychiatry* **145**, 477–486 [529].

ALBERS, J.W., NOSTRANT, T.T. & RIGGS, J.E. (1989) Neurologic manifestations of gastrointestinal disease. In *Neurologic Manifestations of Systemic Disease*, ed. Riggs, J.E. *Neurologic Clinics* **7**, 525–548 [760, 761].

ALBERT, M.L. (1978) Subcortical dementia. In *Alzheimer's Disease: Senile Dementia and Related Disorders, Aging*, Vol. 7, eds Katzman, R., Terry, R.D. & Bick, K.L., pp. 173–180. Raven Press: New York [668].

ALBERT, M.L., FELDMAN, R.G. & WILLIS, A.L. (1974) The 'subcortical dementia' of progressive supranuclear palsy. *Journal of Neurology, Neurosurgery and Psychiatry* **37**, 121–130 [667].

ALBERT, M.S., BUTTERS, N. & BRANDT, J. (1981) Patterns of remote memory in amnesic and demented patients. *Archives of Neurology* **38**, 495–500 [37].

ALBERT, M.S., BUTTERS, N. & LEVIN, J. (1979) Temporal gradients in the retrograde amnesia of patients with alcoholic Korsakoff's disease. *Archives of Neurology* **36**, 211–216 [36].

ALBIN, M.S. & BUNEGIN, L. (1986) An experimental study of craniocerebral trauma during ethanol intoxication. *Critical Care Medicine* **14**, 841–845 [179].

ALDERSON, D., STRONG, A.J., INGHAM, H.R. & SELKON, J.B. (1981) Fifteen-year review of the mortality of brain abscess. *Neurosurgery* **8**, 1–5 [368].

ALEMA, G. (1978) Behçet's disease. Ch. 24 in *Handbook of Clinical Neurology*, Vol. 34. *Infections of the Nervous System*. Pt. 11, eds Vinken, P.J. & Bruyn, G.W. North Holland Publishing Co.: Amsterdam [762, 763].

ALEX, M., BARON, E.K., GOLDENBERG, S. & BLUMENTHAL, H.T. (1962) An autopsy study of cerebrovascular accidents in diabetes mellitus. *Circulation* **25**, 663–673 [538].

ALEXANDER, F. (1939) Emotional factors in essential hypertension. Presentation of a tentative hypothesis. *Psychosomatic Medicine* **1**, 173–179 [398].

ALEXANDER, L. (1938) Clinical and neuropathological aspects of electrical injuries. *Journal of Industrial Hygiene and Toxicology* **20**, 191–243 [765].

ALEXANDER, L. (1940) Wernicke's disease; identity of lesions produced experimentally by B$_1$ avitaminosis in pigeons with haemorrhagic polioencephalitis occurring in chronic alcoholism in man. *American Journal of Pathology* **16**, 61–70 [576].

ALEXANDER, M.P. (1982a) Traumatic brain injury. Ch. 11 in *Psychiatric Aspects of Neurologic Disease*, Vol. 2, eds Benson, D.F. & Blumer, D. Grune & Stratton: New York & London [187].

ALEXANDER, M.P. (1982b) Episodic behaviours due to neurologic disorders other than epilepsy. Ch. 5 in *Pseùdoseizures*, eds Riley, T.L. & Roy, A. Williams & Wilkins: Baltimore & London [291].

ALEXANDER, P.E. & JACKSON, A.H. (1981) Calcium and magnesium: relationship to schizophrenia and neuroleptic-induced extrapyramidal symptoms. Ch. 9 in *Electrolytes and Neuropsychiatric Disorders*, ed. Alexander, P.E. MTP Press: Lancaster [561].

ALFREY, A.C., LE GENDRE, G.R. & KAEHNY, W.D. (1976) The dialysis encephalopathy syndrome. *The New England Journal of Medicine* **294**, 184–188 [558].

ALLEN, I.M. (1930) A clinical study of tumours involving the occipital lobe. *Brain* **53**, 194–243 [227].

ALLEN, J.E. & RODGIN, D.W. (1960) Mental retardation in association with progressive muscular dystrophy. *American Journal of Diseases of Children* **100**, 208–211 [716].

ALLEN, N.H.P., GORDON, S., HOPE, T. & BURNS, A. (1996) Manchester and Oxford universities scale for the psychopathological assessment of dementia (MOUSEPAD). *British Journal of Psychiatry* **169**, 293–307 [125].

ALLENTUCK, S. & BOWMAN, K.M. (1942) The psychiatric aspects of marijuana intoxication. *American Journal of Psychiatry* **99**, 248–250 [612].

ALLISON, R.S. (1961) Chronic amnesic syndromes in the elderly. *Proceedings of the Royal Society of Medicine* **54**, 961–965 [550].

ALLISON, R.S. (1962) *The Senile Brain: a Clinical Study*. Edward Arnold: London [15, 96].

ALLMAN, P. (1991) Emotionalism following brain damage. *Behavioural Neurology* **4**, 57–62 [387].

ALPERS, B.J. (1936) A note on the mental syndrome of corpus callosum tumours. *Journal of Nervous and Mental Disease* **84**, 621–627 [224].

ALPERS, B.J. (1937) Relation of the hypothalamus to disorders of personality. *Archives of Neurology and Psychiatry* **38**, 291–303 [229].

ALPERS, B.J. (1940) Personality and emotional disorders associated with hypothalamic lesions. Ch. 28 in *The Hypothalamus and Central Levels of Autonomic Function*. Research Publications of the Association for Research in Nervous and Mental Disease, Vol. 20. Williams & Wilkins: Baltimore [229].

ALPERS, M. (1969) Kuru: clinical and aetiological aspects. In *Virus Diseases and the Nervous System*, eds Whitty, C.W.M., Hughes, J.T. & MacCallum, F.O. Blackwell Scientific Publications: Oxford [751].

ALSTROM, C.H. (1950) A study of epilepsy in its clinical, social and genetic aspects. *Acta Psychiatrica et Neurologica Scandinavica* **63 (Supplement)**, 5–284 [243, 265, 274].

ALTER, M., NEUGUT, R. & KAHANA, E. (1978) Familial aggregates of Creutzfeldt–Jakob disease (Abstract). *Neurology* **28**, 353 [475].

ALTSHULER, L.L., CUMMINGS, J.L. & MILLS, M.J. (1986) Mutism: review, differential diagnosis, and report of 22 cases. *American Journal of Psychiatry* **143**, 1409–1414 [156].

ALVAREZ, W.C. (1947) The migrainous personality and constitution. The essential features of the disease. A study of 500 cases. *American Journal of the Medical Sciences* **213**, 1–8 [403].

ALVAREZ, W.C. (1966) *Little Strokes*. Lippincott: Philadelphia & Toronto [381, 493].

ALVORD, E.C. JNR, FORNO, L.S., KUSSKE, J.A., KAUFFMAN, R.J., RHODES, J.S. & GOETOWSECI, C.R. (1974) The pathology of Parkinsonism: a comparison of degenerations in cerebral cortex and brain stem. *Advances in Neurology* **5**, 175–193 [655].

ALZHEIMER, A. (1907) Über eine eigenartige Erkrankung der Hirnrinde. *Allgemeine Zeitschrift für Psychiatrie* **64**, 146–148 [437].

ALZHEIMER, A. (1911) Über eigenartige Krankheitsfille des späteren Alters. *Zeitschrift für die gesamte Neurologie und Psychiatrie* **4**, 356–385 [431].

AMADUCCI, L.A., FRATIGLIONI, L., ROCCA, W.A., FIESCHI, C., LIVREA, P., PEDONE, D., BRACCO, L., LIPPI, A., GANDOLFO, C., BINO, G., PRENCIPE, M., BONATTI, M.L., GIROTTI, F., CARELLA, F., TAVOLATO, B., FERLA, S., LENZI, G.L., CAROLEI, A., GAMBI, A., GRIGOLETTO, F. & SCHOENBERG, B.S. (1985) Risk factors for Alzheimer's disease (AD): a case–control study on an Italian population. *Neurology* **35 (Supplement 1)**, 277 [438].

AMBROSE, J. (1973) Computerized transverse axial scanning (tomography). Part 2. Clinical application. *British Journal of Radiology* **46**, 1023–1047 [137].

AMBROSE, J. (1974) Computerized X-ray scanning of the brain. *Journal of Neurosurgery* **40**, 679–695 [137].

AMERICAN PSYCHIATRIC ASSOCIATION (1980) *Diagnostic and Statistical Manual of Mental Disorders* (*DSM-III*), 3rd edn. American Psychiatric Association: Washington, DC [194].

AMERICAN PSYCHIATRIC ASSOCIATION (1987) *Diagnostic and Statistical Manual of Mental Disorders* (*DSM-III-R*), 3rd edn, revised. American Psychiatric Association: Washington DC [194].

AMINOFF, M.J., MARSHALL, J., SMITH, E.M. & WYKE, M.A. (1975)

Pattern of intellectual impairment in Huntington's chorea. *Psychological Medicine* **5**, 169–172 [469].

ANAND, M.P. (1964) Iatrogenic megaloblastic anaemia with neurological complications. *Scottish Medical Journal* **9**, 388–390 [591].

ANASTASI, A. (1982) *Psychological Testing*, 5th edn. Macmillan: New York [122].

ANDERMANN, F. (1994) Brain structure in epilepsy. The crucial role of MRI. Ch. 3 in *Magnetic Resonance Scanning and Epilepsy*, eds Shorvon, S.D., Fish, D.R., Andermann, F., Bydder, G.M. & Stefan, H. Plenum Press: New York & London [289].

ANDERMANN, F., ANDERMANN, E. & GENDRON, D. (1990) Startle disease (hyperekplexia): a hereditary disorder with abnormal startle, falling spells, and attacks of spontaneous clonus. *Cleveland Clinic Journal of Medicine* **57 (Supplement)**, S54–S60 [292].

ANDERMANN, F., KEENE, D.L., ANDERMANN, E. & QUESNEY, L.F. (1980) Startle disease on hyperekplexia. Further delineation of the syndrome. *Brain* **103**, 985–997 [292].

ANDERSON, C. (1942) Chronic head cases. *Lancet* **2**, 1–4 [196].

ANDERSON, E.W. & MALLINSON, W.P. (1941) Psychogenic episodes in the course of major psychoses. *Journal of Mental Science* **87**, 383–396 [480, 481, 482].

ANDERSON, E.W., TRETHOWAN, W.H. & KENNA, J.C. (1959) An experimental investigation of simulation and pseudo-dementia. *Acta Psychiatrica et Neurologica Scandinavica* **132 (Supplement)**, 1–42 [484].

ANDERSON, J. (1968) Psychiatric aspects of primary hyperparathyroidism. *Proceedings of the Royal Society of Medicine* **61**, 1123–1124 [592].

ANDERSON, M. (1993) Virus infections of the nervous system. Ch. 9 in *Brain's Diseases of the Nervous System*, 10th edn. Oxford University Press: Oxford [357, 362, 473].

ANDERSON, V.E. & HAUSER, W.A. (1993) Genetics. Ch. 3 in *A Textbook of Epilepsy*, 4th edn, eds Laidlaw, J., Richens, A. & Chadwick, D. Churchill Livingstone: Edinburgh [247].

ANDERSSON, P.G. (1970) Intracranial tumours in a psychiatric autopsy material. *Acta Psychiatrica Scandinavica* **46**, 213–224 [233].

ANDREASEN, N.C., ARNDT, S., SWAYZE, V., CIZADLO, T., FLAUM, M., O'LEARY, D., EHRHARDT, J.C. & YUH, W.T.C. (1994a) Thalamic abnormalities in schizophrenia visualized through magnetic resonance image averaging. *Science* **266**, 294–298 [85].

ANDREASEN, N.C., CIZADLO, T., HARRIS, G., SWAYZE, V., O'LEARY, D.S., COHEN, G., EHRHARDT, J. & YUH, W.T.C. (1993) Voxl processing techniques for the antemortem study of neuroanatomy and neuropathology using magnetic resonance imaging. *The Journal of Neuropsychiatry and Clinical Neurosciences* **5**, 121–130 [xix, 142].

ANDREASEN, N.C., EHRHARDT, J.C., SWAYZE, V.W., ALLIGER, R.J., YUH, W.T.C., COHEN, G. & ZIEBELL, S. (1990) Magnetic resonance imaging of the brain in schizophrenia. *Archives of General Psychiatry* **47**, 35–44 [85].

ANDREASEN, N.C., FLASHMAN, L., FLAUM, M., ARNDT, S., SWAYZE, V., O'LEARY, D.S., EHRHARDT, J.C. & YUH, W.T.C. (1994b) Regional brain abnormalities in schizophrenia measured with magnetic resonance imaging. *Journal of the American Medical Association* **272**, 1763–1769 [85].

ANDREASEN, N.C., NASRALLAH, H.A., DUNN, V., OLSON, S.C., GROVE, W.M., EHRHARDT, J.C., COFFMAN, J.A. & CROSSETT, J.H.W. (1986) Structural abnormalities in the frontal system in schizophrenia. A magnetic resonance imaging study. *Archives of General Psychiatry* **43**, 136–144 [85].

ANDREASEN, N.C., SMITH, M.R., JACOBY, C.G., DENNERT, J.W. & OLSEN, S.A. (1982) Ventricular enlargement in schizophrenia:

definition and prevalence. *American Journal of Psychiatry* **139**, 292–296 [140].

ANDRÉASSON, S., ALLEBECK, P., ENGSTRÖM, A. & RYDBERG, U. (1987) Cannabis and schizophrenia. A longitudinal study of Swedish conscripts. *Lancet* **2**, 1483–1485 [615].

ANDRÉASSON, S., ALLEBECK, P. & RYDBERG, U. (1989) Schizophrenia in users and non users of cannabis. A longitudinal study in Stockholm County. *Acta Psychiatrica Scandinavica* **79**, 505–510 [615].

ANDREW, J. & NATHAN, P.W. (1964) Lesions of the anterior frontal lobes and disturbances of micturition and defaecation. *Brain* **87**, 233–262 [223].

ANDREW, M. & OWEN, M.J. (1997) Hyperekplexia: abnormal startle response due to glycine receptor mutations. *British Journal of Psychiatry* **170**, 106–108 [292].

ANDREWES, D.G., BULLEN, J.G., TOMLINSON, L., ELWES, R.D.C. & REYNOLDS, E.H. (1986) A comparative study of the cognitive effects of phenytoin and carbamazepine in new referrals with epilepsy. *Epilepsia* **27**, 128–134 [263, 301].

ANDREWS, H. (1996) Magnetoencephalography. Ch. 9 in *Brain Imaging in Psychiatry*, eds Lewis, S. & Higgins, N. Blackwell Science: Oxford [133].

ANNETT, M. (1970) A classification of hand preferences by association analysis. *British Journal of Psychology* **61**, 303–321 [40].

ANTEBI, D. & BIRD, J. (1992) The facilitation and evocation of seizures. *British Journal of Psychiatry* **160**, 154–164 [241, 248].

ANTHONY, J.C., LE RESCHE, L., NIAZ, U., VON KORF, M.R. & FOLSTEIM, M.F. (1982) Limits of the 'Mini-Mental State' as a screening test for dementia and delirium among hospital patients. *Psychological Medicine* **12**, 397–408 [123].

ANTUONO, P., SORBI, S., BRACCO, L., FUSCO, T. & AMADUCCI, L. (1980) A discrete sampling technique in senile dementia of the Alzheimer type and alcoholic dementia: study of cholinergic system. In *Aging of the Brain and Dementia, Aging*, Vol. 13, eds Amaducci, L., Davison, A.N. & Antuono, P. Raven Press: New York [606].

APPENZELLER, O. & SALMON, J.H. (1967) Treatment of parenchymatous degneration of the brain by ventriculo-atrial shunting of the cerebrospinal fluid. *Journal of Neurosurgery* **26**, 478–482 [748].

ARAI, H., KOSAKA, K. & IIZUKA, R. (1984) Changes of biogenic amines and their metabolites in postmortem brains from patients with Alzheimer-type dementia. *Journal of Neurochemistry* **43**, 388–393 [444].

ARDILA, A. & SANCHEZ, E. (1988) Neuropsychologic symptoms in the migraine syndrome. *Cephalgia* **8**, 67–70 [400].

ARENDT, T., ALLEN, Y., SINDEN, J., SCHUGENS, M.M., MARCHBANKS, R.M., LANTOS, P.L. & GRAY, J.A. (1988) Cholinergic-rich brain transplants reverse alcohol-induced memory deficits. *Nature* **332**, 448–450 [26].

ARENDT, T., BIGL, V., ARENDT, A. & TENNSTEDT, A. (1983) Loss of neurons in the nucleus basalis of Meynert in Alzheimer's disease, paralysis agitans and Korsakoff's disease. *Acta Neuropathologica (Berlin)* **61**, 101–108 [26, 607].

ARGYLE, N., JESTICE, S. & BROOK, C.P.B. (1985) Psychogeriatric patients: their supporters problems. *Age and Ageing* **14**, 355–360 [498].

ARIE, T. (1983) Pseudodementia. *British Medical Journal* **286**, 1301–1302 [487].

ARKY, R.A., VEVERBRANTS, E. & ABRAMSON, E.A. (1968) Irreversible hypoglycemia. A complication of alcohol and insulin. *Journal of the American Medical Association* **206**, 575–578 [544, 545].

ARMSTRONG, P. & KEEVIL, S.F. (1991) Magnetic resonance imaging—2: clinical uses. *British Medical Journal* **303**, 105–109 [231, 232, 377, 690].

ARNOLD, O.H. (1949) Untersuchungen zur Frage der akuten tödlichen Katatonien. *Wiener Zeitschrift für Nervenheilkunde und deren Grenzgebiete* **2**, 386–401 [556].

ARNOLD, S.E., HYMAN, B.T., VAN HOESEN, G.W. & DAMASIO, A.R. (1991) Some cytoarchitectural abnormalities of the entorhinal cortex in schizophrenia. *Archives of General Psychiatry* **48**, 625–632 [86].

ARRIA, A.M., TARTER, R.E., WARTY, V. & VAN THIEL, D.H. (1990) Vitamin E deficiency and psychomotor dysfunction in adults with primary biliary cirrhosis. *American Journal of Clinical Nutrition* **52**, 383–390 [565].

ASARE, E.K., GLASS, J.D., LUTHERT, P.J., EVERALL, I.P., DUNN, G., McARTHUR, J. & LANTOS, P.L. (1995) Neuronal pattern differences in HIV-associated dementia. *Neuropathology and Applied Neurobiology* **21**, 151 [323].

ASHER, R. (1949) Myxoedematous madness. *British Medical Journal* **2**, 555–562 [512, 514].

ASHTON, C.H. (1987) Cannabis: dangers and possible uses. *British Medical Journal* **294**, 141–142 [616].

ASHTON, H. (1986) Adverse effects of prolonged benzodiazepine use. *Adverse Drug Reaction Bulletin*, **118 (June)**, 440–443 [609].

ASNIS, G. (1977) Parkinson's disease, depression and ECT. A review and case study. *American Journal of Psychiatry* **134**, 191–195 [656].

ASSO, D., CROWN, S., RUSSELL, J.A. & LOGUE, V. (1969) Psychological aspects of the stereo-tactic treatment of parkinsonism. *British Journal of Psychiatry* **115**, 541–553 [660].

ASTRUP, P. (1972) Some physiological and pathological effects of moderate carbon monoxide exposure. *British Medical Journal* **4**, 447–452 [553].

ATKINS, C.J., KONDON, J.J., QUISMORIO, F.P. & FRIOU, G.J. (1972) The choroid plexus in systemic lupus erythematosus. *Annals of Internal Medicine* **76**, 65–72 [421].

ATKINSON, L. (1991) Concurrent use of the Wechsler Memory Scale—Revised and the WAIS-R. *British Journal of Clinical Psychology* **30**, 87–90 [117].

AVERY, T.L. (1971) Seven cases of frontal tumour with psychiatric presentation. *British Journal of Psychiatry* **119**, 19–23 [223].

AVERY, T.L. (1973) A case of acromegaly and gigantism with depression. *British Journal of Psychiatry* **122**, 599–600 [522].

AVRAHAMI, E., KATZ, A., BORNSTEIN, N. & KORCZYN, A.D. (1987) Computed tomographic findings of brain and skull in myotonic dystrophy. *Journal of Neurology, Neurosurgery, and Psychiatry* **50**, 435–438 [719].

AYLWARD, E., WALKER, E. & BETTES, B. (1984) Intelligence in schizophrenia. Meta-analysis of the research. *Schizophrenia Bulletin* **10**, 430–459 [91].

BABCOCK, H. (1930) An experiment in the measurement of mental deterioration. *Archives of Psychology* **117**, 5–105 [99].

BACH-Y-RITA, G., LION, J.R., CLIMENT, C.E. & ERVIN, F.R. (1971) Episodic dyscontrol: a study of 130 violent patients. *American Journal of Psychiatry* **127**, 1473–1478 [83].

BACH-Y-RITA, G., LION, J.R. & ERVIN, F.R. (1970) Pathological intoxication: clinical and electroencephalographic studies. *American Journal of Psychiatry* **127**, 698–703 [595].

BADDELEY, A.D. (1976) *The Psychology of Memory*. Harper & Row: New York [29].

BADDELEY, A., EMSLIE, H. & NIMMO-SMITH, I. (1992) *The Speed and Capacity of Language-Processing Test*. Thames Valley Test Company: Bury St Edmunds [114].

BADDELEY, A., EMSLIE, H. & NIMMO-SMITH, I. (1993) The Spot-the-Word test: a robust estimate of verbal intelligence based on lexical decision. *British Journal of Clinical Psychology* **32**, 55–65 [114].

BAIL, J.R.B. & LLOYD, J.H. (1971) Myasthenia gravis as hysteria: or sounds of silence. *Medical Journal of Australia* **1**, 1018–1020 [714].

BAILES, D.R., YOUNG, I.R., THOMAS, D.J., STRAUGHAN, K., BYDDER, G.M. & STEINER, R.E. (1982) NMR imaging of the brain using spinecho sequences. *Clinical Radiology* **33**, 395–414 [141].

BAKER, A.B. & KNUTSON, J. (1946) Psychiatric aspects of uraemia. *American Journal of Psychiatry* **102**, 683–687 [556].

BAKER, A.B. & TICHY, F.Y. (1953) The effects of the organic solvents and industrial poisonings on the central nervous system. Ch. 26 in *Metabolic and Toxic Diseases of the Nervous System*, Research Publications of the Association for Research in Nervous and Mental Disease, Vol. 32. Williams & Wilkins: Baltimore [637].

BAKER, L. & BARCAI, A. (1970) Psychosomatic aspects of diabetes mellitus. Ch. 7 in *Modern Trends in Psychosomatic Medicine*, Vol. 2, ed. Hill, O.W. Butterworths: London [535].

BAKER, M. (1973) Psychopathology in systemic lupus erythematosus: 1. Psychiatric observations. *Seminars in Arthritis and Rheumatism* **3**, 95–110 [421].

BAKHEIT, A.M.O. (1990) Drug treatment of Parkinson's disease. *Hospital Update* **June**, 497–504 [649].

BAKHEIT, A.M.O., BEHAN, P.O., DINAN, T.G., GRAY, C.E. & O'KEANE, V. (1992) Possible upregulation of hypothalamic 5-hydroxytryptamine receptors in patients with postural fatigue syndrome. *British Medical Journal* **304**, 1010–1012 [373].

BAKHEIT, A.M.O., KENNEDY, P.G.E. & BEHAN, P.O. (1990) Paraneoplastic limbic encephalitis: clinico-pathological correlations. *Journal of Neurology, Neurosurgery and Psychiatry* **53**, 1084–1088 [742].

BAKIR, F., DAMLUJI, S.F., AMIN-ZAKI, L., MURTADHA, M., KHALIDI, A., AL-RAWI, N.Y., TIKRITI, S., DHAHIR, H.I., CLARKSON, T.W., SMITH, J.C. & DOHERTY, R.A. (1973) Methylmercury poisoning in Iraq. An Inter-University Report. *Science* **181**, 230–240 [635].

BALDESSARINI, R.J. & TARSY, D. (1980) The pathophysiologic basis of tardive dyskinesia. In *Tardive Dyskinesia: Research and Treatment*, eds Fann, W.E., Smith, R.C., Davis, J.M. & Domino, E.F. MTP Press: Lancaster [643].

BALDY, R.E., BRINDLEY, G.S., EWUSI-MENSAH, I., JACOBSON, R.R., REVELEY, M.A., TURNER, S.W. & LISHMAN, W.A. (1986) A fully-automated computer-assisted method of CT brain scan analysis for the measurement of cerebrospinal fluid spaces and brain absorption density. *Neuroradiology* **28**, 109–117 [138].

BALE, R.N. (1973) Brain damage in diabetes mellitus. *British Journal of Psychiatry* **122**, 337–341 [537].

BALL, C.J. (1991) The vascular origins of the Charles Bonnet syndrome: four cases and a review of the pathogenic mechanisms. *International Journal of Geriatric Psychiatry* **6**, 673–679 [296].

BALL, M.J. (1976) Neurofibrillary tangles and the pathogenesis of dementia: a quantitative study. *Neuropathology and Applied Neurobiology* **2**, 395–410 [436].

BALL, M.J. & NUTTALL, K. (1980) Neurofibrillary tangles, granulovacuolar degeneration and neurone loss in Down's syndrome: quantitative comparison with Alzheimer dementia. *Annals of Neurology* **7**, 462–465 [437].

BALLA, J. & IANSEK, R. (1988) Headache arising from disorders of the cervical spine. Ch. 10 in *Headache: Problems in Diagnosis and Management*, ed. Hopkins, A. W.B. Saunders: London [199, 200].

BALLENGER, J.C. & POST, R.M. (1978) Kindling as a model for alcoholic withdrawal syndromes. *British Journal of Psychiatry* **133**, 1–14 [598].

BALTHASAR, K. (1956) Über das anatomische Substrat der generalisierten Tic-krankheit (maladie des tics, Gilles de la Tourette): Entwicklungshemmung des Corpus Striatum. *Archiv für Psychiatrie und Nervenkrankheiten* **195**, 531–549 [685].

BALTIMORE, D. (1995) Lessons from people with nonprogressive HIV infection. *New England Journal of Medicine* **332**, 259–260 [318].

BAMFORD, J., SANDERCOCK, P., DENNIS, M., BURN, J. & WARLOW, C. (1990) A prospective study of acute cerebrovascular disease in the community: the Oxfordshire Community Stroke Project 1981–86. 2. Incidence, case fatality rates and overall outcome at one year of cerebral infarction, primary intracerebral and subarachnoid haemorrhage. *Journal of Neurology, Neurosurgery and Psychiatry* **53**, 16–22 [376].

BAMFORD, J., SANDERCOCK, P., DENNIS, M., WARLOW, C., JONES, L., McPHERSON, K., VESSEY, M., FOWLER, G., MOLYNEUX, A., HUGHES, T., BURN, J. & WADE, D. (1988) A prospective study of acute cerebrovascular disease in the community: the Oxfordshire Community Stroke Project 1981–86. 1. Methodology, demography and incident cases of first-ever stroke. *Journal of Neurology, Neurosurgery and Psychiatry* **51**, 1373–1380 [375].

BANAY, R.S. (1944) Pathologic reaction to alcohol. Review of the literature and original case reports. *Quarterly Journal of Studies on Alcohol* **4**, 580-605 [595].

BANEN, D. (1972) An ergot preparation (hydergine) for relief of symptoms of cerebro-vascular insufficiency. *Journal of the American Geriatrics Society* **20**, 22–24 [502].

BANNISTER, R. (1970) The place of isotope encephalography by the lumbar route in neurological diagnosis. *Proceedings of the Royal Society of Medicine* **63**, 921–925 [136].

BANSAL, B.C., DUA, A., GUPTA, R. & GUPTA, M.S. (1989) Appearing and disappearing CT scan abnormalities in epilepsy in India—an enigma. *Journal of Neurology, Neurosurgery, and Psychiatry* **52**, 1185–1187 [289].

BARBEAU, A. (1971) Long-term side-effects of levodopa. *Lancet* **1**, 395 [658].

BARBIZET, J. (1963) Defect of memorizing of hippocampal-mammillary origin: a review. *Journal of Neurology, Neurosurgery and Psychiatry* **26**, 127–135 [31].

BARCROFT, J. (1920) Anoxemia. *Lancet* **2**, 485–489 [546].

BARCROFT, J. (1925) *The Respiratory Function of the Blood. Part 1: Lessons from high altitudes.* Cambridge University Press: Cambridge [548].

BARCZAK, P., EDMUNDS, E. & BETTS, T. (1988) Hypomania following complex partial seizures. A report of three cases. *British Journal of Psychiatry* **152**, 137–139 [258].

BARD, P. (1928) A diencephalic mechanism for the expression of rage with special reference to the sympathetic nervous system. *American Journal of Physiology* **84**, 490–515 [80].

BARETTE, J. & MARSDEN, C.D. (1979) Attitudes of families to some aspects of Huntington's chorea. *Psychological Medicine* **9**, 327–336 [466].

BARKER, M.G. & LAWSON, J.S. (1968) Nominal aphasia in dementia. *British Journal of Psychiatry* **114**, 1351–1356 [15].

BARKER, W. (1948) Studies in epilepsy: personality pattern, situational stress, and the symptoms of narcolepsy. *Psychosomatic Medicine* **10**, 193–202 [725].

BARKER, W. & WOLF, S. (1947) Studies in epilepsy. *American Journal of the Medical Sciences* **214**, 600–604 [248].

BARLOW, E.D. & DE WARDENER, H.E. (1959) Compulsive water drinking. *Quarterly Journal of Medicine* **28**, 235–258 [525].

BARNES, T.R.E. (1987) The present status of tardive dyskinesia and akathisia in the treatment of schizophrenia. *Psychiatric Developments* **4**, 301–319 [642].

BARNES, T.R.E. (1989) A rating scale for drug-induced akathisia. *British Journal of Psychiatry* **154**, 672–676 [640].

BARNES, T.R.E. & BRAUDE, W.M. (1985) Akathisia variants and tardive dyskinesia. *Archives of General Psychiatry* **42**, 874–878 [640].

BARON, J.A. (1986) Cigarette smoking and Parkinson's disease. *Neurology* **36**, 1490–1496 [661].

BARON, J.C. (1987) Remote metabolic effects of stroke. Ch. 8 in *Impact of Functional Imaging in Neurology and Psychiatry*, eds Wade, J., Knežević, S., Maximilian, V.A., Mubrin, Z., Prohovnik, I. *Current Problems in Neurology* **5** [377].

BARR, A.N., FISCHER, J.H., KOLLER, W.C., SPUNT, A.L. & SINGHAL, A. (1988) Serum haloperidol concentration and choreiform movements in Huntington's disease. *Neurology* **38**, 84–88 [505].

BARRACLOUGH, B. (1981) Suicide and epilepsy. Ch. 7 in *Epilepsy and Psychiatry*, eds Reynolds, E.H. & Trimble, M.R. Churchill Livingstone: Edinburgh & London [286].

BARRETT, K. (1991) Treating organic abulia with bromocriptine and lisuride: four case studies. *Journal of Neurology, Neurosurgery and Psychiatry* **54**, 718–721 [214].

BARRON, S.A., JACOBS, L. & KINKEL, W.R. (1976) Changes in size of normal lateral ventricles during aging determined by computerised tomography. *Neurology* **26**, 1011–1013 [138].

BARTA, P.E., PEARLSON, G.D., POWERS, R.E., RICHARDS, S.S. & TUNE, L.E. (1990) Auditory hallucinations and smaller superior temporal gyral volume in schizophrenia. *American Journal of Psychiatry* **147**, 1457–1462 [85].

BARTH, J.T., ALVES, W.M., RYAN, T.V., MACCIOCCHI, S.N., RIMEL, R.W., JANE, J.A. & NELSON, W.E. (1989) Mild head injury in sports: neuropsychological sequelae and recovery of function. Ch. 17 in *Mild Head Injury*, eds Levin, H.S., Eisenberg, H.M. & Benton, A.L. Oxford University Press: Oxford [184].

BARTHOLOMEW, A.A. & MARLEY, E. (1959) Toxic response to 2-phenyl-3-methyl tetrahydro-1,4-oxazine hydrochloride (Preludin) in humans. *Psychopharmacologia* **1**, 124–139 [617].

BARTLETT, F.C. (1932) *Remembering: A Study in Experimental and Social Psychology.* Cambridge University Press: Cambridge [25].

BARWICK, D.D., OSSELTON, J.W. & WALTON, J.N. (1965) Electroencephalographic studies in hereditary myopathy. *Journal of Neurology, Neurosurgery and Psychiatry* **28**, 109–114 [719].

BATEMAN, D.E., LAWTON, N.F., WHITE, J.E., GREENWOOD, R.J. & WRIGHT, D.J.M. (1988) The neurological complications of Borrelia burgdorferi in the New Forest area of Hampshire. *Journal of Neurology, Neurosurgery and Psychiatry* **51**, 699–703 [369].

BATEMAN, D.E. & WHITE, J.E. (1990) Lyme disease. *Hospital Update* **August**, 677–681 [369].

BATSHAW, M.L., WACHTEL, R.C., DECKEL, A.W., WHITEHOUSE, P.J., MOSES, H., FOCHTMAN, L.J. & ELDRIDGE, R. (1985) Munchausen's syndrome simulating torsion dystonia. *New England Journal of Medicine* **312**, 1437–1439 [680].

BAUER, G., MAYR, U. & PALLUA, A. (1980) Computerised axial tomography in chronic partial epilepsies. *Epilepsia* **21**, 227–233 [289].

BAUER, W.R., TURREL, A.P. & JOHNSON, K.P. (1973) Progressive multifocal leukoencephalopathy and cytarabine: remission with treatment. *Journal of the American Medical Association* **226**, 174–176 [752].

BAXTER, L.R., PHELPS, M.E., MAZZIOTTA, J.C., GUZE, B.H., SCHWARTZ, J.M. & SELIN, C.E. (1987) Local cerebral glucose metabolic rates in obsessive-compulsive disorder. *Archives of General Psychiatry* **44**, 211–218 [145].

BAXTER, L.R., PHELPS, M.E., MAZZIOTTA, J.C., SCHWARTZ, J.M., GERNER, R.H., SELIN, C.E. & SUMIDA, R.M. (1985) Cerebral metabolic rates for glucose in mood disorders. *Archives of General Psychiatry* **42**, 441–447 [145].

BAXTER, L.R., SCHWARTZ, J.M., MAZZIOTTA, J.C., PHELPS, M.E., PAHL, J.J., GUZE, B.H. & FAIRBANKS, L. (1988) Cerebral glucose metabolic rates in nondepressed patients with obsessive-compulsive disorder. *American Journal of Psychiatry* **145**, 1560–1563 [145].

BAXTER, L.R., SCHWARTZ, J.M., PHELPS, M.E., MAZZIOTTA, J.C., GUZE, B.H., SELIN, C.E., GERNER, R.H. & SUMIDA, R.M. (1989) Reduction of prefrontal cortex glucose metabolism common to three types of depression. *Archives of General Psychiatry* **46**, 243–250 [145].

BAY, E. (1953) Disturbances of visual perception and their examination. *Brain* **76**, 515–550 [60].

BAY, E. (1965) The concepts of agnosia, apraxia and aphasia after a history of a hundred years. *Journal of the Mount Sinai Hospital* **32**, 637–650 [60].

BAYLESS, T.M. & KNOX, D.L. (1979) Whipple's disease: a multisystem infection. *New England Journal of Medicine* **300**, 920–921 [760].

BAYLIS, P.H. (1996) Water and sodium homeostasis and their disorders. Section 20.2.1 in *Oxford Textbook of Medicine*, 3rd edn, eds Weatherall, D.J., Ledingham, J.G.G. & Warrell, D.A. Oxford University Press: Oxford [525].

BEAL, M.F., MAZUREK, M.F., TRAN, V.T., CHATTHA, G., BIRD, E.D. & MARTIN, J.B. (1985) Reduced numbers of somatostatin receptors in the cerebral cortex in Alzheimer's disease. *Science* **229**, 289–291 [445].

BEAR, D.M. (1979) Temporal lobe epilepsy—a syndrome of sensory–limbic hyperconnection. *Cortex* **15**, 357–384 [269].

BEAR, D.M. & FEDIO, P. (1977) Quantitative analysis of interictal behaviour in temporal lobe epilepsy. *Archives of Neurology* **34**, 454–467 [267, 269].

BEARD, A.W. (1959) The association of hepatolenticular degeneration with schizophrenia. *Acta Psychiatrica et Neurologica Scandinavica* **34**, 411–428 [665].

BEARDSWORTH, E.D. & ADAMS, C.B.T. (1988) Modified hemispherectomy for epilepsy: early results in 10 cases. *British Journal of Neurosurgery* **2**, 73–84 [313].

BEARN, A.G. (1957) Wilson's disease: an inborn error of metabolism with multiple manifestations. *American Journal of Medicine* **22**, 747–757 [662].

BECK, E., DANIEL, P.M., GAJDUSEK, D.C. & GIBBS, C.J. (1969a) Similarities and differences in the pattern of the pathological changes in scrapie, kuru, experimental kuru and subacute presenile polioencephalopathy. In *Virus Diseases and the Nervous System*, eds Whitty, C.W.M., Hughes, J.T. & MacCallum, F.O. Blackwell Scientific Publications: Oxford [473].

BECK, E., DANIEL, P.M., MATTHEWS, W.B., STEVENS, D.L., ALPERS, M.P., ASHER, D.M., GAJDUSEK, D.C. & GIBBS, C.J. (1969b) Creutzfeldt–Jakob disease: the neuropathology of a transmission experiment. *Brain* **92**, 699–716 [473].

BECK, H.G. (1936) Slow carbon monoxide asphyxiation. *Journal of the American Medical Association* **107(i)**, 1025–1029 [553].

BEDFORD, P.D. (1955) Adverse cerebral effects of anaesthesia on old people. *Lancet* **2**, 259–263 [546].

BEDFORD, P.D. (1958) Discussion: intracranial haemorrhage—diagnosis and treatment. *Proceedings of the Royal Society of Medicine* **51**, 209–213 [411].

BEECH, H.R. (1960) The symptomatic treatment of writer's cramp. In *Behaviour Therapy and the Neuroses*, ed. Eysenck, H.J. Pergamon Press: Oxford [677].

BEELEY, L. (1986) Drug interactions with lithium. *Prescriber's Journal* **26**, 160–163 [626].

BEEVERS, D.G., FAIRMAN, M.J., HAMILTON, M. & HARPUR, J.E. (1973) Antihypertensive treatment and the course of established cerebral vascular disease. *Lancet* **1**, 1407–1409 [389].

BEGLEITER, H., PORJESZ, B. & TENNER, M. (1980) Neuroradiological and neurophysiological evidence of brain deficits in chronic alcoholics. *Acta Psychiatrica Scandinavica* **62** (**Supplement 286**), 3–13, [606].

BEHAN, P.O. & BEHAN, W.M.H. (1979) Possible immunological factors in Alzheimer's disease. Ch. 6 in *Alzheimer's Disease. Early recognition of potentially reversible effects*, eds Glen, A.I.M. & Whalley, L.J. Churchill Livingstone: Edinburgh [447].

BEHAN, P.O. & FELDMAN, R.G. (1970) Serum proteins, amyloid and Alzheimer's disease. *Journal of the American Geriatrics Society* **18**, 792–797 [447].

BEHRMAN, S. (1972) Mutism induced by phenothiazines. *British Journal of Psychiatry* **121**, 599–604 [156, 640].

BEISER, C. (1997) Recent advances. HIV infection—II. *British Medical Journal* **314**, 579–583 [334].

BELL, C.L., PARTINGTON, C., ROBBINS, M., GRAZIANO, F., TURSKI, P. & KORNGUTH, B.S. (1991) Magnetic resonance imaging of central nervous system lesions in patients with lupus erythematosus. Correlation with clinical remission and antineurofilament and anticardiolipin antibody titers. *Arthritis and Rheumatism* **34**, 432–441 [421].

BELL, D.S. (1965) Comparison of amphetamine psychosis and schizophrenia. *British Journal of Psychiatry* **111**, 701–707 [617].

BELL, D.S. (1992) *Medico-legal Assessment of Head Injury*. Charles C. Thomas: Springfield, Illinois [211].

BELL, J. & CARMICHAEL, E.A. (1939) On hereditary ataxia and spastic paraplegia. *The Treasury of Human Inheritance* **4**, 141–281 [705].

BELL, J.I. & HOCKADAY, T.D.R. (1996) Diabetes mellitus. Section 11.11 in *Oxford Textbook of Medicine*, 3rd edn, eds Weatherall, D.J., Ledingham, J.G.G. & Warrell, D.A. Oxford University Press: Oxford [534].

BELL, K., DOONEIEF, G., MARDER, K., MIRABELLO, E., SUN, T-H., STERN, Y. & MAYEUX, R. (1991) Non-drug-induced psychosis in Parkinson's disease. *Neurology*, **41 (Supplement 1)** 191 [657].

BELLAMY, R.J. & KENDALL-TAYLOR, P. (1995) Unrecognized hypocalcaemia diagnosed 36 years after thyroidectomy. *Journal of the Royal Society of Medicine* **88**, 690–691 [531].

BELLER, S.A., OVERALL, J.E. & SWANN, A.C. (1985) Efficacy of oral physostigmine in primary degenerative dementia. *Psychopharmacology* **87**, 147–151 [503].

BELLINGER, D.C., STILES, K.M. & NEEDLEMAN, H.L. (1992) Low-level lead exposure, intelligence and academic achievement: a long-term follow-up study. *Paediatrics* **90**, 855–861 [633].

BELLIVEAU, J.W., KENNEDY, D.N., McKINSTRY, R.C., BUCHBINDER, B.R., WEISSKOFF, R.M., COHEN, M.S., VEVEA, J.M., BRADY, T.J. & ROSEN, B.R. (1991) Functional mapping of the human visual cortex by magnetic resonance imaging. *Science* **254**, 716–719 [143].

BELMAN, A.L. (1994) HIV-1 associated central nervous system disease in infants and children. Ch. 16 in *HIV, AIDS and the Brain*, eds Price, R.W. & Perry, S.W. Association for Research in Nervous and Mental Disease, Vol. 72. Raven Press: New York [327].

BENAZZI, F. & MAZZOLI, M. (1991) Psychiatric illness associated with 'ecstasy'. *Lancet* **338**, 1520 [624].

BENCH, C.J., DOLAN, R.J., FRISTON, K.J. & FRACKOWIAK, R.S.J. (1990) Positron emission tomography in the study of brain metabolism in psychiatric and neuropsychiatric disorders. In *Brain Imaging in*

Psychiatry, ed. Abou-Saleh, M.T. *British Journal of Psychiatry* **157 (Supplement 9)**, 82–95 [87, 144].

BENCH, C.J., FRISTON, K.J., BROWN, R.G., SCOTT, L.C., FRACKOWIAK, R.S.J. & DOLAN, R.J. (1992) The anatomy of melancholia–focal abnormalities of cerebral blood flow in major depression. *Psychological Medicine* **22**, 607–615 [145].

BENDER, L. (1938) *A Visual Motor Gestalt Test and its Clinical Uses*. American Orthopsychiatric Association: New York [112].

BENDER, L. (1942) Post-encephalitic behaviour disorders in childhood. Ch. 8 in *Encephalitis: A Clinical Study*, ed. Neal, J.B. Grune & Stratton: New York [373, 374].

BENDER, L. (1946) *Instructions for the Use of Visual Motor Gestalt Test*. American Orthopsychiatric Association: New York [112].

BENDER, M.B. (1956) Syndrome of isolated episode of confusion with amnesia. *Journal of Hillside Hospital* **5**, 212–215. Quoted by Bender M.B. *(1960), Bulletin of the New York Academy of Medicine* **36**, 197–207 [413].

BENDER, M.B. (1960) Single episode of confusion with amnesia. *Bulletin of the New York Academy of Medicine* **36**, 197–207 [413].

BENDER, M.B. (1969) Disorders of eye movements. Ch. 18 in *Handbook of Clinical Neurology*, Vol. 1, eds Vinken, P.J. & Bruyn, G.W. North-Holland Publishing Co.: Amsterdam [678].

BENEDETTI, G. (1952) *Die Alkoholhalluzinosen*. Thieme: Stuttgart [599].

BENES, F.M. & BIRD, E.D. (1987) An analysis of the arrangement of neurons in the cingulate cortex of schizophrenic patients. *Archives of General Psychiatry* **44**, 608–616 [86].

BENES, F.M., DAVIDSON, J. & BIRD, E.D. (1986) Quantitative cytoarchitectural studies of the cerebral cortex of schizophrenics. *Archives of General Psychiatry* **43**, 31–35 [86].

BENES, F.M., McSPARREN, J., BIRD, E.D., SANGIOVANNI, J.P. & VINCENT, S.L. (1991a) Deficits in small interneurons in prefrontal and cingulate cortices of schizophrenic and schizoaffective patients. *Archives of General Psychiatry* **48**, 996–1001 [86].

BENES, F.M., SORENSON, I. & BIRD, E.D. (1991b) Reduced neuronal size in posterior hippocampus of schizophrenic patients. *Schizophrenia Bulletin* **17**, 597–608 [86, 87].

BENNETT, D.A., WILSON, R.S., GILLEY, D.W. & FOX, J.H. (1990) Clinical diagnosis in Binswanger's disease. *Journal of Neurology, Neurosurgery, and Psychiatry* **53**, 961–965 [459].

BENNETT, R., HUGHES, G.R.V., BYWATERS, E.G.L. & HOLT, P.J.L. (1972) Neuropsychiatric problems in systemic lupus erythematosus. *British Medical Journal* **4**, 342–345 [419, 420, 422].

BENNETT, S.T., LUCASSEN, A.M., GOUGH, S.C.L., POWELL, E.E., UNDLIEN, D.E., PRITCHARD, L.E., MERRIMAN, M.E., KAWAGUCHI, Y., DRONSFIELD, M.J., POCIOT, F., NERUP, J., BOUZEKRI, N., CAMBON-THOMSEN, A., RØNNINGEN, K.S., BARNETT, A.H., BAIN, S.C. & TODD, J.A. (1995) Susceptibility to human type 1 diabetes at *IDDM2* is determined by tandem repeat variation at the insulin gene minisatellite locus. *Nature Genetics* **9**, 284–291 [534].

BENSON, D.F. (1973) Psychiatric aspects of dysphasia. *British Journal of Psychiatry* **123**, 555–566 [54, 108].

BENSON, D.F. (1977) The third alexia. *Archives of Neurology* **34**, 327–331 [54].

BENSON, D.F. (1982) The treatable dementias. Ch. 6 in *Psychiatric Aspects of Neurologic Disease*, eds Benson, D.F. & Blumer, D. Grune & Stratton: New York & London [668].

BENSON, D.F. & ARDILA, A. (1996) *Aphasia. A Clinical Perspective*. Oxford University Press: New York [43, 45, 46, 49, 53, 54, 55].

BENSON, D.F. & CUMMINGS, J.L. (1982) Angular gyrus syndrome simulating Alzheimer's disease. *Archives of Neurology* **39**, 616–620 [493].

BENSON, D.F., DAVIS, R.J. & SNYDER, B.D. (1988) Posterior cortical atrophy. *Archives of Neurology* **45**, 789–793 [754].

BENSON, D.F. & GESCHWIND, N. (1971) Aphasia and related cortical disturbances. In Clinical Neurology, eds Baker A.B. & Baker L.H. *Harper & Row: New York* [51, 54, 102, 103].

BENSON, D.F. & GREENBERG, J.P. (1969) Visual form agnosia. A specific defect in visual discrimination. *Archives of Neurology* **20**, 82–89 [59].

BENSON, D.F., KUHL, D.E., PHELPS, M.E., CUMMINGS, J.L. & TSAI, S.Y. (1982) Positron emission computed tomography in the diagnosis of dementia. *Transactions of the American Neurological Association, 1981* **106**, 68–71 [434, 457].

BENSON, D.F., LEMAY, M., PATTEN, D.H. & RUHENS, A.B. (1970) Diagnosis of normal pressure hydrocephalus. *New England Journal of Medicine* **283**, 609–615 [136].

BENSON, D.F., MARSDEN, C.D. & MEADOWS, J.C. (1974) The amnesic syndrome of posterior cerebral artery occlusion. *Acta Neurologica Scandinavica* **50**, 133–145 [379].

BENSON, D.F. & STUSS, D.T. (1989) Theories of frontal lobe function. In *Neurology and Psychiatry: A Meeting of Minds*, ed. Mueller, J., pp. 266–283. Karger: Basel [76].

BENSON, V.M. (1971) Marihuana 'study' critique. *Journal of the American Medical Association* **217**, 1391 [616].

BENTAL, E. (1958) Acute psychoses due to encephalitis following Asian influenza. *Lancet* **2**, 18–20 [359].

BENTON, A. & SIVAN, A.B. (1993) Disturbances of the body schema. Ch. 6 in *Clinical Neuropsychology*, 3rd edn, eds Heilman, K.M. & Valenstein, E. Oxford University Press: New York [66].

BENTON, A.L. (1955) *The Revised Visual Retention Test: Clinical and Experimental Applications*. The Psychological Corporation: New York [116].

BENTON, A.L. (1959) *Right–Left Discrimination and Finger Localization*. Hoeber: New York [66].

BENTON, A.L. (1961) The fiction of the 'Gerstmann Syndrome'. *Journal of Neurology, Neurosurgery and Psychiatry* **24**, 176–181 [65].

BENTON, A.L. (1963) *The Revised Visual Retention Test: Clinical and Experimental Applications*. The Psychological Corporation: New York [116].

BENTON, A.L. (1967) Problems of test construction in the field of aphasia. *Cortex* **3**, 32–58 [114].

BENTON, A.L. (1968) Differential behavioral effects in frontal lobe disease. *Neuropsychologia* **6**, 53–60 [104].

BENTON, A.L., JENTSCH, R.C. & WAHLER, H.J. (1959) Simple and choice reaction times in schizophrenia. *Archives of Neurology and Psychiatry* **81**, 373–376 [121].

BENTON, A.L. & JOYNT, J. (1959) Reaction time in unilateral cerebral disease. *Confinia Neurologica* **19**, 247–256 [120].

BENTON, A.L. & SPREEN, O. (1961) Visual memory test: the simulation of mental incompetence. *Archives of General Psychiatry* **4**, 79–83 [484].

BENTSON, J., REZA, M., WINTER, J. & WILSON, G. (1978) Steroids and apparent cerebral atrophy on computed tomography scans. *Journal of Computer Assisted Tomography* **2**, 16–23 [141].

BERG, J.M. (1962) Meningitis as a cause of severe mental defect. In *Proceedings of the London Conference on the Scientific Study of Mental Deficiency*, Vol. 1, ed. Richards, B.W. May & Baker: Dagenham, England [365].

BERGER, M., YULE, W. & RUTTER, M. (1975) Attainment and adjustment in two geographical areas. II The prevalence of specific reading retardation. *British Journal of Psychiatry* **126**, 510–519 [47].

BERGIN, J.D. (1957) Rapidly progressing dementia in disseminated sclerosis. *Journal of Neurology, Neurosurgery and Psychiatry* **20**, 285–292 [694].

BERGIN, P.S. & HARVEY, P. (1992) Wernicke's encephalopathy and central pontine myelinolysis associated with hyperemesis gravidarum. *British Medical Journal* **305**, 517–518 [576].

BERGMAN, H., BORG, S., HINDMARSH, T., IDESTRÖM, C.-M. & MÜTZELL, S. (1980a) Computed tomography of the brain and neuropsychological assessment of male alcoholic patients and a random sample from the general male population. *Acta Psychiatrica Scandinavica* **62** (**Supplement 286**), 77–88 [605, 606].

BERGMAN, H., BORG, S., HINDMARSH, T., IDESTRÖM, C.-M. & MÜTZELL, S. (1980b) Computed tomography of the brain and neuropsychological assessment of male alcoholic patients. Ch. 10 in *Addiction and Brain Damage*, ed. Richter, D. Croom Helm: London [605, 606].

BERGMANN, K. (1977) Prognosis in chronic brain failure. *Age and Ageing* **6** (**Supplement**), 61–66 [431].

BERGMANN, K. (1991) Psychiatric aspects of personality in older patients. Ch. 24 in *Psychiatry in the Elderly*, eds Jacoby, R. & Oppenheimer, C. Oxford University Press: Oxford [495].

BERKOVIC, S.F., CARPENTER, S., ANDERMANN, F., ANDERMANN, E. & WOLFE, L.S. (1988) Kuf's disease: a critical reappraisal. *Brain* **111**, 27–62 [759, 760].

BERKOVIC, S.F., McINTOSH, A.M., KALNINS, R.M. & BLADIN, P.F. (1994) Magnetic resonance imaging of hippocampal sclerosis: reliability of visual diagnosis and implications for surgical treatment. Ch. 6 in *Magnetic Resonance Scanning and Epilepsy*, eds Shorvon, S.D., Fish, D.R., Andermann, F., Bydder, G.M. & Stefan, H. Plenum Press: New York [289].

BERLYNE, N. (1972) Confabulation. *British Journal of Psychiatry* **120**, 31–39 [16, 31].

BERMAN, K.F., ILLOWSKY, B.P. & WEINBERGER, D.R. (1988) Physiological dysfunction of dorsolateral prefrontal cortex in schizophrenia. *Archives of General Psychiatry* **45**, 616–622 [87].

BERMAN, K.F., TORREY, E.F., DANIEL, D.G. & WEINBERGER, D.R. (1992) Regional cerebral blood flow in monozygotic twins discordant and concordant for schizophrenia. *Archives of General Psychiatry* **49**, 927–934 [87].

BERNOULLI, C., SEIGFRIED, J., BAUMGARTNER, G., REGLI, F., RABINOWICZ, T., GAJDUSEK, D.C. & GIBBS, Jr, C.J. (1977) Danger of accidental person-to-person transmission of Creutzfeldt–Jakob disease by surgery. *Lancet* **1**, 478–479 [476].

BERNTHAL, P., HAYS, A., TARTER, R.E. VAN THIEL, D., LECKY, J. & HEGEDUS, A. (1987) Cerebral CT scan abnormalities in cholestatic and hepatocellular disease and their relationship to neuropsychologic test performance. *Hepatology* **7**, 107–114 [564].

BERRIOS, G.E. & BROOK, P. (1982) The Charles Bonnet syndrome and the problem of visual perceptual disorders in the elderly. *Age and Ageing* **11**, 17–23 [295].

BERSOFF, D.N. (1970) The revised deterioration formula for the Wechsler Adult Intelligence Scale: a test of validity. *Journal of Clinical Psychology* **26**, 71–73 [111].

BESAG, F.M.C. (1988) Cognitive deterioration in children with epilepsy. Ch. 9 in *Epilepsy, Behaviour and Cognitive Function*, eds Trimble, M.R. & Reynolds, E.H. John Wiley: Chichester [264].

BESSON, J.A.O. (1990) Magnetic resonance imaging and its applications in neuropsychiatry. In *Brain Imaging in Psychiatry*, ed. Abou-Saleh, M.T. *British Journal of Psychiatry* **157** (**Supplement 9**), 25–37 [141].

BESSON, J.A.O., CORRIGAN, F.M., ILJON FOREMAN, E., EASTWOOD, L.M., SMITH, F.W. & ASHCROFT, G.W. (1985) Nuclear magnetic resonance (NMR). II. Imaging in dementia. *British Journal of Psychiatry* **146**, 31–35 [139].

BESSON, J.A.O. & WALKER, L.G. (1983) Hypnotherapy for writer's cramp. *Lancet* **1**, 71–72 [677].

BETTS, T.A. (1974) A follow-up study of a cohort of patients with epilepsy admitted to psychiatric care in an English city. Ch. 56 in *Epilepsy: Proceedings of the Hans Berger Centenary Symposium*, eds Harris, P. & Mawdsley, C. Churchill Livingstone: Edinburgh [285].

BETTS, T.A. (1981) Depression, anxiety and epilepsy. Ch. 6 in *Epilepsy and Psychiatry*, eds Reynolds, E.H. & Trimble, M.R. Churchill Livingstone: Edinburgh [276, 285].

BETTS, T.A. (1982) Psychiatry and epilepsy. In *A Textbook of Epilepsy*, 2nd edn, eds Laidlaw, J. & Richens, A., pp. 227–270. Churchill Livingstone: Edinburgh [264].

BETTS, T. (1990) Pseudoseizures: seizures that are not epilepsy. *Lancet* **336**, 163–164 [292].

BETTS, T.A. (1993) Neuropsychiatry. Ch. 11 in *A Textbook of Epilepsy*, 4th edn, eds Laidlaw, J., Richens, A. & Chadwick, D. Churchill Livingstone: Edinburgh [292].

BETTS, T. & BODEN, S. (1992) Diagnosis, management and prognosis of a group of 128 patients with non epileptic attack disorder. Part I. *Seizure* **1**, 19–26 [292].

BEUMONT, P.J.V., BANCROFT, J.H.J., BEARDWOOD, C.J. & RUSSELL, G.F.M. (1972) Behavioural changes after treatment with testosterone: case report. *Psychological Medicine* **2**, 70–72 [527].

BEWLEY, T.H. (1967) Adverse reactions from the illicit use of lysergide. *British Medical Journal* **3**, 28–30 [622].

BEWSHER, P.D., GARDINER, A.Q., HEDLEY, A.J. & MacLEAN, H.C.S. (1971) Psychosis after acute alteration of thyroid status. *Psychological Medicine* **1**, 260–262 [511].

BHARUCHA, N.E., STOKES, L., SCHOENBERG, B.S., WARD, C., INCE, S., NUTT, J.G., ELDRIDGE, R., CALNE, D.B., MANTEL, N. & DUVOISIN, R. (1986) A case-control study of twin pairs discordant for Parkinson's disease: a search for environmental risk factors. *Neurology* **36**, 284–288 [661].

BHATIA, M.S. (1990) Capgras syndrome in a patient with migraine. *British Journal of Psychiatry* **157**, 917–918 [406].

BICKERSTAFF, E.R. (1961a) Basilar artery migraine. *Lancet* **1**, 15–17 [400].

BICKERSTAFF, E.R. (1961b) Impairment of consciousness in migraine. *Lancet* **2**, 1057–1059 [400, 404].

BICKERSTAFF, E.R. & HOLMES, J.M. (1967) Cerebral arterial insufficiency and oral contraceptives. *British Medical Journal* **1**, 726–729 [401].

BICKFORD, J.A.R. & ELLISON, R.M. (1953) The high incidence of Huntington's chorea in the Duchy of Cornwall. *Journal of Mental Science* **99**, 291–294 [472].

BICKFORD, R.G. & KLASS, D.W. (1966) Acute and chronic EEG findings after head injury. Ch. 6 in *Head Injury: Conference Proceedings*, eds Caveness, W.F. & Walker, A.E. Lippincott: Philadelphia [165].

BICKFORD, R.G., WHELAN, J.L., KLASS, D.W. & CORBIN, K.B. (1956) Reading epilepsy: clinical and electroencephalographic studies of a new syndrome. *Transactions of the American Neurological Association* **81**, 100–102 [241].

BIDSTRUP, P.L., BONNELL, J.A., HARVEY, D.G. & LOCKET, S. (1951) Chronic mercury poisoning in men repairing direct-current meters. *Lancet* **2**, 856–861 [633, 634].

BIGGINS, C.A., BOYD, J.L., HARROP, F.M., MADELEY, P., MINDHAM, R.H.S., RANDALL, J.I. & SPOKES, E.G.S. (1992) A controlled, longitudinal study of dementia in Parkinson's disease. *Journal of Neurology, Neurosurgery, and Psychiatry* **55**, 566–571 [654].

BIGLER, E.D., NELSON, J.E. & SCHMIDT, R.D. (1989) Mamillary body atrophy identified by MRI in alcohol amnesic (Korsakoff's) syndrome. *Neuropsychiatry, Neuropsychology, and Behavioral Neurology* **2**, 189–201 [579].

BINDER, J.R. & RAO, S.M. (1994) Human brain mapping with functional magnetic resonance imaging. Ch. 7 in *Localization and Neuroimaging in Neuropsychology*, ed. Kertesz, A. Academic Press: San Diego [46, 143].

BINDMAN, E. & TIBBETTS, R.W. (1977) Writer's cramp—a rational approach to treatment? *British Journal of Psychiatry* **131**, 143–148, [676].

BINGLEY, T. (1958) Mental symptoms in temporal lobe epilepsy and temporal lobe gliomas. *Acta Psychiatrica et Neurologica Scandinavica* **120 (Supplement)**, 1–151 [224, 225, 226].

BINNIE, C.D., ELWES, R.D.C., POLKEY, C.E. & VOLANS, A. (1994) Utility of stereoelectroencephalography in preoperative assessment of temporal lobe epilepsy. *Journal of Neurology, Neurosurgery, and Psychiatry* **57**, 58–65 [311].

BINNIE, C.D., ROWAN, A.J., OVERWEG, J., MEINARDI, H., WISMAN, T., KAMP, A. & LOPES DA SILVA, F. (1981) Telemetric EEG and video monitoring in epilepsy. *Neurology* **31**, 298–303 [288].

BINSWANGER, O. (1894) Die Abgrenzung der allgemeinen progressiven Paralyse. *Berliner klinische Wochenshrift* **31**, 1137–1139 [458].

BIRD, E.D. & IVERSON, L.L. (1974) Huntington's chorea—postmortem measurement of glutamic acid decarboxylase, choline acetyltransferase and dopamine in basal ganglia. *Brain* **97**, 457–472 [467].

BIRD, E.D., MacKAY, A.V.P., RAYNER, C.N. & IVERSEN, L.L. (1973) Reduced glutamic-acid-decarboxylase activity of post-mortem brain in Huntington's chorea. *Lancet* **1**, 1090–1092 [467].

BIRD, T.D., CEDERBAUM, S., VALPEY, R.W. & STAHL, W.L. (1978) Familial degeneration of the basal ganglia with acanthocytosis: a clinical, neuropathological, and neurochemical study. *Annals of Neurology* **3**, 253–258 [757].

BIRD, T.D., FOLLETT, C. & GRIEP, E. (1983) Cognitive and personality function in myotonic muscular dystrophy. *Journal of Neurology, Neurosurgery, and Psychiatry* **46**, 971–980 [719, 720].

BIRKETT, D.P. (1972) The psychiatric differentiation of senility and arteriosclerosis. *British Journal of Psychiatry* **120**, 321–325 [454].

BIRKETT, D.P., DESOUKY, A., HAN, L. & KAUFMAN, M. (1992) Lewy bodies in psychiatric patients. *International Journal of Geriatric Psychiatry* **7**, 235–240 [450, 452].

BIRLEY, J.L. (1920) The principles of medical science as applied to military aviation. II War flying at high altitude. *Lancet* **1**, 1205–1211 [549].

BISHAI, D.M. & BOZZETTI, L.P. (1986) Current progress toward the prevention of the Wernicke–Korsakoff syndrome. *Alcohol and Alcoholism* **21**, 315–323 [581].

BJÖRKLUND, A. & STENEVI, U. (1977) Reformation of the severed septohippocampal cholinergic pathway in the adult rat by transplanted septal neurons. *Cell and Tissue Research* **185**, 289–302 [505].

BLACK, D.W. (1984) Mental changes resulting from subdural haematoma. *British Journal of Psychiatry* **145**, 200–203 [411].

BLACK, P., JEFFRIES, J.J., BLUMER, D., WELLNER, A. & WALKER, A.E. (1969) The post-traumatic syndrome in children. Ch. 14 in *The Late Effects of Head Injury*, eds Walker, A.E., Caveness, W.F. & Critchley, M. Thomas: Springfield, Illinois [201, 203, 204].

BLACKBURN, H.L. & BENTON, A.L. (1955) Simple and choice reaction times in cerebral disease. *Confinia Neurologica* **15**, 327–338 [120].

BLACKIE, J.D. & LEES, A.J. (1990) Botulinum toxin in the treatment of spasmodic torticollis. *Journal of Neurology, Neurosurgery, and Psychiatry* **53**, 640–643 [675].

BLACKSTOCK, E.E., GATH, D.H., GRAY, B.C. & HIGGINS, G. (1972) The

role of thiamine deficiency in the aetiology of the hallucinatory states complicating alcoholism. *British Journal of Psychiatry* **121**, 357–364 [599].

BLACKWOOD, D.H.R. & MUIR, W.J. (1990) Cognitive brain potentials and their application. In *Brain Imaging in Psychiatry*, ed. Abou-Saleh, M.T. *British Journal of Psychiatry* **157 (Supplement 9)**, 96–101 [132].

BLASS, J.P. & GIBSON, G.E. (1977) Abnormality of a thiamine-requiring enzyme in patients with Wernicke–Korsakoff syndrome. *New England Journal of Medicine* **297**, 1367–1370 [577].

BLAU, A. (1936) Mental changes following head trauma in children. *Archives of Neurology and Psychiatry* **35**, 723–769 [203].

BLAU, J.N. & DAVIS, E. (1970) Small blood vessels in migraine. *Lancet* **2**, 740–742 [402].

BLAU, J.N. & HINTON, J.M. (1960) Hypopituitary coma and psychosis. *Lancet* **1**, 408–409 [523].

BLAUTH, C., SMITH, P., NEWMAN, S., ARNOLD, J., SIDDONS, F., HARRISON, M.J., TREASURE, T., KLINGER, L. & TAYLOR, K.M. (1989) Retinal microembolism and neuropsychological deficit following clinical cardiopulmonary bypass: comparison of a membrane and a bubble oxygenator. A preliminary communication. *European Journal of Cardio-thoracic Surgery* **3**, 135–139 [555].

BLESSED, G. (1980) Clinical aspects of the senile dementias. Ch. 1 in *Biochemistry of Dementia*, ed. Roberts, P.J. John Wiley: Chichester [430, 433].

BLESSED, G., BLACK, S.E., BUTLER, T. & KAY, D.W.K. (1991) The diagnosis of dementia in the elderly. A comparison of CAMCOG (the Cognitive Section of CAMDEX), the AGECAT Program, DSM-III, the Mini-Mental State Examination and some short rating scales. *British Journal of Psychiatry* **159**, 193–198 [124].

BLESSED, G., TOMLINSON, B.E. & ROTH, M. (1968) The association between quantitative measures of dementia and of senile change in the cerebral grey matter of elderly subjects. *British Journal of Psychiatry* **114**, 797–811 [123, 435].

BLESSED, G. & WILSON I.D. (1982) The contemporary natural history of mental disorder in old age. *British Journal of Psychiatry* **141**, 59–67 [435].

BLEULER, E.P. (1924) *Textbook of Psychiatry* (Translated by A.A. Brill). Macmillan: New York. Reissued by Dover Publications, 1951 [490].

BLEULER, M. (1951a) Psychiatry of cerebral diseases. *British Medical Journal* **2**, 1233–1238 [220].

BLEULER, M. (1951b) The psychopathology of acromegaly. *Journal of Nervous and Mental Disease* **113**, 497–511 [521].

BLEULER, M. (1967) Endocrinological psychiatry and psychology. *Henry Ford Hospital Medical Journal* **15**, 309–317 [507, 530].

BLOCK, R.I., FARNHAM, S., BRAVERMAN, K., NOYES, R. & GHONEIM, M.M. (1990) Long-term marijuana use and subsequent effects on learning and cognitive functions related to school achievement: preliminary study. In *Residual Effects of Abused Drugs on Behavior*. National Institute on Drug Abuse Research Monograph, No.101, eds Spencer, J.W. & Boren, J.J., pp. 96–111. U.S. Department of Health and Human Services [616].

BLOOMQUIST, E.R. & COURVILLE, C.B. (1947) The nature and incidence of traumatic lesions of the brain: a survey of 350 cases with autopsy. *Bulletin of the Los Angeles Neurological Society* **12**, 174–183 [163].

BLUESTIEN, H.G. & ZVAIFLER, N.J. (1976) Brain-reactive lymphocytotoxic antibodies in the serum of patients with systemic lupus erythematosus. *Journal of Clinical Investigation* **57**, 509–516 [421].

BLUGLASS, R. (1976) Malingering. In *Encyclopaedic Handbook of*

Medical Psychology, ed. Krauss, S., pp. 280–281. Butterworths: London [484].

BLUMER, D. (1970) Hypersexual episodes in temporal lobe epilepsy. *American Journal of Psychiatry* **126**, 1099–1106 [271, 272].

BLUMER, D. & BENSON, D.F. (1975) Personality changes with frontal and temporal lobe lesions. Ch. 9 in *Psychiatric Aspects of Neurologic Disease*, eds Benson, D.F. & Blumer, D. Grune & Stratton: New York [77].

BOGEN, J.E. (1969) The other side of the brain. I Dysgraphia and dyscopia following cerebral commissurotomy. II An appositional mind. III The corpus callosum and creativity. *Bulletin of the Los Angeles Neurological Society* **34**, 73–105, 135–162 and 191–220 [313].

BOGEN, J.E. & GAZZANIGA, M.S. (1965) Cerebral commissurotomy in man: minor hemisphere dominance for certain visuospatial functions. *Journal of Neurosurgery* **23**, 394–399 [62].

BOGEN, J.E. & VOGEL, P.J. (1962) Cerebral commissurotomy in man. *Bulletin of the Los Angeles Neurological Society* **27**, 169–172 [313].

BOGERTS, B., ASHTARI, M., DEGREEF, G., ALVIR, J., BILDER, R. & LIEBERMAN, J. (1990a) Reduced temporal limbic structure volumes on magnetic resonance images in first episode schizophrenia. *Psychiatry Research* **35**, 1–13 [85].

BOGERTS, B., FALKAI, P., HAUPTS, M., GREVE, B., ERNST, S., TAPERNON-FRANZ, U. & HEINZMANN, U. (1990b) Post-mortem volume measurements of limbic system and basal ganglia structures in chronic schizophrenics. Initial results from a new brain collection. *Schizophrenia Research* **3**, 295–301 [86].

BOGERTS, B., MEERTZ, E. & SCHÖNFELDT-BAUSCH, R. (1985) Basal ganglia and limbic system pathology in schizophrenia. *Archives of General Psychiatry* **42**, 784–791 [86].

BOGOUSSLAVSKI, J., REGLI, F., VAN MELLE, G., PAYOT, M. & USKE, A. (1988) Migraine stroke. *Neurology* **38**, 223–227 [401].

BOHNEN, N., JOLLES, J. & VERHEY, F.R.J. (1993) Persistent neuropsychological deficits in cervical whiplash patients without direct headstrike. *Acta Neurologica Belgica* **93**, 23–31 [200].

BOHNEN, N., TWIJNSTRA, A., WIJNEN, G. & JOLLES, J. (1991) Tolerance for light and sound of patients with persistent post-concussional symptoms 6 months after mild head injury. *Journal of Neurology* **238**, 443–446 [198].

BOLLER, F. & GRAFMAN, J. (1985) Acalculia. Ch. 31 in *Handbook of Clinical Neurology*, Revised Series Vol. 1. *Clinical Neuropsychology*, ed. Frederiks, J.A.M. Elsevier: Amsterdam [66, 67].

BOLLER, F., MIZUTANI, T., ROESSMANN, U. & GAMBETTI, P. (1980) Parkinson disease, dementia and Alzheimer disease: clinicopathological correlations. *Annals of Neurology* **7**, 329–335 [655].

BOLLER, F. & VIGNOLO, L.A. (1966) Latent sensory aphasia in hemisphere damaged patients: an experimental study with the Token Test. *Brain* **89**, 815–830 [113].

BOLT, J.M.W. (1970) Huntington's chorea in the West of Scotland. *British Journal of Psychiatry* **116**, 259–270 [465, 466, 472].

BOLTON, N., BRITTON, P.G. & SAVAGE, R.D. (1966) Some normative data on the WAIS and its indices in an aged population. *Journal of Clinical Psychology* **22**, 184–188 [111].

BOLTON, N., SAVAGE, R.D. & ROTH, M. (1967) The modified word learning test and the aged psychiatric patient. *British Journal of Psychiatry* **113**, 1139–1140 [114].

BOLWIG, T.G. (1968) Transient global amnesia. *Acta Neurologica Scandinavica* **44**, 101–106 [414].

BOND, M.R. (1976) Assessment of the psychosocial outcome of severe head injury. *Acta Neurochirurgica* **34**, 57–70 [172].

BOND, M.R. & BROOKS, D.N. (1976) Understanding the process of recovery as a basis for the investigation of rehabilitation for the brain injured. *Scandinavian Journal of Rehabilitation Medicine* **8**, 127–133 [185].

BONDAREFF, W., BALDY, R. & LEVY, R. (1981a) Quantitative computed tomography in senile dementia. *Archives of General Psychiatry* **38**, 1365–1368 [139].

BONDAREFF, W., MOUNTJOY, C.Q. & ROTH, M. (1981b) Selective loss of neurones of origin of adrenergic projection to cerebral cortex (nucleus locus coeruleus) in senile dementia. *Lancet* **1**, 783–784 [445].

BONDAREFF, W., MOUNTJOY, C.Q. & ROTH, M. (1982) Loss of neurons of origin of the adrenergic projection to cerebral cortex (nucleus locus ceruleus) in senile dementia. *Neurology* **32**, 164–168 [445].

BONDAREFF, W., RAVAL, J., WOO, B., HAUSER, D.L. & COLLETTI, P.M. (1990) Magnetic resonance imaging and the severity of dementia in older adults. *Archives of General Psychiatry* **47**, 47–51 [139].

BONFA, E., GOLOMBEK, S.J., KAUFMAN, L.D., SKELLY, S., WEISSBACH, H., BROT, N. & ELKON, K.B. (1987) Association between lupus psychosis and anti-ribosomal P protein antibodies. *New England Journal of Medicine* **317**, 265–271 [418].

BONHOEFFER, K. (1909) Exogenous psychoses. *Zentralblatt für Nervenheilkunde* **32**, 499–505. Translated by H. Marshall in *Themes and Variations in European Psychiatry*, eds Hirsch, S.R. & Shepherd, M. John Wright: Bristol, 1974 [3].

BONHOEFFER, K. (1910) *Die symptomatischen Psychosen im Gefolge von akuten Infektionen und inneren Erkrankungen*. Deuticke: Leipzig [3].

BONNER, D., RON, M.A., CHALDER, T., BUTLER, S. & WESSELY, S. (1994) Chronic fatigue syndrome: a follow-up study. *Journal of Neurology, Neurosurgery and Psychiatry* **57**, 617–621 [373].

BOOSS, J. & ESIRI, M.M. (1986) *Viral Encephalitis. Pathology, Diagnosis and Management*. Blackwell Scientific Publications: Oxford [348, 356, 359, 360].

BOOTH, G. (1948) Psychodynamics in parkinsonism. *Psychosomatic Medicine* **10**, 1–14 [660, 661].

BOR, R., MILLER, R. & JOHNSON, M. (1991) A testing time for doctors: counselling patients before an HIV test. *British Medical Journal* **303**, 905–907 [333].

BOSHES, B. (1947) Neuropsychiatric manifestations during the course of malaria: experiences in the Mediterranean theater in World War II. *Archives of Neurology and Psychiatry* **58**, 14–27 [370].

BOTEZ, M.I., FONTAINE, F., BOTEZ, T. & BACHEVALIER, J. (1977) Folate-responsive neurological and mental disorders: report of 16 cases. Neuropsychological correlates of computerised transaxial tomography and radionuclide cisternography in folic acid deficiencies. *European Neurology* **16**, 230–246 [592].

BOTTINI, G., CAPPA, S.F., STERZI, R. & VIGNOLO, L.A. (1995) Intramodal somaesthetic recognition disorders following right and left hemisphere damage. *Brain* **118**, 395–399 [65].

BOTTOMLEY, P.A. (1989) Human in vivo NMR spectroscopy in diagnostic medicine: clinical tool or research probe? *Radiology* **170**, 1–15 [143].

BOTTOMLEY, P.A., HARDY, C.J., COUSINS, J., ARMSTRONG, M. & WAGLE, W. (1989) Brain phosphate metabolite concentrations, not ratios, are reduced in AIDS dementia. Book of Abstracts: *Society of Magnetic Resonance in Medicine*, Vol. 1, 369. Berkeley: California [143].

BOTTOMLEY, P.A., HART, H.R., EDELSTEIN, W.A., SCHENCK, J.F., SMITH, L.S., LEUE, W.M., MUELLER, O.M. & REDINGTON, R.W. (1983) NMR imaging/spectroscopy system to study both anatomy and metabolism. *Lancet* **2**, 273–274 [143].

BOTWINICK, J. & BIRREN, J.E. (1951) Differential decline in the Wechsler–Bellevue subtests in the senile psychoses. *Journal of Gerontology* **6**, 365–368 [436].

BOUGHTON, C.R. (1970) Neurological complications of glandular fever. *Medical Journal of Australia* **2**, 573–575 [358].

BOUR, H., TUTIN, N. & PASQUIER, P. (1967) The central nervous system and carbon monoxide poisoning. I: clinical data with reference to 20 fatal cases. In *Carbon Monoxide Poisoning*, eds Bour, H. & Ledingham, I.McA. Progress in Brain Research, Vol. 24. Elsevier: Amsterdam [550, 551].

BOURGEOIS, M., HÉBERT, A. & MAISONDIEU, J. (1970) Depressive senile pseudo-dementia curable by electric shock. *Annales Médico Psychologique* **128**, 751–759 [486].

BOURNE, H.R., BUNNEY, W.E., COLBURN, R.W., DAVIS, J.M., DAVIS, J.N., SHAW, D.M. & COPPEN, A.J. (1968) Noradrenaline, 5-hydroxytryptamine, and 5-hydroxyindoleacetic acid in hindbrains of suicidal patients. *Lancet* **2**, 805–808 [24].

BOVILL, D. (1973) A case of functional hypoglycaemia—a medicolegal problem. *British Journal of Psychiatry* **123**, 353–358 [543].

BOWCOCK, A.M., FARRER, L.A., CAVALLI-SFORZA, L.L., HEBERT, J.M., KIDD, K.K., FRYDMAN, M. & BONNE-TAMIR, B. (1987) Mapping the Wilson disease locus to a cluster of linked polymorphic markers on chromosome 13. *American Journal of Human Genetics* **41**, 27–35 [662].

BOWDEN, S.C. (1990) Separating cognitive impairment in neurology asymptomatic alcoholism from Wernicke–Korsakoff syndrome: is the neuropsychological distinction justified? *Psychological Bulletin* **107**, 355–366 [584].

BOWEN, D.M., SMITH, C.B. & DAVISON, A.N. (1973) Molecular changes in senile dementia. *Brain* **96**, 849–856 [444].

BOWEN, D.M., SPILLANE, J.A., CURZON, G., MEIER-RUGE, W., WHITE, P., GOODHART, M.J., IWANGOFF, D. & DAVISON, A.N. (1979) Accelerated ageing or selective neuronal loss as an important cause of dementia? *Lancet* **1**, 11–14 [444].

BOWER, B. (1978) The treatment of epilepsy in children. *British Journal of Hospital Medicine* **19**, 8–19 [300].

BOWER, H.M. (1967) Sensory stimulation in the treatment of senile dementia. *Medical Journal of Australia* **1**, 1113–1119 [500].

BOWERS, M.B., WOERT, M.V. & DAVIS, L. (1971) Sexual behaviour during L-dopa treatment for parkinsonism. *American Journal of Psychiatry* **127**, 1691–1693 [659].

BOWLING, G. & RICHARDS, N.G. (1961) Diagnosis and treatment of the narcolepsy syndrome. *Cleveland Clinic Quarterly* **28**, 38–45 [723].

BOWMAN, K.M., GOODHART, R. & JOLLIFFE, N. (1939) Observations on the role of vitamin B_1 in the etiology and treatment of Korsakoff psychosis. *Journal of Nervous and Mental Disease* **90**, 569–575 [577].

BOWMAN, M. & LEWIS, M.S. (1980) Sites of subcortical damage in diseases which resemble schizophrenia. *Neuropsychologia* **18**, 597–601 [84].

BOYD, P.R., WALKER, G. & HENDERSON, I.N. (1957) The treatment of tetraethyl lead poisoning. *Lancet* **1**, 181–185 [633].

BRACELAND, F.J. (1942) Mental symptoms following carbon disulphide absorption and intoxication. *Annals of Internal Medicine* **16**, 246–261 [638].

BRACELAND, F.J. & GIFFIN, M.E. (1950) The mental changes associated with multiple sclerosis (an interim report). Ch. 30 in *Multiple Sclerosis and the Demyelinating Diseases*, Research Publications of the Association for Research in Nervous and Mental Disease, Vol. 28. Williams & Wilkins: Baltimore [695, 696, 699].

BRACHA, H.S. (1987) Asymmetric rotational (circling) behavior, a dopamine-related asymmetry: preliminary findings in unmedicated and never-medicated schizophrenic patients. *Biological Psychiatry* **22**, 995–1003 [90].

BRACKEN, P. (1987) Mania following head injury. *British Journal of Psychiatry* **150**, 690–692 [192].

BRADBURY, T.N. & MILLER, G.A. (1985) Season of birth in schizophrenia: a review of evidence, methodology, and etiology. *Psychological Bulletin* **98**, 569–594 [91].

BRADLEY, C. (1979) Life events and the control of diabetes mellitus. *Journal of Psychosomatic Research* **23**, 159–162 [535].

BRADLEY, T.D., BROWN, I.G., GROSSMAN, R.F., ZAMEL, N., MARTINEZ, D., PHILLIPSON, E.A. & HOFFSTEIN, V. (1986) Pharyngeal size in snorers, nonsnorers, and patients with obstructive sleep apnea. *New England Journal of Medicine* **315**, 1327–1331 [730].

BRADLEY, W.G. (1992) Recent advances in magnetic resonance angiography of the brain. *Current Opinion in Neurology and Neurosurgery* **5**, 859–862 [142].

BRADSHAW, J.R., THOMSON, J.L.G. & CAMPBELL, M.J. (1983) Computed tomography in the investigation of dementia. *British Medical Journal* **286**, 277–280 [495].

BRADSHAW, P. & PARSONS, M. (1965) Hemiplegic migraine: a clinical study. *Quarterly Journal of Medicine* **34**, 65–85 [400, 407].

BRADWELL, R.H. (1994) Psychiatric sequelae of organophosphorous poisoning: a case study and review of the literature. *Behavioural Neurology* **7**, 117–122 [637].

BRADY, J.P. (1964) Epilepsy and disturbed behaviour. *Journal of Nervous and Mental Disease* **138**, 468–473 [269].

BRAHAM, J. (1971) Jakob–Creutzfeldt disease: treatment by amantadine. *British Medical Journal* **4**, 212–213 [506].

BRAIN, W.R. (1930) Critical review: disseminated sclerosis. *Quarterly Journal of Medicine* **23**, 343–391 [691, 698].

BRAIN, W.R. (1942) Discussion on rehabilitation after injuries to the central nervous system. *Proceedings of the Royal Society of Medicine* **35**, 302–305 [175].

BRAIN, W.R. (1955) *Diseases of the Nervous System*, 5th edn. Oxford University Press: Oxford [237].

BRAIN, W.R. (1965) *Speech Disorders: Aphasia, Apraxia and Agnosia*, 2nd edn. Butterworths: London [43, 50, 51, 56, 58, 61].

BRAIN, W.R. & ADAMS, R.D. (1965) Epilogue: a guide to the classification and investigation of neurological disorders associated with neoplasms. Ch. 21 in *The Remote Effects of Cancer on the Nervous System*, eds Brain, W.R. & Norris, E.H. Contemporary Neurology Symposia, Vol. 1. Grune & Stratton: New York [739, 740].

BRAIN, W.R., DANIEL, P.M. & GREENFIELD, J.G. (1951) Subacute cortical cerebellar degeneration and its relation to carcinoma. *Journal of Neurology, Neurosurgery and Psychiatry* **14**, 59–75 [739, 740].

BRAIN, W.R., GREENFIELD, J.G. & RUSSELL, D.S. (1943) Discussion on recent experiences of acute encephalomyelitis and allied conditions. *Proceedings of the Royal Society of Medicine* **36**, 319–322 [361].

BRAIN, W.R., GREENFIELD, J.G. & RUSSELL, D.S. (1948) Subacute inclusion encephalitis (Dawson type). *Brain* **71**, 365–385 [361].

BRAIN, W.R., GREENFIELD, J.G. & SUTTON, D. (1951) Epiloia. In *British Encyclopaedia of Medical Practice*, 2nd edn, ed. Lord Horder, Vol. 5, pp. 266–276. Butterworth: London [702].

BRAIN, W.R. & HENSON, R.A. (1958) Neurological syndromes associated with carcinoma. *Lancet* **2**, 971–975 [739, 740].

BRAIN, W.R. & WILKINSON, M. (1965) Subacute cerebellar degeneration in patients with carcinoma. Ch. 3 in *The Remote Effects of Cancer on the Nervous System*, eds Brain, W.R. & Norris, E.H. Contemporary Neurology Symposia, Vol. 1. Grune & Stratton: New York [740].

BRANDT, J. (1988) Malingered amnesia. Ch. 5 in *Clinical Assessment of Malingering and Deception*, ed. Rogers, R. Guilford Press: New York [485].

BRANDT, J. & BUTTERS, N. (1986) The neuropsychology of Huntington's disease. *Trends in Neurosciences* **9**, 118–120 [469].

BRANDT, J., BUTTERS, N., RYAN, C. & BAYOG, R. (1983) Cognitive loss and recovery in long-term alcohol abusers. *Archives of General Psychiatry* **40**, 435–442 [604].

BRANDT, J. & RICH, J.B. (1995) Memory disorders in the dementias. Ch. 10 in *Handbook of Memory Disorders*, eds Baddeley, A.D., Wilson, B.A. & Watts, F.N. John Wiley & Sons: Chichester [469].

BRANDT, J., SPENCER, M., McSORLEY, P. & FOLSTEIN, M.F. (1988) Semantic activation and implicit memory in Alzheimer disease. *Alzheimer's Disease and Associated Disorders* **2**, 112–119 [32].

BRANDT, J., QUAID, K.A., FOLSTEIN, S.E., GARBER, P., MAESTRI, N.E., ABBOTT, M.H., SLAVNEY, P.R., FRANZ, M.L., KASCH, L. & KAZAZIAN, H.H. (1989) Presymptomatic diagnosis of delayed-onset disease with linked DNA markers. The experience in Huntington's disease. *Journal of the American Medical Association* **261**, 3108–3114 [466].

BRAUDE, W.M., BARNES, T.R.E. & GORE, S.M. (1983) Clinical characteristics of akathisia: a systematic investigation of acute psychiatric in-patient admissions. *British Journal of Psychiatry* **143**, 139–150 [640, 644].

BRAVO, E.L. & GIFFORD, R.W. (1984) Phaeochromocytoma: diagnosis, localization, and management. *New England Journal of Medicine* **311**, 1298–1303 [520].

BRAY, P.F. & WISER, W.C. (1965) Evidence for a genetic aetiology of temporal-central abnormalities in focal epilepsy. *New England Journal of Medicine* **271**, 926–933 [247].

BRAYNE, C. (1994) How common are cognitive impairment and dementia? An epidemiological view point. Ch. 9 in *Dementia and Normal Aging*, eds Huppert, F.A., Brayne, C. & O'Connor, D.W. Cambridge University Press: Cambridge [449].

BRAYNE, C.E.G., DOW, L., CALLOWAY, S.P. & THOMPSON, R.J. (1982) Blood creatine kinase isoenzyme BB in boxers. *Lancet* **2**, 1308–1309 [207].

BREITER, H.C., RAUCH, S.L., KWONG, K.K., BAKER, J.R., WEISSKOFF, R.M., KENNEDY, D.N., KENDRICK, A.D., DAVIS, T.L., JIANG A., COHEN, M.S., STERN, C.E., BELLIVEAU, J.W., BAER, L., O'SULLIVAN, R.L., SAVAGE, C.R., JENIKE, M.A. & ROSEN, B.R. (1996) Functional magnetic resonance imaging of symptom provocation in obsessive–compulsive disorder. *Archives of General Psychiatry* **53**, 595–606 [144].

BREITNER, J.C.S. (1994) Genetic factors. Ch. 16 in *Dementia*, eds Burns, A. & Levy, R. Chapman & Hall: London [431].

BREITNER, J.C.S. & FOLSTEIN, M.F. (1984) Familial Alzheimer dementia: a prevalent disorder with specific clinical features. *Psychological Medicine* **14**, 63–80 [431].

BREITNER, J.C.S., GAU, B.A., WELSH, K.A., PLASSMAN, B.L., McDONALD, W.M., HELMS, M.J. & ANTHONY, J.C. (1994) Inverse association of anti-inflammatory treatments and Alzheimer's disease: initial results of a co-twin control study. *Neurology* **44**, 227–232 [447].

BRENNAN, F.N. & LYTTLE, J.A. (1987) Alcohol and seizures: a review. *Journal of the Royal Society of Medicine* **80**, 571–573 [600].

BRENNER, C., FRIEDMAN, A.P., MERRITT, H.H. & DENNY-BROWN, D.E. (1944) Post-traumatic headache. *Journal of Neurosurgery* **1**, 379–391 [174].

BRENTON, D.P. (1996) Inborn errors of amino acid and organic acid metabolism. Section 11.3 in *Oxford Textbook of Medicine*, 3rd edn, eds Weatherall, D.J., Ledingham, J.G.G. & Warrell, D.A. Oxford University Press: Oxford [573].

BRESNIHAN, B., HOHMEISTER, R., CUTTING, J., TRAVERS, R.I., WALD-BURGER, M., BLACK, C., JONES, T. & HUGHES, G.R. (1979) The neuropsychiatric disorder in systemic lupus erythematosus: evidence for both vascular and immune mechanisms. *Annals of the Rheumatic Diseases* **38**, 301–306 [421].

BRETELER, M.M.B., DE GROOT, R.R.M., VAN ROMUNDE, L.K.J. & HOFMAN, A. (1995) Risk of dementia in patients with Parkinson's disease, epilepsy and severe head trauma: a register-based follow-up study. *American Journal of Epidemiology* **142**, 1300–1305 [654].

BRETT, E.M. & LAKE, B.D. (1975) Reassessment of rectal approach to neuropathology in childhood. *Archives of Disease in Childhood* **50**, 753–762 [760].

BREW, B.J., BHALLA, R.B., PAUL, M., SIDTIS, J.J., KEILP, J.J., SADLER, A.E., GALLARDO, H., McARTHUR, J.C., SCHWARTZ, M.K. & PRICE, R.W. (1992) Cerebrospinal fluid β2-microglobulin in patients with AIDS dementia complex: an expanded series including response to zidovudine treatment. *AIDS* **6**, 461–465 [326].

BREW, B.J., SIDTIS, J.J., ROSENBLUM, M. & PRICE, R.W. (1988) AIDS dementia complex. *Journal of the Royal College of Physicians of London* **22**, 140–144 [324].

BREWER, C. (1969) Psychosis due to acute hypothyroidism during the administration of carbimazole. *British Journal of Psychiatry* **115**, 1181–1183 [511].

BREWER, C. (1972) Cerebral atrophy in young cannabis smokers. *Lancet* **1**, 143 [616].

BREWER, C. & PERRETT, L. (1971) Brain damage due to alcohol consumption: an air-encephalographic, psychometric and electroencephalographic study. *British Journal of Addiction* **66**, 170–182 [605].

BRICOLO, A. (1967) Insomnia after bilateral sterotactic thalamotomy in man. *Journal of Neurology, Neurosurgery and Psychiatry* **30**, 154–158 [734].

BRIEG, A., EKBOM, K., GREITZ, T. & KUGELBERG, E. (1967) Hydrocephalus due to elongated basilar artery: a new clinicoradiological syndrome. *Lancet* **1**, 874–875 [746, 749].

BRIERLEY, H. (1967) Treatment of hysterical spasmodic torticollis by behaviour therapy. *Behaviour Research and Therapy* **5**, 139–142 [675].

BRIERLEY, J.B. (1961) Clinico-pathological correlations in amnesia. *Gerontologia Clinica* **3**, 97–109 [32].

BRIERLEY, J.B. (1966) The neuropathology of amnesic states. Ch. 7 in *Amnesia*, eds Whitty, C.W.M. & Zangwill, O.L. Butterworths: London [25].

BRIERLEY, J.B. (1970) Systemic hypotension—neurological and neuropathological aspects, Ch. 9 in *Modern Trends in Neurology*, Vol. 5, ed. Williams, D. Butterworths: London [547, 548].

BRIERLEY, J.B. (1976) Cerebral hypoxia. Ch. 2 in *Greenfield's Neuropathy*, 3rd edn, eds Marks, W. & Corsellis, J.A.N. Edward Arnold: London [548].

BRIERLEY, J.B. (1981) Brain damage due to hypoglycaemia. Ch. 22 in *Hypoglycaemia*, 2nd edn, eds Marks, V. & Rose, F.C. Blackwell Scientific Publications: Oxford [546].

BRIERLEY, J.B., CORSELLIS, J.A.N., HIERONS, R. & NEVIN, S. (1960) Subacute encephalitis of later adult life: mainly affecting the limbic areas. *Brain* **83**, 357–368 [26, 362, 364, 742].

BRILLIANT, P.J. & GYNTHER, M.D. (1963) Relationships between performances on three tests for organicity and selected patient variables. *Journal of Consulting Psychology* **27**, 474–479 [112].

BRIN, M.F., JANKOVIC, J., COMELLA, C., BLITZER, A., TSUI, J. & PULLMAN, S.L. (1995) Treatment of dystonia using botulinum toxin. Ch. 6 in *Treatment of Movement Disorders*, ed. Kurlan, R. J.B. Lippincott: Philadelphia [679].

784   REFERENCES

BRISSAUD, E. (1895) *Leçons sur les Maladies Nerveuses*. Masson: Paris [673].

BRISTOW, M.F. (1991) Posterior fossa tumours presenting to psychiatrists. *Behavioural Neurology* **4**, 249–253 [231, 235].

BRITISH MEDICAL ASSOCIATION (1993) *The Boxing Debate*. British Medical Association Scientific Department: London [206].

BRITISH MEDICAL JOURNAL (1968) Leading article: Nutritional folate deficiency. *British Medical Journal* **2**, 377–378 [590].

BRITISH MEDICAL JOURNAL (1970a) Leading article: Epidemic malaise. *British Medical Journal* **1**, 1–2 [371].

BRITISH MEDICAL JOURNAL (1970b) Correspondence concerning Royal Free Disease. *British Medical Journal* **1**, 170–171 [372].

BRITISH MEDICAL JOURNAL (1971) Leading article: Influenza and the nervous system. *British Medical Journal* **1**, 357–358 [360].

BRITISH MEDICAL JOURNAL (1978) Modified neurosyphilis. *British Medical Journal* **2**, 647–648 [342].

BRITISH MEDICAL JOURNAL (1992) Brazil's mercury poisoning disaster. *British Medical Journal* **304**, 1397 [635].

BROCA, P. (1861) Nouvelle observation d'aphémie produite par une lésion de la moitié postérieure des deuxième et troisième circonvolutions frontales. *Bulletins de la Société Anatomique de Paris* **6**, 398–407 [22].

BROCK, M. (1971) Cerebral blood flow and intracranial pressure changes associated with brain hypoxia. Ch. 2 in *Brain Hypoxia*, eds Brierley, J.B. & Meldrum, B.S. Clinics in Developmental Medicine, No. 39/40. Heinemann: London [548].

BRODERICK, J.P. & SWANSON, J.W. (1987) Migraine-related strokes. Clinical profile and prognosis in 20 patients. *Archives of Neurology* **44**, 868–871 [401].

BRODIE, M.J. (1989a) Epilepsy, anticonvulsants and pregnancy. *Prescribers' Journal* **29**, 251–257 [299].

BRODIE, M.J. (1989b) Management of status epilepticus in adults. *Prescribers' Journal* **29**, 48–56 [306].

BRODIE, M. (1992) Drugs in focus: 1. Vigabatrin. *Prescribers' Journal* **32**, 21–26 [302].

BRODY, H. (1955) Organisation of the cerebral cortex. III. A study of aging in the human cerebral cortex. *Journal of Comparative Neurology*, 511–556 [443].

BRODY, H. (1978) Cell counts in cerebral cortex and brainstem. In *Alzheimer's Disease: Senile Dementia and Related Disorders. Aging*, Vol. 7, eds Katzman, R., Terry, R.D. & Bick, K.L., pp. 345–351. Raven Press: New York [443].

BROLLEY, M. & HOLLENDER, M.H. (1955) Psychological problems of patients with myasthenia gravis. *Journal of Nervous and Mental Disease* **122**, 178–184 [711].

BROMBERG, W. (1934) Marihuana intoxication. *American Journal of Psychiatry* **91**, 303–330 [612, 613].

BRONSTEIN, A.M. & RUDGE, P. (1986) Vestibular involvement in spasmodic torticollis. *Journal of Neurology, Neurosurgery, and Psychiatry* **49**, 290–295 [674].

BRONSTEIN, A.M., RUDGE, P. & BEECHEY, A.H. (1987) Spasmodic torticollis following unilateral VIII nerve lesions: neck EMG modulation in response to vestibular stimuli. *Journal of Neurology, Neurosurgery, and Psychiatry* **50**, 580–586 [674].

BROOK, C.G.D. & EVANS, P.R. (1969) Psychosis in systemic lupus erythematosus and the response to cyclophosphamide. *Proceedings of the Royal Society of Medicine* **62**, 912 [422].

BROOK, P., DEGUN, G. & MATHER, M. (1975) Reality orientation, a therapy for psychogeriatric patients. A controlled study. *British Journal of Psychiatry* **127**, 42–45 [500].

BROOKS, D.J., IBANEZ, V., SAWLE, G.V., QUINN, N., LEES, A.J., MATHIAS, C.J., BANNISTER, R., MARSDEN, C.D. & FRACKOWIAK,

R.S.J. (1990) Differing patterns of striatal F-dopa uptake in Parkinson's disease, multiple system atrophy and progressive supranuclear palsy. *Annals of Neurology* **28**, 547–555 [648].

BROOKS, D.N. (1976) Wechsler Memory Scale performance and its relationship to brain damage after severe closed head injury. *Journal of Neurology, Neurosurgery and Psychiatry* **39**, 593–601 [185].

BROOKS, D.S., MURPHY, D., JANOTA, I. & LISHMAN, W.A. (1987a) Early-onset Huntington's chorea: diagnostic clues. *British Journal of Psychiatry* **151**, 850–852 [xxii, 471].

BROOKS, N. (1984a) Cognitive deficits after head injury. Ch. 4 in *Closed Head Injury. Psychological, Social and Family Consequences*, ed. Brooks, N. Oxford University Press: Oxford [184].

BROOKS, N. (1984b) Head injury and the family. Ch. 7 in *Closed Head Injury. Psychological, Social, and Family Consequences*, ed. Brooks, N. Oxford University Press [216].

BROOKS, N., KUPSHIK, G., WILSON, L., GALBRAITH, S. & WARD, R. (1987b) A neuropsychological study of active amateur boxers. *Journal of Neurology, Neurosurgery, and Psychiatry* **50**, 997–1000 [206].

BROOKS, N., McKINLAY, W., BEATTIE, A. & CAMPSIE, L. (1987c) Return to work within the first seven years of severe head injury. *Brain Injury* **1**, 5–19 [172].

BROOKS, N., SYMINGTON, C., BEATTIE, A., CAMPSIE, L., BRYDEN, J. & McKINLAY, W. (1989) Alcohol and other predictors of cognitive recovery after severe head injury. *Brain Injury* **3**, 235–246 [179].

BROTCHIE, J., BRENNAN, J. & WYKE, M.A. (1985) Temporal orientation in the pre-senium and old age. *British Journal of Psychiatry* **147**, 692–695 [99].

BROUGHTON, R. & GHANEM, Q. (1976) The impact of compound narcolepsy on the life of the patient. Ch. 13 in *Narcolepsy, Advances in Sleep Research*, Vol. III, eds Guilleminault, C., Dement, W.C. & Passouant, P. Spectrum Publications Inc.: New York [728].

BROWN, D.S.O., WILLS, C.E., YOUSEFI, V. & NELL, V. (1991) Neurotoxic effects of chronic exposure to manganese dust. *Neuropsychiatry, Neuropsychology, and Behavioral Neurology* **4**, 238–250 [635].

BROWN, G., CHADWICK, D., SHAFFER, D., RUTTER, M. & TRAUB, M. (1981) A prospective study of children with head injuries: III Psychiatric sequelae. *Psychological Medicine* **11**, 63–78 [203].

BROWN, G.G., LEVINE, S.R., GORELL, J.M., PETTEGREW, J.W., GDOWSKI, J.W., BUERI, J.A., HELPERN, J.A. & WELCH, K.M.A. (1989) In vivo ^{31}P NMR profiles of Alzheimer's disease and multiple subcortical infarct dementia. *Neurology* **39**, 1423–1427 [143].

BROWN, G.W. (1989) Life events and measurement. Ch. 1 in *Life Events and Illness*, eds Brown, G.W. & Harris, T.O. Unwin Hyman: London [700].

BROWN, G.W. & BIRLEY, J.L.T. (1968) Crises and life changes and the onset of schizophrenia. *Journal of Health and Social Behavior* **9**, 203–214 [91].

BROWN, G.W. & HARRIS, T.O. (1978) *Social Origins of Depression. A study of Psychiatric Disorder in Women*. Tavistock: London [700].

BROWN, J. (1992) Pick's disease. Ch. 4 in *Unusual Dementias*, ed. Rossor, M.N. Baillière Tindall: London [461].

BROWN, J.R. & SIMONSON, J. (1957) A clinical study of 100 aphasic patients: Observations on lateralisation and localisation of lesions. *Neurology* **7**, 777–783 [49].

BROWN, P., GOLDFARB, L.G. & GAJDUSEK, D.C. (1991) The new biology of spongiform encephalopathy infectious amyloidoses with a genetic twist. *Lancet* **337**, 1019–1021 [474].

BROWN, P., PREECE, M.A. & WILL, R.G. (1992) 'Friendly fire' in medicine: hormones, homografts, and Creutzfeldt–Jakob disease. *Lancet* **340**, 24–27 [476].

BROWN, R., COLTER, N., CORSELLIS, J.A.N., CROW, T.J., FRITH, C.D., JAGOE, R., JOHNSTONE, E.C. & MARSH, L. (1986) Postmortem evidence of structural brain changes in schizophrenia. *Archives of General Psychiatry* **43**, 36–42 [86].

BROWN, R.G. & MARSDEN, C.D. (1984) How common is dementia in Parkinson's disease? *Lancet* **2**, 1262–1265 [653].

BROWN, R.G., MARSDEN, C.D., QUINN, N. & WYKE, M.A. (1984) Alterations in cognitive performance and affect-arousal state during fluctuations in motor function in Parkinson's disease. *Journal of Neurology, Neurosurgery, and Psychiatry* **47**, 454–465 [650].

BROWN, S.W. & FENWICK, P.B.C. (1989) Evoked and psychogenic epileptic seizures: II. Inhibition. *Acta Neurologica Scandinavica* **80**, 541–547 [309].

BROWN, S.W. & VAUGHAN, M. (1988) Dementia in epileptic patients. Ch. 13 in *Epilepsy, Behaviour and Cognitive Function*, eds Trimble, M.R. & Reynolds, E.H. John Wiley: Chichester [264].

BROWN, W.A. & MUELLER, P.S. (1970) Psychological function in individuals with amyotrophic lateral sclerosis. *Psychosomatic Medicine* **32**, 141–152 [707].

BROWNELL, B. & HUGHES, J.T. (1962) The distribution of plaques in the cerebrum in multiple sclerosis. *Journal of Neurology, Neurosurgery and Psychiatry* **25**, 315–320 [693].

BROWNELL, B. & OPPENHEIMER, D.R. (1965) An ataxic form of subacute presenile polioencephalopathy (Creutzfeldt–Jakob disease). *Journal of Neurology, Neurosurgery and Psychiatry* **28**, 350–361 [479].

BROWNELL, B., OPPENHEIMER, D.R. & HUGHES, J.T. (1970) The central nervous system in motor neurone disease. *Journal of Neurology, Neurosurgery and Psychiatry* **33**, 338–357 [707].

BROWSE, N. (1983) The surgical treatment of cerebrovascular disease. Ch. 21 in *Vascular Disease of the Central Nervous System*, 2nd edn, ed. Russell, R.W.R. Churchill Livingstone: Edinburgh & London [389].

BROZEK, J. & CASTER, W.O. (1957) Psychologic effects of thiamine restriction and deprivation in normal young men. *American Journal of Clinical Nutrition* **5**, 109–120 [572].

BRUCE-JONES, W.D.A., WHITE, P.D., THOMAS, J.M. & CLARE, A.W. (1994) The effect of social adversity on the fatigue syndrome, psychiatric disorders and physical recovery, following glandular fever. *Psychological Medicine* **24**, 651–659 [359].

BRUCHER, J.M. (1967) Neuropathological problems posed by carbon monoxide poisoning and anoxia. In *Carbon Monoxide Poisoning*, eds Bour, H. & Ledingham, I. McA. Progress in Brain Research, Vol. 24. Elsevier: Amsterdam [553].

BRUDER, G., RABINOWICZ, E., TOWEY, J., BROWN, A., KAUFMANN, C.A., AMADOR, X., MALASPINA, D. & GORMAN, J.M. (1995) Smaller right ear (left hemisphere) advantage for dichotic fused words in patients with schizophrenia. *American Journal of Psychiatry* **152**, 932–935 [89].

BRUETSCH, W.L. (1940) Chronic rheumatic brain disease as a possible factor in the causation of some cases of dementia praecox. *American Journal of Psychiatry* **97**, 276–296 [373, 374].

BRUGGER, P., REGARD, M. & LANDIS, T. (1996) Unilaterally felt 'presences': the neuropsychiatry of one's invisible Doppelgänger. *Neuropsychiatry, Neuropsychology, and Behavioral Neurology* **9**, 114–122 [73].

BRUN, A. (1987) Frontal lobe degeneration of non-Alzheimer type. I. Neuropathology. *Archives of Gerontology and Geriatrics* **6**, 193–208 [463].

BRUN, A. & ENGLUND, E. (1981) Regional pattern of degeneration in Alzheimer's disease: neuronal loss and histopathological grading. *Histopathology* **5**, 549–564 [443].

BRUN, A. & ENGLUND, E. (1986) A white matter disorder in dementia

of the Alzheimer type: a pathoanatomical study. *Annals of Neurology* **19**, 253–262 [460].

BRUN, A., ENGLUND, B., GUSTAFSON, L., PASSANT, U., MANN, D.M.A., NEARY, D. & SNOWDEN, J.S. (1994) Clinical and neuropathological criteria for frontotemporal dementia. *Journal of Neurology, Neurosurgery, and Psychiatry* **57**, 416–418 [465].

BRUNO, A., WAGNER, W. & ORRISON, W.W. (1993) Clinical outcome and brain MRI four years after carbon monoxide intoxication. *Acta Neurologica Scandinavica* **87**, 205–209 [552].

BRUTON, C.J. (1988) *The Neuropathology of Temporal Lobe Epilepsy*. Maudsley Monograph No. 31. Oxford University Press: Oxford [246, 270, 312].

BRUTON, C.J., CROW, T.J., FRITH, C.D., JOHNSTONE, E.C., OWENS, D.G.C. & ROBERTS, G.W. (1990) Schizophrenia and the brain: a prospective clinico-neuropathological study. *Psychological Medicine* **20**, 285–304 [86].

BRUUN, R.D. & BUDMAN, C.L. (1992) The natural history of Tourette syndrome. Ch. 1 in *Tourette Syndrome. Genetics, Neurobiology, and Treatment*, eds Chase, T.N., Friedhoff, A.J. & Cohen, D.J. *Advances in Neurology*, Vol. 58. Raven Press: New York [683].

BRUYN, G.W. (1968a) Complicated migraine. Ch. 6 in *Handbook of Clinical Neurology*, Vol. 5, eds Vinkin, P.J. & Bruyn, G.W. North-Holland Publishing Co.: Amsterdam [407].

BRUYN, G.W. (1968b) Huntington's chorea—historical, clinical and laboratory synopsis. Ch. 13 in *Handbook of Clinical Neurology*, Vol. 6, eds Vinken, P.J. & Bruyn, G.W. North-Holland Publishing Co.: Amsterdam [469].

BUCHBINDER, S.P., KATZ, M.H., HESSOL, N.A., O'MALLEY, P.M. & HOLMBERG, S.D. (1994) Long-term HIV-1 infection without immunological progression. *AIDS* **8**, 1123–1128 [317].

BUCHSBAUM, M.S. (1990) The frontal lobes, basal ganglia, and temporal lobes as sites for schizophrenia. *Schizophrenia Bulletin* **16**, 379–389 [87].

BUCHSBAUM, M.S., CARPENTER, W.T., FEDIO, P., GOODWIN, F.K., MURPHY, D.L. & POST, R.M. (1979) Hemispheric differences in evoked potential enhancement by selective attention to hemiretinally presented stimuli in schizophrenic, affective and posttemporal lobectomy patients. In *Hemispheric Asymmetries of Function in Psychopathology*, eds Gruzelier, J. & Flor-Henry, P., pp. 317–328. Elsevier/North-Holland Biochemical Press: Amsterdam [89].

BUCHSBAUM, M.S., INGVAR, D.H., KESSLER, R., WATERS, R.N., CAPPELLETTI, J., VAN KAMMEN, D.P., KING, A.C., JOHNSON, J.L., MANNING, R.G., FLYNN, R.W., MANN, L.S., BUNNEY, W.E. & SOKOLOFF, L. (1982) Cerebral glucography with positron tomography. *Archives of General Psychiatry* **39**, 251–259 [87].

BUCHSBAUM, M.S., RIGAL, F., COPPOLA, R., CAPPELLETTI, J., KING, C. & JOHNSON, J. (1982) A new system for gray-level surface distribution maps of electrical activity. *Electroencephalography and Clinical Neurophysiology* **53**, 237–242 [132].

BUCHWALD, D. (1991) Laboratory abnormalities in chronic fatigue syndrome. Ch. 6 in *Post-viral Fatigue Syndrome*, eds Jenkins, R. & Mowbray, J.F. Wiley & Sons: Chichester [372].

BUCKLEY, P.F. & HUTCHINSON, M. (1995) Neuroleptic malignant syndrome. *Journal of Neurology, Neurosurgery, and Psychiatry* **58**, 271–273 [626, 627].

BUCKLEY, P.F., MOORE, C., LONG, H., LARKIN, C., THOMPSON, P., MULVANY, F., REDMOND, O., STACK, J.P., ENNIS, J.T. & WADDINGTON, J.L. (1994) 1H-magnetic resonance spectroscopy of the left temporal and frontal lobes in schizophrenia: clinical, neurodevelopmental, and cognitive correlates. *Biological Psychiatry* **36**, 792–800 [143].

BUDINGER, T.F. (1981) Nuclear magnetic resonance (NMR) in vivo studies: known thresholds for health effects. *Journal of Computer Assisted Tomography* **5**, 800–811 [142].

BUDKA, H., AGUZZI, A., BROWN, P., BRUCHER, J-M., BUGIANI, O., COLLINGE, J., DIRINGER, H., GULLOTTA, F., HALTIA, M., HAUW, J-J., IRONSIDE, J.W., KRETZSCHMAR, H.A., LANTOS, P.L., MASULLO, C., POCCHIARI, M., SCHLOTE, M., TATEISHI, J. & WILL, R.G. (1995a) Tissue handling in suspected Creutzfeldt–Jakob disease (CJD) and other human spongiform encephalopathies (prion diseases). *Brain Pathology* **5**, 319–322 [476, 477].

BUDKA, H., AGUZZI, A., BROWN, P., BRUCHER, J-M., BUGIANI, O., GULLOTTA, F., HALTIA, M., HAUW, J-J., IRONSIDE, J.W., JELLINGER, K., KRETZSCHMAR, H.A., LANTOS, P.L., MASULLO, C., SCHLOTE, W., TATEISHI, J. & WELLER, R.O. (1995b) Neuropathological diagnostic criteria for Creutzfeldt–Jakob disease (CJD) and other human spongiform encephalopathies (prion diseases). *Brain Pathology* **5**, 459–466 [478].

BUDKA, H., COSTANZI, G., CRISTINA, S., LECHI, A., PARRAVICINI, C., TRABATTONI, R. & VAGO, L. (1987) Brain pathology induced by infection with the human immunodeficiency virus (HIV). A histological, immunocytochemical and electron microscopal study of 100 autopsy cases. *Acta Neuropathologica (Berlin)* **75**, 185–198 [319].

BUDKA, H., WILEY, C.A., KLEIHUES, P., ARTIGAS, J., ASBURY, A.K., CHO, E-S., CORNBLATH, D.R., DAL CANTO, M.C., DEGIROLAMI, U., DICKSON, D., EPSTEIN, L.G., ESIRI, M.M., GIANGASPERO, F., GOSZTONYI, G., GRAY, F., GRIFFIN, J.W., HÉNIN, D., IWASAKI, Y., JANSSEN, R.S., JOHNSON, R.T., LANTOS, P.L., LYMAN, W.D., McARTHUR, J.C., NAGASHIMA, K., PERESS, N., PETITO, C.K., PRICE, R.W., RHODES, R.H., ROSENBLUM, M., SAID, G., SCARAVILLI, F., SHARER, L.R. & VINTERS, H.V. (1991) HIV-associated disease of the nervous system: review of nomenclature and proposal for neuropathology-based terminology. *Brain Pathology* **1**, 143–152 [322, 323].

BUELL, S.J. & COLEMAN, P.D. (1979) Dendritic growth in the aged human brain and failure of growth in senile dementia. *Science* **206**, 854–856 [436, 443, 607].

BUELL, S.J. & COLEMAN, P.D. (1981) Quantitative evidence for selective dendritic growth in normal human ageing but not in senile dementia. *Brain Research* **214**, 23–41 [436, 443, 607].

BUGE, A., SUPINO-VITERBO, V., RANCUREL, G. & PONTES, C. (1981) Epileptic phenomena in bismuth toxic encephalopathy. *Journal of Neurology, Neurosurgery, and Psychiatry* **44**, 62–67 [636, 637].

BUHRICH, N., COOPER, D.A. & FREED, E. (1988) HIV infection associated with symptoms indistinguishable from functional psychosis. *British Journal of Psychiatry* **152**, 649–653 [331].

BULL, J. (1967) The corpus callosum. *Clinical Radiology* **18**, 2–18 [770].

BULL, J. (1969) Massive anuerysms at the base of the brain. *Brain* **92**, 535–570 [412].

BULL, J. (1971) Cerebral atrophy in young cannabis smokers. *Lancet* **2**, 1420 [616].

BULLMORE, E., BRAMMER, M., ALARCON, G. & BINNIE, C. (1992) A new technique for fractal analysis applied to human, intracerebrally recorded, ictal electroencephalographic signals. *Neuroscience Letters* **146**, 227–230 [132].

BULLMORE, E.T., BRAMMER, M.J., ALARCON, G. & BINNIE, C.D. (1994) Synaptic visualisation of brain electrical activity during a cluster of 11 epileptic seizures. In *Fractals in the Natural and Applied Sciences*, ed. Novak, M.M. Elsevier: North Holland [132].

BULLMORE, E., BRAMMER, M., HARVEY, I., MURRAY, R. & RON, M. (1995) Cerebral hemispheric asymmetry revisited: effects of handedness, gender and schizophrenia measured by radius of gyration

in magnetic resonance images. *Psychological Medicine* **25**, 349–363 [89].

BUNDEY, S., CARTER, C.O. & SOOTHILL, J.F. (1970) Early recognition of heterozygotes for the gene for dystrophia myotonica. *Journal of Neurology, Neurosurgery and Psychiatry* **33**, 279–293 [718].

BURDEN, G. (1969) Attitudes towards epilepsy in the U.K. In *Exploring World Attitudes Towards Epilepsy*, Social Studies in Epilepsy No. 7, International Bureau for Epilepsy: London [269].

BURGDORFER, W. (1987) Lyme disease. Ch. 5 in *Oxford Textbook of Medicine*, 2nd edn, eds Weatherall, D.J., Ledingham, J.G.G. & Warrell, D.A., pp. 324–327. Oxford University Press: Oxford [369].

BURGER, P.C. & VOGEL, F.S. (1973) The development of the pathologic changes of Alzheimer's disease and the senile dementia in patients with Down's syndrome. *American Journal of Pathology* **73**, 457–476 [437].

BURGESS, A., FLINT, J. & ADSHEAD, H. (1992) Factor structure of the Wechsler Adult Intelligence Scale—revised (WAIS-R): a clinical sample. *British Journal of Clinical Psychology* **31**, 336–338 [111].

BURGESS, A.P., RICCIO, M., JADRESIC, D., PUGH, K., CATALAN, J., HAWKINS, D.A., BALDEWEG, T., LOVETT, E., GRUZELIER, J. & THOMPSON, C. (1994) A longitudinal study of the neuropsychiatric consequences of HIV-1 infection in gay men. I: Neuropsychological performance and neurological status at baseline and at 12-month follow-up. *Psychological Medicine* **24**, 885–895 [329].

BURKE, C.W. (1983) Adrenocortical diseases. In *Oxford Textbook of Medicine*, Vol. 1, eds Weatherall, D.J., Ledingham, J.G.G. & Warrell, D.A., pp. 10.58–10.69. Oxford University Press [515].

BURKE, R.E., FAHN, S. & GOLD, A.P. (1980) Delayed-onset dystonia in patients with 'static' encephalopathy. *Journal of Neurology, Neurosurgery, and Psychiatry* **43**, 789–797 [669].

BURKE, R.E., FAHN, S., JANKOVIC, J., MARSDEN, C.D., LANG, A.E., GOLLOMP, S. & ILSON, J. (1982) Tardive dystonia: late-onset and persistent dystonia caused by antipsychotic drugs. *Neurology* **32**, 1335–1346 [642].

BURKE, R.E., FAHN, S. & MARSDEN, C.D. (1986) Torsion dystonia: a double-blind, prospective trial of high-dosage trihexyphenidyl. *Neurology* **36**, 160–164 [672].

BURKE, R.E. & KANG, U.J. (1988) Tardive dystonia: clinical aspects and treatment. In *Facial Dyskinesias*, eds Jankovic, J. & Tolosa, E. *Advances in Neurology* **49**, 199–210 [642, 645].

BURKE, R.E., KANG, U.J., JANKOVIC, J., MILLER, L.G. & FAHN, S. (1989) Tardive akathisia: an analysis of clinical features and response to open therapeutic trials. *Movement Disorders* **4**, 157–175 [643, 645].

BURKE, W.H., WESOLOWSKI, M.D. & GUTH, M.L. (1988) Comprehensive head injury rehabilitation: an outcome evaluation. *Brain Injury* **2(4)**, 313–322 [216].

BURKHARDT, C.R., FILLEY, C.M., KLEINSCHMIDT-DE MASTERS, B.K., DE LA MONTE, S., NORENBERG, M.D. & SCHNECK, S.A. (1988) Diffuse Lewy body disease and progressive dementia. *Neurology* **38**, 1520–1528 [451, 452].

BURKLE, F.M. & LIPOWSKI, Z.J. (1978) Colloid cyst of the third ventricle presenting as psychiatric disorder. *American Journal of Psychiatry* **135**, 373–374 [228].

BURKLUND, C.W. & SMITH, A. (1977) Language and the cerebral hemispheres. Observations of verbal and non-verbal responses during 18 months following left ('dominant') hemispherectomy. *Neurology* **27**, 627–633 [42].

BURKS, J.S., ALFREY, A.C., HUDDLESTONE, J., NOVENBERG, M.D. & LEWIN, E. (1976) A fatal encephalopathy in chronic haemodialysis patients. *Lancet* **1**, 764–768 [558].

BURNS, A., JACOBY, R., PHILPOT, M. & LEVY, R. (1991) Computerised tomography in Alzheimer's disease: methods of scan analysis, comparison with normal controls, and clinical/radiological associations. *British Journal of Psychiatry* **159**, 609–614 [139].

BURNS, A. & LEVY, R. (1992) *Clinical Diversity in Late Onset Alzheimer's Disease*, Maudsley Monograph No. 34. Oxford University Press: Oxford [432, 435].

BURNS, A., LUTHERT, P., LEVY, R., JACOBY, R. & LANTOS, P. (1990) Accuracy of clinical diagnosis of Alzheimer's disease. *British Medical Journal* **301**, 1026 [440].

BURNS, A. & PEARLSON, G. (1994) Computed tomography. Ch. 23 in *Dementia*, eds Burns, A. & Levy, R. Chapman & Hall: London [139].

BURNS, A., PHILPOT, M.P., COSTA, D.C., ELL, P.J. & LEVY, R. (1989) The investigation of Alzheimer's disease with single photon emission tomography. *Journal of Neurology, Neurosurgery and Psychiatry* **52**, 248–253 [434].

BURSTEN, B. (1961) Psychoses associated with thyrotoxicosis. *Archives of General Psychiatry* **4**, 267–273 [509].

BURTON, G.V., BULLARD, D.E., WALTHER, P.J. & BURGER, P.C. (1988) Paraneoplastic limbic encephalopathy with testicular carcinoma. A reversible neurologic syndrome. *Cancer* **62**, 2248–2251 [742].

BURTON, R.C., McDUFFIE, F.C. & MULDER, D.W. (1971) Lupus erythematosus: an autoimmune disease of the nervous system. Ch. 12 in *Immunological Disorders of the Nervous System*, Research Publications of the Association for Research in Nervous and Mental Disease, Vol. 49. Williams & Wilkins: Baltimore [420].

BURWELL, C.S., ROBIN, E.D., WHALEY, R.D. & BICKELMANN, A.G. (1956) Extreme obesity associated with alveolar hypoventilation—a Pickwickian syndrome. *American Journal of Medicine* **21**, 811–818 [730].

BUSCH, E. (1940) Physical symptoms in neurosurgical disease. *Acta Psychiatrica et Neurologica Scandinavica* **15**, 257–290 [220].

BUSSE, E.W. (1962) Findings for the Duke Geriatric Research Project: the effects of aging upon the nervous system. In *Medical and Clinical Aspects of Aging*, ed. Blumenthal, H.T., pp. 115–123. Columbia University Press: New York [33].

BUTFIELD, E. & ZANGWILL, O.L. (1946) Re-education in aphasia: a review of 70 cases. *Journal of Neurology, Neurosurgery and Psychiatry* **9**, 75–79 [390].

BUTTERS, N. (1984) Alcoholic Korsakoff's syndrome: an update. *Seminars in Neurology* **4**, 229–247 [583].

BUTTERS, N. (1985) Alcoholic Korsakoff's syndrome: some unresolved issues concerning etiology, neuropathology, and cognitive deficits. *Journal of Clinical and Experimental Neuropsychology* **7**, 181–210 [26].

BUTTERS, N. & ALBERT, M.S. (1982) Processes underlying failures to recall remote events. In *Human Memory and Amnesia*, ed. Cermak, L.S. Lawrence Erlbaum Associates: Hillsdale, New Jersey [37].

BUTTERS, N. & CERMAK, L.S. (1980) *Alcoholic Korsakoff's Syndrome: an Information-Processing Approach to Amnesia*. Academic Press: New York [31, 35, 38, 583, 584].

BUTTERS, N., SAX, D., MONTGOMERY, K. & TARLOW, S. (1978) Comparison of the neuropsychological deficits associated with early and advanced Huntington's disease. *Archives of Neurology* **35**, 585–589 [469].

BUTTERWORTH, R.F., KRIL, J.J. & HARPER, C.G. (1993) Thiamine-dependent enzyme changes in the brains of alcoholics: relationship to the Wernicke–Korsakoff syndrome. *Alcoholism: Clinical and Experimental Research* **17**, 1084–1088 [577].

BUYSSE, D.J., REYNOLDS, C.F., KUPFER, D.J., HOUCK, P.R., HOCH, C.C., STACK, J.A. & BERMAN, S.R. (1988) Electroencephalographic sleep in depressive pseudodementia. *Archives of General Psychiatry* **45**, 568–575 [489].

BYDDER, G.M. & STEINER, R.E. (1982) NMR imaging of the brain. *Neuroradiology* **23**, 231–240 [141].

BYERS, R.K. (1959) Lead poisoning. Review of the literature and report on 45 cases. *Pediatrics* **23**, 585–603 [631, 632].

BYERS, R.K. & LORD, E.E. (1943) Late effects of lead poisoning on mental development. *American Journal of Diseases of Children* **66**, 471–494 [632].

BYRNE, A. (1988) Hypomania following increased epileptic activity. *British Journal of Psychiatry* **153**, 573–574 [258].

BYRNE, E.J., LENNOX, G.G., GODWIN-AUSTEN, R.B., JEFFERSON, D., LOWE, J., MAYER, R.J., LANDON, M. & DOHERTY, F.J. (1991) Dementia associated with cortical Lewy bodies: proposed clinical diagnostic criteria. *Dementia* **2**, 283–284 [451].

BYRNE, E.J., LENNOX, G., LOWE, J. & GODWIN-AUSTEN, R.B. (1989) Diffuse Lewy body disease: clinical features in 15 cases. *Journal of Neurology, Neurosurgery, and Psychiatry* **52**, 709–717 [450].

BYROM, F.B. (1954) The pathogenesis of hypertensive encephalopathy and its relation to the malignant phase of hypertension. Experimental evidence from the hypertensive rat. *Lancet* **2**, 201–211 [399].

BYRON, M.A. & HUGHES, G.R.V. (1983) The connective tissue diseases. In *Oxford Textbook of Medicine*, Vol. 2, eds Weatherall, D.J., Ledingham, J.G.G. & Warrell, D.A., pp. 16.28–16.40. Oxford University Press: Oxford [418].

CAINE, E.D. (1981) Pseudodementia: current concepts and future directions. *Archives of General Psychiatry* **38**, 1359–1364 [488].

CAINE, E.D. (1985) Gilles de la Tourette's syndrome. A review of clinical and research studies and consideration of future directions for investigation. *Archives of Neurology* **42**, 393–397 [685].

CAINE, E.D., McBRIDE, M.C., CHIVERTON, P., BAMFORD, K.A., REDIESS, S. & SHIAO, J. (1988) Tourette's syndrome in Monroe County school children. *Neurology* **38**, 472–475 [682].

CAINE, E.D. & POLINSKY, R.J. (1981) Tardive dyskinesia in persons with Gilles de la Tourette's disease. *Archives of Neurology* **38**, 471–472 [687].

CAIRNS, H. (1950) Mental disorders with tumours of the pons. *Folio Psychiatrica, Neurologica et Neurochirurgica Neerlandica* **53**, 193–203 [231].

CAIRNS, H. & MOSBERG, W.H. (1951) Colloid cysts of the third ventricle. *Surgery, Gynaecology and Obstetrics* **92**, 545–570 [27].

CAIRNS, H., OLDFIELD, R.C., PENNYBACKER, J.B. & WHITTERBRIDGE, D. (1941) Akinetic mutism with an epidermoid cyst of the 3rd ventricle. *Brain* **64** 273–290 [229].

CALA, L.A., JONES, B., WILEY, B. & MASTAGLIA, F.L. (1980) A computerised axial tomographic (CAT) study of alcohol inducedcerebral atrophy—in conjunction with other correlates. *Acta Psychiatrica Scandinavica* **62 (Supplement 286)**, 31–40 [605].

CALDERON, R. (1966) Myotonic dystrophy: a neglected cause of mental retardation. *Journal of Pediatrics* **68**, 423–431 [719].

CALLANAN, M.M., LOGSDAIL, S.J., RON, M.A. & WARRINGTON, E.K. (1989) Cognitive impairment in patients with clinically isolated lesions of the type seen in multiple sclerosis. A psychometric and MRI study. *Brain* **112**, 361–374 [693].

CALNE, D.B. (1995) Selegiline in Parkinson's disease. No neuroprotective effect: increased mortality. *British Medical Journal* **311**, 1583–1584 [650].

CAMERON, D.E. (1963) The process of remembering. *British Journal of Psychiatry* **109**, 325–340 [502].

CAMERON, D.E. (1967) Magnesium pemoline and human performance. *Science* **157**, 958–959 [502].

CAMERON, D.E. & SOLYOM, L. (1961) Effects of ribonucleic acid on memory. *Geriatrics* **16**, 74–81 [502].

CAMERON, D.E., SVED, S., SOLYOM, L., WAINRIB, B. & BARIK, H. (1963) Effects of ribonucleic acid on memory defect in the aged. *American Journal of Psychiatry* **120**, 320–325 [502].

CAMP, W.A. & FRIERSON, J.G. (1962) Sarcoidosis of the central nervous system. *Archives of Neurology* **7**, 432–441 [764].

CAMPBELL, A.C.P. & RUSSELL, W.R. (1941) Wernicke's encephalopathy: the clinical features and their probable relationship to vitamin B deficiency. *Quarterly Journal of Medicine* **34**, 41–64 [576].

CAMPBELL, A.M.G., EVANS, M., THOMSON, J.L.G. & WILLIAMS, M.J. (1971) Cerebral atrophy in young cannabis smokers. *Lancet* **2**, 1219–1224 [616].

CANAVAN, M.M., COBB, S. & DRINKER, C.K. (1934) Chronic manganese poisoning. *Archives of Neurology and Psychiatry* **32**, 501–512 [636].

CANDY, J.M., OAKLEY, A.E., KLINOWSKI, J., CARPENTER, T.A., PERRY, R.H., ATACK, J.R., PERRY, E.K., BLESSED, G., FAIRBAIRN, A. & EDWARDSON, J.A. (1986) Aluminosilicates and senile plaque formation in Alzheimer's disease. *Lancet* **1**, 354–357 [446].

CANTER, A.H. (1951) Direct and indirect measures of psychological deficit in multiple sclerosis. *Journal of General Psychology* **44**, 3–35 and 27–50 [693].

CAPLAN, F., CHEDRU, F., LHERMITTE, F. & MAYMAN, C. (1981) Transient global amnesia and migraine. *Neurology* **31**, 1167–1170 [406].

CAPLAN, L.R. (1980) 'Top of the basilar' syndrome. *Neurology* **30**, 72–79 [379].

CAPLAN, L.R. & SCHOENE, W.C. (1978) Clinical features of subcortical arteriosclerotic encephalopathy (Binswanger disease). *Neurology* **28**, 1206–1215 [458].

CARASSO, R.L., MOSTOFSKY, D.I. & YEHUDA, S. (1992) Aborting seizures by painful stimulation. *Behavioural Neurology* **5**, 107–111 [309].

CARBOTTE, R.M., DENBURG, S.D. & DENBURG, J.A. (1986) Prevalence of cognitive impairment in systemic lupus erythematosus. *Journal of Nervous and Mental Disease* **174**, 357–364 [420].

CARLEN, P.L., WILKINSON, D.A., WORTZMAN, G., HOLGATE, R., CORDINGLEY, J., LEE, M.A., HUZZAR, L., MODDEL, G., SINGH, R., KIRALY, L. & RANKIN, J.G. (1981) Cerebral atrophy and functional deficits in alcoholics without clinically apparent liver disease. *Neurology* **31**, 377–385 [605, 607].

CARLIN, A.S. (1986) Neuropsychological consequences of drug abuse. Ch. 20 in *Neuropsychological Assessment of Neuropsychiatric Disorders*, eds Grant, I. & Adams, K.M. Oxford University Press: New York [612].

CARLSSON, A., ADOLFSSON, R., AQUILONIUS, S.M., GOTTFRIES, C-G., ORELAND, L., SVENNERHOLM, L. & WINBLAD, B. (1980) Biogenic amines in human brain in normal aging, senile dementia, and chronic alcoholism. In *Ergot Compounds and Brain Function: Neuroendocrine and Neuropsychiatric Aspects*, eds Goldstein, M., Calne, D.B., Lieberman, A. & Thorner, M.O., pp. 295–304. Raven Press: New York [606].

CARNALL, D. & WARDEN, J. (1995) Tighter medical controls proposed for boxing. *British Medical Journal* **311**, 1183 [206].

CARNE, C.A., TEDDER, R.S. & SMITH, A. (1985) Acute encephalopathy coincident with seroconversion for anti-HTLV-III. *Lancet* **2**, 1206–1208 [317].

CARNEY, M. (1983) Pseudodementia. *British Journal of Hospital Medicine* **29**, 312–318 [489].

CARNEY, M.W.P. (1967) Serum folate values in 423 psychiatric patients. *British Medical Journal* **4**, 512–516 [590].

CARNEY, M.W.P., CHARY, T.K.N., LAUNDY, M., BOTTIGLIERI, T., CHANARIN, I., REYNOLDS, E.H. & TOONE, B. (1990) Red cell folate concentrations in psychiatric patients. *Journal of Affective Disorders* **19**, 207–213 [590].

CARNEY, M.W.P., RAVINDRAU, A., RINSLER, M.G. & WILLIAMS, D.G. (1982) Thiamine, riboflavin and pyridoxine deficiency in psychiatric in-patients. *British Journal of Psychiatry* **141**, 271–272 [571, 572].

CARNEY, M.W.P. & SHEFFIELD, B.F. (1970) Associations of subnormal serum folate and vitamin B_{12} values and effects of replacement therapy. *Journal of Nervous and Mental Disease* **150**, 404–412 [587, 590].

CARNEY, M.W.P., WIENBREN, I., JACKSON, F. & PURNELL, G.V. (1971) Multiple adenomatosis presenting with psychiatric manifestations. *Postgraduate Medical Journal* **47**, 242–243 [541].

CARNEY, M.W.P., WILLIAMS, D.G. & SHEFFIELD, B.F. (1979) Thiamine-pyridoxine lack in newly-admitted psychiatric patients. *British Journal of Psychiatry* **135**, 249–254 [571, 572].

CAROFF, S.N. (1980) The neuroleptic malignant syndrome. *Journal of Clinical Psychiatry* **41**, 79–83 [626, 627].

CARPENTER, S., KARPATI, G., ANDERMANN, F., JACOB, J.C. & ANDERMANN, E. (1977) The ultrastructural characteristics of the abnormal cytosomes in Batten-Kufs' disease. *Brain* **100**, 137–156 [760].

CARPENTER, W.T. & BUNNEY, W.E. Jr (1971) Behavioral effects of cortisol in man. *Seminars in Psychiatry* **3**, 421–434 [628].

CARR, S.A. (1980) Interhemispheric transfer of stereognostic information in chronic schizophrenics. *British Journal of Psychiatry* **136**, 53–58 [90].

CARROLL, B.A., LANE, B., NORMAN, D. & ENZMANN, D. (1977) Diagnosis of progressive multifocal leukoencephalopathy by computed tomography. *Radiology* **122**, 137–141 [752].

CARROLL, B.J. (1976a) Limbic system-adrenal cortex regulation in depression and schizophrenia. *Psychosomatic Medicine* **38**, 106–121 [507].

CARROLL, B.J. (1976b) Psychoendocrine relationships in affective disorders. Ch. 7 in *Modern Trends in Psychosomatic Medicine*, Vol. 3, ed. Hill, O.W. Butterworths: London [517].

CARROLL, B.J., FINEBERG, M., GREDEN, J.F., TARIKA, J., ALBALA, A.A., HASKETT, R.F., JAMES, N.M., KRONFOL, Z., LOHR, N., STEINER, M., DE VIGNE, J.P. & YOUNG, E. (1981) A specific laboratory test for the diagnosis of melancholia: standardisation, validation, and clinical utility. *Archives of General Psychiatry* **38**, 15–22 [507].

CARTER, A.B. (1972) Clinical aspects of cerebral infarction. Ch. 12 in *Handbook of Clinical Neurology*, Vol. 11, eds Vinken, P.J. & Bruyn, G.W. North-Holland Publishing Co.: Amsterdam [411].

CARTWRIGHT, G.E. (1978) Diagnosis of treatable Wilson's disease. *New England Journal of Medicine* **298**, 1347–1350 [664].

CASELLI, R.J., GRAFF-RADFORD, N.R. & REZAI, K. (1991) Thalamocortical diaschisis: single photon emission tomographic study of cortical blood flow changes after focal thalamic infarction. *Neuropsychiatry, Neuropsychology and Behavioral Neurology* **4**, 193–214 [377].

CASEY, D.E. (1989) Clozapine: neuroleptic-induced EPS and tardive dyskinesia. *Psychopharmacology*, **99**, S47–S53 [645].

CASH, R., L'HEUREUX, R., RAISMAN, R., JAVOY-AGID, F. & SCATTON, B. (1987) Parkinson's disease and dementia: norepinephrine and dopamine in locus caeruleus. *Neurology* **37**, 42–46 [655].

CASSON, I.R., SHAM, R., CAMPBELL, E.A., TARLAU, M. & DI DOMENICO, A. (1982) Neurological and CT evaluation of knocked-out boxers. *Journal of Neurology Neurosurgery and Psychiatry* **45**, 170–174 [205].

CASSON, I.R., SIEGEL, O., SHAM, R., CAMPBELL, E.A., TARLAU, M. & DI DOMENICO, A. (1984) Brain damage in modern boxers. *Journal of the American Medical Association* **251**, 2663–2667 [205].

CASTLE, D.J. & MURRAY, R.M. (1991) The neurodevelopmental basis of sex differences in schizophrenia. *Psychological Medicine* **21**, 565–575 [91].

CATALAN, J. (1991) HIV-associated dementia: review of some conceptual and terminological problems. *International Review of Psychiatry* **3**, 321–330 [324].

CATALAN, J., RICCIO, M. & THOMPSON, C. (1989) HIV disease and psychiatric practice. *Psychiatric Bulletin* **13**, 316–332 [333, 334].

CAUGHEY, J.E. & MYRIANTHOPOULOS, N.C. (1963) *Dystrophia Myotonica and Related Disorders*. Thomas: Springfield, Illinois [717, 720, 721].

CAVENESS, W.F., MEIROWSKY, M., RISH, B.L., MOHR, J.P., KISTLER, J.P., DILLON, J.D. & WEISS, G.H. (1979) The nature of post-traumatic epilepsy. *Journal of Neurosurgery* **50**, 545–553 [245].

CAVENESS, W.F., MERRITT, H.H. & GALLUP, G.H. (1969) Trend in public attitudes towards epilepsy over the past twenty years in the United States. In *Exploring World Attitudes Towards Epilepsy*, Social Studies in Epilepsy No. 7. International Bureau for Epilepsy, London [269].

CAVENESS, W.F. & WALKER, A.E. (1966) Appendix: Head Injury Glossary. In *Head Injury: Conference Proceedings*, eds Caveness, W.F. & Walker, A.E. Lippincott: Philadelphia [167].

CAWLEY, R.H., POST, F. & WHITEHEAD, A. (1973) Barbiturate tolerance and psychological functioning in elderly depressed patients. *Psychological Medicine* **3**, 39–52 [487].

CAWTE, J. (1985) Psychiatric sequelae of manganese exposure in the adult, foetal and neonatal nervous systems. *Australian and New Zealand Journal of Psychiatry* **19**, 211–217 [635].

CELESIA, G.G. & WANAMAKER, W.M. (1972) Psychiatric disturbances in Parkinson's disease. *Diseases of the Nervous System* **33**, 577–583 [653, 656, 657].

CENTERS FOR DISEASE CONTROL (1981) Encephalitis surveillance annual summary 1978. Quoted by Boos, J. & Esiri, M.M. (1986) in *Viral Encephalitis. Pathology, Diagnosis and Management*. Blackwell Scientific Publications: Oxford [346].

CENTERS FOR DISEASE CONTROL (1986) Classification system for human T-lymphotropic virus type III/lymphadenopathy-associated virus infections. *Morbidity and Mortality Weekly Report* **35**, 334–339 [319].

CENTERS FOR DISEASE CONTROL (1987) Classification system for human immunodeficiency virus (HIV) infection in children under 13 years of age. *Morbidity and Mortality Weekly Report* **36**, 225–236 [319].

CENTERS FOR DISEASE CONTROL (1992) 1993 revised classification system for HIV infection and expanded surveillance case definition for AIDS among adolescents and adults. *Morbidity and Mortality Weekly Report*, **41 (No.RR-17)**, 1–19 [319].

CENTERWALL, B.S. & CRIQUI, M.H. (1978) Prevention of the Wernicke–Korsakoff syndrome: a cost–benefit analysis. *New England Journal of Medicine* **299**, 285–289 [581].

CERMAK, L.S. (1982) The long and short of it in amnesia. Ch. 3 in *Human Memory and Amnesia*, ed. Cermak, L.S. Lawrence Erlbaum Associates: Hillsdale, New Jersey [29].

CERMAK, L.S. & BUTTERS, N. (1972) The role of interference and encoding in the short-term memory deficits of Korsakoff patients. *Neuropsychologia* **10**, 89–96 [35].

CHADWICK, D. (1993) Seizures, epilepsy, and other episodic disorders. Ch. 22 in *Brain's Diseases of the Nervous System*, 10th edn, ed. Walton, J. Oxford University Press: Oxford [237, 243, 245].

CHADWICK, D. & REYNOLDS, E.H. (1985) When do epileptic patients need treatment? Starting and stopping medication. *British Medical Journal* **290**, 1885–1888 [299].

CHADWICK, O., RUTTER, M., BROWN, G., SHAFFER, D. & TRAUB, M. (1981) A prospective study of children with head injuries: II Cognitive sequelae. *Psychological Medicine* **11**, 49–61 [202].

CHAFETZ, M.E. (1966) Psychological disturbances in myasthenia gravis. *Annals of the New York Academy of Sciences* **135**, 424–427 [711, 713].

CHAMBERS, W.R. (1955) Neurosurgical conditions masquerading as psychiatric diseases. *American Journal of Psychiatry* **112**, 387–389 [235, 412].

CHAMPAKAM, S., SRIKANTIA, S.G. & GOPALAN, C. (1968) Kwashiorkor and mental development. *American Journal of Clinical Nutrition* **21**, 844–852 [570].

CHANDRA, V., KOKMEN, E., SCHOENBERG, B.S. & BEARD, C.M. (1989) Head trauma with loss of consciousness as a risk factor for Alzheimer's disease. *Neurology* **39**, 1576–1578 [438].

CHANG, K.H., HAN, M.H., KIM, H.S., WIE, B.A. & HAN, M.C. (1992) Delayed encephalopathy after acute carbon monoxide intoxication: MR imaging features and distribution of cerebral white matter lesions. *Radiology* **184**, 117–122 [551].

CHANNON, S., FLYNN, D. & ROBERTSON, M.M. (1992) Attentional deficits in Gilles de la Tourette syndrome. *Neuropsychiatry, Neuropsychology, and Behavioral Neurology* **5**, 170–177 [682].

CHAPEL, J.L., BROWN, N. & JENKINS, R.L. (1964) Tourette's disease: symptomatic relief with haloperidol. *American Journal of Psychiatry* **120**, 608–610 [687].

CHAPMAN, L.F. & WOLFF, H.G. (1959) The cerebral hemispheres and the highest integrative functions of man. *Archives of Neurology* **1**, 357–424 [23, 27].

CHARATAN, F.B. & BRIERLEY, J.B. (1956) Mental disorder associated with primary lung carcinoma. *British Medical Journal* **1**, 765–768 [741].

CHARNESS, M.E. & DELAPAZ, R.L. (1987) Mamillary body atrophy in Wernicke's encephalopathy: antemortem identification using MRI. *Annals of Neurology* **22**, 595–600 [579].

CHARNESS, M.E., SIMON, R.P. & GREENBERG, D.A. (1989) Ethanol and the nervous system. *New England Journal of Medicine* **321**, 442–454 [607].

CHARNEY, D.S., KALES, A., SOLDATOS, C.R. & NELSON, J.C. (1979) Somnambulistic-like episodes secondary to combined lithium-neuroleptic treatment. *British Journal of Psychiatry* **135**, 418–424 [626].

CHARTIER-HARLIN, M.-C., CRAWFORD, F., HOULDEN, H., WARREN, A., HUGHES, D., FIDANI, L., GOATE, A., ROQUES, P., HARDY, J. & MULLAN, M. (1991) Early-onset Alzheimer's disease caused by mutations at codon 717 of the β-amyloid precursor protein gene. *Nature* **353**, 844–846 [448].

CHASE, T.N., FOSTER, N.L., FEDIO, P., BROOKS, R., MANSI, L. & DI CHIRO, G. (1984) Regional cortical dysfunction in Alzheimer's disease as determined by positron emission tomography. *Annals of Neurology* **15 (Supplement)**, S170–S174 [434].

CHASE, T.N., GEOFFREY, V., GILLESPIE, M. & BURROWS, G.H. (1986) Structural and functional studies of Gilles de la Tourette syndrome. *Revue Neurologique* **142**, 851–855 [685].

CHATELLIER, G. & LACOMBLEZ, L. on behalf of Groupe Français d'étude de la tetrahydroaminoacridine (1990) Tacrine (tetrahydroaminoacridine; THA) and lecithin in senile dementia of the Alzheimer type: a multi-centre trial. *British Medical Journal* **300**, 495–499 [504].

CHAUDHRY, M.R. & POND, D.A. (1961) Mental deterioration in epileptic children. *Journal of Neurology, Neurosurgery and Psychiatry* **24**, 213–219 [262, 263].

CHAUDRY, H.R., MOSS, H.B., BASHIR, A. & SULIMAN, T. (1991)

Cannabis psychosis following bhang ingestion. *British Journal of Addiction* **86**, 1075–1081 [614].

CHAUVEL, P., KLIEMANN, F., VIGNAL, J.P., CHODKIEWICZ, J.P., TALAIRACH, J. & BANCAUD, J. (1995) The clinical signs and symptoms of frontal lobe seizures. Phenomenology and classification. Ch. 9 in *Epilepsy and the Functional Anatomy of the Frontal Lobe*, eds Jasper, H.H., Riggio, S. & Goldman-Rakic, P.S. *Advances in Neurology*, Vol. 66. Raven Press: New York [249].

CHAWLUK, J.B., MESULAM, M.-M., HURTIG, H., KUSHNER, M., WEINTRAUB, S., SAYKIN, A., RUBIN, N., ALAVI, A. & REIVICH, M. (1986) Slowly progressive aphasia without generalized dementia: studies with positron emission tomography. *Annals of Neurology* **19**, 68–74 [752].

CHECKLEY, S.A. (1978) Thyrotoxicosis and the course of manic depressive illness. *British Journal of Psychiatry* **133**, 219–223 [509].

CHECKLEY, S. (1992) Neuroendocrinology. Ch. 16 in *Handbook of Affective Disorders*, 2nd edn, ed. Paykel, E.S. Churchill Livingstone: Edinburgh [507].

CHEE, C.P., DAVID, A., GALBRAITH, S. & GILLHAM, R. (1985) Dementia due to meningioma: outcome after surgical removal. *Surgical Neurology* **23**, 414–416 [222].

CHELLY, J., HAMARD, G., KOULAKOFF, A., KAPLAN, J.C., KAHN, A. & BERWALD-NETTER, Y. (1990) Dystrophin gene transcribed from different promoters in neuronal and glial cells. *Nature* **344**, 64–65 [716].

CHENG-MAYER, C. & LEVY, J.A. (1988) Distinct biological and serological properties of human immunodeficiency viruses from the brain. *Annals of Neurology* **23 (Supplement)**, S58–S61 [322].

CHERTKOW, H. & BUB, D. (1994) Functional activation and cognition: the ^{15}O PET subtraction method. Ch. 6 in *Localization and Neuroimaging in Neuropsychology*, ed. Kertesz, A. Academic Press: San Diego [46, 145, 146].

CHESSON, A.L., LEVINE, S.M., KONG, L.-S. & LEE, S.C. (1991) Neuroendocrine evaluation in Kleine–Levin syndrome: evidence of reduced dopaminergic tone during periods of hypersomnolence. *Sleep* **14**, 226–232 [732].

CHICK, J.D., SMITH, M.A., ENGLEMAN, H.M., KEAN, D.M., MANDER, A.J., DOUGLAS, R.H.B. & BEST, J.J.K. (1989) MRI of the brain in alcoholics: cerebral atrophy, lifetime alcoholic consumption, and cognitive deficits. *Alcoholism: Clinical and Experimental Research* **13**, 512–518 [606].

CHOI, D.W. & ROTHMAN, S.M. (1990) The role of glutamate neurotoxicity in hypoxic-ischaemic neuronal death. *Annual Reviews of Neuroscience* **13**, 171–182 [164].

CHOI, I.S. (1983) Delayed neurologic sequelae in carbon monoxide intoxication. *Archives of Neurology* **40**, 433–435 [551].

CHOLLET, F., DI PIERO, V., WISE, R.J.S., BROOKS, D.J., DOLAN, R. & FRACKOWIAK, R.S.J. (1991) The functional anatomy of motor recovery after stroke in humans: a study with positron emission tomography. *Annals of Neurology* **29**, 63–71 [378].

CHOPRA, G.S. & SMITH, J.W. (1974) Psychotic reactions following cannabis use in East Indians. *Archives of General Psychiatry* **30**, 24–27 [614].

CHRISTIANSEN, C., BAASTRUP, P.C. & TRANSÖ, I. (1976) Lithium, hypercalcaemia, hypermagnesaemia, and hyperparathyroidism. *Lancet* **2**, 969 [561].

CHRISTIANSEN, P., DEIGAARD, J. & LUND, M. (1975) Poteus, fertilitet og kønshormonudskillelse hos yugre mandlige epilepsilidende. *Ugeskrift for Laeger* **137**, 2402–2405 (English abstract) [272].

CHRISTIE, A.B. (1994) Survival in Alzheimer's disease. Ch. 6 in *Dementia*, eds Burns, A. & Levy, R. Chapman & Hall: London [435].

CHRISTIE, A.B. & WOOD, E.R.M. (1990) Further change in the pattern of mental illness in the elderly. *British Journal of Psychiatry* **157**, 228–231 [435].

CHRISTIE, J.E., KEAN, D.M., DOUGLAS, R.H.B., ENGLEMAN, H.M., ST CLAIR, D. & BLACKBURN, I.M. (1988) Magnetic resonance imaging in pre-senile dementia of the Alzheimer-type, multi-infarct dementia and Korsakoff's syndrome. *Psychological Medicine* **18**, 319–330 [139].

CHRISTIE BROWN, J. (1975) Late recovery from head injury: case report and review. *Psychological Medicine* **5**, 239–248 [186].

CHRISTISON, G.W., CASANOVA, M.F., WEINBERGER, D.R., RAWLINGS, R. & KLEINMAN, J.E. (1989) A quantitative investigation of hippocampal pyramidal cell size, shape, and variability of orientation in schizophrenia. *Archives of General Psychiatry* **46**, 1027–1032 [87].

CHUI, H.C., MORTIMER, J.A., SLAGER, U., ZAROW, C., BONDAREFF, W. & WEBSTER, D.D. (1986) Pathologic correlates of dementia in Parkinson's disease. *Archives of Neurology* **43**, 991–995 [655].

CHUI, H.C. & PERLMUTTER, L.S. (1992) Pathological correlates of dementia in Parkinson's disease. Ch. 13 in *Parkinson's Disease. Neurobehavioral Aspects*, eds Huber, S.J. & Cummings, J.L. Oxford University Press: Oxford [655].

CHUI, H.C., VICTOROFF, J.I., MARGOLIN, D., JAGUST, W., SHANKLE, R. & KATZMAN, R. (1992) Criteria for the diagnosis of ischemic vascular dementia proposed by the State of California Alzheimer's Disease Diagnostic and Treatment Centers. *Neurology* **42**, 473–480 [457].

CHYNOWETH, R. & FOLEY, J. (1969) Pre-senile dementia responding to steroid therapy. *British Journal of Psychiatry* **115**, 703–708 [425, 426, 506].

CIRAULO, D.A., SHADER, R.I., GREENBLATT, D.J. & CREELMAN, W. (1989) *Drug Interactions in Psychiatry*. Williams & Wilkins: Baltimore [625].

CIRIGNOTTA, F., CICOGNA, P. & LUGARESI, E. (1980a) Epileptic seizures during card games and draughts. *Epilepsia* **21**, 137–140 [248].

CIRIGNOTTA, F., TODESCO, C.V. & LUGARESI, E. (1980b) Temporal lobe epilepsy with ecstatic seizures (so-called Dostoevsky epilepsy). *Epilepsia* **21**, 705–710 [251].

CITRON, B.P., HALPERN, M., McCARRON, M., LUNDBERG, G.D., McCORMICK, R., PINCUS, I.J., TATTER, D. & HAVERBACK, B.J. (1970) Necrotizing angiitis associated with drug abuse. *The New England Journal of Medicine* **283**, 1003–1011 [620].

CLARK, A.F. & DAVISON, K. (1987) Mania following head injury: a report of two cases and a review of the literature. *British Journal of Psychiatry* **150**, 841–844 [192].

CLARK, A.N.G., MANKIKAR, G.D. & GRAY, I. (1975) Diogenes syndrome. A clinical study of gross neglect in old age. *Lancet* **1**, 366–368 [495].

CLARK, D.F. (1966) Behaviour therapy of Gilles de la Tourette's syndrome. *British Journal of Psychiatry* **112**, 771–778 [687].

CLARK, E.C. & BAILEY, A.A. (1956) Neurological and psychiatric signs associated with systemic lupus erythematosus. *Journal of the American Medical Association* **160**, 455–457 [420].

CLARK, E.C. & YOSS, R.E. (1956) Nervous system findings associated with systemic lupus erythematosus. *Minnesota Medicine* **39**, 517–520 [420].

CLARK, R.F. & GOATE, A.M. (1993) Molecular genetics of Alzheimer's disease. *Archives of Neurology* **50**, 1164–1172 [448].

CLARKE, E. & HARRISON, C.V. (1956) Bilateral carotid artery obstruction. *Neurology* **6**, 705–715 [384].

CLAUDE, H., BARUK, H. & LAMACHE, A. (1927) Obsessions-impulsions consécutives à l'encéphalite épidémique. *Encéphale* **22**, 716–720 [352].

CLAYER, J.R. & DUMBRILL, M.N. (1967) Diabetes mellitus and mental illness. *Medical Journal of Australia* 1, 901–904 [536].

CLEARE, A.J., JACOBY, R., TOVEY, S.J. & BERGMANN, K. (1993) Syphilis, neither dead nor buried—a survey of psychogeriatric inpatients. *International Journal of Geriatric Psychiatry* 8, 661–664 [343].

CLECKLEY, H.M., SYDENSTRICKER, V.P. & GEESLIN, L.E. (1939) Nicotinic acid in the treatment of atypical psychotic states associated with malnutrition. *Journal of the American Medical Association* 112(ii), 2107–2110 [574].

CLEGHORN, J.M., GARNETT, E.S., NAHMIAS, C., BROWN, G.M., KAPLAN, R.D., SZECHTMAN, H., SZECHTMAN, B., FRANCO, S., DERMER, S.W. & COOK, P. (1990) Regional brain metabolism during auditory hallucinations in chronic schizophrenia. *British Journal of Psychiatry* 157, 562–570 [88].

CLEGHORN, R.A. (1951) Adrenal cortical insufficiency: psychological and neurological observations. *Canadian Medical Association Journal* 65, 449–454 [519].

CLEGHORN, R.A. (1965) Hormones and humors. In *Hormonal Steroids. Biochemistry, Pharmacology, and Therapeutics*, Vol. 2, eds Martini, L. & Pecile, A. Academic Press: New York [519].

CLEMENTS, J.E., ANDERSON, M.G., ZINC, M.C., JOAG, S.V. & NARAYAN, O. (1994) The SIV model of AIDS encephalopathy. Role of neurotropic viruses in diseases. Ch. 8 in *HIV, AIDS and the Brain*, eds Price, R.W. & Perry, S.W. *Association for Research in Nervous and Mental Disease*, 72. Raven Press: New York [317].

CLEOBURY, J.F., SKINNER, G.R.B., THOULESS, M.E. & WILDY, P. (1971) Association between psychopathic disorder and serum antibody to herpes simplex virus (type 1). *British Medical Journal* 1, 438–439 [358].

CLOAKE, P.C.P. (1951) Certain vascular diseases of the nervous system. Ch. 14 in *Modern Trends in Neurology*, ed. Feiling, A. Butterworths: London [423, 425].

CLOUGH, C. (1987) Restless legs syndrome. *British Medical Journal* 294, 262–263 [640].

CLOW, A., JENNER, P. & MARSDEN, C.D. (1979a) Changes in dopamine mediated behaviour during one year's neuroleptic administration. *European Journal of Pharmacology* 57, 365–375 [644].

CLOW, A., JENNER, P., THEODOROU, A. & MARSDEN, C.D. (1979b) Striatal dopamine receptors become supersensitive while rats are given trifluoperazine for six months. *Nature* 278, 59–61 [644].

CO, B.T., GOODWIN, D.W., GADO, M., MIKHAEL, M. & HILL, S.Y. (1976) Absence of cerebral atrophy in chronic cannabis users. *Journal of the American Medical Association* 237, 1229–1230 [616].

COBB, S. & ROSE, R.M. (1973) Hypertension, peptic ulcer, and diabetes in air traffic controllers. *Journal of the American Medical Association* 224, 489–492 [397].

COBB, W.A. & MORGAN-HUGHES, J.A. (1968) Non-fatal subacute sclerosing leucoencephalitis. *Journal of Neurology, Neurosurgery and Psychiatry* 31, 115–123 [363].

COCHRANE, R. (1969) Neuroticism and the discovery of high blood pressure. *Journal of Pychosomatic Research* 13, 21–25 [398].

COCKBURN, J., WILSON, B., BADDELEY, A. & HIORNS, R. (1990) Assessing everyday memory in patients with dysphasia. *British Journal of Clinical Psychology* 29, 353–360 [117].

COCKBURN, J.J. (1971) Spasmodic torticollis: a psychogenic condition? *Journal of Psychosomatic Research* 15, 471–477 [674].

COHEN, D. & EISDORFER, C. (1980) Serum immunoglobulins and cognitive status in the elderly: 1. A population study. *British Journal of Psychiatry* 136, 33–39 [447].

COHEN, D. & MARKS, F.M. (1977) Gilles de la Tourette's syndrome treated by operant conditioning. *British Journal of Psychiatry* 130, 315 [687].

COHEN, D.J., DETLOR, R.N., YOUNG, G. & SHAYWITZ, B.A. (1980) Clonidine ameliorates Gilles de la Tourette syndrome. *Archives of General Psychiatry* 37, 1350–1357 [687].

COHEN, K.L. & SWIGAR, M.E. (1979) Thyroid function screening in psychiatric patients. *Journal of the American Medical Association* 242, 254–257 [510].

COHEN, N.J. & SQUIRE, L.R. (1981) Retrograde amnesia and remote memory impairment. *Neuropsychologia* 19, 337–356 [30, 36].

COHEN, S. & DITMAN, K.S. (1962) Complications associated with lysergic acid diethylamide (LSD-25). *Journal of the American Medical Association* 181, 161–162 [623].

COHEN, S. & DITMAN, K.S. (1963) Prolonged adverse reactions to lysergic acid diethylamide. *Archives of General Psychiatry* 8, 475–480 [623].

COHEN, S.I. (1980) Cushing's syndrome: a psychiatric study of 29 patients. *British Journal of Psychiatry* 36, 120–124 [516, 517, 518].

COHEN, W. & COHEN, N.H. (1974) Lithium carbonate, haloperidol, and irreversible brain damage. *Journal of the American Medical Association* 230, 1283–1287 [626, 627].

COHN, J.A. (1997) Recent advances. HIV infection—I. *British Medical Journal* 314, 487–491 [335, 336].

COHN, R. (1960) *The Person Symbol in Clinical Medicine*. Thomas: Springfield, Illinois [106].

COID, J. (1979) Mania à potu: a critical review of pathological intoxication. *Psychological Medicine* 9, 709–719 [595].

COLBOURN, C.J. & LISHMAN, W.A. (1979) Lateralisation of function and psychotic illness: a left hemisphere deficit? In *Hemisphere Asymmetries of Function in Psychopathology*, eds Gruzelier, J. & Flor-Henry, P., pp. 539–559. Elsevier/North Holland, Amsterdam [89].

COLE, E.S. (1970) Psychiatric aspects of compensable injury. *Medical Journal of Australia* 1, 93–100 [176].

COLE, G. (1978) Intracranial space-occupying masses in mental hospital patients: necropsy study. *Journal of Neurology, Neurosurgery and Psychiatry* 41, 730–736 [411].

COLE, M., RICHARDSON, E.P. & SEGERRA, J.N. (1964) Central pontine myelinolysis: further evidence relating the lesion to malnutrition. *Neurology* 14, 165–170 [586].

COLEMAN, R.M., ROFFWARG, H.P., KENNEDY, S.J.,GUILLEMINAULT, C., CINQUE, J., COHN, M.A., KARACAN, I., KUPFER, D.J., LEMMI, H., MILES, L.E., ORR, W.C., PHILLIPS, E.R., ROTH, T., SASSIN, J.F., SCHMIDT, H.S., WEITZMAN, E.D. & DEMENT, W.C. (1982) Sleep–wake disorders based on a polysomnographic diagnosis. A national cooperative study. *Journal of the American Medical Association* 247, 997–1003 [729, 731].

COLLEGE OF GENERAL PRACTIONERS REPORT (1960) A survey of the epilepsies in general practice. A report by the research committee of the College of General Practitioners. *British Medical Journal* 2, 416–422 [242, 259].

COLLIGNON, R., BRAYER, R., RECTEM, D., INDEICEU, P. & LATERRE, E.C. (1979) Analyse sémiologique de l'encéphalopathie bismuthique. Confrontation avec sept cas personnels. *Acta Neurologica Belgica* 79, 73–91 [636, 637].

COLLINGE, J., BROWN, J., HARDY, J., MULLAN, M., ROSSOR, M., BAKER, H., CROW, T.J., LOFTHOUSE, R., POULTER, M., RIDLEY, R., OWEN, F., BENNETT, C., DUNN, G., HARDING, A.E., QUINN, N., DOSHI, B., ROBERTS, G.W., HONAVAR, M., JANOTA, I. & LANTOS, P.L. (1992) Inherited prion disease with 144 base pair gene insertion. *Brain* 115, 687–710 [479].

COLLINGE, J., HARDING, A.E., OWEN, F., POULTER, M., LOFTHOUSE, R., BOUGHEY, A.M., SHAH, T. & CROW, T.J. (1989) Diagnosis of Gerstmann–Sträussler syndrome in familial dementia with prion protein gene analysis. *Lancet* **2**, 15–17 [479].

COLLINGE, J., OWEN, F., POULTER, M., LEACH, M., CROW, T.J., ROSSOR, M.N., HARDY, J., MULLAN, M.J., JANOTA, I. & LANTOS, P.L. (1990) Prion dementia without characteristic pathology. *Lancet* **336**, 7–9 [479].

COLLINGE, J. & PALMER, M.S. (1994) Prion diseases. Ch. 53 in *Dementia*, eds Burns, A. & Levy, R. Chapman & Hall: London [475].

COLLINGE, J., PALMER, M.S. & DRYDEN, A.J. (1991) Genetic predisposition to iatrogenic Creutzfeldt–Jakob disease. *Lancet* **337**, 1441–1442 [476].

COLLINGE, J. & ROSSOR, M. (1996) A new variant of prion disease. *Lancet* **347**, 916–917 [475].

COLLINGE, J., SIDLE, K.C.L., MEADS, J., IRONSIDE, J. & HILL, A.F. (1996) Molecular analysis of prion strain variation and the aetiology of 'new variant' CJD. *Nature* **383**, 685–690 [476].

COLLINS, P. (1961) The almoner's role. In *Stroke Rehabilitation*. The Chest and Heart Association: Tavistock Square, London [391].

COLLINS, R.T. (1939) Psychiatric syndromes in myasthenia gravis. *British Medical Journals* **1**, 975–977 [712].

COLLIS, I. & LLOYD, G. (1992) Psychiatric aspects of liver disease. *British Journal of Psychiatry* **161**, 12–22 [563].

COLON, E.J. (1973) The cerebral cortex in presenile dementia. A quantitative analysis. *Acta Neuropathologica (Berlin)* **23**, 281–290 [443].

COLTHEART, M., PATTERSON, K. & MARSHALL, J.C. (eds) (1987) *Deep Dyslexia*, 2nd edn. Routledge & Kegan Paul: London [43].

COMMISSION ON CLASSIFICATION AND TERMINOLOGY OF THE INTERNATIONAL LEAGUE AGAINST EPILEPSY (1981) Proposal for revised clinical and electroencephalographic classification of epileptic seizures. *Epilepsia* **22**, 489–501 [238, 240, 249].

COMMISSION ON CLASSIFICATION AND TERMINOLOGY OF THE INTERNATIONAL LEAGUE AGAINST EPILEPSY (1989) Proposal for revised classification of epilepsy and epileptic syndromes. *Epilepsia* **30**, 389–399 [242].

COMMITTEE ON SAFETY OF MEDICINES (1994) Antidepressant-induced hyponatraemia. *Current Problems in Pharmacovigilance* **20**, 5–6 [526].

COMMUNICABLE DISEASE REPORT (1994a) AIDS and HIV-1 infection worldwide. *Communicable Disease Report* **4**, 221–222 [315, 316].

COMMUNICABLE DISEASE REPORT (1994b) AIDS and HIV-1 infection in the United Kingdom: monthly report. *Communicable Disease Report* **4**, 239–240 [316].

COMMUNICABLE DISEASE REPORT (1995) AIDS and HIV-1 infection in the United Kingdom: monthly report. *Communicable Disease Report* **5**, 13–16 [315].

COMMUNICABLE DISEASE REPORT REVIEW (1993) Unlinked anonymous monitoring of HIV prevalence in England and Wales: 1990–92. *Communicable Disease Report*, **3** (Review No.1), R1-R11 [316].

COMMUNICABLE DISEASE REPORT REVIEW (1994) The changing clinical features of HIV-1 infection in the United Kingdom. *Communicable Disease Report*, **4**, R53-R58 [317, 318].

COMPSTON, A. (1993) Non-infective inflammatory demyelinating, and paraneoplastic diseases of the nervous system. Ch. 10 in *Brain's Diseases of the Nervous System*, 10th edn, ed. Walton, J. Oxford University Press: Oxford [586, 688, 689, 690, 699, 740, 743, 755].

CONCORDE COORDINATING COMMITTEE (1994) Concorde: MRC/ANRS randomised double-blind controlled trial of immediate and deferred zidovudine in symptom-free HIV infection. *Lancet* **343**, 871–881 [336].

CONLON, P., TRIMBLE, M.R. & ROGERS, D. (1990) A study of epileptic psychosis using magnetic resonance imaging. *British Journal of Psychiatry* **156**, 231–235 [281].

CONNELL, P.H. (1958) *Amphetamine Psychosis*. Maudsley Monograph No. 5. Chapman & Hall: London [617].

CONNELL, P.H. (1968) Central nervous system stimulant and antidepressant drugs. Ch. 1 in *Side Effects of Drugs*, eds Meyler, L. & Herxheimer, A. Exerpta Medica: Amsterdam [626].

CONNELL, P.H., CORBETT, J.A., MATHEWS, A.M. & HORNE, D.J. (1967) Drug treatment of adolescent ticquers. A double blind trial of diazepam and haloperidol. *British Journal of Psychiatry* **113**, 375–381 [687].

CONNOLLY, J.F., GRUZELIER, J.H. & MANCHANDA, R. (1983) Electrocortical and perceptual asymmetries in schizophrenia. In *Laterality and Psychopathology*, eds Flor-Henry, P. & Gruzelier, J.J., pp. 363–378. Elsevier: Amsterdam [89].

CONNOLLY, J.H., ALLEN, I.V. & DERMOTT, E. (1988) Transmissible agent in the amyotrophic form of Creutzfeldt–Jakob disease. *Journal of Neurology, Neurosurgery and Psychiatry* **51**, 1459–1460 [479].

CONNOLLY, J.H., ALLEN, I.V., HURWITZ, L.J. & MILLER, J.H.D. (1967) Measles-virus antibody and antigen in subacute sclerosing panencephalitis. *Lancet* **1**, 542–544 [362].

CONRAD, A.J., ABEBE, T., AUSTIN, R., FORSYTHE, S. & SCHEIBEL, A.B. (1991) Hippocampal pyramidal cell disarray in schizophrenia as a bilateral phenomenon. *Archives of General Psychiatry* **48**, 413–417 [86].

CONRAD, A.J. & SCHEIBEL, A.B. (1987) Schizophrenia and the hippocampus: the embryological hypothesis extended. *Schizophrenia Bulletin* **13**, 577–587 [86].

CONSTANTINIDIS, J. (1985) Pick dementia: anatomoclinical correlations and pathophysiological considerations. *Interdisciplinary Topics in Gerontology* **19**, 72–97 [461].

CONSTANTINIDIS, J., GARRONE, G. & AJURIAGUERRA, J. DE (1962) L'hérédité des démences de l'âge avancé. *Encéphale* **51**, 301–344 [430].

CONSTANTINIDIS, J., RICHARD, J. & TISSOT, R. (1974) Pick's disease: histological and clinical correlations. *European Neurology* **11**, 208–217 [462].

CONSTANTINIDIS, J., RICHARD, J. & TISSOT, R. (1977) Maladie de Pick et métabolism du zinc. *Revue Neurologique* **133**, 685–696 [461].

COOK, M.J., FISH, D.R., SHORVON, S.D., STRAUGHAN, K. & STEVENS, J.M. (1992) Hippocampal volumetric and morphometric studies in frontal and temporal lobe epilepsy. *Brain* **115**, 1001–1015 [289].

COOK, R.H., WARD, B.E. & AUSTIN, J.H. (1979) Studies in aging of the brain: IV. Familial Alzheimer's disease: relation to transmissible dementia, aneuploidy, and microtubular defects. *Neurology* **29**, 1402–1412 [437].

COOPER, A.F. & SCHAPIRA, K. (1973) Case report: depression, catatonic stupor, and EEG changes in hyperparathyroidism. *Psychological Medicine* **3**, 509–515 [529, 530].

COOPER, R. (1994a) Normal sleep. Ch. 1 in *Sleep*, ed. Cooper, R. Chapman & Hall: London [725].

COOPER, R. (1994b) Neurology and sleep disorders. Ch. 17 in *Sleep*, ed. Cooper, R. Chapman & Hall: London [726, 729].

COOPER, S.J. (1992) Schizophrenia after prenatal exposure to 1957 A2 influenza epidemic. *British Journal of Psychiatry* **161**, 394–396 [91].

COPE, H. & DAVID, A.S. (1996) Neuroimaging in chronic fatigue syndrome. *Journal of Neurology, Neurosurgery and Psychiatry* **60**, 471–473 [372].

COPE, R.V. & GREGG, E.M. (1983) Neuroleptic malignant syndrome. *British Medical Journal* **286**, 1938 [626].

COPELAND, J.R.M., DAVIDSON, I.A., DEWEY, M.E., GILMORE, C., LARKIN, B.A., McWILLIAM, C., SAUNDERS, P.A., SCOTT, A., SHARMA, V. & SULLIVAN, C. (1992) Alzheimer's disease, other dementias, depression and pseudodementia: prevalence, incidence and three-year outcome in Liverpool. *British Journal of Psychiatry* **161**, 230–239 [124].

COPELAND, J.R.M., DEWEY, M.E. & GRIFFITH-JONES, H.M. (1986) Computerised diagnostic system and case nomenclature for elderly subjects: GMS and AGECAT. *Psychological Medicine* **16**, 89–99 [124].

COPELAND, J.R.M., DEWEY, M.E. & GRIFFITH-JONES, H.M. (1990) Dementia and depression in elderly persons: AGECAT compared with DSM III and pervasive illness. *International Journal of Geriatric Psychiatry* **5**, 47–51 [124].

COPELAND, J.R.M., KELLEHER, M.J., KELLETT, J.M., GOURLAY, A.J., GURLAND, B.J., FLEISS, J.L. & SHARPE, L. (1976) A semi-structured clinical interview for the assessment of diagnosis and mental state in the elderly: the Geriatric Mental State Schedule. *Psychological Medicine* **6**, 439–449 [123, 124].

COPPEN, A. & ABOU-SALEH, M.T. (1982) Plasma folate and affective morbidity during long-term lithium therapy. *British Journal of Psychiatry* **141**, 87–89 [591].

CORBETT, J.A. (1971) The nature of tics and Gilles de la Tourette's syndrome. *Journal of Psychosomatic Research* **15**, 403–409 [683, 684].

CORBETT, J.A., MATHEWS, A.M., CONNELL, P.H. & SHAPIRO, D.A. (1969) Tics and Gilles de la Tourette's syndrome: a follow-up study and critical review. *British Journal of Psychiatry* **115**, 1229–1241 [683, 684].

CORDER, E.H., SAUNDERS, A.M., RISCH, N.J., STRITTMATTER, W.J., SCHMECHEL, D.E., GASKELL, P.C., RIMMLER, J.B., LOCKE, P.A., CON-NEALLY, P.M., SCHMADER, K.E., SMALL, G.W., ROSES, A.D., HAINES, J.L. & PERICAK-VANCE, M.A. (1994) Protective effect of apolipoprotein E type 2 allele for late onset Alzheimer disease. *Nature Genetics* **7**, 180–184 [448].

CORDER, E.H., SAUNDERS, A.M., STRITTMATTER, W.J., SCHMECHEL, D.E., GASKELL, P.C., SMALL, G.W., ROSES, A.D., HAINES, J.L. & PERICAK-VANCE, M.A. (1993) Gene dose of apolipoprotein E type 4 allele and the risk of Alzheimer's disease in late onset families. *Science* **261**, 921–923 [448].

CORDINGLEY, G., NAVARRO, C., BRUST, J.C.M. & HEALTON, E. (1981) Sarcoidosis presenting as senile dementia. *Neurology* **31**, 1148–1151 [764, 765].

COREN, H.Z. & STRAIN, J.J. (1965) A case of narcolepsy with psychosis (paranoid state of narcolepsy). *Comprehensive Psychiatry* **6**, 191–199 [728].

CORKIN, S. (1968) Acquisition of motor skill after bilateral medial temporal lobe excision. *Neuropsychologia* **6**, 255–265 [30].

CORKIN, S. (1982) Some relationships between global amnesias and the memory impairments in Alzheimer's disease. In *Alzheimer's Disease: A Report of Progress in Research, Aging*, Vol. 19, eds Corkin, S., Davis, K.L., Growdon, J.H., Usdin, E. & Wurtman, R.J., pp. 149–164. Raven Press: New York [32].

CORKIN, S., DAVIS, K.L., GROWDON, J.H., USDIN, E. & WURTMAN, R.J. (eds) (1982) *Alzheimer's Disease: A Report of Progress in Research, Aging*, Vol. 19. Raven Press: New York [503].

CORKIN, S., GROWDON, J.H., NISSEN, M.J., HUFP, F.J., FREED, D.M. & SAGAR, H.J. (1984) Recent advances in the neuropsychological study of Alzheimer's disease. In *Alzheimer's Disease: Advances in Basic Research and Therapies. Proceedings of The Third Meeting of the International Study Group on the Treatment of Memory Disorders Associated with Ageing*, eds Wurtman, R.J., Corkin, S. & Growdon, J.H., pp. 75–94. Center for Brain Sciences and Metabolism Charitable Trust [32].

CORKIN, S., ROSEN, J., SULLIVAN, E.V. & CLEGG, R.A. (1989) Penetrating head injury in young adulthood exacerbates cognitive decline in later years. *Journal of Neuroscience* **9**, 3876–3883 [186, 264, 438].

CORSELLIS, J.A.N. (1962) *Mental Illness and the Ageing Brain*. Maudsley Monograph No. 9. Oxford University Press: Oxford [435, 455].

CORSELLIS, J.A.N. (1969a) Subacute encephalitis and malignancy. In *Virus Diseases of the Nervous System*, eds Whitty, C.W.M., Hughes, J.T. & MacCallum, F.O. Blackwell Scientific Publications: Oxford [364].

CORSELLIS, J.A.N. (1969b) The pathology of dementia. *British Journal of Hospital Medicine* **2**, 695–702 [435, 449, 453, 455].

CORSELLIS, J.A.N. (1970) The limbic areas in Alzheimer's disease and in other conditions associated with dementia. In *Alzheimer's Disease and Related Conditions*, CIBA Foundation Symposium, eds Wolstenholme, G.E.W. & O'Connor, M. Churchill: London [32, 440].

CORSELLIS, J.A.N. (1979) On the transmission of dementia: a personal view of the slow virus problem. *British Journal of Psychiatry* **134**, 553–559 [477].

CORSELLIS, J.A.N. (1989) Boxing and the brain. *British Medical Journal* **298**, 105–109 [207].

CORSELLIS, J.A.N. & BRIERLEY, J.B. (1954) An unusual type of presenile dementia (atypical Alzheimer's disease with amyloid vascular change). *Brain* **77**, 571–587 [441].

CORSELLIS, J.A.N. & BRIERLEY, J.B. (1959) Observations on the pathology of insidious dementia following head injury. *Journal of Mental Science* **105**, 714–720 [186].

CORSELLIS, J.A.N., BRUTON, C.J. & FREEMAN-BROWN, E.D. (1973) The aftermath of boxing. *Psychological Medicine* **3**, 270–303 [207].

CORSELLIS, J.A.N. & EVANS, P.H. (1965) The relation of stenosis of the extracranial cerebral arteries to mental disorder and cerebral degeneration in old age. In *Proceedings of the Fifth International Congress of Neuropathology*. Exerpta Medica: Amsterdam [384].

CORSELLIS, J.A.N., GOLDBERG, G.J. & NORTON, A.R. (1968) 'Limbic encephalitis' and its associations with carcinoma. *Brain* **91**, 481–496 [742, 743].

CORSTON, R.N. & GODWIN-AUSTEN, R.B. (1982) Transient global amnesia in four brothers. *Journal of Neurology, Neurosurgery and Psychiatry* **45**, 375–377 [416].

CORWIN, J., SERBY, M., CONRAD, P. & ROTROSEN, J. (1985) Olfactory recognition deficit in Alzheimer's and Parkinsonian dementias. *IRCS Journal of Medical Science* **13**, 260 [441].

COSIN, L.Z., MORT, M., POST, F., WESTROPP, C. & WILLIAMS, M. (1958) Experimental treatment of persistent senile confusion. *International Journal of Social Psychiatry* **4**, 24–42 [500].

COSLETT, B. & SAFFRAN, E. (1991) Simultanagnosia. To see but not two see. *Brain* **114**, 1523–1545 [61].

COSTA, D.C. & ELL, P.J. (1991) *Brain Blood Flow in Neurology and Psychiatry*. Churchill Livingstone: Edinburgh & London [147, 289, 377].

COSTA, D.C., ELL, P.J., BURNS, A., PHILPOT, M. & LEVY, R. (1988) CBF tomograms with $^{99m}T_c$-HMPAO in patients with dementia (Alzheimer type and HIV) and Parkinson's disease—initial results. *Journal of Cerebral Blood Flow and Metabolism*, **8**, S109–S115 [325].

COSTA, D.C., TANNOCK, C. & BROSTOFF, J. (1995) Brainstem perfusion is impaired in chronic fatigue syndrome. *Quarterly Journal of Medicine* **88**, 767–773 [372].

COSTA, L.D. & VAUGHAN, H.G. (1962) Performance of patients with lateralised cerebral lesions, 1: Verbal and perceptual tests. *Journal of Nervous and Mental Disease* **134**, 162–168 [112].

COTTRAUX, J.A., JUENET, C. & COLLET, L. (1983) The treatment of writer's cramp with multimodal behaviour therapy and biofeedback: a study of 15 cases. *British Journal of Psychiatry* **142**, 180–183 [677].

COTTRELL, S.S. & WILSON, S.A.K. (1926) The affective symptomatology of disseminated sclerosis: a study of 100 cases. *Journal of Neurology and Psychopathology* **7**, 1–30 [691, 695, 696].

COUCH, J.R. (1976) Dystonia and tremor in spasmodic torticollis. *Advances in Neurology*, Vol. 14, eds Eldridge, R. & Fahn, S. Raven Press: New York [674].

COUGHLAN, A.K. & HOLLOWS, S.E. (1985) *The Adult Memory and Information Processing Battery*. A.K. Coughlan, Psychology Department, St James University Hospital: Leeds [117].

COUSENS, S.N., ZEIDLER, M., ESMONDE, T.F., DE SILVA, R., WILESMITH, J.W., SMITH, P.G. & WILL, R.G. (1997) Sporadic Creutzfeldt–Jakob disease in the United Kingdom: analysis of epidemiological surveillance data for 1970–96. *British Medical Journal* **315**, 389–395 [475].

COURVILLE, C.B. (1955) *The Effects of Alcohol on the Nervous System of Man*. San Lucas Press: Los Angeles [604].

COWBURN, R., HARDY, J., ROBERTS, P. & BRIGGS, R. (1988a) Presynaptic and postsynaptic glutamatergic function in Alzheimer's disease. *Neuroscience Letters* **86**, 109–113 [445].

COWBURN, R., HARDY, J., ROBERTS, P. & BRIGGS, R. (1988b) Regional distribution of pre- and postsynaptic glutamatergic function in Alzheimer's disease. *Brain Research* **452**, 403–407 [445].

CRAMMER, J. & GILLIES, C. (1981) Psychiatric aspects of diabetes mellitus: diabetes and depression. *British Journal of Psychiatry* **139**, 171–172 [536].

CRAPPER, D.R., KARLIK, S. & DE BONI, U. (1978) Aluminium and other metals in senile (Alzheimer) dementia. In *Alzheimer's Disease: Senile Dementia and Related Conditions, Aging*, Vol. 7, eds Katzman, R., Terry, R.D. & Bick, K.L., pp. 471–485. Raven Press: New York [446].

CRAPPER, D.R., KRISHNAN, S.S. & QUITTKAT, S. (1976) Aluminium, neurofibrillary degeneration and Alzheimer's disease. *Brain* **99**, 67–80 [446].

CRAPPER McLACHLAN, D.R., DALTON, A.J., KRUCK, T.P.A., BELL, M.Y., SMITH, W.L., KALOW, W. & ANDREWS, D.F. (1991) Intramuscular desferrioxamine in patients with Alzheimer's disease. *Lancet* **337**, 1304–1308 [446].

CRAPPER McLACHLAN, D.R. & DE BONI, U. (1980) Etiologic factors in senile dementia of the Alzheimer type. In *Aging of the Brain and Dementia, Aging*, Vol. 13, eds Amaducci, L. & Davidson, A.N., pp. 173–181. Raven Press: New York [447].

CRAUFURD, D. (1989) Progress and problems in Huntington's disease. *International Review of Psychiatry* **1**, 249–258 [466, 467].

CRAUFURD, D.I.O. & HARRIS, R. (1986) Ethics of predictive testing for Huntington's chorea: the need for more information. *British Medical Journal* **293**, 249–251 [467].

CRAUFURD, D. & TYLER, A. (1992) (On behalf of the UK Huntington's Disease Prediction Consortium) Predictive testing for Huntington's disease: protocol of the UK Huntington's Prediction Consortium. *Journal of Medical Genetics* **29**, 915–918 [467].

CRAVIOTO, H., KOREIN, J. & SILBERMAN, J. (1961) Wernicke's encephalopathy: a clinical and pathological study of 28 autopsied cases. *Archives of Neurology* **4**, 510–519 [578, 580].

CRAWFORD, J.R., ALLAN, K.M., BESSON, J.A.O., COCHRANE, R.H.B. & STEWART, L.E. (1990a) A comparison of the WAIS and WAIS-R in matched UK samples. *British Journal of Clinical Psychology* **29**, 105–109 [110].

CRAWFORD, J.R., ALLAN, K.M. & JACK, A.M. (1992a) Short-forms of the UK WAIS-R: regression equations and their predictive validity in a general population sample. *British Journal of Clinical Psychology* **31**, 191–202 [110].

CRAWFORD, J.R., HART, S. & NELSON, H.E. (1990b) Improved detection of cognitive impairment with the NART: an investigation employing hierarchical discriminant function analysis. *British Journal of Clinical Psychology* **29**, 239–241 [111].

CRAWFORD, J.R., MOORE, J.W. & CAMERON, I.M. (1992b) Verbal fluency: a NART-based equation for the estimation of premorbid performance. *British Journal of Clinical Psychology* **31**, 327–329 [112].

CRAWFORD, J.R., PARKER, D.M. & McKINLAY, W.W. (1992c) *A Handbook of Neuropsychological Assessment*. Lawrence Erlbaum: Hove [110].

CRAWLEY, J.W.C., CROW, T.J., JOHNSTONE, E.C., OLDLAND, S.R.D., OWEN, F., OWENS, D.G.C., SMITH, T., VEALL, N. & ZANELLI, G.D. (1986) Uptake of ^{77}Br-spiperone in the striata of schizophrenic patients and controls. *Nuclear Medicine Communications* **7**, 599–607 [88, 148].

CRAWSHAW, J.A. & MULLEN, P.E. (1984) A study of benzhexol abuse. *British Journal of Psychiatry* **145**, 300–303 [658].

CREIGHTON, F.J., BLACK, D.L. & HYDE, C.E. (1991) 'Ecstasy' psychosis and flashbacks. *British Journal of Psychiatry* **159**, 713–715 [624].

CRÉMIEUX, A., ALLIEZ, J., TOGA, M. & PACHE, R. (1959) Sclérose en plaques à début par troubles mentaux. Etude anatomo-clinique. *Revue Neurologique* **101**, 45–51 [697].

CREUTZFELDT, H.G. (1920) Über eine eigenartige herdförmige Erkrankung des Zentralnervensystems. *Zeitschrift für die gesamte Neurologie und Psychiatrie* **57**, 1–18 [473].

CRISP, A.H. & MOLDOFSKY, H. (1965) A psychosomatic study of writer's cramp. *British Journal of Psychiatry* **111**, 841–858 [676].

CRITCHLEY, E.M.R. (1987) *Language and Speech Disorders: A Neurophysiological Approach*. CNS (Clinical Neuroscience) Publishers: London [49].

CRITCHLEY, M. (1931) The neurology of old age. *Lancet* **1**, 1221–1230 [96].

CRITCHLEY, M. (1937) Musicogenic epilepsy. *Brain* **60**, 13–27 [241].

CRITCHLEY, M. (1953) *The Parietal Lobes*. Edward Arnold: London [68, 105].

CRITCHLEY, M. (1954) Discussion on volitional movement. *Proceedings of the Royal Society of Medicine* **47**, 593–599 [675].

CRITCHLEY, M. (1957) Medical aspects of boxing, particularly from a neurological standpoint. *British Medical Journal* **1**, 357–362 [204].

CRITCHLEY, M. (1962) Periodic hypersomnia and megaphagia in adolescent males. *Brain* **85**, 627–656 [732].

CRITCHLEY, M. (1964) Psychiatric symptoms and parietal disease: differential diagnosis. *Proceedings of the Royal Society of Medicine* **57**, 422–428 [69, 227].

CRITCHLEY, M. (1969) Definition of migraine. Ch. 18 in *Background to Migraine*. Third Migraine Symposium, ed. Cochrane, A.L. Heinemann: London [399].

CRITCHLEY, M., COBB, W. & SEARS, T.A. (1959) On reading epilepsy. *Epilepsia* **1**, 403–417 [241].

CRITCHLEY, M. & EARL, C.J.C. (1932) Tuberose sclerosis and allied conditions. *Brain* **55**, 311–346 [702].

CRITCHLEY, P., PEREZ, F.G., QUINN, N., COLEMAN, R., PARKES, D. & MARSDEN, C.D. (1986) Psychosis and the lisuride pump. *Lancet* **2**, 349 [659].

CROCKARD, A., McKEE, H., JOSHI, K. & ALLEN, I. (1980) ICP, CAT scans and psychometric assessment in dementia: a prospective analysis. In *Intracranial Pressure, IV*, eds Shulman, K., Mannsrou,

A., Miller, J.D., Becker, D.P., Hochwald, G.M. & Brock, M., pp. 501–504. Springer-Verlag: Berlin [748].

CROFT, P.B., HEATHFIELD, K.W.G. & SWASH, M. (1973) Differential diagnosis of transient amnesia. *British Medical Journal* **4**, 593–596 [416].

CROFT, P.B. & WILKINSON, M. (1965) The incidence of carcinomatous neuromyopathy with special reference to carcinoma of the lung and breast. Ch. 6 in *The Remote Effects of Cancer on the Nervous System*, eds Brain, W.R. & Norris, F.H. Contemporary Neurology Syraposia, Vol. 1. Grune & Stratton: New York [739].

CRONIN-STUBBS, D., BECKETT, L.A., SCHERR, P.A., FIELD, T.S., CHOWN, M.J., PILGRIM, D.M., BENNETT, D.A. & EVANS, D.A. (1997) Weight loss in people with Alzheimer's disease: a prospective population based analysis. *British Medical Journal* **314**, 178–179 [435].

CROOK, T., BARTUS, R.T., FERRIS, S.H., WHITEHOUSE, P., COHEN, G.D. & GERSHON, S. (1986) Age-associated memory impairment: proposed diagnostic criteria and measures of clinical change—report of a National Institute of Mental Health Work Group. *Developmental Neuropsychology* **2**, 261–276 [432].

CROSS, A.J., CROW, T.J., JOHNSON, J.A., JOSEPH, M.H., PERRY, E.K., PERRY, R.H., BLESSED, G. & TOMLINSON, B.E. (1983) Monoamine metabolism in senile dementia of Alzheimer type. *Journal of the Neurological Sciences* **60**, 383–392 [444].

CROSS, A.J., CROW, T.J., JOHNSON, J.A., PERRY, E.K., PERRY, R.H., BLESSED, G. & TOMLINSON, B.E. (1984) Studies on neurotransmitter receptor systems in neocortex and hippocampus in senile dementia of the Alzheimer-type. *Journal of the Neurological Sciences* **64**, 109–117 [444].

CROSS, A.J., CROW, T.J., PERRY, E.K., PERRY, R.H., BLESSED, G. & TOMLINSON, B.E. (1981) Radical dopamine-beta-hydroxylase activity in Alzheimer's disease. *British Medical Journal* **282**, 93–94 [444].

CROW, T.J. (1978) Viral causes of psychiatric disease. *Postgraduate Medical Journal* **54**, 763–767 [347].

CROW, T.J. (1983a) Discussion: schizophrenic deterioration. *British Journal of Psychiatry* **143**, 80–81 [92].

CROW, T.J. (1983b) Is schizophrenia an infectious disease? *Lancet* **1**, 173–175 [92].

CROW, T.J. (1984) A re-evaluation of the viral hypothesis: is psychosis the result of retroviral integration at a site close to the cerebral dominance gene? *British Journal of Psychiatry* **145**, 243–253 [92].

CROW, T.J. (1986) Left brain, retrotransposons, and schizophrenia. *British Medical Journal* **293**, 3–4 [93].

CROW, T.J. (1987a) Psychosis as a continuum and the virogene concept. *British Medical Bulletin* **43**, 754–767 [93].

CROW, T.J. (1987b) Integrated viral genes as potential pathogens in the functional psychoses. *Journal of Psychiatric Research* **21**, 479–485 [93].

CROW, T.J. (1987c) Mutation and psychosis: a suggested explanation of seasonality of birth. *Psychological Medicine* **17**, 821–828 [93].

CROW, T.J. (1990) Temporal lobe asymmetries as the key to the etiology of schizophrenia. *Schizophrenia Bulletin* **16**, 433–443 [93].

CROW, T.J., BALL, J., BLOOM, S.R., BROWN, R., BRUTON, C.J., COLTER, N., FRITH, C.D., JOHNSTONE, E.C., OWENS, D.G.C. & ROBERTS, G.W. (1989) Schizophrenia as an anomaly of development of cerebral asymmetry. *Archives of General Psychiatry* **46**, 1145–1150 [86].

CROW, T.J. & DONE, D.J. (1992) Prenatal exposure to influenza does not cause schizophrenia. *British Journal of Psychiatry* **161**, 390–393 [91].

CROW, T.J., JOHNSTONE, E.C. & McCLELLAND, H.A. (1976) The coincidence of schizophrenia and parkinsonism: some neurochemical implications. *Psychological Medicine* **6**, 227–233 [657].

CROW, T.J., JOHNSTONE, E.C., OWENS, D.G.C., FERRIER, I.N., MacMILLAN, J.F., PARRY, R.P. & TYRELL, D.A.J. (1979) Characteristics of patients with schizophrenia or neurological disorder and virus-like agent in cerebrospinal fluid. *Lancet* **1**, 842–844 [92].

CROWELL, G.F., STUMP, D.A., BILLER, J., McHENRY, L.C. & TOOLE, J.F. (1984) The transient global amnesia–migraine connection. *Archives of Neurology* **41**, 75–79 [417].

CROWELL, R.M., TEW, J.M. & MARK, V.H. (1973) Aggressive dementia associated with normal pressure hydrocephalus. *Neurology* **23**, 461–464 [745].

CROWN, S. (1971) Psychosomatic aspects of parkinsonism. *Journal of Psychosomatic Research* **15**, 451–459 [660].

CRUICKSHANK, E.K. (1961) Neuropsychiatric disorders in prisoners-of-war. In *Psychiatrie det Gegenwar*, Vol. 3, eds Gruhle, H.W., Jung, R., Mayer-Gross, W. & Muller, M., pp. 807–836. Springer: Berlin [577].

CRUZ-COKE, R. (1960) Environmental influences and arterial blood-pressure. *Lancet* **2**, 885–886 [397].

CRYSTAL, H.A., HOROUPIAN, D.S., KATZMAN, R. & JOTKOWITZ, S. (1982) Biopsy-proved Alzheimer disease presenting as a right parietal lobe syndrome. *Annals of Neurology* **12**, 186–188 [754].

CULEBRAS, A., FELDMAN, R.G. & MERK, F.B. (1973) Cytoplasmic inclusion bodies within neurons of the thalamus in myotonic dystrophy. *Journal of the Neurological Sciences* **19**, 319–329 [719].

CULL, R., GILLIATT, R.W., WILLISON, R.G. & QUY, R. (1982) Prolonged observation and EEG monitoring of epileptic patients. In *A Textbook of Epilepsy*, 2nd edn, eds Laidlaw, J. & Richens, A., pp. 211–226. Churchill Livingstone: Edinburgh & London [288].

CULVER, C.M. & KING, F.W. (1974) Neuropsychological assessment of undergraduate marihuana and LSD users. *Archives of General Psychiatry* **31**, 707–711 [616].

CUMMINGS, J.L. (1982) Cortical dementias. Ch. 5 in *Psychiatric Aspects of Neurologic Disease*, Vol. 2, eds Benson, D.F. & Blumer, D. Grune & Stratton: York [668].

CUMMINGS, J.L. (1992a) Psychosis in neurologic disease. Neurobiology and pathogenesis. *Neuropsychiatry, Neuropsychology, and Behavioral Neurology* **5**, 144–150 [15].

CUMMINGS, J.L. (1992b) Neuropsychiatric complications of drug treatment of Parkinson's disease. Ch. 23 in *Parkinson's Disease. Neurobehavioral Aspects*, eds Huber, S.J. & Cummings, J.L. Oxford University Press: Oxford [658].

CUMMINGS, J.L. & BENSON, D.F. (1992) *Dementia: A Clinical Approach*, 2nd edn. Butterworth-Heinemann: Boston & London [758].

CUMMINGS, J.L. & DUCHEN, L.W. (1981) Klüver-Bucy syndrome in Pick disease: clinical and pathologic correlations. *Neurology* **31**, 1415–1422 [461, 463].

CUMMINGS, J.L. & FRANKEL, M. (1985) Gilles de la Tourette syndrome and the neurological basis of obsessions and compulsions. *Biological Psychiatry* **20**, 1117–1126 [682, 686].

CUMMINGS, J.L., GOSENFELD, L.F., HOULIHAN, J.P. & McCAFFREY, T. (1983) Neuropsychiatric disturbances associated with idiopathic calcification of the basal ganglia. *Biological Psychiatry* **18**, 591–601 [756].

CUMMINGS, J.L. & MAHLER, M.E. (1991) Cerebrovascular dementia. Ch. 7 in *Neurobehavioral Aspects of Cerebrovascular Disease*, eds Bornstein, R.A. & Brown, G. Oxford University Press: Oxford [384].

CURATOLO, P., CUSMAI, R., CORTESI, F., CHIRON, C., JAMBAQUE, I. & DULAC, O. (1991) Neuropsychiatric aspects of tuberous sclerosis. In *Tuberous Sclerosis and Allied Disorders: Clinical, Cellular, and Molecular Studies*, eds Johnson, W.G. & Gomez, M.R. *Annals of the New York Academy of Sciences* **615**, 8–16 [702].

CURCIO, C.A. & KEMPER, T. (1984) Nucleus raphe dorsalis in dementia of the Alzheimer type: neurofibrillary changes and neuronal packing density. *Journal of Neuropathology and Experimental Neurology* **43**, 359–368 [445].

CURRAN, F.J. (1938) The symptoms and treatments of barbiturate intoxication and psychosis. *American Journal of Psychiatry* **95**, 73–85 [608].

CURRAN, F.J. (1944) Current views on neuropsychiatric effects of barbiturates and bromides. *Journal of Nervous and Mental Disease* **100**, 142–169 [608].

CURRIE, S., HEATHFIELD, K.W.G., HENSON, R.A. & SCOTT, D.F. (1971) Clinical course and prognosis of temporal lobe epilepsy—a survey of 666 patients. *Brain* **92**, 173–190 [276].

CURRIER, R.D., LITTLE, S.C., SUESS, J.F. & ANDY, O.J. (1971) Sexual seizures. *Archives of Neurology* **25**, 260–264 [273].

CURTIS, D., ROBERTSON, M.M. & GURLING, H.M.D. (1992) Autosomal dominant gene transmission in a large kindred with Gilles de la Tourette syndrome. *British Journal of Psychiatry* **160**, 845–849 [681, 686].

CUTTING, J. (1978a) Study of anosognosia. *Journal of Neurology, Neurosurgery and Psychiatry* **41**, 548–555 [71].

CUTTING, J. (1978b) The relationship between Korsakov's syndrome and 'alcoholic dementia'. *British Journal of Psychiatry* **132**, 240–251 [584].

CUTTING, J. (1979) Memory in functional psychosis. *Journal of Neurology, Neurosurgery and Psychiatry* **42**, 1031–1037 [34].

CUTTING, J. (1985) *The Psychology of Schizophrenia*. Churchill Livingstone: Edinburgh [75, 89].

CUTTING, J. (1989) Body image disorders: comparison between unilateral hemisphere damage and schizophrenia. *Behavioural Neurology* **2**, 201–210 [75].

CUTTING, J. (1990) *The Right Cerebral Hemisphere and Psychiatric Disorders*. Oxford University Press: Oxford [75, 89].

CUTTING, J. (1992) The role of right hemisphere dysfunction in psychiatric disorders. *British Journal of Psychiatry* **160**, 583–588 [89].

CUTTING, J.C. (1994) Evidence for right hemisphere dysfunction in schizophrenia. Ch. 14 in *The Neuropsychology of Schizophrenia*, eds David, A.S. & Cutting, J.C. Lawrence Erlbaum: Hove, UK [89].

CUTTING, J. & MURPHY, D. (1990) Preference for denotative as opposed to connotative meanings in schizophrenics. *Brain and Language* **39**, 459–468 [89].

CYBULSKA, E. & RUCINSKI, J. (1986) Gross self-neglect in old age. *British Journal of Hospital Medicine* **July**, 21–25 [495].

DALAKAS, M.C. (1994) Post-polio motor neurone disease. Ch. 4 in *Motor Neurone Disease*, ed. Williams, A.C. Chapman & Hall: London [707].

DALAKAS, M.C. & PEZESHKPOUR, G.H. (1988) Neuromuscular diseases associated with human immunodeficiency virus infection. *Annals of Neurology*, **23 (Supplement)**, S38–S48 [327].

DALBY, M.A. (1971) Antiepileptic and psychotropic effect of carbamazepine (tegretol) in the treatment of psychomotor epilepsy. *Epilepsia* **12**, 325–334 [301].

DALLA BARBA, G., CIPOLOTTI, L. & DENES, G. (1990) Autobiographical memory loss and confabulation in Korsakoff's syndrome: a case report. *Cortex* **26**, 525–534 [37].

DALOS, N.P., RABINS, P.V., BROOKS, B.R. & O'DONNELL, P. (1983) Disease activity and emotional state in multiple sclerosis. *Annals of Neurology* **13**, 573–577 [692].

DALSGAARD-NIELSEN, T. (1965) Migraine and heredity. *Acta Neurologica Scandinavica* **41**, 287–300 [402, 403, 404].

DALY, D.D. & BARRY, M.J. (1957) Musicogenic epilepsy. *Psychosomatic Medicine* **19**, 399–408 [241].

DAMAS-MORA, J., SKELTON-ROBINSON, M. & JENNER, F.A. (1982) The Charles Bonnet Syndrome in perspective. *Psychological Medicine* **12**, 251–261 [295].

DAMASIO, A.R. & DAMASIO, H. (1992) Brain and language. *Scientific American* **267**, 89–95 [61].

DAMASIO, A.R., DAMASIO, H. & CHUI, H.C. (1980) Neglect following damage to frontal lobe or basal ganglia. *Neuropsychologia* **18**, 123–132 [68].

DAMASIO, A.R., DAMASIO, H., RIZZO, M., VARNEY, N. & GERSH, F. (1982a) Aphasia with nonhemorrhagic lesions in the basal ganglia and internal capsule. *Archives of Neurology* **39**, 15–20 [46].

DAMASIO, A.R., DAMASIO, H. & VAN HOESEN, G.W. (1982b) Prosopagnosia: anatomic basis and behavioral mechanisms. *Neurology* **32**, 331–341 [60].

DAMASIO, A.R., TRANEL, D. & DAMASIO, H. (1990) Individuals with sociopathic behavior caused by frontal damage fail to respond autonomically to social stimuli. *Behavioural Brain Research* **41**, 81–94 [79, 80].

DANA-HAERI, J., TRIMBLE, M.R. & OXLEY, J. (1983) Prolactin and gonadotrophin changes following generalised and partial seizures. *Journal of Neurology, Neurosurgery and Psychiatry* **46**, 331–335 [290].

DANDONA, P., JAMES, I.M., NEWBURY, P.A., WOOLLARD, M.I. & BECKETT, A.G. (1978) Cerebral blood flow in diabetes mellitus: evidence of abnormal cerebrovascular reactivity. *British Medical Journal* **2**, 325–326 [538].

DANIEL, D.G., WEINBERGER, D.R., BRESLIN, N., JONES, D.W., KLEINMAN, J.E., ZIGUN, J.R., COPPOLA, R., BIGELOW, L.B. & BERMAN, K.F. (1990) The effects of dopamine agonists on CBF (^{133}Xe dynamic SPECT) and negative symptoms in schizophrenia. *Schizophrenia Research* **3**, 28 [87].

DANIELS, L.W. (1934) Narcolepsy. *Medicine* **13**, 1–122 [724, 728].

D'ANTONA, R., BARON, J.C., SAMSON, Y., SERDARU, M., VIADER, F., AGID, Y. & CAMBIER, J. (1985) Subcortical dementia. Frontal cortex hypometabolism detected by positron tomography in patients with progressive supranuclear palsy. *Brain* **108**, 785–799 [666].

DARKINS, A.W., FROMKIN, V.A. & BENSON, D.F. (1988) A characterization of the prosodic loss in Parkinson's disease. *Brain and Language* **34**, 315–327 [647].

DARLEY, F.L. (1982) *Aphasia*. Saunders: Philadelphia [390].

DATHAN, J.G. (1954) Acrodynia associated with excessive intake of mercury. *British Medical Journal* **1**, 247–249 [634].

DAUBE, J. (1965) Sensory precipitated seizures: a review. *Journal of Nervous and Mental Disease* **141**, 524–539 [241, 248].

DAUMAS-DUPORT, C., SCHEITHAUER, B.W., CHODKIEWICZ, J.-P., LAWS, E.R. & VEDRENNE, C. (1988) Dysembrioplastic neuroepithelial tremor: a surgically curable tumour of young patients with intractable partial seizures. Report of thirty-nine cases. *Neurosurgery* **23**, 545–556 [244].

DAVENPORT, R.J., STATHAM, P.F.X. & WARLOW, C.P. (1994) Detection of bilateral isodense subdural haematomas. *British Medical Journal* **309**, 792–794 [412].

DAVID, A.S. (1987) Tachistoscopic tests of colour naming and matching in schizophrenia: evidence for posterior callosum dysfunction? *Psychological Medicine* **17**, 621–630 [90].

DAVID, A.S. (1993) Callosal transfer in schizophrenia: too much or too little? *Journal of Abnormal Psychology* **102**, 573–579 [90].

DAVID, A., BLAMIRE, A. & BREITER, H. (1994) Functional magnetic resonance imaging. A new technique with implications for psychology and psychiatry. *British Journal of Psychiatry* **164**, 2–7 [143, 144].

DAVID, A.S. & CUTTING, J.C. (1990) Affect, affective disorder and schizophrenia. A neuropsychological investigation of right hemisphere function. *British Journal of Psychiatry* **156**, 491–495 [89].

DAVID, A.S. & CUTTING, J.C. (1992) Visual imagery and visual semantics in the cerebral hemispheres in schizophrenia. *Schizophrenia Research* **8**, 263–271 [89].

DAVID, A., FERRY, S. & WESSELY, S. (1997) Gulf war illness. *British Medical Journal* **314**, 239–240 [637].

DAVID, A.S. & GILLHAM, R.A. (1986) Neuropsychological study of motor neurone disease. *Psychosomatics* **27**, 441–445 [708].

DAVID, A.S., WACHARASINDHU, A. & LISHMAN, W.A. (1993) Severe psychiatric disturbance and abnormalities of the corpus callosum: review and case series. *Journal of Neurology, Neurosurgery and Psychiatry* **56**, 85–93 [770].

DAVID, A.S., WOODRUFF, P.W.R., HOWARD, R., MELLERS, J.D.C., BRAMMER, M., BULLMORE, E., WRIGHT, I., ANDREW, C. & WILLIAMS, S.C.R. (1996) Auditory hallucinations inhibit exogenous activation of auditory association cortex. *NeuroReport* **7**, 932–936 [xviii, 88].

DAVID, M. & ASKENASY, H. (1937) Les troubles mentaux dans les meningiomes de la petite aile du sphénoide. *Encéphale* **32(1)**, 169–208 [223].

DAVIDSON, J. (1992) Drug therapy for post-traumatic stress disorder. *British Journal of Psychiatry* **160**, 309–314 [195].

DAVIES, B.M. & MORGANSTERN, F.S. (1960) A case of cysticercosis, temporal lobe epilepsy, and transvestism. *Journal of Neurology, Neurosurgery and Psychiatry* **23**, 247–249 [272, 273].

DAVIES, D.L. (1949a) The intelligence of patients with Friedreich's ataxia. *Journal of Neurology, Neurosurgery and Psychiatry* **12**, 34–38 [705].

DAVIES, D.L. (1949b) Psychiatric changes associated with Friedreich's ataxia. *Journal of Neurology, Neurosurgery and Psychiatry* **12**, 246–250 [706].

DAVIES, D.L. (1949c) *Psychiatric Changes in Friedreich's Ataxia*. Thesis for DM Degree, University of Oxford [706].

DAVIES, G., HAMILTON, S., HENDRICKSON, E., LEVY, R. & POST, F. (1977) The effect of cyclandelate in depressed and demented patients: a controlled study in psychogeriatric patients. *Age and Ageing* **6**, 156–162 [502].

DAVIES, M.G., ROWAN, M.J. & FEELY, J. (1991) Psychometrics in assessing hepatic encephalopathy—a brief review. *Irish Journal of Psychological Medicine* **8**, 144–146 [565].

DAVIES, P. (1977) Cholinergic mechanisms in Alzheimer's disease. *British Journal of Psychiatry* **131**, 318–319 [444].

DAVIES, P., KATZMAN, R. & TERRY, R.D. (1980) Reduced somatostatin-like immunoreactivity in cerebral cortex from cases of Alzheimer disease and Alzheimer senile dementia. *Nature* **288**, 279–280 [445].

DAVIES, P.T.C. & ROSE, F.C. (1987) Headache—including migraine. *Hospital Update* **October**, 763–778 [409].

DAVIES, R.K., TUCKER, G.J., HARROW, M. & DETRE, T.P. (1971) Confusional episodes and antidepressant medication. *American Journal of Psychiatry* **128**, 95–99 [626].

DAVIES-JONES, G.A.B. (1989) Neurological manifestations of hematological disorders. Ch. 12 in *Neurology and General Medicine*, ed. Aminoff, M.J. Churchill Livingstone: New York [589].

DAVIS, J.M., JANICAK, P.G., SAKKAS, P., GILMORE, C. & WANG, Z. (1991) Electroconvulsive therapy in the treatment of the neuroleptic malignant syndrome. *Convulsive Therapy* **7**, 111–120 [627].

DAVIS, K.L. & MOHS, R.C. (1982) Enhancement of memory processes in Alzheimer's disease with multiple-dose intravenous physostigmine. *American Journal of Psychiatry* **139**, 1421–1424 [503].

DAVIS, K.L., THAL, L.J., GAMZU, E.R., DAVIS, C.S., WOOLSON, R.F., GRACON, S.I., DRACHMAN, D.A., SCHNEIDER, L.S., WHITEHOUSE, P.J., HOOVER, T.M., MORRIS, J.C., KAWAS, C.H., KNOPMAN, D.S., EARL, N.L., KUMAR, V., DOODY, R.S. & THE TACRINE COLLABORATIVE STUDY GROUP (1992) A double-blind, placebo-controlled multicenter study of tacrine for Alzheimer's disease. *New England Journal of Medicine* **327**, 1253–1259 [504].

DAVIS, L. & PERRET, G. (1947) Cerebral thrombo-angiitis obliterans. *British Journal of Surgery* **34**, 307–313 [425].

DAVIS, L.E. & SCHMITT, J.W. (1989) Clinical significance of cerebrospinal fluid tests for neurosyphilis. *Annals of Neurology* **25**, 50–55 [343].

DAVIS, P.J., RAPPEPORT, J.R., LUTZ, H. & GREGERMAN, R.I. (1971) Three thyrotoxic criminals. *Annals of Internal Medicine* **74**, 743–745 [511].

DAVIS, R., PETERS, D.H. & McTAVISH, D. (1994) Valproic acid. A reappraisal of its pharmacological properties and clinical efficacy in epilepsy. *Drugs* **47**, 332–372 [302].

DAVIS, R.J., CUMMINGS, J.L. & HIERHOLZER, R.W. (1988) Tardive dystonia: clinical spectrum and novel manifestations. *Behavioural Neurology* **1**, 41–47 [642].

DAVIS-JONES, A., GREGORY, M.C. & WHITTY, C.W.M. (1973) Permanent sequelae in the migraine attack. Ch. 3 in *Background to Migraine*, 5th Migraine Symposium, ed. Cumings, J.N. Heinemann: London [401].

DAVISON, K. (1983) Schizophrenia-like psychoses associated with organic cerebral disorders: a review. *Psychiatric Developments* **1**, 1–34 [84].

DAVISON, K. & BAGLEY, C.R. (1969) Schizophrenia-like psychoses associated with organic disorders of the central nervous system: a review of the literature. In *Current Problems in Neuropsychiatry*, ed. Herrington, R.N. British Journal of Psychiatry Special Publication No. 4. Headley Brothers: Ashford, Kent [84, 190, 191, 225, 230, 234, 282, 284, 354, 387, 657, 665, 697, 706, 708, 716, 728].

DAWSON, J.R. (1933) Cellular inclusions in cerebral lesions of lethargic encephalitis. *American Journal of Pathology* **9**, 7–15 [361].

DAX, M. (1836) Lésions de la moitié gauche de l'encéphale coincidait avec l'oubli des signes de la pensée (Lu à Montpellier en 1836). *Gazette Hebdomadaire de Médecine et de Chirurgie* **33**, 259–262 [22].

DAYAN, A.D. (1969) Progressive multifocal leukoencephalopathy. In *Virus Diseases of the Nervous System*, eds Whitty, C.W.M., Hughes, J.T. & MacCallum, F.O. Blackwell Scientific Publications: Oxford [752].

DE BAETS, M.H. & KUKS, J.J.M. (1993) Immunopathology of myasthenia gravis. Ch. 5 in *Myasthenia Gravis*, eds De Baets, M.H. & Oosterhuis, H.J.G.H. CRC Press: Roca Raton [710].

DE BONI, U. & CRAPPER, D.R. (1978) Paired helical filaments of the Alzheimer type in cultured neurones. *Nature* **271**, 566–568 [447].

DE BOUCAUD, P., VITAL, C.I. & DE BOUCAUD, D. (1968) Thalamic dementia of vascular origin. *Revue Neurologique* **119**, 461–468 [384].

DE BRUIN, V.M.S. & LEES, A.J. (1992) The clinical features of 67 patients with clinically definite Steele–Richardson–Olszewski syndrome. *Behavioural Neurology* **5**, 229–232 [666].

DE JONG, R.N. (1944) Methyl bromide poisoning. *Journal of the American Medical Association* **125(ii)**, 702–703 [637].

DE LA MATA, C., GINGRAS, G. & WITTKOWER, E.D. (1960) Impact of sudden severe disablement of the father upon the family. *Canadian Medical Association Journal* **82**, 1015–1020 [391].

DE LA MONTE, S.M. (1988) Disproportionate atrophy of cerebral white matter in chronic alcoholics. *Archives of Neurology* **45**, 990–992 [604].

DE LA MONTE, S.M., SCHOOLEY, R.T., HIRSCH, M.S. & RICHARDSON, E.P. (1987) Subacute encephalomyelitis of AIDS and its relation to HTLV-III infection. *Neurology* **37**, 562–569 [320].

DE LEON, M.J., FERRIS, S.H., BLAU, I., GEORGE, A.E., REISBERG, B., KRICHEFF, I.I. & GERSHON, S. (1979) Correlations between CT changes and behavioural deficits in senile dementia. *Lancet* **2**, 859–860 [139].

DE MOURA, M.C., CORREIA, J.P. & MADEIRA, F. (1967) Clinical alcohol hypoglycaemia. *Annals of Internal Medicine* **66**, 893–905 [761].

DE RENZI, E. (1982) *Disorders of Space Exploration and Cognition*. John Wiley & Sons: Chichester [63].

DE RENZI, E. & FAGLIONI, P. (1965) The comparative efficiency of intelligence and vigilance tests in detecting hemispheric cerebral damage. *Cortex* **1**, 410–433 [112, 120, 121].

DE RENZI, E. & FAGLIONI, P. (1967) The relationship between visuo-spatial impairment and constructional apraxia. *Cortex* **3**, 327–342 [62].

DE RENZI, E., FAGLIONI, P. & NICHELLI, P. (1991) Apperceptive and associative forms of prosopagnosia. *Cortex* **27**, 213–221 [60].

DE RENZI, E., FAGLIONI, P. & SCOTTI, G. (1971) Judgement of spatial orientation in patients with focal brain damage. *Journal of Neurology, Neurosurgery and Psychiatry* **34**, 485–495 [62].

DE RENZI, E., LIOTTI, M. & NICHELLI, P. (1987) Semantic amnesia with preservation of autobiographic memory: a case report. *Cortex* **23**, 575–597 [37].

DE RENZI, E. & SCOTTI, G. (1970) Autotopagnosia: fiction or reality? *Archives of Neurology* **23**, 221–227 [71].

DE RENZI, E. & VIGNOLO, L.A. (1962) The token test: a sensitive test to detect receptive disturbances in aphasics. *Brain* **85**, 665–678 [113].

DE SMET, Y., RUBERG, M., SERDARU, M., DUBOIS, B., LHERMITTE, F. & AGID, Y. (1982) Confusion, dementia and anticholinergics in Parkinson's disease. *Journal of Neurology, Neurosurgery and Psychiatry* **45**, 1161–1164 [658].

DE VEAUGH-GEISS, J. (1980) Tardive Tourette syndrome. *Neurology* **30**, 562–563 [685].

DE WARDENER, H.E. & LENNOX, B. (1947) Cerebral beri beri (Wernicke's encephalopathy). *Lancet* **1**, 11–17 [577, 579, 581].

DE WIED, D. (1984) The importance of vasopressin in memory. *Trends in Neurosciences* **7**, 62–64 [502].

DE WIED, D., BOHUS, B., GISPEN, W.H., URBAN, I. & VAN WIMERSMA GREIDANUS T.J.B. (1976) Hormonal influences on motivational, learning and memory processes. In *Hormones, Behavior, and Psychopathology*, ed. Sachar, E.J., pp. 1–14. Raven Press: New York [507].

DE WIED, D. & VAN REE, J.M. (1982) Neuropeptides, mental performance, and aging. *Life Sciences* **31**, 709–719 [502].

DEAHL, M. (1991) Cannabis and memory loss. *British Journal of Addiction* **86**, 249–252 [616].

DEAKIN, J.F.W., SLATER, P., SIMPSON, M.D.C. & ROYSTON, C.M. (1990) Disturbed brain glutamate and GABA mechanisms in schizophrenia. *Schizophrenia Research* **3**, 33 [90].

DEARY, I.J. & FRIER, B.M. (1996) Severe hypoglycaemia and cognitive impairment in diabetes. *British Medical Journal* **313**, 767–768 [537].

DEKABAN, R.S. & HERMAN, M.M. (1974) Childhood, juvenile, and adult cerebral lipidoses. *Archives of Pathology* **97**, 65–73 [760].

DeKOSKY, S.T. & SCHEFF, S.W. (1990) Synapse loss in frontal cortex biopsies in Alzheimer's disease: correlation with cognitive severity. *Annals of Neurology* **27**, 457–464 [444].

DEL SER, T., BERMEJO, F., PORTERA, A., ARRENDONDO, J.M., BOURAS, C. & CONSTANTINIDIS, J. (1990) Vascular dementia. A clinicopathological study. *Journal of the Neurological Sciences* **96**, 1–17 [456].

DELALANDE, O., PINARD, J.M., BASDEVANT, C., PLONIN, P. & DULAC, O. (1993) Hemispherotomy: a new procedure for hemispheric disconnection. *Epilepsia*, **34 (Supplement 2)**, 140 (abstract) [313].

DELANEY, P. (1977) Neurologic manifestations in sarcoidosis. *Annals of Internal Medicine* **87**, 336–345 [764].

DELANEY, R.C., ROSEN, A.J., MATTSON, R.H. & NOVELLY, R.A. (1980) Memory function in focal epilepsy: a comparison of non-surgical, unilateral temporal lobe and frontal lobe samples. *Cortex* **16**, 103–117 [261].

DELASNERIE-LAUPRETRE, N., POSER, S., POCCHIARI, M., WIENTJENS, D.P.W.M. & WILL, R. (1995) Creutzfeldt–Jakob disease in Europe. *Lancet* **346**, 898 [475].

DELAY, J., BRION, S. & DEROUESNÉ, C. (1964) Syndrome de Korsakoff et étiologie tumorale. *Revue Neurologique* **111**, 97–133 [227].

DELAY, J., DENIKER, P. & BARANDE, R. (1957) Le suicide des épileptiques. *Encéphale* **46**, 401–436 [286].

DELGADO, J.M.R. (1969) Offensive–defensive behaviour in free monkeys and chimpanzees induced by radio stimulation of the brain. In *Aggressive Behaviour* Proceedings of International Symposium on the Biology of Aggressive Behaviour, eds Garattini, S. & Sigg, E.B. Exerpta Medica: Amsterdam [80].

DELGADO, J.M.R., MARK, V., SWEET, W., ERVIN, F., WEISS, G., BACH-Y-RITA, G. & HAGIWARA, R. (1968) Intracerebral radio stimulation and recording in completely free patients. *Journal of Nervous and Mental Disease* **147**, 329–340 [81–2, 267].

DELGADO, P.L., PRICE, L.H., HENINGER, G.R. & CHARNEY, D.S. (1992) Neurochemistry. Ch. 15 in *Handbook of Affective Disorders*, 2nd edn, ed. Paykel, E.S., pp. 219–253. Churchill Livingstone: Edinburgh [24].

DELGADO-ESCUETA, A.V., MATTSON, R.H., KING, L., GOLDENSOHN, E.S., SPIEGEL, H., MADSEN, J., CRANDALL, P., DREIFUSS, F. & PORTER, R.J. (1981) The nature of aggression during epileptic seizures. *New England Journal of Medicine* **305**, 711–716 [275].

DeLISI, L.E., HOFF, A.L., SCHWARTZ, J.E., SHIELDS, G.W., HALTHORE, S.N., GUPTA, S.M., HENN, F.A. & ANAND, A.K. (1991) Brain morphology in first-episode schizophrenic-like psychotic patients: a quantitative magnetic resonance imaging study. *Biological Psychiatry* **29**, 159–175 [85].

DELLAPORTAS, C.I., WILSON, A. & ROSE, F.C. (1984) Clobazam as adjunctive treatment in chronic epilepsy. In *Advances in Epileptology: XVth Epilepsy International Symposium*, eds Porter, R.J., Mattson, R.H., Ward, A.A. & Dam, M., pp. 363–367. Raven Press: New York [305].

DELMAS-MARSALET, P., VITAL, C., JULIEN, J., BÉRAUD, C., BOURGEOIS, M. & BARGUES, M. (1967) La maladie de Marchiafava et Bignami. *Journal de Médicine de Bordeaux* **144**, 1627–1646 [586].

DEMENT, W.C., RECHTSCHAFFEN, A.R. & GULEVICH, G.D. (1964) A polygraphic study of the narcoleptic sleep attack. *Electroencephalography and Clinical Neurophysiology* **17**, 608–609 [725].

DEMENT, W.C., RECHTSCHAFFEN, A. & GULEVICH, G.D. (1966) The nature of the narcoleptic sleep attack. *Neurology* **16**, 18–33 [725].

DEMETER, S. (1992) Structural imaging in Tourette syndrome. Ch. 24 in *Tourette Syndrome. Genetics, Neurobiology, and Treatment*, eds Chase, T.N., Friedhoff, A.J. & Cohen, D.J. *Advances in Neurology* **Vol. 58**. Raven Press: New York [685].

DENCKER, S.J. (1958) A follow-up study of 128 closed head injuries in twins using co-twins as controls. *Acta Psychiatrica et Neurologica Scandinavica* **123(Supplement)**, 1–125 [173, 198].

DENCKER, S.J. (1960) Closed head injury in twins. *Archives of General Psychiatry* **2**, 569–575 [173, 198].

DENCKER, S.J. & LÖFVING, B. (1958) A psychometric study of identical twins discordant for closed head injury. *Acta Psychiatrica et Neurologica Scandinavica* **122(Supplement)**, 1–50 [184].

DENING, T.R. & BERRIOS, G.E. (1989a) Wilson's disease. Psychiatric symptoms in 195 cases. *Archives of General Psychiatry* **46**, 1126–1134 [664, 665].

DENING, T.R. & BERRIOS, G.E. (1989b) Wilson's disease: a prospective study of psychopathology in 31 cases. *British Journal of Psychiatry* **155**, 206–213 [665].

DENING, T.R. & BERRIOS, G.E. (1990) Wilson's disease: a longitudinal study of psychiatric symptoms. *Biological Psychiatry* **28**, 255–265 [665, 666].

DENING, T.R., BERRIOS, G.E. & WALSHE, J.M. (1988) Wilson's disease and epilepsy. *Brain* **111**, 1139–1155 [662].

DENISON, D.M. (1996) Diving medicine. Section 8.5.5(f) in *Oxford Textbook of Medicine*, 3rd edn, eds Weatherall, D.J., Ledingham, J.G.G. & Warrell, D.A. Oxford University Press: Oxford [766, 769].

DENKO, J.D. & KAELBLING, R. (1962) The psychiatric aspects of hypoparathyroidism. *Acta Psychiatrica Scandinavica* **164(Supplement)**, 1–70 [531, 532, 533].

DENNERLL, R.D. (1964) Cognitive deficits and lateral brain dysfunction in temporal lobe epilepsy. *Epilepsia* **5**, 177–191 [261].

DENNY-BROWN, D. (1945) Disability arising from closed head injury. *Journal of the American Medical Association* **127**, 429–436 [174].

DENNY-BROWN, D. (1948) Primary sensory neuropathy with muscular changes associated with carcinoma. *Journal of Neurology, Neurosurgery and Psychiatry* **11**, 73–87 [739].

DENNY-BROWN, D. & PORTER, H. (1951) The effect of BAL (2, 3-di-mercaptopropanol) on hepatolenticular degeneration (Wilson's disease). *New England Journal of Medicine* **245**, 917–925 [664].

DENNY-BROWN, D. & RUSSELL, W.R. (1941) Experimental cerebral concussion. *Brain* **64**, 93–164 [162].

DES JARLAIS, D.C., FRIEDMAN, S.R., NOVICK, D.M., SOTHERN, J.L., THOMAS, P., YANCOVITZ, S.R., MILDVAN, D., WEBER, J., KREEK, M.J., MASLANSKY, R., BARTELME, S., SPIRA, T. & MARMOR, M. (1989) HIV-1 infection among intravenous drug users in Manhattan, New York City, from 1977 through 1987. *Journal of the American Medical Association* **261**, 1008–1012 [316].

DETRE, T., HIMMELHOCH, J., SWATZBURG, M., ANDERSON, C.M., BYCK, R. & KUPFER, D.J. (1972) Hypersomnia and manic depressive disease. *American Journal of Psychiatry* **128**, 1303–1305 [735].

DEVOUS, M.D. (1989) Imaging brain function by single-photon emission computer tomography. Ch. 4 in *Brain Imaging: Applications in Psychiatry*, ed. Andreasen, N.C. American Psychiatric Press: Washington [148].

DEVOUS, M.D., RAESE, J.D., HERMAN, J.H., PAULMAN, R.G., GREGORY, R.R., RUSH, A.J., CHEHABI, H.H. & BONTE, F.J. (1985) Regional cerebral blood flow in schizophrenic patients at rest and during Wisconsin Card Sort tasks. *Journal of Cerebral Blood Flow and Metabolism* **5**, S201–S202 [148].

DEWAN, M.J., PANDURANGI, A.K., LEE, S.H., RAMACHANDRAM, T., LEVY, B., BOUCHER, M., YOZAWITZ, A. & MAJOR, L.F. (1983) Central brain morphology in chronic schizophrenic patients: a controlled CT study. *Biological Psychiatry* **18**, 1133–1140 [138].

DEWAR, D. & McCULLOCH, J. (1994) Abnormalities in non-cholinergic neurotransmitter systems in Alzheimer's disease. Ch. 11 in *Dementia*, eds Burns, A. & Levy, R. Chapman & Hall: London [445].

DEWEER, B., PILLON, B., MICHON, A. & DUBOIS, B. (1993) Mirror reading in Alzheimer's disease: normal skill learning and acquisition of item-specific information. *Journal of Clinical and Experimental Neuropsychology* **15**, 789–804 [32].

DEWHURST, K. (1969) The neurosyphilitic psychoses today: a survey of 91 cases. *British Journal of Psychiatry* **115**, 31–38 [340, 341, 343, 345].

DEWHURST, K. & BEARD, A.W. (1970) Sudden religious conversions in temporal lobe epilepsy. *British Journal of Psychiatry* **117**, 497–507 [267].

DEWHURST, K. & HATRICK, J.A. (1972) Differential diagnosis and treatment of lysergic acid diethylamide induced psychosis. *Practitioner* **209**, 327–332 [622].

DEWHURST, K., OLIVER, J.E. & McKNIGHT, A.L. (1970) Sociopsychiatric consequences of Huntington's disease. *British Journal of Psychiatry* **116**, 255–258 [472].

DI MAURO, S. & MOSES, L.G. (1992) Mitochondrial encephalomyopathies. *Brain Pathology* **2**, 111–112 [761].

DIAGNOSTIC AND STATISTICAL MANUAL OF MENTAL DISORDERS (1980) *DSM-III*, 3rd edn. American Psychiatric Association: Washington, DC [5, 8].

DIAGNOSTIC AND STATISTICAL MANUAL OF MENTAL DISORDERS (1994) *DSM-IV*, 4th edn. American Psychiatric Association: Washington, DC [5].

DICK, J.P.R., SNOWDEN, J., NORTHEN, B., GOULDING, P.J. & NEARY, D. (1989) Slowly progressive apraxia. *Behavioral Neurology* **2**, 101–114 [754].

DILLER, L. & RIKLAN, M. (1956) Psychosocial factors in Parkinson's disease. *Journal of the American Geriatrics Society* **4**, 1291–1300 [661].

DILLEY, J.W., OCHITILL, H.N., PERL, M. & VOLBERDING, P.A. (1985) Findings in psychiatric consultations with patients with acquired immune deficiency syndrome. *American Journal of Psychiatry* **142**, 82–86 [330].

DILLON, H. & LEOPOLD, R.L. (1961) Children and the post-concussion syndrome. *Journal of the American Medical Association* **175**, 86–92 [203].

DIMOND, S.J., SCAMMELL, R.E., PRYCE, I.G., HUWS, D. & GRAY, C. (1979) Callosal transfer and left-hand anomia in schizophrenia. *Biological Psychiatry* **14**, 735–739 [90].

DIMOND, S.J., SCAMMELL, R., PRYCE, I.J., HUWS, D. & GRAY, C. (1980) Some failures of intermanual and cross-latency transfer in chronic schizophrenia. *Journal of Abnormal Psychology* **89**, 505–509 [90].

DINNICK, O.O. (1964) Deaths associated with anaesthesia: observations on 600 cases. *Anaesthesia* **19**, 536–556 [546].

DIREKZE, M., BAYLISS, S.G. & CUTTING, J.C. (1971) Primary tumours of the frontal lobe. *British Journal of Clinical Practice* **25**, 207–213 [223].

DITCH, M., KELLY, F.J. & RESNICK, O. (1971) An ergot preparation (hydergine) in the treatment of cerebrovascular disorders in the geriatric patient: double-blind study. *Journal of the American Geriatrics Society* **19**, 208–217 [502].

DIVRY, P. (1927) Étude histo-chimique des plaques séniles. *Journal de Neurologie et de Psychiatrie* **27**, 643–657 [441].

DOBROKHOTOVA, T.A. & FALLER, T.O. (1969) Concerning the psychopathological symptomatology in tumours of the posterior brain cavity. *Zhurnal Neuropatologi i Psikhiatrii* **8**, 1225–1230 [231].

DODRILL, C.B. & BATZEL, L.W. (1986) Interictal behavioral features of patients with epilepsy. *Epilepsia* **27**, S64–S76 [266].

DODRILL, C.B. & TROUPIN, A.S. (1977) Psychotropic effects of carbamazepine in epilepsy: a double-blind comparison with phenytoin. *Neurology* **27**, 1023–1028 [301].

DOLAN, R., BENCH, C. & FRISTON, K. (1990) Positron emission tomography in psychopharmacology. *International Review of Psychiatry* **2**, 427–439 [146].

DOLAN, R.J., CALLOWAY, S.P. & MANN, A.H. (1985) Cerebral ventricular size in depressed subjects. *Psychological Medicine* **15**, 873–878 [140].

800   REFERENCES

DOLAN, R.J., CALLOWAY, S.P., THACKER, P.F. & MANN, A.H. (1986) The cerebral cortical appearance in depressed subjects. *Psychological Medicine* **16**, 775–779 [140].

DOLL, E.A. (1947) *Vineland Social Maturity Scale. Manual of Directions.* Educational Test Bureau, Division of American Guidance Service: Minneapolis [125].

DONAGHY, M. (1993) Toxic and environmental disorders. Ch. 15 in *Brain's Diseases of the Nervous System*, 10th edn, ed. Walton, J. Oxford University Press: Oxford [637].

DONGIER, S. (1959) Statistical study of clinical and electroencephalographic manifestations of 536 psychotic episodes occurring in 516 epileptics between clinical seizures. *Epilepsia* **1**, 117–142 [258, 284, 285].

DOOLING, E.C., RICHARDSON, E.P. & DAVIS, K.R. (1980) Computed tomography in Hallervorden-Spatz disease. *Neurology* **30**, 1128–1130 [756].

DOOLING, E.C., SCHOENE, W.C. & RICHARDSON, E.P. (1974) Hallervorden-Spatz syndrome. *Archives of Neurology* **30**, 70–83 [756].

DOOSE, H., BAIER, W. & REINSBERG, E. (1984) Genetic heterogeneity of spike-wave epilepsies. In *Advances in Epileptology: XVth Epilepsy International Symposium*, eds Porter, R.J., Mattson, R.H., Ward, A.A. & Dam, M., pp. 515–519. Raven Press: New York [247].

DOOSE, H., GERKEN, H., HORSTMANN, T. & VÖLZKE, E. (1973) Genetic factors in spike-wave absences. *Epilepsia* **14**, 57–75 [247].

D'ORBÁN, P.T. (1989) Automatism—a medico-legal conundrum. *Irish Journal of Psychological Medicine* **6**, 71–80 [298].

DORFMAN, L.J., MARSHALL, W.H. & ENZMANN, D.R. (1979) Cerebral infarction and migraine: clinical and radiologic correlations. *Neurology* **29**, 317–322 [401].

DORKEN, H. (1958) Normal senescent decline and senile dementia: their differentiation by psychological tests. *Medical Services Journal, Canada, Ottawa* **14**, 18–23 [436].

DORRELL, W. (1973) Myasthenia gravis and schizophrenia. *British Journal of Psychiatry* **123**, 249 [711].

DOTT, N.M. (1938) Surgical aspects of the hypothalamus. In *The Hypothalamus*, eds Clark, W.E.LeG., Beattie, J., Riddoch, G. & Dott, N.M. Oliver & Boyd: Edinburgh [27].

DOUGLAS, N.J. (1994) The sleep apnoea/hypoapnoea syndrome. Ch. 11 in *Sleep*, ed. Cooper, R. Chapman & Hall: London [730].

DOUST, B.C. (1958) Anxiety as a manifestation of phaeochromocytoma. *Archives of Internal Medicine* **102**, 811–855 [521].

DOWNER, J.L. DE C. (1962) Interhemispheric integration in the visual system. Ch. 6 in *Interhemispheric Relations and Cerebral Dominance*, ed. Mountcastle, V.B. Johns Hopkins Press: Baltimore [23, 80].

DRACHMAN, D.A. & ADAMS, R.D. (1962) Herpes simplex and acute inclusion-body encephalitis. *Archives of Neurology* **7**, 45–63 [348, 356].

DRACHMAN, D.A. & ARBIT, J. (1966) Memory and the hippocampal complex. *Archives of Neurology* **15**, 52–61 [30, 104].

DRACHMAN, D.A. & LEAVITT, J. (1974) Human memory and the cholinergic system. *Archives of Neurology* **30**, 113–121 [503].

DRESSER, A.C., MEIROWSKY, A.M., WEISS, G.H., McNEEL, M.L., SIMON, G.A. & CAVENESS, W.F. (1973) Gainful employment following head injury. *Archives of Neurology* **29**, 111–116 [215].

DREW, R.H., TEMPLER, D.I., SCHUYLER, B.A., NEWELL, T.G. & CANNON, W.G. (1986) Neuropsychological deficits in active licensed professional boxers. *Journal of Clinical Psychology* **42**, 520–525 [206].

DREWE, E.A. (1974) The effect of type and area of brain lesion on Wisconsin Card Sorting test performance. *Cortex* **10**, 159–170 [118].

DRIVER, H.S. & SHAPIRO, C.M. (1993) Parasomnias. *British Medical Journal* **306**, 921–924 [736].

DROPCHO, E.J. (1989) The remote effects of cancer on the nervous system. In *Neurologic Manifestations of Systemic Disease*, ed. Riggs, J.E. *Neurologic Clinics* **7**, 579–603 [740, 743].

DRUG AND THERAPEUTICS BULLETIN (1972) *Praxilene (naftidrofuryl)*, Vol. 10, 93–94 and 104 [502].

DRUG AND THERAPEUTICS BULLETIN (1986a) Problems when withdrawing antidepressives. *Drug and Therapeutics Bulletin* **24**, 29–30 [626].

DRUG AND THERAPEUTICS BULLETIN (1986b) The management of multiple sclerosis. *Drug and Therapeutics Bulletin* **24**, 41–44 [690].

DRUG AND THERAPEUTICS BULLETIN (1988a) Naftidrofuryl (Proxilene). *Drug and Therapeutics Bulletin* **26**, 25–27 [503].

DRUG AND THERAPEUTICS BULLETIN (1988b) Oral zinc—when is it useful? *Drug and Therapeutics Bulletin* **26**, 31–32 [561].

DRUG AND THERAPEUTICS BULLETIN (1988c) Treatment of carbon monoxide poisoning. *Drug and Therapeutics Bulletin* **26**, 77–79 [553].

DRUG AND THERAPEUTICS BULLETIN (1989) Withdrawing antiepileptic drugs. *Drug and Therapeutics Bulletin* **27**, 29–31 [299].

DRUG AND THERAPEUTICS BULLETIN (1990) Drugs for Alzheimer's disease. *Drugs and Therapeutics Bulletin* **28**, 42–44 [501].

DRUG AND THERAPEUTICS BULLETIN (1991a) Zidovudine in HIV infection. *Drug and Therapeutics Bulletin* **29**, 81–82 [336].

DRUG AND THERAPEUTICS BULLETIN (1991b) Potassium disorders and cardiac arrhythmias. *Drug and Therapeutics Bulletin* **29**, 73–75 [560].

DRUG AND THERAPEUTICS BULLETIN (1992a) Nimodipine for delayed cerebral ischaemia after subarachnoid haemorrhage. *Drug and Therapeutics Bulletin* **30**, 81–83 [393].

DRUG AND THERAPEUTICS BULLETIN (1992b) Sumatriptan: a new approach to migraine. *Drug and Therapeutics Bulletin* **30**, 85–87 [410].

DRUG AND THERAPEUTICS BULLETIN (1992c) Lamotrigine—an add-on antiepileptic. *Drug and Therapeutics Bulletin* **30**, 75–76 [303].

DSM-III *See* Diagnostic and Statistical Manual of Mental Disorders (1980).

DSM-IV *See* Diagnostic and Statistical Manual of Mental Disorders (1994).

DU BOULAY, G.H., RUIZ, J.S., ROSE, F.C., STEVENS, J.M. & ZILKHA, K.J. (1983) CT changes associated with migraine. *American Journal of Neuroradiology* **4**, 472–473 [401].

DUARA, R., GRADY, C., HAXBY, J., SUNDARAM, M., CUTLER, N.R., HESTON, L., MOORE, A., SCHLAGETER, N., LARSON, S. & RAPOPORT, S.I. (1986) Positron emission tomography in Alzheimer's disease. *Neurology* **36**, 879–887 [434].

DUARA, R., KUSHCH, A., GROSS-GLENN, K., BARKER, W.W., JALLAD, B., PASCAL, S., LOEWENSTEIN, D.A., SHELDON, J., RABIN, M., LEVIN, B. & LUBS, H. (1991) Neuroanatomic differences between dyslexic and normal readers on magnetic resonance imaging scans. *Archives of Neurology* **48**, 410–416 [48].

DUBOIS, B. & PILLON, B. (1992) Biochemical correlates of cognitive changes and dementia in Parkinson's disease. Ch. 14 in *Parkinsons's Disease. Neurobehavioral Aspects*, eds Huber, S.J. & Cummings, J.L. Oxford University Press: Oxford [655].

DUBOIS, E.L. (1966) *Lupus Erythematosus: Review of the Current Status of Discoid and Systemic Lupus Erythematosus and Their Variants*, ed. Dubois, E.L. McGraw Hill: New York [418, 419, 420, 421, 422].

DUBOWITZ, V. (1958) Influenzal encephalitis. *Lancet* **1**, 140–141 [359].

DUBOWITZ, V. (1965) Intellectual impairment in muscular dystrophy. *Archives of Disease in Childhood* **40**, 296–301 [716].

DUBOWITZ, V. (1992) Transferring myoblasts in Duchenne dystrophy. Clinical results are disappointing. *British Medical Journal* **305**, 844–845 [715].

DUFFY, F.H., BURCHFIEL, J.L. & LOMBROSO, C.T. (1979) Brain electrical activity mapping (BEAM): a method for extending the clinical utility of EEG and evoked potential data. *Annals of Neurology* **5**, 309–321 [132].

DUFFY, L. & O'CARROLL, R. (1994) Memory impairment in schizophrenia—a comparison with that observed in the alcoholic Korsakoff syndrome. *Psychological Medicine* **24**, 155–165 [34].

DUFFY, P., WOLF, J., COLLINS, G., DE VOE, A.G., STREETEN, B. & COWEN, D. (1974) Possible person-to-person transmission of Creutzfeldt–Jakob disease. *New England Journal of Medicine* **290**, 692–693 [476].

DUKES, M.N.G. (1992) *Meyler's Side Effects of Drugs. An Encyclopedia of Adverse Reactions and Interactions*, 12th edn. Elsevier: Amsterdam [625].

DULANEY, J.T. & MOSER, H.W. (1978) Sulfatide lipidosis: metachromatic leukodystrophy. Ch. 38 in *The Metabolic Basis of Inherited Disease*, 4th edn, eds Stanbury, J.B., Wyngaarden, J.B. & Frederickson, D.S. McGraw-Hill: New York [758].

DUMAS-DUPORT, C. (1970) *Tumeurs Cerebrales chez les Malades Mentaux*. Thesis for Doctorate of Medicine, Faculté de Médicine de Paris [233, 235].

DUNBAR, G.C. & LISHMAN, W.A. (1984) Depression, recognition memory and hedonic tone: a signal detection analysis. *British Journal of Psychiatry* **144**, 376–382 [25, 34].

DUNBAR, J.M., JAMIESON, W.M., LANGLANDS, J.H.H. & SMITH, G.H. (1958) Encephalitis and influenza. *British Medical Journal* **1**, 913–915 [360].

DUNCAN, D. & TAYLOR, D. (1996) Treatment of psychosis in Parkinson's disease. *Psychiatric Bulletin* **20**, 157–159 [658].

DUNCAN, J.S. (1994) Vigabatrin. Ch. 8 in *New Anticonvulsants. Advances in the Treatment of Epilepsy*, ed. Trimble, M.R. John Wiley & Sons: Chichester [242, 303].

DUNCAN, R., PATTERSON, J., HADLEY, D.M., MacPHERSON, P., BRODIE, M.J., BONE, I., McGEORGE, A.P. & WYPER, D.J. (1990) CT, MR and SPECT imaging in temporal lobe epilepsy. *Journal of Neurology, Neurosurgery and Psychiatry* **53**, 11–15 [289].

DUNLAP, H.F. & MOERSCH, F.P. (1935) Psychic manifestations associated with hyperthyroidism. *American Journal of Psychiatry* **91**, 1215–1238 [509].

DUNNETT, S.B., BADMAN, F., ROGERS, D.C., EVENDEN, J.L. & IVERSEN, S.D. (1988) Cholinergic grafts in the neocortex or hippocampus of aged rats: reduction of delay-dependent deficits in the delayed non-matching to position task. *Experimental Neurology* **102**, 57–64 [505].

DUNNETT, S.B., LOW, W.C., IVERSEN, S.D., STENEVI, U. & BJÖRKLUND, A. (1982) Septal transplants restore maze learning in rats with fornix-fimbria lesions. *Brain Research* **251**, 335–348 [505].

DURELLI, L. (1994) High-dose intravenous immunoglobulin G treatment of myasthenia gravis. Ch. 17 in *Handbook of Myasthenia Gravis and Myasthenic Syndromes*, ed. Lisak, R.P. Marcel Dekker: New York [710].

DUVOISIN, R.C., ELDRIDGE, R., WILLIAMS, A., NUTT, J. & CALNE, D. (1981) Twin study of Parkinson disease. *Neurology* **31**, 77–80 [661].

DUVOISIN, R.C. & KATZ, R. (1968) Reversal of central anticholinergic syndrome in man by physostigmine. *Journal of the American Medical Association* **206**, 1963–1965 [658].

DUVOISIN, R.C. & VINSON, W.M. (1961) Tuberose sclerosis: report of three cases without mental defect. *Journal of the American Medical Association* **175**, 869–873 [702].

DYKEN, M.L., WOLF, P.A., BARNETT, H.J.M., BERGAN, J.J., HASS, W.K., KANNEL, W.B., KULLER, L., KURTZKE, J.F. & SUNDT, T.M. (1984) Risk factors in stroke. A statement for physicians by the subcommittee on risk factors and stroke of the Stroke Council. *Stroke* **15**, 1105–1111 [537].

EADIE, M.J. & SUTHERLAND, J.M. (1964) Arteriosclerosis in parkinsonism. *Journal of Neurology, Neurosurgery and Psychiatry* **27**, 237–240 [646].

EAGGER, S. & LEVY, R. (1992) Serum levels of tacrine in relation to clinical response in Alzheimer's disease. *International Journal of Geriatric Psychiatry* **7**, 115–119 [504].

EAGGER, S.A., LEVY, R. & SAHAKIAN, B.J. (1991a) Tacrine in Alzheimer's disease. *Lancet* **337**, 989–992 [504].

EAGGER, S.A., MORANT, N.J. & LEVY, R. (1991b) Parallel group analysis of the effects of tacrine versus placebo in Alzheimer's disease. *Dementia* **2**, 207–211 [504].

EAGGER, S., MORANT, N., LEVY, R. & SAHAKIAN, B. (1992) Tacrine in Alzheimer's disease. Time course of changes in cognitive function and practice effects. *British Journal of Psychiatry* **160**, 36–40 [504].

EAGLES, J.M., CRAIG, A., RAWLINSON, F., RESTALL, D.B., BEATTIE, J.A.G. & BESSON, J.A.O. (1987) The psychological well-being of supporters of the demented elderly. *British Journal of Psychiatry* **150**, 293–298 [498].

EAMES, P. & WOOD, R. (1985) Rehabilitation after severe brain injury: a follow-up study of a behaviour modification approach. *Journal of Neurology, Neurosurgery and Psychiatry* **48**, 613–619 [214].

EASTWOOD, M.R., RIFAT, S.L., NOBBS, H. & RUDERMAN, J. (1989) Mood disorder following cerebrovascular accident. *British Journal of Psychiatry* **154**, 195–200 [386].

EAYRS, J.T. (1968) Developmental relationships between brain and thyroid. Ch. 14 in *Endocrinology and Human Behaviour*, ed. Michael, R.P. Oxford University Press: Oxford [507].

EBELS, E.J. (1978) How common is Wernicke–Korsakoff syndrome? *Lancet* **2**, 781–782 [576].

EBMEIER, K.P., BESSON, J.A.O., CRAWFORD, J.R., PALIN, A.N., GEMMEL, H.G., SHARP, P.F., CHERRYMAN, G.R. & SMITH, F.W. (1987) Nuclear magnetic resonance imaging and single photon emission tomography with radio-iodine labelled compounds in the diagnosis of dementia. *Acta Psychiatrica Scandinavica* **75**, 549–556 [457, 496].

EBMEIER, K.P., LAWRIE, S.M., BLACKWOOD, D.H.R., JOHNSTONE, E.C. & GOODWIN, G.M. (1995) Hypofrontality revisited: a high resolution single photon emission computed tomography study in schizophrenia. *Journal of Neurology, Neurosurgery and Psychiatry* **58**, 452–456 [87].

ECKER, A. (1954) Emotional stress before strokes: a preliminary report of 20 cases. *Annals of Internal Medicine* **40**, 49–56 [396]

ECKER, A. & KERNOHAN, J.W. (1941) Arsenic as a possible cause of subacute encephalomyelitis. *Archives of Neurology and Psychiatry* **45**, 24–43 [636].

EDEH, J. & TOONE, B.K. (1985) Antiepileptic therapy, folate deficiency, and psychiatric morbidity: a general practice survey. *Epilepsia* **26**, 434–440 [271, 592].

EDEH, J. & TOONE, B. (1987) Relationship between interictal psychopathology and the type of epilepsy. Results of a survey in general practice. *British Journal of Psychiatry* **151**, 95–101 [259, 271].

EDEH, J., TOONE, B.K. & CORNEY, R.H. (1990) Epilepsy, psychiatric morbidity, and social dysfunction in general practice. *Neuropsychiatry, Neuropsychology and Behavioral Neurology* **3**, 180–192 [259].

EDMONDS, C. & BOUGHTON, J. (1985) Intellectual deterioration with excessive diving (punch drunk divers). *Undersea Biomedical Research* **12**, 321–326 [768].

EDWARDS, A.E. & HART, G.M. (1974) Hyperbaric oxygenation and the cognitive functioning of the aged. *Journal of the American Geriatrics Society* **22**, 376–379 [502].

EDWARDS, A.L. (1942) The retention of affective experiences—a criticism and restatement of the problem. *Psychological Review* **49**, 43–53 [25].

EDWARDS, C.R.W. (1996) Adrenocortical diseases. Section 12.7.1 in *Oxford Textbook of Medicine*, 3rd edn, eds Weatherall, D.J., Ledingham, J.G.G. & Warrell, D.A. Oxford University Press: Oxford [519].

EDWARDS, G. (1963) Psychopathology of a drug experience. *British Journal of Psychiatry* **143**, 509–512 [615].

EDWARDS, G. (1974) Drugs, drugs dependence and the concept of plasticity. *Quarterly Journal of Studies on Alcohol* **35**, 176–195 [594].

EDWARDS, G. (1982) *The Treatment of Drinking Problems*. Grant McIntyre: London [602, 603].

EDWARDS, J.G., CANTOPHER, T. & OLIVIERI, S. (1990) Benzodiazepine dependence and the problems of withdrawal. *Postgraduate Medical Journal*, **66 (Supplement 2)**, S27–S35 [611].

EDWARDS, R.H.T., NEWHAM, D.J. & PETERS, T.J. (1991) Muscle pathology and biochemistry. In *Post Viral Fatigue Syndrome*, eds Behan, P.O., Goldberg, D.P. & Mowbray, J.F. *British Medical Bulletin* **47(4)**, 826–837 [372].

EDWARDSON, J.A. & CANDY, J.M. (1990) Aluminium and the aetiopathogenesis of Alzheimer's disease. *Neurobiology of Aging* **11**, 314 [446].

EDWIN, E., HOLTEN, K., NORUM, K.R., SCHRUMPF, A. & SKAUG, O.E. (1965) Vitamin B$_{12}$ hypovitaminosis in mental diseases. *Acta Medica Scandinavica* **177**, 689–699 [587, 588].

EFRON, R. (1957) Conditioned inhibition of uncinate fits. *Brain* **80**, 251–262 [308].

EGGER, M., NEATON, J.D., PHILLIPS, A.N. & SMITH, G.D. (1994) Concorde trial of immediate versus deferred zidovudine. *Lancet* **343**, 1355 [336].

EHYAI, A. & FENICHEL, G.M. (1978) The natural history of acute confusional migraine. *Archives of Neurology* **35**, 368–370 [405].

EIDELBERG, D., DHAWAN, V., MOELLER, J.R., SIDITIS, J.J., GINOS, J.Z., STROTHER, S.C., CEDERBAUM, J., GREENE, P., FAHN, S., POWERS, J.M. & ROTTENBERG, D.A. (1991) The metabolic landscape of cortico-basal ganglionic degeneration: regional asymmetries studied with positron emission tomography. *Journal of Neurology, Neurosurgery and Psychiatry* **54**, 856–862 [668].

EILENBERG, M.D. & WOODS, L.W. (1962) Narcolepsy with psychosis: report of two cases. *Proceedings of the Staff Meetings of the Mayo Clinic* **37**, 561–566 [728].

EISDORFER, C. & COHEN, D. (1980) Serum immunoglobulins and cognitive status in the elderly: 2. An immunological–behavioral relationship? *British Journal of Psychiatry* **136**, 40–45 [447].

EISDORFER, C., COHEN, D. & BUCKLEY, C.E. (1978) Serum immunoglobulins and cognition in the impaired elderly. In *Alzheimer's Disease, Senile Dementia and Related Disorders*, eds Katzman, R., Terry, R.D. & Bick, K.L., pp. 401–407. Raven Press: New York [447].

EISENBERG, H.M. & LEVIN, H.S. (1989) Computed tomography and magnetic resonance imaging in mild to moderate head injury. Ch. 8 in *Mild Head Injury*, eds Levin, H.S., Eisenberg, H.M. & Benton, A.L. Oxford University Press: Oxford [165].

EISENBERG, L., ASCHER, E. & KANNER, L. (1959) A clinical study of Gilles de la Tourette's disease (maladie des tics) in children. *American Journal of Psychiatry* **115**, 715–723 [686].

EITINGER, L. (1959) The importance of atrophy of the brain in psychiatric disease pictures. *Nordisk Medicin* **61**, 301–303 [141].

EKBOM, K., GREITZ, T. & KUGELBERG, E. (1969) Hydrocephalus due to

ectasia of the basilar artery. *Journal of the Neurological Sciences* **8**, 465–477 [746, 749].

ELDRIDGE, R. (1970) The torsion dystonias: literature review and genetic and clinical studies. *Neurology* **20 (part 2)**, 1–78 [670, 672, 674].

ELIAN, M. & BORNSTEIN, B. (1969) The Kline–Levin syndrome with intermittent abnormality in the EEG. *Electroencephalography and Clinical Neurophysiology* **27**, 601–604 [732].

ELIZAN, T.S., HIRANO, A., ABRAMS, B.M., NEED, R.L., VAN NUIS, C. & KURLAND, L.T. (1966) Amyotrophic lateral sclerosis and parkinsonism–dementia complex of Guam. Neurological re-evaluation. *Archives of Neurology* **14**, 356–368 [708].

ELKASHEF, A.M., RUSKIN, P.E., BACHER, N. & BARRETT, D. (1990) Vitamin E in the treatment of tardive dyskinesia. *American Journal of Psychiatry* **147**, 505–506 [645].

ELLINGSON, R.J. (1954) The incidence of EEG abnormality among patients with mental disorders of apparently non-organic origin: a critical review. *American Journal of Psychiatry* **111**, 263–275 [128].

ELLINGTON, E. & MARGOLIS, G. (1969) Block of arachnoid villus by subarachnoid haemorrhage. *Journal of Neurosurgery* **30**, 651–657 [746].

ELLIOTT, F.A. (1969) The corpus callosum, cingulate gyrus, septum pellucidum, septal area and fornix. Ch. 24 in *Handbook of Clinical Neurology*, Vol. 2, eds Vinken, P.J. & Bruyn, G.W. North-Holland Publishing Co.: Amsterdam [224].

ELLIOTT, F.A. (1992) Violence. The neurologic contribution: an overview. *Archives of Neurology* **49**, 595–603 [83].

ELLIOTT, F., GARDNER-THORPE, C., BARWICK, D.D. & FOSTER, J.B. (1974) Jakob–Creutzfeldt disease—modification of clinical and electroencephalographic activity with methylphenidate and diazepam. *Journal of Neurology, Neurosurgery and Psychiatry* **37**, 879–887 [478].

ELLISON, D.W., BEAL, M.F., MAZUREK, M.F., BIRD, E.D. & MARTIN, J.B. (1986) A postmortem study of amino acid neurotransmitters in Alzheimer's disease. *Annals of Neurology* **20**, 616–621 [445].

ELLISON, P.H. & BARRON, K.D. (1979) Clinical recovery from Schilder disease. *Neurology* **29**, 244–251 [700].

ELSASS, P., LUND, Y. & RANEK, L. (1978) Encephalopathy in patients with cirrhosis of the liver. A neuropsychological study. *Scandinavian Journal of Gastroenterology* **13**, 241–247 [565].

ELSOM, K.O., LEWY, F.H. & HEUBLEIN, G.W. (1940) Clinical studies of experimental human vitamin B complex deficiency. *American Journal of the Medical Sciences* **200**, 757–764 [572].

EMERSON, T.R., MILNE, J.R. & GARDNER, A.J. (1981) Cardiogenic dementia—a myth? *Lancet* **2**, 743–744 [431].

EMERY, A.E.H. (1993) *Duchenne Muscular Dystrophy*, 2nd edn. Oxford University Press: Oxford [715, 716].

EMSLEY, R., POTGIETER, A., TALJAARD, F., JOUBERT, G. & GLEDHILL, R. (1989) Water excretion and plasma vasopressin in psychotic disorders. *American Journal of Psychiatry* **146**, 250–253 [526].

ENDERBY, P. & EMERSON, J. (1996) Speech and language therapy: does it work? *British Medical Journal* **312**, 1655–1658 [390].

ENGEL, A.G. (1994) Congenital myasthenia syndromes. Ch. 3 in *Handbook of Myasthenia Gravis and Myasthenic Syndromes*, ed. Lisak, R.P. Marcel Dekker: New York [711].

ENGEL, G.L. (1972) Discussion following paper by Dr. P.B. Storey. In *Physiology, Emotion and Psychosomatic Illness*, Ciba Foundation Symposium 8 (new series). Associated Scientific Publishers: Amsterdam [396].

ENGEL, G.L. & ROMANO, J. (1959) Delirium, a syndrome of cerebral insufficiency. *Journal of Chronic Diseases* **9**, 260–277 [130].

ENGEL, G.L., WEBB, J.P. & FERRIS, E.B. (1945) Quantitative electroencephalographic studies of anoxia in humans; comparison with acute alcoholic intoxication and hypoglycaemia. *Journal of Clinical Investigation* **24**, 691–697 [130].

ENGEL, J. (1993) Update on surgical treatment of the epilepsies. Summary of The Second International Palm Desert Conference on the Surgical Treatment of the Epilepsies (1992). *Neurology* **43**, 1612–1617 [311].

ENGEL, J. Jr, BROWN, W.J., KUHL, D.E., PHELPS, M.E., MAZZIOTTA, J.C. & CRANDALL, P.H. (1982a) Pathological findings underlying focal temporal lobe hypometabolism in partial epilepsy. *Annals of Neurology* **12**, 518–528 [289].

ENGEL, J. Jr, KUHL, D.E., PHELPS, M.E. & MAZZIOTTA, J.C. (1982b) Interictal cerebral glucose metabolism in partial epilepsy and its relation to EEG changes. *Annals of Neurology* **12**, 510–517 [289].

ENGLISH, A., SAVAGE, R.D., BRITTON, P.G., WARD, M.K. & KERR, D.N.S. (1978) Intellectual impairment in chronic renal failure. *British Medical Journal* **1**, 888–890 [558].

ENOCH, M.D., TRETHOWAN, W.H. & BARKER, J.C. (1967) *Some Uncommon Psychiatric Syndromes*. John Wright: Bristol [480].

ENZMANN, D.R. & LANE, B. (1977) Cranial computed tomography findings in anorexia nervosa. *Journal of Computer Assisted Tomography* **1**, 410–414 [141].

EPSTEIN, A.W. (1961) Relationship of fetishism and transvestism to brain and particularly to temporal lobe dysfunction. *Journal of Nervous and Mental Disease* **133**, 247–253 [273].

EPSTEIN, L.G., SHARER, L.R. & GOUDSMIT, J. (1988) Neurological and neuropathological features of human immunodeficiency virus infection in children. *Annals of Neurology* **23 (Supplement)**, S19–S23 [326].

EPSTEIN, M.T., HOCKADAY, J.M. & HOCKADAY, T.D.R. (1975) Migraine and reproductive hormones throughout the menstrual cycle. *Lancet* **1**, 543–548 [402].

ERAUT, D. (1974) Idiopathic hypoparathyroidism presenting as dementia. *British Medical Journal* **1**, 429–430 [532].

ERICKSON, T.C. (1945) Erotomania (nymphomania) as an expression of cortical epileptiform discharge. *Archives of Neurology and Psychiatry* **53**, 226–231 [250].

ERKINJUNTTI, T. & SULKAVA, R. (1991) Diagnosis of multi-infarct dementia. *Alzheimer's Disease and Associated Disorders* **5**, 112–121 [454, 456, 460].

ERLINGTON, G. & NEWSOM-DAVIS, J. (1994) Clinical presentation and current immunology of the Lambert–Eaton myasthenic syndrome. Ch. 5 in *Handbook of Myasthenia Gravis and Myasthenic Syndromes*, ed. Lisak, R.P. Marcel Dekker: New York [711].

ERVIN, F.R., DELGADO, J., MARK, V.H. & SWEET, W.H. (1969) Rage: a paraepileptic phenomenon? *Epilepsia* **10**, 417 [270].

ESCOBAR, A. & ARUFFO, C. (1980) Chronic thinner intoxication: clinico-pathologic report of a human case. *Journal of Neurology, Neurosurgery and Psychiatry* **43**, 986–994 [630].

ESCOBAR, A., ARUFFO, C. & RODRIGUEZ-CARBAJAL, J. (1983) Wernicke's encephalopathy. A case report with neurophysiologic and CT-scan studies. *Acta Vitaminol Enzymol* **5**, 125–131 [579].

ESLINGER, P.J. & DAMASIO, A.R. (1986) Preserved motor learning in Alzheimer's disease: implications for anatomy and behavior. *Journal of Neuroscience* **6**, 3006–3009 [32].

ESLINGER, P.J., WARNER, G.C., GRATTAN, L.M. & EASTON, J.D. (1991) 'Frontal lobe' utilization behavior associated with paramedian thalamic infarction. *Neurology* **41**, 450–452 [79].

ESMONDE, T.F.G., WILL, R.G., SLATTERY, J.M., KNIGHT, R., HARRIES-JONES, R., DE SILVA, R. & MATTHEWS, W.B. (1993) Creutzfeldt–Jakob disease and blood transfusion. *Lancet* **341**, 205–207 [476].

ESPIR, M.L.E. & SPALDING, J.M.K. (1956) Three recent cases of encephalitis lethargica. *British Medical Journal* **1**, 1141–1144 [354].

ESTES, D. & CHRISTIAN, C.L. (1971) The natural history of systemic lupus erythematosus by prospective analysis. *Medicine* **50**, 85–95 [419].

ESTES, J.W., MORLEY, T.J., LEVINE, I.M. & EMERSON, C.P. (1967) A new hereditary acanthocytosis syndrome. *American Journal of Medicine* **42**, 868–881 [757].

ESTRIN, W.J. (1987) Alcoholic cerebellar degeneration is not a dose-dependent phenomenon. *Alcoholism: Clinical and Experimental Research* **11**, 372–375 [586].

ESTROFF, T.W. & GOLD, M.S. (1986) Medical and psychiatric complications of cocaine abuse with possible points of pharmacological treatment. In *Controversies in Alcoholism and Substance Abuse*, ed. Stimmel, B. *Advances in Alcohol and Substance Abuse*, **5 (Nos.1/2)**, 1985–86, 61–76 [618, 620].

ETTLINGER, G. (1956) Sensory deficits in visual agnosia. *Journal of Neurology, Neurosurgery and Psychiatry* **19**, 297–307 [60].

ETTLINGER, G. (1960) The description and interpretation of pictures in cases of brain lesion. *Journal of Mental Science* **106**, 1337–1346 [63].

ETTLINGER, G. (1977) Agenesis of the corpus callosum. Ch. 12 in *Handbook of Clinical Neurology*, Vol. 30, eds Vinken, P.J. & Bruyn, G.W. North-Holland Publishing Co.: Amsterdam [770].

ETTLINGER, G., BLAKEMORE, C.B., MILNER, A.D. & WILSON, J. (1972) Agenesis of the corpus callosum: a behavioural investigation. *Brain* **95**, 327–346 [770].

ETTLINGER, G., BLAKEMORE, C.B., MILNER, A.D. & WILSON, J. (1974) Agenesis of the corpus callosum: a further behavioural investigation. *Brain* **97**, 225–234 [770].

EVANS, J.A., RUBITSKY, H.J., BARTELS, C.C. & BARTELS, E.C. (1951) Re-evaluation of the reliability of pharmacologic and cold pressor studies in hypertension and phaeochromocytoma. *American Journal of Medicine* **11**, 448–460 [520].

EVANS, N.J.R., BALDWIN, J.A. & GATH, D. (1974) The incidence of cancer among in-patients with affective disorders. *British Journal of Psychiatry* **124**, 518–525 [744].

EVERALL, I.P. & LANTOS, P.L. (1991) The neuropathology of HIV: a review of the first 10 years. *International Review of Psychiatry* **3**, 307–320 [320, 322].

EVERALL, I.P., LUTHERT, P.J. & LANTOS, P.L. (1991) Neuronal loss in the frontal cortex in HIV infection. *Lancet* **337**, 1119–1121 [323].

EVERALL, I.P., LUTHERT, P.J. & LANTOS, P.L. (1993a) Neuronal number and volume alterations in the neocortex of HIV infected individuals. *Journal of Neurology, Neurosurgery and Psychiatry* **56**, 481–486 [323].

EVERALL, I., LUTHERT, P. & LANTOS, P. (1993b) A review of neuronal damage in human immunodeficiency virus infection: its assessment, possible mechanism and relationship to dementia. *Journal of Neuropathology and Experimental Neurology* **52**, 561–566 [323].

EVERT, D.L. & OSCAR-BERMAN, M. (1995) Alcohol-related cognitive impairments. An overview of how alcoholism may affect the workings of the brain. *Alcohol Health and Research World* **19**, 89–96 [604].

EWERT, J., LEVIN, H.S., WATSON, M.G. & KALISKY, Z. (1989) Procedural memory during post-traumatic amnesia in survivors of severe closed head injury. Implications for rehabilitation. *Archives of Neurology* **46**, 911–916 [169].

EWING, R., McCARTHY, D., GRONWALL, D. & WRIGHTSON, P. (1980) Persisting effects of minor head injury observable during hypoxic stress. *Journal of Clinical Neuropsychology* **2**, 147–155 [198].

EWUSI-MENSAH, I., SAUNDERS, J.B., WODAK, A.D., MURRAY, R.M. &

WILLIAMS, R. (1983) Psychiatric morbidity in patients with alcoholic liver disease. *British Medical Journal* **287**, 1417–1419 [566].

FABER, R. (1995) Electroconvulsive therapy in Parkinson's disease. Ch. 36 in *Therapy of Parkinson's Disease*, 2nd edn, eds Koller, W.C. & Paulson, G. Marcel Dekker: New York [656].

FABING, H.D. (1946) Narcolepsy: II. Theory of pathogenesis of the narcolepsy–cataplexy syndrome. *Archives of Neurology and Psychiatry* **55**, 353–363 [725].

FABRYKANT, M. (1960) Neuropsychiatric manifestations of somatic disease: a review of nutritional, metabolic and endocrine aspects. *Metabolism* **9**, 413–426 [571].

FADEN, A.I., DEMEDIUK, P., PANTER, S.S. & VINK, R. (1989) The role of excitatory aminoacids and NMDA receptors in traumatic brain injury. *Science* **244**, 798–800 [164].

FAGALY, R.L. (1990) Neuromagnetic instrumentation. Ch. 2 in *Magnetoencephalography*, ed. Sato, S. *Advances in Neurology*, Vol. 54. Raven Press: New York [133].

FAHAL, I.H., SALLOMI, D.F., YAQOOB, M. & BELL, G.M. (1992) Acute renal failure after ecstasy. *British Medical Journal* **305**, 29 [624].

FAHN, S. (1994a) The paroxysmal dyskinesias. Ch. 16 in *Movement Disorders*, Vol. 3, eds Marsden, C.D. & Fahn, S. Butterworth-Heinemann: Oxford [291, 292].

FAHN, S. (1994b) Psychogenic movement disorders. Ch. 18 in *Movement Disorders*, Vol. 3, eds Marsden, C.D. & Fahn, S. Butterworth-Heinemann: Oxford [680].

FAHN, S., MARSDEN, C.D. & CALNE, D.B. (1987) Classification and investigation of dystonia. Ch. 17 in *Movement Disorders*, Vol. 2, eds Marsden, C.D. & Fahn, S. Butterworths: London [669, 679].

FAHN, S., WILLIAMS, D. & RECHES, A. (1983) Hysterical dystonia, a rare disorder: report of five documented cases. *Neurology*, **33 (Supplement 2)**, 161 [680].

FAHY, T.J., IRVING, M.H. & MILLAC, P. (1967) Severe head injuries: a six-year follow-up. *Lancet* **2**, 475–479 [161, 185].

FAIRBURN, C.G., WU, F.C.W., McCULLOCH, D.K., BORSEY, D.Q., EWING, D.J., CLARKE, B.F. & BANCROFT, J.H.J. (1982) The clinical features of diabetic impotence: a preliminary study. *British Journal of Psychiatry* **140**, 447–452 [536].

FAIRHALL, L.T. & NEAL, P.A. (1943) *Industrial Manganese Poisoning*, National Institute of Health Bulletin No. 182. United States Government Printing Office: Washington [635].

FAIRWEATHER, D.S. (1947) Psychiatric aspects of the post-encephalitic syndrome. *Journal of Mental Science* **93**, 201–254 [353].

FALCONER, M.A. (1969) The surgical treatment of temporal lobe epilepsy. Ch. 16 in *Current Problems in Neuropsychiatry*, ed. Herrington, R.N. British Journal of Psychiatry Special Publication No. 4. Headley Brothers: Ashford, Kent [311].

FALCONER, M.A. (1971) Anterior temporal lobectomy for epilepsy. In *Operative Surgery*, Vol. 14, eds Rob, C.G. & Smith, E.R. *Neurosurgery*, ed. Logue, V., pp. 142–149. Butterworths: London [311].

FALCONER, M.A. (1973) Reversibility by temporal lobe resection of the behavioural abnormalities of temporal lobe epilepsy. *New England Journal of Medicine* **289**, 451–455 [270, 281, 312].

FALCONER, M.A. (1974) Mesial temporal (Ammon's horn) sclerosis as a common cause of epilepsy: aetiology, treatment, and prevention. *Lancet* **2**, 767–770 [246].

FALCONER, M.A. & DAVIDSON, S. (1973) Coarse features in epilepsy as a consequence of anticonvulsant therapy. *Lancet* **2**, 1112–1114 [301].

FALCONER, M.A. & TAYLOR, D.C. (1968) Surgical treatment of drug-resistant epilepsy due to mesial temporal sclerosis. Etiology and significance. *Archives of Neurology* **19**, 353–361 [246].

FALCONER, M.A. & TAYLOR, D.C. (1970) Temporal lobe epilepsy: clinical features, pathology, diagnosis, and treatment. Ch. 14 in *Modern Trends in Psychological Medicine*, Vol. 2, ed. Price, J.H. Butterworth: London [266, 294].

FALKAI, P. & BOGERTS, B. (1986) Cell loss in the hippocampus of schizophrenics. *European Archives of Psychiatry and Neurological Sciences* **236**, 154–161 [86].

FALKAI, P., BOGERTS, B., GREVE, B., PFEIFFER, U., MACHUS, B., FÖLSCH-REETZ, B., MAJTENYI, C. & OVARY, I. (1992) Loss of Sylvian fissure asymmetry in schizophrenia. A quantitative post mortem study. *Schizophrenia Research* **7**, 23–32 [86].

FARDE, L., NORDSTRÖM, A.-L., KARLSSON, P., HALLDIN, C. & SEDVALL, G. (1995) Positron emission tomography studies on dopamine receptors in schizophrenia. *Clinical Neuropharmacology*, **18 (Supplement 1)**, S121–S129 [89].

FARDE, L., WIESEL, F.-A., HALL, H., HALLDIN, C., STONE-ELANDER, S. & SEDVALL, G. (1987) No D_2 receptor increase in PET study of schizophrenia. *Archives of General Psychiatry* **44**, 671–672 [88].

FARLOW, M., GRACON, S.I., HERSHEY, L.A., LEWIS, K.W., SADOWSKY, C.H. & DOLAN-URENO, J. FOR THE TACRINE STUDY GROUP (1992) A controlled trial of tacrine in Alzheimer's disease. *Journal of the American Medical Association* **268**, 2523–2529 [504].

FARRELL, D.F. & STARR, A. (1968) Delayed neurological sequelae of electrical injuries. *Neurology* **18**, 601–606 [766].

FARRELL, M.J. & KAUFMAN, M.R. (1943) A compendium on neuropsychiatry in the army. *Army Medical Bulletin* **66**, 1–112 [485].

FAUCI, A.S., HAYNES, B. & KATZ, P. (1978) The spectrum of vasculitis: clinical, pathologic, immunologic and therapeutic considerations. *Annals of Internal Medicine* **89**, 660–676 [425].

FAULSTICH, M.E. (1987) Psychiatric aspects of AIDS. *American Journal of Psychiatry* **144**, 551–556 [330].

FAUST, C. (1955) Zur Symptomatik frischer und alter Stirnhirnverletzungen. *Archiv für Psychiatrie und Nervenkrankheiten* **193**, 78–97 [180].

FAUST, C. (1960) Die psychischen Störungen nach Hirntraumen: Akute traumatische Psychosen und psychische Spätfolgen nach Hirnverletzungen. In *Psychiatrie Der Gegenwart: Forschung Und Praxis*, Vol. 2, eds Gruhle, H.W., Jung, R., Mayer-Gross, W. & Miller, M., pp. 552–645. Springer: Berlin [180].

FAVA, G.A., SONINO, N. & MORPHY, M.A. (1987) Major depression associated with endocrine disease. *Psychiatric Developments* **5**, 321–348 [518, 522].

FAWZY, F.I., FAWZY, N.W. & PASNAU, R.O. (1991) Bereavement in AIDS. *Psychiatric Medicine* **9**, 469–481 [333].

FEELY, M. (1989) Clonazepam and clobazam. *Prescribers' Journal* **29**, 111–115 [305].

FEEMSTER, R.F. (1957) Equine encephalitis in Massachusetts. *New England Journal of Medicine* **257**, 701–704 [348].

FEIDO, P. & MIRSKY, A.F. (1969) Selective intellectual deficits in children with temporal lobe or centrencephalic epilepsy. *Neuropsychologia* **7**, 287–300 [261, 262].

FEIGHNER, J.P., ROBINS, E., GUZE, S.B., WOODRUFF R.A., WINOKUR, G. & MUNOZ, R. (1972) Diagnostic criteria for use in psychiatric research. *Archives of General Psychiatry* **26**, 57–63 [84].

FEINBERG, W.M. & RAPCSAK, S.Z. (1989) 'Peduncular hallucinosis' following paramedian thalamic infarction. *Neurology* **39**, 1535–1536 [388].

FEINDEL, W. & PENFIELD, W. (1954) Localization of discharge in temporal lobe automatism. *Archives of Neurology and Psychiatry* **72**, 605–630 [253, 254].

FEINSTEIN, A. & DOLAN, R. (1991) Predictors of post-traumatic stress disorder following physical trauma: an examination of the stressor criterion. *Psychological Medicine* **21**, 85–91 [195].

FEINSTEIN, A., DU BOULAY, G. & RON, M.A. (1992a) Psychotic illness in multiple sclerosis. A clinical and magnetic resonance imaging study. *British Journal of Psychiatry* **161**, 680–685 [697].

FEINSTEIN, A., KARTSOUNIS, L., MILLER, D., YOUL, B. & RON, M.A. (1992b) Clinically isolated lesions of the type seen in multiple sclerosis followed up: a cognitive, psychiatric and MRI study. *Journal of Neurology, Neurosurgery and Psychiatry* **55**, 869–876 [693].

FEINSTEIN, A., RON, M.A. & WESSELY, S. (1990) Disappearing brain lesions, psychosis and epilepsy: a report of two cases. *Journal of Neurology, Neurosurgery and Psychiatry* **53**, 244–246 [289].

FEINSTEIN, A., YOUL, B. & RON, M. (1992c) Acute optic neuritis. A cognitive and magnetic resonance imaging study. *Brain* **115**, 1403–1415 [693].

FELDMAN, M.H. (1971) Physiological observations in a chronic case of 'locked-in' syndrome. *Neurology* **21**, 459–478 [379].

FELDMAN, R.G. (1982) Neurological manifestations of mercury intoxication. *Acta Neurologica Scandinavica* **66 (Supplement 92)**, 201–209 [635].

FENICHEL, O. (1945) *The Psychoanalytic Theory of Neurosis*. Norton & Co.: New York [684].

FENTON, G.W. (1972) Epilepsy and automatism. *British Journal of Hospital Medicine* **7**, 57–64 [253, 254, 275, 296].

FENTON, G. (1974) The straightforward EEG in psychiatric practice. *Proceedings of the Royal Society of Medicine* **67**, 911–919 [128, 129].

FENTON, G.W. (1978) Epilepsy and psychosis. *Journal of the Irish Medical Association* **71**, 315–324 [256, 285].

FENTON, G.W. (1981) Personality and behavioural disorders in adults with epilepsy. Ch. 8 in *Epilepsy and Psychiatry*, eds Reynolds, E.H. & Trimble, M.R. Churchill Livingstone: London and Edinburgh [267].

FENTON, G. (1983) Epilepsy. Ch. 13 in *Handbook of Psychiatry*, Vol. 2, *Mental Disorders and Somatic Illness*, ed. Lader, M.H. Cambridge Universiy Press: Cambridge [299].

FENTON, G., McCLELLAND, R., MONTGOMERY, A., MacFLYNN, G. & RUTHERFORD, W. (1993) The postconcussional syndrome: social antecedents and psychological sequelae. *British Journal of Psychiatry* **162**, 493–497 [176].

FENTON, T.W. (1987) AIDS-related psychiatric disorder. *British Journal of Psychiatry* **151**, 579–588 [329].

FENWICK, P. (1981a) Precipitation and inhibition of seizures. Ch. 22 in *Epilepsy and Psychiatry*, eds Reynolds, E.H. & Trimble, M.R. Churchill Livingstone: London and Edinburgh [241, 248, 309].

FENWICK, P. (1981b) EEG studies. Ch. 18 in *Epilepsy and Psychiatry*, eds Reynolds, E.H. & Trimble, M.R. Churchill Livingstone: London & Edinburgh [288].

FENWICK, P. (1986) Aggression and epilepsy. Ch. 4 in *Aspects of Epilepsy and Psychiatry*, eds Trimble, M.R. & Bolwig, T.G. John Wiley & Sons Ltd [82, 267].

FENWICK, P. (1987a) Epilepsy and psychiatric disorders. Ch. 18 in *Epilepsy*, ed. Hopkins, A. Chapman & Hall: London [256, 257].

FENWICK, P. (1987b) Somnambulism and the law: a review. *Behavioral Sciences and the Law* **5**, 343–357 [737].

FENWICK, P. (1990a) The use of magnetoencephalography in neurology. Ch. 22 in *Magnetoencephalography*, ed. Sato, S. *Advances in Neurology* **54**. Raven Press: New York [133].

FENWICK, P. (1990b) Automatism, medicine and the law. *Psychological Medicine Monograph Supplement* **17** [298, 736, 737].

FENWICK, P. (1991) Evocation and inhibition of seizures: behavioral treatment. Ch. 11 in *Neurobehavioral Problems in Epilepsy*, eds

Smith, D.B., Treiman, D.M. & Trimble, M.R. *Advances in Neurology* **55**. Raven Press: New York [309].

FENWICK, P. (1993) Brain, mind and behaviour. Some medico-legal aspects. *British Journal of Psychiatry* **163**, 565–573 [298, 737].

FENWICK, P.B.C. & BROWN, S.W. (1989) Evoked and psychogenic epileptic seizures. I. Precipitation. *Acta Neurologica Scandinavica* **80**, 535–540 [248].

FERENCI, P., GRIMM, G., MERYN, S. & GANGL, A. (1989) Successful long-term treatment of portal-systemic encephalopathy by the benzodiazepine antagonist flumazenil. *Gastroenterology* **96**, 240–243 [566].

FERENCZI, S., ABRAHAM, K., SIMMEL, E. & JONES, E. (1921) *Psychoanalysis and the War Neuroses*. International Psychoanalytical Press: London [175].

FERGUSON, D. (1971) An Australian study of telegraphists' cramp. *British Journal of Industrial Medicine* **28**, 280–285 [677].

FERGUSON, S.M. & RAYPORT, M. (1965) The adjustment to living without epilepsy. *Journal of Nervous and Mental Diseases* **140**, 26–37 [270].

FERGUSON, S.M., RAYPORT, M. & CORRIE, W.S. (1985) Neuropsychiatric observations on behavioral consequences of corpus callosum section for seizure control. Ch. 28 in *Epilepsy and the Corpus Callosum*, ed. Reeves, A.G. Plenum Press: New York [313].

FERNER, R.E. (1994) Intellect in neurofibromatosis 1. Ch. 9 in *The Neurofibromatoses*, eds Huson, S.M. & Hughes, R.A.C. Chapman & Hall: London [704].

FERRARO, A. (1934) Histopathological findings in two cases clinically diagnosed dementia praecox. *American Journal of Psychiatry* **90 (part 2)**, 883–903 [701].

FERRARO, A. (1943) Pathological changes in the brain of a case clinically diagnosed dementia praecox. *Journal of Neuropathology and Experimental Neuroloy* **2**, 84–94 [701].

FERRER, I. (1992) Dementia of frontal lobe type and amyotrophy. *Behavioural Neurology* **5**, 87–96 [708].

FERRIER, I.N., CROSS, A.J., JOHNSON, J.A., ROBERTS, G.W., CROW, T.J., CORSELLIS, J.A.N., LEE, Y.C., O'SHAUGHNESSY, D., ADRIAN, T.E., McGREGOR, G.P., BARACESE-HAMILTON, A.J. & BLOOM, S.R. (1983) Neuropeptides in Alzheimer type dementia. *Journal of the Neurological Sciences* **62**, 159–170 [445].

FERRIS, S.H., REISBERG, B., CROOK, T., FRIEDMAN, E., SCHNECK, M.K., MIR, P., SHERMAN, K.A., CORWIN, J., GERSHON, S. & BARTUS, R.T. (1982) Pharmacologic treatment of senile dementia: choline, L-dopa, piracetam, and choline plus piracetam. In *Alzheimer's Disease: A Report of Progress in Research, Aging*, Vol. 19, eds Corkin, S., Davis, K.L., Growdon, J.H. & Wurtman, R.J., pp. 475–481. Raven Press: New York [503].

FESSEL, W.J. & SOLOMON, G.F. (1960) Psychosis and systemic lupus erythematosus: a review of the literature and case reports. *California Medicine* **92**, 266–270 [374, 419].

FEUCHTWANGER, E. (1923) *Die Funktionen des Stirnhirns: ihre Pathologie und Psychologie*. Springer: Berlin [180].

FEUCHTWANGER, E. & MAYER-GROSS, W. (1938) Hirnverletzung und Schizophrenie. *Schweizer Archiv für Neurologie und Pychiatrie* **41**, 17–99 [190].

FEURLE, G.E., VOLK, B. & WALDHERR, R. (1979) Cerebral Whipple's disease with negative jejunal histology. *New England Journal of Medicine* **300**, 907–908 [760, 761].

FIELD, J.H. (1976) *Epidemiology of Head Injuries in England and Wales*. HMSO: London [161, 172].

FIELDS, F.R.J. & FULLERTON, J.R. (1975) Influence of heroin addiction on neuropsychological functioning. *Journal of Consulting and Clinical Psychology* **43**, 114 [612].

806 REFERENCES

FIELDS, W.S. & BLATTNER, R.J. (1958) *Viral Encephalitis* (Fifth Symposium, Houston Neurological Society). Thomas: Springfield, Illinois [26].

FILLEY, C.M., HEATON, R.K., THOMPSON, L.L., NELSON, L.M. & FRANKLIN, G.M. (1990) Effects of disease course on neuropsychological functioning. Ch. 8 in *Neurobehavioral Aspects of Multiple Sclerosis*, ed. Rao, S.M. Oxford University Press: Oxford [693].

FINE, B.D. (1969) Psychoanalytical aspects of head pain. In *Research and Clinical Studies in Headache*, Vol. 2, ed. Friedman, A.P., pp. 169–194. Karger: Basel [403].

FINE, E.W., LEWIS, D., VILLA-LANDA, I. & BLAKEMORE, C.B. (1970) The effect of cyclandelate on mental function in patients with arteriosclerotic brain disease. *British Journal of Psychiatry* **117**, 157–161 [502].

FINELLI, P.F., McENTEE, W.J., LESSELL, S., MORGAN, T.F. & COPETTO, J. (1977) Whipple's disease with predominantly neuroophthalmic manifestations. *Annals of Neurology* **1**, 247–252 [760].

FINLAY-JONES, R. (1986) Should thiamine be added to beer? *Australian and New Zealand Journal of Psychiatry* **20**, 3–6 [581].

FINLEY, K.H. (1958) Postencephalitis manifestations of viral encephalitides. In *Viral Encephalitis*, eds Fields, W.S. & Blattner, R.J. Thomas: Springfield, Illinois [348].

FIORDELLI, E., BEGHI, E., BOGLIUN, G. & CRESPI, V. (1993) Epilepsy and psychiatric disturbance. A cross-sectional study. *British Journal of Psychiatry* **163**, 446–450 [260].

FISCHER, M., KORSKJAER, G. & PEDERSEN, E. (1965) Psychotic episodes in Zarondan treatment. Effects and side-effects in 105 patients. *Epilepsia* **6**, 325–334 [284, 302].

FISCHER, P., JELLINGER, K., GATTERER, G. & DANIELCZYK, W. (1991) Prospective neuropathological validation of Hachinski's ischaemic score in dementias. *Journal of Neurology, Neurosurgery and Psychiatry* **54**, 580–583 [457].

FISCHER-WILLIAMS, M., BOSANQUET, F.D. & DANIEL, P.M. (1955) Carcinomatosis of the meninges. *Brain* **78**, 42–58 [739].

FISCHER-WILLIAMS, M., NIGL, A.J. & SOVINE, D.L. (1981) *A Textbook of Biological Feedback*. Human Sciences Press: New York and London [309, 410, 675].

FISCHL, M.A., RICHMAN, D.D., GRIECO, M.H., GOTTLIEB, M.S., VOLBERDING, P.A., LASKIN, O.L., LEEDOM, J.M., GROOPMAN, J.E., MILDUAN, D., SCHOOLEY, R.T., JACKSON, C.G., DURACK, D.T., KING, D. & THE AZT COLLABORATIVE WORKING GROUP (1987) The efficacy of azidothymidine (AZT) in the treatment of patients with AIDS and AIDS-related complex. *New England Journal of Medicine* **317**, 185–191 [335].

FISCHL, M.A., RICHMAN, D.D., HANSEN, N., COLLIER, A.C., CAREY, J.T., PARA, M.F., HARDY, D., DOLIN, R., POWDERLY, W.G., DAVIS ALLAN, J., WONG, B., MERIGAN, T.C., MCAULIFFE, V.J., HYSLOP, N.E., RHAME, F.S., BALFOUR, H.H., SPECTOR, S.A., VOLBERDING, P., PETTINELLI, C., ANDERSON, J. & THE AIDS CLINICAL TRIALS GROUP (1990) The safety and efficacy of zidovudine (AZT) in the treatment of subjects with mildly symptomatic human immunodeficiency virus type 1 (HIV) infection. *Annals of Internal Medicine* **112**, 727–737 [336].

FISH, B. (1977) Neurobiologic antecedents of schizophrenia in children. *Archives of General Psychiatry* **34**, 1297–1313 [91].

FISH, B., MARCUS, J., HANS, S.L., AUERBACH, J.G. & PERDUE, S. (1992) Infants at risk for schizophrenia: sequelae of a genetic neurointegrative defect. A review and replication. *Archives of General Psychiatry* **49**, 221–235 [91].

FISH, F.J. (1962) *Schizophrenia*. John Wright: Bristol [482].

FISHER, C., KAHN, E., EDWARDS, A. & DAVIS, D.M. (1973) A psychophysiological study of nightmares and night terrors. 1: Physiological aspects of the stage 4 night terror. *Journal of Nervous and Mental Disease* **157**, 75–98 [737].

FISHER, C.M. (1965) Lacunes: small deep cerebral infarcts. *Neurology* **15**, 774–784 [384].

FISHER, C.M. (1968) Dementia in cerebral vascular disease. In *Transactions of the Sixth Conference on Cerebral Vascular Diseases*, American Neurological Association. Grune & Stratton: New York [378, 379, 384].

FISHER, C.M. (1982a) Whiplash amnesia. *Neurology* **32**, 667–668 [200].

FISHER, C.M. (1982b) Lacunar strokes and infarcts: a review. *Neurology* **32**, 871–876 [377, 380, 384].

FISHER, C.M. & ADAMS, R.D. (1958) Transient global amnesia. In *Transactions of the American Neurological Association*, 83rd Annual Meeting, pp. 143–146. William Byrd Press: Richmond, Virginia [413].

FISHER, C.M. & ADAMS, R.D. (1964) Transient global amnesia. *Acta Neurologica Scandinavica* **9 (Supplement)**, 7–83 [413, 414].

FISHER, K. & FINDLEY, L. (1981) Intellectual changes in optimally treated patients with Parkinson's disease. Ch. 8 in *Research in Progress in Parkinson's Disease*, eds Rose, F.C. & Capildeo, R. Pitman Medical: Tunbridge Wells [659].

FISHER, M. (1951) Senile dementia—a new explanation of its causation. *Canadian Medical Association Journal* **65**, 1–7 [384].

FISHER, M. (1954) Occlusion of the carotid arteries: further experiences. *Archives of Neurology and Psychiatry* **72**, 187–204 [384].

FISHER, N.R., COPE, S.J. & LISHMAN, W.A. (1987) Metachromatic leukodystrophy: conduct disorder progressing to dementia. *Journal of Neurology, Neurosurgery and Psychiatry* **50**, 488–489 [xxiii, 759].

FISHMAN, R.A. (1965) Neurological aspects of magnesium metabolism. *Archives of Neurology* **12**, 562–569 [561].

FISMAN, M. (1975) The brain stem in psychosis. *British Journal of Psychiatry* **126**, 414–442 [86].

FITZHUGH, L.C., FITZHUGH, K.B. & REITAN, R.M. (1960) Adaptive abilities and intellectual functioning in hospitalised alcoholics. *Quarterly Journal of Studies on Alcohol* **21**, 414–423 [603].

FITZHUGH, L.C., FITZHUGH, K.B. & REITAN, R.M. (1965) Adaptive abilites and intellectual functioning of hospitalised alcoholics: further considerations. *Quarterly Journal of Studies on Alcohol* **26**, 402–411 [603].

FLAMM, E.S., DEMOPOULOS, H.B., SELIGMAN, M.L., TOMASULA, J.J., DE CRESCITO, V. & RANSOHOFF, J. (1977) Ethanol potentiation of central nervous system trauma. *Journal of Neurosurgery* **46**, 328–335 [179].

FLATAU, E. (1912) Die Migräne. In *Monographien aus dem Gesamtgebiet der Neurologie und Psychiatrie*, eds Alzheimer, A. & Levandowsky, L. Berlin. Quoted by Klee, A. (1968) *A Clinical Study of Migraine with Particular Reference to the Most Severe Cases*. Munksgaard: Copenhagen [407].

FLATEN, T.P. (1986) An investigation of the chemical composition of Norwegian drinking water and its possible relationships with the epidemiology of some diseases. Thesis, Instiutt of Uorganisk Kjem, Norges Teniske Hogskole, Trondheim. Quoted by Rifat, S.L. & Eastwood, M.R. (1994) The role of aluminium in dementia of Alzheimer's type: a review of the hypotheses and summary of the evidence. Ch 15 in *Dementia*, eds Burns, A. & Levy, R. Chapman & Hall Medical: London [446].

FLEMINGER, S. (1991) Left-sided Parkinson's disease is associated with greater anxiety and depression. *Psychological Medicine* **21**, 629–638 [656, 657].

FLEMINGER, S. (1992a) Seeing is believing: the role of 'preconscious' perceptual processing in delusional misidentification. *British Journal of Psychiatry* **160**, 293–303 [12].

FLEMINGER, S. (1992b) Control of simultaneous movements distinguishes depressive motor retardation from Parkinson's disease and neuroleptic parkinsonism. *Brain* **115**, 1459–1480 [647].

FLETCHER, N.A., HARDING, A.E. & MARSDEN, C.D. (1990) A genetic study of idiopathic torsion dystonia in the United Kingdom. *Brain* **113**, 379–395 [670].

FLETCHER, P.C., FRITH, C.D., GRASBY, P.M., SHALLICE, T., FRACK-OWIAK, R.S.J. & DOLAN, R.J. (1995) Brain systems for encoding and retrieval of auditory-verbal memory. An *in vivo* study in humans. *Brain* **118**, 401–416 [28].

FLEWETT, T.H. & HOULT, J.G. (1958) Influenzal encephalopathy and postinfluenzal encephalitis. *Lancet* **2**, 11–15 [359].

FLINK, E.B. (1956) Magnesium deficiency syndrome in man. *Journal of the American Medical Association* **160**, 1406–1409 [561].

FLINK, E.B., STUTZMAN, F.L., ANDERSON, A.R., KONIG, T. & FRASER, F. (1954) Magnesium deficiency after prolonged parenteral fluid administration and after chronic alcoholism complicated by delirium tremens. *Journal of Laboratory and Clinical Medicine* **43**, 169–183 [602].

FLINT, J. & GOLDSTEIN, L.H. (1992) Familial calcification of the basal ganglia: a case report and review of the literature. *Psychological Medicine* **22**, 581–595 [756].

FLOOD, D.G. & COLEMAN, P.D. (1986) Failed compensatory dendritic growth as a pathophysiological process in Alzheimer's disease. *Canadian Journal of Neurological Science* **13**, 475–479 [443, 607].

FLOR-HENRY, P. (1969) Psychosis and temporal lobe epilepsy: a controlled investigation. *Epilepsia* **10**, 363–395 [278, 282, 283, 286].

FLOR-HENRY, P. (1983) *Cerebral Basis of Psychopathology*. John Wright: Bristol [89].

FLOR-HENRY, P., FROMM-AUCH, D. & SCHOPFLOCHER, D. (1983) Neuropsychological dimensions in psychopathology. In *Laterality and Psychopathology*, eds Flor-Henry, P. & Gruzelier, J., pp. 59–82. Elsevier: Amsterdam [89].

FLOR-HENRY, P. & GRUZELIER, J. (eds) (1983) *Laterality and Psychopathology*. Elsevier: Amsterdam [89].

FLOR-HENRY, P. & YEUDALL, L.T. (1979) Neuropsychological investigation of schizophrenia and manic-depressive psychoses. In *Hemisphere Asymmetries of Function in Psychopathology*, eds Gruzelier, J. & Flor-Henry, P., pp. 341–362. Elsevier/North-Holland Biomedical Press: Amsterdam [89].

FLORIAN, V., KATZ, S. & LAHAV, V. (1989) Impact of traumatic brain damage on family dynamics and functioning: a review. *Brain Injury* **3**, 219–233 [172, 216, 217].

FLOURENS, J.P.M. (1824) *Recherches Experimentales sur les Proprietés et les Fonctions du Système Nerveux, dans les Animaux Vertébrés*. Crevot: Paris [21].

FOLKS, D.G. & PETRIE, W.M. (1982) Thyrotoxicosis presenting as depression. *British Journal of Psychiatry* **140**, 432 [511].

FOLSTEIN, M.F., FOLSTEIN, S.E. & McHUGH, P.R. (1975) 'Mini-mental state'. A practical method for grading the cognitive state of patients for the clinician. *Journal of Psychiatric Research* **12**, 189–198 [123].

FOLSTEIN, M.F. & McHUGH, P.R. (1978) Dementia syndrome of depression. In *Alzheimer's Disease: Senile Dementia and Related Disorders, Aging*, Vol. 7, eds Katzman, R., Terry, R.D. & Bick, K.L., pp. 87–93. Raven Press: New York [486].

FOLSTEIN, M.F., MAIBERGER, R. & McHUGH, P.R. (1977) Mood disorder as a specific complication of stroke. *Journal of Neurology, Neurosurgery and Psychiatry* **40**, 1018–1020 [385].

FOLSTEIN, S.E. (1989) *Huntington's Disease. A Disorder of Families*. Johns Hopkins University Press: Baltimore [469].

FOLSTEIN, S.E., ABBOTT, M.H., CHASE, G.A., JENSEN, B.A. & FOLSTEIN, M.F. (1983) The association of affective disorder with Huntington's disease in a case series and in families. *Psychological Medicine* **13**, 537–542 [470].

FOLSTEIN, S.E., LEIGH, R.J., PARHAD, I.M. & FOLSTEIN, M.F. (1986) The diagnosis of Huntington's disease. *Neurology* **36**, 1279–1283 [469, 472].

FONCIN, J.F., GACHES, J., CATHALA, F., EL SHERIF, E. & LE BEAU, J. (1980) Transmission iatrogène interhumaine possible de maladie de Creutzfeldt–Jakob avec atteinte des grains du cervelet. *Revue Neurologique* **136**, 280 [476].

FORD, C.V., BRAY, G.A. & SWERDLOFF, R.S. (1976) A psychiatric study of patients referred with a diagnosis of hypoglycemia. *American Journal of Psychiatry* **133**, 290–294 [543].

FORD, R.G. & SIEKERT, R.G. (1965) Central nervous system manifestations of periarteritis nodosa. *Neurology* **15**, 114–122 [423].

FORNAZZARI, L., WILKINSON, D.A., KAPUR, B.M. & CARLEN, P.L. (1983) Cerebellar, cortical and functional impairment in toluene abusers. *Acta Neurologica Scandinavica* **63**, 319–329 [630].

FORSSMAN, H. (1970) The mental implications of sex chromosome aberrations. The Blake Marsh Lecture for 1970. *British Journal of Psychiatry* **117**, 353–363 [526, 527, 528].

FORSTER, E. (1919) Die psychischen Storungen der Hirnverletzen. *Monatsschrift für Psychiatrie und Neurologie* **46**, 61. Quoted by Tow, M.P. (1955) *Personality Changes Following Frontal Leucotomy*. Oxford University Press: London [180].

FORSTER, F.M. (1969) Clinical therapeutic conditioning in epilepsy. *Wisconsin Medical Journal* **68**, 289–291 [308].

FORSTER, F.M., KLOVE, H., PETERSON, W.G. & BENGZON, A.R.A. (1965) Modification of musicogenic epilepsy by extinction technique. *Transactions of the American Neurological Association* **90**, 179–182 [308].

FORSTER, F.M. & LISKE, E. (1963) Role of environmental clues in temporal lobe epilepsy. *Neurology* **13**, 301–305 [254].

FORSTER, F.M., RICHARDS, J.F., PANITCH, H.S., HUISMAN, R.E. & PAULSEN, R.E. (1975) Reflex epilepsy evoked by decision making. *Archives of Neurology* **32**, 54–56 [248].

FÖRSTL, H., BURNS, A., LUTHERT, P., CAIRNS, N., LANTOS, P. & LEVY, R. (1992) Clinical and neuropathological correlates of depression in Alzheimer's disease. *Psychological Medicine* **22**, 877–884 [443].

FÖRSTL, H., BURNS, A., LUTHERT, P., CAIRNS, N. & LEVY, R. (1993) The Lewy-body variant of Alzheimer's disease: clinical and pathological findings. *British Journal of Psychiatry* **162**, 385–392 [451, 452].

FÖRSTL, H. & LEVY, R. (1991) Classic Text No.5. On certain peculiar diseases of old age, A. Alzheimer, 1911. *History of Psychiatry* **ii**, 71–101 [437].

FÖRSTL, H. & SAHAKIAN, B. (1991) A psychiatric presentation of abulia—three cases of left frontal lobe ischaemia and atrophy. *Journal of the Royal Society of Medicine* **84**, 89–91 [386].

FOURMAN, P., DAVIS, R.H., JONES, K.H., MORGAN, D.B. & SMITH, J.W.G. (1963) Parathyroid insufficiency after thyroidectomy: review of 46 patients with a study of the effects of hypocalcaemia on the electro-encephalogram. *British Journal of Surgery* **50**, 608–619 [532].

FOURMAN, P., RAWNSLEY, K., DAVIS, R.H., JONES, K.H. & MORGAN, D.B. (1967) Effect of calcium on mental symptoms in partial parathyroid insufficiency. *Lancet* **2**, 914–915 [533].

FOWLER, R.C., KRONFOL, Z.A. & PERRY, P.J. (1977) Water intoxication, psychosis, and inappropriate secretion of antidiuretic hormone. *Archives of General Psychiatry* **34**, 1097–1099 [526].

808 REFERENCES

FOX, P.T., MINTUN, M.A., REIMAN, E.M. & RAICHLE, M.E. (1988) Enhanced detection of focal brain responses using intersubject averaging and change-distribution analysis of subtracted PET images. *Journal of Cerebral Blood Flow and Metabolism* **8**, 642–653 [144].

FOX, R.H., WILKINS, D.C., BELL, J.A., BRADLEY, R.D., BROWSE, N.L., CRANSTON, W.I., FOLEY, T.H., GILBY, E.D., HEBDEN, A., JENKINS, B.S. & RAWLINS, M.D. (1973) Spontaneous periodic hypothermia: diencephalic epilepsy. *British Medical Journal* **2**, 693–695 [241].

FRACKOWIAK, R.S.J., LENZI, G.L., JONES, T. & HEATHER, J.D. (1980) Quantitative measurement of regional cerebral blood flow and oxygen metabolism in man using ¹⁵O and positron emission tomography: theory, procedure and normal values. *Journal of Computer Assisted Tomography* **4**, 727–736 [144].

FRACKOWIAK, R.S.J., POZZILLI, C., LEGG, N.J., DU BOULAY, G.H., MARSHALL, J., LENZI, G.L. & JONES, T. (1981) Regional cerebral oxygen supply and utilisation in dementia. A clinical and physiological study with oxygen-15 and positron tomography. *Brain* **104**, 753–778 [434, 457].

FRANCIS, A.F. (1979) Familial basal ganglia calcification and schizophreniform psychosis. *British Journal of Psychiatry* **135**, 360–362 [756].

FRANCIS, A. & FREEMAN, H. (1984) Psychiatric abnormality and brain calcification over four generations. *Journal of Nervous and Mental Diseases* **172**, 166–170 [756].

FRANCIS, J., MARTIN, D. & KAPOOR, W.N. (1990) A prospective study of delirium in hospitalized elderly. *Journal of the American Medical Association* **263**, 1097–1101 [13].

FRANCIS, P.T., BOWEN, D.M., LOWE, S.L., NEARY, D., MANN, D.M.A. & SNOWDEN, J.S. (1987) Somatostatin content and release measured in cerebral biopsies from demented patients. *Journal of the Neurological Sciences* **78**, 1–16 [445].

FRANCIS, P.T., PALMER, A.M., SIMS, N.R., BOWEN, D.M., DAVISON, A.N., ESIRI, M.M., NEARY, D., SNOWDEN, J.S. & WILCOCK, G.K. (1985) Neurochemical studies of early-onset Alzheimer's disease. *New England Journal of Medicine* **313**, 7–11 [444].

FRANKEL, M., CUMMINGS, J.L., ROBERTSON, M.M., TRIMBLE, M.R., HILL, M.A. & BENSON, D.F. (1986) Obsessions and compulsions in Gilles de la Tourette's syndrome. *Neurology* **36**, 378–382 [682].

FRANKLIN, G.M., NELSON, L.M., HEATON, R.K., BURKS, J.S. & THOMPSON, D.S. (1988) Stress and its relationship to acute exacerbations in multiple sclerosis. *Journal of Neurological Rehabilitation* **2**, 7–11 [700].

FRANKLIN, G.M., NELSON, L.M., HEATON, R.K. & FILLEY, C.M. (1990) Clinical perspectives in the identification of cognitive impairment. Ch. 10 in *Neurobehavioral Aspects of Multiple Sclerosis*, ed. Rao, S.M. Oxford University Press: Oxford [692, 693].

FRANKS, S., NABARRO, J.D.N. & JACOBS, H.S. (1977) Prevalence and presentation of hyperprolactinaemia in patients with 'functionless' pituitary tumours. *Lancet* **1**, 778–780 [522].

FRAS, I., LITIN, E.M. & PEARSON, J.S. (1967) Comparison of psychiatric symptoms in carcinoma of the pancreas with those in some other intra-abdominal neoplasms. *American Journal of Psychiatry* **123**, 1553–1562 [744].

FRASER, H.F., WIKLER, A., ESSIG, C.F. & ISBELL, H. (1958) Degree of physical dependence induced by secobarbital or pentobarbital. *Journal of the American Medical Association* **166(i)**, 126–129 [608].

FREDERICKS, E.J. & LAZOR, M.Z. (1963) Recurrent hypoglycaemia associated with acute alcoholism. *Annals of Internal Medicine* **59**, 90–94 [544].

FREDERICKS, R.K., LEFKOWITZ, D.S., CHALLA, V.R. & TROOST, B.T.

(1991) Cerebral vasculitis associated with cocaine abuse. *Stroke* **22**, 1437–1439 [620].

FREDERIKS, J.A.M. (1969) Disorders of the body schema. Ch. 11 in *Handbook of Clinical Neurology*, Vol. 4, eds Vinken, P.J. & Bruyn, G.W. North-Holland Publishing Co.: Amsterdam [58, 59, 66, 67, 70, 74].

FREDERIKS, J.A.M. (1985) Disorders of the body schema. Ch. 25 in *Handbook of Clinical Neurology*, Revised series Vol. 1, *Clinical Neuropsychology*, ed. Frederiks, J.A.M. Elsevier Science Publishers BV: Amsterdam [66, 69, 70, 71, 73].

FREEDMAN, D.X. (1968) On the use and abuse of LSD. *Archives of General Psychiatry* **18**, 330–347 [620, 622].

FREEMON, F.R. (1976) Evaluation of patients with progressive intellectual deterioration. *Archives of Neurology* **33**, 658–659 [490, 491].

FREEMON, F.R. & NEVIS, A.H. (1969) Temporal lobe sexual seizures. *Neurology* **19**, 87–90 [273].

FREUD, S. (1891) On Aphasia: A Critical Study. Translated by Stengel, E. (1953) p. 78. Imago Publishing Co.: London [58].

FREUND, G. (1973) Chronic central nervous system toxicity of alcohol. *Annual Review of Pharmacology* **13**, 217–227 [583].

FRIEDE, R.L. (1961) Experimental concussion acceleration: pathology and mechanics. *Archives of Neurology* **4**, 449–462 [162].

FRIEDE, R.L. (1965) Enzyme histochemical studies of senile plaques. *Journal of Neuropathology and Experimental Neurology* **24**, 477–491 [442].

FRIEDMAN, A.P. (1969) The so-called post traumatic headache. Ch. 5 in *The Late Effects of Head Injury*, eds Walker, A.E., Caveness, W.F. & Critchley, M. Thomas: Springfield, Illinois [197, 215].

FRIEDMAN, A.P., VON STORCH, T.J.C. & MERRITT, H.M. (1954) Migraine and tension headaches. A clinical study of two thousand cases. *Neurology* **4**, 773–788 [409].

FRIEDMAN, E., SHERMAN, K.A., FERRIS, S.H., REISBERG, B., BARTUS, R.T. & SCHNECK, M.K. (1981) Clinical response to choline plus piracetam in senile dementia: relation to red-cell choline levels. *New England Journal of Medicine* **304**, 1490–1491 [503].

FRIEDMAN, J.H. (1994) Clozapine treatment of psychosis in patients with tardive dystonia: report of three cases. *Movement Disorders* **9**, 321–324 [645].

FRIEDMAN, J.H. & FRIEDMAN, H. (1993) Fatigue in Parkinson's disease. *Neurology* **43**, A237 [647].

FRIEDMAN, J.H. & LANNON, M.C. (1989) Clozapine in the treatment of psychosis in Parkinson's disease. *Neurology* **39**, 1219–1221 [658].

FRIEDMAN, S. (1980) Self-control in the treatment of Gilles de la Tourette's syndrome: case study with 18-month follow-up. *Journal of Consulting and Clinical Psychology* **48**, 400–402 [687].

FRISTON, K.J., FRITH, C.D., LIDDLE, P.F. & FRACKOWIAK, R.S.J. (1991) Comparing functional (PET) images: the assessment of significant change. *Journal of Cerebral Blood Flow and Metabolism* **11**, 690–699 [144].

FRISTON, K.J., PASSINGHAM, R.E., NUTT, J.G., HEATHER, J.D., SAWLE, G.V. & FRACKOWIAK, R.S.J. (1989) Localisation in PET images: direct fitting of the intercomissural (AC-PC) line. *Journal of Cerebral Blood Flow and Metabolism* **9**, 690–695 [144].

FRITH, C.D. (1987) The positive and negative symptoms of schizophrenia reflect impairments in the perception and initiation of action. *Psychological Medicine* **17**, 631–648 [146].

FRITH, C.D. (1995) Functional imaging and cognitive abnormalities. *Lancet* **346**, 615–620 [88].

FRITH, C.D., FRISTON, K.J., LIDDLE, P.F. & FRACKOWIAK, R.S.J. (1991)

Willed action and the prefrontal cortex in man: a study with PET. *Proceedings of the Royal Society of London* **244**, 241–246 [87].

FRITSCH, G. & HITZIG, E. (1870) Über dei elektrische Erregbarkeit des Grosshirns. Archiv für Anatomie, Physiologie und wissenschaftliche Medicin, pp. 300–332 [22].

FRÖDERSTRÖM, H. (1912) La dormeuse d'Oknö: 32 ans de stupeur: guérison complète. *Nouvelle Iconographie de la Salpêtrière* **25**, 267–279 [735].

FROMM-REICHMANN, F. (1937) Contribution to the psychogenesis of migraine. *Psychoanalytic Review* **24**, 26–33 [403, 410].

FROSCH, W.A., ROBBINS, E.S. & STERN, M. (1965) Untoward reactions to lysergic acid diethylamide (LSD) resulting in hospitalisation. *New England Journal of Medicine* **273**, 1235–1239 [622, 623].

FRÖSHAUG, H. & YTREHUS, A. (1956) A study of general paresis with special reference to the reasons for the admission of these patients to hospital. *Acta Psychiatrica et Neurologica Scandinavica* **31**, 35–60 [340, 341, 344].

FUEREDI, G.A., CZARNECKI, D.J. & KINDWALL, E.P. (1991) MR findings in the brains of compressed-air tunnel workers: relationship to psychometric results. *American Journal of Neuroradiology* **12**, 67–70 [768].

FUKUDA, K., STRAUS, S.E., HICKIE, T., SHARPE, M.C., DOBBINS, J.G. & KOMAROFF, A.L. (1994) The chronic fatigue syndrome: a comprehensive approach to its definition and study. *Annals of Internal Medicine* **121**, 953–959 [371].

FULLER, G.N., MARSHALL, A., LEWIS, S. & WISE, R.J.S. (1993) Migraine madness: recurrent psychosis following migraine. *Journal of Neurology, Neurosurgery and Psychiatry* **56**, 416–418 [406].

FULTON, J.F. & BAILEY, P. (1929) Tumours in the region of the third ventricle: their diagnosis and relation to pathological sleep. *Journal of Nervous and Mental Disease* **29**, 1–25, 145–164 and 261–277 [228].

FUSTER, J.M. (1989) *The Prefrontal Cortex. Anatomy, Physiology, and Neuropsychology of the Frontal Lobe*, 2nd edn. Raven Press: New York [79].

GADE, A. (1982) Amnesia after operations on aneurysms of the anterior communicating artery. *Surgical Neurology* **18**, 46–49 [394].

GADO, M., HUGHES, C.P., DANZIGER, W., CHI, D., JOST, G. & BERG, L. (1982) Volumetric measurements of the cerebrospinal fluid spaces in demented subjects and controls. *Radiology* **144**, 535–538 [139].

GAGE, F.H., BJÖRKLUND, A., STENEVI, U., DUNNETT, S.B. & KELLY, P.A.T. (1984) Intrahippocampal septal grafts ameliorate learning impairments in aged rats. *Science* **225**, 533–536 [505].

GAJDUSEK, D.C. (1977) Unconventional viruses and the origin and disappearance of Kuru. *Science* **197**, 943–960 [473].

GAJDUSEK, D.C., GIBBS, C.J. & ALPERS, M. (1966) Experimental transmission of a kuru-like syndrome to chimpanzees. *Nature* **209**, 794–796 [751].

GAJDUSEK, D.C., GIBBS, C.J. & ALPERS, M. (1967) Transmission and passage of experimental 'kuru' to chimpanzees. *Science* **155**, 212–214 [751].

GAJDUSEK, D.C., GIBBS, C.J., ASHER, D.M., BROWN, P., DIWAN, A., HOFFMAN P., NEMO, G., ROHWER, R. & WHITE, L. (1977) Precautions in medical care of, and in handling materials from, patients with transmissible virus dementia (Creutzfeldt–Jakob disease). *New England Journal of Medicine* **297**, 1253–1258 [751].

GAJDUSEK, D.C. & ZIGAS, V. (1957) Degenerative disease of the central nervous system in New Guinea. The endemic occurrence of 'kuru' in the native population. *New England Journal of Medicine* **257**, 974–978 [751].

GALABURDA, A.M. (1992) Neurology of developmental dyslexia. *Current Opinion in Neurology and Neurosurgery* **5**, 71–76 [47].

GALABURDA, A.M. & KEMPER, T.L. (1979) Cyto architectonic abnormalities in developmental dyslexia. A case study. *Annals of Neurology* **6**, 94–100 [47].

GALABURDA, A.M., LE MAY, M., KEMPER, T.L. & GESCHWIND, N. (1978) Right–left asymmetries in the brain. *Science* **199**, 852–856 [41].

GALABURDA, A.M., SHERMAN, G.F., ROSEN, G.D., ABOITIZ, F. & GESCHWIND, N. (1985) Developmental dyslexia: four consecutive patients with cortical anomalies. *Annals of Neurology* **18**, 222–233 [47].

GALE, E.A.M. & TATTERSALL, R.B. (1979) Unrecognised nocturnal hypoglycaemia in insulin-treated diabetics. *Lancet* **1**, 1049–1052 [536].

GALLHOFER, B., TRIMBLE, M.R., FRACKOWIAK, R., GIBBS, J. & JONES, T. (1985) A study of cerebral blood flow and metabolism in epileptic psychosis using positron emission tomography and oxygen. *Journal of Neurology, Neurosurgery and Psychiatry* **48**, 201–206 [281].

GALLINECK, A. & KALINOWSKY, L.B. (1958) Psychiatric aspects of multiple sclerosis. *Diseases of the Nervous System* **19**, 77–80 [695, 697].

GALLINEK, A. (1954) Syndrome of episodes of hypersomnia, bulimia and abnormal mental states. *Journal of the American Medical Association* **154**, 1081–1083 [733].

GALLINEK, A. (1962) The Kleine–Levin syndrome: hypersomnia, bulimia, and abnormal mental states. *World Neurology* **3**, 235–243 [733].

GALLUCCI, M., BOZZAO, A., SPLENDIAINI, A., MASCIOCCHI, C. & PASSARIELLO, R. (1990) Wernicke encephalopathy: MR findings in five patients. *American Journal of Neuroradiology* **11**, 887–892 [579].

GALVEZ, S. & CARTIER, L. (1984) Computed tomography findings in 15 cases of Creutzfeldt–Jakob disease with histological verification. *Journal of Neurology, Neurosurgery and Psychiatry* **47**, 1244–1246 [478].

GALVEZ, S., MASTERS, C. & GAJDUSEK, C. (1980) Descriptive epidemiology of Creutzfeldt–Jakob disease in Chile. *Archives of Neurology* **37**, 11–14 [475].

GANSER, S.J.M. (1898) Ueber einen eigenartigen hysterischen Daemmerzustand. *Archiv für Psychiatrie und Nervenkrankheiten* **30**, 633–640. Translated by Schorer, C.E. (1965) in *British Journal of Criminology* **5**, 120–126 [480].

GANZ, V.H., GURLAND, B.J., DEMING, W.E. & FISHER, B. (1972) The study of the psychiatric symptoms of systemic lupus erythematosus: a biometric study. *Psychosomatic Medicine* **34**, 207–220 [420].

GARDNER, D.L. & COWDRY, R.W. (1986) Positive effects of carbamazepine on behavioural dyscontrol in borderline personality disorder. *American Journal of Psychiatry* **143**, 519–522 [298].

GARRON, D.C. & VANDER STOEP, L.R. (1969) Personality and intelligence in Turner's syndrome. A critical review. *Archives of General Psychiatry* **21**, 339–346 [528].

GASCON, G. & BARLOW, C. (1970) Juvenile migraine, presenting as an acute confusional state. *Pediatrics* **45**, 628–635 [405].

GASH, D.M. & THOMAS, G.J. (1983) What is the importance of vasopressin in memory processes? *Trends in Neurosciences* **6**, 197–198 [585].

GASPAR, P. & GRAY, F. (1984) Dementia in idiopathic Parkinson's disease. A neuropathological study of 32 cases. *Acta Neuropathologica* **64**, 43–52 [655].

GASTAUT, H. (1970) Clinical and electroencephalographical classification of epileptic seizures. *Epilepsia* **11**, 102–113 [237].

GASTAUT, H. (1976) Conclusions: computerised transverse axial tomography in epilepsy. *Epilepsia* **17**, 337–338 [289].

GASTAUT, H. & COLLOMB, H. (1954) Étude du comportement sexuel chez les epileptiques psychomoteurs. *Annales Medicopsychologiques* **112(ii)**, 657–696 [271].

GASTAUT, H., COURJON, J., POIRÉ, R. & WEBER, M. (1971) Treatment of status epilepticus with a new benzodiazepine more active than diazepam. *Epilepsia* **12**, 197–214 [306].

GASTAUT, H. & FISCHER-WILLIAMS, M. (1957) Electroencephalographic study of syncope: its differentiation from epilepsy. *Lancet* **2**, 1018–1025 [291].

GASTAUT, H. & GASTAUT, J.L. (1976) Computerised transverse axial tomography in epilepsy. *Epilepsia* **17**, 325–336 [289].

GATES, E.M., KERNOHAN, J.W. & CRAIG, W.M. (1950) Metastatic brain abscess. *Medicine* **29**, 71–98 [368].

GATEWOOD, J.W., ORGAN, C.H. & MEAD, B.T. (1975) Mental changes associated with hyperparathyroidism. *American Journal of Psychiatry* **132**, 129–132 [529].

GATH, A., SMITH, M.A. & BAUM, J.D. (1980) Emotional, behavioural, and educational disorders in diabetic children. *Archives of Disease in Childhood* **55**, 371–375 [536].

GAUTHIER, S., BOUCHARD, R., LAMONTAGNE, A., BAILEY, P., BERGMAN, H., RATNER, J., TESFAYE, Y., SAINT MARTIN, M., BACHER, Y., CARRIER, L., CHARBONNEAU, R., CLARFIELD, A.M., COLLIER, B., DASTOOR, D., GAUTHIER, L., GERMAIN, M., KISSEL, C., KRIEGER, M., KUSHNIR, S., MASSON, H., MORIN, J., NAIR, V., NEIRINCK, L. & SUISSA, S. (1990) Tetrahydroaminoacridine–lecithin combination treatment in patients with intermediate-stage Alzheimer's disease. *New England Journal of Medicine* **322**, 1272–1276 [504].

GAUTIER, J.C. (1983) Cerebral ischaemia in hypertension. Ch. 12 in *Vascular Disease of the Central Nervous System*, 2nd edn, ed. Russell, R.W.R. Churchill Livingstone: Edinburgh & London [380].

GAUTIER-SMITH, P.C. (1965) Neurological complications of glandular fever (infectious mononucleosis). *Brain* **88**, 323–334 [358].

GAWLER, J., BULL, J.W.D., DU BOULAY, G.H. & MARSHALL, J. (1975) Computerized axial tomography: the normal EMI scan. *Journal of Neurology, Neurosurgery and Psychiatry* **38**, 935–947 [137, 138].

GAWLER, J., DU BOULAY, G.H., BULL, J.W.D. & MARSHALL, J. (1974) Computer-assisted tomography (EMI scanner): its place in investigation of suspected cerebral tumours. *Lancet* **2**, 419–423 [137, 138].

GAWLER, J., DU BOULAY, G.H., BULL, J.W.D. & MARSHALL, J. (1976) Computerized tomography (the EMI scanner): a comparison with pneumoencephalography and ventriculography. *Journal of Neurology, Neurosurgery and Psychiatry* **39**, 203–211 [138].

GAY, J.R. & ABBOTT, K.H. (1953) Common whiplash injuries of the neck. *Journal of the American Medical Association* **152**, 1698–1704 [199, 200].

GAZZANIGA, M.S. (1983) Right hemisphere language following brain bisection: a 20-year perspective. *American Psychologist* **38**, 525–537 [42].

GAZZANIGA, M.S. (1985) Some contributions of split-brain studies to the study of human cognition. Ch. 17 in *Epilepsy and the Corpus Callosum*, ed. Reeves, A.G. Plenum Press: New York [42, 313].

GAZZANIGA, M.S., BOGEN, J.E. & SPERRY, R.W. (1965) Observations on visual perception after disconnection of the cerebral hemispheres in man. *Brain* **88**, 221–236 [313].

GAZZANIGA, M.S. & SMYLIE, C.S. (1984) Dissociation of language and cognition. A psychological profile of two disconnected right hemispheres. *Brain* **107**, 145–153 [42].

GAZZANIGA, M.S. & SPERRY, R.W. (1967) Language after section of the cerebral commissures. *Brain* **90**, 131–148 [41].

GEANEY, D.P. & ABOU-SALEH, M.T. (1990) The use and applications of single-photon emission computerised tomography in dementia. In *Brain Imaging in Psychiatry*, ed. Abou-Saleh, M.T. *British Journal of Psychiatry* **157 (Supplement 9)**, 66–75 [457].

GEANEY, D.P., SOPER, N., SHEPSTONE, B.J. & COWEN, P.J. (1990) Effect of central cholinergic stimulation on regional cerebral blood flow in Alzheimer disease. *Lancet* **335**, 1484–1487 [434].

GEBHARDT, C.A., NAESER, M.A. & BUTTERS, N. (1984) Computerised measures of CT scans of alcoholics: thalamic region related to memory. *Alcohol* **1**, 133–140 [606].

GEDYE, J.L., EXTON-SMITH, A.N. & WEDGWOOD, J. (1972) A method for measuring mental performance in the elderly and its use in a pilot clinical trial of meclofenoxate in organic dementia (preliminary communication). *Age and Ageing* **1**, 74–80 [502].

GELARDI, J.A.M. & BROWN, J.W. (1967) Hereditary cataplexy. *Journal of Neurology, Neurosurgery and Psychiatry* **30**, 455–457 [723].

GELENBERG, A.J. (1976) The catatonic syndrome. *Lancet* **1**, 1339–1341 [356].

GELENBERG, A.J. & MANDEL, M.R. (1977) Catatonic reactions to high potency neuroleptic drugs. *Archives of General Psychiatry* **34**, 947–950 [640].

GELINEAU, J.B. (1880) De la narcolepsie. *Gazette des Hôpitaux* **53**, 626–628 and 635–637 [722].

GELLER, T.J. & BELLUR, S.N. (1987) Peduncular hallucinosis: magnetic resonance imaging confirmation of mesencephalic infarction during life. *Annals of Neurology* **21**, 602–604 [388].

GELLERSTEDT, N. (1933) Zur Kenntnis der Hirnveränderungen bei der normaler Altersinvolution. *Upsala lälkareförenings förhandlingar* **38**, 193–404, quoted by Brierley (1966) The neuropathology of amnesic state. Ch. 7 in *Amnesia*, eds Whitty, C.W.M. & Zangwill, O.L. Butterworths: London [33].

GEMMELL, H.G., SHARP, P.F., SMITH, F.W., BESSON, J.A.O., EBMEIER, K.P., DAVIDSON, J., EVANS, N.T.S., ROEDA, D., NEWTON, R. & MALLARD, J.R. (1989) Cerebral blood flow measured by SPET as a diagnostic tool in the study of dementia. *Psychiatry Research* **29**, 327–329 [148, 434, 471].

GENERAL MEDICAL COUNCIL (1988) HIV infection and AIDS: the ethical considerations. *General Medical Council*. London: May 1988 [333, 334].

GENERAL MEDICAL COUNCIL (1993) HIV infection and AIDS: the ethical considerations. *General Medical Council*. London: May 1993 [333, 334].

GENNARELLI, T.A., THIBAULT, L.E., ADAMS, J.H., GRAHAM, D.I., THOMPSON, C.J. & MARCINCIN, R.P. (1982) Diffuse axonal injury and traumatic coma in the primate. *Annals of Neurology* **12**, 564–574 [200].

GEOCARIS, K. (1957) Psychotic episodes heralding the diagnosis of multiple sclerosis. *Bulletin of the Menninger Clinic* **21**, 107–116 [697].

GEORGE, A.E., DE LEON, M.J., CENTES, C.I., MILLER, J., LONDON, E., BUDZILOVICH, G.N., FERRIS, S. & CHASE, N. (1986) Leukoencephalopathy in normal and pathologic aging: 1. CT or brain lucencies. *American Journal of Neuroradiology* **7**, 561–566 [459].

GEORGE, C.F., NICKERSON, P.W., HANLY, P.J., MILLAR, T.W. & KRYGER, M.H. (1987) Sleep apnoea patients have more automobile accidents. *Lancet* **2**, 447 [731].

GERIN, J. (1969) Symptomatic treatment of cerebrovascular insufficiency with Hydergine. *Current Therapeutic Research* **11**, 539–546 [502].

GERIN, J. (1974) Double-blind trial of naftidrofuryl in the treatment of cerebral arteriosclerosis. *British Journal of Clinical Practice* **28**, 177–178 [502].

GERLACH, J. & CASEY, D.E. (1988) Tardive dyskinesia. *Acta Psychiatrica Scandinavica* **77**, 369–378 [644].

GERSHON, S. & SHAW, F.H. (1961) Psychiatric sequelae of chronic exposure to organophosphorus insecticides. *Lancet* 1, 1371–1374 [637].

GERSON, S.N., BENSON, F. & FRAZIER, S.H. (1977) Diagnosis: schizophrenia versus posterior aphasia. *American Journal of Psychiatry* 134, 966–969 [55].

GERSONS, B.P.R. & CARLIER, I.V.E. (1992) Post-traumatic stress disorder: the history of a recent concept. *British Journal of Psychiatry* 161, 742–748 [194].

GERSTENBRAND, F. (1969) Rehabilitation of the head-injured. Ch. 31 in *The Late Effects of Head Injury*, eds Walker, A.E., Caveness, W.F. & Critchley, M. Thomas: Springfield, Illinois [213].

GERSTMANN, J. (1928) Über ein noch nicht beschriebenes Reflexphänomen bei einer Erkrankung des zerebellaren Systems. *Wiener Medizinische Wochenschrift* 78, 906–908 [751].

GERSTMANN, J. (1958) Psychological and phenomenological aspects of disorders of the body image. *Journal of Nervous and Mental Disease* 126, 499–512 [66, 71].

GERSTMANN, J., STRÄUSSLER, E. & SCHEINKER, I. (1936) Über eine eigenartige hereditör-familiäre Erkrankung des Zentralnervensystems. *Zeitschrift für die gesempte Neurologie und Psychiatrie* 154, 736–762 [751].

GESCHWIND, N. (1962) The anatomy of acquired disorders of reading. Ch. 8 in *Reading Disabilities, Progress and Research Needs in Dyslexia*, ed. Money, J. Johns Hopkins Press: Baltimore [19].

GESCHWIND, N. (1965) Disconnexion syndromes in animals and man. *Brain* 88, 237–294 and 585–644 [56, 59].

GESCHWIND, N. (1967) Neurological foundations of language. In *Progress in Learning Disabilities*, ed. Myklebust, H.R., pp. 182–198. Grune & Stratton: New York [44].

GESCHWIND, N. (1968) The mechanism of normal pressure hydrocephalus. *Journal of the Neurological Sciences* 7, 481–493 [749].

GESCHWIND, N. (1979) Behavioural changes in temporal lobe epilepsy. *Psychological Medicine* 9, 217–219 [269].

GESCHWIND, N. & DAMASIO, A.R. (1985) Apraxia. Ch. 28 in *Handbook of Clinical Neurology*, Revised Series Vol. 1, *Clinical Neuropsychology*, ed. Frederiks, J.A.M. Elsevier Science Publishers BV: Amsterdam [55, 57].

GESCHWIND, N. & KAPLAN, E. (1962) A human cerebral deconnection syndrome: a preliminary report. *Neurology* 12, 675–686 [19].

GESCHWIND, N. & LEVITSKY, W. (1968) Human brain: left–right asymmetries in temporal speech region. *Science* 161, 186–187 [41].

GESCHWIND, N., QUADFASEL, F.A. & SEGARRA, J.M. (1968) Isolation of the speech area. *Neuropsychologia* 6, 327–340 [53].

GESSLER, S., CUTTING, J., FRITH, C.D. & WEINMAN, J. (1989) Schizophrenic inability to judge facial emotion: a controlled study. *British Journal of Clinical Psychology* 28, 19–29 [89].

GHODSE, A.H. (1986) Cannabis psychosis. *British Journal of Addiction* 81, 473–478 [614, 615].

GHODSE, H. (1995) *Drugs and Addictive Behaviour. A Guide to Treatment*, 2nd edn. Blackwell Science: Oxford [609, 611, 615, 618, 619, 620].

GIBB, W.R.G. (1989) Dementia and Parkinson's disease. *British Journal of Psychiatry* 154, 596–614 [655].

GIBB, W.R.G. (1990) Cortical Lewy body dementia. *Behavioural Neurology* 3, 189–196 [450].

GIBB, W.R.G., ESIRI, M.M. & LEES, A.J. (1987) Clinical and pathological features of diffuse cortical Lewy body disease (Lewy body dementia). *Brain* 110, 1131–1153 [450].

GIBB, W.R.G. & LEES, A.J. (1987) Dementia in Parkinson's disease. *Lancet* 1, 861 [648].

GIBB, W.R.G. & LEES, A.J. (1989) The significance of the Lewy body in the diagnosis of idiopathic Parkinson's disease. *Neuropathology and Applied Neurobiology* 15, 27–44 [647].

GIBB, W.R.G., LUTHERT, P.J., JANOTA, I. & LANTOS, P.L. (1989a) Cortical Lewy body dementia: clinical features and classification. *Journal of Neurology, Neurosurgery and Psychiatry* 52, 185–192 [450].

GIBB, W.R.G., LUTHERT, P.J. & MARSDEN, C.D. (1989b) Corticobasal degeneration. *Brain* 112, 1171–1192 [668].

GIBBERD, B. (1991) Drug-induced benign intracranial hypertension. *Prescriber's Journal* 31, 118–121 [232].

GIBBERD, F.B. (1973) The diagnosis and investigation of epilepsy. *British Journal of Hospital Medicine* 9, 152–158 [288, 291].

GIBBERD, F.B. & SIMMONDS, J.P. (1980) Neurological disease in ex-Far-East prisoners of war. *Lancet* 2, 135–137 [570].

GIBBS, C.J., AMYX, H.L., BACOTE, A., MASTERS, C.L. & GAJDUSEK, D.C. (1980) Oral transmission of Kuru, Creutzfeldt–Jakob disease, and scrapie to non-human primates. *Journal of Infectious Diseases* 142, 205–208 [475].

GIBBS, C.J., GAJDUSEK, D.C., ASHER, D.M., ALPERS, M.P., BECK, E., DANIEL, P.M. & MATTHEWS, W.B. (1968) Creutzfeldt–Jakcob disease (spongiform encephalopathy): transmission to the chimpanzee. *Science* 161, 388–389 [473].

GIBBS, C.J., JOY, A., HEFFNER, R., FRANKO, M., MIYAZAKI, M., ASHER, D.M., PARISI, J.E., BROWN, P.W. & GAJDUSEK, D.C. (1985) Clinical and pathological features and laboratory confirmation of Creutzfeldt–Jakob disease in a recipient of pituitary-derived human growth hormone. *New England Journal of Medicine* 313, 734–738 [476].

GIBBS, F.A. (1951) Ictal and non-ictal psychiatric disorders in temporal lobe epilepsy. *Journal of Nervous and Mental Disease* 113, 522–528 [266].

GIBBS, F.A. & GIBBS, E.L. (1964) *Atlas of Electroencephalography Volume 3: Neurological and Psychiatric Disorders*. Addison-Wesley Publishing Company: Reading, Massachusetts [266].

GILBERT, G.J. (1964) Periodic hypersomnia and bulimia: the Kleine–Levin syndrome. *Neurology* 14, 844–850 [733].

GILLEARD, C.J. (1984) *Living with Dementia. Community Care of the Elderly Mentally Infirm*. Croom Helm: London [498].

GILLEARD, C.J. (1987) Influence of emotional distress among supporters on the outcome of psychogeriatric day care. *British Journal of Psychiatry* 150, 219–223 [498].

GILLEARD, C.J. & PATTIE, A.H. (1977) The Stockton Geriatric Rating Scale: a shortened version with British normative data. *British Journal of Psychiatry* 131, 90–94 [125].

GILLES DE LA TOURETTE, G. (1855) Étude sur une affection nerveuse charactérisée par de l'incoordination motrice accampagnée d'écholalie et de coprolalie (jumping, latah, myriachit). *Archives de Neurologie* 9, 19–42 and 158–200 [683].

GILLFILLAN, S.C. (1965) Lead poisoning and the fall of Rome. *Journal of Occupational Medicine* 7, 53–60 [630].

GILLHAM, R.A., WILLIAMS, K.D., WIEDMANN, E., BUTLER, E., LARKIN, J.G. & BRODIE, M.J. (1990) Cognitive function in adult epileptic patients established on anticonvulsant monotherapy. *Epilepsy Research* 7, 219–225 [263].

GILLIAM, T.C., BUCAN, M., MacDONALD, M.E., ZIMMER, M., HAINES, J.L., CHENG, S.V., POHL, T.M., MEYERS, R.H., WHALEY, W.L., ALLITTO, B.A., FARYNIARZ, A., WASMUTH, J.J., FRISCHAUF, A., CONNEALLY, P.M., LEHRACH, H. & GUSELLA, J. (1987) A DNA segment encoding two genes very tightly linked to Huntington's disease. *Science* 238, 950–952 [466].

GILLMER, R.E. (1972) Phaeochromocytoma—an interesting psychiatric presentation. *South African Medical Journal* 46, 74–176 [521].

GILMAN, S., ADAMS, K., KOEPPE, R.A., BERENT, S., KLUIN, K.J.,

MODELL, J.G., KROLL, P. & BRUNBERG, J.A. (1990) Cerebellar and frontal hypometabolism in alcoholic cerebellar degeneration studied with PET. *Annals of Neurology* **28**, 775–785 [585].

GILROY, J. & MEYER, J.S. (1969) *Medical Neurology*. Macmillan: London [344].

GINSBERG, M.D. (1985) Carbon monoxide intoxication: clinical features, neuropathology and mechanisms of injury. *Journal of Toxicology—Clinical Toxicology* **23**, 281–288 [553].

GINSBURG, H.M. & NIXON, C.E. (1932) Thallium poisoning. *Journal of the American Medical Association* **98**, 1076–1077 [636].

GITLIN, N., LEWIS, D.C. & HINKLEY, L. (1986) The diagnosis and prevalence of subclinical hepatic encephalopathy in apparently healthy ambulant, non-shunted patients with cirrhosis. *Journal of Hepatology* **3**, 75–82 [565].

GITTLESON, N.L. & RICHARDSON, T.D.E. (1973) Myasthenia gravis and schizophrenia—a rare combination. *British Journal of Psychiatry* **122**, 343–344 [711].

GLADMAN, D.D. (1992) Prognosis of systemic lupus erythematosus and factors that affect it. *Current Opinion in Rheumatology* **4**, 681–687 [418].

GLASER, G.H., NEWMAN, R.J. & SCHAFER, R. (1963) Interictal psychosis in psychomotor-temporal lobe epilepsy: an EEG psychological study. Ch. 14 in *EEG and Behavior*, ed. Glaser, G.H. Basic Books: New York [284].

GLASS, R.M. (1988) AIDS and suicide. *Journal of the American Medical Association* **259**, 1369–1370 [331].

GLATT, M.M. & FRISCH, P. (1969) Chlormethiazole in alcoholism. *Current Psychiatric Therapies*, Vol. 9, ed. Masserman, J.H., pp. 132–135. Grune & Stratton: New York [603].

GLATT, M.M., GEORGE, H.R. & FRISCH, E.P. (1966) Evaluation of chlormethiazole in treatment for alcohol withdrawal syndrome. *Acta Psychiatrica Scandinavica* **192 (Supplement)**, 121–137 [603].

GLAZER, W.M., MORGENSTERN, H., NIEDZWIECKI, D. & HUGHES, J. (1988) Heterogeneity of tardive dyskinesia. A multivariate analysis. *British Journal of Psychiatry* **152**, 253–259 [641].

GLEES, P., COLE, J., WHITTY, C.W.M. & CAIRNS, H. (1950) The effects of lesions in the cingular gyrus and adjacent areas in monkeys. *Journal of Neurology, Neurosurgery and Psychiatry* **13**, 178–190 [23].

GLEES, P. & GRIFFITH, H.B. (1952) Bilateral destruction of hippocampus (cornu Ammonis) in case of dementia. *Monatschrifr für Psychiatrie und Neurologie* **123**, 193–204 [26].

GLEN, A.I.M. & CHRISTIE, J.E. (1979) Early diagnosis of Alzheimer's disease: working definitions for clinical and laboratory criteria. Ch. 26 in *Alzheimer's Disease: Early Recognition of Potentially Reversible Deficits*, eds Glen, A.I.M. & Whalley, L.J. Churchill Livingstone: Edinburgh & London [461].

GLENNER, G.G. & WONG, C.W. (1984) Alzheimer's disease: initial report of the purification and characterisation of a novel cerebrovascular amyloid protein. *Biochemical and Biophysical Research Communications* **120**, 885–890 [442].

GLOOR, P. (1991) Neurobiological substrates of ictal behavioral changes. Ch. 1 in *Neurobehavioral Problems in Epilepsy*, eds Smith, D.B., Trieman, D.M. & Trimble, M.R. *Advances in Neurology*, Vol. 55. Raven Press: New York [241].

GOATE, A., CHARTIER-HARLIN, M.-C., MULLAN, M., BROWN, J., CRAWFORD, F., FIDANI, L., GIUFFRA, L., HAYNES, A., IRVING, N., JAMES, L., MANT, R., NEWTON, P., ROOKE, K., ROQUES, P., TALBOT, C., PERICAK-VANCE, M., ROSES, A., WILLIAMSON, R., ROSSOR, M., OWEN, M. & HARDY, J. (1991) Segregation of a missense mutation in the amyloid precursor protein gene with familial Alzheimer's disease. *Nature* **349**, 704–706 [448].

GODDARD, G.V., McINTYRE, D.C. & LEECH, C.K. (1969) A permanent change in brain function resulting from daily electrical stimulation. *Experimental Neurology* **25**, 295–330 [598].

GODDARD, P. & LOKARE, V.G. (1970) Diazepam in the management of epilepsy. *British Journal of Psychiatry* **117**, 213–214 [306].

GODFREY, P.S.A., TOONE, B.K., CARNEY, M.W.P., FLYNN, T.G., BOTTIGLIERI, T., LAUNDY, M., CHANARIN, I. & REYNOLDS, E.H. (1990) Enhancement of recovery from psychiatric illness by methylfolate. *Lancet* **336**, 392–395 [590].

GOETHE, K.E., MITCHELL, J.E., MARSHALL, D.W., BREY, R.L., CAHILL, W.T., LEGER, D., HOY, L.J. & BOSWELL, R.N. (1989) Neuropsychological and neurological function of human immunodeficiency virus seropositive asymptomatic individuals. *Archives of Neurology* **46**, 129–133 [329].

GOLBE, L.I. (1990) The genetics of Parkinson's disease: a reconsideration. *Neurology* **40 (Supplement 3)**, 7–14 [646].

GOLBE, L.I., CODY, R.A. & DUVOISIN, R.C. (1986) Smoking and Parkinson's disease. Search for a dose response relationship. *Archives of Neurology* **43**, 774–778 [661].

GOLBE, L.I., DI IORIO, G., BONAVITA, V., MILLER, D.C. & DUVOISIN, V. (1990) A large kindred with autosomal dominant Parkinson's disease. *Annals of Neurology* **27**, 276–282 [646].

GOLDBERG, M.A. (1983) The treatment of Kleine–Levin syndrome with lithium. *Canadian Journal of Psychiatry* **28**, 491–493 [733].

GOLDEN, C.J., GRABER, B., COFFMAN, J., BERG, R.A., NEWLIN, D.B. & BLOCH, S. (1981) Structural brain deficits in schizophrenia as identified by CT scan density parameters. *Archives of General Psychiatry* **38**, 1014–1017 [138].

GOLDENBERG, G., PODREKA, I., STEINER, M., WILLMES, K., SUESS, E. & DEECKE, L. (1989a) Regional cerebral blood flow patterns in visual imagery. *Neuropsychologia* **27**, 641–664 [148].

GOLDENBERG, G., PODREKA, I., UHL, F., STEINER, M., WILLMES, K. & DEECKE, L. (1989b) Cerebral correlates of imagining colours, faces and a map—I. SPECT of regional cerebral blood flow. *Neuropsychologia* **27**, 1315–1328 [148].

GOLDFARB, A.I. (1972) Multidimensional treatment approaches. In *Aging and the Brain*, ed. Gaitz, C.M., pp. 179–191. Plenum Press: New York [499].

GOLDFARB, L.G., MITROVA, E., BROWN, P., BAN HOCK TOH & GAJDUSEK, D.C. (1990) Mutation in codon 200 of scrapie amyloid protein gene in two clusters of Creutzfeldt–Jakob disease in Slovakia. *Lancet* **336**, 514–515 [475].

GOLDGABER, D., LERMAN, M.I., McBRIDE, O.W., SAFFIOTTI, U. & GAJDUSEK, D.C. (1987) Characterization and chromosomal localization of a cDNA encoding brain amyloid of Alzheimer's disease. *Science* **235**, 877–880 [447].

GOLDMAN, M.B. & LUCHINS, D.J. (1984) Intermittent neuroleptic therapy and tardive dyskinesia: a literature review. *Hospital and Community Psychiatry* **35**, 1215–1219 [645].

GOLDMAN, M.B., LUCHINS, D.J. & ROBERTSON, G.L. (1988) Mechanisms of altered water metabolism in psychotic patients with polydipsia and hyponatremia. *The New England Journal of Medicine* **318**, 397–403 [526].

GOLDMAN, M.S. (1983) Cognitive impairment in chronic alcoholics. Some cause for optimism. *American Psychologist* **38**, 1045–1054 [604].

GOLDMAN, M.S. (1990) Experience-dependent neuropsychological recovery and the treatment of chronic alcoholism. *Neuropsychology Review* **1**, 75–101 [604].

GOLDMAN, M.S. (1995) Recovery of cognitive functioning in alcoholics. The relationship to treatment. *Alcohol Health and Research World* **19**, 148–154 [604].

GOLDMAN-RAKIC, P.S. (1987) Circuitry of primate prefrontal cortex and regulation of behavior by representational memory. Ch. 9 in *Handbook of Physiology, Section I: The Nervous System*, Vol. 5, Part I, ed. Mountcastle, V.B. American Physiological Society: Bethesda, Maryland [27, 77].

GOLDSMITH, J.R. & LANDAW, S.A. (1968) Carbon monoxide and human health. *Science* **162**, 1352–1359 [553].

GOLDSTEIN, G. & CHOTLOS, J.W. (1965) Dependency and brain damage in alcoholics. *Perceptual and Motor Skills* **21**, 135–150 [603].

GOLDSTEIN, K. (1936) The modifications of behavior consequent to cerebral lesions. *Psychiatric Quarterly* **10**, 586–610 [603].

GOLDSTEIN, K. (1939) *The Organism: A Holistic Approach to Biology Derived from Pathological Data in Man.* American Book Company: New York [14, 22].

GOLDSTEIN, K. (1942) *After Effects of Brain Injuries in War.* Grune & Stratton: New York [14, 97, 177].

GOLDSTEIN, K. (1948) *Language and Language Disturbances.* Grune & Stratton: New York [53].

GOLDSTEIN, K. (1952) The effect of brain damage on the personality. *Psychiatry* **15**, 245–260 [177].

GOLDSTEIN, K. & SHEERER, M. (1941) Abstract and concrete behaviour. An experimental study with special tests. *Psychological Monographs* **53, No. 2**, 1–151 [120].

GOLDSTEIN, L.H. (1990) Behavioural and cognitive-behavioural treatments for epilepsy: a progress review. *British Journal of Clinical Psychology* **29**, 257–269 [309].

GOLDSTEIN, L.H. (1991) Neuropsychological investigation of temporal lobe epilepsy. *Journal of the Royal Society of Medicine* **84**, 460–465 [312].

GOLDSTEIN, L.H., BERNARD, S., FENWICK, P.B.C., BURGESS, P.W. & McNEIL, J. (1993) Unilateral frontal lobectomy can produce strategy application disorder. *Journal of Neurology, Neurosurgery and Psychiatry* **56**, 274–276 [120].

GOLDSTEIN, L.H., CANAVAN, A.G.M. & POLKEY, C.E. (1988) Verbal and abstract designs paired associate learning after unilateral temporal lobectomy. *Cortex* **24**, 41–52 [115, 312].

GOLDSTEIN, L.H., PATEL, V., ASPINALL, P. & LISHMAN, W.A. (1992) The effect of anticonvulsants on cognitive functioning following a probable encephalitic illness. *British Journal of Psychiatry* **160**, 546–549 [262].

GOLDSTEIN, L.H. & POLKEY, C.E. (1992) Everyday memory after unilateral temporal lobectomy or amygdalo-hippocampectomy. *Cortex* **28**, 189–201 [312].

GOLDSTEIN, L.H. & POLKEY, C.E. (1993) Short-term cognitive changes after unilateral temporal lobectomy or unilateral amygdo-hippocampectomy for the relief of temporal lobe epilepsy. *Journal of Neurology, Neurosurgery and Psychiatry* **56**, 135–140 [311].

GOLDSTEIN, N.P., EWERT, J.C., RANDALL, R.V. & GROSS, J.B. (1968) Psychiatric aspects of Wilson's disease: results of psychometric tests during long-term therapy. In *Wilson's Disease*, ed. Bergsma, D. Birth Defects Original Article Series, Vol. 4, No. 2. The National Foundation: New York [666].

GOLDSTEIN, N.P., TAUXE, W.N., McCALL, J.T., RANDALL, R.V. & GROSS, J.B. (1971) Wilson's disease (hepatolenticular degeneration): treatment with penicillamine and changes in hepatic trapping of radioactive copper. *Archives of Neurology* **24**, 391–400 [664].

GOMERSALL, J.D. & STUART, A. (1973) Amitriptyline in migraine prophylaxis. *Journal of Neurology, Neurosurgery and Psychiatry* **36**, 684–690 [410].

GOMEZ, M.R. (1979) Neurologic and psychiatric symptoms. Ch. 6 in *Tuberous Sclerosis*, ed. Gomez, M.R. Raven Press: New York [702].

GOMEZ, M.R. (1991) Phenotypes of tuberous sclerosis complex with a revision of diagnostic criteria. In *Tuberous Sclerosis and Allied Disorders: Clinical, Cellular, and Molecular Studies*, eds Johnson, W.G. & Gomez, M.R. *Annals of the New York Academy of Sciences* **615**, 1–7 [701].

GONEN, J.Y. (1970) The use of Wechsler's deterioration quotient in cases of diffuse and symmetrical cerebral atrophy. *Journal of Clinical Psychology* **26**, 174–177 [111].

GOODE, D.J., PENRY, J.K. & DREIFUSS, F.E. (1970) Effects of paroxysmal spike-wave on continuous visual-motor perfomance. *Epilepsia* **11**, 241–254 [262].

GOODIN, D.S. & AMINOFF, M.J. (1986) Electrophysiological differences between subtypes of dementia. *Brain* **109**, 1103–1113 [132].

GOODIN, D.S., AMINOFF, M.J., CHERNOFF, D.N. & HOLLANDER, H. (1990) Long latency event-related potentials in patients infected with human immunodeficiency virus. *Annals of Neurology* **27**, 414–419 [132].

GOODSTEIN, R. & FERRELL, R.B. (1977) Multiple sclerosis—presenting as depressive illness. *Diseases of the Nervous System* **38**, 127–131 [695].

GOODWIN, D.W., CRANE, J.B. & GUZE, S.B. (1969a) Alcoholic blackouts: a review and clinical study of 100 alcoholics. *American Journal of Psychiatry* **126**, 191–198 [596].

GOODWIN, D.W., CRANE, J.B. & GUZE, S.B. (1969b) Phenomenological aspects of the alcoholic 'blackout'. *British Journal of Psychiatry* **115**, 1033–1038 [596].

GOODWIN, D.W., POWELL, B., BREMER, D., HOINE, H. & STERN, J. (1969c) Alcohol and recall: state-dependent effects in man. *Science* **163**, 1358–1360 [596].

GOODWIN, F.K. (1971) Behavioural effects of L-dopa in man. *Seminars in Psychiatry* **3**, 477–492 [658].

GOPALAN, C. (1970) Some recent studies in the Nutrition Research Laboratories, Hyderabad. *American Journal of Clinical Nutrition* **23**, 35–51 [570].

GORDON, B. & MARIN, O.S.M. (1979) Transient global amnesia: an extensive case report. *Journal of Neurology, Neurosurgery and Psychiatry* **42**, 572–575 [413].

GORDON, B., SELNES, O.A., HART, J., HANLEY, D.F. & WHITLEY, R.J. (1990) Long-term cognitive sequelae of acyclovir-treated herpes simplex encephalitis. *Archives of Neurology* **47**, 646–647 [357].

GORDON, E., KRAIUHIN, C., HARRIS, A., MEARES, R. & HOWSON, A. (1986) The differential diagnosis of dementia using P300 latency. *Biological Psychiatry* **21**, 1123–1132 [132].

GORDON, E.B. (1968) Serial EEG studies in presenile dementia. *British Journal of Psychiatry* **114**, 779–780 [439].

GORDON, E.B. & SIM, M. (1967) The EEG in presenile dementia. *Journal of Neurology, Neurosurgery and Psychiatry* **30**, 285–291 [439, 461].

GORDON, H.W. & BOGEN, J.E. (1974) Hemispheric lateralization of singing after intracarotid sodium amylobarbitone. *Journal of Neurology, Neurosurgery and Psychiatry* **37**, 727–738 [64].

GORDON, M.F. & MERCANDETTI, M. (1989) Carbon monoxide poisoning producing purely cognitive and behavioral sequelae. *Neuropsychiatry, Neuropsychology and Behavioral Neurology* **2**, 145–152 [551].

GORDON, N. & RUSSELL, S. (1958) The problem of unemployment among epileptics. *Journal of Mental Science* **104**, 103–114 [265].

GORDON-SMITH, E.G. & CONTRERAS, M. (1996) Acquired haemolytic anaemia. Section 22.4.13 in *Oxford Textbook of Medicine*, 3rd edn, eds Weatherall, D.J., Ledingham, J.G.G. & Warrell, D.A. Oxford University Press: Oxford [426].

GORE, S.M. (1995) More than happenstance: Creutzfeldt–Jakob disease in farmers and young adults. *British Medical Journal* **311**, 1416–1418 [475].

GOSLING, R.H. (1955) The association of dementia with radiologically demonstrated cerebral atrophy. *Journal of Neurology, Neurosurgery and Psychiatry* **18**, 129–133 [139].

GOSSET, A., PELLISSIER, J.F., DELPUECH, F. & KHALIL, R. (1983) Dégénérescence striato-nigrique associée à une atrophie olivo-ponto-cérébelleuse. *Revue Neurologique* **139**, 125–139 [669].

GOSTLING, J.V.T. (1967) Herpetic encephalitis. *Proceedings of the Royal Society of Medicine* **60**, 693–696 [356].

GOSWAMI, U. & CHANNABASAVANNA, S.M. (1983) Transition from simple writer's cramp to dystonic writer's cramp—a report of two cases from India. *Clinical Neurology and Neurosurgery* **85**, 113–116 [677].

GOTHAM, A.-M., BROWN, R.G. & MARSDEN, C.D. (1986) Depression in Parkinson's disease. A quantitative and qualitative analysis. *Journal of Neurology, Neurosurgery and Psychiatry* **49**, 381–389 [656].

GOTO, K., ISHII, N. & FUKASAWA, H. (1981) Diffuse white-matter disease in the geriatric population. A clinical, neuropathological and CT study. *Radiology* **141**, 687–695 [459].

GOTTEN, N. (1956) Survey of one hundred cases of whiplash injury after settlement of compensation. *Journal of the American Medical Association* **162**, 865–867 [200, 201].

GOTTLIEB, B. (1944) Acute nicotinic acid deficiency (aniacinosis). *British Medical Journal* **1**, 392–393 [574].

GOUDSMIT, J., MORROW, C.H., ASHER, D.M., YANAGIHARA, R.T., MASTERS, C.L., GIBBS, C.J. & GAJDUSEK, D.C. (1980) Evidence for and against the transmissibility of Alzheimer's disease. *Neurology* **30**, 945–950 [446].

GOULATIA, R.K., VERMA, A., MISHRA, N.K. & AHUJA, G.K. (1987) Disappearing CT lesions in epilepsy. *Epilepsia* **28**, 523–527 [289].

GOULDING, P., BURJAN, A., SMITH, R., LAWSON, R., SNOWDEN, J., NORTHEN, B., NEARY, D. & TESTA, H. (1990) Semi-automatic quantification of regional cerebral perfusion in primary degenerative dementia using 99m technetium-hexamethylpropylene amino oxime and single photon emission tomography. *European Journal of Nuclear Medicine* **17**, 77–82 [708].

GOW, J.W., BEHAN, W.M.H., CLEMENTS, G.B., WOODALL, C., RIDING, M. & BEHAN, P.O. (1991) Enteroviral RNA sequences detected by polymerase chain reaction in muscle in patients with postviral fatigue syndrome. *British Medical Journal* **302**, 692–696 [372].

GOWERS, W.R. (1888) *A Manual of Diseases of the Nervous System*, Vol. 2. Churchill: London [407].

GRABSKI, D.A. (1961) Toluene sniffing producing cerebellar degeneration. *American Journal of Psychiatry* **118**, 461–462 [629].

GRADY, C.L., McINTOSH, A.R., HORWITZ, B., MAISOG, J.M., UNGERLEIDER, L.G., MENTIS, M.J., PIETRINI, P., SCHAPIRO, M.B. & HAXBY, J.V. (1995) Age-related reductions in human recognition memory due to impaired encoding. *Science* **269**, 218–221 [33].

GRAF-RADFORD, N.R., ESLINGER, P.J., DAMASIO, A.R. & YAMADA, T. (1984) Nonhaemorrhagic infarction of the thalamus: behavioral, anatomic and physiologic correlates. *Neurology* **34**, 14–23 [384].

GRAFMAN, J. (1988) Acalculia. Ch. 22 in *Handbook of Neuropsychology*, Vol. 1, eds Boller, F. & Grafman, J. Elsevier: Amsterdam [66].

GRAFMAN, J., JONAS, B. & SALAZAR, A. (1990a) Wisconsin Card Sorting Test performance based on location and size of neuroanatomical lesion in Vietnam veterans with penetrating head injury. *Perceptual and Motor Skills* **71**, 1120–1122 [118].

GRAFMAN, J., PASSAFIUME, D., FAGLIONI, P. & BOLLER, F. (1982) Calculation disturbance in adults with focal hemispheric damage. *Cortex* **18**, 37–50 [67].

GRAFMAN, J., RAO, S.M. & LITVAN, I. (1990b) Disorders of memory. Ch. 6 in *Neurobehavioral Aspects of Multiple Sclerosis*, ed. Rao, S.M. Oxford University Press: Oxford [692].

GRAFMAN, J., SALAZAR, A.M., WEINGARTNER, H., VANCE, C. & LUDLOW, C. (1985) Isolated impairment of memory following a penetrating lesion of the fornix cerebri. *Archives of Neurology* **42**, 1162–1168 [27].

GRAHAM, D.I. & ADAMS, J.H. (1971) Ischaemic brain damage in fatal head injury. *Lancet* **1**, 265–266 [163].

GRAHAM, F.K. & KENDALL, B.S. (1960) Memory-for-designs test: revised general manual. *Perceptual and Motor Skills* **11**, 147–188 [116].

GRAHAM, J.D.P. (1945) High blood pressure after battle. *Lancet* **1**, 239–240 [397].

GRAHAM, J.M., BASHIR, A.S., STARK, R.E., SILBERT, A. & WALZER, S. (1988) Oral and written language abilities of XXY boys: implications for anticipatory guidance. *Pediatrics* **81**, 795–806 [526].

GRAHAM, P. & RUTTER, M. (1968) Organic brain dysfunction and child psychiatric disorder. *British Medical Journal* **3**, 695–700 [260, 261, 268].

GRAINGER, D.N. (1992) Rapid development of hyponatraemic seizures in a psychotic patient. *Psychological Medicine* **22**, 513–517 [525, 526].

GRANATO, J.E., STERN, B.J., RINGEL, A., KARIM, A.H., KRUMHOLZ, A., COYLE, J. & ADLER, S. (1983) Neuroleptic malignant syndrome: successful treatment with dantrolene and bromocriptine. *Annals of Neurology* **14**, 89–90 [627].

GRAND ROUNDS, HAMMERSMITH HOPSITAL (1996) Cerebral Whipple's disease. Relapse presenting with spinal myoclonus. *British Medical Journal* **312**, 371–373 [760, 761].

GRANDAS, F., ELSTON, J., QUINN, N. & MARSDEN, C.D. (1988) Blepharospasm: a review of 264 patients. *Journal of Neurology, Neurosurgery and Psychiatry* **51**, 767–772 [678, 679].

GRANT, I. (1987) Alcohol and the brain: neuropsychological correlates. *Journal of Consulting and Clinical Psychology* **55**, 310–324 [604].

GRANT, I., ATKINSON, J.H., HESSELINK, J.R., KENNEDY, C.J., RICHMAN, D.D., SPECTOR, S.A. & McCUTCHAN, J.A. (1987) Evidence for early central nervous system involvement in the acquired immunodeficiency syndrome (AIDS) and other human immunodeficiency virus (HIV) infections. *Annals of Internal Medicine* **107**, 828–836 [328].

GRANT, I., ATKINSON, J.H., HESSELINK, J.R., KENNEDY, C.J., RICHMAN, D.D., SPECTOR, S.A. & McCUTCHAN, J.A. (1988) Human immunodeficiency virus-associated neurobehavioural disorder. *Journal of the Royal College of Physicians of London* **22**, 149–157 [328].

GRANT, I., BROWN, G.W., HARRIS, T., McDONALD, W.I., PATTERSON, T. & TRIMBLE, M.R. (1989) Severely threatening events and marked life difficulties preceding onset or exacerbation of multiple sclerosis. *Journal of Neurology, Neurosurgery and Psychiatry* **52**, 8–13 [700].

GRANT, I., CAUN, K., KINGSLEY, D.P.E., WINER, J., TRIMBLE, M.R. & PINCHING, A.J. (1992) Neuropsychological and NMR abnormalities in HIV infection. The St Mary's-Queen Square study. *Neuropsychiatry, Neuropsychology and Behavioural Neurology* **5**, 185–193 [328].

GRANT, I. & JUDD, L.L. (1976) Neuropsychological and EEG disturbances in polydrug users. *American Journal of Psychiatry* **133**, 1039–1042 [608].

GRANT, I., KYLE, G.C., TEICHMAN, A. & MENDELS, J. (1974) Recent life events and diabetes in adults. *Psychosomatic Medicine* **36**, 121–128 [535].

GRANT, I., MOHNS, L., MILLER, M. & REITAN, R.M. (1976) A neuropsychological study of polydrug users. *Archives of General Psychiatry* **33**, 973–978 [608].

GRANT, I., ROCHFORD, J., FLEMING, T. & STUNKARD, A. (1973) A neuro-psychological assessment of the effects of moderate marihuana use. *Journal of Nervous and Mental Disease* **156**, 278–280 [616].

GRANT, R.H.E. & STORES, O.P.R. (1970) Folic acid in folate-deficient patients with epilepsy. *British Medical Journal* **4**, 644–648 [592].

GRANVILLE-GROSSMAN, K. (1971) *Recent Advances in Clinical Psychiatry*. Churchill: London [628].

GRAVELL, M. (1988) Animal models of AIDS. *Annals of Neurology* **23 (Supplement)**, S213–S214 [317].

GRAVES, A.B., WHITE, E., KOEPSELL, T.D., REIFLER, B.V., VAN BELLE, G., LARSON, E.B. & RASKIND, M. (1990) The association between head trauma and Alzheimer's disease. *American Journal of Epidemiology* **131**, 491–501 [438].

GRAY, F., GENY, C., DOURNON, E., FENELON, G., LIONNET, F. & GHERARDI, R. (1991) Neuropathological evidence that zidovudine reduces incidence of HIV infection of brain. *Lancet* **337**, 852–853 [335].

GRAY, F., GHERARDI, R., KEOHANE, C., FAVOLINI, M., SOBEL, A. & POIRIER, J. (1988) Pathology of the central nervous system in 40 cases of acquired immune deficiency syndrome (AIDS). *Neuropathology and Applied Neurobiology* **14**, 365–380 [320].

GRAY, F., SCARAVILLI, F., EVERALL, I., CHRETIEN, F., AN, S., BOCHE, D., ADLE-BIASSETTE, H., WINGERTSMANN, L., DURIGON, M., HURTREL, B., CHIODI, F., BELL, J. & LANTOS, P. (1996) Neuropathology of early HIV-1 infection. *Brain Pathology* **6**, 1–15 [319].

GRAY, J. & HOFFENBERG, R. (1985) Thyrotoxicosis and stress. *Quarterly Journal of Medicine, New Series* **54**, 153–160 [508].

GREEN, A.R. & GOODWIN, G.M. (1996) Ecstasy and neurodegeneration. *British Medical Journal* **312**, 1493–1494 [625].

GREEN, J., MORRIS, J.C., McKEEL, D.W. & MILLER, J.W. (1990) Progressive aphasia: a precursor of global dementia? *Neurology* **40**, 423–429 [752].

GREEN, M.F., SATZ, P., SMITH, C. & NELSON, L. (1989) Is there atypical handedness in schizophrenia? *Journal of Abnormal Psychology* **98**, 57–61 [89].

GREEN, P. (1978) Defective interhemispheric transfer in schizophrenia. *Journal of Abnormal Psychology* **87**, 472–480 [90].

GREEN, P., HALLETT, S. & HUNTER, M. (1983) Abnormal interhemispheric integration and hemisphere specialisation in schizophrenics and high-risk children. In *Laterality and Psychopathology*, eds Flor-Henry, P. & Gruzelier, J., pp. 443–469. Elsevier: Amsterdam [90].

GREEN, P. & KOTENKO, V. (1980) Superior speech comprehension in schizophrenics under monaural versus binaural listening conditions. *Journal of Abnormal Pychology* **89**, 399–408 [90].

GREEN, S., BUTTRUM, S., MOLLOY, H., STEVENTON, G., STURMAN, S., WARING, R., PALL, H. & WILLIAMS, A. (1991) N-methylation of pyridines in Parkinson's disease. *Lancet* **338**, 120–121 [648].

GREENBAUM, J.V. & LURIE, L.A. (1948) Encephalits as a causative factor in behavior disorders of children. *Journal of the American Medical Association* **136**, 923–930 [347].

GREENBERG, G.D., WATSON, R.K. & DEPTULA, D. (1987) Neuropsychological dysfunction in sleep apnea. *Sleep* **10**, 254–262 [731].

GREENBERG, R. & PEARLMAN, C. (1967) Delirium tremens and dreaming. *American Journal of Psychiatry* **124**, 133–142 [598].

GREENBLATT, M. & SOLOMON, H.C. (1958) Studies of lobotomy. Ch. 11 in *The Brain and Human Behaviour*. Research Publications of the Association for Research in Nervous and Mental Disease, Vol. 36. Williams & Wilkins: Baltimore [77].

GREENFIELD, J.G. & NORMAN, R.M. (1963) Demyelinating diseases. Ch. 8 in *Greenfield's Neuropathology*, 2nd edn, eds Blackwood, W., McMenemey, W.H., Meyer, A., Norman, R.M. & Russell, D.S. Edward Arnold: London [700].

GREENFIELD, R.S. & NELSON, J.S. (1978) Atypical neuronal ceroidlipofuscinosis. *Neurology* **28**, 710–717 [759].

GREENWOOD, J., JEYASINGHAM, M., PRATT, O.E., RYLE, P.R., SHAW, G.K. & THOMSON, A.D. (1984) Heterogeneity of human erythrocyte transketolase: a preliminary report. *Alcohol and Alcoholism* **19**, 123–129 [576].

GREENWOOD, R.J. (1996) Neurosyphilis. Section 24.15.5 in *Oxford Textbook of Medicine*, 3rd edn, eds Weatherall, D.J., Ledingham, J.G.G. & Warrell, D.A. Oxford University Press: Oxford [344].

GREENWOOD, R.J., McMILLAN, T.M., BROOKS, D.N., DUNN, G., BROCK, D., DINSDALE, S., MURPHY, L.D. & PRICE, J.R. (1994) Effects of case management after severe head injury. *British Medical Journal* **308**, 1199–1205 [216].

GREER, H.D., WARD, H.P. & CORBIN, K.B. (1965) Chronic salicylate intoxication in adults. *Journal of the American Medical Association* **193**, 555–558 [628].

GREER, S. & PARSONS, V. (1968) Schizophrenia-like psychosis in thyroid crisis. *British Journal of Psychiatry* **114**, 1357–1362 [509].

GREGORIADIS, A., FRAGOS, E., KAPSLAKIS, Z. & MANDOUVALOS, B. (1971) A correlation between mental disorders and EEG and AEG findings in temporal lobe epilepsy. Abstracts from *5th World Congress of Psychiatry, 1971, Mexico*, p. 325. La Prensa Medica Mexicana: Mexico [282, 286].

GREGSON, R.A.M. & TAYLOR, G.M. (1977) Prediction of relapse in men alcoholics. *Journal of Studies on Alcohol* **38**, 1749–1760 [604].

GREITZ, T. (1969) Effect of brain distension on cerebral circulation. *Lancet* **1**, 863–865 [749].

GRESHAM, G.E., FITZPATRICK, T.E., WOLF, P.A., McNAMARA, P.M., KANNELL, W.B. & DAWBER, T.R. (1975) Residual disability in survivors of stroke. *New England Journal of Medicine* **293**, 954–956 [382].

GREWEL, F. (1969) The acalculias. Ch. 9 in *Handbook of Clinical Neurology*, Vol. 4, eds Vinken, P.J & Bruyn, G.W. North-Holland Publishing Co.: Amsterdam [66].

GREY WALTER, W., COOPER, R., ALDRIDGE, V.J., McCALLUM, W.C. & WINTER, A.L. (1964) Contingent negative variation: an electric sign of sensori-motor association and expectancy in the human brain. *Nature* **203**, 380–384 [132].

GRIFFIN, J.W., WESSELINGH, S.L., GRIFFIN, D.E., GLASS, J.D. & McARTHUR, J.C. (1994) Peripheral nerve disorders in HIV infection: similarities and contrasts with central nervous system disorders. Ch. 9 in *HIV, AIDS and the Brain*, eds Price, R.W. & Perry, S.W. *Association for Research in Nervous and Mental Disease*, **72.** Raven Press: New York [327].

GRINKER, R.R., HAM, G.C. & ROBBINS, F.P. (1950) Some psychodynamic factors in multiple sclerosis. Ch. 31 in *Multiple Sclerosis and the Demyelinating Diseases*. Research Publications of The Association for Research in Nervous and Mental Disease, Vol. 28. Williams & Wilkins: Baltimore [698].

GRINKER, R.R. & SAHS, A.L. (1966) *Neurology*, 6th edn. Thomas: Springfield, Illinois [365, 636, 707].

GRISOLIA, J.S. & WIEDERHOLT, W.C. (1982) CNS cysticercosis. *Archives of Neurology* **39**, 540–544 [370].

GRIST, N.R. (1967) Acute viral infections of the nervous system. *Proceedings of the Royal Society of Medicine* **60**, 696–698 [365].

GROAT, R.A. & SIMMONS, J.Q. (1950) Loss of nerve cells in experimental cerebral concussion. *Journal of Neuropathology and Experimental Neurology* **9**, 150–163 [162].

GROB, D. (1958) Myasthenia gravis: current status of psychogenesis, clinical manifestations and management. *Journal of Chronic Diseases* **8**, 536–566 [713].

GROEN, J.J. & ENDTZ, L.J. (1982) Hereditary Pick's disease. Second re-examination of a large family and discussion of other hereditary cases, with particular reference to electroencephalography and computerised tomography. *Brain* **105**, 443–459 [461, 462].

GRONWALL, D. (1987) Advances in the assessment of attention and information processing after head injury. Ch. 24 in *Neurobehavioral Recovery From Head Injury*, eds Levin, H.S., Grafman, J. & Eisenberg, H.M. Oxford University Press: Oxford [184].

GRONWALL, D. (1989) Cumulative and persisting effects of concussion on attention and cognition. Ch. 10 in *Mild Head Injury*, eds Levin, H.S., Eisenberg, H.M. & Benton, A.L. Oxford University Press: Oxford [184].

GRONWALL, D. & WRIGHTSON, P. (1974) Delayed recovery of intellectual function after minor head injury. *Lancet* **2**, 605–609 [198, 204].

GRONWALL, D. & WRIGHTSON, P. (1975) Cumulative effect of concussion. *Lancet* **2**, 995–997 [183].

GROSS, M.M. & GOODENOUGH, D.R. (1968) Sleep disturbances in the acute alcoholic psychoses. *Psychiatric Research Reports of the American Psychiatric Association* **24**, 132–147 [598].

GROSSMAN, M., GALETTA, S., DING, X.-S., MORRISON, D., D'ESPOSITO, M., ROBINSON, K., JAGGI, J., ALAVI, A. & REIVICH, M. (1996) Clinical and positron emission tomography studies of visual apperceptive agnosia. *Journal of Neuropsychiatry, Neuropsychology, and Behavioral Neurology* **9**, 70–77 [60].

GRUNBERG, F. & POND, D.A. (1957) Conduct disorders in epileptic children. *Journal of Neurology, Neurosurgery and Psychiatry* **20**, 65–68 [268].

GRUNDKE-IQBAL, I., JOHNSON, A.B., WISNIEWSKI, H.M., TERRY, R.D. & IQBAL, K. (1979) Evidence that Alzheimer neurofibrillary tangles originate from neurotubules. *Lancet* **1**, 578–580 [442].

GRUNNET, M. (1963) Cerebrovascular disease: diabetes and cerebral arteriosclerosis. *Neurology* **13**, 486–491 [538].

GRUNNET, M.L. (1969) Changing incidence, distribution, and histopathology of Wernicke's polioencephalopathy. *Neurology* **19**, 1135–1139 [580].

GRUT, A. (1949) *Chronic Carbon Monoxide Poisoning*. Munksgaard: Copenhagen [553].

GRUVSTAD, M., KEBBON, L. & GRUVSTAD, S. (1958) Social and psychiatric aspects of pre-traumatic personality and post-traumatic insufficiency reactions in traumatic head injuries. *Acta Societatis Medicorum Upsaliensis* **63**, 101–113 [174].

GRUZELIER, J. (1979) Synthesis and critical review of the evidence for hemisphere asymmetries of function in psychopathology. In *Hemisphere Asymmetries of Function in Psychopathology*, eds Gruzelier, J. & Flor-Henry, P., pp. 647–672. Elsevier/North Holland, Biomedical Press: Amsterdam [89].

GRUZELIER, J.H. (1981) Cerebral laterality and psychopathology: fact and fiction. *Psychological Medicine* **11**, 219–227 [89].

GRUZELIER, J. & FLOR-HENRY, P. (eds) (1979) *Hemisphere Asymmetries of Function in Psychopathology. Developments in Psychiatry*, Vol. 3. Elsevier/North-Holland, Biomedical Press: Amsterdam [89].

GRUZELIER, J.H. & VENABLES, P. (1974) Bimodality and lateral asymmetry of skin conductance orienting activity in schizophrenics: replication and evidence of lateral asymmetry in patients with depression and disorders of personality. *Biological Psychiatry* **8**, 55–73 [89].

GUBERMAN, A. & STUSS, D. (1983) The syndrome of bilateral paramedian thalamic infarction. *Neurology* **33**, 540–546 [384].

GUDJONSSON, G.H. & SHACKLETON, H. (1986) The pattern of scores on Raven's Matrices during 'faking bad' and 'non-faking' performance. *British Journal of Clinical Psychology* **25**, 35–41 [484].

GUDJONSSON, G.H. & TAYLOR, P.J. (1985) Cognitive deficit in a case

of retrograde amnesia. *British Journal of Psychiatry* **147**, 715–718 [38].

GUDMUNDSSON, G. (1966) Epilepsy in Iceland. A clinical and epidemiological investigation. *Acta Neurologica Scandinavica* **25 (Supplement)**, 7–124 [243, 265, 274].

GUERRANT, J., ANDERSON, W.W., FISCHER, A., WEINSTEIN, M.R., JAROS, R.M. & DESKINS, A. (1962) *Personality in Epilepsy*. Thomas: Springfield, Illinois [261, 265, 266].

GUEY, J., CHARLES, C., COQUERY, C., ROGER, J. & SOULAYROL, R. (1967) Study of psychological effects of ethosuximide (zarontin) on 25 children suffering from petit mal epilepsy. *Epilepsia* **8**, 129–141 [263].

GUILLEMINAULT, C. & ANDERS, T.F. (1976) Sleep disorders in children. *Advances in Paediatrics* **22**, 151–174 [731].

GUILLEMINAULT, C., DEMENT, W.C. & PASSOUANT, P. (eds) (1976) *Narcolepsy: Proceedings of the First International Symposium on Narcolepsy*. Advances in Sleep Research, Vol. 111. Spectrum Publications Inc: New York [722].

GUILLEMINAULT, C. & FAULL, K.F. (1982) Sleepiness in non-narcoleptic, non-sleep apneic EDS patients: the idiopathic CNS hypersomnolence. *Sleep* **5**, S175–S181 [729].

GUILLEMINAULT, C., FAULL, K.F., MILES, L. & VAN DEN HOED, J. (1983) Post traumatic excessive daytime sleepiness: a review of 20 patients. *Neurology* **33**, 1584–1589 [734].

GUILLEMINAULT, C. & MONDINI, S. (1986) Mononucleosis and chronic daytime sleepiness. A long-term follow-up study. *Archives of Internal Medicine* **146**, 1333–1335 [734].

GUISADO, R. & ARIEFF, A.I. (1975) Neurologic manifestations of diabetic comas: correlation with biochemical alterations in the brain. *Metabolism* **24**, 665–679 [538].

GUNN, J.C. (1969) The prevalence of epilepsy among prisoners. *Proceedings of the Royal Society of Medicine* **62**, 60–63 [274].

GUNN, J. (1973) Affective and suicidal symptoms in epileptic prisoners. *Psychological Medicine* **3**, 108–114 [286].

GUNN, J. (1978) Epileptic homicide: a case report. *British Journal of Psychiatry* **132**, 510–513 [274].

GUNN, J. (1993) Non-psychotic violence. Ch. 12 in *Forensic Psychiatry. Clinical, Legal and Ethical Issues*, eds Gunn, J. & Taylor, P.J. Butterworth/Heinemann: Oxford [81].

GUNN, J. & BONN, J. (1971) Criminality and violence in epileptic prisoners. *British Journal of Psychiatry* **118**, 337–343 [274].

GUNN, J. & FENTON, G.W. (1971) Epilepsy, automatism and crime. *Lancet* **1**, 1173–1176 [274].

GUPPY, A. (1994) At what blood alcohol concentration should drink-driving be illegal? *British Medical Journal* **308**, 1055–1056 [595].

GURLAND, B.J., FLEISS, J.L., GOLDBERG, K., SHARPE, L., COPELAND, J.R.M., KELLEHER, M.J. & KELLETT, J.M. (1976) A semistructured clinical interview for the assessment of diagnosis and mental state in the elderly: the Geriatric Mental State Schedule. II A factor analysis. *Psychological Medicine* **6**, 451–459 [124].

GURLAND, B.J., GANZ, V.F., FLEISS, J.L. & ZUBIN, J. (1972) The study of the psychiatric symptoms of systemic lupus erythematosus: a critical review. *Psychosomatic Medicine* **34**, 199–206 [419, 421].

GURLAND, B., KURIANSKY, J., SHARPE, L., SIMON, R., STILLER, P. & BIRKETT, P. (1977) The Comprehensive Assessment and Referral Evaluation (CARE)—rationale, development and reliability. *International Journal of Aging and Human Development* **8**, 9–42 [124].

GURLING, H.M.D., REVELEY, M.A. & MURRAY, R.M. (1984) Increased cerebral ventricular volume in monozygotic twins discordant for alcoholism. *Lancet* **1**, 986–988 [605].

GURNEY, C., HALL, R., HARPER, M., OWEN, S., ROTH, M. & SMART, G.A. (1967) A study of the physical and psychiatric characteristics of women attending an out-patient clinic for investigation for thyrotoxicosis. Communication to the Scottish Society for Experimental Medicine. Glasgow 1967. Quoted Slater, E. & Roth, M. (1969) *Clinical Psychiatry*, 3rd edn. Baillière, Tindall & Cassell: London [508, 510].

GUSELLA, J.F., WEXLER, N.S., CONNEALLY, P.M., NAYLOR, S.L., ANDERSON, M.A., TANZI, R.E., WATKINS, P.C., OTTINA, K., WALLACE, M.R., SAKAGUCHI, A.Y., YOUNG, A.B., SHOULSON, I., BONILLA, E. & MARTIN, J.B. (1983) A polymorphic DNA marker genetically linked to Huntington's disease. *Nature* **306**, 234–239 [466].

GUSTAFSON, L. (1987) Frontal lobe degeneration of non-Alzheimer type. II. Clinical picture and differential diagnosis. *Archives of Gerontology and Geriatrics* **6**, 209–223 [463].

GUSTAFSON, L., BRUN, A. & PASSANT, U. (1992) Frontal lobe degeneration of non-Alzheimer type. Ch. 5 in *Unusual Dementias*, ed. Rossor, M.N. Baillière Tindall: London [463, 464, 465].

GUSTAFSON, L. & NILSSON, L. (1982) Differential diagnosis of presenile dementia on clinical grounds. *Acta Psychiatrica Scandinavica* **65**, 194–209 [439].

GUSTAFSON, L., RISBERG, J., JOHANSON, M., FRANSSON, M. & MAXIMILIAN, V.A. (1978) Effects of Piracetam on regional cerebral blood flow and mental functions in patients with organic dementia. *Psychopharmacology* **56**, 115–117 [503].

GUTHRIE, A. & ELLIOTT, W.A. (1980) The nature and reversibility of cerebral impairment in alcoholism. Treatment implications. *Journal of Studies on Alcohol* **41**, 147–155 [607].

GUTTMANN, E. (1936) On some constitutional aspects of chorea and on its sequelae. *Journal of Neurology and Psychopathology* **17**, 16–26 [373, 374].

GUTTMANN, E. (1946) Late effects of closed head injuries: psychiatric observations. *Journal of Mental Science* **92**, 1–18 [173, 174, 177].

GUTTMANN, E. & HORDER, H. (1943) Head injuries in children and their after-effects. *Archives of Disease in Childhood* **18**, 139–145 [202, 204].

GUZE, B.H. (1991) Magnetic resonance spectroscopy: a technique for functional brain imaging. *Archives of General Psychiatry* **48**, 572–574 [143].

GUZE, S.B. (1967) The occurrence of psychiatric illness in systemic lupus erythematosus. *American Journal of Psychiatry* **123**, 1562–1570 [419, 420, 421].

GYLDENSTED, C. (1977) Measurements of the normal ventricular system and hemispheric sulci of 100 adults with computed tomography. *Neuoradiology* **14**, 183–192 [138].

HABER, S.N., KOWALL, N.W., VON SATTEL, J.P., BIRD, E.D. & RICHARDSON, E.P. (1986) Gilles de la Tourette's syndrome. A postmortem neuropathological and immunohistochemical study. *Journal of the Neurological Sciences* **75**, 225–241 [685].

HABER, S.N. & WOLFER, D. (1992) Basal ganglia peptidergic staining in Tourette syndrome. Ch. 17 in *Tourette Syndrome. Genetics, Neurobiology, and Treatment*, eds Chase, T.N., Friedhoff, A.J. & Cohen, D.J. *Advances in Neurology*, Vol. 58. Raven Press: New York [685].

HABERLAND, C. (1965) Psychiatric manifestations in brain tumours. *Bibliotheca Psychiatrica et Neurologica* **127**, 65–86 [225].

HACHINSKI, V.C., ILIFF, L.D., ZILHKA, E., DU BOULAY, G.H., McALLISTER, V.L., MARSHALL, J., ROSS RUSSELL, R.W. & SYMON, L. (1975) Cerebral blood flow in dementia. *Archives of Neurology* **32**, 632–637 [456, 457].

HACHINSKI, V.C., LASSEN, N.A. & MARSHALL, J. (1974) Multi-infarct dementia: a cause of mental deterioration in the elderly. *Lancet* **2**, 207–210 [453].

HACHINSKI, V.C., POTTER, P. & MERSKEY, H. (1987) Leuko-araiosis. *Archives of Neurology* **44**, 21–23 [459].

HAGEN, A.C. (1969) Communication disorders of the stroke patient. *Clinical Orthopaedics and Related Research* **63**, 102–112 [390].

HAGLUND, Y. & BERGSTRAND, G. (1990) Does Swedish amateur boxing lead to chronic brain damage? 2. A retrospective study with CT and MRI. *Acta Neurologica Scandinavica* **82**, 297–302 [206].

HAGLUND, Y. & PERSSON, H.E. (1990) Does Swedish amateur boxing lead to chronic brain damage? 3. A retrospective clinical neurophysiological study. *Acta Neurologica Scandinavica* **82**, 353–360 [206].

HAHN, R.D. & CLARK, E.G. (1946a) Asymptomatic neurosyphilis: a review of the literature. *American Journal of Syphilis, Gonorrhoea and Venereal Diseases* **30**, 305–316 [337].

HAHN, R.D. & CLARK, E.G. (1946b) Asymptomatic neurosyphilis: prognosis. *American Journal of Syphilis, Gonorrhoea and Venereal Diseases* **30**, 513–548 [337].

HAHN, R.D., WEBSTER, B., WEICKHARDT, G., THOMAS, E., TIMBERLAKE, W., SOLOMON, H., STOKES, J.H., MOORE, J.E., HEYMAN, A., GAMMON, G., GLEESON, G.A., CURTIS, A.C. & CUTLER, J.C. (1959) Penicillin treatment of general paresis (dementia paralytica). *Archives of Neurology and Psychiatry* **81**, 557–590 [340, 344, 345].

HAKIM, A.M. & MATHIESON, G. (1978) Basis of dementia in Parkinson's disease. *Lancet* **2**, 729 [655].

HAKIM, A.M. & MATHIESON, G. (1979) Dementia in Parkinson's disease: a neuropathologic study. *Neurology* **29**, 1209–1214 [655].

HAKIM, S. (1964) *Algunas observaciones sobra la pression del L.C.R. sindrome hidrocefalico en al adulto con 'pression normal' del L.C.R.* Tesis de grado, Universidad Javeriana. Bogota, Columbia, 1964. Quoted by Ojemann, R.G. *et al.* (1969) *Journal of Neurosurgery* **31**, 279–294 [745].

HAKIM, S. & ADAMS, R.D. (1965) The special clinical problem of symptomatic hydrocephalus with normal cerebrospinal fluid pressure: observations on cerebrospinal fluid hydrodynamics. *Journal of the Neurological Sciences* **2**, 307–327 [745, 749].

HALDANE, J.S., KELLAS, A.M. & KENNAWAY, E.L. (1919) Experiments on acclimatisation to reduced atmospheric pressure. *Journal of Physiology* **53**, 181–206 [548].

HALIKAS, J.A. (1974) Marijuana use and psychiatric illness. Ch. 11 in *Marijuana: Effects on Human Behaviour*, ed. Miller, L.L. Academic Press: New York [614].

HALIKAS, J.A., GOODWIN, D.W. & GUZE, S.B. (1972) Marijuana use and psychiatric illness. *Archives of General Psychiatry* **27**, 162–165 [615].

HALL, C.W., POPKIN, M.K., STICKNEY, S.K. & GARDNER, R. (1979) Presentation of the steroid psychoses. *Journal of Nervous and Mental Disease* **167**, 229–236 [628].

HALL, E.D. (1992a) The neuroprotective pharmacology of methylprednisolone. *Journal of Neurosurgery* **76**, 13–22 [165].

HALL, E.D. (1992b) Lazaroids: novel cerebroprotective antioxidants. Ch. 11 in *Emerging Strategies in Neuroprotection*, eds Marangos, P.J. & Lal, H. Birkhäusen: Boston [165].

HALL, P. (1963) Korsakov's syndrome following herpes-zoster encephalitis. *Lancet* **1**, 752 [359].

HALL, R. (1983) Pituitary and hypothalamic disorders. In *Oxford Textbook of Medicine*, 1st edn, Vol. I, eds Weatherall, D.J., Ledingham, J.G.G. & Warrell, D.A., pp. 10.7–10.24. Oxford University Press: Oxford [525].

HALL, R.C.W. (1973) Hypomagnesemia. Physical and psychiatric symptoms. *Journal of the American Medical Association* **224**, 1749–1751 [561].

HALL, S.B. (1929) Mental aspect of epidemic encephalitis. *British Medical Journal* **1**, 444–446 [353].

HALL, T.C., MILLER, A.K.H. & CORSELLIS, J.A.N. (1975) Variations in the human Purkinje cell population according to age and sex. *Neuropathology and Applied Neurobiology* **1**, 267–292 [443].

HALLIDAY, A.M., McDONALD, W.I. & MUSHIN, J. (1973) Visual evoked response in diagnosis of multiple sclerosis. *British Medical Journal* **4**, 661–664 [689].

HALLIDAY, G., ELLIS, J., HEARD, R., CAINE, D. & HARPER, C. (1993) Brainstem serotonergic neurons in chronic alcoholics with and without the memory impairment of Korsakoff's psychosis. *Journal of Neuropathology and Experimental Neurology* **52**, 567–579 [607].

HALLIGAN, P.W., COCKBURN, J. & WILSON, B. (1991) The behavioural assessment of visual neglect. *Neuropsychological Rehabilitation* **1**, 5–32 [113].

HALLIGAN, P.W. & MARSHALL, J.C. (1991) Left neglect for near but not far space in man. *Nature* **350**, 498–500 [62].

HALONEN, P.E., RIMON, R., AROHONKA, K. & JÄNTTI, V. (1974) Antibody levels to herpes simplex type 1, measles and rubella viruses in psychiatric patients. *British Journal of Psychiatry* **125**, 461–465 [358].

HALPERIN, J.J., LANDIS, D.M.D. & KLEINMAN, G.M. (1982) Whipple disease of the nervous system. *Neurology* **32**, 612–617 [760].

HALSTEAD, S., RICCIO, M., HARLOW, P., ORETTI, R. & THOMPSON, C. (1988) Psychosis associated with HIV infection. *British Journal of Psychiatry* **153**, 618–623 [331].

HAMBERT, G. & FREY, T.S. (1964) The electroencephalogram in the Klinefelter syndrome. *Acta Psychiatrica Scandinavica* **40**, 28–36 [527].

HAMBLIN, T.J., HUSSAIN, J., AKBAR, A.N., TANG, Y.C., SMITH, J.L. & JONES, D.B. (1983) Immunological reason for chronic ill health after infectious mononucleosis. *British Medical Journal* **287**, 85–88 [359].

HAMILTON, J.D., HARTIGAN, P.M., SIMBERKOFF, M.S., DAY, P.L., DIAMOND, G.R., DICKINSON, G.M., DRUSANO, G.L., EGORIN, M.J., GEORGE, L., GORDIN, F.M., HAWKES, C.A., JENSEN, P.C., KLIMAS, N.G., LABRIOLA, A.M., LAHART, C.J., O'BRIEN, W.A., OSTER, C.N., WEINHOLD, K.J., WRAY, N.P., ZOLLA-PAZNER, S.B. & THE VETERANS AFFAIRS COOPERATIVE STUDY GROUP ON AIDS TREATMENT (1992) A controlled trial of early versus late treatment with zidovudine in symptomatic human immunodeficiency virus infection. *New England Journal of Medicine* **326**, 437–443 [335].

HAMILTON-DUTOIT, S.J., PALLESEN, G., FRANZMANN, M.B., KARKOV, J., BLACK, F., SKINHOJ, P. & PEDERSEN, C. (1991) AIDS-related lymphoma. Histopathology, immunophenotype, and association with Epstein–Barr virus as demonstrated by in-situ nucleic acid hybridization. *American Journal of Pathology* **138**, 149–163 [321].

HAMMARSTEN, J.F. & SMITH, W.O. (1957) Symptomatic magnesium deficiency in man. *New England Journal of Medicine* **256**, 897–899 [561].

HAMMOND, J.S. & WARD, C.G. (1988) High-voltage electrical injuries: management and outcome of 60 cases. *Southern Medical Journal* **81**, 1351–1352 [765, 766].

HAMMOND, P. & WALLIS, S. (1992) Cerebral oedema in diabetic ketoacidosis. Still puzzling—and often fatal. *British Medical Journal* **305**, 203–204 [538].

HAMOS, J.E., DE GENNARO, L.J. & DRACHMAN, D.A. (1989) Synaptic loss in Alzheimer's disease and other dementias. *Neurology* **39**, 355–361 [443].

HANDLER, C.E. & PERKIN, G.D. (1982) Anorexia nervosa and Wernicke's encephalopathy: an underdiagnosed association. *Lancet* **2**, 771–772 [576].

HANNA, S., HARRISON, M., MacINTYRE, I. & FRASER, R. (1960) The syndrome of magnesium deficiency in man. *Lancet* **2**, 172–176 [561].

HANSEN, L., SALMON, D., GALASKO, D., MASLIAH, E., KATZMAN, R., DETERESA, R., THAL, L., PAY, M.M., HOFSTETTER, R., KLAUBER, M., RICE, V., BUTTERS, N. & ALFORD, M. (1990) The Lewy body variant of Alzheimer's disease. A clinical and pathogenic entity. *Neurology* **40**, 1–8 [450, 451, 452].

HARBAUGH, R.E., ROBERTS, D.W., COOMBS, D.W., SAUNDERS, R.L. & REEDER, T.M. (1984) Preliminary report: intracranial cholinergic drug infusion in patients with Alzheimer's disease. *Neurosurgery* **15**, 514–518 [503].

HARDIE, R.J. (1989) Acanthocytosis and neurological impairment—a review. *Quarterly Journal of Medicine* **71**, 291–306 [757].

HARDIE, R.J., PULLON, H.W.H., HARDING, A.E., OWEN, J.S., PIRES, M., DANIELS, G.L., IMAI, Y., MISRA, V.P., KING, R.H.M., JACOBS, J.M., TIPPETT, P., DUCHEN, L.W., THOMAS, P.K. & MARSDEN, C.D. (1991) Neuroacanthocytosis: a clinical, haematological and pathological study of 19 cases. *Brain* **114**, 13–49 [757].

HARDING, A.E. (1993a) Movement disorders. Ch. 11 in *Brain's Diseases of the Nervous System*, 10th edn, ed. Walton, J. Oxford University Press: Oxford [648, 662, 663, 671].

HARDING, A.E. (1993b) Neurocutaneous disorders and degenerative diseases of the spinal cord and cerebellum. Ch. 12 in *Brain's Diseases of the Nervous System*, 10th edn, ed. Walton, J. Oxford University Press [705, 707].

HARE, E.H. (1959) The origin and spread of dementia paralytica. *Journal of Mental Sciences* **105**, 594–626 [339].

HARE, E.H. (1973) The duration of the fortification spectrum in migraine. Ch. 12 in *Background to Migraine*, 5th Migraine Symposium, ed. Cumings, J.N. Heinemann: London [400].

HARE, E.H. (1987) Epidemiology of schizophrenia and affective psychosis. *British Medical Bulletin* **43**, 514–530 [91].

HARE, E. (1988) Temporal factors and trends, including birth seasonality and the viral hypothesis. Ch. 15 in *Nosology, Epidemiology and Genetics of Schizophrenia*, eds Tsuang, M.T. & Simpson, J.C. *Handbook of Schizophrenia*, Vol. 3. Series editor Nasrallah, H.A. Elsevier: Amsterdam [91].

HARE, M. (1978) Clinical check list for diagnosis of dementia. *British Medical Journal* **2**, 266–267 [433].

HARGREAVES, M.M., RICHMOND, H. & MORTON, R. (1948) Presentation of two bone marrow elements: the 'tart' cell and the 'L.E.' cell. *Proceedings of the Staff Meetings of the Mayo Clinic* **23**, 25–28 [417].

HARLEY, H.G., BROOK, J.D., RUNDLE, S.A., CROW, S., REARDON, W., BUCKLER, A.J., HARPER, P.S., HOUSMAN, D.E. & SHAW, D.J. (1992a) Expansion of an unstable DNA region and phenotypic variation in myotonic dystrophy. *Nature* **355**, 545–546 [717].

HARLEY, H.G., RUNDLE, S.A., REARDON, W., MYRING, J., CROW, S., BROOK, J.D., HARPER, P.S. & SHAW, D.J. (1992b) Unstable DNA sequence in myotonic dystrophy. *Lancet* **339**, 1125–1128 [717].

HARPER, C. (1979) Wernicke's encephalopathy: a more common disease than realised. A neuropathological study of 51 cases. *Journal of Neurology, Neurosurgery and Psychiatry* **42**, 226–231 [581].

HARPER, C. (1983) The incidence of Wernicke's encephalopathy in Australia—a neuropathological study of 131 cases. *Journal of Neurology, Neurosurgery and Psychiatry* **46**, 593–598 [581, 582].

HARPER, C. (1989) Brain damage and alcohol misuse. *Current Opinion in Psychiatry* **2**, 434–438 [607].

HARPER, C.G. & BLUMBERGS, P.C. (1982) Brain weights in alcoholics. *Journal of Neurology, Neurosurgery and Psychiatry* **45**, 838–840 [604, 607].

HARPER, C. & CORBETT, D. (1990) Changes in the basal dendrites of cortical pyramidal cells from alcoholic patients—a quantitative Golgi study. *Journal of Neurology, Neurosurgery and Psychiatry* **53**, 856–861 [604].

HARPER, C., FORNES, P., DUYCKAERTS, C., LECOMTE, D. & HAUW, J.-J. (1995) An international perspective on the prevalence of the Wernicke–Korsakoff syndrome. *Metabolic Brain Disease* **10**, 17–24 [576].

HARPER, C.G., GILES, M. & FINLAY-JONES, R. (1986) Clinical signs in the Wernicke–Korsakoff complex: a retrospective analysis of 131 cases diagnosed at necropsy. *Journal of Neurology, Neurosurgery and Psychiatry* **49**, 341–345 [578].

HARPER, C., GOLD, J., RODRIGUEZ, M. & PERDICES, M. (1989) The prevalence of the Wernicke–Korsakoff syndrome in Sydney, Australia: a prospective necropsy study. *Journal of Neurology, Neurosurgery and Psychiatry* **52**, 282–285 [576].

HARPER, C. & KRIL, J. (1985) Brain atrophy in chronic alcoholic patients—a quantitative pathological study. *Journal of Neurology, Neurosurgery and Psychiatry* **48**, 211–217 [604, 607].

HARPER, C.G. & KRIL, J.J. (1988) Corpus callosum thickness in alcoholics. *British Journal of Addiction* **83**, 577–580 [604].

HARPER, C.G. & KRILL, J.J. (1990) Neuropathology of alcoholism. *Alcohol and Alcoholism* **25**, 207–216 [607].

HARPER, C., KRIL, J. & DALY, J. (1987) Are we drinking our neurones away? *British Medical Journal* **294**, 534–536 [604].

HARPER, C.G., KRIL, J.J. & HOLLOWAY, R.L. (1985) Brain shrinkage in chronic alcoholics: a pathological study. *British Medical Journal* **290**, 501–504 [604].

HARPER, M. & ROTH, M. (1962) Temporal lobe epilepsy and the phobic anxiety-depersonalization syndrome. *Comprehensive Psychiatry* **3**, 129–151 and 215–226 [294].

HARPER, P.S. (1986) The prevention of Huntington's chorea. *Journal of the Royal College of Physicians of London* **20**, 7–14 [466].

HARPER, P.S. (1989) *Myotonic Dystrophy*, 2nd edn. W.B. Saunders: London [717, 718, 721].

HARPER, P.S. (1993) A specific mutation for Huntington's disease. *Journal of Medical Genetics* **30**, 975–977 [466].

HARPER, P.S. & MORRIS, M.R. (1991) Introduction: a historical background. Ch. 1 in *Huntington's Disease*, ed. Harper, P.S. W.B. Saunders: London [465].

HARPER, P.S., TYLER, A., SMITH, S. & JONES, P. (1981) Decline in the predicted incidence of Huntington's chorea associated with systematic genetic counselling and family support. *Lancet* **2**, 411–413 [466].

HARRINGTON, C.R., LOUWAGIE, J., ROUSSAU, R., VANMECHELEN, E., PERRY, R.H., PERRY, E.K., XUEREB, J.H., ROTH, M. & WISCHIK, C.M. (1994) Influence of apolipoprotein E genotype on senile dementia of the Alzheimer and Lewy body types. *American Journal of Pathology* **145**, 1472–1484 [442, 448].

HARRINGTON, C.R. & WISCHIK, C.M. (1994) Molecular pathobiology of Alzheimer's disease. Ch. 13 in *Dementia*, eds Burns, A. & Levy, R. Chapman & Hall: London [442].

HARRINGTON, J.A. & LETEMENDIA, F.J.J. (1958) Persistent psychiatric disorders after head injuries in children. *Journal of Mental Science* **104**, 1205–1218 [203].

HARRIS, A.I., COX, E. & SMITH, C.R.W. (1971) *Handicapped and Impaired in Great Britain, Part 1*. Office of Population Censuses and Surveys, H.M.S.O.: London [375].

HARRIS, M.J., JESTE, D.V., GLEGHORN, A. & SEWELL, D.D. (1991) New-onset psychosis in HIV-infected patients. *Journal of Clinical Psychiatry* **52**, 369–376 [331].

HARRIS, R. (1982) Genetics of Alzheimer's disease. *British Medical Journal* **284**, 1065–1066 [447].

HARRIS, T., CREED, F. & BRUGHA, T.S. (1992) Stressful life events and Graves' disease. *British Journal of Psychiatry* **161**, 535–541 [508].

HARRISON, M.J.G., ROBERT, C.M. & UTTLEY, D. (1974) Benign aqueduct stenosis in adults. *Journal of Neurology, Neurosurgery and Psychiatry* **37**, 1322–1328 [750].

HARRISON, M.J.G., THOMAS, D.J., DU BOULAY, G.H. & MARSHALL, J. (1979) Multi-infarct dementia. *Journal of the Neurological Sciences* **40**, 97–103 [454, 456, 457].

HARRISON, M.S. (1956) Notes on the clinical features and pathology of post-concussional vertigo, with especial reference to positional nystagmus. *Brain* **79**, 474–486 [197].

HARRISON, P.J. & ROBERTS, G.W. (1991) Life, Jim, but not as we know it? Transmissible dementias and the prion protein. *British Journal of Psychiatry* **158**, 457–470 [475].

HARRISON, P.J. & ROBERTS, G.W. (1992) How now mad cow? The science progresses, but the risk to humans remains uncertain. *British Medical Journal* **304**, 929–930 [475].

HARROWER, M.R. (1950) The results of psychometric and personality tests in multiple sclerosis. Ch. 32 in *Multiple Sclerosis and the Demyelinating Diseases*. Research Publications of the Association for Research in Nervous and Mental Disease, Vol. 28. Williams & Wilkins: Baltimore [696].

HARROWER, M. (1954) Psychological factors in multiple sclerosis. *Annals of the New York Academy of Sciences* **58**, 715–719 [696].

HARTMAN, D.E. (1988) *Neuropsychological Toxicology: Identification and Assessment of Human Neurotoxic Syndromes*. Pergamon Press: Oxford [610, 631, 634, 637, 638].

HARTMANN, E.L. (1965) The D-state. A review and discussion of studies on the physiologic state concomitant with dreaming. *New England Journal of Medicine* **273**, 30–35 and 87–92 [725].

HARVEY, I., PERSAUD, R., RON, M.A., BAKER, G. & MURRAY, R.M. (1994) Volumetric MRI measurements in bipolars compared with schizophrenics and healthy controls. *Psychological Medicine* **24**, 689–699 [85].

HARVEY, I., RON, M.A., DU BOULAY, G., WICKS, D., LEWIS, S.W. & MURRAY, R.M. (1993) Reduction of cortical volume in schizophrenia on magnetic resonance imaging. *Psychological Medicine* **23**, 591–604 [85].

HASSLER, R. & DIECKMANN, G. (1970) Traitement stéréotaxique des tics et cris inarticulés ou coprolaliques considérés comme phénomène d'obsession motrice au cours de la maladie de Gilles de la Tourette. *Revue Neurologique* **123**, 89–100 [687].

HASSLER, R. & DIECKMANN, G. (1973) Relief of obsessive–compulsive disorders, phobias and tics by stereotactic coagulation of the rostral intralaminar and medial-thalamic nuclei. Ch. 19 in *Surgical Approaches in Psychiatry*, eds Laitinen, L.V. & Livingston, K.E. Medical and Technical Publishing Co.: Lancaster [687].

HATA, T., MEYER, J.S., TANAHASHI, N., ISHIKAWA, Y., IMAI, A., SHINOHARA, T., VELEZ, M., FANN, W.E., KANDULA, P. & SAKAI, F. (1987) Three-dimensional mapping of local cerebral perfusion in alcoholic encephalopathy with and without Wernicke–Korsakoff syndrome. *Journal of Cerebral Blood Flow and Metabolism* **7**, 35–44 [579, 606].

HATRICK, J.A. & DEWHURST, K. (1970) Delayed psychosis due to LSD. *Lancet* **2**, 742–744 [622].

HAUG, G. (1977) Age and sex dependence of the size of normal ventricles on computed tomography. *Neuroradiology* **14**, 201–204 [138].

HAUG, J.O. (1962) Pneumoencephalographic studies in mental disease. *Acta Psychiatrica Scandinavica* **165 (Supplement)**, 1–104 [139].

HAUG, J.O. (1968) Pneumoencephalographic evidence of brain damage in chronic alcoholics. *Acta Psychiatrica Scandinavica* **203 (Supplement)**, 135–143 [605].

HAUSER, R.A., FREEMAN, T.B. & OLANOW, C.W. (1995) Surgical therapies for Parkinson's disease. Ch. 2 in *Treatment of Motor Disorders*, ed. Kurlan, R. J.B. Lippincott: Philadelphia [652].

HAUSER, W.A., ANNEGERS, J.F., ANDERSON, E. & KURLAND, L.T. (1985) The risk of seizure disorders among relatives of children with febrile convulsions. *Neurology* **35**, 1268–1273 [247].

HAUW, J.-J., DE BAECQUE, C., HAUSSER-HAUW, C. & SERDARU, M. (1988) Chromatolysis in alcoholic encephalopathies. *Brain* **111**, 843–857 [575].

HAWKES, C. (1996) A gene for Parkinson's disease? Evidence for genetic linkage in a family with autosomal dominant disease. *British Medical Journal* **313**, 1278 [646].

HAWKES, C.H., CAVANAGH, J.B. & FOX, A.J. (1989) Motoneuron disease: a disorder secondary to solvent exposure. *Lancet* **1**, 73–75 [707].

HAWKINS, C.P., MUNRO, P.M.G., MacKENZIE, F., KESSELRING, J., TOFTS, P.S., DU BOULAY, E.P.G.H., LANDON, D.N. & McDONALD, W.I. (1990) Duration and selectivity of blood-brain barrier breakdown in chronic relapsing experimental allergic encephalomyelitis studied by gadolinium-DTPA and protein markers. *Brain* **113**, 365–378 [142].

HAWKINS, R.A., MAZZIOTTA, J.C. & PHELPS, M.E. (1987) Wilson's disease studied with FDG and positron emission tomography. *Neurology* **37**, 1707–1711 [662].

HAWKINS, T.D. & MARTIN, L. (1965) Incidence of hyperostosis frontalis interna in patients at a general hospital and at a mental hospital. *Journal of Neurology, Neurosurgery and Psychiatry* **28**, 171–174 [769].

HAWTON, K., FAGG, J. & MARSACK, P. (1980) Association between epilepsy and attempted suicide. *Journal of Neurology, Neurosurgery and Psychiatry* **43**, 168–170 [286].

HAXBY, J.V., GRADY, C.L., KOSS, E., HORWITZ, B., HESTON, L., SCHAPIRO, M., FRIEDLAND, R.P. & RAPOPORT, S.I. (1990) Longitudinal study of cerebral metabolic asymmetries and associated neuropsychological patterns in early dementia of the Alzheimer type. *Archives of Neurology* **47**, 753 [434].

HAXBY, J.V., GRADY, C.L., KOSS, E., HORWITZ, B., SCHAPIRO, M., FRIEDLAND, R.P. & RAPOPORT, S.I. (1988) Heterogeneous anterior-posterior metabaolic patterns in dementia of the Alzheimer type. *Neurology* **38**, 1853–1863 [434].

HAXBY, J.V., GRADY, C.L., UNGERLEIDER, L.G. & HORWITZ, B. (1991) Mapping the functional neuroanatomy of the intact human brain with brain work imaging. *Neuropsychologia* **29**, 539–555 [145, 146].

HAY, W.J., RICKARDS, A.G., McMENEMY, W.H. & CUMINGS, J.N. (1963) Organic mercurial encephalopathy. *Journal of Neurology, Neurosurgery and Psychiatry* **26**, 199–202 [635].

HAYASHI, R., HAYASHI, K., INOUE, K. & YANAGISAWA, N. (1993) A serial computerized tomographic study of the interval form of co-poisoning. *European Neurology* **33**, 27–29 [551].

HAYDEN, M.R. (1981) *Huntington's Chorea*. Springer-Verlag: New York [471].

HAYES, F.A., GREEN, A.A., SENZER, N. & PRATT, C.B. (1979) Tetany: a complication of cis-dichlorodiammineplatinum (11) therapy. *Cancer Treatment Reports* **63**, 547–548 [561].

HAYES, R.L., LYETH, B.G. & JENKINS, L.W. (1989) Neurochemical mechanisms of mild and moderate head injury: implications for treatment. Ch. 5 in *Mild Head Injury*, eds Levin, H.S., Eisenberg, H.M. & Benton, A.L. Oxford University Press: Oxford [164].

HAYES, R.L., LYETH, B.G., JENKINS, L.W., ZIMMERMAN, R., McINTOSH, T.K., CLIFTON, G.L. & YOUNG, H.F. (1990) Possible protective effect of endogenous opioids in traumatic brain injury. *Journal of Neurosurgery* **72**, 252–261 [165].

HAYMAN, M. (1941) Myasthenia gravis and psychosis: report of a case with observations on its psychosomatic implications. *Psychosomatic Medicine* **3**, 120–137 [711].

HAYS, P., KRIKLER, B., WALSH, L.S. & WOOLFSON, G. (1966) Psychological changes following surgical treatment of parkinsonism. *American Journal of Psychiatry* **123**, 657–663 [660].

HEAD, H. (1920) *Studies in Neurology*, Vol. 2. Oxford University Press: Oxford [67].

HEADACHE CLASSIFICATION COMMITTEE OF THE INTERNATIONAL HEADACHE SOCIETY (1988) Classification and diagnostic criteria for headache disorders, cranial neurologies and facial pain. *Cephalgia* **8 (Supplement 7)**, 1–96 [399].

HEALY, D. & EVANS, J. (1993) Creutzfeldt–Jakob disease after pituitary gonadotrophins. *British Medical Journal* **307**, 517–518 [476].

HEATH, R.G., MONROE, R.R. & MICKLE, W.A. (1955) Stimulation of the amygdaloid nucleus in a schizophrenic patient. *American Journal of Psychiatry* **111**, 862–863 [81, 267].

HEATHFIELD, K.W.G. (1967) Huntington's chorea. *Brain* **90**, 203–232 [466, 468, 506].

HEATHFIELD, K.W.G., CROFT, P.B. & SWASH, M. (1973) The syndrome of transient global amnesia. *Brain* **96**, 729–736 [415].

HEATON, R.K., NELSON, L.M., THOMPSON, D.S., BURKS, J.S. & FRANKLIN, G.M. (1985) Neuropsychological findings in relapsing–remitting and chronic–progressive multiple sclerosis. *Journal of Consulting and Clinical Psychology* **53**, 103–110 [692].

HÉCAEN, H. (1962) Clinical symptomatology in right and left hemisphere lesions. Ch. 10 in *Interhemispheric Relations and Cerebral Dominance*, ed. Mountcastle, V.B. Johns Hopkins Press: Baltimore [63].

HÉCAEN, H. (1969) Aphasic, apraxic and agnosic syndromes in right and left hemisphere lesions. Ch. 15 in *Handbook of Clinical Neurology*, Vol. 4, eds Vinken, P.J. & Bruyn, G.W. North-Holland Publishing Co.: Amsterdam [67].

HÉCAEN, H. & AJURIAGUERRA, J. DE (1956) *Troubles Mentaux au cours des Tumeurs Intracraniennes*. Masson: Paris [218, 220, 221, 222, 224, 225, 226, 227, 231].

HÉCAEN, H. & ALBERT, M.L. (1975) Disorders of mental functioning related to frontal lobe pathology. Ch. 8 in *Psychiatric Aspects of Neurologic Disease*, eds Benson, D.F. & Blumer, D. Grune & Stratton: New York [76].

HÉCAEN, H. & ANGELERGUES, R. (1962) Agnosia for faces (prosopagnosia). *Archives of Neurology* **7**, 24–32 [60].

HECK, A.W. & PHILLIPS, L.H. (1989) Sarcoidosis of the nervous system. In *Neurologic Manifestations of Systemic Disease*, ed. Riggs, J.E. *Neurologic Clinics* **7**, 641–654 [764].

HECK, L.L., HOFFER, P.B. & GOTTSHALK, A. (1971) Brain-scanning successes, limitations, and future developments. Ch. 17 in *Clinical Neurosurgery*, Proceedings of the Congress of Neurological Surgeons, Vol. 18. Williams & Wilkins: Baltimore [135].

HECKERS, S., HEINSEN, H., GEIGER, B. & BECKMANN, H. (1991) Hippocampal neuron number in schizophrenia. A stereological study. *Archives of General Psychiatry* **48**, 1002–1008 [86].

HEIKKLA, R.E., MANZINO, L., CABBAT, F.S. & DUVOISIN, R.C. (1984) Protection against the dopaminergic neurotoxicity of 1-methyl-4-phenyl-1,2,5,6-tetrahydropyridine by monoamine oxidase inhibitors. *Nature* **311**, 467–469 [650].

HEILMAN, K.M., SCHOLES, R. & WATSON, R.T. (1975) Auditory affective agnosia. Disturbed comprehension of affective speech. *Journal of Neurology, Neurosurgery and Psychiatry* **38**, 69–72 [65].

HEILMAN, K.M., VALENSTEIN, E. & WATSON, R.T. (1985) The neglect syndrome. Ch.12 in *Handbook of Clinical Neurology*, Revised Series,

Vol. 1. *Clinical Neuropsychology*, ed. Frederiks, J.A.M. Elsevier Science Publishers BV: Amsterdam [62].

HEIMBURGER, R.F., DEMYER, W. & REITAN, R.M. (1964) Implications of Gerstmann's syndrome. *Journal of Neurology, Neurosurgery and Psychiatry* **27**, 52–57. [65].

HEINE, B.E. (1969) Psychiatric aspects of systemic lupus erythematosus. *Acta Psychiatrica Scandinavica* **45**, 307–326 [419, 420].

HEINE, B.E., SAINSBURY, P. & CHYNOWETH, R.C. (1969) Hypertension and emotional disturbance. *Journal of Psychiatric Research* **7**, 119–130 [397].

HEINZ, E.R., MARTINEZ, J. & HAENGGELI, A. (1977) Reversibility of cerebral atrophy in anorexia nervosa and Cushing's syndrome. *Journal of Computer Assisted Tomography* **1**, 415–418 [141, 517].

HEISKANEN, O. & SIPPONEN, P. (1970) Prognosis of severe brain injury. *Acta Neurologica Scandinavica* **46**, 343–348 [174].

HELWEG-LARSEN, P., HOFFMEYER, H., KIELER, J., THAYSEN, E.H., THAYSEN, J.H., THYGESEN, P. & WULFF, M.H. (1952) Famine disease in German concentration camps: complications and sequels. *Acta Psychiatrica et Neurologica Scandinavica* **83 (Supplement)**, 1–460 [570].

HEMMINGSEN, R. & KRAMP, P. (1988) Delirium tremens and related clinical states: psychopathology, cerebral pathophysiology and psychochemistry: a two-component hypothesis concerning etiology and pathogenesis. *Acta Psychiatrica Scandinavica* **78 (Supplement 345)**, 94–107 [598].

HEMMINGSEN, R., VORSTRUP, S., CLEMMESEN, L., HOLM, S., TFELT-HANSEN, P., SØRENSEN, A.S., HANSEN, C., SOMMER, W. & BOLWIG, T.G. (1988) Cerebral blood flow during delirium tremens and related clinical states studied with xenon-133 inhalation tomography. *American Journal of Psychiatry* **145**, 1384–1390 [602].

HEMPHILL, R.E. & STENGEL, E. (1940) A study on pure word-deafness. *Journal of Neurology, Neurosurgery and Psychiatry* **3**, 251–262 [49].

HEMSI, L.K., WHITEHEAD, A. & POST, F. (1968) Cognitive functioning and cerebral arousal in elderly depressives and dements. *Journal of Psychosomatic Research* **12**, 145–156 [487].

HENDERSON, A.S., DUNCAN-JONES, P. & FINLAY-JONES, R.A. (1983) The reliability of the Geriatric Mental State Examination. Community survey version. *Acta Psychiatrica Scandinavica* **67**, 281–289 [124].

HENDERSON, G., TOMLINSON, B.E. & GIBSON, P.H. (1980) Cell counts in human cerebral cortex in normal adults throughout life using an image analysing computer. *Journal of the Neurological Sciences* **46**, 113–136 [443].

HENDERSON, J.G., STRACHAN, R.W., BECK, J.S., DAWSON, A.A. & DANIEL, M. (1966) The antigastric-antibody test as a screening procedure for vitamin B$_{12}$ deficiency in psychiatric practice. *Lancet* **2**, 809–813 [587, 588, 589].

HENDRICK, E.B. (1993) Results of treatment in infants and children. Ch. 7 in *Hydrocephalus*, eds Schurr, P.H. & Polkey, C.E. Oxford University Press: Oxford [748].

HENDRICK, I. (1928) Encephalitis lethargica and the interpretation of mental disease. *American Journal of Psychiatry* **7**, 989–1014 [349].

HENDRICKSON, E., LEVY, R. & POST, F. (1979) Average evoked responses in relation to cognitive and affective state of elderly psychiatric patients. *British Journal of Psychiatry* **134**, 494–501 [487].

HENKIN, R.I., PATTEN, B.M., RE, P.K. & BRONZERT, D.A. (1975) A syndrome of acute zinc loss. Cerebellar dysfunction, mental changes, anorexia and taste and smell dysfunction. *Archives of Neurology* **32**, 745–751 [562].

HENKIN, R.I., SCHECHTER, P.J., HOYLE, R. & MATTERN, C.F.T. (1971) Idiopathic hypogeusia with dysgeusia, hyposmia, and dysosmia. A new syndrome. *Journal of the American Medical Association* **217**, 434–440 [562].

HENRIKSEN, B., JUUL-JENSEN, P. & LUND, M. (1970) The mortality of epileptics. In *Life Assurance Medicine: Proceedings of the 10th International Conference of Life Assurance Medicine*, ed. Brackenridge, R.D.C. Pitman: London [286].

HENRIKSEN, L. (1984) Evidence suggestive of diffuse brain damage following cardiac operations. *Lancet* **1**, 816–820 [554].

HENRY, G.W. (1932) Mental phenomena observed in cases of brain tumour. *American Journal of Psychiatry* **89**, 415–473 [219].

HENRY, J.A. (1992) Ecstasy and the dance of death. Severe reactions are unpredictable. *British Medical Journal* **305**, 5–6 [624].

HENRY, J.A. & WOODRUFF, G.H.A. (1978) A diagnostic sign in states of apparent unconsciousness. *Lancet* **2**, 920–921 [294].

HENRYK-GUTT, R. & REES, W.L. (1973) Psychological aspects of migraine. *Journal of Psychosomatic Research* **17**, 141–153 [403, 404].

HENSON, R.A. (1966) The neurological aspects of hypercalcaemia: with special reference to primary hyperparathyroidism. *Journal of the Royal College of Physicians, London* **1**, 41–50 [530].

HENSON, R.A. (1985) Amusia. Ch. 32 in *Handbook of Clinical Neurology*, Revised Series, Vol. 1. *Clinical Neuropsychology*, ed. Frederiks, J.A.M. Elsevier Science Publishers BV: Amsterdam [64, 65].

HENSON, R.A. (1988) Maurice Ravel's illness: a tragedy of lost creativity. *British Medical Journal* **296**, 1585–1588 [752].

HENSON, R.A. & URICH, H. (1982) *Cancer and the Nervous System*. Blackwell Scientific Publications: Oxford [739, 743].

HERHOLZ, K., ADAMS, R., KESSLER, J., SZELIES, B., GROND, M. & HEISS, W.-D. (1990) Criteria for the diagnosis of Alzheimer's disease with positron emission tomography. *Dementia* **1**, 156–164 [457].

HERMAN, J.P., GUILLONEAU, D., DANTZER, R., SCATTON, B., SEMERDJIAN-ROUQUIER, L. & LE MOAL, M. (1982) Differential effects of inescapable footshocks and of stimuli previously paired with inescapable footshocks on dopamine turnover in cortical and limbic areas of the rat. *Life Sciences* **30**, 2207–2214 [92].

HERMAN, M.N. & SANDOK, B.A. (1967) Conversion symptoms in a case of multiple sclerosis. *Military Medicine* **132**, 816–818 [698].

HERMANN, B.P. & RIEL, P. (1981) Interictal personality and behavioral traits in temporal lobe and generalised epilepsy. *Cortex* **17**, 125–128 [268].

HERMANN, B.P., WYLER, A.R., BLUMER, D. & RICHEY, E.T. (1992) Ictal fear: lateralizing significance and implications for understanding the neurobiology of pathological fear states. *Neuropsychiatry, Neuropsychology, and Behavioral Neurology* **5**, 205–210 [251].

HERNING, R.I., GLOVER, B.J., KOEPPL, B., WEDDINGTON, W. & JAFFE, J.H. (1990) Cognitive deficits in abstaining cocaine abuse. In *Residual Effects of Abused Drugs on Behavior*. National Institute on Drug Abuse Research Monograph, No. 101, eds Spencer, J.W. & Boren, J.J., pp. 167–178. US Department of Health and Human Services, National Institute on Drug Abuse: Rockville, Maryland [619].

HERRIDGE, C.F. & ABEY-WICKRAMA, I. (1969) Acute iatrogenic hypothyroid psychosis. *British Medical Journal* **3**, 154 [511].

HERRINGTON, R.N. (1969) The personality in temporal lobe epilepsy. Ch. 11 in *Current Problems in Neuropsychiatry*, ed. Herrington, R.N. British Journal of Psychiatry Special Publication No. 4. Headley Brothers: Ashford, Kent [266].

HERRMANN, C., MULDER, D.G. & FONKALSRUD, E.W. (1963) Thymectomy for myasthenia gravis. *Annals of Surgery* **158**, 85–92 [710].

HERRMANN, N., SADAVOY, J. & STEINGART, A. (1987) Oral tetrahydroaminoacridine in the treatment of senile dementia, Alzheimer's type. *New England Journal of Medicine* **316**, 1603–1604 [503].

HERSHEY, L.A., GADO, M.H. & TROTTER, J.L. (1979) Computerised tomography in the diagnostic evaluation of multiple sclerosis. *Annals of Neurology* **5**, 32–39 [690].

HERSHEY, L.A. & TROTTER, J.L. (1979) The use and abuse of the cerebrospinal fluid IgG profile in the adult: a practical evaluation. *Annals of Neurology* **8**, 426–434 [689].

HERSOV, L.A. & RODNIGHT, R. (1960) Hartnup disease in psychiatric practice: clinical and biochemical features of three cases. *Journal of Neurology, Neurosurgery and Psychiatry* **23**, 40–45 [574].

HERTZ, P.E., NADAS, E. & WOJTKOWSKI, H. (1955) Cushing's syndrome and its management. *American Journal of Psychiatry* **112**, 144–145 [518].

HERZ, E. & GLASER, G.H. (1949) Spasmodic torticollis: II Clinical evaluation. *Archives of Neurology and Psychiatry* **61**, 227–239 [674].

HERZ, E. & HOEFER, P.F.A. (1949) Spasmodic torticollis: I Physiologic analysis of involuntary motor activity. *Archives of Neurology and Psychiatry* **61**, 129–136 [674].

HESTON, L.L. (1978) The clinical genetics of Pick's disease. *Acta Psychiatrica Scandinavica* **57**, 202–206 [461].

HESTON, L.L., MASTRI, A.R., ANDERSON, E. & WHITE, J. (1981) Dementia of the Alzheimer type. Clinical genetics, natural history and associated conditions. *Archives of General Psychiatry* **38**, 1085–1090 [430, 435, 437, 440, 447, 448].

HEYGSTER, H. (1949) Über doppelseitige Stirnhirnverletzungen. *Pychiatrie, Neurologie und Medizinische Psychologie* **1**, 114–123 [180].

HEYINK, J., TYMSTRA, T., SLOOFF, M.J.H. & KLOMPMAKER, I. (1990) Liver transplantation—psychosocial problems following the operation. *Transplantation* **49**, 1018–1019 [566].

HEYMAN, A., WILKINSON, W.E., HURWITZ, B.J., SCHMECHEL, D., SIGMON, A.H., WEINBERG, T., HELMS, M.J. & SWIFT, M. (1983) Alzheimer's disease: Genetic aspects and associated clinical disorders. *Annals of Neurology* **14**, 507–515 [437, 447].

HEYMAN, A., WILKINSON, W.E., STAFFORD, J.A., HELMS, M.J., SIGMON, A.H. & WEINBERG, T. (1984) Alzheimer's disease: a study of epidemiological aspects. *Annals of Neurology* **15**, 335–341 [437, 438, 447].

HICKMAN, J.W., ATKINSON, R.P., FLINT, L.D. & HURXTHAL, L.M. (1961) Transient schizophrenic reaction as a major symptom of Cushing's syndrome. *New England Journal of Medicine* **264**, 797–800 [518].

HIERONS, R., JANOTA, I. & CORSELLIS, J.A.N. (1978) The late effects of necrotising encephalitis of the temporal lobes and limbic areas: a clinico-pathological study of 10 cases. *Psychological Medicine* **8**, 21–42 [357].

HIERONS, R. & SAUNDERS, M. (1966) Impotence in patients with temporal lobe lesions. *Lancet* **2**, 761–764 [271].

HILL, A.F., ZEIDLER, M., IRONSIDE, J. & COLLINGE, J. (1997) Diagnosis of new variant Creutzfeldt–Jakob disease by tonsil biopsy. *Lancet* **349**, 99–100 [496].

HILL, D. (1944) Cerebral dysrhythmia; its significance in aggressive behaviour. *Proceedings of the Royal Society of Medicine* **37**, 317–328 [82].

HILL, D. (1948) The relationship between epilepsy and schizophrenia: EEG studies. *Folia Psychiatrica, Neurologica et Neurochirurgica Neerlandica*, Congresnummer, 3–19 [278].

HILL, D. (1952) EEG in episodic psychotic and psychopathic behaviour. *Electroencephalography and Clinical Neurophysiology* **4**, 419–442 [128].

HILL, D. (1953) Psychiatric disorders of epilepsy. *Medical Press* **229**, 473–475 [266, 279].

HILL, D. (1957a) Electroencephalogram in schizophrenia. In *Schizophrenia: Somatic Aspects*, ed. Richter, D. Pergamon: London [128, 278].

HILL, D. (1957b) Epilepsy. *British Encyclopaedia of Medical Practice* 86–99 [279].

HILL, D. (1958) Indications and contra-indications to temporal lobectomy. *Proceedings of the Royal Society of Medicine* **51**, 610–613 [312].

HILL, D. (1963a) The EEG in psychiatry. Ch. 12 in *Electroencephalography*, 2nd edn, eds Hill, D. & Parr, G. Macdonald: London [128].

HILL, D. (1963b) Epilepsy: clinical aspects. Ch. 9 in *Electroencephalography*, 2nd edn, eds Hill, D. & Parr, G. Macdonald: London [247].

HILL, D. & MITCHELL, W. (1953) Epileptic anamnesis. *Folia Psychiatrica, Neurologica et Neurochirurgica Neerlandica* **56**, 718–725 [252].

HILL, D. & POND, D.A. (1952) Reflections on one hundred capital cases submitted to electroencephalography. *Journal of Mental Science* **98**, 23–43 [274].

HILL, D., POND, D.A., MITCHELL, W. & FALCONER, M.A. (1957) Personality changes following temporal lobectomy for epilepsy. *Journal of Mental Science* **103**, 18–27 [270].

HILL, D. & WATTERSON, D. (1942) Electroencephalographic studies of psychopathic personalities. *Journal of Neurology, Neurosurgery and Psychiatry* **5**, 47–65 [128].

HILL, P. (1989) Psychiatric aspects of children's head injury. Ch. 11 in *Children's Head Injury. Who Cares?* eds Johnson, D.A., Uttley, D. & Wyke, M. Taylor & Francis: London [204].

HILL, S.Y., REYES, R.B., MIKHAEL, M. & AYRE, F. (1979) A comparison of alcoholics and heroin abusers: computerized transaxial tomography and neuropsychological functioning. *Currents in Alcoholism* **5**, 187–205 [612].

HILLBOM, E. (1951) Schizophrenia-like psychoses after brain trauma. *Acta Pychiatrica et Neurologica Scandinavica* **60** (**Supplement**), 36–47 [181, 191].

HILLBOM, E. (1960) After-effects of brain-injuries. *Acta Psychiatrica et Neurologica Scandinavica* **142** (**Supplement**), 1–195 [173, 177, 181, 182, 192, 196].

HILLBOM, M. & HOLM, L. (1986) Contribution of traumatic head injury to neuropsychological deficits in alcoholics. *Journal of Neurology, Neurosurgery and Psychiatry* **49**, 1348–1353 [179].

HIMMELHOCH, J., PINCUS, J., TUCKER, G. & DETRE, T. (1970) Subacute encephalitis: behavioural and neurological aspects. *British Journal of Psychiatry* **116**, 531–538 [362, 363, 364].

HINGE, H.-H., JENSEN, T.S., KJAER, M., MARQUARDSEN, J. & OLIVARIUS, B. de F. (1986) The prognosis of transient global amnesia. Results of a multicenter study. *Archives of Neurology* **43**, 673–676 [416].

HINKLE, L.E. & WOLF, S. (1952a) Importance of life stress in course and management of diabetes mellitus. *Journal of the American Medical Association* **148**, 513–520 [534].

HINKLE, L.E. & WOLF, S. (1952b) A summary of experimental evidence relating life stress to diabetes mellitus. *Journal of the Mount Sinai Hospital* **19**, 537–570 [534, 535].

HINTON, J. & WITHERS, E. (1971) The usefulness of the clinical tests of the sensorium. *British Journal of Psychiatry* **119**, 9–18 [98, 100].

HIRANO, A., MALAMUD, N., ELIZAN, T.S. & KURLAND, L.T. (1966) Amyotrophic lateral sclerosis and parkinsonism–dementia complex on Guam: further pathologic studies. *Archives of Neurology* **15**, 35–51 [709].

HIRANO, A., MALAMUD, N. & KURLAND, L.T. (1961) Parkinsonism–dementia complex, an endemic disease on the island of Guam. II: Pathological features. *Brain* **84**, 662–679 [709].

HIRSCH, S.R. & PURI, B.K. (1993) Clozapine: progress in treating refractory schizophrenia. *British Medical Journal* **306**, 1427–1428 [643].

HISHIKAWA, Y. & KANEKO, Z. (1965) Electroencephalographic study on narcolepsy. *Electroencephalography and Clinical Neurophysiology* **18**, 249–259 [725].

HISHIKAWA, Y., NANNO, H., TACHIBANA, M., FURUYA, E., KOIDA, H. & KANEKO, Z. (1968) The nature of sleep attack and other symptoms of narcolepsy. *Electroencephalography and Clinical Neurophysiology* **24**, 1–10 [725].

HITCH, G.J. (1984) Working memory. Editorial in *Psychological Medicine* **14**, 265–271 [29].

HITCHCOCK, E. (1992) Neural implants and recovery of function: human work. In *Recovery from Brain Damage. Reflections and Directions*, eds Rose, F.D. & Johnson, D.A., pp. 67–78. Plenum Press: New York [652].

HITCHCOCK, E., ASHCROFT, G.W., CAIRNS, V.M. & MURRAY, L.G. (1972) Preoperative and postoperative assessment and management of psychosurgical patients. Ch. 14 in *Psychosurgery*, eds Hitchcock, E., Laitinen, L. & Vaernet, K. Proceedings of the Second International Conference on Psychosurgery. Thomas: Springfield, Illinois [82].

HITCHCOCK, E. & CAIRNS, V. (1973) Amygdalotomy. *Postgraduate Medical Journal* **49**, 894–904 [267, 314].

HJERN, B. & NYLANDER, I. (1962) Late prognosis of severe head injuries in childhood. *Archives of Disease in Childhood* **37**, 113–116 [201].

HO, D.D., ROTA, T.R., SCHOOLEY, R.T., KAPLAN, J.C., DAVIS-ALLAN, J., GROOPMAN, J.E., RESNICK, L., FELSENSTEIN, D., ANDREWS, C.A. & HIRSCH, M.S. (1985) Isolation of HTLV-III from cerebrospinal fluid and neural tissues of patients with neurologic syndromes related to the acquired immunodeficiency syndrome. *New England Journal of Medicine* **313**, 1493–1497 [319, 327].

HOCKADAY, J.M. & WHITTY, C.W.M. (1969) Factors determining the electroencephalogram in migraine: a study of 560 patients, according to clinical type of migraine. *Brain* **92**, 769–788 [405].

HOCKADAY, J.M., WILLIAMSON, D.H. & ALBERTI, K.G.M.M. (1973) Effects of intravenous glucose on some blood metabolites and hormones in migraine subjects. Ch. 13 in *Background to Migraine*, Fifth Migraine Symposium, ed. Cumings, J.N., Heinemann: London [402].

HOCKADAY, J.M., WILLIAMSON, D.H. & WHITTY, C.W.M. (1971) Blood-glucose levels and fatty-acid metabolism in migraine related to fasting. *Lancet* **1**, 1153–1156 [402].

HOCKADAY, T.D.R., KEYNES, W.M. & McKENZIE, J.K. (1966) Catatonic stupor in elderly woman with hyperparathyroidism. *British Medical Journal* **1**, 85–87 [529].

HODGES, H., ALLEN, Y., SINDEN, J., MITCHELL, S.N., ARENDT, T., LANTOS, P.L. & GRAY, J.A. (1991) The effects of cholinergic drugs and cholinergic-rich foetal neural transplants on alcoholinduced deficits in radial maze performance in rats. *Behavioural Brain Research* **43**, 7–28 [26].

HODGES, J.R. (1991) *Transient Amnesia: Clinical and Neuropsychological Aspects*. W.B. Saunders: London [413, 414, 415, 416, 417].

HODGES, J.R. (1995) Retrograde amnesia. Ch. 4 in *Handbook of Memory Disorders*, eds Baddeley, A.D., Wilson, B.A. & Watts, F.N. John Wiley: Chichester [37].

HODGES, J.R. & CARPENTER, K. (1991) Anterograde amnesia with fornix damage following removal of IIIrd ventricle colloid cyst. *Journal of Neurology, Neurosurgery and Psychiatry* **54**, 633–638 [27].

HODGES, J.R. & OXBURY, S.M. (1990) Persistent memory impairment following transient global amnesia. *Journal of Clinical and Experimental Neuropsychology* **12**, 904–920 [415].

HODGES, J.R., PATTERSON, K., OXBURY, S. & FUNNELL, E. (1992) Semantic dementia. Progressive fluent aphasia with temporal lobe atrophy. *Brain* **115**, 1783–1806 [753, 754].

HODGES, J.R. & WARD, C.D. (1989) Observations during transient

global amnesia. A behavioural and neuropsychological study of five cases. *Brain* **112**, 595–620 [413, 414].

HOEHN, M.M. & YAHR, M.D. (1967) Parkinsonism: onset, progression and mortality. *Neurology* **17**, 427–442 [646, 647].

HOFF, E.C., GRENELL, R.G. & FULTON, J.F. (1945) Histopathology of the central nervous system after exposure to high altitudes, hypoglycaemia and other conditions associated with central anoxia. *Medicine* **24**, 161–217 [548].

HOFFMAN, E.P., BROWN, R.H. & KUNKEL, L.M. (1987) Dystrophin: the protein product of the Duchenne muscular dystrophy locus. *Cell* **51**, 919–928 [715].

HOFFMAN, E.P., FISCHBECK, K.H., BROWN, R.H., JOHNSON, M., MEDORI, R., LOIKE, J.D., HARRIS, J.B., WATERSTON, R., BROOKE, M., SPECHT, L., KUPSKY, W., CHAMBERLAIN, J., CASKEY, C.T., SHAPIRO, F. & KUNKEL, L.M. (1988) Characterization of dystrophin in muscle-biopsy specimens from patients with Duchenne's or Becker's muscular dystrophy. *New England Journal of Medicine* **318**, 1363–1368 [715].

HOGG, K.E., GOLDSTEIN, L.H. & LEIGH, P.N. (1994) The psychological impact of motor neurone disease. *Psychological Medicine* **24**, 625–632 [707].

HOHEISEL, H.P. & WALCH, R. (1952) Über manisch-depressive und verwandte Verstimmungszustände nach Hirnverletzung. *Archiv für Psychiatrie und Nervenkrankheiten* **188**, 1–25 [180, 191].

HOHENSCHUTZ, C., EICH, P., FRIEDL, W., WAHEED, A., CONZELMANN, E. & PROPPING, P. (1989) Pseudodeficiency of arylsulfatase A: a common genetic polymorphism with possible disease implications. *Human Genetics* **82**, 45–48 [759].

HOLBOURN, A.H.S. (1943) Mechanics of head injuries. *Lancet* **2**, 438–441 [162].

HOLBROOK, M. (1982) Stroke: social and emotional outcome. *Journal of the Royal College of Physicians, London* **16**, 100–104 [391].

HOLLANDER, D. & STRICH, S.J. (1970) Atypical Alzheimer's disease with congophilic angiopathy, presenting with dementia of acute onset. In *Alzheimer's Disease and Related Conditions*, eds Wolstenholme, G.E.W. & O'Connor, M. Ciba Foundation Symposium. Churchill: London [438].

HOLLANDER, H. & STRINGARI, S. (1987) Human immunodeficiency virus-associated meningitis. Clinical course and correlations. *American Journal of Medicine* **83**, 813–816 [327].

HOLLON, T.H. (1973) Behaviour modification in a community hospital rehabilitation unit. *Archives of Physical Medicine and Rehabilitation* **54**, 65–68 [214].

HOLMAN, B.L., GIBSON, R.E., HILL, T.C., ECKELMAN, W.C., ALBERT, M. & REBA, R.C. (1985) Muscarinic acetylcholine receptors in Alzheimer's disease: in vivo imaging with iodine 123-labelled 3-quinuclidinyl-4-iodobenzilate and emission tomography. *Journal of the American Medical Association* **254**, 3063–3066 [148].

HOLMES, G.L., McKEEVER, M. & ADAMSON, M. (1987) Absence seizures in children: clinical and electroencephalic features. *Annals of Neurology* **21**, 268–273 [238].

HOLMES, G.P., KAPLAN, J.E., GANTZ, N.M., KOMAROFF, A.L., SCHONBERGER, L.B., STRAUSS, S.E., JONES, J.F., DUBOIS, R.E., CUNNINGHAM-RUNDLES, C., PAHWA, S., TOSATO, G., ZEGANS, L.S., PURTILLO, D.T., BROWN, N., SCHOOLEY, R.T. & BUS, I. (1988) Chronic fatigue syndrome: a working case definition. *Annals of Internal Medicine* **108**, 387–389 [371].

HOLMES, J.M. (1956) Cerebral manifestations of vitamin B_{12} deficiency. *British Medical Journal* **2**, 1394–1398 [587].

HOLT, E.K. & TEDESCHI, C. (1943) Cerebral patchy demyelination. *Journal of Neuropathology and Experimental Neurology* **2**, 306–314 [701].

824 REFERENCES

HOLTZMAN, J. (1985) The integrity of attentional control following commissural section. Ch. 19 in *Epilepsy and the Corpus Callosum*, ed. Reeves, A.G. Plenum Press: New York [313].

HONER, W.G., HURWITZ, T., LI, D.K.B., PALMER, M. & PATY, D.W. (1987) Temporal lobe involvement in multiple sclerosis patients with psychiatric disorders. *Archives of Neurology* **44**, 187–190 [695].

HONOVAR, M., JANOTA, I. & POLKEY, C.E. (1992) Rasmussen's encephalitis in surgery for epilepsy. *Developmental Medicine and Child Neurology* **34**, 3–14 [313].

HOOK, O. (1954) Sarcoidosis with involvement of the nervous system. Report of nine cases. *Archives of Neurology and Psychiatry* **71**, 554–575 [764].

HOOPER, R.S., McGREGOR, J.M. & NATHAN, P.W. (1945) Explosive rage following head injury. *Journal of Mental Science* **91**, 458–471 [188].

HOOSHMAND, H. & BRAWLEY, B.W. (1969) Temporal lobe seizures and exhibitionism. *Neurology* **19**, 1119–1124 [273].

HOOSHMAND, H., ESCOBAR, M.R. & KOPF, S.W. (1972) Neurosyphilis. A study of 241 patients. *Journal of the American Medical Association* **219**, 726–729 [342].

HOPE, T. & FAIRBURN, C.G. (1992) The present behavioural examination (PBE): the development of an interview to measure current behavioural abnormalities. *Psychological Medicine* **22**, 223–230 [125].

HOPKINSON, N.D., BENDALL, P. & POWELL, R.J. (1992) Screening of acute psychiatric admissions for previously misdiagnosed systemic lupus erythematosus. *British Journal of Psychiatry* **161**, 107–110 [419].

HORN, S. (1974) Some psychological factors in parkinsonism. *Journal of Neurology, Neurosurgery and Psychiatry* **37**, 27–31 [656].

HORNYKIEWICZ, O., KISH, S.J., BECKER, L.E., FARLEY, I. & SHANNAK, K. (1986) Brain neurotransmitters in dystonia musculorum deformans. *New England Journal of Medicine* **315**, 347–353 [671].

HOROWITZ, M.J. (1969) Flashbacks: recurrent intrusive images after the use of LSD. *American Journal of Psychiatry* **126**, 565–569 [623].

HOROWITZ, M.J., COHEN, F.M., SAUNDERS, F.A. & SKOLNIKOFF, A.Z. (1970) *Psychosocial Function in Epilepsy*. Thomas: Springfield, Illinois [270].

HORST, D., GRACE, N.D., CONN, H.O., SCHIFF, E., SCHENKER, S., VITERI, A., LAW, D. & ATTERBURY, C.E. (1984) Comparison of dietary protein with an oral, branched chain-enriched amino acid supplement in chronic post-systemic encephalopathy: a randomized controlled trial. *Hepatology* **4**, 279–287 [566].

HORTA-BARBOSA, L., FUCCILLO, D.A., LONDON, W.T., JABBOUR, J.T., ZEMAN, W. & SEVER, J.L. (1969) Isolation of measles virus from brain cell cultures of two patients with subacute sclerosing panencephalitis. *Proceedings of the Society for Experimental Biology and Medicine* **132**, 272–277 [362].

HORVATH, T.B. (1975) Clinical spectrum and epidemiological features of alcoholic dementia. In *Alcohol, Drugs and Brain Damage*, ed. Rankin, J.G. Addiction Research Foundation of Ontario: Toronto [603].

HOTOPF, M.H., POLLOCK, S. & LISHMAN, W.A. (1994) An unusual presentation of multiple sclerosis. *Psychological Medicine* **24**, 525–528 [xxiii, 694].

HOTSON, J.R. (1989) Neurological sequelae of cardiac surgery. Ch. 3 in *Neurology and General Medicine*, ed. Aminoff, M.J. Churchill Livingstone: New York [553].

HOTSON, J.R. & PEDLEY, T.A. (1976) The neurological complications of cardiac transplantation. *Brain* **99**, 673–694 [555].

HOUNSFIELD, G.N. (1973) Computerized transverse axial scanning (tomography) Part 1. Description of system. *British Journal of Radiology* **46**, 1016–1022 [137].

HOUPT, J.L., GOULD, B.S. & NORRIS, F.H. (1977) Psychological characteristics of patients with amyotrophic lateral sclerosis (ALS). *Psychosomatic Medicine* **39**, 299–303 [707].

HOUSE, A., DENNIS, M., MOGRIDGE, L., HAWTON, K. & WARLOW, C. (1990a) Life events and difficulties preceding stroke. *Journal of Neurology, Neurosurgery and Psychiatry* **53**, 1024–1028 [375].

HOUSE, A., DENNIS, M., MOGRIDGE, L., WARLOW, C., HAWTON, K. & JONES, L. (1991) Mood disorders in the year after first stroke. *British Journal of Psychiatry* **158**, 83–92 [385, 388].

HOUSE, A., DENNIS, M., MOLYNEUX, A., WARLOW, C. & HAWTON, K. (1989) Emotionalism after stroke. *British Medical Journal* **298**, 991–994 [387].

HOUSE, A., DENNIS, M., WARLOW, C., HAWTON, K. & MOLYNEUX, A. (1990b) Mood disorders after stroke and their relation to lesion location. *Brain* **113**, 1113–1129 [386].

HOUSER, O.W. & McLEOD, R.A. (1979) Roentgenographic experience at the Mayo Clinic. Ch. 3 in *Tuberous Sclerosis*, ed. Gomez, M.R. Raven Press: New York [702].

HOUSER, O.W., SHEPHARD, C.W. & GOMEZ, M.R. (1991) Imaging and intracranial tuberous sclerosis. In *Tuberous Sclerosis and Allied Disorders: Clinical, Cellular, and Molecular Studies*, eds Johnson, W.G. & Gomez, M.R. *Annals of the New York Academy of Sciences* **615**, 81–93 [702].

HOWARD, R.S. & MILLER, D.H. (1995) The persistent vegetative state. Information on prognosis allows decisions to be made on management. *British Medical Journal* **310**, 341–342 [183].

HOWELLS, R. (1994) Neuroleptic malignant syndrome. Don't confuse with anticholinergic intoxication. *British Medical Journal* **308**, 200–201 [627].

HSIAO, K., BAKER, H.F., CROW, T.J., POULTER, M., OWEN, F., TERWILLIGER, J.D., WESTAWAY, D., OTT, J. & PRUSINER, S.D. (1989) Linkage of a prion protein missense variant to Gersmann–Sträussler syndrome. *Nature* **338**, 342–345 [474].

HSIAO, K., MEINER, Z., KAHANA, E., CASS, C., KAHANA, I., AVRAHAMI, A., SCARLATO, G., ABRAMSKY, O., PRUSINER, S.B. & GABIZON, R. (1991) Mutation of the prion protein in Libyan Jews with Creutzfeldt–Jakob disease. *New England Journal of Medicine* **324**, 1091–1097 [475].

HSIAO, K. & PRUSINER, S.B. (1990) Inherited human prion diseases. *Neurology* **40**, 1820–1827 [751].

HSIAO, K.K., SCOTT, M., FOSTER, D., GROTH, D.F., DEARMOND, S.J. & PRUSINER, S.B. (1990) Spontaneous neurodegeneration in transgenic mice with mutant prion protein. *Science* **250**, 1587–1590 [475].

HSICH, G., KENNEY, K., GIBBS, C.J., LEE, K.H. & HARRINGTON, M.G. (1996) The 14-3-3 brain protein in cerebrospinal fluid as a marker for transmissible spongiform encephalopathies. *New England Journal of Medicine* **335**, 924–930 [478].

HUANG, C.-C., CHU, N.-S., LU, C.-S., WANG, J.-D., TSAI, J.-L., TZENG, J.-L., WOLTERS, E.C. & CALNE, D.B. (1989) Chronic manganese intoxication. *Archives of Neurology* **46**, 1104–1106 [635].

HUAPAYA, L. (1979) Seven cases of somnambulism induced by drugs. *American Journal of Psychiatry* **136**, 985–986 [736].

HUBBARD, B.M. & ANDERSON, J.M. (1981) Age, senile dementia, and ventricular enlargement. *Journal of Neurology, Neurosurgery and Psychiatry* **44**, 631–635 [139].

HUBER, G. (1957) *Pneumoencephalographische und Psychopathologische Bilder bei Endogenen Psychosen*. Monographien aus dem Gesamtgebiete der Neurologie und Psychiatrie. Springer: Berlin [140].

HUBER, G., GROSS, G. & SCHÜTTLER, R. (1975) A long-term follow-up study of schizophrenia: psychiatric course of illness and prognosis. *Acta Psychiatrica Scandinavica* **52**, 49–57 [140].

HUBER, S.J. & GLATT, S.L. (1992) Neuroimaging correlates of dementia in Parkinson's disease. Ch. 12 in *Parkinson's Disease. Neurobehavioral Aspects*, eds Huber, S.J. & Cummings, J.L. Oxford University Press: Oxford [655].

HUBER, S.J., SHUTTLEWORTH, E.C., CHRISTY, J.A., CHAKERES, D.W., CURTIN, A. & PAULSON, G.W. (1989) Magnetic resonance imaging in dementia of Parkinson's disease. *Journal of Neurology, Neurosurgery and Psychiatry* **52**, 1221–1227 [655].

HUDSON, A.J. (1981) Amyotrophic lateral sclerosis and its association with dementia, parkinsonism and neurological disorders: a review. *Brain* **104**, 217–247 [707, 708].

HUDSON, H.S. & WALKER, H.I. (1961) Withdrawal symptoms following ethchlorvynol (placidyl) dependence. *American Journal of Psychiatry* **118**, 361 [628].

HUGHES, A.J., BISHOP, S., KLEEDORFER, B., TURJANSKI, N., FERNANDEZ, W., LEES, A.J. & STERN, G.M. (1993) Subcutaneous apomorphine in Parkinson's disease: response to chronic administration for up to five years. *Movement Disorders* **8**, 105–170 [651].

HUGHES, A.J., DANIEL, S.E., KILFORD, L. & LEES, A.J. (1992) Accuracy of clinical diagnosis of idiopathic Parkinson's disease: a clinicopathological study of 100 cases. *Journal of Neurology, Neurosurgery and Psychiatry* **55**, 181–184 [649].

HUGHES, G.V. (1974) Systemic lupus erythematosus. *British Journal of Hospital Medicine* **12**, 309–319 [419].

HUGHES, R.A.C. (1994) Neurological complications of neurofibromatosis 1. Ch. 8 in *The Neurofibromatosus*, eds Huson, S.M. & Hughes, R.A.C. Chapman & Hall: London [704].

HUMPHREYS, P., KAUFMANN, W.E. & GALABURDA, A.M. (1990) Developmental dyslexia in women: neuropathological findings in three patients. *Annals of Neurology* **28**, 727–738 [47].

HUMPHRIES, S.R. & DICKINSON, P.S. (1988) Hypomania following complex partial seizures. *British Journal of Psychiatry* **152**, 571–572 [258].

HUNDER, G.G., AREND, W.P., BLOCH, D.A., CALABRESE, L.H., FAUCI, A.S., FRIES, J.F., LEAVITT, R.Y., LIE, J.T., LIGHTFOOT, R.W. Jr, MASI, A.T., McSHANE, D.J., MICHEL, B.A., MILLS, J.A., STEVENS, M.B., WALLACE, S.L. & SZVIFLER, N.J. (1990) The American College of Rheumatology 1990 criteria for the classification of vasculitis. *Arthritis and Rheumatism* **33**, 1065–1067 [425].

HUNGERFORD, G.D., DU BOULAY, G.H. & ZILKHA, K.J. (1976) Computerised axial tomography in patients with severe migraine: a preliminary report. *Journal of Neurology, Neurosurgery and Psychiatry* **39**, 990–994 [401].

HUNT, H.F. (1973) The differentiation of malingering, dissimulation, and pathology. Ch. 24 in *Psychopathology: Contributions from the Social, Behavioral and Biological Sciences*, eds Hammer, M., Salzinger, K. & Sutton, S. John Wiley & Sons: New York [484].

HUNTER, D. (1959) *Health in Industry*. Penguin Books: Harmondsworth [631].

HUNTER, D. (1978) *The Diseases of Occupations*, 6th edn. Hodder & Stoughton: London [553, 635, 638].

HUNTER, R., BLACKWOOD, W. & BULL, J. (1968a) Three cases of frontal meningiomas presenting psychiatrically. *British Medical Journal* **3**, 9–16 [222, 223, 234, 235].

HUNTER, R. & JONES, M. (1966) Acute lethargica-type encephalitis. *Lancet* **2**, 1023–1024 [355].

HUNTER, R., JONES, M. & COOPER, F. (1968b) Modified lumbar air encephalography in the investigation of long-stay psychiatric patients. *Journal of the Neurological Sciences* **6**, 593–596 [140].

HUNTER, R., JONES, M., JONES, T.G. & MATTHEWS, D.M. (1967a) Serum B$_{12}$ and folate concentrations in mental patients. *British Journal of Psychiatry* **113**, 1291–1295 [588, 590].

HUNTER, R., JONES, M. & MALLESON, A. (1969) Abnormal cerebrospinal fluid total protein and gamma-globulin levels in 256 patients admitted to a psychiatric unit. *Journal of the Neurological Sciences* **9**, 11–38 [355].

HUNTER, R., JONES, M. & MATTHEWS, D.M. (1967b) Postgastrectomy vitamin-B$_{12}$ deficiency in psychiatric practice. *Lancet* **1**, 47 [589].

HUNTER, R., LOGUE, V. & McMENEMY, W.H. (1963) Temporal lobe epilepsy supervening on longstanding transvestism and fetishism. A case report. *Epilepsia* **4**, 60–65 [272, 273].

HUNTER, R., McLUSKIE, R., WYPER, D., PATTERSON, J., CHRISTIE, J.E., BROOKS, D.N., McCULLOCH, J., FINK, G. & GOODWIN, G.M. (1989) The pattern of function-related regional cerebral blood flow investigated by single photon emission tomography with ^{99m}Tc-HMPAO in patients with presenile Alzheimer's disease and Korsakoff's psychosis. *Psychological Medicine* **19**, 847–855 [582].

HUNTINGTON, G. (1872) On chorea. *Medical and Surgical Reporter (Philadelphia)* **26**, 317–321 [465].

HUNTINGTON, G. (1910) Recollections of Huntington's chorea as I saw it at East Hampton, Long Island, during my boyhood. *Journal of Nervous and Mental Disease* **37**, 255–257 [470].

HUNTINGTON'S DISEASE COLLABORATIVE RESEARCH GROUP (1993) A novel gene containing a trinucleotide repeat that is expanded and unstable on Huntington's disease chromosomes. *Cell* **72**, 971–983 [466].

HUPPERT, F.A. (1994) Memory function in dementia and normal aging—dimension or dichotomy? Ch. 15 in *Dementia and Normal Aging*, eds Huppert, F.A., Brayne, C. & O'Connor, D.W. Cambridge University Press: Cambridge [33].

HUPPERT, F.A. & KOPELMAN, M.D. (1989) Rates of forgetting in normal ageing: a comparison with dementia. *Neuropsychologia* **27**, 849–860 [33, 437].

HUPPERT, F.A. & PIERCY, M. (1978) Dissociation between learning and remembering in organic amnesia. *Nature* **275**, 317–318 [35, 38].

HUPPERT, F.A. & PIERCY, M. (1979) Normal and abnormal forgetting in organic amnesia: effect of locus of lesion. *Cortex* **15**, 385–390 [35, 38].

HURDLE, A.D.F. & PICTON-WILLIAMS, T.C. (1966) Folic acid deficiency in elderly patients admitted to hospital. *British Medical Journal* **2**, 202–205 [590].

HURWITZ, L.J. & ADAMS, G.F. (1972) Rehabilitation of hemiplegia: indices of assessment and prognosis. *British Medical Journal* **1**, 94–98 [375, 381, 383, 389].

HURWITZ, T.A., CALNE, D.B. & WATERMAN, K. (1988) Treatment of dopaminomimetic psychosis in Parkinson's disease with electroconvulsive therapy. *Canadian Journal of Neurological Science* **15**, 32–34 [658].

HUSON, S.M. (1994) Neurofibromatosis 1: a clinical and genetic overview. Ch. 7 in *The Neurofibromatoses*, eds Huson, S.M. & Hughes, R.A.C. Chapman & Hall: London [703].

HUSON, S.M., HARPER, P.S. & COMPSTON, D.A.S. (1988) Von Recklinghausen neurofibromatosis. A clinical and population study in south-east Wales. *Brain* **111**, 1355–1381 [704].

HUTCHINSON, E.C. (1983) Management of cerebral infarction. Ch. 10 in *Vascular Disease of the Central Nervous System*, 2nd edn, ed. Russell, R.W.R. Churchill Livingstone: Edinburgh & London [389].

HUTCHISON, G.B., EVANS, J.A. & DAVIDSON, D.C. (1958) Pitfalls in the diagnosis of phaeochromocytoma. *Annals of Internal Medicine* **48**, 300–309 [520].

HUTT, S.J., JACKSON, P.M., BELSHAM, A. & HIGGINS, G. (1968) Perceptual-motor behaviour in relation to blood phenobarbitone level: a preliminary report. *Developmental Medicine and Child Neurology* **10**, 626–632 [263].

HUTT, S.J., NEWTON, J. & FAIRWEATHER, H. (1977) Choice reaction time and EEG activity in children with epilepsy. *Neuropsychologia* **15**, 257–267 [262].

HYDE, T.M., ZIEGLER, J.C. & WEINBERGER, D.R. (1992) Psychiatric disturbances in metachromatic leukodystrophy. Insights into the neurobiology of psychosis. *Archives of Neurology* **49**, 401–406 [758].

HYND, G.W. & HIEMENZ, J.R. (1997) Dyslexia and gyral morphology variation. Ch. 3 in *Dyslexia: Biology, Cognition and Intervention*, eds Hulme, C. & Snowling, M. Whurr Publishers: London [48].

HYND, G.W., SEMRUD-CLIKEMAN, M., LORYS, A.R., NOVEY, E.S. & ELIOPULOS, D. (1990) Brain morphology in developmental dyslexia and attention deficit disorder/hyperactivity. *Archives of Neurology* **47**, 919–926 [48].

HYSLOP, G.H. (1949) Torticollis of central origin. *Medical Clinics of North America* **25**, 747–754 [673].

ICD-10 *See* World Health Organization (1992, 1993).

IGARASHI, H., SAKAI, F., KAN, S., OKADA, J. & TAZAKI, Y. (1991) Magnetic resonance imaging of the brain in patients with migraine. *Cephalgia* **11**, 69–74 [401, 402].

ILLIS, L.S. & MERRY, R.T. (1972) Treatment of herpes simplex encephalitis. *Journal of the Royal College of Physicians of London* **7**, 34–44 [357].

ILLOWSKY, B.P. & KIRCH, D.G. (1988) Polydipsia and hyponatremia in psychiatric patients. *American Journal of Psychiatry* **145**, 675–683 [525, 526, 559].

INGLIS, J. (1959) A paired-associate learning test for use with elderly psychiatric patients. *Journal of Mental Science* **105**, 440–443 [114].

INGVAR, D.H. (1970) Cerebral blood flow in organic dementia. In *Research on the Cerebral Circulation*, eds Meyer, J.S., Reivich, M., Lechner, H. & Eichhorn, O. Thomas: Springfield, Illinois [434].

INGVAR, D.H. & FRANZEN, G. (1974) Abnormalities of cerebral blood flow distribution in patients with chronic schizophrenia. *Acta Psychiatrica Scandinavica* **50**, 425–462 [87].

INGVAR, D.H. & LASSEN, N.A. (1961) Quantitative determination of regional cerebral blood-flow in man. *Lancet* **2**, 806–807 [147].

INOSE, T. (1968) Neuropsychiatric manifestations in Wilson's disease: attacks of disturbance of consciousness. In *Wilson's Disease*, ed. Bergsma, D., Birth Defects Original Article Series, Vol. 4, No. 2. The National Foundation: New York [665].

INTERNATIONAL STUDY GROUP OF BEHÇET'S DISEASE (1990) Criteria for diagnosis of Behçet's disease. *Lancet* **335**, 1078–1080 [762].

INZITARI, D., DIAZ, F., FOX, A., HACHINSKI, V.C., STENGART, A., LAU, C., DONALD, A., WADE, J., MULIC, H. & MERSKEY, H. (1987) Vascular risk factors and leuko-araiosis. *Archives of Neurology* **44**, 42–47 [459].

IQBAL, K., GRUNDKE-IQBAL, I., WISNIEWSKI, H.K. & TERRY, R.D. (1978) Neurofibers in Alzheimer's disease and other conditions. In *Alzheimer's Disease: Senile Dementia and Related Diseases, Aging*, Vol. 7, eds Katzman, R., Terry, R.D. & Bick, K.L., pp. 409–420. Raven Press: New York [442].

IRVING, G., ROBINSON, R.A. & McADAM, W. (1970) The validity of some cognitive tests in the diagnosis of dementia. *British Journal of Psychiatry* **117**, 149–156 [99, 100, 112, 114].

ISAACS, B. (1971) Identification of disability in the stroke patient. *Modern Geriatrics* **1**, 390–402 [389].

ISAACS, B. (1973) Stroke. In *Textbook of Geriatric Medicine and Gerontol-* *ogy*, ed. Brocklehurst, J.C. Churchill Livingstone: Edinburgh [389].

ISAACS, B. & WALKEY, F.A. (1964) A simplified paired-associate test for elderly hospital patients. *British Journal of Psychiatry* **110**, 80–83 [104, 114].

ISBELL, H., ALTSCHUL, S., KORNETSKY, C.H., EISENMAN, A.J., FLANARY, H.G. & FRASER, H.F. (1950) Chronic barbiturate intoxication. *Archives of Neurology and Psychiatry* **64**, 1–28 [608, 609].

ISBELL, H., BELLEVILLE, R.E., FRASER, H.F., WIKLER, A. & LOGAN, C.R. (1956) Studies on lysergic acid diethylamide (LSD-25): 1. Effects in former morphine addicts and development of tolerance during chronic intoxication. *Archives of Neurology and Psychiatry* **76**, 468–478 [620, 621].

ISBELL, H., FRASER, H.F., WICKLER, A., BELLEVILLE, R.E. & EISENMAN, A.J. (1955) An experimental study of aetiology of 'rum fits' and delirium tremens. *Quarterly Journal of Studies on Alcohol* **16**, 1–33 [595, 597, 602].

ISBELL, H., GORODETZKY, C.W., JASINSKI, D., CLAUSSEN, U., SPULAK, F. VON & KORTE, F. (1967) Effects of (—) 9-trans-tetrahydrocannabinol in man. *Psychopharmacologia* **11**, 184–188 [613].

ISHERWOOD, I. (1983) Principles of neuroradiology. In *Oxford Textbook of Medicine*, Vol. 2, eds Weatherall, D.J., Ledingham, J.G.G. & Warrell, D.A., pp. 21.4–21.9. Oxford University Press: Oxford [136].

ISHII, N. & NISHIHARA, Y. (1981) Pellagra among chronic alcoholics: clinical and pathological study of 20 necropsy cases. *Journal of Neurology, Neurosurgery and Psychiatry* **44**, 209–215 [575].

ISHII, T. & HAGA, S. (1976) Immuno-electron microscopic localisation of immunoglobulins in amyloid fibrils of senile plaques. *Acta Neuropathologica* **36**, 243–249 [447].

ISHIKAWA, Y., MEYER, J.S., TANAHASHI, N., HATA, T., VELEZ, M., FANN, W.E., KANDULA, P., MOTEL, K.F. & ROGERS, R.L. (1986) Abstinence improves cerebral perfusion and brain volume in alcoholic neurotoxicity without Wernicke–Korsakoff syndrome. *Journal of Cerebral Blood Flow in Metabolism* **6**, 86–94 [606].

IVES, E.R. (1963) Mental aberrations in diabetic patients. *Bulletin of the Los Angeles Neurological Society* **28**, 279–285 [537].

IVNIK, R.J. (1978) Neuropsychological stability in multiple sclerosis. *Journal of Consulting and Clinical Psychology* **46**, 913–923 [693].

JABLENSKY, A., JANOTA, I. & SHEPHERD, M. (1970) Neuropsychiatric illness and neuropathological findings in a case of Klinefelter's syndrome. *Psychological Medicine* **1**, 18–19 [527].

JACKSON, J.H. (1869) Certain points in the study and classification of diseases of the nervous system (Goulstonian Lectures). *Lancet* **1**, 307, 344, 379. Reprinted (1932) in *Selected Writings of John Hughlings Jackson*, Vol. 2, ed. Taylor, J., p. 246. Hodder & Stoughton: London [22].

JACKSON, J.H. (1889) On a particular variety of epilepsy ('intellectual aura'): one case with symptoms of organic brain disease. *Brain* **11**, 179–207 [254].

JACOBS, E.A., WINTER, P.M., ALVIS, H.J. & SMALL, S.M. (1969) Hyperoxygenation effect on cognitive functioning in the aged. *New England Journal of Medicine* **281**, 753–757 [502].

JACOBS, L. & GOSSMAN, M.D. (1980) Three primitive reflexes in normal adults. *Neurology* **30**, 184–188 [96].

JACOBS, L., KINKEL, W.R., PAINTER, F., MURAWSKI, J. & HEFFNER, R.R. (1978) Computerised tomography in dementia with special reference to changes in size of normal ventricles during aging and normal pressure hydrocephalus. In *Alzheimer's Disease: Senile Dementia and Related Disorders Aging*, Vol. 7, eds Katzman, R., Terry, R.D. & Bick, K.L., pp. 241–260. Raven Press: New York [138].

JACOBSEN, C.F. (1935) Functions of frontal association area in primates. *Archives of Neurology and Psychiatry* **33**, 558–569 [77].

JACOBSON, R.R. (1986) The contribution of sex and drinking history to the CT brain scan changes in alcoholics. *Psychological Medicine* **16**, 547–559 [605].

JACOBSON, R.R. (1987) *CT Scan, Psychometric and Clinical Studies of the Wernicke–Korsakoff Syndrome*. MD thesis: University of Cambridge. Quoted Lishman, W.A. (1990) Alcohol and the brain. *British Journal of Psychiatry* **156**, 635–644 [581].

JACOBSON, R.R. (1989) Alcoholism, Korsakoff's syndrome and the frontal lobe. *Behavioural Neurology* **2**, 25–38 [582].

JACOBSON, R.R. (1995) The post-concussional syndrome: physiogenesis, psychogenesis and malingering. An integrative model. *Journal of Psychosomatic Research* **39**, 675–693 [199].

JACOBSON, R.R., ACKER, C.F. & LISHMAN, W.A. (1990) Patterns of neuropsychological deficit in alcoholic Korsakoff's syndrome. *Psychological Medicine* **20**, 321–334 [583].

JACOBSON, R.R. & LISHMAN, W.A. (1987) Selective memory loss and global intellectual deficits in alcoholic Korsakoff's syndrome. *Psychological Medicine* **17**, 649–655 [584].

JACOBSON, R.R. & LISHMAN, W.A. (1990) Cortical and diencephalic lesions in Korsakoff's syndrome: a clinical and CT scan study. *Psychological Medicine* **20**, 63–75 [582].

JACOBSON, R.R., TURNER, S.W., BALDY, R.E. & LISHMAN, W.A. (1985) Densitometric analysis of scans: important sources of artefact. *Psychological Medicine* **15**, 879–889 [138].

JACOBY, R. (1996) Managing the financial affairs of mentally disordered persons in the UK. Ch. 41B in *Psychiatry of the Elderly*, 2nd edn, eds Jacoby, R. & Oppenheimer, C. Oxford University Press: Oxford [498].

JACOBY, R. & BERGMANN, K. (1996) Testamentary capacity. Ch. 41A in *Psychiatry of the Elderly*, 2nd edn, eds Jacoby, R. & Oppenheimer, C. Oxford University Press: Oxford [498].

JACOBY, R.J., DOLAN, R.J., LEVY, R. & BALDY, R. (1983) Quantitative computed tomography in elderly depressed patients. *British Journal of Psychiatry* **143**, 124–127 [487].

JACOBY, R.J. & LEVY, R. (1980a) Computed tomography in the elderly. 2. Senile dementia: diagnosis and functional impairment. *British Journal of Psychiatry* **136**, 256–269 [139].

JACOBY, R.J. & LEVY, R. (1980b) Computed tomography in the elderly. 3. Affective disorder. *British Journal of Psychiatry* **136**, 270–275 [140, 487].

JACOBY, R.J., LEVY, R. & BIRD, J.M. (1981) Computed tomography and the outcome of affective disorder: a follow-up study of elderly patients. *British Journal of Psychiatry* **139**, 288–292 [140].

JACOME, D.E. (1987) EEG in whiplash: a reappraisal. *Clinical Electroencephalography* **18**, 41–45 [200].

JACQUES, A. (1988) *Understanding Dementia*. Churchill Livingstone: Edinburgh [498].

JADRESIC, D.P. (1990) Psychiatric aspects of hyperthyroidism. *Journal of Psychosomatic Research* **34**, 603–615 [508].

JADRESIC, D., RICCIO, M., HAWKINS, D.A., WILSON, B., SHANSON, D.C. & THOMPSON, C. (1994) Long-term impact of HIV diagnosis on mood and substance use—St Stephen's cohort study. *International Journal of STD and AIDS* **5**, 248–252 [330].

JAHANSHAHI, M. & MARSDEN, C.D. (1988) Personality in torticollis: a controlled study. *Psychological Medicine* **18**, 375–387 [674].

JAKOB, A. (1921) Über eigenartige Erkrankungen des Zentralnerven-systems mit bemerkenswertem anatomischen Befunde. *Zeitschrift für die gesamte Neurologie und Psychiatrie* **64**, 147–228 [473].

JAKOB, H. & BECKMANN, H. (1989) Gross and histological criteria for developmental disorders in brains of schizophrenics. *Journal of the Royal Society of Medicine* **82**, 466–469 [86].

JAMAL, G.A. (1991) Neurophysiological findings in the post-viral fatigue syndrome (myalgic encephalomyelitis). Ch. 9 in *Post-viral Fatigue Syndrome*, eds Jenkins, R. & Mowbray, J.F. Wiley & Sons: Chichester [372].

JAMAL, G.A., HANSEN, S., APARTOPOULOS, F. & PEDEN, A. (1996) The 'Gulf War syndrome'. Is there evidence of dysfunction in the nervous system? *Journal of Neurology, Neurosurgery and Psychiatry* **60**, 449–451 [637].

JAMES, G. (1992) Treatment of sarcoidosis. *Prescribers' Journal* **32**, 9–14 [763].

JAMES, I.P. (1960) Temporal lobectomy for psychomotor epilepsy. *Journal of Mental Science* **106**, 543–558 [270, 285].

JANA, D.K. & ROMANO-JANA, L. (1973) Hypernatremic psychosis in the elderly: case reports. *Journal of the American Geriatrics Society* **21**, 473–477 [559].

JANKOVIC, J., KIRKPATRIC, J.B., BLOMQUIST, K.A., LANGLAIS, P.J. & BIRD, E.D. (1985) Late-onset Hallervorden–Spatz disease presenting as familial parkinsonism. *Neurology* **35**, 227–234 [756].

JANKOWIAK, J. & ALBERT, M.L. (1994) Lesion localization in visual agnosia. Ch. 14 in *Localization and Neuroimaging in Neuropsychology*, ed. Kertesz, A. Academic Press: San Diego [60].

JANKOWSKI, K. (1963) A case of Schilder's diffuse sclerosis diagnosed clinically as schizophrenia. *Acta Neuropathologica* **2**, 302–305 [701].

JANOTA, I. (1981) Dementia, deep white matter damage and hypertension: Binswanger's disease. *Psychological Medicine* **11**, 39–48 [460].

JANOTA, I., MIRSEN, T.R., HACHINSKI, V.C., LEE, D.H. & MERSKEY, H. (1989) Neuropathologic correlates of leuko-araiosis. *Archives of Neurology* **46**, 1124–1128 [460].

JANSSEN, R.S., SAYKIN, A.J., CANNON, L., CAMPBELL, J., PINSKY, P.F., HESSOL, N.A., O'MALLEY, P.M., LIFSON, A.R., DOLL, L.S., RUTHERFORD, G.W. & KAPLAN, J.E. (1989) Neurological and neuropsychological manifestations of HIV-1 infection: association with AIDS-related complex but not asymptomatic HIV-1 infection. *Annals of Neurology* **26**, 592–600 [329].

JANSSEN, R.S., SAYKIN, A.J., KAPLAN, J.E., SPIRA, T.J., PINSKY, P.F., SPREHN, G.C., HOFFMAN, J.C., MAYER, W.B. Jr & SCHONBERGER, L.B. (1988) Neurological symptoms and neuropsychological abnormalities in lymphadenopathy syndrome. *Annals of Neurology* **23 (Supplement)**, S17–S18 [318].

JARVIE, H. (1954) Frontal lobe wounds causing disinhibition: a study of six cases. *Journal of Neurology, Neurosurgery and Psychiatry* **17**, 14–32 [174].

JARVIK, L.F., YEN, F.-S. & GOLDSTEIN, F. (1974a) Chromosomes and mental status. *Archives of General Psychiatry* **30**, 186–190 [431].

JARVIK, L.F., YEN, F.-S. & MORALISHVILI, E. (1974b) Chromosome examinations in ageing institutionalized women. *Journal of Gerontology* **29**, 269–276 [431].

JASKIW, G.E., JULIANO, D.M., GOLDBERG, T.E., HERTZMAN, M., UROW-HAMELL, E. & WEINBERGER, D.R. (1994) Cerebral ventricular enlargement in schizophreniform disorder does not progress. A seven year follow-up study. *Schizophrenia Research* **14**, 23–28 [85].

JASPER, H.H. (1964) Some physiological mechanisms involved in epileptic automatisms. *Epilepsia* **5**, 1–20 [254].

JASPERS, K. (1963) *General Psychopathology*. Translated from the German 7th edn by Hoenig, J. & Hamilton, M.W. Manchester University Press: Manchester [4].

JAYAKUMAR, P.N., TALY, A.B., ARYA, B.Y.T. & NAGARAJ, D. (1988) Computed tomography in subacute sclerosing panencephalitis: report of 15 cases. *Acta Neurologica Scandinavica* **77**, 328–330 [362].

828   REFERENCES

JEAVONS, P.M. & HARDING, G.F.A. (1970) Television epilepsy. *Lancet* **2**, 926 [241].

JEEVES, M.A. (1965) Psychological studies of three cases of congenital agenesis of the corpus callosum. In *Functions of the Corpus Callosum*, Ciba Foundation Study Group No. 20, eds Ettlinger, E.G., de Reuck, A.V.S. & Porter, R., pp. 73–94. J. & A. Churchill: London [770].

JEEVES, M.A. (1969) A comparison of interhemispheric transmission times in acallosals and normals. *Psychonomic Science* **16**, 245–246 [770].

JEEVES, M.A. & TEMPLE, C.M. (1987) A further study of language function in callosal agenesis. *Brain and Language* **32**, 325–335 [770].

JEFFCOATE, W.J., SILVERSTONE, J.T., EDWARDS, C.R.W. & BESSER, G.M. (1979) Psychiatric manifestations of Cushing's syndrome: response to lowering of plasma cortisol. *Quarterly Journal of Medicine* **191**, 465–472 [516, 518].

JEFFERSON, G. (1955) *The Invasive Adenomas of the Anterior Pituitary*. The Sherrington Lectures, No. 3, University Press of Liverpool [230].

JEFFERSON, M. (1957) Sarcoidosis of the nervous system. *Brain* **80**, 540–556 [764].

JEFFREYS, R.V. (1993) Investigation and management of hydrocephalus in adults. Ch. 8 in *Hydrocephalus*, eds Schurr, P.H. & Polkey, C.E. Oxford University Press: Oxford [746, 748].

JEFFREYS, R.V. & WOOD, M.M. (1978) Adult non-tumourous dementia and hydrocephalus. *Acta Neurochirurgica* **45**, 103–114 [748].

JELLINEK, E.H. (1962) Fits, faints, coma and dementia in myxoedema. *Lancet* **2**, 1010–1012 [513, 515].

JELLINEK, E.H. & KELLY, R.E. (1960) Cerebellar syndrome in myxoedema. *Lancet* **2**, 225–227 [513].

JELLINEK, E.M. (1952) Phases of alcohol addiction. *Quarterly Journal of Studies on Alcohol* **13**, 673–684 [596].

JELLINGER, K. & RIEDERER, P. (1984) Dementia in Parkinson's disease and (pre)senile dementia of Alzheimer type: morphological aspects and changes in the intracerebral MAO activity. *Advances in Neurology* **40**, 199–210 [655].

JELLINGER, K. & SEITELBERGER, F. (1969) Protracted post-traumatic encephalopathy: pathology and clinical implications. Ch. 18 in *The Late Effects of Head Injury*, eds Walker, A.E., Caveness, W.F. & Critchley, M. Thomas: Springfield, Illinois [164].

JENIKE, M.A. & PATO, C. (1986) Disabling fear of AIDS responsive to imipramine. *Psychosomatics* **27**, 143–144 [332].

JENKINS, A., HADLEY, D.M., TEASDALE, G.M., CONDON, B., MacPHERSON, P. & PATTERSON, J. (1988) Magnetic resonance imaging of acute subarachnoid haemorrhage. *Journal of Neurosurgery* **68**, 731–736 [393].

JENKINS, A., TEASDALE, G., HADLEY, M.D.M., MacPHERSON, P. & ROWAN, J.O. (1986) Brain lesions detected by magnetic resonance imaging in mild and severe head injuries. *Lancet* **2**, 445–446 [166].

JENKINS, R. (1991) Assessment and diagnosis of ME in the psychiatric clinic. Ch. 16 in *Post-viral Fatigue Syndrome*, eds Jenkins, R. & Mowbray, J.F. Wiley & Sons: Chichester [371].

JENKINS, R.B. & GROH, R.H. (1970) Mental symptoms in parkinsonian patients treated with L-dopa. *Lancet* **2**, 177–180 [658].

JENNEKENS, F.G.I., VELDMAN, H. & WOKKE, J.H.J. (1993) Histology and pathology of the human neuromuscular junction with a description of the clinical features of the myasthenic syndromes. Ch. 4 in *Myasthenia Gravis*, eds De Baets, M.H. & Oosterhuis, H.J.G.H. CRC Press: Boca Raton [710].

JENNETT, W.B. (1962) *Epilepsy After Blunt Head Injuries*. Heinemann: London [177, 178].

JENNETT, W.B. (1969) Early traumatic epilepsy. *Lancet* **1**, 1023–1025 [244].

JENNETT, B. (1975) *Epilepsy After Non-missile Head Injuries*, 2nd edn. Heinemann: London [165, 244].

JENNETT, B. (1986) *High Technology Medicine—Costs and Benefits*. Quoted by Mendelow, A.D. Ch. 5 in *Brain's Diseases of the Nervous System*, 10th edn, 1993, ed. Walton, J. Oxford University Press: Oxford [161].

JENNETT, B. & BOND, M. (1975) Assessment of outcome after severe brain damage: a practical scale. *Lancet* **1**, 480–484 [183, 185].

JENNETT, B. & PLUM, F. (1972) Persistent vegetative state after brain damage. A syndrome in search of a name. *Lancet* **1**, 734–737 [183].

JENNETT, B., SNOEK, J., BOND, M.R. & BROOKS, N. (1981) Disability after severe head injury: observations on the use of the Glasgow Coma Scale. *Journal of Neurology, Neurosurgery and Psychiatry* **44**, 285–293 [172, 185, 216].

JENNETT, B., TEASDALE, G., GALBRAITH, S., PICKARD, J., GRANT, H., BRAAKMAN, R., AVEZAAT, C., MAAS, A., MINDERHOUD, J., VECHT, C.J., HEIDEN, J., SMALL, R., CATON, W. & KURZE, T. (1977) Severe head injuries in three countries. *Journal of Neurology, Neurosurgery and Psychiatry* **40**, 291–298 [167, 185].

JENNETT, B., TEASDALE, G.M. & KNILL-JONES, R.P. (1975) Predicting outcome after head injury. *Journal of the Royal College of Physicians* **9**, 231–237 [167].

JENNINGS, W.G. (1972) An ergot alkaloid preparation (hydergine) versus placebo for treatment of symptoms of cerebrovascular insufficiency: double-blind study. *Journal of the American Geriatrics Society* **20**, 407–412 [502].

JENSEN, I. & LARSEN, J.K. (1979a) Mental aspects of temporal lobe epilepsy: follow-up of 74 patients after resection of a temporal lobe. *Journal of Neurology, Neurosurgery and Psychiatry* **42**, 256–265 [270, 312].

JENSEN, I. & LARSEN, J.K. (1979b) Psychoses in drug-resistant temporal lobe epilepsy. *Journal of Neurology, Neurosurgery and Psychiatry* **42**, 948–954 [282, 312].

JENSEN, R., BRINCK, T. & OLESEN, J. (1994) Sodium valproate has a prophylactic effect in migraine without aura: a triple-blind, placebo-controlled crossover study. *Neurology* **44**, 647–651 [410].

JERNIGAN, T.L., BUTTERS, N., DITRAGLIA, G., SCHAFER, K., SMITH, T., IRWIN, M., GRANT, I., SCHUCKIT, M. & CERMAK, L.S. (1991a) Reduced cerebral grey matter observed in alcoholics using MRI. *Alcoholism: Clinical and Experimental Research* **15**, 418–427 [605].

JERNIGAN, T.L., SALMON, D.P., BUTTERS, N. & HESSELINK, J.R. (1991b) Cerebral structure on MRI. Part II: Specific changes in Alzheimer's and Huntington's diseases. *Biological Psychiatry* **29**, 68–81 [470].

JERNIGAN, T.L., SCHAFER, K., BUTTERS, N. & CERMAK, L.S. (1991c) Magnetic resonance imaging of alcoholic Korsakoff patients. *Neuropsychopharmacology* **4**, 175–186 [582].

JERNIGAN, T.L., ZATZ, L.M. & NAESER, M.A. (1979) Semiautomated methods for quantitating CSF volume on cranial computed tomography. *Radiology* **132**, 463–466 [138].

JERVIS, G.A. (1948) Early senile dementia in mongoloid idiocy. *American Journal of Psychiatry* **105**, 102–106 [437].

JESTE, D.V. & LOHR, J.B. (1989) Hippocampal pathologic findings in schizophrenia. *Archives of General Psychiatry* **46**, 1019–1024 [86].

JOBST, K.A., SMITH, A.D., SZATMARI, M., ESIRI, M.M., JASKOWSKI, A., HINDLEY, N., McDONALD, B. & MOLYNEUX, A.J. (1994) Rapidly progressing atrophy of medical temporal lobe in Alzheimer's disease. *Lancet* **343**, 829–830 [449].

JOBST, K.A., SMITH, A.D., SZATMARI, M., MOLYNEUX, A.J., ESIRI, M.M.,

KING, E., SMITH, A., JASKOWSKI, A., McDONALD, B. & WALD, N. (1992) Detection in life of confirmed Alzheimer's disease using a simple measurement of medial temporal lobe atrophy by computed tomography. *Lancet* **340**, 1179–1183 [434].

JOFFE, R., BLACK, M.M. & FLOYD, M. (1968) Changing clinical picture of neurosyphilis: report of seven unusual cases. *British Medical Journal* **1**, 211–212 [343].

JOFFE, R.T., LIPPERT, G.P., GRAY, T.A., SAWA, G. & HORVATH, Z. (1987) Mood disorder and multiple sclerosis. *Archives of Neurology* **44**, 376–378 [695].

JOHANNESSON, G., HAGBERG, B., GUSTAFSON, L. & INGVAR, D.H. (1979) EEG and cognitive impairment in presenile dementia. *Acta Neurologica Scandinavica* **59**, 225–240 [461].

JOHNS, R.J. & McQUILLEN, M.P. (1966) Syndromes simulating myasthenia gravis: asthenia with anticholinesterase tolerance. *Annals of the New York Academy of Sciences* **135**, 385–397 [713].

JOHNSON, A.M. & DE COCK, K.M. (1994) What's happening to AIDS? *British Medical Journal* **309**, 1523–1524 [316].

JOHNSON, D.A.W. (1968) The evaluation of routine physical examination in psychiatric cases. *Practitioner* **200**, 686–691 [95].

JOHNSON, J. (1967) Myotonia congenita (Thomsen's disease) and hereditary psychosis. *British Journal of Psychiatry* **113**, 1025–1030 [721].

JOHNSON, J. (1969) Organic psychosyndromes due to boxing. *British Journal of Psychiatry* **115**, 45–53 [205, 207].

JOHNSON, J. (1975) Schizophrenia and Cushing's syndrome cured by adrenalectomy. *Psychological Medicine* **5**, 165–168 [516].

JOHNSON, J. (1982) Stupor: its diagnosis and management. *British Journal of Hospital Medicine* **27**, 530–532 [156].

JOHNSON, J. & LUCEY, P.A. (1987) Encephalitis lethargica, a contemporary cause of catatonic stupor. A report of two cases. *British Journal of Psychiatry* **151**, 550–552 [355].

JOHNSON, R.T. & RICHARDSON, E.P. (1968) The neurological manifestations of systemic lupus erythematosus: a clinical-pathological study of 24 cases and review of the literature. *Medicine* **47**, 337–369 [419, 420, 421].

JOHNSON, W.O. (1928) Psychosis and hyperthyroidism. *Journal of Nervous and Mental Disease* **67**, 558–566 [509].

JOHNSTONE, E.C., CROW, T.J., FRITH, C.D., HUSBAND, J. & KREEL, L. (1976) Cerebral ventricular size and cognitive impairment in chronic schizophrenia. *Lancet* **2**, 924–926 [140].

JOHNSTONE, E.C., CROW, T.J., FRITH, C.D., STEVENS, M., KREEL, L. & HUSBAND, J. (1978) The dementia of dementia praecox. *Acta Psychiatrica Scandinavica* **57**, 305–324 [140].

JOHNSTONE, E.C., OWENS, D.G.C., CROW, T.J., FRITH, C.D., ALEXANDROPOLIS, K., BYDDER, G. & COLTER, N. (1989) The structure as determined by nuclear magnetic resonance in schizophrenia and bipolar affective disorder. *Journal of Neurology, Neurosurgery and Psychiatry* **52**, 736–741 [85].

JOHNSTONE, J.A., ROSS, C.A.C. & DUNN, M. (1972) Meningitis and encephalitis associated with mumps infection. A 10 year survey. *Archives of Disease in Childhood* **47**, 647–651 [358].

JOLLIFFE, N., BOWMAN, K.M., ROSENBLUM, L.A. & FEIN, H.D. (1940) Nicotinic acid deficiency encephalopathy. *Journal of the American Medical Association* **114**, 307–312 [574].

JOLLIFFE, N., GOODHART, R., GENNIS, J. & CLINE, J.K. (1939) Experimental production of vitamin B_1 deficiency in normal subjects; dependence of urinary excretion of thiamin on dietary intake of vitamin B_1. *American Journal of the Medical Sciences* **198**, 198–211 [572].

JOLLIFFE, N., WORTIS, H. & FEIN, H.D. (1941) The Wernicke syndrome. *Archives of Neurology and Psychiatry* **46**, 569–597 [576].

JONES, B. & PARSONS, O.A. (1971) Impaired abstracting ability in chronic alcoholics. *Archives of General Psychiatry* **24**, 71–75 [604].

JONES, D.P. & NEVIN, S. (1954) Rapidly progressive cerebral degeneration (subacute vascular encephalopathy) with mental disorder, focal disturbances and myoclonic epilepsy. *Journal of Neurology, Neurosurgery and Psychiatry* **17**, 148–159 [479].

JONES, P.B., OWEN, M.J., LEWIS, S.W. & MURRAY, R.M. (1993) A case-control study of family history and cerebral cortical abnormalities in schizophrenia. *Acta Psychiatrica Scandinavica* **87**, 6–12 [85].

JONES, P., RODGERS, B., MURRAY, R. & MARMOT, M. (1994) Child developmental risk factors for adult schizophrenia in the British 1946 birth cohort. *Lancet* **344**, 1398–1402 [91].

JONES, R.K. (1974) Assessment of minimal head injuries: indications for in-hospital care. *Surgical Neurology* **2**, 101–104 [197].

JONES-GOTMAN, M. & MILNER, B. (1977) Design fluency: the invention of nonsense drawings after focal cortical lesions. *Neuropsychologia* **15**, 653–654 [104].

JORDAN, B.D. & ZIMMERMAN, R.D. (1988) Magnetic resonance imaging in amateur boxers. *Archives of Neurology* **45**, 1207–1208 [206].

JORDAN, B.D. & ZIMMERMAN, R.D. (1990) Computed tomography and magnetic resonance imaging comparisons in boxers. *Journal of the American Medical Association* **263**, 1670–1674 [206].

JORDAN, R.M., KAMMER, H. & RIDDLE, M.R. (1977) Sulfonylurea-induced factitious hypoglycaemia: a growing problem. *Archives of Internal Medicine* **137**, 390–393 [544].

JORGE, R.E., ROBINSON, R.G., ARNDT, S.V., FORRESTER, A.W., GEISLER, F. & STARKSTEIN, S.E. (1993) Comparison between acute- and delayed-onset depression following traumatic brain injury. *Journal of Neuropsychiatry and Clinical Neurosciences* **5**, 43–49 [191].

JOSE, C.J., BARTON, J.L. & PEREZ-CRUET, J. (1979) Hyponatraemic seizures in psychiatric patients. *Biological Psychiatry* **14**, 839–843 [525, 526].

JOSEPHSON, A.M. & MACKENZIE, T.B. (1980) Thyroid-induced mania in hypothyroid patients. *British Journal of Psychiatry* **137**, 222–228 [515].

JOUSSE, A.T., GEISLER, W.O. & WYNNE-JONES, M. (1969) Motivation in rehabilitation. Ch. 30 in *The Late Effects of Head Injury*, eds Walker, A.E., Caveness, W.F. & Critchley, M. Thomas: Springfield, Illinois [213].

JOYCE, E.M. (1992) The relevance to psychiatry of recent advances in functional imaging. *Journal of Neurology, Neurosurgery and Psychiatry* **55**, 427–430 [146].

JOYCE, E.M., RIO, D.E., RUTTIMANN, U.E., ROHRBAUGH, J.W., MARTIN, P.R., RAWLINGS, R.R. & ECKARDT, M.J. (1994) Decreased cingulate and precuneate glucose utilization in alcoholic Korsakoff's syndrome. *Psychiatry Research* **54**, 225–239 [582].

JOYCE, E.M. & ROBBINS, T.W. (1991) Frontal lobe function in Korsakoff and non-Korsakoff alcoholics: planning and spatial working memory. *Neuropsychologia* **29**, 709–723 [583].

JOYCE-CLARK, N. & MOLTENO, A.C.B. (1978) Modified neurosyphilis in the Cape peninsula. *South African Medical Journal* **53**, 10–16 [342].

JOYSTON-BECHAL, M.P. (1966) The clinical features and outcome of stupor. *British Journal of Psychiatry* **117**, 967–981 [155, 156].

JUDELSOHN, F.A. (1970) Depression and carcinoma. *British Journal of Psychiatry* **117**, 119–121 [744].

JUDGE, T.G. (1968) Quoted by Ferguson Anderson, W. in The interrelationship between physical and mental disease in the elderly. Ch. 11 in *Recent Developments in Psychogeriatrics*, eds Kay, D.W.K. & Walk, A., British Journal of Psychiatry Special Publication No. 6. Headley Brothers: Ashford, Kent 1971 [560].

JUDGE, T.G. & URQUHART, A. (1972) Naftidrofuryl—a double blind cross-over study in the elderly. *Current Medical Research and Opinion* **1**, 166–172 [502].

JUS, A. & JUS, K. (1962) Retrograde amnesia in petit mal. *Archives of General Psychiatry* **6**, 163–167 [262].

JUUL-JENSEN, P. (1964) Epilepsy: a clinical and social analysis of 1020 adult patients with epileptic seizures. *Acta Neurologica Scandinavica* **5 (Supplement)**, 1–148 [243, 274].

KACZMAREK, M.J. & NIXON, P.F. (1983) Variants of transketolate from human erythrocytes. *Clinica Chimica Acta* **130**, 349–356 [576].

KAELEN, C., HARPER, C. & VIEIRA, B.I. (1986) Acute encephalopathy and death due to petrol sniffing: neuropathological findings. *Australian and New Zealand Journal of Medicine* **16**, 804–807 [630].

KAHANA, E., ALTER, M., BRAHAM, J. & SOFER, D. (1974) Creutzfeldt–Jakob disease: focus among Libyan Jews in Israel. *Science* **183**, 90–91 [475].

KAHANA, E., LEIBOWITZ, U. & ALTER, M. (1971) Cerebral multiple sclerosis. *Neurology* **21**, 1179–1185 [695].

KALES, A. & KALES, J.D. (1974) Sleep disorders: recent findings in the diagnosis and treatment of disturbed sleep. *New England Journal of Medicine* **290**, 487–499 [736, 737].

KALES, A., SOLDATOS, C.R., CALDWELL, A.B., KALES, J.D., HUMPHREY, F.J., CHARNEY, D.S. & SCHWEITZER, P.K. (1980) Somnambulism: clinical characteristics and personality patterns. *Archives of General Psychiatry* **37**, 1406–1410 [736, 737].

KALES, A., SOLDATOS, C.R. & KALES, J.D. (1987) Sleep disorders: insomnia, sleepwalking, night terrors, nightmares, and enuresis. *Annals of Internal Medicine* **106**, 582–592 [735, 737].

KALINOWSKY, L.B. & KENNEDY, F. (1943) Observations in electric shock therapy applied to problems in epilepsy. *Journal of Nervous and Mental Disease* **98**, 56–67 [310].

KALLMANN, F.J. (1956) Genetic aspects of mental disorders in later life. Ch. 3 in *Mental Disorders in Later Life*, ed. Kaplan, O.J. Stanford University Press: Stanford [430].

KALSBEEK, W.D., McLAURIN, R.L., HARRIS, B.S.H. & MILLER, J.D. (1980) The national head and spinal cord injury survey: major findings. *Journal of Neurosurgery* **53**, S19–S31 [161].

KAMINSKI, H.J. & RUFF, R.L. (1989) Neurologic complications of endocrine diseases. In *Neurologic Manifestations of Systemic Disease*, ed. Riggs, J.E. *Neurologic Clinics* **7**, 489–508 [509, 513].

KAMO, H., McGEER, P.L., HARROP, R., McGEER, E.G., CALNE, D.B., MARTIN, W.R.W. & PATE, B.D. (1987) Positron emission tomography and histopathology in Pick's disease. *Neurology* **37**, 439–445 [462].

KANDEL, E.R. & HAWKINS, R.D. (1992) The biological basis of learning and individuality. *Scientific American* **267**, 78–86 [24].

KANG, J., LEMAIRE, H.G., UNTERBECK, A., SALBAUM, J.M., MASTERS, C.L., GRZESCHIK, K.-H., MULTHAUP, G., BEYREUTHER, K. & MÜLLER-HILL, B. (1987) The precursor of Alzheimer's disease amyloid A_4 protein resembles a cell-surface receptor. *Nature* **325**, 733–736 [442, 447].

KANG, U.J., BURKE, R.E. & FAHN, S. (1986) Natural history and treatment of tardive dystonia. *Movement Disorders* **1**, 193–208 [642, 645].

KANIS, J.A. (1996) Disorders of calcium metabolism. Section 12.6 in *Oxford Textbook of Medicine*, 3rd edn, eds Weatherall, D.J., Ledingham, J.G.G. & Warrell, D.A. Oxford University Press: Oxford [531].

KANNEL, W.B. & McGEE, D.L. (1979) Diabetes and cardiovascular disease. The Framingham study. *Journal of the American Medical Association* **241**, 2035–2038 [537].

KANNEL, W.B. & WOLF, P.A. (1983) Epidemiology of cerebrovascular disease. Ch. 1 in *Vascular Disease of the Central Nervous System*, 2nd edn, ed. Russell, R.W.R. Churchill Livingstone: Edinburgh & London [376].

KANNER, L. (1957) *Child Psychiatry*, 3rd edn. Blackwell Scientific Publications: Oxford [681].

KAPILA, C.C., KAUL, S., KAPUR, S.C., KALAYANAM, T.S. & BANERJEE, D. (1958) Neurological and hepatic disorders associated with influenza. *British Medical Journal* **2**, 1311–1314 [360].

KAPLAN, E., GOODGLASS, H. & WEINTRAUB, S. (1983) *Boston Naming Test*. Lea & Febiger: Philadelphia [113].

KAPLAN, R.D., SZECHTMAN, H., FRANCO, S., SZECHTMAN, B., NAHMIAS, C., GARNETT, E.S., LIST, S. & CLEGHORN, J.M. (1993) Three clinical syndromes of schizophrenia in untreated subjects: relation to brain glucose activity measured by positron emission tomography (PET). *Schizophrenia Research* **11**, 47–54 [88].

KAPPAS, A., SASSA, S., GALBRAITH, R.A. & NORDMANN, Y. (1989) The porphyrias. Ch. 52 in *The Metabolic Basis of Inherited Disease*, 6th edn, eds Scriver, C.R., Beaudet, A.L., Sly, W.S. & Valle, D. McGraw-Hill: New York [567, 568, 569].

KAPUR, N. & COUGHLAN, A.K. (1980) Confabulation and frontal lobe dysfunction. *Journal of Neurology, Neurosurgery and Psychiatry* **43**, 461–463 [31].

KAPUR, N., ELLISON, D., SMITH, M.P., McLELLAN, D.L. & BURROWS, E.H. (1992) Focal retrograde amnesia following bilateral temporal lobe pathology. *Brain* **115**, 73–85 [37].

KAPUR, N., HEATH, P., MEUDELL, P. & KENNEDY, P. (1986) Amnesia can facilitate memory performance: evidence from a patient with dissociated retrograde amnesia. *Neuropsychologia* **24**, 215–221 [37].

KAPUR, N., TURNER, A. & KING, C. (1988) Reduplicative paramnesia: possible anatomical and neuropsychological mechanisms. *Journal of Neurology, Neurosurgery and Psychiatry* **51**, 579–581 [12].

KAPUR, N., YOUNG, A., BATEMAN, D. & KENNEDY, P. (1989) Focal retrograde amnesia: a longterm clinical neuropsychological follow-up. *Cortex* **25**, 387–402 [37].

KARAGULLA, S. & ROBERTSON, E.E. (1955) Psychical phenomena in temporal lobe epilepsy and the psychoses. *British Medical Journal* **1**, 748–752 [295].

KARHUNEN, P.J., ERKINJUNTTI, T. & LAIPPALA, P. (1994) Moderate alcohol consumption and loss of cerebellar Purkinje cells. *British Medical Journal* **308**, 1663–1667 [586].

KARK, R.A.P., POSKANZER, D.C., BULLOCK, J.D. & BOYLEN, G. (1971) Mercury poisoning and its treatment with n-acetyl-d, l-penicillamine. *New England Journal of Medicine* **285**, 10–16 [634].

KARPATI, G. & FRAME, B. (1964) Neuropsychiatric disorders in primary hyperparathyroidism: clinical analysis with review of the literature. *Archives of Neurology* **10**, 387–397 [529, 530, 531].

KASTE, M., VILLKE, J., SAINIO, K., KUURNE, T., KATEVUO, K. & MEURALA, H. (1982) Is chronic brain damage in boxing a hazard of the past? *Lancet* **2**, 1186–1188 [204, 205].

KASTELEIJN-NOLST TRENITÉ, D.G.A., BAKKER, D.J., BINNIE, C.D., BUERMAN, A. & VAN RAAIJ, M. (1988) Psychological effects of subclinical epileptiform EEG discharges. I. Scholastic skills. *Epilepsy Research* **2**, 111–116 [262].

KASZNIAK, A.W., FOX, J., GADELL, D.L., GARRON, D.C., HUCKMAN, M.S. & RAMSEY, R.G. (1978) Predictors of mortality in presenile and senile dementia. *Annals of Neurology* **3**, 246–252 [433].

KASZNIAK, A.W., GARRON, D.C. & FOX, J. (1979) Differential effects of age and cerebral atrophy upon span of immediate recall and paired associated learning in older patients suspected of dementia. *Cortex* **15**, 285–295 [32].

KATHOL, R.G., TURNER, R. & DELAHUNT, J. (1986) Depression and anxiety associated with hyperthyroidism: response to antithyroid therapy. *Psychosomatics* **27**, 501–505 [508, 511].

KATZ, A., AWAD, I.A., KONG, A.K., CHELUNE, G.J., NAUGLE, R.I., WYLIE, E., BEAUCHAMP, G. & LUDERS, H. (1989) Extent of resection in temporal lobectomy for epilepsy. II. Memory changes and neurologic complications. *Epilepsia* **30**, 763–771 [312].

KATZMAN, R. (1976) The prevalence and malignancy of Alzheimer's disease. *Archives of Neurology* **33**, 217–218 [429].

KAUFMAN, D.M., ZIMMERMAN, R.D. & LEEDS, N.E. (1979) Computed tomography in herpes simplex encephalitis. *Neurology* **29**, 1392–1396 [357].

KAWAMURA, M., SHIOTA, J., YAGISHITA, T. & HIRAYAMA, K. (1985) Marchiafava–Bignami disease: computed tomographic scan and magnetic resonance imaging. *Annals of Neurology* **18**, 103–104 [586].

KAY, D.W.K., BEAMISH, P. & ROTH, M. (1964) Old age mental disorders in Newcastle upon Tyne. Part 1: a study of prevalence. *British Journal of Psychiatry* **110**, 146–158 [429].

KAY, D.W.K., BERGMANN, K., FOSTER, E.M., McKECHNIE, A.A. & ROTH, M. (1970) Mental illness and hospital usage in the elderly: a random sample followed up. *Comprehensive Psychiatry* **11**, 26–35 [429].

KAY, D.W.K., KERR, T.A. & LASSMAN, L.P. (1971) Brain trauma and the postconcussional syndrome. *Lancet* **2**, 1052–1055 [198].

KAYE, W.H., WEINGARTNER, H., GOLD, P., EBERT, M.H., GILLIN, J.C., SITARAM, N. & SMALLBERG, S. (1982) Cognitive effects of cholinergic and vasopressin-like agents in patients with primary degenerative dementia. In *Alzheimer's Disease: a Report of Progress in Research, Aging, Vol. 19*, eds Corkin, S., Davis, K.L., Growden, J.H., Usdin, E., Wurtman, R.J., pp. 433–442. Raven Press: New York [502].

KAZNER, E., LANKSCH, W., STEINHOFF, H. & WILSKE, J. (1975) Die axiale Computer-Tomographie des Gehirnschädels—Anwendungsmöglichkeiten und klinische Ergebnisse. *Fortschritte der Neurologie-Psychiatrie* **75**, 487–574 [137].

KAZUI, H., TANABE, H., IKEDA, M., NAKAGAWA, Y., SHIRAISHI, J. & HASHIKAWA, K. (1995) Memory and cerebral blood flow in cases of transient global amnesia during and after the attack. *Behavioural Neurology* **8**, 93–101 [413, 417].

KEARNEY, T.R. (1964) Parkinson's disease presenting as a depressive illness. *Journal of the Irish Medical Association* **54**, 117–119 [656].

KEARSLEY, J.H. & MUSSO, A.F. (1980) Hypothermia and coma in the Wernicke–Korsakoff syndrome. *Medical Journal of Australia* **2**, 504–506 [578].

KEDDIE, K.M.G. (1965) Toxic psychosis following mumps. *British Journal of Psychiatry* **111**, 691–696 [358].

KEELER, M.H., REIFLER, C.B. & LIPTZIN, M.B. (1968) Spontaneous recurrence of marihuana effect. *American Journal of Psychiatry* **125**, 384–386 [613].

KELLAM, A.M.P. (1987) Neuroleptic malignant syndrome, so-called. A survey of the world literature. *British Journal of Psychiatry* **150**, 752–759 [626, 627].

KELLER, J.M., EDWARDS, F.M. & RUNDLE, R. (1981) Automatic outlining of regions on CT scans. *Journal of Computer Assisted Tomography* **5**, 240–265 [138].

KELLEY-GERACHTY, D.C. & JUBELT, B. (1994) Viruses and motor neurone disease: the viral hypothesis lives. Ch. 27 in *Motor Neurone Disease*, ed. Williams, A.C. Chapman & Hall: London [707].

KELLY, A.B., ZIMMERMAN, R.D., SNOW, R.B., GANDY, S.E., HEIER, L.A. & DECK, M.D. (1988) Head trauma: comparison of MR and CT-experience in 100 patients. *American Journal of Neuroradiology* **9**, 699–708 [166, 412].

KELLY, M., MYRSTEN, A-L. & GOLDBERG, L. (1971) Intravenous vitamins in acute alcoholic intoxication: effects on physiological and psychological functions. *British Journal of Addiction* **66**, 19–30 [597].

KELLY, R. & SMITH, B.N. (1981) Post-traumatic syndrome: another myth discredited. *Journal of the Royal Society of Medicine* **74**, 275–277 [177].

KELLY, W.F., CHECKLEY, S.A., BENDER, D.A. & MASHITER, K. (1983) Cushing's syndrome and depression—a prospective study of 26 patients. *British Journal of Psychiatry* **142**, 16–19 [517, 518].

KEMP, P.M., HOUSTON, A.S., MacLEOD, M.A. & PETHYBRIDGE, R.J. (1995) Cerebral perfusion and psychometric testing in military amateur boxers and controls. *Journal of Neurology, Neurosurgery and Psychiatry* **59**, 368–374 [206].

KEMP, P.M., MacLEOD, M.A., JENKINS, L., HOUSTON, A.S. & TOMS, L. (1991) Abstract: Cerebral perfusion in amateur boxers. Is there evidence of brain damage? *Nuclear Medicine Communications* **12**, 279 [206].

KENDALL, B.E. (1980) The detection of intracranial tumours. *British Journal of Hospital Medicine* **23**, 116–133 [137, 231].

KENDELL, R.E. (1967) Psychiatric sequelae of benign myalgic encephalomyelitis. *British Journal of Psychiatry* **113**, 833–840 [371].

KENDELL, R.E. (1974) The stability of psychiatric diagnoses. *British Journal of Psychiatry* **124**, 352–356 [486].

KENDELL, R.E., JUSZCZAK, E. & COLE, S.K. (1996) Obstetric complications and schizophrenia: a case control study based on standardised obstetric records. *British Journal of Psychiatry* **168**, 556–561 [91].

KENDRICK, D.C. (1967) A cross-validation study of the use of the SLT and DCT in screening for diffuse brain pathology in elderly subjects. *British Journal of Medical Psychology* **40**, 173–178 [115].

KENDRICK, D.C., GIBSON, A.J. & MOYES, I.C.A. (1979) The revised Kendrick battery: clinical studies. *British Journal of Social and Clinical Psychology* **18**, 329–340 [115].

KENDRICK, D.C., PARBOOSINGH, R-C. & POST, F. (1965) A synonym learning test for use with elderly psychiatric subjects: a validation study. *British Journal of Social and Clinical Psychology* **4**, 63–71 [114, 115].

KENDRICK, D.C. & POST, F. (1967) Differences in cognitive status between healthy, psychiatrically ill, and diffusely brain-damaged elderly subjects. *British Journal of Psychiatry* **113**, 75–81 [112, 115].

KENNARD, C. & SWASH, M. (1981) Acute viral encephalitis: its diagnosis and outcome. *Brain* **104**, 129–148 [346, 360].

KENNEDY, A. (1959a) Psychological factors in confusional states in the elderly. *Gerontologia Clinica* **1**, 71–82 [499, 500].

KENNEDY, A. & NEVILLE, J. (1957) Sudden loss of memory. *British Medical Journal* **2**, 428–433 [483, 485].

KENNEDY, A. & SCHON, F. (1991) Epilepsy: disappearing lesions appearing in the United Kingdom. *British Medical Journal* **302**, 933–935 [289].

KENNEDY, A.C., LINTON, A.L., LUKE, R.G. & RENFREW, S. (1963) Electroencephalographic changes during haemodialysis. *Lancet* **1**, 408–411 [558].

KENNEDY, C. (1968) A ten-year experience with subacute sclerosing panencephalitis. *Neurology* **18 (Supplement)**, 58–59 [362].

KENNEDY, G.C., GERMAN, M.S. & RUTTER, W.J. (1995) The minisatellite in the diabetes susceptibility locus IDDM2 regulates insulin transcription. *Nature Genetics* **9**, 293–298 [534].

KENNEDY, J., PARBHOO, S.P., MacGILLIVRAY, B. & SHERLOCK, S. (1973) Effect of extracorporeal liver perfusion on the electroencephalogram of patients in coma due to acute liver failure. *Quarterly Journal of Medicine* **42**, 549–561 [564].

KENNEDY, W. & SECCOMBE, B. (1959) Quoted by James, I.P. (1960) *Journal of Mental Science* **106**, 543–558 [265].

KENNEDY, W.A. (1959b) Clinical and electroencephalographic aspects of epileptogenic lesions of the medial surface and superior border of the cerebral hemisphere. *Brain* **82**, 147–161 [250].

KERMODE, A.G., THOMPSON, A.J., TOFTS, P., MacMANUS, D.G., KENDALL, B.E., KINGSLEY, D.P.E., MOSELEY, I.F., RUDGE, P. & McDONALD, W.I. (1990) Breakdown of the blood–brain barrier precedes symptoms and other magnetic resonance imaging signs of new lesions in multiple sclerosis. *Brain* **113**, 1477–1489 [690].

KERR, T.A., KAY, D.W.K. & LASSMAN, L.P. (1971) Characteristics of patients, type of accident, and mortality in a consecutive series of head injuries admitted to a neurosurgical unit. *British Journal of Preventive and Social Medicine* **25**, 179–185 [174].

KERR, T.A., SCHAPIRA, K. & ROTH, M. (1969) The relationship between premature death and affective disorders. *British Journal of Psychiatry* **115**, 1277–1282 [744].

KERSHAW, P.W. (1967) Blood thiamine and nicotinic acid levels in alcoholism and confusional states. *British Journal of Psychiatry* **113**, 387–393 [602].

KERTESZ, A. & BENSON, D.F. (1970) Neologistic jargon: a clinico-pathological study. *Cortex* **6**, 362–386 [54].

KERTESZ, A. & NAESER, M.A. (1994) Anatomical asymmetries and cerebral lateralization. Ch. 8 in *Localization of Neuroimaging in Neuropsychology*, ed. Kertesz, A. Academic Press: San Diego [41].

KERWIN, R. (1990) The neurochemical anatomy of the hippocampus in post-mortem schizophrenic brain. *Schizophrenia Research* **3**, 33–34 [90].

KERWIN, R.W., PATEL, S., MELDRUM, B.S., CZUDEK, C. & REYNOLDS, G.P. (1988) Asymmetrical loss of glutamate receptor subtype in left hippocampus in schizophrenia. *Lancet* **1**, 583–584 [90].

KESCHNER, M., BENDER, M.B. & STRAUSS, I. (1936) Mental symptoms in cases of tumour of the temporal lobe. *Archives of Neurology and Psychiatry* **35**, 572–596 [223, 224, 225, 226].

KESCHNER, M., BENDER, M.B. & STRAUSS, I. (1937) Mental symptoms in cases of subtentorial tumour. *Archives of Neurology and Psychiatry* **37**, 1–15 [219, 230].

KESCHNER, M., BENDER, M.B. & STRAUSS, I. (1938) Mental symptoms associated with brain tumour: a study of 530 verified cases. *Journal of the American Medical Association* **110**, 714–718 [218, 220, 221, 226].

KESHAVAN, M.S. (1993) Magnetic resonance spectroscopy. *Schizophrenia Monitor* **3 (3)**, 1–3 [143].

KESHAVAN, M.S., CHANNABASAVANNA, S.M. & REDDY, G.M. (1981) Post-traumatic psychiatric disturbances: patterns and predictors of outcome. *British Journal of Psychiatry* **138**, 157–160 [198].

KESHAVAN, M.S., DAVID, A.S., NARAYANEN, H.S. & SATISH, P. (1986) 'On-off' phenomena and manic-depressive mood shifts: case report. *Journal of Clinical Psychiatry* **47**, 93–94 [651].

KESHAVAN, M.S., DAVID, A.S., STEINGARD, S. & LISHMAN, W.A. (1992) Musical hallucinations: a review and synthesis. *Neuropsychiatry, Neuropsychology, and Behavioral Neurology* **5**, 211–223 [291].

KESHAVAN, M.S., KAPUR, S. & PETTEGREW, J.W. (1991a) Magnetic resonance spectroscopy in psychiatry: potential, pitfalls and promise. *American Journal of Psychiatry* **148**, 976–985 [143].

KESHAVAN, M.S., KUMAR, Y.V. & CHANNABASAVANNA, S.M. (1979) A critical evaluation of infantile reflexes in neuropsychiatric diagnosis. *Indian Journal of Psychiatry* **21**, 267–270 [96].

KESHAVAN, M.S. & LISHMAN, W.A. (1986) Prolonged depersonalization following cannabis abuse. *British Journal of Addiction* **81**, 140–142 [615].

KESHAVAN, M.S., LISHMAN, W.A. & HUGHES, J.T. (1987) Psychiatric presentation of Creutzfeldt–Jakob disease. *British Journal of Psychiatry* **151**, 260–263 [477].

KESHAVAN, M.S., PETTEGREW, J.W. & PANCHALIN-GAM, K.S. (1991b) Phosphorus 31 magnetic resonance spectroscopy detects altered brain metabolism before onset of schizophrenia. *Archives of General Psychiatry* **48**, 1112–1113 [143].

KESSELRING, J., MILLER, D.H., ROBB, S.A., KENDALL, B.E., MOSELEY, I.F., KINGSLEY, D., DU BOULAY, G.H. & McDONALD, I. (1990) Acute disseminated encephalomyelitis. MRI findings and the distinction from multiple sclerosis. *Brain* **113**, 291–302 [361].

KESSLAK, J.P., NALCIOGLU, O. & COTMAN, C.W. (1991) Quantification of magnetic resonance scans for hippocampal and parahippocampal atrophy in Alzheimer's disease. *Neurology* **41**, 51–54 [434].

KESSLER, R.M., PARKER, E.S., CLARK, C.M., MARTIN, P.R., GEORGE, D.T., WEINGARTNER, H., SOKOLOFF, L., EBERT, M.H. & MISHKIN, M. (1984) Regional cerebral glucose metabolism in patients with alcoholic Korsakoff's syndrome. *Society for Neuroscience* **10**, 541 (Abstract) [582].

KEW, J.J.M., GOLDSTEIN, L.H., LEIGH, P.N., ABRAHAMS, S., COSGRAVE, N., PASSINGHAM, R.E., FRACKOWIAK, R.S.J. & BROOKS, D.J. (1993b) The relationship between abnormalities of cognitive function and cerebral activation in amyotrophic lateral sclerosis. A neuropsychological and positron emission tomographic study. *Brain* **116**, 1399–1423 [708].

KEW, J. & LEIGH, N. (1992) Dementia with motor neurone disease. Ch. 7 in *Unusual Dementias*, ed. Rossor, M.N. Ballière Tindall: London [708].

KEW, J.J.M., LEIGH, P.N., PLAYFORD, E.D., PASSINGHAM, R.E., GOLDSTEIN, L.H., FRACKOWIAK, R.S.J. & BROOKS, D.J. (1993c) Cortical function in amyotrophic lateral sclerosis. A positron emission tomographic study. *Brain* **116**, 655–680 [708].

KEW, J., MORRIS, C., AIHIE, A., FYSH, R., JONES, S. & BROOKS, D. (1993a) Arsenic and mercury intoxication due to Indian ethnic remedies. *British Medical Journal* **306**, 506–507 [633, 636].

KHAMNEI, A.K. (1984) Psychosis, inappropriate antidiuretic hormone secretion, and water intoxication. *Lancet* **1**, 963 [525, 526].

KHANNA, S., AMMINI, A., SAXENA, S. & MOHAN, D. (1988) Hypopituitarism presenting as delirium. *International Journal of Psychiatry in Medicine* **18**, 89–92 [524].

KIBRICK, S. & GOODING, G.W. (1965) Pathogenesis of infection with herpes simplex virus with special reference to nervous tissue. In *Slow, Latent and Temperate Virus Infections*, eds Gajdusek, D.C., Gibbs, C.J. & Alpers, M., pp. 143–154. National Institute of Neurological Diseases and Blindness Monograph No. 2: Washington [356].

KIDD, M. (1963) Pathology; paired helical filaments in electron microscopy of Alzheimer's disease. *Nature* **197**, 192–193 [442].

KIDGER, T., BARNES, R.E., TRAUER, T. & TAYLOR, P.J. (1980) Subsyndromes of tardive dyskinesia. *Psychological Medicine* **10**, 513–520 [640].

KIDSON, M.A. (1973) Personality and hypertension. *Journal of Psychosomatic Research* **17**, 35–41 [398].

KIEBURTZ, K., ZETTELMAIER, A.E., KETONEN, L., TUITE, M. & CAINE, E.D. (1991) Manic syndrome in AIDS. *American Journal of Psychiatry* **148**, 1068–1070 [331].

KIEV, A., CHAPMAN, L.F., GUTHRIE, T.C. & WOLFF, H.G. (1962) The highest integrative functions and diffuse cerebral atrophy. *Neurology* **12**, 385–393 [139].

KIHLBOM, M. (1969) Psychopathology of Turner's syndrome. *Acta Paedopsychiatrica* **36**, 75–81 [528].

KILOH, L.G. (1961) Pseudo-dementia. *Acta Psychiatrica Scandinavica* **37**, 336–351 [480, 486, 489].

KILOH, L.G., McCOMAS, A.J., OSSLETON, J.W. & UPTON, A.R.M. (1981) *Clinical Electroencephalography*, 4th edn. Butterworths: London [128, 129, 131, 231, 239, 412, 433].

KIMBERLIN, R.H. (1986) Scrapie: how much do we really understand? *Neuropathology and Applied Neurobiology* **12**, 131–147 [474].

KIMURA, D. (1961) Some effects of temporal lobe damage on auditory perception. *Canadian Journal of Psychology* **15**, 156–165 [64].

KIMURA, D. (1963) Right temporal lobe damage: perception of unfamiliar stimuli after damage. *Archives of Neurology* **8**, 264–271 [63].

KIMURA, D. (1964) Left–right differences in the perception of melodies. *Quarterly Journal of Experimental Psychology* **16**, 355–358 [64].

KIND, H. (1958) Die Psychiatrie der Hypophyseninsuffienz speziell der Simmondsschen Krankheit. *Fortschritte der Neurologie-Psychiatrie* **26**, 501–563 [523].

KING, M.A., HUNTER, B.E. & WALKER, D.W. (1988) Alterations and recovery of dendritic spine density in rat hippocampus following long-term ethanol ingestion. *Brain Research* **459**, 381–385 [607].

KING, M.B. (1989) Psychological status of 192 out-patients with HIV infection and AIDS. *British Journal of Psychiatry* **154**, 237–242 [330].

KING, M.B. (1993) *AIDS, HIV and Mental Health*. Cambridge University Press: Cambridge [329, 330, 331, 332, 333].

KING, M.D., DAY, R.E., OLIVER, J.S., LUSH, M. & WATSON, J.M. (1981) Solvent encephalopathy. *British Medical Journal* **283**, 663–665 [629, 630].

KINKEL, W.R., JACOBS, L., POLACHINI, I., BATES, V. & HEFFNER, R.R. (1985) Subcortical arteriosclerotic encephalopathy (Binswanger's disease). *Archives of Neurology* **42**, 951–959 [460].

KINSBOURNE, M. & WARRINGTON, E.K. (1962a) A disorder of simultaneous form perception. *Brain* **85**, 461–486 [61].

KINSBOURNE, M. & WARRINGTON, E.K. (1962b) A study of finger agnosia. *Brain* **85**, 47–66 [66, 106].

KINSBOURNE, M. & WARRINGTON, E.K. (1963) The localizing significance of limited simultaneous visual form perception. *Brain* **86**, 697–702 [61].

KINSBOURNE, M. & WARRINGTON, E.K. (1964) Disorders of spelling. *Journal of Neurology, Neurosurgery and Psychiatry* **27**, 224–228 [66].

KIRKPATRICK, J.B. & HAYMAN, L.A. (1987) White matter lesions of MR imaging of clinically healthy brains of elderly subjects: possible pathologic basis. *Neuroradiology* **162**, 509–511 [460].

KIRSHNER, H.S., TANRIDAG, O., THURMAN, L. & WHETSELL, W.O. (1987) Progressive aphasia without dementia: two cases with focal spongiform degeneration. *Annals of Neurology* **22**, 527–534 [752].

KIRSHNER, H.S., WEBB, W.G., KELLY, M.P. & WELLS, C.E. (1984) Language disturbance: an initial symptom of cortical degenerations and dementia. *Archives of Neurology* **41**, 491–496 [752].

KLABER, M. & LACEY, J. (1968) Epidemic of glandular fever. *British Medical Journal* **3**, 124 [358].

KLATZO, I., WIŚNIEWSKI, H. & STREICHER, E. (1965) Experimental production of neurofibrillary degeneration. *Journal of Neuropathology and Experimental Neurology* **24**, 187–199 [446].

KLAWANS, H.L. (1988) Psychiatric side effects during the treatment of Parkinson's disease. *Journal of Neural Transmission* **27 (Supplement)**, 117–122 [658].

KLAWANS, H.L., GOETZ, C.G., PAULSON, G.W. & BARBEAU, A. (1980) Levodopa and pre-symptomatic detection of Huntington's disease—eight-year follow-up. *New England Journal of Medicine* **302**, 1090 [467].

KLAWANS, H.L., PAULSON, G.W., RINGEL, S.P. & BARBEAU, A. (1973) The use of L-dopa in the presymptomatic detection of Huntington's chorea. In *Advances in Neurology, Vol. 1, Huntington's Chorea,* 1872–1972, eds Barbeau, A., Chase, T.N. & Paulson, G.W. Raven Press: New York [467].

KLEE, A. (1968) *A Clinical Study of Migraine with Particular Reference to the Most Severe Cases*. Munksgaard: Copenhagen [404, 405, 407].

KLEE, A. & WILLANGER, R. (1966) Disturbances of visual perception in migraine. *Acta Neurologica Scandinavica* **42**, 400–414 [407].

KLEIN, D. (1959) Ten years' inquiries about myotonic dystrophy in Swizerland (1945–1956). In *First International Congress of Neurological Sciences*, Vol. 1, eds van Bogaert, L. & Radermecker, J., pp. 318–319. Pergamon: London [719].

KLEIN, R. (1952) Immediate effects of leucotomy on cerebral functions and their significance. *Journal of Mental Science* **98**, 60–65 [27].

KLEIN, R. & DUMBLE, L.J. (1993) Transmission of Creutzfeldt–Jakob disease by blood transfusion. *Lancet* **341**, 768 [476].

KLEIN, R. & MAYER-GROSS, W. (1957) *The Clinical Examination of Patients with Organic Cerebral Disease*. Cassell: London [100].

KLEINE, W. (1925) Periodische Schlafsucht. *Monatsschrift für Psychiatrie und Neurologie* **57**, 285–320 [732].

KLEINFELD, M., PETER, S. & GILBERT, G.M. (1984) Delirium as the predominant manifestation of hyperparathyroidism. *Journal of the American Geriatric Society* **32**, 689–690 [529].

KLEIST, K. (1934) *Kriegverletzungen des Gehirns in ihrer Bedeutung für Hirnlokalisation und Hirnpathologie*. Barth: Leipzig. Quoted by Tow, P.M. (1955) *Personality Changes Following Frontal Leucotomy*. Oxford University Press: Oxford [180].

KLEIST, K. (1937) Bericht über die Gehirnpathologie in ihrer Bedeutung für Neurologie und Psychiatrie. *Zeitschrift für die gesamte Neurologie und Psychiatrie* **158**, 159–192 [22].

KLIGMAN, D. & GOLDBERG, D.A. (1975) Temporal lobe epilepsy and aggression. *Journal of Nervous and Mental Disease* **160**, 324–341 [267].

KLONOFF, H., LOW, M.D. & CLARK, C. (1977) Head injuries in children: a prospective five year follow-up. *Journal of Neurology, Neurosurgery and Psychiatry* **40**, 1211–1219 [202].

KLOTZ, M. (1957) Incidence of brain tumours in patients hospitalised for chronic mental disorders. *Psychiatric Quarterly* **31**, 669–680 [233].

KLÜVER, H. & BUCY, P.C. (1939) Preliminary analysis of functions of the temporal lobes in monkeys. *Archives of Neurology and Psychiatry* **42**, 979–1••• [23, 80].

KLUZNIK, J.C., SPEED, N., VAN VALKENBURG, C. & MAGRAW, R. (1986) Forty-year follow-up of United States prisoners of war. *American Journal of Psychiatry* **143**, 1443–1446 [195].

KNAPP, M.J., KNOPMAN, D.S., SOLOMON, P.R., PENDLEBURY, W.W., DAVIS, C.S. & GRACON, S.I. (1994) A 30-week randomized controlled trial of high-dose tacrine in patients with Alzheimer's disease. *Journal of the American Medical Association* **271**, 985–991 [504].

KNAUTH, M., RIES, S., POHIMANN, S., KERBY, T., FORSTING, M., DAFFERTSHOFER, M., HENNERICI, M. & SARTOR, K. (1997) Cohort study of multiple brain lesions in sport divers: role of a patent foramen ovale. *British Medical Journal* **314**, 701–705 [768].

KNEHR, C.A. & BEARN, A.G. (1956) Psychological impairment in Wilson's disease. *Journal of Nervous and Mental Disease* **124**, 251–255 [665].

KNOX, J.W. & NELSON, J.R. (1966) Permanent encephalopathy from toluene inhalation. *New England Journal of Medicine* **275**, 1494–1496 [629].

KNOX, S.J. (1968) Epileptic automatism and violence. *Medicine, Science and the Law* **8**, 96–104 [253, 275].

KNUPFER, L. & SPIEGEL, R. (1986) Differences in olfactory test performance between normal aged, Alzheimer and vascular type dementia individuals. *International Journal of Geriatric Psychiatry* **1**, 3–14 [441].

KOCH, T.K., BERG, B.O., DE ARMOND, S.J. & GRAVINA, R.F. (1985) Creutzfeldt–Jakob disease in a young adult with idiopathic hypopituitarism: possible relation to the administration of cadaveric human growth hormone. *New England Journal of Medicine* **313**, 731–733 [476].

KOEHLER, K. & JAKUMEIT, U. (1976) Subacute sclerosing panencephalitis presenting as Leonhard's speech-prompt catatonia. *British Journal of Psychiatry* **129**, 29–31 [362].

KOENIG, H. (1968) Dementia associated with the benign form of multiple sclerosis. *Transactions of the American Neurological Association* **93**, 227–231 [694].

KOENIG, M., HOFFMAN, E.P., BERTELSON, C.J., MONACO, A.P., FEENER, C. & KUNKEL, L.M. (1987) Complete cloning of the Duchenne muscular dystrophy (DMD) cDNA and preliminary genomic organisation of the DMD gene in normal and affected individuals. *Cell* **50**, 509 [715].

KOENIG, S., GENDELMAN, H.E., ORENSTEIN, J.M., DAL CANTO, M.C., PEZESHKPOUR, G.H., YUNGBLUTH, M., JANOTTA, F., AKSAMIT, A., MARTIN, M.A. & FAUCI, A.S. (1986) Detection of AIDS virus in macrophages in brain tissue from AIDS patients with encephalopathy. *Science* **233**, 1089–1093 [322].

KOFMAN, O. & HYLAND, H.H. (1959) Tuberose sclerosis in adults with normal intelligence. *Archives of Neurology and Psychiatry* **81**, 43–48 [702].

KOGEORGOS, J., FONAGY, P. & SCOTT, D.F. (1982) Psychiatric symptom patterns of chronic epileptics attending a neurological clinic: a controlled investigation. *British Journal of Psychiatry* **140**, 236–243 [276].

KOGEORGOS, J. & SCOTT, D.F. (1981) Biofeedback and its clinical applications. *British Journal of Hospital Medicine* **25**, 601–603 [309, 410].

KOLANSKY, H. & MOORE, W.T. (1971) Effects of marihuana on adolescents and young adults. *Journal of the American Medical Association* **216**, 486–492 [615].

KOLANSKY, H. & MOORE, W.T. (1972) Toxic effects of chronic marihuana use. *Journal of the American Medical Association* **222**, 35–41 [615, 616].

KOLARSKY, A., FREUND, K., MACHEK, J. & POLAK, O. (1967) Male sexual deviation. Association with early temporal lobe damage. *Archives of General Psychiatry* **17**, 735–743 [272].

KOLLER, W.C., GLATT, S., WILSON, R.S. & FOX, J.H. (1982) Primitive reflexes and cognitive function in the elderly. *Annals of Neurology* **12**, 302–304 [96].

KOLODNY, R.C. (1971) Sexual dysfunction in diabetic females. *Diabetes* **20**, 557–559 [536].

KOLODNY, R.C., KAHN, C.B., GOLDSTEIN, H.H. & BARNETT, D.M. (1974) Sexual dysfunction in diabetic men. *Diabetes* **23**, 306–309 [536].

KONDO, R., WAKAMATSU, N., YOSHINO, H., FUKUHARA, N., MIYATAKE, T. & TSUJI, S. (1991) Identification of a mutation in the arylsulfatase A gene of a patient with adult-type metachromatic leukodystrophy. *American Journal of Human Genetics* **48**, 971–978 [759].

KOPELMAN, M.D. (1985a) Rates of forgetting in Alzheimer-type dementia and Korsakoff's syndrome. *Neuropsychologia* **23**, 623–638 [32, 35, 437].

KOPELMAN, M.D. (1985b) Multiple memory deficits in Alzheimer-type dementia: implications for pharmacotherapy. *Psychological Medicine* **15**, 527–541 [32, 39].

KOPELMAN, M.D. (1986) The cholinergic neurotransmitter system in human memory and dementia: a review. *Quarterly Journal of Experimental Psychology* **38A**, 535–573 [32].

KOPELMAN, M.D. (1987a) Two types of confabulation. *Journal of Neurology, Neurosurgery and Psychiatry* **50**, 1482–1487 [31].

KOPELMAN, M.D. (1987b) Amnesia: organic and psychogenic. *British Journal of Psychiatry* **150**, 428–442 [33, 38, 39].

KOPELMAN, M. (1987c) Oral tetrahydroaminoacridine in the treatment of senile dementia, Alzheimer's type. *New England Journal of Medicine* **316**, 1604 [503].

KOPELMAN, M.D. (1989) Remote and autobiographical memory, temporal context memory and frontal atrophy in Korsakoff and Alzheimer patients. *Neuropsychologia* **27**, 437–460 [36, 37].

KOPELMAN, M.D. (1991) Frontal dysfunction and memory deficits in the alcoholic Korsakoff syndrome and Alzheimer-type dementia. *Brain* **114**, 117–137 [27, 37].

KOPELMAN, M.D. (1995) The Korsakoff syndrome. *British Journal of Psychiatry* **166**, 154–173 [25, 583].

KOPELMAN, M.D., CHRISTENSEN, H., PUFFETT, A. & STANHOPE, N. (1994a) The great escape: a neuropsychological study of psychogenic amnesia. *Neuropsychologia* **32**, 675–691 [34].

KOPELMAN, M.D. & CORN, T.H. (1988) Cholinergic 'blockade' as a model for cholinergic depletion: a comparison of the memory deficits with those of Alzheimer-type dementia and the alcoholic Korsakoff syndrome. *Brain* **111**, 1079–1110 [32, 504].

KOPELMAN, M.D., GREEN, R.E.A., GUINAN, E.M., LEWIS, P.D.R. & STANHOPE, N. (1994b) The case of the amnesic intelligence officer. *Psychological Medicine* **24**, 1037–1045 [33].

KOPELMAN, M.D. & LISHMAN, W.A. (1986) Pharmacological treatments of dementia (non-cholinergic). *British Medical Bulletin* **42**, 101–105 [501].

KOPELMAN, M.D., WILSON, B.A. & BADDELEY, A.D. (1989) The autobiographical and personal semantic memory in amnesic patients. *Journal of Clinical and Experimental Neuropsychology* **11**, 724–744 [36].

KOPPEL, B.S., WORMSER, G.P., TUCHMAN, A.J., MAAYAN, S., HEWLETT, D. Jr & DARAS, M. (1985) Central nervous system involvement in patients with acquired immune deficiency syndrome (AIDS). *Acta Neurologica Scandinavica* **71**, 337–353 [320].

KORAN, L.M., SOX, H.C., MARTON, K.I., MOLTZEN, S., SOX, C.H., KRAEMER, H.C., IMAI, K., KELSEY, T.G., ROSE, T.G., LEVIN, L.C. & CHANDRA, S. (1989) Medical evaluation of psychiatric patients. *Archives of General Psychiatry* **46**, 733–740 [95].

KOREIN, J. & BRUDNY, J. (1976) Integrated EMG feedback in the management of spasmodic torticollis and focal dystonia: a prospective study of 80 patients. In *The Basal Ganglia*. Association for Research in Nervous and Mental Disease 55, ed. Yahr, M.D., pp. 385–424. Raven Press: New York [675].

KORMAN, M., TRIMBOLI, F. & SEMLER, I. (1980) A comparative evaluation of 162 inhalant users. *Addictive Behaviors* **5**, 143–152 [630].

KOROLENKO, C.P., YEVSEYEVA, T.A. & VOLKOV, P.P. (1969) Data for a comparative account of toxic psychoses of various aetiologies. *British Journal of Psychiatry* **115**, 273–779 [631].

KORSAKOFF, S.S. (1887) Disturbance of psychic function in alcoholic paralysis and its relation to the disturbance of the psychic sphere in multiple neuritis of non-alcoholic origin. *Vestnik Psichiatrii*, Vol. IV, fasicle 2. Quoted by Victor, M., Adams, R.D. & Collins, G.H. (1971) *The Wernicke–Korsakoff Syndrome*. Blackwell Scientific Publications: Oxford [577].

KOSAKA, K., MATSUSHITA, M., IIZUKA, R. & MEHRAEIN, P. (1982) Pick's disease and head trauma. *Folia Psychiatrica et Neurologica Japonica* **36**, 125–136 [461].

KOSTEN, T.R. (1990) Neurobiology of abused drugs. Opioids and stimulants. *Journal of Nervous and Mental Disease* **178**, 217–227 [611, 620].

KOVANEN, J., HALTIA, M. & CANTELL, K. (1980) Failure of interferon to modify Creutzfeldt–Jakob disease. *British Medical Journal* **280**, 902 [506].

KOVELMAN, J.A. & SCHEIBEL, A.B. (1984) A neurohistological correlate of schizophrenia. *Biological Psychiatry* **19**, 1601–1621 [86].

KOZOL, H.L. (1945) Pretraumatic personality and sequelae of head injury. *Archives of Neurology and Psychiatry* **53**, 358–364 [173, 174].

KOZOL, H.L. (1946) Pretraumatic personality and psychiatric sequelae of head injury. *Archives of Neurology and Psychiatry* **56**, 245–275 [174].

KRAEPELIN, E. (1896) *Psychiatrie*, 5th edn. Barth: Leipzig [507].

KRAEPELIN, E. (1910) *Psychaitrie, Vol. 2: Klinische Psychiatrie.* Barth: Leipzig [755].

KRAFT, E., FINBY, N. & SCHILLINGER, A. (1963) Routine skull roentgenography of psychiatric hospital admissions. *American Journal of Roentgenography* **89**, 1212–1219 [233].

KRAFT, E., SCHILLINGER, A., FINBY, N. & HALPERIN, M. (1965) Routine skull radiography in a neuropsychiatric hospital. *American Journal of Psychiatry* **121**, 1011–1012 [135, 233].

KRAL, V.A. (1959) Amnesia and the amnestic syndrome. *Canadian Psychiatric Association Journal* **4**, 61–68 [38].

KRAL, V.A. (1962) Senescent forgetfulness: benign and malignant. *Canadian Medical Association Journal* **86**, 257–260 [431].

KRAL, V.A. (1978) Benign senescent forgetfulness. In *Alzheimer's Disease: Senile Dementia and Related Disorders, Aging*, Vol. 7, eds Katzman, R., Terry, R.D. & Bick, K.L., pp. 47–51. Raven Press: New York [432].

KRAL, V.A. (1983) The relationship between senile dementia (Alzheimer type) and depression. *Canadian Journal of Psychiatry* **28**, 304–306 [487].

KRAL, V.A. & DUROST, H.B. (1953) A comparative study of the amnesic syndrome in various organic conditions. *American Journal of Psychiatry* **110**, 41–47 [27].

KRAMER, P.L., DE LEON, D., OZELIUS, L., RISCH, N., BRESSMAN, S.B., BRIN, M.F., SCHUBACK, D.E., BURKE, R.E., KWIATKOWSKI, D.J., SHALE, H., GUSELLA, J.F., BREAKFIELD, X.O. & FAHN, S. (1990) Dystonia gene in Ashkenazi Jewish population is located on chromosome 9$_q$32–34. *Annals of Neurology* **27**, 114–120 [671].

KRAPF, E.E. (1957) On the pathogenesis of epileptic and hysterical seizures. *Bulletin of the World Health Organization* **16**, 749–762 [252, 293].

KRÄUPL-TAYLOR, F. (1966) *Psychopathology: Its Causes and Symptoms.* Butterworths: London [485].

KRAUSS, S. (1946) Post-choreic personality and neurosis. *Journal of Mental Sciences* **92**, 75–95 [374].

KRAUSS, S. (1957) Schizophreniform psychoses in the later lives of encephalopathic persons. *Report of Second International Congress of Psychiatry, Zurich*, Vol. 2, 100–103 [374].

KRAWIECKI, J.A., COUPER, L. & WALTON, D. (1957) The efficacy of parentrovite in the treament of a group of senile psychotics. *Journal of Mental Science* **103**, 601–605 [501].

KREISLER, O., LIBERT, E. & HORWITT, M.K. (1948) Psychiatric observations on induced vitamin B complex deficiency in psychotic patients. *American Journal of Psychiatry* **105**, 107–110 [572].

KREMER, M. (1943) Discussion on disorders of personality after head injury. *Proceedings of the Royal Society of Medicine* **37**, 564–566 [178].

KRETSCHMER, E. (1949) Die Orbitalhirn-und Zwischenhirnsyndrome nach Schädelbasisfrakturen. *Allgemeine Zeitschrift für Psychiatrie* **124**, 358–360 [180].

KRETSCHMER, E. (1956) Lokalisation und Beurteilung psychophysischer Syndrome bei Hirnverletzten. In *Das Hirntrauma*, ed. Rehwald, E., pp. 155–158. Thieme: Stuttgart [180].

KRETSCHMER, H. (1968) Zur Klinik des Balkensyndroms. *Archiv für Psychiatrie und Nervenkrankheiten* **211**, 250–265 [770].

KRIL, J.J. & HARPER, C.G. (1989) Neuronal counts from four cortical regions of alcoholic brains. *Acta Neuropathologica* **79**, 200–204 [604].

KRISTENSEN, O. & SINDRUP, E.H. (1978a) Psychomotor epilepsy and psychosis. I. Physical aspects. *Acta Neurologica Scandinavica* **57**, 361–369 [281, 283, 284].

KRISTENSEN, O. & SINDRUP, E.H. (1978b) Psychomotor epilepsy and psychosis. II. Electroencephalographic findings (sphenoidal electrode recordings). *Acta Neurologica Scandinavica* **57**, 370–379 [282, 283].

KRONFOL, Z., GREDEN, J. & CARROLL, B. (1981) Psychiatric aspects of diabetes mellitus: diabetes and depression. *British Journal of Psychiatry* **139**, 172–173 [536].

KRONFOL, Z., HAMSHER, K. DE S., DIGRE, K. & WAZIRI, R. (1978) Depression and hemispheric functions: changes associated with unilateral ECT. *British Journal of Psychiatry* **132**, 560–567 [89].

KRYNICKI, V.E. (1978) Cerebral dysfunction in repetitively assaultive adolescents. *Journal of Nervous and Mental Disease* **166**, 59–67 [83].

KUEHNLE, J., MENDELSON, J.H., DAVIS, K.R. & NEW, P.F.J. (1977) Computed tomographic examination of heavy marijuana smokers. *Journal of the American Medical Association* **237**, 1231–1232 [616].

KUGLER, J. (1964) *Electroencephalography in Hospital and General Consulting Practice: An Introduction.* Elsevier: Amsterdam [129, 357, 433].

KUHL, D.E., MARKHAM, C.H., METTER, E.J., RIEGE, W.H., PHELPS, M.E. & MAZZIOTTA, J.C. (1985a) Local cerebral glucose utilization in symptomatic and presymptomatic Huntington's disease. In *Brain Imaging and Brain Function*, ed. Sokoloff, L. Association for Research in Nervous and Mental Disease, Vol. 63, pp. 199–209. Raven Press: New York [470].

KUHL, D.E., METTER, E.J. & RIEGE, W.H. (1985b) Patterns of cerebral glucose utilization in depression, multiple infarct dementia, and Alzheimer's disease. In *Brain Imaging and Brain Function*, ed. Sokoloff, L. Association for Research in Nervous and Mental Disease, Vol. 63, pp. 211–226. Raven Press: New York [457].

KUHL, D.E., PHELPS, M.E., MARKHAM, C.H., METTER, J., RIEGE, W.H. & WINTER, J. (1982) Cerebral metabolism and atrophy in Huntington's disease determined by ^{18}FDG and computed tomographic scan. *Annals of Neurology* **12**, 425–434 [470].

KUKS, J.B.M., COOK, M.J., FISH, D.R., STEVENS, J.M. & SHORVON, S.D. (1993) Hippocampal sclerosis in epilepsy and childhood febrile seizures. *Lancet* **342**, 1391–1394 [246].

KUNZE, K. & LEITENMAIER, K. (1976) Vitamin B$_{12}$ deficiency and subacute combined degeneration of the spinal cord. Ch. 6 in *Handbook of Clinical Neurology*, Vol. 28, *Metabolic and Deficiency Diseases of the Nervous System, Part II*, eds Vinken, P.J. & Bruyn, G.W. North-Holland Publishing Co.: Amsterdam [589].

KUPFER, D.J., HIMMELHOCH, J.M., SWARTZBURG, M., ANDERSON, C., BUICK, R. & DETRE, T.P. (1972) Hypersomnia in manic-depressive disease (a preliminary report). *Diseases of the Nervous System* **33**, 720–724 [735].

KURIANSKY, J.B., GURLAND, B.J. & FLEISS, J.L. (1976) The assessment of self-care capacity in geriatric psychiatric patients by objective and subjective methods. *Journal of Clinical Psychology* **32**, 95–102 [125].

KURLAN, R., EAPEN, V., McDERMOTT, M.P. & ROBERTSON, M.M. (1994)

Bilineal transmission in Tourette's syndrome families. *Neurology* **44**, 2336–2342 [681].

KURLAN, R. & TRINIDAD, K.S. (1995) Treatment of tics. Ch. 9 in *Treatment of Movement Disorders*, ed. Kurlan, R. J.B. Lippincott: Philadelphia [687].

KURLAND, G.S., HAMOLSKY, M.W. & FREEDBERG, A.S. (1955) Studies in non-myxoedematous hypometabolism. I: The clinical syndrome and the effect of triiodothyronine, alone or combined with thyroxine. *Journal of Clinical Endocrinology and Metabolism* **15**, 1354–1366 [514].

KURLAND, L.T., FARO, S.N. & SIEDLER, H. (1960) The outbreak of a neurologic disorder in Minamata, Japan, and its relationship to the ingestion of seafood contaminated by mercuric compounds. *World Neurology* **1**, 370–395 [635].

KURLAND, L.T. & MULDER, D.W. (1954) Epidemiologic investigations of amyotrophic lateral sclerosis. *Neurology* **4**, 355–378 and 438–448 [708].

KURLAND, L.T., RADHAKRISHNAN, K., WILLIAMS, D.B. & WARING, S.C. (1994) Amyotrophic lateral sclerosis–parkinsonism–dementia complex on Guam: epidemiologic and etiological perspectives. Ch. 5 in *Motor Neurone Disease*, ed. Williams, A.C. Chapman & Hall: London [709].

KURLAND, M.L. (1965) Gilles de la Tourette's syndrome: the psychotherapy of two cases. *Comprehensive Psychiatry* **6**, 298–305 [686].

KUZNIECKY, R. (1994) Focal cortical dysplasia in temporal lobe epilepsy: the role of magnetic resonance imaging. Ch. 20 in *Magnetic Resonance Scanning and Epilepsy*, eds Shorvon, S.D., Fish, D.R., Andermann, F., Bydder, G.M. & Stefan, H. Plenum Press: New York & London [246].

KUZNIECKY, R., DE LA SAYETTE, V., ETHIER, R., MELANSON, D., ANDERMANN, F., BERKOVIC, S., ROBITAILLE, Y., OLIVIER, A., PETERS, T. & FEINDEL, W. (1987) Magnetic resonance imaging in temporal lobe epilepsy: pathological correlations. *Annals of Neurology* **22**, 341–347 [289].

KWONG, K.K., BELLIVEAU, J.W., CHESLER, D.A., GOLDBERG, I.E., WEISSKOFF, R.M., PONCELET, B.P., KENNEDY, D.N., HOPPEL, B.E., COHEN, M.S., TURNER, R., CHENG, H.-M., BRADY, T.J. & ROSEN, B.R. (1992) Dynamic magnetic resonance imaging of human brain activity during primary sensory stimulation. *Proceedings of the National Academy of Sciences* **89**, 5675–5679 [143].

LADURNER, G., ILIFF, L.D. & LECHNER, H. (1982) Clinical factors associated with dementia in ischaemic stroke. *Journal of Neurology, Neurosurgery and Psychiatry* **45**, 97–101 [383].

LAGENSTEIN, I., WILLIG, R.P. & KUHNE, D. (1979) Reversible cerebral atrophy caused by corticotrophin. *Lancet* **1**, 1246–1247 [141].

LAHEY, F.H. (1931) Non-activated (apathetic) type of hyperthyroidism. *New England Journal of Medicine* **204**, 747–748 [511].

LAMBERTI, J.S. & BELLNIER, T. (1993) Clozapine and tardive dystonia. *Journal of Nervous and Mental Disease* **181**, 137–138 [645].

LAMPERT, P., TOM, M.I. & CUMINGS, J.N. (1962) Encephalopathy in Whipple's disease. A histochemical study. *Neurology* **12**, 65–71 [760].

LAMPERT, P.W. & HARDMAN, J.M. (1984) Morphological changes in brains of boxers. *Journal of the American Medical Association* **251**, 2676–2678 [207].

LANCE, J.W. (1993) *Mechanism and Management of Headache*, 5th edn. Butterworth Heinemann: Oxford [399, 402, 403, 409, 410].

LANCET (1950) Death of a mind: a study of disintegration by an anonymous author. *Lancet* **1**, 1012–1015 [499].

LANCET (1966a) Leading article: Encephalitis of lethargica type in a mental hospital. *Lancet* **2**, 1014–1015 [351].

LANCET (1966b) Leading article: Polyoma virus and leucoencephalopathy. *Lancet* **1**, 353–354 [752].

LANCET (1970) Annotation: a new line on age pigment? *Lancet* **2**, 451–452 [502].

LANCET (1971) Annotation: cannabis encephalopathy. *Lancet* **2**, 1240–1241 [616].

LANCET (1973) Zinc deficiency in man. Lancet **1**, 299–300 [563].

LANCET (1977) Cardiogenic dementia. *Lancet* **1**, 27–28 [431].

LANCET (1978) Factitious hypoglycaemia. *Lancet* **1**, 1293 [544].

LANCET (1989) SPET and PET in epilepsy. *Lancet* **1**, 135–137 [289].

LANCET (1990a) Editorial: zidovudine for symptomless HIV infection. *Lancet* **335**, 821–822 [336].

LANCET (1990b) Editorial: BSE in perspective. *Lancet* **335**, 1252–1253 [475].

LANDFIELD, P.W., CADWALLADER, L.B. & VINSANT, S. (1988) Quantitative changes in hippocampal structure following long-term exposure of Δ^9-tetrahydrocannabinol: possible mediation by glucocorticoid systems (BRE 13333). *Brain Research* **443**, 47–62 [612].

LANDOLT, H. (1958) Serial electroencephalographic investigations during psychotic episodes in epileptic patients and during schizophrenic attacks. Ch. 3 in *Lectures on Epilepsy*, ed. Lorentz de Haas, A.M. Elsevier: Amsterdam [256, 257, 284].

LANDRIGAN, P.J. (1997) Illness in Gulf war veterans. Causes and consequences. *Journal of the American Medical Association* **277**, 259–261 [637].

LANG, A.E., QUINN, N., BRINCAT, S., MARSDEN, C.D. & PARKES, J.D. (1982) Pergolide in late-stage Parkinson's disease. *Annals of Neurology* **12**, 243–247 [659].

LANGAN, S.J., DEARY, I.J., HEPBURN, D.A. & FRIER, B.M. (1991) Cumulative cognitive impairment following recurrent severe hypoglycaemia in adult patients with insulin-treated diabetes mellitus. *Diabetalogia* **34**, 337–344 [537].

LANGFITT, T.W., OBRIST, W.D., ALAVI, A., GROSSMAN, R.I., ZIMMERMAN, R., JAGGI, J., UZZELL, B., REIVICH, M. & PATTON, D.R. (1986) Computerized tomography, magnetic resonance imaging, and positron emission tomography in the study of brain trauma. *Journal of Neurosurgery* **64**, 760–767 [166].

LANGLAIS, P.J. (1995) Alcohol-related thiamine deficiency. Impact on cognitive and memory functioning. *Alcohol Health and Research World* **19**, 113–121 [576].

LANGSTON, J.W., BALLARD, P., TETRUD, J.W. & IRWIN, I. (1983) Chronic parkinsonism in humans due to a product of mepiridine-analog synthesis. *Science* **219**, 979–980 [648].

LANGWORTHY, O.R. (1936) Neurological abnormalities produced by electricity. *Journal of Nervous and Mental Disease* **84**, 13–26 [765].

LANGWORTHY, O.R. & BETZ, B.J. (1944) Narcolepsy as a type of response to emotional conflicts. *Psychosomatic Medicine* **6**, 211–226 [725].

LANSDELL, H. & MIRSKY, A.F. (1964) Attention in focal and centrencephalic epilepsy. *Experimental Neurology* **9**, 463–469 [262].

LANSDOWN, R.G., SHEPHERD, J., CLAYTON, B.E., DELVES, H.T., GRAHAM, P.J. & TURNER, W.C. (1974) Blood-lead levels, behaviour and intelligence. A population study. *Lancet* **1**, 538–541 [632].

LANTOS, P.L. (1988) The neuropathology of schizophrenia: a critical review of recent work. Ch. 7 in *Schizophrenia. The Major Issues*, eds Bebbington, P. & McGuffin, P., pp. 73–89. Heinemann: Oxford [86].

LANTOS, P.L. (1992a) The neuropathology of unusual dementias: an overview. Ch. 2 in *Unusual Dementias*, ed. Rossor, M.N. Ballière Tindall: London [462].

LANTOS, P.L. (1992b) From slow virus to prion: a review of transmissible spongiform encephalopathies. *Histopathology* **20**, 1–11 [473, 478].

LANTOS, P.L. & CAIRNS, N.J. (1994) The neuropathology of Alzheimer's disease. Ch. 12 in *Dementia*, eds Burns, A. & Levy, R. Chapman & Hall: London [441, 442].

LANTOS, P.L., McLAUGHLIN, J.E., SCHOLTZ, C.L., BERRY, C.L. & TIGHE, J.R. (1989) Neuropathology of the brain in HIV infection. *Lancet* **1**, 309–310 [320].

LANTOS, P.L. & PAPP, M.I. (1994) Cellular pathology of multiple system atrophy: a review. *Journal of Neurology, Neurosurgery and Psychiatry* **57**, 129–133 [669].

LAPRESLE, J. & FARDEAU, M. (1967) The central nervous system and carbon monoxide poisoning, II: Anatomical study of brain lesions following intoxication with carbon monoxide (22 cases). In *Carbon Monoxide Poisoning*, eds Bour, H. & Ledingham, I.McA. Progress in Brain Research, Vol. 24. Elsevier: Amsterdam [552].

LARGEN, J.W. Jr, CALDERON, M. & SMITH, R.C. (1983) Asymmetries in the densities of white and gray matter in the brains of schizophrenic patients. *American Journal of Psychiatry* **140**, 1060–1062 [138].

LARSBY, H. & LINDGREN, E. (1940) Encephalographic examinations of 125 institutionalised epileptics. *Acta Psychiatrica et Neurologica* **15**, 337–352 [139].

LARSEN, J.P., HØIEN, T., LUNDBERG, I. & ØDEGAARD, H. (1990) MRI evaluation of the size and symmetry of the planum temporale in adolescents with developmental dyslexia. *Brain and Language* **39**, 289–301 [48].

LARSSON, T., SJÖGREN, T. & JACOBSON, G. (1963) Senile dementia: a clinical, sociomedical and genetic study. *Acta Psychiatrica Scandinavica* **167 (Supplement)**, 1–259 [430, 431, 456].

LASHLEY, K.S. (1929) *Brain Mechanisms and Intelligence*. University of Chicago Press. Reissued 1963, Dover Publications: New York [21].

LAURENT, J., DEBRY, G. & FLOQUET, J. (1971) *Hypoglycaemic Tumours*. Excerpta Medica: Amsterdam [545].

LAURITZEN, M. (1987) Controversial aspects of brain imaging of migraine. Ch. 11 in *Impact of Functional Imaging in Neurology and Psychiatry*, eds Wade, J., Knežević, S., Maximilian, V.A., Mubrin, S. & Prohovnik, I. *Current Problems in Neurology* **5** [402].

LAUTER, H. & MEYER, J.E. (1968) Clinical and nosological concepts of senile dementia. In *Senile Dementia: Clinical and Therapeutic Aspects*, eds Müller, C.H. & Ciompi, L. Huber: Bern [430, 433, 438, 449].

LAVENDER, A. (1981) A behavioural approach to the treatment of epilepsy. *Behavioural Psychotherapy* **9**, 231–243 [309].

LAW, W.R. & NELSON, E.R. (1968) Gasoline-sniffing by an adult: report of a case with the unusual complication of lead encephalopathy. *Journal of the American Medical Association* **204**, 1002–1004 [630].

LAWSON, I.R. & MacLEOD, R.D.M. (1969) The use of imipramine ('Tofranil') and other psychotrophic drugs in organic emotionalism. *British Journal of Psychiatry* **115**, 281–285 [392].

LAY, C. & WOODS, B. (1989) *Caring for the Person with Dementia: A Guide for Families and Other Carers*, 2nd edn. Alzheimer's Disease Society: London [498].

LE BOEUF, A., LODGE, J. & EAMES, P.G. (1978) Vasopressin and memory in Korsakoff syndrome. *Lancet* **2**, 1370 [585].

LE FEUVRE, C.M., ISAACS, A.J. & FRANK, O.S. (1982) Bromocriptine-induced psychosis in acromegaly. *British Medical Journal* **285**, 1315 [522].

LE MAY, M. (1976) Morphological cerebral asymmetries and modern man, fossil man, and non-human primate. *Annals of the New York Academy of Sciences* **280**, 349–366 [41, 89].

LE MAY, M. (1977) Asymmetries of the skull and handedness. *Journal of the Neurological Sciences* **32**, 243–253 [41, 89].

LE MAY, M. & GESCHWIND, N. (1978) Asymmetries of the human cerebral hemispheres. Ch. 15 in *Language Acquisition and Language Breakdown: Parallels and Divergencies*, eds Caramazza, A. & Zurif, E.B. Johns Hopkins University Press: Baltimore and London [41].

LE MAY, M., STAFFORD, J.L., SANDOR, T., ALBERT, M., HAYKAL, H. & ZAMANI, A. (1986) Statistical assessment of perceptual CT scan ratings in patients with Alzheimer type dementia. *Journal of Computer Assisted Tomography* **10**, 802–809 [434].

LEBENSOHN, Z.M. & JENKINS, R.B. (1975) Improvement in parkinsonism in depressed patients treated with ECT. *American Journal of Psychiatry* **132**, 283–285 [656].

LEBOWITZ, H.E. (1965) Endocrine-metabolic syndromes associated with neoplasms. Ch. 11 in *The Remote Effects of Cancer on the Nervous System*, eds Brain, W.R. & Norris, F.H. Contemporary Neurology Symposia, Vol. 1. Grune & Stratton: New York [743].

LECHE, P. (1972) Speech therapy and the treatment of cerebrovascular diseases. *Proceedings of the Royal Society of Medicine* **65**, 85–88 [390].

LECKMAN, J., ANANTH, J.V., BAN, T.A. & LEHMANN, H.E. (1971) Pentylenetetrazol in the treatment of geriatric patients with disturbed memory function. *Journal of Clinical Pharmacology* **11**, 301–303 [502].

LECKMAN, J.F., PRICE, R.A., WALKUP, J.T., ORT, S., PAULS, D.L. & COHEN, D.J. (1987) Nongenetic factors in Gilles de la Tourette's syndrome. *Archives of General Psychiatry* **44**, 100 [686].

LEDINGHAM, J.G.G. (1983) Water and sodium homeostasis. In *Oxford Textbook of Medicine*, 1st edn, Vol. 2, eds Weatherall, D.J., Ledingham, J.G.G. & Warrell, D.A., pp. 18.19–18.28. Oxford University Press: Oxford [525].

LEDOUX, J.E., WILSON, D.H. & GAZZANIGA, M.S. (1977) Manipulospatial aspects of cerebral lateralization: clues to the origin of lateralization. *Neuropsychologia* **15**, 743–750 [62].

LEE, K., MOLLER, L., HARDT, F., HAUBER, A. & JENSEN, E. (1979) Alcohol-induced brain damage and liver damage in young males. *Lancet* **2**, 759–761 [607].

LEE, M.S. & MARSDEN, C.D. (1994) Neurological sequelae following carbon monoxide poisoning. Clinical course and outcome according to clinical types and brain computed tomography scan findings. *Movement Disorders* **9**, 550–558 [551, 552].

LEE, W.R. (1981) What happens in lead poisoning? *Journal of the Royal College of Physicians of London* **15**, 48–54 [631].

LEES, A.J. (1985) *Tics and Related Disorders*. Churchill Livingstone: Edinburgh [680, 681].

LEES, A.J. (1995) on behalf of the Parkinson's Disease Research Group of the United Kingdom. Comparison of therapeutic effects and mortality data of levodopa and levodopa combined with selegiline in patients with early, mild Parkinson's disease. *British Medical Journal* **311**, 1602–1607 [650].

LEES, A.J., ROBERTSON, M., TRIMBLE, M.R. & MURRAY, N.M.F. (1984) A clinical study of Gilles de la Tourette syndrome in the United Kingdom. *Journal of Neurology, Neurosurgery and Psychiatry* **47**, 1–8 [685].

LEES, A.J. & SMITH, E. (1983) Cognitive deficits in the early stages of Parkinson's disease. *Brain* **106**, 257–270 [654].

LEES, F. (1970) *The Diagnosis and Treatment of Diseases Affecting the Nervous System*, Vols 1 and 2. Staples Press: London [358, 373].

LEGG, N.J. (1967) Virus antibodies in subacute sclerosing panencephalitis: a study of 22 patients. *British Medical Journal* **3**, 350–352 [362].

LEGROS, J.J., GILOT, P., SERON, X., CLAESSENS, J., ADAM, A., MOEGLEN, J.M., AUDIBERT, A. & BERCHIER, P. (1978) Influence of vasopressin on learning and memory. *Lancet* **1**, 41–42 [585].

LEHMANN, H.E. & BAN, T.A. (1968) Studies with new drugs in the treatment of convulsive disorders. *International Journal of Clinical Pharmacology, Therapy and Toxicology* **1**, 230–234 [306].

LEHMANN, H.J. & LAMPE, H. (1970) Observations on the inter-hemispheric transmission of information in 9 patients with corpus callosum defect. *European Neurology* **4**, 129–147 [770].

LEHRICH, J.R., KATZ, M., RORKE, L.B., BARBANTI-BRODANO, G. & KOPROWSKI, H. (1970) Subacute sclerosing panencephalitis. Encephalitis in hamsters produced by viral agents isolated from human brain cells. *Archives of Neurology* **23**, 97–102 [362].

LEIDER, W., MAGOFFIN, R.L., LENNETTE, E.H. & LEONARDS, L.N.R. (1965) Herpes-simplex-virus encephalitis: its possible association with reactivated latent infection. *New England Journal of Medicine* **273**, 341–347 [356, 357].

LEIGH, A.D. (1946) Infections of the nervous system occurring during an epidemic of influenza B. *British Medical Journal* **2**, 936–938 [354].

LEIGH, D. (1951) Subacute necrotizing encephalomyelopathy in an infant. *Journal of Neurology, Neurosurgery and Psychiatry* **14**, 216–221 [587].

LEIGH, D. (1952) Pellagra and the nutritional neuropathies: a neuropathological review. *Journal of Mental Science* **98**, 130–142 [573].

LEIGH, H. & KRAMER, S.I. (1984) The psychiatric manifestations of endocrine disease. *Advances in Internal Medicine* **29**, 413–445 [519].

LEIGH, P.N. (1994) Ubiquitin. Ch. 16 in *Motor Neurone Disease*, ed. Williams, A.C. Chapman & Hall: London [707].

LEIGH, P.N., ANDERTON, B.H., DODSON, A., GALLO, J.-M., SWASH, M. & POWER, D.M. (1988) Ubiquitin deposits in anterior horn cells in motor neurone disease. *Neuroscience Letters* **93**, 197–203 [707].

LENNOX, B. & PRITCHARD, S. (1950) The association of bronchial carcinoma and peripheral neuritis. *Quarterly Journal of Medicine* **19**, 97–109 [739].

LENNOX, G. (1992) Lewy body dementia. Ch. 9 in *Unusual Dementias*, ed. Rossor, M.N. Baillière Tindall: London [451, 452, 505].

LENNOX, G., LOWE, J., BYRNE, E.J., LANDON, M., MAYER, R.J. & GODWIN-AUSTEN, R.B. (1989a) Diffuse Lewy body disease. *Lancet* **1**, 323–324 [452].

LENNOX, G., LOWE, J., MORRELL, K., LANDON, M. & MAYER, J. (1989b) Anti-ubiquitin immunocytochemistry is more sensitive than conventional techniques in the detection of diffuse Lewy body disease. *Journal of Neurology, Neurosurgery and Psychiatry* **52**, 67–71 [452].

LENNOX, W.G. (1960) *Epilepsy and Related Disorders*, Vols 1 and 2. Churchill: London [238, 241, 253, 261].

LEONARD, B.E. (1986) Is ethanol a neurotoxin?: the effects of ethanol on neuronal structure and function. *Alcohol and Alcoholism* **21**, 325–338 [607].

LEREBOULLET, J., PLUVINAGE, R. & AMSTUTZ, A. (1956) Aspects cliniques et électroencéphalographiques des atrophies cérébrales alcooliques. *Revue Neurologique* **94**, 674–682 [605].

LESLIE, K.O., ROBERTSON, A.S. & NORENBERG, M.D. (1980) Central pontine myelinolysis: an osmotic gradient pathogenesis. *Journal of Neuropathy and Experimental Neurology* **39**, 370 [586].

LESSELL, S., HIRANO, A., TORRES, J. & KURLAND, L.T. (1962) Parkinsonism–dementia complex. *Archives of Neurology* **7**, 377–385 [708].

LESSER, R. & REICH, S. (1982) Language disorders. Ch. 5 in *The Pathology and Psychology of Cognition*, ed. Burton, A. Methuen: London [43].

LESSER, R.P., MODIC, M.T., WEINSTEIN, M.A., DUCHESNEAU, P.M., LÜDERS, H., DINNER, D.S., MORRIS III, H.H., ESTES, M., CHOU, S.M. & HAHN, J.F. (1986) Magnetic resonance imaging (1.5 tesla) in patients with intractable focal seizures. *Archives of Neurology* **43**, 367–371 [289].

LETEMENDIA, F. & PAMPIGLIONE, G. (1958) Clinical and electroencephalographic observations in Alzheimer's disease. *Journal of Neurology, Neurosurgery and Psychiatry* **21**, 167–172 [439].

LETEMENDIA, F.J.J., PROWSE, A. & SOUTHMAYD, S. (1981) Diagnostic use of sleep deprivation. *British Journal of Psychiatry* **138**, 352 [489].

LEVIN, E. (1991) Carers—problems, strains, and services. Ch. 8B in *Psychiatry in the Elderly*, eds Jacoby, R. & Oppenheimer, C. Oxford University Press: Oxford [498].

LEVIN, E., MORIARTY, J. & GORBACH, P. (1994) *Better for the Break*. HMSO: London [498].

LEVIN, H.S. (1989) Memory deficit after closed head injury. *Journal of Clinical and Experimental Neuropsychology* **12**, 129–153 [169].

LEVIN, H.S., AMPARO, E., EISENBERG, H.M., WILLIAMS, D.H., HIGH, W.M., McARDLE, C.B., & WEINER, R.L. (1987a) Magnetic resonance imaging and computerized tomography in relation to the neurobehavioural sequelae of mild and moderate head injuries. *Journal of Neurosurgery* **66**, 706–713 [166].

LEVIN, H.S., HIGH, W.M. & EISENBERG, H.M. (1988) Learning and forgetting during post-traumatic amnesia in head injured patients. *Journal of Neurology, Neurosurgery and Psychiatry* **51**, 14–20 [169].

LEVIN, H.S., HIGH, W.M., MEYERS, C.A., VON LAUFEN, A., HAYDEN, M.E. & EISENBERG, H.M. (1985) Impairment of remote memory after closed head injury. *Journal of Neurology, Neurosurgery and Psychiatry* **48**, 556–563 [169].

LEVIN, H.S., LIPPOLD, S.C., GOLDMAN, A., HANDEL, S., HIGH, W.M., EISENBERG, H.M. & ZELITT, D. (1987b) Neurobehavioral functioning and magnetic resonance imaging findings in young boxers. *Journal of Neurosurgery* **67**, 657–667 [206].

LEVIN, H.S., MATTIS, S., RUFF, R.M., EISENBERG, H.M., MARSHALL, L.F., TABADDOR, K., HIGH, W.M. & FRANKOWSKI, R.F. (1987c) Neurobehavioral outcome following minor head injury: a three-center study. *Journal of Neurosurgery* **66**, 234–243 [182].

LEVIN, H.S., RODNITZKY, R.L. & MICK, D.L. (1976) Anxiety associated with exposure to organophosphate compounds. *Archives of General Psychiatry* **33**, 225–228 [637].

LEVIN, M. (1935) The pathogenesis of cataplexy on anger. *Journal of Neurology and Psychopathology* **16**, 140–143 [725].

LEVIN, M. (1936) Periodic somnolence and morbid hunger: a new syndrome. *Brain* **59**, 494–504 [732].

LEVIN, M. (1953) Aggression, guilt and cataplexy. *Archives of Neurology and Psychiatry* **69**, 224–235 [727].

LEVIN, M.E. (1960) 'Metabolic insufficiency': a double-blind study using triiodothyronine, thyroxine and a placebo: psychometric evaluation of the hypometabolic patient. *Journal of Clinical Endocrinology and Metabolism* **20**, 106–115 [514].

LEVIN, S. (1952) Epileptic clouded states. A review of 52 cases. *Journal of Nervous and Mental Disease* **116**, 215–225 [257].

LEVINE, D.N. & FINKLESTEIN, S. (1982) Delayed psychosis after right temporoparietal stroke or trauma: relation to epilepsy. *Neurology* **32**, 267–273 [388].

LEVINE, I.M., ESTES, J.W. & LOONEY, J.M. (1968) Hereditary neurological disease with acanthocytosis. *Archives of Neurology* **19**, 403–409 [757].

LEVINSON, D.F. & SIMPSON, G.M. (1986) Neuroleptic-induced extrapyramidal symptoms with fever. *Archives of General Psychiatry* **43**, 839–848 [627].

LEVY, A. & LIGHTMAN, S.S. (1994) Diagnoses and management of pituitary tumours. *British Medical Journal* **308**, 1087–1091 [232].

LEVY, R. (1970) Hanover's complaint. Review of *George III and the Mad-Business* by Macalpine, I. and Hunter, R. *British Journal of Psychiatry* **117**, 106–107 [567].

LEVY, R. (1994) Cholinergic treatment of Alzheimer's disease. Ch. 29 in *Dementia*, eds Burns, A. & Levy, R. Chapman & Hall: London [503].

LEVY, R., EAGGER, S., GRIFFITHS, M., PERRY, E., HONOVAR, M., DEAN, A. & LANTOS, P. (1994) Lewy bodies and response to tacrine in Alzheimer's disease. *Lancet* **343**, 176 [505].

LEVY, R., ISAACS, A. & BEHRMAN, J. (1971) Neurophysiological correlates of senile dementia: II. The somatosensory evoked response. *Psychological Medicine* **1**, 159–165 [431].

LEVY, R., ISAACS, A. & HAWKS, G. (1970) Neurophysiological correlates of senile dementia: I. Motor and sensory nerve conduction velocity. *Psychological Medicine* **1**, 40–47 [431].

LEVY, R.M., BREDESEN, D.E. & ROSENBLUM, M.L. (1985) Neurological manifestations of the acquired immunodeficiency syndrome (AIDS): experience at UCSF and review of the literature. *Journal of Neurosurgery* **62**, 475–495 [319, 324].

LEVY, R.M., BREDESEN, D.E. & ROSENBLUM, M.L. (1988) Opportunistic central nervous system pathology in patients with AIDS. *Annals of Neurology* **23 (Supplement)**, S7–S12 [319, 320].

LEVY, R.M., ROSENBLOOM, S. & PERRETT, L.V. (1986) Neuroradiologic findings in AIDS: a review of 200 cases. *American Journal of Radiology* **147**, 977–983 [320, 325].

LEVY-LAHAD, E., WASCO, W., POORKAJ, P., ROMANO, D.M., OSHIMA, J., PETTINGELL, W.H., YU, C.-E., JONDRO, P.D., SCHMIDT, S.D., WANG, K., CROWLEY, A.C., FU, Y.-H., GUENETTE, S.Y., GALAS, D., NEMENS, E., WIJSMAN, E.M., BIRD, T.D., SCHELLENBERG, G.D. & TANZI, R.E. (1995a) Candidate gene for the chromosome 1 familial Alzheimer's disease locus. *Science* **269**, 973–977 [448].

LEVY-LAHAD, E., WIJSMAN, E.M., NEMENS, E., ANDERSON, L., GODDARD, K.A.B., WEBER, J.L., BIRD, T.D. & SCHELLENBERG, G.D. (1995b) A familial Alzheimer's disease locus on chromosome 1. *Science* **269**, 970–973 [448].

LEWIN, W. (1959) The management of prolonged unconsciousness after head injury. *Proceedings of the Royal Society of Medicine* **52**, 880–884 [167].

LEWIN, W. (1966) *The Management of Head Injuries*. Baillière, Tindall & Cassell: London [161, 212].

LEWIN, W. (1968) Rehabilitation after head injury. *British Medical Journal* **1**, 465–470 [212].

LEWIN, W. (1970) Rehabilitation needs of the brain-injured patient. *Proceedings of the Royal Society of Medicine* **63**, 28–32 [244].

LEWIS, A.J. (1938) Some recent aspects of dementia. In *Festskrift tillägnad Olof Kinberg*, pp. 238–244. Asbrink: Stockholm [211].

LEWIS, A.J. (1942) Discussion on differential diagnosis and treatment of post-contusional states. *Proceedings of the Royal Society of Medicine* **35**, 607–614 [173, 196].

LEWIS, A.J. (1956) Psychological medicine. Section 19 in *Price's Textbook of the Practice of Medicine*, 9th edn, ed. Hunter, D. Oxford University Press: Oxford [373].

LEWIS, A.J. & MINSKI, L. (1935) Chorea and psychosis. *Lancet* **1**, 536–538 [374].

LEWIS, J.D., MORITZ, D. & MELLIS, L.P. (1981) Long-term toluene abuse. *American Journal of Psychiatry* **138**, 368–370 [629].

LEWIS, S.A., OSWALD, I. & DUNLEAVY, D.L.F. (1971) Chronic fenfluramine administration: some cerebral effects. *British Medical Journal* **3**, 67–70 [617].

LEWIS, S.W. (1989) Congenital risk factors for schizophrenia. *Psychological Medicine* **19**, 5–13 [92].

LEWIS, S.W. (1990) Computerised tomography in schizophrenia 15 years on. In *Brain Imaging in Psychiatry*, ed. Abou-Saleh, M.T. *British Journal of Psychiatry* **157 (Supplement 9)**, 16–24 [85].

LEZAK, M.D. (1978) Living with the characterologically altered brain injured patient. *Journal of Clinical Psychiatry* **39**, 592–598 [217].

LEZAK, M.D. (1995) *Neuropsychological Assessment*, 3rd edn. Oxford University Press: New York [64, 104, 108, 110, 112, 113, 115, 116, 118, 120, 485].

LHERMITTE, F. (1983) 'Utilization behaviour' and its relation to lesions of the frontal lobes. *Brain* **106**, 237–255 [106].

LHERMITTE, F. (1986) Human autonomy and the frontal lobes. Part II: Patient behavior in complex and social situations: the environmental dependency syndrome. *Annals of Neurology* **19**, 335–343 [79].

LHERMITTE, F., PILLON, B. & SERDARU, M. (1986) Human autonomy and the frontal lobes. Part I: Imitation and utilization behavior: a neuropsychological study of 75 patients. *Annals of Neurology* **19**, 326–334 [106].

LHERMITTE, F. & SIGNORET, J.L. (1972) Analyse neuropsychologique et différénciation des symptomes amnesiques. *Revue Neurologique* **126**, 161–178 [38].

LHERMITTE, J. (1922) Syndrome de la calotte du pédoncule cérébral. Les troubles psycho-sensoriels dans les lésions du mésocéphale. *Revue Neurologique* **38**, 1359–1365 [388].

LHERMITTE, J. (1932) L'hallucinose pédonculaire. *Encéphale* **27**, 422–435 [388].

LIDDELL, D.W. (1953) Observations on epileptic automatism in a mental hospital population. *Journal of Mental Science* **99**, 732–748 [265].

LIDDELL, D.W. (1958) Investigations of EEG findings in presenile dementia. *Journal of Neurology, Neurosurgery and Psychiatry* **21**, 173–176 [439].

LIDDLE, P.F. (1987) The symptoms of chronic schizophrenia: a re-examination of the positive–negative dichotomy. *British Journal of Psychiatry* **151**, 145–151 [146].

LIDDLE, P.F., FRISTON, K.J., FRITH, C.D., HIRSCH, S.R., JONES, T. & FRACKOWIAK, R.S.J. (1992) Patterns of cerebral blood flow in schizophrenia. *British Journal of Psychiatry* **160**, 179–186 [87].

LIDVALL, H.F., LINDEROTH, B. & NORLIN, B. (1974) Causes of the post-concussional syndrome. *Acta Neurologica Scandinavica* **56 (Supplement)**, 1–144 [197, 198].

LIEBERMAN, A., DZIATOLOWSKI, M., KUPERRSMITH, M., SERBY, M., GOODGOLD, A., KOREIN, J. & GOLDSTEIN, M. (1979) Dementia in Parkinson disease. *Annals of Neurology* **6**, 355–359 [653].

LIGNELLI, G.J. & BUCHHEIT, W.A. (1971) Angiitis in drug abusers. *New England Journal of Medicine* **284**, 112–113 [620].

LILLY, R., CUMMINGS, J.L., BENSON, F. & FRANKEL, M. (1983) The human Klüver–Bucy syndrome. *Neurology* **33**, 1141–1145 [23].

LIM, L., RON, M.A., ORMEROD, I.E.C., DAVID, J., MILLER, D.H., LOGSDAIL, S.J., WALPORT, M.J. & HARDING, A.E. (1988) Psychiatric and neurological manifestations in systemic lupus erythematosus. *Quarterly Journal of Medicine* **66 (249)**, 27–38 [419, 420, 421].

LINDBOE, C.F. & LØBERG, E.M. (1989) Wernicke's encephalopathy in non-alcoholics. An autopsy study. *Journal of the Neurological Sciences* **90**, 125–129 [576].

LINDENBERG, W. (1951) Hirnverletzung, organische Wesensänderung, Neurose. *Nervenarzt* **22**, 254–260 [180].

LINDGREN, S.A. (1961) A study of the effect of protracted occupational exposure to carbon monoxide. *Acta Medica Scandinavica* **356 (Supplement)**, 1–135 [553].

LINDQVIST, G. & NORLÉN, G. (1966) Korsakoff's syndrome after operation on ruptured aneurysm of the anterior communicating artery. *Acta Psychiatrica Scandinavica* **42**, 24–34 [394].

LINDSAY, J., OUNSTED, C. & RICHARDS, P. (1979a) Long-term

outcome in children with temporal lobe seizures: 1. Social outcome and childhood factors. *Developmental Medicine and Child Neurology* **21**, 285–298 [266].

LINDSAY, J., OUNSTED, C. & RICHARDS, P. (1979b) Long-term outcome in children with temporal lobe seizures. Marriage, parenthood and sexual indifference. *Developmental Medicine and Child Neurology* **21**, 433–440 [272].

LINDSAY, J., OUNSTED, C. & RICHARDS, P. (1979c) Long-term outcome in children with temporal lobe epilepsy. III. Psychiatric aspects in childhood and adult life. *Developmental Medicine and Child Neurology* **21**, 610–636 [282].

LINDVALL, O. (1994) Transplantation—the clinical position. Ch. 12 in *Movement Disorders*, Vol. 3, eds Marsden, C.D. & Fahn, S. Butterworth-Heinemann: Oxford [652].

LIPOWSKI, Z.J. (1967) Delirium, clouding of consciousness and confusion. *Journal of Nervous and Mental Disease* **145**, 227–255 [4].

LIPOWSKI, Z.J. (1980a) *Delirium: Acute Brain Failure in Man.* Charles C. Thomas: Springfield, Illinois [5, 8, 10].

LIPOWSKI, Z.J. (1980b) A new look at organic brain syndromes. *American Journal of Psychiatry* **137**, 674–678 [8].

LIPOWSKI, Z.J. (1990) *Delirium: Acute Confusional States*, 2nd edn. Oxford University Press: Oxford [10, 131, 625].

LIPPMAN, C.W. (1952) Certain hallucinations peculiar to migraine. *Journal of Nervous and Mental Disease* **116**, 346–351 [406].

LIPPMAN, C.W. (1953) Hallucinations of physical duality in migraine. *Journal of Nervous and Mental Disease* **117**, 345–350 [407].

LIPPMANN, S., MANSHADI, M., BALDWIN, H., DRASIN, G., RICE, J. & ALRAJEH, S. (1982) Cerebellar vermis dimensions on computerised tomographic scans of schizophrenic and bipolar patients. *American Journal of Psychiatry* **139**, 667–668 [140].

LIPSEY, J.R., ROBINSON, R.G., PEARLSON, G.D., RAO, K. & PRICE, T.R. (1983) Mood change following bilateral hemisphere brain injury. *British Journal of Psychiatry* **143**, 266–273 [386].

LIPSEY, J.R., ROBINSON, R.G., PEARLSON, G.D., RAO, K. & PRICE, T.R. (1984) Nortriptyline treatment of post-stroke depression: a double-blind study. *Lancet* **1**, 297–300 [392].

LIPTZIN, B. & LEVKOFF, S.E. (1992) An empirical study of delirium subtypes. *British Journal of Psychiatry* **161**, 843–845 [5].

LISHMAN, W.A. (1968) Brain damage in relation to psychiatric disability after head injury. *British Journal of Psychiatry* **114**, 373–410 [171, 178, 181, 196, 198].

LISHMAN, W.A. (1969) Split minds: a review of the results of brain bisection in man. *British Journal of Hospital Medicine* **2**, 477–484 [313].

LISHMAN, W.A. (1971) Emotion, consciousness and will after brain bisection in man. *Cortex* **7**, 181–192 [313].

LISHMAN, W.A. (1972) Selective factors in memory. Part 1: age, sex and personality attributes. *Psychological Medicine* **2**, 121–138 [25].

LISHMAN, W.A. (1973) The psychiatric sequelae of head injury: a review. *Psychological Medicine* **3**, 304–318 [175, 188, 193].

LISHMAN, W.A. (1974) The speed of recall of pleasant and unpleasant experiences. *Psychological Medicine* **4**, 212–218 [25].

LISHMAN, W.A. (1978) Psychiatric sequelae of head injuries: problems in diagnosis. *Journal of the Irish Medical Association* **71**, 306–314 [189, 196].

LISHMAN, W.A. (1981) Cerebral disorder in alcoholism: syndromes of impairment. *Brain* **104**, 1–20 [575, 580, 582, 603].

LISHMAN, W.A. (1983a) The apparatus of mind: brain structure and function in mental disorder. *Psychosomatics* **24**, 699–720 [85].

LISHMAN, W.A. (1983b) *Brain Damage and Psychiatric Disability.* Royal Hospital and Home for Incurables, Booklet 1/83: Putney, London [215].

LISHMAN, W.A. (1986) Alcoholic dementia: a hypothesis. *Lancet* **1**, 1184–1186 [607].

LISHMAN, W.A. (1988) Physiogenesis and psychogenesis in the 'post-concussional syndrome'. *British Journal of Psychiatry* **153**, 460–469 [175, 197, 198, 199].

LISHMAN, W.A. (1990) Alcohol and the brain. *British Journal of Psychiatry* **156**, 635–644 [583, 607].

LISHMAN, W.A. (1991) The evolution of research into the dementias. *Dementia* **2**, 177–185 [448].

LISHMAN, W.A. (1992) Neuropsychiatry. A delicate balance. *Psychosomatics* **33**, 4–9 [95, 149].

LISHMAN, W.A. (1994) The history of research into dementia and its relationship to current concepts. Ch. 3 in *Dementia and Normal Aging*, eds Huppert, F.A., Brayne, C. & O'Connor, D.W. Cambridge University Press: Cambridge [441, 448].

LISHMAN, W.A. (1995) Psychiatry and neuropathology: the maturing of a relationship. *Journal of Neurology, Neurosurgery and Psychiatry* **58**, 284–292 [91].

LISHMAN, W.A., JACOBSON, R.R. & ACKER, C. (1987) Brain damage in alcoholism: current concepts. In *Alcohol, Brain Damage and Cardiovascular Disease*, ed. Hillbom, M. Third International Magnus Huss Symposium. *Acta Medica Scandinavica* **717** (**Supplement**), 5–17 [605, 606].

LISHMAN, W.A. & McMEEKAN, E.R.L. (1977) Handedness in relation to direction and degree of cerebral dominance for language. *Cortex* **13**, 30–43 [40].

LISHMAN, W.A., SYMONDS, C.P., WHITTY, C.W.M. & WILLISON, R.G. (1962) Seizures induced by movement. *Brain* **85**, 93–108 [241, 291].

LISHMAN, W.A. & WHITTY, C.W.M. (1965) Seizures induced by movement. *Rivista di Patologia nervosa e mentale* **86**, 237–243 [291].

LISSAUER, H. (1890) Ein Fall von Seelenblindheit nebst einem Beitrage zur Theorie derselben. *Archiv für Psychiatrie und Nervenkrankheiten* **21**, 222–270 [58].

LIST, S.J. & CLEGHORN, J.M. (1993) Implications of positron emission tomography research for the investigation of the actions of antipsychotic drugs. *British Journal of Psychiatry* **163** (**Supplement 22**), 25–30 [147].

LISTER, R.G. (1985) The amnesic action of benzodiazepines in man. *Neuroscience and Biobehavioral Reviews* **9**, 87–94 [610].

LISTON, E.H. & LA RUE, A. (1983) Clinical differentiation of primary degenerative and multi-infarct dementia: a critical review of the evidence. Part II: pathological studies. *Biological Psychiatry* **18**, 1467–1484 [453].

LITTLE, A., LEVY, R., CHUAQUI-KIDD, P. & HAND, D. (1985) A double-blind, placebo controlled trial of high-dose lecithin in Alzheimer's disease. *Journal of Neurology, Neurosurgery and Psychiatry* **48**, 736–742 [503].

LITVAN, I., GRAFMAN, J., GOMEZ, C. & CHASE, T.N. (1989) Memory impairment in patients with progressive supranuclear palsy. *Archives of Neurology* **46**, 765–767 [666].

LIU, M.C. (1960) General paralysis of the insane in Peking between 1933 and 1943. *Journal of Mental Science* **106**, 1082–1092 [340].

LIU, M.C. (1966) Clinical experience with sulthiame (ospolot). *British Journal of Psychiatry* **112**, 621–628 [305].

LIVERSEDGE, L.A. (1969) Involuntary movements. Ch. 10 in *Handbook of Clinical Neurology*, Vol. 1, eds Vinken, P.J. & Bruyn, G.W. North-Holland Publishing Company: Amsterdam [676].

LIVERSEDGE, L.A. & SYLVESTER, J.D. (1955) Conditioning techniques in the treatment of writer's cramp. *Lancet* **1**, 1147–1149 [677].

LIVINGSTON, G.A., SAX, K.B., McCLENAHAN, Z., BLUMENTHAL, E., FOLEY, K., WILLISON, J., MANN, A.H. & JAMES, I.M. (1991) Acetyl-l-carnitine in dementia. *International Journal of Geriatric Psychiatry* **6**, 853–860 [503].

LIVINGSTON, K.E. (1977) Limbic system dysfunction induced by 'kindling': its significance for psychiatry. In *Neurosurgical Treatment in Psychiatry, Pain, and Epilepsy*, eds Sweet, W.H., Obrador, S. & Martin-Rodriguez, J.G., pp. 63–75. University Park Press: Baltimore [283].

LIVINGSTONE, M.S., ROSEN, G.D., DRISLANE, F.W. & GALABURDA, A.M. (1991) Physiological and anatomical evidence for a magnocellular defect in developmental dyslexia. *Proceedings of the National Academy of Sciences* **88**, 7943–7947 [48].

LLOYD, E.A. & CLARK, L.D. (1959) Convulsions and delirium incident to glutethimide (doriden) withdrawal. *Diseases of the Nervous System* **20**, 524–526 [628].

LLOYD, G.G. & LISHMAN, W.A. (1975) Effect of depression on the speed of recall of pleasant and unpleasant experiences. *Psychological Medicine* **5**, 173–180 [34].

LLOYD-STILL, R.M. (1958) Psychosis following Asian influenza in Barbados. *Lancet* **2**, 20–21 [359].

LOCK, T., ABOU-SALEH, M.T. & EDWARDS, R.H.T. (1990) Psychiatry and the new magnetic resonance era. *British Journal of Psychiatry* **157 (Supplement 9),** 38–55 [143].

LOESER, J.D. & ALVORD, E.C. *(1968)* Clinicopathological correlations in agenesis of the corpus callosum. *Neurology* **18**, 745–756 [770].

LOFTUS, L.S. & ARNOLD, W.N. (1991) Vincent van Gogh's illness: acute intermittent porphyria? *British Medical Journal* **303**, 1589–1591 [567].

LOGSDAIL, S.J. & TOONE, B.K. (1988) Post-ictal psychoses. A clinical and phenomenological description. *British Journal of Psychiatry* **152**, 246–252 [257].

LOGUE, V., DURWARD, M., PRATT, R.T.C., PIERCY, M. & NIXON, W.L.B. (1968) The quality of survival after rupture of an anterior cerebral aneurysm. *British Journal of Psychiatry* **114**, 137–160 [393, 394, 395].

LOIZOU, L.A., KENDALL, B.E. & MARSHALL, J. (1981) Subacute arteriosclerotic encephalopathy: a clinical and radiological investigation. *Journal of Neurology, Neurosurgery and Psychiatry* **44**, 294–304 [458, 459].

LÖKEN, A.C. (1959) The pathologic–anatomical basis for late symptoms after brain injuries in adults. *Acta Psychiatrica et Neurologica Scandinavica* **137 (Supplement)**, 30–42 [163, 164].

LOMBES, A., BONILLA, E. & DIMAURO, S. (1989) Mitochondrial encephalomyopathies. *Revue Neurologique* **145**, 671–689 [761].

LOMBROSO, C. (1911) *Crime: Its Causes and Remedies*. Translated by Horton, H.P. (1918). Little, Brown & Co.: Boston [273].

LONDON, P.S. (1967) Some observations on the course of events after severe injury of the head. *Annals of the Royal College of Surgeons of England* **41**, 460–479 [161].

LONG, J.A. & McLACHLAN, J.F.C. (1974) Abstract reasoning and perceptual-motor efficiency in alcoholics: impairment and reversibility. *Quarterly Journal of Studies on Alcohol* **35**, 1220–1229 [604].

LORANGER, A.W., GOODELL, H., LEE, J.E. & McDOWELL, F. (1972a) Levodopa treatment of Parkinson's syndrome: improved intellectual functioning. *Archives of General Psychiatry* **26**, 163–168 [659].

LORANGER, A.W., GOODELL, H., McDOWELL, F.H., LEE, J.E. & SWEET, R.D. (1972b) Intellectual impairment in Parkinson's syndrome. *Brain* **95**, 405–412 [659].

LORBER, J. (1961) Long-term follow-up of 100 children who recovered from tuberculous meningitis. *Pediatrics* **28**, 778–791 [367].

LORENTZ DE HAAS, A.M. & MAGNUS, O. (1958) Clinical and electroencephalographic findings in epileptic patients with episodic mental disorders. Ch. 4 in *Lectures on Epilepsy*, ed. Lorentz de Haas, A.M. Elsevier: Amsterdam [285].

LOU, H.O.C.L. (1968) Repeated episodes of transient global amnesia. *Acta Neurologica Scandinavica* **44**, 612–618 [415].

LOUDON, J.B. & WARING, H. (1976) Toxic reactions to lithium and haloperidol. *Lancet* **2**, 1088 [626].

LOURIA, D.B. (1968) Lysergic acid diethylamide. *New England Journal of Medicine* **278**, 435–438 [620, 622].

LOVELAND, N., SMITH, B. & FORSTER, F.M. (1957) Mental and emotional changes in epileptic patients on continuous anticonvulsant medication. *Neurology* **7**, 856–865 [263].

LOWENSTEIN, D.H., MASSA, S.M., ROWBOTHAM, M.C., COLLINS, S.D., McKINNEY, H.E. & SIMON, R.P. (1987) Acute neurologic and psychiatric complications associated with cocaine abuse. *American Journal of Medicine* **83**, 841–846 [619].

LUCAS, P. (1994) Episodic dyscontrol: a look back at anger. *Journal of Forensic Psychiatry* **5**, 371–407 [83].

LUCAS, R.N. & FALKOWSKI, W. (1973) Ergotamine and methysergide abuse in patients with migraine. *British Journal of Psychiatry* **122**, 199–203 [410].

LUCAS, S.B., HOUNNOU, A., PEACOCK, C., BEAUMEL, A., DJOMAND, G., N'GBICHI, J.-M., YEBOUE, K., HONDÉ, M., DIOMANDE, M., GIORDANO, C., DOORLY, R., BRATTEGAARD, K., KESTENS, L., SMITHWICK, R., KADIO, A., NIAMKEY, E., YAPI, A. & DE COCK, K.M. (1993) The mortality and pathology of HIV infection in a West African city. *AIDS* **7**, 1569–1579 [318].

LUCCHELLI, F., MUGGIA, S. & SPINNLER, H. (1995) The 'Petites Madeleines' phenomenon in two amnesic patients. Sudden recovery of forgotten memories. *Brain* **118**, 167–183 [39].

LUCHINS, D.J., SHERWOOD, P.M., GILLIN, J.C., MENDELSON, W.B. & WYATT, R.J. (1978) Filicide during psychotropic-induced somnambulism: a case report. *American Journal of Psychiatry* **135**, 1404–1405 [736].

LUCHINS, D.J., WEINBERGER, D.R. & WYATT, R.J. (1979) Schizophrenia. Evidence of a subgroup with reversed cerebral asymmetry. *Archives of General Psychiatry* **36**, 1309–1311 [89].

LUCHINS, D.J., WEINBERGER, D.R. & WYATT, R.J. (1982) Schizophrenia and cerebral asymmetry detected by computed tomography. *American Journal of Psychiatry* **139**, 753–757 [89].

LUCKI, I., RICKELS, K. & GELLER, A.M. (1986) Chronic use of benzodiazepines and psychomotor and cognitive test performance. *Psychopharmacology* **88**, 426–433 [610].

LUDOLPH, A.C., LANGEN, K.J., REGARD, M., HERZOG, H., KEMPER, B., KUWERT, T., BÖTTGER, I.G. & FEINENDEGEN, L. (1992) Frontal lobe function in amyotrophic lateral sclerosis: a neuropsychologic and positron emission tomography study. *Acta Neurologica Scandinavica* **85**, 81–89 [708].

LUGARESI, E., MEDORI, R., MONTAGNA, P., BARUZZI, A., CORTELLI, P., LUGARESI, A., TINUPER, P., ZUCCONI, M. & GAMBETTI, P. (1986) Fatal familial insomnia and dysautonomia with selective degeneration of thalamic nuclei. *New England Journal of Medicine* **315**, 997–1003 [734].

LUKIANOWICZ, N. (1958) Autoscopic phenomena. *Archives of Neurology and Psychiatry* **80**, 199–220 [73].

LUKIANOWICZ, N. (1967) 'Body image' disturbances in psychiatric disorders. *British Journal of Psychiatry* **113**, 31–47 [72, 73, 74].

LUND, M. & TROLLE, E. (1973) Clonazepam in the treatment of epilepsy. *Acta Neurologica Scandinavica* **53 (Supplement)**, 82–90 [302].

LUNDERVOLD, A., REFSUM, S. & JACOBSEN, W. (1969) The EEG in dystrophia myotonica. *European Neurology* **2**, 279–284 [719].

LUNDQUIST, G. (1961) Delirium tremens: a comparative study· of pathogenesis, course, and prognosis with delirium tremens. *Acta Psychiatrica Scandinavica* **36**, 443–466 [602].

LURIA, A.R. (1964) Neuropsychology in the local diagnosis of brain damage. *Cortex* **1**, 3–18 [22].

LURIA, A.R. (1966) *Higher Cortical Functions in Man.* Tavistock Publications: London [78, 79, 106].

LURIA, A.R. & HOMSKAYA, E.D. (1964) Disturbance in the regulative role of speech with frontal lobe lesions. Ch. 17 in *The Frontal Granular Cortex and Behaviour*, eds Warren, J.M. & Akert, K. McGraw-Hill: New York [78, 118].

LURIA, A.R., KARPOV, B.A. & YARBUSS, A.L. (1966) Disturbances of active visual perception with lesions of the frontal lobes. *Cortex* **2**, 202–212 [78].

LURIA, A.R., PRAVDINA-VINARSKAYA, E.N. & YARBUSS, A.L. (1963) Disorders of ocular movement in a case of simultanagnosia. *Brain* **86**, 219–228 [61].

LUXON, L., LEES, A.J. & GREENWOOD, R.J. (1979) Neurosyphilis today. *Lancet* **1**, 90–93 [342].

LYCKE, E., NORRBY, R. & ROOS, B. (1974) A serological study on mentally ill patients: with particular reference to the prevalence of herpes virus infections. *British Journal of Psychiatry* **124**, 273–279 [358].

LYLE, O.E. & GOTTESMAN, I.I. (1977) Premorbid psychometric indicators of the gene for Huntington's disease. *Journal of Consulting and Clinical Psychology* **45**, 1011–1022 [467].

LYLE, O. & QUAST, W. (1976) The Bender Gestalt: use of clinical judgement versus recall scores in prediction of Huntington's disease. *Journal of Consulting and Clinical Psychology* **44**, 229–232 [467].

LYNCH, M.J.G. (1960) Brain lesions in chronic alcoholism. *Archives of Pathology* **69**, 342–353 [604].

LYON, R.L. (1962) Huntington's chorea in the Moray Firth area. *British Medical Journal* **1**, 1301–1306 [465, 468].

MAAS, O. & PATERSON, A.S. (1937) Mental changes in families affected by dystrophia myotonica. *Lancet* **1**, 21–23 [719, 720].

MABILLE, H. & PITRES, A. (1913) Sur un cas d'amnésie de fixation post-apoplectique ayant persisté pendant vingt-trois ans. *Revue de Médicine* **33**, 257–279 [27].

MACALPINE, I. & HUNTER, R. (1966) The 'insanity' of King George III: a classic case of porphyria. *British Medical Journal* **1**, 65–71 [567].

MACALPINE, I. & HUNTER, R. (1969) *George III and the Mad-Business.* Allen Lane, The Penguin Press: London [567].

MACALPINE, I., HUNTER, R. & RIMINGTON, C. (1968) Porphyria in the royal houses of Stuart, Hanover, and Prussia: a follow-up study of George III's illness. *British Medical Journal* **1**, 7–18 [567].

McARDLE, B. (1964) Metabolic and endocrine myopathies. Ch. 15 in *Disorders of Voluntary Muscle*, ed. Walton, J.N. Churchill: London [721].

McARTHUR, J.C. (1987) Neurologic manifestations of AIDS. *Medicine (Baltimore)* **66**, 407–437 [325].

McARTHUR, J.C., COHEN, B.A., FARZEDEGAN, H., CORNBLATH, D.R., SELNES, O.A., OSTROW, D., JOHNSON, R.T., PHAIR, J. & POLK, B.F. (1988) Cerebrospinal fluid abnormalities in homosexual men with and without neuropsychiatric findings. *Annals of Neurology* **23 (Supplement)**, S34–S37 [319].

McARTHUR, J.C., COHEN, B.A., SELNES, O.A., KUMAR, A.J., COOPER, K., McARTHUR, J.H., SOUCY, G., CORNBLATH, D.R., CHMIEL, J.S., WANG, M.-C., STARKEY, D.L., GINZBURG, H., OSTROW, D.G., JOHNSON, R.T., PHAIR, J.P. & POLK, B.F. (1989) Low prevalence of neurological and neuropsychological abnormalities in otherwise healthy HIV-1-infected individuals: results from the multicenter AIDS cohort study. *Annals of Neurology* **26**, 601–611 [329].

McARTHUR, J.C., SELNES, O.A., GLASS, J.D., HOOVER, D.R. & BACELLAR, H. (1994) HIV dementia: incidence and risk factors. Ch. 14 in *HIV, AIDS, and the Brain*, eds Price, R.W. & Perry, S.W. *Association for Research in Nervous and Mental Disease* **72**. Raven Press: New York [319, 325, 326].

McCARLEY, R.W., SHENTON, M.E., O'DONNELL, B.F., FAUX, S.I., KININIS, R., NESTOR, G. & JOLESZ, F.A. (1993) Auditory P300 abnormalities and left posterior superior temporal gyrus volume reduction in schizophrenia. *Archives of General Psychiatry* **50**, 190–197 [132].

McCARTHY, M.M. (1994) Molecular aspects of sexual differentiation of the rodent brain. *Psychoneuroendocrinology* **19**, 415–427 [507].

McCLELLAND, H.A. (1986) Psychiatric reactions to psychotropic drugs. *Adverse Drug Reaction Bulletin* **119**, 444–447 [626].

McCLELLAND, H.A., METCALFE, A.V., KERR, T.A., DUTTA, D. & WATSON, P. (1991) Facial dyskinesia: a 16-year follow-up study. *British Journal of Psychiatry* **158**, 691–696 [642].

McCOLL, K.E.L., DOVER, S., FITZSIMONS, E. & MOORE, M.R. (1996) Porphyrin metabolism and the porphyrias. Section 11.5 in *Oxford Textbook of Medicine*, 3rd edn, Vol. 2, eds Weatherall, D.J., Ledingham, J.G.G. & Warrell, D.A. Oxford University Press: Oxford [567, 568, 569].

McCONAGHY, N., CATTS, S.V., MICHIE, P.T., FOX, A., WARD, P.B. & SHELLEY, A. (1993) P300 indexes thought disorder in schizophrenics, but allusive thinking in normal subjects. *Journal of Nervous and Mental Diseases* **181**, 176–182 [132].

McCONKEY, B. & DAWS, R.A. (1958) Neurological disorders associated with Asian influenza. *Lancet* **2**, 15–17 [359].

McCORMICK, G.F., ZEE, C.-S. & HEIDEN, J. (1982) Cysticercosis cerebri. *Archives of Neurology* **39**, 534–539 [370].

McCORMICK, H.M. & NEUBERGER, K.T. (1958) Giant-cell arteritis involving small meningeal and intracerebral vessels. *Journal of Neuropathology and Experimental Neurology* **17**, 471–478 [423].

McCUNE, W.J. & GOLBUS, J. (1988) Neuropsychiatric lupus. *Rheumatic Disease Clinics of North America* **14**, 149–167 [419, 420, 422].

McDANIEL, K.D., CUMMINGS, J.L. & SHAIN, S. (1989) The 'yips'. A focal dystonia of golfers. *Neurology* **39**, 192–195 [677].

McDERMOTT, J.R., FRASER, H. & DICKINSON, A.G. (1978a) Reduced choline-acetyltransferase activity in scrapie mouse brain. *Lancet* **2**, 318–319 [446].

McDERMOTT, J.R., SMITH, A.I., WARD, M.K., PARKINSON, I.S. & KERR, D.N.S. (1978b) Brain-aluminium concentration in dialysis encephalopathy. *Lancet* **1**, 901–904 [558].

McDONALD, C. (1969) Clinical heterogeneity in senile dementia. *British Journal of Psychiatry* **115**, 267–271 [433].

MacDONALD, J.M. (1969) *Psychiatry and the Criminal*, 2nd edn. Thomas: Springfield, Illinois [275].

McDONALD, W.I. (1967) Recurrent cholesterol embolism as a cause of fluctuating cerebral symptoms. *Journal of Neurology, Neurosurgery and Psychiatry* **30**, 489–496 [377].

McDONALD, W.I. (1995) New treatments for multiple sclerosis. *British Medical Journal* **310**, 345–346 [690].

McDOWELL, J.R. & LE BLANC, H.J. (1984) Computed tomographic findings in Wernicke–Korsakoff syndrome. *Archives of Neurology* **41**, 453–454 [579].

MACE, C.J. (1987) Brittle diabetes in a drug and alcohol abuser. *British Journal of Addiction* **82**, 931–934 [537].

MACE, C.J. (1993) Epilepsy and schizophrenia. *British Journal of Psychiatry* **163**, 439–445 [282].

MACE, C.J. & TRIMBLE, M.R. (1991) Psychosis following temporal lobe surgery: a report of six cases. *Journal of Neurology, Neurosurgery and Psychiatry* **54**, 639–644 [313].

MACE, N.L. & RABINS, P.V. (1981) *The 36-hour Day: A Family Guide to*

Caring for Persons with Alzheimer's Disease, Related Dementing Illnesses, and Memory Loss in Later Life. Johns Hopkins University Press: Baltimore and London [498].

McENTEE, W.J. & MAIR, R.G. (1978) Memory impairment in Korsakoff's psychosis: a correlation with brain noradrenergic activity. *Science* **202**, 905–907 [585].

McENTEE, W.J. & MAIR, R.G. (1980) Memory enhancement in Korsakoff's psychosis by clonidine: further evidence for a noradrenergic defect. *Annals of Neurology* **7**, 466–470 [585].

McENTEE, W.J., MAIR, R.G. & LANGLAIS, J. (1984) Neurochemical pathology in Korsakoff's psychosis: implications for other cognitive disorders. *Neurology* **34**, 648–652 [585].

McEVEDY, C.P. & BEARD, A.W. (1970a) Royal Free epidemic of 1955: a reconsideration. *British Medical Journal* **1**, 7–11 [372].

McEVEDY, C.P. & BEARD, A.W. (1970b) Concept of benign myalgic encephalomyelitis. *British Medical Journal* **1**, 11–15 [372].

McEVEDY, C.P. & BEARD, A.W. (1973) A controlled follow-up of cases involved in an epidemic of 'benign myalgic encephalomyelitis'. *British Journal of Psychiatry* **122**, 141–150 [372].

McFARLAND, H.R. (1963) Addison's disease and related psychoses. *Comprehensive Psychiatry* **4**, 90–95 [519].

McFARLAND, R.A. (1932) The psychological effects of oxygen deprivation (anoxaemia) on human behaviour. *Archives of Psychology* **145** [548].

McFARLAND, R.A. (1937) Psycho-physiological studies at high altitudes in the Andes; mental and psychosomatic responses during gradual adaptation. *Journal of Comparative Psychology* **24**, 147–188 [548].

MacFARLANE, A.B. (1988) Patients and Powers of Attorney. *Bulletin of the Royal College of Psychiatrists* **12**, 181–182 [498].

McFARLANE, A.C. (1989) The aetiology of post-traumatic morbidity: predisposing, precipitating and perpetuating factors. *British Journal of Psychiatry* **154**, 221–228 [195].

MACFIE, A.M.C. (1972) *A Study of Ancillary Investigations in Clinical Psychiatric Practice.* Dissertation for M.Phil. (Psychiatry): University of London [126].

McFIE, J. (1960) Psychological testing in clinical neurology. *Journal of Nervous and Mental Disease* **131**, 383–393 [63, 109, 111].

McFIE, J. & PIERCY, F.M. (1952) The relation of literality of lesion to performance on Weigl's sorting test. *Journal of Mental Science* **98**, 299–305 [27].

MacFLYNN, G., MONTGOMERY, E.A., FENTON, G.W. & RUTHERFORD, W. (1984) Measurement of reaction time following minor head injury. *Journal of Neurology, Neurosurgery and Psychiatry* **47**, 1326–1331 [198].

McGEER, P.L. (1986) Brain imaging in Alzheimer's disease. *British Medical Bulletin* **42**, 24–28 [434].

McGEER, P.L., McGEER, E.G., SUZUKI, J., DOLMAN, C.E. & NAGAI, T. (1984) Aging, Alzheimer's disease, and the cholinergic system of the basal forebrain. *Neurology* **34**, 741–745 [444].

McGILCHRIST, I., GOLDSTEIN, L.H., JADRESIC, D. & FENWICK, P. (1993) Thalamo-frontal psychosis: a case report. *British Journal of Psychiatry* **163**, 113–115 [387].

McGINN, N.F., HAMBURG, E., JULIUS, S. & McLEOD, J.M. (1964) Psychological correlates of blood pressure. *Psychological Bulletin* **61**, 209–219 [397].

McGOVERN, G.P., MILLER, D.H. & ROBERTSON, E.E. (1959) A mental syndrome associated with lung carcinoma. *Archives of Neurology and Psychiatry* **81**, 341–347 [741].

McGRATH, S.D. & McKENNA, J. (1961) The Ganser syndrome: a critical review. *Proceedings of the Third World Congress of Psychiatry*, Vol. 1, pp. 156–161, Montreal [482].

McGREGOR, A.M. (1996) The thyroid gland and disorders of thyroid function. Section 12.4 in *Oxford Textbook of Medicine*, 3rd edn, eds Weatherall, D.J., Ledingham, J.G.G. & Warrell, D.A. Oxford University Press: Oxford [510, 513].

MacGREGOR, M.I., BLOCK, A.J. & BALL, W.C. (1970) Serious complications and sudden death in the Pickwickian syndrome. *Johns Hopkins Medical Journal* **126**, 279–295 [731].

McGUIRE, P.K. (1995) The brain in obsessive-compulsive disorder. *Journal of Neurology, Neurosurgery and Psychiatry* **59**, 457–459 [145].

McGUIRE, P.K., BENCH, C.J., FRITH, C.D., MARKS, I.M., FRACKOWIAK, R.S.J. & DOLAN, R.J. (1995a) Functional anatomy of obsessive-compulsive phenomena. *British Journal of Psychiatry* **164**, 459–468 [145].

McGUIRE, P.K., COPE, H. & FAHY, T. (1994a) Diversity of psychiatric morbidity associated with use of 3,4-methylenedioxymethamphetamine (ecstasy). *British Journal of Psychiatry* **165**, 391–395 [624].

McGUIRE, P. & FAHY, T. (1991) Chronic paranoid psychosis after misuse of MDMA ('ecstasy'). *British Medical Journal* **302**, 697 [624].

McGUIRE, P.K., JONES, P., HARVEY, I., BEBBINGTON, P., TOONE, B., LEWIS, S. & MURRAY, R.M. (1994b) Cannabis and acute psychosis. *Schizophrenia Research* **13**, 161–168 [614].

McGUIRE, P.K., SHAH, G.M.S. & MURRAY, R.M. (1993) Increased blood flow in Broca's area during auditory hallucinations in schizophrenia. *Lancet* **342**, 703–706 [88, 148].

McGUIRE, P.K., SILBERSWEIG, D.A., MURRAY, R.M., DAVID, A.S., FRACKOWIAK, R.S.J. & FRITH, C.D. (1996) Functional anatomy of inner speech and auditory verbal imagery. *Psychological Medicine* **26**, 29–38 [88].

McGUIRE, P.K., SILBERSWEIG, D.A., WRIGHT, I., MURRAY, R.M., DAVID, A.S., FRACKOWIAK, R.S.J. & FRITH, C.D. (1995b) Abnormal monitoring of inner speech: a physiological basis for auditory hallucinations. *Lancet* **346**, 596–600 [88].

MACHIN, S.J. (1996) Purpura. Section 22.6.3 in *Oxford Textbook of Medicine*, 3rd edn, eds Weatherall, D.J., Ledingham, J.G.G. & Warrell, D.A. Oxford University Press: Oxford [426].

MACHLE, W.F. (1935) Tetra-ethyl lead intoxication and poisoning by related compounds of lead. *Journal of the American Medical Association* **105**, 578–585 [633].

McHUGH, P.R. (1964) Occult hydrocephalus. *Quarterly Journal of Medicine* **33**, 279–308 [750].

McHUGH, P.R. (1966) Hydrocephalic dementia. *Bulletin of the New York Academy of Medicine* **42**, 907–917 [747, 748].

McHUGH, P.R. & FOLSTEIN, M.F. (1975) Psychiatric syndromes of Huntington's chorea. Ch. 13 in *Psychiatric Aspects of Neurologic Disease*, eds Benson, D.F. & Blamer, D. Grune & Stratton: New York [469, 470].

McINTYRE, H.D. & McINTYRE, A.P. (1942) The problem of brain tumour in psychiatric diagnosis. *American Journal of Psychiatry* **98**, 720–726 [235].

McKANN C.F. (1932) Lead poisoning in children: the cerebral manifestations. *Archives of Neurology and Psychiatry* **27**, 294–304 [632].

MacKAY, A. (1979) Self-poisoning—a complication of epilepsy. *British Journal of Psychiatry* **134**, 277–282 [286].

MacKAY, M.E., McLARDY, T. & HARRIS, C. (1950) A case of periarteritis nodosa of the central nervous system. *Journal of Mental Science* **96**, 470–475 [423].

McKEE, A.C., LEVINE, D.N., KOWALL, N.W. & RICHARDSON, E.P. (1990) Peduncular hallucinosis associated with isolated infarction of the substantia nigra pars reticulata. *Annals of Neurology* **27**, 500–504 [388].

McKEITH, I.G., BARTHOLOMEW, P.H., IRVINE, E.M., COOK, J., ADAMS, R. & SIMPSON, A.E.S. (1993) Single photon emission computerised tomography in elderly patients with Alzheimer's disease and multi-infarct dementia. Regional uptake of technetium-labelled HMPAO related to clinical measurements. *British Journal of Psychiatry* **163**, 597–603 [434].

McKEITH, I.G., GALASKO, D., WILCOCK, G.K. & BYRNE, E.J. (1995) Lewy body dementia—diagnosis and treatment. *British Journal of Psychiatry* **167**, 709–717 [450, 505].

McKEITH, I.G., PERRY, R.H., FAIRBAIRN, A.F., JABEEN, S. & PERRY, E.K. (1992) Operational criteria for senile dementia of Lewy body type (SDLT). *Psychological Medicine* **22**, 911–922 [450, 451].

McKENNA, D.J. & PEROUTKA, S.J. (1990) Neurochemistry and neurotoxicity of 3,4-methylenedioxymethamphetamine (MDMA, 'ecstasy'). *Journal of Neurochemistry* **54**, 14–22 [625].

McKENNA, P., CLARE, L. & BADDELEY, A.D. (1995) Schizophrenia. Ch. 11 in *Handbook of Memory Disorders*, eds Baddeley, A.D., Wilson, B.A. & Watts, F.N. John Wiley: Chichester [34].

McKENNA, P. & WARRINGTON, E.K. (1983) *Graded Naming Test*. NFER-Nelson: Windsor [113].

McKENNA, P.J., KANE, J.M. & PARRISH, K. (1985) Psychotic syndromes in epilepsy. *American Journal of Psychiatry* **142**, 895–904 [282].

McKENNA, P.J., TAMLYN, D., LUND, C.E., MORTIMER, A.M., HAMMOND, S. & BADDELEY, A.D. (1990) Amnesic syndrome in schizophrenia. *Psychological Medicine* **20**, 967–972 [34].

MacKENZIE, K.R., MARTIN, M.J. & HOWARD, F.M. (1969) Myasthenia gravis: psychiatric concomitants. *Canadian Medical Association Journal* **100**, 988–991 [710, 711, 712].

McKEON, J., McGUFFIN, P. & ROBINSON, P. (1984) Obsessive-compulsive neurosis following head injury. A report of four cases. *British Journal of Psychiatry* **144**, 190–192 [196].

McKHANN, G., DRACHMAN, D., FOLSTEIN, M., KATZMAN, R., PRICE, D. & STADLAN, E.M. (1984) Clinical diagnosis of Alzheimer's disease: report of the NINCDS-ADRDA work group under the auspices of Department of Health and Human Services Task Force on Alzheimer's disease. *Neurology* **34**, 939–944 [439].

McKINLAY, W.W., BROOKS, D.N., BOND, M.R., MARTINAGE, D.P. & MARSHALL, M.M. (1981) The short-term outcome of severe blunt head injury as reported by relatives of the injured persons. *Journal of Neurology, Neurosurgery and Psychiatry* **44**, 527–533 [172, 217].

McLARTY, D.G., RATCLIFFE, W.A., RATCLIFFE, J.G., SHIMMINS, J.G. & GOLDBERG, A. (1978) A study of thyroid function in psychiatric in-patients. *British Journal of Psychiatry* **133**, 211–218 [508].

McLATCHIE, G., BROOKS, N., GALBRAITH, S., HUTCHISON, J.S.F., WILSON, L., MELVILLE, I. & TEASDALE, E. (1987) Clinical neurological examination, neuropsychology, electroencephalography and computed tomographic head scanning in active amateur boxers. *Journal of Neurology, Neurosurgery and Psychiatry* **50**, 96–99 [206].

MacLEAN, P.D. (1955) The limbic system ('visceral brain') and emotional behaviour. *Archives of Neurology* **73**, 130–134 [23].

McLESTER, J.S. (1943) *Nutrition and Diet in Health and Disease*, 4th edn. Saunders: Philadelphia [573].

McLOUGHLIN, D. & McKEON, P. (1991) Bipolar disorder and cerebral sarcoidosis. *British Journal of Psychiatry* **158**, 410–413 [764].

McMAHON, W.M., LEPPERT, M., FILLOUX, F., VAN DE WETERING, J.M. & HASSTEDT, S. (1992) Tourette symptoms in 161 related family members. Ch. 19 in *Tourette Syndrome. Genetics, Neurobiology, and Treatment*, eds Chase, T.N., Friedhoff, A.J. & Cohen, D.J. *Advances in Neurology* **58**. Raven Press: New York [681, 686].

McMENEMEY, W.H. (1941) A critical review: dementia in middle age. *Journal of Neurology, Neurosurgery and Psychiatry* **4**, 48–79 [234].

McMENEMEY, W.H. (1963a) Alzheimer's disease: problems concerning its concept and nature. *Acta Neurologica Scandinavica* **39**, 369–380 [437].

McMENEMEY, W.H. (1963b) The dementia and progressive diseases of the basal ganglia. Ch. 9 in *Greenfield's Neuropathology*, 2nd edn, eds Blackwood, W., McMenemey, W.H., Meyer, A., Norman, R.M. & Russell, D.S. Edward Arnold: London [755].

MACMILLAN, D. (1960) Preventive geriatrics: opportunities of a community mental health service. *Lancet* **2**, 1439–1441 [498].

McMILLAN, J.J. & WILLIAMS, B. (1977) Aqueduct stenosis. *Journal of Neurology, Neurosurgery and Psychiatry* **40**, 521–532 [750].

McMILLAN, T.M. (1991) Post-traumatic stress disorder and severe head injury. *British Journal of Psychiatry* **159**, 431–433 [195].

McMILLAN, T.M. & GLUCKSMAN, E.E. (1987) The neuropsychology of moderate head injury. *Journal of Neurology, Neurosurgery and Psychiatry* **50**, 393–397 [198].

McMILLAN, T.M., GREENWOOD, R.J., MORRIS, J.R., BROOKS, D.N., MURPHY, L. & DUNN, G. (1988) An introduction to the concept of head injury case management with respect to the need for service provision. *Clinical Rehabilitation* **2**, 319–322 [216].

McMULLEN, P.A., SAINT-CYR, J.A. & CARLEN, P.L. (1984) Morphological alterations in rat CA1 hippocampal pyramid cell dendrites resulting from chronic ethanol consumption and withdrawal. *Journal of Comparative Neurology* **225**, 111–118 [607].

McNALLY, R.J. (1992) Psychopathology of post-traumatic stress disorder (PTSD): boundaries of the syndrome. Ch. 10 in *Torture and Its Consequences*, ed. Başoğ, M. Cambridge University Press: Cambridge [194].

McNALLY, R.J., KASPI, S.P., RIEMANN, B.C. & ZEITLIN, S.B. (1990) Selective processing of threat cues in post-traumatic stress disorder. *Journal of Abnormal Psychology* **99**, 398–402 [194].

McNEIL, J.E. & WARRINGTON, E.K. (1991) Prosopagnosia: a reclassification. *Quarterly Journal of Experimental Psychology* **43A**, 267–287 [60].

McNEIL, J.E. & WARRINGTON, E.K. (1993) Prosopagnosia: a face-specific disorder. *Quarterly Journal of Experimental Psychology*, **46A**, 1–10 [60].

McNICHOL, R.W. (1970) *The Treatment of Delirium Tremens and Related States*. Thomas: Springfield, Illinois [600].

McQUILLEN, M.P. & JOHNS, R.J. (1963) Asthenic syndrome: anticholinesterase tolerance in nonmyasthenic patients. *Archives of Neurology* **8**, 382–387 [713].

McRAE, D.L., BRANCH, C.L. & MILNER, B. (1968) The occipital horns and cerebral dominance. *Neurology* **18**, 95–98 [41].

MADDEN, S. (1990) Effects of drugs of dependence. Ch. 2 in *Substance Abuse and Dependence*, eds Ghodse, H. & Maxwell, D. Macmillan Press: London [612].

MADELEY, P., BIGGINS, C.A., BOYD, J.L., MINDHAM, R.H.S. & SPOKES, E.G.S. (1992) Emotionalism in Parkinson's disease. *Irish Journal of Psychological Medicine* **9**, 24–25 [657].

MADGE, N., DIAMOND, J., MILLER, D., ROSS, E., McMANUS, C., WADSWORTH, J. & YULE, W. (1993) The National Childhood Encephalopathy Study: a 10-year follow-up. A report on the medical, social, behavioural and educational outcomes after serious, acute, neurological illness in early childhood. *Developmental Medicine and Child Neurology (London)* **35 (Supplement 68)**, 1–117 [348].

MADOW, L. & ALPERS, B.J. (1951) Encephalitic form of metastatic carcinoma. *Archives of Neurology and Psychiatry* **65**, 161–173 [738].

MAHADIK, S.P. (1992) Gangliosides: new generation of neuroprotective agents. Ch. 10 in *Emerging Strategies in Neuroprotection*, eds Marangos, P.J. & Lal, H. Birkhäuser: Boston [165].

MAHENDRA, B. (1981) Where have all the catatonics gone? *Psychological Medicine* **11**, 669–671 [355].

MAHER, E.R. & LEES, A.J. (1986) The clinical features and natural history of the Steele–Richardson–Olszewski syndrome (progressive supranuclear palsy). *Neurology* **36**, 1005–1008 [666].

MAHLER, M. & RANGELL, L. (1943) A psychosomatic study of maladies des tics (Gilles de la Tourette's disease). *Psychiatric Quarterly* **17**, 579–603 [684, 686].

MAHLER, M.E. & BENSON, D.F. (1990) Cognitive dysfunction in multiple sclerosis: a subcortical dementia? Ch. 5 in *Neurobehavioral Aspects of Multiple Sclerosis*, ed. Rao, S.M. Oxford University Press: Oxford [693].

MAHLER, M.S. & LUKE, J.A. (1946) Outcome of the tic syndrome. *Journal of Nervous and Mental Disease* **103**, 433–445 [686].

MAHORNEY, S.L. & CAVENAR, J.O. (1988) A new and timely delusion: the complaint of having AIDS. *American Journal of Psychiatry* **145**, 1130–1132 [332].

MAIER, M. (1995) *In vivo* magnetic resonance spectroscopy. Applications in psychiatry. *British Journal of Psychiatry* **167**, 299–306 [143].

MAIER, M., RON, M.A., BARKER, G.J. & TOFTS, P.S. (1995) Proton magnetic resonance spectroscopy: an *in vivo* method of estimating hippocampal neuronal depletion in schizophrenia. *Psychological Medicine* **25**, 1201–1209 [86, 143].

MAIMARIS, C. (1989) Neck sprains after car accidents. *British Medical Journal* **299**, 123 [200].

MAIMARIS, C., BARNES, M.R. & ALLEN, M.J. (1988) 'Whiplash injuries' of the neck: a retrospective study. *Injury* **19**, 393–396 [201].

MAIR, R.G. & McENTEE, W.J. (1986) Cognitive enhancement in Korsakoff's psychosis by clonidine: a comparison with L-dopa and ephedrine. *Psychopharmacology* **88**, 374–380 [585].

MAIR, W.G.P., WARRINGTON, E.K. & WEISKRANTZ, L. (1979) Memory disorder in Korsakoff's psychosis: a neuropathological and neuropsychological investigation of two cases. *Brain* **102**, 749–783 [25].

MAJ, M. (1990) Psychiatric aspects of HIV-1 infection and AIDS. *Psychological Medicine* **20**, 547–563 [329, 331, 332].

MALAMUD, N. (1964) Neuropathology. In *Mental Retardation: A Review of Research*, eds Stevens, H.A. & Hexer, R. University of Chicago Press: Chicago [437].

MALAMUD, N. (1967) Psychiatric disorder with intracranial tumours of limbic system. *Archives of Neurology* **17**, 113–123 [234].

MALAMUD, N. (1972) Neuropathology of organic brain syndromes associated with aging. In *Aging and the Brain*, ed. Gaitz, C.M. Plenum Press: New York [437].

MALAMUD, N. & SKILLICORN, S.A. (1956) Relationship between the Wernicke and the Korsakoff syndrome. *Archives of Neurology and Psychiatry* **76**, 585–596 [577].

MALETZKY, B.M. (1973) The episodic dyscontrol syndrome. *Diseases of the Nervous System* **34**, 178–185 [83, 297].

MALETZKY, B.M. (1976) The diagnosis of pathological intoxication. *Journal of Studies on Alcohol* **37**, 1215–1228 [595].

MALLOY, P., CIMINO, C. & WESTLAKE, R. (1992) Differential diagnosis of primary and secondary Capgras delusions. *Neuropsychiatry, Neuropsychology, and Behavioral Neurology* **5**, 83–96 [15].

MALLOY, P., MISHRA, S.K. & ADLER, S.H. (1990) Neuropsychological deficits in myotonic muscular dystrophy. *Journal of Neurology, Neurosurgery and Psychiatry* **53**, 1011–1013 [719].

MALONE, W.H. (1937) Psychosis with multiple sclerosis. *Medical Bulletin of the Veterans' Administration* **14**, 113–117 [696].

MALTBY, N., BROE, G.A., CREASEY, H., JORM, A.F., CHRISTENSEN, H. & BROOKS, W.S. (1994) Efficacy of tacrine and lecithin in mild to moderate Alzheimer's disease: double blind trial. *British Medical Journal* **308**, 879–883 [504].

MANCHANDA, R., MILLER, H. & McLACHLAN, R.S. (1993) Post-ictal psychosis after right temporal lobectomy. *Journal of Neurology, Neurosurgery and Psychiatry* **56**, 277–279 [313].

MANDELBROTE, B.M. & WITTKOWER, E.D. (1955) Emotional factors in Grave's disease. *Psychosomatic Medicine* **17**, 109–123 [508].

MANDLEBERG, I.A. & BROOKS, D.N. (1975) Cognitive recovery after severe head injury. I. Serial testing on the Wechsler Adult Intelligence Scale. *Journal of Neurology, Neurosurgery and Psychiatry* **38**, 1121–1126 [185].

MANJI, H. & CONNOLLY, S. (1992) AIDS and the central nervous system: part 2. *Hospital Update* **January 1992**, 28–38 [325, 334].

MANN, A.H. (1972) *A Follow-up Study of Psychiatric Patients Shown to Have Cortical Atrophy by Air Encephalography*. Dissertation for M.Phil. (Psychiatry): University of London [141].

MANN, A.H. (1973) Cortical atrophy and air encephalography: a clinical and radiological study. *Psychological Medicine* **3**, 374–378 [141].

MANN, A.H. (1977) Psychiatric morbidity and hostility in hypertension. *Psychological Medicine* **7**, 653–659 [398].

MANN, A.H. (1981) Factors affecting psychological state during one year on a hypertension trial. *Clinical and Investigative Medicine* **4**, 197–200 [398].

MANN, A.H. (1984) Hypertension: psychological aspects and diagnostic impact in a clinical trial. *Psychological Medicine Monograph Supplement* **5** [398].

MANN, D.M.A. (1985) The neuropathology of Alzheimer's disease: a review with pathogenetic, aetiological and therapeutic considerations. *Mechanisms of Ageing and Development* **31**, 213–255 [443].

MANN, D.M.A., LINCOLN, J., YATES, P.O., STAMP, J.E. & TOPER, S. (1980) Changes in the monoamine containing neurones of the human CNS in senile dementia. *British Journal of Psychiatry* **136**, 533–541 [444].

MANN, D.M.A., SOUTH, P.W., SNOWDEN, J.S. & NEARY, D. (1993) Dementia of frontal lobe type: neuropathology and immunohistochemistry. *Journal of Neurology, Neurosurgery and Psychiatry* **56**, 605–614 [465].

MANN, D.M.A., YATES, P.O. & MARCYNIUK, B. (1984) A comparison of changes in the nucleus basalis and locus caeruleus in Alzheimer's disease. *Journal of Neurology, Neurosurgery and Psychiatry* **47**, 201–203 [444].

MANN, D.M.A., YATES, P.O. & MARCYNIUK, B. (1985) Some morphometric observations on the cerebral cortex and in hippocampus in presenile Alzheimer's disease, senile dementia of Alzheimer type and Down's syndrome in middle age. *Journal of the Neurological Sciences* **69**, 135–159 [443].

MANOACH, D.S., MAHER, B.A. & MANSCHRECK, T.C. (1988) Left-handedness and thought disorder in schizophrenias. *Journal of Abnormal Psychology* **97**, 97–99 [89].

MANSCHRECK, T.C., ALLEN, D.F. & NEVILLE, M. (1987) Freebase psychosis: cases from a Bahamian epidemic of cocaine abuse. *Comprehensive Psychiatry* **28**, 555–564 [619].

MAPOTHER, E. (1937) Mental symptoms associated with head injury: the psychiatric aspect. *British Medical Journal* **2**, 1055–1061 [178].

MAPOU, R.L. & KAPLAN, E. (1991) Neuropsychological improvement from chelation after long-term exposure to lead: case study. *Neuropsychiatry, Neuropsychology, and Behavioral Neurology* **4**, 224–237 [631, 632].

MARCHAND, M.L. (1953) A propos des azotémies dites extra-rénales au cours des affections neuro-mentales aiguës. *Annales Medicopsychologiques* **111(ii)**, 203–207 [556].

MARCHUK, D.A. & COLLINS, F.S. (1994) Molecular genetics of neurofibromatosis 1. Ch. 2 in *The Neurofibromatoses*, eds Huson, S.M. & Hughes, R.A.C. Chapman & Hall: London [703].

MARDER, K., MAESTRE, G., COTE, L., MEJIA, H., ALFARO, B., HALIM, A., TANG, M., TYCKO, B. & MAYEUX, R. (1994) The apolipoprotein $_e4$ allele in Parkinson's disease with and without dementia. *Neurology* **44**, 1330–1331 [448].

MARDER, K., STERN, Y., MALOUF, R., TANG, M.-X., BELL, K., DOONEIEF, G., EL-SADR, W., GOLDSTEIN, S., GORMAN, J., RICHARDS, M., SANO, M., SORRELL, S., TODAK, G., WILLIAMS, J.B.W., EHRHARDT, A. & MAYEUX, R. (1992) Neurologic and neuropsychological manifestations of human immunodeficiency virus infection in intravenous drug users without acquired immunodeficiency syndrome. *Archives of Neurology* **49**, 1169–1175 [329].

MARGERISON, J.H. & LIDDELL, D.W. (1961) The incidence of temporal lobe epilepsy among a hospital population of long-stay female epileptics. *Journal of Mental Science* **107**, 909–920 [265].

MARGO, A. (1981) Acromegaly and depression. *British Journal of Psychiatry* **139**, 467–468 [522].

MARGOLIN, D.I., PATE, D.S., FRIEDRICH, F.J. & ELIA, E. (1990) Dysnomia in dementia and in stroke patients: different underlying cognitive deficits. *Journal of Clinical and Experimental Neuropsychology* **12**, 597–612 [113].

MARK, A.S. & ATLAS, S.W. (1989) Progressive multifocal leukoencephalopathy in patients with AIDS: appearance on MR images. *Radiology* **173**, 517–520 [321].

MARK, V.H. & ERVIN, F.R. (1970) *Violence and the Brain*. Harper and Row: New York [83].

MARK, V.H., SWEET, W.H. & ERVIN, F.R. (1972) The effect of amygdalotomy on violent behavior in patients with temporal lobe epilepsy. Ch. 12 in *Psychosurgery*, eds Hitchcock, E., Laitinen, L. & Vaernet, K. Proceedings of the Second International Conference on Psychosurgery. Thomas: Springfield, Illinois [82].

MARKAND, O.N., WHEELER, G.L. & POLLACK, S.L. (1978) Complex partial status epilepticus (psychomotor status). *Neurology* **28**, 189–196 [256].

MARKHAM, C.H., TRECIOKAS, L.J. & DIAMOND, S.G. (1974) Parkinson's disease and levodopa: a five-year follow-up and review. *Western Journal of Medicine* **121**, 188–206 [659].

MARKOWITZ, A.M., SLANETZ, C.A. & FRANTZ, V.K. (1961) Functioning islet cell tumours of the pancreas: twenty-five year follow up. *Annals of Surgery* **154**, 877–844 [545].

MARKS, I.M. (1969) *Fears and Phobias*. Heinemann: London [277].

MARKS, V. (1981a) Symptomatology. Ch. 5 in *Hypoglycaemia*, 2nd edn, eds Marks, V. & Rose, F.C. Blackwell Scientific Publications: Oxford [539, 544].

MARKS, V. (1981b) Pancreatic hypoglycaemia (hyperinsulinism). Ch. 7 in *Hypoglycaemia*, 2nd edn, eds Marks, V. & Rose, F.C. Blackwell Scientific Publications: Oxford [540].

MARKS, V. (1981c) The investigation of hypoglycaemia. Ch. 19 in *Hypoglycaemia*, 2nd edn, eds Marks, V. & Rose, F.C. Blackwell Scientific Publications: Oxford [541].

MARLOWE, W.B., MANCALL, E.L. & THOMAS, J.J. (1975) Complete Kluver–Bucy syndrome in man. *Cortex* **11**, 53–59 [23].

MARNEROS, A. (1983) Adult onset of Tourette's syndrome: a case report. *American Journal of Psychiatry* **140**, 924–925 [681].

MARQUARDSEN, J. (1969) The natural history of acute cerebrovascular disease. A retrospective study of 769 patients. *Acta Neurologica Scandinavica* **38 (Supplement)**, 1–192 [381].

MARQUARDSEN, J. (1983) Natural history and prognosis of cerebrovascular disease. Ch. 2 in *Vascular Disease of the Central Nervous System*, 2nd edn, ed. Russell, R.W.R. Churchill Livingstone: Edinburgh & London [375].

MARRIOTT, P.J., O'BRIEN, M.D., MacKENZIE, I.C.K. & JANOTA, I. (1975) Progressive multifocal leucoencephalopathy: remission with cytarabine. *Journal of Neurology, Neurosurgery and Psychiatry* **38**, 205–209 [752].

MARSAN, C.A. & ZIVIN, L.S. (1970) Factors related to the occurrence of typical paroxysmal abnormalities in the EEG records of epileptic patients. *Epilepsia* **11**, 361–381 [288].

MARSDEN, C.D. (1976a) The problem of adult-onset idiopathic torsion dystonia and other isolated dyskinesias in adult life (including blepharospasm, oromandibular dystonia, dystonic writer's cramp, and torticollis, or axial dystonia). In *Dystonia*, eds Eldridge, R. & Fahn, S. *Advances in Neurology* **14**, 259–276. Raven Press: New York [678].

MARSDEN, C.D. (1976b) Blepharospasm-oromandibular dystonia syndrome (Brueghel's syndrome). A variant of adult-onset torsion dystonia? *Journal of Neurology, Neurosurgery and Psychiatry* **39**, 1204–1209 [678, 679].

MARSDEN, C.D. (1982) Basal ganglia and disease. *Lancet* **2**, 1141–1146 [467].

MARSDEN, C.D. (1990) Parkinson's disease. *Lancet* **335**, 948–952 [648].

MARSDEN, C.D. & HARRISON, M.J.G. (1972) Outcome of investigation of patients with presenile dementia. *British Medical Journal* **2**, 249–252 [490, 491].

MARSDEN, C.D. & JENNER, P. (1980) The pathophysiology of extrapyramidal side-effects of neuroleptic drugs. *Psychological Medicine* **10**, 55–72 [640, 643].

MARSDEN, C.D. & PARKES, J.D. (1976) 'On–off' effects in patients with Parkinson's disease on chronic levodopa therapy. *Lancet* **1**, 292–296 [650].

MARSDEN, C.D. & PARKES, J.D. (1977) Success and problems of long-term levodopa therapy in Parkinson's disease. *Lancet* **1**, 345–349 [650].

MARSDEN, C.D. & QUINN, N.P. (1990) The dystonias. Neurological disorders affecting 20 000 people in Britain. *British Medical Journal* **300**, 139–144 [669, 672].

MARSDEN, C.D. & REYNOLDS, E.H. (1982) Neurology. Ch. 4 Part 1 in *A Textbook of Epilepsy*, 2nd edn, eds Laidlaw, J. & Richens, A. Churchill Livingstone: Edinburgh and London [238].

MARSDEN, C.D. & SHEEHY, M.P. (1990) Writer's cramp. *Trends in Neurosciences* **13**, 148–153 [675, 676, 677].

MARSDEN, C.D., TARSY, D. & BALDESSARINI, R.J. (1975) Spontaneous and drug-induced movement disorders in psychotic patients. Ch. 12 in *Psychiatric Aspects of Neurologic Disease*, eds Benson, D.F. & Blumer, D. Grune & Stratton: New York [640].

MARSHALL, D.W., BREY, R.L., CAHILL, W.T., HOUK, R.W., ZAJAC, R.A. & BOSWELL, R.N. (1988) Spectrum of cerebrospinal fluid findings in various stages of human immunodeficiency virus infection. *Archives of Neurology* **45**, 954–958 [327].

MARSHALL, E.J., SYED, G.M.S., FENWICK, P.B.C. & LISHMAN, W.A. (1993) A pilot study of schizophrenia-like psychosis in epilepsy using single photon emission computerised tomography. *British Journal of Psychiatry* **163**, 32–36 [281].

MARSHALL, J. (1964) The natural history of transient ischaemic cerebrovascular attacks. *Quarterly Journal of Medicine* **33**, 309–324 [381].

MARSHALL, J.C. & NEWCOMBE, F. (1973) Patterns of paralexia: a psycholinguistic approach. *Journal of Psycholinguistic Research* **2**, 175–199 [43].

MARSHALL, L.F. (1990) Current head injury research. *Current Opinion in Neurology and Neurosurgery* **3**, 4–9 [164].

MARSON, A.G., KADIR, Z.A. & CHADWICK, D.W. (1996) New antiepileptic drugs: a systematic review of their efficacy and tolerability. *British Medical Journal* **313**, 1169–1174 [304].

MARTIN, A.J., FRISTON, K.J., COLEBATCH, J.G. & FRACKOWIAK, R.S.J. (1991) Decreases in regional cerebral blood flow with normal aging. *Journal of Cerebral Blood Flow and Metabolism* **11**, 684–689 [434].

MARTIN, J.J., YAP, M., NEI, I.P. & TAN, T.E. (1983) Selective thalamic degeneration—report of a case with memory and mental disturbances. *Clinical Neuropathology* **2**, 156–162 [755].

MARTIN, J.M. (1982) Chromosome loss and senescence. *Psychological Medicine* **12**, 231–233 [431].

MARTIN, J.M., KELLETT, J.M. & KHAN, J. (1981) Aneuploidy in cultured human lymphocytes: II a comparison between senescence and dementia. *Age and Ageing* **10**, 24–28 [431].

MARTIN, M.J. (1966) Tension headache: a psychiatric study. *Headache* **6**, 47–54 [409].

MARTIN, P.R., ADINOFF, B., ECKARDT, M.J., STAPLETON, J.M., BONE, G.A.H., RUBINOW, D.R., LANE, E.A. & LINNOILA, M. (1989) Effective pharmacotherapy of alcoholic amnestic disorder with fluvoxamine. *Archives of General Psychiatry* **46**, 617–621 [585].

MARTIN, P.R., WEINGARTNER, H., GORDON, E.K., BURNS, R.S., LINNOILA, M., KOPIN, I.J. & EBERT, M.H. (1984) Central nervous system catecholamine metabolism in Korsakoff's psychosis. *Annals of Neurology* **15**, 184–187 [585].

MARTINDALE, B. & BOTTOMLEY, V. (1980) The management of families with Huntington's chorea: a case study to illustrate some recommendations. *Journal of Child Psychology and Psychiatry* **21**, 343–351 [499].

MARTINOT, J.-L., PAILLÈRE-MARTINOT, M.L., LOC'H, C., LECRUBIER, Y., DAO-CASTELLANA, M.H., AUBIN, F., ALLILAIRE, J.F., MAZOYER, B., MAZIÈRE, B. & SYROTA, A. (1994) Central D$_2$ receptors and negative symptoms of schizophrenia. *British Journal of Psychiatry* **164**, 27–34 [88].

MARTINOT, J.-L., PERON-MAGNAN, P., HURET, J.-D., MAZOYER, B., BARON, J.-C., BOULENGER, J.-P., LOC'H, C., MAZIÈRE, B., CAILLARD, V., LOO, H. & SYROTA, A. (1990) Striatal D$_2$ dopaminergic receptors assessed with positron emission tomography and [^{76}Br] bromospiperone in untreated schizophrenic patients. *American Journal of Psychiatry* **147**, 44–50 [88].

MARTLAND, H.S. (1928) Punch drunk. *Journal of the American Medical Association* **91**, 1103–1107 [204].

MARTTILA, R.J. & RINNE, U.K. (1976) Dementia in Parkinson's disease. *Acta Neurologica Scandinavica* **54**, 431–441 [653].

MARTYN, C.N., BARKER, D.J.P., OSMOND, C., HARRIS, E.C., EDWARDSON, J.A. & LACEY, R.F. (1989) Geographical relation between Alzheimer's disease and aluminium in drinking water. *Lancet* **1**, 59–62 [446].

MARZUK, P.M. (1991) Suicidal behavior and HIV illness. *International Review of Psychiatry* **3**, 365–371 [331].

MARZUK, P.M., TIERNEY, H., TARDIFF, K., GROSS, E.M., MORGAN, E.B., HSU, M.-A. & MANN, J.J. (1988) Increased risk of suicide in persons with AIDS. *Journal of the American Medical Association* **259**, 1333–1337 [331].

MASH, D.C., FLYNN, D.D. & POTTER, L.T. (1985) Loss of M$_2$ muscarine receptors in the cerebral cortex in Alzheimer's disease and experimental cholinergic denervation. *Science* **228**, 1115–1117 [444].

MASLIAH, E., ACHIM, C.L., GE, N., DETERESA, R. & WILEY, C.A. (1994) Cellular neuropathy in HIV encephalitis. Ch. 6 in *HIV, AIDS, and the Brain*, eds Price, R.W. & Perry, S.W. *Association for Research in Nervous and Mental Disease* **72**. Raven Press: New York [323].

MASON, J.C. & WALPORT, M.J. (1992) Giant cell arteritis. Probably underdiagnosed and overtreated. *British Medical Journal* **305**, 68–69 [424].

MASTER, D.R. & LISHMAN, W.A. (1984) Seizures, dyslexia, and dysgraphia of psychogenic origin. *Archives of Neurology* **41**, 889–890 [55].

MASTER, D.R., LISHMAN, W.A. & SMITH, A. (1983) Speed of recall in relation to affective tone and intensity of experience. *Psychological Medicine* **13**, 325–331 [25].

MASTER, D.R., THOMPSON, C., DUNN, G. & LISHMAN, W.A. (1986) Memory selectivity and unilateral cerebral dysfunction. *Psychological Medicine* **16**, 781–788 [25].

MASTER, D.R., TOONE, B.K. & SCOTT, D.F. (1984) Interictal behaviour in temporal lobe epilepsy. In *Advances in Epileptology: XVth Epilepsy International Symposium*, eds Porter, R.J., Mattson, R.H., Ward, A.A. & Dam, M. Raven Press: New York [268].

MASTERS, C.L., HARRIS, J.O., GAJDUSEK, D.C., GIBBS, C.J., BERNOULLI, C. & ASHER, D.M. (1979) Creutzfeldt–Jakob disease: patterns of worldwide occurrence and the significance of familial and sporadic clustering. *Annals of Neurology* **5**, 177–188 [473, 476].

MASTERS, C.L., SIMMS, G., WEINMAN, N.A., MULTHAUP, G., McDONALD, B.L. & BEYREUTHER, K. (1985) Amyloid plaque core protein in Alzheimer disease and Down syndrome. *Proceedings of the National Academy of Science* **82**, 4245–4249 [442].

MATHEW, N.T. & MEYER, J.S. (1974) Pathogenesis and natural history of transient global amnesia. *Stroke* **5**, 303–311 [415, 416].

MATHEW, N.T., MEYER, J.S., WELSCH, K.M. & NEBLETT, C.R. (1977) Abnormal CT scans in migraine. *Headache* **16**, 272–279 [401].

MATSUDA, L.A., LOLAIT, S.J., BROWNSTEIN, M.J., YOUNG, A.C. & BONNER, T.I. (1990) Structure of a cannabinoid receptor and functional expression of the cloned cDNA. *Nature* **346**, 561–564 [612].

MATSUMOTO, J. & HALLETT, M. (1994) Startle syndromes. Ch. 21 in *Movement Disorders*, Vol. 3, eds Marsden, C.D. & Fahn, S. Butterworth-Heinemann: Oxford [292].

MATTHEWS, W.B. (1965) Sarcoidosis of the nervous system. *Journal of Neurology, Neurosurgery and Psychiatry* **28**, 23–29 [764].

MATTHEWS, W.B. (1975) Epidemiology of Creutzfeldt–Jakob disease in England and Wales. *Journal of Neurology, Neurosurgery and Psychiatry* **38**, 210–213 [475].

MATTHEWS, W.B. (1979) Multiple sclerosis presenting with acute remitting psychiatric symptoms. *Journal of Neurology, Neurosurgery and Psychiatry* **42**, 859–863 [697].

MATTHEWS, W.B. (1981) Slow virus infections. *Journal of the Royal College of Physicians of London* **15**, 109–112 [479].

MATTHEWS, W.B. (1982) Spongiform virus encephalopathy. In *Recent Advances in Clinical Neurology*, Vol. 3, eds Matthews, W.B. & Glaser, G.H. Churchill Livingstone: Edinburgh [479].

MATTSON, R.H. (1991) Emotional effects on seizure occurrence. Ch. 28 in *Neurobehavioral Problems in Epilepsy*, eds Smith, D.B., Treiman, D.M. & Trimble, M.R. *Advances in Neurology*, Vol. 55. Raven Press: New York [248].

MAUDSLEY, H. (1873) *Body and Mind*. Macmillan & Co.: London [274].

MAUDSLEY, H. (1906) *Responsibility in Mental Disease*. Kegan Paul, Trench, Trübner & Co.: London [274].

MAUGHAN, B. & YULE, W. (1994) Reading and other learning disabilities. Ch. 36 in *Child and Adolescent Psychiatry. Modern Approaches*, 3rd edn, eds Rutter, M., Taylor, E. & Hersov, L. Blackwell Science Ltd: Oxford [47].

MAURI, M., SINFORIANI, E., BONO, G., VIGNATI, F., BERSELLI, M.E., ATTANASIO, R. & NAPPI, G. (1993) Memory impairment in Cushing's disease. *Acta Neurologica Scandinavica* **87**, 52–55 [517].

MAURICE-WILLIAMS, R.S. (1974) Micturition symptoms in frontal tumours. *Journal of Neurology, Neurosurgery and Psychiatry* **37**, 431–436 [223].

MAURICE-WILLIAMS, R.S. (1987) *Subarachnoid Haemorrhage: Aneurysms and Vascular Malformations of the Central Nervous System*, pp. 49–145. Wright: Bristol [393].

MAURICE-WILLIAMS, R.S. & DUNWOODY, G. (1988) Late diagnosis of frontal meningiomas presenting with psychiatric symptoms. *British Medical Journal* **296**, 1785–1788 [234].

MAURICE-WILLIAMS, R.S. & SINAR, E.J. (1984) Depression caused by an intracranial meningioma relieved by leucotomy prior to diagnosis of the tumour. *Journal of Neurology, Neurosurgery and Psychiatry* **47**, 844–885 [235].

MAWDSLEY, C. (1961) Epilepsy and television. *Lancet* **1**, 190–191 [241].

MAWDSLEY, C. (1972) Neurological complications of haemodialysis. *Proceedings of the Royal Society of Medicine* **65**, 871–873 [556, 558].

MAWDSLEY, C. & FERGUSON, F.R. (1963) Neurological disease in boxers. *Lancet* **2**, 795–801 [204].

MAXWELL, D.L., POLKEY, M.I. & HENRY, J.A. (1993) Hyponatraemia and catatonic stupor after taking 'ecstasy'. *British Medical Journal* **307**, 1399 [624].

MAY, P.R.A. & EBAUGH, F.G. (1953) Pathological intoxication, alcoholic hallucinosis, and other reactions to alcohol: a clinical study. *Quarterly Journal of Studies on Alcohol* **14**, 200–227 [595].

MAY, R.H., VOEGELE, G.E. & PAOLINO, A.F. (1960) The Ganser syndrome: a report of 3 cases. *Journal of Nervous and Mental Disease* **130**, 331–339 [481].

MAY, W.W. (1968) Creutzfeldt–Jakob disease. *Acta Neurologica Scandinavica* **44**, 1–32 [478].

MAYBERG, H.S., PARIKH, R.M., MORRIS, P.L.P. & ROBINSON, R.G. (1991) Spontaneous remission of post-stroke depression and temporal changes in cortical S₂-serotonin receptors. *Clinical and Research Reports* **3**, 80–83 [386].

MAYBERG, H.S., ROBINSON, R.G., WONG, D.F., PARIKH, R.M., BOLDUC, P., STARKSTEIN, S.E., PRICE, T., DANNALS, R.F., LINKS, J.M., WILSON, A.A., RAVERT, H.T. & WAGNER, H.N. (1988) PET imaging of cortical S₂ serotonin receptors after stroke: lateralized changes and relationship to depression. *American Journal of Psychiatry* **145**, 937–943 [386].

MAYES, A.R. (1988) *Human Organic Memory Disorders*. Cambridge University Press: Cambridge [27].

MAYES, A.R., MEUDELL, P.R. & PICKERING, A. (1985) Is organic amnesia caused by a selective deficit in remembering contextual information? *Cortex* **21**, 167–202 [27].

MAYEUX, R., STERN, Y., COTE, L. & WILLIAMS, J.B.W. (1984) Altered serotonin metabolism in depressed patients with Parkinson's disease. *Neurology* **34**, 642–646 [657].

MAYEUX, R., STERN, Y., ROSEN, J. & LEVENTHAL, J. (1981) Depression, intellectual impairment, and Parkinson's disease. *Neurology* **31**, 645–650 [656].

MAYEUX, R., STERN, Y., ROSENSTEIN, R., MARDER, K., HAUSER, A., COTE, L. & FAHN, S. (1988a) An estimate of the prevalence of dementia in idiopathic Parkinson's disease. *Archives of Neurology* **45**, 260–262 [654].

MAYEUX, R., STERN, Y., SANO, M., WILLIAMS, J.B.W. & COTE, L.J. (1988b) The relationship of serotonin to depression in Parkinson's disease. *Movement Disorders* **3**, 237–244 [657].

MAYOU, R. (1986) The psychiatric and social consequences of coronary artery surgery. *Journal of Psychosomatic Research* **30**, 255–271 [554].

MAYOU, R., BRYANT, B. & DUTHIE, R. (1993) Psychiatric consequences of road traffic accidents. *British Medical Journal* **307**, 647–651 [194, 195, 201].

MAZZIOTTA, J.C., PHELPS, M.E., PAHL, J.J., HUANG, S., BAXTER, L.R.,

RIEGE, W.H., HOFFMAN, J.M., KUHL, D.E., LANTO, A.B., WAPENSKI, J.A. & MARKHAM, C.H. (1987) Reduced cerebral glucose metabolism in asymptomatic subjects at risk for Huntington's disease. *New England Journal of Medicine* **316**, 357–362 [470].

MAZZUCCHI, A., MORETTI, G., CAFFARA, P. & PARMA, M. (1980) Neuropsychological functions in the follow-up of transient global amnesia. *Brain* **103**, 161–178 [415].

MEADER, H. & VELLA, M. (1992) Hypercalcaemia is an essential diagnosis. *Geriatric Medicine* **22(1)**, 16–19 [560].

MEARES, R. (1971a) Natural history of spasmodic torticollis, and effect of surgery. *Lancet* **2**, 149–150 [673].

MEARES, R. (1971b) Features which distinguish groups of spasmodic torticollis. *Journal of Psychosomatic Research* **15**, 1–11 [673].

MEARES, R. (1971c) An association of spasmodic torticollis and writer's cramp. *British Journal of Psychiatry* **119**, 441–442 [677].

MEARES, R. (1973) Spasmodic torticollis. *British Journal of Hospital Medicine* **9**, 235–241 [675].

MEDALIA, A., ISAACS-GLABERMAN, K. & SCHEINBERG, H. (1988) Neuropsychological impairment in Wilson's disease. *Archives of Neurology* **45**, 502–504 [665].

MEDICAL DISABILITY SOCIETY (1988) *The Management of Traumatic Brain Injury*. Development Trust for the Young Disabled: London [215].

MEDICAL RESEARCH COUNCIL (1977) *Senile and Presenile Dementias*. A report of the MRC Subcommittee, compiled by Lishman, W.A. Medical Research Council: London [441].

MEDORI, R., MONTAGNA, P., TRITSCHLER, H.J., LEBLANC, A., CORTELLI, P., TINUPER, P., LUGARESI, E. & GAMBETTI, P. (1992a) Fatal familial insomnia: a second kindred with mutation of prion protein gene at codon 178. *Neurology* **42**, 669–670 [734].

MEDORI, R., TRITSCHLER, H.J., LEBLANC, A., VILLARE, F., MANETTO, V., CHEN, H.Y., XUE, R., LEAL, S., MONTAGNA, P., CORTELLI, P., TINUPER, P., AVONI, P., MOCHI, M., BARUZZI, A., HAUW, J.J., OTT, J., LUGARESI, E., AUTILIO-GAMBETTI, L. & GAMBETTI, P. (1992b) Fatal familial insomnia, a prion disease with a mutation at codon 178 of the prion protein gene. *New England Journal of Medicine* **326**, 444–449 [734].

MEDUNA, L.J. (1937) *Die Konvulsiontherapie der Schizphrenie*. Marhold: Halle [279].

MEER, B. & BAKER, J.A. (1966) The Stockton Geriatric Rating Scale. *Journal of Gerontology* **21**, 393–403 [125].

MEHTA, S., TEJA, J.S., WIG, N.N., THUKRAL, S. & PASRICHA, S. (1975) Protein calorie malnutrition: a follow-up study. *Indian Journal of Medical Research* **64**, 576–582 [570].

MEHTA, T. (1965) Subdural haematoma. *Journal of the Indian Medical Association* **44**, 635–641 [412].

MELAMED, E. (1979) Neurological disorders related to folate deficiency. Ch. 38 in *Folic Acid in Neurology, Psychiatry, and Internal Medicine*, eds Botez, M.I. & Reynolds, E.H. Raven Press: New York [591].

MELDRUM, B. & GARTHWAITE, J. (1990) Excitatory amino acid neurotoxicity and neurodegenerative disease. *Trends in Pharmacological Sciences* **11**, 379–387 [164].

MELDRUM, B.S., HORTON, R.W. & BRIERLEY, J.B. (1974) Epileptic brain damage in adolescent baboons following seizures induced by allylglycine. *Brain* **97**, 407–418 [246].

MELDRUM, B.S., VIGOUROUX, R.A. & BRIERLEY, J.B. (1973) Systemic factors and epileptic brain damage: prolonged seizures in paralyzed artificially ventilated baboons. *Archives of Neurology* **29**, 82–87 [246].

MELGAARD, B., HENRIKSEN, L., AHLGREN, P., DANIELSEN, U.T., SØRENSEN, H. & PAULSON, O.B. (1990) Regional CBF in chronic alcoholics measured by single photon emission computerized tomography. *Acta Neurologica Scandinavica* **82**, 87–93 [606].

MELLERS, J.D.C., ADACHI, N., TAKEI, N., CLUCKEY, A., TOONE, B.K. & LISHMAN, W.A. (1996) A SPET study of word generation in schizophrenia and epilepsy (Abstract). *Schizophrenia Research* **18**, 193–194 [281].

MENDELOW, A.D. (1993) Raised intracranial pressure, cerebral oedema, hydrocephalus, and intracranial tumours. Ch. 4 in *Brain's Diseases of the Nervous System*, 10th edn, ed. Walton, J. Oxford University Press: Oxford [231, 232, 746].

MENDELSON, G. (1982) Not 'cured by verdict'. Effect of legal settlement on compensation claims. *Medical Journal of Australia* **2**, 132–134 [177].

MENDEZ, M.F. & DOSS, R.C. (1995) Neurobehavioral aspects of the delayed encephalopathy of carbon monoxide intoxication: case report and review. *Behavioural Neurology* **8**, 47–52 [551].

MENDEZ, M.F., GRAU, R., DOSS, R.C. & TAYLOR, J.L. (1993) Schizophrenia in epilepsy: seizure and psychosis variables. *Neurology* **43**, 1073–1077 [279].

MENDHIRATTA, S.S., WIG, N.N. & VERMA, S.K. (1978) Some psychological correlates of long-term heavy cannabis users. *British Journal of Psychiatry* **132**, 482–486 [616].

MENNINGER, K.A. (1924) Paranoid psychosis with uraemia. *Journal of Nervous and Mental Disease* **60**, 26–34 [556].

MENON, D.K., BAUDOUIN, C.J., TOMLINSON, D. & HOYLE, C. (1990) Proton MR spectroscopy and imaging of the brain in AIDS: evidence of neuronal loss in regions that appear normal with imaging. *Journal of Computer Assisted Tomography* **14**, 882–885 [325].

MENON, R.R., BARTA, P.E., AYLWARD, E.H., RICHARDS, S.S., VAUGHN, D.D., TIEN, A.Y., HARRIS, G.J. & PEARLSON, G.D. (1995) Posterior superior temporal gyrus in schizophrenia: grey matter changes and clinical correlates. *Schizophrenia Research* **16**, 127–135 [85].

MERIKANGAS, K.R., ANGST, J. & ISLER, H. (1990) Migraine and psychopathology. Results of the Zurich cohort study of young adults. *Archives of General Psychiatry* **47**, 849–853 [404].

MERLIS, J.K. (1970) Proposal for an international classification of the epilepsies. *Epilepsia* **11**, 114–119 [237].

MERLIS, J.K. (1974) Reflex epilepsy. Ch. 25 in *Handbook of Clinical Neurology, Vol. 15: The Epilepsies*, eds Vinken, P.J. & Bruyn, G.W. North-Holland Publishing Co.: Amsterdam [241].

MERRIN, E.L. (1981) Schizophrenia and brain asymmetry. An evaluation of evidence for dominant lobe dysfunction. *Journal of Nervous and Mental Disease* **169**, 405–416 [89].

MERRITT, H.H. (1979) *A Textbook of Neurology*, 6th edn. Lea and Febiger: Philadelphia [770].

MERSKEY, H. & WOODFORDE, J.M. (1972) Psychiatric sequelae of minor head injury. *Brain* **95**, 521–528 [177].

MESSERT, B. & BAKER, N.H. (1966) Syndrome of progressive spastic ataxia and apraxia associated with occult hydrocephalus. *Neurology* **16**, 440–452 [749].

MESSERT, B., HENKE, T.K. & LANGHEIM, W. (1966) Syndrome of akinetic mutism associated with obstructive hydrocephalus. *Neurology* **16**, 635–649 [749].

MESULAM, M.-M. (1982) Slowly progressive aphasia without generalised dementia. *Annals of Neurology* **11**, 592–598 [752].

MESULAM, M.-M., WAXMAN, S.G., GESCHWIND, N. & SABIN, T.D. (1976) Acute confusional states with right middle cerebral artery infarctions. *Journal of Neurology, Neurosurgery and Psychiatry* **39**, 84–89 [378].

MESULAM, M.-M. & WEINTRAUB, S. (1992) The spectrum of primary progressive aphasia. Ch. 6 in *Unusual Dementias*, ed. Rossor, M.N. Ballière Tindall: London [752, 753].

METCALF, D.R. & HOLMES, J.H. (1969) EEG, psychological, and neurological alterations in humans with organophosphorus exposure. *Annals of the New York Academy of Science* **160**, 357–365 [637].

METRAKOS, J.D. & METRAKOS, K. (1960) Genetics of convulsive disorders. 1: Introduction, problems, methods, baselines. *Neurology* **10**, 228–240 [261].

METRAKOS, J.D. & METRAKOS, K. (1961) Genetics of convulsive disorders. II: Genetic and electroencephalographic studies in centrencephalic epilepsy. *Neurology* **11**, 474–483 [247].

METRAKOS, J.D. & METRAKOS, K. (1970) Genetic factors in epilepsy. *Modern Problems in Pharmacopsychiatry* **4**, 71–86 [247].

METTER, E.J. & HANSON, W.R. (1994) Use of positron emission tomography to study aphasia. Ch. 5 in *Localization and Neuroimaging in Neuropsychology*, ed. Kertesz, A. Academic Press: San Diego [45].

METTER, E.J., KUHL, D.E. & RIEGE, W.H. (1990) Brain glucose metabolism in Parkinson's disease. In *Parkinson's Disease: Anatomy, Pathology, and Therapy*, eds Streffler, M.B., Korczyn, A.D., Melamed, E. & Youdm, M.B.H. *Advances in Neurology* **53**, 135–139. Raven Press: New York [655].

MEUDELL, P.R. (1992) Irrelevant, incidental and core features in the retrograde amnesia associated with Korsakoff's psychosis: a review. *Behavioural Neurology* **5**, 67–74 [37].

MEUDELL, P.R., NORTHERN, B., SNOWDEN, J.S. & NEARY, D. (1980) Long-term memory for famous voices in amnesic and normal subjects. *Neuropsychologia* **18**, 133–139 [36].

MEYER, E. (1966) Psychological disturbances in myasthenia gravis: a predictive study. *Annals of the New York Academy of Sciences* **135**, 417–423 [710, 712].

MEYER, J.S. & GOTOH, F. (1960) Metabolic and electroencephalographic effects of hyperventilation. *Archives of Neurology* **3**, 539–552 [127].

MEYER, J.S., SHINOHARA, T., IMAI, A., KOBARI, M., SAKAI, F., HATA, T., ORAVEZ, W.T., TINIPE, G.M., DEVILLE, T. & SOLOMON, E. (1988) Imaging local cerebral blood flow by xenon-enhanced computed tomography—technical optimization procedures. *Neuroradiology* **30**, 283–292 [138].

MEYER, J.S., TANAHASHI, N., ISHIKAWA, Y., HATA, T., VELEZ, M., FANN, W.E., KANDULA, P., MORTEL, K.F. & ROGERS, R.L. (1985) Cerebral atrophy and hypoperfusion improve during treatment of Wernicke–Korsakoff syndrome. *Journal of Cerebral Blood Flow and Metals* **5**, 376–385 [579].

MICHAEL, R.P. (1957) Treatment of a case of compulsive swearing. *British Medical Journal* **1**, 1506–1508 [686].

MICHAEL, R.P. & GIBBONS, J.L. (1963) Interrelationships between the endocrine system and neuropsychiatry. *International Review of Neurobiology* **5**, 243–302 [514, 516, 519].

MICHEL, P.H., COMMENGES, D., DARTIGUES, J.F. & GAGNON, M. & THE PAQUID RESEARCH GROUP (1990) Study of the relationship between Alzheimer's disease and aluminium in drinking water. *Neurobiology of Aging* **11**, 264 [446].

MIELKE, R., HERHOLZ, K., GROND, M., KESSLER, J. & HEISS, W.-D. (1991) Differences of regional cerebral glucose metabolism between presenile and senile dementia of Alzheimer-type. *Neurobiology of Aging* **13**, 93–98 [449].

MIKKELSEN, B. & BIRKET-SMITH, E. (1973) A clinical study of the benzodiazepine Ro 5–4023 (clonazepam) in the treatment of epilepsy. *Acta Neurologica Scandinavica* **53 (Supplement)**, 91–96 [302].

MIKKELSON, E.J. & REIDER, A.A. (1979) Post-parathyroidectomy psychosis: clinical and research implications. *Journal of Clinical Psychiatry* **40**, 352–358 [531].

MILLER, D., ACTON, T.M.G. & HEDGE, B. (1988) The worried well:

their identification and management. *Journal of the Royal College of Physicians of London* **22**, 158–165 [332].

MILLER, D. & RICCIO, M. (1990) Non-organic psychiatric and psychosocial syndromes associated with HIV-1 infection and disease. *AIDS* **4**, 381–388 [330].

MILLER, D.H., RUDGE, P., JOHNSON, G., KENDALL, B.E., MACMANUS, D.G., MOSELEY, I.F., BARNES, D. & McDONALD, W.I. (1988) Serial gadolinium enhanced magnetic resonance imaging in multiple sclerosis. *Brain* **111**, 927–939 [690].

MILLER, E. (1973) Short- and long-term memory in patients with presenile dementia. *Psychological Medicine* **3**, 221–224 [32].

MILLER, E. (1974) Dementia as accelerated ageing of the nervous system: some psychological and methodological considerations. *Age and Ageing* **3**, 197–202 [436].

MILLER, E. (1977) *Abnormal Ageing: The Psychology of Senile and Presenile Dementia.* John Wiley: London [436, 501].

MILLER, E.N., SELNES, O.A., McARTHUR, J.C., SATZ, P., BECKER, J.T., COHEN, B.A., SHERIDAN, K., MACHADO, A.M., VAN GORP, W.G. & VISSCHER, B. (1990) Neuropsychological performance in HIV-1-infected homosexual men: the Multicenter AIDS Cohort Study (MACS). *Neurology* **40**, 197–203 [329].

MILLER, H. (1961) Accident neurosis. *British Medical Journal* **1**, 919–925 and 992–998 [174, 176].

MILLER, H. (1966a) Mental after-effects of head injury. *Proceedings of the Royal Society of Medicine* **59**, 257–261 [175, 176].

MILLER, H. (1966b) Neurological manifestations of collagen-vascular disease. *Journal of the Royal College of Physicians of London* **1**, 15–19 [426].

MILLER, H. (1969) Problems of medicolegal practice. Ch. 42 in *The Late Effects of Head Injury*, eds Walker, A.E., Caveness, W.F. & Critchley, M. Thomas: Springfield, Illinois [177, 209].

MILLER, H. & CARTLIDGE, N. (1972) Simulation and malingering after injuries to the brain and spinal cord. *Lancet* **1**, 580–585 [208, 209].

MILLER, H. & STERN, G. (1965) The long-term prognosis of severe head injury. *Lancet* **1**, 225–229 [185].

MILLER, J.W., PETERSEN, R.C., METTER, E.J., MILLIKAN, C.H. & YANAGIHARA, T. (1987) Transient global amnesia: clinical characteristics and prognosis. *Neurology* **37**, 733–737 [414, 416, 417].

MILLICHAP, J.G. (1974) Metabolic and endocrine factors. Ch. 19 in *Handbook of Clinical Neurology, Vol. 15, The Epilepsies*, eds Vinken, P.J. & Bruyn, G.W. North Holland: Amsterdam [513].

MILLMAN, P.P., FOGEL, B.S., McNAMARA, M.E. & CARLISLE, C.C. (1989) Depression as a manifestation of obstructive sleep apnoea: reversal with nasal continuous positive airway pressure. *Journal of Clinical Psychiatry* **50**, 348–351 [731].

MILNER, B. (1958) Psychological defects produced by temporal lobe excision. Ch. 8 in *The Brain and Human Behavior*, Research Publications of the Association for Research in Nervous and Mental Disease, Vol. 36. Williams & Wilkins: Baltimore [63, 261].

MILNER, B. (1962) Laterality effects in audition. Ch. 9 in *Interhemispheric Relations and Cerebral Dominance*, ed. Mountcastle, V. Johns Hopkins Press: Baltimore [64, 261].

MILNER, B. (1963) Effects of different brain lesions on card sorting. *Archives of Neurology* **9**, 90–100 [77, 118].

MILNER, B. (1964) Some effects of frontal lobectomy in man. Ch. 15 in *The Frontal Granular Cortex and Behaviour*, eds Warren, J.M. & Akert, K. McGraw-Hill: New York [77, 78, 118].

MILNER, B. (1966) Amnesia following operation on the temporal lobes. Ch. 5 in *Amnesia*, eds Whitty, C.W.M. & Zangwill, O. Butterworths: London [26, 30, 100].

MILNER, B. (1969) Residual intellectual and memory deficits after head injury. Ch. 7 in *The Late Effects of Head Injury*, eds Walker, A.E.,

Caveness, W.F. & Critchley, M. Thomas: Springfield, Illinois [116, 118].

MILNER, D. (1983) Neuropsychological studies of callosal agenesis. *Psychological Medicine* **13**, 721–725 [770].

MINDEN, S.L. & SCHIFFER, R.B. (1990) Affective disorders in multiple sclerosis. Review and recommendations for clinical research. *Archives of Neurology* **47**, 98–104 [694].

MINDHAM, R.H.S. (1970) Psychiatric symptoms in parkinsonism. *Journal of Neurology, Neurosurgery and Psychiatry* **33**, 188–191 [653, 656, 657].

MINDHAM, R.H.S. (1974) Psychiatric aspects of Parkinson's disease. *British Journal of Hospital Medicine* **11**, 411–414 [656].

MINSKI, L. (1933) The mental symptoms associated with 58 cases of cerebral tumour. *Journal of Neurology and Psychopathology* **13**, 330–343 [219, 235].

MINSKI, L. & GUTTMANN, E. (1938) Huntington's chorea: a study of thirty-four families. *Journal of Mental Science* **84**, 21–96 [472].

MIRSEN, T.R. & MERSKEY, H. (1994) Leukoaraiosis. Ch. 39 in *Dementia*, eds Burns, A. & Levy, R. Chapman & Hall: London [460].

MISHKIN, M. (1978) Memory in monkeys severely impaired by combined but not separate removal of amygdala and hippocampus. *Nature* **273**, 297–298 [26].

MISRA, P.C. & HAY, G.G. (1971) Encephalitis presenting as acute schizophrenia. *British Medical Journal* **1**, 532–533 [347].

MITCHELL, J.R.A., SURRIDGE, D.H.C. & WILLISON, R.G. (1959) Hypothermia after chlorpromazine in myxoedematous psychosis. *British Medical Journal* **2**, 932–933 [515].

MITCHELL, K.R. (1971) A psychological approach to the treatment of migraine. *British Journal of Psychiatry* **119**, 533–534 [410].

MITCHELL, W., FALCONER, M.A. & HILL, D. (1954) Epilepsy with fetishism relieved by temporal lobectomy. *Lancet* **2**, 626–630 [272].

MITCHELL, W. & FELDMAN, F. (1968) Neuropsychiatric aspects of hypokalaemia. *Canadian Medical Association Journal* **98**, 49–51 [560].

MIYASAKI, J.M. & LANG, A.E. (1995) Treatment of drug-induced movement disorders. Ch. 11 in *Treatment of Movement Disorders*, ed. Kurlan, R.J.B. Lippincott: Philadelphia [627, 640, 643].

MJÖNES, H. (1949) Paralysis agitans: a clinical and genetic study. *Acta Psychiatrica et Neurologica* **54 (Supplement)**, 1–195 [652, 657].

MODY, C.K., MILLER, B.L., McINTYRE, H.B., COBB, S.K. & GOLDBERG, M.A. (1988) Neurologic complications of cocaine abuse. *Neurology* **38**, 1189–1193 [617].

MOELI, C. (1888) Ueber ihre Verbrecher. Quoted by Enoch, M.D., Trethowan, W.H. & Barker, J.C. (1967) In *Some Uncommon Psychiatric Syndromes*. John Wright: Bristol [480].

MOERSCH, F.P. (1924) Psychic manifestations in migraine. *American Journal of Psychiatry* **80**, 697–716 [291, 407].

MOFFATT, W.R., SIDDIQUI, A.R. & MacKAY, D.N. (1970) The use of sulthiame with disturbed mentally subnormal patients. *British Journal of Psychiatry* **117**, 673–678 [305].

MOFFOOT, A., O'CARROLL, R.E., MURRAY, C., DOUGALL, N., EBMEIER, K. & GOODWIN, G.M. (1994) Clonidine infusion increases uptake of 99mTc-Exametazime in anterior cingulate cortex in Korsakoff's psychosis. *Psychological Medicine* **24**, 53–61 [585].

MOHR, J.A., GRIFFITHS, W., JACKSON, R., SAADAH, H., BIRD, P. & RIDDLE, J. (1976) Neurosyphilis and penicillin levels in cerebrospinal fluid. *Journal of the American Medical Association* **236**, 2208–2209 [344].

MOHS, R.C., BREITNER, J.C.S., SILVERMAN, J.M. & DAVIS, K.L. (1987) Alzheimer's disease. Morbid risk among first-degree relatives approximates 50% by 90 years of age. *Archives of General Psychiatry* **44**, 405–408 [431].

MOHS, R.C., DAVIS, K.L., TINKLENBERG, J.R., PFEFFERBAUM, A., HOLLISTER, L.E. & KOPELL, B.S. (1979) Cognitive effects of physostigmine and choline chloride in normal subjects. In *Brain Acetylcholine and Neuropsychiatric Disease*, eds Davis, K.L. & Berger, P.A. Plenum Press: New York [503].

MÖLSÄ, P.K., PALJARVI, L., RINNE, J.O., RINNE, U.K. & SÄKÖ, E. (1985) Validity of clinical diagnosis in dementia: a prospective clinicopathological study. *Journal of Neurology, Neurosurgery and Psychiatry* **48**, 1085–1090 [457].

MOMOSE, K.J., KJELLBERG, R.N. & KLIMAN, B. (1971) High incidence of cortical atrophy of the cerebral and cerebellar hemispheres in Cushing's disease. *Radiology* **99**, 341–348 [517].

MONEY, J. (1963) Cytogenetic and psychosexual incongruities with a note on space-form blindness. *American Journal of Psychiatry* **119**, 820–827 [528].

MONEY, J. (1964) Two cytogenetic syndromes: psychologic comparisons. 1. Intelligence and specific-factor quotients. *Journal of Psychiatric Research* **2**, 223–231 [528].

MONEY, J. & EHRHARDT, A.A. (1968) Prenatal hormonal exposures: possible effects on behaviour in man. Ch. 1 in *Endocrinology and Human Behaviour*, ed. Michael, R.P. Oxford University Press: London [507].

MONPETIT, V.J.A., ANDERMANN, F., CARPENTER, S., FAWCETT, J.S., ZBOROWSKA-SLUIS, D. & GIBERSON, H.R. (1971) Subacute necrotizing encephalomyelopathy. A review and a study of two families. *Brain* **94**, 1–30 [587].

MONTALDI, D., BROOKS, D.N., McCOLL, J.H., WYPER, D., PATTERSON, J., BARRON, E. & McCULLOCH, J. (1990) Measurements of regional cerebral blood flow and cognitive performance in Alzheimer's disease. *Journal of Neurology, Neurosurgery and Psychiatry* **53**, 33–38 [434].

MONTGOMERY, A., FENTON, G.W. & McCLELLAND, R.J. (1984) Delayed brainstem conduction time in post-concussional syndrome. *Lancet* **1**, 1011 [198].

MONTGOMERY, E.A., FENTON, G.W., McCLELLAND, R.J., MacFLYNN, G. & RUTHERFORD, W.H. (1991) The psychobiology of minor head injury. *Psychological Medicine* **21**, 375–384 [198].

MONTGOMERY, M.A., CLAYTON, P.J. & FRIEDHOFF, A.J. (1982) Psychiatric illness in Tourette syndrome patients and first-degree relatives. In *Gilles de la Tourette Syndrome*, eds Friedhoff, A.J. & Chase, T.N. *Advances in Neurology* **35**, 335–339. Raven Press: New York [682].

MOON, R.E., CAMPORESI, E.M. & KISSLO, J.A. (1989) Patent foramen ovale and decompression sickness in divers. *Lancet* **1**, 513–514 [769].

MOORE, B.E. & RUESCH, J. (1944) Prolonged disturbances of consciousness following head injury. *New England Journal of Medicine* **230**, 445–452 [168].

MOORE, J.W., DUNK, A.A., CRAWFORD, J.R., DEANS, H., BESSON, J.A.O., DE LACEY, G., SINCLAIR, T.S., MOWAT, N.A.G. & BRUNT, P.W. (1989) Neuropsychological deficits and morphological MRI brain scan abnormalities in apparently healthy non-encephalopathic patients with cirrhosis. *Journal of Hepatology* **9**, 319–325 [564].

MOORE, M.R. & DISLER, P.B. (1988) Drug-sensitive diseases—1: acute porphyrias. *Adverse Drug Reaction Bulletin* **129**, 484–487 [568].

MORBIDITY AND MORTALITY WEEKLY REPORT (1995) Update: acquired immunodeficiency syndrome—United States, 1994. *Morbidity and Mortality Weekly Report* **44**, 64–67 [315, 316].

MORGAN, H.G. (1968) Acute neuropsychiatric complications of chronic alcoholism. *British Journal of Psychiatry* **114**, 85–92 [599].

MORGAN, M.Y. (1982) Alcohol and the endocrine system. In *Alcohol and Disease*, ed. Sherlock, S. *British Medical Bulletin* **38**, 35–42 [515].

MORGANSTERN, F.S. (1964) The effects of sensory input and concentration on post-amputation phantom limb pain. *Journal of Neurology, Neurosurgery and Psychiatry* **27**, 58–65 [74].

MORGANSTERN, H. & GLAZER, W.M. (1993) Identifying risk factors for tardive dyskinesia among long-term outpatients maintained with neuroleptic medications. *Archives of General Psychiatry* **50**, 723–733 [642].

MORIARTY, J., CAMPOS COSTA, D., SCHMITZ, B., TRIMBLE, M.R., ELL, P.J. & ROBERTSON, M.M. (1995) Brain perfusion abnormalities in Gilles de la Tourette's syndrome. *British Journal of Psychiatry* **167**, 249–254 [685].

MORIHISA, J.M. (1989) Computerized EEG and evoked potential mapping. Ch. 3 in *Brain Imaging: Applications in Psychiatry*, ed. Andreasen, N.C. American Psychiatric Press: Washington [132].

MORLEY, J.B. (1967) Unruptured vertebro-basilar aneurysms. *Medical Journal of Australia* **2**, 1024–1027 [412].

MOROZOV, G.V., KACHAEV, A.K. & LUKACHER, C.I. (1973) The pathogenesis of pathological inebriation. *Zhurnal Neuropatologii i Psikhiatrii Korsakova* **73**, 1196–1199 [595].

MORPHEW, J.A. (1988) Hypomania following complex partial seizures. *British Journal of Psychiatry* **152**, 572 [258].

MORPHEW, J.A. & SIM, M. (1969) Gilles de la Tourette's syndrome: a clinical and psychopathological study. *British Journal of Medical Psychology* **42**, 293–301 [684].

MORRELL, F., ROBERTS, L. & JASPER, H.H. (1956) Effect of focal epileptogenic lesions and their ablation upon conditioned electrical responses of the brain in the monkey. *Electroencephalography and Clinical Neurophysiology* **8**, 217–236 [262].

MORRELL, F., WHISLER, W.W. & BLECK, T.P. (1989) Multiple subpial transection: a new approach to the treatment of focal epilepsy. *Journal of Neurosurgery* **70**, 231–239 [314].

MORRIS, G.O. & SINGER, M.T. (1966) Sleep deprivation: the content of consciousness. *Journal of Nervous and Mental Disease* **143**, 291–304 [149].

MORRIS, J.S., FRITH, C.D., PERRETT, D.I., ROWLAND, D., YOUNG, A.W., CALDER, A.J. & DOLAN, R.J. (1996) A differential neural response in the human amygdala to fearful and happy facial expressions. *Nature* **383**, 812–815 [60].

MORRIS, M.R. & TYLER, A. (1991) Management and Therapy. Ch. 7 in *Huntington's Disease*, ed. Harper, P.S. W.B. Saunders: London [506].

MORRIS, P.L.P., ROBINSON, R.G. & RAPHAEL, B. (1992) Lesion location and depression in hospitalized stroke patients. Evidence supporting a specific relationship in the left hemisphere. *Neuropsychiatry, Neuropsychology and Behavioural Neurology* **5**, 75–82 [386].

MORRIS, P.L.P., ROBINSON, R.G., RAPHAEL, B. & BISHOP, D. (1991) The relationship between the perception of social support and post-stroke depression in hospitalized patients. *Psychiatry* **54**, 306–315 [386].

MORRIS, R.G., DOWNES, J.J., SAHAKIAN, B.J., EVENDEN, J.L., HEALD, A. & ROBBINS, T.W. (1988) Planning and spatial working memory in Parkinson's disease. *Journal of Neurology, Neurosurgery and Psychiatry* **51**, 757–766 [122].

MORRIS, R.G., EVENDEN, J.L., SAHAKIAN, B.J. & ROBBINS, T.W. (1987) Computer-aided assessment of dementia: comparative studies of neuropsychological deficits in Alzheimer-type dementia and Parkinson's disease. Ch. 2 in *Cognitive Neurochemistry*, eds Stahl, S.M., Iversen, S.D. & Goodman, E.C. Oxford University Press: Oxford [122].

MORROW, R.S. & COHEN, J. (1954) The psycho-social factors in muscular dystrophy. *Journal of Child Psychiatry* **3**, 70–80 [716].

MORTIMER, J.A. (1994) What are the risk factors for dementia? Ch.

852   REFERENCES

10 in *Dementia and Normal Aging*, eds Huppert, F.A., Brayne, C. & O'Connor, D.W. Cambridge University Press: Cambridge [438].

MORTIMER, J.A., FRENCH, L.R., HUTTON, J.T. & SCHUMAN, L.M. (1985) Head trauma as a risk factor of Alzheimer's disease. *Neurology* **35**, 264–267 [438].

MORTIMER, J.A., VAN DUIJN, C.M., CHANDRA, V., FRATIGLIONI, L., GRAVES, A.B., HEYMAN, A., JORM, A.F., KOKMEN, E., KONDO, K., ROCCA, W.A., SHALAT, S.L., SONINEN, H. & HOFMAN, A FOR THE EURODEM RISK FACTORS RESEARCH GROUP (1991) Head trauma as a risk factor for Alzheimer's disease: a collaborative re-analysis of case-control studies. EURODEM Risk Factors Research Group. *International Journal of Epidemiology* **20 (Supplement 2)**, S28–S35 [438].

MOSCOWITZ, M.A., WINICKOFF, R.N. & HEINZ, E.R. (1971) Familial calcification of the basal ganglions. A metabolic and genetic study. *New England Journal of Medicine* **285**, 72–77 [756].

MOSELEY, I. (1981) Aneurysms of the cerebral arteries. *British Journal of Hospital Medicine* **26**, 613–618 [393].

MOSELEY, I. (1994) Safety and magnetic resonance imaging. *British Medical Journal* **308**, 1181–1182 [142].

MOSER, H.W., MOSER, A.E., SINGH, I. & O'NEILL, B.P. (1984) Adrenoleukodystrophy: survey of 303 cases: biochemistry, diagnosis, and therapy. *Annals of Neurology* **16**, 628–641 [755].

MOUNTJOY, C.Q., ROTH, M., EVANS, N.J.R. & EVANS, H.M. (1983) Cortical neuronal counts in normal elderly controls and demented patients. *Neurobiology of Aging* **4**, 1–11 [443].

MOURE, J.M.B. (1967) The electroencephalogram in hypercalcemia. *Archives of Neurology* **17**, 34–51 [530].

MOWBRAY, J. (1991) Enteroviruses and Epstein-Barr virus in ME. Ch. 3 in *Post-viral Fatigue Syndrome*, eds Jenkins, R. & Mowbray, J.F. Wiley & Sons: Chichester [372].

MUELLER, J. & AMINOFF, M.J. (1982) Tourette-like syndrome after long-term neuroleptic drug treatment. *British Journal of Psychiatry* **141**, 191–193 [685].

MUHLEMANN, M.F. (1992) Uncommon infections: 3. Lyme disease. *Prescribers Journal* **32**, 77–82 [369].

MUKAETOVA-LADINSKA, E.B., HARRINGTON, C.R., ROTH, M. & WISCHIK, C.M. (1993) Biochemical and anatomical redistribution of tau protein in Alzheimer's disease. *American Journal of Pathology* **143**, 565–578 [442].

MUKHERJEE, A.B., SVORONOS, S., GHAZANFARI, A., MARTIN, P.R., FISHER, A., ROECKLEIN, B., RODBARD, D., STATON, R., BEHAR, D., BERG, C.J. & MANJUNATH, R. (1987) Transketolase abnormality in cultured fibroblasts from familial chronic alcoholic men and their male offspring. *Journal of Clinical Investigation* **79**, 1039–1043 [577].

MULLAN, M. (1992) Familial Alzheimer's disease: second gene locus located. *British Medical Journal* **305**, 1108–1109 [448].

MULLAN, M., HOULDEN, H., WINDELSPECHT, M., FIDANI, L., LOMBARDI, C., DIAZ, P., ROSSOR, M., CROOK, R., HARDY, J., DUFF, K. & CRAWFORD, F. (1992) A locus for familial early-onset Alzheimer's disease on the long arm of chromosome 14, proximal to the alpha 1-antichymotrypsin gene. *Nature Genetics* **2**, 340–342 [448].

MULLAN, S. & PENFIELD, W. (1959) Illusions of comparative interpretation and emotion. *Archives of Neurology and Psychiatry* **81**, 269–284 [251].

MULLER, D.J. (1971) ECT in LSD psychosis: a report of three cases. *American Journal of Psychiatry* **128**, 351–352 [622].

MULLER, R., NYLANDER, I., LARSSON, L.-E., WIDEN, L. & FRANKENHAEUSER, M. (1958) Sequelae of primary aseptic meningo-encephalitis. *Acta Psychiatrica et Neurologica Scandinavica* **126 (Supplement)**, 1–115 [366].

MUNGAS, D. (1982) Interictal behavior abnormality in temporal lobe epilepsy. *Archives of General Psychiatry* **39**, 108–111 [268].

MUR, J., KÜMPEL, G. & DOSTAL, S. (1966) An anergic phase of disseminated sclerosis with psychotic course. *Confinia Neurologica* **28**, 37–49 [697].

MURELIUS, O. & HAGLUND, Y. (1991) Does Swedish amateur boxing lead to chronic brain damage? 4. A retrospective neuropsychological study. *Acta Neurologica Scandinavica* **83**, 9–13 [206].

MURPHY, D. & CUTTING, J. (1990) Prosodic comprehension and expression in schizophrenia. *Journal of Neurology, Neurosurgery and Psychiatry* **53**, 727–730 [89].

MURPHY, D.G.M., DECARLI, C., DALY, E., HAXBY, J.V., ALLEN, G., WHITE, B.J., McINTOSH, A.R., POWELL, C.M., HORWITZ, B., RAPOPORT, S.I. & SCHAPIRO, M.B. (1993) X-chromosome effects on female brain: a magnetic resonance imaging study of Turner's syndrome. *Lancet* **342**, 1197–1200 [528].

MURPHY, L.D., McMILLAN, T.M., GREENWOOD, R.J., BROOKS, D.N., MORRIS, J.R. & DUNN, G. (1990) Services for severely head-injured patients in North London and environs. *Brain Injury* **4**, 95–100 [216].

MURPHY, S.M., OWEN, R.T. & TYRER, P.J. (1984) Withdrawal symptoms after six weeks' treatment with diazepam. *Lancet* **2**, 1389 [611].

MURPHY, T.L., CHALMERS, T.C., ECKHARDT, R.D. & DAVIDSON, C.S. (1948) Hepatic coma: clinical and laboratory observations on forty patients. *New England Journal of Medicine* **239**, 605–612 [564].

MURRAY, D. & HODGSON, R. (1991) Polycythaemia rubra vera, cerebral ischaemia and depression. *British Journal of Psychiatry* **158**, 842–844 [426].

MURRAY, R.M. (1994) Neurodevelopmental schizophrenia: the rediscovery of dementia praecox. *British Journal of Psychiatry* **165 (Supplement 25)**, 6–12 [91].

MURRAY, R.M., GREENE, J.G. & ADAMS, J.H. (1971) Analgesic abuse and dementia. *Lancet* **2**, 242–245 [628].

MURRAY, R.M., LEWIS, S.W., OWEN, M.J. & FOERSTER, A. (1988) The neurodevelopmental origins of dementia praecox. Ch. 8 in *Schizophrenia. The Major Issues*, eds Bebbington, P. & McGuffin, P. Heinemann: Oxford [91, 92].

MUSALEK, M., PODREKA, I., WALTERS, H., SUESS, E., PASSWEG, V., NUTZINGER, D., STROBL, R. & LESCH, O.M. (1989) Regional brain function in hallucinations: a study of regional cerebral blood flow with 99m-Tc-HMPAO-SPECT in patients with auditory hallucinations, tactile-hallucinations, and normal controls. *Comprehensive Psychiatry* **30**, 99–108 [148].

MUTSCHLER, D. (1956) Neurosebildende Faktoren bei Hirnverletzten. In *Das Hirntrauma*, ed. Rehwald, E. Thieme: Stuttgart [180].

MYERS, R.H., GROWDON, J.H., BIRD, E.D., FELDMAN, R.G. & MARTIN, J.B. (1982) False-negative results with levodopa for early detection of Huntington's disease. *New England Journal of Medicine* **307**, 561–562 [467].

MYRIANTHOPOULOS, N.C. (1966) Huntington's chorea. *Journal of Medical Genetics* **3**, 298–314 [465, 467, 469].

NADEEM, A.A. & YOUNIS, Y.O. (1977) Physical illness and psychiatric disorders in Tigani El-Mahi Psychiatric Hospital (Sudan). *East African Medical Journal* **54**, 207–210 [370].

NADEL, C. (1981) Somnambulism, bed-time medication and overeating. *British Journal of Psychiatry* **139**, 79 [736].

NADVORNIK, P., SRAMKA, M., LISY, L. & SVICKA, I. (1972) Experiences with dentatotomy. *Confinia Neurologica* **34**, 320–324 [687].

NAESER, M.A., ALEXANDER, M.P., HELM-ESTABROOKS, N., LEVINE, H.L., LAUGHLIN, S.A. & GESCHWIND, N. (1982) Aphasia with predominantly subcortical lesion sites. Description of three capsular putaminal aphasia syndromes. *Archives of Neurology* **39**, 2–14 [47].

NAESER, M.A., GEBHARDT, C. & LEVINE, H.L. (1980) Decreased computerised tomography numbers in patients with presenile dementia. Detection in patients with otherwise normal scans. *Archives of Neurology* **37**, 401–409 [139].

NAG, T.K. & FALCONER, M.A. (1966) Non-tumoral stenosis of the aqueduct in adults. *British Medical Journal* **2**, 1168–1170 [750].

NAGUIB, M. & LEVY, R. (1982a) Prediction of outcome in senile dementia—a computed tomography study. *British Journal of Psychiatry* **140**, 263–267 [433].

NAGUIB, M. & LEVY, R. (1982b) CT scanning in senile dementia. A follow-up of survivors. *British Journal of Psychiatry* **141**, 618–620 [139].

NAGUIB, M. & LEVY, R. (1987) Late paraphrenia: neuropsychological impairment and structural brain abnormalities on computed tomography. *International Journal of Geriatric Psychiatry* **2**, 83–90 [489].

NAHEEDY, M.H., HAAG, J.R., AZAR-KIA, B., MAFEE, M.F. & ELIAS, D.A. (1987) MRI and CT of sellar and parasellar disorders. *Radiologic Clinics of North America* **25**, 819–847 [232, 522].

NANDY, K. (1968) Further studies on the effects of centrophenoxine on the lipofuscin pigment in the neurones of senile guinea pigs. *Journal of Gerontology* **23**, 82–92 [502].

NANDY, K. (ed.) (1978) *Senile Dementia: A Biomedical Approach.* Developments in Neuroscience, Vol. 3. Elsevier/North-Holland, Biomedical Press: Amsterdam [447].

NANDY, K. (1981) Senile dementia: a possible immune hypothesis. Ch. 5 in *The Epidemiology of Dementia*, eds Mortimer, J.A. & Schuman, L.M. Oxford University Press: Oxford [447].

NANDY, K. & BOURNE, G.H. (1966) Effect of centrophenoxine on the lipofuscin pigments in the neurones of senile guinea-pigs. *Nature* **210**, 313–314 [502].

NARABAYASHI, H., NAGAO, T., SAITO, Y., YOSHIDA, M. & NAGAHATA, M. (1963) Stereotaxic amygdalotomy for behaviour disorders. *Archives of Neurology* **9**, 1–16 [82].

NARABAYASHI, H. & UNO, M. (1966) Long range results of stereotaxic amygdalotomy for behaviour disorders. *Confinia Neurologica* **27**, 168–171 [82].

NASRALLAH, H.A. (1990) Brain structure and function in schizophrenia: evidence for fetal neurodevelopmental impairment. *Current Opinion in Psychiatry* **3**, 75–78 [85].

NASRALLAH, H.A., JACOBY, C.G., McCALLEY-WHITTERS, M. & KUPERMAN, S. (1982a) Cerebral ventricular enlargement in subtypes of chronic schizophrenia. *Archives of General Psychiatry* **39**, 774–777 [140].

NASRALLAH, H.A., McCALLEY-WHITTERS, M. & JACOBY, C.G. (1982b) Cerebral ventricular enlargement in young manic males. A controlled CT study. *Journal of Affective Disorders* **4**, 15–19 [140].

NATH, F.P., BEASTAL, G. & TEASDALE, G.M. (1986) Alcohol and traumatic brain damage. *Injury* **17**, 150–153 [179].

NATIONAL HEAD INJURY FOUNDATION (1992) *The Silent Epidemic.* Framingham: Massachusetts. Quoted Wesolowski, M.D. & Zenicus, A.H. (1994) *A Practical Guide to Head Injury Rehabilitation.* Plenum Press: New York & London [161].

NAUSIEDA, P.A., GROSSMAN, B.J., KOLLER, W.C., WEINER, W.J. & KLAWANS, H.L. (1980) Sydenham chorea: an update. *Neurology* **30**, 331–334 [373, 374].

NAVIA, B.A., CHO, E.-S., PETITO, C.K. & PRICE, R.W. (1986b) The AIDS dementia complex: II. Neuropathology. *Annals of Neurology* **19**, 525–535 [324, 325].

NAVIA, B.A., JORDAN, B.D. & PRICE, R.W. (1986a) The AIDS dementia complex: I. Clinical features. *Annals of Neurology* **19**, 517–524 [324, 325].

NAVIA, B.A. & PRICE, R.W. (1987) The acquired immunodeficiency syndrome dementia complex as the presenting or sole manifestation of human immunodeficiency virus infection. *Archives of Neurology* **44**, 65–69 [325].

NEARY, D. (1976) Neuropsychiatric sequelae of renal failure. *British Journal of Hospital Medicine* **15**, 122–130 [557].

NEARY, D., SNOWDEN, J.S., BOWEN, D.M., SIMS, N.R., MANN, D.M.A., YATES, P.O. & DAVISON, A.N. (1986a) Cerebral biopsy in the investigation of presenile dementia due to cerebral atrophy. *Journal of Neurology, Neurosurgery and Psychiatry* **49**, 157–162 [496].

NEARY, D., SNOWDEN, J.S. & MANN, D.M.A. (1993a) Familial progressive aphasia: its relationship to other forms of lobor atrophy. *Journal of Neurology, Neurosurgery and Psychiatry* **56**, 1122–1125 [753].

NEARY, D., SNOWDEN, J.S. & MANN, D.M.A. (1993b) The clinical pathological correlates of lobor atrophy. *Dementia* **4**, 154–159 [753].

NEARY, D., SNOWDEN, J.S. & MANN, D.M.A. (1994) Dementia of frontal lobe type. Ch. 51 in *Dementia*, eds Burns, A. & Levy, R. Chapman & Hall Medical: London [464].

NEARY, D., SNOWDEN, J.S., MANN, D.M.A., BOWEN, D.M., SIMS, N.R., NORTHEN, B., YATES, P.O. & DAVISON, A.N. (1986b) Alzheimer's disease: a correlative study. *Journal of Neurology, Neurosurgery and Psychiatry* **49**, 229–237 [443].

NEARY, D., SNOWDEN, J.S., MANN, D.M.A., NORTHEN, B., GOULDING, P.J. & MacDERMOTT, N. (1990) Frontal lobe dementia and motor neurone disease. *Journal of Neurology, Neurosurgery and Psychiatry* **53**, 23–32 [708].

NEARY, D., SNOWDEN, J.S., NORTHEN, B. & GOULDING, P. (1988) Dementia of frontal lobe type. *Journal of Neurology, Neurosurgery and Psychiatry* **51**, 353–361 [463, 464].

NEARY, D., SNOWDEN, J.S., SHIELDS, R.A., BURJAN, A.W.I., NORTHEN, B., MacDERMOTT, N., PRESCOTT, M.C. & TESTA, H.J. (1987) Single photon emission tomography using 99mTc-HM-PAO in the investigation of dementia. *Journal of Neurology, Neurosurgery and Psychiatry* **50**, 1101–1109 [465].

NEE, L.E., POLINSKY, R.J. & EBERT, M.H. (1982) Tourette syndrome: clinical and family studies. In *Gilles de la Tourette Syndrome*, eds Friedhoff, A.J. & Chase, T.N. Raven Press: New York [682].

NEEDLEMAN, H.L. (1982) The neuropsychiatric implications of low level exposure to lead. *Psychological Medicine* **12**, 461–463 [632].

NEEDLEMAN, H.L., GUNNOE, C., LEVITON, A., REED, R., PERESIE, H., MAHER, C. & BARRETT, P. (1979) Deficits in psychologic and classroom performance of children with elevated dentine lead levels. *New England Journal of Medicine* **300**, 689–695 [632].

NEEDLEMAN, H.L., SCHELL, A., BELLINGER, D., LEVITON, A. & ALLRED, E.N. (1990) The long-term effects of exposure to low doses of lead in childhood. An 11-year follow-up report. *New England Journal of Medicine* **322**, 83–88 [633].

NELSON, H.E. (1976) A modified card sorting test sensitive to frontal lobe defects. *Cortex* **12**, 313–324 [118].

NELSON, H.E. (1982) *The National Adult Reading Test Manual.* NFER-Nelson: Windsor, England [111].

NELSON, H.E. & McKENNA, P. (1975) The use of current reading ability in the assessment of dementia. *British Journal of Social and Clinical Psychology* **14**, 759–267 [111].

NELSON, H.E. & O'CONNELL, A. (1978) Dementia: the estimation of premorbid intelligence levels using the new adult reading test. *Cortex* **14**, 234–244 [111].

NELSON, H.E. & WILLISON, J.R. (1991) *National Adult Reading Test*, 2nd edn. NFER-Nelson: Windsor [111, 112].

NELSON, L.D., GREEN, P.S., GREEN, M. & CICCHETTI, D. (1993) Re-examining handedness in schizophrenia: now you see it—now you don't! *Journal of Clinical and Experimental Neuropsychology* **152**, 149–158 [89].

NERI, L.C. & HEWITT, D. (1991) Aluminium, Alzheimer's disease, and drinking water. *Lancet* **338**, 390 [446].

NESHIGE, R., BARRETT, G. & SHIBASAKI, H. (1988) Auditory long latency event related potentials in Alzheimer's disease and multi-infarct dementia. *Journal of Neurology, Neurosurgery and Psychiatry* **51**, 1120–1125 [132].

NESTOR, P.G., SHENTON, M.E., McCARLEY, R.W., HAIMSON, J., SMITH, S., O'DONNELL, B., KIMBLE, M., KIKINIS, R. & JOLESZ, F.A. (1993) Neuropsychological correlates of MRI temporal lobe abnormalities in schizophrenia. *American Journal of Psychiatry* **150**, 1849–1855 [85].

NETLEY, C. & ROVET, J. (1982a) Verbal deficits in children with 47,XXY and 47,XXX karyotypes: a descriptive and experimental study. *Brain and Language* **17**, 58–72 [526].

NETLEY, C. & ROVET, J. (1982b) Handedness in 47,XXY males. *Lancet* **2**, 267 [527].

NEUBERGER, K.T. (1957) The changing neuropathological picture of chronic alcoholism. *Archives of Pathology* **63**, 1–6 [604].

NEUGUT, R.H., NEUGUT, A.I., KAHANA, E., STEIN, Z. & ALTER, M. (1979) Creutzfeldt–Jakob disease: familial clustering among Libyan-born Israelis. *Neurology* **29**, 225–231 [475].

NEUMANN, M.A. & COHN, R. (1967) Progressive subcortical gliosis: a rare form of presenile dementia. *Brain* **90**, 405–417 [462].

NEUROMUSCULAR DISORDERS: GENE LOCATION (1992) *Neuromuscular Diseases* **2**, 431–434 [720, 721].

NEVILLE, B.G.R. (1993) Paediatric neurology. Ch. 13 in *Brain's Diseases of the Nervous System*, 10th edn, ed. Walton, J. Oxford University Press: Oxford [242, 770].

NEVIN, S. (1967) On some aspects of cerebral degeneration in later life. *Proceedings of the Royal Society of Medicine* **60**, 517–526 [479].

NEVIN, S., McMENEMEY, W.H., BEHRAM, S. & JONES, D.P. (1960) Subacute spongiform encephalopathy—a subacute form of encephalopathy attributable to vascular dysfunction (spongiform cerebral atrophy). *Brain* **83**, 519–564 [476].

NEWCOMBE, F. (1969) *Missile Wounds of the Brain: A Study of Psychological Deficits*. Oxford University Press: Oxford [46, 63, 118, 184].

NEWCOMBE, F. (1983) The psychological consequences of closed head injury: assessment and rehabilitation. *Injury* **14**, 111–136 [184, 213].

NEWCOMBE, F. (1996) Very late outcome after focal wartime brain wounds. *Journal of Clinical and Experimental Neuropsychology* **18**, 1–23 [186].

NEWCOMBE, F., BROOKS, N. & BADDELEY, A. (1980) Rehabilitation after brain damage: an overview. *International Rehabilitation Medicine* **2**, 133–137 [212].

NEWCOMBE, F. & MARSHALL, J.C. (1981) On psycholinguistic classifications of the acquired dyslexias. *Bulletin of the Orton Society* **31**, 29–46 [43].

NEWCOMBE, F.B., OLDFIELD, R.C. & WINGFIELD, A. (1965) Object naming by dysphasic patients. *Nature* **207**, 1217–1718 [103].

NEWMAN, P.K. (1990) Whiplash injury. *British Medical Journal* **301**, 395–396 [201].

NEWMAN, P.K. & SAUNDERS, M. (1979) Lithium neurotoxicity. *Postgraduate Medical Journal* **55**, 701–703 [626].

NEWMAN, S., KLINGER, L., VENN, G., SMITH, P., HARRISON, M. & TREASURE, T. (1990) The persistence of neuropsychological deficits twelve months after coronary artery bypass surgery. In *Impact of Cardiac Surgery on the Quality of Life*, eds Wilner, A. & Rodewald, G., pp. 173–179. Plenum Press: New York [555].

NEWMAN, S., SMITH, P., TREASURE, T., JOSEPH, P., ELL, P. & HARRISON, M. (1987) Acute neuropsychological consequences of coronary artery bypass surgery. *Current Psychological Research and Reviews* **6**, 115–124 [554].

NEWMARK, J. & HOCHBERG, F.H. (1987) Isolated painless manual incoordination in 57 musicians. *Journal of Neurology, Neurosurgery and Psychiatry* **50**, 291–295 [678].

NEWTON, M.R., GREENWOOD, R.J., BRITTON, K.E., CHARLESWORTH, M., NIMMON, C.C., CARROLL, M.J. & DOLKE, G. (1992) A study comparing SPECT with CT and MRI after closed head injury. *Journal of Neurology, Neurosurgery and Psychiatry* **55**, 92–94 [166].

NGIM, C.H., FOO, S.C., BOEY, K.W. & JEYARATNAM, J. (1992) Chronic neurobehavioural effects of elemental mercury in dentists. *British Journal of Industrial Medicine* **49**, 782–790 [634].

NICKLAS, W.J., VYAS, I. & HEIKKILA, R.E. (1985) Inhibition of NADH-linked oxidation in brain mitochondria by 1-methyl-4-phenyl-pyridine, a metabolite of the neurotoxin, 1-methyl-4-phenyl-1,2,5,6-tetrahydropyridine. *Life Sciences* **36**, 2503–2508 [648].

NIEDERMEYER, E. & KHALIFEH, R. (1965) Petit mal status: an electro-clinical approach. *Epilepsia* **6**, 250–262 [256].

NIEDERMEYER, E., ZELLWEGER, H. & ALEXANDER, T. (1965) Central nervous system manifestations in myopathies. In *Eighth International Congress of Neurology*, International Congress Series No. 94, pp. 67–68. Exerpta Medica Foundation [716].

NIELSEN, J. (1968) Chromosomes in senile dementia. *British Journal of Psychiatry* **114**, 303–309 [431].

NIELSEN, J. (1969) Klinefelter's syndrome and the XYY syndrome. *Acta Psychiatrica Scandinavica* **209 (Supplement)**, 1–353 [527].

NIELSEN, J. (1970a) Chromosomes in senile, presenile, and arteriosclerotic dementia. *Journal of Gerontology* **25**, 312–315 [431].

NIELSEN, J. (1970b) Turner's syndrome in medical neurological and psychiatric wards. *Acta Psychiatrica Scandinavica* **46**, 286–310 [528].

NIELSEN, J.M. (1930) Migraine equivalent. *American Journal of Psychiatry* **9**, 637–641 [406].

NIELSEN, J.M. (1958) *Memory and Amnesia*. San Lucas Press: Los Angeles [291, 406, 407].

NIEMAN, E.A. (1991) Neurosyphilis yesterday and today. *Journal of the Royal College of Physicians of London* **25**, 321–324 [321, 337, 338, 344].

NIETO, D. & ESCOBAR, A. (1972) Major psychoses. Section 189 in *Pathology of the Nervous System*, Vol. 3, ed. Minckler, J., pp. 2654–2665. McGraw-Hill: New York [86].

NIH CONSENSUS DEVELOPMENT CONFERENCE (1988) Neurofibromatosis. Conference statement. *Archives of Neurology* **45**, 575–578 [703].

NISIJIMA, K. & ISHIGURO, T. (1990) Neuroleptic malignant syndrome: a study of CSF monoamine metabolism. *Biological Psychiatry* **27**, 280–288 [627].

NISSENBAUM, H., QUINN, N.P., BROWN, R.G., TOONE, B., GOTHAM, A.-M. & MARSDEN, C.D. (1987) Mood swings associated with the 'on–off' phenomenon in Parkinson's disease. *Psychological Medicine* **17**, 899–904 [650, 651].

NIXON, P.F. (1984) Is there a genetic component to the pathogenesis of the Wernicke–Korsakoff syndrome? *Alcohol and Alcoholism* **19**, 219–221 [577].

NOBLE, P. (1974) Depressive illness and hyperparathyroidism. *Proceedings of the Royal Society of Medicine* **67**, 1066–1067 [531].

NODINE, J.H., SHULKIN, M.W., SLAP, J.W., LEVINE, M. & FREIBERG, K. (1967) A double-blind study of the effect of ribonucleic acid in senile brain disease. *American Journal of Psychiatry* **123**, 1257–1259 [502].

NOGUCHI, H. & MOORE, J.W. (1913) A demonstration of treponema pallidum in the brain in cases of general paralysis. *Journal of Experimental Medicine* **17**, 232–238 [339].

NORDBERG, A., ADOLFSSON, R., AQUILONIUS, S.-M., MARKLUND, S., ORELAND, L. & WINBLAD, B. (1980) Brain enzymes and acetylcholine receptors in dementia of Alzheimer type and chronic alcohol abuse. In *Aging of the Brain and Dementia, Aging*, Vol. 13, eds Amaducci, L., Davison, A.N. & Antuono, P. Raven Press: New York [606].

NORDENSON, I., ADOLFSSON, R., BECKMAN, G., BUCHT, G. & WINBLAD, B. (1980) Chromosomal abnormality in dementia of Alzheimer type. *Lancet* **1**, 481–482 [437].

NORDIC MEDICAL RESEARCH COUNCIL'S HIV THERAPY GROUP (1992) Double blind dose–response study of zidovudine in AIDS and advanced HIV infection. *British Medical Journal* **304**, 13–17 [336].

NORMAN, E.H. & BORDLEY, W.C. (1995) Lead toxicity intervention in children. *Journal of the Royal Society of Medicine* **88**, 121–124 [632].

NORRIS, J.W. & PRATT, R.F. (1971) A controlled study of folic acid in epilepsy. *Neurology* **21**, 659–664 [592].

NORRMAN, B. & SVAHN, K. (1961) A follow-up study of severe brain injuries. *Acta Psychiatrica Scandinavica* **37**, 236–264 [178, 198].

NOSEWORTHY, J.H., MILLER, J., MURRAY, T.J. & REGAN, D. (1981) Auditory brainstem responses in post concussion syndrome. *Archives of Neurology* **38**, 275–278 [198].

NOTES ON ELICITING AND RECORDING CLINICAL INFORMATION (1973) The Department of Psychiatry Teaching Committee, The Institute of Psychiatry, London. Oxford University Press: London [98].

NOTES ON ELICITING AND RECORDING CLINICAL INFORMATION IN PSYCHIATRIC PATIENTS (1987) 2nd edn. The Departments of Psychiatry and Child Psychiatry, The Institute of Psychiatry and the Maudsley Hospital, London. Oxford University Press: London [94, 98, 123].

NOTT, P.N. & FLEMINGER, J.J. (1975) Presenile dementia: the difficulties of early diagnosis. *Acta Psychiatrica Scandinavica* **51**, 210–217 [486, 492].

NUFFIELD, E.J.A. (1961) Neuro-physiology and behaviour disorders in epileptic children. *Journal of Mental Science* **107**, 438–458 [265].

NUMANN, P.J., TORPPA, A.J. & BLUMETTI, A.E. (1984) Neuropsychologic deficits associated with primary hyperparathyroidism. *Surgery* **96**, 1119–1123 [529].

NNUWER, M.R. (1982) Coprolalia as an organic symptom. In *Gilles de la Tourette Syndrome*, eds Friedhoff, A.J. & Chase, T.N. *Advances in Neurology* **35**, 363–368. Raven Press: New York [681].

NYGAARD, T.G., MARSDEN, C.D. & DUVOISIN, R.C. (1988) Dopa-responsive dystonia. In *Dystonia, 2*, eds Fahn, S., Marsden, C.D. & Calne, D.B. *Advances in Neurology* **50**, 377–384. Raven Press: New York [671].

NYGAARD, T.G., MARSDEN, C.D. & FAHN, S. (1991) Dopa-responsive dystonia: long-term treatment response and prognosis. *Neurology* **41**, 174–181 [671].

OAKLEY, D.P. (1965) Senile dementia: some aetiological factors. *British Journal of Psychiatry* **111**, 414–419 [433].

OATES, J.K. (1979) Serological tests for syphilis and their clinical use. *British Journal of Hospital Medicine* **21**, 612–617 [343].

OBESO, J.A., ROTHWELL, J.C. & MARSDEN, C.D. (1981) Simple tics in Gilles de la Tourette's syndrome are not prefaced by a normal pre-movement EEG potential. *Journal of Neurology, Neurosurgery and Psychiatry* **44**, 735–738 [685].

OBRECHT, R., OKHOMINA, F.O.A. & SCOTT, D.F. (1979) Value of EEG in acute confusional states. *Journal of Neurology, Neurosurgery and Psychiatry* **42**, 75–77 [130].

O'BRIEN, J.T., BEATS, B., HILL, K., HOWARD, R., SAHAKIAN, B. & LEVY, R. (1992) Do subjective memory complaints precede dementia? A three-year follow-up of patients with supposed 'benign senescent forgetfulness'. *International Journal of Geriatric Psychiatry* **7**, 481–486 [432].

O'BRIEN, M.D. (1994a) Vascular dementia: definitions, epidemiology and clinical features. Ch. 38 in *Dementia*, eds Burns, A. & Levy, R. Chapman and Hall: London [454, 457].

O'BRIEN, M.D. & GILMOUR-WHITE, S. (1993) Epilepsy and pregnancy. *British Medical Journal* **307**, 492–495 [299].

O'BRIEN, M.D. & HARRIS, P.W.R. (1968) Cerebral-cortex perfusion-rates in myxoedema. *Lancet* **1**, 1170–1172 [514].

O'BRIEN, W.A. (1994b) Genetic and biologic basis of HIV-1 neurotropism. Ch. 2 in *HIV, AIDS, and the Brain*, eds Price, R.W. & Perry, S.W. *Association for Research in Nervous and Mental Disease* **72**. Raven Press: New York [322].

O'CARROLL, R.E., MASTERTON, G., DOUGALL, N., EBMEIER, K.P. & GOODWIN, G.M. (1995a) The neuropsychiatric sequelae of mercury posioning. The Mad Hatter's disease revisited. *British Journal of Psychiatry* **167**, 95–98 [634].

O'CARROLL, R.E., MOFFOOT, A.P.R., EBMEIER, K.P. & GOODWIN, G.M. (1994) Effects of fluvoxamine treatment on cognitive functioning in the alcoholic Korsakoff syndrome. *Psychopharmacology* **116**, 85–88 [585].

O'CARROLL, R.E., MOFFOOT, A., EBMEIER, K.P., MURRAY, C. & GOODWIN, G.M. (1993) Korsakoff's syndrome, cognition and clonidine. *Psychological Medicine* **23**, 341–347 [585].

O'CARROLL, R.E., PRENTICE, N., MURRAY, C., VAN BECK, M., EBMEIER, K.P. & GOODWIN, G.M. (1995b) Further evidence that reading ability is not preserved in Alzheimer's disease. *British Journal of Psychiatry* **167**, 659–662 [111].

O'CONNELL, S. (1995) Lyme disease in the United Kingdom. *British Medical Journal* **310**, 303–308 [369].

O'CONNOR, J.F. (1959) Psychoses associated with disseminated lupus erythematosus. *Annals of Internal Medicine* **51**, 526–536 [420].

O'CONNOR, J.F. & MUSHER, D.M. (1966) Central nervous system involvement in systemic lupus erythematosus. *Archives of Neurology* **14**, 157–164 [419, 420, 421].

ODDY, M. (1984) Head injury and social adjustment. Ch. 6 in *Closed Head Injury: Psychological, Social, and Family Consequences*, ed. Brooks, N. Oxford University Press: Oxford [216].

ODDY, M. & HUMPHREY, M. (1980) Social recovery during the year following severe head injury. *Journal of Neurology, Neurosurgery and Psychiatry* **43**, 798–802 [217].

ODDY, M., HUMPHREY, M. & UTTLEY, D. (1978) Stress upon the relatives of head-injured patients. *British Journal of Psychiatry* **133**, 507–513 [217].

OGAWA, S., TANK, D.W., MENON, R., ELLERMAN, J.M., KIM, S., MERKLE, H. & UGURBIL, K. (1992) Intrinsic signal changes accompanying sensory stimulation: functional brain mapping with magnetic resonance imaging. *Proceedings of the National Academy of Science* **89**, 5951–5955 [143].

OGURA, C., OKUMA, T., NAKAZAWA, K. & KISHIMOTO, A. (1976) Treatment of periodic somnolence with lithium carbonate. *Archives of Neurology* **33**, 143 [733].

OJEMANN, J.G., OJEMANN, G.A. & LETTICH, E. (1992) Neuronal activity related to faces and matching in human right nondominant temporal cortex. *Brain* **115**, 1–13 [60].

OJEMANN, R.G. (1971) Normal pressure hydrocephalus. Ch. 16 in *Clinical Neurosurgery*, Proceedings of the Congress of Neurological

Surgeons, Vol. 18. Williams & Wilkins: Baltimore [745, 746, 748, 749].

OJEMANN, R.G., FISHER, C.M., ADAMS, R.D., SWEET, W.H. & NEW, P.J.F. (1969) Further experience with the syndrome of 'normal' pressure hydrocephalus. *Journal of Neurosurgery* **31**, 279–294 [748, 750].

OKAMURA, T., FUKAI, M., YAMADORI, A., HIDARI, M., ASABA, H. & SAKAI, T. (1993) A clinical study of hypergraphia in epilepsy. *Journal of Neurology, Neurosurgery and Psychiatry* **56**, 556–559 [268].

OKASHA, A., SADEK, A. & MONEIM, S.A. (1975) Psychosocial and electroencephalographic studies of Egyptian murderers. *British Journal of Psychiatry* **126**, 34–40 [128].

OKAZAKI, H., LIPKIN, L.E. & ARONSON, S.M. (1961) Diffuse intracytoplasmic gangliotic inclusions (Lewy-type) associated with progressive dementia and quadriparesis in flexion. *Journal of Neuropathology and Experimental Neurology* **20**, 237–244 [450].

OLDENDORF, W.H. (1980) *The Quest for an Image of Brain.* Raven Press: New York [144].

OLESEN, J. & JORGENSEN, M.B. (1986) Leao's spreading depression in the hippocampus explains transient global amnesia. A hypothesis. *Acta Neurologica Scandinavica* **73**, 219–220 [417].

OLIN, H.S. & WEISMAN, A.D. (1964) Psychiatric misdiagnosis in early neurological disease. *Journal of the American Medical Association* **189**, 533–538 [235, 236].

OLIVARUS, B. DE F. & RÖDER, E. (1970) Reversible psychosis and dementia in myxoedema. *Acta Psychiatrica Scandinavica* **46**, 1–13 [513].

OLIVER, J.E. (1970) Huntington's chorea in Northamptonshire. *British Journal of Psychiatry* **116**, 241–253 [465, 472].

OLIVER, J. & DEWHURST, K. (1969) Childhood and adolescent forms of Huntington's disease. *Journal of Neurology, Neurosurgery and Psychiatry* **32**, 455–459 [471].

OLSEN, S. (1961) The brain in uraemia. *Acta Psychiatrica et Neurologica Scandinavica* **156 (Supplement)**, 1–129 [558].

OLSEN, W.L., LONGO, F.M., MILLS, C.M. & NORMAN, D. (1988) White matter disease in AIDS: findings at MR imaging. *Radiology* **169**, 445–448 [325].

OLSON, L., NORDBERG, A., VON HOLST, H., BÄCKMAN, L., EBENDAL, T., ALAFUZOFF, I., AMBERLA, K., HARTVIG, P., HERLITZ, A., LILJA, A., LUNDQVIST, H., LÅNGSTRÖM, B., MEYERSON, B., PERSSON, A., VIITANEN, M., WINBLAD, B. & SEIGER, A. (1992) Nerve growth factor affects ^{11}C-nicotine binding, blood flow, EEG, and verbal episodic memory in an Alzheimer patient. *Journal of Neural Transmission—Parkinson's Disease and Dementia Section* **4**, 79–95 [505].

OLSON, L.C., BUESCHER, E.L., ARTENSTEIN, M.S. & PARKMAN, P.D. (1967) Herpes virus infections of the human central nervous system. *New England Journal of Medicine* **277**, 1271–1277 [357].

OLSON, M.I. & SHAW, C.M. (1969) Presenile dementia and Alzheimer's disease in mongolism. *Brain* **92**, 147–156 [437].

OLSZEWSKI, J. (1962) Subcortical arteriosclerotic encephalopathy: review of the literature on the so-called Binswanger's disease and presentation of two cases. *World Neurology* **3**, 359–375 [458].

O'MALLEY, S.S. & GAWIN, F.H. (1990) Abstinence symptomatology and neuropsychological impairment in chronic cocaine abusers. In *Residual Effects of Abused Drugs on Behavior.* National Institute on Drug Abuse Research Monograph No. 101, eds Spencer, J.W. & Boren, J.J., pp. 179–190. US Department of Health and Human Services, National Institute on Drug Abuse: Rockville, Maryland [619].

OMBREDANE, A. (1929) Sur les troubles mentaux de la sclérose en plaques. Thèse de Paris. Quoted Surridge, D. (1969) *British Journal of Psychiatry* **115**, 749–764 [691].

OMMAYA, A.K., FAAS, F. & YARNELL, P. (1968) Whiplash injury and brain damage. An experimental study. *Journal of the American Medical Association* **204**, 285–289 [200].

O'NEILL, S., TIPTON, K.F., PRITCHARD, J.S. & QUINLAN, A. (1984) Survival after high blood alcohol levels. Association with first-order elimination kinetics. *Archives of Internal Medicine* **144**, 641–642 [597].

ONO, S., INOUE, K., MANNEN, T., KANDA, F., JINNAI, K. & TAKAHASHI, K. (1987) Neuropathological changes of the brain in myotonic dystrophy—some new observations. *Journal of the Neurological Sciences* **81**, 301–320 [719].

OOSTERHUIS, H.J.G.H. & WILDE, G.J.S. (1964) Psychiatric aspects of myasthenia gravis. *Pychiatria, Neurologia, Neurochirurgia* **67**, 484–496 [711, 712, 713, 714].

OPPENHEIMER, D.R. (1976) Diseases of the basal ganglia, cerebellum and motor neurons. Ch. 14 in *Greenfield's Neuropathology*, 3rd edn, eds Blackwood, W. & Corsellis, J.A.N. Edward Arnold: London [705].

OPPENHEIMER, D.R. (1979) Brain lesions in Friedrich's ataxia. *Canadian Journal of Neurological Sciences* **6**, 173–176 [705].

ORBAN, T. (1957) Experiences with a follow-up of 200 tabetic patients. *Acta Psychiatrica et Neurologica Scandinavica* **32**, 89–102 [338].

O'REGAN, J.B. (1974) Hypersomnia and MAOI antidepressants. *Canadian Medical Association Journal* **111**, 213 [735].

ORMEROD, I.E.C., MILLER, D.H., McDONALD, W.I., DU BOULAY, E.P.G.H., RUDGE, P., KENDALL, B.E., MOSELEY, I.F., JOHNSON, G., TOFTS, P.S., HALLIDAY, A.M., BRONSTEIN, A.M., SCARAVILLI, F., HARDING, A.E., BARNES, D. & ZILKHA, K.J. (1987) The role of NMR imaging in the assessment of multiple sclerosis and isolated neurological lesions. *Brain* **110**, 1579–1616 [690].

ORRELL, M. & SAHAKIAN, B. (1995) Education and dementia. Research evidence supports the concept 'use it or lose it'. *British Medical Journal* **310**, 951–952 [449].

ORRELL, M.W., SAHAKIAN, B.J. & BERGMANN, K. (1989) Self-neglect and frontal lobe dysfunction. *British Journal of Psychiatry* **155**, 101–105 [495].

ORRELL, R.W., LANE, R.J.M. & GUILOFF, R.J. (1994) Recent developments in the drug treatment of motor neurone disease. *British Medical Journal* **309**, 140–141 [707].

ORWIN, A., JAMES, S.R.N. & TURNER, R.K. (1974) Sex chromosome abnormalities, homosexuality and psychological treatment. *British Journal of Psychiatry* **124**, 293–295 [527].

OSBORNE, J.P., MUNSON, P. & BURMAN, D. (1982) Huntington's chorea. Report of 3 cases and review of the literature. *Archives of Disease of Childhood* **57**, 99–103 [471].

OSCAR-BERMAN, M., HUTNER, N. & BONNER, R.T. (1992) Visual and auditory spatial and nonspatial delayed-response performance by Korsakoff and non-Korsakoff alcoholic and aging individuals. *Behavioral Neuroscience* **106**, 613–622 [583].

O'SHEA, B. & FALVEY, J. (1991) Juvenile Huntington's disease. *Irish Journal of Psychological Medicine* **8**, 149–153 [471].

O'SHEA, H.E., ELSOM, K.O. & HIGBE, R.V. (1942) Studies of B-vitamins in the human subject: IV. Mental changes in experimental deficiency. *American Journal of the Medical Sciences* **203**, 388–397 [572].

OSTERRIETH, P.-A. (1944) Le test de copie d'une figure complexe. Contribution à l'étude de la perception et de la mémoire. *Archives de Psychologie* **30**, 206–353 [116].

OSTFELD, A.M. & LEBOVITS, B.Z. (1958) A comparison of the effects of psychological stress in renal and essential hypertension. *Psychosomatic Medicine* **20**, 414 [398].

OSTROV, F.G., QUENCER, R.M., GAYLIS, N.B. & ALTMAN, R.D. (1982) Cerebral atrophy in systemic lupus erythematosus: steroid- or disease-induced phenomenon? *American Journal of Neuroradiology* **3**, 21–23 [421].

OSTROW, D.G. (1990) *Psychiatric Aspects of Human Immunodeficiency Virus Infection*. The Upjohn Company: Kalamazoo, Michigan [330].

OSWALD, I. & EVANS, J. (1985) On serious violence during sleepwalking. *British Journal of Psychiatry* **147**, 688–691 [737].

OSWALD, I. & PRIEST, R.G. (1965) Five weeks to escape the sleeping-pill habit. *British Medical Journal* **2**, 1093–1095 [609].

OSWALD, I. & THACORE, V.R. (1963) Amphetamine and phenmetrazine addiction. *British Medical Journal* **2**, 427–431 [617].

OTA, Y. (1969) Psychiatric studies on civilian head injuries. Ch. 9 in *The Late Effects of Head Injury*, eds Walker, A.E., Caveness, W.F. & Critchley, M. Thomas: Springfield, Illinois [182, 193].

OTT, A., BRETELER, M.M.B., VAN HARSKAMP, F., CLAUS, J.J., VAN DER CAMMEN, T.J.M., GROBBEE, D.E. & HOFMAN, A. (1995) Prevalence of Alzheimer's disease and vascular dementia: association with education. The Rotterdam study. *British Medical Journal* **310**, 970–973 [449].

OTTOSSON, J.-O. & RAPP, W. (1971) Serum levels of phenylalanine and tyrosine in Huntington's chorea. *Acta Psychiatrica Scandinavica* **221 (Supplement)**, 89–102 [467].

OUNSTED, C. (1955) The hyperkinetic syndrome in epileptic children. *Lancet* **2**, 303–311 [266, 271].

OUNSTED, C., HUTT, S.J. & LEE, D. (1963) The retrograde amnesia of petit mal. *Lancet* **1**, 671 [262].

OUNSTED, C., LINDSAY, J. & NORMAN, R. (1966) *Biological Factors in Temporal Lobe Epilepsy*. Heinemann: London [246, 261].

OVERGAARD, J. & TWEED, W.A. (1974) Cerebral circulation after head injury. Part 1: cerebral blood flow and its regulation after closed head injury with emphasis on clinical correlations. *Journal of Neurosurgery* **41**, 531–541 [165].

OVERS, R.P. & HEALY, J.R. (1973) Stroke patients: their spouses, families and the community. Ch. 5 in *Medical and Psychological Aspects of Disability*, ed. Cobb, A.B. Thomas: Springfield, Illinois [391].

OVSIEW, F. & SCHNEIDER, J. (1993) Schizophrenia and atypical motor features in a case of progressive supranuclear palsy (the Steele–Richardson–Olszewski syndrome). *Behavioural Neurology* **6**, 243–247 [666].

OWEN, A.T. & TYRER, P. (1983) Benzodiazepine dependence: a review of the evidence. *Drugs* **25**, 385–398 [611].

OWEN, F., POULTER, M., LOFTHOUSE, R., COLLINGE, J., CROW, T.J., RISBY, D., BAKER, H.F., RIDLEY, R.M., HSAIO, K. & PRUSINER, S.B. (1989) Insertion in prion protein gene in familial Creutzfeldt–Jakob disease. *Lancet* **1**, 51–52 [474].

OWEN, M.J., LEWIS, S.W. & MURRAY, R.M. (1988) Obstetric complications and schizophrenia: a computed tomographic study. *Psychological Medicine* **18**, 331–339 [85, 91].

OWEN, M., LIDDELL, M. & McGUFFIN, P. (1994) Alzheimer's disease. An association with apolipoprotein E_4 may help unlock the puzzle. *British Medical Journal* **308**, 672–673 [448].

OWENS, D.G.C. (1990) Dystonia—a potential psychiatric pitfall. *British Journal of Psychiatry* **156**, 620–634 [669].

OXBURY, J.M. & ADAMS, C.B.T. (1989) Neurosurgery for epilepsy. *British Journal of Hospital Medicine* **41**, 372–377 [311].

OXBURY, J.M. & MacCALLUM, F.O. (1973) Herpes simplex virus encephalitis: clinical features and residual damage. *Postgraduate Medical Journal* **49**, 387–389 [357].

OZELIUS, L., KRAMER, P.L., MOSKOWITZ, C.B., KWIATKOWSKI, D.J., BRIN, M.F., BRESSMAN, S.B., SCHUBACK, D.E., FALK, C.T.,

RISCH, N., DE LEON, D., BURKE, R.E., HAINES, J., GUSELLA, J.F., FAHN, S. & BREAKFIELD, X.O. (1989) Human gene for torsion dystonia located on chromosome 9q32-q34. *Neuron* **2**, 1427–1434 [671].

PAI, M.N. (1945) Change in personality after cerebrospinal fever. *British Medical Journal* **1**, 289–293 [365].

PAILLAS, J.-E. & TAMALET, J. (1950) Les tumeurs temporales. *Presse Medicale* **58**, 550–554 [226].

PAKALNIS, A., DRAKE, M.E., JOHN, K. & KELLUM, J.B. (1987) Forced normalisation. Acute psychosis after seizure control in seven patients. *Archives of Neurology* **44**, 289–292 [284].

PALAZIDOU, E., ROBINSON, P. & LISHMAN, W.A. (1990) Neuroradiological and neuropsychological assessment in anorexia nervosa. *Psychological Medicine* **20**, 521–527 [141].

PALLIS, C. & LEWIS, P.D. (1980) Neurology of gastrointestinal disease. Ch. 21 in *Handbook of Clinical Neurology, Vol. 39, Neurological Manifestations of Systemic Diseases, Part II*, eds Vinken, P.J. & Bruyn, C.W. North-Holland Publishing Co.: Amsterdam [760].

PALLIS, C. & LOUIS, S. (1961) Television-induced seizures. *Lancet* **1**, 188–190 [241].

PALLIS, C.A. (1971) Parkinsonism: natural history and clinical features. *British Medical Journal* **3**, 683–690 [646].

PALLIS, C.A. & FUDGE, B.J. (1956) The neurological complications of Behcet's syndrome. *Archives of Neurology and Psychiatry* **75**, 1–14 [762].

PALMER, A.C., CALDER, I.M. & HUGHES, J.T. (1987) Spinal cord degeneration in divers. *Lancet* **2**, 1365–1366 [767].

PALMER, A.C., CALDER, I.M. & YATES, P.O. (1992) Cerebral vasculopathy in divers. *Neuropathology and Applied Neurobiology* **18**, 113–124 [767, 768].

PALMER, A.M., STRATMANN, G.C., PROCTER, A.W. & BOWEN, D.M. (1988) Possible neurotransmitter basis of behavioral changes in Alzheimer's disease. *Annals of Neurology* **23**, 616–620 [444].

PALMER, M.S., DRYDEN, A.J., HUGHES, J.T. & COLLINGE, J. (1991) Homozygous prion protein genotype predisposes to sporadic Creutzfeldt–Jakob disease. *Nature* **352**, 340–342 [475].

PAMPIGLIONE, G. & FALCONER, M.A. (1960) Electrical stimulation of the hippocampus in man. Ch. 57 in *Handbook of Physiology, Section 1: Neurophysiology*, Vol. 2, ed. Field, J. (Section ed. Magoun, H.W.) American Physiological Society: Washington, DC [269].

PANAYIOTOPOULOS, C.P., SHAROQI, I.A. & AGATHONIKOU, A. (1997) Occipital seizures imitating migraine aura. *Journal of the Royal Society of Medicine* **90**, 255–257 [291].

PANG, A. & LEWIS, S.W. (1996) Bipolar affective disorder minus left prefrontal cortex equals schizophrenia. *British Journal of Psychiatry* **168**, 647–650 [85].

PANKRATZ, L. (1988) Malingering on intellectual and neuropsychological measures. Ch. 10 in *Clinical Assessment of Malingering and Deception*, ed. Rogers, R. Guilford Press: New York [485].

PAPEZ, J.W. (1937) A proposed mechanism of emotion. *Archives of Neurology and Psychiatry* **38**, 725–743 [23, 38].

PARDO, J.V., PARDO, P.J., JANER, K.W. & RAICHLE, M.E. (1990) The anterior cingulate cortex mediates processing selection in the Stroop attention of conflict paradigm. *The Proceedings of the National Academy of Sciences* **87**, 256–259 [118, 146].

PARE, C.M.B., YEUNG, D.P.H., PRICE, K. & STACEY, R.S. (1969) 5-Hydroxytryptamine, noradrenaline, and dopamine in brain stem, hypothalamus, and caudate nucleus of controls and of patients committing suicide by coal-gas poisoning. *Lancet* **2**, 133–135 [24].

PARKER, N. (1956) Disseminated sclerosis presenting as schizophrenia. *Medical Journal of Australia* **1**, 405–407 [697].

PARKER, N. (1957) Manic-depressive psychosis following head injury. *Medical Journal of Australia* **2**, 20–22 [191].

PARKER, S.A. & SERRATS, A.F. (1976) Memory recovery after traumatic coma. *Acta Neurochirurgica* **34**, 71–77 [185].

PARKES, J.D. (1985) *Sleep and its Disorders*. W.B. Saunders: London [722, 724, 725, 726, 730, 731, 732, 737].

PARKES, J.D. (1986a) Sleep disorders. *Progress in Clinical Neurosciences* **2**, 1–22 [640, 723, 724, 726, 732].

PARKES, J.D. (1986b) The parasomnias. *Lancet* **2**, 1021–1025 [736].

PARKIN, A.J. (1987) *Memory and Amnesia: An Introduction*. Basil Blackwell: Oxford [29, 38].

PARKINSON, I.S., WARD, M.K., FEEST, T.G., FAWCETT, R.W.P. & KERR, D.N.S. (1979) Fracturing dialysis osteodystrophy and dialysis encephalopathy. An epidemiological survey. *Lancet* **1**, 406–409 [558].

PARKINSON, J. (1817) *An Essay on the Shaking Palsy*. Sherwood: London [646].

PARKINSON STUDY GROUP (1989) Effect of deprenyl on the progression of disability in early Parkinson's disease. *New England Journal of Medicine* **321**, 1364–1371 [650].

PARRY, G.J. (1988) Peripheral neuropathies associated with human immunodeficiency virus infection. *Annals of Neurology* **23 (Supplement)**, S49–S53 [327].

PARRY, J. (1968) *Contribution à l'étude des manifestations des lesions expansives observées dans un hôpital psychiatrique*. Thesis, Faculté de Médicine de Paris [218, 221].

PARSONAGE, M. (1973) The differential diagnosis of seizures. *Journal of the Royal College of Physicians of London* **7**, 213–233 [288].

PARSONS, O.A. (1987) Intellectual impairment in alcoholics: persistent issues. *Acta Medica Scandinavica* **717 (Supplement)**, 33–46 [604].

PARSONS-SMITH, B.G., SUMMERSKILL, W.H.J., DAWSON, A.M. & SHERLOCK, S. (1957) The encephalograph in liver disease. *Lancet* **2**, 867–871 [564].

PARTRIDGE, M. (1950) *Prefontal Leucotomy*. Blackwell Scientific Publications: Oxford [77].

PASAMANICK, B. & KAWI, A. (1956) A study of the association of prenatal and paranatal factors with the development of tics in children. *Journal of Pediatrics* **48**, 596–601 [685].

PASQUALINI, R.Q., VIDAL, G. & BUR, G.E. (1957) Psychopathology of Klinefelter's syndrome. Review of thirty-one cases. *Lancet* **2**, 164–167 [526, 527].

PASSOUANT, P., CADILHAC, J. & BALDY-MOULINIER, M. (1967) Physiopathologie des hypersomnies. *Revue Neurologique* **116**, 585–629 [733].

PATERSON, M.T. (1945) Spasmodic torticollis: results of psychotherapy in twenty-one cases. *Lancet* **2**, 556–559 [674, 675].

PATRICK, M. & HOWELLS, R. (1990) Barbiturate-assisted interviews in modern clinical practice. *Psychological Medicine* **20**, 763–765 [488].

PATTEN, B.M. & PAGES, M. (1984) Severe neurological disease associated with hyperparathyroidism. *Annals of Neurology* **15**, 453–456 [530].

PATTERSON, A. & ZANGWILL, O.L. (1944) Recovery of spatial orientation in the post-traumatic confusional state. *Brain* **67**, 54–68 [11].

PATTERSON, M.B. & MACK, J.L. (1985) Neuropsychological analysis of a case of reduplicative paramnesia. *Journal of Clinical and Experimental Neuropsychology* **7**, 111–121 [12].

PATTERSON, R.M., BAGGHI, B.K. & TEST, A. (1948) The prediction of Huntington's chorea. An electroencephalographic and genetic study. *American Journal of Psychiatry* **104**, 786–797 [467].

PATTERSON, R.M. & LITTLE, S.C. (1943) Spasmodic torticollis. *Journal of Nervous and Mental Disease* **98**, 571–599 [672, 673].

PATTIE, A.H. & GILLEARD, C.J. (1975) A brief psychogeriatric assessment schedule. Validation against psychiatric diagnosis and discharge from hospital. *British Journal of Psychiatry* **127**, 489–493 [125].

PATTIE, A.H. & GILLEARD, C.J. (1976) The Clifton Assessment Schedule—further validation of a psychogeriatric assessment schedule. *British Journal of Psychiatry* **129**, 68–72 [125].

PATTIE, A.H. & GILLEARD, C.J. (1978) The two-year predictive validity of the Clifton Assessment Schedule and the Shortened Stockton Geriatric Rating Scale. *British Journal of Psychiatry* **133**, 457–460 [125].

PATTON, R.B. & SHEPPARD, J.A. (1956) Intracranial tumors found at autopsy in mental patients. *American Journal of Psychiatry* **113**, 319–324 [233].

PAULESU, E., FRITH, C.D. & FRACKOWIAK, R.S.J. (1993) The neural correlates of the verbal component of working memory. *Nature* **362**, 342–345 [48, 88].

PAULESU, E., FRITH, U., SNOWLING, M., GALLAGHER, A., MORTON, J., FRACKOWIAK, R.S.J. & FRITH, C.D. (1996) Is developmental dyslexia a disconnection syndrome? Evidence from PET scanning. *Brain* **119**, 143–157 [xvii, 48, 49].

PAULSON, G.W. (1971) The neurological examination in dementia. Ch. 2 in *Dementia*, ed. Wells, C.E. Blackwell Scientific Publications: Oxford [96].

PAWLIKOWSKA, T., CHALDER, T., HIRSCH, S.R., WALLACE, P., WRIGHT, D.J.M. & WESSELY, S.C. (1994) Population based study of fatigue and psychological distress. *British Medical Journal* **308**, 763–766 [373].

PAXTON, R. & AMBROSE, J. (1974) The EMI scanner: a brief review of the first 650 patients. *British Journal of Radiology* **47**, 530–565 [137].

PEABODY, C.A., DAVIES, H., BERGER, P.A. & TINKLENBERG, J.R. (1986) Desamino-D-arginine-vasopressin (DDAVP) in Alzheimer's disease. *Neurobiology of Ageing* **7**, 301–303 [502].

PEARCE, J.M.S. (1969) *Migraine: Clinical Features, Mechanisms and Management*. Thomas: Springfield, Illinois [399, 402].

PEARCE, J.M.S. (1989) Whiplash injury: a reappraisal. *Journal of Neurology, Neurosurgery and Psychiatry* **52**, 1329–1331 [201].

PEARCE, J.M.S. (1992) *Parkinson's Disease and its Management*. Oxford University Press: Oxford [646].

PEARCE, J.M.S. & MILLER, E. (1973) *Clinical Aspects of Dementia*. Baillière Tindall: London [438, 501].

PEARLSON, G.D. & VEROFF, A.E. (1981) Computerised tomographic scan changes in manic-depressive illness. *Lancet* **2**, 470 [140].

PEARSON, R.C.A., ESIRI, M.M., HIORNS, R.W., WILCOCK, G.K. & POWELL, T.P.S. (1985) Anatomical correlates of the distribution of the pathological changes in the neocortex in Alzheimer disease. *Proceedings of the National Academy of Science, USA* **82**, 4531–4534 [441].

PEDERSEN, K.K. (1980) Migraene og demens. *Ugeskrift for Laeger* **142**, 1346–1347 [407].

PEDLEY, T.A. & GUILLEMINAULT, C. (1977) Episodic nocturnal wanderings responsive to anticonvulsant drug therapy. *Annals of Neurology* **2**, 30–35 [296].

PELLIZARI, C.A., CHEN, G.T.Y., SPELBRING, D.R., WEICHSELBAUM, R.R. & CHEN, C.J. (1989) Accurate three-dimensional registration of CT, PET, and/or MR images of the brain. *Journal of Computer Assisted Tomography* **13**, 20–26 [144].

PELTONEN, L. (1962) Pneumoencephalographic studies on the third ventricle of 644 neuropsychiatric patients. *Acta Psychiatrica Scandinavica* **38**, 15–34 [140].

PENALVER, R. (1955) Manganese poisoning. *Industrial Medicine and Surgery* **24**, 1–7 [635, 636].

PENFIELD, W. (1968) Engrams in the human brain. *Proceedings of the Royal Society of Medicine* **61**, 831–840 [24].

PENFIELD, W. & PEROT, P. (1963) The brain's record of auditory and visual experience. A final summary and discussion. *Brain* **86**, 595–696 [251].

PENN, R.D., BELANGER, M.G. & YASNOFF, W.A. (1978) Ventricular volume in man computed from CAT scans. *Annals of Neurology* **3**, 216–223 [138].

PENROSE, R.J.J. (1972) Life events before subarachnoid haemorrhage. *Journal of Psychosomatic Research* **16**, 329–333 [396].

PENROSE, R. & STOREY, P.B. (1970) Emotional disturbance and subarachnoid haemorrhage. *Psychotherapy and Psychosomatics* **18**, 321–325 [396].

PENTLAND, B., JONES, P.A., ROY, C.W. & MILLER, J.D. (1986) Head injury in the elderly. *Age and Ageing* **15**, 193–202 [174].

PENTLAND, B. & MAWDSLEY, C. (1982) Wernicke's encephalopathy following hunger strike. *Postgraduate Medical Journal* **58**, 427–428 [576].

PENTLAND, B., MITCHELL, J.D., CULL, R.E. & FORD, M.J. (1985) Central nervous system sarcoidosis. *Quarterly Journal of Medicine* **56**, 457–465 [764, 765].

PEPPARD, R.F., MARTIN, W.R.W., CARR, G.D., GROCHOWSKI, E., SCHULZER, M., GUTTMAN, M., McGEER, P.L., PHILLIPS, A.G., TSUI, K.C. & CALNE, D.B. (1992) Cerebral glucose metabolism in Parkinson's disease with and without dementia. *Archives of Neurology* **49**, 1262–1268 [655].

PERANI, D., VALLAR, G., CAPPA, S., MESSA, C. & FAZIO, F. (1987) Aphasia and neglect after subcortical stroke. A clinical/cerebral perfusion correlation study. *Brain* **110**, 1211–1229 [46].

PEREZ, M.M., TRIMBLE, M.R., MURRAY, N.N.F. & REIDER, I. (1985) Epileptic psychosis: an evaluation of PSE profiles. *British Journal of Psychiatry* **146**, 155–163 [280, 281, 282, 286].

PERICAK-VANCE, M.A., BEBOUT, J.L., GASKELL, P.C., YAMAOKA, L.H., HUNG, W.-Y., ALPERTS, M.J., WALKER, A.P., BARTLETT, R.J., HAYNES, C.A., WELSH, K.A., EARL, N.L., HEYMAN, A., CLARK, C.M. & ROSES, A.D. (1991) Linkage studies in familial Alzheimer disease: evidence for chromosome 19 linkage. *American Journal of Human Genetics* **48**, 1034–1050 [448].

PERK, D. (1947) Cerebral symptoms in thrombo-angiitis obliterans. *Journal of Mental Science* **93**, 748–755 [425].

PERKS, W.H., HORROCKS, P.M., COOPER, R.A., BRADBURY, S., ALLEN, A., BALDOCK, N., PROWSE, K. & VAN'T HOFF, W. (1980) Sleep apnoea in acromegaly. *British Medical Journal* **280**, 894–897 [522].

PERL, D.P. & BRODY, A.R. (1980) Alzheimer's disease: X-ray spectrometric evidence of aluminium accumulation in neurofibrillary tangle-bearing neurones. *Science* **208**, 297–299 [446].

PERLMUTER, L.C., HAKAMI, M.K., HODGSON-HARRINGTON, C., GINSBERG, J., KATZ, J., SINGER, D.E. & NATHAN, D.M. (1984) Decreased cognitive function in aging non-insulin-dependent diabetic patients. *American Journal of Medicine* **77**, 1043–1048 [538].

PERLSTEIN, M. & ATTALA, R. (1966) Neurologic sequelae of plumbism in children. *Clinical Pediatrics* **5**, 292–298 [632].

PERLSTEIN, M.A., GIBBS, F.A., GIBBS, E.L. & STEIN, M.D. (1960) Electroencephalogram and myopathy. Relation between muscular dystrophy and related diseases. *Journal of the American Medical Association* **173**, 1329–1333 [716].

PERRET, E. (1974) The left frontal lobe of man and the suppression of habitual responses in verbal categorical behaviour. *Neuropsychologia* **12**, 323–330 [104].

PERRON, M., VEILLETTE, S. & MATHIEU, J. (1989) La dystrophie myotonique: 1. caractéristiques socio-économiques et résidentielles des malades. *The Canadian Journal of Neurological Sciences* **16**, 109–113 [720].

PERRONE, P., CANDELISE, L., SCOTTI, G., DE GRANDI, C. & SCIALFA, G. (1979) CT evaluation in patients with transient ischaemic attack. Correlation between clinical and angiographic findings. *European Neurology* **18**, 217–221 [380].

PERRY, E.K., CURTIS, M., DICK, D.J., CANDY, J.M., ATACK, J.R., BLOXHAM, C.A., BLESSED, G., FAIRBAIRN, A., TOMLINSON, B.E. & PERRY, R.H. (1985) Cholinergic correlates of cognitive impairment in Parkinson's disease: comparisons with Alzheimer's disease. *Journal of Neurology, Neurosurgery and Psychiatry* **48**, 413–421 [655].

PERRY, E.K., GIBSON, P.H., BLESSED, G., PERRY, R.H. & TOMLINSON, B.E. (1977) Neurotransmitter enzyme abnormalities in senile dementia. Choline acetyltransferase and glutamic acid decarboxylase activities in necropsy brain tissue. *Journal of the Neurological Sciences* **34**, 247–265 [444].

PERRY, E.K., KERWIN, J., PERRY, R.H., IRVING, D., BLESSED, G. & FAIRBAIRN, A. (1990a) Cerebral cholinergic activity is related to the incidence of visual hallucinations in senile dementia of Lewy body type. *Dementia* **1**, 2–4 [452].

PERRY, E.K., MARSHALL, E., KERWIN, J., SMITH, C.J., JABEEN, S., CHENG, A.V. & PERRY, R.H. (1990b) Evidence of a monoaminergic-cholinergic imbalance related to visual hallucinations in Lewy body dementia. *Journal of Neurochemistry* **55**, 1454–1456 [452].

PERRY, E.K., MARSHALL, E., PERRY, R.H., IRVING, D., SMITH, C.J., BLESSED, G. & FAIRBAIRN, A.F. (1990c) Cholinergic and dopaminergic activities in senile dementia of Lewy body type. *Alzheimer Disease and Associated Disorders* **4**, 87–95 [452].

PERRY, E.K., SMITH, C.J., PERRY, R.H., JOHNSON, M. & FAIRBAIRN, A.F. (1989) Nicotinic (^{3}H-Nicotine) receptor binding in human brain: characterization and involvement in cholinergic neuropathology. *Neurosciences Research Communications* **5**, 117–124 [444].

PERRY, E.K., TOMLINSON, B.E., BLESSED, G., BERGMANN, K., GIBSON, P.H. & PERRY, R.H. (1978) Correlation of cholinergic abnormalities with senile plaques and mental test scores in senile dementia. *British Medical Journal* **2**, 1457–1459 [444].

PERRY, J.C. & JACOBS, D. (1982) Overview: clinical applications of the amytal interview in psychiatric emergency settings. *American Journal of Psychiatry* **139**, 552–559 [488].

PERRY, R.H., IRVING, D., BLESSED, G., FAIRBAIRN, A. & PERRY, E.K. (1990d) Senile dementia of Lewy body type. A clinically and neuropathologically distinct form of Lewy body dementia in the elderly. *Journal of the Neurological Sciences* **95**, 119–139 [450, 452].

PERRY, R.H., IRVING, D., BLESSED, G., PERRY, E.K., SMITH, C.J. & FAIRBAIRN, A.F. (1990e) Dementia in old age: identification of a clinically and pathologically distinct disease category. *Advances in Neurology* **51**, 41–46 [452].

PERRY, S.W. (1994) HIV-related depression. Ch. 12 in *HIV, AIDS, and the Brain*, eds Price, R.W. & Perry, S.W. *Association for Research in Nervous and Mental Disease*, Vol. 72. Raven Press: New York [330].

PERRY, S., JACOBSBERG, L. & FISHMAN, B. (1990f) Suicidal ideation and HIV testing. *Journal of the American Medical Association* **263**, 679–682 [331].

PERRY, S.W., JACOBSBERG, L.B., FISHMAN, B., WEILER, P.H., GOLD, J.W.M. & FRANCES, A.J. (1990g) Psychological responses to serological testing for HIV. *AIDS* **4**, 145–152 [330].

PERRY, S. & JACOBSEN, P. (1986) Neuropsychiatric manifestations of AIDS-spectrum disorders. *Hospital and Community Psychiatry* **37**, 135–142 [325].

PERRY, T.L., HANSEN, S., DIAMOND, S. & STEDMAN, D. (1969) Plasma-aminoacid levels in Huntington's chorea. *Lancet* **1**, 806–808 [467].

PERRY, T.L., HANSEN, S. & KLOSTER, M. (1973) Huntington's chorea: deficiency of g-aminobutyric acid in brain. *New England Journal of Medicine* **288**, 337–342 [467].

PERSSON, G., BERG, S., NILSSON, L. & SVANBORG, A. (1991) Subclinical dementia. Relation to cognition, personality and psychopathology: a nine-year prospective study. *International Journal of Geriatric Psychiatry* **6**, 239–247 [432].

PERSSON, G. & SKOOG, I. (1992) Subclinical dementia: relevance of cognitive symptoms and signs. *Journal of Geriatric Psychiatry and Neurology* **5**, 172–178 [432].

PETERS, W.J. (1983) Lightning injury. *Canadian Medical Association Journal* **128**, 148–150 [766].

PETERSEN, P. (1968) Psychiatric disorders in primary hyperparathyroidism. *Journal of Clinical Endocrinology and Metabolism* **28**, 1491–1495 [529, 530, 561].

PETERSEN, S.E., FOX, P.T., POSNER, M.I., MINTUN, M. & RAICHLE, M.E. (1988) Positron emission tomographic studies of the cortical anatomy of single-word processing. *Nature* **331**, 585–589 [45, 146].

PETERSON, H. DE C. & SWANSON, A.G. (1964) Acute encephalopathy occurring during haemodialysis. *Archives of Internal Medicine* **113**, 877–880 [558].

PETITO, C.K. (1988) Review of central nervous system pathology in human immunodeficiency virus infection. *Annals of Neurology* **23 (Supplement)**, S54–S57 [323, 326].

PETITO, C.K., CHO, E.-S., LEMANN, W., NAVIA, B.A. & PRICE, R.W. (1986) Neuropathology of acquired immunodeficiency syndrome (AIDS): An autopsy review. *Journal of Neuropathology and Experimental Neurology* **45**, 635–646 [320].

PETITO, C.K., NAVIA, B.A., CHO, E.-S., JORDAN, B.D., GEORGE, D.C. & PRICE, R.W. (1985) Vacuolar myelopathy pathologically resembling subacute combined degeneration in patients with the acquired immunodeficiency syndrome. *New England Journal of Medicine* **312**, 874–879 [323, 326].

PETTEGREW, J.W., KESHAVAN, M.S. & MINSHEW, N.J. (1993) ^{31}P nuclear magnetic resonance spectroscopy: neurodevelopment and schizophrenia. *Schizophrenia Bulletin* **19**, 35–53 [143].

PETTEGREW, J.W., KESHAVAN, M.S., PANCHALINGAM, K., STRYCHOR, S., KAPLAN, D.B., TRETTA M.G. & ALLEN, M. (1991) Alterations in brain high-energy phosphate and membrane phospholipid metabolism in first-episode, drug-naive schizophrenics: a pilot study of the dorsal prefrontal cortex by in vivo phosphorus 31 nuclear magnetic resonance spectroscopy. *Archives of General Psychiatry* **48**, 563–568 [143].

PETTEGREW, J.W., MOOSSY, J., WITHERS, G., McKEAG, D. & PANCHALINGAM, K. (1988) ^{31}P nuclear magnetic resonance study of the brain in Alzheimer's disease. *Journal of Neuropathology and Experimental Neurology* **47**, 235–248 [143].

PETTY, R.K.H., HARDING, A.E. & MORGAN-HUGHES, J.A. (1986) The clinical features of mitochondrial myopathy. *Brain* **109**, 915–938 [761].

PEYSER, J.M., EDWARDS, K.R. & POSER, C.M. (1980a) Psychological profiles in patients with multiple sclerosis. A preliminary investigation. *Archives of Neurology* **37**, 437–440 [692].

PEYSER, J.M., EDWARDS, K.R., POSER, C.M. & FILSKOV, S.B. (1980b) Cognitive function in patients with multiple sclerosis. *Archives of Neurology* **37**, 577–579 [692].

PFEFFERBAUM, A., ZIPURSKY, R.B., LIM, K.O., ZATZ, L.M., STAHL, S.M. & JERNIGAN, T.L. (1988) Computed tomographic evidence for generalized sulcal and ventricular enlargement in schizophrenia. *Archives of General Psychiatry* **45**, 633–640 [140].

PHELPS, C. (1898) *Traumatic Injuries of the Brain and its Membranes*. Kimpton: London [180].

PHELPS, M.E., HUANG, S.C., HOFFMAN, E.J., SELIN, C., SOKOLOFF, L. & KUHL, D.E. (1979) Tomographic measurement of local cerebral glucose metabolic rate in humans with (F-18) 2-fluoro-2-deoxy-D-glucose: validation of method. *Annals of Neurology* **6**, 371–388 [144].

PHELPS, M.E. & MAZZIOTTA, J.C. (1985) Positron emission tomography: human brain function and biochemistry. *Science* **228**, 799–809 [145].

PHILIPPOPOULOS, G.S., WITTKOWER, E.D. & COUSINEAU, A. (1958) The etiologic significance of emotional factors in onset and exacerbation of multiple sclerosis. *Psychosomatic Medicine* **20**, 458–474 [699].

PHILLIPS, A.N., SABIN, C.A., ELFORD, J., BOFILL, M., JANOSSY, G. & LEE, C.A. (1994) Use of CD_4 lymphocyte count to predict long-term survival free of AIDS after HIV infection. *British Medical Journal* **309**, 309–313 [318].

PICK, A. (1892) Ueber die Beziehungen der senilen Hirnatrophie zur Aphasie. *Prager Medizinische Wochenschrift* **17**, 165–167 [461].

PICKARD, J.D. (1982) Adult communicating hydrocephalus. *British Journal of Hospital Medicine* **27**, 35–44 [748].

PICKETT, J.B.E., LAYZER, R.B., LEVIN, S.R., SCHNEIDER, V., CAMPBELL, M.J. & SUMNER, A.J. (1975) Neuromuscular complications of acromegaly. *Neurology* **25**, 638–645 [522].

PIERCY, M. (1959) Testing for intellectual impairment—some comments on the tests and the testers. *Journal of Mental Science* **105**, 489–495 [108, 109].

PIERCY, M. (1964) The effects of cerebral lesions on intellectual function: a review of current research trends. *British Journal of Psychiatry* **110**, 310–352 [40, 43, 46, 62, 183].

PIERCY, M. (1977) Experimental studies of the organic amnesic syndrome. Ch. 1 in *Amnesia: Clinical, Psychological and Medicolegal Aspects*, 2nd edn, eds Whitty, C.W.M. & Zangwill, O.L. Butterworths: London [35].

PIERCY, M. & SMYTH, V.O.G. (1962) Right hemisphere dominance for certain non-verbal intellectual skills. *Brains* **85**, 775–790 [112].

PIKE, M. & STORES, G. (1994) Kleine–Levin syndrome: a cause of diagnostic confusion. *Archives of Disease in Childhood* **71**, 355–357 [732, 733].

PILLERI, G. (1966) The Klüver–Bucy syndrome in man: a clinico-anatomical contribution to the function of the medial temporal lobe structures. *Psychiatria et Neurologia* **152**, 65–103 [23].

PILOWSKY, I. (1985) Cryptotrauma and 'accident neurosis'. *British Journal of Psychiatry* **147**, 310–311 [175].

PILOWSKY, L.S. (1996) Imaging receptors in psychiatry. Ch. 7 in *Brain Imaging in Psychiatry*, eds Lewis, S. & Higgins, N. Blackwell Science: Oxford [146].

PILOWSKY, L.S., COSTA, D.C., ELL, P.J., VERHOEFF, N.P.L.G., MURRAY, R.M. & KERWIN, R.W. (1994) D_2 dopamine receptor binding in the basal ganglia of antipsychotic-free schizophrenic patients an ^{123}I-IBZM single photon emission computerised tomography study. *British Journal of Psychiatry* **164**, 16–26 [88, 148].

PINCHING, A.J. (1996) Managing HIV disease after Delta. *British Medical Journal* **312**, 521–522 [336].

PINCUS, J.H. (1972) Subacute necrotizing encephalomyelopathy (Leigh's disease): a consideration of clinical features and etiology. *Developmental Medicine and Child Neurology* **14**, 87–101 [587].

PINCUS, J.H., COOPER, J.R., ITOKAWA, Y. & GUMBINAS, M. (1971) Subacute necrotizing encephalomyelopathy: effects of thiamine and thiamine propyl disulfide. *Archives of Neurology* **24**, 511–517 [586].

PINTO, R. (1972) A case of movement epilepsy with agarophobia treated successfully by flooding. *British Journal of Psychiatry* **121**, 287–288 [276].

PIROZZOLO, F.J., BASKIN, D.S., SWIHART, A.A. & APPEL, S.H. (1987) Oral tetrahydroaminoacridine in the treatment of senile dementia, Alzheimer's type. *New England Journal of Medicine* **316**, 1603 [503].

PIZZO, P.A., EDDY, J., FALLOON, J., BALIS, F.M., MURPHY, R.F., MOSS, H., WOLTERS, P., BROUWERS, P., JAROSINSKI, P., RUBIN, M., BRODER, S., YARCHOAN, R., BRUNETTI, A., MAHA, M., NUSINOFF-LEHRMAN, S. & POPLACK, D.G. (1988) Effect of continuous intravenous infusion of zidovudine (AZT) in children with symptomatic HIV infection. *New England Journal of Medicine* **319**, 889–896 [335].

PLAITAKIS, A., WHETSELL, W.O., COOPER, J.R. & YAHR, M.D. (1980) Chronic Leigh disease: a genetic and biochemical study. *Annals of Neurology* **7**, 304–310 [587].

PLUM, F. (1972) Prospects for research on schizophrenia. 3: Neuropsychology. Neuropathological findings. *Neurosciences Research Program Bulletin* **10**, 384–388 [86].

PLUM, F. & POSNER, J.B. (1972) *Diagnosis of Stupor and Coma*, 2nd edn. Davis: Philadelphia [379].

PLUM, F., POSNER, J.B. & HAIN, R.F. (1962) Delayed neurological deterioration after anoxia. *Archives of Internal Medicine* **110**, 18–25 [551].

POECK, K. (1969) Pathophysiology of emotional disorders associated with brain damage. Ch. 20 in *Handbook of Clinical Neurology*, Vol. 3, eds Vinken, P.J. & Bruyn, G.W. North-Holland Publishing Company: Amsterdam [81].

POEWE, W., BENKE, T.H., FELBER, S.T. & AICHNER, F. (1989) Symptomatic blepharospasm accompanying the paramedian diencephalic syndrome: report of a case. *Behavioural Neurology* **2**, 143–151 [679].

POEWE, W., KARAMAT, E., KEMMLER, G.W. & GERSTENBRAND, F. (1990) The premorbid personality of patients with Parkinson's disease: a comparative study with healthy controls and patients with essential tremor. In *Parkinson's Disease: Anatomy, Pathology, and Therapy*, eds Streifler, M.B., Korczyn, A.D., Melamed, E. & Youdin, M.B.H. *Advances in Neurology*, Vol. 53, pp. 339–342. Raven Press: New York [661].

POIRER, J., DAVIGNON, J., BOUTHILLIER, D., KOGAN, S., BERTRAND, P. & GAUTHIER, S. (1993) Apolipoprotein E polymorphism and Alzheimer's disease. *Lancet* **342**, 697–699 [448].

POKLIS, A. & BURKETT, C.D. (1977) Gasoline sniffing: a review. *Clinical Toxicology* **11**, 35–41 [630].

POLKEY, C.E. & BINNIE, C.D. (1993) Neurosurgical treatment of epilepsy. Ch. 16 in *A Textbook of Epilepsy*, 4th edn, eds Laidlaw, J., Richens, A. & Chadwick, D. Churchill Livingstone: Edinburgh [311, 312].

POLKINGHORNE, P.J., SEHMI, K., CROSS, M.R., MINASSIAN, D. & BIRD, A.C. (1988) Ocular fundus lesions in divers. *Lancet* **2**, 1381–1383 [767].

POLLARD, A.J., PRENDERGAST, M., AL-HAMMOURI, F., RAYNER, P.H.W. & SHAW, N.J. (1994) Different subtypes of pseudohypoparathyroidism in the same family with an unusual psychiatric presentation of the index case. *Archives of Disease in Childhood* **70**, 99–102 [533].

POLLOCK, M. & HORNABROOK, R.W. (1966) The prevalence, natural history and dementia of Parkinson's disease. *Brain* **89**, 429–448 [653, 661].

POLSON, R.J., ROLLES, K., CALNE, R.Y., WILLIAMS, R. & MARSDEN, D. (1987) Reversal of severe neurological manifestations of Wilson's disease following orthotopic liver transplantation. *Quarterly Journal of Medicine* **64**, 685–691 [664].

POMEROY, J.C. (1980) Klinefelter's syndrome and schizophrenia. *British Journal of Psychiatry* **136**, 597–599 [527].

POND, D.A. (1952a) Psychiatric aspects of epilepsy in children. *Journal of Mental Science* **98**, 404–410 [265].

POND, D.A. (1952b) Narcolepsy: a brief critical review and study of eight cases. *Journal of Mental Science* **98**, 595–604 [727].

POND, D.A. (1957) Psychiatric aspects of epilepsy in children. *Journal of the Indian Medical Profession* **3**, 1441–1451 [249, 257, 265, 275, 284, 295].

POND, D.A. (1961) Psychiatric aspects of epileptic and brain-damaged children. *British Medical Journal* **2**, 1377–1382 and 1454–1459 [262, 271].

POND, D.A. (1962) Discussion following 'The schizophrenia-like psychoses of epilepsy'. *Proceedings of the Royal Society of Medicine* **55**, 316 [282, 283].

POND, D.A. & BIDWELL, B.H. (1960) A survey of epilepsy in fourteen general practices. II: Social and psychological aspects. *Epilepsia* **1**, 285–299 [259, 265, 266].

POND, D.A., BIDWELL, B.H. & STEIN, L. (1960) A survey of epilepsy in fourteen general practices. 1: Demographic and medical data. *Psychiatria, Neurologia, Neurochirurgia* **63**, 217–236 [242, 243, 259].

POPPEN, J.L. & MARTINEZ-NIOCHET, A. (1951) Spasmodic torticollis. *Surgical Clinics of North America* **31**, 883–890 [674].

PORJESZ, B. & BEGLEITER, H. (1987) Evoked brain potentials and alcoholism. In *Neuropsychology of Alcoholism: Implications for Diagnosis and Treatment*, eds Parsons, O.A., Butters, N. & Nathan, P.E., pp. 45–63. Guilford Press: New York [606].

PORTEGIES, P., DEGANS, J., LANGE, J.M.A., DERIX, M.M.A., SPEELMAN, H., BAKKER, M., DANNER, S.A. & GOUDSMIT, J. (1989) Declining incidence of AIDS dementia complex after introduction of zidovudine treatment. *British Medical Journal* **299**, 819–821 [335].

PORTEGIES, P., ENTING, R.H., DE GANS, J., ALGRA, P.R., DERIX, M.M.A., LANGE, J.M.A. & GOUDSMIT, J. (1993) Presentation and course of AIDS dementia complex: 10 years of follow-up in Amsterdam, the Netherlands. *AIDS* **7**, 669–675 [335].

PORTEOUS, H.B. & ROSS, D.N. (1956) Mental symptoms in parkinsonism following benzhexol hydrochloride therapy. *British Medical Journal* **2**, 138–140 [657].

POSER, C.M. (1990) Notes on the pathogenesis of subacute sclerosing panencephalitis. *Journal of the Neurological Sciences* **95**, 219–224 [361].

POSER, C.M., HUNTLEY, C.J. & POLAND, J.D. (1969) Para-encephalitic parkinsonism. Report of an acute case due to coxsackie virus type B2 and re-examination of the etiologic concepts of post-encephalitic parkinsonism. *Acta Neurologica Scandinavica* **45**, 199–215 [349].

POSER, C.M. & ZIEGLER, D.K. (1960) Temporary amnesia as a manifestation of cerebrovascular insufficiency. In *Transactions of the American Neurological Association*, ed. Yahr, M.D., pp. 221–223. Springer: New York [413].

POST, F. (1944) Some problems arising from a study of mental patients over the age of sixty years. *Journal of Mental Science* **90**, 554–565 [433].

POST, F. (1962) *The Significance of Affective Symptoms in Old Age*. Oxford University Press: London [487].

POST, F. (1965) *The Clinical Psychiatry of Late Life*. Pergamon: Oxford [114, 123, 486, 487].

POST, F. (1968) The development and progress of senile dementia in relationship to the functional psychiatric disorders of later life. In *Senile Dementia: Clinical and Therapeutic Aspects*, eds Müller, Ch. & Ciompi, L. Huber: Bern [433].

POST, R.M., DELISI, L.E., HOLCOMB, H.H., UHDE, T.W., COHEN, R. & BUCHSBAUM, M.S. (1987) Glucose utilization in the temporal cortex of affectively ill patients: positron emission tomography. *Biological Psychiatry* **22**, 545–553 [145].

POTAMIANOS, G. & KELLETT, J.M. (1982) Anti-cholinergic drugs and memory: the effects of benzhexol on memory in a group of geriatric patients. *British Journal of Psychiatry* **140**, 470–472 [625].

POTTER, J.M. (1969) Clinical aspects of herpes simplex encephalitis. In *Virus Diseases and the Nervous System*, eds Whitty, C.W.M., Hughes, J.T. & MacCallum, F.O. Blackwell Scientific Publications: Oxford [357].

POVLISHOCK, J.T. & COBURN, T.H. (1989) Morphopathological change associated with mild head injury. Ch. 4 in *Mild Head Injury*, eds Levin, H.S., Eisenberg, H.M. & Benton, A.L. Oxford University Press: New York [163].

POWELL, E.E., PENDER, M.P., CHALK, J.B., PARKIN, P.J., STRONG, R., LYNCH, S., KERLIN, P., COOKSLEY, W.G., CHENG, W. & POWELL, L.W. (1990) Improvement in chronic hepatocerebral degeneration following liver transplantation. *Gastroenterology* **98**, 1079–1082 [566].

POWELL, G.E. (1981) *Brain Function Therapy*. Gower Publishing Co.: Aldershot, Hants [309].

POWELL, G.E., POLKEY, C.E. & CANAVAN, A.G.M. (1987) Lateralisation of memory functions in epileptic patients by use of the sodium amytal (Wada) technique. *Journal of Neurology, Neurosurgery and Psychiatry* **50**, 665–672 [312].

POWELL-JACKSON, J., WELLER, R.O., KENNEDY, P., PREECE, M.A., WHITCOMBE, E.M. & NEWSOM-DAVIS, J. (1985) Creutzfeldt–Jakob disease after administration of human growth hormone. *Lancet* **2**, 244–246 [476].

POWELL-PROCTOR, L. & MILLER, E. (1982) Reality orientation: a critical appraisal. *British Journal of Psychiatry* **140**, 457–463 [500].

PRAKASH, C. & STERN, G. (1973) Neurological signs in the elderly. *Age and Ageing* **2**, 24–27 [96].

PRATT, O.E., JEYASINGHAM, M., SHAW, G.K. & THOMSON, A.D. (1985) Transketolase variant enzymes and brain damage. *Alcohol and Alcoholism* **20**, 223–232 [576].

PRATT, R.T.C. (1951) An investigation of the psychiatric aspects of disseminated sclerosis. *Journal of Neurology, Neurosurgery and Psychiatry* **14**, 326–335 [696, 698, 699].

PRATT, R.T.C. (1967) *The Genetics of Neurological Disorders*. Oxford University Press: Oxford [437].

PRATT, R.T.C. & WARRINGTON, E.K. (1972) The assessment of cerebral dominance with unilateral ECT. *British Journal of Psychiatry* **121**, 327–328 [40].

PRESS, G.A., AMARAL, D.G. & SQUIRE, L.R. (1989) Hippocampal abnormalities in amnesic patients revealed by high-resolution magnetic resonance imaging. *Nature* **341**, 54–57 [27].

PRICE, J. & KERR, R. (1985) Some observations on the Wernicke–Korsakoff syndrome in Australia. *British Journal of Addiction* **80**, 69–76 [576].

PRICE, J., KERR, R., HICKS, M. & NIXON, P.F. (1987) The Wernicke–Korsakoff syndrome: a reappraisal in Queensland with special reference to prevention. *Medical Journal of Australia* **147**, 561–565 [581].

PRICE, R.A., KIDD, K.K., COHEN, D.J., PAULS, D.L. & LECKMAN, J.F. (1985) A twin study of Tourette syndrome. *Archives of General Psychiatry* **42**, 815–820 [686].

PRICE, R.W. (1994) Understanding the AIDS dementia complex: the challenge of HIV and its effects on the central nervous system. Ch. 1 in *HIV, AIDS, and the Brain*, eds Price, R.W. & Perry, S.W. *Association for Research in Nervous and Mental Disease* **72**. Raven Press: New York [322, 325, 326].

PRICE, R.W., BREW, B., SIDTIS, J., ROSENBLUM, M., SCHECK, A.C. & CLEARY, P. (1988) The brain in AIDS: central nervous system HIV-1 infection and AIDS dementia complex. *Science* **239**, 586–592 [326].

PRICE, R.W., SIDTIS, J.J. & BREW, B.J. (1991) AIDS dementia complex and HIV-1 infection: a view from the clinic. *Brain Pathology* **1**, 155–162 [326].

PRIEN, R.F. (1973) Chemotherapy in chronic organic brain syndrome—a review of the literature. *Psychopharmacology Bulletin* **9**, 5–20 [502].

PRIEST, R.G., TARIGHATI, S. & SHARIATMADARI, M.E. (1969) A brief test of organic brain disease validation in a mental hospital population. *Acta Psychiatrica Scandinavica* **45**, 347–354 [114].

PROBST, F.P. (1973) Congenital defects of the corpus callosum. Morphology and encephalographic appearances. *Acta Radiologica; Diagnosis* **Supplement 331**, 1–152 [770].

PRUDHOMME, C. (1941) Epilepsy and suicide. *Journal of Nervous and Mental Disease* **94**, 722–731 [286].

PRUITT, B.A. & MASON, A.D. (1996) Lightning and electric shock. Section 8.5.5(g) in *Oxford Textbook of Medicine*, 3rd edn, eds Weatherall, D.J., Ledingham, J.G.G. & Warrell, D.A. Oxford University Press: Oxford [766].

PRUSINER, S.B. (1982) Novel proteinaceous infectious particles cause scrapie. *Science* **216**, 136–144 [474].

PRUSINER, S.B. (1987) Prions and neurodegenerative diseases. *New England Journal of Medicine* **317**, 1571–1581 [474].

PRUSINER, S.B. (1991) Molecular biology of prion diseases. *Science* **252**, 1515–1522 [474].

PRUSINER, S.B., SCOTT, M., FOSTER, D., PAN, K., GROTH, D., MIRENA, C., TORCHIA, M., YANG, S., SERBAN, D., CARLSON, G.A., HOPPE, P.C., WESTAWAY, D. & DE ARMOND, S.J. (1990) Transgenetic studies implicate interactions between homologous PrP isoforms in scrapie prion replication. *Cell* **63**, 673–686 [474].

PUDENZ, R.H. & SHELDEN, C.H. (1946) The lucite calvarium—a method for direct observation of the brain. *Journal of Neurosurgery* **3**, 487–505 [162].

PUGH, L.G.C. & WARD, M.P. (1956) Some effects of high altitude on man. *Lancet* **2**, 1115–1121 [549].

PUGSLEY, W., KLINGER, L., PASCHALIS, C., TREASURE, T., HARRISON, M. & NEWMAN, S. (1994) The impact of microemboli during cardiopulmonary bypass on neuropsychological functioning. *Stroke* **25**, 1393–1399 [555].

PUJOL, J., LEAL, S., FLUVIA, X. & CONDE, C. (1989) Psychiatric aspects of normal pressure hydrocephalus. A report of five cases. *British Journal of Psychiatry* **154 (Supplement 4)**, 77–80 [747].

PUTNAM, C.E. (1974) Morgagni syndrome and hyperostosis frontalis interna. *Lancet* **2**, 1331–1332 [769].

PYCOCK, C.J., KERWIN, R.W. & CARTER, C.J. (1980) Effect of lesion of cortical dopamine terminals on subcortical dopamine receptors in rats. *Nature* **286**, 74–77 [92].

PYE, I.F. & ABBOTT, R. (1983) Bromocriptine induced psychosis in acromegaly. *British Medical Journal* **286**, 50–51 [522].

QUADFASEL, A.F. & PRUYSER, P.W. (1955) Cognitive deficit in patients with psychomotor epilepsy. *Epilepsia* **4**, 80–90 [261].

QUARRELL, O.W.J. & HARPER, P.S. (1991) The clinical neurology of Huntington's disease. Ch. 2 in *Huntington's Disease*, ed. Harper, P.S. W.B. Saunders: London [469, 473].

QUIGLEY, B.J. & KOWALL, N.W. (1991) Substance P-like immunoreactive neurons are depleted in Alzheimer's disease cerebral cortex. *Neuroscience* **41**, 41–60 [445].

QUINN, N. (1989) Multiple system atrophy—the nature of the beast. *Journal of Neurology, Neurosurgery and Psychiatry* **52 (Special Supplement),** 78–89 [669].

QUINN, N. (1995) Drug treatment of Parkinson's disease. *British Medical Journal* **310**, 575–579 [649, 650, 659, 669].

QUINN, N.P., TOONE, B., LANG, A.E., MARSDEN, C.D. & PARKES, J.D. (1983) Dopa dose-dependent sexual deviation. *British Journal of Psychiatry* **142**, 296–298 [659].

RABINS, P.V. (1990) Euphoria in multiple sclerosis. Ch. 11 in *Neurobehavioural Aspects of Multiple Sclerosis*, ed. Rao, S.M. Oxford University Press: Oxford [695].

RABINS, P.V., BROOKS, B.R., O'DONNELL, P., PEARLSON, G.D., MOBERG, P., JUBELT, B., COYLE, P., DALOS, N. & FOLSTEIN, M.F. (1986) Structural brain correlates of emotional disorder in multiple sclerosis. *Brain* **109**, 585–597 [695].

RABINS, P.V., MERCHANT, A. & NESTADT, G. (1984) Criteria for diagnosing reversible dementia caused by depression. Validation by 2-year follow-up. *British Journal of Psychiatry* **144**, 488–492 [486].

RABINS, P.V., STARKSTEIN, S.E. & ROBINSON, R.G. (1991) Risk factors for developing atypical (schizophreniform) psychosis following stroke. *Journal of Neuropsychiatry and Clinical Neurosciences* **3**, 6–9 [388].

RADANOV, B.P., STURZENEGGER, M., DE STEFANO, G. & SCHNIDRIG, A. (1994) Relationship between early somatic radiological, cognitive and psychosocial findings and outcome during a one-year follow-up in 117 patients suffering from common whiplash. *British Journal of Rheumatology* **33**, 442–448 [200, 201].

RADERMECKER, J. & DUMON, J. (1969) Genetic epilepsies. Ch. 3 in *The Physiopathogenesis of the Epilepsies*, eds Gastaut, H., Jasper, H., Bancaud, J. & Waltregny, A. Thomas: Springfield, Illinois [247].

RADUE, E.W., DU BOULAY, G.H., HARRISON, M.J.G. & THOMAS, D.J. (1978) Comparison of angiographic and CT findings between patients with multi-infarct dementia and those with dementia due to primary neuronal degeneration. *Neuroradiology* **16**, 113–115 [454, 456].

RAFFLE, P.A.B. (1989) Interrelation between alcohol and accidents. *Journal of the Royal Society of Medicine* **82**, 132–138 [179].

RAGHEB, S. & LISAK, R.P. (1994) The immunopathogenesis of acquired (autoimmune) myasthenia gravis. Ch. 12 in *Handbook of Myasthenia Gravis and Myasthenic Syndromes*, ed. Lisak, R.P. Marcel Dekker: New York [710].

RAICHLE, M.E., MARTIN, W.R.W., HERSCOVITCH, M.P., MINTUN, M.A. & MARKHAM, J. (1983) Brain blood flow measured with intravenous H$_2$^{15}O. II Implementation and validation. *Journal of Nuclear Medicine* **24**, 790–798 [144].

RAIL, D., SCHOLTZ, C. & SWASH, M. (1981) Post-encephalitic parkinsonism: current experience. *Journal of Neurology, Neurosurgery and Psychiatry* **44**, 670–676 [355].

RAIL, D.L. & PERKIN, G.D. (1980) Computerized tomographic appearance of hypertensive encephalopathy. *Archives of Neurology* **37**, 310–311 [399].

RAINEY, J.M., ALEEM, A., ORTIZ, A., YERAGANI, V., POHL, R. & BERCHOU, R. (1987) A laboratory procedure for the induction of flashbacks. *American Journal of Psychiatry* **144**, 1317–1319 [194].

RAJPUT, A.H., OFFORD, K., BEARD, C.M. & KURLAND, L.T. (1984) Epidemiological survey of dementia in parkinsonism and control population. In *Parkinson-Specific Motor and Mental Disorders*, eds

Hassler, R.G. & Christ, J.F. *Advances in Neurology* **40**, 229–234. Raven Press: New York [654].

RAJSHEKHAR, V. & ABRAHAM, J. (1990) Disappearing CT lesions in Indian patients with epilepsy. *Journal of Neurology, Neurosurgery and Psychiatry* **53**, 818 [289].

RAMANI, S.V. (1981) Psychosis associated with frontal lobe lesions in Schilder's cerebral sclerosis. *Journal of Clinical Psychiatry* **42**, 250–252 [701].

RAMIREZ, G., KHAMASHTA, M.A. & HUGHES, G.R. (1990) The ANCA test: its clinical relevance. *Annals of the Rheumatic Diseases* **49**, 741–742 [425].

RAMSAY, A.M. (1973) Benign myalgic encephalomyelitis. *British Journal of Psychiatry* **122**, 618–619 [372].

RAMSAY, R.E. (1994) Clinical efficacy and safety of gabapentin. *Neurology* **44 (Supplement 5)**, S23–S30 [304].

RANDALL, R.E., ROSSMEISL, E.C. & BLEIFER, K.H. (1959) Magnesium depletion in man. *Annals of Internal Medicine* **50**, 257–287 [561].

RAO, D.B. & NORRIS, J.R. (1972) A double-blind investigation of hydergine in the treatment of cerebrovascular insufficiency in the elderly. *Johns Hopkins Medical Journal* **130**, 317–324 [502].

RAO, M.L., STEFAN, H. & BAUER, J. (1989) Epileptic but not psychogenic seizures are accompanied by simultaneous, elevation of serum pituitary hormones and cortisol levels. *Neuroendocrinology* **49**, 33–39 [290].

RAO, N.S. & PEARCE, J. (1971) Hypothalamic-pituitary-adrenal axis studies in migraine with special reference to insulin sensitivity. *Brain* **94**, 289–298 [402].

RAO, S.M. (1986) Neuropsychology of multiple sclerosis: a cortical review. *Journal of Clinical and Experimental Neuropsychology* **8**, 502–542 [692, 693].

RAO, S.M. (1990) Neuroimaging correlates of cognitive dysfunction. Ch. 7 in *Neurobehavioral Aspects of Multiple Sclerosis*, ed. Rao, S.M. Oxford University Press: Oxford [693].

RAO, S.M., LEO, G.J., HAUGHTON, V.M., ST AUBIN-FAUBERT, P. & BERNARDIN, L. (1989) Correlation of magnetic resonance imaging with neuropsychological testing in multiple sclerosis. *Neurology* **39**, 161–166 [693].

RAPHAEL, B. (1981) Personal disaster. *Australian and New Zealand Journal of Psychiatry* **15**, 183–198 [195].

RASKIN, N. (1956) Intracranial neoplasms in psychotic patients. *American Journal of Psychiatry* **112**, 481–484 [233, 234].

RASKIN, N.H. (1989) Neurological aspects of renal failure. Ch. 14 in *Neurology and General Medicine*, ed. Aminoff, M.J. Churchill Livingstone: New York [556, 557].

RASMUSSEN, K.G. & ABRAMS, R. (1992) The role of electroconvulsive therapy in Parkinson's disease. Ch. 19 in *Parkinson's Disease. Neurobehavioral Aspects*, eds Huber, S.J. & Cummings, J.L. Oxford University Press: Oxford [656].

RASMUSSEN, T. & MILNER, B. (1977) The role of early left-brain injury in determining lateralization of cerebral speech functions. *Annals of New York Academy of Sciences* **299**, 355–369 [40].

RASMUSSEN, T., OLSZEWSKI, J. & LLOYD-SMITH, D. (1958) Focal seizures due to chronic localized encephalitis. *Neurology* **8**, 435–445 [313].

RATCLIFF, G. & NEWCOMBE, F. (1973) Spatial orientation in man: effects of left, right, and bilateral posterior cerebral lesions. *Journal of Neurology, Neurosurgery and Psychiatry* **36**, 448–454 [63].

RATCLIFFE, J., RITTMAN, A., WOLF, S. & VERITY, M.A. (1975) Creutzfeldt–Jakob disease with focal onset unsuccessfully treated with amantadine. *Bulletin of the Los Angeles Neurological Society* **40**, 18–20 [506].

864   REFERENCES

RAUSCHER, H., POPP, W. & ZWICK, H. (1993) Model for investigating snorers with suspected sleep apnoea. *Thorax* **48**, 275–279 [731].

RAUTONEN, J., KOSKINIEMI, M. & VAHERI, A. (1991) Prognostic factors in childhood acute encephalitis. *The Pediatric Infectious Disease Journal* **10(6)**, 441–446 [348].

RAVEN, J.C. (1958a) *Guide to the Standard Progressive Matrices.* H.K. Lewis: London [112].

RAVEN, J.C. (1958b) *Guide to using the Mill Hill Vocabulary Scale and the Progressive Matrices Scales.* H.K. Lewis: London [112].

RAVEN, J.C. (1965) *Guide to Using the Coloured Progressive Matrices.* H.K. Lewis: London [112].

RAVEN, J.C. (1982) *Revised Manual for Raven's Progressive Matrices and Vocabulary Scale.* NFER-Nelson: Windsor [112].

RAVEN, J.C., COURT, J.H. & RAVEN, J. (1984) *Manual for Raven's Progressive Matrices and Vocabulary Scales. Section 2: Coloured Progressive Matrices.* H.K. Lewis: London [112].

RAVEN, J.C., COURT, J.H. & RAVEN, J. (1992) *Manual for Raven's Progressive Matrices and Vocabulary Scales. Section 3: Standard Progressive Matrices.* H.K. Lewis: London [112].

RAVITS, J., HALLETT, M., BAKER, M. & WILKINS, D. (1985) Primary writing tremor and myoclonic writer's cramp. *Neurology* **35**, 1387–1391 [676].

RAYMOND, A.A., COOK, M., FISH, D.R. & SHORVON, S.D. (1994a) Cortical dysgenesis in adults with epilepsy. Ch. 16 in *Magnetic Resonance Scanning and Epilepsy*, eds Shorvon, S.D., Fish, D.R., Andermann, F., Bydder, G.M. & Stefan, H. Plenum Press: New York & London [244].

RAYMOND, A.A., FISH, D.R., SISODIYA, S.M., ALSANJARI, N., STEVENS, J.M. & SHORVON, S.D. (1995) Abnormalities of gyration, heterotopias, tuberous sclerosis, focal cortical dysplasia, microdysgenesis, dysembryoplastic neuroepithelial tumour and dysgenesis of the archicortex in epilepsy. Clinical, EEG and neuroimaging features in 100 adult patients. *Brain* **118**, 629–660 [244].

RAYMOND, A.A., FISH, D.R., STEVENS, J.M., COOK, M.J., SISODIYA, S.M. & SHORVON, S.D. (1994b) Association of hippocampal sclerosis with cortical dysgenesis in patients with epilepsy. *Neurology* **44**, 1841–1845 [246].

RAYMOND, A.A., HALPIN, S.F.S., ALSANJARI, N., COOK, M.J., KITCHEN, N.D., FISH, D.R., STEVENS, J.M., HARDING, B.N., SCARAVILLI, F., KENDALL, B., SHORVON, S.D. & NEVILLE, B.G.R. (1994c) Dysembryoplastic neuroepithelial tumour. Features in 16 patients. *Brain* **117**, 461–475 [244].

RAYMOND, R.W. & WILLIAMS, R.L. (1948) Infectious mononucleosis with psychosis; report of case. *New England Journal of Medicine* **239**, 542–544 [358].

READ, A.E., GOUGH, K.R., PARDOE, J.L. & NICHOLAS, A. (1965) Nutritional studies on the entrants to an old people's home, with particular reference to folic acid deficiency. *British Medical Journal* **2**, 843–848 [590, 591].

READ, A.E., SHERLOCK, S., LAIDLAW, J. & WALKER, J.G. (1967) The neuropsychiatric syndromes associated with chronic liver disease and an extensive portal-systemic collateral circulation. *Quarterly Journal of Medicine* **36**, 135–150 [564].

REAVLEY, W. (1975) The use of biofeedback in the treatment of writer's cramp. *Journal of Behaviour Therapy and Experimental Psychiatry* **6**, 335–338 [677].

REBEIZ, J.J., KOLODNY, E.H. & RICHARDSON, E.P. (1968) Corticodentatonigral degeneration with neuronal achromasia. *Archives of Neurology* **18**, 20–33 [668].

RECHTSCHAFFEN, A.R., WOLPERT, E.A., DEMENT, W.C., MITCHELL, S.A. & FISHER, C. (1963) Nocturnal sleep of narcoleptics.

Electroencephalography and Clinical Neurophysiology **15**, 599–609 [725].

REDING, M., HAYCOX, J. & BLASS, J. (1985) Depression in patients referred to a dementia clinic. A three-year prospective study. *Archives of Neurology* **42**, 894–896 [487].

REED, D., CRAWLEY, J., FARO, S.N., PIEPER, S.J. & KURLAND, L.T. (1963) Thallotoxosis. *Journal of the American Medical Association* **183(I)**, 516–522 [636].

REED, R.J. & GRANT, I. (1990) The long-term neurobehavioral consequences of substance abuse: conceptual and methodological challenges for future research. In *Residual Effects of Abused Drugs on Behavior*, eds Spencer, J.W. & Boren, J.J. National Institute on Drug Abuse Research Monograph No. 101, pp. 10–56. US Department of Health and Human Services, National Institute on Drug Abuse: Rockville, Maryland [616].

REED, T.E. & CHANDLER, J.H. (1958) Huntington's chorea in Michigan. I: Demography and genetics. *American Journal of Human Genetics* **10**, 201–225 [470].

REES, L.H. (1981) Brain opiates and corticotrophin-related peptides. The Goulstonian Lecture, 1980. *Journal of the Royal College of Physicians of London* **15**, 130–134 [507].

REES, W.L. (1961) Fundamentals in the psychological background. In *Stroke Rehabilitation*, pp. 12–15. The Chest and Heart Association: Tavistock Square, London [388].

REES, W.L. (1971) Psychiatric and psychological factors in migraine. Ch. 6 in *Background to Migraine*, Fourth Migraine Symposium, ed. Cumings, J.N. Heinemann: London [404].

REEVE, A., ROSE, D.F. & WEINBERGER, D.R. (1989) Magnetoencephalography. Applications in psychiatry. *Archives of General Psychiatry* **46**, 573–576 [133].

REEVES, A.G. (1991) Behavioral changes following callosotomy. Ch. 18 in *Neurobehavioural Problems in Epilepsy*, eds Smith, D.B., Treiman, D.M. & Trimble, M.R. *Advances in Neurology* **55**. Raven Press: New York [313].

REEVES, A.G. & PLUM, F. (1969) Hyperphagia, rage and dementia accompanying a ventromedial hypothalamic neoplasm. *Archives of Neurology* **20**, 616–624 [229].

REFSUM, S., ENGESET, A. & LONNUM, A. (1959) Pneumoencephalographic changes in dystrophia myotonica. *Acta Psychiatrica et Neurologica Scandinavica* **137 (Supplement)**, 98–99 [720].

REFSUM, S., LONNUM, A., SJAASTAD, O. & ENGESET, A. (1967) Dystrophia myotonica: repeated pneumoencephalographic studies in ten patients. *Neurology* **17**, 345–348 [720].

REGARD, M., OELZ, O., BRUGGER, P. & LANDIS, T. (1989) Persistent cognitive impairment in climbers after repeated exposure to extreme altitude. *Neurology* **39**, 210–213 [549].

REICHLIN, S. (1968) Neuroendocrinology. Ch. 12 in *Textbook of Endocrinology*, 4th edn, ed. Williams, R.H. Saunders: Philadelphia [519].

REIFLER, B.V., LARSON, E. & HANLEY, R. (1982) Coexistence of cognitive impairment and depression in geriatric outpatients. *American Journal of Psychiatry* **139**, 623–636 [486].

REIMAN, E.M., RAICHLE, M.E., BUTLER, F.K., HERSCOVITCH, P. & ROBINS, E. (1984) A focal brain abnormality in panic disorder, a severe form of anxiety. *Nature* **310**, 683–685 [145].

REIMAN, E.M., RAICHLE, M.E., ROBINS, E., BUTLER, F.K., HERSCOVITCH, P., FOX, P. & PERLMUTTER, J. (1986) The application of positron emission tomography to the study of panic disorder. *American Journal of Psychiatry* **143**, 469–477 [145].

REIMAN, E.M., RAICHLE, M.E., ROBINS, E., MINTUN, M.A., FUSSELMAN, M.J., FOX, P.T., PRICE, J.L. & HACKMAN, K.A. (1989) Neuroanatomical correlates of a lactate-induced anxiety attack. *Archives of General Psychiatry* **46**, 493–500 [145].

REIO, L. & WETTERBERG, L. (1969) False porphobilinogen reactions in the urine of mental patients. *Journal of the American Medical Association* **207**, 148–150 [568].

REISBERG, B., FERRIS, S.H. & GERSHON, S. (1981) An overview of pharmacologic treatment of cognitive decline in the aged. *American Journal of Psychiatry* **138**, 593–600 [503].

REISER, M.F., ROSENBAUM, M. & FERRIS, E.B. (1951) Psychologic mechanisms in malignant hypertension. *Psychosomatic Medicine* **13**, 147–159 [397].

REITAN, R.M. (1958) Validity of the trail making test as an indicator of organic brain damage. *Perceptual and Motor Skills* **8**, 271–276 [120].

REITAN, R.M. (1966) A research program on the psychological effects of brain lesions in human beings. In *International Review of Research in Mental Retardation*, Vol. 1, ed. Ellis, N.R. Academic Press: New York [121].

REITE, M. (1990) Magnetoencephalography in the study of mental illness. Ch. 17 in *Magnetoencephalography*, ed. Sato, S. *Advances in Neurology* **54**. Raven Press: New York [133].

RELMAN, D.A., SCHMIDT, T.M., MacDERMOTT, R.P. & FALKOW, S. (1992) Identification of the uncultured bacillus of Whipple's disease. *New England Journal of Medicine* **327**, 293–301 [760].

REMINGTON, F.B. & RUBERT, S.L. (1962) Why patients with brain tumours come to a psychiatric hospital. *American Journal of Psychiatry* **119**, 256–257 [233].

RENNIE, T.A.C. & HOWARD, J.E. (1942) Hypoglycaemia and tension-depression. *Psychosomatic Medicine* **4**, 273–282 [543].

REPORT OF A WORKING GROUP OF THE AMERICAN ACADEMY OF NEUROLOGY AIDS TASK FORCE (1991) Nomenclature and research case definitions for neurologic manifestations of human immunodeficiency virus-type 1 (HIV-1) infection. *Neurology* **41**, 778–785 [324].

REPORT OF THE BOARD OF SCIENCE AND EDUCATION WORKING PARTY (1984) *Boxing*. British Medical Association: London [206].

RESKE-NIELSEN, E., CHRISTENSEN, A.-L. & NIELSEN, J. (1982) A neuropathological and neuropsychological study of Turner's syndrome. *Cortex* **18**, 181–190 [528].

RESKE-NIELSEN, E. & LUNDBAEK, K. (1963) Diabetic encephalopathy: diffuse and focal lesions of the brain in long-term diabetes. *Acta Neurologica Scandinavica* **4 (Supplement)**, 273–290 [538].

RESNICK, J.S., ENGEL, W.K. & SEVER, J.L. (1968) Subacute sclerosing panencephalitis. *New England Journal of Medicine* **279**, 126–129 [362].

REUL, J., WEIS, J., JUNG, A., WILLMES, K. & THRON, A. (1995) Central nervous system lesions and cervical disc herniations in amateur divers. *Lancet* **345**, 1403–1405 [768].

REULER, J.B., GIRARD, D.E. & COONEY, T.G. (1985) Medical intelligence: current concepts. Wernicke's encephalopathy. *New England Journal of Medicine* **312**, 1035–1039 [581].

REVELEY, A.M. & REVELEY, M.A. (1983) Aqueduct stenosis and schizophrenia. *Journal of Neurology, Neurosurgery and Psychiatry* **46**, 18–22 [750].

REVELEY, A.M., REVELEY, M.A., CLIFFORD, C.A. & MURRAY, R.M. (1982) Cerebral ventricular size in twins discordant for schizophrenia. *Lancet* **1**, 540–541 [85].

REVELEY, A.M., REVELEY, M.A. & MURRAY, R.M. (1984) Cerebral ventricular enlargement in non-genetic schizophrenia: a controlled twin study. *British Journal of Psychiatry* **144**, 89–93 [85, 138].

REVELEY, M.A. (1985) CT scans in schizophrenia. *British Journal of Psychiatry* **146**, 367–371 [85].

REVELEY, M.A., REVELEY, A.M. & BALDY, R. (1987) Left cerebral hemisphere hypodensity in discordant schizophrenic twins. *Archives of General Psychiatry* **44**, 625–632 [138].

REY, A. (1941) L'examen psychologique dans les cas d'encéphalopathie traumatique. *Archives de Pathologie* **28**, 286–340 [116].

REYNOLDS, C.F., KUPFER, D.J., HOUCK, P.R., HOCH, C.C., STACK, J.A., BERMAN, S.R. & ZIMMER, B. (1988) Reliable discrimination of elderly depressed and demented patients by electroencephalographic sleep data. *Archives of General Psychiatry* **45**, 258–264 [489].

REYNOLDS, E.H. (1967a) Effects of folic acid on the mental state and fit frequency of drug-treated epileptic patients. *Lancet* **1**, 1086–1088 [271, 592].

REYNOLDS, E.H. (1967b) Scizophrenia-like psychoses of epilepsy and disturbances of folate and vitamin B_{12} metabolism induced by anticonvulsant drugs. *British Journal of Psychiatry* **113**, 911–919 [285, 592].

REYNOLDS, E.H. (1968) Epilepsy and schizophrenia: relationship and biochemistry. *Lancet* **1**, 398–401 [285].

REYNOLDS, E.H. (1973) Anticonvulsants, folic acid, and epilepsy. *Lancet* **1**, 1376–1378 [592].

REYNOLDS, E.H. (1975) Chronic antiepileptic toxicity: a review. *Epilepsia* **16**, 319–352 [301].

REYNOLDS, E.H. (1981) The management of seizures associated with psychological disorders. Ch. 3 in *Epilepsy and Psychiatry*, eds Reynolds, E.H. & Trimble, M.R. Churchill Livingstone: Edinburgh & London [301].

REYNOLDS, E.H. (1982) The pharmacological management of epilepsy associated with psychological disorders. *British Journal of Psychiatry* **141**, 549–557 [299, 300, 301].

REYNOLDS, E.H. (1983) Interictal behaviour in temporal lobe epilepsy. *British Medical Journal* **286**, 918–191 [267].

REYNOLDS, E.H. (1991) Interictal psychiatric disorders: neurochemical aspects. Ch. 3 in *Neurobehavioral Problems in Epilepsy*, eds Smith, D.B., Treiman, D.M. & Trimble, M.R. *Advances in Neurology* **55**. Raven Press: New York [591, 592].

REYNOLDS, E.H., CARNEY, M.W.P. & TOONE, B.K. (1984) Methylation and mood. *Lancet* **2**, 196–198 [591].

REYNOLDS, E.H., CHANARIN, I., MILNER, G. & MATTHEWS, D.M. (1966a) Anticonvulsant therapy, folic acid and vitamin B_{12} metabolism and mental symptoms. *Epilepsia* **7**, 261–270 [592].

REYNOLDS, E.H., MILNER, G., MATTHEWS, D.M. & CHANARIN, I. (1966b) Anticonvulsant therapy, megaloblastic haemopoeisis and folic acid metabolism. *Quarterly Journal of Medicine* **35**, 521–537 [592].

REYNOLDS, E.H., PREECE, J.M., BAILEY, J. & COPPEN, A. (1970) Folate deficiency in depressive illness. *British Journal of Psychiatry* **117**, 287–292 [591].

REYNOLDS, E.H., PREECE, J. & CHANARIN, I. (1969) Folic acid and anticonvulsants. *Lancet* **1**, 1264–1265 [592].

REYNOLDS, E.H., PREECE, J. & JOHNSON, A.L. (1971a) Folate metabolism in epileptic and psychiatric patients. *Journal of Neurology, Neurosurgery and Psychiatry* **34**, 726–732 [592].

REYNOLDS, E.H., ROTHFELD, P. & PINCUS, J.H. (1973) Neurological disease associated with folate deficiency. *British Medical Journal* **2**, 398–400 [591].

REYNOLDS, E.H. & SHORVON, S.D. (1982) Monotherapy or polytherapy for epilepsy? *Epilepsia* **22**, 1–10 [299].

REYNOLDS, E.H. & TRAVERS, R.D. (1974) Serum anticonvulsant

concentrations in epileptic patients with mental symptoms: a pre-liminary report. *British Journal of Psychiatry* **124**, 440–445 [263, 271].

REYNOLDS, E.H., WRIGHTON, R.J., JOHNSON, A.L., PREECE, J. & CHANARIN, I. (1971b) Interrelations of folic acid and vitamin B_{12} in drug-treated epileptic patients. *Epilepsia* **12**, 165–171 [593].

REYNOLDS, G.P. (1983) Increased concentrations and lateral asymmetry of amygdala dopamine in schizophrenia. *Nature* **305**, 527–529 [90].

REYNOLDS, G.P. (1988) The post-mortem neurochemistry of schizophrenia. *Psychological Medicine* **18**, 793–797 [90].

REYNOLDS, G.P., ARNOLD, L., ROSSOR, M.N., IVERSEN, L.L., MOUNT-JOY, C.Q. & ROTH, M. (1984) Reduced binding of [^{3}H] ketanserin to cortical 5-HT$_2$ receptors in senile dementia of the Alzheimer-type. *Neuroscience Letters* **44**, 47–51 [444].

REYNOLDS, G.P. & CZUDEK, C. (1990) Neurochemical pathology in schizophrenia: limbic deficits in GABA systems. *Schizophrenia Research* **3**, 34 [90].

RICAURTE, G.A., FORNO, L.S., WILSON, M.A., DELANNEY, L.E., IRWIN, I., MOLLIVER, M.E. & LANGSTON, J.W. (1988) (±)3,4-Methylene-dioxymethamphetamine selectively damages central serotonergic neurons in nonhuman primates. *Journal of the American Medical Association* **260**, 51–55 [625].

RICCARDI, V.M. (1981) Von Recklinghausen neurofibromatosis. *New England Journal of Medicine* **305**, 1617–1627 [703, 704].

RICCIO, M., PUGH, K., JADRESIC, D., BURGESS, A., THOMPSON, C., WILSON, B., LOVETT, E., BALDEWEG, T., HAWKINS, D.A. & CATALAN, J. (1993) Neuropsychiatric aspects of HIV-1 infection in gay men: controlled investigation of psychiatric, neuropsychological and neurological status. *Journal of Psychosomatic Research* **37**, 819–830 [329].

RICE, E. & GENDELMAN, S. (1973) Psychiatric aspects of normal pressure hydrocephalus. *Journal of the American Medical Association* **223**, 409–412 [747].

RICH, S.S., ANNEGERS, J.F., HAUSER, W.A. & ANDERSON, V.E. (1987) Complex segregation analysis of febrile convulsions. *American Journal of Human Genetics* **41**, 249–257 [247].

RICHARDSON, E.P. (1961) Progressive multifocal leucoencephalo-pathy. *New England Journal of Medicine* **265**, 815–823 [751].

RICHARDSON, E.P. (1968) Progressive multifocal leucoencephalo-pathy. Ch. 2 in *The Remote Effects of Cancer on the Nervous System*, eds Brain, W.R. & Norris, F.H. Contemporary Neurology Symposia, Vol. I. Grune & Stratton: New York [751].

RICHARDSON, J.C., CHAMBERS, R.A. & HEYWOOD, P.M. (1959) Encephalopathies of anoxia and hypoglycaemia. *Archives of Neurology* **1**, 178–190 [546, 548, 551].

RICHENS, A. & PERUCCA, E. (1993) Clinical pharmacology and medical treatment. Ch. 15 in *A Textbook of Epilepsy*, 4th edn, eds Laidlaw, J., Richens, A. & Chadwick, D. Churchill Livingstone: Edinburgh [299].

RICHET, G., LOPEZ DE NOVALES, E. & VERROUST, P. (1970) Drug intoxication and neurological episodes in chronic renal failure. *British Medical Journal* **1**, 394–395 [557].

RICHET, G. & VACHON, F. (1966) Troubles neuro-psychiques de l'urémie chronique. *Présse Medicale* **74**, 1177–1182 [557].

RIDDLE, M.A., RASMUSSON, A.M., WOODS, S.W. & HOFFER, P.B. (1992) SPECT imaging of cerebral blood flow in Tourette syndrome. Ch. 25 in *Tourette Syndrome. Genetics, Neurobiology and Treatment*, eds Chase, T.N., Friedhoff, A.J. & Cohen, D.J. *Advances in Neurology* **58**. Raven Press: New York [685].

RIDDOCH, G. (1936) Progressive dementia, without headache or

changes in the optic discs, due to tumours of the third ventricle. *Brain* **59**, 225–233 [749].

RIFAT, S.L. & EASTWOOD, M.R. (1994) The role of aluminium in dementia of Alzheimer's type: a review of the hypotheses and summary of the evidence. Ch. 15 in *Dementia*, eds Burns, A. & Levy, R. Chapman & Hall: London [446].

RIGG, G.A. & BERCU, B.A. (1967) Hypoglycaemia-a complication of haemodialysis. *New England Journal of Medicine* **277**, 1139–1140 [558].

RIGGIO, S. & HARNER, R.N. (1992) Frontal lobe epilepsy. *Neuropsychiatry, Neuropsychology and Behavioral Neurology* **5**, 283–293 [249].

RIGGS, J.E. (1989) Neurologic manifestations of fluid and electrolyte disturbances. In *Neurologic Manifestations of Systemic Disease*, ed. Riggs, J.E. *Neurologic Clinics* **7**, 509–523 [559, 561].

RIGGS, J.E., GRIGGS, R.C. & MOXLEY, R.T. (1977) Acetazolamide-induced weakness in paramyotonia congenita. *Annals of Internal Medicine* **86**, 169–173 [721].

RIKLAN, M. & LEVITA, E. (1970) Psychological studies of thalamic lesions in humans. *Journal of Nervous and Mental Disease* **150**, 251–265 [660].

RIKLAN, M., WEINER, H. & DILLER, L. (1959) Somato-psychologic studies in Parkinson's disease. 1: An investigation into the relationship of certain disease factors to psychological functions. *Journal of Nervous and Mental Disease* **129**, 263–272 [653].

RIKLAN, M., ZAHN, T.P. & DILLER, L. (1962) Human figure drawings before and after chemosurgery of the basal ganglia in parkinsonism. *Journal of Nervous and Mental Disease* **135**, 500–506 [660].

RILEY, D.E., LANG, A.E., LEWIS, A., RESCH, L., ASHBY, P., HORNYKIEWICZ, O. & BLACK, S. (1990) Cortical-basal ganglionic degeneration. *Neurology* **40**, 1203–1212 [668].

RILEY, J.N. & WALKER, D.W. (1978) Morphological alterations in hippocampus after long-term alcohol consumption in mice. *Science* **201**, 646–648 [607].

RILEY, T.L. (1982) Syncope and hyperventilation. Ch. 3 in *Pseudoseizures*, eds Riley, T.L. & Roy, A. Williams & Wilkins: Baltimore & London [290, 291].

RIMALOVSKI, A.B. & ARONSON, S.M. (1966) Pathogenic observations in Wernicke–Korsakoff encephalopathy. *Transactions of the American Neurological Association* **91**, 29–31 [576].

RIMON, R. & HALONEN, P. (1969) Herpes simplex virus infection and depressive illness. *Diseases of the Nervous System* **30**, 338–340 [358].

RINCK, P.A., SVIHUS, R. & DE FRANCISCO, P. (1991) MR imaging of the central nervous system in divers. *Journal of Magnetic Resonance Imaging* **1**, 293–299 [768].

RINNE, J.O., RUMMUKAINEN, J., PALJÄRUI, L. & RINNE, U.K. (1989) Dementia in Parkinson's disease is related to neuronal loss in the medial substantia nigra. *Annals of Neurology* **26**, 47–50 [654].

RISBERG, J. & BERGLUND, M. (1987) Cerebral blood flow and metabolism in alcoholics. In *Neuropsychology of Alcoholism: Implications for Diagnosis and Treatment*, eds Parsons, O.A., Butters, N. & Nathan, P.E., pp. 64–75. Guilford Press: New York [606].

RISK, W.S., HADDAD, F.S. & CHEMALI, P. (1978) Substantial spontaneous long-term improvement in subacute sclerosing panencephalitis. Six cases from the Middle East and a review of the literature. *Archives of Neurology* **35**, 494–502 [362].

RIVEST, J., LEES, A.J. & MARSDEN, C.D. (1991) Writer's cramp: treatment with botulinum toxin injections. *Movement Disorders* **6**, 55–59 [677].

RIX, K.J.B. (1978) Alcohol withdrawal states. *Hospital Update* **July**, 403–407 [602].

RIZZO, L., DANION, J.-M., VAN DER LINDEN, M. & GRANGÉ, D. (1996) Patients with schizophrenia remember that an event has occurred, but not when. *British Journal of Psychiatry* **168**, 427–431 [34].

ROBBINS, F.C. (1958) The clinical and laboratory diagnosis of viral infections of the central nervous system. In *Viral Encephalitis*, eds Fields, W.C. & Blattner, R.J. Thomas: Springfield, Illinois [347].

ROBBINS, L.R. & VINSON, D.B. (1960) Objective psychologic assessment of the thyrotoxic patient and the response to treatment: preliminary report. *Journal of Clinical Endocrinology and Metabolism* **20**, 120–129 [508].

ROBBINS, T.W., JAMES, M., OWEN, A.M., SAHAKIAN, B.J., McINNES, L. & RABBITT, P. (1994) Cambridge neuropsychological test automated battery (CANTAB): a factor analytic study of a large sample of normal elderly volunteers. *Dementia* **5**, 266–281 [122].

ROBERTS, A.H. (1969) *Brain Damage in Boxers.* Pitman: London [204, 206].

ROBERTS, A.H. (1976) Sequelae of closed head injuries. *Proceedings of the Royal Society of Medicine* **69**, 137–141 [172, 186, 188].

ROBERTS, A.H. (1979) *Severe Accidental Head Injury: An Assessment of Long-term Prognosis.* Macmillan: London [186, 188, 195].

ROBERTS, D.W. (1991) Corpus callosum section. Ch. 8 in *Surgery for Epilepsy*, eds Spencer, S.S. & Spencer, D.D. Blackwell Scientific Publications: Oxford [313].

ROBERTS, G.W. (1988) Immunocytochemistry of neurofibrillary tangles in dementia pugilistica and Alzheimer's disease: evidence for common genesis. *Lancet* **2**, 1456–1458 [207].

ROBERTS, G.W., ALLSOP, D. & BRUTON, C. (1990a) The occult aftermath of boxing. *Journal of Neurology, Neurosurgery and Psychiatry* **53**, 373–378 [207].

ROBERTS, G.W. & BRUTON, C.J. (1990) Notes from the graveyard: neuropathology and schizophrenia. *Neuropathology and Applied Neurobiology* **16**, 3–16 [86].

ROBERTS, G.W., COLTER, N., LOFTHOUSE, R., JOHNSTONE, E.C. & CROW, T.J. (1987) Is there gliosis in schizophrenia? Investigation of the temporal lobe. *Biological Psychiatry* **22**, 1459–1468 [86].

ROBERTS, G.W. & CROW, T.J. (1987) The neuropathology of schizophrenia—a progress report. *British Medical Bulletin* **43**, 599–615 [86].

ROBERTS, G.W., DONE, D.J., BRUTON, C.J. & CROW, T.J. (1990b) A 'mock-up' of schizophrenia: temporal lobe epilepsy and schizophrenia-like psychosis. *Biological Psychiatry* **28**, 127–143 [281].

ROBERTS, G.W., GENTLEMAN, S.M., LYNCH, A. & GRAHAM, D.I. (1991) βA_4 amyloid protein deposition in brain after head trauma. *Lancet* **338**, 1422–1423 [438].

ROBERTS, J.K.A. & LISHMAN, W.A. (1984) The use of the CAT head scanner in clinical psychiatry. *British Journal of Psychiatry* **145**, 152–158 [126].

ROBERTS, J.K.A., ROBERTSON, M.M. & TRIMBLE, M.R. (1982) The lateralising significance of hypergraphia in temporal lobe, epilepsy. *Journal of Neurology, Neurosurgery and Psychiatry* **45**, 131–138 [268].

ROBERTS, M.A. & CAIRD, F.I. (1976) Computerised tomography and intellectual impairment in the elderly. *Journal of Neurology, Neurosurgery and Psychiatry* **39**, 986–989 [139].

ROBERTS, M.C. & EMSLEY, R.A. (1992) Psychiatric manifestations of neurosyphilis. *South African Medical Journal* **82**, 335–337 [343].

ROBERTSON, E.E., LE ROUX, A. & BROWN, J.H. (1958) The clinical differentiation of Pick's disease. *Journal of Mental Science* **104**, 1000–1024 [461].

ROBERTSON, E.G. (1954) Photogenic epilepsy: self-precipitated attacks. *Brain* **77**, 232–251 [241].

ROBERTSON, M.M. (1983) *Depression in patients with epilepsy.* Thesis for MD Degree, University of Cape Town, South Africa [283, 286].

ROBERTSON, M.M. (1985) Depression in patients with epilepsy: an overview and clinical study. Ch. 5 in *The Psychopharmacology of Epilepsy*, ed. Trimble, M.R. John Wiley & Sons Ltd: Chichester [285, 310].

ROBERTSON, M.M. (1989) The Gilles de la Tourette syndrome: the current status. *British Journal of Psychiatry* **154**, 147–169 [680, 682, 686, 687].

ROBERTSON, M.M. (1992) Self-injurious behavior and Tourette syndrome. Ch. 13 in *Tourette Syndrome. Genetics, Neurobiology, and Treatment*, eds Chase, T.H., Friedhoff, A.J. & Cohen, D.J. *Advances in Neurology* **58**. Raven Press: New York [682].

ROBERTSON, M.M. (1994) Annotation: Gilles de la Tourette syndrome—an update. *Journal of Child Psychology and Psychiatry* **35**, 597–611 [680, 685].

ROBERTSON, M.M. (1997) Structural neuroimaging in Gilles de la Tourette syndrome. Due to appear in *Neuroimaging in Child Psychiatric Disorders*, ed. Garrean, B. Springer Verlag: Berlin [685].

ROBERTSON, M.M., CHANNON, S., BAKER, J. & FLYNN, D. (1993) The psychopathology of Gilles de la Tourette's syndrome. A controlled study. *British Journal of Psychiatry* **162**, 114–117 [682].

ROBERTSON, M.M. & GOURDIE, A. (1990) Familial Tourette's syndrome in a large British pedigree. Associated psychopathology severity, and potential for linkage analysis. *British Journal of Psychiatry* **156**, 515–521 [681].

ROBERTSON, M.M. & TRIMBLE, M.R. (1983) Depressive illness in patients with epilepsy: a review. *Epilepsia* **24 (Supplement 2)**, S109–S116 [285].

ROBERTSON, M. & TRIMBLE, M.R. (1988) Some personality variables in functional neurological disorders. *Behavioural Neurology* **1**, 23–28 [674].

ROBERTSON, M.M., TRIMBLE, M.R. & LEES, A.J. (1988) The psychopathology of the Gilles de la Tourette syndrome. A phenomenological analysis. *British Journal of Psychiatry* **152**, 383–390 [692].

ROBINS, A.H. (1976) Depression in patients with parkinsonism. *British Journal of Psychiatry* **128**, 141–145 [656].

ROBINSON, J.O. (1963) A study of neuroticism and casual arterial blood pressure. *British Journal of Social and Clinical Psychology* **2**, 56–64 [397, 398].

ROBINSON, J.O. (1969) Symptoms and the discovery of high blood pressure. *Journal of Psychosomatic Research* **13**, 157–161 [399].

ROBINSON, J.T., CHITHAM, R.G., GREENWOOD, R.M. & TAYLOR, J.W. (1974) Chromosome aberrations and LSD: a controlled study in 50 psychiatric patients. *British Journal of Psychiatry* **125**, 238–244 [620].

ROBINSON, J.T. & McQUILLAN, J. (1951) Schizophrenic reaction associated with the Kleine–Levin syndrome. *Journal of the Royal Army Medical Corps* **96**, 377–381 [733].

ROBINSON, K.C., KALLBERG, M.H. & CROWLEY, M.F. (1954) Idiopathic hypoparathyroidism presenting as dementia. *British Medical Journal* **2**, 1203–1206 [532].

ROBINSON, R.A. (1961) Some problems of clinical trials in elderly people. *Gerontologia Clinica* **3**, 247–257 [124].

ROBINSON, R.A. (1977) Differential diagnosis and assessment in brain failure. *Age and Ageing* **Supplementary Issue 1977**, 42–49 [124].

ROBINSON, R.G. (1979) Differential behavioural and biochemical effects of right and left hemispheric cerebral infarction in the rat. *Science* **205**, 707–710 [386].

ROBINSON, R.G. & COYLE, J.T. (1980) The differential effect of right versus left hemisphere cerebral infarction on catecholamines and behavior in the rat. *Brain Research* **188**, 63–78 [386].

ROBINSON, R.G., KUBOS, K.L., STARR, L.B., RAO, K. & PRICE, T.R. (1984) Mood disorders in stroke patients. Importance of location of lesion. *Brain* **107**, 81–93 [385, 386].

ROBINSON, R.G. & PRICE, T.R. (1982) Post-stroke depressive disorders: a follow-up study of 103 patients. *Stroke* **13**, 635–641 [385].

ROBINSON, R.G. & SZETELA, B. (1981) Mood change following left hemisphere brain injury. *Annals of Neurology* **9**, 447–453 [385, 386].

ROBINSON, R.O. (1978) Tetraethyl lead poisoning from gasoline sniffing. *Journal of American Medical Association* **240**, 1373–1374 [630].

ROCHFORD, G. & WILLIAMS, M. (1962) Studies in the development and breakdown of the use of names. *Journal of Neurology, Neurosurgery and Psychiatry* **25**, 222–233 [52].

ROCHFORD, G. & WILLIAMS, M. (1965) Studies in the development and breakdown of the use of names. *Journal of Neurology, Neurosurgery and Psychiatry* **28**, 407–413 [52].

RODGERS, T.S., PECK, J.R.S. & JUPE, M.H. (1934) Lead poisoning in children. *Lancet* **2**, 129–133 [631].

RODZILSKY, B., CUMINGS, J.N. & HUSTON, A.F. (1968) Hallervorden–Spatz disease—late infantile and adult types, report of two cases. *Acta Neuropathologica* **10**, 1–16 [756].

ROELTGEN, D.P., SEVUSH, S. & HEILMAN, K.M. (1983) Pure Gerstmann's syndrome from a focal lesion. *Archives of Neurology* **40**, 46–47 [65].

ROGER, J., GRANGEON, H., GUEY, J. & LOB, H. (1968) Incidences psychiatriques et psychologiques du traitement par l'éthosuccimide chez les épileptiques. *L'Encéphale* **57**, 407–438 [284].

ROGERS, J., KIRBY, L.C., HEMPELMAN, S.R., BERRY, D.L., McGEER, D.L., KASZNIAK, A.W., ZALINSKI, J., COFIELD, M., MANSUKHANI, L., WILLSON, P. & KOGAN, F. (1993) Clinical trial of indomethacin in Alzheimer's disease. *Neurology* **43**, 1609–1611 [502].

ROGERS, R.S. (1979) Dermatologic manifestations. Ch. 7 in *Tuberous Sclerosis*, ed. Gomez, M.R. Raven Press: New York [701].

ROGERS, S.L., FRIEDHOFF, L.T. & THE DONEPEZIL STUDY GROUP (1996) The efficacy and safety of donepezil in patients with Alzheimer's disease: results of a US multicentre, randomised, double-blind placebo-controlled trial. *Dementia* **7**, 293–303 [504].

ROIZIN, L., MORIARTY, J.D. & WEIL, A.A. (1945) Schizophrenic reaction syndrome in course of acute demyelination of central nervous system: clinicopathological report of a case, with brief review of the literature. *Archives of Neurology and Psychiatry* **54**, 202–211 [701].

ROLAND, P.E. & FRIBERG, L. (1985) Localization of cortical areas activated by thinking. *Journal of Neurophysiology* **53**, 1219–1243 [148].

ROMÁN, G.C. (1987) Senile dementia of the Binswanger type. A vascular form of dementia in the elderly. *Journal of the American Medical Association* **258**, 1782–1788 [460].

ROMÁN, G.C., TATEMICHI, T.K., ERKINJUNTTI, T., CUMMINGS, J.L., MASDEU, J.C., GARCIA, J.H., AMADUCCI, L., ORGOGOZO, J.-M., BRUN, A., HOFMAN, A., MOODY, D.M., O'BRIEN, M.D., YAMAGUCHI, T., GRAFMAN, J., DRAYER, B.P., BENNETT, D.A., FISHER, M., OGATA, J., KOKMEN, E., BERMEJO, F., WOLF, P.A., GORELICK, P.B., BICK, K.L., PAJEAU, A.K., BELL, M.A., DECARLI, C., CULEBRAS, A., KORCZYN, A.D., BOGOUSSLAVSKY, J., HARTMANN, A. & SCHEIN-

BERG, P. (1993) Vascular dementia: diagnostic criteria for research studies. Report of the NINDS-AIREN International Workshop. *Neurology* **43**, 250–260 [454, 457].

ROMANELLI, M.F., MORRIS, J.C., ASHKIN, K. & COBEN, L.A. (1990) Advanced Alzheimer's disease is a risk factor for late-onset seizures. *Archives of Neurology* **47**, 847–850 [245].

ROMANO, J. & COON, G.P. (1942) Physiologic and psychologic studies in spontaneous hypoglycaemia. *Psychosomatic Medicine* **4**, 283–300 [541].

ROMANO, J. & ENGEL, G.L. (1944) Delirium: I, EEG data. *Archives of Neurology and Psychiatry* **51**, 356–392 [130].

ROMANUL, F.C.A., RADVANY, J. & ROSALES, R.K. (1977) Whipple's disease confined to the brain: a case studied clinically and pathologically. *Journal of Neurology, Neurosurgery and Psychiatry* **40**, 901–909 [760].

RON, M.A. (1977) Brain damage in chronic alcoholism: a neuropathological, neuroradiological and psychological review. *Psychological Medicine* **7**, 103–112 [605].

RON, M.A. (1983) The alcoholic brain: CT scan and psychological findings. *Psychological Medicine Monograph Supplement* **3** [605].

RON, M.A. (1986) Volatile substance abuse: a review of possible long-term neurological, intellectual and psychiatric sequelae. *British Journal of Psychiatry* **148**, 235–246 [630].

RON, M.A., ACKER, W. & LISHMAN, W.A. (1980) Morphological abnormalities in the brains of chronic alcoholics. A clinical, psychological and computerised axial tomographic study. *Acta Psychiatrica Scandinavica* **62 (Supplement 286)**, 41–46 [605].

RON, M.A., ACKER, W., SHAW, G.K. & LISHMAN, W.A. (1982) Computerised tomography of the brain in chronic alcoholism. A survey and follow-up study. *Brain* **105**, 497–514 [605].

RON, M.A. & FEINSTEIN, A. (1992) Multiple sclerosis and the mind. *Journal of Neurology, Neurosurgery and Psychiatry* **55**, 1–3 [692].

RON, M.A. & LOGSDAIL, S.J. (1989) Psychiatric morbidity in multiple sclerosis: a clinical and MRI study. *Psychological Medicine* **19**, 887–895 [692].

RON, M.A., TOONE, B.K., GARRALDA, M.E. & LISHMAN, W.A. (1979) Diagnostic accuracy in presenile dementia. *British Journal of Psychiatry* **134**, 161–168 [486, 492].

RÖNTY, H., AHONEN, A., TOLONEN, U., HEIKKILÄ, J. & NIEMELÄ, O. (1993) Cerebral trauma and alcohol abuse. *European Journal of Clinical Investigation* **23**, 182–187 [179].

ROOS, R.P. (1981) Alzheimer's disease and the lessons of transmissible virus dementia. Ch. 4 in *The Epidemiology of Dementia*, eds Mortimer, J.A. & Schuman, L.M. Oxford University Press: Oxford [475].

RÖPER, E. (1917) Zur Prognose der Hirnschüsse. *Meunchener Medizinische Wochenschrift* **64(i)**, 121–125. Quoted by Tow, P.M. (1955) in *Personality Changes Following Frontal Leucotomy*. Oxford University Press: London [180].

ROSE, F.C. (1981) Electroencephalography. Ch. 20 in *Hypoglycaemia*, 2nd edn, eds Marks, V. & Rose, F.C. Blackwell Scientific Publications: Oxford [542].

ROSE, F.C. & SYMONDS, C.P. (1960) Persistent memory defect following encephalitis. *Brain* **83**, 195–212 [26, 357].

ROSEBUSH, P.I., STEWART, T.D. & GELENBERG, A.J. (1989) Twenty neuroleptic rechallenges after neuroleptic malignant syndrome in 15 patients. *Journal of Clinical Psychiatry* **50**, 295–298 [627].

ROSEN, D.R., SIDDIQUE, T., PATTERSON, D., FIGLEWICZ, D.A., SAPP, P., HENTATI, A., DONALDSON, D., GOTO, J., O'REGAN, J.P., DENG,

H.-X., RAHMANI, Z., KRIZUS, A., McKENNA-YASEK, D., CAYABYAB, A., GASTON, S.M., BERGER, R., TANZI, R.E., HALPERIN, J.J., HERZFELDT, B., VAN DEN BERGH, R., MULDER, D.W., SMYTH, C., LAING, N.G., SORIANO, E., PERICAK-VANCE, M.A., HAINES, J., ROULEAU, G.A., GUSELLA, J.S., HORVITZ, H.R. & BROWN, R.H. Jr (1993) Mutations in Cu/Zn superoxide dismutase gene are associated with familial amyotrophic lateral sclerosis. *Nature* **362**, 59–62 [707].

ROSEN, J.A. (1964) Paroxysmal choreoathetosis: associated with perinatal hypoxic encephalopathy. *Archives of Neurology* **11**, 385–387 [291].

ROSEN, J.A. (1968) Dilantin dementia. *Transactions of the American Neurological Association* **93**, 273 [263].

ROSEN, W.G., TERRY, R.D., FULD, P.A., KATZMAN, R. & PECK, A. (1980) Pathological verification of ischaemic score in differentiation of dementias. *Annals of Neurology* **7**, 486–488 [457].

ROSENBAUM, M. & NAJENSON, T. (1976) Changes in life patterns and symptoms of low mood as reported by wives of severely brain-injured soldiers. *Journal of Consulting and Clinical Psychology* **44**, 881–888 [217].

ROSENBERG, G.A. & APPENZELLER, O. (1988) Amantadine, fatigue, and multiple sclerosis. *Archives of Neurology* **45**, 1104–1106 [690].

ROSENBLUM, M.L., LEVY, R.M., BREDESEN, D.E., SO, Y.T., WARA, W. & ZIEGLER, J.L. (1988) Primary central nervous system lymphomas in patients with AIDS. *Annals of Neurology* **23 (Supplement)**, S13–S16 [321].

ROSENTHAL, S.H. (1964) Persistent hallucinosis following repeated administration of hallucinogenic drugs. *American Journal of Psychiatry* **121**, 238–244 [623].

ROSMAN, N.P. & KAKULAS, B.A. (1966) Mental deficiency associated with muscular dystrophy: a neuropathological study. *Brain* **89**, 769–787 [716, 719].

ROSMAN, N.P. & PEARCE, J. (1967) The brain in multiple neurofibromatosis (von Recklinghausen's disease): a suggested neuropathological basis for the associated mental defect. *Brain* **90**, 829–838 [704].

ROSS, E.D. (1981) The aprosodias: functional-anatomic organisation of the affective components of language in the right hemisphere. *Archives of Neurology* **38**, 561–569 [42].

ROSS, E.D. & MESULAM, M.-M. (1979) Dominant language functions of the right hemisphere. Prosody and emotional gesturing. *Archives of Neurology* **36**, 144–148 [42].

ROSS, E.J. (1972a) Clinical aspects of phaeochromocytoma. *Proceedings of the Royal Society of Medicine* **65**, 792–793 [520].

ROSS, E.J. (1972b) Diseases of the adrenal medulla. *Medicine (monthly add-on series 1972-3)* **2**, 157–160. Medical Education (International) Ltd: London [520, 521].

ROSS, G.W., MAHLER, M.E. & CUMMINGS, J.L. (1992) The dementia syndromes of Parkinson's disease: cortical and subcortical features. Ch. 11 in *Parkinson's Disease. Neurobehavioral Aspects*, eds Huber, S.J. & Cummings, J.L. Oxford University Press: Oxford [654, 655].

ROSS, J.L., MacKENZIE, T.B., HANSON, D.R. & CHARLES, C.R. (1987) Diltiazem for tardive dyskinesia. *Lancet* **1**, 268 [645].

ROSS, R.J., COLE, M., THOMPSON, J.S. & KIM, K.H. (1983) Boxers—computed tomography, EEG and neurological evaluation. *Journal of the American Medical Association* **249**, 211–213 [205].

ROSSER, R. (1976) Depression during renal dialysis and following transplantation. *Proceedings of the Royal Society of Medicine* **69**, 832–834 [556].

ROSSOR, M.N. (1981) Parkinson's disease and Alzheimer's disease as disorders of the isodendritic core. *British Medical Journal* **283**, 1588–1590 [445].

ROSSOR, M. (1987) Alzheimer's disease: neurobiochemistry. Ch. 8 in *Dementia*, ed. Pitt, B. Churchill Livingstone: Edinburgh & London [445].

ROSSOR, M.N., GARRETT, N.J., JOHNSON, A.L., MOUNTJOY, C.Q., ROTH, M. & IVERSEN, L.L. (1982) A post-mortem study of the cholinergic and GABA systems in senile dementia. *Brain* **105**, 313–330 [445].

ROSSOR, M.N., IVERSEN, L.L., JOHNSON, A.J., MOUNTJOY, C.Q. & ROTH, M. (1981) Cholinergic deficit in frontal cerebral cortex in Alzheimer's disease is age dependent. *Lancet* **2**, 1422 [445].

ROSSOR, M.N., IVERSEN, L.L., REYNOLDS, G.P., MOUNTJOY, C.Q. & ROTH, M. (1984) Neurochemical characteristics of early and late onset types of Alzheimer's disease. *British Medical Journal* **288**, 961–964 [445].

ROSVOLD, H.E., MIRSKY, A.F., SARASON, I., BRANSOME, E.D. & BECK, L.H. (1956) A continuous performance test of brain damage. *Journal of Consulting Psychology* **20**, 343–350 [121].

ROSZELL, D.K., CALSYN, D.A. & CHANEY, E.F. (1986) Alcohol use and psychopathology in opioid addicts on methadone maintenance. *American Journal of Drug and Alcohol Abuse* **12**, 269–278 [612].

ROTH, B. (1980) *Narcolepsy and Hypersomnia*. Translated by Schierlova, M. Revised and edited by Broughton, R. Basel: Karger [722, 723, 724, 728, 729, 734, 735].

ROTH, B. & BRUHOVA, S. (1969) Dreams in narcolepsy, hypersomnia and dissociated sleep disorders. *Experimental Medicine and Surgery* **27**, 187–209 [723, 726].

ROTH, B., NEVSIMALOVA, S. & RECHTSCHAFFEN, A. (1972) Hypersomnia with sleep drunkenness. *Archives of General Psychiatry* **26**, 456–462 [729, 730].

ROTH, M. (1955) The natural history of mental disorder in old age. *Journal of Mental Science* **101**, 281–301 [455].

ROTH, M. (1968) Cerebral disease and mental disorders of old age as causes of antisocial behaviour. In *The Mentally Abnormal Offender*, eds Rueck, A.V.S. & Porter, R. Ciba Foundation Symposium. Churchill: London [275].

ROTH, M. (1971) Classification and aetiology in mental disorders of old age: some recent developments. Ch. 1 in *Recent Developments in Psychogeriatrics*, eds Kay, D.W.K. & Walk, A. British Journal of Psychiatry Special Publication No. 6. Headley Brothers: Ashford, Kent [435, 456].

ROTH, M. (1981) The diagnosis of dementia in late and middle life. Ch. 7 in *The Epidemiology of Dementia*, eds Mortimer, J.A. & Schuman, L.M. Oxford University Press: Oxford [151, 489, 494].

ROTH, M., HUPPERT, F.A., TYM, E. & MOUNTJOY, C.Q. (1988) *CAMDEX. The Cambridge Examination for Mental Disorders of the Elderly*. Cambridge University Press: Cambridge [124].

ROTH, M. & MYERS, D.H. (1969) The diagnosis of dementia. *British Journal of Hospital Medicine* **2**, 705–717 [15, 151, 487].

ROTH, M., TOMLINSON, B.E. & BLESSED, G. (1967) The relationship between quantitative measures of dementia and of degenerative changes in the cerebral grey matter of elderly subjects. *Proceedings of the Royal Society of Medicine* **60**, 254–259 [435].

ROTH, M., TYM, E., MOUNTJOY, C.Q., HUPPERT, F.A., HENDRIE, H., VERMA, S. & GODDARD, R. (1986) CAMDEX: a standardised instrument for the diagnosis of mental disorder in the elderly with special reference to the early detection of dementia. *British Journal of Psychiatry* **149**, 698–709 [124].

ROTH, N. (1945) The neuropsychiatric aspects of porphyria. *Psychosomatic Medicine* **7**, 291–301 [568].

870   REFERENCES

ROTHSCHILD, D. (1956) Senile psychoses and psychoses with cerebral arteriosclerosis. In *Mental Disorders in Later Life*, ed. Kaplan, O.J. Stanford University Press: Stanford [435].

ROTTENBERG, D.A., MOELLER, J.R., STROTHER, S.C., SIDTIS, J.J., NAVIA, B.A., DHAWAN, V., GINOS, J.Z. & PRICE, R.W. (1987) The metabolic pathology of the AIDS dementia complex. *Annals of Neurology* **22**, 700–706 [325].

ROUBICEK, J., GEIGER, C. & ABT, K. (1972) An ergot alkaloid preparation (hydergine) in geriatric therapy. *Journal of the American Geriatrics Society* **20**, 222–229 [502].

ROULEAU, G.A. (1994) Molecular genetic studies of neurofibromatosis 2. Ch. 3 in *The Neurofibromatoses*, eds Huson, S.M. & Hughes, R.A.C. Chapman & Hall: London [703].

ROULEAU, G.A., WERTELECKI, W., HAINES, J.L., HOBBS, W.J., TROFATTER, J.A., SEIZINGER, B.R., MARTUZA, R.L., SUPERNEAU, D.W., CONNEALLY, P.M. & GUSELLA, J.F. (1987) Genetic linkage of bilateral acoustic neurofibromatosis to a DNA marker on chromosome 22. *Nature* **329**, 246–248 [703].

ROUSE, I.L. & ARMSTRONG, B.K. (1988) Thiamin and alcoholic beverages: to add or not to add? *Medical Journal of Australia* **148**, 605–607 [581].

ROVIRA, M., ROMERO, F., TORRENT, O. & IBARRA, B. (1980) Study of tuberculous meningitis by CT. *Neuroradiology* **19**, 137–141 [366].

ROWE, M.J. & CARLSON, C. (1980) Brainstem auditory evoked potentials in postconcussion dizziness. *Archives of Neurology* **37**, 679–683 [198].

ROWLAND, L.P. (1955) Prostigmine-responsiveness and the diagnosis of myasthenia gravis. *Neurology* **5**, 612–624 [713, 714].

ROY, A. (1976) Psychiatric aspects of narcolepsy. *British Journal of Psychiatry* **128**, 562–565 [727].

ROY, A. (1979) Hysterical seizures. *Archives of Neurology* **36**, 447–448 [294].

ROY, A. (1981) Schizophrenia and Klinefelter's syndrome. *Canadian Journal of Psychiatry* **26**, 262–264 [527].

ROYAL COLLEGE OF PHYSICIANS (1981) Organic mental impairment in the elderly: implications for research, education and the provision of services. Report of the Royal College of Physicians by the College Committee on Geriatrics. *Journal of the Royal College of Physicians of London* **15**, 141–167 [429, 441].

ROYAL COLLEGE OF PHYSICIANS OF LONDON (1986) Physical disability in 1986 and beyond. *Journal of the Royal College of Physicians of London* **20**, 3–37 [215].

ROZEWICZ, L., LANGDON, D.W., DAVIE, C.A., THOMPSON, A.J. & RON, M. (1996) Resolution of left hemisphere cognitive dysfunction in multiple sclerosis with magnetic resonance correlates: a case report. *Cognitive Neuropsychiatry* **1**, 17–25 [693].

RUBIN, R.T. & RUBIN, L.E. (1966) Skull roentgenography in hospitalised psychiatric patients. *American Journal of Psychiatry* **122**, 1028–1032 [135].

RUDELLI, R., STROM, J.O., WELCH, P.T. & AMBLER, M.W. (1982) Post traumatic premature Alzheimer's disease. *Archives of Neurology* **39**, 570–575 [186].

RUDGE, P. & WARRINGTON, E.K. (1991) Selective impairment of memory and visual perception in splenial tumours. *Brain* **114**, 349–360 [27, 224].

RUESCH, J. & BOWMAN, K.M. (1945) Prolonged post-traumatic syndromes following head injury. *American Journal of Psychiatry* **102**, 145–163 [173, 176, 194].

RUFF, R.M., BUCHSBAUM, M.S., TRÖSTER, A.I., MARSHALL, L.F., LOTTENBERG, S., SOMERS, L.M. & TOBIAS, M.D. (1989) Computerized tomography, neuropsychology, and positron emission tomogra-

phy in the evaluation of head injury. *Neuropsychiatry, Neuropsychology, and Behavioral Neurology* **2**, 103–123 [166].

RUMBAUGH, C.L., BERGERON, R.T., FANG, H.C. & McCORMICK, R. (1971) Cerebral angiographic changes in the drug abuse patient. *Radiology* **101**, 335–344 [620].

RUNGE, W. (1928) Psychische Störungen bei multipler Sklerose. In *Handbuch der Geisteskrankheiten*, Vol. 7, Special Part 3, ed. Bumke, O. Springer: Berlin [691].

RUSH, A.J., SCHLESSER, M.A., STOKELY, E., BONTE, F.R. & ALTSHULLER, K.Z. (1982) Cerebral blood flow in depression and mania. *Psychopharmacological Bulletin* **18(3)**, 6–7 [148].

RUSK, H.A., BLOCK, J.M. & LOWMAN, E.W. (1969) Rehabilitation of the brain-injured patient: a report of 157 cases with long-term follow-up of 118. Ch. 29 in *The Late Effects of Head Injury*, eds Walker, A.E., Caveness, W.F. & Critchley, M. Thomas: Springfield, Illinois [216].

RUSKIN, A., BEARD, O.W. & SCHAFFER, R.L. (1948) 'Blast hypertension': elevated arterial pressures in victims of the Texas City disaster. *American Journal of Medicine* **4**, 228–236 [397].

RUSSELL, E.W., NEURINGER, C. & GOLDSTEIN, G. (1970) *Assessment of Brain Damage*. Wiley: New York [121].

RUSSELL, R.W.R. (1959) Giant cell arteritis. A review of 35 cases. *Quarterly Journal of Medicine* **28**, 471–489 [424].

RUSSELL, R.W.R. (1963) Observations on intracerebral aneurysms. *Brain* **86**, 425–442 [376].

RUSSELL, R.W.R. (ed.) (1983) Transient cerebral ischaemia. Ch. 11 in *Vascular Disease of the Central Nervous System*, 2nd edn. Churchill Livingstone: Edinburgh & London [380, 381].

RUSSELL, R.W.R. & GRAHAM, E.M. (1988) Giant cell arteritis. Ch. 8 in *Headache. Problems in Diagnosis and Management*, ed. Hopkins, A. W.B. Saunders: London [424].

RUSSELL, R.W.R. & PENNYBACKER, J.B. (1961) Craniopharyngioma in the elderly. *Journal of Neurology, Neurosurgery and Psychiatry* **24**, 1–13 [228].

RUSSELL, W.R. (1932) Cerebral involvement in head injury. *Brain* **55**, 549–603 [171, 174].

RUSSELL, W.R. (1935) Amnesia following head injuries. *Lancet* **2**, 762–763 [168].

RUSSELL, W.R. (1951) Disability caused by brain wounds. *Journal of Neurology, Neurosurgery and Psychiatry* **14**, 35–39 [171].

RUSSELL, W.R. & NATHAN, P.W. (1946) Traumatic amnesia. *Brain* **69**, 280–300 [170, 171].

RUSSELL, W.R. & SCHILLER, F. (1949) Crushing injuries to the skull. *Journal of Neurology, Neurosurgery and Psychiatry* **12**, 52–60 [162, 171].

RUSSELL, W.R. & SMITH, A. (1961) Post-traumatic amnesia in closed head injury. *Archives of Neurology* **5**, 4–17 [171].

RUSSELL, W.R. & WHITTY, C.W.M. (1952) Studies in traumatic epilepsy. 1: Factors influencing the incidence of epilepsy after brain wounds. *Journal of Neurology, Neurosurgery and Psychiatry* **15**, 93–98 [244].

RUTHERFORD, G. (1994) Long term survival in HIV-1 infection. *British Medical Journal* **309**, 283–284 [317].

RUTHERFORD, W.H. (1989) Postconcussion symptoms: relationship to acute neurological indices, individual differences, and circumstances of injury. Ch. 14 in *Mild Head Injury*, eds Levin, H.S., Eisenberg, H.M. & Benton, A.L. Oxford University Press: Oxford [177].

RUTHERFORD, W.H., MERRETT, J.D. & McDONALD, J.R. (1977) Sequelae of concussion caused by minor head injuries. *Lancet* **1**, 1–4 [198].

RUTTER, M. (1978) Prevalence and types of dyslexia. Ch. 1 in *Dyslexia.*

An Appraisal of Current Knowledge, eds Benton, A.L. & Pearl, D. Oxford University Press: New York [47].

RUTTER, M. (1980) Raised lead levels and impaired cognitive/behavioural functioning: a review of the evidence. *Developmental Medicine and Child Neurology* **22 (Supplement 42)**, 1–26 [632, 633].

RUTTER, M. (1993) An overview of developmental neuropsychiatry. In *The Brain and Behaviour: Organic Influences on the Behaviour of Children*, eds Besag, F.M. & Williams, R.T. *Educational and Child Psychology* **10**, 4–11 [201].

RUTTER, M., GRAHAM, P. & YULE, W. (1970) A neuropsychiatric study in childhood. *Clinics in Developmental Medicine* **Nos 35/36**. Spastics International Medical Publications/Heinemann: Philadelphia [47].

RUTTER, M., TIZARD, J., YULE, W., GRAHAM, P. & WHITMORE, K. (1976) Research report: Isle of Wight Studies 1964–1974. *Psychological Medicine* **6**, 313–332 [47].

RUTTER, M. & YULE, W. (1975) The concept of specific reading retardation. *Journal of Child Psychology and Psychiatry* **16**, 181–197 [47].

RYAN, C. & BUTTERS, N. (1980) Further evidence for a continuum-of-impairment encompassing male alcoholic Korsakoff patients and chronic alcoholic men. *Alcoholism: Clinical and Experimental Research* **4**, 190–198 [583, 604].

RYBACK, R.S. (1971) The continuity and specificity of the effects of alcohol on memory. *Quarterly Journal of Studies on Alcohol* **32**, 995–1016 [583].

RYDING, E., ROSÉN, I., ELMQVIST, D. & INGVAR, D.H. (1988) SPECT measurements with ^{99m}Tc-HM-PAO in focal epilepsy. *Journal of Cerebral Blood Flow and Metabolism* **8**, S95–S100 [289].

RYLANDER, G. (1939) Personality changes after operations on the frontal lobes: a clinical study of 32 cases. *Acta Psychiatrica et Neurologica Scandinavica* **20 (Supplement)**, 1–327 [77].

RYLANDER, G. (1943) Mental changes after excision of cerebral tissue. *Acta Psychiatrica et Neurologica Scandinavica* **25 (Supplement)**, 1–81 [77].

RYN, Z. (1988) Psychopathology in mountaineering—mental disturbances under high-altitude stress. *International Journal of Sports Medicine* **9**, 163–169 [549].

SABERS, A. & GRAM, L. (1994) Oxcarbazepine. Ch. 7 in *New Anticonvulsants. Advances in the Treatment of Epilepsy*, ed. Trimble, M.R. John Wiley & Sons: Chichester [304].

SABOT, L.M., GROSS, M.M. & HALPERT, E. (1968) A study of acute alcoholic psychoses in women. *British Journal of Addiction* **63**, 29–49 [599].

SACHS, E. (1950) Meningiomas with dementia as the first and presenting failure. *Journal of Mental Science* **96**, 998–1007 [222].

SACKHEIM, H.A., PROHOVNIK, I., MOELLER, J.R., BROWN, R.P., APTER, S., PRUDIC, J., DEVANAND, D.P. & MUKHERJEE, S. (1990) Regional cerebral blood flow in mood disorders: 1. Comparison of major depressives and normal controls at rest. *Archives of General Psychiatry* **47**, 60–70 [148].

SACKNER, M.A., LANDA, J., FORREST, T. & GREENELTCH, D. (1975) Periodic sleep apnea: chronic sleep deprivation related to intermittent upper airway obstruction and central nervous system disturbance. *Chest* **67**, 164–171 [731].

SACKS, O.W. (1970) *Migraine: The Evolution of a Common Disorder*. Faber: London [399, 403, 405, 407, 408, 410].

SACKS, O. (1973) *Awakenings*. Duckworth: London [353, 660].

SACKS, O.W., AGUILAR, M.J. & BROWN, W.J. (1966) Hallervorden Spatz disease. Its pathogenesis and place among the axonal dystrophies. *Acta Neuropathologica* **6**, 164–174 [756].

SACKS, O.W., KOHL, M.S., MESSELOFF, C.R. & SCHWARTZ, W.F. (1972) Effects of levodopa in parkinsonian patients with dementia. *Neurology* **22**, 516–519 [659].

SACKS, O.W., MESSELOFF, C., SCHWARTZ, W., GOLDFARB, A. & KOHL, M. (1970) Effects of L-dopa in patients with dementia. *Lancet* **1**, 1231 [659].

SAGAR, H.J. & OXBURY, J.M. (1987) Hippocampal neuron loss in temporal lobe epilepsy: correlation with early childhood convulsions. *Annals of Neurology* **22**, 334–340 [246].

SAHAKIAN, B., JOYCE, E. & LISHMAN, W.A. (1987) Cholinergic effects on constructional abilities and on mnemonic processes: a case report. *Psychological Medicine* **17**, 329–333 [754].

SAHAKIAN, B.J., MORRIS, R.G., EVENDEN, J.L., HEALD, A., LEVY, R., PHILPOT, M. & ROBBINS, T.W. (1988) A comparative study of visuospatial memory and learning in Alzheimer-type dementia and Parkinson's disease. *Brain* **111**, 695–718 [122].

SAHAKIAN, B.J. & OWEN, A.M. (1992) Computerized assessment in neuropsychiatry using CANTAB: discussion paper. *Journal of the Royal Society of Medicine* **85**, 399–402 [122].

SAINSBURY, P. (1964) Neuroticism and hypertension in an out-patient population. *Journal of Psychosomatic Research* **8**, 235–238 [398].

SAINSBURY, P., COSTAIN, W.R. & GRAD, J. (1965) The effects of community service on the referral and admission rates of elderly psychiatric patients. In *Psychiatric Disorders of the Aged*, Report on Symposium held by the World Psychiatric Association, pp. 23–37. Geigy (UK) Ltd: Manchester [431].

ST CLAIR, D. & WHALLEY, L.J. (1983) Hypertension, multi-infarct dementia and Alzheimer's disease. *British Journal of Psychiatry* **143**, 274–276 [453].

ST GEORGE-HYSLOP, P.H., HAINES, J.L., FARRIER, L.A., POLINSKY, R.J., VAN BROECKHOVEN, C., GOATE, A., CRAPPER McLACHLAN, D.R., ORR, H., BRUNI, A.C., SORBI, S., RAINERO, I., FONCIN, J.F., POLLEN, D., CANTU, J.-M., TUPLER, R., VOSKRESENSKAYA, N., MAYEUX, R., GROWDEN, J., FRIED, V.A., MYERS, R.H., NEE, L., BACKHOVENS, H., MARTIN, J.J., ROSSOR, M., OWEN, M.J., MULLAN, M., PERCY, M.E., KARLINSKY, H., RICH, S., HESTON, L., MONTESI, M., MORTILLA, M., NACMIAS, N., GUSELLA, J.F. & HARDY, J.A. (1990) Genetic linkage studies suggest that Alzheimer's disease is not a single homogeneous disorder. *Nature* **347**, 194–197 [448].

ST GEORGE-HYSLOP, P.H., TANZI, R.E., POLINSKY, R.J., HAINES, J.L., NEE, L., WATKINS, P.C., MYERS, R.H., FELDMAN, R.G., POLLEN, D., DRACHMAN, D., GROWDON, J., BRUNI, A., FONCIN, J.-F., SALMON, D., FROMMELT, P., AMADUCCI, L., SORBI, S., PIACENTINI, S., STEWART, G.D., HOBBS, W.J., CONNEALLY, P.M. & GUSELLA, J.F. (1987) The genetic defect causing familial Alzheimer's disease maps on chromosome 21. *Science* **235**, 885–890 [447].

SAITO, I., UEDA, Y. & SANO, K. (1977) Significance of vasospasm in the treatment of ruptured intracranial aneurysms. *Journal of Neurosurgery* **47**, 412–429 [392].

SALGADO, E.D., WEINSTEIN, M., FURLAN, A.J., MODIC, M.T., BECK, G.J., ESTES, M., AWAD, I. & LITTLE, J.R. (1986) Proton magnetic resonance imaging in ischaemic cerebrovascular disease. *Annals of Neurology* **20**, 502–507 [380].

SALIB, E.A. (1988) Subacute sclerosing panencephalitis (SSPE) presenting at the age of 21 as a schizophrenia-like state with bizarre dysmorphophobic features. *British Journal of Psychiatry* **152**, 709–710 [362].

SALMON, E. & FRANCK, G. (1989) Positron emission tomographic study in Alzheimer's disease and Pick's disease. *Archives of Gerontology and Geriatrics* **1 (Supplement)**, 241–247 [462].

SALMON, J.H. (1971) Surgical treatment of severe post-traumatic encephalopathy. *Surgery, Gynaecology and Obstetrics* **133**, 634–636 [748].

SALMON, J.H. & ARMITAGE, J.L. (1968) Surgical treatment of hydrocephalus ex-vacuo: ventriculoatrial shunt for degenerative brain disease. *Neurology* **18**, 1223–1226 [748].

SALMON, J.H., GONEN, J.Y. & BROWN, L. (1971) Ventriculoatrial shunt for hydrocephalus ex-vacuo: psychological and clinical evaluation. *Diseases of the Nervous System* **32**, 299–307 [748].

SALMONS, P.H. (1980) Psychological aspects of chronic renal failure. *British Journal of Hospital Medicine* **23/6**, 617–622 [557].

SALT COLLABORATIVE GROUP (1991) Swedish aspirin low-dose trial (SALT) of 75 mg aspirin as secondary prophylaxis after cerebrovascular ischaemic events. *Lancet* **338**, 1345–1349 [381, 389].

SAMARA, K., RIKLAN, M., LEVITA, E., ZIMMERMAN, J., WALTZ, J.M., BERGMANN, L. & COOPER, I.S. (1969) Language and speech correlates of anatomically verified lesions in thalamic surgery for parkinsonism. *Journal of Speech and Hearing Research* **12**, 510–540 [660].

SAMUELSSON, B. (1981) *Neurofibromatosis (v. Recklinghausen's Disease). A Clinical-Psychiatric and Genetic Study.* Thesis, translated by Jacobs, A., Psychiatric Department, University of Göteborg, Sweden [704].

SAND, P.L. & CARLSON, C. (1973) Failure to establish control over tics in the Gilles de la Tourette syndrome with behaviour therapy techniques. *British Journal of Psychiatry* **122**, 665–670 [687].

SANDER, J.W.A.S., HART, Y.M., JOHNSON, A.L. & SHORVON, S.D. FOR THE NGPSE (1990) National General Practice Study of Epilepsy: newly diagnosed epileptic seizures in a general population. *Lancet* **336**, 1267–1271 [246].

SANDER, J.W.A.S., HART, Y.M., TRIMBLE, M.R. & SHORVON, S.D. (1991) Vigabatrin and psychosis. *Journal of Neurology, Neurosurgery and Psychiatry* **54**, 435–439 [284, 303].

SANDERCOCK, P., MOLYNEUX, A. & WARLOW, C. (1985) Value of computed tomography in patients with stroke: Oxfordshire Community Stroke Project. *British Medical Journal* **290**, 193–197 [138].

SANDERS, H.I. & WARRINGTON, E.K. (1971) Memory for remote events in amnesic patients. *Brain* **94**, 661–668 [36].

SANDERS, W.L. (1979) Creutzfeldt–Jakob disease treated with amantadine. *Journal of Neurology, Neurosurgery and Psychiatry* **42**, 960–961 [506].

SANDERS, W.L. & DUNN, T.L. (1973) Creutzfeldt–Jakob disease treated with amantadine. *Journal of Neurology, Neurosurgery and Psychiatry* **36**, 581–584 [506].

SANDIFER, M.G. (1983) Hyponatraemia due to psychotropic drugs. *Journal of Clinical Psychiatry* **44**, 301–303 [526].

SANDS, I.J. (1928) The acute psychiatric type of epidemic encephalitis. *American Journal of Psychiatry* **7**, 975–987 [350].

SANDS, I.R. (1942) The type of personality susceptible to Parkinson disease. *Journal of the Mount Sinai Hospital* **9**, 792–794 [660].

SANDYK, R. (1984) Aggressive dementia in normal-pressure hydrocephalus. *South African Medical Journal* **65**, 114 [745].

SANO, K., SEKINO, H. & MAYANAGI, Y. (1972) Results of stimulation and destruction of the posterior hypothalamus in cases with violent, aggressive, or restless behaviors. Ch. 5 in *Psychosurgery*, eds Hitchcock, E., Laitinen, L. & Vaernet, K. Proceedings of the Second International Conference on Psychosurgery. Thomas: Springfield, Illinois [82].

SANO, K., YOSHIOKA, M., OGASHIWA, M., ISHIJIMA, B. & OHYE, C. (1966) Postero-medial hypothalamotomy in the treatment of aggressive behaviors. *Confinia Neurologica* **27**, 164–167 [82].

SANTA, T., ENGEL, A.G. & LAMBERT, E.H. (1972) Histometric study of neuromuscular junction ultrastructure. 1: Myasthenia gravis. *Neurology* **22**, 71–82 [710]..

SAPHIR, W. (1945) Chronic hypochloremia simulating psychoneurosis. *Journal of the American Medical Association* **129**, 510–512 [559].

SARGENT, J.D., LAWSON, R.C., SOLBACH, P. & COYNE, L. (1979) Use of CT scan in an out-patient headache population: an evaluation. *Headache* **19**, 388–390 [401].

SARIN, S.K., SACHDEV, G., JILOHA, R.C., BHATT, A. & MUNJAL, G.C. (1988) Pattern of psychiatric morbidity and alcohol dependence in patients with alcoholic liver disease. *Digestive Diseases and Sciences* **33**, 443–448 [566].

SATO, T., UCHIUMI, T., OZAWA, T., KIKUCHI, M., NAKANO, M., KOMINAMI, R. & ARAKAWA, L.M. (1991) Autoantibodies against ribosomal proteins found with high frequency in patients with systemic lupus erythematosus with active disease. *Journal of Rheumatology* **18**, 1681–1684 [418].

SATZ, P., ACHENBACH, K. & FENNELL, E. (1967) Correlations between assessed manual laterality and predicted speech laterality in a normal population. *Neuropsychologia* **5**, 295–310 [40].

SAUER, D., MASSIEU, L., ALLEGRINI, P.R., AMACKER, H., SCHMUTZ, M. & FAGG, G.E. (1992) Excitotoxicity, cerebral ischaemia, and neuroprotection by competitive NMDA receptor antagonists. Ch. 6 in *Emerging Strategies in Neuroprotection*, eds Marangos, P.J. & Lal, H. Birkhäuser: Boston [164].

SAUGET, J., BENTON, A.L. & HÉCAEN, H. (1971) Disturbances of the body schema in relation to language impairment and hemispheric locus of lesion. *Journal of Neurology, Neurosurgery and Psychiatry* **34**, 496–501 [66].

SAUL, L. (1939) Hostility in cases of essential hypertension. *Psychosomatic Medicine* **1**, 153–161 [398].

SAVARD, G., ANDERMANN, F., TEITELBAUM, J. & LEHMANN, H. (1988) Epileptic Munchausen's syndrome: a form of pseudoseizures distinct from hysteria and malingering. *Neurology* **38**, 1628–1629 [293].

SAVIC, I., PERSSON, A., ROLAND, P., PAULI, S., SEDVALL, G. & WIDÉN, L. (1988) In-vivo demonstration of reduced benzodiazepine receptor binding in human epileptic foci. *Lancet* **2**, 863–866 [289].

SAWLE, G.V., BROOKS, D.J., IBANEZ, V. & FRACKOWIAK, R.S.J. (1990) Striatal D2 receptor density is inversely proportional to dopa uptake in untreated hemi-Parkinson's disease: a positron emission tomography study. Proceedings of the Association of British Neurologists, London, 28–30 September 1989. *Journal of Neurology, Neurosurgery and Psychiatry* **53**, 177 [648].

SAWLE, G.V., BROOKS, D.J., MARSDEN, C.D. & FRACKOWIAK, R.S.J. (1991) Corticobasal degeneration. A unique pattern of regional cortical oxygen, hypometabolism and striatal fluorodopa uptake demonstrated by positron emission tomography. *Brain* **114**, 541–556 [668].

SAYKIN, A.J., GUR, R.C., GUR, R.E., MOZLEY, P.D., MOZLEY, L.H., RESNICK, S.M., KESTER, B. & STAFINIAK, P. (1991) Neuropsychological function in schizophrenia, selective impairment in memory and learning. *Archives of General Psychiatry* **48**, 618–624 [34].

SCARLETT, J.A., MAKO, M.E., RUBENSTEIN, A.H., BLIX, P.M., GOLDMAN, J., HORWITZ, D.L., TAGER, H., JASPAN, J.B., STJERNHOLM, M.R. & OLEFSKY, J.M. (1977) Factitious hypoglycemia. Diagnosis by measurement of serum C-peptide immunoreactivity and insulin binding antibodies. *New England Journal of Medicine* **297**, 1029–1032 [544].

SCARONE, S., CAZZULLO, C.L. & GAMBINI, O. (1987) Asymmetry of lateralised hemispheric function in schizophrenia. Influence of clinical and epidemiological characteristics on quality extinction test performance. *British Journal of Psychiatry* **151**, 15–17 [89].

SCHÄCHTER, F., FAURE-DELANEF, L., GUÉNOT, F., ROUGER, H., FROGUEL, P., LESUER-GINOT, L. & COHEN, D. (1994) Genetic associations with human longevity at the APOE and ACE loci. *Nature Genetics* **6**, 29–32 [448].

SCHACTER, D.L. (1987) Memory, amnesia, and frontal lobe dysfunction. *Psychobiology* **15**, 21–36 [27].

SCHACTER, D.L., WANG, P.L., TULVING, E. & FREEDMAN, M. (1982) Functional retrograde amnesia: a quantitative case study. *Neuropsychologia* **20**, 523–532 [33].

SCHADY, W. & MEARA, R.J. (1988) Hereditary progressive chorea without dementia. *Journal of Neurology, Neurosurgery and Psychiatry* **51**, 295–297 [473].

SCHAPIRA, A.H.V., COOPER, J.M., DEXTER, D., CLARK, J.B., JENNER, P. & MARSDEN, C.D. (1990a) Mitochondrial Complex I deficiency in Parkinson's disease. *Journal of Neurochemistry* **54**, 823–827 [648].

SCHAPIRA, A.H.V., COOPER, J.M., DEXTER, D., JENNER, P., CLARK, J.B. & MARSDEN, C.D. (1989) Mitochondrial Complex I deficiency in Parkinson's disease. *Lancet* **1**, 1269 [648].

SCHAPIRA, A.H.V., MANN, V.M., COOPER, J.M., DEXTER, D., DANIEL, S.E., JENNER, P., CLARK, J.B. & MARSDEN, C.D. (1990b) Anatomic and disease specificity of NADH CoQ$_1$ reductase (Complex I) deficiency in Parkinson's disease. *Journal of Neurochemistry* **55**, 2142–2145 [648].

SCHAUMBERG, H.H. & SUZUKI, K. (1968) Non-specific familial presenile dementia. *Journal of Neurology, Neurosurgery and Psychiatry* **31**, 479–486 [755].

SCHEFF, S.W., DE KOSKY, S.T. & PRICE, D.A. (1990) Quantitative assessment of cortical synaptic density in Alzheimer's disease. *Neurobiological Aging* **11**, 29–37 [444].

SCHEFFER, I.E., BHATIA, K.P., LOPES-CENDES, I., FISH, D.R., MARSDEN, C.D., ANDERMANN, E., ANDERMANN, F., DESBIENS, R., KEENE, D., CENDES, F., MANSON, J.I., CONSTANTINOU, J.E.C., McINTOSH, A. & BERKOVIC, S.F. (1995) Autosomal dominant nocturnal frontal lobe epilepsy. A distinctive clinical disorder. *Brain* **118**, 61–73 [247].

SCHEIBEL, A.B. (1978) Structural aspects of the aging brain: spine systems and the dendritic arbor. In *Alzheimer's Disease: Senile Dementia and Related Disorders, Aging*, Vol. 7, eds Katzman, R., Terry, R.D. & Bick, K.L., pp. 353–373. Raven Press: New York [436, 443].

SCHEIBEL, A.B. (1991) Are complex partial seizures a sequela of temporal lobe dysgenesis? Ch. 4 in *Neurobehavioral Problems in Epilepsy*, eds Smith, D.B., Treiman, D.M. & Trimble, M.R. *Advances in Neurology* **55**. Raven Press: New York [246].

SCHEIBEL, A.B. & TOMIYASU, U. (1978) Dendritic sprouting in Alzheimer's presenile dementia. *Experimental Neurology* **60**, 1–8 [443].

SCHEINBERG, I.H. & GITLIN, D. (1952) Deficiency of ceruloplasmin in patients with hepatolenticular degeneration (Wilson's disease). *Science* **116**, 484–485 [663].

SCHEINBERG, I.H., STERNLIEB, I. & RICHMAN, J. (1968) Psychiatric manifestations in patients with Wilson's disease. In *Wilson's Disease*, ed. Bergsma, D., Birth Defects Original Article Series, Vol. 4, No. 2. The National Foundation: New York [665, 666].

SCHEINBERG, P. (1951) Cerebral blood flow and metabolism in pernicious anaemia. *Blood* **6**, 213–227 [589].

SCHEINBERG, P., STEAD, E.A., BRANNON, E.S. & WARREN, J.V. (1950) Correlative observations on cerebral metabolism and cardiac output in myxoedema. *Journal of Clinical Investigation* **29**, 1139–1146 [514].

SCHELLENBERG, G.D., BIRD, T.D., WIJSMAN, E.M., ORR, H.T., ANDERSON, L., NEMENS, E., WHITE, J.A., BONNYCASTLE, L., WEBER, J.L., ALONSO, M.E., POTTER, H., HESTON, L.L. & MARTIN, G.M. (1992) Genetic linkage evidence for a familial Alzheimer's disease locus on chromosome 14. *Science* **258**, 668–671 [448].

SCHENCK, C.H., BUNDLIE, S.R., ETTINGER, M.G. & MAHOWALD, M.W. (1986) Chronic behavioral disorders of human REM sleep: a new category of parasomnia. *Sleep* **9**, 293–308 [737].

SCHENCK, C.H., BUNDLIE, S.R., PATTERSON, A.L. & MAHOWALD, M.W. (1987) Rapid eye movement sleep behavior disorder. A treatable parasomnia affecting older adults. *Journal of the American Medical Association* **257**, 1786–1789 [737, 738].

SCHENCK, C.H. & MAHOWALD, M.W. (1990) Polysomnographic, neurologic, psychiatric, and clinical outcome report on 70 consecutive cases with REM sleep behavior disorder (RBD): sustained clonazepam efficacy in 89.5% of 57 treated patients. *Cleveland Clinic Journal of Medicine* **57 (Supplement),** S9–S23 [738].

SCHENCK, C.H. & MAHOWALD, M.W. (1992) Motor dyscontrol in narcolepsy: rapid-eye-movement (REM) sleep without atonia and REM sleep behavior disorder. *Annals of Neurology* **32**, 3–10 [738].

SCHIAVI, R.C., THEILGAARD, A., OWEN, D.R. & WHITE, D. (1984) Sex chromosome anomalies, hormones, and aggressivity. *Archives of General Psychiatry* **41**, 93–99 [527].

SCHIFFER, R.B. & BABIGIAN, H.M. (1984) Behavioral disorders in multiple sclerosis, temporal lobe epilepsy, and amyotrophic lateral sclerosis. An epidemiologic study. *Archives of Neurology* **41**, 1067–1069 [695].

SCHIFFER, R.B., CAINE, E.D., BAMFORD, K.A. & LEVY, S. (1983) Depressive episodes in patients with multiple sclerosis. *American Journal of Psychiatry* **140**, 1498–1500 [695].

SCHIFFER, R.B., HERNDON, R.M. & RUDICK, R.A. (1985) Treatment of pathological laughing and weeping with amitriptyline. *New England Journal of Medicine* **312**, 1480–1482 [392].

SCHIFFER, R.B., KURLAN, R., RUBIN, A. & BOER, S. (1988) Evidence for atypical depression in Parkinson's disease. *American Journal of Psychiatry* **145**, 1020–1022 [656].

SCHIFFER, R.B., WINEMAN, N.M. & WEITKAMP, L.R. (1986) Association between bipolar affective disorder and multiple sclerosis. *American Journal of Psychiatry* **143**, 94–95 [695].

SCHILDER, P. (1935) *The Image and Appearance of the Human Body: Studies in the Constructive Energies of the Psyche*. Psyche Monographs No. 4. Kegan Paul, Trench, Trubner: London [67].

SCHILDER, P. (1938) The organic background of obsessions and compulsions. *American Journal of Psychiatry* **94**, 1397–1413 [352].

SCHLAUG, G., JÄNCKE, L., HUANG, Y. & STEINMETZ, H. (1995) In vivo evidence of structural brain asymmetry in musicians. *Science* **267**, 699–701 [64].

SCHLESINGER, B. (1950) Mental changes in intracranial tumours, and related problems. *Confinia Neurologica* **10**, 225–263 and 322–355 [223, 224].

SCHMID, B. (1969) Occupational rehabilitation of the brain-injured worker. Ch. 34 in *The Late Effects of Head Injury*, eds Walker, A.E., Caveness, W.F. & Critchley, M. Thomas: Springfield, Illinois [215].

SCHMIDTKE, K. (1993) Wernicke–Korsakoff syndrome following attempted hanging. *Revue Neurologique* **149**, 213–216 [576].

SCHMITT, F.A., BIGLEY, J.W., McKINNIS, R., LOGUE, P.E., EVANS, R.W., DRUCKER, J.L. & THE AZT COLLABORATIVE WORKING GROUP (1988)

Neuropsychological outcome of zidovudine (AZT) treatment of patients with AIDS and AIDS-related complex. *New England Journal of Medicine* **319**, 1573–1578 [335].

SCHOTT, G.D. (1985) The relationship of peripheral trauma and pain to dystonia. *Journal of Neurology, Neurosurgery and Psychiatry* **48**, 698–701 [669].

SCHOTT, G.D., McLEOD, A.A. & JEWITT, D.E. (1977) Cardiac arrhythmias that masquerade as epilepsy. *British Medical Journal* **1**, 1454–1457 [291].

SCHOU, M. (1984) Long-lasting neurological sequelae after lithium intoxication. *Acta Psychiatrica Scandinavica* **70**, 594–602 [626].

SCHRAMM, J., BEHRENS, E. & ENTZIAN, W. (1995) Hemispherical deafferentation: an alternative to functional hemispherectomy. *Neurosurgery* **36**, 509–516 [313].

SCHROTH, G., NAEGELE, T., KLOSE, U., MANN, K. & PETERSON, D. (1988) Reversible brain shrinkage in abstinent alcoholics, measured by MRI. *Neuroradiology* **30**, 385–389 [605].

SCHULSINGER, F., PARNAS, J., PETERSEN, E.T., SCHULSINGER, H., TEASDALE, T.W., MEDNICK, S.A., MØLLER, L. & SILVERTON, L. (1984) Cerebral ventricular size in the offspring of schizophrenic mothers. *Archives of General Psychiatry* **41**, 602–606 [85].

SCHWAB, R.S., FABING, H.D. & PRICHARD, J.S. (1951) Psychiatric symptoms and syndromes in Parkinson's disease. *American Journal of Psychiatry* **107**, 901–907 [352].

SCHWAB, R.S. & PERLO, V.P. (1966) Syndromes simulating myasthenia gravis. *Annals of the New York Academy of Sciences* **135**, 350–366 [713].

SCHWANDT, P., RICHTER, W. & WILKENING, J. (1979) Chronic insulin overtreatment. *Lancet* **2**, 261–262 [536].

SCHWARTZ, C.J. & MITCHELL, J.R.A. (1961) Atheroma of the carotid and vertebral arterial systems. *British Medical Journal* **2**, 1057–1063 [384].

SCHWARTZ, M.S. & SCOTT, D.F. (1971) Isolated petit-mal status presenting de novo in middle age. *Lancet* **2**, 1399–1401 [256].

SCHWARTZ, R.H., GRUENEWALD, P.J., KLITZNER, M. & FEDIO, P. (1989) Short-term memory impairment in cannabis-dependent adolescents. *American Journal of Diseases of Childhood* **143**, 1214–1219 [616].

SCHWEITZER, L. (1982) Evidence of right cerebral hemisphere dysfunction in schizophrenic patients with left hemisphere overactivation. *Biological Psychiatry* **17**, 655–673 [89].

SCOTT, D.F. (1982a) Recognition and diagnostic aspects of nonepileptic seizures. Ch. 2 in *Pseudoseizures*, eds Riley, T.L. & Roy, A. Williams & Wilkins: Baltimore & London [293, 294].

SCOTT, D.F. (1982b) The use of EEG in pseudoseizures. Ch. 6 in *Pseudoseizures*, eds Riley, T.L. & Roy, A. Williams & Wilkins: Baltimore & London [294].

SCOTT, J. (1993) Apolipoprotein E and Alzheimer's disease. *Lancet* **342**, 696 [448].

SCOTT, M. (1970) Transitory psychotic behaviour following operation for tumours of the cerebello-pontine angle. *Psychiatria, Neurologia, Neurochirurgia* **73**, 37–48 [231].

SCOTT, M.L., GOLDEN, C.J., RUEDRICH, S.L. & BISHOP, R.J. (1983) Ventricular enlargement in major depression. *Psychiatry Research* **8**, 91–93 [140].

SCOTT, P.D. (1965) The Ganser syndrome. *British Journal of Criminology* **5**, 127–131 [481, 482].

SCOURFIELD, J., SOLDAN, J., GRAY, J., HOULIHAN, G. & HARER, P.S. (1997) Huntington's disease: psychiatric practice in molecular genetic prediction and diagnosis. *British Journal of Psychiatry* **170**, 146–149 [467].

SCOVILLE, W.B. (1954) The limbic lobe in man. *Journal of Neurosurgery* **11**, 64–66 [26].

SCOVILLE, W.B. & MILNER, B. (1957) Loss of recent memory after bilateral hippocampal lesions. *Journal of Neurology, Neurosurgery and Psychiatry* **20**, 11–21 [26].

SCREATON, G.R., SINGER, M., CAIRNS, H.S., THRASHER, A., SARNER, M. & COHEN, S.L. (1991) Hyperpyrexia and rhabdomyolysis after MDMA ('ecstasy') abuse. *Lancet* **339**, 677–678 [624].

SCRIMA, L., HARTMAN, P.G., JOHNSON, F.H. Jr & HILLER, F.C. (1989) Efficacy of gamma-hydroxybutyrate versus placebo in treating narcolepsy-cataplexy: double-blind subjective measures. *Biological Psychiatry* **26**, 331–343 [727].

SCRIMA, L., HARTMAN, P.G., JOHNSON, F.H., THOMAS, E.E. & HILLER, F.C. (1990) The effects of g-hydroxybutyrate on the sleep of narcolepsy patients: a double-blind study. *Sleep* **13**, 479–490 [727].

SEAB, J.P., JAGUST, W.J., WONG, S.T.S., ROOS, M.S., REED, B.R. & BUDINGER, T.F. (1988) Quantitative NMR measurements of hippocampal atrophy in Alzheimer's disease. *Magnetic Resonance in Medicine* **8**, 200–208 [434].

SEARLEMAN, A. (1977) A review of right hemisphere linguistic capabilities. *Psychological Bulletin* **84**, 503–528 [42].

SEGARRA, J.M. (1970) Cerebral vascular disease and behavior. 1 The syndrome of the mesencephalitic artery (basilar artery bifurcation). *Archives of Neurology* **22**, 408–418 [156].

SEGGEV, J., SHAPIRO, M.S., LEVIN, S. & SCHEY, G. (1986) Alveolar hypoventilation and daytime hypersomnia in acromegaly. *European Journal of Respiratory Diseases* **68**, 381–383 [522].

SELBY, G. (1968) Cerebral atrophy in Parkinsonism. *Journal of the Neurological Sciences* **6**, 517–559 [655].

SELBY, G. (1990) Clinical features. Ch. 12 in *Parkinson's Disease*, ed. Stern, G.M. Chapman & Hall: London [646].

SELBY, G. & LANCE, J.W. (1960) Observations on 500 cases of migraine and allied vascular headache. *Journal of Neurology, Neurosurgery and Psychiatry* **23**, 23–32 [403, 404].

SELECKI, B.R. (1964) Cerebral mid-line tumours involving the corpus callosum among mental hospital patients. *Medical Journal of Australia* **2**, 954–960 [224].

SELECKI, B.R. (1965) Intracranial space-occupying lesions among patients admitted to mental hospitals. *Medical Journal of Australia* **1**, 383–390 [412].

SELLERS, J., TYRER, P., WHITELEY, A., BANKS, D.C. & BARER, D.H. (1982) Neurotoxic effects of lithium with delayed rise in serum lithium levels. *British Journal of Psychiatry* **140**, 623–625 [626].

SELLS, C.J., CARPENTER, R.L. & RAY, C.G. (1975) Sequelae of central-nervous-system enterovirus infections. *New England Journal of Medicine* **293**, 1–4 [349].

SELNES, O.A., McARTHUR, J.C., ROYAL, W. III, UPDIKE, M.L., NANCE-SPROSON, T., CONCHA, M., GORDON, B., SOLOMON, L. & VLAHOV, D. (1992) HIV-1 infection and intravenous drug use: longitudinal neuropsychological evaluation of asymptomatic subjects. *Neurology* **42**, 1924–1930 [329].

SELNES, O.A., MILLER, E., McARTHUR, J., GORDON, B., MUÑOZ, A., SHERIDAN, K., FOX, R., SAAH, A.J. & THE MULTICENTER AIDS COHORT STUDY (1990) HIV-1 infection: no evidence of cognitive decline during the asymptomatic stages. *Neurology* **40**, 204–208 [329].

SELTZER, B. & SHERWIN, I. (1983) A comparison of clinical features in early- and late-onset primary degenerative dementia. *Archives of Neurology* **40**, 143–146 [433, 440, 450].

SELZER, M.L., ROGERS, J.E. & KERN, S. (1968) Fatal accidents: the role of psychopathology, social stress, and acute disturbances. *American Journal of Psychiatry* **124**, 1028–1036 [176].

SEMMES, J., WEINSTEIN, S., GHENT, L. & TEUBER, H.-L. (1955) Spatial orientation in man after cerebral injury. 1: Analyses by locus of lesion. *Journal of Psychology* **39**, 227–244 [63].

SENSENBACH, W., MADISON, L., EISENBERG, S. & OCHS, L. (1954) The cerebral circulation and metabolism in hypothyroidism and myxoedema. *Journal of Clinical Investigation* **33**, 1434–1440 [514].

SENSKY, T., WILSON, A., PETTY, R., FENWICK, P.B.C. & ROSE, F.C. (1984) The interictal personality traits of temporal lobe epileptics: religious belief and its association with reported mystical experiences. In *Advances in Epileptology, XVth Epilepsy International Symposium*, eds Porter, R.J., Mattson, R.H., Ward, A.A. & Dam, M. Raven Press: New York [268].

SERAFETINIDES, E.A. (1965) Aggressiveness in temporal lobe epileptics and its relation to cerebral dysfunction and environmental factors. *Epilepsia* **6**, 33–42 [266].

SERAFETINIDES, E.A. & FALCONER, M.A. (1962a) Some observations on memory impairment after temporal lobectomy for epilepsy. *Journal of Neurology, Neurosurgery and Psychiatry* **25**, 251–255 [26].

SERAFETINIDES, E.A. & FALCONER, M.A. (1962b) The effects of temporal lobectomy in epileptic patients with psychosis. *Journal of Mental Science* **108**, 584–593 [285].

SERAFETINIDES, E.A. & FALCONER, M.A. (1963) Speech disturbances in temporal lobe seizures: a study in 100 epileptic patients submitted to anterior temporal lobectomy. *Brain* **86**, 333–346 [251].

SERBY, M., CORWIN, J., CONRAD, P. & ROTROSEN, J. (1985) Olfactory dysfunction in Alzheimer's disease and Parkinson's disease. *American Journal of Psychiatry* **142**, 781–782 [441].

SERDAROĞLU, P., YAZICI, H., OZDEMIR, C., YURDAKUL, S., BAHAR, S. & AKTIN, E. (1989) Neurologic involvement in Behçet's syndrome. *Archives of Neurology* **46**, 265–269 [763].

SERDARU, M., HAUSSER-HAUW, C., LAPLANE, D., BUGE, A., CASTAIGNE, P., GOULON, M., LHERMITTE, F. & HAUW, J.-J. (1988) The clinical spectrum of alcoholic pellagra encephalopathy. A retrospective analysis of 22 cases studied pathologically. *Brain* **111**, 829–842 [575].

SERGENT, J. (1994) Cognitive and neural structures in face processing. Ch. 15 in *Localization and Neuroimaging in Neuropsychology*, ed. Kertesz, A. Academic Press: San Diego [60].

SERRA CATAFAU, J., RUBIO, F. & PERRES SERRA, J. (1992) Peduncular hallucinosis associated with posterior thalamic infarction. *Journal of Neurology* **239**, 89–90 [388].

SERVIT, Z., MACHEK, J., STERCOVA, A., KRISTOF, M., CERVENKOVA, V. & DUDAS, D. (1963) Reflex influences in the pathogenesis of epilepsy in the light of clinical statistics. In *Reflex Mechanisms in the Genesis of Epilepsy*, ed. Servit, Z. Elsevier: Amsterdam [248].

SETHURAJAN, C., CROFT, P.B. & WILKINSON, M. (1967) Bronchial neoplasm with endocrine, metabolic, and neurological manifestations. *Neurology* **17**, 1169–1173 [743].

SEVERINGHAUS, J.W. & MITCHELL, R.A. (1962) Ondine's curse: failure of respiratory centre automaticity while awake. *Clinical Research* **10**, 122 [730].

SHAGASS, C. (1965) The EEG in affective psychosis. In *Applications of Electroencephalography in Psychiatry*, ed. Wilson, W.P. Duke University Press: Durham, North Carolina [129].

SHAGASS, C., ROEMER, R.A. & STRAUMANIS, J.J. (1983) Evoked potential studies of topographic correlates of psychopathology. In *Laterality and Psychopathology*, eds Flor-Henry, P. & Gruzelier, J., pp. 395–408. Elsevier: Amsterdam [89].

SHAGASS, C., ROEMER, R.A., STRAUMANIS, J.J. & AMADEO, M. (1979) Evoked potential evidence of lateralised hemispheric dysfunction in psychoses. In *Hemisphere Asymmetries of Function in Psychopathology*, eds Gruzelier, J. & Flor-Henry, P., pp. 293–316. Elsevier/North-Holland Biomedical Press: Amsterdam [89].

SHAH, K.V., BANK, G.D. & MERSKEY, H. (1969) Survival in atherosclerotic and senile dementia. *British Journal of Psychiatry* **115**, 1283–1286 [435, 455].

SHALLICE, T. (1982) Specific impairments of planning. In *The Neuropsychology of Cognitive Function*, eds Broadbent, D.E. & Weiskrantz, L., pp. 199–209. The Royal Society: London [120].

SHALLICE, T. & BURGESS, P.W. (1991) Deficits in strategy application following frontal lobe damage in man. *Brain* **114**, 727–741 [119].

SHALLICE, T. & EVANS, M.E. (1978) The involvement of the frontal lobes in cognitive estimation. *Cortex* **14**, 294–303 [119].

SHALLICE, T. & WARRINGTON, E.K. (1987) Single and multiple component central dyslexic syndromes. Ch. 5 in *Deep Dyslexia*, 2nd edn, eds Coltheart, M., Patterson, K. & Marshall, J.C. Routledge & Kegan Paul: London [43].

SHAM, P. (1995) Schizophrenia and maternal influenza: where we stand now. *Schizophrenia Monitor* **5**, 1–5 [91].

SHANKWEILER, D. (1966) Effects of temporal-lobe damage on perception of dichotically presented melodies. *Journal of Comparative and Physiological Psychology* **62**, 115–119 [64].

SHANSKE, S. (1992) Mitochondrial encephalomyopathies: defects of nuclear DNA. *Brain Pathology* **2**, 159–162 [761].

SHAPIRO, A.K. & SHAPIRO, E. (1982) Clinical efficacy of haloperidol, pimozide, penfluridol, and clonidine in the treatment of Tourette syndrome. In *Gilles de la Tourette Syndrome*, eds Friedhoff, A.J. & Chase, T.N. *Advances in Neurology* **35**, 383–386. Raven Press: New York [687].

SHAPIRO, A.K., SHAPIRO, E.S., BRUUN, R.D. & SWEET, R.D. (1978) *Gilles de la Tourette Syndrome*. Raven Press: New York [680, 681, 683, 685].

SHAPIRO, A.K., SHAPIRO, E., WAYNE, H. & CLARKIN, J. (1972) The psychopathology of Gilles de la Tourette's syndrome. *American Journal of Psychiatry* **129**, 427–434 [684].

SHAPIRO, A.K., SHAPIRO, E., WAYNE, H. & CLARKIN, J. (1973a) Organic factors in Gilles de la Tourette's syndrome. *British Journal of Psychiatry* **122**, 659–664 [685].

SHAPIRO, A.K., SHAPIRO, E., WAYNE, H.L., CLARKIN, J. & BRUUN, R.D. (1973b) Tourette's syndrome: summary of data on 34 patients. *Psychosomatic Medicine* **35**, 419–435 [682, 685].

SHAPIRO, B.E., GROSSMAN, M. & GARDNER, H. (1981) Selective musical processing deficits in brain damaged populations. *Neuropsychologia* **19**, 161–169 [64].

SHAPIRO, L.B. (1939) Schizophrenia-like psychosis following head injury. *Illinois Medical Journal* **76**, 250–254 [191].

SHAPIRO, M.B., POST, F., LÖFVING, B. & INGLIS, J. (1956) 'Memory function' in psychiatric patients over sixty; some methodological and diagnostic implications. *Journal of Mental Science* **102**, 233–246 [98, 100, 112].

SHAPIRO, S.K. (1959) Psychosis due to bilateral carotid artery occlusion. *Minnesota Medicine* **42**, 25–27 [388].

SHAPLESKE, J., McKAY, A.P. & McKENNA, P.J. (1996) Successful treatment of tardive dystonia with clozapine and clonazepam. *British Journal of Psychiatry* **168**, 516–518 [645].

SHARMA, O.P. (1975) *Sarcoidosis: A Clinical Approach*. Charles C. Thomas: Springfield, Illinois [763].

SHARMAN, M.G., WATT, D.C., JANOTA, I. & CARRASCO, L.H. (1979) Alzheimer's disease in a mother and identical twin sons. *Psychological Medicine* **9**, 771–774 [437].

SHARPE, M.C., ARCHARD, L.C., BANATVALA, J.E., BORYSIEWICZ, L.K., CLARE, A.W., DAVID, A.S., EDWARDS, R.H.T., HAWTON, K.E.H., LAMBERT, H.P., LANE, R.J.M., McDONALD, E.M., MOWBRAY, J.F., PEARSON, D.J., PETO, T.E.A., PREEDY, V.R., SMITH, A.P., SMITH, D.G., TAYLOR, D.J., TYRELL, D.A.J., WESSELY, S. & WHITE, P.D. (1991) A report—chronic fatigue syndrome: guidelines for research. *Journal of the Royal Society of Medicine* **84**, 118–121 [371].

SHARPE, M., HAWTON, K., HOUSE, A., MOLYNEUX, A., SANDERCOCK, P., BAMFORD, J. & WARLOW, C. (1990) Mood disorders in long-term survivors of stroke: associations with brain lesion location and volume. *Psychological Medicine* **20**, 815–828 [386].

SHARPE, M., HAWTON, K., SEAGROATT, V., BAMFORD, J., HOUSE, A., MOLYNEUX, A., SANDERCOCK, P. & WARLOW, C. (1994) Depressive disorders in long-term survivors of stroke: associations with demographic and social factors, functional status, and brain lesion volume. *British Journal of Psychiatry* **164**, 380–386 [386].

SHARPE, M., HAWTON, K., SIMKIN, S., SURAWY, C., HACKMANN, A., KLIMES, I., PETO, T., WARRELL, D. & SEAGROATT, V. (1996) Cognitive behaviour therapy for the chronic fatigue syndrome: a randomised controlled trial. *British Medical Journal* **312**, 22–26 [373].

SHARPE, M., PEVELER, R. & MAYOU, R. (1992) The psychological treatment of patients with functional somatic symptoms: a practical guide. *Journal of Psychosomatic Research* **36**, 515–529 [373].

SHAW, D. & HILL, D. (1947) A case of musicogenic epilepsy. *Journal of Neurololgy, Neurosurgery and Psychiatry* **10**, 107–117 [241].

SHAW, G.M., HARPER, M.E., HAHN, B.H., EPSTEIN, L.G., GAJDUSEK, D.C., PRICE, R.W., NAVIA, B.A., PETITO, C.K., O'HARA, C.J., GROOPMAN, J.E., CHO, E.-S., OLESKE, J.M., WONG-STAAL, F. & GALLO, R.C. (1985) HTLV-III infection in brains of children and adults with AIDS encephalopathy. *Science* **227**, 177–182 [322].

SHAW, P.J., BATES, D., CARTLIDGE, N.E.F., FRENCH, J.M., HEAVISIDE, D., JULIAN, D.G. & SHAW, D.A. (1986) Early intellectual dysfunction following coronary bypass surgery. *Quarterly Journal of Medicine, New Series* **58**, 59–68 [554].

SHAW, P.J., BATES, D., CARTLIDGE, N.E.F., HEAVISIDE, D., JULIAN, D.G. & SHAW, D.A. (1985) Early neurological complications of coronary artery bypass surgery. *British Medical Journal* **291**, 1384–1386 [554].

SHEARD, M.H. (1971) Effect of lithium on human aggression. *Nature* **230**, 113–114 [298].

SHEARER, M.L. & FINCH, S.M. (1964) Periodic organic psychosis associated with recurrent herpes simplex. *New England Journal of Medicine* **271**, 494–497 [357].

SHEARMAN, J.D., CHAPMAN, R.W.G., SATSANGI, J. & RYLEY, N.G. (1992) Misuse of ecstasy. *British Medical Journal* **305**, 309 [624].

SHEDLACK, K.J., HUNTER, R., WYPER, D., McLUSKIE, R., FINK, G. & GOODWIN, G.M. (1991) The pattern of cerebral activity underlying verbal fluency shown by split-dose single photon emission tomography (SPET or SPECT) in normal volunteers. *Psychological Medicine* **21**, 687–696 [148].

SHEEHAN, H.L. & SUMMERS, V.K. (1949) The syndrome of hypopituitrism. *Quarterly Journal of Medicine* **18**, 319–378 [523, 524].

SHEEHY, M.P. & MARSDEN, C.D. (1980) Trauma and pain in spasmodic torticollis. *Lancet* **1**, 777–778 [672].

SHEEHY, M.P. & MARSDEN, C.D. (1982) Writer's cramp—a focal dystonia. *Brain* **105**, 461–480 [676].

SHEEHY, M.P., ROTHWELL, J.C. & MARSDEN, C.D. (1988) Writer's cramp. *Advances in Neurology* **50**, 457–472 [676, 677, 678].

SHEFER, V.F. (1973) Absolute number of neurones and thickness of the cerebral cortex during aging, senile and vascular dementia, and Pick's and Alzheimer's diseases. *Neuroscience and Behavioral Physiology* **6**, 319–324 [443].

SHENTON, M.E., KIKINIS, R., JOLESZ, F.A., POLLAK, S.D., LEMAY, M., WIBLE, C.G., HOKAMA, H., MARTIN, J., METCALF, D., COLEMAN, M. & McCARLEY, R.W. (1992) Abnormalities of the left temporal lobe and thought disorder in schizophrenia. A quantitative magnetic resonance imaging study. *New England Journal of Medicine* **327**, 604–612 [83].

SHEPHERD, R.H. & WADIA, N.H. (1956) Some observations on atypical features in acoustic neuromas. *Brain* **79**, 282–318 [231].

SHERLOCK, S. & DOOLEY, J. (1993) *Diseases of the Liver and Biliary System*, 9th edn. Blackwell Scientific Publications: Oxford [564, 565, 566].

SHERWIN, I. (1980) Specificity of psychopathology in epilepsy: significance of lesion laterality. In *Limbic Epilepsy and the Dyscontrol Syndrome*, eds Girgis, M. & Kiloh, L.G. *Developments in Psychiatry*, Vol. 4. Elsevier/North-Holland Biomedical Press: Amsterdam [266].

SHERWIN, I. (1981) Psychosis associated with epilepsy: significance of the laterality of the epileptogenic lesion. *Journal of Neurology, Neurosurgery and Psychiatry* **44**, 83–85 [282].

SHERWOOD, S.L. (1962) Self-induced epilepsy. *Archives of Neurology* **6**, 49–65 [241].

SHILLITO, F.H., DRINKER, C.K. & SHAUGHNESSY, T.J. (1936) The problem of nervous and mental sequelae in carbon monoxide poisoning. *Journal of the American Medical Association* **106**, 669–674 [550, 551].

SHILS, M.E. (1969) Experimental human magnesium depletion. *Medicine* **48**, 61–85 [651].

SHIMAMURA, A.P., JERNIGAN, T.L. & SQUIRE, L.R. (1988) Korsakoff's syndrome: radiological (CT) findings and neuropsychological correlates. *Journal of Neuroscience* **8**, 4400–4410 [582].

SHIMAMURA, A.P., SALMON, D.P., SQUIRE, L.R. & BUTTERS, N. (1987) Memory dysfunction and word priming in dementia and amnesia. *Behavioral Neuroscience* **101**, 347–351 [32].

SHORVON, S. (1995) Epilepsy and driving. British regulations have recently been eased. *British Medical Journal* **310**, 885–886 [307].

SHORVON, S.D., CARNEY, M.W.P., CHANARIN, I. & REYNOLDS, E.H. (1980) The neuropsychiatry of megaloblastic anaemia. *British Medical Journal* **281**, 1036–1038 [590, 592].

SHORVON, S.D. & REYNOLDS, E.H. (1979) Reduction of polypharmacy for epilepsy. *British Medical Journal* **2**, 1023–1025 [299].

SHOULSON, I. & PLASSCHE, W. (1980) Huntington disease: the specificity of computed tomography measurements. *Neurology* **30**, 382–383 [470].

SHUKLA, G.D. & KATIYAR, B.C. (1980) Psychiatric disorders in temporal lobe epilepsy: the laterality effect. *British Journal of Psychiatry* **137**, 181–182 [276].

SHUKLA, G.D., SRIVASTAVA, O.N. & KATIYAR, B.C. (1979) Sexual disturbances in temporal lobe epilepsy: a controlled study. *British Journal of Psychiatry* **134**, 288–292 [271, 272].

SHUKLA, S., COOK, B.L., MUKHERJEE, S., GOODWIN, C. & MILLER, M.G. (1987) Mania following head trauma. *American Journal of Psychiatry* **144**, 93–96 [192].

SHULMAN, R. (1967a) A survey of vitamin B$_{12}$ deficiency in an elderly psychiatric population. *British Journal of Psychiatry* **113**, 241–251 [587, 589, 590].

SHULMAN, R. (1967b) Vitamin B$_{12}$ deficiency and psychiatric illness. *British Journal of Psychiatry* **113**, 252–256 [588].

SHULMAN, R. (1967c) Psychiatric aspects of pernicious anaemia: a prospective controlled investigation. *British Medical Journal* **3**, 266–270 [588].

SIAKOTOS, A.N. (1981) Neuronal ceroid lipofuscinosis, adult (Kufs); Neuronal ceroid lipofuscinosis, adult (Parry). In *Handbook of Clinical Neurology*, Vol. 42, Part 1. *Neurogenetic Directory*, eds Vinken, P.J. & Bruyn, G.W., pp. 465–468. North-Holland Publishing Company: Amsterdam [759].

SIDTIS, J.J. (1985) Bilateral language and commisurotomy: interactions between the hemispheres with and without the corpus callosum. Ch. 20 in *Epilepsy and the Corpus Callosum*, ed. Reeves, A.G. Plenum Press: New York [313].

SIDTIS, J.J., GATSONIS, C., PRICE, R.W., SINGER, E.J., COLLIER, A.C., RICHMAN, D.D., HIRSCH, M.S., SCHAERF, F.W., FISCHL, M.A., KIEBURTZ, K., SIMPSON, D., KOCH, M.A., FEINBERG, J., DAFNI, U., & THE AIDS CLINICAL TRIALS GROUP (1993) Zidovudine treatment of the AIDS dementia complex: results of a placebo-controlled trial. *Annals of Neurology* **33**, 343–349 [335].

SIEDLER, H. & MALAMUD, N. (1963) Creutzfeldt–Jakob's disease: clinicopathologic report of 15 cases and review of the literature. *Journal of Neuropathology and Experimental Neurology* **22**, 381–402 [473].

SIEGEL, R.K. (1978) Cocaine hallucinations. *American Journal of Psychiatry* **135**, 309–314 [619].

SIEKERT, R.G. & CLARK, E.C. (1955) Neurologic signs and symptoms as early manifestations of systemic lupus erythematosus. *Neurology* **5**, 84–88 [419].

SIGAL, L.H. (1987) The neurologic presentation of vasculitic and rheumatologic syndromes. *Medicine* **66**, 157–180 [424, 425].

SIGNORET, J.P. & BALTHAZART, J. (1994) Preface. Proceedings of the International Conference on hormones, brain, and behaviour. (Tours, France, August 24–27, 1993). *Psychoneuroendocrinology* **19**, 403–406 [507].

SILBERBERG, D.H. (1989) Sarcoidosis of the nervous system. Ch. 39 in *Neurology and General Medicine*, ed. Aminoff, M.J., pp. 701–712. Churchill Livingstone: New York [764].

SILINKOVA-MALKOVA, E. & MALEK, J. (1965/66) Endocraniosis. *Neuroendrocrinology* **1**, 68–82 [769].

SILLANPÄÄ, M. (1981) Carbamazepine. Pharmacology and clinical uses. *Acta Neurologica Scandinavica* **64 (Supplement 88)**, 1–202 [301].

SILVERMAN, C.S., BRENNER, J. & MURTAGH, F.R. (1993) Hemorrhagic necrosis and vascular injury in carbon monoxide poisoning: MR demonstration. *American Journal of Neuroradiology* **14**, 168–170 [553].

SILVERMAN, M. (1949) Paranoid reaction during the phase of recovery from subarachnoid haemorrhage. *Journal of Mental Science* **95**, 706–708 [395].

SILVERMAN, M. (1964) Organic stupor subsequent to a severe head injury treated with ECT. *British Journal of Psychiatry* **110**, 648–650 [214].

SILVERSIDES, J. (1964) The neurological sequelae of electrical injury. *The Canadian Medical Association Journal* **91**, 195–204 [766].

SILVERSTEIN, A., FEVER, M.M. & SILTZBACH, L.E. (1965) Neurologic sarcoidosis. *Archives of Neurology* **12**, 1–11 [764].

SILVERSTEIN, A., GILBERT, H. & WASSERMAN, L.R. (1962) Neurologic complications of polycythaemia. *Annals of Internal Medicine* **57**, 909–916 [426].

SIM, M., TURNER, E. & SMITH, W.T. (1966) Cerebral biopsy in the investigation of presenile dementia: I, clinical aspects. *British Journal of Psychiatry* **112**, 119–125 [438, 439].

SIMARD, D. (1971) Regional cerebral blood flow and its regulation in dementia. In *Brain and Blood Flow*, ed. Russell, R.W.R. Pitman: London [434].

SIMON, A. & CAHAN, R.B. (1963) The acute brain syndrome in geriatric patients. *Psychiatric Research Reports* **16**, 8–21 [95].

SIMON, R.P. (1985) Neurosyphilis. *Archives of Neurology* **42**, 606–613 [344].

SIMPSON, B.R., WILLIAMS, M., SCOTT, J.F. & SMITH, A.C. (1961) The effects of anaesthesia and elective surgery on old people. *Lancet* **2**, 887–893 [546].

SIMPSON, J.A. (1964) Myasthenia gravis and myasthenic syndromes. Ch. 13 in *Disorders of Voluntary Muscle*, ed. Walton, J.N. Churchill. London [709, 710, 711, 712, 713].

SIMPSON, J.A. (1968) Myasthenia gravis: clinical aspects. *Proceedings of the Rayal Society of Medicine* **61**, 757–759 [711].

SIMPSON, S.A. & HARDING, A.E. (1993) Predictive testing for Huntington's disease: after the gene. *Journal of Medical Genetics* **30**, 1036–1038 [467].

SIMS, N.R., BOWEN, D.M., SMITH, C.C.T., FLACK, R.H.A., DAVISON, A.N., SNOWDEN, J.S. & NEARY, D. (1980) Glucose metabolism and acetylcholine synthesis in relation to neuronal activity in Alzheimer's disease. *Lancet* **1**, 333–335 [444].

SINFORIANI, E., MAURO, M., BONO, G., MURATORI, S., ALESSI, E. & MINOLI, L. (1991) Cognitive abnormalities and disease progression in a selected population of asymptomatic HIV-positive subjects. *AIDS* **5**, 1117–1120 [329].

SINGER, H.S. (1992) Neurochemical analysis of postmortem cortical and striatal brain tissue in patients with Tourette syndrome. Ch. 16 in *Tourette Syndrome. Genetics, Neurobiology, and Treatment*, eds Chase, T.N. Friedhoff, A.J. & Cohen, D.J. *Advances in Neurology* **58**. Raven Press: New York [685].

SINGER, H.S., HAHN, I.-H. & MORAN, T.H. (1991) Abnormal dopamine uptake sites in postmortem striatum from patients with Tourette's syndrome. *Annals of Neurology* **30**, 558–562 [685].

SINGH, S., PADI, M.H., BULLARD, H. & FREEMAN, H. (1985) Water intoxication in psychiatric patients. *British Journal of Psychiatry* **146**, 127–131 [525].

SINYOR, D., JACQUES, P., KALOUPEK, D.G., BECKER, R., GOLDENBERG, M. & COOPERSMITH, H. (1986) Post stroke depression and lesion location. An attempted replication. *Brain* **109**, 537–546 [386].

SIROTA, P., EVIATAR, J. & SPIVAK, B. (1989) Neurosyphilis presenting as psychiatric disorders. *British Journal of Psychiatry* **155**, 559–561 [343].

SITARAM, N., WEINGARTNER, H. & GILLIN, J.C. (1978) Human serial learning enhancement with arecholine and choline. Impairment with scopamine. *Science* **201**, 274–276 [503].

SIVA, A., NECDET, V., YURDAKUL, S., YARDIM, M., DENKTAŞ, H. & YAZICI, H. (1991) Neuroradiological findings in neuro–Behçet's syndrome. Ch. 46 in *Behçet's Disease. Basic and Clinical Aspects*, eds O'Duffy, J.D. & Kokmen, E. Marcel Dekker: New York [763].

SIVAKUMAR, K. & OKOCHA, C.I. (1992) Neurosyphilis and schizophrenia. *British Journal of Psychiatry* **161**, 251–254 [343].

SIVAKUMAR, K. & WILLIAMS, M. (1991) Psychiatric aspects of acromegaly—a review and case report. *Irish Journal of Psychological Medicine* **8**, 55–56 [522].

SIVAN, A.B. (1992) *Benton Visual Retention Test*, 5th edn. The Psychological Corporation: San Antonio, Texas [116].

SJÖGREN, T. (1943) Klinische und erbbiologische Untersuchungen über die Heredoataxien. *Acta Psychiatrica et Neurologica Scandinavica* **27 (Supplement)**, 1–200. Quoted by Davies, D.L. (1949) *Journal of Neurology, Neurosurgery and Psychiatry* **12**, 34–38 [705].

SJÖGREN, T., SJÖGREN, H. & LINDGREN, A.G.H. (1952) Morbus Alzheimer and morbus Pick. A genetic, clinical and pathoanatomical study. *Acta Psychiatrica et Neurologica Scandinavica* **82 (Supplement)**, 1–152 [437, 438, 461, 463].

SKEGG, K. (1993) Multiple sclerosis presenting as a pure psychiatric disorder. *Psychological Medicine* **23**, 909–914 [698].

SKILLICORN, S. (1955) Presenile cerebellar ataxia in chronic alcoholics. *Neurology* **5**, 527–534 [586].

SKINHOJ, E. & STRANDGAARD, S. (1973) Pathogenesis of hypertensive encephalopathy. *Lancet* **1**, 461–462 [399].

SKÖLDENBERG, B., FORSGREN, M., ALESTIG, K., BERGSTRÖM, T., BURMAN, L., NORLIN, K., NORRBY, R., OLDING-STENKVIST, E., STIERNSTEDT, G., UHNOO, I. & DE VAHL, K. (1984) Acyclovir versus vidarabine in herpes simplex encephalitis. Randomised multicentre study in consecutive Swedish patients. *Lancet* **2**, 707–711 [357].

SLADE, P.D. & RUSSELL, G.F.M. (1971) Developmental dyscalculia: a brief report of four cases. *Psychological Medicine* **1**, 292–298 [213].

SLATER, E. (1942) Psychosis associated with vitamin B deficiency. *British Medical Journal* **1**, 257–258 [575].

SLATER, E. (1943) The neurotic constitution: a statistical study of 2000 neurotic soldiers. *Journal of Neurology and Psychiatry* **6**, 1–16 [173, 193].

SLATER, E., BEARD, A.W. & GLITHERO, E. (1963) The schizophrenia-like psychoses of epilepsy. *British Journal of Psychiatry* **109**, 95–150 [279, 280, 282, 283, 284].

SLATER, E. & COWIE, V. (1971) *The Genetics of Mental Disorders*. Oxford University Press: Oxford [247, 467].

SLATER, E. & ROTH, M. (1969) *Clinical Psychiatry*, 3rd edn. Baillière, Tindall & Cassell: London [276, 287, 295, 310, 353, 368, 547, 553].

SLATER, E.T.O. (1962) Psychological aspects. In *Modern Views on 'Stroke' Illness*. The Chest and Heart Association: Tavistock Square, London [385].

SMALL, G.W., KUHL, D.E., RIEGE, W.H., FUJIKAWA, D.G., ASHFORD, J.W., METTER, J. & MAZZIOTTA, J.C. (1989) Cerebral glucose metabolic patterns in Alzheimer's disease. *Archives of General Psychiatry* **46**, 527–532 [449].

SMALL, G.W., SPAR, J.E. & PLOTKIN, D.A. (1987) Oral tetrahydroaminoacridine in the treatment of senile dementia, Alzheimer's type. *New England Journal of Medicine* **316**, 1604 [503].

SMALL, J.G., MILSTEIN, V. & STEVENS, J.R. (1962) Are psychomotor epileptics different? *Archives of Neurology* **7**, 187–194 [266].

SMALL, J.G., SMALL, I.F. & HAYDEN, M.P. (1966) Further psychiatric investigations of patients with temporal and non-temporal lobe epilepsy. *American Journal of Psychiatry* **123**, 303–310 [266, 282].

SMALS, A.G., KLOPPENBORG, P.W., NJO, K.T., KNOBEN, J.M. & RUTLAND, C.M. (1976) Alcohol-induced Cushingoid syndrome. *British Medical Journal* **2**, 1298 [515].

SMITH, A. (1961) Duration of impaired consciousness as an index of severity in closed head injuries: a review. *Diseases of the Nervous System* **2**, 69–74 [171].

SMITH, A. (1962) Ambiguities in concepts and studies of 'brain damage' and 'organicity'. *Journal of Nervous and Mental Disease* **135**, 311–326 [108].

SMITH, A. (1966a) Speech and other functions after left (dominant) hemispherectomy. *Journal of Neurology, Neurosurgery and Psychiatry* **29**, 467–471 [42].

SMITH, A. (1966b) Intellectual functions in patients with lateralised frontal tumours. *Journal of Neurology, Neurosurgery and Psychiatry* **29**, 52–59 [222].

SMITH, A. (1972) Dominant and non-dominant hemispherectomy. Ch. 3 in *Drugs, Development and Cerebral Function*, ed. Smith, W.L. Thomas: Springfield, Illinois [42].

SMITH, A. (1978) Lenneberg, Locke, Zangwill, and the neuropsychology of language and language disorders. Ch. 7 in *Psychology and Biology of Language and Thought*, eds Lenneberg, E., Brown, R. & Miller, G. Academic Press: New York [49].

SMITH, A.D.M. (1960) Megaloblastic madness. *British Medical Journal* **2**, 1840–1845 [587].

SMITH, C.M. (1958) Comments and observations on psychogenic hypersomnia. *Archives of Neurology and Psychiatry* **80**, 619–624 [735].

SMITH, C.M. & HAMILTON, J. (1959) Psychological factors in the narcolepsy–cataplexy syndrome. *Psychosomatic Medicine* **21**, 40–49 [727].

SMITH, C.M. & SWASH, M. (1980) Effects of cholinergic drugs on memory in Alzheimer's disease. In *Aging of the Brain and Dementia, Aging*, Vol. 13, eds Amaducci, L., Davison, A.N. & Antuono, P. Raven Press: New York [503].

SMITH, D.B. (1991) Cognitive effects of antiepileptic drugs. Ch. 13 in *Neurobehavioral Problems in Epilepsy*, eds Smith, D.B., Treiman, D.M. & Trimble, M.R. *Advances in Neurology* **55**. Raven Press: New York [263].

SMITH, D.B. & OBBENS, E.A.M.T. (1979) Antifolate–antiepileptic relationships. Ch. 28 in *Folic Acid in Neurology, Psychiatry, and Internal Medicine*, eds Botez, M.I. & Reynolds, E.H. Raven Press: New York [592].

SMITH, F.W., BESSON, J.A.O., GEMMELL, H.G. & SHARP, P.F. (1988) The use of technetium-99m-HMPAO in the assessment of patients with dementia and other neuropsychiatric conditions. *Journal of Cerebral Blood Flow and Metabolism* **8**, S116–S122 [148, 471].

SMITH, H.V. & SPALDING, J.M.K. (1959) Outbreak of paralysis in Morocco due to *ortho*-cresyl phosphate poisoning. *Lancet* **2**, 1019–1021 [637].

SMITH, J.B., WESTMORELAND, B.F., REAGAN, T.J. & SANDOK, B.A. (1975) A distinctive clinical EEG profile in herpes simplex encephalitis. *Mayo Clinic Proceedings* **50**, 469–474 [357].

SMITH, J.S. & BRANDON, S. (1970) Acute carbon monoxide poisoning—3 years experience in a defined population. *Postgraduate Medical Journal* **46**, 65–70 [550, 551].

SMITH, J.S. & BRANDON, S. (1973) Morbidity from acute carbon monoxide poisoning at three-year follow-up. *British Medical Journal* **1**, 318–321 [551, 552].

SMITH, J.S. & KILOH, L.G. (1981) The investigation of dementia: results in 200 consecutive admissions. *Lancet* **1**, 824–827 [490, 491].

SMITH, J.W., BURT, D.W. & CHAPMAN, R.F. (1973) Intelligence and brain damage in alcoholics: a study in patients of middle and upper social class. *Quarterly Journal of Studies on Alcohol* **34**, 414–422 [604].

SMITH, M.G., LENNETTE, E.M. & REAMES, H.R. (1941) Isolation of the virus of herpes simplex and the demonstration of intranuclear inclusions in a case of acute encephalitis. *American Journal of Pathology* **17**, 55–68 [356].

SMITH, P.E.M., ZEIDLER, M., IRONSIDE, J.W., ESTIBEIRO, P. & MOSS, T.H. (1995) Creutzfeldt–Jakob disease in a dairy farmer. *British Medical Journal* **346**, 898 [475].

SMITH, P.L.C., TREASURE, T., NEWMAN, S.P., JOSEPH, P., ELL, P.J., SCHNEIDAU, A. & HARRISON, M.J.G. (1986) Cerebral consequences of cardiopulmonary bypass. *Lancet* **1**, 823–825 [554].

SMITH, R. (1982a) The world's best system of compensating injury? *British Medical Journal* **284**, 1243–1245 [207].

SMITH, R. (1982b) Problems with a no-fault system of accident compensation. *British Medical Journal* **284**, 1323–1325 [207].

SMITH, R. & OLIVER, R.A.M. (1967) Sudden onset of psychosis in association with vitamin-B_{12} deficiency. *British Medical Journal* **3**, 34 [588].

SMITH, S.J.M. & KOCEN, R.S. (1988) A Creutzfeldt–Jakob like syndrome due to lithium toxicity. *Journal of Neurology, Neurosurgery and Psychiatry* **51**, 120–123 [626].

SMITH, W.T. (1976) Intoxications, poisons and related metabolic disorders. Ch. 4 in *Greenfield's Neuropathology*, 3rd edn, eds Blackwood, W. & Corsellis, J.A.N. Edward Arnold: London [663].

SMYTH, G.E. & STERN, K. (1938) Tumours of the thalamus—a clinicopathological study. *Brain* **61**, 339–374 [228].

SMYTHIES, J.R. (1967) The previous personality in parkinsonism. *Journal of Psychosomatic Research* **11**, 169–171 [661].

SNAITH, M.L. & ISENBERG, D.A. (1996) Systemic lupus erythematosus and related disorders. Section 18.11.3 in *Oxford Textbook of Medicine*, 3rd edn, eds Weatherall, D.J., Ledingham, J.G.G. & Warrell, D.A. Oxford University Press: Oxford [422].

SNAITH, R.P., MEHTA, S. & RABY, A.H. (1970) Serum folate and vitamin B_{12} in epileptics with and without mental illness. *British Journal of Psychiatry* **116**, 179–183 [592].

SNEATH, P., CHANARIN, I., HODKINSON, H.M., McPHERSON, C.K. & REYNOLDS, E.H. (1973) Folate status in a geriatric population and its relation to dementia. *Age and Ageing* **2**, 177–182 [592].

SNEDDON, J. (1980) Myasthenia gravis: a study of social, medical, and emotional problems in 26 patients. *Lancet* **1**, 526–528 [711, 712].

SNIDER, W.D., SIMPSON, D.M., NIELSEN, S., GOLD, W.M., METROKA, C.E. & POSNER, J.B. (1983) Neurological complications of acquired immune deficiency syndrome: analysis of 50 patients. *Annals of Neurology* **14**, 403–418 [319, 324].

SNOWDEN, J.S., GOULDING, P.J. & NEARY, D. (1989) Semantic dementia: a form of circumscribed cerebral atrophy. *Behavioural Neurology* **2**, 167–182 [753].

SNOWDEN, J., GRIFFTHS, H. & NEARY, D. (1994) Semantic dementia: autobiographical contribution to preservation of meaning. *Cognitive Neuropsychology* **11**, 265–288 [753].

SNOWDEN, J.S., NEARY, D., MANN, D.M.A., GOULDING, P.J. & TESTA, H.J. (1992) Progressive language disorder due to lobar atrophy. *Annals of Neurology* **31**, 174–183 [752].

SNOWLING, M.J. (1996) Dyslexia: a hundred years on. A verbal not a visual disorder, which responds to early intervention. *British Medical Journal* **313**, 1096–1097 [48].

SNOWLING, M., GOULANDRIS, N. & STACKHOUSE, J. (1994) Phonological constraints on learning to read: evidence from single-case studies of reading difficulty. Ch. 6 in *Reading Development and Dyslexia*, eds Hulme, C. & Snowling, M. Whurr Publishers Ltd: London [48].

SOFFER, L.J., IANNACCONE, A. & GABRILOVE, J.L. (1961) Cushing's syndrome. A study of fifty patients. *American Journal of Medicine* **30**, 129–146 [517].

SOGES, L.J., CACAYORIN, E.D., PETRO, G.R. & RAMACHANDRAN, T.S. (1988) Migraine: evaluation by MR. *American Journal of Neuroradiology* **9**, 425–429 [401].

SOHLBERG, M.M. & MATEER, C.A. (1987) Effectiveness of an attention-training program. *Journal of Clinical and Experimental Neuropsychology* **9**, 117–130 [213].

SOLOMON, S. (1954) A critical review of the Morgagni–Stewart–Morel syndrome. *New York State Journal of Medicine* **54**, 629–648 [769].

SOLOWIJ, N., MICHIE, P.T. & FOX, A.M. (1991) Effects of long-term cannabis use on selective attention: an event-related potential study. *Pharmacology, Biochemistry and Behavior* **40**, 683–688 [616].

SOMERVILLE, R.A. (1985) Ultrastructural links between scrapie and Alzheimer's disease. *Lancet* **1**, 504–506 [474].

SOOD, G.K., SARIN, S.K., MAHAPTRA, J. & BROOR, S.L. (1989) Comparative efficacy of psychometric tests in detection of subclinical hepatic encephalopathy in non-alcoholic cirrhotics: search for a rational approach. *American Journal of Gastroenterology* **84**, 156–159 [565].

SOTANIEMI, K.A., MONONEN, H. & HOKKANEN, T.E. (1986) Long-term cerebral outcome after open-heart surgery. A five year neuropsychological follow-up study. *Stroke* **17**, 410–416 [554].

SOURANDER, P. & SJÖGREN, H. (1970) The concept of Alzheimer's disease and its clinical implications. In *Alzheimer's Disease*, Ciba Foundation Symposium, eds Wolstenholme, G.E.W. & O'Connor, M. Churchill: London [433, 435, 439, 449].

SOURS, J.A. (1963) Narcolepsy and other disturbances in the sleep–waking rhythm: a study of 115 cases with review of the literature. *Journal of Nervous and Mental Disease* **137**, 525–542 [726, 734].

SOURS, J.A., FRUMKIN, P. & INDERMILL, R.R. (1963) Somnambulism: its clinical significance and dynamic meaning in late adolescence and adulthood. *Archives of General Psychiatry* **9**, 400–413 [727, 736].

SPEED, N., ENGDAHL, B., SCHWARTZ, J. & EBERLY, R. (1989) Post traumatic stress disorder as a consequence of the POW experience. *Journal of Nervous and Mental Diseases* **177**, 147–153 [195].

SPENCE, S. (1995) The psychopathology of acromegaly. *Irish Journal of Psychological Medicine* **12**, 142–144 [522].

SPENCE, S.A., TAYLOR, D.G. & HIRSCH, S.R. (1995) Depressive disorder due to craniopharyngioma. *Journal of the Royal Society of Medicine* **88**, 637–638 [234].

SPENCER, D.J. (1970) Cannabis induced psychosis. *West Indian Medical Journal* **19**, 228–230 [614].

SPENCER, S.S., SPENCER, D.D., WILLIAMSON, P.D. & MATTSON, R.H. (1983) Sexual automatisms in complex partial seizures. *Neurology* **33**, 527–533 [273].

SPERLING, M. (1953) Psychodynamics and treatment of petit mal in children. *International Journal of Psychoanalysis* **34**, 248–252 [307].

SPERLING, M. (1964) A further contribution to the psychoanalytic study of migraine and psychogenic headaches. *International Journal of Psychoanalysis* **45**, 549–557 [403, 410].

SPERRY, R.W. (1966) Brain bisection and consciousness. Ch. 13 in *Brain and Conscious Experience*, ed. Eccles, J.C. Springer: Berlin [41].

SPERRY, R.W. & GAZZANIGA, M.S. (1967) Language following surgical disconnection of the hemispheres. In *Brain Mechanisms Underlying Speech and Language*, ed. Darley, F.L. Grune & Stratton: New York [41, 313].

SPIEGEL, A.M. (1989) Pseudohypoparathyroidism. Ch. 79 in *The Metabolic Basis of Inherited Disease*, 6th edn, eds Scriver, C.R., Beaudet, A.L., Sly, W.S. & Valle, D. McGraw-Hill: New York [531].

SPIEGEL, L.A. & OBERNDORF, C.P. (1946) Narcolepsy as a psychogenic symptom. *Psychosomatic Medicine* **8**, 28–35 [735].

SPIELMEYER, G. (1969) Causation in German law. Ch. 45 in *The Late Effects of Head Injury*, eds Walker, A.E., Caveness, W.F. & Critchley, M. Thomas: Springfield, Illinois [210].

SPIERS, J. & HIRSCH, S.R. (1978) Severe lithium toxicity with 'normal' serum concentrations. *British Medical Journal* **1**, 815–816 [626].

SPIES, T.D., ARING, C.D., GELPERIN, J. & BEAN, W.B. (1938) The mental symptoms of pellagra: their relief with nicotinic acid. *American Journal of the Medical Sciences* **196**, 461–475 [573].

SPILLANE, J.A., WHITE, P., GOODHARDT, M.J., FLACK, R.H.A., BOWEN, D.M. & DAVISON, A.N. (1977) Selective vulnerability of neurones in organic dementia. *Nature* **266**, 558–559 [444].

SPILLANE, J.D. (1947) *Nutritional Disorders of the Nervous System*. Livingstone: Edinburgh [573, 576].

SPILLANE, J.D. (1951) Nervous and mental disorders in Cushing's syndrome. *Brain* **74**, 72–94 [517].

SPILLANE, J.D. (1962) Five boxers. *British Medical Journal* **2**, 1205–1210 [204].

SPITTLE, B. & PARKER, J. (1993) Wernicke's encephalopathy complicating schizophrenia. *Australia and New Zealand Journal of Psychiatry* **27**, 638–682 [576].

SPITZER, R.L., ENDICOTT, J. & ROBINS, E. (1975) Clinical criteria for psychiatric diagnosis and DSM-III. *American Journal of Psychiatry* **132**, 1187–1192 [84].

SPITZER, R.L., FLEISS, J.L., BURDOCK, E.I. & HARDESTY, A.S. (1964) The mental status schedule: rationale, reliability and validity. *Comprehensive Psychiatry* **5**, 384–395 [123].

SPOKES, E.G.S. (1980) Neurochemical alterations in Huntington's chorea: a study of post-mortem brain tissue. *Brain* **103**, 179–210 [467].

SPRATLING, W.P. (1902) Epilepsy in its relation to crime. *Journal of Nervous and Mental Disease* **29**, 481–496 [255].

SPRING, G.K. (1979) Neurotoxicity with combined use of lithium and thioridazine. *Journal of Clinical Psychiatry* **40**, 135–138 [626].

SPROFKIN, B.E. & SCIARRA, D. (1952) Korsakoff psychosis associated with cerebral tumours. *Neurology* **2**, 427–434 [227].

SQUIRE, L.R. (1981) Two forms of human amnesia: an analysis of forgetting. *The Journal of Neuroscience* **1**, 635–640 [38].

SQUIRE, L.R. (1982) The neuropsychology of human memory. *Annual Review of Neuroscience* **5**, 241–273 [38].

SQUIRE, L.R. (1986) Mechanisms of memory. *Science* **232**, 1612–1619 [29].

SQUIRE, L.R. (1987) Memory: neural organization and behavior. Ch. 8 in *Handbook of Physiology—Section I: The Nervous System V*, Vol. 5, Part I, ed. Mountcastle, V.B., pp. 295–371. American Physiological Society: Bethesda, Maryland [24, 25, 29].

SQUIRE, L.R., AMARAL, D.G. & PRESS, G.A. (1990) Magnetic resonance imaging of the hippocampal formation and mammillary nuclei distinguish medial temporal lobe and diencephalic amnesia. *Journal of Neuroscience* **10**, 3106–3117 [27].

SQUIRE, L.R. & COHEN, N.J. (1982) Remote memory, retrograde amnesia, and the neuropsychology of memory. In *Human Memory and Amnesia*, ed. Cermak, L.S. Lawrence Erlbaum Associates: Hillsdale, New Jersey [36].

SQUIRE, L.R. & MOORE, R.Y. (1979) Dorsal thalamic lesion in a noted case of human memory dysfunction. *Annals of Neurology* **6**, 503–506 [25].

SQUIRE, L.R., OJEMANN, J.G., MIEZEN, F.M., PETERSEN, S.E., VIDEEN, T.O. & RAICHLE, M.E. (1992) Activation of the hippocampus in normal humans: a functional anatomical study of memory. *Proceedings of the National Academy of Science, USA* **89**, 1837–1841 [28].

SQUIRE, L.R., SHIMAMURA, A.P. & GRAF, P. (1987) Strength and duration of priming effects in normal subjects and amnesic patients. *Neuropsychologia* **25**, 195–210 [30].

SQUIRE, L.R. & SLATER, P.C. (1975) Forgetting in very long-term memory as assessed by an improved questionnaire technique. *Journal of Experimental Psychology: Human Learning and Memory* **104**, 50–54 [36].

SROKA, H., ELIZAN, T.S., YAHR, M.D., BURGER, A. & MENDOZA, M.R. (1981) Organic mental syndrome and confusional states in Parkinson's disease. Relationship to computerised tomographic signs of cerebral atrophy. *Archives of Neurology* **38**, 339–342 [655].

STACY, M. & JANKOVIC, J. (1992) Clinical and neurobiological aspects of Parkinson's disease. Ch. 2 in *Parkinson's Disease: Neurobehavioral Aspects*, eds Huber, S.J. & Cummings, J.L. Oxford University Press: New York [648].

STAFFORD-CLARK, D. & TAYLOR, F.H. (1949) Clinical and electro-encephalographic studies of prisoners charged with murder. *Journal of Neurology, Neurosurgery and Psychiatry* **12**, 325–330 [128, 274].

STANDAGE, K.F. & FENTON, G.W. (1975) Psychiatric symptom profiles of patients with epilepsy: a controlled investigation. *Psychological Medicine* **5**, 152–160 [276].

STANLEY, J.A., WILLIAMSON, P.C., DROST, D.J., CARR, T., RYLETT, J. & MERSKEY, H. (1992) In vivo proton magnetic resonance spectroscopy in never treated schizophrenics. *New Research Abstracts* **10**. American Psychiatric Association: Washington [143].

STANLEY, J.A., WILLIAMSON, P.C., DROST, D.J., CARR, T., RYLETT, J. & MERSKEY, H. (1993) The study of schizophrenia via in vivo ^{31}P and ^{1}H MRS. *Schizophrenia Research* **9**, 210 [143].

STANOVICH, K.E. (1991) The theoretical and practical consequences of discrepancy definitions of dyslexia. Ch. 9 in *Dyslexia, Integrating Theory and Practice*, eds Snowling, M. & Thomson, M. Whurr Publishers: London [48].

STARKMAN, M.N., GEBARSKI, S.S., BERENT, S. & SCHTEINGART, D.E. (1992) Hippocampal formation volume, memory dysfunction, and cortisone levels in patients with Cushing's syndrome. *Biological Psychiatry* **32**, 756–765 [518].

STARKMAN, M.N., SCHTEINGART, D.E. & SCHORK, M.A. (1981) Depressed mood and other psychiatric manifestations of Cushing's syndrome: relationship to hormone levels. *Psychosomatic Medicine* **43**, 3–18 [516].

STARKSTEIN, S.E., BOSTON, J.D. & ROBINSON, R.G. (1988) Mechanisms of mania after brain injury. 12 case reports and review of the literature. *Journal of Nervous and Mental Disease* **176**, 87–100 [192, 235, 258, 387].

STARKSTEIN, S.E., ESTEGUY, M., BERTHIER, M.L., GARCIA, H. & LEIGUARDA, R. (1989) Evoked potentials, reaction time and cognitive performance in on and off phases of Parkinson's disease. *Journal of Neurology, Neurosurgery and Psychiatry* **52**, 338–340 [132].

STARKSTEIN, S.E., FEDOROFF, J.P., PRICE, T.R., LEIGUARDA, R. & ROBINSON, R.G. (1992) Anosognosia in patients with cerebrovascular lesions. A study of causative factors. *Stroke* **23**, 1446–1453 [70, 388].

STARKSTEIN, S.E., ROBINSON, R.G. & PRICE, T.R. (1987) Comparison of cortical and subcortical lesions in the production of post-stroke mood disorders. *Brain* **110**, 1045–1059 [386].

STAROSTA-RUBINSTEIN, S. (1995) Treatment of Wilson's disease. Ch. 4 in *Treatment of Movement Disorders*, ed. Kurlan, R. Lippincott: Philadelphia [663, 664].

STARR, A. & PHILLIPS, L. (1970) Verbal and motor memory in the amnestic syndrome. *Neuropsychologia* **8**, 75–88 [30].

STATON, M.A., DONALD, A.G. & GREEN, G.B. (1976) Zinc deficiency presenting as schizophrenia. *Current Concepts in Psychiatry* **2**, 11–14 [562].

STAUDER, K.H. (1934) Die tödliche Katatonie. *Archiv für Psychatrie und Nervenkrankheiten* **102**, 614–634 [556].

STEADMAN, J.H. & GRAHAM, J.G. (1970) Head injuries: an analysis and follow-up study. *Proceedings of the Royal Society of Medicine* **63**, 23–28 [171, 177, 178, 209].

STEBBINS, G.T. & TANNER, C.M. (1992) Behavioral effects of intrastriatal adrenal medullary surgery in Parkinson's disease. Ch. 24 in *Parkinson's Disease. Neurobehavioral Aspects*, eds Huber, S.J. & Cummings, J.L. Oxford University Press: Oxford [652].

STEEL, R. (1960) GPI in an observation ward. *Lancet* **1**, 121–123 [343].

STEELE, J.C. (1972) Progressive supranuclear palsy. *Brain* **95**, 693–704 [666].

STEELE, J.C., RICHARDSON, J.C. & OLSZEWSKI, J. (1964) Progressive supranuclear palsy. *Archives of Neurology* **10**, 333–359 [666].

STEENLAND, K. (1996) Chronic neurological effects of organophosphate pesticides. *British Medical Journal* **312**, 1312–1313 [637].

STEHLING, M.K., TURNER, R. & MANSFIELD, P. (1991) Echo-planar imaging: magnetic resonance imaging in a fraction of a second. *Science* **254**, 43–50 [142].

STEIN, G. (1993) Drug treatment of the personality disorder. Ch. 11 in *Personality Disorder Reviewed*, eds Tyrer, P. & Stein, G. Gaskell: London [298].

STEIN, J.A. & TSCHUDY, D.P. (1970) Acute intermittent porphyria. A Clinical and biochemical study of 46 patients. *Medicine* **49**, 1–16 [567].

STEINBERG, D., HIRSCH, S.R., MARSTON, S.D., REYNOLDS, K. & SUTTON, R.N.P. (1972) Influenza infection causing manic psychosis. *British Journal of Psychiatry* **120**, 531–535 [360].

STEINGART, A., HACHINSKI, V.C., LAU, C., FOX, A.J., DIAZ, F., CAPE, R., LEE, D., INZITARI, D. & MERSKEY, H. (1987a) Cognitive and neurologic findings in subjects with diffuse white matter lucencies on computed tomographic scan (leuko-araiosis). *Archives of Neurology* **44**, 32–35 [459].

STEINGART, A., HACHINSKI, V.C., LAU, C., FOX, A.J., FOX, H., LEE, D., INZITARI, D. & MERSKEY, H. (1987b) Cognitive and neurologic findings in demented patients with diffuse white matter lucencies on computed tomographic scan (leuko-araiosis). *Archives of Neurology* **44**, 36–39 [459].

STEINMETZ, E.F. & VROOM, F.Q. (1972) Transient global amnesia. *Neurology* **22**, 1193–1200 [415].

STELL, R., THOMPSON, P.D. & MARSDEN, C.D. (1988) Botulinum toxin in spasmodic torticollis. *Journal of Neurology, Neurosurgery and Psychiatry* **51**, 920–923 [675].

STENBÄCK, A. & HAAPANEN, E. (1967) Azotaemia and psychosis. *Acta Psychiatrica Scandinavica* **197 (Supplement)**, 1–65 [555].

STENGEL, E. (1941) On the aetiology of the fugue states. *Journal of Mental Science* **87**, 572–599 [297].

STENGEL, E. (1943a) Further studies on pathological wandering (fugues with the impulse to wander). *Journal of Mental Science* **89**, 224–241 [297].

STENGEL, E. (1943b) A study on the symptomatology and differential diagnosis of Alzheimer's disease and Pick's disease. *Journal of Mental Science* **89**, 1–20 [463].

STENGEL, E. (1964) Psychopathology of dementia. *Proceedings of the Royal Society of Medicine* **57**, 911–914 [15].

STENGEL, E. (1965) Pain and the psychiatrist. *British Journal of Psychiatry* **111**, 795–802 [74].

STEPHENS, D.A. (1967) Psychotoxic effects of benzhexol hydrochloride (artane). *British Journal of Psychiatry* **113**, 213–218 [658].

STERKY, G. (1963) Diabetic schoolchildren. *Acta Paediatrica Scandinavica* **144 (Supplement)**, 1–39 [536].

STERN, B.J., KRUMHOLZ, A., JOHNS, C., SCOTT, P. & NISSIM, J. (1985) Sarcoidosis and its neurological manifestations. *Archives of Neurology* **42**, 909–917 [763, 764].

STERN, K. (1939) Severe dementia associated with bilateral symmetrical degeneration of the thalamus. *Brain* **62**, 157–171 [755].

STERN, Y. & MARDER, K. (1991) The neurology and neuropsychology of HIV infection. Ch. 12 in *Handbook of Neuropsychology*, Vol. 5, eds Boller, F. & Grafman, J. Elsevier Science Publications: Holland [321, 328].

STERN, Y., MARDER, K., BELL, K., CHEN, J., DOONEIEF, G., GOLDSTEIN, S., MINDRY, D., RICHARDS, M., SANO, M., WILLIAMS, J., GORMAN, J., EHRHARDT, A. & MAYEUX, R. (1991) Multidisciplinary baseline assessment of homosexual men with and without human immunodeficiency virus infection. III. Neurologic and neuropsychological findings. *Archives of General Psychiatry* **48**, 131–138 [328].

STERNBERG, D.E. (1986) Neuroleptic malignant syndrome: the pendulum swings. *American Journal of Psychiatry* **143**, 1273–1275 [627].

STERNER, R.T. & PRICE, W.R. (1973) Restricted riboflavin: within-subject behavioral effects in humans. *American Journal of Clinical Nutrition* **26**, 150–160 [571].

STERNS, R.H., RIGGS, J.E. & SCHOCHET, S.S. (1986) Osmotic demyelination syndrome following correction of hyponatremia. *New England Journal of Medicine* **314**, 1535–1542 [586].

STEVENS, H. (1966a) Paroxysmal choreo-athetosis. *Archives of Neurology* **14**, 415–421 [291].

STEVENS, J.R. (1959) Emotional activation of the electroencephalogram in patients with convulsive disorders. *Journal of Nervous and Mental Disease* **128**, 339–351 [248].

STEVENS, J.R. (1966b) Psychiatric implications of psychomotor epilepsy. *Archives of General Psychiatry* **14**, 461–471 [253, 266, 282].

STEVENS, J.R. (1982) Neuropathology of schizophrenia. *Archives of General Psychiatry* **39**, 1131–1139 [86].

STEVENS, J.R. (1990) Psychiatric consequences of temporal lobectomy for intractable seizures: a 20–30-year follow-up of 14 cases. *Psychological Medicine* **20**, 529–545 [313].

STEVENS, J.R. (1991) Psychosis and the temporal lobe. Ch. 5 in *Neurobehavioral Problems in Epilepsy*, eds Smith, D.B., Treiman, D.M. & Trimble, M.R. *Advances in Neurology* **55**. Raven Press: New York [282].

STEVENS, J.R. (1992) Abnormal reinnervation as a basis for schizophrenia: a hypothesis. *Archives of General Psychiatry* **49**, 238–243 [283].

STEVENS, J.R. & HERMANN, B.P. (1981) Temporal lobe epilepsy, psychopathology, and violence: the state of the evidence. *Neurology* **31**, 1127–1132 [266, 267].

STEVENS, M. (1979) Famous personality test: a test for measuring remote memory. *Bulletin of the British Psychological Society* **32**, 211 [36].

STEVENSON, J.F. (1967) M.Sc. Thesis, University of Cambridge. Quoted by Warrington, E.K. (1970) in *The Psychological Assessment of Mental and Physical Handicaps*, ed. Mittler, P. Methuen: London [106].

STEVENTON, G.B., HEAFIELD, M.T.E., WARING, R.H. & WILLIAMS, A.C. (1989) Xenobiotic metabolism in Parkinson's disease. *Neurology* **39**, 883–887 [648].

STEWART, I.McD.G. (1953) Headache and hypertension. *Lancet* **1**, 1261–1266 [398].

STIBE, C.M.H., LEES, A.J., KEMPSTER, P.A. & STERN, G.M. (1988) Subcutaneous apomorphine in Parkinsonian on-off oscillations. *Lancet* **1**, 403–406 [651].

STORES, G. (1978) School-children with epilepsy at risk for learning and behaviour problems. *Developmental Medicine and Child Neurology* **20**, 502–508 [261].

STORES, G. (1981) Problems of learning and behaviour in children with epilepsy. Ch. 4 in *Epilepsy and Psychiatry*, eds Reynolds, E.H. & Trimble, M.R. Churchill Livingstone: Edinburgh and London [264].

STORES, G., ZAIWALLA, Z. & BERGEL, N. (1991) Frontal lobe complex partial seizures in children: a form of epilepsy at particular risk of misdiagnosis. *Developmental Medicine and Child Neurology* **33**, 998–1009 [249].

STOREY, P.B. (1966) Lumbar air encephalography in chronic schizophrenia: a controlled experiment. *British Journal of Psychiatry* **112**, 135–144 [140].

STOREY, P.B. (1967) Psychiatric sequelae of subarachnoid haemorrhage. *British Medical Journal* **3**, 261–266 [393].

STOREY, P.B. (1969) The precipitation of subarachnoid haemorrhage. *Journal of Psychosomatic Research* **13**, 175–182 [396].

STOREY, P.B. (1970) Brain damage and personality change after subarachnoid heamorrhage. *British Journal of Psychiatry* **117**, 129–142 [393, 395].

STOREY, P.B. (1972) Emotional disturbances before and after subarachnoid haemorrhage. In *Physiology, Emotion and Psychosomatic Illness*, Ciba Foundation Symposium No. 8 (new series), eds Porter, R. & Knight, J., pp. 337–343. Associated Scientific Publishers: Amsterdam [393, 395, 396].

STORM-MATHISEN, A. (1969) General paresis. A follow up study of 203 patients. *Acta Psychiatrica Scandinavica* **45**, 118–132 [342].

STORM VAN LEEUWEN, W., BICKFORD, R., BRAZIER, M., COBB, W.A., DONDEY, M., GASTAUT, H., GLOOR, P., HENRY, C.E., HESS, R., KNOTT, J.R., KUGLER, J., LAIRY, G.C., LOEB, C., MAGNUS, O., OLLER DAU-RELLA, L., PETSCHE, H., SCHWAB, R., WALTER, W.G. & WIDÉN, L. (1966) Proposal for an EEG terminology by the terminology committee of the international federation for electroencephalography and clinical neurophysiology. *Electroencephalography and Clinical Neurophysiology* **20**, 306–310 [127].

STRACHAN, R.W. & HENDERSON, J.G. (1965) Psychiatric syndromes due to avitaminosis B$_{12}$ with normal blood and marrow. *Quarterly Journal of Medicine* **34**, 303–317 [588, 589].

STRACHAN, R.W. & HENDERSON, J.G. (1967) Dementia and folate deficiency. *Quarterly Journal of Medicine* **36**, 189–204 [591].

STRANG, J., GRIFFITHS, P., ABBEY, J. & GOSSOP, M. (1994) Survey of use of injected benzodiazepines among drug users in Britain. *British Medical Journal* **308**, 1082 [610].

STRANG, J., JOHNS, A. & CAAN, W. (1993) Cocaine in the UK—1991. *British Journal of Psychiatry* **162**, 1–13 [620].

STRAUSS, I. & KESCHNER, M. (1935) Mental symptoms in cases of tumour of the frontal lobe. *Archives of Neurology and Psychiatry* **33**, 986–1005 [222, 223].

STRECKER, E.A. & EBAUGH, F.G. (1924) Neuropsychiatric sequelae of cerebral trauma in children. *Archives of Neurology and Psychiatry* **12**, 443–453 [203].

STREICHER, H.Z., GABOW, P.A., MOSS, A.H., KONO, D. & KAEHNY, W.D. (1981) Syndromes of toluene sniffing in adults. *Annals of Internal Medicine* **94**, 758–762 [630].

STRICH, S.J. (1956) Diffuse degeneration of the cerebral white matter in severe dementia following head injury. *Journal of Neurology, Neurosurgery and Psychiatry* **19**, 163–185 [163].

STRICH, S.J. (1969) The pathology of brain damage due to blunt head injuries. Ch. 51 in *The Late Effects of Head Injury*, eds Walker, A.E., Caveness, W.F. & Critchley, M. Thomas: Springfield, Illinois [163, 186].

STRITTMATTER, W.J., SAUNDERS, A.M., SCHMECHEL, D., PERICAK-VANCE, M., ENGHILD, J., SALVESEN, G.S. & ROSES, A.D. (1993) Apolipoprotein E: high-avidity binding to β-amyloid and increased frequency of type 4 allele in late-onset familial Alzheimer disease. *Proceedings of the National Academy of Science* **90**, 1977–1981 [448].

STROBOS, R.R.J. (1953) Tumours of temporal lobe. *Neurology* **3**, 752–760 [225, 226].

STROOP, J.R. (1935) Studies of interference in serial verbal reactions. *Journal of Experimental Psychology* **18**, 643–662 [118].

STUDDY, P.R. (1996) Sarcoidosis. Section 17.10.10 in *Oxford Textbook of Medicine*, 3rd edn, eds Weatherall, D.J., Ledingham, J.G.G. & Warrell, D.A. Oxford University Press: Oxford [763].

STUSS, D.T., ALEXANDER, M.P., LIEBERMAN, A. & LEVINE, H. (1978) An extraordinary form of confabulation. *Neurology* **28**, 1166–1172 [31].

STUSS, D.T. & BENSON, D.F. (1986) *The Frontal Lobes*. Raven Press: New York [79].

STUSS, D.T., STETHEM, L.L., HUGENHOLTZ, H., PICTON, T., PIVIK, J. & RICHARDS, M.T. (1989) Reaction time after head injury: fatigue, divided and focused attention, and consistency of performance. *Journal of Neurology, Neurosurgery and Psychiatry* **52**, 742–748 [184].

STUTEVILLE, P. & WELCH, K. (1958) Subdural haematoma in the elderly person. *Journal of the American Medical Association* **168**, 1445–1449 [411, 412].

SUBIRANA, A. (1969) Handedness and Cerebral dominance. Ch. 13 in *Handbook of Clinical Neurology*, Vol. 4, eds Vinken, P.J. & Bruyn, G.W. North-Holland Publishing Co.: Amsterdam [40].

SUDDATH, R.L., CASANOVA, M.F., GOLDBERG, T., DANIEL, D.G., KELSOE, J.R. & WEINBERGER, D.R. (1989) Temporal lobe pathology in schizophrenia: a quantitative magnetic resonance imaging study. *American Journal of Psychiatry* **146**, 464–472 [85].

SUDDATH, R.L., CHRISTISON, G.W., TORREY, E.F., CASANOVA, M.F. & WEINBERGER, D.R. (1990) Anatomical abnormalities in the brain of monozygotic twins discordant for schizophrenia. *New England Journal of Medicine* **322**, 789–794 [85].

SUMMERS, W.K., MAJOUSKI, L.V., MARSH, G.M., TACHIKI, K. & KLING, A. (1986) Oral tetrahydroaminoacridine in long-term treatment of senile dementia, Alzheimer type. *New England Journal of Medicine* **315**, 1241–1245 [503].

SUMMERSKILL, W.H.J., DAVIDSON, E.A., SHERLOCK, S. & STEINER, R.E. (1956) The neuropsychiatric syndrome associated with hepatic cirrhosis and an extensive portal collateral circulation. *Quarterly Journal of Medicine* **25**, 245–266 [563, 565].

SUMNER, D. (1969) The diagnosis of intracranial tumours. *British Journal of Hospital Medicine* **2**, 489–494 [231, 233].

SURRIDGE, D. (1969) An investigation into some psychiatric aspects of multiple sclerosis. *British Journal of Psychiatry* **115**, 749–764 [691, 694, 695, 696].

SURRIDGE, D.H.C., ERDAHL, D.L.W., LAWSON, J.S., DONALD, M.W., MONGA, T.N., BIRD, C.E. & LETEMENDIA, F.J.J. (1984) Psychiatric aspects of diabetes mellitus. *British Journal of Psychiatry* **145**, 269–276 [536].

SUSSER, E.S. & LIN, S.P. (1992) Schizophrenia after prenatal exposure to the Dutch Hunger Winter of 1944–1945. *Archives of General Psychiatry* **49**, 983–988 [91].

SUTHERLING, W.W. & BARTH, D.S. (1990) Magnetoencephalography in clinical epilepsy studies: the UCLA experience. Ch. 19 in *Magnetoencephalography*, ed. Sato, S. *Advances in Neurology* **54**. Raven Press: New York [133].

SUTTON, S., BRAREN, M., ZUBIN, J. & JOHN, E.R. (1965) Evoked-potential correlates of stimulus uncertainty. *Science* **150**, 1187–1188 [132].

SUTULA, T.P., SACKELLARES, J.C., MILLER, J.Q. & DREIFUSS, F.E. (1981) Intensive monitoring in refractory epilepsy. *Neurology* **31**, 243–247 [288].

SWAIN, J.M. (1959) Electroencephalographic abnormalities in pre-senile atrophy. *Neurology* **9**, 722–727 [439, 461].

SWANSON, D.W. & STIPES, A.H. (1969) Psychiatric aspects of Kline-felter's syndrome. *American Journal of Psychiatry* **126**, 814–822 [526, 527].

SWEDO, S.E., RAPOPORT, J.L., CHESLOW, D.L., LEONARD, H.L., AYOUB, E.M., HOSIER, D.M. & WALD, E.R. (1989) High prevalence of obses-sive–compulsive symptoms in patients with Sydenham's chorea. *American Journal of Psychiatry* **146**, 246–249 [374].

SWEENEY, D.F. (1990) Alcoholic blackouts: legal implications. *Journal of Substance Abuse Treatment* **7**, 155–159 [596].

SWEET, R.A. & ZUBENKO, G.S. (1994) Peripheral markers in Alzheimer's disease. Ch. 22 in *Dementia*, eds Burns, A. & Levy, R. Chapman & Hall: London [447].

SWEET, R.D., McDOWELL, F.H., FEIGENSON, J.S., LORANGER, A.W. & GOOD, H. (1976) Mental symptoms in Parkinson's disease during chronic treatment with levodopa. *Neurology* **26**, 305–310 [658, 659].

SWEET, R.D., SOLOMON, G.E., WAYNE, H., SHAPIRO, E. & SHAPIRO, A.K. (1973) Neurological features of Gilles de la Tourette's syn-drome. *Journal of Neurology, Neurosurgery and Psychiatry* **36**, 1–9 [685].

SWEET, W.H., ERVIN, F. & MARK, V.H. (1969) The relationship of violent behaviour to focal cerebral disease. In *Aggressive Behaviour*, Proceedings of International Symposium on the Biology of Aggressive Behaviour, eds Garattini, S. & Sigg, E.B. Exerpta Medica: Amsterdam [81, 82, 189].

SWEET, W.H., TALLAND, G.A. & BALLANTINE, H.T. (1966) A memory and mood disorder associated with ruptured anterior communi-cating aneurysm. *Transactions of the American Neurological Association* **91**, 346–348 [394].

SWIFT, C.R., SEIDMAN, F. & STEIN, H. (1967) Adjustment problems in juvenile diabetes. *Psychosomatic Medicine* **29**, 555–571 [536].

SYDENSTRICKER, V.P. (1943) Psychic manifestations of nicotinic acid deficiency. *Proceedings of the Royal Society of Medicine* **36**, 169–171 [574].

SYLVESTER, J.D. & LIVERSEDGE, L.A. (1960) A follow-up study of patients treated for writer's cramp by conditioning techniques. In *Behaviour Therapy and the Neuroses*, ed. Eysenck, H.J. Pergamon Press: Oxford [677].

SYMONDS, C.P. (1937) Mental disorder following head injury. *Pro-ceedings of the Royal Society of Medicine* **30**, 1081–1092 [191].

SYMONDS, C. (1951) Migrainous variants. *Transactions of the Medical Society of London* **67**, 237–250 [407].

SYMONDS, C. (1959) Excitation and inhibition in epilepsy. *Brain* **82**, 133–146 [248].

SYMONDS, C. (1962a) Concussion and its sequelae. *Lancet* **1**, 1–5 [170].

SYMONDS, C.P. (1962b) Discussion following 'The schizophrenia-like psychoses of epilepsy'. *Proceedings of the Royal Society of Medicine* **55**, 314–315 [282, 283].

SYMONDS, C.P. (1966) Disorders of memory. *Brain* **89**, 625–644 [36].

SYMONDS, C.P. & RUSSELL, W.R. (1943) Accidental head injuries. *Lancet* **1**, 7–10 [171, 173].

SYPERT, G.W., LEFFMAN, H. & OJEMANN, G.A. (1973) Occult normal pressure hydrocephalus manifested by Parkinsonism–dementia complex. *Neurology* **23**, 234–239 [747].

SZE, G., BRANT-ZAWADZKI, N., NORMAN, D. & NEWTON, T.H. (1987) The neuroradiology of AIDS. *Seminars in Roentgenology* **22**, 42–53 [321].

SZE, G. & ZIMMERMAN, R.D. (1988) The magnetic resonance imaging of infections and inflammatory diseases. *Radiologic Clinics of North America* **26**, 839–859 [368].

SZYMANSKI, H.V. (1981) Prolonged depersonalization after mari-juana use. *American Journal of Psychiatry* **138**, 231–233 [615].

TABATON, M., CAMMARATA, S., MANCARDI, G.L., CORDONE, G., PERRY, G. & LOEB, C. (1991) Abnormal tau-reactive filaments in olfactory mucosa in biopsy specimens of patients with probable Alzheimer's disease. *Neurology* **41**, 391–394 [441].

TAGLIAVINI, F. & PILLERI, G. (1983) Neuronal counts in basal nucleus of Meynert in Alzheimer's disease and in simple senile dementia. *Lancet* **1**, 469–470 [445].

TAKEUCHI, T., ETO, N. & ETO, K. (1979) Neuropathology of childhood cases of methylmercury poisoning (Minamata disease) with pro-longed symptoms, with particular reference to the decortication syndrome. *Neurotoxicology* **1**, 1–20 [635].

TALAMO, B.R., RUDEL, R.A., KOSIK, K.S., LEE, V.M.-Y., NEFF, S., ADELMAN, L. & KAUER, J.S. (1989) Pathological changes in olfac-tory neurons in patients with Alzheimer's disease. *Nature* **337**, 736–739 [441].

TALBOTT, J.A. & TEAGUE, J.W. (1969) Marihuana psychosis. *Journal of the American Medical Association* **210**, 299–302 [614].

TALLAND, G.A. (1965) *Deranged Memory: A Psychonomic Study of the Amnesic Syndrome*. Academic Press: New York [30, 31].

TALLAND, G.A., SWEET, W.H. & BALLANTYNE, H.T. (1967) Amnesic syndrome with anterior communicating artery aneurysm. *Journal of Nervous and Mental Disease* **145**, 179–192 [394].

TALLEY, B.J. & FABER, R. (1989) Mitochondrial encephalomyopathic dementia in a young adult. *Neuropsychiatry, Neuropsychology and Behavioral Neurology* **2**, 49–60 [761].

TAMERIN, J.S., WEINER, S., POPPEN, R., STEINGLASS, P. & MENDELSON, J.H. (1971) Alcohol and memory: amnesia and short-term memory function during experimentally induced into-xication. *American Journal of Psychiatry* **127**, 1659–1664 [596].

TAMLYN, D., McKENNA, P.J., MORTIMER, A.M., LUND, C.E., HAMMOND, S. & BADDELEY, A.D. (1992) Memory impairment in schizophre-nia: its extent, affiliations and neuropsychological character. *Psy-chological Medicine* **22**, 101–115 [34].

TANELI, B., OZASKINLI, S., KIRLI, S., ERDEN, G. & BORA, I. (1986) Bromocriptine-induced schizophrenic syndrome. *American Journal of Psychiatry* **143**, 935 [659].

TANZI, R.E., ST GEORGE-HYSLOP, P.H., HAINES, J.L., POLINSKY, R.J., NEE, L., FONCIN, J.-F., NEVE, R.L., McCLATCHEY, A.I., CONNEALLY, P.M. & GUSELLA, J.F. (1987) The genetic defect in familial Alzheimer's disease is not tightly linked to the amyloid β-protein gene. *Nature* **329**, 156–157 [448].

TARACHOW, S. (1939) The Korsakoff psychosis in spontaneous subarachnoid haemorrhage. *American Journal of Psychiatry* **95**, 887–899 [394].

TARIOT, P.N. & CAINE, E.D. (1987) Oral tetrahydroaminoacridine in the treatment of senile dementia, Alzheimer's type. *New England Journal of Medicine* **316**, 1604–1605 [503].

TARIOT, P.N., COHEN, R.M., SUNDERLAND, T., NEWHOUSE, P.A., YOUNT, D., MELLOW, A.M., WEINGARTNER, H., MUELLER, E.A. & MURPHY, D.L. (1987) Preliminary evidence for behavioral change with monoamine oxidase B inhibition. *Archives of General Psychiatry* **44**, 427–433 [502].

TARLOV, E. (1970) On the problem of the pathology of spasmodic tor-ticollis in man. *Journal of Neurology, Neurosurgery and Psychiatry* **33**, 457–463 [674].

TARSH, M.J. & ROYSTON, C. (1985) A follow-up study of accident neurosis. *British Journal of Psychiatry* **146**, 18–25 [176].

TARTER, R.E. & EDWARDS, K.L. (1985) Neuropsychology of alcoholism. Ch. 8 in *Alcohol and the Brain: Chronic Effects*, eds Tarter, R.E. & van Thiel, D.H. Plenum Medical Books: London [604].

TARTER, R.E., HAYS, A.L., SANDFORD, S.S. & VAN THIEL, D.H. (1986a) Cerebral morphological abnormalities associated with non-alcoholic cirrhosis. *Lancet* **2**, 893–895 [564].

TARTER, R.E., HEGEDUS, A.M., VAN THIEL, ˙D.H., GAVALER, J.S. & SCHADE, R.R. (1986b) Hepatic dysfunction and neuropsychological test performance in alcoholics with cirrhosis. *Journal of Studies on Alcohol* **47**, 74–77 [565].

TARTER, R.E. & SCHNEIDER, D.U. (1976) Blackouts: relationship with memory capacity and alcoholism history. *Archives of General Psychiatry* **33**, 1492–1496 [596].

TARTER, R.E., VAN THIEL, D.H., ARRIA, A.M., CARRA, J. & MOSS, H. (1988) Impact of cirrhosis on the neuropsychological test performance of alcoholics. *Alcoholism* **12**, 619–621 [565].

TASK FORCE ON LATE NEUROLOGICAL EFFECTS OF ANTIPSYCHOTIC DRUGS (1980) Tardive dyskinesia: summary of a task force report of the American Psychiatric Association. *American Journal of Psychiatry* **137**, 1163–1172 [641, 642, 645].

TATTERSALL, R.B. (1981) Psychiatric aspects of diabetes—a physician's view. *British Journal of Psychiatry* **139**, 485–493 [534, 535].

TAYLOR, A.R. & BELL, T.K. (1966) Slowing of cerebral circulation after concussional head injury. *Lancet* **2**, 178–180 [198].

TAYLOR, C.P. (1994) Emerging perspectives on the mechanism of action of gabapentin. *Neurology* **44 (Supplement 5)**, S10–S16 [304].

TAYLOR, D.C. (1969a) Aggression and epilepsy. *Journal of Psychosomatic Research* **13**, 229–236 [266].

TAYLOR, D.C. (1969b) Sexual behaviour and temporal lobe epilepsy. *Archives of Neurology* **21**, 510–516 [270, 271, 272, 273].

TAYLOR, D.C. (1972) Mental state and temporal lobe epilepsy: a correlative account of 100 patients treated surgically. *Epilepsia* **13**, 727–765 [281].

TAYLOR, D.C. (1975) Factors influencing the occurrence of schizophrenia-like psychosis in patients with temporal lobe epilepsy. *Psychological Medicine* **5**, 249–254 [281, 282].

TAYLOR, D.C. & FALCONER, M.A. (1968) Clinical, socioeconomic, and psychological changes after temporal lobectomy for epilepsy. *British Journal of Psychiatry* **114**, 1247–1261 [262, 268, 269, 270, 312].

TAYLOR, D.C. & MARSH, S.M. (1977) Implications of long-term follow-up studies in epilepsy: with a note on the cause of death. In *Epilepsy: The Eighth International Symposium*, ed. Penry, J.K., pp. 27–34. Raven Press: New York [312].

TAYLOR, E. (1991) Toxins and allergens. Ch. 8 in *Biological Risk Factors for Psychosocial Disorders*, eds Rutter, M. & Casaer, P. Cambridge University Press: Cambridge [632, 633].

TAYLOR, J.W. (1975) Depression in thyrotoxicosis. *American Journal of Psychiatry* **132**, 552–553 [511].

TAYLOR, M.A. & ABRAMS, R. (1987) Cognitive impairment patterns in schizophrenia and affective disorder. *Journal of Neurology, Neurosurgery and Psychiatry* **50**, 895–899 [89].

TAYLOR, P.J. (1987) Hemispheric lateralization and schizophrenia. In *Biological Perspectives of Schizophrenia*, eds Helmchen, H. & Henn, F.A., pp. 213–236. John Wiley & Sons Ltd: Chichester [89].

TAYLOR, P., DALTON, R. & FLEMINGER, J.J. (1982a) Handedness and schizophrenic symptoms. *British Journal of Medical Psychology* **55**, 287–291 [89].

TAYLOR, P.J., DALTON, R., FLEMINGER, J.J. & LISHMAN, W.A. (1982b) Differences between two studies of hand preference in psychiatric patients. *British Journal of Psychiatry* **140**, 166–173 [89].

TAYLOR, P.J. & KOPELMAN, M.D. (1984) Amnesia for criminal offences. *Psychological Medicine* **14**, 581–588 [39].

TCHICALOFF, M. & GAILLARD, F. (1970) Quelques effets indésirables des médicaments antiépileptiques sur les rendements intellectuels. *Revue de Neuropsychiatrie Infantile* **18**, 599–603 [263].

TEASDALE, G. & JENNETT, B. (1974) Assessment of coma and impaired consciousness: a practical scale. *Lancet* **2**, 81–84 [167].

TEASDALE, G. & MENDELOW, D. (1984) Pathophysiology of head injuries. Ch. 2 in *Closed Head Injury. Psychological, Social and Family Consequences*, ed. Brooks, N. Oxford University Press: Oxford [163].

TEMPLE, C.M., JEEVES, M.A. & VILARROYA, O. (1989) Ten pen men: rhyming skills in two children with callosal agenesis. *Brain and Language* **37**, 548–564 [770].

TENNENT, T. (1937) Discussion on mental disorder following head injury. *Proceedings of the Royal Society of Medicine* **30**, 1092–1093 [190].

TEOH, R. (1988) Tardive dyskinesia. *Adverse Drug Reaction Bulletin* **132** (October 1988), 496–499 [645].

TERI, L., LARSON, E.B. & REIFLER, B.V. (1988) Behavioral disturbance in dementia of the Alzheimer's type. *Journal of the American Geriatrics Society* **36**, 1–6 [432].

TERRY, R.D. (1979) Morphological changes in Alzheimer's disease—senile dementia: ultrastructural changes and quantitative studies. In *Congenital and Acquired Disorders*, ed. Katzman, R. Research Publications: Association for Research in Nervous and Mental Disease, Vol. 57, pp. 99–105. Raven Press: New York [443].

TERRY, R.D., FITZGERALD, C., PECK, A., MILLNER, J. & FARMER, P. (1977) Cortical cell counts in senile dementia. *Journal of Neuropathology and Experimental Neurology* **36**, 633 [443].

TERRY, R.D. & KATZMAN, R. (1983) Senile dementia of the Alzheimer type. *Annals of Neurology* **14**, 497–506 [429, 436, 443, 449].

TERRY, R.D., PECK, A., DE TERESA, R., SCHECHTER, R. & HOROUPIAN, D.S. (1981) Some morphometric aspects of the brain in senile dementia of the Alzheimer type. *Annals of Neurology* **10**, 184–192 [436, 443].

TERRY, R.D. & WISNIEWSKI, H. (1970) The ultrastructure of the neurofibrillary tangle and the senile plaque. In *Alzheimer's Disease and Related Conditions*, eds Wolstenholme, G.E.W. & O'Connor, M. Ciba Foundation Symposium. Churchill: London [441, 442].

TERRY, R.D. & WISNIEWSKI, H.M. (1972) Ultrastructure of senile dementia and of experimental analogs. In *Aging and the Brain*, ed. Gaitz, C.M. Plenum Press: New York and London [442].

TERZANO, M.G., MONTANARI, E., CALZETTI, S., MANCIA, D. & LECHI, A. (1983) The effect of amantadine on arousal and EEG patterns in Creutzfeldt–Jakob disease. *Archives of Neurology* **40**, 555–559 [506].

TETRUD, J.W. & LANGSTON, J.W. (1989) The effect of deprenyl (Selegiline) on the natural history of Parkinson's disease. *Science* **245**, 519–522 [650].

TEUBER, H.-L. (1959) Some alterations in behaviour after cerebral lesions in man. In *Evolution of Nervous Control*, ed. Bass, A.D. Publication No. 52 of the American Association for the Advancement of Science: Washington [180, 183].

TEUBER, H.-L. (1962) Effects of brain wounds implicating right or left hemisphere in man. In *Interhemispheric Relations and Cerebral Dominance*, ed. Mountcastle, V.B. Johns Hopkins Press: Baltimore [180, 183].

TEUBER, H.-L. (1964) The riddle of frontal lobe function in man. Ch. 20 in *The Frontal Granular Cortex and Behaviour*, eds Warren, J.M. & Akert, K. McGraw-Hill: New York [76, 78].

TEUBER, H.-L. & MILNER, B. (1968) Alteration of perception and memory in man: reflection on methods. Ch. 11 in *Analysis of Behavioural Change*, ed. Weiskrantz, L. Harper & Row: New York [116].

TEUBER, H.-L., MILNER, B. & VAUGHAN, H.G. (1968) Persistent anterograde amnesia after stab wound of the basal brain. *Neurophsychologia* **6**, 267–282 [116].

TEUBER, H.-L. & RUDEL, R.G. (1962) Behaviour after cerebral lesions in children and adults. *Developmental Medicine and Child Neurology* **4**, 3–20 [201, 202].

TEUBER, H.-L. & WEINSTEIN, S. (1956) Ability to discover hidden figures after cerebral lesions. *Archives of Neurology and Psychiatry* **76**, 369–379 [46].

TEUNISSE, S., BOLLEN, A.E., VAN GOOL, W.A. & WALSTRA, G.J.M. (1996) Dementia and subnormal levels of vitamin B_{12}: effects of replacement therapy on dementia. *Journal of Neurology* **243**, 522–529 [588].

THACORE, V.R. (1973) Bhang psychosis. *British Journal of Psychiatry* **123**, 225–229 [615].

THAKER, G.K., NGUYEN, J.A., STRAUSS, M.E., JACOBSON, R., KAUP, B.A. & TAMMINGA, C.A. (1990) Clonazepam treatment of tardive dyskinesia: a practical GABAminetic strategy. *American Journal of Psychiatry* **147**, 445–451 [645].

THAL, L.J., FULD, P.A., MASUR, D.M. & SHARPLESS, N.S. (1983) Oral physostigmine and lecithin improve memory in Alzheimer's disease. *Annals of Neurology* **13**, 491–496 [503].

THEANDER, S. & GRANHOLM, L. (1967) Sequelae after spontaneous subarachnoid haemorrhage, with special reference to hydrocephalus and Korsakoff's syndrome. *Acta Neurologica Scandinavica* **43**, 479–488 [394, 395].

THIGPEN, C.H. & MOSS, B.F. (1955) Unusual paranoid manifestations in a case of psychomotor epilepsy and narcolepsy. *Journal of Nervous and Mental Disease* **122**, 381–385 [728].

THOMAS, C.J. (1979) Brain damage with lithium/haloperidol. *British Journal of Psychiatry* **134**, 552 [626].

THOMAS, C.S. & SZABADI, E. (1987) Paranoid psychosis as the first presentation of a fulminating lethal case of AIDS. *British Journal of Psychiatry* **151**, 693–695 [331].

THOMAS, F.B., MAZZAFERI, E.L. & SKILLMAN, T.G. (1970) Apathetic thyrotoxicosis: in a distinctive clinical and laboratory entity. *Annals of Internal Medicine* **72**, 679–685 [511].

THOMAS, P.K. (1993) The chronic fatigue syndrome: what do we know? *British Medical Journal* **306**, 1557–1558 [373].

THOMASEN, E. (1948) *Myotonia: Thomsen's Disease (Myotonia Congenita), Paramyotonia, and Dystrophia Myotonica*. Universitetsforlaget: Aarhus [719, 720, 721].

THOMPSON, C. & CHECKLEY, S. (1981) Short term memory deficit in a patient with cerebral sarcoidosis. *British Journal of Psychiatry* **139**, 160–161 [764].

THOMPSON, C., DENT, J. & SAXBY, P. (1988) Effects of thallium poisoning on intellectual function. *British Journal of Psychiatry* **153**, 396–399 [636].

THOMPSON, L.W., DAVIS, G.C., OBRIST, W.D. & HEYMAN, A. (1976) Effects of hyperbaric oxygen on behavioral and physiological measures in elderly demented patients. *Journal of Gerontology* **31**, 23–28 [502].

THOMPSON, P.D. & MARSDEN, C.D. (1992) Corticobasal degeneration. In *Unusual Dementias*, ed. Rossor, M.N. Baillière Tindall: London [668].

THOMPSON, P.J., HUPPERT, F. & TRIMBLE, M. (1980) Anticonvulsant drugs, cognitive function and memory. *Acta Neurologica Scandinavica* **62 (Supplement 80)**, 75–81 [300].

THOMPSON, P.J. & TRIMBLE, M.R. (1982) Anticonvulsant drugs and cognitive functions. *Epilepsia* **23**, 531–544 [263].

THOMPSON, P.J. & TRIMBLE, M.R. (1983) Anticonvulsant serum levels: relationship to impairments of cognitive functioning. *Journal of Neurology, Neurosurgery and Psychiatry* **46**, 227–233 [263].

THOMPSON, R.H.S. (1967) The value of blood pyruvate determination in the diagnosis of thiamine deficiency. In *Thiamine Deficiency*, Ciba Foundation Study Group No. 28, eds Wolstenholme, G.E.W. & O'Connor, M. Churchill: London [572].

THOMPSON, T.L., FILLEY, C.M., MITCHELL, W.D., CULIG K.M., LoVERDE, M. & BYYNY, R.L. (1990) Lack of efficacy of hydergine in patients with Alzheimer's disease. *New England Journal of Medicine* **323**, 445–448 [502].

THOMSEN, I.V. (1974) The patient with severe head injury and his family: a follow-up study of 50 patients. *Scandinavian Journal of Rehabilitation Medicine* **6**, 180–183 [172, 216, 217].

THOMSEN, I.V. (1984) Late outcome of very severe blunt head trauma: a 10–15 year second follow-up. *Journal of Neurology, Neurosurgery and Psychiatry* **47**, 260–268 [167].

THOMSEN, J. (1876) Tonische Krämpfe in willkürlich beweglichen Muskeln in Folge von ererbter psychischer Disposition. *Arkiv für Psychiatrie und Nervenkrankheiten* **6**, 702–718. Quoted by Johnson, J. (1967) *British Journal of Psychiatry* **113**, 1025–1030 [720, 721].

THORNDIKE, E.L. & LORGE, I. (1944) *The Teacher's Word Book of 30 000 Words*. Teachers' College Press, Columbia University: New York [103].

THYGESEN, P., HERMANN, K. & WILLANGER, R. (1970) Concentration camp survivors in Denmark. Persecution, disease, disability, compensation. A 23-year follow-up. A survey of the long-term effects of severe environmental stress. *Danish Medical Bulletin* **17**, 65–108 [570].

TIBBETTS, R.W. (1971) Spasmodic torticollis. *Journal of the Pychosomatic Research* **15**, 461–469 [672, 673, 674].

TINKLENBERG, J.R., MELGES, F.T., HOLLISTER, L.E. & GILLESPIE, H.K. (1970) Marihuana and immediate memory. *Nature* **226**, 1171–1172 [613].

TISSENBAUM, M.J., HARTER, H.M. & FRIEDMAN, A.P. (1951) Organic neurological syndromes diagnosed as functional disorders. *Journal of the American Medical Association* **147**, 1519–1521 [688].

TITUS, F., MONTALBÁN, J., MOLINS, A., GILI, J., LOPEZ, M. & CODINA, A. (1989) Migraine-related stroke: brain infarction in superior cerebellar artery territory demonstrated by nuclear magnetic resonance. *Acta Neurologica Scandinavica* **79**, 357–360 [401].

TIZARD, B. & MARGERISON, J.H. (1964) Psychological functions during wave-spike discharge. *British Journal of Social and Clinical Psychology* **3**, 6–15 [262].

TODD, J. (1989) AIDS as a current psychopathological theme: a report on five heterosexual patients. *British Journal of Psychiatry* **154**, 253–255 [332].

TODNEM, K., NYLAND, H., KAMBESTAD, B.K. & AARLI, J.A. (1990) Influence of occupational diving upon the nervous system: an epidemiological study. *British Journal of Industrial Medicine* **47**, 708–714 [768].

TODNEM, K., SKEIDSVOLL, H., SVIHUS, R., RINCK, P., RIISE, T., KAMBESTAD, B.K. & AARLI, J.A. (1991) Electroencephalography, evoked potentials and MRI brain scans in saturation divers. An epidemiological study. *Electroencephalography and Clinical Neurophysiology* **79**, 322–329 [768].

TOGLIA, J.U. (1969) Dizziness after whiplash injury of the neck and closed head injury: electronystagmographic correlations. Ch. 6 in *The Late Effects of Head Injury*, eds Walker, A.E., Caveness, W.F. & Critchley, M. Thomas: Springfield, Illinois [197].

TOLOSA, E. & MARTÍ, M.J. (1988) Blepharospasm–oromandibular dystonia syndrome (Meige's syndrome): clinical aspects. In *Facial Dyskinesias*, eds Jankovic, J. & Tolosa, E. *Advances in Neurology* **49**, 73–84. Raven Press: New York [678].

TOMLINSON, B.E. (1979) The ageing brain. Ch. 6 in *Recent Advances in Neuropathology*, eds Smith, W.T. & Cavanah, J.B. Churchill Livingstone: Edinburgh & London [443].

TOMLINSON, B.E. (1982) Plaques, tangles and Alzheimer's disease. *Psychological Medicine* **12**, 449–459 [436].

TOMLINSON, B.E., BLESSED, G. & ROTH, M. (1968) Observations on the brains of non-demented old people. *Journal of the Neurological Sciences* **7**, 331–356 [435].

TOMLINSON, B.E., BLESSED, G. & ROTH, M. (1970) Observations on the brains of demented old people. *Journal of the Neurological Sciences* **11**, 205–242 [430, 435, 441, 453, 456].

TOMLINSON, B.E., IRVING, D. & BLESSED, D.G. (1981) Cell loss in the locus coeruleus in senile dementia of Alzheimer type. *Journal of the Neurological Sciences* **49**, 419–428 [444].

TONER, H.L. (1987) Effectiveness of a written guide for carers of dementia sufferers. *British Journal of Clinical and Social Psychiatry* **5**, 24–26 [498].

TONER, I., PEDEN, C.J., HAMID, S.K., NEWMAN, S., TAYLOR, K.M. & SMITH, P.L.C. (1994) Magnetic resonance imaging and neuropsychological changes after coronary artery bypass graft surgery: preliminary findings. *Journal of Neurosurgical Anesthesiology* **6**, 163–169 [555].

TONG, S., BAGHURST, P., McMICHAEL, A., SAWYER, M. & MUDGE, J. (1996) Lifetime exposure to environmental lead and children's intelligence at 11–13 years: the Port Pirie cohort study. *British Medical Journal* **312**, 1569–1575 [633].

TONKONOGY, J.M. (1991) Violence and temporal lobe lesion: head CT and MRI data. *Journal of Neuropsychiatry and Clinical Neuroscience* **3**, 189–196 [81].

TONKS, C.M. (1964) Mental illness in hypothyroid patients. *British Journal of Psychiatry* **110**, 706–710 [514, 515].

TOONE, B.K. (1981) Psychoses of epilepsy. Ch. 10 in *Epilepsy and Psychiatry*, eds Reynolds, E.H. & Trimble, M.R. Churchill Livingstone: Edinburgh & London [256, 310].

TOONE, B. (1984) The electroencephalogram. Ch. 2 in *The Scientific Principles of Psychopathology*, eds McGuffin, P., Shanks, M.F. & Hodgson, R.J. Grune & Stratton: London [127, 128].

TOONE, B.K., DAWSON, J. & DRIVER, M.V. (1982a) Psychoses of epilepsy: a radiological evaluation. *British Journal of Psychiatry* **140**, 244–248 [281].

TOONE, B.K., EDEH, J., FENWICK, P., GRANT, R., NANJEE, M., PURCHES, A.C. & WHEELER, M. (1984) Hormonal and behavioural changes in male epileptics. In *Advances in Epileptology: XVth Epilepsy International Symposium*, eds Porter, R.J., Mattson, R.H., Ward, A.A. & Dam, M. Raven Press: New York [272].

TOONE, B.K., EDEH, J., NANJEE, M.N. & WHEELER, M. (1989) Hyposexuality and epilepsy: a community survey of hormonal and behav-ioural changes in male epileptics. *Psychological Medicine* **19**, 937–943 [272].

TOONE, B.K. & FENTON, G.W. (1977) Epileptic seizures induced by psychotropic drugs. *Psychological Medicine* **7**, 265–270 [245].

TOONE, B.K., GARRALDA, M.E. & RON, M.A. (1982b) The psychoses of epilepsy and the functional psychoses: a clinical and phenomenological comparison. *British Journal of Psychiatry* **141**, 256–261 [280, 281, 282, 285].

TOONE, B.K., WHEELER, M., NANJEE, M., FENWICK, P. & GRANT, R. (1983) Sex hormones, sexual activity and plasma anticonvulsant levels in male epileptics. *Journal of Neurology, Neurosurgery and Psychiatry* **46**, 824–826 [272].

TORNATORE, F.L., SRAMEK, J.J., OKEYA, B.L. & PI, E.H. (1987) *Reactions to Psychotropic Medication*. Plenum Medical Book Co.: New York [625].

TORRES, F. & SHAPIRO, S.K. (1961) Electroencephalograms in whiplash injury. A comparison of electroencephalographic abnormalities with those present in closed head injuries. *Archives of Neurology* **5**, 28–35 [200].

TORVIK, A., LINDBOE, C.F. & ROGDE, S. (1982) Brain lesions in alcoholics. A neuropathological study with clinical correlations. *Journal of the Neurological Sciences* **56**, 233–248 [604, 607].

TOW, P.M. (1955) *Personality Changes Following Frontal Leucotomy*. Oxford University Press: Oxford [77].

TOWNES, B.D., HORNBEIN, T.F., SCHOENE, R.B., SARNQUIST, F.H. & GRANT, I. (1984) Human cerebral function at extreme altitude. Ch. 3 in *High Altitude and Man*, eds West, J.B. & Lahiri, S. American Physiological Society: Bethesda [549].

TOWNSEND, J.J., BARINGER, J.R., WOLINSKY, J.S., MALAMUD, N., MEDNICK, J.P., PANITCH, H.S., SCOTT, R.A.T., OSHIRO, L.S. & CREMER, N.E. (1975) Progressive rubella panencephalitis. Late onset after congenital rubella. *New England Journal of Medicine* **292**, 990–993 [363].

TOWNSEND, J.J., WOLINSKY, J.S. & BARINGER, J.R. (1976) The neuropathology of progressive rubella panencephalitis of late onset. *Brain* **99**, 81–90 [363].

TRAMONT, E.C. (1976) Persistence of *Treponema pallidum* following penicillin G therapy. *Journal of American Medical Association* **236**, 2206–2207 [344].

TRANEL, D. & DAMASIO, A.D. (1995) Neurobiological foundations of human memory. Ch. 2 in *Handbook of Memory Disorders*, eds Baddeley, A.D., Wilson, B.A. & Watts, F.N. John Wiley: Chichester [24].

TRAUB, R., GAJDUSEK, D.C. & GIBBS, C.J. (1977) Transmissible virus dementia: the relation of transmissible spongiform encephalopathy to Creutzfeldt–Jakob disease. Ch. 5 in *Aging and Dementia*, eds Lynn Smith, W. & Kinsbourne, M. Spectrum Publications: New York [446].

TRAVIESA, D.C. (1974) Magnesium deficiency: a possible cause of thiamine refractoriness in Wernicke–Korsakoff encephalopathy. *Journal of Neurology, Neurosurgery and Psychiatry* **37**, 959–962 [582].

TREASURE, T., SMITH, P.L.C., NEWMAN, S., SCHNEIDAU, A., JOSEPH, P., ELL, P. & HARRISON, M.J.G. (1989) Impairment of cerebral function following cardiac and other major surgery. *European Journal of Cardiothoracic Surgery* **3**, 216–221 [554].

TREFFERT, D.A. (1963) The psychiatric patient with an EEG temporal lobe focus. *American Journal of Psychiatry* **120**, 765–771 [267, 295].

TREISMAN, G., FISHMAN, M., LYKETSOS, C. & McHUGH, P.R. (1994) Evaluation and treatment of psychiatric disorders associated with HIV infection. Ch. 13 in *HIV, AIDS, and the Brain*, eds Price, R.W. & Perry, S.W. *Association for Research in Nervous and Mental Disease* **72**. Raven Press: New York [331].

TRENERRY, M.R., CROSSON, B., DEBOE, J. & LEBER, W.R. (1989) *Stroop Neuropsychological Screening Test Manual*. Psychological Assessment Resources Inc: Florida [119].

TRETHOWAN, W.H. & COBB, S. (1952) Neuropsychiatric aspects of Cushing's syndrome. *Archives of Neurology and Psychiatry* **67**, 281–309 [516, 517].

TREUTING, T.F. (1962) The role of emotional factors in the etiology and course of diabetes mellitus: a review of the recent literature. *American Journal of the Medical Sciences* **244**, 93–109 [534, 535].

TRIBOLETTI, F. & FERRI, H. (1969) Hydergine for treatment of symptoms of cerebrovascular insufficiency. *Current Therapeutic Research* **11**, 609–620 [502].

TRIMBLE, M.R. (1978) Serum prolactin in epilepsy and hysteria. *British Medical Journal* **2**, 1682 [290].

TRIMBLE, M.R. (1981a) *Post-Traumatic Neurosis: from Railway Spine to the Whiplash*. John Wiley & Sons: Chichester [210].

TRIMBLE, M.R. (1981b) Psychotropic drugs in the management of epilepsy. Ch. 24 in *Epilepsy and Psychiatry*, eds Reynolds, E.H. & Trimble, M.R. Churchill Livingstone: Edinburgh & London [310].

TRIMBLE, M.R. (1982) Anticonvulsant drugs and hysterical seizures. Ch. 9 in *Pseudoseizures*, eds Riley, T.L. & Roy, A. Williams & Wilkins: Baltimore [293].

TRIMBLE, M.R. (1983) Pseudoseizures. *British Journal of Hospital Medicine* **29**, 326–333 [294].

TRIMBLE, M.R. (1986) Hysteria, hystero-epilepsy and epilepsy. Ch. 17 in *What is Epilepsy. The Clinical and Scientific Basis of Epilepsy*, eds Trimble, M.R. & Reynolds, E.H. Churchill Livingstone: Edinburgh & London [292].

TRIMBLE, M.R. (1991) *The Psychoses of Epilepsy*. Raven Press: New York [278, 282, 284, 310, 312].

TRIMBLE, M.R. (1992) Behaviour changes following temporal lobectomy, with special reference to psychosis. *Journal of Neurology, Neurosurgery and Psychiatry* **55**, 89–91 [312, 313].

TRIMBLE, M.R., CORBETT, J.A. & DONALDSON, D. (1980) Folic acid and mental symptoms in children with epilepsy. *Journal of Neurology, Neurosurgery and Psychiatry* **43**, 1030–1034 [263].

TRIMBLE, M.R. & REYNOLDS, E.H. (1976) Anticonvulsant drugs and mental symptoms: a review. *Psychological Medicine* **6**, 169–178 [263].

TRIMBLE, M.R. & REYNOLDS, E.H. (1984) Neuropsychiatric toxicity of anticonvulsant drugs. Ch. 12 in *Recent Advances in Clinical Neurology, No. 4*, eds Matthews, W.B. & Glaser, G.H. Churchill Livingstone: Edinburgh & London [263, 271].

TROUSSEAU, A. (1868) *Lectures on Clinical Medicine*, Vol. 35, p. 453. New Sydenham Society, London. Quoted by Williams, M. & Smith, H.V. (1954) *Journal of Neurology, Neurosurgery and Psychiatry* **17**, 173–182 [366].

TRUITT, C.J. (1955) Personal and social adjustments of children with muscular dystrophy. *American Journal of Physical Medicine* **34**, 124–128 [716].

TRZEPACZ, P.T., BRENNER, R. & VAN THIEL, D.H. (1989) A psychiatric study of 247 liver transplantation candidates. *Psychosomatics* **30**, 147–153 [567].

TRZEPACZ, P.T., HERTWECK, M., STARRATT, C., ZIMMERMAN, L. & ADATEPE, M.H. (1992) The relationship of SPECT scans to behavioral dysfunction in neuropsychiatric patients. *Psychosomatics* **33**, 62–71 [148].

TRZEPACZ, P.T., McCUE, M., KLEIN, I., GREENHOUSE, J. & LEVEY, G.S. (1988) Psychiatric and neuropsychological response to propanolol in Graves' disease. *Biological Psychiatry* **23**, 678–688 [511].

TSUI, J.K.C., EISEN, A., STOESSL, A.J., CALNE, S. & CALNE, D.B. (1986) Double-blind study of botulinum toxin in spasmodic torticollis. *Lancet* **2**, 245–247 [675].

TUCCI, J.R. (1981) Neuropsychiatric syndromes of electrolyte imbalance. Ch. 1 in *Electrolytes and Neuropsychiatric Disorders*, ed. Alexander, P.E. MTP Press: Lancaster [561].

TUCKER, D.M., ROELTGEN, D.P., TULLY, R., HARTMANN, J. & BOXELL, C. (1988) Memory dysfunction following unilateral transection of the fornix: a hippocampal disconnection syndrome. *Cortex* **24**, 465–472 [27].

TUCKER, D.M., ROELTGEN, D.P., WANN, P.D. & WERTHEIMER, R.I. (1988) Memory dysfunction in myasthenia gravis: evidence for central cholinergic effects. *Neurology* **38**, 1173–1177 [712].

TULVING, E. (1972) Episodic and semantic memory. Ch. 10 in *Organisation of Memory*, eds Tulving, E. & Donaldson, W. Academic Press: New York [29].

TULVING, E., KAPUR, S., CRAIK, F.I.M., MOSCOVITCH, M. & HOULE, S. (1994) Hemispheric encoding/retrieval asymmetry in episodic memory: positron emission tomography findings. *Proceedings of the National Academy of Science, USA* **91**, 2016–2020 [28].

TUNE, L.E., HOLLAND, A., FOLSTEIN, M.F., DAMLOUJI, N.F., GARDENER, T.J. & COYLE, J.T. (1981) Association of post-operative delirium with raised serum levels of anticholinergic drugs. *Lancet* **2**, 651–652 [625].

TUPIN, J.P., SMITH, D.B., CLANON, T.L., KIM, L.I., NUGENT, A. & GROUPE, A. (1973) The long-term use of lithium in aggressive prisoners. *Comprehensive Psychiatry* **14**, 311–317 [298].

TUREK, I., KURLAND, A.A., OTA, K.Y. & HANLON, T.E. (1969) Effects of pipradol hydrochloride on geriatric patients. *Journal of the American Geriatrics Society* **17**, 408–413 [502].

TURLAND, D.N. & STEINHARD, M. (1969) The efficiency of the Memory-For-Designs Test. *British Journal of Social and Clinical Psychology* **8**, 44–49 [116].

TURNER, E.A. (1969) A surgical approach to the treatment of symptoms in temporal lobe epilepsy. Ch. 17 in *Current Problems in Neuropsychiatry*, ed. Herrington, R.N. British Journal of Psychiatry Special Publication No. 4. Headley Brothers: Ashford, Kent [82, 314].

TURNER, E.A. (1972) Operations for aggression: bilateral temporal lobotomy and posterior cingulectomy. Ch. 18 in *Psychosurgery*, eds Hitchcock, E., Laitinen, L. & Vaernet, K. Proceedings of the Second International Conference on Psychosurgery. Thomas: Springfield, Illinois [82].

TURNER, R.C. (1996) Hypoglycaemia. Section 11.12 in *Oxford Textbook of Medicine*, 3rd edn, eds Weatherall, D.J., Ledingham, J.G.G. & Warrell, D.A. Oxford University Press: Oxford [541].

TURNER, S., DANIELS, L. & GREER, S. (1989) Wernicke's encephalopathy in an 18-year-old woman. *British Journal of Psychiatry* **154**, 261–262 [576].

TURNER, S.W., TOONE, B.K. & BRETT-JONES, J.R. (1986) Computerized tomographic scan changes in early schizophrenia—preliminary findings. *Psychological Medicine* **16**, 219–225 [85].

TURNER, T.H., COOKSON, J.C., WASS, J.A.H., DRURY, P.L., PRICE, P.A. & BESSER, G.M. (1984) Psychotic reactions during treatment of pituitary tumours with dopamine agonists. *British Medical Journal* **289**, 1101–1103 [522, 523, 659].

TYLER, A., BALL, D. & CRAUFURD, D. (1992a) Presymptomatic testing for Huntington's disease in the United Kingdom. *British Medical Journal* 304, 1593–1596 [466].

TYLER, A., MORRIS, M., LAZAROU, L., MEREDITH, L., MYRING, J. & HARPER, P. (1992b) Presymptomatic testing for Huntington's disease in Wales, 1987–90. *British Journal of Psychiatry* 161, 481–488 [466].

TYLER, H.R. (1968) Neurologic disorders in renal failure. *American Journal of Medicine* 44, 734–748 [557].

TYRER, P., OWEN, R. & DAWLING, S. (1983) Gradual withdrawal of diazepam after long-term therapy. *Lancet* 1, 1402–1406 [611].

TYRER, P., RUTHERFORD, D. & HUGGETT, T. (1981) Benzodiazepine withdrawal symptoms and propanolol. *Lancet* 1, 520–522 [611].

TYRRELL, D.A.J., PARRY, R.P., CROW, T.J., JOHNSTONE, E. & FERRIER, I.N. (1979) Possible virus in schizophrenia and some neurological disorders. *Lancet* 1, 839–841 [92].

TYRRELL, P.J. & ROSSOR, M.N. (1994) Progressive aphasia and other focal symptoms. In *Dementia*, eds Burns, A. & Levy, R. Chapman Hall: London [754].

TYRRELL, P.J., WARRINGTON, E.K., FRACKOWIAK, R.S.J. & ROSSOR, M.N. (1990) Heterogeneity in progressive aphasia due to focal cortical atrophy. *Brain* 113, 1321–1336 [752].

UDAKA, F., YAMAO, S., NAGATA, H., NAKAMURA, S. & KAMEYAMA, M. (1984) Pathological laughing and crying treated with levodopa. *Archives of Neurology* 41, 1095–1097 [392].

ULLMAN, M. (1962) *Behavioural Changes in Patients Following Strokes*. Thomas: Springfield, Illinois [385, 388, 389, 396].

ULLMAN, M., ASHENHURST, E.M., HURWITZ, L.J. & GRUEN, A. (1960) Motivational and structural factors in the denial of hemiplegia. *Archives of Neurology* 3, 306–318 [70].

UNDERWOOD, M.J. & MORE, R.S. (1994) The aspirin papers. *British Medical Journal* 308, 71–72 [389].

UNGERLEIDER, J.T., FISHER, D.D. & FULLER, M. (1966) The dangers of LSD. *Journal of the American Medical Association* 197, 389–392 [621, 622].

UNTERHANSCHEIDT, F., JACHNIK, D. & GÖTT, H. (1968) *Der Balkenmangel Vol. 128, Monographien aus dem Gesamtgebiete der Neurologie und Psychiatrie (Berlin)*. Quoted by Ettlinger, G. (1977) Agencies of the corpus callosum. Ch. 12 in *Handbook of Clinical Neurology*, Vol. 30, eds Vinken, P.J. & Bruyn, G.W. North-Holland Publishing Co.: Amsterdam [770].

VAERNET, K. (1972) Stereotaxic amygdalotomy in temporal lobe epilepsy. *Confinia Neurologica* 34, 176–180 [314].

VAERNET, K. & MADSEN, A. (1970) Stereotaxic amygdalotomy and baso-frontal tractotomy in psychotics with aggressive behaviour. *Journal of Neurology, Neurosurgery and Psychiatry* 33, 858–863 [82].

VAGUS NERVE STIMULATION STUDY GROUP (1995) A randomized controlled trial of chronic vagus nerve stimulation for treatment of medically intractable seizures. *Neurology* 45, 224–230 [314].

VALENSTEIN, E., BOWERS, D., VERFAELLIE, M., HEILMAN, K.M., DAY, A. & WATSON, R.T. (1987) Retrosplenial amnesia. *Brain* 110, 1631–1646 [27].

VALENTINE, A.R., MOSELEY, I.F. & KENDALL, B.E. (1980) White matter abnormality in cerebral atrophy: clinico-radiological correlations. *Journal of Neurology, Neurosurgery and Psychiatry* 43, 139–142 [459].

VALLAR, G. & PAPAGNO, C. (1995) Neuropsychological impairments of short-term memory. Ch. 6 in *Handbook of Memory Disorders*, eds Baddeley, A.D., Wilson, B.A. & Watts, F.N. John Wiley: Chichester [29].

VALLEE, B.L., WACKER, W.E.C. & ULMER, D.D. (1960) The magnesium-deficiency tetany syndrome in man. *New England Journal of Medicine* 262, 155–161 [561].

VAN AMBERG, R.J. (1942) Prognosis of carbon monoxide poisoning in 15 patients, previously mentally ill. *Psychiatric Quarterly* 16, 668–680 [551].

VAN BOCKXMEER, F.M. (1994) ApoE and ACE genes: impact on human longevity. *Nature Genetics* 6, 4–5 [448].

VAN BOGAERT, L. (1925) Les troubles mentaux dans la sclérose latérale amyotrophique. *Encéphale* 20, 27–47 [708].

VAN BOGAERT, L. (1945) Une leuco-encéphalite sclérosante subaigue. *Journal of Neurology, Neurosurgery and Psychiatry* 8, 101–120 [361].

VAN DER KNAAP, M.S., VAN DER GROND, J., LUYTEN, P.R., DEN HOLLANDER, J.A., NAUTA, J.J.P. & VALK, J. (1992) ^{1}H and ^{31}P magnetic resonance spectroscopy of the brain in degenerative cerebral disorders. *Annals of Neurology* 31, 202–211 [143].

VAN DER LUGT, P.J.M. & DE VISSER, A.P. (1967) Two patients with a vital expansive syndrome following a cerebrovascular accident. *Psychiatria, Neurologia, Neurochirurgia* 70, 349–359 [387].

VAN GORP, W.G., SATZ, P., KIERSCH, M.E. & HENRY, R. (1986) Normative data on the Boston Naming Test for a group of normal older adults. *Journal of Clinical and Experimental Neuropsychology* 8, 702–705 [113].

VAN LIERE, E.J. & STICKNEY, J.C. (1963) *Hypoxia*. University of Chicago Press: Chicago [548].

VAN ROOIJEN, L.A.A., MacDONALD, G. & HULLA, F. (1995) Nimodipine in the treatment of senile dementia. Ch. 7 in *Developments in Dementia and Functional Disorders in the Elderly*, eds Levy, R. & Howard, R. Wrightson: Petersfield [502].

VAN WAGENEN, W.P. & HERREN, R.Y. (1940) Surgical division of commissural pathways in the corpus callosum. Relation to spread of an epileptic attack. *Archives of Neurology and Psychiatry* 44, 740–759 [313].

VAN ZOMEREN, A.H., BROUWER, W.H. & DEELMAN, B.G. (1984) Attentional deficits: the riddles of selectivity, speed, and alertness. Ch. 5 in *Closed Head Injury. Psychological, Social and Family Consequences*, ed. Brooks, N. Oxford University Press: Oxford [184].

VARGHA-KHADEM, F., ISAACS, E.B., PAPALELOUDI, H., POLKEY, C.E. & WILSON, J. (1991) Development of language in six hemispherectomized patients. *Brain* 114, 473–495 [42].

VARGHA-KHADEM, F. & POLKEY, C.E. (1992) A review of cognitive outcome after hemidecortication in humans. Ch. 5 in *Recovery from Brain Damage. Reflections and Directions*, eds Rose, F.D. & Johnson, D.A. Plenum Press: New York & London [202].

VARMA, L.P. (1952) The incidence and clinical features of general paresis. *Indian Journal of Neurology and Psychiatry* 3, 141–163 [340].

VAUGHN, C. & LEFF, J.P. (1976) The influence of family and social factors on the course of psychiatric illness. *British Journal of Psychiatry* 129, 125–137 [91].

VAUHKONEN, K. (1959) Suicide among the male disabled with war injuries to the brain. *Acta Psychiatrica et Neurologica Scandinavica* 137 **(Supplement)**, 90–91 [192].

VENABLES, P.J.W. (1993) Diagnosis and treatment of systemic lupus erythematosus. *British Medical Journal* 307, 663–666 [418, 422].

VEREKER, R. (1952) The psychiatric aspects of temporal arteritis. *Journal of Mental Science* 98, 280–286 [423].

VESSIE, R.P. (1932) On the transmission of Huntington's chorea for 300 years—the Bures family group. *Journal of Nervous and Mental Disease* 76, 553–573 [465].

VICTOR, M. (1964) Observations on the amnestic syndrome in man and its anatomical basis. In *Brain Function, Vol. II: RNA and Brain Function, Memory and Learning*, ed. Brazier, M.A.B. University of California Press: Berkeley and Los Angeles [25, 30, 580].

VICTOR, M. (1966) Treatment of alcoholic intoxication and the withdrawal syndrome. *Psychosomatic Medicine* **28**, 636–650 [600].

VICTOR, M. & ADAMS, R.D. (1953) The effect of alcohol on the nervous system. Ch. 28 in *Metabolic and Toxic Diseases of the Nervous System*. Research Publications of the Association for Research in Nervous and Mental Disease, Vol. 32. Williams & Wilkins: Baltimore [597, 598, 600, 601].

VICTOR, M. & ADAMS, R.D. (1962) The acute confusional states. Ch. 38 in *Principles of Internal Medicine*, eds Harrison, T.R., Adams, R.D., Bennett, I.L., Resnick, W.H., Thorn, G.W. & Wintrobe, M.M. McGraw-Hill: New York [4].

VICTOR, M. & ADAMS, R.D. (1985) The alcoholic dementias. Ch. 22 in *Handbook of Clinical Neurology, Series 2*, Vol. 46, *Neurobehavioural Disorders*, eds Vinken, P.J., Bruyn, G.W. & Klawans, H.L. Elsevier: Amsterdam [607].

VICTOR, M., ADAMS, R.D. & COLE, M. (1965) The acquired (non-Wilsonian) type of chronic hepatocerebral degeneration. *Medicine* **44**, 345–396 [563, 566].

VICTOR, M., ADAMS, R.D. & COLLINS, G.H. (1971) *The Wernicke–Korsakoff Syndrome*. Blackwell Scientific Publications: Oxford [31, 576, 578, 579, 580, 582, 583, 584].

VICTOR, M., ADAMS, R.D. & COLLINS, G.H. (1989) *The Wernicke–Korsakoff Syndrome and Related Neurologic Disorders due to Alcoholism and Malnutrition*, 2nd edn. F.A. Davis: Philadelphia [578, 579, 580, 586, 607].

VICTOR, M., ADAMS, R.D. & MANCALL, E.L. (1959) A restricted form of cerebellar cortical degeneration occurring in alcoholic patients. *Archives of Neurology* **1**, 579–688 [585].

VICTOR, M., ANGEVINE, J.B., MANCALL, E.L. & FISHER, C.M. (1961) Memory loss with lesions of hippocampal formation. *Archives of Neurology* **5**, 244–263 [26, 379].

VICTOR, M. & HOPE, J.M. (1958) The phenomenon of auditory hallucinations in chronic alcoholism. A critical evaluation of the status of alcoholic hallucinosis. *Journal of Nervous and Mental Disease* **126**, 451–481 [599, 600].

VICTORATOS, G.C., LENMAN, J.A.R. & HERZBERG, L. (1977) Neurological investigation of dementia. *British Journal of Psychiatry* **130**, 131–133 [490, 491].

VIEWEG, W.V.R., DAVID, J.J., ROWE, W.T., WAMPLER, C.J., BURNS, W.J. & SPRADLIN, W.W. (1985) Death from self-induced water intoxication among patients with schizophrenic disorders. *Journal of Nervous and Mental Disease* **173**, 161–165 [525].

VIGNOLO, L.A. (1969) Auditory agnosia: a review and report of recent evidence. Ch. 7 in *Contributions to Clinical Neuropsychology*, ed. Benton, A.L. Aldine Publishing Company: Chicago [64].

VILLA, J.L. & CIOMPI, L. (1968) Therapeutic problems of senile dementia. In *Senile Dementia: Clinical and Therapeutic Aspects*, eds Müller, Ch. & Giompi, L. Huber: Bern [502].

VILLEMURE, J.-G., ADAMS, B.T., HOFFMAN, H.J. & PEACOCK, W.J. (1993) Hemispherectomy. Ch. 42 in *Surgical Treatment of the Epilepsies*, 2nd edn, ed. Engel, J. Raven Press: New York [313].

VILLIERS, J.C. DE (1966) Intracranial haemorrhage in patients treated with monoamine oxidase inhibitors. *British Journal of Psychiatry* **112**, 109–118 [392].

VINCENT, A. & NEWSOM-DAVIS, J. (1985) Acetylcholine receptor antibody as a diagnostic test for myasthenia gravis: results in 153 validated cases and 2967 diagnostic assays. *Journal of Neurology, Neurosurgery and Psychiatry* **48**, 1246–1252 [710].

VISLIE, H. & HENRIKSEN, G.F. (1958) Psychic disturbances in epileptics. Ch. 2 in *Lectures on Epilepsy*, ed. Lorentz de Haas, A.M. Elsevier: Amsterdam [260, 261].

VOGEL-SCIBILIA, S.E., MULSANT, B.H. & KESHAVAN, M.S. (1988) HIV infection presenting as psychosis: a critique. *Acta Psychiatrica Scandinavica* **78**, 652–656 [331].

VOGT, C. & VOGT, O. (1952) Altérations anatomiques de la schizophrénie et d'autres psychoses dites fonctionelles. *First International Congress of Neuropathology* **1**, 515–532 [86].

VOLBERDING, P.A., LAGAKOS, S.W., KOCH, M.A., PETTINELLI, C., MYERS, M.W., BOOTH, D.K., BALFOUR, H.H., REICHMAN, R.C., BARTLETT, J.A., HIRSCH, M.S., MURPHY, R.L., HARDY, W.D., SOEIRO, R., FISCHL, M.A., BARTLETT, J.G., MERIGAN, T.C., HYSLOP, N.E., RICHMAN, D.D., VALENTINE, F.T., COREY, L. & THE AIDS CLINICAL TRIALS GROUP OF THE NATIONAL INSTITUTE OF ALLERGY AND INFECTIOUS DISEASES (1990) Zidovudine in asymptomatic human immunodeficiency virus infection. A controlled trial in persons with fewer than 500 CD_4-positive cells per cubic millimetre. *New England Journal of Medicine* **322**, 941–949 [336].

VOLKOW, N.D., TANCREDI, L.R., GRANT, C., GILLESPIE, H., VALENTINE, A., MULLANI, N., WANG, G.-J. & HOLLISTER, L. (1995) Brain glucose metabolism in violent psychiatric patients: a preliminary study. *Psychiatry Research: Neuroimaging* **61**, 243–253 [83].

VOLPE, B.J. (1985) Observation of motor control in patients with partial and complete callosal section: implications for current theories of apraxia. Ch. 21 in *Epilepsy and the Corpus Callosum*, ed. Reeves, A.G. Plenum Press: New York [313].

VON BOSE, M.J. & ZAUDIG, M. (1991) Encephalopathy resembling Creutzfeldt–Jakob disease following oral, prescribed doses of bismuth nitrate. *British Journal of Psychiatry* **158**, 278–280 [637].

VON ECONOMO, C. (1929) *Encephalitis Lethargica: Its Sequelae and Treatment*. First published 1929. Translated by Newman, K.O. (1931). Oxford University Press [349, 350, 351, 354].

VON KNORRING, L. (1983) Interhemispheric EEG differences in affective disorders. In *Laterality and Psychopathology*, eds Flor-Henry, P. & Gruzelier, J., pp. 315–326. Elsevier: Amsterdam & London [89].

WADA, J. & RASMUSSEN, T. (1960) Intracarotid injection of sodium amytal for the lateralization of cerebral speech dominance: experimental and clinical observations. *Journal of Neurosurgery* **17**, 266–282 [40].

WADDELL, P.A. & GRONWALL, D.M.A. (1984) Sensitivity to light and sound following minor head injury. *Acta Neurologica Scandinavica* **69**, 270–276 [198].

WADDINGTON, J.L. & YOUSSEF, H.A. (1986) An unusual cluster of tardive dyskinesia in schizophrenia: association with cognitive dysfunction and negative symptoms. *American Journal of Psychiatry* **143**, 1162–1165 [642].

WADDY, H.M., FLETCHER, N.A., HARDING, A.E. & MARSDEN, C.D. (1991) A genetic study of idiopathic focal dystonias. *Annals of Neurology* **29**, 320–324 [670].

WADE, D.T., LANGTON HEWER, R., SKILBECK, C.E. & DAVID, R.M. (1985) *Stroke. A Critical Approach to Diagnosis, Treatment and Management*. Chapman & Hall: London [389, 390, 391].

WADE, J.P., MIRSEN, T.R., HACHINSKI, V.C., FISMAN, M., LAU, C. & MERSKEY, H. (1987) The clinical diagnosis of Alzheimer's disease. *Archives of Neurology* **44**, 24–29 [457].

WADIA, N. & WILLIAMS, E. (1957) Behçet's syndrome with neurological complications. *Brain* **80**, 59–71 [763].

WADIA, R.S., MAKHALE, C.N., KELKAR, A.V. & GRANT, K.B. (1987)

Focal epilepsy in India with special reference to lesions showing ring or disc-like enhancement on contrast computed tomography. *Journal of Neurology, Neurosurgery and Psychiatry* **50**, 1298–1301 [289].

WAITZKIN, L. (1966a) A survey for unknown diabetics in a mental hospital: I. Men under age fifty. *Diabetes* **15**, 97–104 [536].

WAITZKIN, L. (1966b) A survey for unknown diabetics in a mental hospital. II. Men from age fifty. *Diabetes* **15**, 164–172 [536].

WAKELING, A. (1972) Comparative study of psychiatric patients with Klinefelter's syndrome and hypogonadism. *Psychological Medicine* **2**, 139–154 [526, 527].

WALCH, R. (1956) Orbitalhirn und Charakter. In *Das Hirntrauma*, ed. Rehwald, E., pp. 203–213. Thieme: Stuttgart [180].

WALINDER, J. (1977) Hyperostosis frontalis interna and mental morbidity. *British Journal of Psychiatry* **131**, 155–159 [769].

WALKER, A.E. (1961) Murder or epilepsy? *Journal of Nervous and Mental Disease* **133**, 430–437 [275].

WALKER, A.E. & BLUMMER, D. (1989) The fate of World War II veterans with post-traumatic seizures. *Archives of Neurology* **46**, 23–26 [186].

WALKER, A.E. & ERCULEI, F. (1969) *Head Injured Men Fifteen Years Later*. Thomas: Springfield, Illinois [174, 197].

WALKER, A.E. & JABLON, S. (1959) A follow-up of head-injured men of World War II. *Journal of Neurosurgery* **16**, 600–610 [178].

WALKER, A.E. & JABLON, S. (1961) *A Follow-up Study of Head Wounds in World War II*. Veterans Administration Medical Monograph No. 5: Washington, DC [244].

WALKER, D.W., BARNES, D.E., RILEY, J.N., HUNTER, B.E. & ZORNETZER, S.F. (1980a) Neurotoxicity of chronic alcohol consumption: an animal model. In *Psychopharmacology of Alcohol*, ed. Sandler, M. Raven Press: New York [607].

WALKER, D.W., BARNES, D.E., ZORNETZER, S.F., HUNTER, B.E. & KUBANIS, P. (1980b) Neuronal loss in hippocampus induced by prolonged ethanol consumption in rats. *Science* **209**, 711–713 [607].

WALKER, E. (1993) Neurodevelopmental aspects of schizophrenia. *Schizophrenia Research* **9**, 151–152 [91].

WALKER, F.O., YOUNG, A.B., PENNEY, J.B., DOVORINI-ZIS, K. & SHOULSON, I. (1984) Benzodiazepine and GABA receptors in early Huntington's disease. *Neurology* **34**, 1237–1240 [467].

WALLACE, M.R., MARCHUK, D.A., ANDERSEN, L.B., LETCHER, R., ODEH, H.M., SAULINO, A.M., FOUNTAIN, J.W., BRERETON, A., NICHOLSON, J., MITCHELL, A.L., BROWNSTEIN, B.H. & COLLINS, F.S. (1990) Type 1 neurofibromatosis gene: identification of a large transcript disrupted in three NFI patients. *Science* **249**, 181–186 [703].

WALLACE, S.J. (1994) Lamotrigine—a clinical overview. *Seizure* **3 (Supplement A)**, 47–51 [242].

WALLER, J.A. (1968) Holiday drinking and highway fatalities. *Journal of the American Medical Association* **206**, 2693–2697 [179].

WALSER, R.L. & ACKERMAN, L.V. (1977) Determination of volume from computerised tomograms: finding the volume of fluid-filled brain cavities. *Journal of Computer Assisted Tomography* **1**, 117–130 [138].

WALSH, A.C. (1969a) Arterial insufficiency of the brain: progression prevented by long-term anticoagulant therapy in eleven patients. *Journal of the American Geriatrics Society* **17**, 93–104 [502].

WALSH, A.C. (1969b) Prevention of senile and presenile dementia by bishydroxycoumarin (dicumarol) therapy. *Journal of the American Geriatrics Society* **17**, 477–487 [502].

WALSH, K. (1994) *Neuropsychology. A Clinical Approach*, 3rd edn. Churchill Livingstone: Edinburgh [60].

WALSHE, F.M.R. (1958) The role of injury, of the law and of the doctor in the aetiology of the so-called traumatic neurosis. *Medical Press* **239**, 493–496 [198].

WALSHE, J.M. (1968) Some observations on the treatment of Wilson's disease with penicillamine. In *Wilson's Disease*, ed. Bergsma, D. Birth Defects Original Article Series, Vol. 4, No. 2. The National Foundation: New York [664].

WALSHE, J.M. (1986) Wilson's disease. Ch. 12 in *Handbook of Clinical Neurology. Extrapyramidal Disorders*, Vol. 5(49), eds Vinken, P.J., Bruyn, G.W. & Klawans, H.L. Elsevier Science Publishers: Amsterdam [664].

WALSTRA, G.J.M., TEUNISSE, S., VAN GOOL, W.A. & VAN CREVEL, H. (1997a) Reversible dementia in elderly patients referred to a memory clinic. *Journal of Neurology* **244**, 17–22 [491].

WALSTRA, G.J.M., TEUNISSE, S., VAN GOOL, W.A. & VAN CREVEL, H. (1997b) Symptomatic treatment of elderly patients with early Alzheimer's disease at a memory clinic. *Journal of Geriatric Psychiatry and Neurology* **10**, 33–38 [491].

WALTON, D. & BLACK, D.A. (1957) The validity of a psychological test of brain damage. *British Journal of Medical Psychology* **30**, 270–279 [115].

WALTON, J.N. (1952) The late prognosis of subarachnoid haemorrhage. *British Medical Journal* **2**, 802–808 [393, 395].

WALTON, J.N. (1953) The Korsakoff syndrome in spontaneous subarachnoid haemorrhage. *Journal of Mental Science* **99**, 521–530 [394, 395].

WALTON, J.N. (1956) *Subarachnoid Haemorrhage*. Livingstone: Edinburgh and London [392, 393].

WALTON, J.N. (1977) *Brain's Diseases of the Nervous System*, 8th edn. Oxford University Press: Oxford [373, 676].

WALTON, J. (1982) *Essentials of Neurology*, 5th edn. Pitman: London [377].

WALTON, J. (1993a) Disorders of function in the light of anatomy and physiology. Ch. 1 in *Brain's Diseases of the Nervous System*, 10th edn, ed. Walton, J. Oxford University Press: Oxford [133, 134].

WALTON, J. (1993b) The neurology of some general (internal) medical disorders. Ch. 17 in *Brain's Diseases of the Nervous System*, 10th edn, ed. Walton, J. Oxford University Press: Oxford [426].

WALTON, J. (1993c) Disorders of muscle. Ch. 19 in *Brain's Diseases of the Nervous System*, 10th edn, ed. Walton, J. Oxford University Press: Oxford [709, 710, 714, 715].

WALTON, J.N., KILOH, L.G., OSSELTON, J.W. & FARRALL, J. (1954) The electroencephalogram in pernicious anaemia and subacute combined degeneration of the cord. *Electroencephalography and Clinical Neurophysiology* **6**, 45–64 [589].

WALTON, J.N. & NATTRASS, F.J. (1954) On the classification, natural history and treatment of the myopathies. *Brain* **77**, 169–231 [714, 719].

WALTZ, G., HARIK, S.I. & KAUFMAN, B. (1987) Adult metachromatic leukodystrophy. Value of computed tomographic scanning and magnetic resonance imaging of the brain. *Archives of Neurology* **44**, 225–227 [759].

WARBURTON, J.W. (1967) Depressive symptoms in Parkinson patients referred for thalamotomy. *Journal of Neurology, Neurosurgery and Psychiatry* **30**, 368–370 [656].

WARD, A.A. (1948) The cingular gyrus: area 24. *Journal of Neurophysiology* **11**, 13–22 [23].

WARD, A.A. (1966) The physiology of concussion. Ch. 16 in *Head Injury: Conference Proceedings*, eds Caveness, W.F. & Walker, A.E. Lippincott: Philadelphia [162, 164].

WARD, C.D., DUVOISIN, R.C., INCE, S.E., NUTT, J.D., ELDRIDGE, R., CALNE, D.B. & DAMBROSIA, J. (1984) Parkinson's disease in twins.

In *Parkinson-Specific Motor and Mental Disorders*, eds Hassler, R.G. & Christ, J.F. *Advances in Neurology* **40**, 341–344. Raven Press: New York [661].

WARDEN, D.L., LABBATE, L.A., SALAZAR, A.M., NELSON, R., SHELEY, E., STAUDENMEIER, J. & MARTIN, E. (1997) Posttraumatic stress disorder in patients with traumatic brain injury and amnesia for the event? *Journal of Neuropsychiatry and Clinical Neurosciences* **9**, 18–22 [195].

WARDEN, J. (1996a) When MPs chicken out over beef. *British Medical Journal* **312**, 1502 [476].

WARDEN, J. (1996b) Pesticide link with the Gulf War syndrome. *British Medical Journal* **313**, 897 [637].

WARDEN, J. (1997) Call for inquiry into CJD cluster. *British Medical Journal* **315**, 331 [476].

WARKANY, J. & HUBBARD, D.M. (1951) Adverse mercurial reactions in the form of acrodynia and related conditions. *American Journal of Diseases of Children* **81**, 335–373 [633, 634].

WARKENTIN, S., NILSSON, A., RISBERG, J. & KARLSON, S. (1989) Absence of frontal lobe activation in schizophrenia. *Journal of Cerebral Blood Flow and Metabolism* **9 (Supplement 1)**, S354 [87].

WARREN, L.P., DJANG, W.T., MOON, R.E., CAMPORESI, E.M., SALLEE, D.S., ANTHONY, D.C., MASSEY, E.W., BURGER, P.C. & HEINZ, E.R. (1988) Neuroimaging of scuba diving injuries to the CNS. *American Journal of Radiology* **151**, 1003–1008 [768].

WARREN, S., GREENHILL, S. & WARREN, K.G. (1982) Emotional stress and the development of multiple sclerosis: case-control evidence of a relationship. *Journal of Chronic Diseases* **35**, 821–831 [699].

WARRINGTON, E.K. (1970) Neurological deficits. Ch. 9 in *The Psychological Assessment of Mental and Physical Handicaps*, ed. Mittler, P. Methuen: London [62, 66, 67, 104].

WARRINGTON, E.K. (1971) Neurological disorders of memory. *British Medical Bulletin* **27**, 243–247 [35].

WARRINGTON, E.K. (1974) Deficient recognition memory in organic amnesia. *Cortex* **10**, 289–291 [115].

WARRINGTON, E.K. (1975) The selective impairment of semantic memory. *Quarterly Journal of Experimental Psychology* **27**, 635–657 [753].

WARRINGTON, E.K. (1982) The fractionation of arithmetical skills: a single case study. *Quarterly Journal of Experimental Psychology* **34A**, 31–51 [67].

WARRINGTON, E.K. (1984) *Manual for Recognition Memory Test for Words and Faces*. NFER-Nelson: Windsor [115].

WARRINGTON, E.K. (1985) Agnosia: the impairment of object recognition. Ch. 23 in *Handbook of Clinical Neurology*, Revised Series, Vol. 1, *Clinical Neuropsychology*, ed. Frederiks, J.A.M. Elsevier Science Publishers BV: Amsterdam [59, 60].

WARRINGTON, E.K. & JAMES, M. (1967a) An experimental investigation of facial recognition in patients with unilateral cerebral lesions. *Cortex* **3**, 317–326 [60].

WARRINGTON, E.K. & JAMES, M. (1967b) Tachistoscopic number estimation in patients with unilateral cerebral lesions. *Journal of Neurology, Neurosurgery and Psychiatry* **30**, 468–474 [62].

WARRINGTON, E.K. & JAMES, M. (1967c) Disorders of visual perception in patients with localised cerebral lesions. *Neuropsychologia* **5**, 253–266 [63].

WARRINGTON, E.K. & JAMES, M. (1988) Visual apperceptive agnosia: a clinico-anatomical study of three cases. *Cortex* **24**, 13–32 [59].

WARRINGTON, E.K. & JAMES, M. (1991) *The Visual Object and Space Perception Battery*. Thames Valley Test Company: Bury St Edmunds [112].

WARRINGTON, E.K., LOGUE, V. & PRATT, R.T.C. (1971) The anatomical localisation of selective impairment of auditory verbal short-term memory. *Neuropsychologia* **9**, 377–387 [53].

WARRINGTON, E.K. & PRATT, R.T.C. (1973) Language laterality in left handers assessed by unilateral ECT. *Neuropsychologia* **11**, 423–428 [40].

WARRINGTON, E.K. & PRATT, R.T.C. (1981) The significance of laterality effects. *Journal of Neurology, Neurosurgery and Psychiatry* **44**, 193–196 [40].

WARRINGTON, E.K. & SHALLICE, T. (1969) The selective impairment of auditory verbal short-term memory. *Brain* **92**, 885–896 [53].

WARRINGTON, E.K. & WEISKRANTZ, L. (1968) New method of testing long-term retention with special reference to amnesic patients. *Nature* **217**, 972–974 [35].

WARRINGTON, E.K. & WEISKRANTZ, L. (1970) Amnesic syndrome-consolidation or retrieval? *Nature* **228**, 628–630 [35].

WARRINGTON, E.K. & WEISKRANTZ, L. (1978) Further analysis of the prior learning effect in amnesic patients. *Neuropsychologia* **16**, 169–177 [35].

WASMUTH, J.J., HEWITT, J., SMITH, B., ALLARD, D., HAINES, J.L., SKARECKY, D., PARTLOW, E. & HAYDEN, M.R. (1988) A highly polymorphic locus very tightly linked to the Huntington's disease gene. *Nature* **332**, 734–736 [466].

WASS, J.A.H. (1993) Acromegaly: treatment after 100 years. *British Medical Journal* **307**, 1505–1506 [522].

WATERS, W.E. (1971) Migraine: intelligence, social class and familial prevalence. *British Medical Journal* **2**, 77–81 [402, 403].

WATSON, C.G. (1965) WAIS profile patterns of hospitalised brain-damaged and schizophrenic patients. *Journal of Clinical Psychology* **21**, 294–295 [111].

WATSON, C.G., KUCALA, T., MANIFOLD, V., VASSAR, P. & JUBA, M. (1988) Differences between post traumatic stress disorder patients with delayed and undelayed onset. *Journal of Nervous and Mental Diseases* **176**, 568–572 [195].

WATSON, J.D.G. (1991) The current state of positron emission tomography. *British Journal of Hospital Medicine* **46**, 163–166 [144].

WATSON, J.D.G., MYERS, R., FRACKOWIAK, R.S.J., HAJNAL, J.V., WOODS, R.P., MAZZIOTTA, J.C., SHIPP, S. & ZEKI, S. (1993) Area V5 of the human brain: evidence from a combined study using positron emission tomography and magnetic resonance imaging. *Cerebral Cortex* **3**, 79–94 [144].

WATSON, J.M. (1979a) Glue sniffing: two case reports. *Practitioner* **222**, 845–847 [629].

WATSON, J.M. (1979b) Morbidity and mortality statistics on solvent abuse. *Medicine, Science and the Law* **19**, 246–252 [629].

WATSON, L. (1968) Clinical aspects of hyperparathyroidism. *Proceedings of the Royal Society of Medicine* **61**, 1123 [529].

WATSON, L. (1972) Diseases of the parathyroid glands. *Medicine (monthly add-on series, 1972-3)* **2**, 148–156. Medical Education (International) Ltd: London [533].

WATSON, M.R., FENTON, G.W., McCLELLAND, R.J., LUMSDEN, J., HEADLEY, M. & RUTHERFORD, W.H. (1995) The post-concussional state: neurophysiological aspects. *British Journal of Psychiatry* **167**, 514–521 [198].

WATSON, R.T. & HEILMAN, K.M. (1979) Thalamic neglect. *Neurology* **29**, 690–694 [68].

WATSON, R.T., VALENSTEIN, E. & HEILMAN, K.M. (1981) Thalamic neglect. Possible role of the medial thalamus and nucleus reticularis in behaviour. *Archives of Neurology* **38**, 501–506 [68].

WATT, D.C. & SELLER, A. (1993) A clinico-genetic study of psychiatric disorder in Huntington's chorea. *Psychological Medicine Monograph Supplement* **23**, 1–43 [470, 472].

WATTS, R.L., MIRRA, S.S. & RICHARDSON, E.P. (1994) Corticobasal ganglionic degeneration. Ch. 14 in *Movement Disorders*, Vol. 3, eds Marsden, C.D. & Fahn, S. Butterworth-Heinemann: Oxford [668].

WAXMAN, S.G. & GESCHWIND, N. (1974) Hypergraphia in temporal lobe epilepsy. *Neurology* 24, 629–636 [267].

WAXMAN, S.G. & GESCHWIND, N. (1975) The interictal behavior syndrome of temporal lobe epilepsy. *Archives of General Psychiatry* 32, 1580–1586 [267, 269].

WAYNE, E.J. (1960) Clinical and metabolic studies in thyroid disease. *British Medical Journal* 1, 1–11 and 78–90 [510].

WEATHERALL, D.J. (1996) Polycythaemia vera. Section 22.3.8 in *Oxford Textbook of Medicine*, 3rd edn, eds Weatherall, D.J., Ledingham, J.G.G. & Warrell, D.A. Oxford University Press: Oxford [426].

WEBB, D.W. & OSBORNE, J.P. (1992) New research in tuberous sclerosis. *British Medical Journal* 304, 1647–1648 [701].

WEBB, M. & KIRKER, J.G. (1981) Severe post-traumatic insomnia treated with L-5-hydroxytryptophan. *Lancet* 1, 1365–1366 [734].

WEBSTER, J.E. & GURDJIAN, E.S. (1943) Acute physiological effects of gunshot and other penetrating wounds of the brain. *Journal of Neurophysiolgy* 6, 255–262 [162].

WECHSLER, A.F. (1977) Presenile dementia presenting as aphasia. *Journal of Neurology, Neurosurgery and Psychiatry* 40, 303–305 [752].

WECHSLER, A.F., VERITY, A., ROSENSCHEIN, S., FRIED, I. & SCHEIBEL, A.B. (1982) Pick's disease: a clinical, computed tomographic, and histologic study with golgi impregnation observations. *Archives of Neurology* 39, 287–290 [752].

WECHSLER, B., DORMONT, D., LUBETZKI, C., LYON-CAEN, O., CHIRAS, J., BORIES, J. & GODEAU, P. (1991) Magnetic resonance imaging in Behçet's disease. Ch. 47 in *Behçet's Disease. Basic and Clinical Aspects*, eds O'Duffy, J.D. & Kokmen, E. Marcel Dekker: New York [763].

WECHSLER, B. & PIETTE, J.C. (1992) Behçet's disease. Retains most of its mysteries. *British Medical Journal* 304, 1199–1200 [762, 763].

WECHSLER, B., VIDAILHET, M., PIETTE, J.C., BOUSSER, M.G., ISOLA, B.D., BLETRY, O. & GODEAU, P. (1992) Cerebral venous thrombosis in Behçet's disease: clinical study and long-term follow-up of 25 cases. *Neurology* 42, 614–618 [762].

WECHSLER, D. (1945) A standardised memory scale for clinical use. *Journal of Psychology* 19, 87–95 [116].

WECHSLER, D. (1958) *The Measurement and Appraisal of Adult Intelligence*, 4th edn. Williams and Wilkins: Baltimore [111].

WECHSLER, D. (1981) *Wechsler Adult Intelligence Scale—Revised*. The Psychological Corporation: New York [110].

WECHSLER, D. (1987) *Wechsler Memory Scale—Revised Manual*. The Psychological Corporation: San Antonio, Texas [116].

WECHSLER, D. & STONE, C.P. (1945) *Wechsler Memory Scale Manual*. The Psychological Corporation: New York [116].

WECHSLER, I.S. & DAVISON, C. (1932) Amyotrophic lateral sclerosis with mental symptoms. *Archives of Neurology and Psychiatry* 27, 859–880 [708].

WEDDELL, R., ODDY, M. & JENKINS, D. (1980) Social adjustment after rehabilitation: a two year follow-up of patients with severe head injury. *Psychological Medicine* 10, 257–263 [217].

WEIL, M.L., ITABASHI, H.H., CREMER, N.E., OSHIRO, L.S., LENNETTE, E.H. & CARNAY, L. (1975) Chronic progressive panencephalitis due to rubella virus simulating subacute sclerosing panencephalitis. *New England Journal of Medicine* 292, 994–998 [363].

WEILLER, C., CHOLLET, F., FRISTON, K.J., WISE, R.J.S. & FRACKOWIAK, R.S.J. (1992) Functional reorganization of the brain in recovery striatocapsular infarction in man. *Annals of Neurology* 31, 463–472 [378].

WEILLER, C., RAMSAY, S.C., WISE, R.J.S., FRISTON, K.J. & FRACKOWIAK, R.S.J. (1993) Individual patterns of functional reorganization in the human cerebral cortex after capsular infarction. *Annals of Neurology* 33, 181–189 [378].

WEINBERGER, D.R. (1987) Implications of normal brain development for the pathogenesis of schizophrenia. *Archives of General Psychiatry* 44, 660–669 [91, 92].

WEINBERGER, D.R. (1995) From neuropathology to neurodevelopment. *Lancet* 346, 552–557 [91].

WEINBERGER, D.R., BERMAN, K.F. & DANIEL, D.G. (1991a) Prefrontal cortex dysfunction in schizophrenia. Ch. 14 in *Frontal Lobe Function and Dysfunction*, eds Levin, H.S., Eisenberg, H.M. & Benton, A.L. Oxford University Press: New York [87].

WEINBERGER, D.R., BERMAN, K.F., IADAROLA, M., DRIESEN, N. & ZEC, R.F. (1988a) Prefrontal cortical blood flow and cognitive function in Huntington's disease. *Journal of Neurology, Neurosurgery and Psychiatry* 51, 94–104 [87].

WEINBERGER, D.R., BERMAN, K.F. & ILLOWSKY, B.P. (1988b) Physiological dysfunction of dorsolateral prefrontal cortex in schizophrenia. *Archives of General Psychiatry* 45, 609–615 [87].

WEINBERGER, D.R., BERMAN, K.F. & ZEC, R.F. (1986) Physiologic dysfunction of dorsolateral prefrontal cortex in schizophrenia. *Archives of General Psychiatry* 43, 114–124 [87].

WEINBERGER, D.R., DeLISI, L.E., NEOPHYTIDES, N. & WYATT, R.J. (1981) Familial aspects of CT scan abnormalities in chronic schizophrenic patients. *Psychiatry Research* 4, 65–71 [85].

WEINBERGER, D.R., DELISI, L.E., PERMAN, G.P., TARGUM, S. & WYATT, R.J. (1982) Computed tomography in schizophreniform disorder and other acute psychiatric disorders. *Archives of General Psychiatry* 39, 778–783 [85].

WEINBERGER, D.R., GIBSON, R., COPPOLA, R., JONES, D.W., MOLCHAN, S., SUNDERLAND, T., BERMAN, K.F. & REBA, R.C. (1991b) The distribution of cerebral muscarinic acetylcholine receptors in vivo in patients with dementia: a controlled study with ^{123}IQNB and single photon emission computed tomography. *Archives of Neurology* 48, 169–176 [148].

WEINBERGER, D.R., TORREY, E.F., NEOPHYTIDES, N. & WYATT, R.J. (1979a) Lateral cerebral ventricular enlargement to chronic schizophrenia. *Archives of General Psychiatry* 36, 735–739 [140].

WEINBERGER, D.R., TORREY, E.F., NEOPHYTIDES, N. & WYATT, R.J. (1979b) Structural abnormalities in the cerebral cortex of chronic schizophrenic patients. *Archives of General Psychiatry* 36, 935–939 [140].

WEINBERGER, D.R., TORREY, E.F. & WYATT, R.J. (1979c) Cerebellar atrophy in chronic schizophrenia. *Lancet* 1, 718 [140].

WEINBERGER, D.R., WAGNER, R.L. & WYATT, R.J. (1983) Neuropathological studies of schizophrenia: a selective review. *Schizophrenia Bulletin* 9, 193–212 [85].

WEINSTEIN, E.A. & COLE, M. (1963) Concepts of anosognosia. In *Problems of Dynamic Neurology*, ed. Halpern, L. Hadassah Medical School: Jerusalem [70].

WEINSTEIN, E.A. & KAHN, R.L. (1950) The syndrome of anosognosia. *Archives of Neurology and Psychiatry* 64, 772–791 [70].

WEINSTEIN, E.A. & KAHN, R.L. (1955) *Denial of Illness: Symbolic and Physiological Aspects*. Thomas: Springfield, Illinois [70].

WEINSTEIN, E.A., KAHN, R.L., MALITZ, S. & ROZANSKI, J. (1954) Delusional reduplication of parts of the body. *Brain* 77, 45–60 [73].

WEINSTEIN, E.A., LYERLY, O.G., COLE, M. & OZER, M.N. (1966) Meaning in jargon aphasia. *Cortex* 2, 165–187 [54].

WEINSTEIN, M.C. (1978) Prevention that pays for itself. *New England Journal of Medicine* 299, 307–308 [581].

WEINSTEIN, S., TEUBER, H.-L., GHENT, L. & SEMMES, J. (1955)

Complex visual task performance after penetrating brain injury in man. *American Psychologist* **10**, 408 [46].

WEINTRAUB, S., RUBIN, N.P. & MESULAM, M.-M. (1990) Primary progressive aphasia. Longitudinal course, neuropsychological profile, and language features. *Archives of Neurology* **47**, 1329–1335 [752].

WEISBERG, L.A. (1982) Lacunar infarcts. Clinical and computed tomographic correlations. *Archives of Neurology* **39**, 37–40 [384].

WEISS, R.D., MIRIN, S.M. & BARTEL, R.L. (1994) *Cocaine*, 2nd edn. American Psychiatric Press: Washington [619].

WEISSENBORN, K., SCHOLZ, M., HINRICHS, H., WILTFANG, J., SCHMIDT, F.W. & KÜNKEL, H. (1990) Neurophysiological assessment of early hepatic encephalopathy. *Electroencephalography and Clinical Neurophysiology* **75**, 289–295 [565].

WEISSMANN, C. (1991a) The prion's progress. *Nature* **349**, 569–571 [474].

WEISSMANN, C. (1991b) A 'unified theory' of prion propagation. *Nature* **352**, 679–682 [474].

WEIZMAN, A., ELDAR, M., SHOENFELD, Y., HIRSHORN, M., WIJSEN-BEEK, W. & PINKHAS, J. (1979) Hypercalcaemia-induced psychopathology in malignant diseases. *British Journal of Psychiatry* **135**, 363–366 [561].

WELLER, I.V.D., CONLON, C.P. & PETO, T.E.A. (1996) HIV infection and AIDS. Section 7.10.29 in *Oxford Textbook of Medicine*, 3rd edn, eds Weatherall, D.J., Ledingham, J.G.G. & Warrell, D.A. Oxford University Press: Oxford [333].

WELLER, M. & KORNHUBER, J. (1992) Clozapine rechallenge after an episode of 'neuroleptic malignant syndrome'. *British Journal of Psychiatry* **161**, 855–856 [627].

WELLER, M.P.I. (1988) Neuropsychiatric symptoms following bismuth intoxication. *Postgraduate Medical Journal* **64**, 308–310 [636].

WELLS, C.E. (1971b) The clinical management of the patient with dementia. Ch. 11 in *Dementia*, ed. Wells, C.E. Blackwell Scientific Publications: Oxford [499].

WELLS, C.E. (1978) Chronic brain disease; an overview. *American Journal of Psychiatry* **135**, 1–12 [491].

WELLS, C.E. (1979) Pseudodementia. *American Journal of Psychiatry* **136**, 895–900 [487].

WELLS, C.E. (1982) Pseudodementia and the recognition of organicity. Ch. 8 in *Psychiatric Aspects of Neurologic Disease*, Vol. 2, eds Benson, D.F. & Blumer, D. Grune & Stratton: New York [487].

WELLS, C.E.C. (1971a) Neurological complications of so-called influenza. A winter study in South-east Wales. *British Medical Journal* **1**, 369–373 [359].

WELMAN, A.J. (1969) Right-sided unilateral visual spatial agnosia, asomatognosia and anosognosia with left hemisphere lesions. *Brain* **92**, 571–580 [383].

WERNICKE, C. (1874) *Der aphaisische Symptomencomplex. Eine psychologische Studie auf anatomischer Basis.* Cohn & Weigert: Breslau [22, 45].

WERNICKE, C. (1881) *Lehrbuch der Gehirnkrankheiten*, Part 2, p. 229. Kassel: Berlin [576].

WESSELY, S., BUTLER, S., CHALDER, T. & DAVID, A. (1991) The cognitive behavioural management of the post-viral fatigue syndrome. Ch. 22 in: *Post-viral Fatigue Syndrome*, eds Jenkins, R. & Mowbray, J.F. Wiley & Sons Ltd: Chichester [373].

WESSELY, S., DAVID, A., BUTLER, S. & CHALDER, T. (1989) Management of chronic (post-viral) fatigue syndrome. *Journal of the Royal College of General Practitioners* **January**, 26–29 [373].

WEST, J.B. (1986) Do climbs to extreme altitude cause brain damage? *Lancet* **2**, 387–388 [549].

WEST, J.R., LIND, M.D., DEMUTH, R.M., PARKER, E.S., ALKANA, R.L.,

CASSELL, M. & BLACK, A.C. (1982) Lesion-induced sprouting in the rat dentate gyrus is inhibited by repeated ethanol administration. *Science* **218**, 808–810 [179, 607].

WESTLAKE, E.K., SIMPSON, T. & KAYE, M. (1955) Carbon dioxide narcosis in emphysema. *Quarterly Journal of Medicine* **24**, 155–173 [563].

WESTMORELAND, B.F. (1979) Electroencephalographic experience at the Mayo Clinic. Ch. 4 in *Tuberous Sclerosis*, ed. Gomez, M.R. Raven Press: New York [702].

WESTON, M.J. & WHITLOCK, F.A. (1971) The Capgras' syndrome following head injury. *British Journal of Psychiatry* **119**, 25–31 [169].

WHALLEY, L.J. & BAILEY, S. (1994) Non-cholinergic therapies of dementia. Ch. 28 in *Dementia*, eds Burns, A. & Levy, R. Chapman & Hall: London [501, 502].

WHEATLEY, D., BALTER, M., LEVINE, J., LIPMAN, R., BAUER, M.L. & BONATO, R. (1975) Psychiatric aspects of hypertension. *British Journal of Psychiatry* **127**, 327–336 [397].

WHELAN, T.B., SCHTEINGART, D.E., STARKMAN, M.N. & SMITH, A. (1980) Neuropsychological deficits in Cushing's syndrome. *Journal of Nervous and Mental Disease* **168**, 753–757 [517].

WHILES, W.H. (1940) Treatment of spasmodic torticollis by psychotherapy. *British Medical Journal* **1**, 969–971 [675].

WHITAKER-AZMITIA, P.M. & ARONSON, T.A. (1989) 'Ecstasy' (MDMA)-induced panic. *American Journal of Psychiatry* **146**, 119 [624].

WHITE, J.C. & COBB, S. (1955) Psychological changes associated with giant pituitary neoplasms. *Archives of Neurology and Psychiatry* **74**, 383–396 [230].

WHITE, P., HILEY, C.R., GOODHARDT, M.J., CARRASCO, L.H., KEET, J.P., WILLIAMS, I.E.I. & BOWEN, D.M. (1977) Neocortical cholinergic neurons in elderly people. *Lancet* **1**, 668–670 [444].

WHITE, P.D. (1990) Fatigue and chronic fatigue syndromes. Ch. 5 in *Somatization: Physical Symptoms and Psychological Illness*, ed. Bass, C. Blackwell Scientific Publications: Oxford [370].

WHITE, P.D., GROVER, S.A., KANGRO, H.O., THOMAS, J.M., AMESS, J. & CLARE, A.W. (1995b) The validity and reliability of the fatigue syndrome that follows glandular fever. *Psychological Medicine* **25**, 917–924 [359].

WHITE, P.D. & LEWIS, S.W. (1987) Delusional depression after infectious mononucleosis. *British Medical Journal* **295**, 97–98 [359].

WHITE, P.D., THOMAS, J.M., AMESS, J., GROVER, S.A., KANGRO, H.O. & CLARE, A.W. (1995a) The existence of a fatigue syndrome after glandular fever. *Psychological Medicine* **25**, 907–916 [359].

WHITE, S.J., McLEAN, A.E.M. & HOWLAND, C. (1979) Anticonvulsant drugs and cancer. A cohort study in patients with severe epilepsy. *Lancet* **2**, 458–461 [286].

WHITEHOUSE, A.M. & DUNCAN, J.M. (1987) Ephedrine psychosis rediscovered. *British Journal of Psychiatry* **150**, 258–261 [617].

WHITEHOUSE, P.J., PRICE, D.L., STRUBLE, R.G., CLARK, A.W., COYLE, J.T. & DELONG, M.R. (1982) Alzheimer's disease and senile dementia: loss of neurons in the basal forebrain. *Science* **215**, 1237–1239 [444].

WHITLEY, R.J., ALFORD, C.A., HIRSCH, M.S., SCHOOLEY, R.T., LUBY, J.P., AOKI, F.Y., HANLEY, D., NAHMIAS, A.J. & SOONG, S.-J. (1986) Vidarabine versus acyclovir therapy in herpes simplex encephalitis. *New England Journal of Medicine* **314**, 144–149 [357].

WHITLOCK, F.A. (1967a) The aetiology of hysteria. *Acta Psychiatrica Scandinavica* **43**, 144–162 [196].

WHITLOCK, F.A. (1967b) The Ganser syndrome. *British Journal of Psychiatry* **113**, 19–29 [480, 481].

WHITLOCK, F.A. (1978) Suicide, cancer and depression. *British Journal of Psychiatry* **132**, 269–274 [744].

WHITLOCK, F.A. & SISKIND, M.M. (1980) Depression as a major symptom of multiple sclerosis. *Journal of Neurology, Neurosurgery and Psychiatry* **43**, 861–865 [695, 697].

WHITLOCK, F.A., STOLL, J.R. & REKHDAHL, R.J. (1977) Crisis, life events and accidents. *Australian and New Zealand Journal of Psychiatry* **11**, 127–132 [176].

WHITMAN, S., COLEMAN, T.E., PATMON, C., DESAI, B.T., COHEN, R. & KING, L.N. (1984) Epilepsy in prison: elevated prevalence and no relationship to violence. *Neurology* **34**, 775–782 [274].

WHITTY, C.W.M. (1953) Familial hemiplegic migraine. *Journal of Neurology, Neurosurgery and Psychiatry* **16**, 172–177 [400].

WHITTY, C.W.M. (1956) Mental changes as a presenting feature in subcortical cerebral lesions. *Journal of Mental Science* **102**, 719–725 [230].

WHITTY, C.W.M. (1958) Neurologic implications of Behçet's syndrome. *Neurology* **8**, 369–373 [762].

WHITTY, C.W.M. & HOCKADAY, J.M. (1968) Migraine: a follow-up study of 92 patients. *British Medical Journal* **1**, 735–736 [401].

WHITTY, C.W.M., HOCKADAY, J.M. & WHITTY, M.M. (1966) The effect of oral contraceptives on migraine. *Lancet* **1**, 856–859 [399, 401].

WHITTY, C.W.M. & LEWIN, W. (1960) A Korsakoff syndrome in the post-cingulectomy confusional state. *Brain* **83**, 648–653 [27, 582].

WHITTY, C.W.M., LISHMAN, W.A. & FITZGIBBON, J.P. (1964) Seizures induced by movement: a form of reflex epilepsy. *Lancet* **1**, 1403–1405 [241].

WHITTY, C.W.M., STORES, G. & LISHMAN, W.A. (1977) Amnesia in cerebral disease. Ch. 2 in *Amnesia: Clinical, Psychological and Medicolegal Aspects*, 2nd edn, eds Whitty, C.W.M. & Zangwill, O.L., pp. 52–92. Butterworths: London [255, 541].

WHITTY, C.W.M. & ZANGWILL, O.L. (1966) Traumatic amnesia. Ch. 4 in *Amnesia*, eds Whitty, C.W.M. & Zangwill, O.L. Butterworths: London [170].

WHYBROW, P.C. & HURWITZ, T. (1976) Psychological disturbances associated with endocrine disease and hormone therapy. In *Hormones, Behavior and Psychopathology*, ed. Sachar, E.J. Raven Press: New York [516].

WHYBROW, P.C., PRANGE, A.J. & TREADWAY, C.R. (1969) Mental changes accompanying thyroid gland dysfunction. *Archives of General Psychiatry* **20**, 48–63 [508].

WHYTE, K.F., ALLEN, M.B., JEFFREY, A.A., GOULD, G.A. & DOUGLAS, N.J. (1989) Clinical features of the sleep apnoea/hypopnoea syndrome. *Quarterly Journal of Medicine* **72**, 659–666 [730, 731].

WIECK, A., HARRINGTON, R., MARKS, I. & MARSDEN, C.D. (1988) Writer's cramp: a controlled trial of habit reversal treatment. *British Journal of Psychiatry* **153**, 111–115 [677].

WIEDERHOLT, W.C. & SIEKERT, R.G. (1965) Neurological manifestations of sarcoidosis. *Neurology* **15**, 1147–1154 [764].

WIESTLER, O.D. & RADNER, H. (1994) Pathology of neurofibromatosis 1 and 2. Ch. 6 in *The Neurofibromatoses*, eds Huson, S.M. & Hughes, R.A.C. Chapman & Hall: London [704].

WIJMENGA, C., FRANTS, R.R., BROUWER, O.F., MOERER, P., WEBER, J.L. & PADBERG, G.W. (1990) Location of facioscapulohumeral muscular dystrophy gene on chromosome 4. *Lancet* **336**, 651–653 [715].

WIK, G., BORG, S., SJÖGREN, I., WIESEL, F.A., BLOMQVIST, G., BORG, J., GREIT, Z.T., NYBÄCK, H., SEDVALL, G., STONE-ELANDER, S. & WIDEN, L. (1988) PET determination of regional cerebral glucose metabolism in alcohol-dependent men and healthy controls using ^{11}C-glucose. *Acta Psychiatrica Scandinavica* **78**, 234–241 [606].

WILCOCK, G.K. & ESIRI, M.M. (1982) Plaques, tangles, and dementia: a quantitative study. *Journal of the Neurological Sciences* **56**, 343–356 [436, 441].

WILCOCK, G.K., ESIRI, M.M., BOWEN, D.M. & SMITH, C.C.T. (1982) Alzheimer's disease. Correlations of cortical choline acetyltransferase activity with the severity of dementia and histological abnormalities. *Journal of the Neurological Sciences* **57**, 407–417 [436, 444].

WILCOCK, G.K., SURMON, D.J., SCOTT, M., BOYLE, M., MULLIGAN, K., NEUBAUER, K.A., O'NEILL, D. & ROYSTON, V.H. (1993) An evaluation of the efficacy and safety of tetrahydroaminoacridine (THA) without lecithin in the treatment of Alzheimer's disease. *Age and Ageing* **22**, 316–324 [504].

WILES, C.M. (1993a) The meninges: bacterial (excluding spirochaetal disease) and fungal meningitis; intracranial abscess. Ch. 7 in: *Brain's Diseases of the Nervous System*, 10th edn, ed. Walton, J. Oxford University Press: Oxford [366, 367].

WILES, C.M. (1993b) Spirochaetal diseases, some other specific infections and intoxications and their neurological complications. Ch. 8 in: *Brain's Diseases of the Nervous System*, 10th edn, ed. Walton, J. Oxford University Press: Oxford [339].

WILEY, C.A., MASLIAH, E., MOREY, M., LEMERE, C., DETERESA, R., GRAFE, M., HANSEN, L. & TERRY, R. (1991) Neocortical damage during HIV infection. *Annals of Neurology* **29**, 651–657 [323].

WILKIE, F.L., EISDORFER, C., MORGAN, R., LOEWENSTEIN, D.A. & SZAPOCZNIK, J. (1990) Cognition in early human immunodeficiency virus infection. *Archives of Neurology* **47**, 433–440 [328].

WILKINSON, A.E. (1972) Problems in the treatment of venereal disease: bacterial resistance: treatment. *Journal of the Royal College of Physicians of London* **6**, 175–180 [336].

WILKINSON, D.G. (1981) Psychiatric aspects of diabetes mellitus. *British Journal of Psychiatry* **138**, 1–9 [534].

WILKINSON, H.A., LEMAY, M. & DREW, J.H. (1966) Adult aqueductal stenosis. *Archives of Neurology* **15**, 643–648 [750].

WILKINSON, P., KORNACZEWSKI, A., RANKIN, J.G. & SANTAMARIA, J.N. (1971) Physical disease in alcoholism: initial survey of 1000 patients. *Medical Journal of Australia* **1**, 1217–1223 [603].

WILL, A.M. & McLAREN, E.H. (1981) Reversible renal damage due to glue sniffing. *British Medical Journal* **283**, 525–526 [630].

WILL, R.G. (1993) Epidemiology of Creutzfeldt–Jakob disease. *British Medical Bulletin* **49**, 960–970 [473].

WILL, R.G., IRONSIDE, J.W., ZEIDLER, M., COUSENS, S.N., ESTIBEIRO, K., ALPEROVITCH, A., POSER, S., POCCHIARI, M., HOFMAN, A. & SMITH, P.G. (1996) A new variant of Creutzfeldt–Jakob disease in the UK. *Lancet* **347**, 921–925 [475, 476, 478].

WILL, R.G. & MATTHEWS, W.B. (1982) Evidence for case-to-case transmission of Creutzfeldt–Jakob disease. *Journal of Neurology, Neurosurgery and Psychiatry* **45**, 235–238 [476].

WILL, R.G., YOUNG, J.P.R. & THOMAS, D.J. (1988) Kleine–Levin syndrome: report of two cases with onset of symptoms precipitated by head trauma. *British Journal of Psychiatry* **152**, 410–412 [732].

WILLANGER, R., THYGESEN, P., NIELSEN, R. & PETERSEN, O. (1968) Intellectual impairment and cerebral atrophy: a psychological, neurological and radiological investigation. *Danish Medical Bulletin* **15**, 65–93 [138, 139].

WILLIAMS, D. (1956) The structure of emotions reflected in epileptic experiences. *Brain* **79**, 29–67 [251].

WILLIAMS, D. (1963) The psychiatry of the epileptic. *Proceedings of the Royal Society of Medicine* **56**, 707–710 [264, 268].

WILLIAMS, D. (1966) Temporal lobe epilepsy. *British Medical Journal* **1**, 1439–1442 [252].

WILLIAMS, D. (1969) Neural factors related to habitual aggression: consideration of the differences between those habitual aggressives and others who have committed crimes of violence. *Brain* **92**, 503–520 [83].

WILLIAMS, D.G. (1976) Methods for the estimation of three vitamin dependent red cell enzymes. *Clinical Biochemistry* **9**, 252–255 [572].

WILLIAMS, D.T., MEHL, R., YUDOFSKY, S., ADAMS, D. & ROSEMAN, B. (1982) The effect of propanolol on uncontrolled rage outbursts in children and adolescents with organic brain dysfunction. *Journal of the American Academy of Child Psychiatry* **21**, 129–135 [298].

WILLIAMS, F.J.B. & WALSHE, J.M. (1981) Wilson's disease. An analysis of the cranial computerised tomographic appearances found in 60 patients and the changes in response to treatment with chelating agents. *Brain* **104**, 735–752 [662].

WILLIAMS, M. (1956) Studies of perception in senile dementia; cue-selection as a function of intelligence. *British Journal of Medical Psychology* **29**, 270–279 [499].

WILLIAMS, M. (1968) The measurement of memory in clinical practice. *British Journal of Social and Clinical Psychology* **7**, 19–34 [99].

WILLIAMS, M. & PENNYBACKER, J. (1954) Memory disturbances in third ventricle tumours. *Journal of Neurosurgery and Psychiatry* **17**, 115–123 [227].

WILLIAMS, M. & SMITH, H.V. (1954) Mental disturbances in tuberculous meningitis. *Journal of Neurology, Neurosurgery and Psychiatry* **17**, 173–182 [25, 366, 367].

WILLIAMS, R.D., MASON, H.L., POWER, M.H. & WILDER, R.M. (1943) Induced thiamine (vitamin B_1) deficiency in man. *Archives of Internal Medicine* **71**, 38–53 [572].

WILLIAMS, R.D., MASON, H.L., WILDER, R.M. & SMITH, B.F. (1940) Observations on induced thiamine (vitamin B_1) deficiency in man. *Archives of Internal Medicine* **66**, 785–799 [572].

WILLIAMSON, J., STOKOE, I.H., GRAY, S., FISHER, M., SMITH, A., McGHEE, A. & STEPHENSON, E. (1964) Old people at home. Their unreported needs. *Lancet* **1**, 1117–1120 [429].

WILLIAMSON, P.D. (1995) Frontal lobe epilepsy. Some clinical characteristics. Ch. 10 in *Epilepsy and the Functional Anatomy of the Frontal Lobe*, eds Jasper, H.H., Riggio, S. & Goldman-Rakic, P.S. *Advances in Neurology* **66**. Raven Press: New York [249].

WILLIAMSON, P.D. & SPENCER, S.S. (1986) Clinical and EEG features of complex partial seizures of extratemporal origin. *Epilepsia* **27** (Supplement 2), S46–S63 [253].

WILLIAMSON, P.D., SPENCER, D.D., SPENCER, S.S., NOVELLY, R.A. & MATTSON, R.H. (1985) Complex partial seizures of frontal lobe origin. *Annals of Neurology* **18**, 497–504 [250, 254].

WILLISON, J.R., DU BOULAY, G.H., PAUL, E.A., RUSSELL, R.W.R., THOMAS, D.J., MARSHALL, J., PEARSON, T.C., SYMON, L. & WETHERLEY-MEIN, G. (1980) Effects of high haematocrit on alertness. *Lancet* **1**, 846–848 [426].

WILMSHURST, P. (1997) Brain damage in divers. Diving itself may cause brain damage — but we need more evidence. *British Medical Journal* **314**, 689–690 [766, 768].

WILMSHURST, P.T., BYRNE, J.C. & WEBB-PEPLOE, M.M. (1989) Relation between interatrial shunts and decompression sickness in divers. *Lancet* **2**, 1302–1306 [769].

WILNER, E. & BRODY, J.A. (1968) Prognosis of general paresis after treatment. *Lancet* **2**, 1370–1371 [346].

WILSON, A., HICKIE, I., LLOYD, A., HADZI-PAVLOVIC, D., BOUGHTON, C., DWYER, J. & WAKEFIELD, D. (1994) Longitudinal study of outcome of chronic fatigue syndrome. *British Medical Journal* **308**, 756–759 [373].

WILSON, B. (1982) Success and failure in memory training following a cerebral vascular accident. *Cortex* **18**, 581–594 [391].

WILSON, B.A. (1987) *Rehabilitation of Memory*. Guilford Press: New York [117, 391].

WILSON, B.A., COCKBURN, J. & BADDELEY, A. (1991) *The Rivermead Behavioural Memory Test*, 2nd edn. Thames Valley Test Company: Bury St Edmunds [117].

WILSON, B.A., COCKBURN, J. & HALLIGAN, P. (1987) *Behavioural Inattention Test*. Thames Valley Test Company: Fareham, Hants [113].

WILSON, B.A. & MOFFAT, N. (1984) *Clinical Management of Memory Problems*. Croom Helm: London [391].

WILSON, D.H., REEVES, A.G. & GAZZANIGA, M.S. (1982) 'Central' commissurotomy for intractable generalised epilepsy: series two. *Neurology* **32**, 687–697 [313].

WILSON, E.A. & BRODIE, M.J. (1997) Severe persistent visual field constriction associated with vigabatrin. Chronic refractory epilepsy may have a role in causing these unusual lesions. *British Medical Journal* **314**, 1693 [303].

WILSON, G. & RUPP, C. (1946) Mental symptoms associated with extramedullary posterior fossa tumours. In *Transactions of the American Neurological Association*, 71st Annual Meeting, pp. 104–107. William Byrd Press: Richmond, Virginia [230].

WILSON, J.T.L., WIEDMANN, K.D., HADLEY, D.M., CONDON, B., TEASDALE, G. & BROOKS, D.N. (1988) Early and late magnetic resonance imaging and neuropsychological outcome after head injury. *Journal of Neurology, Neurosurgery and Psychiatry* **51**, 391–396 [166].

WILSON, L.G. (1976) Viral encephalopathy mimicking functional psychosis. *American Journal of Psychiatry* **133**, 165–170 [347].

WILSON, P.J.E. (1970) Cerebral hemispherectomy for infantile hemiplegia. *Brain* **93**, 147–180 [270].

WILSON, R.S., KASZNIAK, A.W. & FOX, J.H. (1981) Remote memory in senile dementia. *Cortex* **17**, 41–48 [32, 37].

WILSON, S.A.K. (1912) Progressive lenticular degeneration: a familial nervous disease associated with cirrhosis of the liver. *Brain* **34**, 295–509 [661, 665].

WILSON, S.A.K. (1940) *Neurology*. Edward Arnold: London [339, 340, 341, 665, 673, 698].

WINDEBANK, A.J. & McEVOY, K.M. (1989) Diabetes and the nervous system. Ch. 17 in *Neurology and General Medicine*, ed. Aminoff, M.J. Churchill Livingstone: New York [534, 538].

WINDLE, W.F., GROAT, R.A. & FOX, C.A. (1944) Experimental structural alterations in the brain during and after concussion. *Surgery Gynaecology and Obstetrics* **79**, 561–572 [162].

WING, J.K., BIRLEY, J.L.T., COOPER, J.E., GRAHAM, P. & ISAACS, A.D. (1967) Reliability of a procedure for measuring and classifying 'present psychiatric state'. *British Journal of Psychiatry* **113**, 499–515 [84, 123].

WING, J.K., COOPER, J.E. & SARTORIUS, N. (1974) *The Measurement and Classification of Psychiatric Symptoms. An Instruction Manual for the PSE and Catego Program.* Cambridge University Press: Cambridge [84].

WINICK, M. (1976) *Malnutrition and Brain Development*. Oxford University Press: Oxford [570].

WINICK, M. (ed.) (1979) Malnutrition and mental development. Ch. 2 in *Nutrition: Pre- and Post-natal Development*. Plenum Press: New York [570].

WINNACKER, J.L., BECKER, K.L. & KATZ, S. (1968) Endocrine aspects of sarcoidosis. *New England Journal of Medicine* **278**, 483–492 [764].

WINSTOCK, A.R. (1991) Chronic paranoid psychosis after misuse of MDMA. *British Medical Journal* **302**, 1150–1151 [624].

WISCHIK, C.M., NOVAK, M., EDWARDS, P.C., KLUG, A., TICHELLAR, W. & CROWTHER, R.A. (1988a) Structural characterization of the core of the paired helical filament of Alzheimer disease. *Proceedings of the National Academy of Sciences of the USA* **85**, 4884–4888 [442].

WISCHIK, C.M., NOVAK, M., THØGERSEN, H.C., EDWARDS, P.C., RUNSWICK, M.J., JAKES, R., WALKER, J.E., MILSTEIN, C., ROTH, M. & KLUG, A. (1988b) Isolation of a fragment of tau derived from the core of the paired helical filament of Alzheimer disease. *Proceedings of the National Academy of Sciences of the USA* **85**, 4506–4510 [442].

WISE, M.P., BLUNT, S. & LANE, R.J.M. (1995) Neurological presentations of hypothyroidism: the importance of slow relaxing reflexes. *Journal of the Royal Society of Medicine* **88**, 272–274 [513].

WISE, R., CHOLLET, F., HADAR, U., FRISTON, K., HOFFNER, E. & FRACKOWIAK, R. (1991) Distribution of cortical neural networks involved in word comprehension and word retrieval. *Brain* **114**, 1803–1817 [45].

WISE, R.J.S., BERNARDI, S., FRACKOWIAK, R.S.J., LEGG, N.J. & JONES, T. (1983a) Serial observations of the pathophysiology of acute stroke: the transition from ischaemia to infarction as reflected in regional oxygen extraction. *Brain* **106**, 197–222 [377].

WISE, R.J.S., RHODES, C.G., GIBBS, J.M., HATAZAWA, J., PALMER, T., FRACKOWIAK, R.S.J. & JONES, T. (1983b) Disturbance of oxidative metabolism of glucose in recent human cerebral infarcts. *Annals of Neurology* **14**, 627–637 [377].

WISNA, B., ADAMI, H.-O., BERGSTRÖM, R., GAMSTEDT, A., DAHLBERG, P.A., ADAMSON, U., JANSSON, R. & KARLSSON, A. (1991) Stressful life events and Graves' disease. *Lancet* **338**, 1475–1479 [508].

WISNIEWSKI, H.M., BRUCE, M.E. & FRASER, H. (1975) Infectious aetiology of neuritic (senile) plaques in mice. *Science* **190**, 1108–1110 [446].

WISNIEWSKI, K., HOWE, J., WILLIAMS, D.G. & WISNIEWSKI, H.M. (1978) Precocious aging and dementia in patients with Down's syndrome. *Biological Psychiatry* **13**, 619–627 [437].

WISNIEWSKI, H.M. & KOZLOWSKI, P.B. (1982) Evidence for blood–brain barrier changes in senile dementia of the Alzheimer type (SDAT). *Annals of the New York Academy of Science* **396**, 119–129 [447].

WITELSON, S.F. (1991) Neural sexual mosaicism: sexual differentiation of the human temporo-parietal region for functional asymmetry. *Psychoneuroendocrinology* **16**, 131–153 [41].

WITELSON, S.F. & KIGAR, D.L. (1988) Asymmetry in brain function follows asymmetry in anatomical form: gross, microscopic, postmortem and imaging studies. Ch. 6 in *Handbook of Neuropsychology*, Vol. 1, eds Boller, F. & Graffman, J. Elsevier: Amsterdam [41].

WITTENBORN, J.R. (1981) Pharmacotherapy for age-related behavioural deficiencies. *Journal of Nervous and Mental Disease* **169**, 139–156 [502].

WOLF, J.K., SANTANA, H.B. & THORPY, M. (1979) Treatment of 'emotional incontinence' with levodopa. *Neurology* **29**, 1435–1436 [392].

WOLF, P. (1982) Manic episodes in epilepsy. In *Advances in Epileptology, XIIIth Epilepsy International Symposium*, eds Akimoto, H., Kazamatsuri, H., Seino, M. & Ward, A.A., pp. 237–240. Raven Press: New York [285].

WOLF, P. (1991) Acute behavioral symptomatology at disappearance of epileptiform EEG abnormality: paradoxical or 'forced' normalization. Ch. 8 in *Neurobehavioral Problems of Epilepsy*, eds Smith, D.B., Treiman, D.M. & Trimble, M.R. *Advances in Neurology* **55**. Raven Press: New York [284].

WOLF, P. & TRIMBLE, M.R. (1985) Biological antagonism and epileptic psychosis. *British Journal of Psychiatry* **146**, 272–276 [278].

WOLF, S.M., SCHOTLAND, D.L. & PHILLIPS, L.L. (1965) Involvement of nervous system in Behçet's syndrome. *Archives of Neurology* **12**, 315–325 [762, 763].

WOLF-KLEIN, G.P. & SILVERSTONE, F.A. (1994) Weight loss in Alzheimer's disease: an international review of the literature. *International Psychogeriatrics* **6**, 135–142 [435].

WOLFF, H.G. (1937) Personality features and reactions of subjects with migraine. *Archives of Neurology and Psychiatry* **37**, 895–921 [403].

WOLFF, H.G. (ed.) (1963) The relation of life situations, personality features, and reactions to the migraine syndrome. Ch. 11 in *Headache and Other Head Pain*, 2nd edn. Oxford University Press: New York [403].

WOLKOWITZ, O.M., WEINGARTNER, H., THOMPSON, K., PICKAR, D., PAUL, S.M. & HOMMER, D.W. (1987) Diazepam-induced amnesia: a neuropharmological model of an 'organic amnesic syndrome'. *American Journal of Psychiatry* **144**, 25–29 [610].

WONG, D.F., WAGNER, H.N., TUNE, L.E., DANNALS, R.F., PEARLSON, G.D., LINKS, J.M., TAMINGA, C.A., BROUSSOLLE, F.P., RAUERT, H.T., WILSON, A.A., TOUNG, J.K.T., MALAT, J., WILLIAMS, J.A., O'TUAMA, L.A., SNYDER, S.H., KUHAR, M.T. & GJEDDE, A. (1986) PET reveals elevated D_2 dopamine receptors in drug-naive schizophrenics. *Science* **234**, 1558–1563 [88].

WONG, I.C.K., MAWER, C.E. & SANDER, J.W.A.S. (1997) Severe persistent visual field constriction associated with vigabatrin. Reaction might be dose dependent. *British Medical Journal* **314**, 1693–1694 [303].

WONG, K.L., WOO, E.K.W., YU, Y.L. & WONG, R.W.S. (1991) Neurologic manifestations of systemic lupus erythematosus: a prospective study. *Quarterly Journal of Medicine* **81**, 857–870 [422].

WOOD, R.L. (1984a) Behaviour disorders following severe brain injury: their presentation and psychological management. Ch. 10 in *Closed Head Injury. Psychological, Social and Family Consequences*, ed. Brooks, N. Oxford University Press: Oxford [214].

WOOD, R.L. (1984b) Management of attention disorders following brain injury. Ch. 8 in *Clinical Management of Memory Problems*, eds Wilson, B.A. & Moffat, N. Croom Helm: London [213].

WOOD, R. & EAMES, P. (1981) Application of behaviour modification in the treatment of traumatically brain-injured adults. Ch. 4 in *Applications of Conditioning Theory*, ed. Davey, G. Methuen: London [214].

WOODCOCK, S.M. (1967) Mental symptoms in patients with acoustic neuromas. *Journal of Neurology, Neurosurgery and Psychiatry* **30**, 587 [231].

WOODRUFF, P.W.R., McMANUS, I.C. & DAVID, A.S. (1995) Meta-analysis of corpus callosum size in schizophrenia. *Journal of Neurology, Neurosurgery and Psychiatry* **58**, 457–461 [86].

WOODRUFF, P.W.R., PEARLSON, G.D., GEER, M.J., BARTA, P.E. & CHILCOAT, H.D. (1993) A computerized magnetic resonance imaging study of corpus callosum morphology in schizophrenia. *Psychological Medicine* **23**, 45–56 [86].

WOODS, R.T. (1979) Reality orientation and staff attention: a controlled study. *British Journal of Psychiatry* **134**, 502–507 [500].

WOODS, R.T. & BRITTON, P.G. (1977) Psychological approaches to the treatment of the elderly. *Age and Ageing* **6**, 104–112 [501].

WOODS, R.T. & PIERCY, M. (1974) A similarity between amnesic memory and normal forgetting. *Neuropsychologia* **12**, 437–445 [35].

WORDEN, D.K. & VIGNOS, P.J. (1962) Intellectual function in childhood progressive muscular dystrophy. *Pediatrics* **29**, 968–977 [716].

WORKING GROUP OF THE RESEARCH COMMITTEE OF THE ROYAL COLLEGE OF PSYCHIATRISTS (1991) Services for brain injured adults. *Bulletin of the Royal College of Psychiatrists* **15**, 513–518 [215].

WORKING GROUP REPORT (1993) The incidence and prevalence of AIDS and other severe HIV disease in England and Wales for 1992–1997: projections using data to the end of June 1992. *Communicable Disease Report* **3** (**Supplement 1**), S1–S17 [316].

WORLD FEDERATION OF NEUROLOGY: RESEARCH COMMITTEE RESEARCH GROUP ON HUNTINGTON'S CHOREA (1989) Ethical issues policy statement on Huntington's disease molecular genetic predictive test. *Journal of Neurological Science* **94**, 327 [467].

WORLD FEDERATION OF NEUROLOGY: RESEARCH GROUP ON HUNTINGTON'S CHOREA (1990) Ethical issues policy statement—predictive test. *Journal of Medical Genetics* **27**, 34–38 [467].

WORLD HEALTH ORGANIZATION (1990a) *Report of the second consultation on the neuropsychiatric aspects of HIV-1 infection, Global Programme on AIDS, Geneva, Annex 3*. Ref. No. WHO/GPA/MNH 90.1. World Health Organization: Geneva [324].

WORLD HEALTH ORGANIZATION (1990b) *Suicidal Behaviour Among People with HIV and AIDS*. Report on a WHO consultation. WHO Regional Office for Europe: Copenhagen [331].

WORLD HEALTH ORGANIZATION (1992) *The ICD-10 Classification of Mental and Behavioural Disorders: Clinical Descriptions and Diagnostic Guidelines*. World Health Organization: Geneva [5, 8].

WORLD HEALTH ORGANIZATION (1993) *The ICD-10 Classification of Mental and Behavioural Disorders: Diagnostic Criteria for Research*. World Health Organization: Geneva [7].

WORLD HEALTH ORGANIZATION REPORT (1955) Alcohol and alcoholism. *World Health Organization Technical Report Series*, No. 94. World Health Organization: Geneva [596].

WORRAL, E.P. & DEWHURST, D. (1979) Manipulating central cholinergic functions: studies with deanol and physostigmine. Ch. 37 in *Alzheimer's Disease: Early Recognition of Potentially Reversible Deficits*, eds Glen, A.I.M. & Whalley, L.J. Churchill Livingstone: Edinburgh & London [503].

WORTIS, S.B., HERMAN, M. & LONDON, J. (1943) Mental changes in patients with subdural haematomas. Ch. 11 in *Trauma of the Central Nervous System*, Research Publications of the Association for Research in Nervous and Mental Disease, Vol. 24. Williams & Wilkins: Baltimore [412].

WREDLING, R., LEVANDER, S., ADAMSON, U. & LINS, P.E. (1990) Permanent neuropsychological impairment after recurrent episodes of severe hypoglycaemia in man. *Diabetalogia* **33**, 152–157 [537].

WRIGHT, C.E., HARDING, G.F.A. & ORWIN, A. (1984) Presenile dementia—the use of the flash and pattern VEP in diagnosis. *Electroencephalography and Clinical Neurophysiology* **57**, 405–415 [131].

WRIGHT, J., JOHNS, R., WATT, I., MELVILLE, A. & SHELDON, T. (1997) Health effects of obstructive sleep apnoea and the effectiveness of continuous positive airways pressure: a systematic review of the research evidence. *British Medical Journal* **314**, 851–860 [731].

WYATT, G.B. (1992) Malaria, the mimic. *Journal of the Medical Defence Union* **3**, 54–55 [370].

WYKE, B. (1963) *Brain Function and Metabolic Disorders*. Butterworths: London [562].

WYKE, M. (1968) The effect of brain lesions in the performance of an arm–hand precision task. *Neuropsychologia* **6**, 125–134 [58].

WYKE, M.A. (1977) Musical ability: a neuropsychological interpretation. Ch. 10 in *Music and the Brain*, eds Critchley, M. & Henson, R.A. Heinemann: London [64].

WYSE, D.G. (1973) Deliberate inhalation of volatile hydrocarbons: a review. *Canadian Medical Association Journal* **108**, 71–74 [630].

WYSZYNSKI, B., MERRIAM, A., MEDALIA, A. & LAWRENCE, C. (1989) Choreoacanthocytosis. Report of a case with psychiatric features. *Neuropsychiatry, Neuropsychology, and Behavioral Neurology* **2**, 137–144 [757].

YAHR, M.D., DUVOISIN, R.C. & COWEN, D. (1965) Encephalopathy associated with carcinoma. *Transactions of the American Neurological Association* **90**, 80–86 [742].

YAHR, M.D., DUVOISIN, R.C., SCHEAR, M.J., BARRETT, R.E. & HOEHN, M.M. (1969) Treatment of parkinsonism with levodopa. *Archives of Neurology* **21**, 343–354 [659].

YAKOVLEV, P.I. (1947) Paraplegias of hydrocephalics. *American Journal of Mental Deficiency* **51**, 561–576 [749].

YAKOVLEV, P.I. & RAKIC, P. (1966) Patterns of decussation of bulbar pyramids and distribution of pyramidal tracts on two sides of the spinal cord. *Transactions of the American Neurological Association* **91**, 366–367 [41].

YAMAMOTO, T. & HIRANO, A. (1985) Nucleus raphe dorsalis in Alzheimer's disease: neurofibrillary tangles and loss of large neurons. *Annals of Neurology* **17**, 573–577 [445].

YANKNER, B.A., DUFFY, L.K. & KIRSCHNER, D.A. (1990) Neurotrophic and neurotoxic effect of amyloid β protein: reversal by tachykinin neuropeptides. *Science* **250**, 279–282 [443].

YAP, P.M. (1952) The Latah reaction: its pathodynamics and nosological position. *Journal of Mental Science* **98**, 515–564 [683].

YARCHOAN, R., BERG, G., BROUWERS, P., FISCHL, M.A., SPITZER, A.R., WICHMAN, A., GRAFMAN, J., THOMAS, R.V., SAFAI, B., BRUNETTI, A., PERNO, C.F., SCHMIDT, P.J., LARSON, S.M., MYERS, C.E. & BRODER, S. (1987) Response of human-immunodeficiency-virus-associated neurological disease to 3'-azido-3'-deoxythymidine. *Lancet* **1**, 132–135 [335].

YARCHOAN, R., THOMAS, R.V., GRAFMAN, J., WICHMAN, A., DALAKAS, M., McATEE, N., BERG, G., FISCHL, M., PERNO, C.F., KLECKER, R.W., BUCHBINDER, A., TAY, S., LARSON, S.M., MYERS, C.E. & BRODER, S. (1988) Long-term administration of 3'-azido-2',3'-dideoxythymidine to patients with AIDS-related neurological disease. *Annals of Neurology* **23** (**Supplement**), S82–S87 [335].

YASE, Y., MATSUMOTO, N., AZUMA, K., NAKAI, Y. & SHIRAKI, H. (1972) Amyotrophic lateral sclerosis: association with schizophrenic symptoms and showing Alzheimer's tangles. *Archives of Neurology* **21**, 118–128 [709].

YASSA, R., NAIR, V. & SCHWARTZ, G. (1984) Tardive dyskinesia and the primary psychiatric diagnosis. *Psychosomatics* **25**, 135–138 [642].

YATES, A. (1958) The application of learning theory to the treatment of tics. *Journal of Abnormal and Social Psychology* **56**, 175–182 [684, 687].

YATES, A.J. (1954) The validity of some psychological tests of brain damage. *Psychological Bulletin* **51**, 359–379 [108].

YATES, A.J. (1966) Psychological deficit. *Annual Review of Psychology* **17**, 111–144 [108, 116].

YATES, C.M., SIMPSON, J., MALONEY, A.F.J. & GORDON, A. (1980b) Neurochemical observations in a case of Pick's disease. *Journal of the Neurological Sciences* **48**, 257–263 [461].

YATES, C.M., SIMPSON, J., MALONEY, A.F.J., GORDON, A. & REID, A.H. (1980a) Alzheimer-like cholinergic deficiency in Down syndrome. *Lancet* **2**, 979 [437].

YESAVAGE, J.A., TINKLENBERG, J.R., HOLLISTER, L.E. & BERGER, P.A.

(1979) Vasodilators in senile dementias. *Archives of General Psychiatry* **36**, 220–223 [502].

YONAS, H., GUR, D., LATCHAW, R.E. & OBRIST, W. (1987) Stable xenon in computerized tomography imaging of cerebral blood flow. Ch. 2 in *Impact of Functional Imaging in Neurology and Psychiatry*, eds Wade, J., Knežvić, S., Maximilian, V.A., Mubrin, Z. & Prohovnik, I. *Current Problems in Neurology*, Vol. 5. John Libbey: London [138].

YOSS, R.E. (1970) The inheritance of diurnal sleepiness as measured by pupillography. *Proceedings of the Staff Meetings of the Mayo Clinic* **45**, 426–437 [726].

YOSS, R.E. & DALY, D.D. (1957) Criteria for the diagnosis of the narcoleptic syndrome. *Proceedings of the Staff Meetings of the Mayo Clinic* **32**, 320–328 [722].

YOSS, R.E. & DALY, D.D. (1960a) Hereditary aspects of narcolepsy. In *Transactions of the American Neurological Association*, ed. Yahr, M.D., pp. 239–240. Springer: New York [726].

YOSS, R.E. & DALY, D.D. (1960b) Narcolepsy. *Medical Clinics of North America* **44**, 953–968 [722, 723].

YOUNG, A.C., SAUNDERS, J. & PONSFORD, J.R. (1976) Mental change as an early feature of multiple sclerosis. *Journal of Neurology, Neurosurgery and Psychiatry* **39**, 1008–1013 [694].

YOUNG, I.R., BAILES, D.R., BURE, M., COLLINS, A.G., SMITH, D.T., McDONNELL, M.J., ORR, J.S., BANKS, L.M., BYDDER, G.M., GREENSPAN, R.H. & STEINER, R.E. (1982) Initial clinical evaluation of a whole body nuclear magnetic resonance (NMR) tomograph. *Journal of Computer Assisted Tomography* **6**, 1–18 [141].

YOUNG, I.R., HALL, A.S., PALLIS, C.A., BYDDER, G.M., LEGG, N.J. & STEINER, R.E. (1981) Nuclear magnetic resonance imaging of the brain in multiple sclerosis. *Lancet* **2**, 1063–1066 [690].

YOUNG, J., HALL, P. & BLAKEMORE, C. (1974) Treatment of the cerebral manifestions of arteriosclerosis with cyclandelate. *British Journal of Psychiatry* **124**, 177–180 [502].

YOZAWITZ, A., BRUDER, G., SUTTON, S., SHARPE, L., GURLAND, B., FLEISS, J. & COSTA, L. (1979) Dichotic perception: evidence for right hemisphere dysfunction in affective psychosis. *British Journal of Psychiatry* **135**, 224–237 [89].

YULE, W. (1973) Differential prognosis of reading backwardness and specific reading retardation. *The British Journal of Educational Psychology* **43**, 244–248 [47].

YULE, W., LANSDOWN, R., MILLAR, I.B. & URBANOWICZ, M.-A. (1981) The relationship between blood lead concentrations, intelligence and attainment in a school population: a pilot study. *Developmental Medicine and Child Neurology* **23**, 567–576 [633].

YUNUS, M.B. & ALDAG, J.C. (1996) Restless legs syndrome and leg cramps in fibromyalgia syndrome: a controlled study. *British Medical Journal* **312**, 1339 [640].

ZAGAMI, A.S., LETHLEAN, A.K. & MELLICK, R. (1993) Delayed neurological deterioration following carbon monoxide poisoning: MRI findings. *Journal of Neurology* **240**, 113–116 [551].

ZAIDEL, E. (1977) Unilateral auditory language comprehension on the token test following cerebral commissurotomy and hemispherectomy. *Neuropsychologia* **15**, 1–18 [42].

ZAIDEL, E. (1978) Auditory language comprehension in the right hemisphere following cerebral commissurotomy and hemispherectomy: a comparison with child language and aphasia. In *Language Acquisition and Language Breakdown*, eds Caramazza, A. & Zurif, E. Johns Hopkins University Press: Baltimore [42].

ZANGWILL, O.L. (1946) Some qualitative observations on verbal memory in cases of cerebral lesion. *British Journal of Psychology* **37**, 8–19 [100].

ZANGWILL, O.L. (1947) Psychological aspects of rehabilitation in cases of brain injury. *British Journal of Psychology* **37**, 60–69 [213].

ZANGWILL, O.L. (1961) Psychological studies of amnesic states. *Proceedings of the Third World Congress of Psychiatry*, Vol. III, pp. 219–222. McGill University Press: Montreal [39].

ZANGWILL, O.L. (1966) The amnesic syndrome. Ch. 3 in *Amnesia*, eds Whitty, C.W.M. & Zangwill, O.L. Butterworths: London [31].

ZANGWILL, O.L. (1967) The Grunthal–Störring case of amnesic syndrome. *British Journal of Psychiatry* **113**, 113–128 [33].

ZANGWILL, O.L. (1969) Intellectual status in aphasia. Ch. 6 in *Handbook of Clinical Neurology*, Vol. 4, *Disorders of Speech, Perception, and Symbolic Behaviour*, eds Vinken, P.J. & Bruyn, G.W. North-Holland Publishing Co.: Amsterdam [46].

ZARCONE, V. (1973) Narcolepsy. *England Journal of Medicine* **288**, 1156–1166 [722, 723, 725, 727].

ZATORRE, R.J., EVANS, A.C. & MEYER, E. (1994) Neural mechanisms underlying melodic perception and memory for pitch. *Journal of Neuroscience* **14**, 1908–1919 [64].

ZATZ, L.M., JERNIGAN, T.L. & AHUMADA, A.J. (1982) White matter changes in cerebral computed tomography related to aging. *Journal of Computer Assisted Tomography* **6**, 19–23 [139].

ZEIFERT, M., PENNELL, W.H., FINLEY, K.H. & RIGGS, N. (1962) The electro-encephalogram following Western and St Louis encephalitis. *Neurology* **12**, 311–319 [348].

ZEITLIN, C. & ODDY, M. (1984) Cognitive impairment in patients with severe migraine. *British Journal of Clinical Psychology* **23**, 27–35 [407].

ZEKI, S., WATSON, J.D.G., LUECK, C.J., FRISTON, K.J., KENNARD, C. & FRACKOWIAK, R.S.J. (1991) A direct demonstration of functional specialisation in human visual cortex. *Journal of Neuroscience* **11**, 641–649 [145].

ZELLWEGER, H. & IONASESCU, V. (1973) Myotonic dystrophy and its differential diagnosis. *Acta Neurologica Scandinavica* **55 (Supplement)**, 5–28 [719, 721].

ZEMAN, W. & DYKEN, P. (1968) Dystonia musculorum deformans. Ch. 21 in *Handbook of Clinical Neurology*, Vol. 6, eds Vinken, P.J. & Bruyn, G.W. North-Holland Publishing Co.: Armsterdam [677].

ZEMCOV, A., BARCLAY, L. & BLASS, J.P. (1984) Regional decline of cerebral blood flow with age in cognitively intact subjects. *Neurobiology of Aging* **5**, 1–6 [434].

ZENEROLI, M.L., CIONI, G., VEZZELLI, C., GRANDI, S., CRISI, G., LUZETTI, R. & VENTURA, E. (1987) Prevalence of brain atrophy in liver cirrhosis patients with chronic persistent encephalopathy. Evaluation by computed tomography. *Journal of Hepatology* **4**, 283–292 [564].

ZENEROLI, M.L., PINELLI, G., GOLLINI, G., PENNE, A., MESSORI, E., ZANI, G. & VENTURA, E. (1984) Visual evoked potential: a diagnostic tool for the assessment of hepatic encephalopathy. *Gut* **25**, 291–299 [565].

ZEUMER, H., SCHONSKY, B. & STURM, K.W. (1980) Predominent white matter involvement in subcortical arteriosclerotic encephalopathy (Binswanger's disease). *Journal of Computer Assisted Tomography* **4**, 14–19 [459].

ZIEGLER, D.K., BATNITZKY, S., BARTER, R. & McMILLAN, J.H. (1991) Magnetic resonance image abnormality in migraine with aura. *Cephalgia* **11**, 147–150 [401].

ZIEGLER, L.H. (1930) Psychotic and emotional phenomena associated with amyotrophic lateral sclerosis. *Archives of Neurology and Psychiatry* **24**, 930–936 [707].

ZIMMERMAN, R.D., RUSSELL, E.J., LEEDS, N.E. & KAUFMAN, D. (1980) CT in the early diagnosis of herpes simplex encephalitis. *American Journal of Roentgenology* **134**, 61–66 [357].

ZIPURSKY, R.B., LIM, K.O., SULLIVAN, E.V., BROWN, B.W. & PFEFFERBAUM, A. (1992) Widespread cerebral gray matter volume deficits in schizophrenia. *Archives of General Psychiatry* **49**, 195–205 [85, 87].

ZLOTLOW, M. & KLEINER, S. (1965) Catatonic schizophrenia associated with tuberose sclerosis. *Psychiatric Quarterly* **39**, 466–475 [702].

ZOLA-MORGAN, S., SQUIRE, L.R. & AMARAL, D.G. (1986) Human amnesia and the medial temporal region: enduring memory impairment following a bilateral lesion limited to field CAI of the hippocampus. *Journal of Neuroscience* **6**, 2950–2967 [26].

ZORUMSKI, C.F. & OLNEY, J.W. (1992) Excitotoxicity and neurodegenerative disorders. Ch. 17 in *Emerging Strategies in Neuroprotection*, eds Marangos, P.J. & Lal, H. Birkhäuser: Boston [445].

ZUCKER, D.K., LIVINGSTON, R.L., NAKRA, R. & CLAYTON, P.J. (1981) B_{12} deficiency and psychiatric disorders: case report and literature review. *Biological Psychiatry* **16**, 197–205 [587].

ZUCKERMAN, M. (1964) Perceptual isolation as a stress situation. *Archives of General Psychiatry* **11**, 255–276 [149].

ZUGER, A. & O'DOWD, M.A. (1992) The Baron has AIDS: a case of factitious human immunodeficiency virus infection and review. *Clinical Infectious Diseases* **14**, 211–216 [332].

ZÜLCH, K.-J. (1969) Medical causation. Ch. 46 in *The Late Effect of Head Injury*, eds Walker, A.E., Caveness, W.F. & Critchley, M. Thomas: Springfield, Illinois [210].

ZUMWALT, R.E., McFEELEY, P.J. & MAITO, J. (1987) Fraudulent AIDS. *Journal of the American Medical Association* **257**, 3231 [332].

Index